Jeffcoate's

Principles of

GYNAECOLOGY

Jeffcoate's Principles of GYNAECOLOGY

TENTH INTERNATIONAL EDITION

Revised, updated and edited by

Editor

Muralidhar V Pai

MD FRCOG FICOG FKCOG FICMCH
Pro Vice Chancellor
Sikkim Manipal University, Sikkim
Dean and Professor
Department of Obstetrics and Gynaecology
Sikkim Manipal Institute of Medical Sciences
Gangtok, Sikkim, India

Foreword

Sir Sabaratnam Arulkumaran

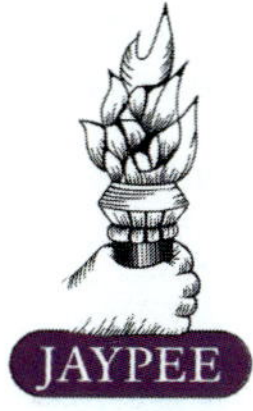

JAYPEE BROTHERS MEDICAL PUBLISHERS

The Health Sciences Publisher

New Delhi | London

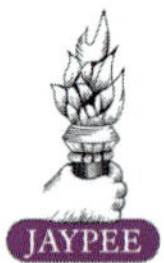

Jaypee Brothers Medical Publishers (P) Ltd

Headquarters
EMCA House, 23/23-B
Ansari Road, Daryaganj
New Delhi 110 002, India
Landline: +91-11-23272143, +91-11-23272703
+91-11-23282021, +91-11-23245672
e-mail: jaypee@jaypeebrothers.com

Corporate Office
4838/24, Ansari Road, Daryaganj
New Delhi 110 002, India
Phone: +91-11-43574357
Fax: +91-11-43574314
e-mail: jaypee@jaypeebrothers.com

Overseas Office
JP Medical Ltd.
83, Victoria Street, London
SW1H 0HW (UK)
Phone: +44-20 3170 8910
e-mail: info@jpmedpub.com

EU GPSR Authorised Representative
Logos Europe, 9 rue Nicolas Poussin
17000, La Rochelle, France
Phone: +33 (0) 6 67 93 73 78
e-mail: contact@logoseurope.eu

Website: www.jaypeebrothers.com
Website: www.jaypeedigital.com

Inquiries for bulk sales may be solicited at: jaypee@jaypeebrothers.com

Jeffcoate's Principles of Gynaecology

Ninth Edition: 2019

Tenth Edition: **2026**

ISBN: 978-93-5696-808-0

Printed in India

Dedication

I dedicate this book to my family, teachers and students.

Contributors

Akhila Vasudeva
MD (Obs & Gyne) DNB FRCOG
Professor and Head
Department of Obstetrics and Gynaecology
Kasturba Medical College
Manipal, Karnataka, India

Anjali Mundkur
MBBS MS DNB MRCOG FRM
Associate Professor
Department of Reproductive Medicine and Surgery
Kasturba Medical College
Udupi, Karnataka, India

Argyia Desouza MD (Obs & Gyne)
Assistant Professor
Department of Obstetrics and Gynaecology
Kasturba Medical College
Manipal, Karnataka, India

Brihathi Pranavi Dasari
MS (Obs & Gyne) DNB (Obs & Gyne)
Senior Resident
Department of Obstetrics and Gynaecology
Kasturba Medical College
Manipal, Karnataka, India

Chaitanya Nagori
MD (Obstetrics and Gynaecology) DGO
Director
Dr Nagori's Institute for Infertility and IVF
Ahmedabad, Gujarat, India

Chandra Mithila MBBS MS
Fellow in Urogynaecology
Department of Obstetrics and Gynaecology
Kasturba Medical College
Manipal, Karnataka, India

Deepa Reddy MBBS MS
Assistant Professor
Department of Obstetrics and Gynaecology
Kasturba Medical College
Manipal, Karnataka, India

Deepak Goenka MBBS MD FIAOG FICOG
Director
Department of Obstetrics and Gynaecology, Infertility
Institute of Human Reproduction
Guwahati, Assam, India

Divyashree Bhat MBBS MS DNB
Senior Resident
Department of Obstetrics and Gynaecology
Kasturba Medical College
Manipal, Karnataka, India

Ektha M Shetty MBBS MS (Obs & Gyne)
Assistant Professor
Department of Obstetrics and Gynaecology
Father Muller Medical College Hospital
Mangaluru, Karnataka, India

Jayaraman Nambiar M MBBS MD
Professor
Department of Obstetrics and Gynaecology
Kasturba Medical College
Manipal, Karnataka, India

Jyothi Shetty MBBS MD
Professor
Department of Obstetrics and Gynaecology
Kasturba Medical College
Manipal, Karnataka, India

Kaushik Naik V MBBS MS (Obs & Gyne)
Assistant Professor
Department of Obstetrics and Gynaecology
Kasturba Medical College
Manipal, Karnataka, India

Kavisha Bhat MBBS DGO DNB
Senior Resident
Department of Obstetrics and Gynaecology
Kasturba Medical College
Manipal, Karnataka, India

Kavitha D Nayak
MBBS MS (Obs & Gyne) DNB
Senior Resident
Department of Obstetrics and Gynaecology
Kasturba Medical College
Manipal, Karnataka, India

Krupa Hitesh Shah
MD FICOG Fellowship in Clinical Genetics
Associate Professor
Department of Obstetrics and Gynaecology
Kasturba Medical College
Manipal, Karnataka, India

Latha V Kharka MBBS DNB (Obs & Gyne)
Associate Professor
Department of Obstetrics and Gynaecology
Sikkim Manipal Institute of Medical Sciences
Gangtok, Sikkim, India

Mahesh C Koregol
MBBS MS (Obs & Gyne) FIAGE Fellowship in Reproductive Medicine (RGUHS)
Senior Clinical Director and Consultant
Department of Reproductive Medicine
NOVA IVF Fertility
Bengaluru, Karnataka, India

Meghna A Nayak
MBBS MS (Obs & Gyne) FRM MRCOG
Specialist in Reproductive Medicine
Newcastle Fertility Centre
Newcastle Upon Tyne Hospital Trust
NHS, England, Stockton on Tees TS160FL

Muralidhar V Pai
MD FRCOG FICOG FKCOG FICMCH
Pro Vice Chancellor
Sikkim Manipal University, Sikkim
Dean and Professor
Department of Obstetrics and Gynaecology
Sikkim Manipal Institute of Medical Sciences
Gangtok, Sikkim, India

Mythreyi Kadambi
MS DNB FMIGS (RGUHS)
Fellow
Department of Minimally Invasive Surgery
Radhakrishna Multispecialty Hospital and IVF Centre
Bengaluru, Karnataka, India

Nikil Shetty MBBS MS (Obs & Gyne)
Professor
Department of Obstetrics and Gynaecology
Kasturba Medical College, Mangaluru
Manipal Academy of Higher Education
Manipal, Karnataka, India

Niraj Jadav MBBS DGO
Private Practitioner
Department of Obstetrics and Gynaecology
Sankalp Maternity Home
Surat, Gujarat, India

Nithesh Prabhu MBBS MS (Obs & Gyne)
Assistant Professor
Department of Obstetrics and Gynaecology
Kasturba Medical College
Manipal, Karnataka, India

Pesona Grace Lucksom
MS (Obs & Gyne) Fellowship in Gynaecology Oncology PGDME PhD
Professor
Department of Obstetrics and Gynaecology
Sikkim Manipal Institute of Medical Sciences
Gangtok, Sikkim, India

Pooja HN MBBS MS
Assistant Professor
Department of Obstetrics and Gynaecology
Kasturba Medical College
Manipal, Karnataka, India

Poonam Mishra
MBBS DNB (Obs & Gyne) FAM FCG FSRM
Director
Department of Obstetrics and Gynaecology
Manns Hospital
Lucknow, Uttar Pradesh, India

Pralhad Kushtagi MD DNB FICOG
Former Professor
Department of Obstetrics and Gynaecology
Kasturba Medical College, Manipal
Mangalore Campuses
Bengaluru, Karnataka, India

Pratik Kumar Chatterjee
MBBS MD PGDBEME PDCR FAGE
Associate Professor
Department of Physiology
Kasturba Medical College, Mangaluru
Manipal Academy of Higher Education
Manipal, Karnataka, India

Pratik Tambe
MD FICOG FICRM FICMCH FIAOG
ART Consultant, Gynec Endoscopic Surgeon
Ashirwad IVF
Mumbai, Maharashtra, India
Governing Council Member, ICOG and ICRM
Managing Committee Member, MOGS, ISAR, MSR

Priti Venkatesh
MBBS DGO MD (Obs & Gyne)
Consultant (Fetal Medicine)
Department of Obstetrics and Gynaecology
Karnataka, India

Priya Ballal K MD (Obs & Gyne)
Professor
Department of Obstetrics and Gynaecology
Kasturba Medical College, Mangaluru
Manipal Academy of Higher Education
Manipal, Karnataka, India

Priya Ganeshkumar
MBBS MD DGO (MUM) DGO (CPS) DFP FICOG
Medical Director
Department of Gynaecology
SaiNiwas Health Care
Thane, Maharashtra, India

Priya SP Patil
MS (Obs & Gyne) FMIS (RGUHS) Fellowship in Cosmetic Gynaecology
Clinical Director and Consultant
Department of Obstetrics and Gynaecology
Altius Hospitals
Bengaluru, Karnataka, India

Priyankur Roy
MBBS MS (Obs & Gyne) DRM FAGE
Senior Consultant Gynecologist
Department of Reproductive Medicine and Surgery
Roy's Clinic and Multispecialty Hospital
Siliguri, West Bengal, India

Rajani Upadhyaya MBBS MS
Assistant Professor
Department of Obstetrics and Gynaecology
Kasturba Medical College
Manipal, Karnataka, India

Rajeshwari G Bhat
MBBS MD (Obs & Gyne)
Professor
Department of Obstetrics and Gynaecology
Kasturba Medical College
Manipal, Karnataka, India

Rani Akhil Bhat
MBBS MS FRCOG (UK) Fellowship in Gynea-Oncology (SIngapore) Fellowship in Gynea-Oncology & Robotic Surgeon (Hong Kong) Diploma in Gynecological Operative Endoscopy (France)
Head and Senior Consultant
Division of Gynecological Oncology
Apollo Hospitals
Bengaluru, Karnataka, India

Rekha Upadhya
DNB (Obs & Gyne) Certificate Course in Gynecological Oncology FMAS DMAS (World Lap Hospital)
Associate Professor
Department of Obstetrics and Gynaecology
Kasturba Medical College
Manipal, Karnataka, India

Roopa PS MBBS MS MRCOG
Additional Professor
Department of Obstetrics and Gynaecology
Kasturba Medical College
Manipal, Karnataka, India

Sanjay Kumar KR MBBS DGO DNB
Associate Professor
Department of Obstetrics and Gynaecology
Melaka-Manipal Medical College
Manipal, Karnataka, India

Saritha Shamsunder
MBBS MD FICOG FRCOG
Professor
Department of Obstetrics and Gynaecology
Vardhman Mahavir Medical College and Safdarjung Hospital
New Delhi, India

Shamantaka Somayaji
MBBS DGO Fellowship in Reproductive Medicine
Consultant
Department of Infertility and Assisted Reproduction
Institute of Human Reproduction
Guwahati, Assam, India

Shashikala K Bhat
MBBS MD (Obs & Gyne) FICOG
Professor and Head
Department of Obstetrics and Gynaecology
Dr TMA Pai Hospital, Udupi
Melaka Manipal Medical College
Manipal, Karnataka, India

Shivani Verma MBBS MS DNB
Senior Resident
Department of Obstetrics and Gynaecology
Vardhman Mahavir Medical College and Safdarjung Hospital
New Delhi, India

Shobha N Gudi MD DNB FICOG CIMP
Professor and Head
Department of Obstetrics and Gynaecology
St Philomenas Hospital
Bengaluru, Karnataka, India

Shripad Hebbar MBBS MD
Professor and Head
Department of Obstetrics and Gynaecology
Kasturba Medical College
Manipal, Karnataka, India

Shyamala Guruvare MBBS MD
Professor
Department of Obstetrics and Gynaecology
Kasturba Medical College
Manipal, Karnataka, India

Shyjus P MBBS MS FMAS DMAS FICOG
Centre Head and Consultant
Department of Obstetrics and Gynaecology
Birla's Amala Institute of Medical Sciences (ARMC) and Kannur Institute of Medical Science and Technology (KIMST) Hospitals
Kannur, Kerala, India

Sonal Panchal
MBBS MD (Radiodiagnosis) PhD
Consultant Sonography Specialist
Dr Nagori's Institute for Infertility and IVF
Ahmedabad, Gujarat, India

Soumya Mahesh Koregol
MBBS MS (Obs & Gyne)
Senior Consultant
Department of Reproductive Medicine
Shreshtha Women's and Fertility Clinic
Bengaluru, Karnataka, India

Sourjya Banerjee MBBS MD
Additional Professor
Department of Radiation Oncology
Kasturba Medical College, Mangaluru
Manipal Academy of Higher Education
Manipal, Karnataka, India

Srirama Bhat M
MS (Surgery) FRCS (Glasgow)
Professor
Department of Surgery
Kasturba Medical College, Mangaluru
Manipal Academy of Higher Education
Manipal, Karnataka, India

Sufian Zaheer MBBS MD (Pathology)
Professor
Department of Pathology
Vardhman Mahavir Medical College and Safdarjung Hospital
New Delhi, India

Sujatha BS MS (Obs & Gyne)
Associate Professor
Department of Obstetrics and Gynaecology
Kasturba Medical College
Manipal, Karnataka, India

Suprajna Shetty MBBS MS
Assistant Professor
Department of Obstetrics and Gynaecology
Kasturba Medical College
Mangaluru, Karnataka, India

Vidya Bhat MBBS MD DNB MNAMS FICOG
Medical Director
Department of Gynaecology Endoscopy and Reproductive Medicine
Radhakrishna Multispecialty Hospital and IVF Centre
Bengaluru, Karnataka, India

Vidya Thobbi MD FICOG
Professor
Department of Obstetrics and Gynaecology
Alameen Medical College
Bengaluru, Karnataka, India

Vidyashree G Poojari
MS (Obs & Gyne) DNB MNAMS FRM
Associate Professor
Department of Reproductive Medicine and Surgery
Kasturba Medical College
Manipal, Karnataka, India

Foreword

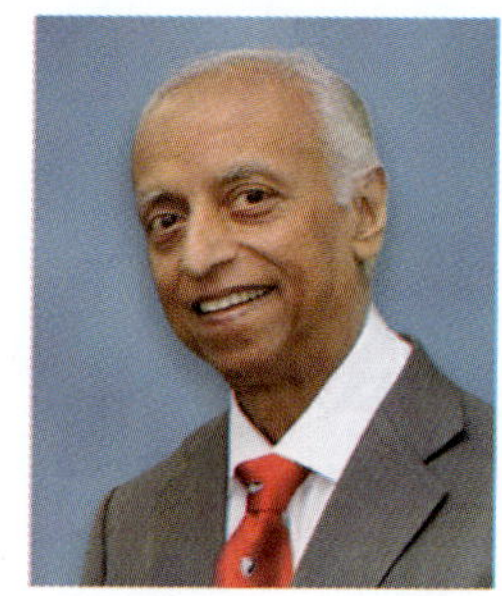

It was a pleasure to read the classic textbook *Jeffcoate's Principles of Gynaecology*, 10th edition, edited by Professor Dr Muralidhar V Pai, Pro Vice Chancellor, Sikkim Manipal University; Dean and Professor, Department of Obstetrics and Gynaecology, Sikkim Manipal Institute of Medical Sciences, Gangtok, Sikkim, India. This textbook has withstood the passage of time over a century as one of the most sorted after book because of the strenuous work by the editors who have kept pace with the evidence-based advancing knowledge, new surgical techniques, advancing technology and new modalities of imaging. The editor's effort to keep the book up-to-date is reflected by the fact that of the 66 chapters in the book 44 are co-authored by the editor—a tremendous task to keep a watchful eye. This has helped to maintain the style and consistency of the chapters.

The chapters are well-illustrated with colour photographs, figures, tables, flowcharts, bullet points, and have suitable headings and subheadings in each chapter to make the reader navigate and understand the chapter easily. This is a reflection of the knowledge, experience and wisdom of the authors who are senior academic clinicians. Several chapters are co-authored by the editor who has helped to maintain the consistency of the book and for easy reading.

The first chapter by the editor on the different aspects of clinical examination in gynaecology provides important aspects of various types of examination and investigations that are usually performed and concludes with list of articles for further reading. This format is maintained for each chapter for easy reading and clear understanding of the theory and practice of gynaecology. The 66 chapters provide information on development and function of the urogenital tract, anomalies of the development/structure and function; reproductive endocrinology including adolescent issues, menstrual disturbances, PCOS/hirsutism, advances in contraception, issues related to subfertility and modern management of climacteric and menopause. Benign gynaecological problems are the common reason for attendance to outpatient clinic, and this area is well covered with inclusion of endometriosis, adenomyosis, benign reproductive tract tumours (e.g., fibroids) and pelvic inflammatory disease. In the reproductive age, women face the issues of miscarriage (some have recurrent), ectopic pregnancy and rarely hydatidiform mole and choriocarcinoma. Useful information is given as to how to make the diagnosis, manage and provide appropriate follow-up. Presentation of history, clinical features, investigation findings and clinical management of gynaecological malignancy of each reproductive tract organ is covered, i.e., of the cervix, body of the uterus, ovary, vulva, vagina, and the fallopian tubes. Surgical management of each malignancy is included within each chapter, but additional chapters deal with the principles and application of chemotherapy, radiotherapy and immunotherapy. Pelvic floor disorders and urinary incontinence are explained in detail. To the editor's credit, areas of general interest like application of laser in gynaecology, genetics, nutrition and exercise, ultrasound, robotic surgery, endoscopic surgery and instruments in gynaecological procedures are tackled in individual chapters.

The book is a compilation of all what you need to know in gynaecology and is highly recommended for practicing clinicians, trainees and members of allied specialty who help to manage gynaecological patients. It would be an advantage to have a copy in the library, gynaecological clinic and theatre in addition to your personal copies. My sincere congratulations to the editor, the authors and the publishers for producing this excellent book.

Sir Sabaratnam Arulkumaran
MBBS DCH MD PhD DSc FRCS FRCOG
Professor Emeritus of Obstetrics and Gynaecology
City St George's University of London
Foundation Professor of Obstetrics and Gynaecology, University of Nicosia
Visiting Professor, Institute of Global Health, Imperial College, London
Past President of the RCOG, BMA and FIGO

Preface to the Tenth International Edition

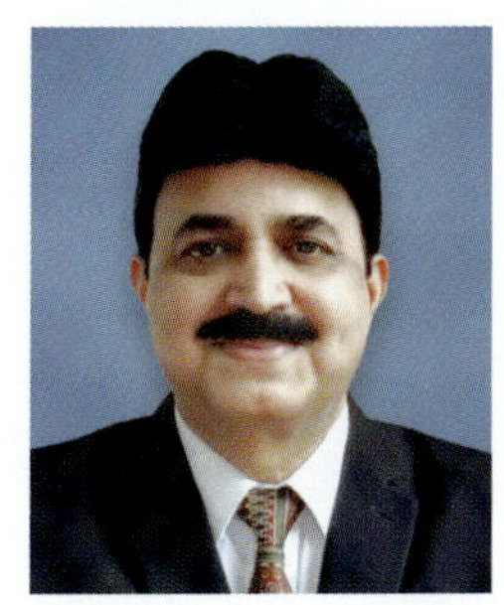

It is an honor for me to edit this prestigious *Textbook of Gynaecology*, originally authored by Professor Jeffcoate. I thoroughly enjoyed reading this book during my postgraduate days, and it has evolved through many editions since then. While emulating the writing style of the original author is a challenging task, in this edition, we have strived to maintain a clinically oriented approach.

What makes this edition unique is that it has been updated not only with recent advances but also with the latest international guidelines. The illustrations, tables, and flowcharts have all been carefully revised to enhance clarity and facilitate understanding. This edition provides comprehensive coverage of all areas in gynaecology, including adolescence, reproductive endocrinology, menopause, urogynaecology, gynaecological oncology, gynaecological imaging, contraception, and surgical aspects, including robotics.

Experts in each of these subspecialities have been invited to contribute to the chapters, ensuring that the content is both lucid and engaging.

I sincerely hope that this edition will be embraced with the same enthusiasm and recognition as its esteemed predecessors.

Muralidhar V Pai
Editor

Extracts from the Preface to the First Edition

The book is meant to add to rather than replace clinical and tutorial instruction, so those matters which can best be taught beside the patient, or which are easy for any student to learn and understand from other sources, receive little attention. In planning the text, I recalled those subjects which I myself found (and still do find) difficult to master, or on which I had to search far and long for information, and gave them disproportionate emphasis. This and other considerations resulted in a disregard for the relative importance, as judged by their clinical frequency, of different conditions. Indeed, the reader will find that quite rare conditions are mentioned, illustrated or described at length; and that all manner of asides—even some with an obstetrical flavour—creep in. This is partly because they are of special interest to me but mainly because they appeared to offer scope for presenting an attitude of mind; for discouraging loose thinking and empiricism; for inculcating a scientifically and ethically honest outlook; for emphasising the art as well as the science of gynaecology.

I have not played safe by stating only generally accepted views, nor have I played fair by giving the differing views of various authorities. Instead, after weighing the evidence, I have attempted to reach a conclusion which satisfies me as being as rational as present knowledge allows. Without intended disrespect, mention by name of authors and workers has been avoided as a rule; references clutter up the text, destroy continuity and are hardly ever used properly. On the other hand, I have not hesitated to give my own views and have, at times, been more dogmatic than clinical experience ever really justifies. I have even gone so far as to enunciate ideas which in many respects are conjectural, if not fanciful. I do not expect these all to be accepted; if they are I shall be disappointed because their object is to provoke trains of thought and discussion.

In offering this book to fellow students, I remember with affection and gratitude William Blair-Bell, one of the great gynaecologists of this century. He not only taught me gynaecology and a particular approach to it, he taught me to think and to write. He, more than anyone else, provided me with the stimulus and the opportunity to obtain the experience which has led to this work.

Norman Jeffcoate

Acknowledgements

I can never thank Professor Jeffcoate enough for writing the original book and for inspiring successive Editors to update and refine it through the years. His contribution to the field of gynaecology has been monumental, and this textbook stands as a testament to his vision.

I would also like to express my heartfelt gratitude to all the contributors of this edition, as well as to those who have contributed to the previous editions. Their expertise and dedication have played a crucial role in shaping this work into what it is today.

A special note of thanks goes to Pragati Singh (Senior Development Editor), Kritika Dua (Manager–Content Acquisition & Business Development), Mr Ankit Vij (Managing Director), Mr Sabyasachi Hazra (Associate Director–Publishing and Digital Sales), and the entire team at M/s Jaypee Brothers Medical Publishers (P) Ltd, New Delhi, India. Their hard work and commitment behind the scenes have been instrumental in bringing this edition to fruition on time.

Thank you all for your invaluable contributions to this important work.

Muralidhar V Pai

Contents

1. A Clinical Approach to Gynaecology **1**

Shripad Hebbar, Divyashree Bhat, Muralidhar V Pai

- Psychosomatic and Sociological Aspects of Gynaecology *1*
- Clinical Methods *2*
- Physical Examination *6*
- Special Tests and Accessory Aids to Diagnosis *12*
- Endometrial Sampling Procedures *13*
- Transvaginal Sonography *16*
- Transrectal Sonography *16*
- Colour Doppler *16*
- Endoscopy *17*
- Laparoscopy *17*
- Hysteroscopy *19*
- Robotic Surgery *20*
- Computed Tomography *21*
- Magnetic Resonance Imaging *22*
- Positron Emission Tomography Scan *23*

2. Anatomy **26**

Argyia Desouza, Muralidhar V Pai

- Vulva *26*
- Vagina *30*
- Uterus *35*
- Fallopian Tubes *40*
- Ovary *41*
- Urethra and Bladder *43*
- Ureter *47*
- Sigmoid Colon *48*
- Rectum and Anus *48*
- Pelvic Peritoneum and Ligaments *49*
- Pelvic Musculature *51*
- Pelvic Fascia and Cellular Tissue *52*
- The Supports of the Genital Organs *52*
- Blood Vessels of the Pelvis *53*
- Lymphatic Drainage *57*
- Innervation of Pelvic Organs *57*

3. Ovarian Functions **61**

Priya SP Patil, Muralidhar V Pai

- Production of OVA *62*
- Ovarian Hormones *75*
- Pituitary Hormones *81*

- Pituitary–Hypothalamic Relations *82*
- Pituitary–Ovarian Relations (Control of Ovulation) *85*
- Hormone Levels and Assays *86*

4. Menstruation and Other Cyclical Phenomena 88

Deepa Reddy, Muralidhar V Pai

- Normal Menstrual Cycle *88*
- Endometrial Cycle *88*
- Correlation of Endometrial and Ovarian Cycle *92*
- Uterine Bleeding *94*
- Myometrial Cycle *98*
- Cyclical Changes in the Tube *98*
- Cervical Cycle *99*
- Vaginal Cycle *99*
- Cyclical, Metabolic, Vascular and Psychological Changes *99*

5. Clinical Aspects of Menstruation and Ovulation 101

Nithesh Prabhu, Muralidhar V Pai

- Menstruation *101*
- The Menopause and the Climacteric *106*
- Abnormal Menopause *119*
- Ovulation *120*

6. Puberty and Adolescent Gynaecology 132

Roopa PS, Muralidhar V Pai

- Puberty and Adolescence *132*
- Abnormalities of Puberty and Adolescence *136*
- Prolactin *144*
- Puberty Menorrhagia *146*

7. Conception 150

Akhila Vasudeva, Muralidhar V Pai

- Process *150*
- Early Development of the Ovum *152*
- Formation of Foetus and Membranes *155*
- Hormonal Control of Early Pregnancy *158*

8. Spontaneous Abortions (Including Recurrent Loss) 162

Akhila Vasudeva, Muralidhar V Pai

- Spontaneous Abortions *162*
- Recurrent Early Pregnancy Loss *169*

9. Ectopic Pregnancy and Pregnancy of Unknown Location 179

Shripad Hebbar, Kavisha Bhat, Muralidhar V Pai

Ectopic Pregnancy 179

- Frequency of Ectopic Pregnancy *179*
- Sites of Ectopic Pregnancy *179*
- Aetiology of Ectopic Pregnancy *180*
- Ectopic Pregnancy in Fallopian Tubes *181*
- Management and Treatment Options of Ectopic Pregnancy *192*

- Expectant Management *193*
- Medical Management *194*
- Surgical Management *194*
- Complications of Ectopic Pregnancy *200*
- Ovarian Pregnancy *200*
- Cornual Pregnancy *201*
- Cervical Pregnancy *202*
- Caesarean Scar Pregnancy *202*
- Abdominal Pregnancy *203*
- Interstitial Pregnancy *204*
- Intraligamentary Pregnancy *205*

Pregnancy of Unknown Location 205
- Outcome of Ectopic Pregnancy *206*
- Diagnosis *207*
- Management of Pregnancy of Unknown Location *207*

10. Gestational Trophoblastic Disease 214

Priya Ballal K, Suprajna Shetty
- Types of Tumours *214*
- Aetiology *215*
- Pathology *215*
- Clinical Features *218*
- Evaluation and Treatment *218*
- Postmolar Surveillance *219*
- Persistent Trophoblastic Disease *219*
- Classification and Staging of Gestational Trophoblastic Disease *221*
- Treatment of Gestational Trophoblastic Tumours *222*
- Management of Metastasis *223*
- Postchemotherapy Surveillance for High-risk Gestational Trophoblastic Tumours *223*

11. Breast Function and its Disorders 225

Shripad Hebbar, Rajani Upadhyaya, Muralidhar V Pai
- Breast Development *225*
- Developmental Anomalies of the Breast *227*
- Breastfeeding and Lactation *231*
- Endocrine Disorders (Galactorrhoea and Breast Atrophy) *232*
- Benign Breast Condition *237*
- Screening for Breast Diseases *240*
- Benign Breast Disease *241*
- Breast Cancer *245*
- Epidemiology *245*

12. Development of the Urogenital System 252

Latha Kharka, Muralidhar V Pai
- Gonad *253*
- Wolffian System *253*
- Müllerian Ducts *255*

- Mesenteries and Ligaments *255*
- Development of the Vagina, Bladder and Urethra *257*
- Development of the Vulva *257*

13. Malformations and Maldevelopments of the Genital Tract.......... 259
Priyankur Roy, Muralidhar V Pai
- Causes of Malformations *259*
- Cytogenetics *260*
- Uterine Anomalies *263*
- Ovary *276*
- Fallopian Tube *277*
- Uterus *277*
- Conical Cervix and Pinhole Ostium *278*
- Vagina *279*
- Vulva *282*
- Errors Arising in Connection with the Cloaca *283*
- Malformations of the Urinary Tract *284*

14. Disorders of Sex Differentiation 287
Rajeshwari G Bhat, Muralidhar V Pai
- Factors Responsible for Normal Sexual Patterns *287*
- Turner Syndrome 45, XO *292*
- Triple X Syndrome (47, XXX) (From Old Jeffcoate's) *293*
- Klinefelter Syndrome (47, XXY) (From Old Jeffcoate's) *294*
- YY Syndrome *294*
- Disorders of Sex Development with Normal Sex Chromosomes *295*
- Approach to a Neonate with Atypical Genitalia *300*
- Intersex Developing after Birth *303*

15. Injuries 312
Kavitha D Nayak, Muralidhar V Pai
- Different Types of Injuries *312*

16. Female Genital Mutilation.......... 318
Rajeshwari G Bhat, Muralidhar V Pai
- Classification of Female Genital Mutilation *318*
- Prevalence of Female Genital Mutilation *318*
- Indications *320*
- Complications *320*
- Diagnosis *322*
- Management in Obstetric and Gynaecological Practice *322*
- Management of Short-term Complications *322*
- Management during the Antenatal Period *323*
- Management during the Intrapartum Period *323*
- Postnatal Care *324*
- Eradication *324*

17. Pelvic Organ Prolapse.......... 327
Rajeshwari G Bhat, Muralidhar V Pai
- Uterine and Vaginal Prolapse *327*
- Prolapse of the Ovaries *347*

18. **Other Displacements of the Uterus** 348
Jyothi Shetty, Muralidhar V Pai
- Upward Displacement of the Uterus *348*
- Lateral Displacement of the Uterus *348*
- Forward Displacement of the Uterus *348*
- Backward Displacement of the Uterus *349*
- Retroverted Gravid Uterus *353*
- Inversion of the Uterus *355*
- Chronic Inversion *356*

19. **Torsion of Pelvic Organs** 359
Latha V Khakra, Muralidhar V Pai
- Torsion in Normal and Abnormal Uterus *359*
- Aetiology *361*
- Differential Diagnosis *362*
- Treatment *363*

20. **Infections Including Sexually Transmitted Diseases** 364
Jayaraman Nambiar M, Muralidhar V Pai
- Natural Defences of the Genital Tract *364*
- Variations in the Efficiency of Defence Mechanisms *364*
- Types of Infecting Organisms *365*
- Sexually Transmitted Diseases *366*
- Genital Tuberculosis *382*
- Sarcoidosis *389*
- Actinomycosis *389*
- Schistosomiasis (Bilharzia) *390*
- Amoebiasis *390*

21. **Infections as They Affect Individual Organs** 391
Jayaraman Nambiar M, Muralidhar V Pai
- Vulvitis *391*
- Bartholinitis *395*
- Vaginitis *396*
- Cervicitis *404*
- Endometritis *406*
- Metritis *407*
- Salpingo-Oophoritis *407*
- Oophoritis *413*
- Pelvic Peritonitis *413*
- Pelvic Cellulitis *414*
- Chronic Cellulitis *415*
- Pelvic Inflammatory Disease *416*
- Suppurative Thrombophlebitis of the Pelvic Veins *417*

22. **Genital Tuberculosis** 419
Pesona Grace Lucksom, Latha V Kharka, Muralidhar V Pai
- Clinical Profile *419*
- Classification *420*

- Diagnosis *421*
- Management *430*
- Pathology of Pelvic Organs *431*

23. Endometriosis and Chronic Pelvic Pain 433
Anjali Mundkur, Muralidhar V Pai

Endometriosis and Allied States 433
- Endometriosis and Adenomyosis *433*
- Adenomyosis *454*
- Endosalpingiosis *455*
- Cervical Endometriosis *455*
- Causes in the Genital Tract *456*
- Extragenital Causes *457*
- Management and Treatment *459*

Chronic Pelvic Pain 459
- General Considerations *459*
- Step-wise Evaluation of Chronic Pelvic Pain *460*
- Examination *460*
- Diagnostic Investigations *460*
- Management *460*

24. Polycystic Ovary Syndrome 463
Meghna A Nayak
- Oligomenorrhoea and Anovulation: Definition *464*
- Hyperandrogenism (Clinical and/or Biochemical) *464*
- Polycystic Ovaries on Ultrasound or Elevated Serum Anti-Müllerian Hormone *464*
- Pathophysiology *464*
- Ovarian and Other Endocrine Aspects of Polycystic Ovary Syndrome *465*
- Metabolic Component of Polycystic Ovary Syndrome *467*
- Pathology *469*
- Clinical, Biochemical and Metabolic Features of Polycystic Ovary Syndrome *469*
- Ultrasonographic Examination *470*
- Puberty and Polycystic Ovary Syndrome *471*
- Management *471*
- Infertility *473*
- Weight Loss *473*
- Summaries *476*

25. Hirsutism 478
Deepak Goenka, Shamantaka Somayaji, Muralidhar V Pai
- Types of Hair *478*
- Physiology of Hair Growth *478*
- Androgens Physiology *479*
- Aetiology *480*
- Diagnosis of Hyperandrogenism *482*
- Laboratory Evaluation *482*
- Treatment *484*

26. Epithelial Abnormalities of the Genital Tract 487

Shyamala Guruvare, Muralidhar V Pai

- Senile Atrophy *487*
- Lichen Sclerosus *488*
- Aetiology *489*
- Symptoms *490*
- Diagnosis *490*
- Treatment *490*
- Vulvar and Oral Epithelial Abnormalities *492*
- Vulvar Intraepithelial Neoplasia *492*
- Vagina *496*
- Cervix *497*
- Uterine Corpus *509*
- Fallopian Tube *512*

Annexures 514

- Annexure 1: Flowcharts for Screen-and-Treat Strategies (Negative or Unknown Human Immunodeficiency Virus Status) *514*
- Annexure 2: Flowcharts for Screen-and-Treat Strategies (Human Immunodeficiency Virus-Positive Status or Unknown Human Immunodeficiency Virus Status in Areas with High Endemic Human Immunodeficiency Virus Infection) *518*

27. Genital Cancers 522

Shyamala Guruvare, Muralidhar V Pai

- Significance of Genital Cancer *522*
- Treatment and Results *523*
- Prevention of Pelvic Cancer *523*
- Early Diagnosis *524*
- General Management of the Cancer Patient *528*
- Management of Advanced Pelvic Cancer *529*

28. Tumours of the Vulva 536

Rekha Upadhya, Muralidhar V Pai

- Swellings of the Vulva *536*
- Varicose Veins *537*
- Oedema *537*
- Retention Cysts *537*
- Benign Neoplasms *538*
- Malignant Neoplasms of Vulva *542*
- Tumours of Bartholin's Gland *550*
- Urethral Tumours *551*
- Tumours of the Inguinal Canal *555*

29. Tumours of the Vagina 557

Rekha Upadhya, Muralidhar V Pai

- Swellings of the Vagina *557*
- Vaginal Cysts *557*
- Benign Neoplasms *558*
- Malignant Neoplasms *563*

30. Tumours of the Cervix Uteri 570

Priya Ganeshkumar

- Benign Neoplasms of the Cervix *570*
- Benign Tumours of the Cervix *570*
- Carcinoma of the Cervix *572*
- Screening for Cervical Cancer *576*
- Other Malignant Tumours of the Cervix *595*

31. Tumours of the Corpus Uteri 596

Saritha Shamsunder, Sufian Zaheer, Shivani Verma

- Enlargement of the Uterus *596*
- Uterine Polyps *597*
- Benign Neoplasms *597*
- Malignant Neoplasms *616*
- Molecular Classification *624*
- Adjuvant Treatment *628*
- Endometrial Stromal Tumours *632*

32. Adenomyosis 636

Anjali Mundkur, Muralidhar V Pai

- Associated Pathology *636*
- Aetiology *636*
- Diagnosis *637*
- Differential Diagnosis *638*
- Management *638*
- Complications *640*

33. Tumours of the Fallopian Tubes 642

Sanjay Kumar KR, Muralidhar V Pai

- Benign Neoplasms *642*
- Primary Malignant Neoplasms *642*
- Secondary Malignant Neoplasms *648*
- Prevention of Fallopian Tube Cancer *648*
- Recurrent Disease *648*
- Coping with Disease *648*

34. Tumours of the Pelvic Ligaments 649

Sanjay Kumar KR, Muralidhar V Pai

- Cysts of the Broad Ligament and Associated Structures *649*
- Neoplasms of the Pelvic Ligaments and Connective Tissues *650*
- Neoplasms of the Peritoneum *652*

35. Tumours of the Ovary 654

Pralhad Kushtagi

- Clinical Diagnosis of Ovarian Tumours *654*
- Complications of Ovarian Tumours *655*
- Features Suggestive of Malignancy in Ovarian Tumour *656*
- Pathology of Ovarian Tumours *658*
- Non-neoplastic Ovarian 'Tumours' *658*

- Neoplastic Ovarian Tumours 663
- Staging 668
- Nonepithelial Ovarian Tumours 674
- Germ Cell Tumours 677
- Treatment of Malignant Germ Cell Tumours 681

36. Chemotherapy in Gynaecological Malignancies 686

Sourjya Banerjee, Pratik Kumar Chatterjee

- Chemotherapy and the Cell Cycle 686
- Therapeutic Agents Used in the Treatment of Gynaecological Cancer 687
- Chemotherapy Toxicity 688
- Systemic Therapy in Gynaecological Malignancies 688
- Assessment of Response to Chemotherapy 693

37. Radiotherapy in Gynaecological Malignancies 695

Sourjya Banerjee, Pratik Kumar Chatterjee

- Biological basis of Radiotherapy Treatment 695
- Radiation Dosage 695
- Therapeutic Ratio 696
- Radiotherapy Machines 696
- Brachytherapy 696
- Radiotherapy in Carcinoma of the Cervix 696
- Radiotherapy in Endometrial Cancer 697
- Radiotherapy in Vulvar Cancer 698
- Brachytherapy in Carcinoma of the Cervix 699
- Chemoradiation in Locally Advanced Carcinoma of the Cervix 700
- Radiotherapy in Vaginal Cancer 700

38. Immunotherapy in Obstetrics and Gynaecology 701

Pralhad Kushtagi

- Immune System—Some Basics 701
- Immunotherapy in Gynaecologic Cancers 702
- Immunotherapy in Reproductive Medicine 709
- Immunotherapy in Other Situations 714
- Immunotherapy in Pregnancy 714

39. Amenorrhoea, Hypomenorrhoea, and Oligomenorrhoea 718

Pratik Tambe, Muralidhar V Pai

- Amenorrhoea 718
- Aetiology 718
- Treatment 735
- Hypomenorrhoea 738
- Oligomenorrhoea 741

40. Abnormal and Excessive Uterine Bleeding 743

Jayaraman Nambiar M, Muralidhar V Pai

- Terminology in Abnormal Uterine Bleeding 743
- Palm-Coein Classification of Abnormal Uterine Bleeding 744
- Causes of Abnormal Uterine Bleeding—Palm-Coein 744

- Wamsteker Classification *746*
- STEPW Classification of Myoma *746*
- Approach to a Patient with Abnormal Uterine Bleeding *749*
- Special Clinical Types of Bleeding *750*

41. Dysmenorrhoea 754

Brihathi Pranavi Dasari, Muralidhar V Pai

- Primary Dysmenorrhoea *754*
- Secondary Dysmenorrhoea *758*
- Membranous Dysmenorrhoea *760*
- Other Conditions Simulating Dysmenorrhoea *760*

42. Premenstrual Syndrome and Other Menstrual Phenomena 762

Kaushik Naik V, Muralidhar V Pai

- Clinical Features *762*
- Natural History *762*
- Laboratory Findings *763*
- Aetiology *763*
- Differential Diagnosis *764*
- Treatment *764*
- Menstrual Migraine *766*
- Premenstrual Mastalgia *767*
- Recurrent (Cyclical) Buccal and Vulvar Ulceration *768*
- Pelvic Allergy *769*
- Vicarious Menstruation *770*
- Cyclical Haemothorax and Pneumothorax *770*
- Menstrual Epilepsy *771*

43. Hormone Therapy in Gynaecology 772

Vidyashree G Poojari, Muralidhar V Pai

- Oestrogens *772*
- Antioestrogens *778*
- Progestogens *779*
- Antiprogestogens *782*
- Androgens *783*
- Antiandrogens *785*
- Types of Gonadotrophins *785*
- Antigonadotrophins *787*
- Hypothalamic Hormones *790*

44. Vaginal Discharge 792

Sujatha BS, Muralidhar V Pai

- General Considerations *792*
- Causes of Physiological Discharge *792*
- Prognosis *797*
- Risk Factors *797*
- Diagnosis *797*
- Management *799*
- Therapy *800*
- Prevention *802*

45. Pruritus Vulvae and Vulvodynia 804

Sujatha BS, Muralidhar V Pai

- Definition and Incidence *804*
- Pathophysiology *804*
- Natural Defence Mechanisms *804*
- Aetiological Classification of Pruritus Vulvae *805*
- Causes of Pruritus According to Age Groups *805*
- Evaluation of Patient with Pruritus *805*
- Investigations *805*
- General Measures for Women with Pruritus *805*
- Differential Diagnosis of Pruritus *807*
- Treatment *812*
- Results *813*
- Vulvodynia *813*
- Management *815*

46. Problems of Sex and Marriage 818

Niraj Jadav, Poonam Mishra

- Physical Sex—Coitus *819*
- Consummation of Marriage *819*
- Annulment of Marriage *820*
- Unconsummated Marriages *820*
- Coital Difficulties in the Male *821*
- Homosexuality *825*
- Marriage and Sexual Problems in Females: Understanding, Challenges and Solutions *826*
- Female Sexual Interest/Arousal Disorder *826*
- Female Orgasmic Disorder *829*
- Genito-Pelvic Pain/Penetration Disorder *832*
- Vaginismus *833*

47. Male and Female Infertility Overview 840

Mahesh C Koregal, Muralidhar V Pai, Soumya Mahesh Koregal

- Infertility *840*
- Frequency *840*
- Concept of Fertility *840*
- Causes of Infertility *841*
- Investigation of Infertility *846*
- Treatment *858*

48. Assisted Reproductive Technology 869

Mahesh C Koregol, Soumya Mahesh Koregol, Muralidhar V Pai

- In Vitro Fertilisation and Embryo Transfer *869*
- Controlled Ovarian Hyperstimulation *869*
- Oocyte Retrieval *870*
- Insemination *870*
- Embryo Transfer *872*
- Outcome *872*
- Cryopreservation *873*
- Oocyte Donation *873*

- Embryo Donation *874*
- Surrogacy *874*
- Intrauterine Insemination *875*
- Donor Insemination *877*
- Other Assisted Reproductive Technology Methods *878*
- Results of Treating Infertility *879*
- Dangers of Investigating and Treating Infertility *880*
- Complications of Assisted Reproductive Technology *880*
- Adoption *881*

49. Instruments in Gynaecological Procedures 884

Shripad Hebbar, Pooja HN, Muralidhar V Pai

- Instruments *884*
- Gynaecological Procedures *892*

50. Ultrasonography in Gynaecology 896

Priti Venkatesh

- Indications for Ultrasound in Gynaecology *896*
- Techniques *896*
- Normal Female Pelvic Anatomy *897*
- Uterus *897*
- Myometrium *911*
- Adenomyosis *919*
- Endometrium *926*
- Cervix *939*
- Adnexa *943*
- Polycystic Ovary *953*
- Ovarian Malignant Lesions *953*
- Fallopian Tubes *959*
- Endometriosis *960*
- Ultrasound Imaging in Gynaec Emergencies *962*

51. Ultrasound in Infertility 970

Vidyashree G Poojari, Muralidhar V Pai

- Method *971*
- Uterine Abnormalities *971*
- Cycle Assessment Consisting of Baseline Scan, Preovulatory Scan and Secretory Scan *991*

52. Ultrasound in Menopause 1001

Priti Venkatesh

- Normal Uterus in Menopause *1001*
- Ultrasound Evaluation of the Endometrium in Postmenopausal Women *1002*
- Postmenopausal Bleeding *1002*
- Hormone Replacement Therapy and Tamoxifen *1003*
- Incidental Finding of Thick Endometrium *1005*
- Normal Atrophic Ovary *1006*
- Fluid in Pouch of Douglas *1006*
- Ovary and Ovarian Cancer Screening *1006*

53. **Robotic Surgery** **1011**
Rani Akhil Bhat
- About da Vinci Surgical System *1011*
- Distinguishing Laparoscopy from Robotic Surgery: Unveiling Contrasts in Minimally Invasive Techniques *1014*
- Robotic Surgery Considerations for Patients *1016*
- Robotic Surgery Considerations for Doctors *1016*
- Introduction of da Vinci Robotic in Gynaecology *1016*
- Revolutionising Medicine: The Future Horizons of Robotic Surgery Innovation *1018*

54. **Endoscopic Surgery in Gynaecology** **1019**
Vidya Bhat, Mythreyi Kadambi

Laparoscopic Surgery 1019
- Surgical Equipment *1019*
- Indications *1026*
- Contraindications to Laparoscopy *1030*
- Preoperative Preparation *1030*
- Surgical Steps *1032*
- Postoperative Care *1034*
- Advantages *1035*
- Disadvantages *1035*
- Complications *1035*

Hysteroscopic Surgery 1037
- Surgical Equipment *1037*
- Indications *1041*
- Preoperative Preparation *1044*
- Surgical Steps *1044*
- Postoperative Care *1046*
- Advantages *1047*
- Disadvantages *1048*
- Complications *1048*
- Conclusion *1052*
- Hysteroscopic Resectoscope *1052*
- Slim Resectoscope *1052*
- Hysteroscopic Morcellator *1052*

Laparoendoscopic Single-site Surgery 1053
- Surgical Equipment *1053*
- Indications *1055*
- Laparoendoscopic Single-site Surgical Techniques *1055*
- Advantages *1057*
- Complications *1057*
- Conclusion *1057*
- Robotic Surgery *1057*

55. Contraception **1061**

Shobha N Gudi

- General Consideration *1061*
- Epidemiology *1061*
- Impact of Contraception Throughout the World *1062*
- Efficacy of Contraception *1062*
- Indications for Contraception *1063*
- Criteria for the Use of Various Contraceptive Methods *1064*
- Contraceptive Methods *1064*
- Natural Family Planning Method *1064*
- Barrier Methods *1068*
- Intrauterine Contraceptive Devices *1075*
- Hormonal Contraception Methods *1092*
- Progestogen-only Contraception *1105*
- Emergency Postcoital Contraception (Morning After Pills) *1115*
- Other Methods of Contraception *1117*
- Choice of Methods *1123*
- Contraception Choice for Older Women *1124*
- Contraception and Litigation *1124*

56. Sterilisation and Termination of Pregnancy **1128**

Priya Ballal K, Nikil Shetty, Ektha M Shetty

- Sterilisation *1128*
- Female Sterilisation *1129*
- Male Sterilisation *1131*
- Termination of Pregnancy *1133*

57. Urinary Incontinence **1140**

Shripad Hebbar, Muralidhar V Pai, Chandra Mithila

- Bladder Dysfunction *1140*
- Urethral Sphincter Dysfunction *1143*
- Investigation of Urinary Problems *1145*
- Treatment of Urinary Problems *1148*
- Incontinence of Urine *1149*
- Management *1153*
- Overview of Surgical Management *1155*
- Enuresis *1163*
- Urinary Retention and Difficulty in Micturition *1164*

58. Urinary Tract Infection **1170**

Shripad Hebbar, Chandra Mithila, Muralidhar V Pai

- Aetiology *1173*
- Diagnosis *1173*
- Investigations *1173*
- Management *1174*
- Treatment *1175*
- Complications *1177*
- Clinical Pearls *1178*
- Evidence-Based Medicine *1179*

59. Menopause 1181

Shyjus P

- History *1181*
- Definitions and Staging of Menopause *1181*
- Physiology of Menopause *1183*
- Problems Associated with Menopause *1185*
- Effect of Oestrogen Deficiency *1186*
- Menstrual Problems *1195*
- Management of Menopause *1196*
- Symptoms of Menopause *1196*
- Various Types of Hormonal and Nonhormonal Pharmacological Agents Available *1198*
- Use of Progesterones in Menopausal Hormone Therapy *1200*
- Hormone Therapy in Special Circumstances *1201*
- Androgens in Menopause *1202*

60. Hysterectomy and its Aftermath 1204

Shashikala K Bhat, Muralidhar V Pai

- History *1204*
- Types of Hysterectomy *1204*
- Preoperative Preparation *1205*
- Abdominal Hysterectomy—Operative Steps *1207*
- Minimally Invasive Hysterectomy Procedures *1208*
- Total Laparoscopic Hysterectomy in Special Situations *1212*
- Vaginal Hysterectomy *1212*
- Complications of Hysterectomy *1214*

61. Conditions of the Lower Intestinal Tract 1216

Srirama Bhat M

- Rectal Prolapse *1216*
- Incontinence of Faeces and Flatus *1223*
- Diarrhoea *1224*
- Difficult Evacuation *1225*
- Irritable Bowel Syndrome *1226*
- Pruritus Ani *1227*
- Pilonidal Sinus (Jeep Bottom; Driver's Bottom) Pilus—Hair; Nidus—Nest *1228*
- Rectal and Anal Pain *1228*
- External Pile/Haemorrhoids *1234*
- Anorectal Abscess *1234*
- Fistula-In-Ano *1235*
- Proctitis *1238*
- Endometriosis *1238*
- Neoplasm of the Anal Canal *1239*

62. Preoperative and Postoperative Management and Postoperative Complications 1241

Srirama Bhat M

- Fluid and Electrolytes *1241*
- Preoperative Management *1246*
- Postoperative Management *1249*
- Fast-track Protocol *1254*

- Postoperative Examination *1254*
- Postoperative Complications *1255*
- Deep Venous Thrombosis *1262*
- Pulmonary Embolism *1268*
- Pulmonary Complications *1271*

63. Nutrition and Exercise in Women 1274

Vidya Thobbi

Nutrition in Women 1274

- Maternal, Infant and Young Child Nutrition and Sustainable Goals *1275*
- Nutrition Basics *1275*
- Micronutrients *1275*
- Macronutrients *1275*
- Energy *1280*
- Adolescents Nutrition *1280*
- Nutrition During the Preconception Period *1285*
- Nutritional Requirements in Midlife *1285*

Exercise and Physiotherapy in Gynaecology 1287

- Active Muscle Exercises *1287*
- Electrical Stimulation of Pelvic Muscles *1289*
- Short-wave Therapy *1289*
- Infrared Radiation *1290*
- Transcutaneous Electric Nerve Stimulation *1290*
- Ultrasound *1290*

64. Applications of Lasers in Gynaecology 1292

Vidya Bhat, Mythreyi Kadambi

- History *1292*
- Laser Physics *1292*
- Types of Lasers *1293*
- Laser Safety *1294*
- Extraperitoneal Laser Surgery *1294*
- Clinical Applications of Lasers in Intra-abdominal Gynaecological Surgery *1295*
- Other Clinical Applications of Lasers in Gynaecology and Reproductive Medicine *1297*
- Novel Concepts—Lasers in Cosmetic Gynaecology *1298*

65. Genetics in Gynaecology 1300

Krupa Hitesh Shah, Muralidhar V Pai

- Genetics of Gynaecological Cancers *1300*
- Genetics of Common Benign Condition *1302*
- Genetic Testing *1304*
- Genetic Counselling *1304*

66. Artificial Intelligence in Gynaecology 1306

Sonal Panchal, Chaitanya Nagori

- How Artificial Intelligence Works? *1307*
- Artificial Intelligence Applications in Gynaecology *1307*

- Imaging *1308*
- Role of Artificial Intelligence in Benign Gynaecology *1308*
- Role of Artificial Intelligence in Gynaecological Cancers *1309*
- Role of Artificial Intelligence in Gynaecological Surgery *1310*
- Artificial Intelligence in In Vitro Fertilisation *1310*
- Embryology *1311*
- Urogynaecology *1311*
- Drug Research *1312*
- Artificial Intelligence Limitations *1312*
- Challenges *1312*

Index 1315

1

CHAPTER

A Clinical Approach to Gynaecology

Shripad Hebbar, Divyashree Bhat, Muralidhar V Pai

Chapter Outline

- Psychosomatic and Sociological Aspects of Gynaecology
- Clinical Methods
- Physical Examination
- Special Tests and Accessory Aids to Diagnosis
- Endometrial Sampling Procedures
- Transvaginal Sonography
- Transrectal Sonography
- Colour Doppler
- Endoscopy
- Laparoscopy
- Hysteroscopy
- Robotic Surgery
- Computed Tomography
- Magnetic Resonance Imaging
- Positron Emission Tomography Scan

"Mulier est hominis confusio—Madame, this Latin sentence means, "Woman is man's joye and all his bliss."

—Chaucer

INTRODUCTION

Gynaecology (from the Greek *gyne*, woman and *logos*, discourse) is the study of woman. But in medicine, usage restricts it mainly to the study of anatomy and physiology of the female organs of reproduction and their diseases. This is convenient, although the dividing line between gynaecology and other branches of medicine is ill-defined and varies from time to time and from clinic to clinic according to advances in knowledge, custom and local working conditions. At one time, the breasts were wholly within the domain of the gynaecologist, but now the general surgeon deals with certain breast disorders and the gynaecologist and obstetrician with the others. The genital tract is so closely linked, embryologically and anatomically, with the urinary tract and the large bowel that certain conditions of the urethra, bladder, and rectum come to a greater or lesser extent within the province of the gynaecologist. The whole endocrine system is concerned with the control of genital functions and birth of a baby. The psyche and sex are also inseparable from endocrine control. It may be added that, according to definition, obstetrics is the study of childbirth and its disorders. It is another aspect of gynaecology and, in practice, both go side by side. That is why, a clinician is addressed as obstetrician and gynaecologist.

These points merely serve to emphasise that it is impossible to consider the reproductive system separately from the remainder of the body and that it is necessary to interpret gynaecology in the wider sense. A woman is much more than just a caisson for a uterus and ovaries or a thingamabob for birthing. The woman who seeks advice for discomforts related to genital organs needs to be understood as a whole, i.e. her outlook, her achievements, her failures and her domestic, social, and sexual problems. Her ailment is to be addressed in highly specialised ways and with a lot of sensitivity.

The care of the whole woman will be threatened by the development of subspecialties, such as gynaecological endocrinology, foetal medicine, gynaecological oncology and gynaecological urology, endoscopy, infertility and assisted reproduction unless proper basic training in obstetrics and gynaecology remains a prerequisite to subspecialisations. These developments are justified only in a few centres to promote the growth of knowledge and expertise; otherwise, they deprive the woman of the person she can look for help at any time, one whom she knows has a personal interest in, and responsibility for, her welfare.

Although covering all aspects of the physiology of the female genital tract, gynaecology is basically a clinical discipline, and gynaecologists need to be primarily clinicians.

PSYCHOSOMATIC AND SOCIOLOGICAL ASPECTS OF GYNAECOLOGY

Environment can cause or aggravate physical and mental ill health; the psyche influences the development of organic diseases in all parts of the body; illness begets anxiety and this in turn begets illness; the reactions of doctor, relatives and friends to illness can determine recovery or chronic invalidism. These are not new discoveries but are as old as the practice of medicine. Psychosomatic medicine and social medicine are merely new names for old arts, which are practised almost automatically by the good doctor, and which find an important place in gynaecology.

Thus, menstruation can be inhibited for many months by a subconscious need to attract attention, by a desire for pregnancy, by a change in occupation or in living conditions and by extreme stress. On the other hand, menstruation may be precipitated by excitement and can become regularly excessive in response to nervous tension and domestic disharmony. A woman may develop pelvic symptoms to escape the advances of her husband. Painful menstruation, painful coitus and the like frequently have fear, resentment or guilt over genital functions as their basis, inculcated possibly by impressions and experiences gained during childhood. Social taboos also influence psyche. Obesity is much more likely to be a manifestation of an anxiety state or unhealthy lifestyle than evidence of endocrine disturbance. Many women, when worried, find solace in eating and drinking; if they are sleepless, they have longer hours in which to solace themselves.

A woman faced with unwanted responsibilities, or with any distasteful situation, may try to escape by blaming her genital organs about which there remains an air of mystery, which secures for her the sympathy of other women and of the oversolicitous husband. A gynaecologist must be a psychologist and a good counsellor although not necessarily a trained psychiatrist. If the part played by emotional and environmental factors in pelvic disease is recognised, only experience and wisdom are required to elicit them.

The majority of women are unconscious of these factors in their illness, and when made aware of them by sympathetic explanation, encouragement and tact, can adjust themselves to ensure a cure. There are a few, however, who deliberately set out to deceive and go to such lengths to achieve their objective that they are not easily found out.

Take for example the following rare case—a married woman aged 30 years, with two children, complained of recurrent and persistent vaginal bleeding which failed to respond to several lines of treatment. Ultimately, her uterus was removed, whereupon the bleeding continued and was found to be coming from vaginal ulcers which refused to heal even when repeatedly excised. It was then proved that she deliberately injured the vagina to make it bleed.

Rather than confining psychosomatic gynaecology to a single chapter, the aim in this book is to include it wherever it belongs, in the hope of placing it in its proper context. If the psychological aspects of gynaecology suffered from neglect in the past, there is now some danger of their being exaggerated. In clinical practice, the golden rule is that it should be made a rule never to diagnose neurosis or a psychogenic basis for symptoms until organic disease is excluded for certain clinically as well as on investigations.

CLINICAL METHODS

The handling and examination of the patient can only be properly taught and learned in the consulting room and at the bedside, and there is more than one way of doing them well. A systematic account of clinical methods is as wearisome to the writer as it is unprofitable to the reader. In this chapter, it is proposed to comment only on certain general principles and to offer suggestions for overcoming common difficulties.

The correct diagnosis of the cause of the patient's ailments depends on a process of detection. Some clues are worthless and misleading, and others are small but important. The good clinician is one who quickly realises what is significant and what is not, one who will not dismiss evidence, bizarre though it may appear, if it does not fit in with preconceived ideas. Clinical intuition is no more than the capacity to take intelligent notice (sometimes almost subconsciously) of small points **(Flowchart 1)**.

History

It is essential for the physician to communicate with a patient in a manner that allows her to continue to seek appropriate medical attention. It is necessary that a doctor listens to a patient completely, and if there is a good ear to listen the diagnosis will be made easy. Not only the words used, but also the patterns of speech, the manner in which the words are delivered, even body language and eye contact are important aspects of the patient–physician interaction.

The most important evidence is always provided by the history which the patient or her relatives can give, if allowed to do so. The diagnosis can nearly always be made or reduced to one of two or three possibilities based on the history without any physical examination.

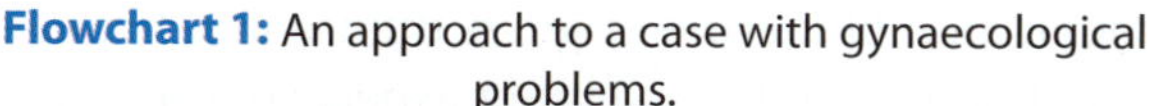

Flowchart 1: An approach to a case with gynaecological problems.

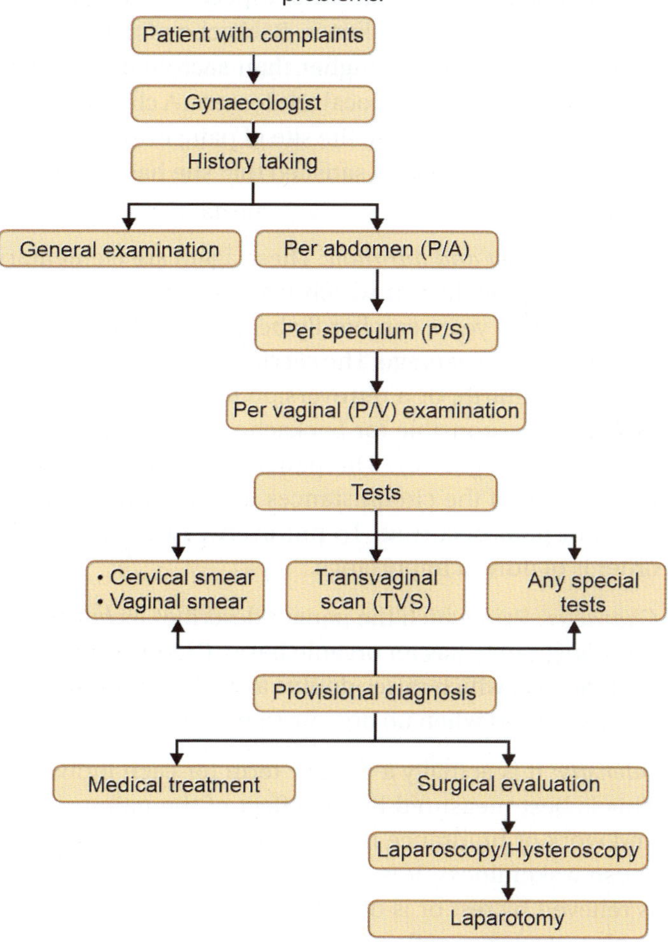

Physical signs are reliable and should mainly be used as confirmatory evidence. It is good practice never to examine the patient without taking history and having a provisional diagnosis in mind.

The previous medical history, family history and the account of symptoms as given by the woman can be boring, but scrupulous attention to them saves time, trouble and mistakes. She appreciates the opportunity to tell her story, and amongst irrelevances, invariably gives vital clues. Moreover, many irrelevances can be avoided by skilful guidance and by the occasional leading question.

An interesting incident will explain this; a garrulous old woman aged 80 years was admitted to the hospital as an emergency case with a history of a sudden onset of lower abdominal pain following a fall on getting out of bed. A few leading questions did not reveal typical features of any of the ordinary abdominal crises and, as the physical signs were not remarkable, she was kept under observation for 10 days during which time her discomfort subsided. She then appeared well and was prepared for discharge home. On the day, the patient was due to leave the hospital, as a final check, she was referred for the opinion of a gynaecologist. She was then, for the first time, allowed to tell her own story, from which it became clear that the sequence of events was—sudden lower abdominal pain, getting out of bed and faintness causing her to fall on floor—becoming unconsciousness on the floor for a few minutes and then residual abdominal pain and tenderness. All that remained necessary was to recognise a faint bruise around the umbilicus as *Cullen's sign*, and the picture of intraperitoneal haemorrhage was sufficiently complete to justify laparotomy. The laparotomy revealed the cause to be a small and previously nonpalpable sarcoma in the fundus of the uterus, which had caused intraperitoneal bleed. Her symptoms were being taken in the light of her age.

Thus, successful interrogation requires an inquisitive outlook. Why has this woman come to see me today and not 6 months ago? Why has she not had children during 3 years of marriage? What was the illness, which confined her to bed for 3 months in childhood, and what were its symptoms and treatment? At what time in pregnancy did the two abortions occur? How long did she breastfeed the last baby? Did she suffer from fever after any of the pregnancies? How old is her husband? Is she only child? Have her aunts got hairy faces? What operation was carried out 5 years ago? What were her symptoms at the time and what was she told? What is her lifestyle? What is her job? Does she go out to work and who looks after the children while she does? Why is she worrying about a trivial symptom or is her mother worrying on her behalf? Is she afraid of cancer or of a sexually transmitted disease? Is she stressed or appears to be depressed? So, as a good learned clinician, one has to address all this smoothly, sensibly and with utmost sensitivity and care.

History taking also requires tact, for it is concerned with details of what some women regard as highly embarrassing topics. It calls for privacy, kindness, courtesy, and a deferment of more personal questions until confidence is established. Previous illness and confinements are usually safe grounds, although caution is necessary if a baby has been lost. A woman may find it easier to talk about menstruation than about discharge, while marital and domestic problems should come last. A matter of fact and coldly scientific attitude is the one most likely to encourage the patient to discuss intimate matters without embarrassment. Attention to dress, avoidance of jokes, formal behaviour and concentration on the patient and her problems are especially important to maintain the right atmosphere in a teaching clinic.

Importance should be given to the patient–physician relationship. One needs to listen more and talk less. Encourage the pursuit of topics important to patients. It is necessary to realise that one should minimise controlling speech habits, such as interrupting, issuing commands and lecturing. Care should be taken to understand the discomfort of certain issues and become aware of discomfort in an interview, recognise when it originates in an attempt by the physician to take control and redirect that attempt. The confidence one gives by assuring patients that they have the opportunity to discuss their problems fully is very important. Sometimes, all that is necessary is to be there as a compassionate human being. If clinical findings or confirmatory testing strongly suggest a serious condition such as malignancy, the gravity and urgency of this situation must be conveyed in a manner that does not unduly alarm or frighten the individual. Honest answers without false hopes should be provided to any specific questions the patient may want to discuss.

Often during the course of examination, some fact of which the patient is ashamed comes to light. Perhaps, she is pregnant, has been pregnant, or has had a sexually transmitted disease. Such confidential disclosures are to be received impassively and naturally, without a sign of approval or disapproval, and the patient should not see that any record is made of them. Such records can be made in medical language.

Symptoms

Trivial Symptoms

Whenever the symptom appears inadequate or atypical, suspect that it is a cloak for another worry. The recently married woman who complains of long-standing dysmenorrhoea is probably suffering from dyspareunia. The woman without children after several years of marriage is often complains of infertility whatever other symptoms she has. Vague pains or insignificant discharge may denote cancer phobia. Malaise and general weakness, which may be taken as due to overwork, are actually may be due to hypothyroid or deficiency of vitamin D.

Pain

Exact site and radiation: Ovarian and tubal pain is felt *low* in the abdomen, usually immediately above the inguinal ligament. Pain of uterine origin is diffuse and hypogastric in site, often referred to the inner aspects of the thighs but not extending below the knees. Backache of pelvic origin is in the midline, never higher than sacroiliac (SI) level. It is not accompanied by local tenderness. A clinician must ask the patient to indicate the site of pain; even if she fails to do so, at least she feels satisfied that she has told all her problems.

Nature of onset and duration: These again are elementary matters, the neglect of which leads to errors. The pain present for 10 years can hardly be attributed to an event that occurred 2 years ago. The cervical laceration sustained during childbirth, or a retroversion following pregnancy, cannot be responsible for backache, which commenced during the pregnancy. The patient should have a clear recollection of the circumstances under which a sudden onset of pain occurred. To put events in chronological order is of utmost importance.

Character: Pain which the patient describes as *burning* or *throbbing* rarely has an organic basis. *Excruciating* is also an adjective, which raises doubts as to the genuineness of the discomfort when no organic signs are evident.

Intensity: It is actually a relative term for each individual. This is best measured by the effect of the pain on sleep and work or hindrance in her daily routine. If it does not cause wakefulness, it is either caused by a lesion, which is relieved by rest or is of little consequence. Severe pain is almost always reflected in the patient's manner and demeanour. A good clinician should realise that woman of healthy appearance who describes her agony with a smile, and whose attention is easily distracted from it, is overstating her case.

Relationships: In a female patient complaining of pain, the clinician should try and establish its relationship to the menstruation.

Menstruation: Women may try to link discomfort with menstruation and persuade themselves, if not the observer, that an association exists. There is always a lowering of pain threshold before and during menstruation, so that even toothache feels worse at that time. Fact is that nearly every condition affecting the lower part of the body exhibits a premenstrual exacerbation, e.g. irritable bowel syndrome, SI, lumbosacral strain. Care is, therefore, necessary to ensure that pain is truly associated with menstruation and, if it is, to know its exact relationship to the occurrence of the flow. Like in endometriosis, there is a very specific relationship of pain with menses. A chronic dull pelvic pain becomes worse with start of bleeding and lingers on even after stoppage of flow. Spasmodic dysmenorrhoea presents differently.

When there is dysmenorrhoea that is painful menses, the history should be in more detail as follows.

As there are two types of dysmenorrhoea (spasmodic and congestive), a careful history is needed to differentiate the same. Spasmodic or primary dysmenorrhoea has no obvious cause and is seen on day 1 or 2 of the menstruation, whereas congestive or the secondary dysmenorrhoea is due to some pathology in the gynaecological organs, and the pain may be premenstrual, menstrual or postmenstrual in nature. When a girl or a woman gets secondary-type congestive dysmenorrhoea, it is necessary to ask whether the pain is relieved on menstruation and if so the reason may be pelvic inflammatory disease (PID), whereas if the pain is more after menstruation, it is usually due to endometriosis (ectopic menstruation). Menstrual type of dysmenorrhoea is usually due to fibroid of uterus (benign tumours of uterus) or adenomyosis (ectopic endometrium in the myometrium). Triple dysmenorrhoea (premenstrual, menstrual, and postmenstrual) is typical of endometriosis.

- *Coitus:* Dyspareunia is specific in some diseases such as endometriosis.
- *Micturition:* Dysuria or painful micturition is also important.
- *Defaecation:* Tenesmus is present in cases of endometriosis and in the presence of ovarian cysts.
- *Eating:* This pain may indicate its bowel origin.
- *Posture and movement:* Recognition of the relationship between exercise and rest prevents many types of backache from being attributed to a pelvic lesion. In fact, a backache, which worsens by the evening, is most often the result of strain imposed by a lax protuberant abdominal wall and the consequent compensatory lumbar lordosis. It is also important to rule out pelvic pathology.

Menstrual Function

Menarche and Standard Menstrual Habit

It is necessary to know the age of the menarche and the cycle, which is normal for the particular individual. Knowledge of the latter provides a standard with which to compare symptoms. Women are often treated for *heavy periods* without it being recognised that their menstrual function has never changed. Leading questions are sometimes helpful.

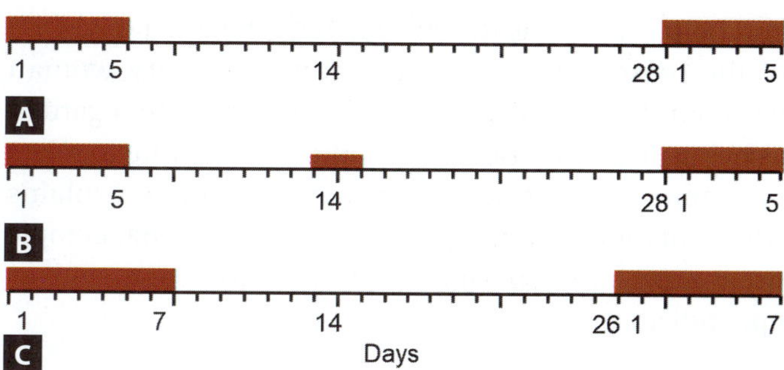

Figs. 1A to C: Examples of misinterpretation of the menstrual cycle. (A) This represents a normal situation in which bleeding occurs for 5 days every 28 days; (B) A normal cycle with a short loss at the time of ovulation, described by the patient as menstruation every 2 weeks;(C) An essentially normal cycle (7/26), described by the patient as having two periods in 1 month or bleeding every 19 days.

Menstrual Symptoms

Patients unwittingly mislead themselves and the observer about the cycle. They say they menstruate *twice a month* when periods begin on the 2nd and 28th day of the same month (i.e. a 26-day cycle). They say they menstruate every 3 weeks when they mean that they are *free* from bleeding for 3 weeks **(Figs. 1A to C)**. Many keep no record of the dates of menstruation.

When there is no urgency, ask the patient to keep a menstrual calendar for 3 months; she is often surprised at the regularity which this reveal. The amount of bleeding can be judged by the number of sanitary pads or tampons used, by interference with work or other pursuits, and by the presence of anaemia. In difficult and doubtful cases, the woman should be kept under observation throughout a certain period.

Abnormal menstrual cycles deserve close analysis. It is not enough to know whether the loss is profuse or slight; its exact duration and periodicity must be determined. Indeed, a clear menstrual history of bleeding days, amount of bleeding and interval is important.

Last Menstrual Period

Knowledge of the date of the first day of the last menstrual period and in many cases the date of the preceding one is vital from the standpoints of diagnosis and treatment. The woman may say she does not know or may use some vague expression such as *2 weeks ago* but, with encouragement and help, can nearly always calculate the exact day. One of the reasons for knowing this is that every woman between the ages of 15 and 50 years should be regarded as being pregnant until proven otherwise. Failure to relate symptoms to the time in the menstrual cycle explains why ovulation pain, corpus luteum haematoma, ectopic pregnancy and endometriosis are misdiagnosed as appendicitis.

Associated Symptoms

In a condition such as endometriosis, a girl or woman may have all of the following symptoms or none of them or some of them.

It is important to remember the five *Ds:*

1. Dysmenorrhoea
2. Disorders of menstruation
3. Dyspareunia (painful coitus)
4. Dyschezia (pain during defecation)
5. Dull aching pain in the abdomen (due to distortion of pelvic anatomy)

Infertility will be an additional problem in cases of endometriosis.

PHYSICAL EXAMINATION

General

A full general examination is as important in gynaecology as in any other branches of medicine, more important than in some others. Note the general appearance and behaviour of the patient. Does she show evidence of anaemia, dehydration, wasting, obesity or hirsutism? The neck may reveal enlargement of the thyroid gland or of lymph nodes. Disease of the heart and lungs must be excluded and in certain conditions, chest radiography may be required. Examination of the mouth, hands, arms, legs and feet may precede or follow examination of the abdomen.

Breasts

While examining the heart and lungs, the breasts can be inspected to assess their development and to exclude those changes indicative of early pregnancy without the patient realising that pregnancy is suspected. This is particularly true for the young unmarried girl. In all women and especially in those aged 30 years and more, the breasts should be palpated routinely to exclude tumour formation. Galactorrhoea should be looked for in women who are infertile and in those who have oligomenorrhoea.

Abdomen

It is necessary to understand that by a proper examination with the patient being comfortable, we will be able to get the right findings which will give the path to the right diagnosis. With the patient in the supine position, an attempt should be made to have the patient relax as much as possible. Her head should be leaned back and supported gently by a pillow so that she does not tense her abdominal muscles.

The abdomen should be inspected for signs of an intra-abdominal mass, organomegaly or distention that would, for example, suggest ascites or intestinal obstruction. Initial palpation of the abdomen is performed to evaluate the size and configuration of the liver, spleen and other abdominal contents. Evidence of fullness or mass effect should be noted. This is particularly important in evaluating patients who may have a pelvic mass and in determining the extent of omental involvement, for example with metastatic ovarian cancer. A fullness in the upper abdomen could be consistent with an *omental cake*. All quadrants should be carefully palpated for any evidence of mass, firmness, irregularity, or distention. A systematic approach should be used (e.g. clockwise, starting in the right upper quadrant). Percussion should be used to measure the dimensions of the liver. The patient should be asked to inhale and exhale during palpation of the edge of the liver.

Omission to carry out an abdominal examination *before* a pelvic one results in many errors. The following are some points deserving emphasis:

- No one is, nor should be, better than the gynaecologist at palpation, for she/he is dependent on a highly developed and regularly used sense of touch for work in the antenatal clinic and in the delivery room and for pelvic examination in general.
- The lighter the palpation and the more the hand is kept on the flat, the easier it is to define tumours.
- Every tumour in the lower abdomen should be suspected as being a full bladder, and this condition can sometimes only be excluded for certain by passing a catheter. Otherwise, the most common mass is a pregnant uterus.
- The clinician should rub his hands to make it warmth before touching the patient's abdomen.
- Take notice of any rigidity and guarding if present.
- Percussion of the abdomen can be even more valuable than palpation in the diagnosis of abdominal tumour in distinguishing it from ascites and in deciding their origin whether it is intraperitoneal or retroperitoneal.

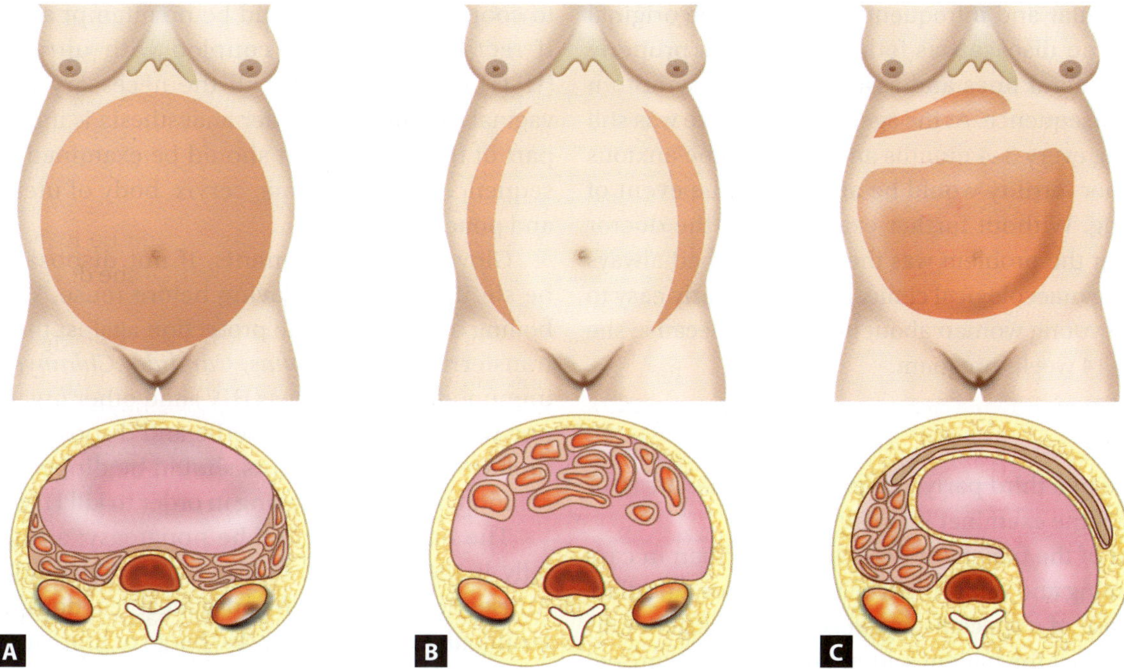

Figs. 2A to C: Percussion of the abdomen in the diagnosis of tumours. Dullness is indicated by shaded areas. (A) An ovarian or uterine tumour; (B) Ascites; (C) A retroperitoneal tumour and a large hydronephrosis.

Except when a loop of bowel is adherent, all tumours arising from the pelvic organs are uniformly dull to percussion. A retroperitoneal tumour (including one of renal origin) almost always has one or more loops of bowel in front, which is shown by resonance **(Figs. 2A to C)**. Pseudocyesis and phantom tumours provide no problem to the doctor who percusses.

Whenever an abdominal tumour is found, examine especially for ascites and enlargement of the liver.

Examination of a Mass Per Abdomen

Inspection

Note the abdomen for the shape or contour and any evidence of distension, scar, stria and loosening and presence of dilated veins. Umbilicus is seen for eversion and herniation.

On Palpation

Note the size, shape, consistency, margins and mobility of mass—unilateral or bilateral. It is important to differentiate between benign ovarian tumours and fibroid uterus. When a suprapubic mass is palpable, it is necessary to find out whether we can put our hands below the lower border or not. This is called getting below the mass. If so, the diagnosis is a benign ovarian tumour since the mass is pushed up because of the long pedicle an ovarian tumour has. If we cannot get below the lower border, then the diagnosis is usually fibroid of uterus and the mass is described as *arising from the pelvis or uterus*. However, if the problem is of malignant ovarian tumour, then because of the spread of the disease, the mass will be of variegated consistency, margins not clear, fixed or restricted mobility, and there may be the presence of ascites too. However, all the malignant tumours do not have ascites, as only epithelial ovarian malignancy produces ascites.

Percussion

Fluid thrill and shifting dullness should be tested for to rule out ascites.

Pelvic Examination

Pelvic examination is the last part of a gynaecological examination, its main purpose being to confirm a diagnosis already made or suspected from the history and symptoms and by abdominal inspection. It should be repeated from time to time when an illness is long lasting for the situation may change. One of the common traps is illustrated by the following case.

A young single woman was attended on and off for many years by an excellent general practitioner because she had irregular and infrequent periods. At the original assessment, no disease was found so she was properly treated on general lines and assured that her symptom was of no consequence. At the age of 23 years, she was still menstruating every 3–4 months and had become anxious to know if her fertility would be affected in the event of her marrying. Without further examination, the doctor assumed that the problem was the same as it had always been. At the gynaecological clinic, it was singularly easy to reassure the young woman about her fertility because she was already 14 weeks pregnant.

Prerequisites

- Presence of a third party, preferably a female nurse or relative, if the examiner is a male.
- Consent of the patient or her parent, guardian in case she is young and unmarried, of her parent or guardian.
- In the case of a specialist gynaecologist, it is generally accepted that the patient's attendance implies consent to a pelvic examination.
- The patient's bladder must be empty.
- The rectum and pelvic colon too should preferably be empty. If loaded, it may be wise to ask the patient to return after the bowel has been cleared by a laxative.
- A good light which is well situated.

Vaginal Examination

Vaginal examination is usually more informative than rectal examination and is possible in most women. If the patient is virginal, the opening in the hymen may be wide enough to allow a one-finger or narrow speculum examination without pain or injury, especially if she is in the habit of using a tampon to control the menstrual discharge. A decision about attempting a vaginal examination in any case must be based on the previous assessment of the circumstances and the likely reaction of a given patient. In this connection, it is necessary to recognise the customs and religious beliefs of different countries. In the East and Middle East, for example, vaginal examination of the unmarried woman is generally never attempted for it may prejudice her prospects of marriage. Unless a bride can prove her virginity by an intact and unstretched hymen, the marriage may be annulled. For such reasons, it is not unknown for parents to refuse to allow their daughters to be treated for imperforate hymen causing haematocolpos. Whenever a tentative approach makes it clear that the patient is averse to the examination and that she is unlikely to cooperate, there should be no attempt at persuasion. If rectal examination coupled with ultrasonography (USG) does not supply all the necessary information, vaginal examination under anaesthesia is indicated. Each part of the genital tract should be examined in a logical sequence—vulva, vagina, cervix, body of uterus, adnexa and pouch of Douglas.

Gloves and instruments, if not disposable, should be sterilised by autoclaving before reuse. Washing and boiling offer inadequate protection against the real risk of transferring *Trichomonas*, *Candida*, *Chlamydia*, human immunodeficiency virus (HIV) and other organisms from one woman to another. Sterile and disposable gloves are preferred. All instruments should be dipped in a bleach solution before autoclaving in order to kill HIV.

The lubricant should be nongreasy; a water-soluble jelly is the best and, failing that, a cetrimide solution. Antiseptic creams often cause local reactions and lanolin is difficult to remove. Any discharge or lubricant left on the vulva at the end of the examination should be swabbed away for the patient's comfort.

Local inspection should precede per speculum examination and palpation.

Speculum examination of the vagina should usually *precede* bimanual examination for the following reasons:

- Vaginal discharge can be seen and removed for examination before it is contaminated with the lubricant.
- The cellular debris from the cervix and uterus is undisturbed and can be obtained for cytological study.
- Bimanual examination may make some lesions of cervix and vagina bleed, which can compromise further examination.

Size of speculum should be carefully chosen as it may cause pain during insertion; however, any difficulty in insertion can usually be overcome by careful appraisal of the introitus.

A Sims' **(Figs. 3A and B)** or bivalve speculum **(Fig. 4)** should not be inserted straight away; actually, these instruments are designed for direct application after separation of the labia with the fingers of the opposite hand. The vagina is, in any case, wider from side to side than from front to back. Speculum is inserted in longitudinal fashion and then rotated in vagina to push away the anterior and posterior vaginal walls to show cervix.

For palpation, first insert one finger into the vagina; insert the second finger only when the patient relaxes the muscles around the vagina and when it is clear that a

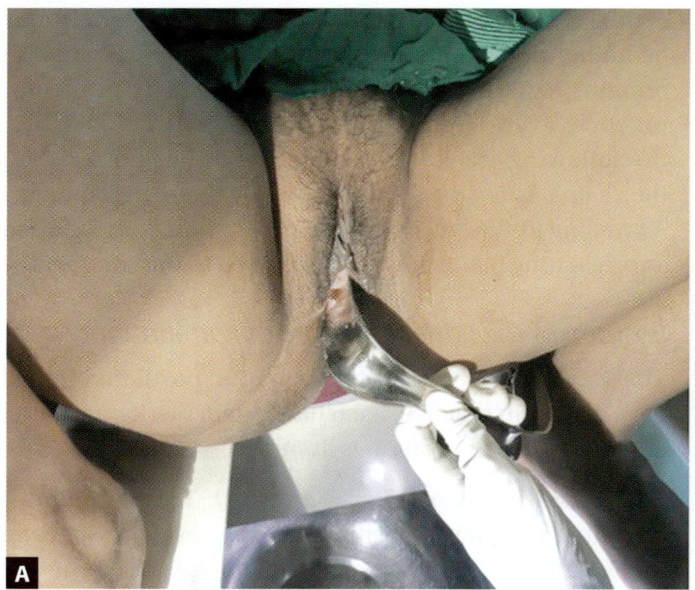

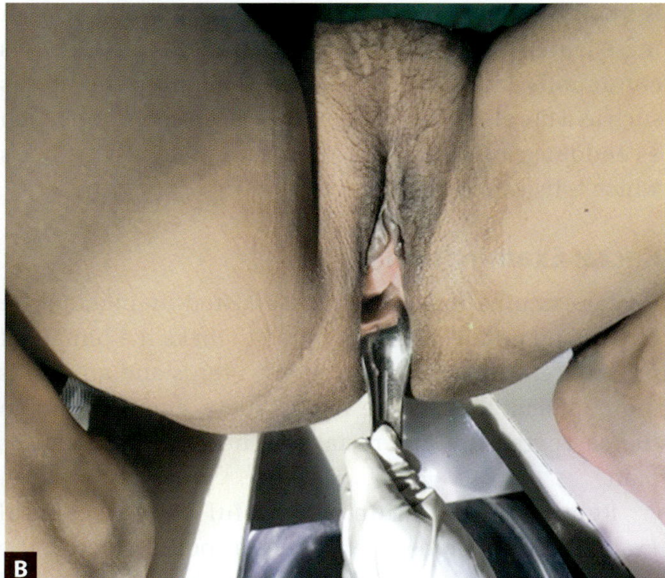

Figs. 3A and B: Insertion of Sims' speculum for examination.

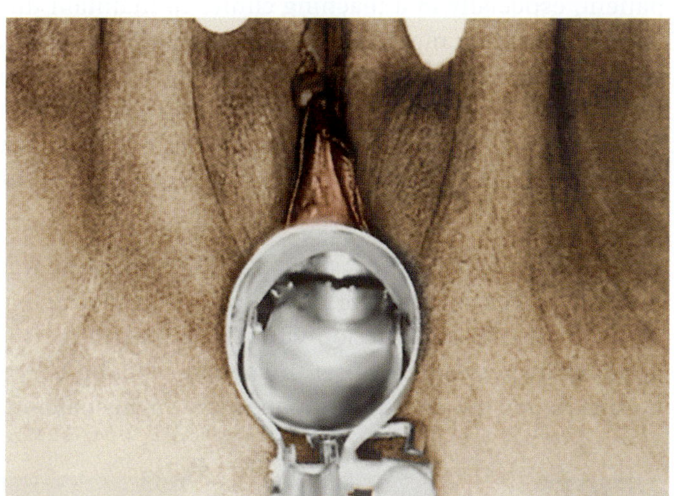

Fig. 4: The Cusco's speculum is introduced directly in the transverse axis of vagina.

two-finger examination is possible without causing pain. Avoid the sensitive vestibule and urethral orifice, and remember that the vagina slopes upwards and backwards. Insert and withdraw fingers slowly.

The secret of bimanual examination is to use the abdominal hand more than the vaginal fingers. It is the former which must bring the various organs within comfortable reach. The beginner always thinks that shortness of the fingers accounts for inaptitude, whereas it is failure to use the abdominal hand correctly. To feel the uterus, the vaginal fingers should move the cervix as far backwards as possible to rotate the fundus downwards and forwards. The abdominal hand is then placed just below the umbilicus (not suprapubically) and gradually moved lower until the fundus is caught and pressed against the fingers in the anterior fornix. The uterus, which is not felt, is lying above and behind the abdominal hand.

The points to be determined with regard to the cervix and the uterus are the size, shape, position, mobility, consistency and tenderness caused by pressure or movement. The normal uterus is tender when squeezed between the two hands. The position and direction of the cervix are the guides to the body of the uterus; for this reason, mere inspection of the cervix usually indicates whether the uterus is anteverted or retroverted.

How do we describe the size of a uterus?

A bulky uterus (corresponding to 6 weeks' pregnant size) is just bigger than normal. When the uterine enlargement fills the fornices, then the size of uterus is equivalent to 12 weeks gravid uterus. When the fornices are not full, the size can be <12 weeks' size. In between, the size could be between 8 and 10 weeks' size.

The following points are noted: Size of the uterus, anteverted or retroverted, mobile uterus, restricted mobility or fixed uterus. The adnexa are palpable for any masses or tenderness. If there is a mass felt, its relation to the uterus is noted like whether the mass is felt separate to the uterus or felt continuous with the uterus. When the mass is felt separate from the uterus, the origin of the mass is from the adnexa or broad ligament such as the ovarian mass and broad ligament masses, whereas if the mass is continuous with the uterus, it is arising from the uterus such as a fibroid of the uterus. However, in conditions such as endometriosis and PIDs, the adnexa may have a mass which is fixed and tender.

Rectal Examination

Rectal examination too can be assisted by placing the other hand on the lower abdomen to make it a bimanual procedure. Palpation of the cervix, uterus and adnexa is more difficult than by the vaginal route, and pressure on the cervix through the rectal wall nearly always causes pain.

Rectal examination is useful when vaginal examination is impossible and has a special place in the pelvic investigation of babies and children, especially if ultrasound is not possible. It is also a useful adjunct to vaginal examination and is the best approach for feeling the uterosacral ligaments, pouch of Douglas and the outer parts of the broad ligaments; it is, therefore, used for assessing the extent of a growth arising in the cervix.

Combined Rectal and Vaginal Palpation

It is extremely helpful to insert the index finger into the vagina and the middle finger into the rectum. This combined method has a special value in determining whether a lesion is situated within the bowel or between the bowel and the genital tract.

Findings

The student new to gynaecology is often depressed at being unable to palpate the uterus and adnexa. It should be explained that it usually takes 1 month's work in a clinic before one can expect to feel the uterus bimanually in a reasonably cooperative unanaesthetised patient. In more difficult cases, the uterus can be felt only if the patient is anaesthetised and not always even then. The expert gynaecologist who confidently states that the uterus is normal in all respects sometimes does so without actually defining it. If honest, he or she will admit that often the findings are deduced by noting the position and mobility of the cervix and by knowing that the uterus would be felt if it were enlarged.

Normal tubes are never palpable, even in the anaesthetised patient. Palpation of the ovaries is largely a matter of chance, but if they are not felt, the gynaecologist can be reasonably certain they are not enlarged. It may be added that even an expert at bimanual examination remains expert only so long as he or she is in regular practice; even 1 month's holiday reduces one's skill in the following week. A swelling, which lies posterior to the vagina, is nearly always caused by the rectal contents. A swelling in the left side of the pelvis should be regarded as originating in the bowel until proved to the contrary.

Position of the Patient for Pelvic Examination

There are several possible examination positions, and all have a place in practice. Each has certain merits, and strict adherence to one position is limiting.

Full dorsal position ***(Figs. 5 and 6A)****:* This is the most commonly employed position. It is the best for inspection of the vulva and for bimanual palpation of the uterus and adnexa. It is not as good as the lateral position for inspecting the vaginal walls. Moreover, it can be embarrassing for the patient, especially in a teaching clinic. To maintain this position, nothing more than a firm couch is necessary, the examiner standing on the right side. The woman feels much less exposed if the thighs and knees are kept partly covered. Some gynaecologists prefer a short couch with footrests, and they then stand directly in front of the patient.

Sims' semiprone position ***(Fig. 7)****:* This position was devised by Marion Sims for operations on vesicovaginal fistulas. Used in conjunction with Sims' speculum, it is good for inspecting the anterior vaginal wall and cervix because when the introitus is opened, the vagina balloons

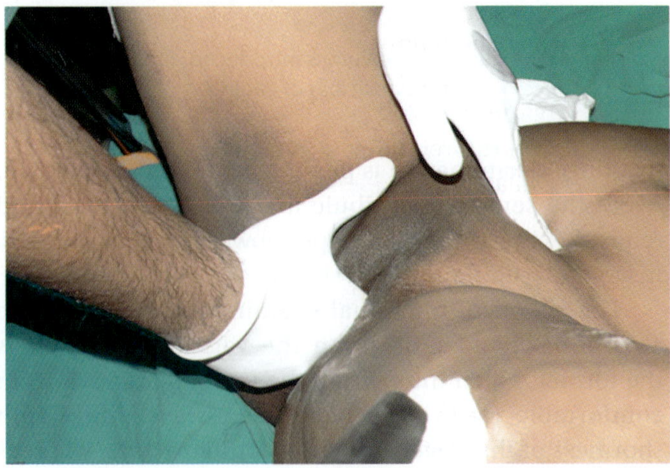

Fig. 5: Bimanual examination in the full dorsal position. Keeping the knees covered makes the patient feel less exposed.

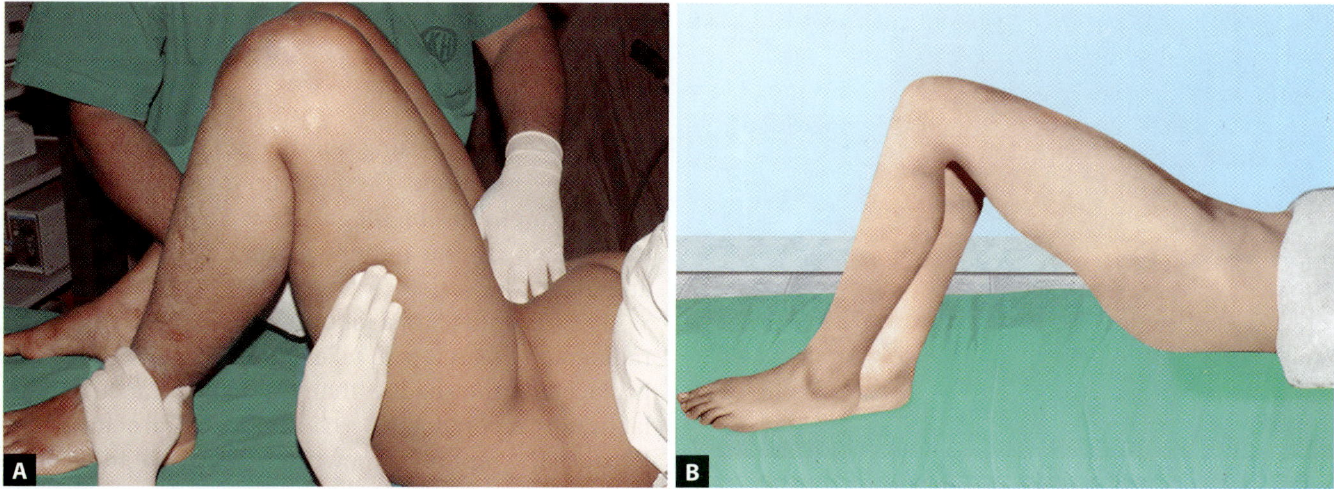

Figs. 6A and B: (A) Bimanual examination with the patient in the full dorsal position; (B) The attitude which the patient should adopt when examination is difficult. Use of the extensor muscles of the trunk ensures relaxation of the abdominal muscles; abduction of the thighs encourages relaxation of the pelvic floor. Tilting of the pelvis brings the pelvic organs within easier access of the abdominal hand.

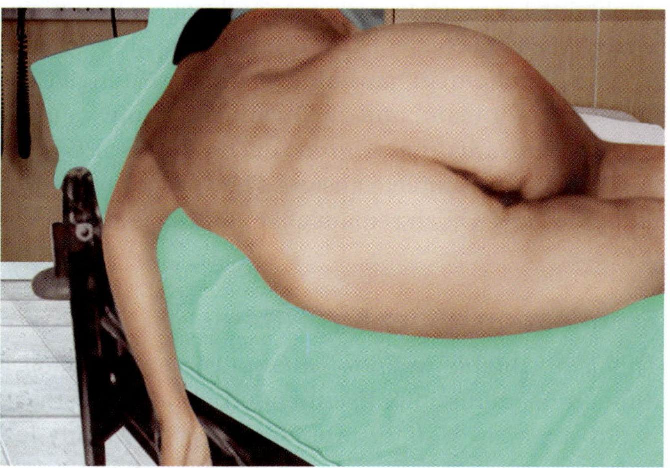

Fig. 7: Sims' semiprone position.

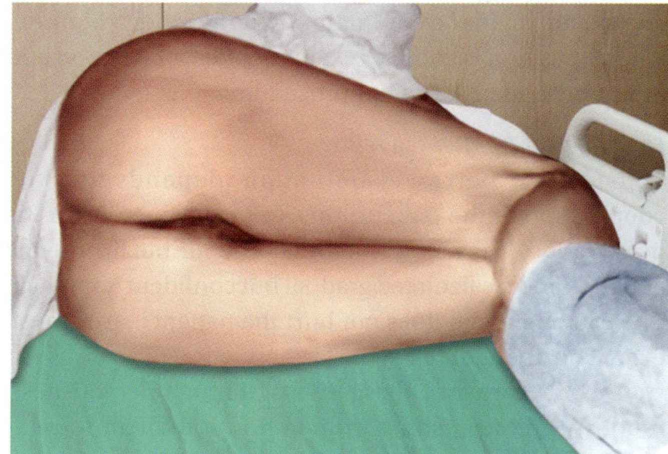

Fig. 8: Lateral position.

with air. The patient finds this position least embarrassing, but movement is limited by the position of the left arm, and the abdomen is not easily accessible to the examiner's left hand. It is, therefore, rarely used, especially nowadays with the availability of sophisticated operating tables.

Modified Sims' or lateral position ***(Fig. 8)****:* Here, the patient keeps her left arm in front and she lies more on her side. It causes little embarrassment but allows good inspection of the anus, perineum and posterior parts of the vulva, vagina and cervix. It may be used for demonstrating prolapse during coughing and straining and for minor operations on the cervix of the unanaesthetised woman. Bimanual examination is possible, but it is generally not as satisfactory as in the dorsal position.

Lithotomy position ***(Fig. 9)****:* This is usually used for vaginal operations and for examination under anaesthesia.

Knee-chest position: This allows the vagina to balloon with air, encourages the intestines to fall away from the pelvis and is ideal for visualising the cervix and anterior vaginal wall. The patient finds it objectionable; however, it is rarely used. It was previously used for certain operations, such as the insertion of radium or caesium, repair of a vesicovaginal fistula and culdoscopy.

Bearing in mind the advantages and disadvantages, one should make it a practice to examine the patient in the full dorsal position. This allows inspection of the introitus, testing for prolapse, inspection of vagina and cervix and taking of swabs and smears. After speculum examination,

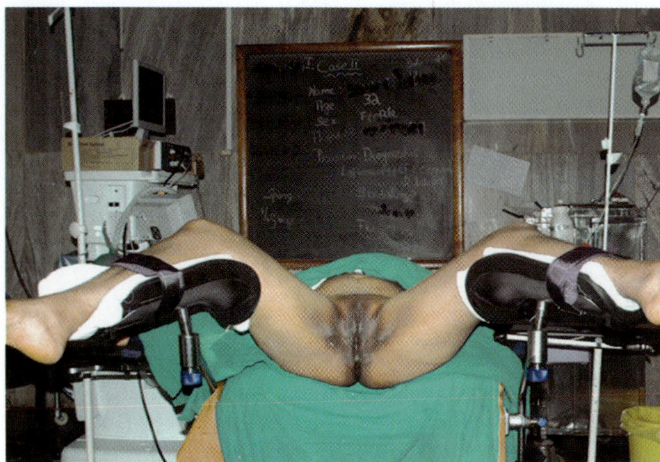

Fig. 9: Lithotomy position.

first one and then two fingers are inserted into the vagina and bimanual examination is conducted. Combined rectal and vaginal examination is done when required. Lateral position is good for examining the anal region and lithotomy is ideal for minor procedures.

How to get the patient to relax?

Satisfactory pelvic examination depends on the cooperation of the patient; this, in turn, depends on the personality of the medical attendant, gentle but firm laying of hands and a calculated gradual but confident approach. The examiner who does not hurt the patient learns most, even if he does not reach the farthest.

Despite care over these points, through nervousness, modesty and fear, some women find it difficult to relax the muscles of the abdomen and pelvic floor to allow bimanual examination. In these circumstances, it is generally advised that the patient should flex the thighs on the abdomen and breathe deeply through the mouth, a procedure which is not always effective.

The best way to obtain relaxation of the abdominal muscles in the dorsal position is for the patient to arch her back (without assistance from attendants) and to support herself on her shoulders and feet **(Fig. 6B)**. Strong action of the extensor muscles of the trunk ensures complete and automatic relaxation of the flexors. This method also helps with the insertion of a bivalve speculum in the dorsal position. Moreover, in this position, the pelvis rotates to bring the uterus nearer to the abdominal wall. Relaxation of the levators and other muscles around the vagina is secured by the patient deliberately abducting the thighs or by bearing down as in defaecation.

SPECIAL TESTS AND ACCESSORY AIDS TO DIAGNOSIS

Ancillary Services

With the ever-increasing number of laboratory tests and other investigations, the paramount value of ordinary clinical methods of diagnosis is in danger of being overlooked by the patient as well as by the medical attendant.

It is easier to fill in a request form for blood analysis or radiography than it is to take a full history. More reliance is placed on the shadow than on the substance and on a laboratory report than on a clinical appraisal of the patient. Because the report is typewritten, many fail to recognise that. It is no more than an opinion and sometimes the opinion of a relatively inexperienced technician. It is useful but often not any more than the opinion of the doctor at the bedside. Information about hormones can be obtained at much less expense and trouble by noticing their effect on the patient's own genital tract.

The biochemist, pathologist and radiologist are members of a team, and each can contribute valuable evidence towards the solution of the problem but not necessarily the complete answer. They should be used to fill in the gaps, which remain after clinical assessment of the case.

Examination Under Anaesthesia

This is a valuable weapon when pelvic examination is difficult or impossible. Examination under anaesthesia is not the answer to all problems; it is frequently less satisfactory than examination without anaesthesia, can be frankly misleading and in certain conditions, e.g. ectopic pregnancy, is dangerous. Its great disadvantage is that the all-important sign of tenderness is lost. Whenever this examination is carried out, anaesthesia must be sufficient to ensure complete relaxation of the abdominal muscles. To obtain the maximum information, the examination should generally include measurement of the cavity of the uterus and endometrial sampling. Hysteroscopy may sometimes give additional information. This procedure is not required in current facilities. However, hysteroscopy is a minimally invasive procedure requiring anaesthesia and imaging studies such as high resolution transvaginal ultrasound, magnetic resonance imaging (MRI), imaging will give equally good information. When additional procedure is required, e.g. polypectomy, septal resection, then diagnostic and therapeutic hysteroscopy may be helpful to the patient.

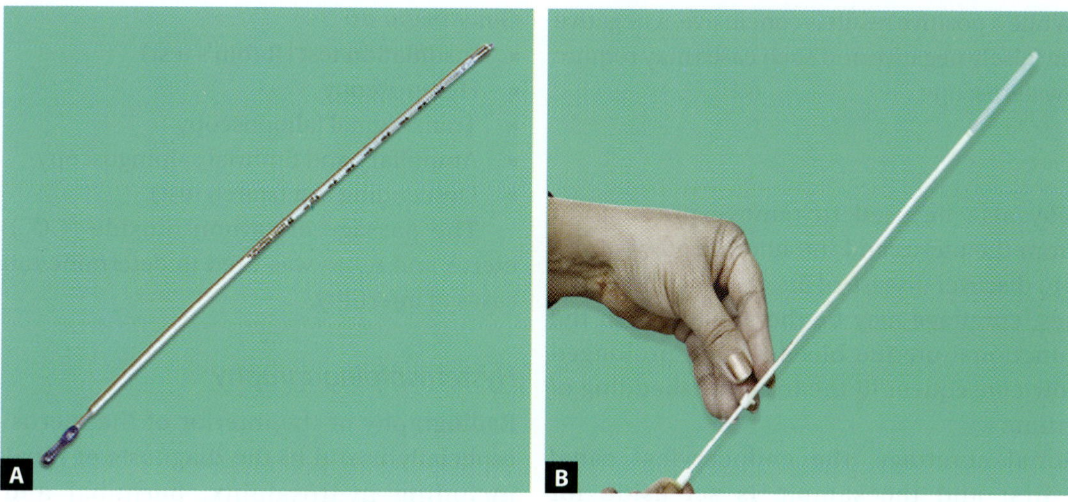

Figs. 10A and B: Endometrial aspiration cannula.

ENDOMETRIAL SAMPLING PROCEDURES

Endometrial Biopsy

Outpatient (Office) Curettage

The term endometrial biopsy is, by custom, applied to the incomplete diagnostic curettage carried out without anaesthesia. By means of a narrow biopsy curette, one or two strips of endometrium are obtained for histological study.

Endometrial sampling suction devices are made up of a plunger enclosed in a sheath. The plunger is retracted to create negative pressure when the sheath is placed within the uterus, which pushes tissue into the sample device. The majority of suction sampling methods work at low pressure.

The most widely used technique for endometrial sampling is the use of low-pressure devices, such as Pipelle and Endocell.

Higher pressure devices, such as the Karman cannula and Vabra aspirator, are used less commonly because patients generally feel less comfortable with them.

This method is only used to determine the reactions of the endometrium to ovarian stimulation or the presence of infective pathology, e.g. tuberculosis.

Endometrial Aspiration

Endometrial aspiration is an extension of the biopsy. It allows more thorough evaluation and can be used to diagnose or exclude certain types of endometrial disease as an outpatient procedure, e.g. hyperplasia and tuberculosis, to determine the response of the endometrium to endogenous hormones and thereby assess ovarian function, including ovulation. A special narrow cannula **(Figs. 10A and B)** curette is inserted into the uterus, and the endometrial tissue is extracted by electric suction or suction by the cannula itself. A 4-mm Karman-type cannula **(Fig. 11)** to which is attached a 20-mL syringe can be used instead with similar results. Suction is maintained for 2 minutes. This detaches the endometrium, following which the curette is gently rotated in all directions, and the endometrium is sucked out. Endometrial aspiration is essentially a diagnostic procedure, and any material obtained by it must always be submitted to histological, and often to bacteriological, examination. Its indications are definite, and it should never be carried out without a clear reason and for want of something better to do. Since dilatation of the cervix is not required, no anaesthesia, or at most local infiltration of the paracervical nerve plexuses, is necessary, and the patient feels little discomfort. This procedure is now used instead of endometrial biopsy or curettage, except in select cases where curettage is done for therapeutic indications. Endometrial aspiration coupled with endocervical curettage can be used instead of fractional curettage in women with postmenopausal bleeding to diagnose malignancy in the uterus or

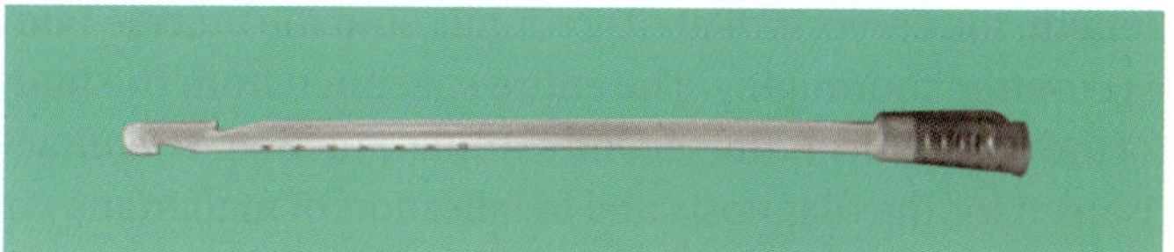

Fig. 11: 4-mm Karman cannula.

endocervix. While a positive result is conclusive, a negative result could be falsely negative and such cases may require curettage or hysteroscopy.

Curettage

Curettage may also be used to remove products of conception from the uterus and intrauterine polyps from the uterus or to discover disease of the endometrium.

Sometimes, curettage may be therapeutic as in the case of dysfunctional uterine bleeding and prolonged menstrual flow consequent to the irregular shedding of the endometrium.

In fractional curettage, the endocervical canal is curetted first and the sample is set aside for histopathological examination. Next, the sound is passed gently into the uterine cavity to assess the direction and length, the cervix is dilated gradually, and the uterine body is curetted thoroughly. The entire specimen from the body of the uterus forms the second sample. Fractional curettage is used for the diagnosis and localisation of malignancy in the uterine corpus or cervix.

All curettage procedures require some form of anaesthesia. They also carry a higher risk of complications such as perforation and injury to the cervical os and, therefore, aspiration procedures are generally preferred.

Now, procedures such as fractional curettage are not preferred unless in rural settings; otherwise, hysteroscopy is ideal, and biopsy is taken under vision.

Culdocentesis and Culdotomy

Culdocentesis is a procedure wherein the needle is put through the posterior fornix into the pouch of Douglas, and culdotomy is a procedure where a transverse incision is put in the posterior fornix. However, culdocentesis was done for diagnosis of ruptured ectopic pregnancy or pelvic abscess but is no more done as there are better diagnostic modalities. Colpotomy is rarely done in cases of pelvic abscess drainage.

Tubal Patency Tests

Tubal patency assessment is a necessary part of a thorough infertility evaluation.

The commonly used tests are:

- Hysterosalpingogram
- Sonosalpingogram
- Laparoscopy chromotubation.

Other methods:

- Insufflation test (Rubin's test)
- Hysteroscopy
- Transvaginal falloposcopy
- Ampullary and fimbrial salpingoscopy
- Descending test (starch test).

The passage of carbon dioxide (CO_2) through the uterus and tubes was used to determine tubal patency in cases of infertility.

Hysterosalpingography

Radiography of the interior of the uterus and tubes is especially useful in the diagnosis of tubal obstruction, including hydrosalpinx, peritubal and intrapelvic adhesions, malformation of the uterus, small intracavitary tumours causing dysmenorrhoea and menorrhagia, and a defective internal cervical os causing abortion or premature labour.

Hysterosalpingography is valuable in the diagnosis of tubal disease such as tuberculosis. However, in the presence of active disease, it can lead to dissemination or activation of the disease and prove dangerous.

Sonosalpingography

- Also known as Sion test, it is a diagnostic procedure primarily used for evaluating the patency of fallopian tubes.
- It was introduced as a screening procedure for infertility investigation and is becoming popular due to the absence of side effects.

Under ultrasonography scanning, a slow injection of 200 mL of physiologic saline into the uterine cavity is accomplished via Foley catheter. By visualising the flow of saline along the tube and observing it as a shower at fimbrial end, tubal patency can be tested. Also, the presence of fluid in the pouch of Douglas confirms tubal patency.

Laparoscopic Chromotubation

- It is a procedure usually done during a laparoscopy to visualise the fallopian tube to see if it is patent.
- It is a procedure where a coloured dye, diluted methylene blue, is passed through the fallopian tube via cervix to confirm that it is patent.
- This is ideal as a tubo-ovarian relationship can also be seen.

Ultrasonography

Ultrasonography or sonar (sound navigation and ranging) was originally used to detect submarines by means of ultrasonic echo sounding. Highly sophisticated apparatus working on this principle is now the most valuable diagnostic tool in a wide range of obstetrical and gynaecological conditions. Ultrasound waves of very high frequency (3.5–5 MHz) generated by passing electric current through a piezoelectric crystal are passed through the abdominal wall, which has been smeared with jelly to secure acoustic coupling. Solid tissues reflect the ultrasound beam while liquids allow it to pass through. The echoes, which are reflected back to the crystal, are converted to electrical energy. The images thus vary according to the character of the tissues encountered by the entering beam. By photographic recording of the echoes, a picture of the tumour or tissue under study is obtained. *Real-time* imaging allows one to see the scanned object in motion by processing numerous pictures like a movie. The higher the wavelength used, the less the depth of penetration. Ultrasound permits the diagnosis of pregnancy (and of multiple pregnancies) and can determine its viability by 6–8 weeks. It can also identify the placental site and detect foetal abnormalities. In gynaecology, it distinguishes between ascites and abdominal tumours and between uterine leiomyomas, ovarian cysts (benign or malignant) and other masses such as pyosalpinx. The interactivity of ultrasound makes it an extension of clinical examination. Probe palpation can be used to assess tenderness, movement and compressibility.

Ultrasound is a reliable and acceptable method of distinguishing between hydatidiform mole and normal pregnancy **(Figs. 12A and B)**. It is routinely used in the management of infertility to detect the ripening of Graafian follicles, for confirmation of ovulation and for ovum pickup in cases of in vitro fertilisation. Ultrasound-guided biopsies and cyst aspiration can also be done.

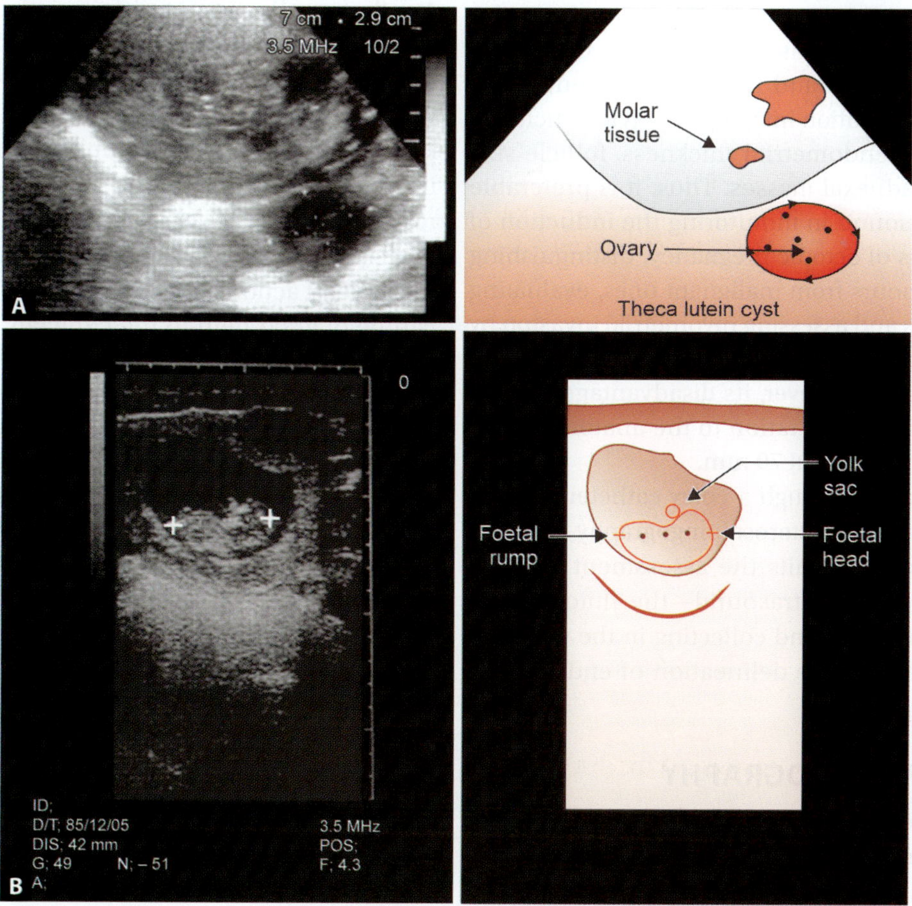

Figs. 12A and B: (A) This ultrasonic scan shows the typical molar tissue filling the uterus and below and to the lower right there is a theca lutein cyst; (B) This shows a normal foetus in its sac with the +mark indicating the crown–rump length of an 11–12-week-old foetus.

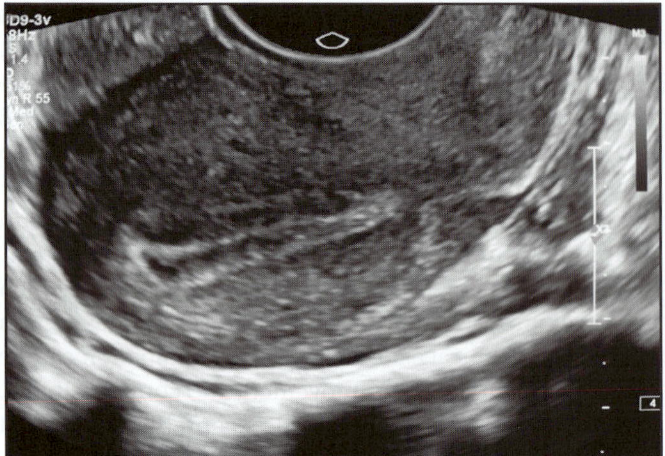

Fig. 13: Transvaginal sonogram with a 7.0-MHz probe showing the uterus in longitudinal section with a central endometrial echo.

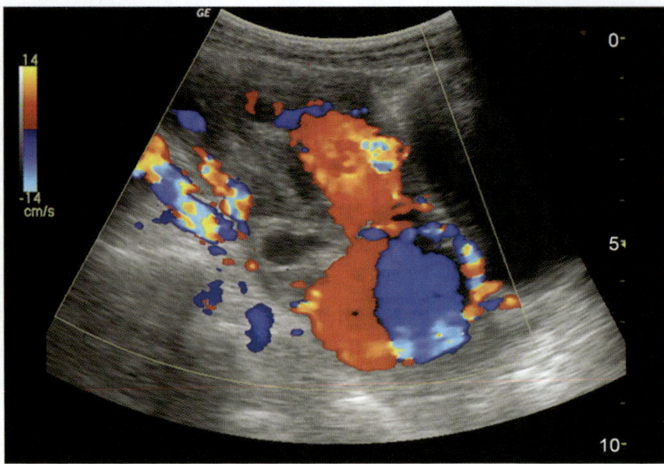

Fig. 14: Sagittal sonogram showing enlarged vessels within the myometrium. After a dilatation and curettage, an arteriovenous malformation developed; the extensive colour signal is seen on axial power Doppler imaging.

TRANSVAGINAL SONOGRAPHY

Transvaginal sonography (TVS) is a valuable adjunct in gynaecology **(Fig. 13)**. The TVS probe generates waves of a higher frequency, i.e. 5.5–7.5 MHz. The closer the probe is to the area which has to be scanned, the higher is the frequency required and the less the attenuation. TVS allows higher resolution imaging of pelvic structures, especially to assess endometrial thickness, follicle size and evaluation of adnexal masses. Thus, it is preferable to abdominal ultrasound in monitoring the induction of ovulation, diagnosis of ectopic pregnancy, distinguishing benign ovarian tumours from malignant ones, evaluating endometrial lesions and assessing myometrial invasion by endometrial cancer. A major advantage is that it does not require a full bladder. However, its disadvantages are an initial lack of observer orientation to the anatomy and a depth of view limited to about 70 mm.

Instillation of saline through a Foley catheter into the endometrial cavity (sonohysterosalpingography or saline infusion sonography) permits the assessment of tubal patency by transvaginal ultrasound—the fluid is seen passing through the tubes and collecting in the pouch of Douglas. It also permits the delineation of endometrial lesions.

TRANSRECTAL SONOGRAPHY

The transrectal probe is of particular benefit in the evaluation of cervical lesions and assessment of parametrial extension of cervical cancers. It is also useful in patients with vaginal stenosis in whom the TVS probe cannot be inserted.

COLOUR DOPPLER

Another application of ultrasonic is the Doppler device which detects movement—for example the flow of blood, and translates it into sound **(Fig. 14)**. Strictly speaking, Doppler is not ultrasound because it usually falls within the audible range. The Doppler principle uses the shift in frequency of the sound wave, as the source moves relative to the observer to determine its velocity. Using this principle, it requires a relatively simple apparatus to detect foetal heart action by the 10th week of pregnancy, and this can be of great help to the clinician. More sophisticated apparatus is able to quantitate blood flow through vessels, e.g. uterine artery, umbilical artery, foetal aorta, carotid and cerebral arteries, and is important in managing cases of intrauterine growth restriction and preeclampsia. In gynaecology, it is used to diagnose the occurrence of deep venous thrombosis in the lower limbs. The Doppler gate is superimposed on a real-time scan that allows the target to be pinpointed.

Commonly used indices of pulsatility in Doppler ultrasound are as follows:

- *Systolic/diastolic ratio:* It is the ratio of peak systolic to end-diastolic.
- Doppler shift frequencies
- *Resistance index (RI) (Pourcelot index):* It is the difference of maximum and minimum Doppler shifts divided by the maximum.
- *Pulsatility index (PI):* It is the difference between maximum and minimum values divided by mean

values of the waveform. This value is independent of the Doppler angle, i.e. the angle between the ultrasound beam and the axis of the blood vessel.

Transvaginal colour Doppler blood flow studies are useful in predicting whether tumours are benign or malignant. Malignant cell growth is accompanied by neovascularisation and angiogenesis. These vessels are thin-walled and, therefore, have low impedance. Thus, benign ovarian cystic tumours may be avascular or relatively avascular and record moderate velocity and high-resistance flow with an RI of about 0.525. The RI falls to 0.322–0.255 in malignant ovarian tumours due to high-velocity and low-resistance blood flow, while the PI is <1. Low-resistance flows are also seen in the placenta, corpus luteum and inflammation.

ENDOSCOPY

Visualisation of the pelvic organs by way of endoscopes has been employed sporadically since the beginning of the 20th century, but these diagnostic procedures achieved wide popularity only with the development of modern apparatus which ensures adequate lighting without dangerous heating of the peritoneal cavity.

Endoscopy is now so simple and efficient that there is danger of its being used too freely, to the neglect of standard clinical methods of diagnosis. Instead of analysing symptoms and signs, it is tempting to look and see.

LAPAROSCOPY

Laparoscopy uses apparatus which incorporates a fibre-optic lighting system for complex inspection of the pelvic organs and for several surgical procedures. In many countries, the earliest laparoscopic procedures were sterilisation operations, which involved destruction of part of the fallopian tubes by diathermy. Later, application of rings or clips was adopted as these destroyed smaller segments of the tubes, offering better prognosis for recanalisation operations, if required. These procedures were and still are done using single-puncture laparocators.

Subsequently, diagnostic laparoscopy was developed. This is almost always done using two or more ports, the additional ports allowing the use of a grasper, biopsy forceps or a cannula for suction and irrigation. Diagnostic laparoscopy is used for the investigation of unexplained infertility, to detect small islands of endometriosis, streak gonads, small ovarian tumours, polycystic ovaries, and pelvic adhesions. When tubal patency is in question, the passage of an aqueous solution of methylene blue injected via the cervix demonstrates the presence and site of the block.

Operative procedures, which can be undertaken simultaneously laparoscopically, include ovarian biopsy and cystectomy, aspiration of cyst fluid, the division of peritubal and periovarian adhesions, fimbrioplasty and drainage of hydrosalpinx, ovarian drilling in polycystic ovaries, ablation of endometrial deposits, excision of endometriomata, laparoscopic uterosacral nerve ablation (LUNA), management of ectopic pregnancy and even myomectomy. Advanced operative laparoscopic work includes laparoscopy-assisted vaginal hysterectomy, lymphadenectomy in cases of malignancy, urogynaecologic procedures, etc. Gamete or zygote intrafallopian transfer is done laparoscopically as well.

The procedure involves the insertion of a laparoscope under general anaesthesia through the abdominal wall **(Figs. 15A to D)**. For this to be done safely, the peritoneal cavity has first to be distended with CO_2. The gas, of which as much as several litres may be required, is introduced through a Veress needle inserted in the abdominal wall by way of a tiny transverse incision, usually on the lower rim of the umbilicus. The trocar with its sleeve is inserted through this and made to enter the tense peritoneal cavity just below the umbilicus. The trocar is then replaced by the endoscope. To bring the organs into better view, the uterus can be manipulated by means of a uterine elevator placed in the cervix.

The operator must be reasonably certain that the gut is not adherent to the anterior abdominal wall at the site of entry of the trocar. If there is a previous scar near the umbilicus, access can be sought through the left upper quadrant first in the midclavicular line below the 9th rib (Palmer's point) and the trocar inserted under vision. Alternatively, the open laparoscopy technique can be used. Additional ports are located in the iliac fossa medial to the inferior epigastric vessels or suprapubically to permit the insertion of various instruments. Hundreds of instruments have now been designed to facilitate all types of surgery laparoscopically **(Fig. 16A)**. Monitors with built-in controls permit autoregulation of gas flow rates, intra-abdominal pressure, etc., to increase safety. The use of a camera and video monitor allows the entire team to visualise the procedure **(Fig. 16B)**. The proceedings can also be recorded. For tissue division, scissors, electrodiathermy or

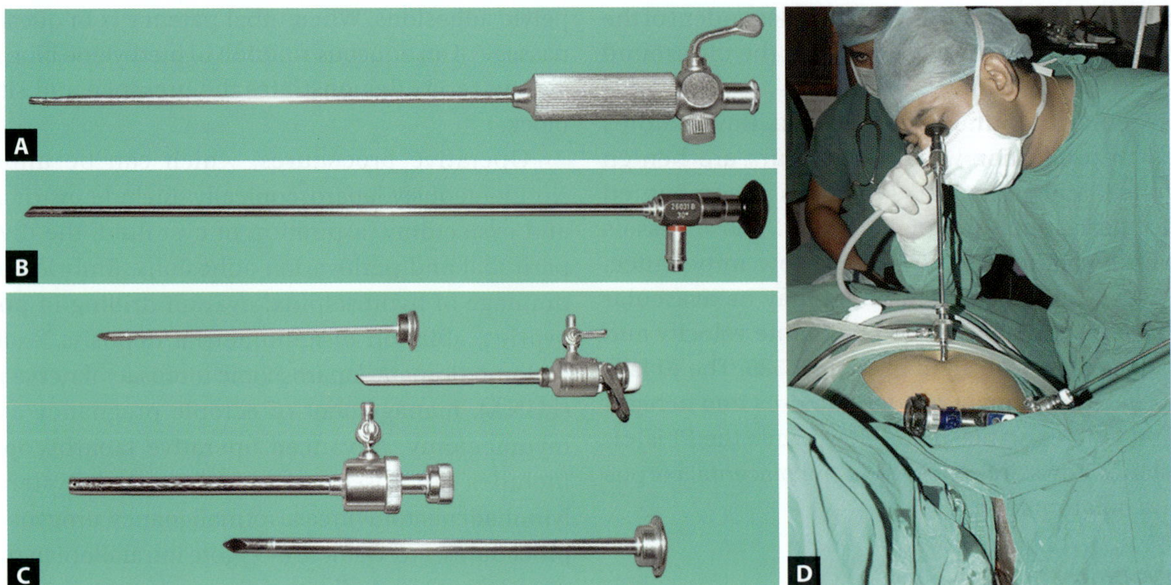

Figs. 15A to D: Laparoscopy. (A) Veress insufflation needle for creating a pneumoperitoneum with carbon dioxide; (B) The simple laparoscope with its trocar and cannula (photographs presented by Down Bros and Mayer and Phelps Ltd); (C) Trocars and cannulas; (D) The laparoscope in place with the patient in the Trendelenburg position. The laparoscope has been inserted through a small incision along the lower rim of the umbilicus. Bipolar grasping forceps have been inserted through a small suprapubic incision and are being used to manipulate the pelvic organs. A camera attachment over the eyepiece, if available, permits viewing on a monitor.

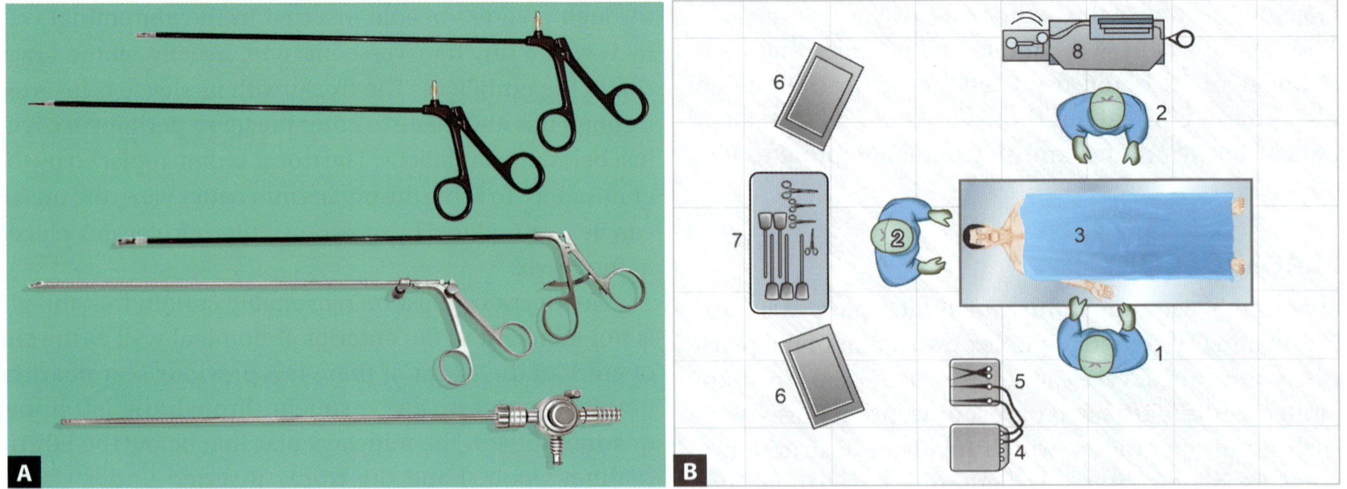

Figs. 16A and B: (A) Instruments for operative laparoscopy (from above down): Serrated edged grasper without lock, pointed atraumatic grasper, serrated edged grasper with lock, curved scissor and irrigation aspiration suction cannula; (B) Operating room layout: (1) Surgeon, (2) assistant scrub nurse, (3) patient table with stirrups (arms are placed as indicated), (4) electrosurgical cart, (5) surgeon's instrument trolleys, (6) video display monitors with videocassette recorder (VCR) power source, (7) operating instruments table, and (8) endoscopic supply cart with carbon dioxide (CO_2) insufflator and suction machine.

laser can be used. Various lasers currently in use include the CO_2, neodymium-doped yttrium-aluminium-garnet (Nd:YAG), potassium titanyl phosphate (KTP), argon and holmium. Each has its own cutting and coagulating abilities, and the choice of laser depends on the task at hand. Suturing with barbed suture material, which does not require knotting, is now available and stapling devices can be used as required.

At the conclusion of the operation, the gas is expressed from the abdomen by way of the cannula. The skin incision is closed with one or two clips or sutures which are removed 5 days later.

The complication rate of laparoscopy depends on the experience of the surgeon but for large series, it is about 0.1–0.2%. Some patient-related parameters such as obesity and a prior history of abdominal surgery may increase the incidence of complications. Complications of laparoscopic surgery can be divided into two phases—the first is the creation of the pneumoperitoneum and the second is the operation itself. The insertion of the Veress needle and the first trocar is carried out blind and is the most hazardous part. Injury to major blood vessels, bowel or bladder may ensue. Damage by the lateral trocars can result in damage to the inferior epigastric vessels, haematoma formation or incisional hernia if a 10-mm port is used. CO_2 embolism can be fatal. Ureteric damage, pulmonary embolism and infection can also occur. Burn injury is more likely from monopolar than from bipolar coagulation. To increase the safety of the procedure, special sheathed trocars have been devised. In the alternative system of open laparoscopy, the rectus sheath is incised and the peritoneum is opened under direct vision. However, some bowel injury can still occur.

Gasless laparoscopy is done using mechanical abdominal wall elevators placed through one or more openings in the abdomen. These use simple suspensory chains on sophisticated equipment. This avoids the complications of CO_2 insufflation and may be useful in combined laparovaginal procedures. However, there is a risk of trauma and pressure ischaemia to the abdominal wall; visualisation of the lateral pelvic wall is impaired by the triangular shape of cavity distension; lack of abdominal pressure allows the bowel to come into the operative field.

Laparoscopy is contraindicated in severe cardiorespiratory disease, massive intra-abdominal haemorrhage, acute intestinal obstruction, severe intra-abdominal adhesions, very large intra-abdominal masses and untreated advanced malignancy.

HYSTEROSCOPY

It is possible to visualise the cavity of the uterus with hysteroscopes incorporating fibre-optics **(Figs. 17A and B)**. Several media have been used to distend the uterine cavity: 32% dextran, 5% dextrose in water, normal saline, CO_2 and 1.5% glycine.

While any of the media may be used for diagnostic hysteroscopy, operative hysteroscopy which uses electrocautery, is done using 1.5% glycine, i.e. a nonelectrolyte solution, as the distension medium. Hysteroscopy is used to exclude intrauterine pathology as a cause of abnormal bleeding or infertility, such as myomas, polyps and foreign bodies, e.g. misplaced intrauterine contraceptive devices (IUCDs) and bony fragments following incomplete abortion. It also offers an opportunity for their removal. In the diagnosis of endometrial carcinoma, it may be used for taking a guided biopsy, but there is a theoretical risk of disseminating malignant cells into the peritoneal cavity. Women with oligomenorrhoea or amenorrhoea may be found to have intrauterine synechiae, atrophic endometrium or chronic endometritis. Synechiae can be divided under hysteroscopic guidance. Other hysteroscopic procedures include endometrial ablation, resection of intrauterine septa and proximal fallopian tube cannulation. Hysteroscopic sterilisation using

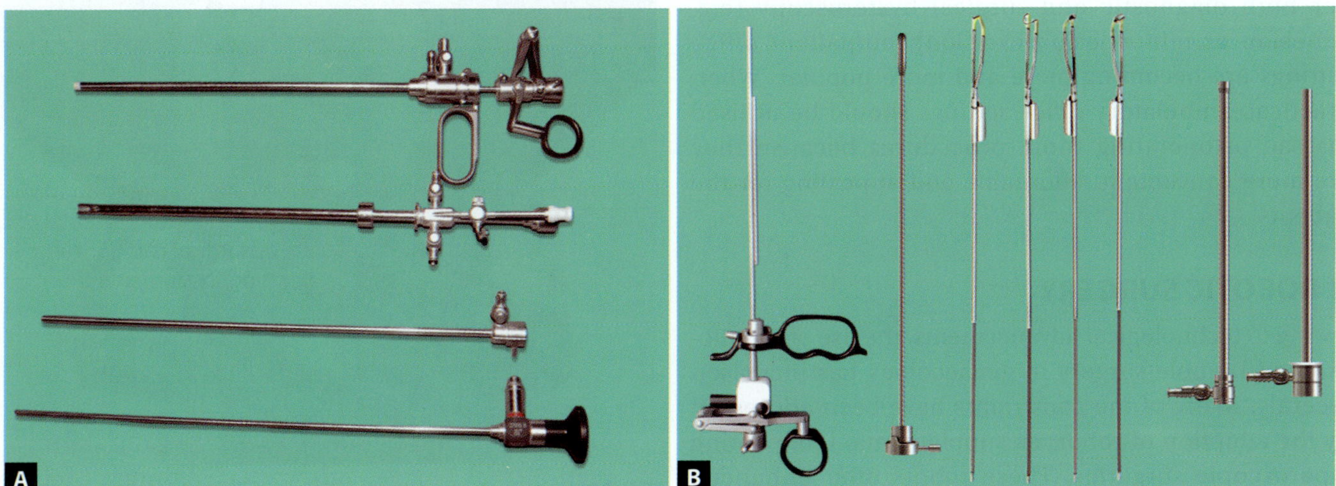

Figs. 17A and B: (A) Diagnostic hysteroscope (4 mm) with sheath and pressure bag; (B) Instruments for operative hysteroscopy: Resectoscope with obturator, wire loop electrode, Collin's knife, roller ball electrodes, sheaths dioxide and 1.5% glycine.

sclerosing chemicals (quinacrine, methyl cyanoacrylate and silver nitrate), injectable chemicals (silicone rubber), mechanical devices and electrocautery has been tried but has not been universally accepted.

The procedure involves dilatation of the cervix followed by introduction of the hysteroscope. The hysteroscope has a side channel which permits the passage of the distension medium. For operative hysteroscopy, an additional channel permits the introduction of the resectoscope, roller ball or laser fibre. An outflow tract allows the fluid passing out to be collected in a bottle. Special collecting bags have been devised which are placed under the patient's buttocks to collect any fluid leaking out of the vagina to allow as accurate an estimation as possible of the fluid deficit and thus prevent fluid overload. Office hysteroscopy is a diagnostic procedure done under local anaesthesia using a hysteroscope of smaller diameter (<4 mm) so that cervical dilatation is not required.

Complications of hysteroscopy include uterine perforation, haemorrhage, mechanical or burn injury to intra-abdominal viscera and vessels, and fluid overload, especially with the use of nonelectrolyte solutions. Delayed complications include infection, secondary haemorrhage, haematometra, cyclical pain and treatment failure with recurrence of symptoms. Hysteroscopy is contraindicated in the presence of infection (except in the case of a misplaced IUCD), in pregnancy and in cervical malignancy. In the presence of bleeding, it may pose some difficulty, especially to the novice.

Outpatient Hysteroscopy

For both diagnostic and surgical hysteroscopy (e.g. adhesion or minor lesion excision), outpatient office settings are becoming more and more popular. When practical, ambulatory office settings should be utilised instead of operating room procedures because they are more convenient, affordable and appealing for the patients.

ROBOTIC SURGERY

Owing to technological advancements, the use of robotic-assisted keyhole surgery in gynaecology has increased recently. Many of the constraints have been addressed by the adoption of robots as supplemental tools during laparoscopic surgeries. These robots offer enhanced dexterity, natural movement, 3D vision, better ergonomics, independent camera control and a reduced learning curve.

Some of the limitations associated with robotic surgery are lack of tactile feedback, operating surgeon's remote position, and expense, which remain a contentious issue. Since the early 2000s, more advanced surgical robots are available in the market; nonetheless, only one device—the da Vinci Surgical System (Intuitive Surgical, Sunnyvale, CA)—has seen widespread use in gynaecologic surgery.

Equipment

The four parts of the Da Vinci surgical system are:

1. *Surgeon console:* The surgeon performs robot-assisted laparoscopic surgery while seated at the surgeon console, also referred to as the workstation or cockpit, and watching high-definition 3D views of the operating field **(Fig. 18)**.
2. *Patient-side cart:* This one attaches itself straight to the patient and has four robotic arms fixed to either a rotating boom (Xi system) or a stationary column (Si system) that moves in response to commands given by the surgeon at the console **(Fig. 19)**.
3. EndoWrist instruments have 90° of articulation and seven degrees of motion, which are intended to allow for fluidity and dexterity. Cutting, dissecting, clamping, coagulating, suturing and tissue manipulation are among the unique tasks for which each EndoWrist device is made **(Fig. 20)**.
4. *Vision system:* High-definition images of the operating field are supplied to the surgeon's station by the 3D endoscope.

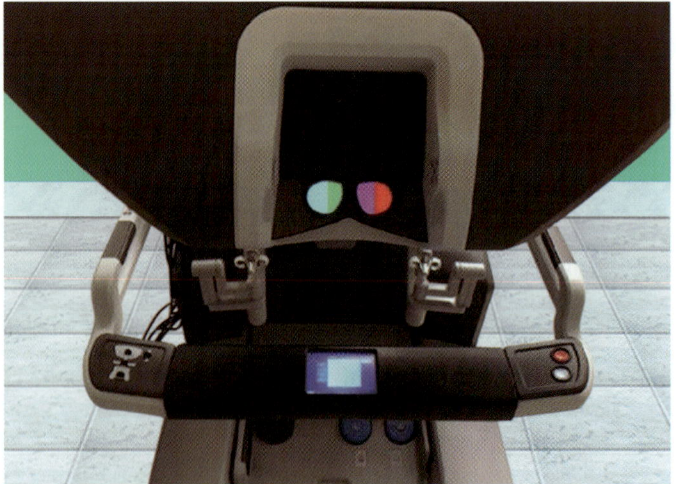

Fig. 18: Surgeon's console.
Source: Handa VL, Van Le L. Te Linde's Operative Gynecology, 12th edition. Philadelphia: Wolters Kluwer; 2019.

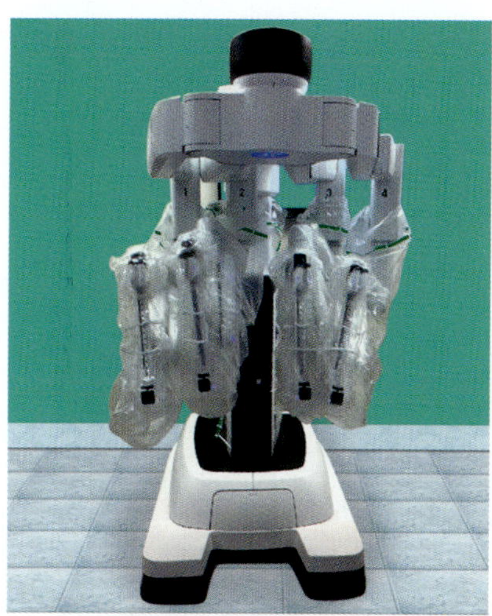

Fig. 19: Patient-side cart with draped robotic arms (Xi platform). *Source:* Handa VL, Van Le L. Te Linde's Operative Gynecology, 12th edition. Philadelphia: Wolters Kluwer; 2019.

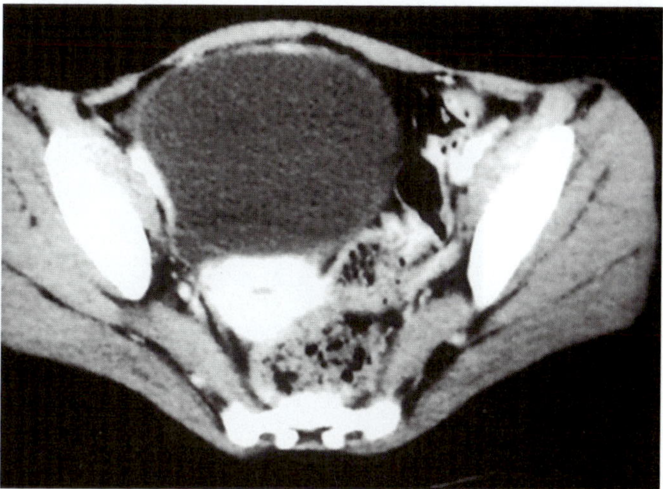

Fig. 21: Axial contrast-enhanced CT showing a simple cyst in the right adnexal region and anterior to the uterus.

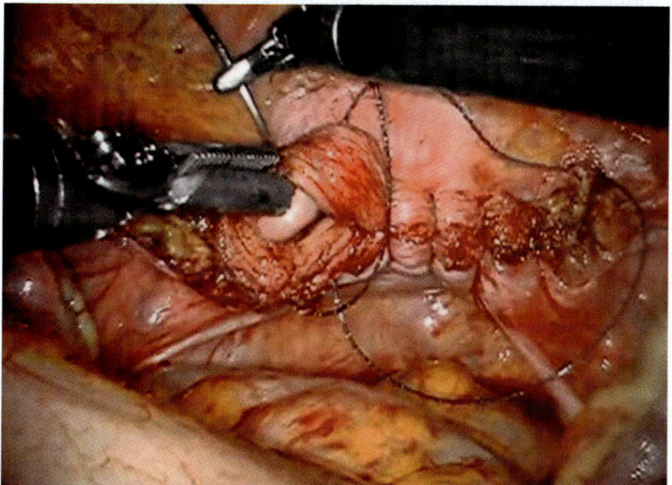

Fig. 20: Example of EndoWrist instruments (Cobra Grasper and Mega SutureCut Needle Driver) used for vaginal cuff closure. *Source:* Handa VL, Van Le L. Te Linde's Operative Gynecology, 12th edition. Philadelphia: Wolters Kluwer; 2019.

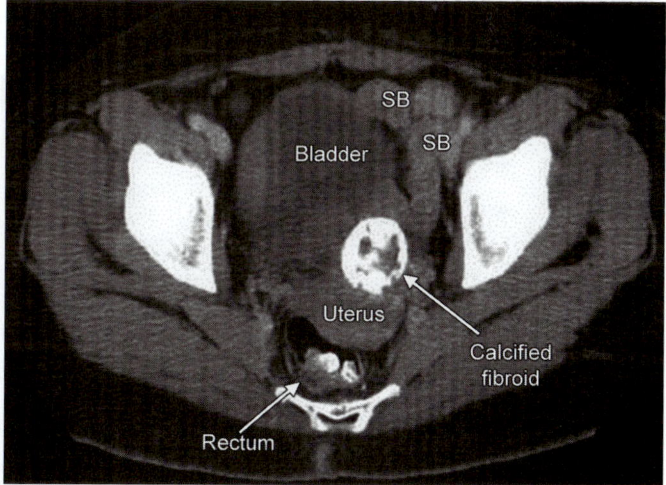

Fig. 22: CT showing a calcified fibroid.

Robotics has improved a surgeon's toolkit in many ways, particularly in terms of its capacity to influence patient outcomes and increase the range of treatment alternatives. After mastering this technique, gynaecological surgeons have tried to use it for a range of treatments that take advantage of aspects that can help overcome constraints and challenges that are frequently related to traditional laparoscopy.

COMPUTED TOMOGRAPHY

Computed tomography (CT) is able to demonstrate the pelvic anatomy very clearly. Contrast enhancement is the standard technique—opacification of the gastrointestinal tract with oral contrast and of the bladder and blood vessels with intravenously administered contrast enables the pelvic organs to be delineated clearly. Scanning begins at the level of the iliac crest and moves to the symphysis or ischial tuberosities. The thickness of each slice is 5–10 mm and the procedure is usually done in the supine position using axial scanning.

Computed tomography scanning is especially useful in the evaluation of pelvic masses to identify the organ of origin, to stage pelvic cancer (supplemented by abdominal CT) and in the follow-up of cancers to detect recurrence of disease **(Figs. 21 to 23)**. Lymph node involvement and uterine lesions are well demonstrated. However, cervical

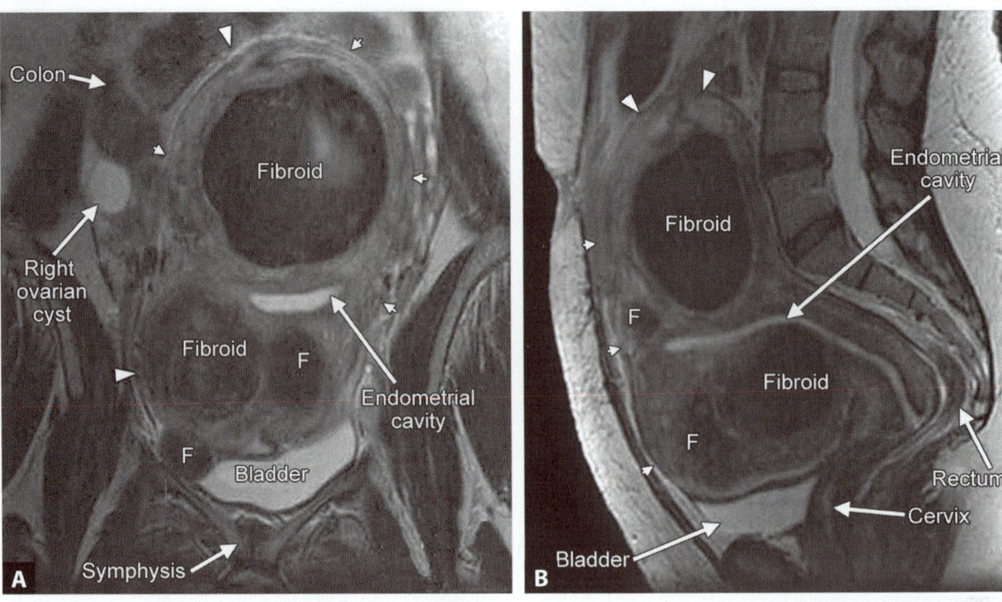

Figs. 23A and B: CT scans showing multiple uterine fibroids in different views on the same patient. Note that arrowheads point to the uterine counter.

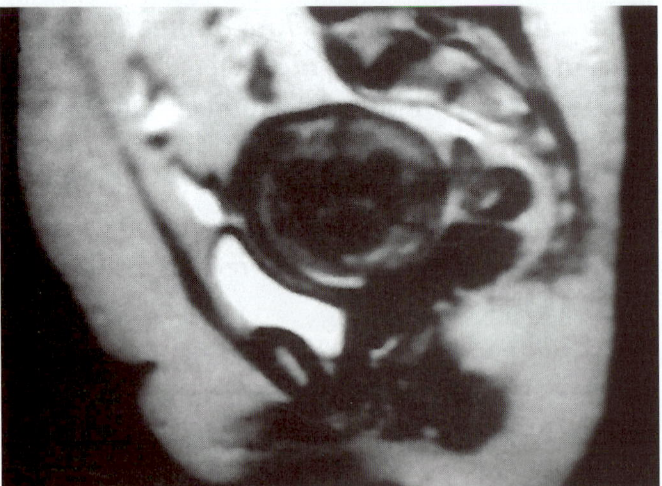

Fig. 24: T2-weighted sagittal MRI showing a large hypointense uterine fundal leiomyoma.

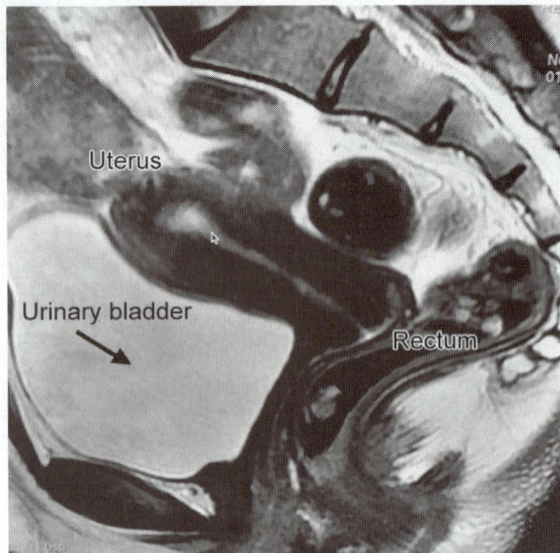

Fig. 25: T2-weighted sagittal MRI showing normal pelvis.

cancers and parametrial invasion are not accurately evaluated. Tumours <2 cm in size may not be detected and normal ovaries may not be identified routinely. CT-guided procedures such as biopsy or aspiration are sometimes done for diagnostic or therapeutic purposes.

MAGNETIC RESONANCE IMAGING

Magnetic resonance imaging is the latest addition to the armamentarium of diagnostic modalities, but it is still not available in most parts of the developing world. It uses the property of nuclear magnetic resonance (NMR).

Certain atomic nuclei, when placed within a magnetic field and stimulated by radiowaves of a specific frequency, will absorb and then re-emit some of this energy as a radiosignal **(Figs. 24 to 28)**. Data for each set of images is accumulated over about 5 minutes and patients need to remain still for this period. The total process can take 30–60 minutes. The female pelvis is particularly suitable for MRI because it does not move with respiration. Congenital anomalies of the uterus and lesions of the myometrium and endometrium can be most accurately demonstrated by MRI.

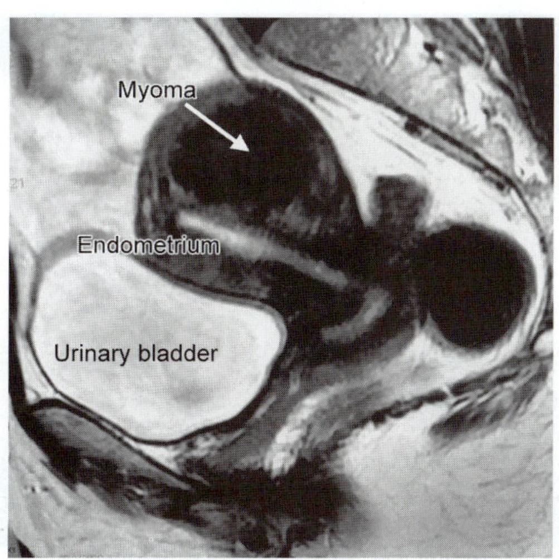

Fig. 26: T2-weighted sagittal MRI showing a hypointense uterine posterior wall leiomyoma.

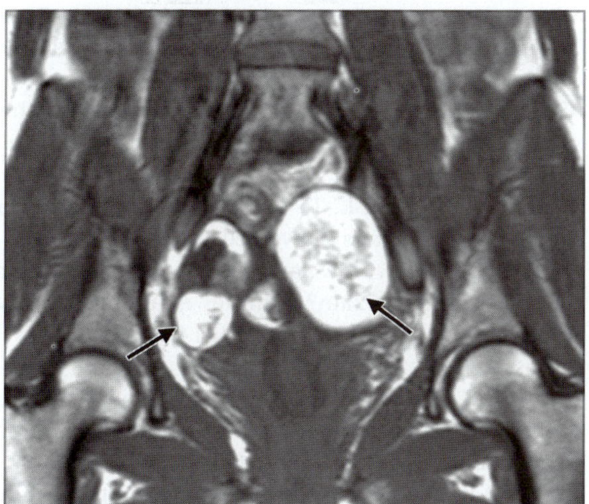

Fig. 27: T1-weighted sagittal MRI showing a mature teratoma.

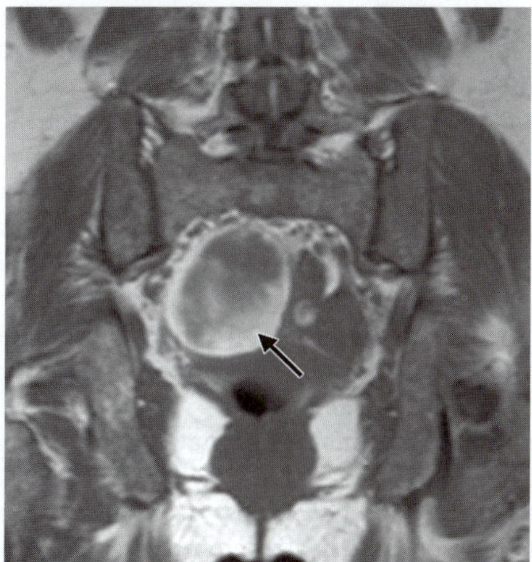

Fig. 28: MRI showing endometrioma.

Magnetic resonance imaging has several advantages over CT scan; there is no radiation exposure; imaging is multiplanar; hence, pictures can be obtained in sagittal, oblique or other planes; contrast is not required; soft-tissue contrast resolution is superior to CT. Thus, it is more useful in patients with tumours. However, it cannot be used in patients with pacemakers or metallic implants; interventional procedures cannot be performed; the costs are higher; time taken is longer, and this is particularly a problem for those who feel claustrophobic in confined spaces. Absence of signals from bony structures means that certain characteristic features such as teeth in a dermoid cyst, which can be picked up on a straight X-ray, will be missed on MRI.

POSITRON EMISSION TOMOGRAPHY SCAN

Positron emission tomography (PET) scans are often used to diagnose a condition or to track how it is developing. It can be used with CT or MRI; it shows how a part of the body is working. PET scans **(Figs. 29A and B)** demonstrate the physical state and function of body organs.

In a PET scan, a machine detects radiation that is emitted by a radiotracer or radioactive substance that is tagged to a natural chemical, such as glucose. This radiotracer is injected into the body, where it travels to cells that use glucose for energy. The more energy a group of cells needs, the more the radiotracer will build up in that location. This will show up on images that are reconstructed by a computer. The cells, or activity, will show up as *hot spot* if over activity and *cold spot* if less uptake of glucose. Malignant cells usually are overactive and take up more energy and present like hot spot. PET scans can reveal the presence and stage of a cancer, show whether and where it has spread and help doctors decide on treatment. A PET scan can give an idea of response to chemotherapy, and it can detect a recurring tumour sooner than other techniques. PET is complimentary to CT and MRI, completing the picture. Very rarely, an individual may have an allergic reaction to the tracer.

CONCLUSION

Gynaecology and obstetrics is a very intriguing branch of medical science, which is dedicated to women's reproductive health and childbirth. A clinician has to respect a woman's privacy and sensitivity. If a proper stepwise clinical approach is taken, diagnosis can be reached at and confirmed with tests. Ultrasound is very

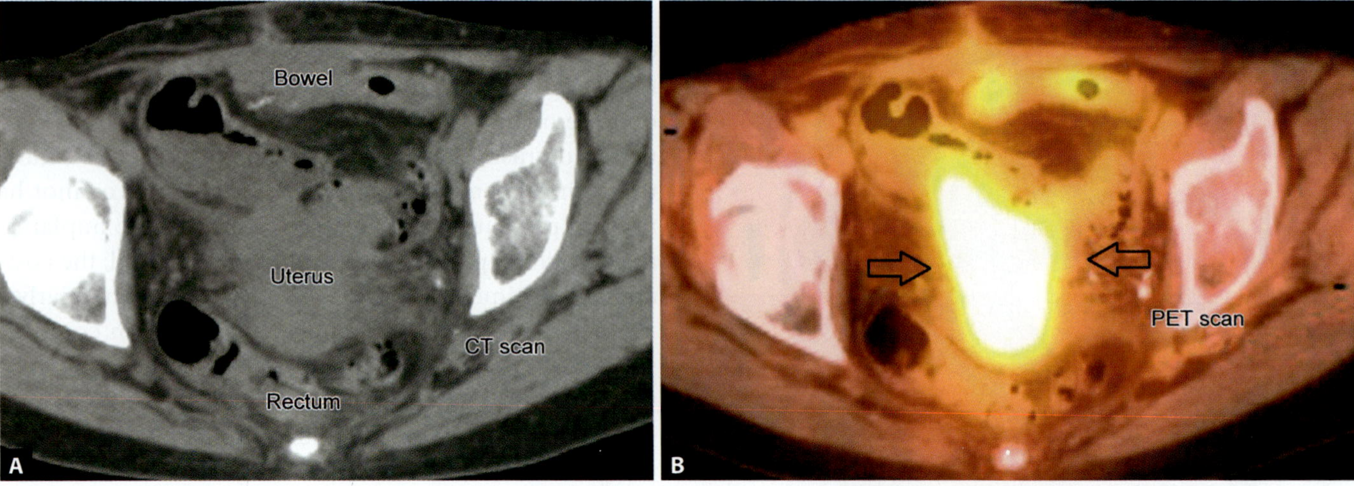

Figs. 29A and B: Hot spot in the uterus showing malignancies.

helpful, and all should be well versed with basic scans. Most of the minor procedures such as endometrial biopsy, colposcopy and diagnostic hysteroscopy can now be performed in clinic setups.

SUGGESTED READING

1. ACOG committee opinion no. 373: sexual misconduct. Obstet Gynecol. 2007;110(2):441-4.
2. ACOG committee opinion no. 483: primary and preventive care: periodic assessments. Obstet Gynecol. 2011;117(4):1008-15.
3. Bates B. A Guide to Physical Examination and History Taking, 6th edition. Philadelphia: J B Lippincott & Co.; 1995.
4. Bayer SR, DeCherney AH. Clinical manifestations and treatment of dysfunctional uterine bleeding. JAMA. 1993;269:1823-8.
5. Bhangu AA. Please don't touch me there: the ethics of intimate examinations: consent is crucial—but don't go too far, for students' and patients' sakes. BMJ. 2003;326(7402):1326.
6. Bradley LD. (2024). Hysteroscopy: Instruments and procedure. [online] Available from https://www.uptodate.com/contents/hysteroscopy-instruments-and-procedure#:~:text=A%20hysteroscope%20is%20a%20telescope,for%20diagnostic%20or%20therapeutic%20indications. [Last accessed April, 2025].
7. Carr SE, Carmody D. Outcomes of teaching medical students core skills for women's health: the pelvic examination educational program. Am J Obstet Gynecol. 2004;190(5):1382-7.
8. Chuong CJ, Brenner PF. Management of abnormal uterine bleeding. Am J Obstet Gynecol. 1996;175(3):787-92.
9. Committee opinion no. 534: well-woman visit. Obstet Gynecol. 2012;120(2 Pt 1):421-4.
10. Gupta S, Hogan R, Kirkman RJ. Experience of the first pelvic examination. Eur J Contracept Reprod Health Care. 2001;6(1):34-8.
11. Handa VL, Van Le L. Te Linde's Operative Gynecology. Philadelphia: Wolters Kluwer; 2020.
12. Hughes B. (2003). How can I make a woman comfortable during a pelvic exam? [online] Available from www.medscape.com/viewarticle/461420?form=fpf. [Last accessed April, 2025].
13. Lyons MS, Lindsell CJ, Trott AT. Emergency department pelvic examination and Pap testing: addressing patient misperceptions. Acad Emerg Med. 2004;11(4):405-8.
14. Nestel D, Kneebone R. Please don't touch me there: the ethics of intimate examinations: integrated approach to teaching and learning clinical skills. BMJ. 2003;326(7402):1327.
15. Petravage JB, Reynolds LJ, Gardner HJ, Reading JC. Attitudes of women toward the gynecologic examination. J Fam Pract. 1979;9(6):1039-45.
16. Priore GD. (2024). Office-based endometrial sampling procedure. [online] Available from https://www.uptodate.com/contents/office-based-endometrial-sampling-procedures#:~:text=Equipment%20and%20techniques%20for%20office,hyperplasia%2C%20and%20other%20endometrial%20pathology. [Last accessed April, 2025].
17. Selby M. Please don't touch me there: the ethics of intimate examinations: informed consent failed to protect me. BMJ. 2003;326(7402):1326.
18. Singer PA. Intimate examinations and other ethical challenges in medical education. BMJ. 2003;326(7380):62-3.
19. Soto E, Lo Y, Friedman K, Soto C, Nezhat F, Chuang L, et al. Total laparoscopic hysterectomy versus da Vinci robotic

hysterectomy: is using the robot beneficial? J Gynecol Oncol. 2011;22:253-9.

20. Stewart FH, Harper CC, Ellertson CE, Grimes DA, Sawaya GF, Trussell J. Clinical breast and pelvic examination requirements for hormonal contraception: current practice vs evidence. JAMA. 2001;285(17):2232-9.
21. Stormo AR, Hawkins NA, Cooper CP, Saraiya M. The pelvic examination as a screening tool: practices of US physicians. Arch Intern Med. 2011;171(22):2053-4.
22. Supe AN, Kulkarni GV, Supe PA. Ergonomics in laparoscopic surgery. J Minim Access Surg. 2010;6(2):31-6.
23. Ueland FR, Depriest PD, Desimone CP, Pavlik EJ, Lele SM, Kryscio RJ, et al. The accuracy of examination under anesthesia and transvaginal sonography in evaluating ovarian size. Gynecol Oncol. 2005;99(2):400-3.
24. Workowski KA, Berman S. Sexually transmitted diseases treatment guidelines, 2010. MMWR Recomm Rep. 2010;59(RR-12):1-110.

2

CHAPTER

Anatomy

Argyia Desouza, Muralidhar V Pai

Chapter Outline

- Vulva
- Vagina
- Uterus
- Fallopian Tubes
- Ovary
- Urethra and Bladder
- Ureter
- Sigmoid Colon
- Rectum and Anus
- Pelvic Peritoneum and Ligaments
- Pelvic Musculature
- Pelvic Fascia and Cellular Tissue
- The Supports of the Genital Organs
- Blood Vessels of the Pelvis
- Lymphatic Drainage
- Innervation of Pelvic Organs

INTRODUCTION

It is essential to realise that nothing is more fundamental to the knowledge base of the practicing gynaecologist than an understanding of the anatomy of the female pelvis. Although the basic facts of anatomy and their relevance to gynaecologic practice do not change with time, our understanding of specific anatomic relationships and the development of new clinical and surgical correlations continues to evolve. It is essential to review relevant anatomy before each surgical procedure. We need to study the gynaecologic literature on an ongoing basis—numerous publications have documented the evolution of newer concepts regarding anatomic issues such as pelvic support.

VULVA

The vulva is a composite name for the external genitalia **(Fig. 1)**. It includes the mons veneris, the labia majora and minora, the clitoris, the entrance to the vagina, the hymen and the vestibule; but the term is ill-defined and many regard it as covering deeper structures such as the vestibular bulbs and Bartholin's glands as well. Some gynaecologists regard the perineum as part of the vulva, and many include under this term the perineal body (central tendon of the perineum) as well as the overlying skin. To anatomists, 'perineum' means all structures within the bony outlet of the pelvis. For convenience, the perineum is considered with the vulva.

Individual Structures

Mons Veneris and Labia Majora

The mons is the hair-bearing skin and the fatty pad, which overlie the upper part of the symphysis pubis and the lower abdominal muscles; it acts as a coital buffer. Extending backwards from the mons, on either side of the vaginal orifice, are the labia majora which are folds of skin with underlying deposits of fat. These are homologous to the scrotum. Posteriorly, they merge into each other and the perineal skin. Their outer aspects are covered with hair, their inner aspects are smooth and moistened by the

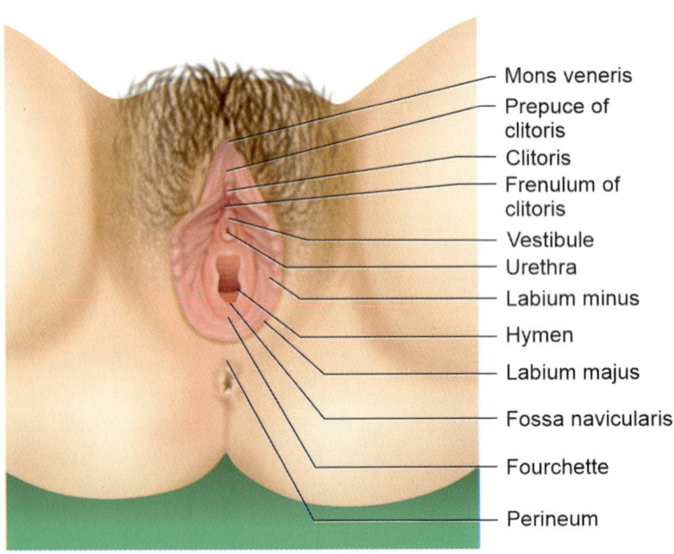

Fig. 1: The virginal vulva.

secretions of sebaceous and other glands. Except where the labia minora intervene, the inner surfaces ordinarily lie in contact with each other, and thus close the entrance to the vagina.

The mons and labia majora are covered with coarse skin, which contains hair follicles, sebaceous glands and sweat glands. Some of the latter are large, coiled and specialised and are known as apocrine glands; these are only found in certain areas of the body such as the axilla and vulva, and their secretion (when modified by bacteria) gives rise to a characteristic odour, which is of sexual significance.

In view of their structure, the mons and labia majora are exposed to ordinary diseases of the skin including conditions, such as psoriasis, sebaceous cysts, boils and carbuncles and new growths. Because the underlying connective tissue is very loose, the labia readily become oedematous.

Perineum

The perineum is a diamond-shaped structure inferior to pelvic diaphragm between the symphysis pubis and the coccyx. Its bony boundaries include a lower margin of pubic symphysis anteriorly, tip of coccyx posteriorly and ischial tuberosities laterally. It is divided into anterior urogenital triangle and the posterior anal triangle by imaginary line joining both ischial tuberosities **(Fig. 2)**.

Urogenital triangle includes external genital structures called vulva and the urethral opening.

Anal triangle includes lower end of the anal canal.

Labia Minora

The labia minora are delicate flaps of soft skin lying within the labia majora, one on each side of the vaginal orifice, and are homologous to the ventral shaft of the penis in male. They vary considerably in size and may be hidden by the labia majora or may project between them. Ordinarily, their inner surfaces lie in contact with each other, and their outer surfaces are in contact with the labium majus on the same side. Anteriorly, the labia minora join together and, in so doing, split to provide the clitoris with a prepuce and frenulum. They join posteriorly to form a sharp fold of skin, the fourchette and they also merge into the labia majora. The fourchette is nearly always injured during childbirth, and sometimes suffers slight tearing during initial attempts at coitus. The depression between the fourchette and hymen which is found in virgins is the fossa navicularis.

The labia minora each consists of two layers of non-keratinised skin with some intervening loose connective tissue. The latter is devoid of fat but is so vascular that it enables the labia to become turgid under conditions of sexual excitement. They also contain sebaceous glands, especially near their bases, but few, if any, sweat glands.

Clitoris

The clitoris is the homologue of the penis and is a small structure lying on the front of the symphysis almost hidden by the foreparts of the labia majora. It has a glans, prepuce, body and two crura (corpora cavernosa), which attach it to the pubic bones. The clitoris consists of erectile

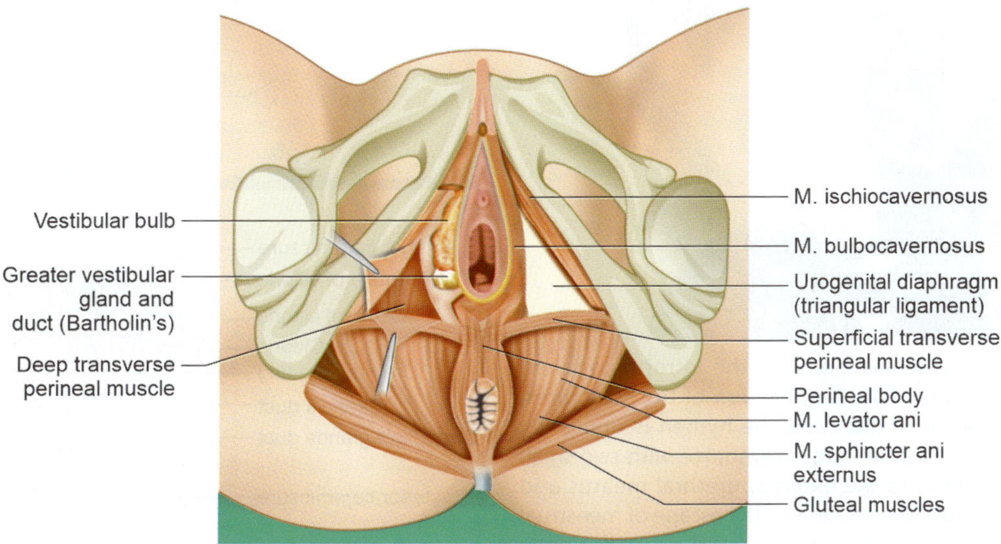

Fig. 2: The urogenital diaphragm (triangular ligament) and associated structures as seen here.

tissue richly supplied with nerves which make it the most erotically sensitive part of the vulva. Smegma is secreted beneath the prepuce. Only the glans and prepuce are visible, but the body is palpable against the symphysis pubis as a small cord-like structure approximately 2 cm in length.

Vestibule

The definition of vestibule (from the Latin *vestibulum* meaning a forecourt or a hall next to the entrance) varies, but generally the term is applied only to the area of smooth skin lying within the labia minora and in front of the vaginal orifice. The urethra opens onto it. On either side of the urethral meatus are tiny depressions called paraurethral pouches with adjacent insignificant folds—the urethral labia.

Hymen

The hymen is a delicate incomplete membrane guarding the entrance to the vagina prior to maturity and sexual experience **(Figs. 3 and 4)**. It has one or more apertures to allow the outflow of menstrual blood and, according to their number and shape, is described as being annular, crescentic, septate or cribriform.

Unless the opening is unusually large, and the hymen itself particularly elastic, coitus nearly always causes tearing. The tear is most commonly found posteriorly or posterolaterally. It is one of the signs of loss of virginity, but is not a very reliable one because injuries may be caused by operations, digital interference or the insertion of tampons or menstrual cup to contain the menstrual discharge. Moreover, coitus can take place without a tear as well. Inspection alone is often insufficient to permit a conclusion that a hymen is intact and unstretched a better clinical test is to feel gently for its resistant edge with the tip of the finger.

The hymen is relatively avascular so its tearing usually causes only a slight loss of blood. During childbirth the hymen is destroyed, its remains as being a few tags around the vaginal orifice—Carunculae myrtiformes.

Vestibular Bulb

The two bulbs are collections of erectile tissue, which together are homologous to the corpus spongiosum in the male.

Fig. 3: The normal vulva (shaved) with the introitus opened to show an intact hymen. For identification of the structures, compare with **Figure 1**. In this case, the hymen is unusually well developed to form a thick tough membrane with two small openings (posterolateral to the external urethral meatus and indicated by white arrows) which allowed the escape of menstrual blood. This so-called septate hymen would probably have hindered consummation of marriage.

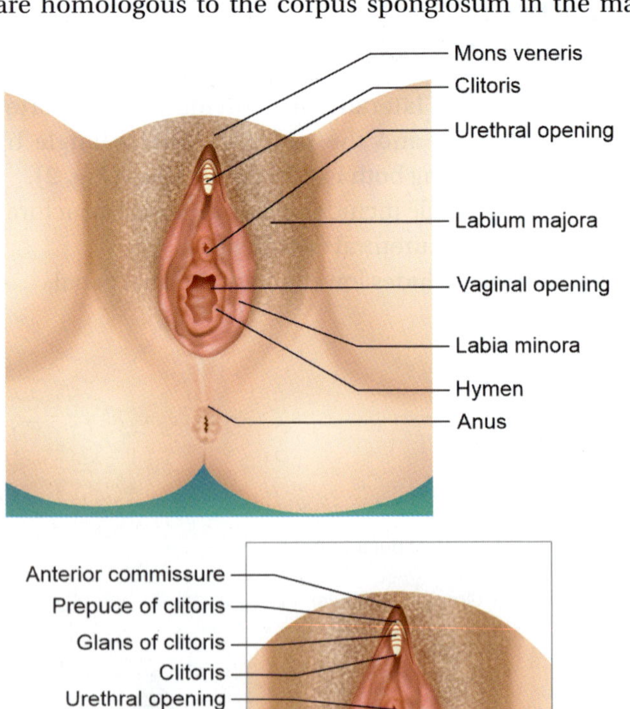

Fig. 4: Anatomy of the external genital organs.

Each passes backwards from the root of the clitoris, lying deep to the bulbospongiosus (bulbocavernosus) muscle (sphincter vaginae) but superficial to the lower layer of the triangular ligament (urogenital diaphragm), the compressor urethrae (external urethral sphincter) and the deep transverse perineal muscles **(Fig. 2)**.

Bartholin's Glands (Greater Vestibular Glands)

Bartholin's glands are two in number and are homologous to Cowper's glands in the male. They lie posterolaterally to the vaginal orifice, embedded in the posterior part of the vestibular bulb, one on either side **(Fig. 2)**. Each gland is oval in shape and approximately the size of a pea but is not palpable unless hardened or enlarged by infection. Its duct is 1.25–2 cm in length, and runs downwards and inwards to open at the introitus below the hymen but above the attachment of the posterior end of the labium minus **(Fig. 2)**. The orifice of the duct is not normally visible but, when the duct and gland are infected, may be indicated by a small red area.

The gland is lobulated and racemose, the acini being lined by a single layer of low columnar or cuboidal cells **(Fig. 5)**. The duct is lined by multilayered columnar cells and not by transitional epithelium, as is usually stated. The impression of the latter is created by a study of pathological states. Thus, the surface columnar cells become flattened when the duct is distended to form a cyst, and infection may sometimes result in metaplasia.

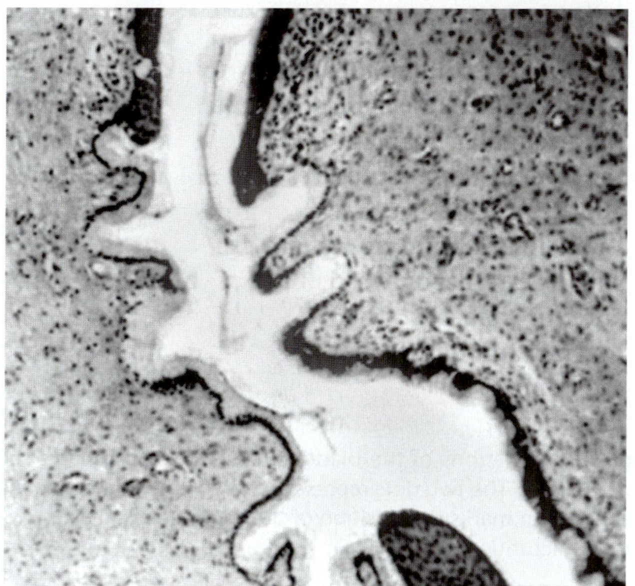

Fig. 5: The duct of Bartholin's gland, at the top, joining the gland lined by columnar epithelium. The duct is lined by immature metaplastic squamous epithelium. When the duct is distended by cyst formation, this can become flattened to give a false impression of its true morphology.

The secretion of the gland is colourless and mucoid and has a characteristic odour. It is produced mainly in response to sexual excitement when considerable amounts are poured onto the vulva to act as a lubricant for coitus. The gland continues limited activity after the menopause.

Changes in the Vulva with Age and Parity

The tissues of the vulva are sensitive to sex hormones, especially oestrogens, so their anatomy and function change with reproductive age and the endocrine environment. In infancy and childhood, the mons veneris and labia majora are devoid of hair. In the very young baby, the labia majora are under the influence of maternal hormones and tend to obscure the tiny labia minora, but the vaginal orifice is seen surprisingly easily when the legs are abducted. Later, the labia lose their fat, so the labia minora and the clitoris are relatively prominent and protruding. During childhood the skin of all the tissues is thin and delicate and that of the vestibule reddish in colour. Fat reappears in the mons and labia majora as part of sexual development in adolescence, and the labia minora and vaginal orifice then become hidden. The growth of pubic hair known as pubarche is an early sign of puberty.

The effect of coitus on the hymen has already been described. The fourchette and the perineum are frequently torn during childbirth and thereafter appear scarred. Deep tearing may leave the perineum shorter than it was originally; the vaginal orifice then becomes wider and more exposed because of separation of the posterior parts of the labia majora.

In old age, all the tissues atrophy and the skin becomes drier, thinner and glazed. The subcutaneous fat is lessened except in obese women. The labia minora shrink and may almost disappear. The vaginal orifice tends to contract. Pubic hair becomes sparse.

Relations

An understanding of the relations of the vulva rests on an appreciation of the position of its component parts in relation to the bony pelvis, and this is illustrated in **Figures 2 and 6**.

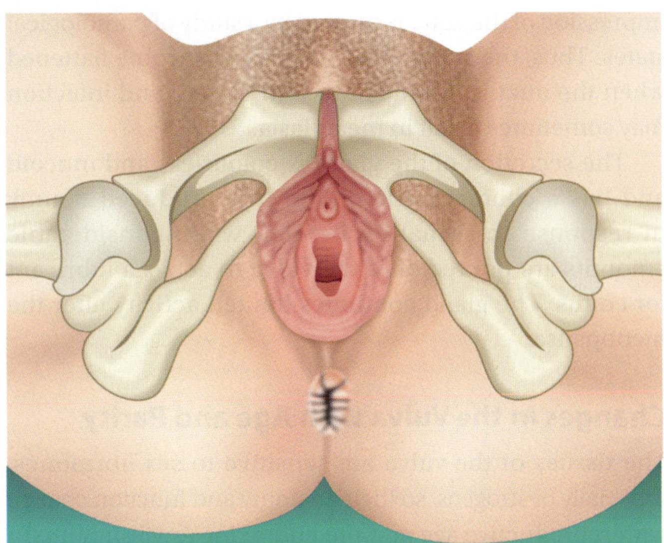

Fig. 6: The relation of the tissues of the vulva to the bones of the pelvis. Note that the clitoris lies relatively high on the symphysis pubis. The introitus is depicted as multiparous and gapes to show rugae and a central column on the anterior vaginal wall.

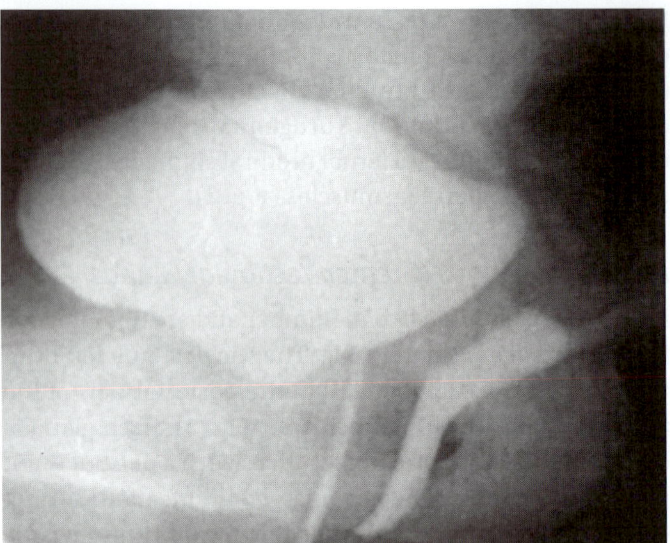

Fig. 7: Lateral urethrocystograph and colpograph in a normal multiparous woman sitting at ease. The urethra is straight and joins a relatively flat bladder base to produce what appear in silhouette as clearly defined 'angles' in front of, and behind, the urethrovesical junction. The vagina is not straight but slightly angulated to conform to the anatomy of the urethrovesical junction.
Source: With permission from the Editor, J Obstet Gynaecol Br Empire.

Vascular Connections

All the tissues of the vulva are extremely vascular, so even a minor operation in that area should not be attempted except in well-equipped surroundings.

Arterial: The vulva is mainly supplied by branches of the internal pudendal artery, which is one of the two terminal branches of the internal iliac artery, but its foreparts are also served by the superficial external pudendal artery.

Venous: Some veins accompany corresponding arteries to the internal pudendal vein; those of the clitoris and bulb link with the vesical and vaginal plexuses. The long saphenous vein also takes a share of the venous return; ligating it can improve vulvar varicosities.

Lymphatic: Drainage is mainly to the superficial inguinal nodes, and thence to the deep inguinal and external iliac nodes. Lymphatics from the deep tissues accompany the internal pudendal vessels to the internal iliac nodes.

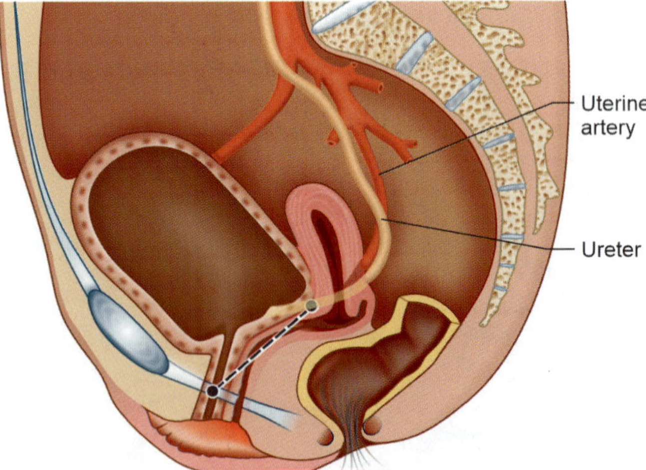

Fig. 8: The relations of the bladder, urethra and vagina as seen from the side. The two dots represent fixed points; the broken line joining them marks the position of the trigone and urethral floor during micturition.

VAGINA

General Description

The vagina is a hollow elastic fibromuscular canal extending upwards and backwards from the vulva at an angle of 60–70° to the horizontal, although it is not straight as is generally supposed but angled backwards **(Figs. 7 to 9)**. This is also demonstrated by colpographs as well as by taking the casts of vagina in the living woman. The vagina pierces the triangular ligament and the pelvic diaphragm, the level of these structures being approximately 1 and 2.5 cm, respectively, from its lower end. The vagina has a

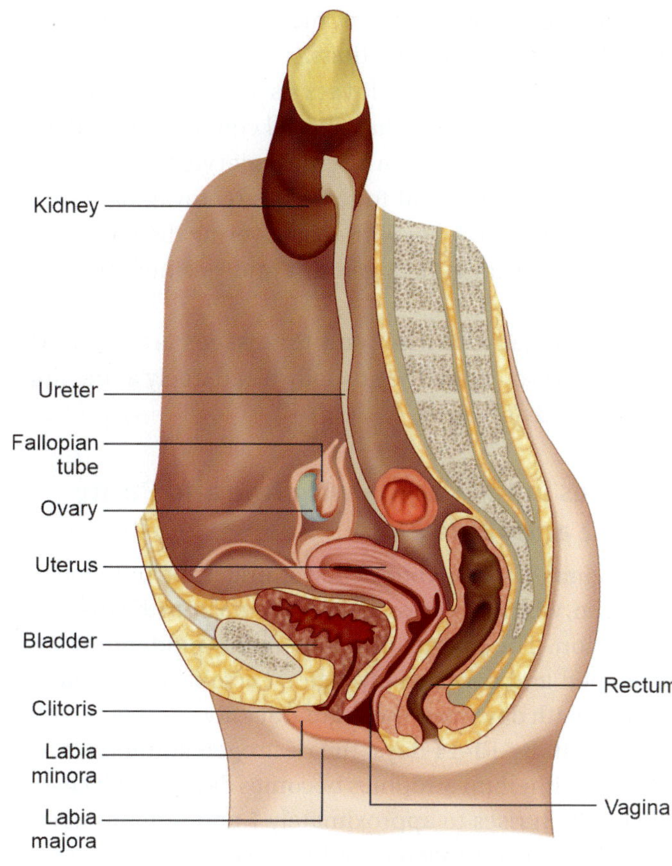

Fig. 9: Female genital system.

blind upper end except for the cervix with its external os, which projects through its upper anterior wall.

The vault of the vagina that is the upper part is divided into four areas according to their relations to the cervix: The posterior fornix which is capacious, the anterior fornix which is shallow, and two lateral fornices. Because the cervix is inserted below the vault, the posterior vaginal wall is approximately 10 cm, whereas the anterior wall is approximately 8 cm, in length.

The introitus is functionally closed by the labia which are in contact with each other. Moreover, the lumen of the vagina is ordinarily obliterated by the anterior and posterior walls lying in apposition. In its lower part, it appears H-shaped on cross section with lateral recesses anteriorly and posteriorly. When, however, a woman is in the knee-chest, Sims' or kneeling position and the labia are separated, the vagina balloons out. This is the result of a negative intra-abdominal pressure transmitted to the vagina, causing the entry of air. Exceptionally, such air can enter the uterus, tubes and peritoneal cavity.

If the walls are separated, the vagina of the nulliparous married woman has a diameter of approximately 4–5 cm at its lower end and is twice as wide at its upper end. Although the width and length of the vagina show considerable individual variations, anatomical shortness or narrowness is rarely a cause of difficulty or pain on coitus because the vagina is distensible and accommodates itself. The functional width is determined to a large extent by the tone and contractions of surrounding muscles.

A raised double column formed by underlying fascia can often be seen running sagittally down the anterior wall, and there is a less definite median ridge on the posterior wall. Running circumferentially from these columns are folds of epithelium (rugae), which account in part for the ability of the vagina to distend during labour **(Fig. 6)**.

Structure

Epithelium

The vagina is lined by stratified squamous epithelium, which also extends onto and covers the vaginal cervix as far as the external os **(Fig. 10)**. The surface is normally devoid of keratin but is capable of becoming keratinised if it becomes exposed to the air as in prolapse. The epithelium is many layered, the basal cuboidal cells being the source of a continuous production of the squamous cells above. The cells in the middle and superficial zones contain glycogen, which explains why the vagina stains deep brown with iodine. It shows cyclical histological changes in association with menstruation. The epithelium does not contain glands of any kind and does not secrete in the ordinary sense of the word. The frequently used term vaginal mucosa is, therefore, strictly incorrect. Although it may in part represent a transudate (globules of fluid, the sweating phenomenon, are said to collect on the surface during coitus and sexual excitation), the vaginal 'secretion' arises mainly from the constant breakdown of superficial epithelial cells. This breakdown liberates the contained glycogen which is acted upon by the lactobacillus (Doderlein's bacillus), a normal inhabitant of the vagina, to produce lactic acid. The vaginal 'secretion', therefore, consists of tissue fluids, epithelial debris, electrolytes, proteins and lactic acid. The amount of the lactic acid is governed by the glycogen content of the epithelium and the presence of lactobacilli but, in the adult healthy vagina, is in a concentration of 0.75%.

The pH varies with the level of the vagina, being the highest in the upper part because of an admixture of

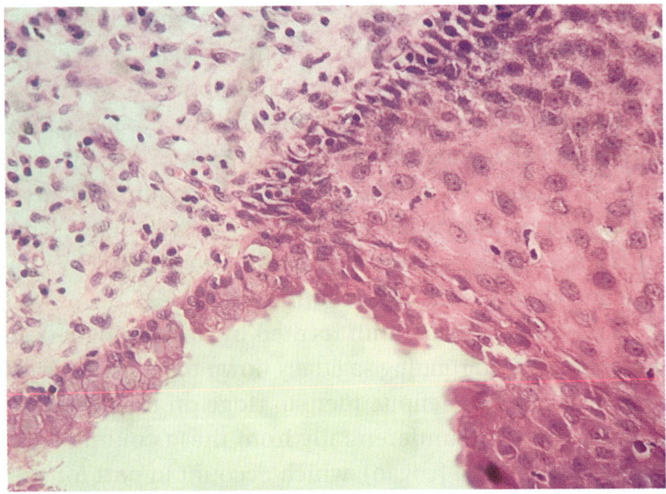

Fig. 10: Cervix, squamocolumnar junction. The section shows the abrupt transition from the single layer of endocervical mucus-secreting epithelium to the mature, multilayered squamous epithelium of the ectocervix (H&E 400×).

alkaline cervical mucus. Estimates also vary, according to the method used for its determination. Some authorities give the normal range for the adult nonpregnant woman as from 3.5 to 4.2, but the generally accepted figures are from 4.0 to 5.5 with an average of 4.5. The level varies with the time in the menstrual cycle and the effects of ovarian hormones on the vaginal epithelium and the cervical secretion. During menstruation the flow of alkaline blood raises the vaginal pH to levels ranging from 5.8 to 6.8.

The acidity of the vagina is of great practical importance for it explains the resistance of the mature vagina to pyogenic organisms.

The vagina not only 'secretes', but also absorbs water, electrolytes and substances of low molecular weight. This property is utilized when therapeutic agents, such as oestrogens and glucose are administered locally, and can be a nuisance in that it permits the absorption of medicaments such as mercurials and arsenicals to cause systemic reactions. Absorption and reabsorption are believed to occur mainly in the lateral recesses of the lower vagina.

Fascia and Muscle

The epithelium rests on a subepithelial connective layer which contains elastic tissue. Outside this are muscle coats in which the fibres are nearly all arranged in a criss-cross spiral fashion. The muscle of the vaginal wall is involuntary in type although there are sometimes a few intermingling voluntary fibres contributed by muscles such as the levator ani at the sites of their insertions.

Outside the muscle layers is a strong sheath of connective tissue, which has special condensations down the anterior wall to form the pubocervical fascia, and down the posterior wall to form the rectovaginal fascia. This fascial sheath fuses with that covering the levator ani muscles, the triangular ligament and perineal muscles **(Fig. 11)**.

The vaginal wall itself and the tissues around it are extremely vascular, so they usually bleed freely at the time of injury and operation.

Changes in the Vagina with Age and Parity (Fig. 12 and Table 1)

The vagina of the newborn child is under the influence of oestrogen, which has crossed the placenta from the maternal circulation. The epithelium is therefore moderately well developed and contains glycogen. Lactobacilli appear by the 3rd or 4th day when the vaginal acidity approaches that of an adult. By 10–14 days, the oestrogen stimulus is lost and the epithelium atrophies becomes devoid of glycogen. The pH then rises to approximately 7 and remains at that level until the approach of puberty when, with the onset of full ovarian function, the vagina assumes the features already described. Throughout childhood, lactobacilli are present in small numbers but after puberty, they are the predominant organism. During pregnancy the amount of glycogen is increased to a maximum and the acidity of the vagina is high (pH 3.5–4.5). After the menopause, the epithelium atrophies and loses its glycogen. Lactobacilli are found in fewer numbers and the pH rises to a range of 6–8. In some women menopausal atrophy is slow to develop, possibly because of the peripheral conversion of androgens produced by the adrenal cortex to oestrone.

Regular coitus result in some stretching of the vaginal walls, and this is increased by childbearing. Repeated childbirth leads to obliteration of the rugae and the vagina becomes a smooth-walled and rather patulous canal. After the menopause, it undergoes contracture in length and width, but this change is to some extent counteracted by the continuance of regular coitus. The fornices become shallow, however, and the cervix no longer projects far into the vault. When these changes are extreme the vagina is said to become tent-shaped. Even in nulliparous women, the vagina loses its rugae after the climacteric.

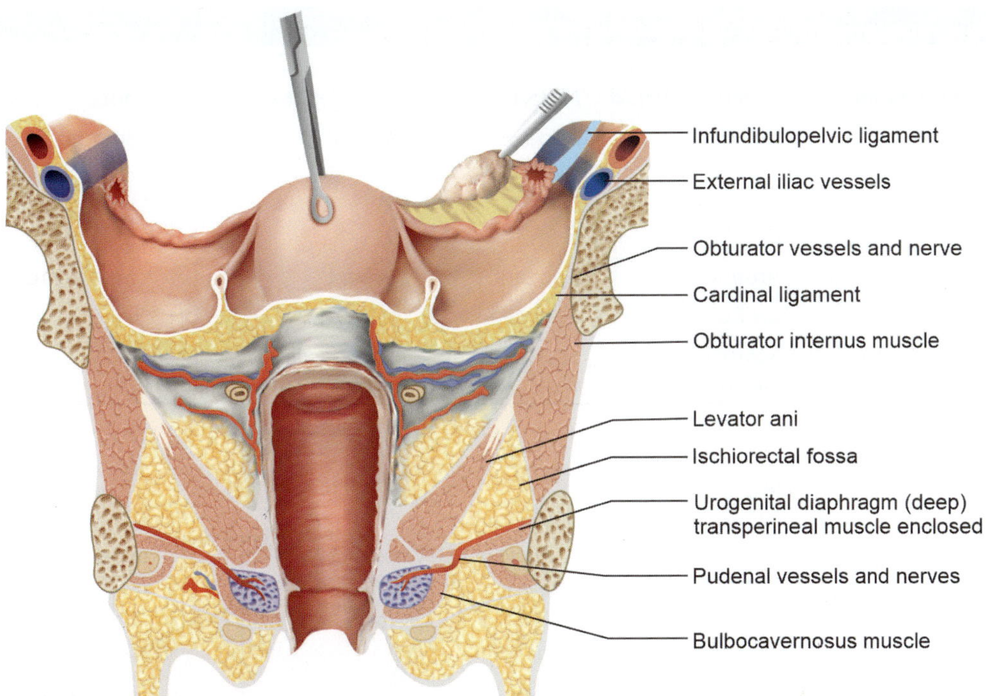

Fig. 11: The pelvic muscles, ligaments and fascia as seen from the front.

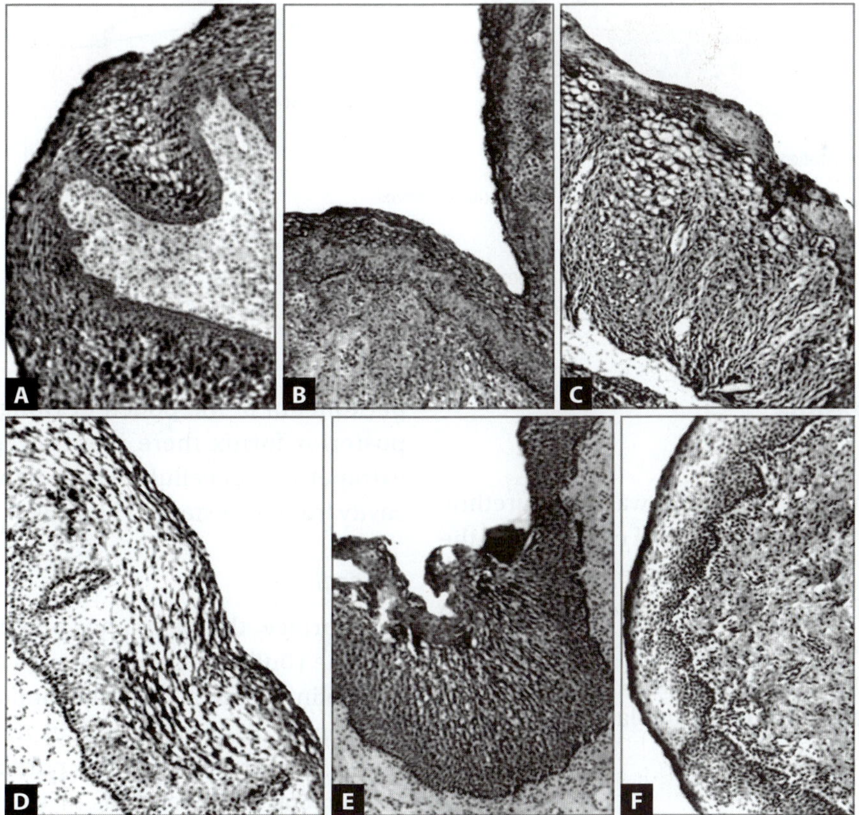

Figs. 12A to F: The characteristics of the vagina at different ages.
Courtesy: By permission of the late Mr RL Hartley.

TABLE 1: Changes in various vaginal parameters at different ages in a female.

	Newborn infant	*6-week-old child*	*Puberty*	*Sexual maturity*	*Pregnancy*	*Late postmenopausal*
Oestrogenic hormone stimulus	Present	Negligible	Appears	Present	Large amount	Small amount
Epithelium	A	B	C	D	E	F
Glycogen	Present	Absent	Appears	Present	Large amount	Small amount
Acidity	pH 4.5–7.0	pH 7.0	alkaline → acid	pH 4.0–5.5	pH 3.5–4.5	pH 6–8
Flora	Sterile → Lactobacilli	Sparse coccal varied flora	Sparse coccal flora	Lactobacilli	Lactobacilli	Varied flora

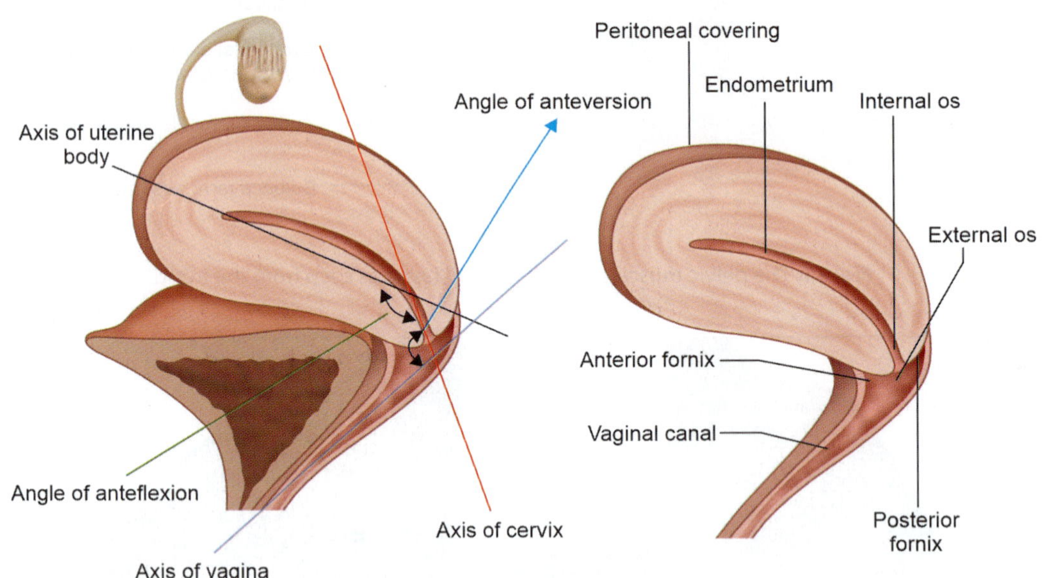

Fig. 13: Anteverted and anteflexed uterus.
Image courtesy: Dr Harshith Kramadhari.

Relations of the Vagina

Anterior

Embedded in the lower anterior vaginal wall is the urethra. Its muscles fuse with those of the vaginal coat without the intervention of fascia, so it is difficult to separate from the vagina at the time of operation. In close connection too are Skene's tubules which open into the urethra. Above the urethra, the vagina is directly related to the bladder, separated from it by fascia and loose areolar tissue **(Fig. 8)**.

Posterior

From below upwards the vaginal wall is in relation to the perineal body, the ampulla of the rectum and the peritoneum of the pouch of Douglas. At the level of the posterior fornix there is only vaginal wall, fascia and extraperitoneal cellular tissue separating the peritoneal cavity from the exterior **(Fig. 13)**.

Lateral

At its orifice, the vagina has on either side the sphincter vaginae (bulbospongiosus) muscle, the vestibular bulb, Bartholin's gland and its duct and the triangular ligament (urogenital diaphragm) with its muscles. At a higher level is the levator ani with the paracolpos above, and the ischiorectal fossa below its insertion. The lateral fornix is related to the lower parts of the cardinal ligament which are inserted into it **(Fig. 11)**.

Superior

The cervix dips into the upper and anterior part of the vagina; above this is the uterus itself. Overlying the lateral fornix and situated only 1-2 cm away is the ureter with the uterine vessels immediately above. These lie in the cellular tissue of the base of the broad ligament, which is also an important relation. The uterosacral ligaments are just above the posterior fornix; between and above them is the peritoneal pouch of Douglas containing loops of intestine. Above and to the side are the fallopian tube and ovary **(Fig. 11)**.

Vascular Connections

Arterial: These are: The vaginal artery mainly, branches of the uterine artery; branches of the internal pudendal artery; and twigs from the middle and inferior rectal arteries also supply the vagina.

Venous: A plexus of veins around the vagina connects with those around the bladder and rectum, and ultimately drains into the internal iliac veins by branches which mainly accompany corresponding arteries.

Lymphatic: The lymphatics of the lower vagina accompany those of the vulva to the inguinal nodes. The drainage of the upper vagina is the same as that of the cervix to the internal iliac (hypogastric), external iliac, obturator and sacral nodes.

UTERUS

General Description

The uterus is a thick-walled, fibromuscular, hollow organ shaped like a pear, its tapering end being the cervix which projects into the upper vagina. The measurements were formerly given as 3 × 2 × 1 inch but these understate its size. Its dimensions vary but the nulliparous organ measures approximately 8 cm (3.25 inches) in overall length, 6 cm (2.5 inches) across its widest part and 4 cm (1.5 inches) from before backwards in its thickest part. It weighs 45-55 g. The wall is 1-2 cm thick, so the length of the normal uterine cavity, including the cervical canal, is not <7 cm and may be 7.5-8.0 cm.

The uterus is made up of a body or corpus, isthmus and cervix. The part of the body situated above the level of insertion of the fallopian tubes is described separately as the fundus, especially during pregnancy. The area of insertion of each fallopian tube is termed as the cornu.

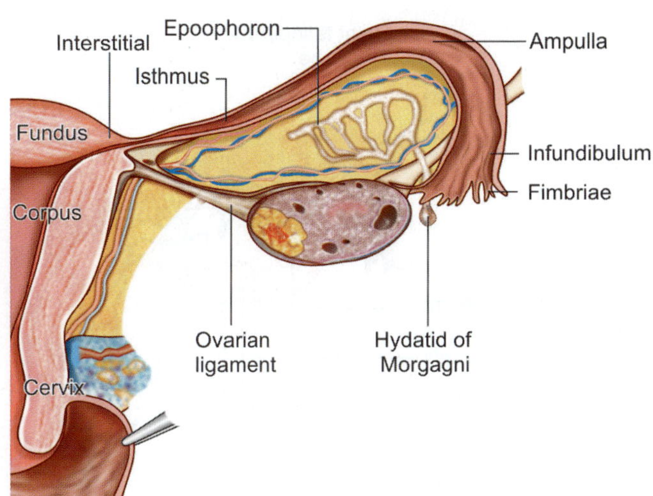

Fig. 14: The uterus and broad ligament from behind.

The opening of the cervix into the vagina is the external os uteri. The layers of uterus corpus and isthmus from outside to inside: Serosa/perimetrium, myometrium and endometrium.

The cavity of the uterus is triangular in shape when seen from the front **(Fig. 14)**, but is no more than a slit when seen from the side **(Fig. 13)**. It communicates with the vagina through the cervical canal, and with the lumen of each fallopian tube at the cornua.

Structure

The whole of the fundus, the anterior wall as low as the isthmus and the posterior wall as low as the attachment of the vagina to the cervix are covered with visceral peritoneum, which is so intimately connected with the underlying muscle that it cannot be stripped away **(Figs. 13 and 15)**. The sides of the uterus between the attachment of the two leaves of the broad ligament, the lower anterior uterine wall and the whole of the cervix except for the posterior aspect of its supravaginal part, are devoid of peritoneum. The main mass of the wall is composed of involuntary muscle fibres which for the most part run obliquely in a criss-cross spiral fashion. The more superficial fibres, however, are arranged longitudinally and are continuous with those forming the outer coats of the tubes and vagina. Fibrous and elastic tissues are mixed with the muscle in varying amounts. Internal to the muscle layers is a mucous membrane which is directly applied to the muscle without an intervening submucosa, so its glands often dip into the fibromuscular tissue.

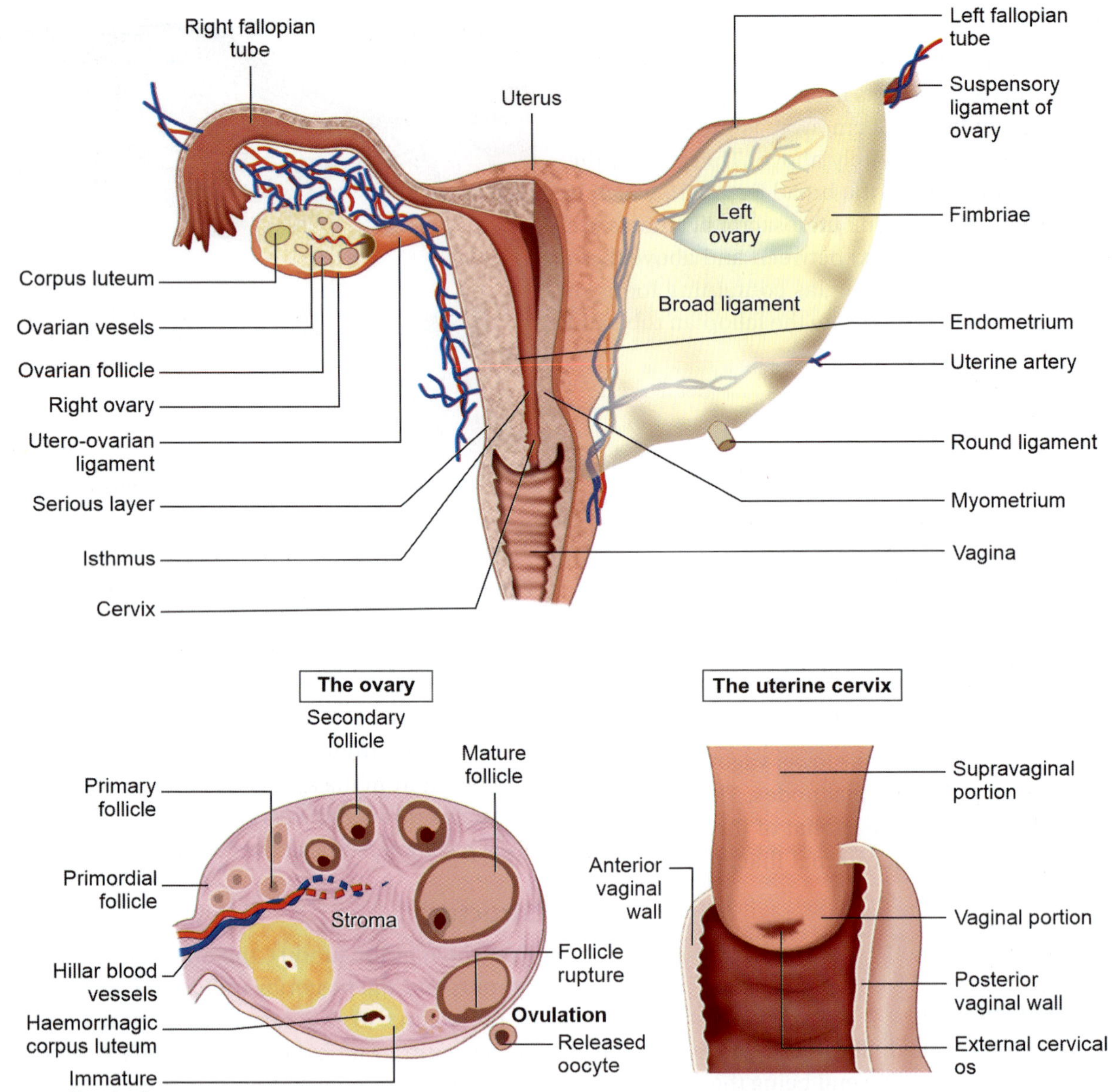

Fig. 15: Anatomy of the internal genital organs.

Special Features of Each Part of the Uterus

Corpus (Including Fundus)

The corpus makes up two-thirds or three-quarters of the uterus of the mature woman. The main muscle coat (myometrium) is lined by endometrium—a specialised form of mucous membrane. The latter varies in thickness from 1 mm to 10 mm according to the phase of the menstrual cycle. It is covered by a single layer of columnar epithelium which dips into form simple unbranched tubular or spiral glands, some of which are so long that they extend from the surface to the myometrium. The epithelium is ciliated on the surface but not in the glands. The cilia are lost once menstrual shedding starts at puberty. The glands lie in a stroma which is made up of loosely arranged immature connective tissue cells, amongst which can be seen blood vessels, lymphatics and leucocytes. Stromal cells are spindle or star-shaped with little cytoplasm so, in microscopic sections, it is the darkly staining, small round or oval nuclei, rather than the cell outlines, which are seen **(Figs. 16A and B)**.

The endometrium and, to a lesser extent, the myometrium show cyclical histological and functional changes related to menstruation. These are described in Chapter 4: Menstruation and Other Cyclical Phenomena.

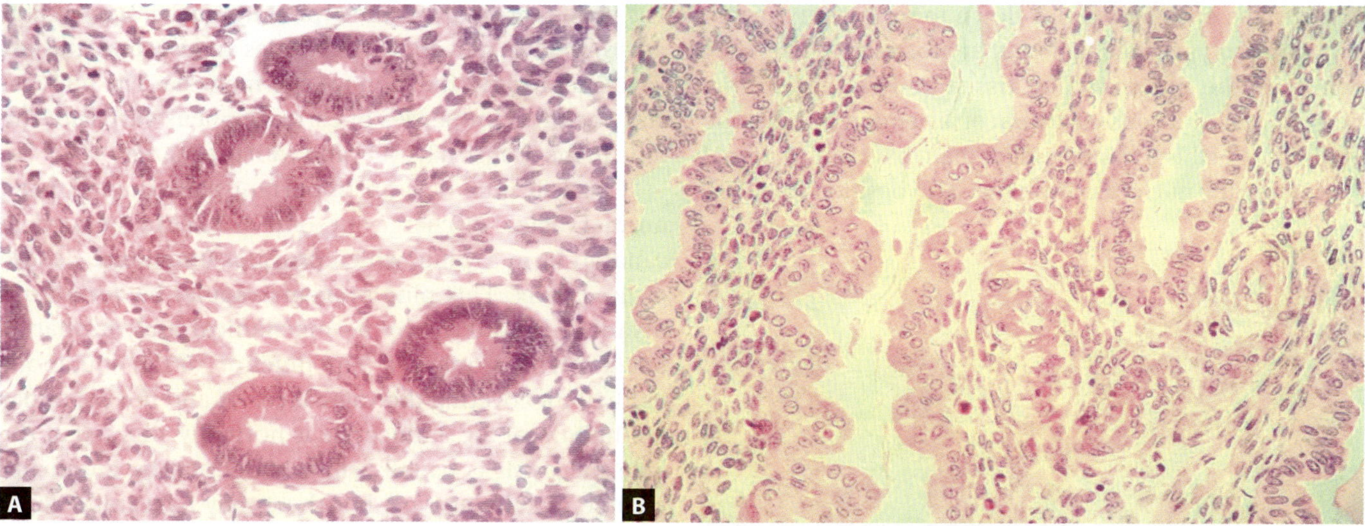

Figs. 16A and B: (A) Proliferative endometrium; (B) Secretory endometrium.

Isthmus

The isthmus is an annular zone, no >0.1–0.5 cm from top to bottom in the nonpregnant uterus, which lies between the cervix and the corpus **(Fig. 13)**. The obvious constriction between the uterine cavity and the cervical canal is the *anatomical internal os* and the isthmus is below this. The junction between the isthmus and the cervical canal proper, which is only recognised microscopically, is the *internal os*. The mucous membrane of the isthmus is intermediate in structure and function between that of the corpus and that of the cervix. The importance of the isthmus is that it is the area which, during late pregnancy and labour, becomes the lower uterine segment.

Cervix

The cervix is barrel-shaped, measuring 2.5–3.5 cm from above downwards. Half of it projects into the vagina (vaginal cervix or portio vaginalis) while half is above the vaginal attachment (supravaginal cervix) **(Figs. 13 and 14)**. The vaginal part is covered with squamous epithelium continuous with that of the vagina. The supravaginal part is surrounded by pelvic fascia except on its posterior aspect where it is covered with the peritoneum of the pouch of Douglas. A spindle-shaped canal, disposed centrally, connects the uterine cavity with the vagina. The upper part of the cervix is composed mainly of involuntary muscle, many of the fibres being continuous with those in the corpus. The lower half has a thin peripheral layer of muscle (the external cervical muscle) but is otherwise entirely composed of fibrous and collagenous tissues. The mucous membrane lining the canal (endocervix) is thrown into folds, which consist of anterior and posterior columns from which radiate circumferential folds to give the appearance of tree trunk and branches, hence the name *arbor vitae* **(Fig. 17)**. This arrangement is most obvious in the young nullipara in whom the irregularity of surface can make the passage of a sound difficult. Histologically, the endocervix differs considerably from the endometrium. It is covered by a single layer of tall columnar epithelial cells which, on the tops of the folds but not in the crypts and glands, are ciliated. Beneath this is a layer of more cubical 'basal' or 'reserve' cells from which new surface cells are believed to develop and undergo squamous metaplasia.

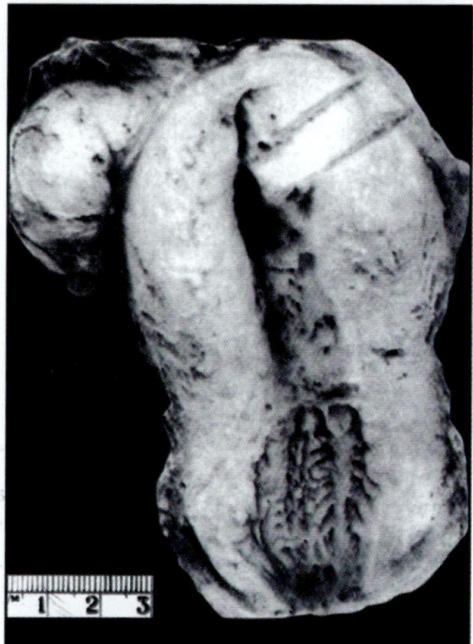

Fig. 17: The arbor vitae in the cervix. The specimen otherwise shows generalised hypertrophy of the uterus which was associated with pelvic adhesions and which resulted in menorrhagia.

The surface epithelium dips down to form complicated glands and crypts which number approximately 100. They penetrate the fibromuscular tissue and lie in a stroma more fibrous and dense than that of the endometrium. The epithelium of these glands is taller than that of endometrial glands and the nuclei are always basal in position **(Fig. 18)**.

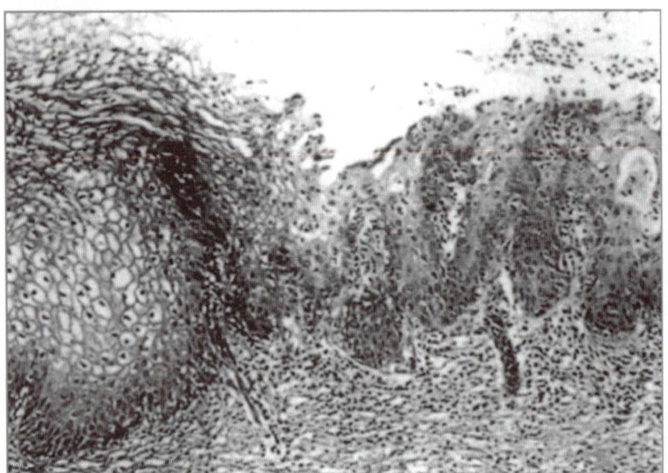

Fig. 18: Cervix, transformation zone. To the left, is seen the mature, well-glycogenated squamous epithelium of the ectocervix, and to the right, the immature metaplastic squamous epithelium of the transformation zone (Photomicrograph 120×).

The acini secrete an alkaline (pH 7.8) mucus, a gel rich in mucoproteins, mucopolysaccharides and fructose, the last having a nutritive function for spermatozoa. The physical and chemical properties of cervical mucus vary with the time in the menstrual cycle and with pregnancy.

Cervical mucus is an important constituent of the normal vaginal discharge but some of it lies in the cervical canal to form a 'plug', which provides functional closure of the cervix. This plug prevents vaginal bacteria from invading the uterus by its mechanical and, probably, bacteriolytic properties. The junction of the squamous epithelium covering the vaginal cervix and the columnar epithelium of the endocervix is normally situated at the external os. It is usually sharply defined by an abrupt change in cellular type, but there may be a transitional zone 1–10 mm in width with variable histological features **(Figs. 10 and 18)**.

Changes in the Uterus with Age and Parity

In childhood, the cervix is longer than the corpus uteri, the proportions being 2:1. At one stage in intrauterine development the proportions are 5:1 or 6:1 **(Figs. 19A and B)**. At and after puberty, however, the corpus grows faster than the cervix and the latter represents only

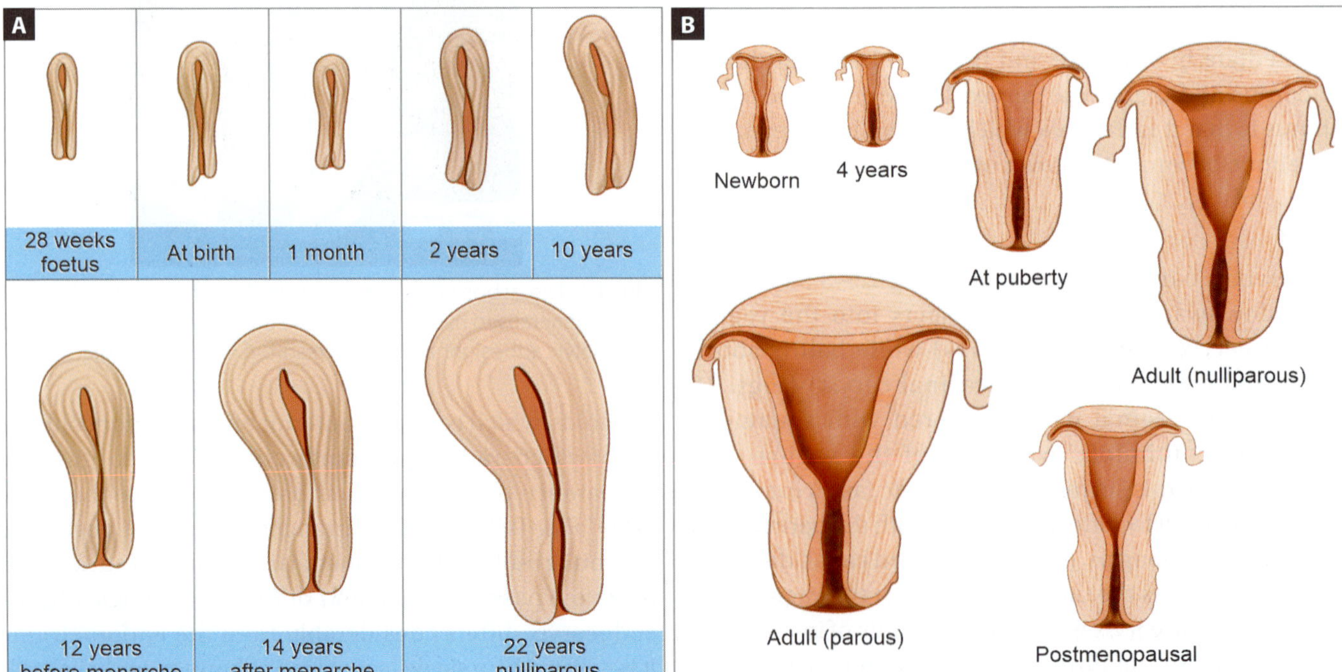

Figs. 19A and B: The relative sizes of the uterus at different ages. The size at birth is greater than in a child aged 1 month because of the effect of oestrogen circulating in the foetus in utero. Note also that the length of the cervix in relation to that of the corpus diminishes with increasing development, and anteflexion of the uterus only appears at puberty.

one-third of the total length of the mature uterus; indeed, it is sometimes only one-quarter of the parous uterus. After the climacteric the uterus atrophies, its overall length is reduced and its walls become thinner, less muscular and more fibrous. The cervix shrinks so the vaginal portion no longer projects and the external os becomes more or less flush with the vaginal wall.

In infancy, the epithelium covering the vaginal cervix and the adjacent vaginal walls lies in folds to give it a puckered appearance. The endometrium and endocervix are thin and inactive, with only a few small superficial glands. Their development at puberty and subsequent cyclical behavior during the reproductive age are described in Chapter 4: Menstruation and Other Cyclical Phenomena and Chapter 11: Breast Function and its Disorders.

In old age, both the endometrium and the endocervix become grossly atrophic; their glands are sparse and inactive.

The uterus hypertrophies during pregnancy and involutes afterwards, but never returns completely to its former state. The body of the uterus remains somewhat larger and its structure is slightly modified in that elastic tissue, deposited in and around blood vessels during pregnancy, is not reabsorbed. The amount of elastic tissue found in any myometrium is therefore proportional to the number of pregnancies previously experienced. Repeated childbearing and advancing years may also lead to a relative increase of fibrous tissue in the myometrium and a consequent increased risk of spontaneous rupture of the uterus during labour.

The cervix is modified by childbearing because, during its dilatation in labour, it always suffers some degree of tearing and injury. The nulliparous external os is circular in shape and gives to the examining finger the same sensation as that obtained by feeling the tip of a nose. The multiparous external os appears as a transverse slit and feels somewhat similar to pursed lips.

Position of the Uterus

When viewed from the side, the adult uterus is bent forwards on itself in an attitude of *anteflexion.* The bend is situated about the level of the internal os **(Fig. 13)**.

In addition, the axis of the cervix is inclined forwards at an angle of approximately 90° to the axis of the vagina, giving rise to a state of *anteversion;* when a woman is standing, the cavity of the uterus is therefore more horizontal than vertical. Version and flexion are not always in the forward direction and approximately 15% of women have uteri, which are retroverted or retroflexed or both; such states are not usually pathological (refer to Chapter 18: Other Displacements of the Uterus).

The uterus is normally moderately mobile, its most fixed part being the supravaginal cervix where the strong supporting ligaments are attached. The fundus can therefore rotate around this point, and the degree of anteflexion and anteversion is influenced by the state of adjacent organs. Thus, a full bladder rotates the uterus backwards and also reduces anteflexion.

The height of the uterus in the pelvis varies with posture and other factors (refer to Chapter 18: Other Displacements of the Uterus) but, in the standing woman, the internal os is approximately level with the upper border of the symphysis pubis, and the external os is opposite the tip of the ischial spine. It follows that the body of the uterus lies normally above the level of the symphysis pubis so, in the thin woman with relaxed abdominal muscles and an empty bladder; it is possible to feel it on abdominal examination.

Relations of the Uterus

Anterior

The upper part of the uterus has the uterovesical pouch of peritoneum and either intestines or bladder in front of it. The lower part is closely associated with the base of the bladder from which it is separated only by loose connective tissue.

Posterior

Posteriorly lies the peritoneum flap pouch of Douglas (uterorectal pouch) with coils of intestine. The vaginal cervix also has the posterior fornix behind it.

Lateral

Lateral to the uterus is the broad ligament and its contents, especially the uterine artery, which runs up the side of the uterus, giving off branches at different levels. As it passes forward to reach the base of the bladder the ureter lies only 1-2 cm to the side of the supravaginal cervix—an extremely important point for the surgeon **(Fig. 20)**.

Vascular Connections

Arterial:

- Uterine artery
- Ovarian artery

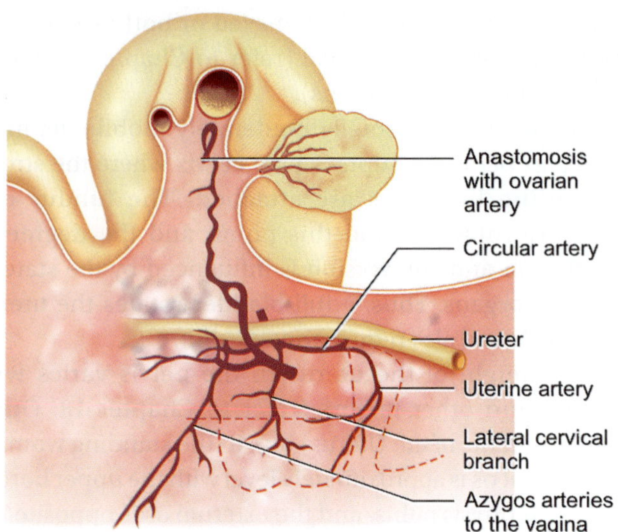

Fig. 20: The broad ligament from the side showing the relation of the ureter to the uterine artery, and how the latter supplies branches to the corpus, cervix and vagina.

Venous:
- Pampiniform plexus in broad ligament
- Uterine vein
- Ovarian vein
- Vaginal plexus
- Vertebral plexus

Lymphatic
- *Cervix:*
  - Paracervical plexus
  - Obturator nodes
  - External iliac and internal iliac (hypogastric) nodes
  - Sacral nodes
- *Corpus:* The same as the cervix. Also, the aortic nodes (via lymphatics accompanying the ovarian vessels) and the superficial inguinal nodes (via lymphatics in the round ligament).

FALLOPIAN TUBES

General Description

The two fallopian tubes are oviducts, which extend from the ovaries to the cornua of the uterus, one on either side. They are somewhat tortuous and their outer parts curve backwards **(Fig. 11)**. Each lies in the free upper border of the broad ligament and, when straightened, is 10 cm in length. Its lumen communicates with the uterine cavity at its inner end and with the peritoneal cavity at its outer, and thus provides the final section of an open, or potentially open, canal which leads from the exterior to the abdominal cavity.

The fallopian tube is divided into four parts **(Fig. 14)** as discussed here.

Interstitial or Intramural Part

This is only 1–2 cm in length and is the part which traverses the uterine wall. It has a very narrow lumen (1 mm in diameter) and is different from the remainder of the tube in that it is without a peritoneal coat, and in that the outer longitudinal muscle has disappeared to cover the uterus.

Isthmus

This is the straight and narrow portion adjacent to the uterus and measures 2–3 cm. It has thick walls but the lumen is so narrow that it will only admit the finest probe (1–2 mm in diameter).

Ampulla

This is the wider, thin-walled and tortuous outer portion, approximately 5 cm in length, which leads to the infundibulum.

Infundibulum

This is the trumpet-shaped outer end with an opening into the peritoneal cavity (abdominal ostium). The latter is surrounded by fronds or fimbriae, one of which is longer than the others and is directed towards the ovary (fimbria ovarica). The fimbriated extremity is free of the broad ligament and curls back on itself so that its fimbriae aim to embrace the ovary like the tentacles of an octopus; this is important to fertility.

Structure

Except for a narrow strip opposite to its attachment to the broad ligament, the extrauterine part of the fallopian tube is covered with peritoneum. Beneath this are an outer longitudinal layer and an inner circular layer of involuntary muscle. The muscle zone is thick at the isthmus and thin at the ampulla. It is separated from the mucosa lining the lumen (endosalpinx) by a delicate connective tissue submucosa. The mucous membrane is arranged in the interstitial and isthmic portions of the tube in four or five main longitudinal ridges, but these develop subsidiary folds or plicae to form a very complicated arborescence in the ampullary portion. It is lined by columnar epithelium supported by a thin stroma **(Figs. 21 and 22)**. About half

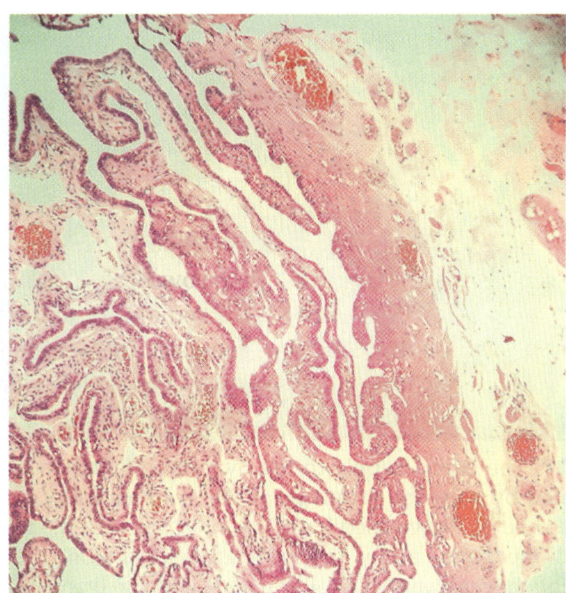

Fig. 21: Photomicrograph showing the mucosa of the fallopian tube 100×.

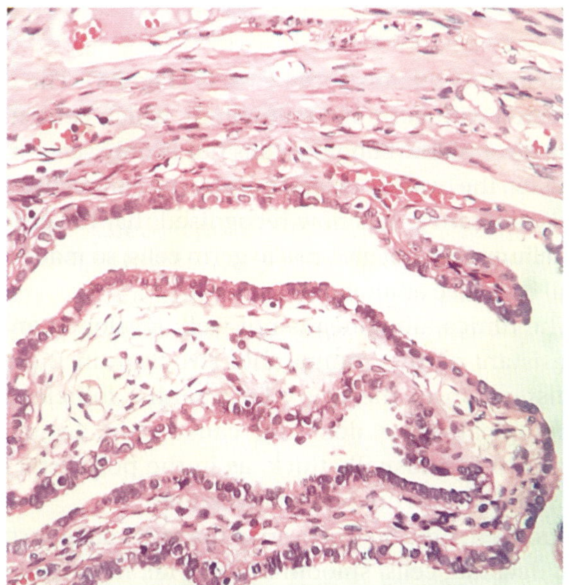

Fig. 22: A higher magnification of the endosalpinx showing ciliated cells, secretory cells and 'peg' cells.

the epithelial cells, especially in the outer parts of the tube, are ciliated and create a current. This, combined with peristaltic action of the muscle, propels the ovum towards the uterus.

This is in accord with the general view that the peristaltic wave is towards the uterus. Yet observations on the tube in situ indicate that the contraction wave is variable and sometimes in reverse. Most of the other epithelial cells have a secretory function, which is achieved by cytoplasmic and nuclear extrusion. The resulting product is a serous fluid, rich in protein, which may be nutritive to the fertilised ovum. A third type of epithelial cell is 'peg-shaped'; its function is doubtful and it may represent an immature or senile form of the others. Another suggestion is that the 'peg' cell is merely a secretory (goblet) cell which has discharged its secretion.

Both the muscular and secretory activities of the tube are under the influence of ovarian hormones and therefore show cyclical changes during the menstrual life of a woman. Before puberty and after the menopause, the tube is functionally quiet.

Relations

Superior

Above the fallopian tubes lie coils of intestine and the omentum, with the appendix and caecum on the right side and the pelvic colon on the left.

Inferior

The broad ligament and its contents, and particularly the mesosalpinx with the epoophoron, paroophoron and Gartner's duct **(Figs. 14 and 23)** lie below. So do the ovary and mesovarium, but on a more posterior plane.

Posterior

Behind the fallopian tubes are the ovaries and the uterorectal pouch with its contents.

Anterior

To the front lie the top of the bladder and the uterovesical pouch.

Lateral

On either side is the lateral pelvic wall with the structures thereon.

Vascular Connections and Innervation

The vascular connections and innervation are similar to those of the ovary.

OVARY

General Description

The two ovaries are mainly solid ovoid structures, approximately 3.5 cm in length and 1.5–2.5 cm in

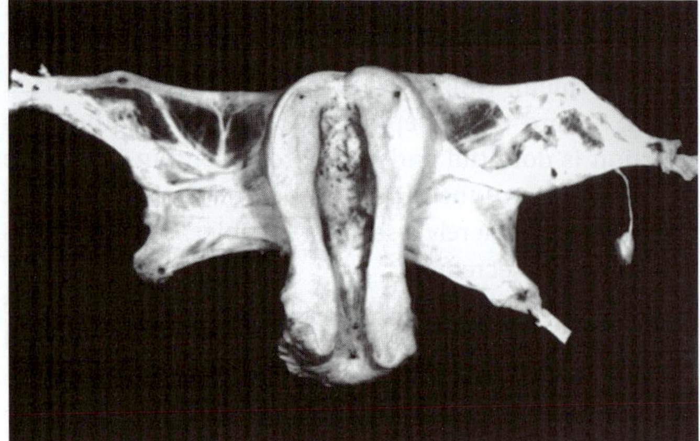

Fig. 23: Gartner's duct and other vestigial structures in the broad ligament. These are easily seen, because the specimen was obtained from a senile woman in whom the fat and the connective tissue of the broad ligament had atrophied. The ovaries are equally atrophic. The structures can be identified by comparison with **Figure 12**. The dependent small cyst on the right is the hydatid of Morgagni. The fundus of the uterus contains an early endometrial carcinoma.

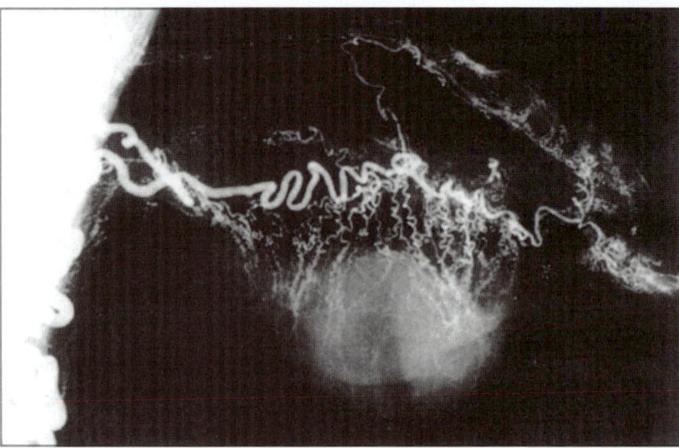

Fig. 24: The blood supply to the ovary and fallopian tube as revealed by a uterine arteriogram. The ovarian artery was not injected but is shown filled from its connection with the terminal part of the uterine artery. The spiral arterioles entering the ovary through the mesovarium are well shown, and also branches to the fallopian tube with a continuous vessel running just below and parallel to it.

thickness. Each weighs 4–8 g, the right tending to be larger than the left. They are attached to the back of the broad ligament by the mesovarium, one on either side of the uterus **(Fig. 14)**. Each is suspended from the cornu of the uterus by an ovarian ligament. The surface of the adult active ovary is corrugated, and is pale except where there happens to be some structure such as a corpus luteum. The ovary is the only organ in the abdomen which is not covered by peritoneum. The part of the ovary attached to the mesovarium is the hilum and all nerves and vessels enter and leave at this point. In the hilum and adjacent mesovarium are small collections of hilus cells which may be homologous to the interstitial cells of the testis.

Structure

Mainly composed of the ovarian parenchyma and the stroma.

The ovarian parenchyma has three layers: *Albuginea* (hypocellular fibrotic most superficial layer), *cortex* (outer zone) and *medulla* (inner zone), but these are not clearly defined. Both areas have a connective tissue stroma in which can be found blood vessels, nerves and Graafian follicles in varying stages of development together with their derivatives, the corpora lutea and corpora albicantia (refer to Chapter 3: Ovarian Functions). Primordial follicles are mostly found in the cortex, the medulla is more vascular and contains spiral vessels **(Fig. 24)**. The cortex is covered with germinal epithelium, which consists of a single layer of low cuboidal cells but is only seen in early life. Later, the ovary is coated only by the connective tissue tunica albuginea. It is now recognised that the germinal epithelium does not give rise to germ cells, so many prefer to call it surface epithelium.

The tunica albuginea is not well developed and not as resistant as the comparable structure in the testis. So distension of the ovary by ripening follicles or by pathological states does not cause pain. Even when the tunica is unusually thick, as in the polycystic ovary syndrome, it does not prevent ovulation.

Stroma has the bulk of ovarian tissue. It contains stromal cells, decidual cells, smooth muscle, fat, neuroendocrine cells and endometrial stroma-like cells.

Relations

These are similar to those of the fallopian tube. Indeed, the tube and ovary and their mesenteries are so closely related anatomically that they are often collectively called the *adnexum* (plural = adnexa). The exact position of the ovary and tube varies considerably; they are sometimes near the pelvic brim, at other times in the uterorectal pouch.

The ovary usually lies against the lateral wall of the pelvis in a depression called the ovarian fossa. The fossa is bounded by the external iliac vessels above, anteriorly and inferiorly by broad ligament and by the internal iliac vessels and the ureter behind the obturator nerve crosses the floor of the fossa.

Changes with Age and Parity

In infancy and childhood, the ovary is a tiny elongated structure with a smooth surface, situated near the pelvic brim, and packed with primary oocytes. Although in the newborn baby it may show small follicular cysts resulting from the stimulation by chorionic gonadotrophins, it later contains only primordial or atretic follicles.

After the menopause, the ovary becomes smaller in size and shriveled in appearance; these changes are the results of atrophy of the medulla, and not of scarring following repeated ovulation as is sometimes stated. At a later stage, the surface becomes smooth again as in childhood. No follicles are found in old age. The spiral shape of the arterioles in the medulla is seen only in the reproductive years and appears to be controlled by oestrogen.

Vascular Connections

The **Flowchart 1** is given below.

URETHRA AND BLADDER

General Description

The external urinary meatus is in the vestibule, outside the hymen, and enclosed by the foreparts of the labia minora. The urethra itself runs upwards and backwards, being partly incorporated in the anterior vaginal wall. It is short and straight, measuring only 2–4 cm in length. It joins the bladder base to form what appear on radiographic silhouettes as clearly defined angles. These are present in both lateral and anteroposterior views, and there is no such thing as a 'bladder neck' in the female **(Figs. 7, 8, and 25)**. On the floor of the urethra at its lower end are tiny openings of Skene's tubules, which drain two small collections of periurethral or paraurethral glands. These are rudimentary structures homologous to the prostate in the male. They resemble this organ in that they are sites for chronic infection.

Flowchart 1: Vascular connections of the ovary.

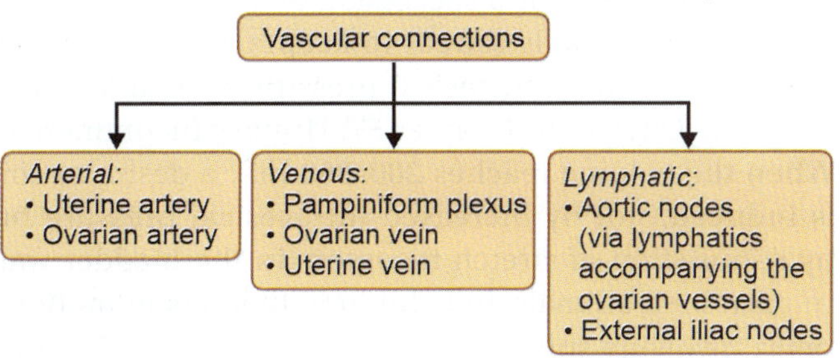

The bladder is a hollow muscular organ with a capacity of 300–600 mL but with such powers of distension that, in conditions of prolonged retention, it can accommodate several litres of fluid. The base of the full bladder is comparatively flat and, when viewed from the side, occupies a plane which runs from the middle of the back of the symphysis pubis to the fourth sacral vertebra **(Figs. 7, 8, and 25)**. The shape and position of the fundus of the bladder vary with the volume of the contents; the top can extend as high as the umbilicus (refer to Chapter 18: Other Displacements of the Uterus).

The ureters enter the bladder on the posterior aspect of its base, piercing the bladder wall obliquely, one on either side of the middle line. The obliquity acts as a valve in that it prevents reflux of urine into the ureter when the bladder is full. The ridge joining the internal orifices is the *interureteric (Mercier's) bar,* and the smooth triangular area bounded by the ureteric openings and the internal urethral meatus is the *trigone.*

Structure

Only the fundus of the bladder has a peritoneal covering. Elsewhere, the muscle is coated with fascia only.

Except for the external meatus, which has true stratified epithelium, the bladder and urethra are lined by transitional epithelium, which is supported by a thin layer of connective tissue. Beneath this is a complicated pattern of involuntary muscle, which is continued from the bladder into the urethra. An intricate decussation at the urethrovesical junction has the effect of forming anterior and posterior slings, which function as an internal sphincter **(Figs. 26A and B)**. The muscle of the trigone is an insignificant structure in women.

The wall of the urethra is made up entirely of involuntary muscle, the fibres of which are mainly disposed in the form of crossed spirals. When these are closely coiled, they have a circular arrangement which provides good urethral tone and resistance. When they are drawn out their resistance is lowered and the urethra can dilate **(Figs. 26A and B)**. Indeed, the bladder and urethra have a polarity similar to that of the uterus; when the bladder detrusor contracts, it opens the urethra from above downwards by pulling on the spiral framework.

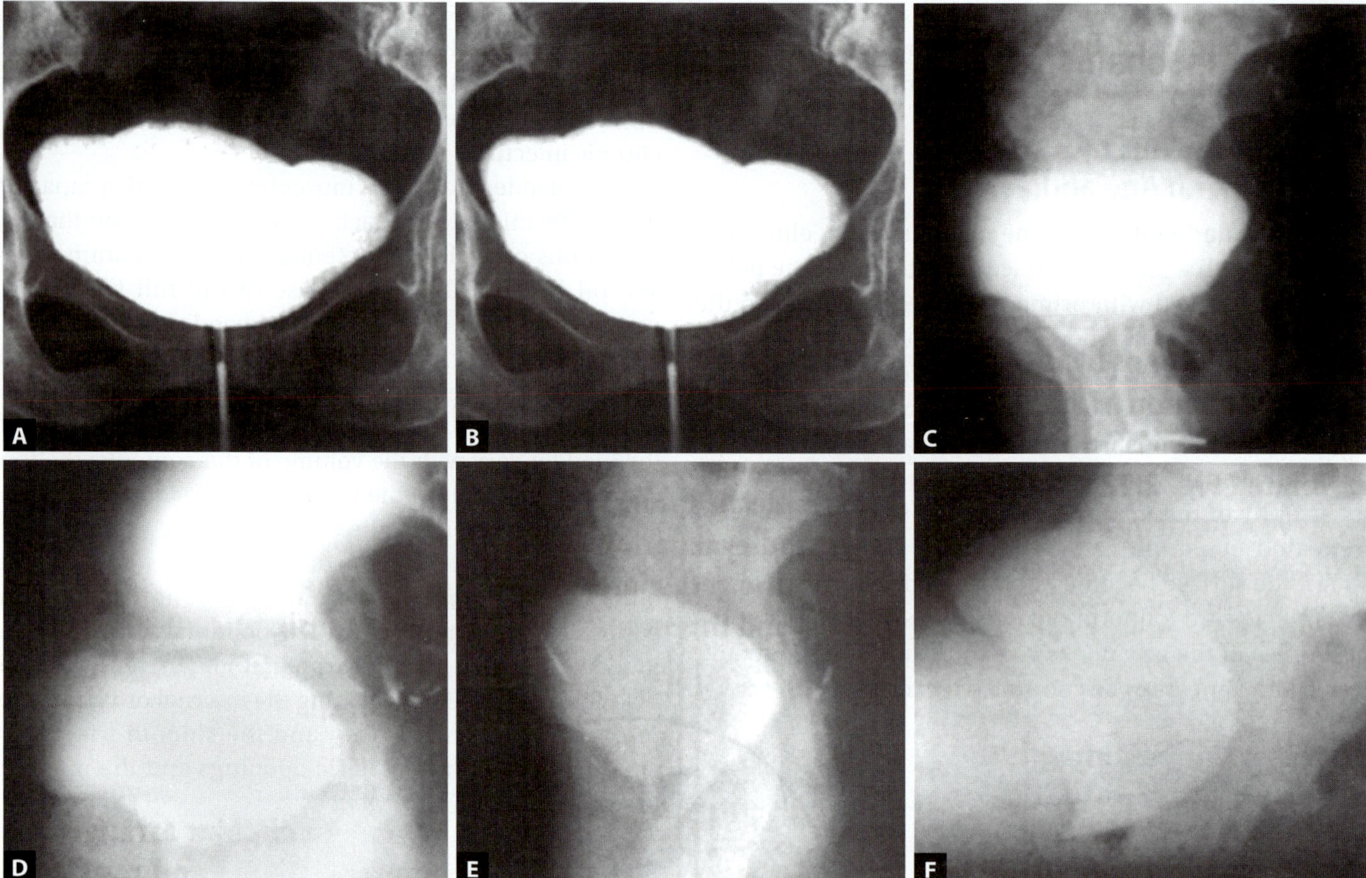

Figs. 25A to F: The anatomy and function of the bladder and urethra as revealed by lateral urethrocystography. (A) Normal nulliparous woman at ease with the bladder made radio-opaque with a solution of sodium iodide. The urethra is outlined by a soft and pliable catheter filled with radio-opaque fluid; (B) Normal nulliparous woman resting easily, anteroposterior view; what appears to be the urethrovesical junction is not so because, as shown in (A), this is at a higher level than part of the bladder base; (C) Normal nulliparous woman raising her intravesical pressure by bearing down; there is no change in the anatomy of the urethrovesical junction; (D) Commencing voiding. The catheter has been removed and the urethra is opening from above downwards, the floor of the urethra coming into line with the trigone of the bladder (disappearance of the posterior urethrovesical angle). This reflects opening of the internal urethral sphincter brought about by contraction of the bladder detrusor muscle, which is manifested by the crenated outline of the posterior bladder wall; (E) Voiding is now well established. The urethra is dilated, the 'posterior angle' is obliterated and the bladder base and upper urethra have rotated slightly backwards and downwards. Active contraction of the bladder is indicated by its ovoid shape and fluffy outline; (F) Micturition inhibited by voluntary contraction of the external urethral sphincter (compressor urethrae). The bladder is still contracting but the woman has shut off the stream at the lower end of the urethra.
Source: With permission from Mr H Robert and the Editor, J Obstet Gynaecol Br Emp.

The urethra itself is devoid of true anatomical sphincters but the tone and elasticity of its involuntary muscles keep it closed except during micturition. Where it pierces the triangular ligament, approximately 1 cm from its lower end, it is encompassed by the voluntary compressor urethra which is sometimes called the external sphincter. The urethra probably does not receive voluntary fibres from the levator ani, as is sometimes suggested; the inner parts of the puborectalis pass well to the side to be inserted into the vagina **(Fig. 27)**.

Sphincter Mechanism

As the bladder fills by a succession of drops of urine from the ureters, its walls retreat to keep a constant muscle tone, so that the intravesical pressure is maintained at <10 cmH_2O (refer to Chapter 57: Urinary Incontinence). When the volume reaches 200–300 mL, a desire to void is induced, not by increased intravesical pressure but by stimulation of stretch receptors in the bladder wall. In untrained animals and children, this sets in motion a reflex involving spinal roots S2, S3 and S4, which results

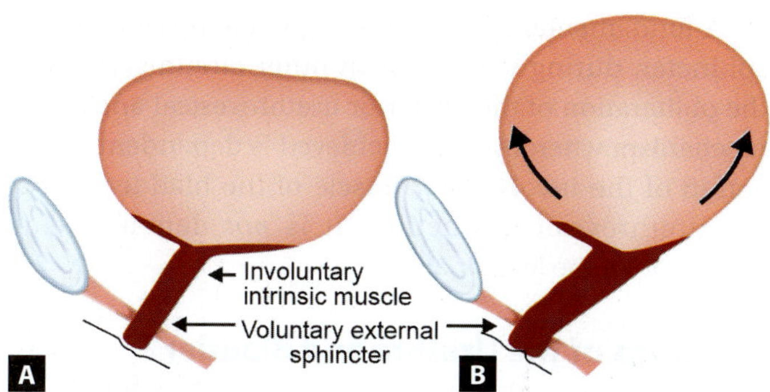

Figs. 26A and B: The involuntary intrinsic muscle in the urethra is distributed in the form of crossed spirals, the fibres being continuous with those of the bladder detrusor. Their decussation at the urethrovesical junction, with a suggestion of the formation of slings, constitutes the internal urethral sphincter. The external voluntary sphincter lies outside the intrinsic muscle, between the layers of the urogenital diaphragm. (A) Detrusor inactive so the spirals in the urethra are closely coiled to bring the walls in apposition; (B) When the detrusor muscle contracts, as in voiding, the spirals in the urethra are pulled out with consequent loss of resistance. The urethra then opens from above downwards, the trigone coming into line with the floor of the urethra.

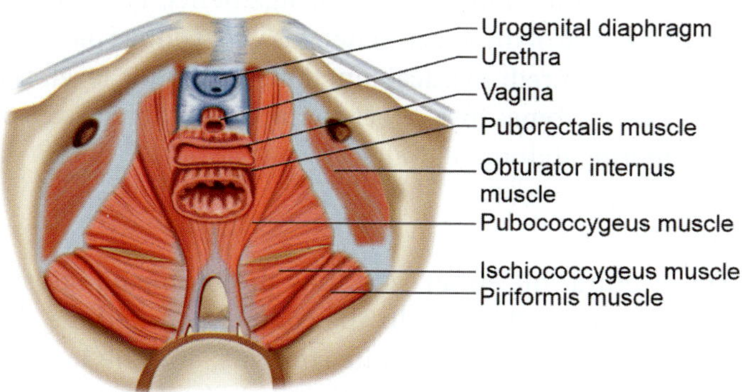

Fig. 27: The levator ani muscles from above.

in automatic contraction of the detrusor muscle and evacuation of the bladder. In the adult, however, the reflex arc is subservient to the hypothalamus, and this in turn to higher areas of the brain, notably the anterior parts of the frontal lobes **(Fig. 28)**. Action of the detrusor muscle can therefore be voluntarily inhibited and the urge resisted until it is convenient to void. When this happens the bladder distends further, but there is still no appreciable rise in the intravesical pressure until the limit of bladder capacity is approached. The slight increase at that time is the result of the detrusor escaping from inhibition and is accompanied by an intense and irresistible urge to void.

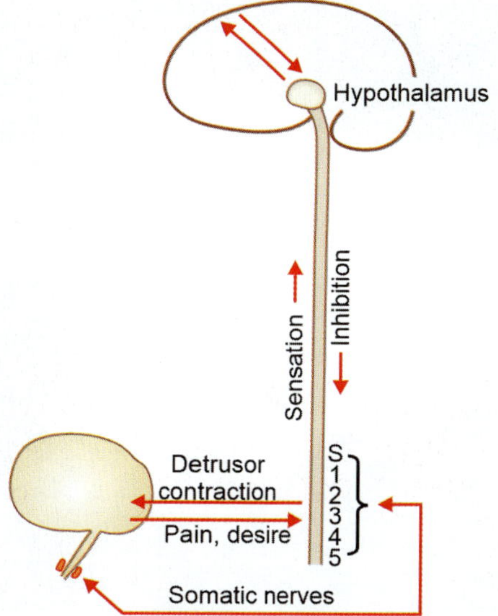

Fig. 28: The nervous control of bladder filling and emptying. Stretch receptors in the bladder wall transmit sensation of fullness to the spinal cord. A basic reflex then provides for stimulation of the involuntary detrusor muscle of the bladder to produce automatic emptying. This reflex is controlled in trained animals by central inhibition, the centres involved being the cortex and the hypothalamus. The external sphincter is voluntarily controlled by the central nervous system.

During micturition, the pressure rises to 30 or 50 cmH_2O as a result of the contraction of the bladder wall, and can be raised to a total of 100 cmH_2O by voluntary contraction of the abdominal muscles. Except during micturition, the urethra is always empty, even if the intravesical pressure is raised to 50 or 70 cmH_2O by coughing or other strong effort. Continence is therefore normally maintained at the urethrovesical junction, by the involuntary internal sphincter. This fundamental fact explains why an urethrovaginal fistula, unless it involves the uppermost part of the urethra, does not result in incontinence of urine, neither does surgical removal of the lower half of the urethra.

The urethral resistance as a whole, which is offered by the inherent tone and elasticity of the intrinsic involuntary muscle, provides a second, although not very efficient, line of defence when a weak internal sphincter allows urine to enter the lumen. The compressor urethrae enables a woman voluntarily to arrest the flow of urine, even during voiding, and its action can be demonstrated radiologically **(Figs. 25F and 29)**. It can always be brought into play in an emergency. Otherwise, the action of these urethral and periurethral muscles is to empty the urethra at the conclusion of micturition.

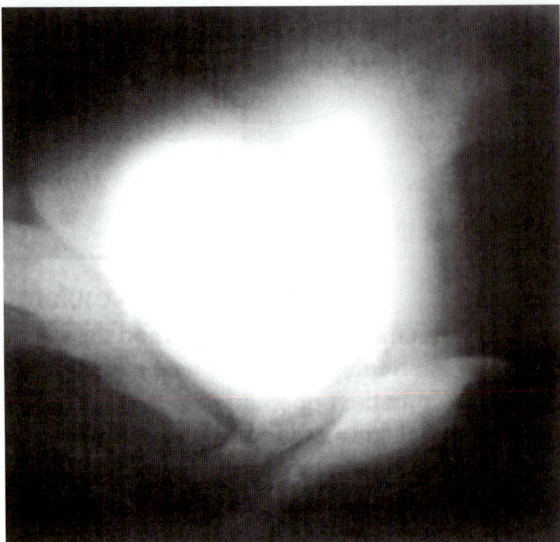

Fig. 29: The voluntary arrest of micturition shown by a double exposure of the same film. The vagina as well as the bladder contains radio-opaque material. The fainter shadows illustrate the situation during voiding: The deeper ones the effect of deliberate stoppage of the act. The flow down the urethra is arrested by the external sphincter, and the urethra then closes from below upwards returning to the bladder any fluid within it unless it involves the uppermost part of the urethra, which does not result in incontinence of urine; neither does surgical removal of the lower half of the urethra.

The process of micturition is illustrated in **Figures 8 and 25** and is as follows:

- Bearing-down effort accompanied by relaxation of the pelvic diaphragm.
- Descent of the bladder base with rotation of the upper urethra around a fixed point at the triangular ligament.
- Contraction of the detrusor muscle is now released from inhibition.
- Dilatation of the urethra from above downwards.
- The characteristic feature of opening of the internal sphincter, as seen on lateral radiographs, is the coming into line of the trigone and the floor of the urethra. This results in the radiological sign of 'disappearance of the posterior urethrovesical angle', the 'anterior angle' being maintained.
- During voiding, and especially if the woman under study is nervous, detrusor activity can be intermittent and this shows by periodic partial closure of the internal sphincter with consequent periodic partial restoration of the posterior angle.
- At the end of micturition, the urethra closes from below upwards and any remaining drops of urine are returned to the bladder.

A fundamental radiographic sign of a relaxed internal sphincter, during voiding or in other circumstances, is the obliteration of the posterior urethrovesical angle. The mechanism whereby this is achieved is dependent on the action of the involuntary muscle of the bladder and of the urethrovesical junction. It is *not* dependent on relaxation of the levator ani.

Relations of the Urethra and Bladder

Posterior

Behind the urethra are Skene's tubules and the vaginal wall but no intervening fascia. The base of the bladder is separated from the upper anterior vaginal wall by the pubocervical fascia. Above this the bladder comes into relation with the supravaginal cervix, the isthmus of the uterus, and the uterovesical pouch of peritoneum containing intestine.

Anterior

In front of the urethra and bladder, and separating them from the pubic bones and their ligaments, is the loose cellular tissue of the space of Retzius with venous plexuses marking the urethrovesical junction. Above this level, the full bladder comes into direct contact with the muscles of the anterior abdominal wall.

Lateral

The urethra, on either side, has the bulbospongiosus muscle, the vestibular bulb, the compressor urethrae, the urogenital diaphragm and its contents, and the inferior pubic ramus. The levator ani muscle (puborectalis) is a lateral relation as it sweeps backwards to be inserted partly into the side of the vagina **(Fig. 27)**. The tendinous foreparts of this muscle also lie below and to the side of the bladder.

Vascular Connections

Arterial:

- *Bladder*: Superior and inferior vesical arteries from the internal iliac artery
- *Urethra*: Inferior vesical artery and branches of the internal pudendal artery.

Venous: Vesical and vaginal plexuses and hence to the internal iliac veins.

Lymphatic: Lymphatics accompany blood vessels to the internal iliac (hypogastric) and external iliac nodes. The external urethral meatus drains with the vulva to the inguinal nodes.

Innervation: See **Figure 28**.

URETER

General Description

The ureter is 25 cm long and is lined by transitional epithelium and its main coat consists of involuntary muscle which has a peristaltic action to propel urine from the kidney to the bladder. It lies behind the peritoneum, but it is closely adherent to it. In its pelvic course, the ureter has such close relations to the genital organs that it may be obstructed by their diseases and is always at risk of injury during pelvic surgeries.

Relations

As it enters the pelvis, the ureter lies anterior to the sacroiliac joint although separated from it by muscles, ligaments and the common iliac artery and vein. It crosses in front of these vessels at the point where they bifurcate into external and internal branches, and then turns downwards into the pelvis, running along the front of the internal iliac artery but on the medial side of the branches of this artery. At the pelvic brim the ureter is in relation to the ovarian vessels which cross it anteriorly and, on the left side, to the pelvic mesocolon and its vessels **(Fig. 30)**.

In the true pelvis, it turns inwards and forwards towards the bladder, running lateral to the uterosacral ligament. It crosses the base of the broad ligament lying below and at right angles to the uterine artery **(Fig. 20)**. In the latter part of its course, the ureter lies 1 cm to the side of the supravaginal cervix and 1 cm above the lateral vaginal fornix. At this point it pierces the cardinal ligament of the uterus which is condensed around to form the ureteric canal.

The ureter is the most exposed to surgical injury: At the pelvic brim when the ovarian vessels are ligated; during division and ligature of the lower part of the broad ligament; during removal of broad ligament, which displace it from its normal position; during peritonization of the pelvis when, being adherent to the posterior leaf, it may be included in a suture; and when the cardinal ligaments are tightened to cure uterine prolapse.

About 75% of all iatrogenic injuries to the ureter result from gynaecologic procedures, most commonly abdominal hysterectomy. Distortions of pelvic anatomy, including adnexal masses, endometriosis, other pelvic adhesive disease or fibroids, may increase susceptibility to injury

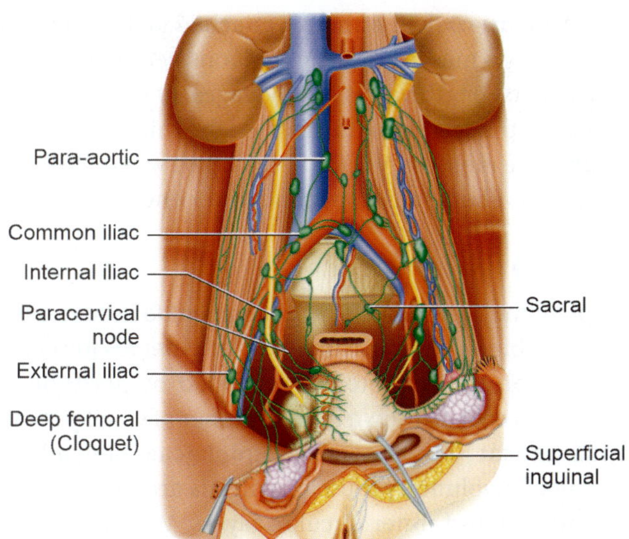

Fig. 30: The lymphatic drainage of the internal pelvic organs together with the main arteries and veins. The paracervical node is rarely present; usually, there is merely a plexus of lymph vessels at this site. The lettering applies to lymph nodes, not blood vessels.

by displacement or alteration of usual anatomy. Even with severe intraperitoneal disease, however, the ureter can always be identified using a retroperitoneal approach and noting fundamental landmarks and relationships.

Vascular Connections

Arterial

Special branches from:

- Renal artery
- Ovarian artery
- Internal iliac or common iliac artery
- Uterine artery
- Inferior vesical artery

Venous: Veins accompany arteries.

Lymphatic:

- Para-aortic nodes
- Internal iliac nodes

Interference with all the arterial supplies, or stripping of the outer vascular coat, such as may occur during extensive pelvic operations, results in ischaemic necrosis of the ureter with consequent fistula formation.

SIGMOID COLON

General Description

The sigmoid (pelvic) colon is the continuation of the descending colon, the arbitrary dividing line being the brim of the true pelvis. Although attached to the left side of the pelvis by a mesentery, it lies in loops behind the broad ligament. Its length varies but averages 40 cm, and it terminates in the rectum at the level of the third piece of the sacrum. The mesentery is the longest part where the colon loops, but is short at its upper and lower ends.

Structure

Except for the narrow line of its attachment to its mesentery, where the blood vessels, lymphatics and nerves join it, the pelvic colon is completely surrounded by peritoneum. This serous coat is thrown into a number of small pouches containing fat—the appendices epiploicae. Beneath it is the wall of involuntary muscle, which is arranged in outer longitudinal and inner circular, layers. Within this, and separated by areolar tissue, is the inner lining of mucous membrane. The latter is covered by a single layer of nonciliated columnar cells. These dip down in the form of simple tubules to form glands, which secrete mucus and also absorb fluid.

Relations

Anterior

These are mainly the broad ligament and all the organs associated with it, including the uterus.

Posterior

Behind and to the left lies the rectum, the posterior and left walls of the pelvis, together with the retroperitoneal structures. The latter include the left common and external iliac vessels, the left ureter, the left sacral plexus and pyriformis muscle.

Vascular Connections

Arterial:

- Inferior mesenteric artery
- Left colic artery

Venous: Veins corresponding to arteries

Lymphatic: Preaortic nodes around the origins of the inferior mesenteric vessels.

Innervation:

- This is entirely autonomic by way of parasympathetic nerves from the preaortic plexuses.
- These are motor and sensory and accompany blood vessels.

RECTUM AND ANUS

General Description

The importance of the rectum and anus lies in their close proximity to the genital organs, and their consequent involvement in the same diseases and in injuries during childbirth and gynaecological operations. The rectum commences at the level of the S3 vertebrae and is 12–15 cm in length. It curves twice on the left and once to the right as it passes down to end in the anal canal which is approximately 2–3 cm in length. The ampulla bulges forward against the posterior vaginal wall and the anal canal is directed backwards, almost at right angles to the ampulla **(Fig. 8)**. This angulation is at the site of the insertion of fibres of the puborectalis muscle.

Structure

Only the anterior and lateral aspects of the upper rectum are covered with peritoneum. Beneath this are the outer longitudinal and inner circular muscle coats. The lining is mucus-secreting tall columnar epithelium with a complicated glandular pattern, except for the lowermost part of the anal canal which has a stratified squamous covering continuous with the skin. The mucous membrane is exuberant and ridged and is also raised to form the three valves of Houston.

The anal canal has internal (involuntary) and external (voluntary) sphincters, but its control is also dependent on the levator ani, the inner parts of which surround it and are inserted into its outer wall **(Figs. 27 and 31)**.

Relations

Anterior

In front of the upper part of the rectum lies the uterorectal pouch of peritoneum, which often contains loops of small or large bowel. Anterior to this is the uterus with the broad ligaments and adnexa. Below the pelvic peritoneum the anterior wall of the rectum comes into close association with the middle part of the posterior vaginal wall, being separated from it only by rectovaginal fascia and connective tissues. Interposed between the anal canal and lower vagina is the perineal body.

Posterior

Behind the rectum are loose connective tissue, sacral nerve trunks, the middle sacral vessels, the sacrum and the coccyx.

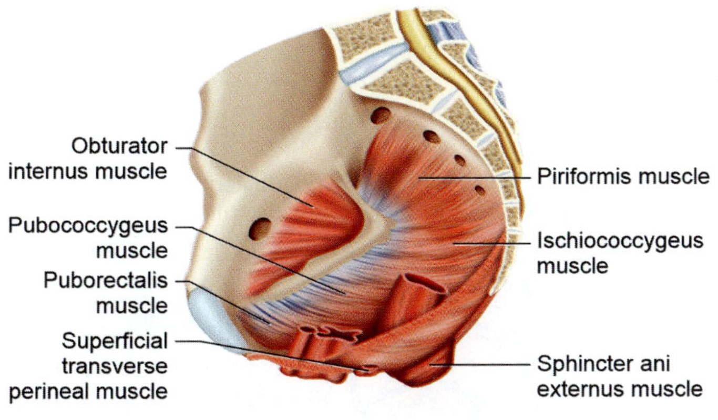

Fig. 31: The levator ani and the urogenital diaphragm on the right side of the pelvis viewed from the left.

Lateral

On either side are the uterosacral ligament, the pelvic plexus of autonomic nerves and the ureter. At a lower level is the levator ani muscle, which is in part inserted into the rectum and anus **(Figs. 27 and 31)**. Below and lateral to this muscle are the fat and areolar tissue of the ischiorectal fossa.

Vascular Connections

Arterial:

- Superior rectal branch of the inferior mesenteric artery
- Middle rectal branch of the internal iliac artery
- Inferior rectal branch of the pudendal artery

Venous: Veins accompanying arteries, the superior rectal draining to the portal circulation. The junction of the portal and systemic venous drainages in the anal canal marks the site of haemorrhoid formation.

Lymphatic:

- Internal iliac nodes mainly, also sacral and para-aortic
- Superficial inguinal nodes (anus only).

Innervation: The anus and voluntary external sphincter have a somatic sensory and motor innervation from S4 and S5 roots via the sacral plexus **(Figs. 32A to D)**. The rectum and anal canal otherwise have only an autonomic supply (sensory and motor) from the preaortic, superior hypogastric and pelvic plexuses.

PELVIC PERITONEUM AND LIGAMENTS

Peritoneal Pouches

The peritoneum of the anterior abdominal wall is reflected onto the fundus of the bladder to which it is adherent. As it approaches the uterovesical pouch the attachment is loose and this allows accommodation for filling of the bladder. From the uterovesical pouch, the peritoneum is reflected onto the uterus at the level of the isthmus. It covers the fundus and back of the uterus, the posterior aspect of the supravaginal cervix and the posterior vaginal fornix. It then passes backwards to cover the upper rectum and the posterior wall of the pelvis **(Fig. 13)**.

The small peritoneal pouch lying between the rectum and the posterior vaginal fornix and bounded laterally by the uterosacral ligaments is the rectovaginal pouch, or pouch of Douglas, or cul-de-sac. In practice, however, the *whole uterorectal pouch* (the space between the uterus and the broad ligaments in front and the rectum and pelvic wall behind), is often referred to as the pouch of Douglas. This pouch is protected from the exterior only by the vaginal wall and a layer of extraperitoneal fat and connective tissue. This arrangement offers opportunities for injury and infection of the peritoneal cavity by instruments such as douche nozzles inserted into the vagina; as well as easy access for diagnosis, for drainage of a pelvic abscess or haematoma, and for other operations.

Broad Ligament

Each broad ligament consists of a raised fold of peritoneum and subperitoneal fibromuscular tissue stretching across from the uterus to the side wall of the true pelvis.

It contains fallopian tubes, ovaries, ovarian arteries, uterine arteries, round ligament, infundibulopelvic ligaments and ovarian ligaments.

The fallopian tube is enclosed in its free upper edge and the mesentery of the ovary (mesovarium) is attached to its posterior leaf. The portion of the broad ligament which lies between the outer end (infundibulum) of the fallopian tube and the pelvic wall is the infundibulopelvic ligament; the part between the fallopian tube and level of the attachment of the ovary is the mesosalpinx.

The lower part of the broad ligament is wider from front to back than is the upper, the anterior leaf turning forwards into the uterovesical pouch while the posterior leaf continues downwards to a lower level before turning to form the uterorectal pouch. It contains loose cellular tissue and fat, endopelvic fascia condensed to form the cardinal ligaments, the terminal part of the ureter and the paracervical nerve and lymphatic plexuses **(Fig. 20)**.

The upper part of the broad ligament contains the fallopian tube and below this the ovarian vessels and

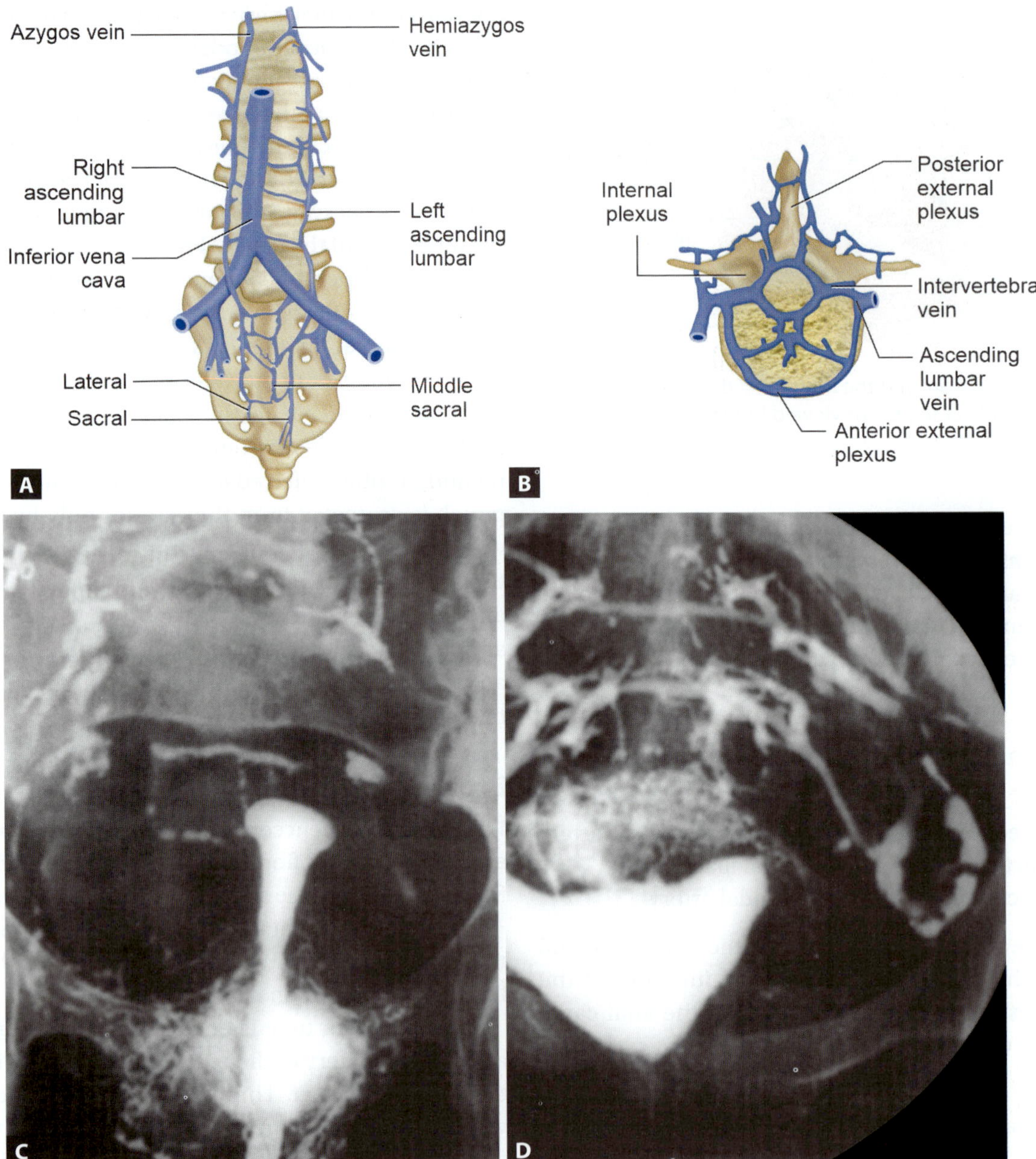

Figs. 32A to D: The vertebral venous plexus responsible for some return of blood from the pelvic organs. (A and B) Diagrammatic representations of the anatomy; (C) Intravasation at the level of the cervix during hysterography, with entry of the medium into the presacral venous plexus, the ascending lumbar and the intervertebral veins. Radiograph obtained in an apparently normal woman lying quietly; (D) Intravasation of the fundus with entry of the medium into veins which communicate with the presacral plexus.
Source: Figure 32A, B and C with permission from the Editor, J Obstet Gynaecol Br Emp.

nerves which enter the infundibulopelvic ligament to reach the mesovarium. Also lying in the mesosalpinx are the vestigial Gärtner's duct, paroophoron, epoophoron (organ of Rosenmuller), Kobelt's tubules and the hydatid of Morgagni **(Figs. 14 and 20)**. Gärtner's duct runs inwards below the fallopian tube until it approaches the uterus when it turns downwards to lie anterolateral to the uterus, cervix and vagina, ultimately disappearing near the lower end of the vagina or in the region of the external urethral meatus.

Three other paired ligaments closely associated with the broad ligament are described separately.

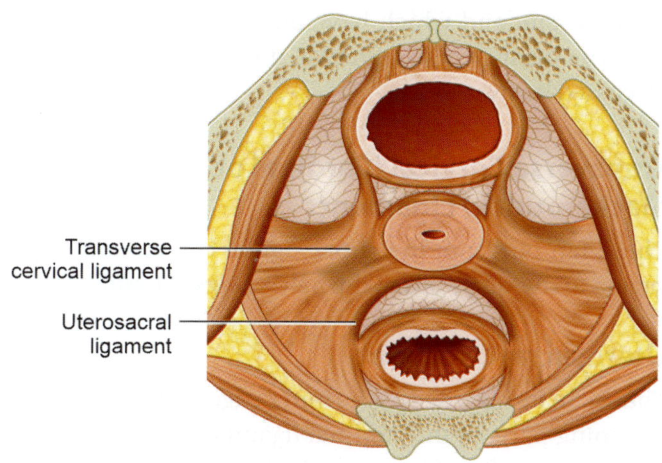

Fig. 33: The main supporting ligaments of the uterus viewed from above.

Round Ligament

The round ligament is a fibromuscular cord of varying strength and thickness, which raises a peritoneal fold on the front of each broad ligament. It extends from the cornu of the uterus to the internal abdominal ring through which it enters the inguinal canal to be inserted in the subcutaneous tissue of the foreparts of the labium majus.

The round ligament is weakly contractile at all times in the mature woman, but especially in late pregnancy and the puerperium.

Ovarian Ligament

The ovarian ligament is a cord-like fibromuscular structure, which links the inner pole of the ovary to the cornu of the uterus **(Fig. 14)**. It lies on the posterior leaf of the broad ligament but is embryologically continuous with the round ligament. These two ligaments are the homologues of the gubernaculum testis.

Uterosacral Ligament

Each uterosacral ligament represents a condensation of endopelvic fascia to form a band, which passes backwards beside the rectum from the supravaginal cervix to the sacrum **(Fig. 33)**. It contains cellular tissue and is also rich in nerves which use it as a route from the pelvic plexus to the pelvic viscera.

PELVIC MUSCULATURE

The *pelvic floor* consists of all tissues lying between the pelvic cavity and the surface of the vulva and perineum.

It includes the pelvic peritoneum, extraperitoneal fat and cellular tissue, the levator ani and their fascial coats, the urogenital diaphragm (triangular ligament), the muscles of the perineum and their aponeuroses, subcutaneous fascia and fat, and finally the skin. The most important of these structures are the levator ani muscles, which together with the fascia covering their upper and lower surfaces, are collectively called the pelvic diaphragm. Sometimes the term pelvic floor is inaccurately used to mean only the perineum and the muscle underlying it: hence the 'pelvic floor repair' operation.

Levator Ani

The levator ani is a broad sheet of muscle, which stretches from the back of the body of the pubis to the sacrum and coccyx and to the anococcygeal raphe, one on each side **(Fig. 31)**. It is attached laterally to the fascia over the obturator internus (at the 'white line') and to the ischial spine. It sweeps downwards and inwards to meet its fellow from the opposite side and to form a diaphragm which is not complete in that the urethra, vagina and rectum pass through it. Some of its inner fibres are inserted into the vagina and rectum, but not into the bladder and urethra as is sometimes stated. The fascia covering it fuses with vaginal and rectal fascia. Although the muscle functions as a whole, it is divided into three parts, as given below.

Pubococcygeus

This is the inner and main part of the muscle sheet and is slung from the pubis to the coccyx. Some fibres are inserted into the vaginal and rectal walls and these are sometimes separately defined as pubovaginalis and puborectalis muscles. It is also inserted into the perineal body which it supports.

Iliococcygeus

This extends from the 'white line' of fascia of obturator internus muscle to the sacrum, coccyx, anococcygeal raphe and perineal body.

Ischiococcygeus (Coccygeus)

This is the portion arising from the ischial spine and inserted into the sacrum and coccyx. Together with the iliococcygeus it forms a sloping roof to the ischiorectal fossa **(Fig. 11)**.

Pelvic Part of Piriformis Muscle

This is sometimes regarded as part of the levator ani; at least it functions with it.

The levator ani is a voluntary muscle supplied by branches of the pudendal nerve, and possibly by fibres coming directly from S3 and S4 roots. It is relaxed during evacuation of the bladder and bowel, which is during a bearing-down effort, but is contracted when the pelvic floor is lifted at the conclusion of such efforts. It is also contracted as part of a protective mechanism during coughing or other sudden strains which increase intra-abdominal pressure.

Perineal Muscles and Triangular Ligament

At a lower level in the pelvis is the urogenital diaphragm as described earlier (triangular ligament) with its two layers stretching between and attached to the inferior pubic rami **(Fig. 2)**. It is pierced by the dorsal vein of the clitoris, which joins the retropubic urethrovesical plexus, by the urethra and by the vagina. Between its fascial layers lie the compressor urethrae and the deep transverse perineal muscles; also branches of the internal pudendal vessels and the pudendal nerve. The deep transverse perineal muscle arises from the ramus of the ischium and is inserted partly into the side walls of the vagina and partly into the perineal body. On the under surface of the urogenital diaphragm are the vestibular bulb and Bartholin's gland, and immediately superficial to these are the sphincter vaginae (bulbospongiosus), ischiocavernosus and superficial transverse perineal muscles. Then comes the superficial fascia and skin.

The perineal body (central tendon of the perineum) includes the insertions of the anterior fibres of the levator ani, transverse perineal (superficial and deep), sphincter vaginae and external sphincter ani muscles.

PELVIC FASCIA AND CELLULAR TISSUE

All the spaces between organs and between muscles in the pelvis are filled with areolar tissue and with fat which is continuous with the extraperitoneal fat on the abdominal wall. These tissues are especially noticeable in the bases of the broad ligaments (parametrium), beneath the uterovesical pouch, in the uterosacral ligaments and around the upper vagina (*paracolpos*).

In certain places, and especially around blood vessels and nerves, connective tissue is condensed to form *fascial* ligaments, which contain some involuntary muscle and elastic tissue and which have an important supporting role. The most clearly defined of these condensations are discussed below.

Transverse Cervical (Cardinal or Mackenrodt's) Ligaments

These fan out from the supravaginal cervix, and upper vagina to the side walls of the pelvis **(Figs. 11 and 33)**.

Uterosacral Ligament

These can be regarded as the inner edges of the backward-sweeping parts of the cardinal ligaments **(Fig. 33)**. They consist of two firm fibromuscular bands passing from the cervix and upper end of the vagina to the lower end of the sacrum. They form two ridges, one on either side of the pouch of Douglas.

Pubocervical Fascia

This extends from the supravaginal cervix (where it fuses with the cardinal ligaments) down the anterior vaginal wall beneath the base of the bladder. It splits around the urethra and turns forwards to be inserted into the body of the pubis and the upper layer of the triangular ligament.

All the pelvic muscles have aponeuroses on both aspects and these too are designated fascia, as are the connective tissue sheaths of the vagina, bladder and rectum. These and the fascial ligaments mentioned above are directly continuous wherever they come in contact **(Figs. 11 and 33)**.

The specially named fascial layers and ligaments described above are best regarded as part of a continuous connective tissue framework, collectively known as endopelvic fascia, which extends throughout the pelvis. Their demonstration at operations is often the result of artificial dissection; indeed, it has been suggested that the pubocervical fascia cannot be identified unless it is hypertrophied as a result of the stress imposed by prolapse of the anterior vaginal wall.

THE SUPPORTS OF THE GENITAL ORGANS

Uterus

The uterus is held in a position of anteflexion and anteversion by its weight, by the round ligaments which hold the fundus forwards, and by the uterosacral ligaments which keep the supravaginal cervix far back in the pelvis. To appreciate these actions, it is necessary to envisage the uterus rotating around an axis situated at the level of the internal os. The broad ligaments and their cellular tissue also have a steadying effect on the uterus.

The round and broad ligaments do not, however, have any significant action in preventing descent of the uterus.

Anteflexion function is performed almost entirely by the transverse cervical ligaments and their posterior extensions—the uterosacral ligaments. Individual strands of these ligaments are likened to the spokes of a bicycle wheel. Each is weak, but together they form a strong mechanism. These are inserted not only in the supravaginal cervix but also into the upper vagina, and their support of the vaginal vault is also important in preventing uterine prolapse.

Vagina

The vagina is supported in its upper part by the lower components of the transverse cervical ligaments which fuse with its fascial sheath. Below this it is held by the fibres of the levator ani which are inserted into its side walls, by the urogenital diaphragm, and by the perineal muscles. The anterior vaginal wall, urethra and bladder base are supported by the pubocervical fascia and also, it is said, by the posterior vaginal wall and perineal body on which they rest when the woman is standing. The posterior vaginal wall rests on the rectovaginal fascia and perineal body. The perineal body supports the vaginal walls where the pelvic diaphragm offers an elastic foundation to which the important inelastic ligaments are attached.

However, by themselves the perineum and the levator muscles are insignificant as supporting structures. This fact can be demonstrated at operation. If they are divided, there is no effect on the downward mobility of the uterus. Moreover, complete disruption of the perineum in childbirth, with consequent divarication of the levator ani, usually does not result in the later development of either uterine or vaginal prolapse nor even rectocele. This clinical observation was made many centuries ago. Occasionally, disruption of the perineal body leads to a situation where contraction of the levator ani widens the hiatus rather than tightening it. Such patients may even develop cystocele and, in extreme cases, may have prolapse of the uterus and rectum as well.

The idea that the vagina is supported by the perineum and the uterus by the vagina still lingers in the minds of gynaecologists and explains why so many take the view that no operation for any type of genital prolapse is complete unless perineorrhaphy be included, and that vaginal hysterectomy must always be followed by tightening of the posterior vaginal wall and perineum to avoid subsequent vault prolapse. In fact, the avoidance of posterior colpoperineorrhaphy in those who have no evidence of vaginal or perineal body descent generally has no untoward effects and has many advantages.

BLOOD VESSELS OF THE PELVIS

The pelvic vasculature is a high-volume, high-flow system with enormous expansive capabilities throughout reproductive life. Blood flow through the uterine arteries increases to about 500 mL/minute in late pregnancy. In nonpregnant women, certain conditions, such as uterine fibroids or malignant neoplasms, may be associated with neovascularisation and hypertrophy of existing vessels and a corresponding increase in pelvic blood flow. It is necessary to understand the system of blood flow since a knowledge of the volume and flow characteristics of the pelvic vasculature in different clinical situations will enable the surgeon to anticipate problems and take appropriate preoperative and intraoperative measures (including blood and blood product availability) to prevent or manage haemorrhage. The collaterals in the pelvis are extensive.

The pelvic vasculature is supplied with an extensive network of collateral connections that provides a rich anastomotic communication between different major vessel systems. This degree of redundancy is important to ensure an adequate supply of oxygen and nutrients in the event of major trauma or other vascular compromise. Hypogastric artery ligation continues to be used as a strategy for management of massive pelvic haemorrhage when other measures have failed. Bilateral hypogastric artery ligation, particularly when combined with ovarian artery ligation, dramatically reduces pulse pressure in the pelvis, converting flow characteristics from that of an arterial system to a venous system and allowing the use of collateral channels of circulation to continue blood supply to pelvic structures. The significance of collateral blood flow is demonstrated by reports of successful pregnancies occurring after bilateral ligation of both hypogastric and ovarian arteries.

Arteries

Ovarian Artery

The ovarian artery branches from the aorta at approximately the same level as the renal artery. It runs

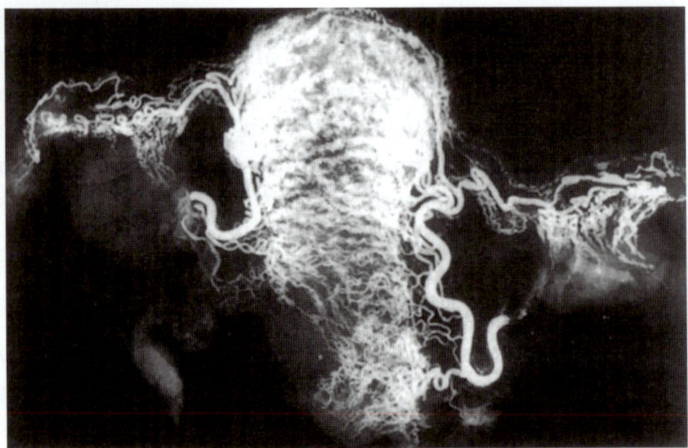

Fig. 34: A radiograph of the uterus and ovaries, showing the uterine arteries injected with radio-opaque material. The right uterine artery was damaged and displaced during hysterectomy, but the descending cervical branch is well seen on the left side. Note the characteristic spiral shape of the coronary arteries in the myometrium and of the arterioles in the ovary. The ovarian arteries were not injected and the radiograph indicates the free anastomosis between the uterine and ovarian vessels. This component of the blood supply can be diminished after panhysterectomy and explains the early cessation of menstrual function in some of these women.

downwards and laterally retroperitoneally, and crosses the ureter to reach the brim of the pelvis where it enters the infundibulopelvic ligament **(Fig. 30)**. Here it divides to send main branches to the ovary through the mesovarium. These, together with their tributaries within the ovary, are coiled **(Figs. 24 and 34)**.

One branch, if not the continuation of the parent trunk, runs towards the cornu of the uterus lying parallel to and just below the fallopian tube, and makes an end-to-end anastomosis with the terminal part of the uterine artery. There is thus a continuous arterial arch, and it is impossible to define the limits of the ovarian and uterine contributions. From the arch in the mesosalpinx, vessels run off to supply the round ligament and tube.

The anastomosis is so free that fluid injected into the uterine artery alone passes easily into the vessels within the substance of the ovary **(Fig. 34)**. On embryological grounds, it is reasonable to suppose that the tube is supplied by the uterine artery. In fact, it can be equally well maintained by the ovarian vessels.

Common Iliac Artery

The two common iliac arteries **(Fig. 30)** result from the terminal bifurcation of the aorta on the left side of the fourth lumbar vertebra. Each runs downwards and outwards for a distance of 4 or 5 cm (depending on the side) before dividing into the external and internal iliac arteries. At the point of division, the ureter lies in front and the sacroiliac joint behind.

Behind the right common iliac artery are the terminations of the two common iliac veins and the lowermost part of the inferior vena cava. The right common iliac vein lies to its outer side at a lower level.

The artery on the left side has the superior rectal (haemorrhoidal) artery as an anterior relation; the left common iliac vein is partly behind and partly medial to it.

External Iliac Artery

The external iliac artery **(Fig. 30)** runs downwards and outwards from the common iliac artery towards the thigh and, on passing under the inguinal ligament, becomes the femoral artery. It lies at the brim of the pelvis, on the medial border of the psoas muscle, and immediately beneath the peritoneum. Numerous lymphatic vessels and nodes are associated with it. Its main branches are the inferior (deep) epigastric and deep circumflex iliac arteries.

The anterior relations are the ovarian vessels and the round ligament. The external iliac vein lies behind the artery in its upper part but becomes medial at a lower level. As the external iliac artery becomes the femoral artery, the femoral nerve lies on its outer, and the femoral vein on its inner side.

Internal Iliac Artery

The internal iliac artery **(Fig. 30)** arises from the bifurcation of the common iliac artery and, in the foetus, is the umbilical (hypogastric) artery. After birth, all except some of the pelvic portion becomes obliterated.

From its origin, the internal iliac artery descends into the pelvis as far as the greater sciatic foramen where it divides into anterior and posterior trunks. The ureter runs down its front of the internal iliac artery and, behind it, are the internal iliac vein(s), the lumbosacral nerve trunk and the pyriformis muscle. On its outer side is the external iliac vein and, lower down, the obturator nerve.

The posterior division passes through the foramen to supply the muscles of the buttock. The anterior division supplies the internal pelvic organs and terminates as the internal pudendal artery (see further).

The branches of the *anterior* division of the internal iliac artery are the following arteries: Obturator, umbilical (remnant of foetal umbilical artery), superior vesical; inferior vesical; middle rectal; uterine; vaginal; internal pudendal and inferior gluteal (sciatic). The last two are its terminal branches.

The branches of the posterior division are the iliolumbar artery, the lateral sacral arteries and the superior gluteal artery.

Ligation of the internal iliac artery is often resorted to in the management of postpartum haemorrhage. Physiologically active anastomoses develop soon after between the systemic and pelvic arteries, leading to the formation of a collateral circulation. The iliolumbar, lateral sacral and middle rectal arteries anastomose with the lumbar, middle sacral and superior rectal arteries, respectively (the lumbar and middle sacral arteries arise from the aorta and the superior rectal artery arises from the inferior mesenteric artery). The correct point for internal iliac ligation is, therefore, not immediately after the bifurcation of the common iliac, but immediately below the last branch of the posterior division. This point also preserves and bypasses the anastomosis of the superior gluteal artery and profunda femoris which may be vital to the survival of the leg where the external iliac artery has been damaged by disease or become spastic consequent to operative manipulation.

Uterine Artery

The uterine artery arises from the anterior division of the internal iliac artery, either directly or as a branch of the superior vesical artery, the distal part of which is obliterated in the adult. It runs forwards and inwards in the base of the broad ligament, crossing above and almost at right angles to the ureter, and approaches the uterus at the level of the internal os **(Fig. 20)**. Here it gives off a descending branch to supply the lower cervix, and a circular branch (the circular artery of the cervix) from which arise the anterior and posterior azygos arteries to the vagina. There are also subsidiary branches to the lower end of the ureter, to the bladder and the vagina. The main trunk is coiled and tortuous and turns upwards beside the uterus. It supplies the uterus at all levels and ends by anastomosing with the ovarian artery to form a continuous arterial arch **(Fig. 34)**.

The main branches to the uterus each divide into anterior and posterior arcuate arteries, which are disposed circumferentially in the myometrium and anastomose with those from the opposite side **(Fig. 34)**. The uterus is therefore least vascular in the middle line, which becomes the natural site for an incision.

The arcuate arteries give off serosal branches and radial arteries, which penetrate the myometrium to end as basal arteries, which supply the endometrium. Arcuate and radial arteries are also coiled and the purpose of this is to reduce arterial pressure without reducing the flow, an important matter in pregnancy. The coiling of the main uterine artery may have a similar purpose although it is also suggested that this is to allow lengthening and accommodation of the vessel to the enlarging uterus during pregnancy.

Vaginal Artery

The vaginal artery is usually a separate branch (or branches) of the internal iliac artery but may come off the first part of the uterine artery. It passes forwards and inwards low in the broad ligament to reach the lateral vaginal fornix. In the vaginal wall, it anastomoses with the azygos branches of the circular artery of the cervix. The lower vagina is supplied from the middle and inferior rectal vessels and by branches from the internal pudendal artery.

Internal Pudendal Artery

The internal pudendal artery is the terminal branch of the internal iliac artery, it exits pelvis through the greater sciatic notch, curls round the ischial spine and returns to the lateral wall of the ischiorectal fossa through the lesser sciatic notch. At this point, it lies 4 cm above the ischial tuberosity. Together with the pudendal nerve, it runs forward in Alcock's canal under the lee of the inferior pubic ramus and then enters between the layers of the triangular ligament to give branches to the labia, vagina, bulbs of the vestibule, perineum and various muscles. It ends as the dorsal artery of the clitoris **(Fig. 35)**.

Superficial and Deep External Pudendal Arteries

These are branches of the femoral artery which come off just below the inguinal ligament and turn inwards to supply the foreparts of the vulva.

Veins

The veins of the pelvis normally accompany the arteries and have the same names. Sometimes there are two veins to one artery, not an uncommon finding in the case of the uterine and internal iliac vessels. In the broad ligament near the mesovarium, there is a pampiniform plexus of veins which drains into the ovarian and uterine trunks. It is

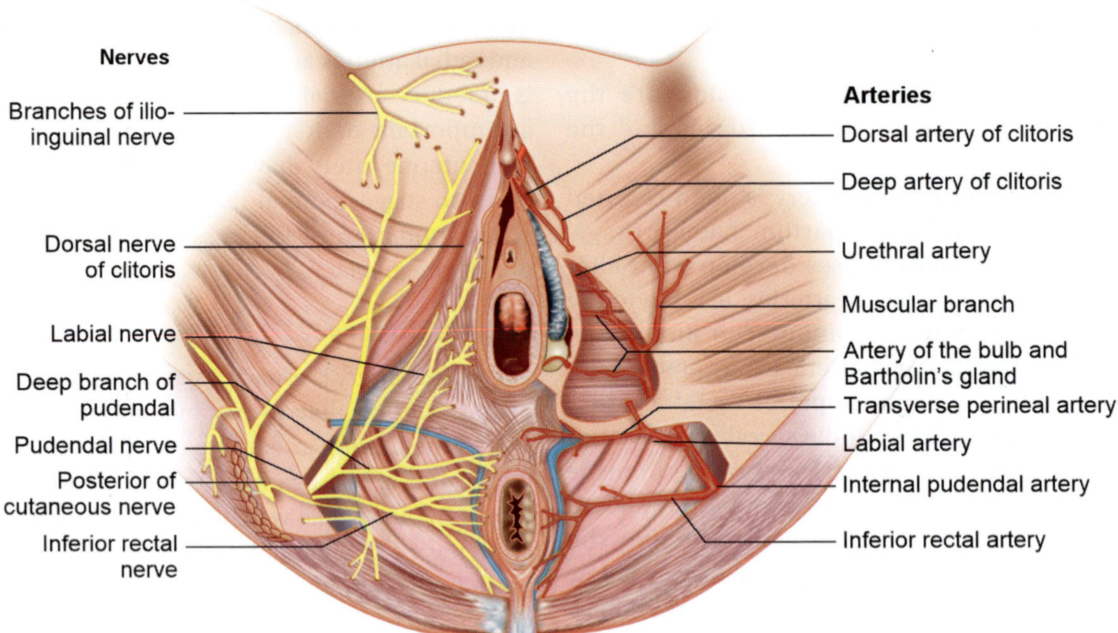

Fig. 35: The blood vessels and nerves of the vulva and perineum.

this plexus which sometimes becomes varicose and gives rise to a pelvic. The uterine veins also communicate with the vaginal or broad ligament varicocele. The right ovarian vein joins the inferior vena cava, but the left usually drains into the left renal vein.

There are plexuses of veins around the vagina, the urethrovesical junction and the anorectal junction, and all ultimately drain into the internal iliac veins. The venous return from the rectum and pelvic colon enters the portal system by way of the inferior mesenteric vein.

The uterine vein also communicates with the vaginal plexuses and this accounts for vaginal metastases in cancer of the body of the uterus. The vessels of the bulb and clitoris link with the vesical and vaginal plexuses.

The pelvic plexuses and veins also have communications with the presacral and lumbar channels of the vertebral plexus, and in this way, it is possible for blood, tissue cells, emboli and organisms to travel to remote parts of the body without passing through the heart and lungs **(Figs. 32 and 36)**. This is probably the explanation for the occurrence of metastatic growths in the spine and brain when the primary is in the uterus.

This collateral pathway is especially important in late pregnancy when the large uterus always obstructs the inferior vena cava of the woman lying on her back. It is mainly when this alternative venous return route is inadequate that she suffers the supine hypotension, or vena caval syndrome.

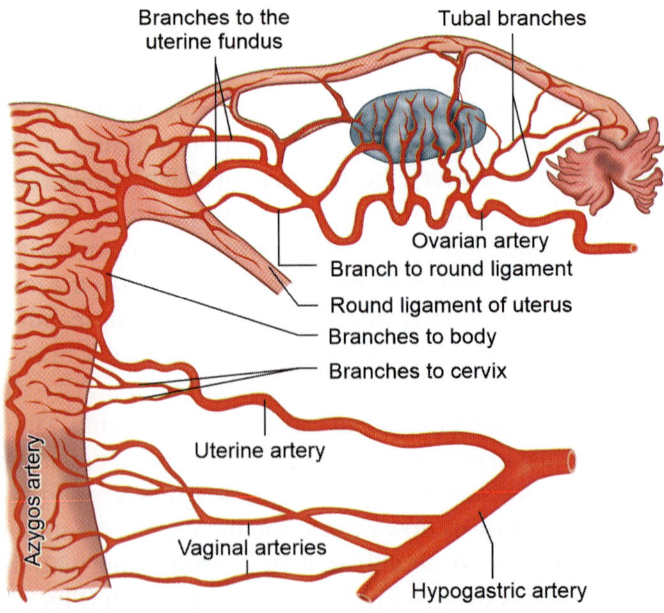

Fig. 36: Blood supply of the internal genital organs.

LYMPHATIC DRAINAGE

The pelvic lymph nodes are generally arranged in groups or chains and follow the course of the larger pelvic vessels for which they are usually named. Smaller nodes that lie close to the visceral structures are usually named for those organs. Lymph nodes in the pelvis receive afferent lymphatic vessels from pelvic and perineal visceral and parietal structures and send efferent lymphatics to more proximal nodal groups. The number of lymph nodes and their exact location is variable; however, certain nodes tend to be relatively constant:

- Obturator node in the obturator foramen, close to the obturator vessels and nerve.
- Nodes at the junction of the internal and external iliac veins.
- Ureteral node in the broad ligament near the cervix, where the uterine artery crosses over the ureter.
- The Cloquet or Rosenmüller node—the highest of the deep inguinal nodes that lies within the opening of the femoral canal.

Vulva and Perineum

The lymphatics of the vulva pass forwards to the mons veneris and the subcutaneous tissues of the lower abdominal wall to enter the medial group of the superficial inguinal nodes. These connect with the deep inguinal (femoral) groups from which lymphatics pass to the external, and ultimately to the common iliac lymph nodes **(Fig. 30)**. The deep femoral node of Cloquet, which lies beneath the inner end of the inguinal ligament, is said to drain the clitoris directly, thus accounting for carcinoma of the clitoris supposedly having a poor prognosis; but this is probably not true.

Lymphatics from the deep tissues of the vulva accompany the internal pudendal vessels to the internal iliac nodes.

Vagina

The lower vagina drains to the inguinal and femoral nodes in the same way as the vulva. The drainage of the middle and upper vagina is the same as that of the cervix.

Cervix

Lymphatics from the cervix run in the uterosacral ligaments and the cellular tissue beneath these to the obturator, external and internal iliac and sacral nodes. There is a plexus of lymphatic vessels, and rarely one node, in the broad ligament beside the cervix. The internal and external iliac nodes communicate with those around the common iliac vessels and ultimately with the para-aortic groups **(Fig. 30)**.

Corpus Uteri

The lower part of the body of the uterus has the same lymphatic connections as the cervix. The fundus has an additional drainage by lymphatics which accompany the ovarian vessels, and by others which accompany the round ligament to the abdominal wall and thence to the superficial inguinal nodes.

Fallopian Tube and Ovary

The tube drains in part with the fundus of the uterus but mainly with the ovary. Lymphatics from the ovary accompany the ovarian vessels to reach the aortic nodes **(Fig. 30)**. They are said to communicate with those from the opposite gonad by crossing the fundus uteri; this is doubtful but is put forwards as one explanation of the tendency for ovarian cancer to be bilateral.

Urethra and Bladder

The external urethral meatus drains with the vulva to the inguinal nodes. The remainder of the urethra, together with the bladder, has lymph vessels which go to the external, internal and common iliac nodes.

Sigmoid Colon

From this organ, lymphatics accompany the inferior mesenteric vessels to the preaortic nodes.

Anus and Rectum

The anal orifice drains to the superficial inguinal nodes; the anal canal to the internal iliac (along with the internal pudendal vessels). The lower rectum also drains to the internal inguinal nodes, the lymph channels accompanying the inferior rectal and internal pudendal vessels. That of the upper rectum is to the preaortic nodes, the lymph channels being associated with the superior rectal vessels.

INNERVATION OF PELVIC ORGANS

Somatic Nerves

The skin of the mons veneris and the foreparts of the vulva are supplied by the ilioinguinal nerve and the genital branch of the genitofemoral nerve, both arising from the L1 and L2 roots of the lumbar plexus.

The outer parts of the labia posteriorly and the perineum receive some sensory fibres from the perineal branch of the posterior cutaneous nerve of the thigh **(Fig. 35)**.

The main somatic supply to the pelvic organs is, however, the *pudendal nerve,* which is both motor and sensory and is formed from the S2, S3 and S4 roots of the sacral plexus. This leaves the pelvis through the greater sciatic notch, curls round the ischial spine and, in company with the internal pudendal vessels, re-enters through the lesser sciatic notch to lie on the outer wall of the ischiorectal fossa in Alcock's canal. Its branches run forwards and inwards between the two layers of the triangular ligament.

The pudendal nerve supplies sensory fibres to the skin of the vulva, external urethral meatus, clitoris, perineum and the *lower* vagina. It provides motor fibres to all the voluntary muscles, including the compressor urethrae, sphincter vaginae, levator ani and external anal sphincter. Pudendal block **(Fig. 37)** is carried out by injecting a local anaesthetic solution around the nerve as it circles the ischial spine and comes to lie on the medial aspect of the inferior pubic ramus. In order to obtain complete anaesthesia of the vulva, the other cutaneous nerves require to be injected. Relaxation of the levator ani needs direct injection of the muscle and its fascial coats, probably because the muscle is partly innervated from above by fibres arising directly from the S3 and S4 roots.

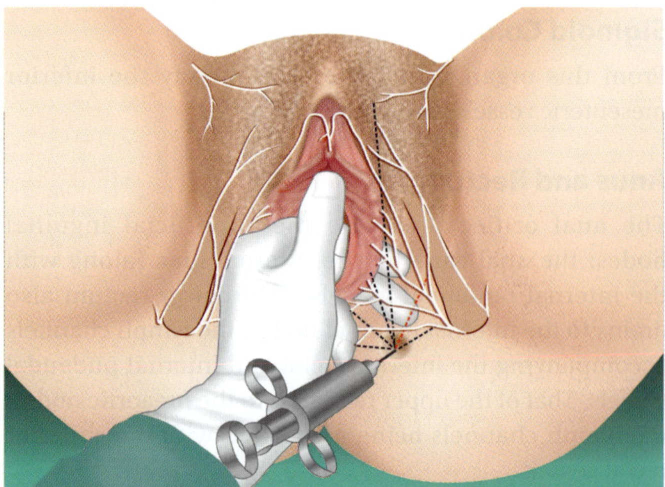

Fig. 37: The surface anatomy of pudendal block and local vulvar anaesthesia. Some surgeons prefer to inject the pudendal nerves by a direct approach through the side walls of the vagina; a specially devised and guarded needle is available for this technique.
Source: With permission from the Editor, BMJ.

Pudendal block anaesthesia carries a slight but definite risk of injury to the internal pudendal vessels with consequent haematoma formation. In obstetric practice, it is rarely necessary since local infiltration of the perineum, the adjacent vaginal wall and the levator ani muscles suffices for all except the more difficult operations.

The skin of the vulva is very sensitive and perineal injuries are especially painful. The discomfort which results from perineorrhaphy or episiotomy, however, is mostly due to spasm in the underlying muscles.

Except in its lower part, the vagina is remarkably insensitive to ordinary stimuli. Diseases such as vaginitis, ulcers, cancer and injuries, including burns, do not cause pain. Vaginal surgery can be carried out with minimal infiltration of local anaesthetic, provided the perineum and introitus are avoided. This insensitivity is explained by the fact that most of the vagina is supplied by autonomic and not somatic nerves given in the diagram below.

Autonomic Nerves

All the internal organs of reproduction, including the upper vagina, together with the urinary apparatus, rectum and colon, have only an autonomic innervation. The blood vessels are controlled by their own intrinsic nerves; what follows concerns other tissues. The autonomic nerves to these carry both sensory and motor fibres, adrenergic and cholinergic.

Sympathetic

Sympathetic nerves, arising from segments T5 and T6 in the case of motor nerves and from segments T10 to L1 in the case of sensory nerves, pass down from the coeliac plexus through the intermesenteric plexus, lying retroperitoneally on the front of the abdominal aorta. Over the bifurcation of the aorta and the promontory of the sacrum is a complicated network lying just beneath the peritoneum; this is called the superior hypogastric plexus or presacral nerve **(Fig. 38B)**. From this, two main chains (hypogastric nerves) run outwards and downwards, one on each side wall of the pelvis. These join the pelvic (inferior hypogastric) plexuses which lie on either side of the ampulla of the rectum extending forwards beneath the uterosacral and broad ligaments. The forward extension of the pelvic plexus is often called the Lee-Frankenhäuser plexus.

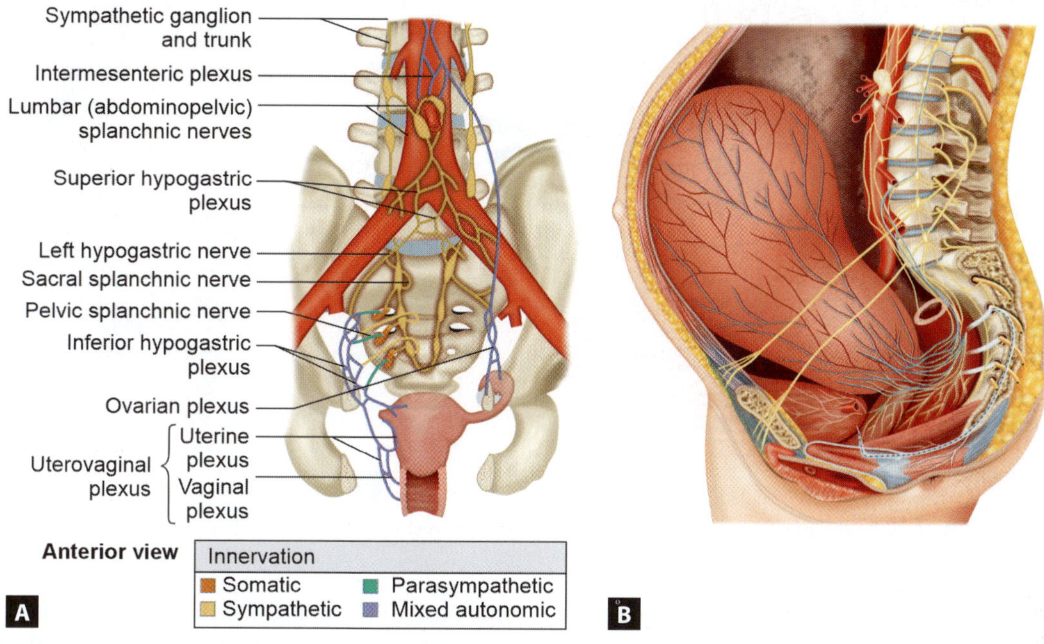

Figs. 38A and B: The autonomic innervation of the internal genitalia. (A) Nerves to the tubes and ovaries travel with the ovarian vessels directly from the preaortic plexuses; (B) The uterus and upper vagina is supplied from the hypogastric plexus which is composed of fibres from the superior hypogastric plexus (presacral nerves) together with a contribution from S2, S3 and S4 nerve roots.

Parasympathetic

The pelvic plexus also receives important motor and sensory fibres from S2, S3 and S4 nerve roots. Amongst other functions, they probably carry sensation from the cervix and lower uterus and thus mediate the low backache which is sometimes a feature of lesions in these organs.

With the exception of the fallopian tube and ovary, the pelvic plexuses supply sympathetic and parasympathetic nerves to all the pelvic organs, including the bladder and bowel. Those to the cervix and uterus pass through the paracervical ganglia in the bases of the broad ligaments.

The fundus of the uterus probably receives additional twigs from nerves which accompany the ovarian vessels **(Figs. 39A and B)**.

Sympathetic nerves of the uterus are sensory and possibly motor but their functions are not well understood; and there is doubt whether the uterus, except in its lower part, receives parasympathetic nerves. A motor function for such nerves, and an inhibitory action by sympathetic nerves, although often postulated, has not been demonstrated in the human being. Stimulation of the autonomic system produces uterine responses which vary from animal to animal.

In women, division of all uterine nerves, or of the spinal cord at very high levels, does not appear to affect myometrial contractility, not even in labour. Moreover, presacral neurectomy alone does not abolish the pain of labour, even though it may sometimes improve dysmenorrhoea. To remove all sensation from the uterus and other pelvic organs, it is necessary to divide every nervous connection (including the parasympathetic) or to block the spinal pathway above the level of T10.

The cervix and body of the uterus are relatively insensitive to touching, cutting and burning and can be operated on without any form of anaesthesia. Abdominal hysterotomy, e.g. can be performed under local infiltration anaesthesia of the abdominal wall alone; cauterisation of the external aspect of the cervix of the conscious woman causes little discomfort. The application of a vulsellum to the cervix sometimes causes a momentary stab of pain; touching the internal os with a sound and scratching the endometrium with a curette also cause fleeting discomfort. When the cervix is unusually sensitive, it often betokens chronic cervicitis with associated parametritis.

Despite what is said above, touching the cervix or the introduction of an instrument into its canal, especially in a woman under emotional tension, can cause severe vasovagal collapse. Sudden death from this cause is a remote but real possibility.

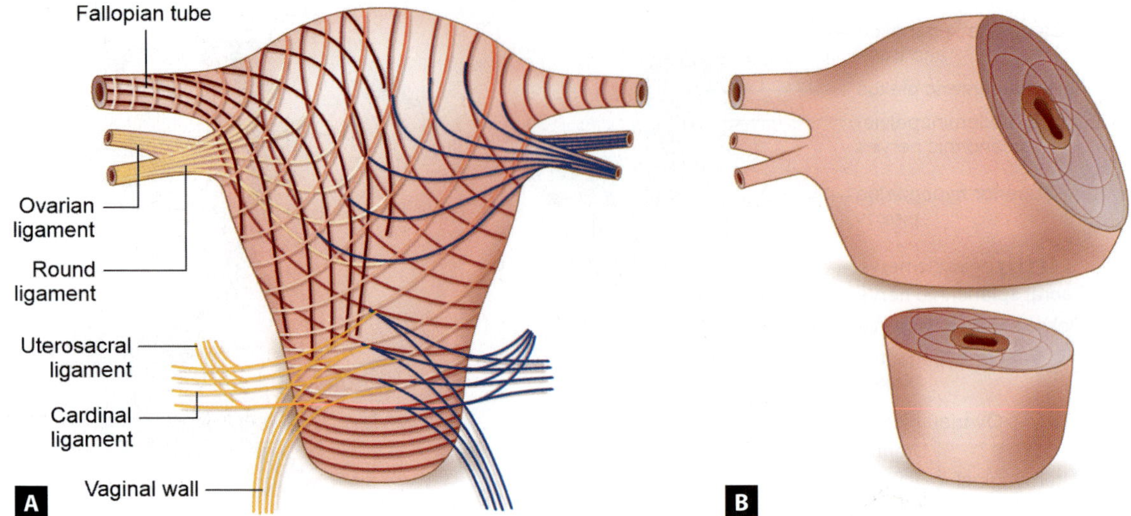

Figs. 39A and B: (A) Scheme of uterine musculature; (B) Diagram to show how spiral fibres into wall and interface.

Distension of the uterus or dilatation of the cervical canal causes intense colicky pain or a sickening deep-seated ache in the hypogastrium, iliac fossae and the sacral area.

The bladder is also innervated from the pelvic plexus. Motor parasympathetic nerves are responsible for the contraction of the detrusor muscle. It is doubtful whether there is a sympathetic motor supply, if there is, its function is to inhibit the detrusor muscle and contract the sphincter mechanism of the urethrovesical junction. This is the hypothetical basis for the administration of ephedrine in the treatment of enuresis and other conditions in which bladder control is poor. Bladder sensation is conveyed mainly not only by sympathetic but also by the parasympathetic nerves **(Fig. 28)**.

Presacral neurectomy does not usually cause more than temporary disturbance of micturition, but blocking or sectioning of the nerve trunks leading from the pelvic plexus to the floor of the bladder abolishes or diminishes sensation and detrusor activity.

The urethra is under the same nervous control as the bladder, except for the voluntary external sphincter muscle which is motivated by branches of the pudendal nerve.

Fallopian Tubes and Ovaries

The fallopian tubes and ovaries are supplied by parasympathetic and sympathetic nerves which accompany the ovarian vessels and come directly from the preaortic plexuses **(Fig. 38A)**. They are both motor and sensory. The segmental supply is T10 or T11 for the ovary and T11 or T12 for the tube. Pain from the adnexa is usually referred to the lower abdominal wall on one or other side but can be central.

The ovary is insensitive except to squeezing on bimanual examination. The fallopian tube, however, is unlike other viscera in that it is sensitive to cutting, crushing and touching, as can be demonstrated during sterilisation operations carried out under local analgesia.

ACKNOWLEDGMENT

Thanks to Dr Apoorva Kanthaje for the histopathology images and Dr Harshith Kramadhari for the artwork.

SUGGESTED READING

1. Anson BJ (Ed). An atlas of Human Anatomy. Philadelphia: WB Saunders; 1950. p. 241.
2. Kumar P, Malhotra N (Eds). Jeffcoate's Principles of Gynaecology, 7th edition. New Delhi: Jaypee Brothers Medical Publishers (P) Ltd.; 2008.
3. Milloy FJ, Anson BJ, McAfee DK. The rectus abdominis muscle and the epigastric arteries. Surg Gynecol Obstet. 1960;110:293-302.
4. Moore KL, Dalley AF, Agur AMR (Eds). Clinically Oriented Anatomy, 6th edition. Philadelphia: Lippincott Williams & Wilkins; 2010.
5. Padubidri VG, Daftary SN (Eds). Shaw's Textbook of Gynaecology, 14th edition. New Delhi: Elsevier; 2008.
6. Rock JA, Jones HW (Eds). TeLinde's Operative Gynecology, 10th edition. Philadelphia: Lippincott Williams & Wilkins; 2008.
7. Snell RS (Ed). Clinical Anatomy by Regions, 8th edition. Philadelphia: Lippincott Williams & Wilkins; 2008.

3

CHAPTER

Ovarian Functions

Priya SP Patil, Muralidhar V Pai

Chapter Outline

- Production of Ova
- Ovarian Hormones
- Pituitary Hormones
- Pituitary–Hypothalamic Relations
- Pituitary–Ovarian Relations (Control of Ovulation)
- Hormone Levels and Assays

INTRODUCTION

Neuroendocrinology is a dynamic process, and it represents facets of two traditional fields of medicine: Endocrinology, which is the study of hormones (i.e. substances secreted into the bloodstream that have diverse actions at sites remote from the point of secretion), and neuroscience, which is the study of the action of neurons. It is interesting to know that the discovery of neurons that transmit impulses and secrete their products into the vascular system to function as hormones themselves, a process known as neurosecretion, demonstrates that the two systems are intimately linked. For instance, the menstrual cycle is regulated through the feedback of hormones on the neural tissue of the central nervous system (CNS). The hypothalamic neuron-derived factors influence the target organs directly through hormones or indirectly through hormone-releasing factors.

The phases of the ovarian cycle are characterised as follows:

- *Follicular phase:* Hormonal feedback promotes the orderly development of a single dominant follicle, which should be mature at mid-cycle and prepared for ovulation through the stages of the preantral, antral and preovulatory follicle **(Fig. 1)**. The average length of the human follicular phase ranges from 10 to 14 days, and variability in this length is responsible for most variations in total cycle length.
- *Ovulation:* The preovulatory follicle produces its own ovulatory stimulation by raising oestradiol levels. Luteinising hormone (LH) surge occurs through a unique neuroendocrine phenomenon along with ovarian factors. Ovulation occurs approximately 10–12 hours LH peak and 24–36 hours of the oestradiol peak.
- *Luteal phase:* Luteinisation of corpus luteum occurs due to the continued tonic LH secretion with optimum preovulatory follicular development. The time from ovulation to the onset of menses with an average length of 14 days.
- *Luteal–follicular transition:* Decline of oestradiol, progesterone and inhibin leads to regression of corpus luteum to corpus albicans. The interval extending from luteal decline to selection of the dominant follicle is marked by the onset of menses.

The extremes of reproductive life (after menarche and perimenopause) are characterised by a higher percentage of anovulatory or irregularly timed cycles.

At the beginning of each monthly menstrual cycle, levels of gonadal steroids are low and have been decreasing since the end of the luteal phase of the previous cycle.

With the demise of the corpus luteum, follicle-stimulating hormone (FSH) levels begin to rise and a cohort of growing follicles is recruited. These follicles each secrete increasing levels of oestrogen as they grow in the follicular phase. This, in turn, stimulates the uterine endometrial proliferation. With the rising oestrogen levels, the same provide negative feedback on pituitary FSH secretion, which begins to wane by the midpoint of the follicular phase. Conversely, LH initially decreases in response to rising oestradiol levels, but late in the follicular phase, the LH level is increased dramatically (biphasic response). At the end of the follicular phase (just prior to ovulation), FSH-induced LH receptors are present on granulosa cells and, with LH stimulation, modulate the secretion of progesterone. After a sufficient degree of oestrogenic stimulation, the pituitary LH surge is triggered, which is the proximate cause of ovulation that occurs approximately 36 hours later. Ovulation triggers

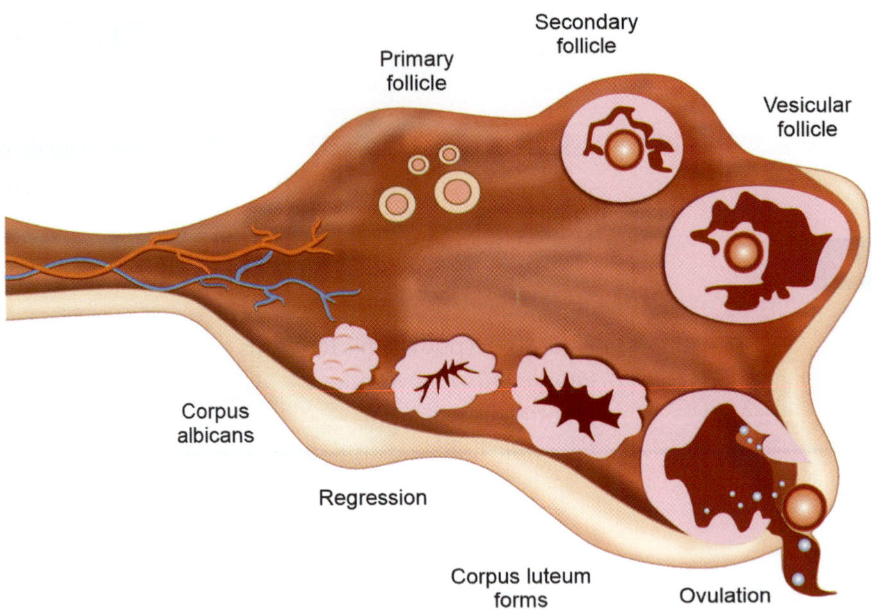

Fig. 1: Ovulation.

the transition to the luteal-secretory phase. The oestrogen level decreases through the early luteal phase from just before ovulation until the mid-luteal phase, when it begins to rise again as a result of corpus luteum secretion. Progesterone levels rise precipitously after ovulation and can be used as a presumptive sign that ovulation has occurred. Both oestrogen and progesterone levels remain elevated through the lifespan of the corpus luteum and then wane with its demise, thereby setting the stage for the next cycle.

The regulation of ovarian function occurs through autocrine, paracrine and endocrine mechanisms. The growth and differentiation of ovarian cells are particularly influenced by the insulin-like growth factors (IGFs). The IGF amplifies the actions of gonadotrophin hormones on autocrine and paracrine growth factors found in the ovary. IGF-2 is the principal growth factor found in follicular fluid, although other factors, including IGF-1, tumour necrosis factor-α (TNF-α), TNF-β and epidermal growth factor (EGF), also play important roles. Disruption of these autocrine and paracrine intraovarian pathways may be the basis of polycystic ovarian disease and disorders of ovulation.

The main compartment of the ovary is the follicle. Their quantity and health define the capacity for reproduction and length of reproductive life. The two ovaries function as one, and between them, one normally sheds only one ovum at a time. Moreover, they do not necessarily take it in turn to ovulate. If one ovary is removed, the other maintains a full function, ovulating every month according to Lipschutz's 'Law of Follicular Constancy', which was established at the beginning of the last century. The same is true of a portion of one ovary, but if the remaining fragment is very small, it may prove inadequate.

The ovaries have two functions: (1) The production of ova and (2) the production of hormones. The latter is secondary to the former and is present to a limited extent for a few years before regular ovulation is established and for some time after ovulation ceases. Both these functions are controlled through the hypothalamic-pituitary-ovarian axis by endocrine, paracrine and autocrine pathways.

PRODUCTION OF OVA

The primordial germ cells originate in the endoderm of the yolk sac, allantois and hindgut of the embryo and migrate to the genital ridge where the ovary is formed. Oogenesis **(Fig. 2)** begins in the ovary at 6–8 weeks' gestation. Mitotic division of the germ cells results in the formation of oogonia, which reaches a maximum number of 6–7 million oogonia in a 16–20-week-old foetus. By 11–12 weeks, the transformation of oogonia to oocytes has begun and there is a steady decline in the numbers. The oocytes enter the first meiotic phase and arrest in prophase.

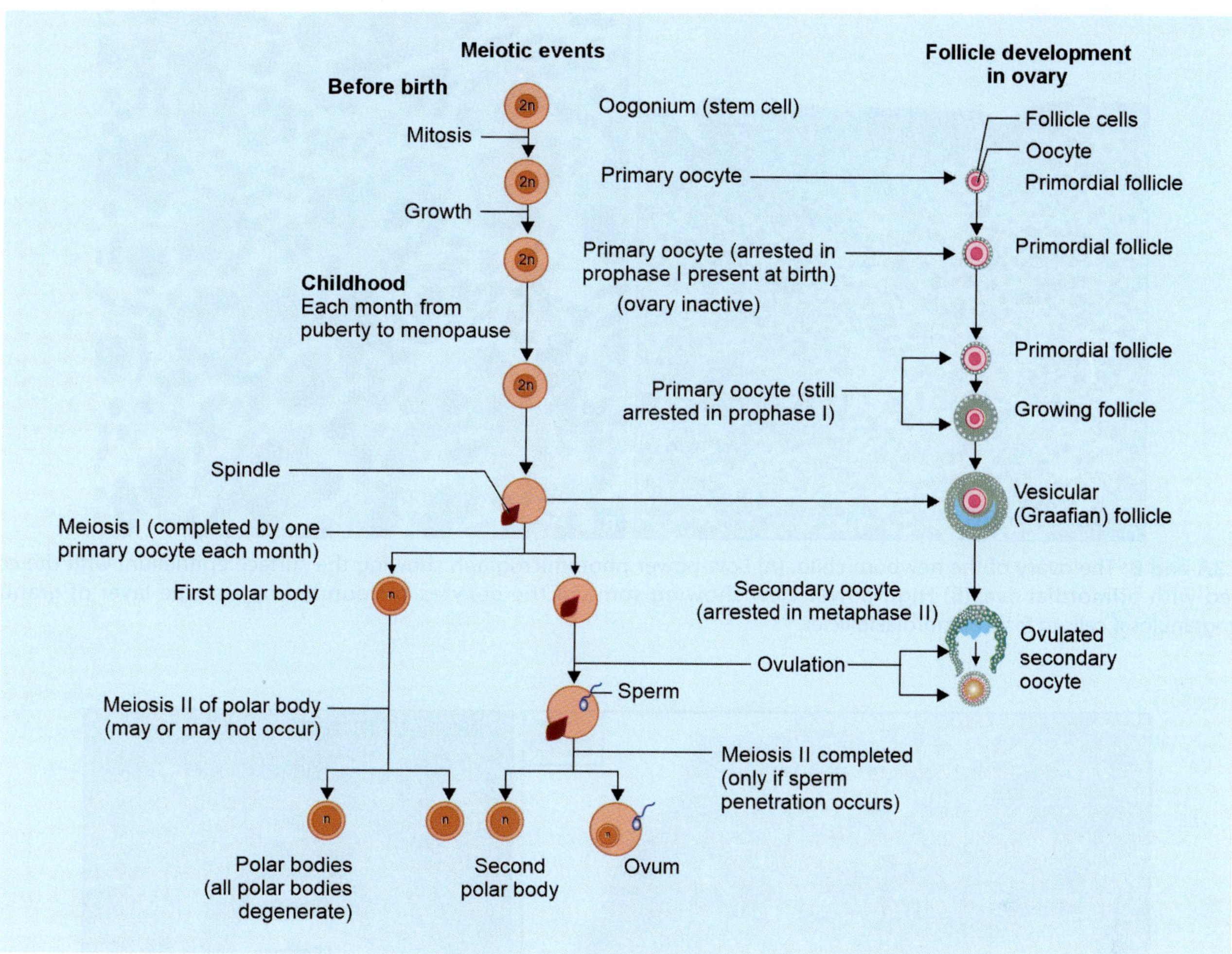

Fig. 2: Oogenesis.

The ovary of the female child at birth contains all the primary oocytes, which it will ever possess, and these are scattered amongst the mesenchymal stroma cells of the medulla and cortex **(Figs. 3A and B)**. The total content of both ovaries at birth is estimated at 2 million. It is further reduced during childhood so that at puberty the figure is about 300,000–500,000. Of these, not >500 are destined to mature during the individual's lifetime, and the remainder will be lost by some form of degenerative process. Each primordial follicle consists of an oocyte surrounded by a single layer of granulosa or pregranulosa cells, which are specially differentiated stromal cells. A number of follicles (which depends on the residual number of follicles in the ovary but is generally <12 in each ovary) may develop several layers of granulosa cells and even show some luteinisation and liquor folliculi formation during the weeks preceding birth. These changes probably reflect the action of placental gonadotrophin and they soon disappear in infancy, as do multiovular follicles and multinucleated ova also found in the foetus at term. The occasional persistence of multiovular follicles to adult life may account for certain cases of multiple pregnancy.

During childhood, the ovary grows in size by an increase of stroma but is relatively quiescent. Nevertheless, ova do attempt to ripen from time to time, but they fail to complete the process and become blighted **(Figs. 4A and B)**.

Ovulation is the process by which an ovum, in the form of a secondary oocyte **(Fig. 5)**, is discharged from the ovary to become a gamete. The ovary probably first sheds an ovum about the time of the onset of menstruation, but ovulation is not usually established as a regular phenomenon until 2–3 years after the menarche. It then continues until the age of 45–50 years, although it may

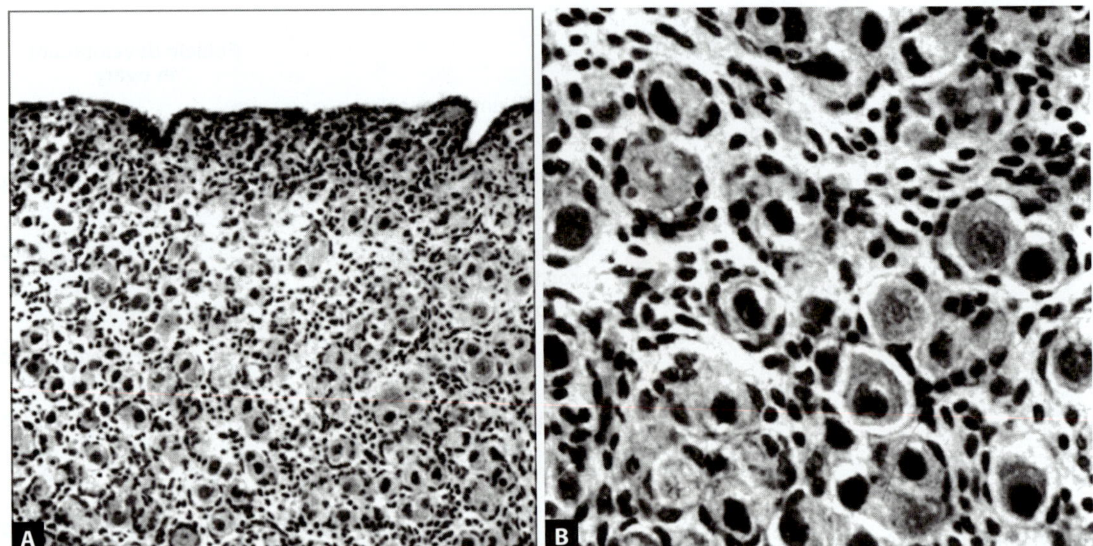

Figs. 3A and B: The ovary of the newborn child. (A) Low-power photomicrograph showing the surface epithelium with the cortex packed with primordial ova; (B) High-power view showing some of the oocytes surrounded by a single layer of granulosa (or pregranulosa) cells to form primordial follicles.

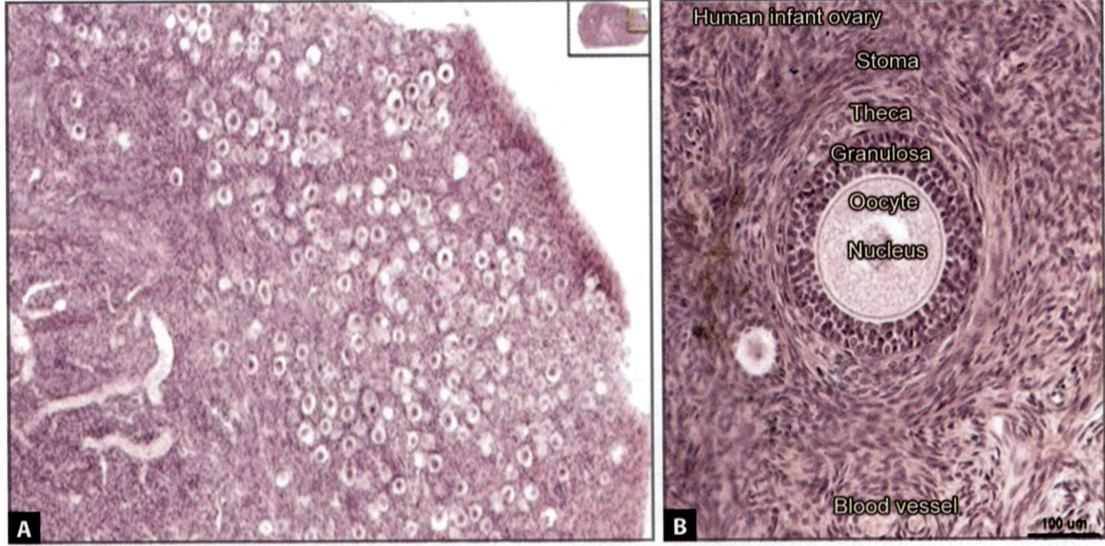

Figs. 4A and B: The ovary of the newborn child. (A) Low-power photomicrograph showing the surface epithelium with the cortex packed with primordial ova; (B) A region (see inset) of the infant ovary cortex. There are a large number of developing oocytes that will eventually form a dense primordial germ layer at the ovary periphery. Later stages of follicle development are completely absent and will begin to appear just prior to puberty.

get less frequent and less regular after the age of 40 years. Ovulation occasionally precedes the establishment of menstruation and sometimes occurs even after the cessation of menstrual periods. This accounts for the rare cases of pregnancy reported to have occurred before the menarche and after menopause.

The adult ovary goes through a cycle of activity, which occupies approximately 28 days. The cycle commences on the first day of menstruation and has two phases: (1) The ripening of an ovum, which occupies the first 14 days—the follicular phase; and (2) the formation, activity, function and degeneration of the corpus luteum, which occupies

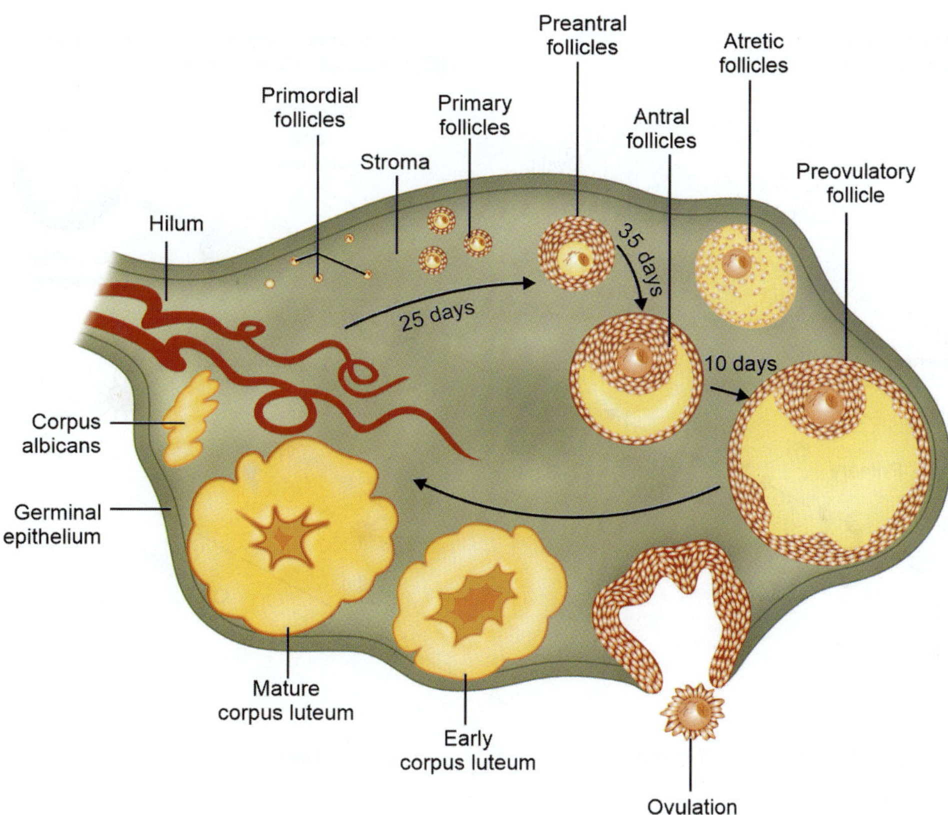

Fig. 5: Several follicle units propelled to varying degrees of maturity, advancing to ovulation.

the second 14 days—the luteal phase. These two phases are separated by ovulation. The duration of the luteal phase is more constant than that of the follicular phase and is generally reckoned as 14 ± 2 days. Nevertheless, it is subject to variations.

Primordial Follicles

The initial recruitment and growth of the primordial follicles is gonadotrophin-independent and affects a cohort over several months. However, the stimuli responsible for the recruitment of a specific cohort of follicles in each cycle are unknown. At the primordial follicle stage, shortly after initial recruitment, FSH assumes control of follicular differentiation and growth and allows a cohort of follicles to continue differentiation. This process signals the shift from gonadotrophin-independent to gonadotrophin-dependent growth. The first changes seen are the growth of the oocyte and expansion of the single layer of follicular granulosa cells into a multilayer of cuboidal cells. The decline in luteal phase progesterone and inhibin production by the now-fading corpus luteum from the previous cycle allows the increase in FSH that stimulates this follicular growth.

Preantral Follicle

During the several days following the breakdown of the corpus luteum, growth of the cohort of follicles continues, driven by the stimulus of FSH. The enlarging oocyte then secretes a glycoprotein-rich substance, the zona pellucida, which separates it from the surrounding granulosa cells (except for the aforementioned gap junction). With the transformation from a primordial to a preantral follicle, there is continued mitotic proliferation of the encompassing granulosa cells. Simultaneously, theca cells in the stroma bordering the granulosa cells proliferate. Both cell types function synergistically to produce oestrogens that are secreted into the systemic circulation. At this stage of development, each of the seemingly identical cohort members must either be selected for dominance or undergo atresia. It is likely that the follicle destined to ovulate has been selected prior to this point, although the mechanism for selection remains obscure **(Figs. 6 and 7)**.

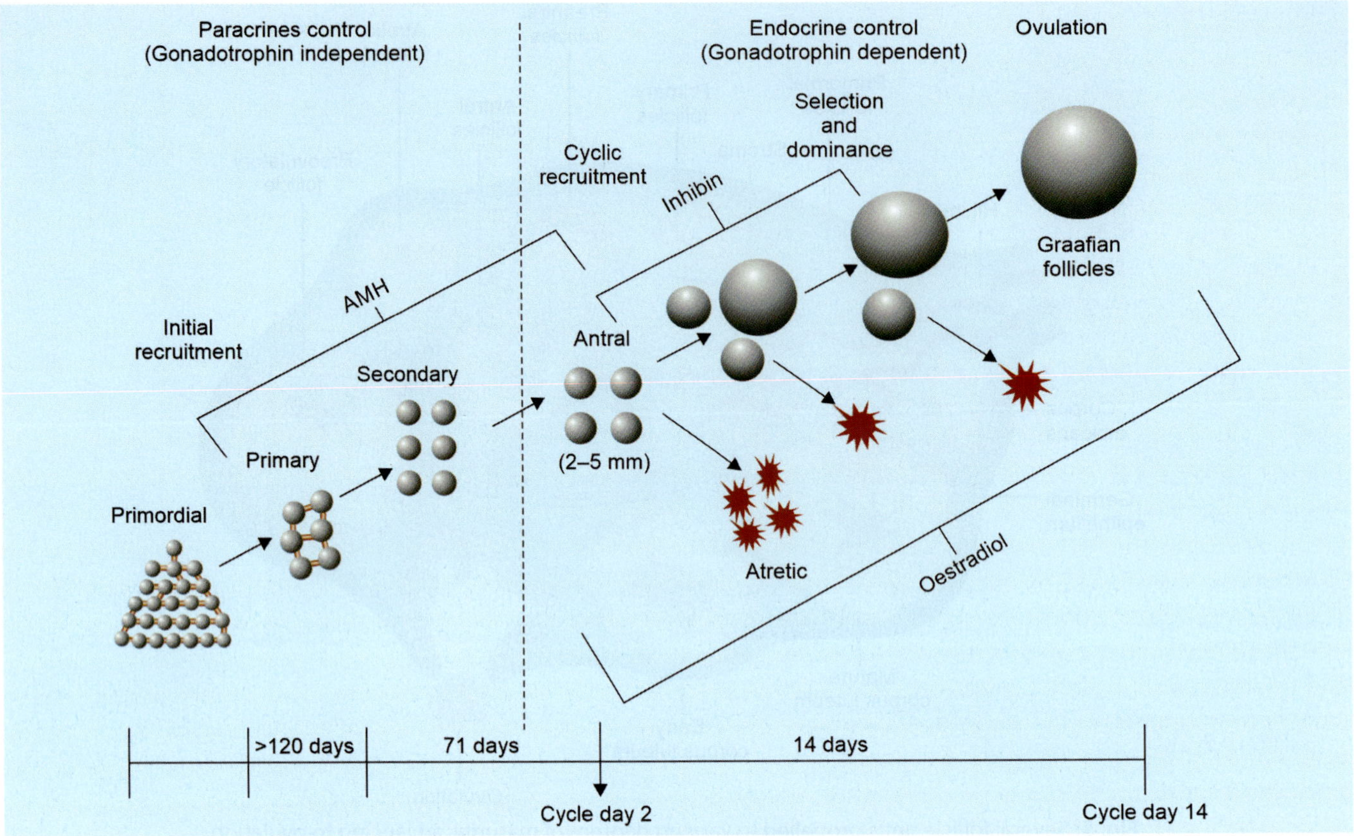

Paracrines control
(Gonadotrophin independent)
Endocrine control
(Gonadotrophin dependent)
Ovulation
Selection
and
dominance
Cyclic
recruitment
Inhibin
AMH
Initial
recruitment
Graafian
follicles
Antral
Secondary
Primary
(2–5 mm)
Primordial
Atretic
Oestradiol
>120 days
71 days
14 days
Cycle day 2
Cycle day 14

Fig. 6: Follicular, recruitment and dominance. (AMH: anti-Müllerian hormone)

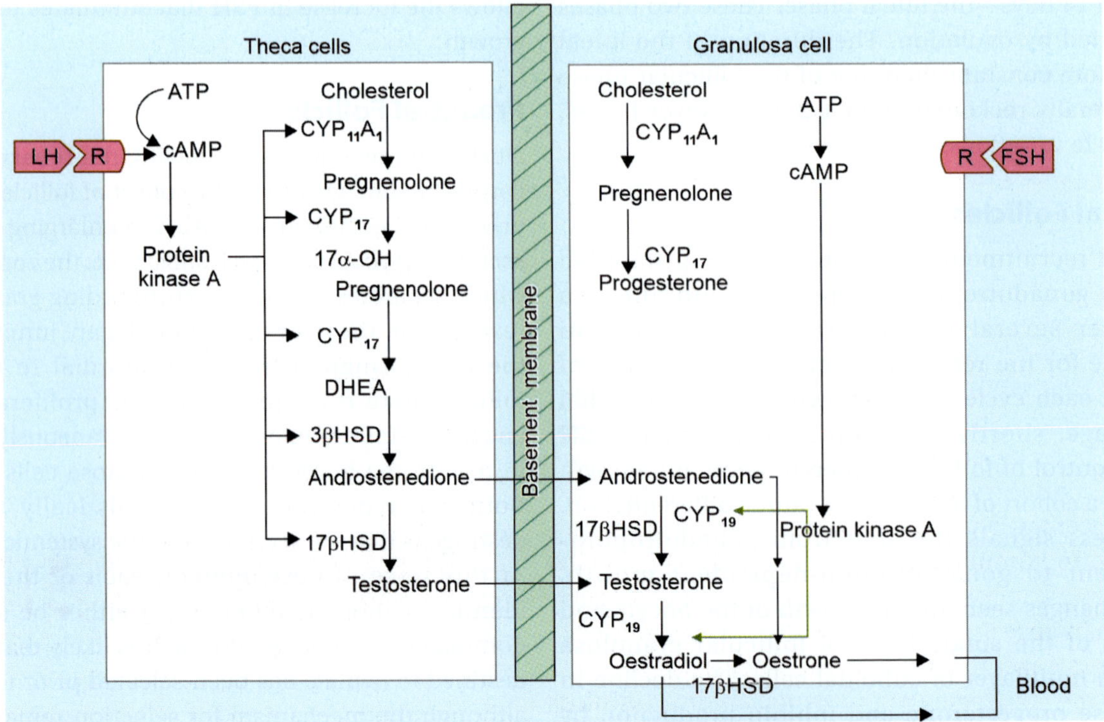

Fig. 7: Two-cell, two-gonadotrophin theory. (ATP: adenosine triphosphate; DHEA: dehydroepiandrosterone; HSD: hydroxysteroid dehydrogenase)

Two-cell, Two-gonadotrophin Theory

The fundamental information of follicular development is the two-cell, two-gonadotrophin theory. This theory states that there is a subdivision and compartmentalisation of steroid hormone synthesis activity in the developing follicle. In general, most aromatase activity (for oestrogen production) is in the granulosa cells. Aromatase activity is enhanced by FSH stimulation of specific receptors on these cells. However, granulosa cells lack several enzymes that occur earlier in the steroidogenic pathway and require androgens as a substrate for aromatisation. Androgens, in turn, are synthesised primarily in response to stimulation by LH, and the theca cells possess most of the LH receptors at this stage. Therefore, a synergistic relationship must exist: LH stimulates the theca cells to produce androgens (primarily androstenedione) which, in turn, are transferred to the granulosa cells for FSH-stimulated aromatisation into oestrogens. These locally produced oestrogens create a microenvironment within the follicle that is favourable for continued growth and nutrition. Both FSH and local oestrogens serve to further stimulate oestrogen production, FSH receptor synthesis and expression and granulosa cell proliferation and differentiation **(Fig. 10)**.

Follicular Phase

There are three phases of oocyte maturation, which are mentioned in **Figure 8**.

As shown in **Figure 7**, to get one dominant follicle, the process starts several weeks before. It starts with the recruitment of the follicles, and then at the time of menstruation, selection of a cohort of follicles is done from which one becomes a dominant follicle. Hence, to get one dominant follicle, so many follicles are activated, but many of them become atretic.

In a Graafian follicle, there are different functions in granulosa cells (inner cell layer) and theca cells (outer cell layer), and hence, two-cell theory for gonadotrophins has been described **(Fig. 9)**. Androgens have two different regulatory roles in follicular development. At low concentrations (i.e. in the early preantral follicle), they serve to stimulate aromatase activity via specific receptors in granulosa cells. At higher levels of androgens, there is an intense 5α-reductase activity that converts the androgens to forms that cannot be aromatised.

Thus, the androgenic microenvironment inhibits the expression of FSH receptors on the granulosa cells, thereby inhibiting aromatase activity and setting the

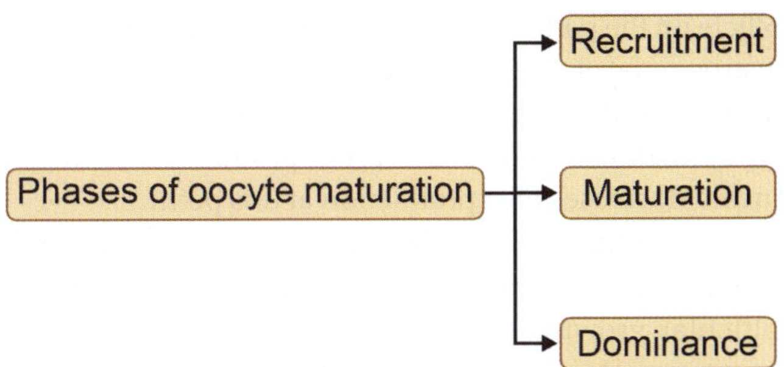

Fig. 8: Phase of oocyte maturation.

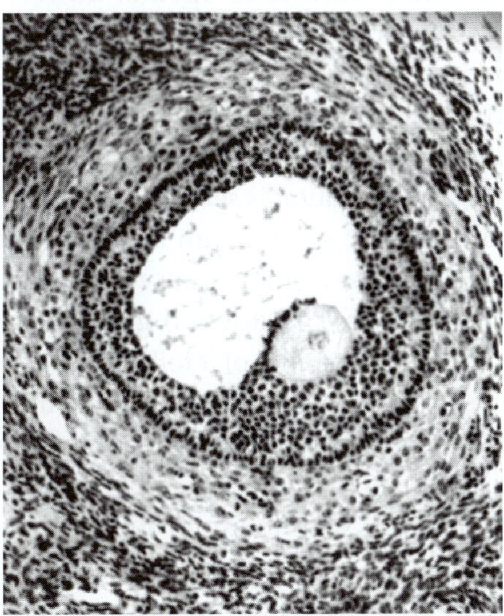

Fig. 9: A ripening Graafian follicle. The granulosa cells are many layers thick, and liquor folliculi form one central pool. The ovum is in the discus proligerus. Outside the membrana granulosa is the active theca interna layer.

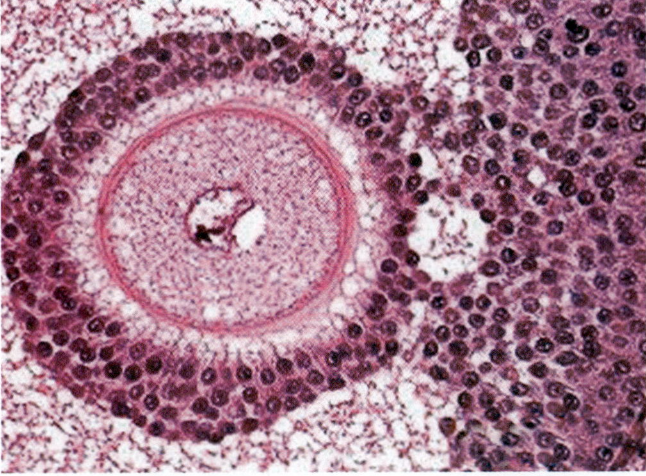

Fig. 10: The wall of a ripe Graafian follicle lined by granulosa cells with theca interna within and externa without. Tangential cutting of the section has resulted in the omission of the attachment of the discus proligerus to the wall of the follicle.

follicle on the path to atresia. Meanwhile, as the peripheral oestrogen level rises, the circulating FSH levels decrease because of the negative feedback on the pituitary and hypothalamus. Increased ovarian production of inhibin further decreases FSH production at this point.

The falling FSH level that occurs with the progression of the follicular phase represents a threat to continued follicular growth. The dominant follicle has the most receptors and has the rich oestrogenic microenvironment. As it grows and develops, the follicle continues to produce oestrogen, which results in further lowering of the circulating FSH and creating a more adverse environment for competing follicles. This process continues until the cohort of follicles undergoes atresia, other than the dominant follicle. With the increasing oestrogen, the LH surge occurs and ovulation is seen.

The normal state of an ovum awaiting release from the adult ovary is that of a primary oocyte surrounded by one or two layers of flattened granulosa cells. The commencement of ripening of a follicle is heralded by an increase in size of the ovum and of its nucleus. Thereafter, the surrounding granulosa cells become cuboidal and multiply quickly to become many layered. At the same time, they begin to secrete liquor folliculi, a colourless viscid alkaline fluid, which contains proteins, globules of fat and small amounts of the various ovarian hormone products, which form small pools separating groups of cells. These pools (Call-Exner bodies) later run together to form a single lake, and the system becomes a Graafian follicle **(Figs. 9 to 11 and 22)**. This cystic structure is lined by several layers of granulosa cells, which are collectively called the membrana granulosa. At one point, they project into the cyst as the discus proligerus (cumulus oophorus). This clump of cells contains the ovum itself, which at this stage is surrounded by a pale-staining noncellular, porous area of glycoproteins—the zona pellucida. Between the ovum and the zona pellucida is the perivitelline space.

The granulosa cells immediately around the ovum constitute the corona radiata. Outside the membrane granulosa, the stroma cells become differentiated (possibly as a result of a stimulus provided by granulosa cells) into a vascular layer of spindle-shaped cells—the theca interna. Outside this again, the stroma cells are compressed and modified to form a false capsule; this is called the theca externa **(Fig. 12)**.

During the process of ripening, the Graafian follicle, by asymmetrical development seen particularly in the form of

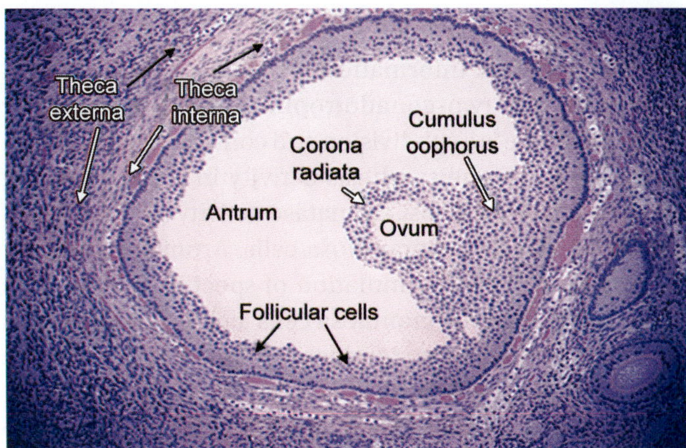

Fig. 11: Graffian follicle, 25×.

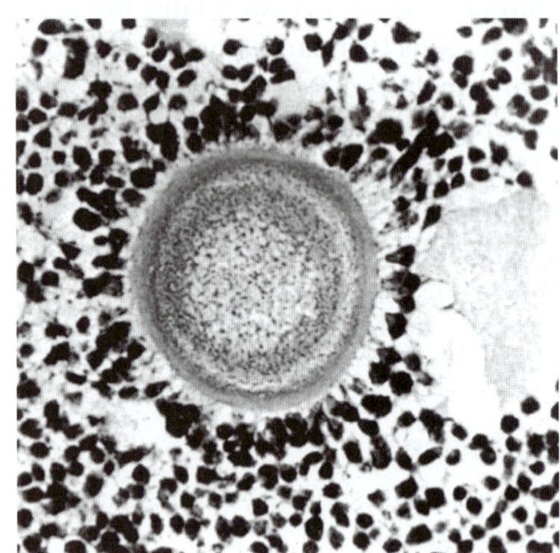

Fig. 12: A high-power view of the ovum seen in Figure 11: The zona pellucida and its surrounding corona radiata of granulosa cells are well shown. The space on the right of the ovum represents the preatrium.

a cone-shaped theca interna **(Fig. 13)**, makes its way to the surface of the ovary, easily piercing the tunica albuginea. It thus arranges itself so that the discus proligerus with the ovum lies on the side of the follicle adjacent to the peritoneal cavity.

- The final stage of development is the Graafian or mature follicle. The antral cavity is now complete, and the ovum is only attached by the cumulus oophorus. It is as if the follicle was a water-filled basketball, and the ovum was a ping pong ball, wrapped in paper and then glued to the inside of the basketball by some of the paper around it.
- Ovulation appears to be brought on by an LH surge, amongst other unknown things. The follicle bulges

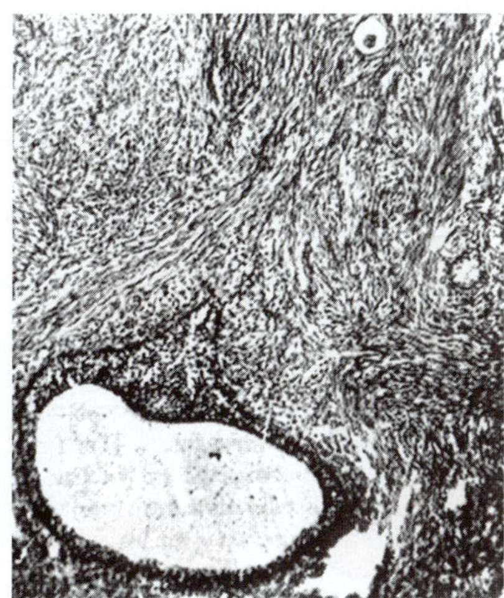

Fig. 13: The theca cone is said to be found on one side of a ripening Graafian follicle. The membrana granulosa also streams into the cone. This asymmetrical development may explain how the ripening follicle finds its way to the surface of the ovary.

against the wall of the ovary, attenuating it and making it look translucent. This is called the stigma. Production of the follicular fluid increases, causing the follicle to swell and burst, releasing the ovum with its corona radiata.

The hormonal changes which bring about this development are as follows.

At the beginning of a cycle, several ova in both ovaries begin to ripen independently of hormonal influence. A rise in FSH levels stimulates the growth of follicles to the preantral stage. While FSH receptors are present only on the granulosa cells, LH receptors are present exclusively on the theca cells. In response to LH, thecal cells are stimulated to produce androgens. In the granulosa cells, these androgens are converted to oestrogens by FSH-induced aromatisation. Thus, FSH alone will lead to folliculogenesis but the presence of LH is also essential for steroidogenesis. This is called the 'two-cell, two-gonadotropin' theory **(Fig. 7)**.

Consequent to selection of the dominant follicle, peripheral levels of oestradiol begin to rise significantly by day 7. The rising levels of oestradiol so produced exert negative feedback on the pituitary secretion of FSH. Autocrine and paracrine regulation also suppresses FSH. Inhibin is an important inhibitor of FSH secretion, while follistatin suppresses FSH activity by binding activin, which is thought to be a stimulatory peptide. The decline in FSH leads to a decline in aromatase activity, which leads to atresia of the lesser follicles (apoptosis or naturally programmed cell death). Only the dominant follicle, which is the largest with more granulosa cells and FSH receptors, can maintain its growth at the low FSH levels. FSH stimulates the production of oestrogen from the follicle, which further maintains its growth by paracrine action. Thus, through a variety of mechanisms, only one ovum matures and is discharged each month **(Fig. 14)**.

Androgens have positive regulatory roles in follicular development—promote granulosa cell proliferation, aromatase activity and inhibit apoptosis of these cells. Chronic elevation of androgens suppresses the hypothalamic-pituitary secretion of FSH, thereby making it unsuitable for the growth and maturation of dominant follicle resulting in anovulation, as seen in polycystic ovarian syndrome (PCOS).

The mid-follicular rise in oestradiol exerts a positive feedback effect on LH secretion. The steady rise in LH levels during the late follicular phase stimulates androgen production in the theca cells, which results in further oestrogen production in the granulosa cells of the dominant follicle. Once a threshold concentration of oestradiol is achieved, it induces the LH surge.

Luteinising hormone initiates progesterone production in the granulosa layer. The preovulatory rise in progesterone facilitates the positive feedback action of oestradiol and induces a mid-cycle FSH peak. A mid-cycle increase in androgens also occurs; these are derived from the thecal tissue of lesser, unsuccessful follicles.

In the presence of FSH, oestrogen becomes the dominant substance in the follicular fluid, whereas androgen dominates in the absence of FSH. LH is not normally present in follicular fluid until the mid-cycle. In the presence of prematurely elevated LH in plasma and antral fluid, mitotic activity in the granulosa cells decreases, degenerative changes ensue and the intrafollicular androgen level rises. This is the picture seen, e.g. in the polycystic ovary syndrome. Antral follicles with the highest oestrogen concentration and the lowest androgen: Oestrogen ratios are most likely to contain a healthy oocyte.

Follicular ripening does not take place at an even rate throughout the earlier 14 days, and the major histological changes only appear within the last few hours or days. An immature follicle is only 0.03 mm (30 μm) in diameter. A ripe follicle is 5–8 mm in diameter and may reach 16–24 mm immediately before rupture, so it is visible to the naked eye.

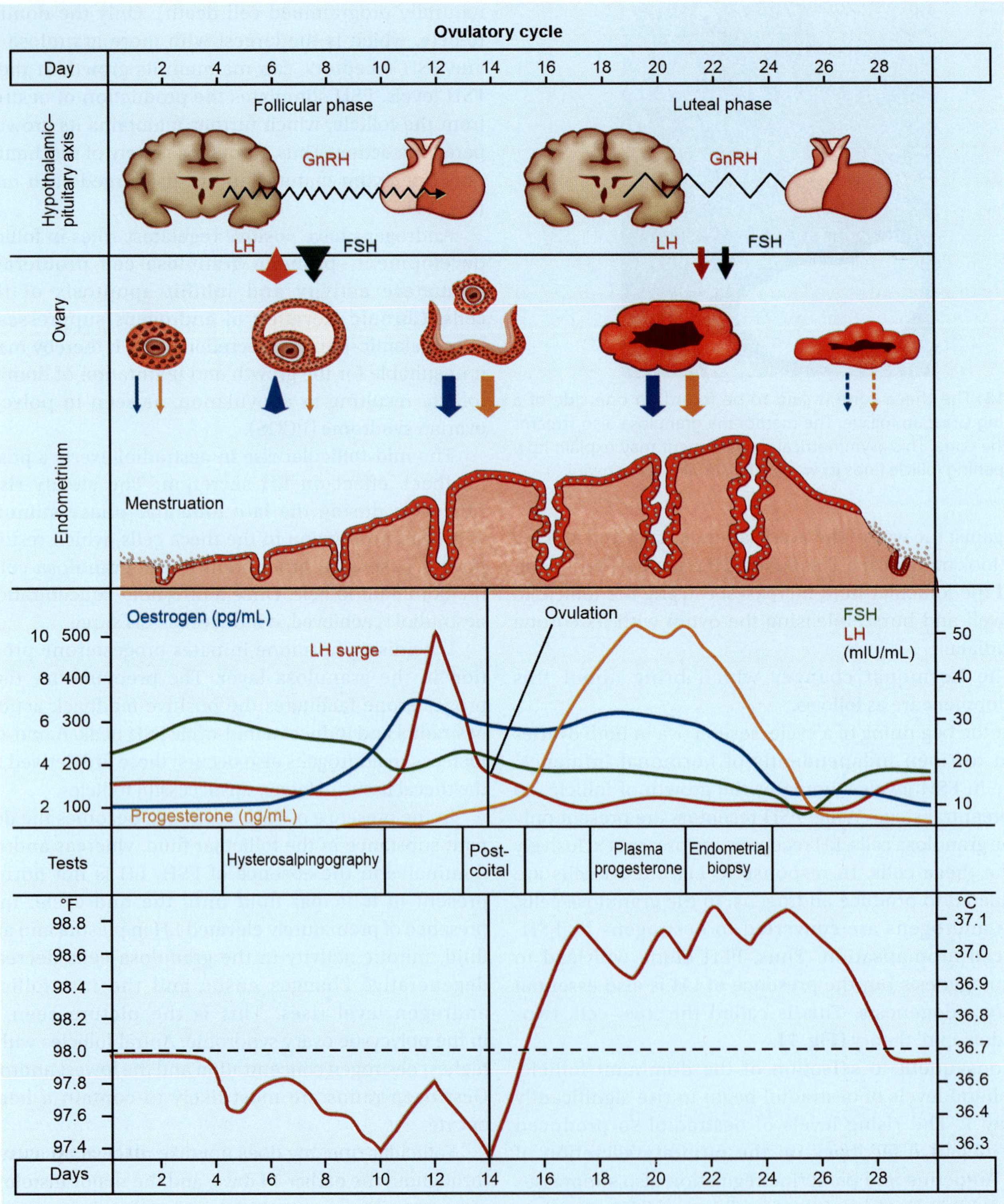

Fig. 14: Hormone levels and peripheral effects. (FSH: follicle-stimulating hormone; GnRH: gonadotrophin-releasing hormone; LH: luteinising hormone)

Preovulatory follicles are characterised by a fluid-filled antrum that is composed of plasma with granulosa-cell secretions. The oocyte remains connected to the follicle by a stalk of specialised granulosa known as the cumulus oophorus.

Rising oestrogen levels have a negative feedback effect on FSH secretion. Conversely, LH undergoes biphasic regulation by circulating oestrogens. At lower concentrations, oestrogens inhibit LH secretion. At higher levels, however, oestrogen enhances LH release. This stimulation requires a sustained high level of oestrogen (200 pg/mL) for >48 hours. Once the rising oestrogen level produces positive feedback, there is an LH surge. In the dominant follicle, LH receptors are induced in the granulosa cells. Thus, exposure to high levels of LH results in luteinisation of the granulosa cells, production of progesterone and initiation of ovulation. In general, ovulation will occur in the single mature, or Graafian, follicle 10–12 hours after the LH peak or 34–36 hours after the initial rise in mid-cycle LH.

The sex steroids and one of the peptides inhibin are involved in the regulation of follicular development. Inhibin is secreted in two forms: (1) Inhibin A and (2) inhibin B. Inhibin B is secreted primarily in the follicular phase and is stimulated by FSH, whereas inhibin A is mainly active in the luteal phase. Both forms act to inhibit FSH synthesis and release. The second peptide, activin and stimulates FSH release from the pituitary gland and potentiates its action in the ovary. It is likely that there are numerous other intraovarian regulators similar to inhibin and activin, each of which may play a key role in promoting the normal ovulatory process. Some of these include insulin-like growth factor 1 (ILF-1), EGF/transforming growth factor (TGF)-α, TGF-β1, β-fibroblast growth factor (FGF), interleukin-1 (IL-1), TNF-α, oocyte maturation inhibitor (OMI) and renin angiotensin.

Maturation of the Ovum

Meiotic Arrest of Oocyte and Resumption

Meiosis (the germ cell process of reduction division) is commonly divided into four phases: (1) Prophase, (2) metaphase, (3) anaphase and (4) telophase. The prophase of meiosis I is further divided into five stages: (1) Leptotene, (2) zygotene, (3) pachytene, (4) diplotene and (5) diakinesis.

Oogonia differs from spermatogonia in that only one final daughter cell (oocyte) forms from each precursor cell, with the excess genetic material discarded in two polar bodies. When the developing oogonia begin to enter meiotic prophase I, they are known as primary oocytes. This process begins at roughly 8 weeks of gestation. Only those oogonia that enter meiosis will survive the wave of atresia that sweeps the foetal ovary before birth. The oocytes arrested in prophase (in the late diplotene or 'dictyate' stage) will remain so until the time of ovulation, when the process of meiosis resumes. The mechanism for this mitotic stasis is believed to be an OMI produced by granulosa cells. This inhibitor gains access to the oocyte via gap junctions connecting the oocyte and its surrounding cumulus of granulosa. With the mid-cycle LH surge, the gap junctions are disrupted, granulosa cells are no longer connected to the oocyte and meiosis I is allowed to resume.

All the primary oocytes in the ovary of a newborn baby are already in the early stages of the meiotic (reduction) division. The process becomes arrested in the late prophase stage and remains dormant (diplotene stage) until follicular ripening is established. Then, as a result of the mid-cycle pre-ovulatory LH surge, meiosis is resumed and is completed within 35–45 hours prior to the ovum leaving the follicle. This first maturation division, during which the number of chromosomes in the nucleus is halved, results in the formation of a secondary oocyte and a polar body.

The latter comes to lie in the perivitelline space of the oocyte. The second division, which results in the oocyte casting off another polar body and in the first polar body dividing into two (to make three in all), only occurs after the ovum is liberated and probably only after it is fertilised.

During maturation, the ovum increases in diameter from 0.02 to 0.1 mm and, in the end, its nucleus is off-centre and displays a prominent nucleolus.

Rupture of the Follicle—Ovulation

The word rupture implies an explosive or dramatic occurrence, but the discharge of the ovum from the follicle is a comparatively gradual process occupying many seconds, if not minutes during which the ovum, still surrounded by a corona radiata of variable thickness, oozes out.

It occurs as a result of thinning and degeneration of the cyst wall, this being associated with the production of proteolytic enzymes, the activity of which is enhanced by progesterone.

- Under the influence of LH surge, meiosis in the oocyte continues, luteinisation of granulosa and synthesis of progesterone and prostaglandins within the follicle occurs.
- The progesterone-induced mid-cycle rise in FSH also serves to free the oocyte from its follicular attachments. Plasminogen activators activate plasmin, which generates active collagenase, leading to degeneration of the collagen in the cell wall, especially at the follicular apex or stigma.
- The exit of the ovum may possibly be encouraged by contraction of micromuscle cells present in the theca externa and the stroma, these being activated by prostaglandins, which are said to be essential to follicle rupture and the ovarian content of which is increased by the action of LH.

The follicular fluid escapes with the ovum and, occasionally, slight bleeding takes place from the site of rupture. As the time for ovulation approaches, the outer end of the fallopian tube moves towards the ovary so that the fimbriae tend to embrace it and are ready to catch the ovum. Peritoneal currents also tend to waft the ovum into the tube, so it rarely gets free into the peritoneal cavity. This 'pick up' function of the tube is vital to fertility.

Unless fertilised, the ovum survives only 12–24 hours and then disintegrates in the tube without leaving any trace. Nevertheless, ova have been recovered from the fimbria and from the lumen of the tube 2–4 days after ovulation and from the uterus 4–5 days after ovulation. Such, if not already fertilised, probably degenerate and certainly are not capable of being fertilised.

Luteal Phase

Immediately after the ovum is discharged, profound changes take place in the wall of the follicle. The cyst collapses and the lining cells undergo *luteinisation,* a process in which they enlarge by imbibing fluid **(Figs. 15 to 18)**. Their bloatedness causes them to become closely packed and makes their nuclei look relatively small. Luteinisation, which is brought about by enzyme action, affects both the granulosa layer (granulosa lutein cells) and the theca interna (theca lutein cells), the latter being more prominent in the early stages and the former in the later stages. Indeed, luteinisation of the theca is often apparent before ovulation occurs. Apart from increasing in size, the cells also proliferate and the total effect is to enlarge the original follicle until the new structure, the corpus luteum, is 1–2 cm in diameter and projects from the surface of the ovary **(Figs. 19 and 20)**. Some of the expansion is taken up by the layers of cells folding into the old cavity, and this gives the corpus luteum its characteristic crenated shape on section **(Fig. 21)**. The fluid within the

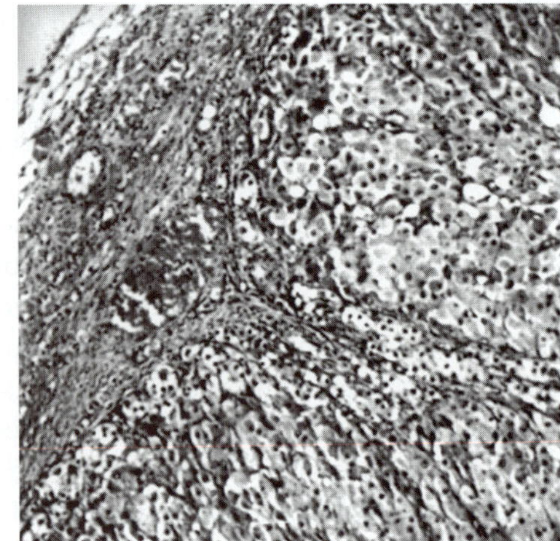

Fig. 15: The edge of an active corpus luteum, with connective tissue containing blood vessels running between two folds.

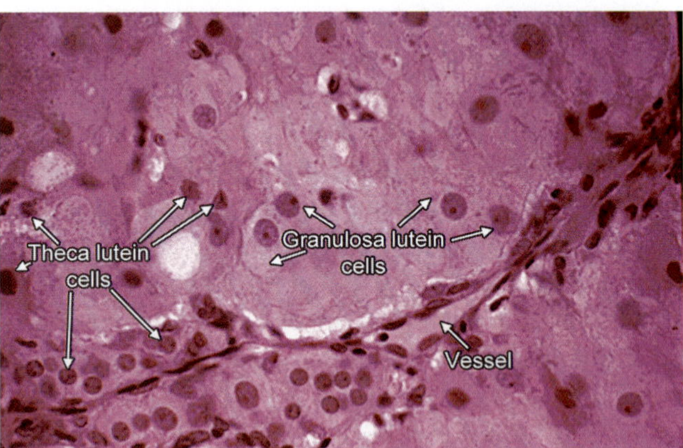

Fig. 16: Corpus luteum, 100×. Higher power reveals the cell types of the corpus luteum. The theca lutein cells are small and have dark staining. They secrete androstenedione. They are derived from the theca interna, which invades the granulosa cells. The vessel is probably derived from theca interna as well. The granulosa lutein cells are pale-staining, large, and hypertrophied granulosa cells. They produce progesterone as well as oestrogen.

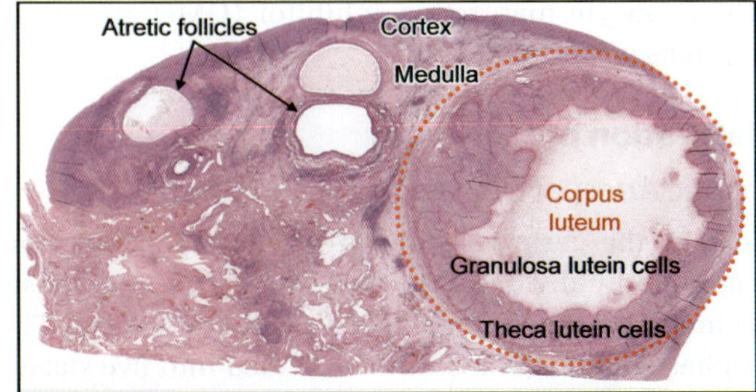

Fig. 17: Ovary showing corpus luteum and atretic follicles. Histological image, H&E stained. (H&E: haematoxylin and eosin)
Source: UNSW Embryology; https://embryology.med.unsw.edu.au/embryology/index.php?title=File:Ovary_corpus_luteum.jpg

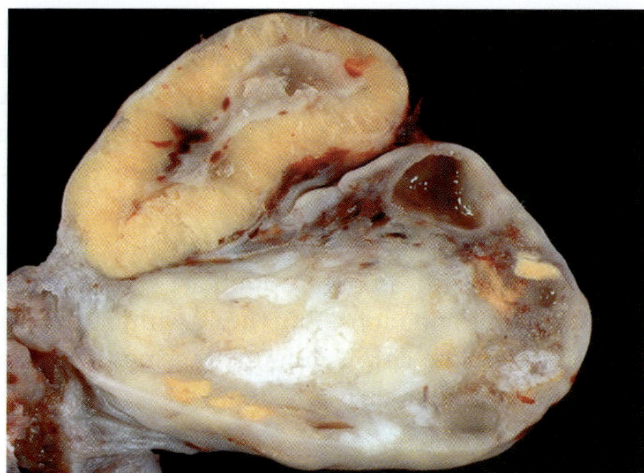

Fig. 18: Corpus luteum in cut section of ovary.

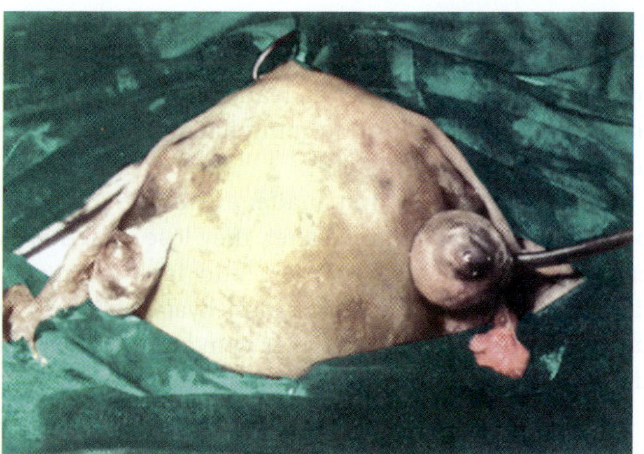

Fig. 19: Two recent corpora lutea, one in each ovary, found at the operation. This indicates the simultaneous ripening of two ova, a phenomenon that is unusual but explains binovular twinning. The uterus is enlarged by multiple myomas.

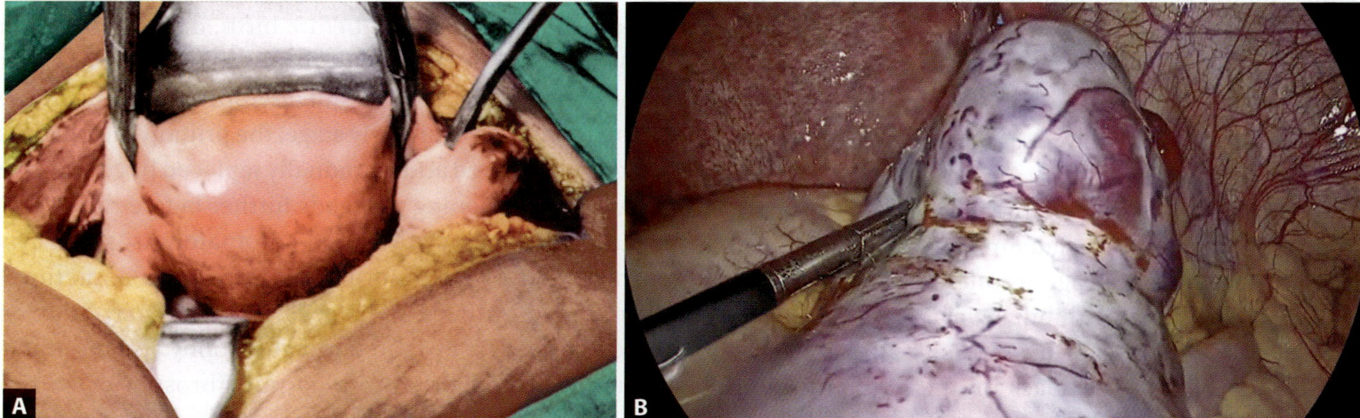

Figs. 20A and B: (A) A single corpus luteum associated with an 8-week pregnancy (10-week amenorrhoea). Photograph taken prior to Wertheim's operation for carcinoma of the cervix; (B) A corpus luteal cyst associated with a 9-week pregnancy with ovarian torsion. Photograph taken prior to detorsion and cystectomy done via laparoscopy.

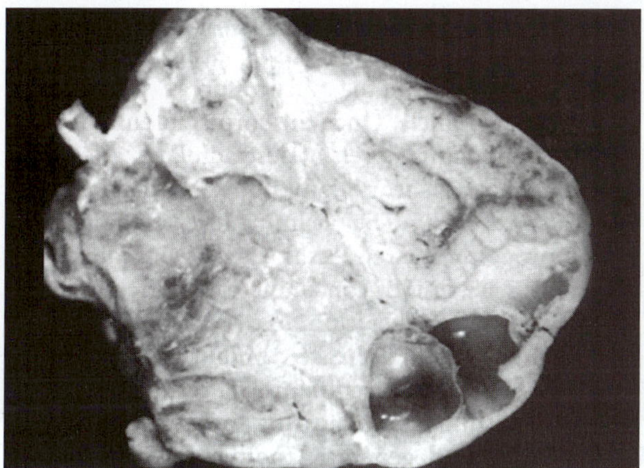

Fig. 21: A normal ovary cut across to show a recent corpus luteum, which is situated above two atretic follicles.

cells is rich in phospholipid, cholesterol and carotene. The mature structure has a yellow colour on naked-eye examination because of the presence of lipoids. In its early stages, the corpus luteum is grey or greyish-yellow.

Within 2–3 days of ovulation, the corpus luteum becomes supplied with blood vessels that grow down the core of each invagination from the theca interna. During this process, there is often a little bleeding into the cavity where the blood mixes with remaining liquor to form a pale red coagulum and makes the whole structure appear red or orange—the 'corpus haemorrhagicum'. The development of the corpus luteum is completed in 5 days, during which time, it is already functioning. Its activity is at a maximum during the following 3 or 4 days but wanes thereafter as degenerative changes commence

4–6 days before the next menstrual period. This is another example of apoptosis. It maybe very rarely complicated by rupture of corpus luteum, leading to bleeding filling in the central cavity and forming haemorrhagic corpus luteal cyst.

Degeneration is first made evident by the cells becoming vacuolated; thereafter, they lose their staining capacity. Colloid degeneration and fatty change are described, but these are followed by hyalinisation so that ultimately the corpus luteum is converted into hyaline tissue. It is then known as a corpus albicans.

Although yellow staining may linger for a long time, the typical corpus albicans is white and structureless. However, it preserves the crenated outline **(Fig. 22)**. It is absorbed over the course of 6–12 months, a process so slow that an ovary, on section, always shows several corpora albicantia in varying stages of dissolution. Thus, the life cycle of a corpus luteum has four stages: (1) Proliferation, (2) vascularisation, (3) maturity and (4) degeneration.

The mid-cycle rise in FSH ensures sufficient LH receptors and is, therefore, essential for normal luteal function. In the luteal phase, progesterone acts centrally and within the ovary to suppress the growth of the new follicle. Once the corpus luteum degenerates, circulating levels of oestradiol, progesterone and inhibin decline. With the decline in inhibin levels, FSH starts rising. The declining levels of oestradiol and progesterone release the negative feedback on the pituitary resulting in an increase in the frequency of gonadotrophin-releasing hormone (GnRH) pulsatile secretion. As a result of increased GnRH pulses and decreased inhibin and oestradiol, there is a greater secretion of FSH compared to LH. Thus, within a few days of the corpus luteum beginning to degenerate, another follicular phase commences in the ovary, and the whole process is repeated.

If the ovum, which is discharged into the tube, happens to be fertilised, its trophoblast starts secreting human chorionic gonadotrophin (hCG) within 7 days, and this ensures that the corpus luteum does not degenerate and that the ovarian cycle is arrested.

Follicular Atresia

Most of the primary oocytes are destined never to mature, and they all disappear by the time of the menopause or soon after. Their loss is accounted for mainly by atresia of the follicles, a process that occurs throughout life and is particularly noticeable before birth, during childhood and in pregnancy. During these stages, there is what appears to be an unsuccessful attempt at ripening. If the ovum is blighted at an early stage, the primordial follicle is merely obliterated and is gradually replaced by connective tissue. If the ripening proceeds further before the oocyte disintegrates by pyknosis and chromatolysis, small cyst forms lined by granulosa cells, which are sometimes surrounded by theca lutein cells, and these may function for a few days. They then undergo atrophy and the whole structure is converted to a corpus fibrosum or corpus atreticum, which ultimately reverts to stromal connective tissue **(Figs. 23 to 27)**.

Fig. 22: A corpus albicans of homogeneous hyaline tissue, which still preserves the crenated outline characteristic of the corpus luteum.

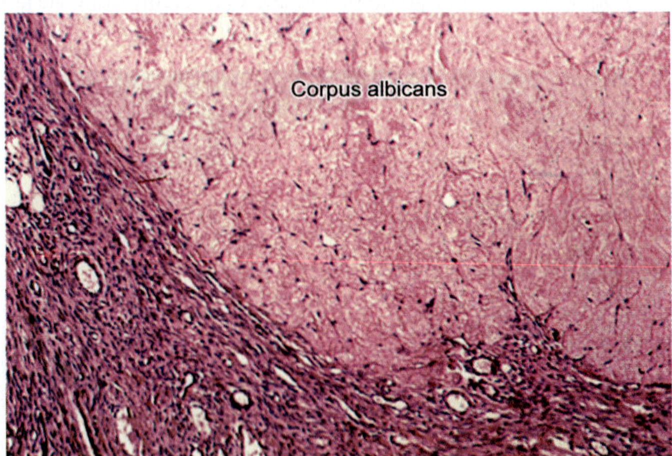

Fig. 23: Corpus albicans, 35×. Atretic follicles and the degenerating corpus luteum form a connective tissue scar called the corpus albicans. It resembles the luteum but has a fibrous, not cellular nature.

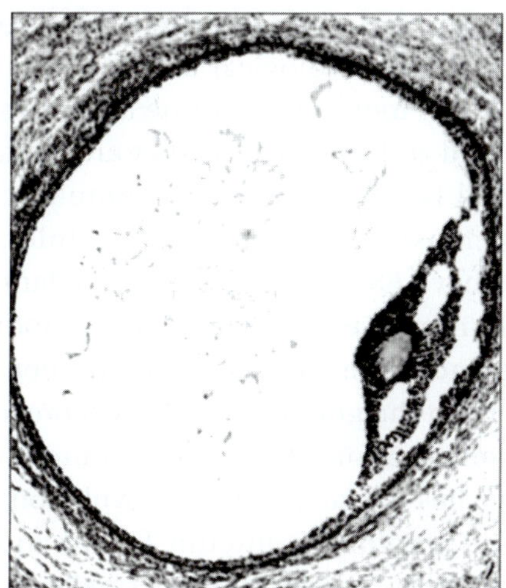

Fig. 24: A Graafian follicle in the early stages of atresia. This is a biopsy specimen taken from a woman suffering from amenorrhoea caused by an androgenic adrenal cortical tumour.

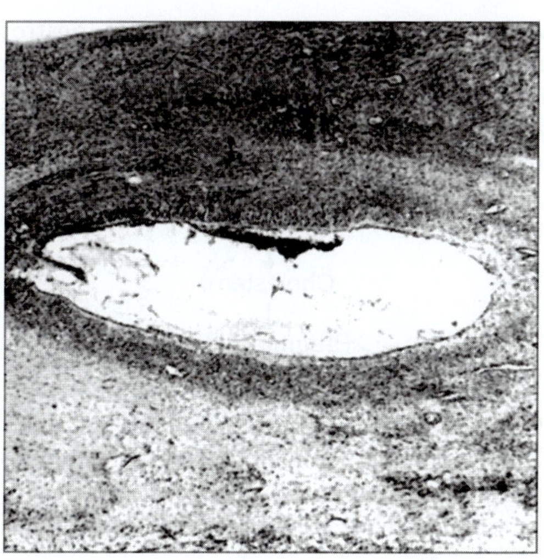

Fig. 26: A cyst representing the late stage of atresia of a follicle.

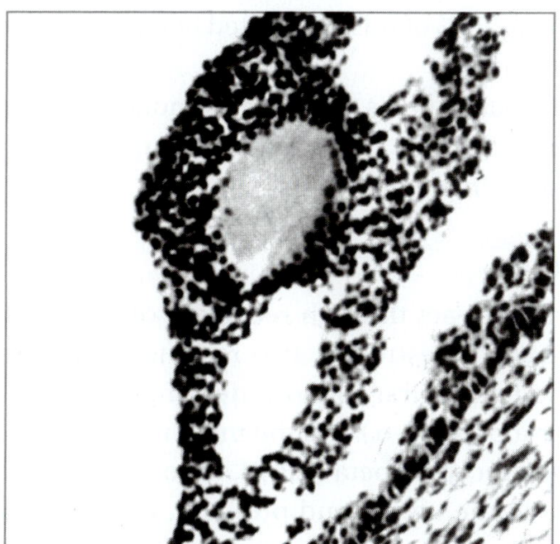

Fig. 25: An enlargement of one part of Figure 24 showing the discus proligerus with degenerative changes in the ovum.

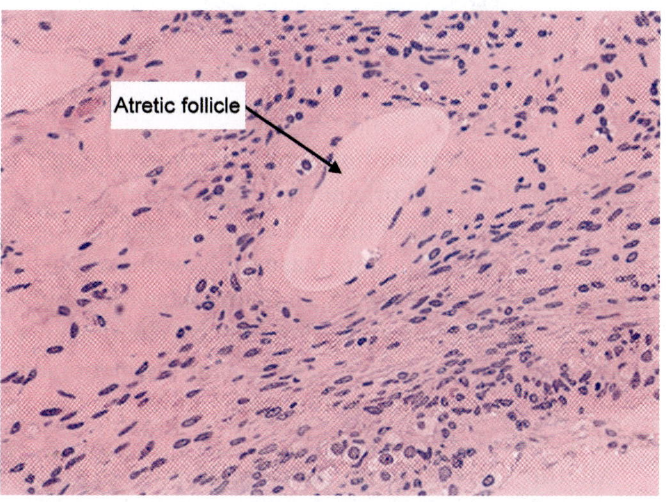

Fig. 27: Atretic follicle.

The lining consists of a single layer of low cuboidal cells.

Atresia accounts for the 'cystic' ovaries commonly seen in children, and even in newly born babies, as well as many of those which are seen in adults. It has no pathological significance. The occurrence of atresia, however, is probably of some importance because it may be a means whereby the ovary produces hormones in small amounts in individuals who are neither ovulating nor menstruating. The theca lutein cells of atretic follicles, e.g. are possible sources of the oestrogen produced by the ovary during the few years preceding puberty.

OVARIAN HORMONES

The endocrine activity of the ovary is mainly concerned not only with the production of oestrogens and progesterones but also results in the liberation of androgens. The gonad, such as the adrenal, is bisexual.

In the adult woman, both the ovary and the adrenal cortex produce, directly or indirectly, 0.05–0.2 mg testosterone in 24 hours as well as weaker androgens such as androstenedione and dehydroepiandrosterone. The plasma testosterone levels of normal females range from 20 to 80 ng/dL, compared with values of 280–840 ng/dL for normal males.

Flowchart 1: The several pathways whereby oestrogens are synthesised from cholesterol, via progesterone and androgens. This represents the normal metabolism and interchangeability of steroid hormones in the ovary and testis, and probably in the adrenal cortex too.

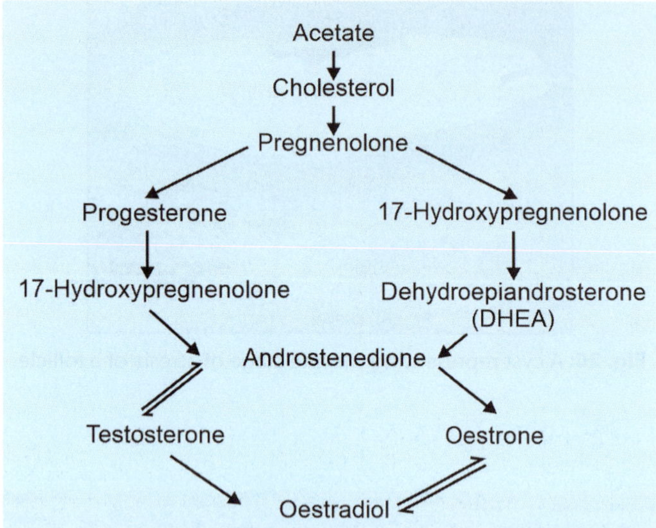

Each of the ovarian hormones was once thought to have a specific tissue origin: Oestrogens from granulosa cells, progesterone from thecal lutein cells and androgens from thecal cells. It is now reasonably well established that any of the special tissues, all of which have a common mesenchymal origin, can, under different circumstances, produce any of the hormones. Even after the menopause, steroidogenesis may be continued at a low level by the stromal or hilus cells of the ovary.

All the steroid hormones are chemically interchangeable and, in both the ovary and the adrenal cortex, are metabolised from cholesterol **(Flowchart 1)**. Cholesterol is converted to progesterone, which can change to oestradiol and oestrone, intermediate products being androstenedione and testosterone.

Oestrogens

Production

The main and most powerful oestrogen produced by the ovary is oestradiol, but the less active oestrone is also secreted, and both are found in circulation. They are inactivated by the liver, and their metabolites are excreted in the urine and faeces. When liver function is impaired, the amount of active oestrogen in circulation is increased, and excessive menstrual bleeding can result. The most important metabolite is oestriol, which has a low degree of biological activity. This and many other oestrogens found in the urine are conjugated with glucuronic acid and, in this form, they are inert.

Oestradiol is produced by the granulosa and theca cells in increasing amounts as the follicle ripens. The former have FSH receptors, and the latter have LH receptors. In response to LH, thecal cells produce androstenedione and testosterone. These are then converted to oestrogens in the granulosa cells by a process of FSH-induced aromatisation. Production, at first moderate in amount, reaches a peak just before ovulation; thereafter, it falls until the corpus luteum forms and becomes active to give rise to a second but smaller peak. When the corpus luteum degenerates, the output falls sharply **(Fig. 28)**.

The total quantity of oestradiol formed during one cycle (almost entirely by the ovulating ovary) is estimated to be 10 mg. 25% of this is excreted in the urine in the form of metabolites.

While oestradiol is the chief hormone in the reproductive years, oestrone is the main hormone in menopause and oestriol in pregnancy.

Receptors

All hormones act through receptors on the cell surface. In the case of oestrogen, two receptors have now been identified: the first is now designated as oestrogen receptor-alpha (ER-α) and the more recently identified as oestrogen receptor-beta (ER-β). ER-α is the predominant subtype in the uterus and pituitary. ER-β seems to be a weak trans-activator. It is present in significant numbers in the ovary, testis and prostate, and also in the brain, blood vessels and bone. There is a differential expression of these receptor subtypes in different target tissues, e.g. both ER-α and ER-β in the breast but only ER-β in the brain and cardiovascular system. Different oestrogens also bind differentially, e.g. phytoestrogens preferentially bind ER-β rather than ER-α. Even within the same receptor type, different molecules, e.g. oestradiol, tamoxifen and raloxifene, produce different conformational shapes and, therefore, different effects, which are not just positive or negative effects but a whole spectrum of agonistic and antagonistic actions.

This is the basis of developing selective oestrogen receptor modulators (SERMs), which will produce the desired action without the side effects.

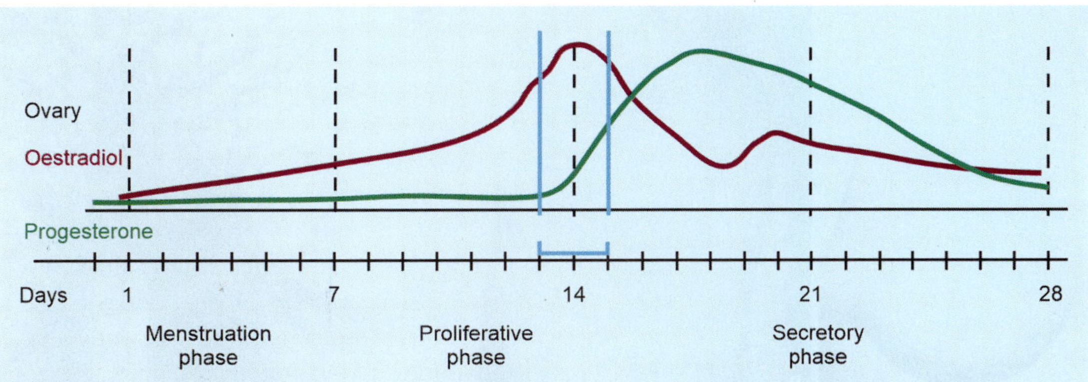

Fig. 28: Plasma levels of oestradiol and progesterone in relation to the menstrual cycle. The basic level of oestradiol in the plasma starts to rise on about the eighth and ninth days to reach a peak in mid-cycle, just before the gonadotrophin peaks. A second oestrogen peak, which is broader and more variable, occurs in the second half of the cycle and reflects corpus luteum activity. The plasma level of progesterone during the follicular phase is low. It rises mainly after ovulation as a result of corpus luteum activity and falls 2–3 days before the onset of menstruation.

Actions

Oestrus: The characteristic action of oestrogen is that it induces sexual heat or oestrus in 'lower animals'. In women, it plays only a small part in determining sexual desire, the basis for which is neurological as much as endocrinological. Even in other animals, the effect of oestrogen on behaviour such as migration and mating is mediated through the CNS.

Secondary sex characters: It was formerly thought that oestrogen was the sole cause of female physical and mental characteristics, and so it was regarded as the female sex hormone. Even though it is now recognised that several other hormones play a part, oestrogen has a major role in determining feminine sensitivity and shyness, feminine curves, soft skin and luxuriant scalp hair. It is of prime importance to the development of the breasts at puberty but not so much to the growth of body hair, not even the so-called female pattern of hair on the lower abdomen and pubes. The development of axillary and pubic hair in both sexes is governed more by androgens, which, in the female, are probably of adrenal origin. In male animals, including human beings, oestrogens tend to induce feminine characteristics.

Secondary sex organ: The main action of oestrogens is stimulation of the development of the secondary sex organs—vulva, vagina, uterus, fallopian tubes and breasts **(Figs. 29 and 30)**. Their action is selective, being mediated through special receptors and having the effect of stimulating local cell division and metabolism by way of specific ribonucleic acid (RNA) synthesis.

Vulva and vagina: The vulva and vagina are developed and maintained by oestrogens, and the same is true of the involuntary muscular and fascial tissues associated with them. Oestrogens increase their vascularity and stimulate epithelial activity. It is responsible for the deposition of glycogen in the vaginal epithelium and therefore for vaginal acidity, it encourages cornification of superficial vaginal cells to give a characteristic vaginal smear.

Uterus: The primary effect of oestrogens on the uterus is to increase its vascularity and because of this, as well as its direct action on tissue cells, it leads to hypertrophy of the myometrium and the endometrium. Oestrogens change the uterus from the infantile to the adult form and the withdrawal of their influence at menopause leads to atrophy of all elements. In the absence of oestrogens, the myometrium loses its power to contract; in their presence, it contracts regularly and forcefully and is sensitive to oxytocic drugs.

Oestrogens cause proliferation of endometrial glands and growth and compaction of the stroma. They restore the endometrium, including its coiled arteries, after menstruation, but do not induce the glands to secrete. An endometrium suddenly deprived of an oestrogen influences break down and bleeds.

The cervix also hypertrophies under the influence of oestrogens and atrophies when they are withdrawn. The growth and secretory activity of cervical epithelium is determined, at least in part, by oestrogens.

Fallopian tubes: These respond to oestrogens by increased vascularity, hypertrophy and peristaltic movements of

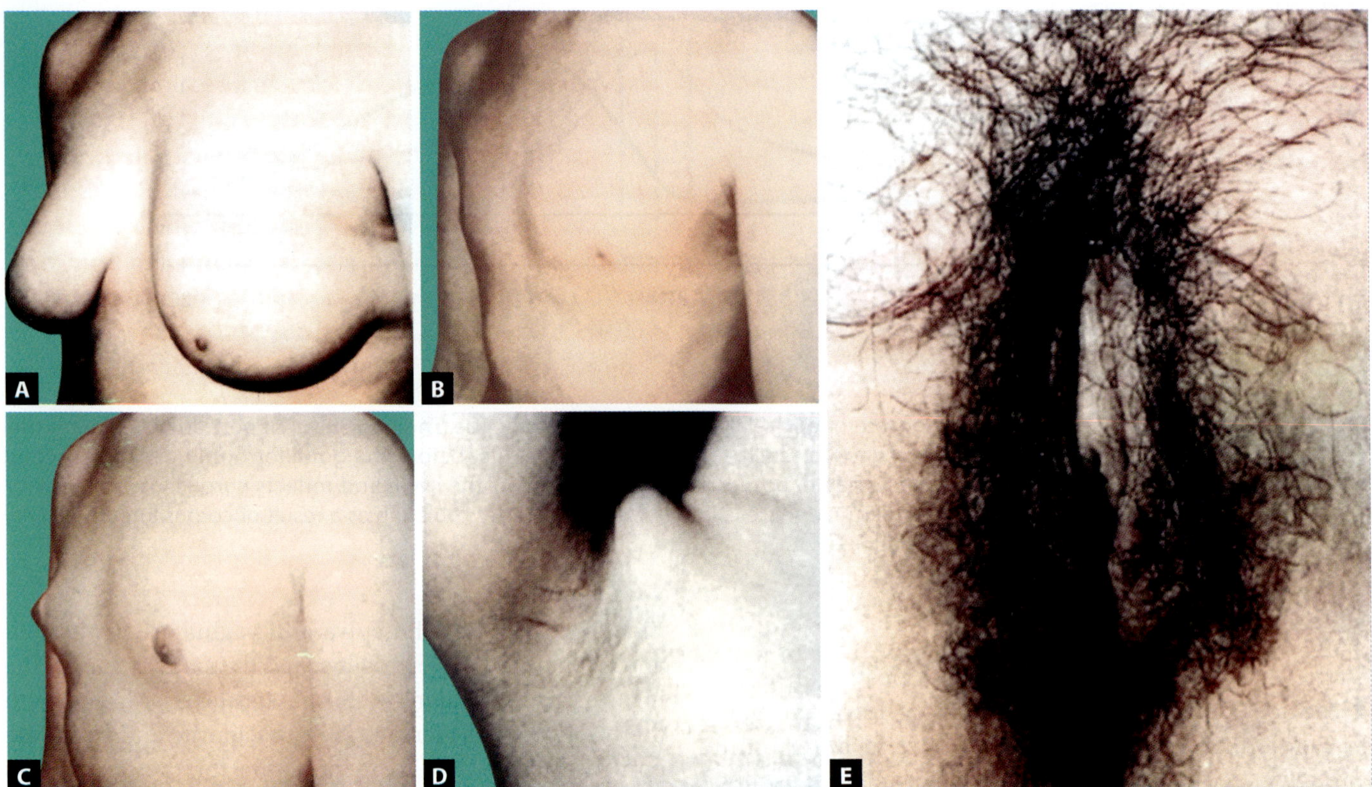

Figs. 29A to E: The part played by the gonad in the development of secondary sex characters. (A) The bust of a girl aged 18 years who had both ovaries removed at the age of 15 years. By that time, the breasts had developed and deprival of ovarian function did not lead to their becoming smaller. The tiny nipples, however, are evidence of atrophy of the duct and glandular systems; (B) Hypoplasia of the breasts of a girl aged 19 years who had both ovaries removed at the age of 12 years, that is, before the breasts had developed; (C) The same pattern as (B) with the breasts developing as the result of oestrogen therapy; (D) The same patient as (B) and before hormone therapy, axillary hair is well grown despite the absence of ovarian function; (E) The vulva of a girl aged 18 years who had ovarian function destroyed at the age of 10 years and who had no replacement therapy. Despite this, the pubic hair was formed quite well. Pubic and axillary hair reflect adrenal rather than gonadal activity.
Courtesy: Editor, J Obstet Gynaecol Br Commonw

the muscle and by the enhanced cilial and secretory activity of the endosalpinx.

Breasts: The breasts also respond to oestrogens by increased vascularity, enlargement, pigmentation of the areola and epithelial growth; the last is seen mainly in the lacteal ducts and nipple, rather than in the acini. No matter how great the stimulus is, oestrogens do not cause lactation in women, they inhibit it.

Endocrine system: By controlling the releasing factors of the hypothalamus, oestrogens depress the output of FSH, but stimulate the production of LH and adrenocorticotrophic hormone (ACTH). Oestrogens inhibit follicular activity in the ovary, indirectly through the hypothalamus and pituitary and directly by autocrine mechanisms, on the granulosa cell itself. Oestrogens, by increasing the amounts of binding globulins in circulation, also raise the blood levels of protein-bound iodine and protein-bound cortisol. They decrease glucose tolerance.

Skeletal system: Oestrogens act on both osteoblasts and osteoclasts. They conserve calcium and phosphorus. They also inhibit IL-1, TNF and IL-6, which are potent stimulators of osteoclastogenesis and bone resorption. The net result is that they encourage bone formation. At puberty, they first give rise to a growth spurt. Removal of both ovaries in childhood results in stunted growth. Closure of epiphyses and limitation of stature are mostly the effects of androgens of adrenal origin. After the menopause, lack of oestrogens leads to osteoporosis.

Urinary tract: Oestrogen receptors are found in the urethra and bladder. Oestrogens promote urethral resistance and thus improve urethral continence. By maintaining the thickness of the urinary tract epithelium and urethral

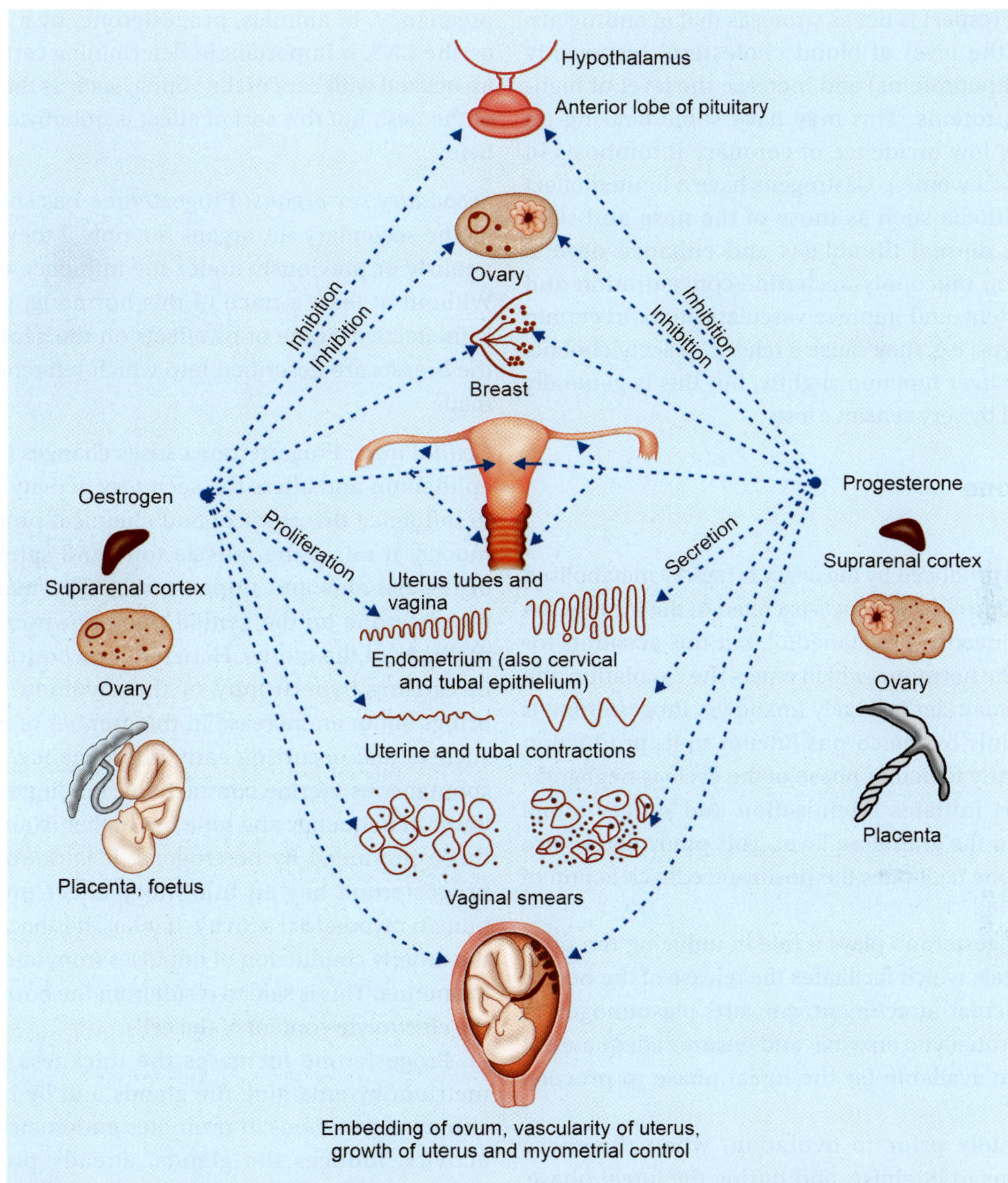

Fig. 30: Diagrammatic representation of the sources and main actions of oestrogens and progesterone. The inhibitory action of oestrogen on the anterior pituitary is probably mainly mediated through the hypothalamus. Although shown here, progesterone has a slight, if any, inhibitory effect on the hypothalamic–pituitary system, and then only when large doses are administered, or when a protestant is metabolised to an oestrogen.

collagen, as well as by their effect on the vaginal pH, they protect against urinary tract infection. They may also have an action on the sensory threshold of the lower urinary tract. Lowering of this threshold in hypoestrogenism may lead to urge incontinence and nocturia as seen in postmenopausal women.

Blood: Oestrogens increase the coagulability of the blood by raising the levels of fibrinogen and of factors VII, VIII and X and by increasing the adhesiveness of platelets.

General: Oestrogens, such as other steroids, encourage nitrogen, sodium and fluid retention in the body, but their action in this respect is not as strong as that of androgens. They lower the level of blood cholesterol (especially low-density lipoproteins) and increase the level of high-density lipoproteins. This may have some bearing on the relatively low incidence of coronary thrombosis in premenopausal women. Oestrogens have a limited effect on other epithelia such as those of the nose and skin. They act on dermal fibroblasts and enhance dermal water content, mucopolysaccharide concentration and collagen content, and improve vascularisation. In certain sites, the uterus, e.g. they cause a release of acetylcholine. They modify liver function slightly, but this is generally only revealed by very sensitive tests.

Progesterone

Production

Progesterone produced by the ovary is rapidly metabolised by the liver. One of its products excreted in the urine is the biologically inactive pregnanediol, but this accounts for only 10% of the hormone, which enters the circulation, the fate of the remainder is largely unknown. Progesterone is secreted mainly by the corpus luteum so its production during the early follicular phase of the cycle is negligible. However, LH initiates luteinisation and progesterone production in the granulosa layer. This preovulatory rise in progesterone facilitates the positive feedback action of oestrogen.

Thus, progesterone plays a role in inducing the mid-cycle FSH peak, which facilitates the release of the oocyte from its follicular attachment, converts plasminogen to plasmin, a proteolytic enzyme, and ensures adequate LH receptors are available for the luteal phase to proceed normally.

Immediately prior to ovulation, when the theca interna begins to luteinise, and during the luteal phase, the plasma progesterone level rises from 6 to 63 nmol/L, falling in the next follicular phase to 1.3–6 nmol/L **(Fig. 28)**. The total amount of progesterone produced by the ovary during one menstrual cycle is 300–400 mg.

Actions (Fig. 30)

Pregnancy, maternal instinct: Progesterone is essential to the maintenance of pregnancy in animals, hence its name. This may also be true for women but in this case, the hormone is produced by the placenta rather than the corpus luteum during all except the early days of pregnancy. In animals, progesterone, by a direct action on the CNS, is important in determining certain activities associated with care of the young, such as the preparation of the nest, but this sort of effect is not obvious in human beings.

Secondary sex organs: Progesterone has some effect on all the secondary sex organs but only if they are simultaneously or previously under the influence of oestrogen. Without at least a trace of this hormone, progesterone is ineffective. Some of its effects on the genital tract and the breasts are described into which reference should be made.

Genital tract: Progesterone causes changes in the vaginal epithelium and alters the secretory activity of the cervix to influence the physical and chemical properties of its mucus. It raises the muscle tone and sphincter action of the isthmus and upper cervix. The main effects of progesterone on the genital tract, however, are seen in the body of the uterus. Here it assists oestrogen not only in causing hypertrophy of the myometrium but also brings about an increase in the number of muscle fibres such as that occurring early in pregnancy. It influences spontaneous uterine contractions, tending to make them lower in frequency and tone but higher in amplitude than those produced by oestrogens. It is doubtful whether progesterone has an inhibitory effect on established human myometrial activity. If it has, it is because it blocks the orderly conduction of impulses from one muscle fibre to another. This is said to result from the hormone altering the electrolyte content of the cells.

Progesterone increases the thickness of the endometrium by enlarging the glands and by rendering the stroma oedematous. It promotes endometrial enzymatic activity, induces the glands, already proliferated by oestrogen, to secrete and brings about a decidual reaction in the stroma. The last is seen mostly in stromal cells near the endometrial surface, especially if they are simultaneously or subsequently exposed to a mechanical stimulus such as is provided by implantation of an ovum. Decidual reaction is characterised by the cells imbibing fluid so that they swell to reveal the cytoplasm and cell walls previously not obvious. The loose network of the endometrial stroma is thus replaced by closely packed polyhedral cells with relatively small nuclei **(Fig. 31)**. An endometrium that is suddenly deprived of a progesterone influence disintegrates on its surface and bleeds.

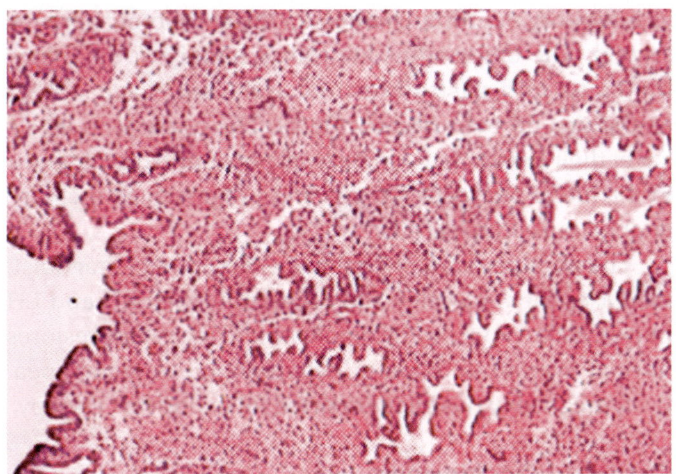

Fig. 31: Endometrium in the late secretory phase. The glands have become serrated, the stroma in the upper part of the field shows the changes of a predecidua, and the spiral arteries, which lie between the glands, are well-muscularised and surrounded by a mantle of decidualised cells (photomicrograph, 95x).

Breasts: Progesterone acts in conjunction with oestrogen in producing breast development at puberty and during pregnancy. It stimulates the epithelium of the acini rather than that of the ducts but does not induce lactation.

Endocrine system: At low levels, progesterone in the presence of oestrogen exerts positive feedback on the pituitary and is responsible for the FSH surge and for LH secretion. The increased levels of progesterone in the luteal phase exert negative feedback or the hypothalamus to inhibit GnRH production and consequent gonadotrophin release. High levels of progesterone can inhibit ovulation by this mechanism.

General: The sodium- and fluid-retaining effects of progesterone are similar to those of other steroids. Progesterone promotes the secretion of sebum by the skin and makes scalp hair more greasy; this may explain premenstrual acne and hair changes during pregnancy. Progesterone is thermogenic and raises the body temperature by 0.2–0.5°C (0.4–0.8°F). Progesterone relaxes smooth muscle throughout the body—in the ureters, blood vessels and alimentary tract; this probably accounts for the occurrence of hydroureter, varicose veins, haemorrhoids and constipation during pregnancy.

Relaxin

Relaxin is a peptide hormone produced by the corpus luteum of pregnancy and perhaps by the human placenta, chorion and decidua as well. It congests and softens the ligaments controlling the joints of the pelvis and lower spine; this allows increased movement during pregnancy and labour. Relaxin has been shown to produce cervical ripening in in vitro studies of human cervical stromal cells; in the future, recombinant relaxin may be available as a cervical ripening agent.

Inhibin, Activin and Follistatin

Inhibin, activin and follistatin are peptides with paracrine functions secreted by granulosa cells into the follicular fluid, by the placenta and also in other tissues in the body. These peptides are secreted in response to FSH; in turn, they exert feedback on FSH secretion. As the name suggests, inhibin inhibits FSH secretion while activin stimulates it. Follistatin suppresses FSH activity through hypothalamic GnRH activity.

PITUITARY HORMONES

The functions of the genital organs and breasts are controlled by hormones released from the pituitary gland. The output of these is, in turn, determined by the hypothalamus (*see further*), so the pituitary acts to some extent as a storehouse or reservoir.

Posterior Lobe Hormones

The posterior pituitary (neurohypophysis) discharges oxytocin and vasopressin (antidiuretic hormone), both of which cause smooth muscle to contract. Oxytocin stimulates particularly the muscle of the uterus and that of the myoepithelial cells in the breasts even in a pure synthetic form and has slight vasopressor and antidiuretic effects. Vasopressin maintains blood pressure by controlling arteriolar resistance, stimulates smooth muscle of the bowel and is strongly antidiuretic. It also, even in its pure synthetic form, has a slight oxytocic action.

Anterior Lobe Hormones

The anterior pituitary (adenohypophysis) secretes at least six hormones: (1) FSH, (2) LH, (3) prolactin, (4) ACTH, (5) growth hormone (GH) and (6) thyroid-stimulating hormone (TSH). Melanocyte-stimulating hormone (MSH) is thought to be secreted by the middle lobe. FSH and LH are collectively called gonadotrophins. FSH acts on the granulosa cells in the female and on the Sertoli cells in the male. LH acts on the preovulatory follicle and corpus luteum in the female and on the Leydig cells in the male. The basophil (β) cells of the adenohypophysis are credited with the production of FSH and LH, the acidophil (α) cells with the production of prolactin and GH. The chromophobe cells may represent a state in which, having discharged their secretion, they are temporarily without a capacity to take up stains. Another view is that chromophobes are undifferentiated cells that can give rise to acidophils or basophils.

Follicle-stimulating Hormone

Follicle-stimulating hormone is a glycoprotein, which is responsible for the formation and ripening of the Graafian follicle and for stimulating it to secrete oestrogen, although in these functions it requires the help of LH. By itself, it certainly cannot bring about ovulation. The level of FSH in the plasma shows cyclical changes with peaks when follicular ripening is being initiated and also immediately before ovulation **(Fig. 32)**. They play an important role in the menstrual cycle through an inhibitory effect on hypothalamic GnRH secretion. Other pituitary hormones are also modulated by opiates. There are essentially three classes of opioids: (1) The endorphins, (2) the enkephalins and (3) the dynorphins. The endorphins are generated mainly in the anterior and middle lobes of the pituitary gland, but also in the hypothalamus and other areas of the brain, in the sympathetic nervous system and in peripheral tissues including the gonads, lungs, placenta and the gastrointestinal tract.

The enkephalins are produced in the posterior pituitary, the brain and spinal cord, adrenal medulla and the gastrointestinal tract and play an important role as inhibitory neurotransmitters in the autonomic nervous system. The dynorphins are found mainly in the hypothalamus and gastrointestinal tract and have potent analgesic and behavioural effects. The endorphin levels are at their lowest in the menstrual phase and their highest in the luteal phase. Oestrogen and progesterone increase endogenous opiate levels.

The administration of naloxone, an opioid antagonist, increases the frequency and amplitude of GnRH and LH pulses. Naltrexone, which blocks opioid receptors, restores normal ovarian function in hypothalamic amenorrhoea. Even pregnancy has been reported following this therapy.

Catechol Oestrogens

Catechol Oestrogens are formed in the hypothalamus by the conversion of oestrogens by the 2-hydroxylase enzymes. They have a catechol and an oestrogen side and can therefore interact with both systems. Thus, they can increase and decrease catecholamine levels. Their exact mode of action has not been defined but it is postulated that there may be a link between catecholamines and GnRH secretion.

PITUITARY–HYPOTHALAMIC RELATIONS

There are close anatomical and functional links between the pituitary gland and the hypothalamus. The hypothalamus in humans is the area of the forebrain situated above the pituitary gland and forming the anteroinferior wall and floor of the third ventricle.

It is bounded laterally by the optic tracts and cerebral peduncles and anteriorly by the optic chiasma. The

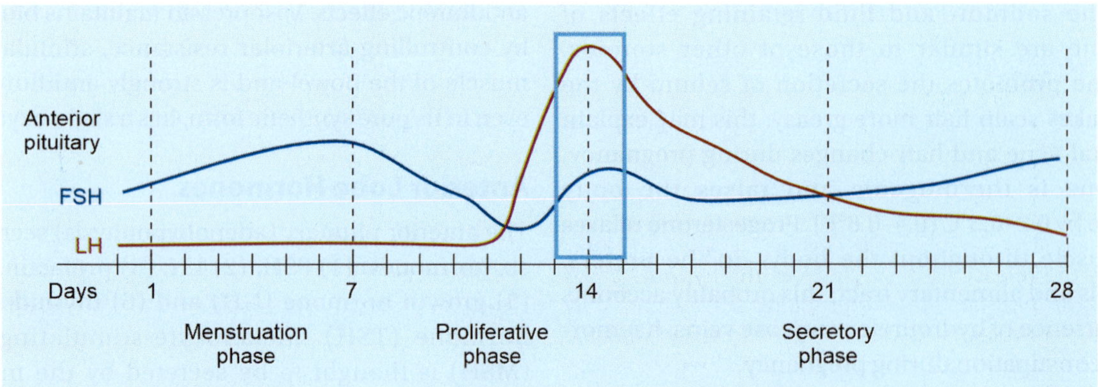

Fig. 32: Plasma levels of follicle-stimulating hormone (FSH) and luteinising hormone (LH) in relation to the menstrual cycle. The heights of the mid-cycle peaks, which are related to ovulation, vary, but that of LH is always more pronounced than that of FSH. During the rest of the cycle, the plasma levels of both hormones are fairly constant, although sometimes an extra pre-ovulatory peak of FSH is demonstrable.

neurohypophysis differs from the adenohypophysis in that it is a secretory and storage unit composed of neural tissue. Anatomically, it consists of the supraoptic and paraventricular nuclei of the hypothalamus, in which the synthesis of vasopressin and oxytocin occurs. The hypothalamo–hypophyseal tract, which conveys the hormones, is controlled by nerve impulses, and the hormones are secreted directly into the capillary plexus of veins draining into the cavernous sinus and jugular veins in response to physiological stimuli **(Fig. 33)**.

The hypothalamic control of the anterior lobe is achieved via the hypophyseal portal venous system; secretion and synthesis of each anterior pituitary hormone are controlled by releasing and release-inhibiting hormones from the hypothalamic nuclei, which pass down the portal system of capillaries to the adenohypophysis. Secretion of the released hormones is controlled by direct feedback or by influences, which act via the higher centres. Feedback control is usually inhibitory (negative), i.e. depressing both the releasing hormone production and the trophic hormone secretions from the anterior lobe. Positive feedback (stimulatory) is less common but is involved in the secretion of LH in response to high levels of oestrogen and progesterone. The feedback is indirect if it operates on the pituitary via the hypothalamus and direct if the effect is on the anterior lobe itself.

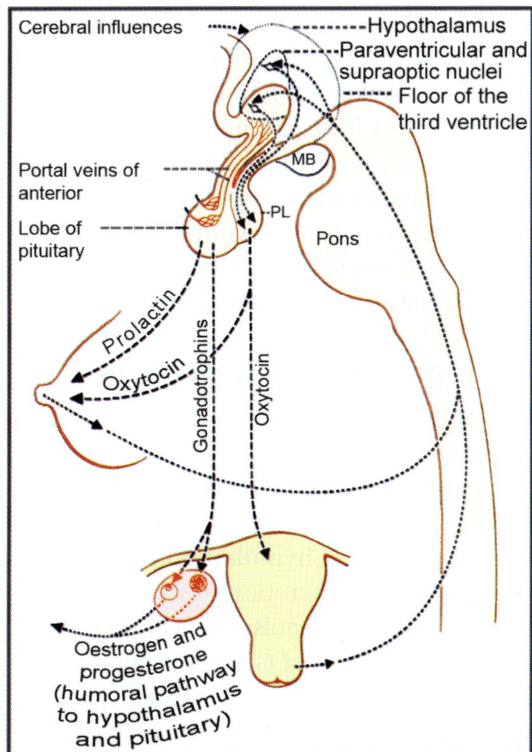

Fig. 33: Diagrammatic representation of the hypothalamic–hypophyseal relations. Nerve reflexes from the nipple and cervix can stimulate the release of oxytocin from the hypothalamus and the posterior pituitary via neuron pathways, and possibly the production of prolactin. Ovarian hormones travel through the bloodstream to exert their influence on the hypothalamic–pituitary axis. Releasing factors or hormones from the hypothalamus to the anterior pituitary via the portal veins. Their secretion is also modulated by the inputs from the cerebral cortex. (MB: mammillary body, which is not part of the hypothalamus; PL: posterior lobe of the pituitary).

Some of the releasing hormones have been synthesised. A list of the releasing hormones and inhibiting hormones is given in **Table 1**.

Within the CNS, the control of the releasing factors is mediated by the local synthesis of neurotransmitters dopamine, serotonin and noradrenaline. These neurotransmitters, apart from controlling hypothalamic neurohormone secretion, are also concerned at other sites including regulation of sexual function, behaviour and mood. There are many other peptides that also function as neurotransmitters with local regulatory autocrine and paracrine roles. These include neurotensin, which alters pituitary hormone release; vasoactive intestinal peptide, which increases prolactin secretion; angiotensin II, which controls gonadotrophin and prolactin secretion; endothelins, which cause release of gonadotropins and inhibit prolactin; somatostatin, which inhibits the release of GH, prolactin and TSH; neuropeptide Y, which is increased in undernutrition, anorexia and

TABLE 1: Pituitary–hypothalamic hormones.

Hypothalamic-releasing hormone	***Hormone released***
Gonadotrophin-releasing hormone (GnRH)	LH and FSH
Corticotrophin-releasing hormone (CRH)	ACTH
Growth hormone-releasing hormone [(GHRH) (SRH)]	GH (somatotrophin)
Thyrotrophin-releasing hormone (TRH)	TSH
Hypothalamic-inhibiting hormone	Hormone inhibited
Prolactin-inhibiting factor (PIF)	Prolactin
Growth hormone release inhibiting hormone [(GHRIH) (somatostatin)]	GH (somatotrophin)

(ACTH: adrenocorticotropic hormone; FSH: follicle-stimulating hormone; GH: growth hormone; LH: luteinising hormone; SRH: somatotropin-releasing hormone; TSH: thyroid-stimulating hormone)

bulimia nervosa and may be a link between nutrition and reproductive function; growth factors, which modulate pituitary hormone production and secretion; activin, which augments the secretion of FSH and inhibits prolactin and GHs; inhibin, which selectively inhibits FSH, but not LH secretion; follistatin, which decreases the activity of activin; galanin, the endogenous opiates, etc. The response to the neurotransmitters can be modified by various pharmacological preparations.

In exciting or inhibiting the output of pituitary hormones, the hypothalamus can be influenced by higher centres in the brain, especially those in the temporal lobes. So, emotional upsets can encourage or depress pituitary and, therefore, ovarian and menstrual functions.

The hypothalamus is also affected by environmental factors, and this is especially evident in animals. Thus, increasing or decreasing hours of daylight affects gonadal activity in many species and can be used to induce or inhibit ovulation. In birds especially, daylight operates via the eyes along a chain which consists of retina → brain → hypothalamus → pituitary → gonad. Exposure to continuous daylight can so disturb the hypothalamic clock in female rats as to bring about persistent oestrus associated with cystic ovaries.

It also appears that the hypothalamus, and indeed the brain, is sexually differentiated in some if not all species. The discharge of gonadotropins from the male hypothalamic-pituitary system is, excluding hourly variations, continuous and not cyclical. If it were otherwise, spermatogenesis in men would wax and wane. It might be attributable to the fact that testosterone is not so inhibitory to hypothalamic-pituitary activity as are oestrogens. The phenomenon may also reflect a sexual difference in the CNS. In some animals, not including human beings, so far as is known, sexual differentiation of this system is determined by the influence of gonadal hormones before or shortly after birth. Thus, if a newborn female rat is given a single injection of testosterone, or if its brain is directly exposed to this hormone, the subsequent discharge of gonadotropins by its hypothalamic-pituitary system in later life is continuous and not cyclical or intermittent. Moreover, the animal's sexual and other behaviour becomes male rather than female.

There are many loops for control of ovulation. It starts from the hypothalamus, which has multiple interconnections with other regions in the brain. Many of these pathways form feedback loops to areas supplying neural input to the hypothalamus.

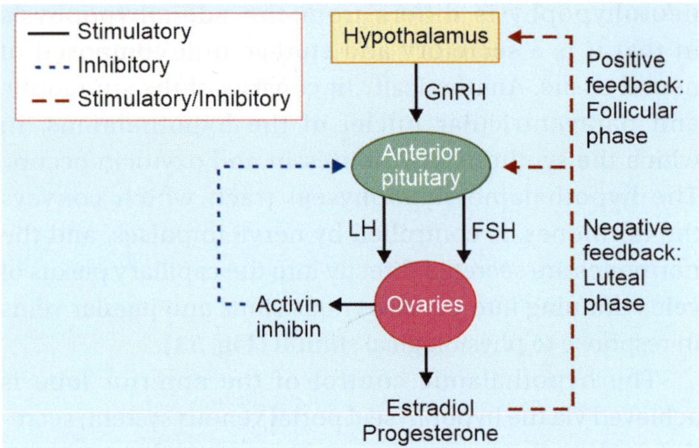

Fig. 34: Feedback loops. (FSH: follicle-stimulating hormone; GnRH: gonadotrophin-releasing hormone; LH: luteinising hormone)

The feedback loops **(Fig. 34)** to the hypothalamus exist and are known as the long, short and ultrashort feedback loops. The long feedback loop is composed of endocrine input from circulating hormones, just as feedback of androgens and oestrogens. Similarly, pituitary hormones may feedback to the hypothalamus and serve important regulatory functions in short-loop feedback. Finally, hypothalamic secretions may directly feedback to the hypothalamus, itself, in an ultrashort feedback loop.

Gonadotrophin-releasing Hormone

Gonadotrophin-releasing hormone [also called luteinising hormone-releasing hormone (LHRH)] is the controlling factor for gonadotrophin secretion. It is a decapeptide produced by neurons with cell bodies primarily in the arcuate nucleus of the hypothalamus. GnRH simultaneously regulates the secretion of two hormones—FSH and LH. It is secreted in a pulsatile fashion to be effective, and the pulsatile release of GnRH influences the release of the two gonadotrophins. Continual administration does not result in gonadotrophin secretion, and in fact, it suppresses the release of FSH and LH. The pituitary gets suppressed with the continuous exposure of GnRH. Hence, a continual exposure of the pituitary gonadotroph to GnRH results in a phenomenon called down-regulation, through which the number of gonadotroph cell surface GnRH receptors is decreased. Similarly, intermittent exposure to GnRH will 'upregulate' or 'autoprime' the gonadotroph to increase its number of GnRH receptors. This allows the cell to have a greater response to subsequent GnRH exposure. The continual pulsatile secretion of GnRH is necessary because GnRH has an extremely short half-life (only 2–4 minutes).

When the amplitude of the GnRH secretion is seen in the follicular phase, it is characterised by frequent, small-amplitude pulses of GnRH secretion. In the late follicular phase, there is an increase in both frequency and amplitude of pulses. During the luteal phase, however, there is a progressive lengthening of the interval between pulses as well as a decrease in the amplitude. This variation in pulse amplitude and frequency is directly responsible for the magnitude and relative proportions of gonadotrophin secretion from the pituitary.

Over the years, the structure of the GnRH molecule has been changed and made into a more useful molecule for the management of infertility and other gynaecological conditions. Additional modification of the GnRH molecule results in an analogue that has no intrinsic activity but competes with GnRH for the same receptor site. These GnRH antagonists produce a competitive blockade of GnRH receptors, preventing stimulation by endogenous GnRH and causing an immediate fall in gonadotrophin and sex steroid secretion. Antagonists have the advantage of not suppressing the required FSH in the beginning phase of the follicular development unlike the GnRH-a, which suppresses both FSH and LH. Compared with that of GnRH agonists, this action greatly reduces the time for therapy to become effective. Thus, as with constant GnRH exposure, downregulation occurs. GnRH agonists are now widely used to treat disorders that are dependent on ovarian hormones. They are used to control ovulation induction cycles and to treat precocious puberty, ovarian hyperandrogenism, leiomyomas, endometriosis and hormonally dependent cancers. The development of GnRH antagonists proved more difficult, in that a molecule was needed that maintained the binding and degradation resistance of agonists but failed to activate the receptor.

PITUITARY–OVARIAN RELATIONS (CONTROL OF OVULATION)

The neurohormonal connections are again illustrated by the control of ovulation in certain animals such as the rabbit. In these, follicular ripening proceeds spontaneously but ovulation only occurs as a result of coitus. This acts by mechanical stimulation of the cervix. From the cervix, nerve impulses travel through the spinal cord to the hypothalamic–pituitary system, which liberates LH to cause ovulation 18 hours after the initial stimulus. In women, ovulation ordinarily occurs independent of coitus and is spontaneous, but this does not exclude the possibility that it may sometimes be determined by outside influences. It is timed in relation to the next menstrual period which it precedes by 14 ± 2 days—this means that the luteal phase in the ovary is relatively constant in duration, whereas the length of the follicular phase varies with the total length of the cycle.

The onset and duration of these phases are determined by a cyclical and sequential discharge of gonadotrophins by the hypothalamic–pituitary system.

Gonadotrophins are found only in small quantities in the anterior pituitary of the foetus and child; significant amounts do not become demonstrable in the urine until the age of 10–12 years. The relative quiet of the ovary during childhood is therefore partly explained by failure of the pituitary to put out gonadotrophins. This in turn is almost certainly because the hypothalamus does not release GnRH, the evidence being the fact that the administration of this factor to a child results in the secretion of FSH and LH by the pituitary. It follows that the awakening of ovarian function at puberty has a hypothalamic basis.

The cyclical production of FSH and LH in the adult woman is itself largely controlled by the ovarian cycle. This is by way of a feedback mechanism that operates through the hypothalamus and which can be explained in a simplified form as follows. This discharge of FSH (and a little LH) from the pituitary, initiated by the hypothalamus, causes a follicle in the ovary to ripen and secrete oestrogen. A resulting high level of oestrogen in circulation increases GnRH-receptor concentration.

A surge in GnRH accompanies the LH surge. A high level of LH induces ovulation and corpus luteum formation with a consequent increase in the secretion of progesterone.

The negative feedback on the pituitary operates at both the hypothalamus and anterior pituitary. Oestrogen exerts inhibitory effects at both levels, decreasing GnRH pulsatile secretion and GnRH pituitary response. Progesterone also exerts its inhibitory action at the hypothalamic level. The degeneration of the corpus luteum results in a fall in the level of both oestrogen and progesterone in the circulation then stimulates the hypothalamus to put out GnRH to start the next cycle.

The details of this feedback mechanism are complicated, operating on the pituitary and the hypothalamus. Moreover, oestrogen and progesterone, in different amounts and circumstances, exert either positive or negative effects on the hypothalamus and/or pituitary. Progesterone can first stimulate and then inhibit the production of GnRH. All actions are receptor mediated.

There is evidence to show that a 'short-loop feedback' mechanism also operates between the pituitary and the hypothalamus, so that levels of different gonadotrophins influence the discharge of releasing hormone by the hypothalamus. Thus, a high level of LH in the circulation may inhibit the output of GnRH.

The balance between the actions of the hypothalamic–pituitary complex and the ovary is well demonstrated by the fact that, when ovarian function is feeble, the gonadotrophic activity of the pituitary becomes excessive. When both ovaries are removed from an adult woman, the outpouring of gonadotropins (mainly FSH but also some LH) into the blood and urine continues without break for many months and may even be 5–20 times greater than the peak excretion in the normal menstruating woman.

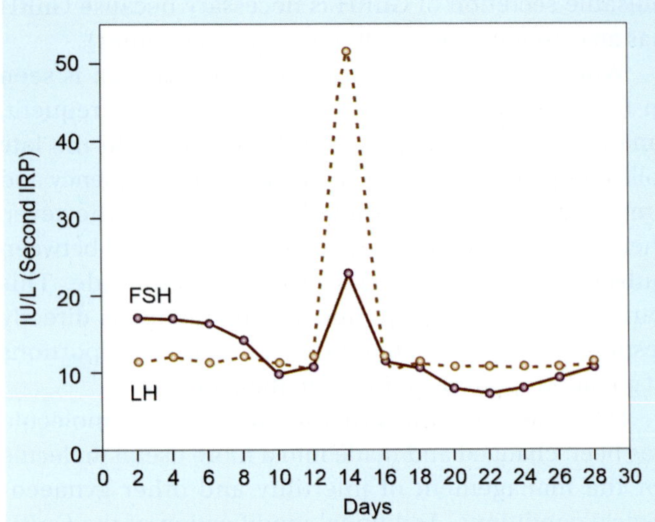

Fig. 35: Cyclical variations in levels of follicle-stimulating hormone (FSH) and luteinising hormone (LH). (IRP: international reference preparation)

HORMONE LEVELS AND ASSAYS

The quantitative assay of many of the hormones and their metabolites in blood and urine was difficult till the development of specific and reliable radioimmunoassay techniques. The tests are still relatively expensive and should only be carried out for specific diagnostic and therapeutic indications. The ability to measure circulating steroid hormones has almost eliminated the need for measuring the urinary metabolic products.

The steroid hormones, their fractions and metabolites found in the blood are assayed by mass. For plasma assays, the general rule is to give the amount per millilitre in picograms (pg), nanograms (ng) and micrograms (μg) as well as milligrams (1.0 ng/mL is equivalent to 0.1 μg/100 mL and 1.0 μg/L), or in mIU/mL or IU/L.

The cyclical variations of the mean plasma levels of FSH and LH are shown in **Figure 35**. However, there are wide variations from one woman to another and from 1 day to another. In practice, therefore, single assays are of little value in monitoring patients but may help diagnostically, such as in PCOS where the ratio of LH:FSH is reversed and may reach as high as 2 and 3 wherein usually it is between 1 and 2.

The picture is also complicated by the fact that the adrenal cortex produces oestrogens, progesterone and intermediate substances, as well as androgens. Once secreted into the circulation, the fate of the hormone is related to the nature of the steroid and not to the source. The excretion of pregnanediol and oestrogens by post-menopausal women, e.g. reflects adrenal rather than ovarian activity. In the male, oestrogens are secreted by both the testes and the adrenal cortex. Hormone excretion products such as 17-ketosteroids are almost entirely indicative of adrenal cortical function.

Pregnanetriol, an excretion product of 17α-hydroxyprogesterone, comes partly from the adrenal and partly from the ovary. Its urinary levels, therefore, show cyclical variations, and these persist in some measure in women subjected to bilateral adrenalectomy.

Adult women produce 300 mg testosterone in 24 hours, half of it coming from the adrenals and half from the ovaries. Adult men produce 7,000 mg in 24 hours, 500 mg from the adrenals and 6,500 mg from the testes. Testosterone contributes only 100 mg of the total urinary 17-ketosteroids in women. The fact that the testosterone contribution is so small probably explains why androgenic tumours of the ovary do not usually result in significant increases in the output of 17-ketosteroids. Plasma testosterone levels in these conditions are raised.

The range of total serum testosterone in women is 0.2–0.6 ng/mL compared with that of 4–8 ng/mL for men. There is little variation in women throughout the menstrual cycle save for a slight increase during the LH rise at mid-cycle. Unlike testosterone, androstenedione levels are higher in women, 1.5–2.0 ng/mL compared to 0.8–1.2 ng/mL in men. There is a slight rise mid-cycle, and the androstenedione levels are always slightly higher in the luteal phase. The peripheral conversion of androstenedione to oestrogens in nonpregnant women and in men is an important factor in hormonal status physiologically as well as in pathological states or conditions. Studies have indicated that there is diurnal variation of testosterone, with peak early in the morning and gradually decline during the day. There is always some variation in level from one laboratory to the other, so each laboratory must provide its reference range along with the report.

Hence, to summarise the whole event of ovarian cycle, GnRH is produced in the arcuate nucleus of the hypothalamus and secreted in a pulsatile fashion into the portal circulation, where it travels to the anterior pituitary. A change in ovarian follicular development moves from a period of gonadotrophin independence to a phase of FSH dependence. As the corpus luteum of the previous cycle degenerates, luteal production of progesterone and inhibin A decreases, allowing FSH levels to rise. In response to FSH stimulus, the follicles grow and differentiate and secrete increasing amounts of oestrogen. Oestrogens stimulate growth and differentiation of the functional layer of the endometrium, which prepares for implantation. Oestrogens work with FSH in stimulating follicular development.

The two-cell, two-gonadotrophin theory dictates that with LH stimulation, the ovarian theca cells will produce androgens that are converted by the granulosa cells into oestrogens under the stimulus of FSH. Rising oestrogen levels negatively feedback on the pituitary gland and hypothalamus and decrease the secretion of FSH. The one follicle destined to ovulate each cycle is called the dominant follicle. It has relatively more FSH receptors and produces a larger concentration of oestrogens than the follicles that will undergo atresia. It can grow despite falling FSH levels. Sustained high oestrogen levels cause a surge in pituitary LH secretion that triggers ovulation, progesterone production and shift to the secretory, or luteal, phase. Luteal function is dependent on the presence of LH. Without continued LH secretion, the corpus luteum will regress after 12–16 days. In the event of pregnancy, the embryo secretes hCG, which mimics the action of LH by sustaining the corpus luteum. Subsequently, the corpus luteum continues to secrete progesterone and supports the secretory endometrium, allowing the pregnancy to continue to develop.

SUGGESTED READING

1. de Kretser DM, Hedger MP, Loveland KL, Phillips DJ. Inhibins, activins and follistatin in reproduction. Hum Reprod Update. 2002;8(6):529-41.
2. Ecochard R, Gougeon A. Side of ovulation and cycle characteristics in normally fertile women. Hum Reprod. 2000;15(4):752-5.
3. England MA. Life Before Birth, 2nd edition. St. Louis, MO: Mosby-Wolfe; 1996.
4. Fortune JE. Ovarian follicular growth and development in mammals. Biol Reprod. 1994;50(2):225-32.
5. Menstruation in girls and adolescents: using the menstrual cycle as a vital sign (committee opinion no. 65). Obstet Gynecol. 2015;126:e143-6.
6. Muttukrishna S, Tannetta D, Groome N, Sargent I. Activin and follistatin in female reproduction. Mol Cell Endocrinol. 2004;225(1-2):45-56.
7. Ringler GE, Strauss JF. Recent advances in understanding the process of implantation. Curr Opin Obstet Gynecol. 1990;2(5):703-8.
8. Sherman BM, Korenman SG. Hormonal characteristics of the human menstrual cycle throughout reproductive life. J Clin Invest. 1975;55(4):699-706.
9. Speroff L, Glass RH, Kase NG. Clinical Gynecologic Endocrinology and Infertility, 5th edition. Baltimore: Williams and Wilkins; 1994.
10. Tsafriri A, Chun SY, Reich R. Follicular rupture and ovulation. In: Adashi EY, Leung PC (Eds). The Ovary, 1st edition. New York: Raven Press; 1993. p. 227.
11. Westergaard L, Christensen IJ, McNatty KP. Steroid levels in ovarian follicular fluid related to follicle size and health status during the normal menstrual cycle in women. Hum Reprod. 1986;1(4):227-32.

4

CHAPTER

Menstruation and Other Cyclical Phenomena

Deepa Reddy, Muralidhar V Pai

Chapter Outline

- Normal Menstrual Cycle
- Endometrial Cycle
- Correlation of Endometrial and Ovarian Cycle
- Uterine Bleeding
- Myometrial Cycle
- Cyclical Changes in the Tube
- Cervical Cycle
- Vaginal Cycle
- Cyclical, Metabolic, Vascular and Psychological Changes

NORMAL MENSTRUAL CYCLE

Menstruation is the periodic and cyclical sloughing of uterine inner lining (endometrium) in response to interactions between hormones produced by the hypothalamus, pituitary and ovaries. A menstrual cycle takes place at approximately 28-day intervals although a normal cycle can be anywhere between 24 and 38 days, with 2–8 days of flow and blood loss of 20–60 mL. Menstruation begins at menarche and stops at menopause.

There are five phases in the normal cycle as mentioned in **Flowchart 1**.

The normal human menstrual cycle can be divided into two segments: (1) The ovarian cycle and (2) the uterine cycle. There is orderly cyclic hormone production accompanied by the simultaneous proliferation of uterine endometrium in the respective segments. The ovarian cycle may be further divided into follicular and luteal phases, whereas the uterine cycle is divided into corresponding proliferative and secretory phases.

Flowchart 1: Five phases of normal cycle.

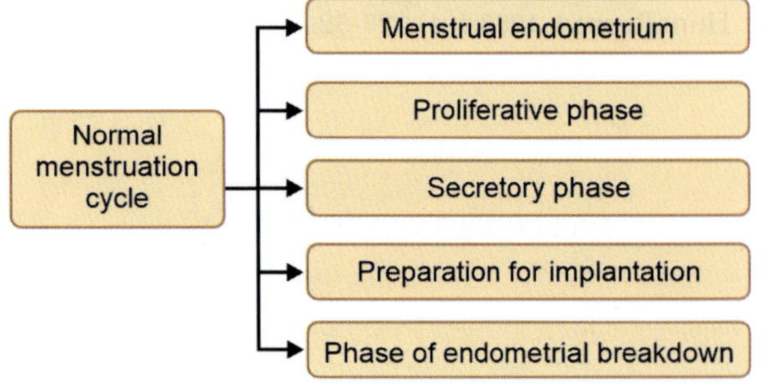

ENDOMETRIAL CYCLE

The cyclic histologic changes in the adult human endometrium proceed in an orderly fashion in response to cyclic hormonal production by the ovaries. Histologic cycling of the endometrium can be best viewed in two parts: (1) The endometrial glands and (2) the surrounding stroma. The superficial two thirds of the endometrium is the zone that proliferates and is ultimately shed with each cycle if pregnancy does not occur. This cycling portion of the endometrium is known as the decidua functionalis and is composed of a deeply situated intermediate zone (stratum spongiosum) and a superficial compact zone (stratum compactum). The decidua basalis is the deepest region of the endometrium. It does not undergo significant monthly proliferation but, instead, is the source of endometrial regeneration after each menses.

In a 28-day cycle, the first 4 days are occupied with menstruation when two thirds to four fifths of the endometrium is shed. During the remaining 24 days, the histological cycle consists basically of a proliferative and a secretory phase.

Menstrual Endometrium

The first day of vaginal bleeding is conventionally dated as day 1 of menstruation. Menstrual endometrium is dense tissue composed of nonfunctioning basalis and variable stratum spongiosum. Menstrual endometrium represents a transitional state between proliferative and exfoliative endometrium. As much as two thirds of the functioning endometrium is lost during menstruation.

Proliferative Phase

At the conclusion of menses or vaginal bleeding, the remaining endometrium is necrotic, disorganised and devoid of surface epithelium; sometimes only the basal layer remains. The glands are macerated and broken; the stroma is infiltrated with red and white blood corpuscles **(Figs. 1 and 2)**. Repair proceeds quickly, and the surface is re-covered with epithelium, which grows from the glands and the stroma, within hours of the completion of the menstrual phase. Vascular endothelial growth factor (VEGF) is a highly potent endothelial mitogen produced by the endometrium in response to oestrogen and hypoxia. It plays a role in angiogenesis and endometrial repair. By the end of 2 or 3 days, the surface is intact, new vessels are growing from the stumps of the old, and the glands and stroma are reformed. At this stage, the glands are small and lined by cuboidal epithelium; they have a regular outline and tend to lie parallel to the surface **(Figs. 3 and 4)**. Thereafter proliferation proceeds slowly at first but then quickly, the glands increasing in size and becoming

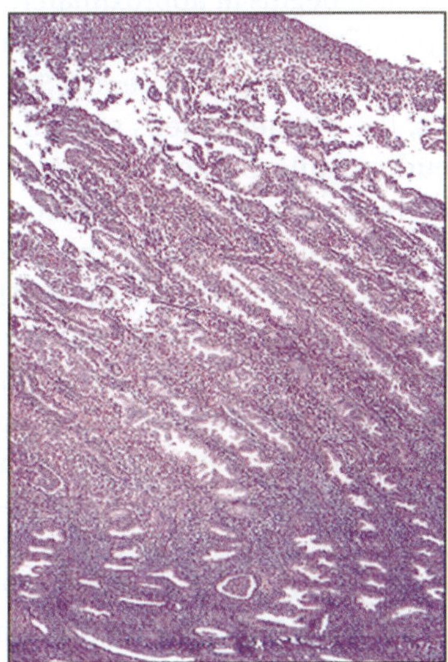

Fig. 1: A low-power view of a menstrual endometrium showing the unresponsive basalis in the lower part of the photomicrograph and the functionalis disintegrating near the surface.

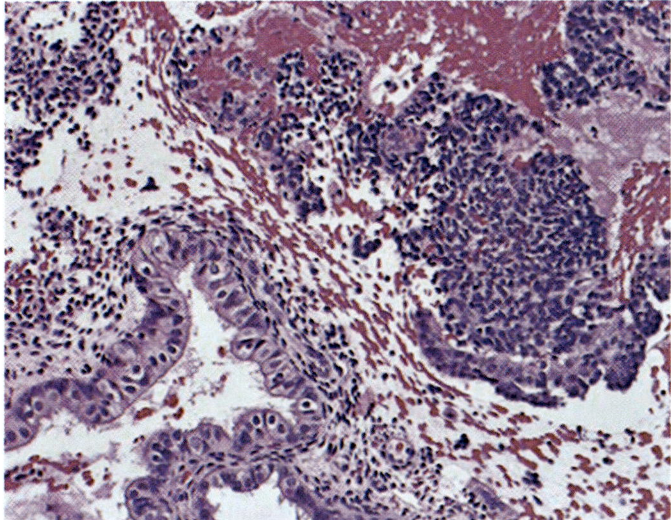

Fig. 2: Menstrual endometrium, secretory glands and detached stromal aggregate ('blue ball').

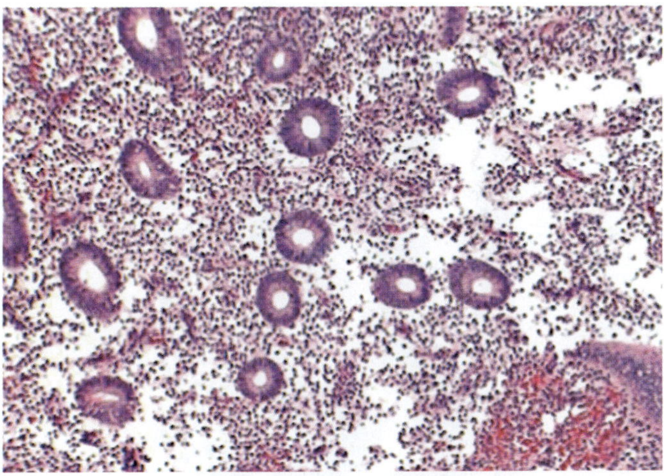

Fig. 3: Early proliferative endometrium. In cross section, the glands look like blue donuts.

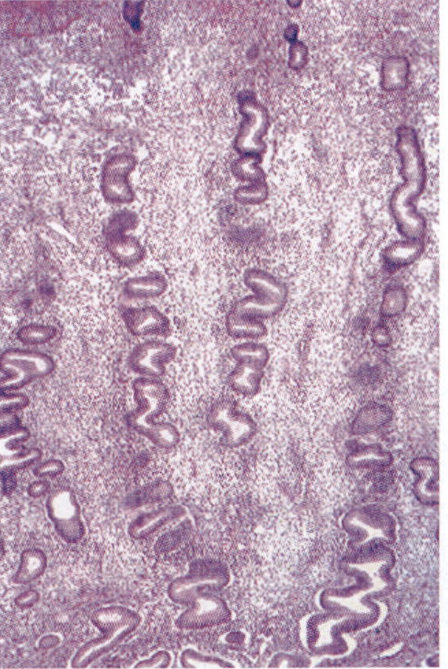

Fig. 4: Midproliferative endometrium. Note the early coiling and synchronously developed glands.

perpendicular to the surface **(Figs. 5 to 7)**. Mitoses are common in epithelial and stromal cells. The epithelial cells become columnar with their nuclei situated basally, but they show no evidence of secretory activity. The stromal cells become spindle-shaped and assume a compact arrangement.

At the beginning of the proliferative phase, the endometrium is thin and measures about 1–2 mm, whereas at the end of it, i.e. on day 14, it measures around 8 mm. The predominant change seen at the beginning of the proliferative phase during this time is the evolution of the initially straight, narrow and short endometrial glands into longer, tortuous structures. Histologically, these proliferating glands have multiple mitotic cells and their organisation changes from a low columnar pattern in the early proliferative period to a pseudostratified pattern before ovulation. The stroma is a dense compact layer throughout this time.

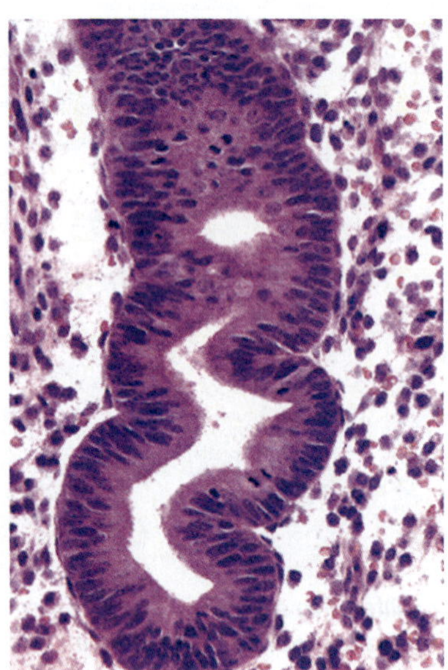

Fig. 5: High-power view of a proliferative phase gland. The constituent cells are pseudostratified, and the characteristically elongated glandular nuclei have dense chromatin.

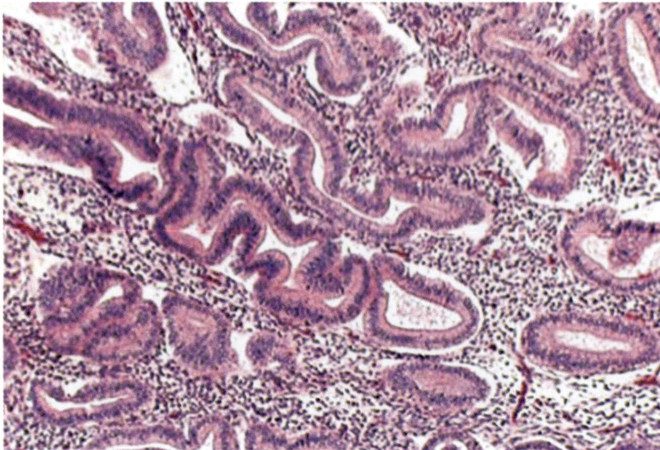

Fig. 6: Late proliferative endometrium showing extensive coiling of glands. This can appear as numerous glands in cross section and should not be interpreted as glandular crowding or hyperplasia.

Secretory Phase

The secretory phase begins at approximately the 14th day of a 28-day cycle. During this phase, the endometrium continues to grow to reach a thickness of 5–7 mm. During the first 3 days, the epithelial cells still undergo mitosis and show pseudostratification of their nuclei. Thereafter, mitosis ceases in the glandular epithelium but can be seen in the stromal cells. The glands increase in size and become actively secretory **(Figs. 7 to 9)**. The secretion collects first as a globule at the base of the cell to give rise to the appearance of subnuclear vacuolation. The globule is later seen on both sides of the nucleus but eventually collects near the lumen of the glands acinus and pushes the nucleus to the base of the cell. At the end of 5–8 days (19th to the 22nd day of the cycle), the secretion enters the gland lumen on its way to the uterine cavity, leaving the cells with their edges frayed **(Figs. 10A and B)**. This secretion, rich in glycogen, fructose and glucose, has a nutritive function for any fertilised ovum reaching the uterus. The secretory phase is also characterised by a change in the

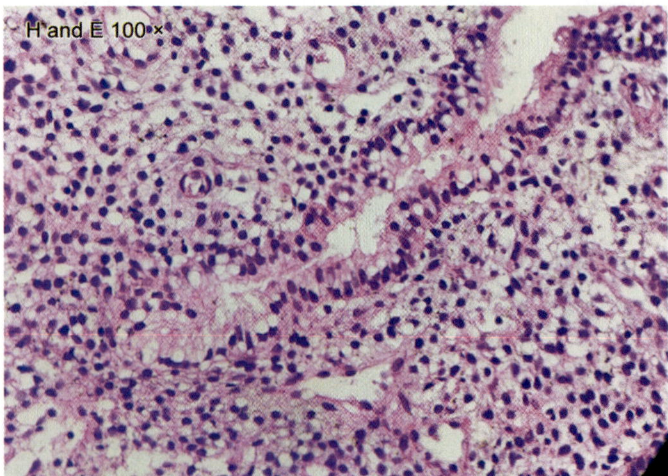

Fig. 7: The early secretory phase. The glands are larger and less regular in outline. The lining cells show globules of secretion lying basal to the nuclei, the so-called subnuclear vacuolation (photomicrograph 100×).
Courtesy: Dr Megha Murali, Assistant Professor, KMC, Manipal.

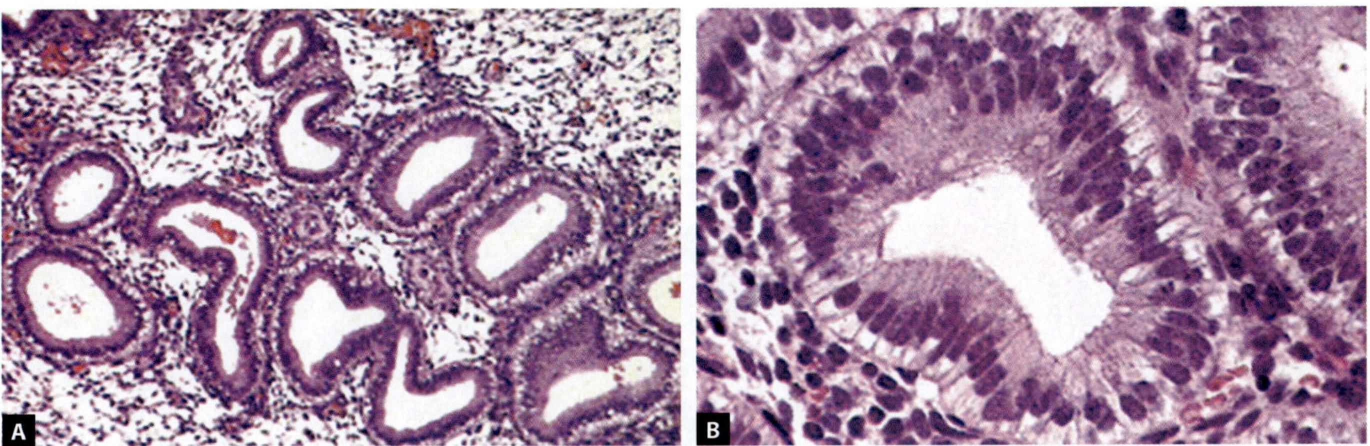

Figs. 8A and B: Early secretory endometrium with subnuclear vacuoles. The nuclei retain the dense chromatin of the proliferative phase. Uniformly present cytoplasmic vacuoles are the most useful marker of the first third of the secretory phase.

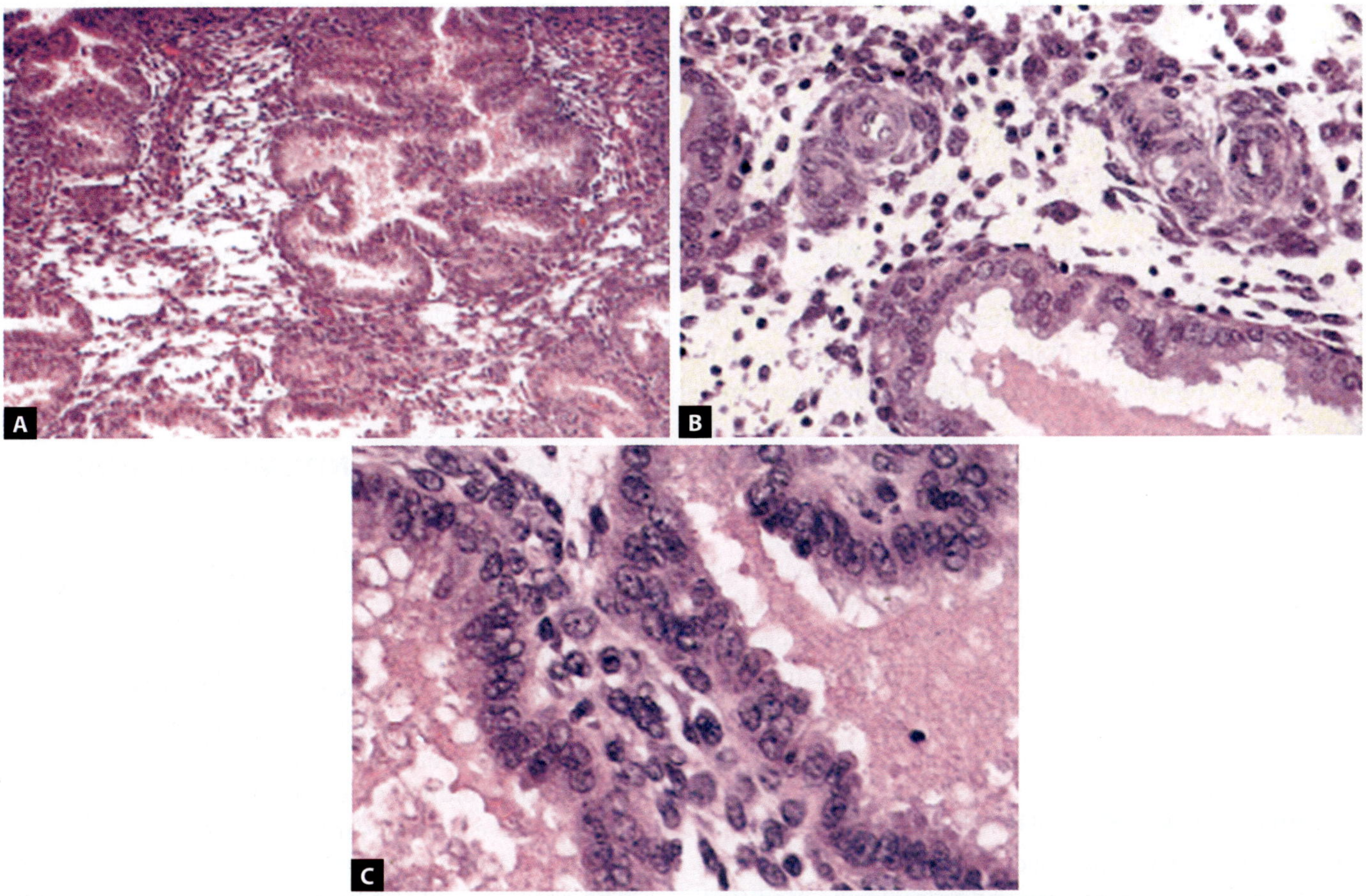

Figs. 9A to C: Midsecretory endometrium. The hallmarks of this period can be seen in these three photomicrographs. At low magnification (A), extreme glandular coiling and stromal oedema are apparent. At a somewhat higher magnification (B), the coiled spiral arteries are seen within an oedematous stroma. Perivascular predecidual reaction has not occurred. At yet higher magnification (C), the characteristically round vesicular nuclei of the midsecretory endometrium are apparent.

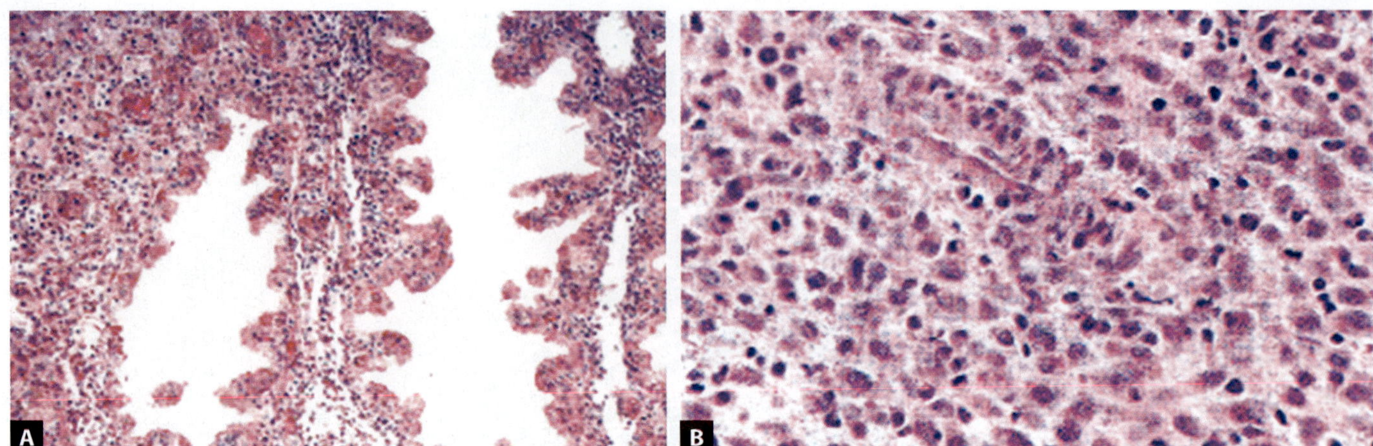

Figs. 10A and B: Late secretory endometrium. At low magnification (A), the serrated appearance of the gland reflects its coiled state. The stroma cells have undergone predecidual reaction (B). Predecidual reaction begins around the spiral arteries, and this reaction serves to distinguish midsecretory endometria from late secretory endometria.

shape of the glands. As the glands and cells increase in size, and possibly also because of increased pressure from the surrounding stroma, the gland walls infold so that, on cross section, they are crenated instead of round, and on longitudinal section, they appear 'corkscrew' and finally 'saw-toothed'. Meanwhile, the stroma as a whole becomes more vascular and oedematous. These changes give the stroma a reticular appearance although near the surface it shows a decidual reaction which makes it compact. The latter keeps the necks of the glands narrow and straight. Decidual reaction also occurs in the vicinity of blood vessels **(Table 1 and Figs. 11A and B)**. During its secretory phase, the endometrium shows three layers:

1. A superficial compact zone consisting of stroma (with decidual reaction) surrounding the mouths of the glands
2. A middle spongy functional layer—spongy because of the numerous dilated glands and oedematous stroma
3. An inactive basal layer that shows little secretory response. This is not shed during menstruation and from it the new endometrium is formed after each period.

Preparation for Implantation

On days 21–22 of the cycle, oedema of endometrial stroma occurs secondary to oestrogen and progesterone-mediated increase in prostaglandin production by the endometrium. Implantation requires endometrial haemostasis, and the maternal uterus requires resistance to invasion.

Phase of Endometrial Breakdown

Endometrial growth ceases 5 or 6 days before menstruation (22nd or 23rd day), and within 1 or 2 days, shrinkage is apparent. This occurs as a result of dehydration of the stroma, decreased blood flow and discharge of secretion from the glands. The stroma becomes infiltrated with leucocytes and some red blood cells. Menstruation is heralded by extravasations of serum and blood, which collect in small pools near the endometrial surface. These fragment the new necrotic endometrium and break through the surface epithelium, carrying pieces of it away in the bloody discharge, which is the menstrual flow. Loss of tissue occurs mainly on the 2nd and 3rd days.

CORRELATION OF ENDOMETRIAL AND OVARIAN CYCLE

By the end of, if not just before the onset of, a menstrual period, a new follicle is beginning to ripen in the ovary; endometrial proliferation therefore occurs during the follicular phase in the ovary and is the direct result of a mounting oestrogen influence **(Figs. 11A and B)**.

Ovulation marks the changeover from the proliferative to the secretory phase in the endometrium. Secretory activity and decidual reaction are manifestations of the luteal phase in the ovary and are brought about by progesterone acting in the presence of oestrogens.

The shrinkage of the endometrium premenstrually coincides with the commencement of the failure of corpus luteum activity and is the direct result of the withdrawal of the supporting effect of oestrogens and progesterone.

TABLE 1: Main histologic features of the menstrual cycle. Histologic classification stages, according to a 28-day idealised cycle in which day 1 is the first day of clinical menses and ovulation occurs on day 14.

Endometrial phase					***Secretory***				
		Menstrual	***Proliferative***	***'Interval'***	***Early***		***Mid***	***Late***	
Day of 28 days cycle (ovulation on D14)		1–3	4–15	-16	17	18	19–21	22–24	25–28
Key feature		Stromal crumbling	Mitoses	Subnuclear vacuoles, staggered, with mitoses	Subnuclear vacuoles, regular with mitoses	• Subnuclear and supranuclear vacuoles • No mitoses	Stromal oedema	Focal predecidua around spiral arteries	Predecidua involves surface
Microscopic features of functional zone	Stroma	• Stromal aggregates • "Blue balls" haemorrhage	• Loose stroma • Mitoses	• Loose stroma • Mitoses	Loose stroma, scanty mitoses	Loose stroma, scanty mitoses	Stromal oedema increases from D19–21	Perivascular "naked nuclei" (D22) from predecidual cuffs (D23) that bridge vessels (D24)	• Focal (D25) then extensive (D26) surface predecidua extends downward (D26-28) • Prominent granulated lymphocytes
	Glands	Collapsed epithelium and displaced secretory glands	• Straight to tightly coiled tubules • Mitoses	• Some staggered subnuclear vacuoles • Many mitoses	• "Piano key" subnuclear vacuoles • Some mitoses	• Some staggered subnuclear vacuoles • No mitoses	• Dilated glands with irregular outlines • Luminal secretion	"Saw tooth" glands	Prominent "saw tooth" glands
Appearances		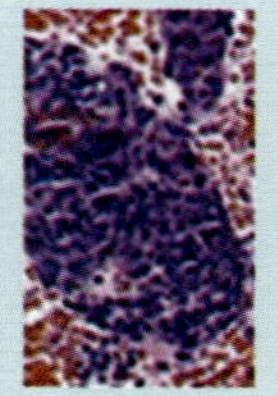	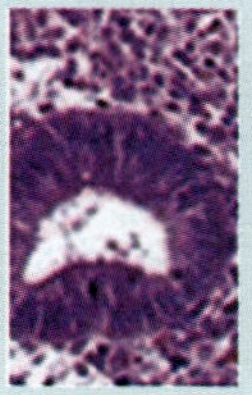	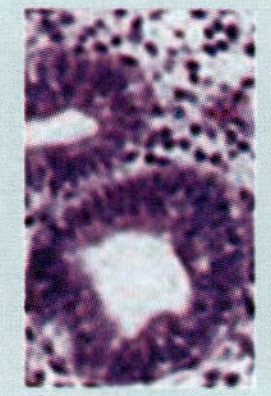	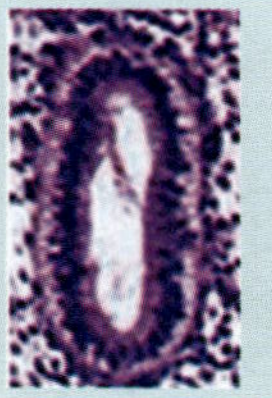	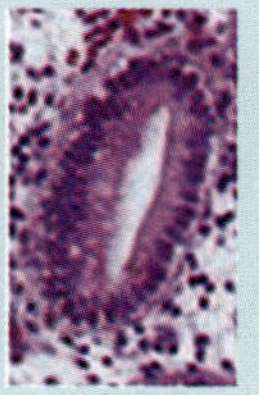	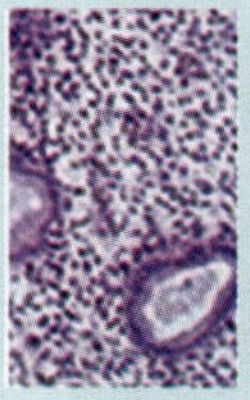	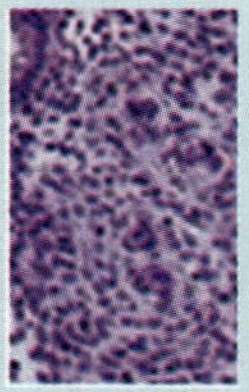	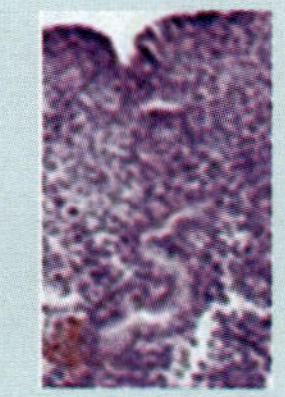

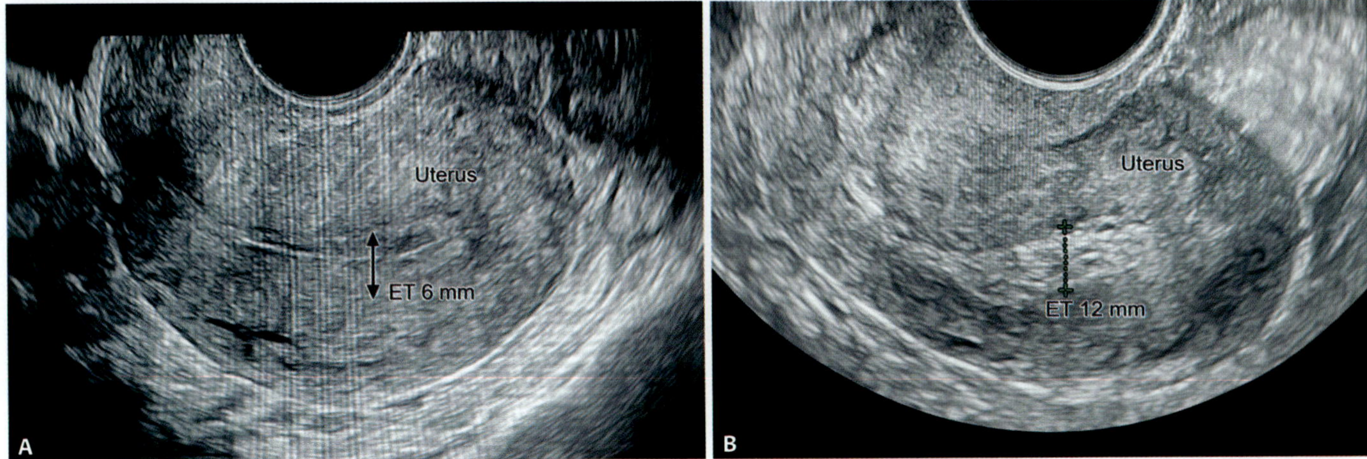

Figs. 11A and B: Ultrasonography (USG) images of endometrium: (A) Proliferative phase and (B) secretory phase. (ET: endometrial thickness)

These are the fundamental correlations with ovarian activity, although the timing of the histological cycle does not exactly match the rise and fall of hormone levels in the plasma **(Fig. 12)**.

Hormonal Variations

The relative pattern of ovarian, uterine and hormonal variation along the normal menstrual cycle is seen.

At the beginning of each monthly menstrual cycle, levels of gonadal steroids are low and have been decreasing since the end of the luteal phase of the previous cycle.

With the demise of the corpus luteum, follicle-stimulating hormone (FSH) levels begin to rise, and a cohort of growing follicles is recruited. These follicles each secrete increasing levels of oestrogen as they grow in the follicular phase. This, in turn, is the stimulus for uterine endometrial proliferation. Rising oestrogen levels provide negative feedback on pituitary FSH secretion, which begins to reduce by the midpoint of the follicular phase. Late in the follicular phase the luteinising hormone (LH) level is increased dramatically (biphasic response). At the end of the follicular phase (just prior to ovulation), FSH-induced LH receptors are present on granulosa cells and, with LH stimulation, modulate the secretion of progesterone.

With the oestrogen rising to a peak, the pituitary LH surge is triggered, which induces ovulation 24–36 hours later. Ovulation is the beginning of the transition to the luteal phase of the ovary or the secretory phase of the endometrium. The oestrogen level decreases through the early luteal phase from just before ovulation until the midluteal phase, when it begins to rise again as a result of corpus luteum secretion. Progesterone levels rise precipitously after ovulation and can be used as a presumptive sign that ovulation has occurred. Both oestrogen and progesterone levels remain elevated through the lifespan of the corpus luteum and then wane with its demise, thereby setting the stage for the next cycle **(Fig. 12 and Table 2)**.

UTERINE BLEEDING

The phenomenon of uterine bleeding is best considered from the experimental aspect.

- If a woman without ovaries but possessing a normal uterus is given large doses of oestrogens for a few weeks and the administration is then suddenly discontinued, uterine haemorrhage always occurs 2–10 days later. This is termed *oestrogen withdrawal bleeding*.
- If progesterone is substituted for oestrogen in this experiment, then, provided the uterus has been previously primed with oestrogens, *progesterone withdrawal bleeding* occurs within 2–5 days of suspension of medication.
- A mixture of oestrogens and progesterone has a similar effect.
- If large doses of oestrogens are given first and then replaced by progesterone, no bleeding occurs on withholding the oestrogen. It is deferred until the progesterone is withdrawn. Progesterone is an adequate substitute for oestrogen but the converse is not true.
- If, in the first type of experiment, only a small dose of oestrogen is administered, no effect is seen when it is withdrawn.
- If, however, a moderate dose of oestrogen is given, then bleeding sometimes occurs intermittently, even while treatment is in progress.

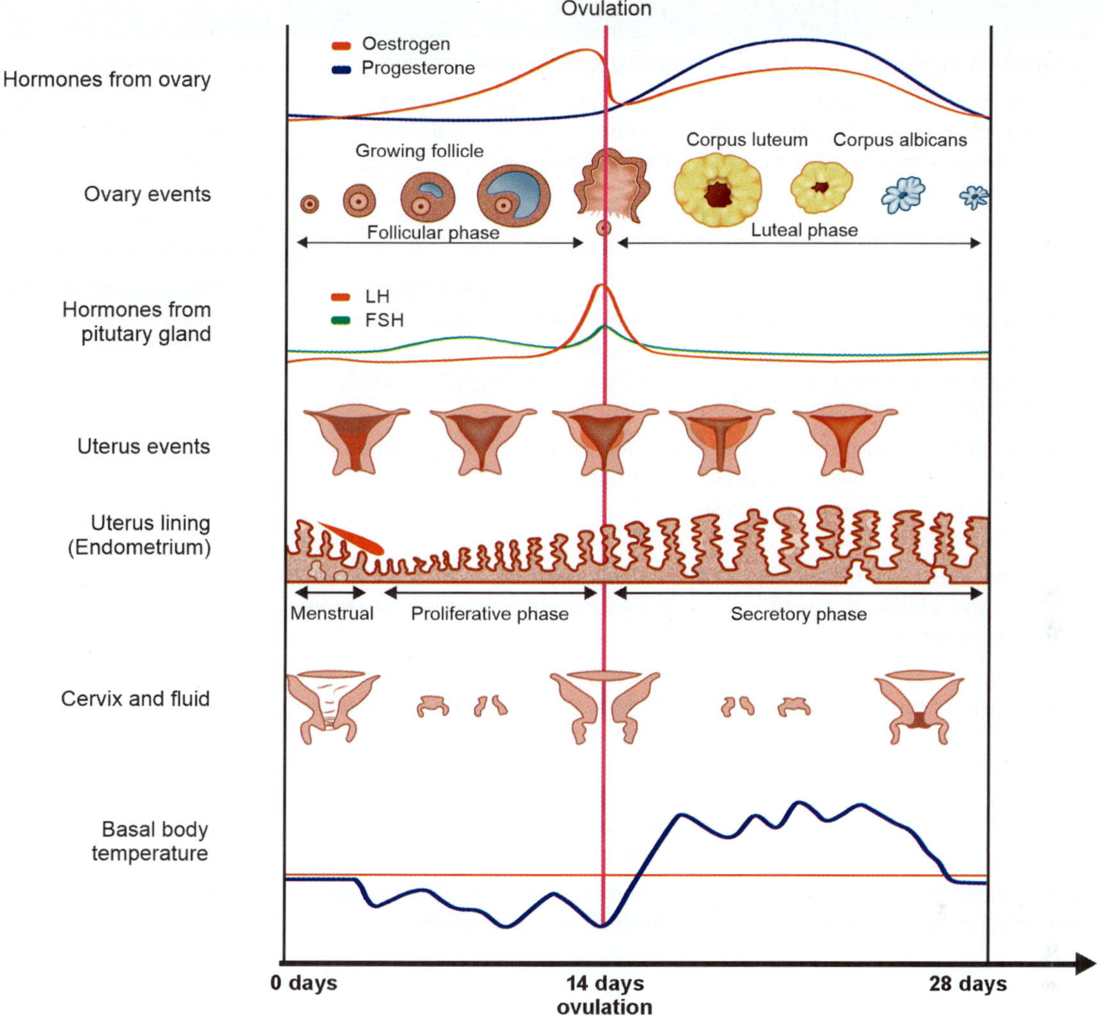

Fig. 12: Diagrammatic representation of the hormonal control of the ovarian and endometrial cycles. (FSH: follicle-stimulating hormone; LH: luteinising hormone)

Observations such as these have given rise to a concept of a *bleeding threshold* level of oestrogens in the bloodstream. The quantitative value of this level is unknown, and its existence is hypothetical. Nevertheless, the idea is of practical value and is illustrated in **Figure 13**. If the critical level is not reached, that is, if the amount of oestrogen administered is too small, no bleeding occurs. If the oestrogen level is pushed above the threshold, then no bleeding takes place so long as it remains above, but once it drops to and below the threshold, haemorrhage occurs. If, however, the amount of oestrogen administered is such as to keep the blood level at or about the threshold, then bleeding may occur even while oestrogen is being given. This is generally called 'breakthrough' bleeding.

The above observations explain why removal of an ovary, or of the corpus luteum, at operation is often followed by uterine bleeding 2 or 3 days later.

Menstruation

As a result of the ovarian cycle, the uterus is subjected to the influence first of oestrogens and then of a combination of oestrogens and progesterone. Both are withdrawn when the corpus luteum degenerates and menstruation occurs within a few days, that is, as soon as their levels fall to, and below, the bleeding threshold. There is some dispute as to whether the period represents oestrogen deprival haemorrhage or progesterone deprival haemorrhage, but this is an academic argument.

TABLE 2: Female reproductive cycle.

Days	*Changes in the ovary*	*Changes in the endometrium*	*Hormonal changes*
1–5	*Follicular phase:* Follicles further develop and compete for dominance; one outgrows the others. The other follicles become atretic	*Menstruation phase:* The endometrium breaks and is shed as menstruation	Luteinising hormone (LH) and follicle-stimulating hormone (FSH) (hormones secreted from the anterior pituitary) act on ovaries to stimulate follicular growth. The follicles secrete oestrogen and progesterone
6–11	*Follicular phase:* A single dominant follicle continues to grow The oocyte inside is maturing and begins producing oestrogen	*Proliferative phase:* Oestrogen secreted from the growing follicle causes the endometrium to grow and thicken, thereby preparing for implantation	The follicles continue to secrete oestrogen and progesterone
12–13	*Follicular phase:* LH surge occurs. The rise in LH causes the follicle to rupture over the next 24–36 hours and release a mature oocyte	*Proliferative phase:* The endometrium continues to grow	Rising levels of oestrogen reach a point that causes a rapid rise in LH
14	*Ovulation phase:* The follicle wall ruptures and releases the mature oocyte from the ovary	*Proliferative phase:* The endometrium continues to grow	
15–20	*Luteal phase:* The remains of the follicle that released the oocyte form a structure called the *corpus luteum*	*Secretory phase:* Progesterone from *the corpus luteum* brings about secretory changes in the uterus and prepares it for implantation Progesterone also raises basal body temperature (BBT)	Corpus luteum secretes progesterone
21–28 If the oocyte was fertilised	*Luteal phase:* The corpus luteum continues to secrete progesterone	*Secretory phase:* After about 9 days, the embryo gets implanted	• The embryo releases human chorionic gonadotrophin (hCG) • Corpus luteum produces progesterone until 11 weeks of pregnancy, when the uteroplacental shift takes place
21–28 If the egg was NOT fertilised	*Luteal phase:* The corpus luteum transforms into the *corpus albicans*	*Secretory phase:* Without progesterone from the corpus luteum, the endometrium begins to break up and is eventually shed again (a new cycle begins)	Hormones fall back to their original levels

The fundamental cause of menstruation is degeneration of the corpus luteum, and this only degenerates if the ovum is not fertilised. Menstruation represents the breaking down and casting off of an endometrium prepared for a pregnancy, which does not materialise, and so is sometimes described as 'the weeping of a disappointed uterus.'

With the withdrawal of sex steroids, there is a profound spiral artery vascular spasm that ultimately leads to endometrial ischaemia. Simultaneously, there is a breakdown of lysosomes and a release of proteolytic enzymes, which further promote local tissue destruction. This layer of endometrium is then shed, leaving the decidua basalis as the source of subsequent endometrial growth. Prostaglandins are produced throughout the menstrual cycle and are at their highest concentration during menses. Prostaglandin $F_{2\alpha}$ ($PGF_{2\alpha}$) is a potent vasoconstrictor, causing further arteriolar vasospasm and endometrial ischaemia. $PGF_{2\alpha}$ also produces myometrial contractions that decrease local uterine wall blood flow and may serve to physically expel sloughing endometrial tissue from the uterus.

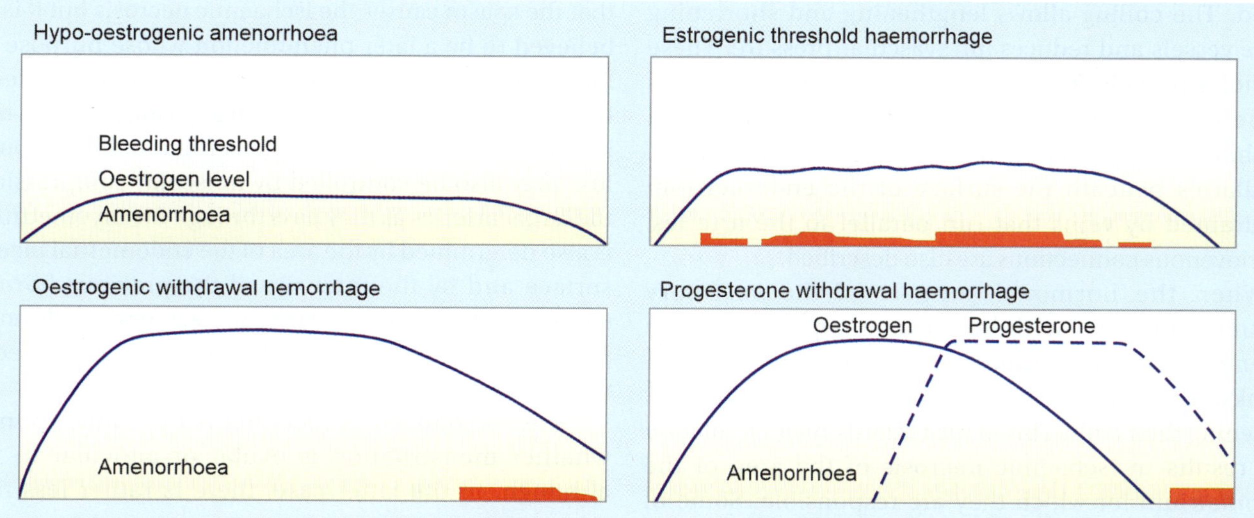

Fig. 13: The theoretical concept of a blood threshold level of hormones to account for different types of uterine bleeding. The black areas on the baseline indicate episodes of bleeding.

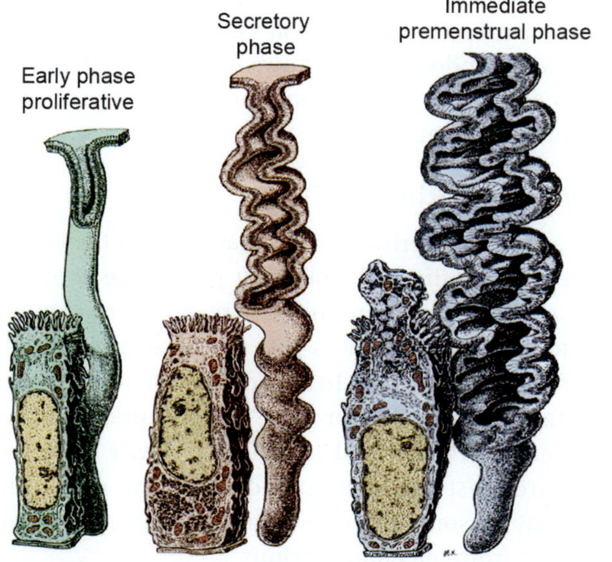

Fig. 14: Diagrammatic representation of the endometrial glands and arterioles throughout the menstrual cycle. The veins are omitted for simplicity. The endometrium deep to the dotted line is relatively insensitive to hormones and is not shed during menstruation; its viability is maintained by special branches from the straight portions of the arterioles.

Anovular Menstruation

Degeneration of the corpus luteum was suggested as the cause of menstruation long before ovarian hormones and their effects were discovered, but the idea was always questioned because it was noted that sometimes there is no sign of a recent corpus luteum in the ovary when the abdomen is opened during a menstrual period. This observation is now explained by the phenomenon of *anovular menstruation*. Sometimes, a follicle ripens but fails to rupture and is not converted to a corpus luteum. After a phase of activity, the follicle degenerates, and there is thus a rise and fall in oestrogen production, the latter giving rise to oestrogen withdrawal haemorrhage. This can be completely cyclical and is outwardly indistinguishable from normal menstruation. It can, however, be recognised by histological examination of the endometrium, which remains proliferative or hyperplastic but never secretory. Anovular menstruation is also always painless and unaccompanied by the usual menstrual molimina.

Anovular menstruation occurs occasionally in all women. It is probably not uncommon during the first 2 or 3 years of menstrual life and after the age of 40 years, the incidence may rise to as high as 1 in 4 cycles. In the active reproductive period, however, not more than 1 in 10 to 1 in 50 regular cycles is anovular. For practical purposes, regular menstruation in mature women means regular ovulation.

Mechanism of Bleeding from the Endometrium

The main arteries supplying the endometrium lie where the muscle mucosal elements of the uterus intermingle, and they run parallel to the endometrium. Arterioles from these basal arteries come off at right angles and are directed towards the uterine cavity **(Fig. 14)**. In the first part of their course, they are straight, but more superficially they are coiled. The coiling allows lengthening and shortening of the vessels and reduces intravascular pressure. These arterioles provide for the middle and superficial layers of the endometrium, each supplying a limited area and having very little communication with its fellows. Capillaries beneath the surface of the endometrium are drained by veins that run parallel to the arteries. Arteriovenous connections are also described.

When the hormonal support of the secretory endometrium is withdrawn consequent to the degeneration of the corpus luteum, the endometrium shrinks and the vessels have to shorten by increasing and tightening their coils. This in turn retards their circulation and results in ischaemic necrosis of the area of the endometrium for which they are responsible. Some of the capillary stasis and other changes such as leucocytic infiltration of the stroma are caused by haemodynamic factors, which are not understood, but some authorities believe that there is an arteriovenous shunt. Increased premenstrual permeability of the capillary reflects an oestrogen influence.

The breakdown does not occur simultaneously in all parts of the endometrium and each microscopic area bleeds intermittently for short periods, but the endometrium oozes from one part or another for a total of 3–5 days. The bleeding itself occurs from broken arteries, veins and capillaries, and from haematomas, which form in the stroma in the immediate premenstrual phase.

Having entered the uterine cavity, the blood coagulates, but the clot is mostly dissolved by thrombolysis released from the endometrium. Proactivator of plasminogen is present in the endometrium at all times and, with the approach of menstruation, is converted to activator, probably as a result of anoxia or breakdown of tissue. Fibrin degradation products therefore circulate in increased amounts during menstruation, and especially high levels are found in the uterine veins.

As a result of fibrinolysis, the effluent from the uterus consists of altered blood, rich in calcium but deficient in prothrombin and fibrinogen. The expulsion of this, together with fragments of endometrium, is brought about by uterine contractions.

The occurrence of spasm in the straight stems of the endometrial arterioles is very important. This is seen about the time that bleeding commences and may be the result of the action of the $PGF_{2\alpha}$ released from the degenerating surface of the endometrium. It was at one time thought that the spasm causes the ischaemic necrosis but it is now believed to be a later phenomenon whose purpose is to limit the amount of bleeding from the arteriole. Indeed, it is alleged that but for this protective spasm, a woman might bleed to death as a result of menstruation. The amount of loss may also be controlled by muscular compression of the larger arteries as they pass through the myometrium. It is also determined by the area of the endometrial bleeding surface and by the intensity of the previous hormone stimulus. Other vasoconstrictors, e.g. endothelium and platelet-activating factor (PAF) have been identified but their exact role is unclear.

The mechanism of bleeding is the same no matter whether menstruation is ovular or anovular in type, although, in the latter case, there is rather less tissue destruction.

When the endometrium breaks down, the basal layers are not involved because they are supplied by blood vessels, which come off the main arteriole proximal to the part affected by coiling and spasm **(Fig. 13)**. Postmenstrually, new arterioles grow from the old stumps just as the endometrium grows from its basal layer. They do so as a result of the oestrogen stimulus from the next ripening Graafian follicle.

MYOMETRIAL CYCLE

The activity of uterine muscle changes with the menstrual cycle. During the early follicular phase, the contractions are small and frequent and the response to oxytocics is limited. Activity increases with the oestrogen stimulus of approaching ovulation. In the premenstrual and menstrual phases, the contractions are less frequent but are of greater amplitude, and muscle sensitivity is increased. The strongest contractions occur during menstruation and may, to some extent, be stimulated by *prostaglandins* released from the endometrium.

CYCLICAL CHANGES IN THE TUBE

The muscle of the fallopian tube behaves like the myometrium in that it shows increased movement about the time of ovulation. This is an oestrogen effect, as is the increased cilial activity at that time. These changes are timed to propel the ovum towards the uterus.

The follicular phase is marked by slight proliferation, with minimal mitotic activity of the mucosa, and this continues up to the premenstrual phase when it regresses. During menstruation, there is further shrinkage and slight shedding of the surface epithelium; occasionally, the endosalpinx may even menstruate.

The secretory activity of the tube is also cyclical, being highest just before ovulation and in response to oestrogen. Progesterone may also play a part in this, but the consensus of opinion is that this hormone reduces the amount of secretion.

CERVICAL CYCLE

Progesterone raises the tone of the muscles of the isthmus and internal os, so the cervical 'sphincter' is tighter and more competent during the luteal than during the follicular phase. The glandular elements of the cervix proliferate during the follicular phase, and the epithelial cells become taller. Under the influence of oestrogens, the glands also actively secrete mucus which will stretch into threads measuring >6.5 cm, and even 10–15 cm, at the time of ovulation. This property of 'spinnbarkeit' is the basis of the thread test for oestrogen in circulation. During the follicular phase, the cervical mucus absorbs water and salts and, when allowed to dry, deposits crystals of sodium chloride and potassium chloride in a characteristic pattern that suggests the fronds of a fern (*see* **Fig. 3** in **Chapter 5**). At the time of ovulation, the secretion is so profuse that it may be noticeable as a vaginal discharge—the 'ovulation cascade.' Its special character at this time makes for its easy penetration by spermatozoa. This property is related to its low content of protein.

During the luteal phase, the cervical glands become more branched and their secretion changes its physical and chemical properties. The mucus becomes more viscous and forms a more secure cervical plug. It loses its ability to stretch without breaking and resists penetration by spermatozoa. These changes are brought about by progesterone and are related to an increase in the amount of protein in the mucus and to the presence of phospholipids.

Progesterone also reduces the electrolyte content of the mucus, so by the 22nd day of the cycle, its property of ferning or arborisation on drying is lost.

During menstruation, the cervical glands collapse and may show slight desquamation with loss of blood.

VAGINAL CYCLE

Cyclical histological changes occur in the vaginal epithelium, but they are not clearly defined in tissue sections. They are better seen in smears of desquamated cells. The unstimulated vagina shows relatively small basal-type cells with healthy nuclei. These and intermediate basophil forms are also seen in vaginal smears taken in the early follicular phase. The fully oestrogenic smear, evident during the late follicular phase, contains a preponderance of large cornified epithelial cells with pyknotic nuclei. These stain pink with eosin. During the luteal phase, the smear shows evidence of increased desquamation, many of the cells having rolled edges, and is characterised by the reappearance of clumps of intermediate cells and the presence of leucocytes.

The *maturation index*, which is the percentage of superficial, intermediate and parabasal cells in a vaginal smear, is used as a measure of the levels of hormones in circulation. It is a useful guide, but it is not as precise as assaying the hormones in blood.

CYCLICAL, METABOLIC, VASCULAR AND PSYCHOLOGICAL CHANGES

These are discussed in detail in **Chapter 5** (Section on Menstruation) and **Chapter 42**.

SUGGESTED READING

1. American College of Obstetricians and Gynaecologists. Menstruation in girls and adolescents: using the menstrual cycle as a vital sign (Committee opinion No. 65). Obstet Gynecol. 2015;126:e143-6. Reaffirmed 2021.
2. Munro MG, Critchley HOD, Fraser IS; FIGO Menstrual Disorders Committee. The two FIGO systems for normal and abnormal uterine bleeding symptoms and classification of causes of abnormal uterine bleeding in the reproductive years: 2018 revisions. Int J Gynaecol Obstet. 2018;143(3):393-408.
3. Reed BF, Carr BR. The normal menstrual cycle and the control of ovulation. In: Feingold KR, Ahmed SF, Anawalt B, Blackman MR, Boyce A, Chrousos G, Corpas E, de Herder WW, Dhatariya K, Dungan K, Hofland J, Kalra S, Kaltsas G, Kapoor N, Koch C, Kopp P, Korbonits M, Kovacs CS, Kuohung W, Laferrère B, Levy M, McGee EA, McLachlan R, Muzumdar R, Purnell J, Rey R, Sahay R, Shah AS, Singer F, Sperling MA, Stratakis CA, Trence DL, Wilson DP (Eds). Endotext (Review). South Dartmouth (MA): MDText.com, Inc.; 2018.
4. Salamonsen LA. Women in reproductive science: Understanding human endometrial function. Reproduction (Review). 2019;158(6):F55-F67.
5. Menstruation and the Menstrual Cycle Fact Sheet. Office of Women's Health. US Department of Health and Human Services; 2014.

6. Liu AY, Petit MA, Prior JC. Exercise and the hypothalamus: ovulatory adaptations. In: Hackney AC, Constantini NW (Eds). Endocrinology of Physical Activity and Sport. Contemporary Endocrinology. New York: Springer International Publishing. pp. 124-47.
7. Finn CA. Menstruation: a nonadaptive consequence of uterine evolution. Q Rev Biol (Review). 1998;73(2): 163-73.
8. Diaz A, Laufer MR, Breech LL. Menstruation in girls and adolescents: using the menstrual cycle as a vital sign. Pediatrics. 2006;118(5):2245-50.
9. Ecochard R, Gougeon A. Side of ovulation and cycle characteristics in normally fertile women. Hum Reprod. 2000;15(4):752-5.
10. Hall JE, Hall ME (Eds). Guyton and Hall Textbook of Medical Physiology, 14th edition. Elsevier - Health Science; 2021.

5

CHAPTER

Clinical Aspects of Menstruation and Ovulation

Nithesh Prabhu, Muralidhar V Pai

Chapter Outline

- Menstruation
- The Menopause and the Climacteric
- Abnormal Menopause
- Ovulation

INTRODUCTION

Menstruation is a regular, cyclical process that marks an important aspect of the female reproductive system. It involves shedding of the endometrial lining from the uterus, usually occurring every 21 to 35 days, and is regulated by a complex interplay of hormones. Menstruation begins during menarche and continues till menopause. Abnormal menstruation may reflect the various pathologies in the anatomy of the reproductive organs and hormonal imbalance within the body. It also plays a key role in infertility. This chapter will guide you through basics of the menstrual cycle, its hormonal control, normal and abnormal variations, its causes, clinical concerns and the treatment.

MENSTRUATION

General Description

Menstruation is the cyclic, orderly sloughing of the uterine lining, in response to the interactions of hormones produced by the hypothalamus, pituitary and ovaries.

The menarche is quite a late feature of puberty. The first period may be short or long; thereafter, the cycle is often irregular, with periods occurring sometimes every few months, sometimes too frequently. A more or less regular rhythm is usually established within 2–3 years. It begins at puberty, ranging from the ages of 10–16, and ends at menopause at an average age of 51 years.

Normal menstrual cycle is a tightly co-ordinated cycle of stimulatory and inhibitory effects that results in the release of a single mature oocyte from a pool of hundreds of thousands of primordial oocytes. Various changes occur at the endometrial and ovarian levels at the same time in order to ovulate and implant the egg if fertilised in that cycle. The cyclic changes in the major pituitary and gonadal hormones are responsible for menstruation **(Fig. 1)**.

During the active reproductive era, menstruation occurs at approximately 28-day intervals. Each woman

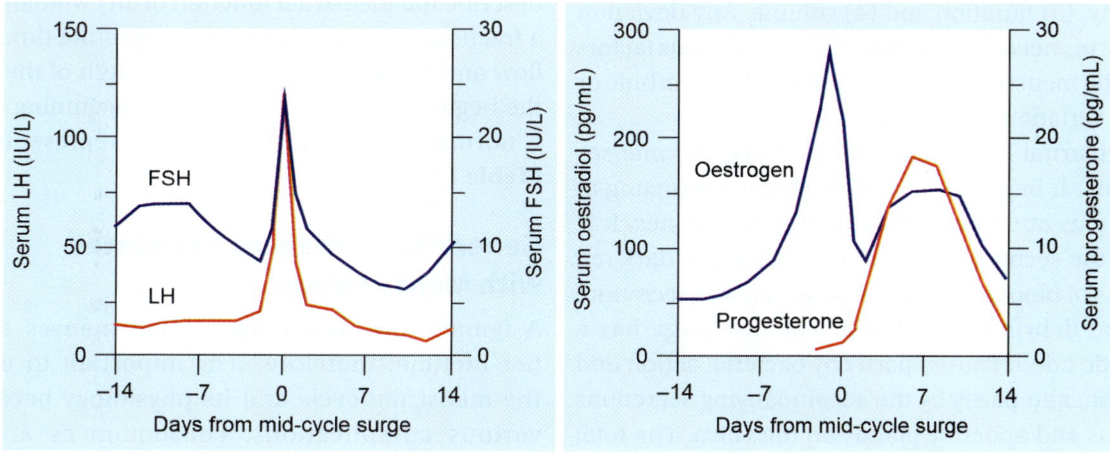

Fig. 1: Hormonal changes during menstruation. (FSH: follicle-stimulating hormone; LH: luteinizing hormone)

TABLE 1: Suggested normal limits for menstrual parameters in the mid-reproductive years.

Clinical dimensions of menstruation and menstrual cycle	*Descriptive terms*	*Normal limits (5th–95th percentiles)*
Frequency of menses (days)	Frequent	<24
	Normal	24–38
	Infrequent	>38
Regularity of menses (cycle-to-cycle variation over 12 months in days)	Absent	—
	Regular	Variation ±2 to 20
	Irregular	Variation >20
Duration of flow (days)	Prolonged	>8.0
	Normal	4.5–8.0
	Shortened	<4.5
Volume of monthly blood loss (mL)	Heavy	>80
	Normal	5–80
	Light	<5

Source: Hallberg L, Högdahl AM, Nilsson L, Rybo G. Menstrual blood loss—a population study. Variation at different ages and attempts to define normality. Acta Obstet Gynecol Scand. 1966;45(3):320-51.

tends to have her own rhythm, although it may change after marriage or childbearing. Any regular cycle of 3–5 weeks is arbitrarily accepted as normal, but some women menstruate less frequently than this and still have good health and fertility. Those women who allege that their menstrual function is always completely regular delude themselves, if not others: If records are kept, all can be shown to have occasional cycles which vary by at least 2 days less or more than 28 days.

In the same way, there are wide variations in the duration and amount of blood loss. The duration is most often from 3 to 5 days, but anything between 2 and 7 days is accepted as normal; even these limits need to be extended in individual cases. Hence, there are four parameters used to define normal uterine bleeding—(1) frequency, (2) regularity, (3) duration and (4) volume. Any deviation from the norms needs evaluation. There are various factors that affect the menstrual cycle including cultural, ethnic or geographic variation components.

The menstrual flow is sometimes called the menses or catamenia. It begins as a pink discharge consisting of cervical mucus and blood and is rich in leucocytes. It is heavier on the second and third days when it is dark red and consists of blood, endometrial and cervical secretion, endometrial debris and bacteria. The discharge has a characteristic odour caused partly by bacterial action and degeneration, and partly by the accompanying secretions of sebaceous and apocrine glands on the vulva. The total loss of blood is difficult to estimate but is said normally to vary from 5 to 60 or 80 mL, with an average of 35–45 mL. This is equivalent to an average daily loss of 0.6–0.7 mg iron throughout each month.

Menstrual blood is chiefly arterial, with only 25% of the blood being venous blood. It contains prostaglandins, tissue debris and relatively large amounts of fibrinolysis from endometrial tissue. Normally, high fibrinolytic activity makes the menstrual efflux mainly fluid; small clots are noticed occasionally by 50% of women. The passage of large clots usually means that the bleeding is so abnormally heavy as to defeat the process of fibrinolysis.

The length of a menstrual cycle is the number of days between the first day of menstrual bleeding of one cycle to the onset of menses of the next cycle. It is convenient to describe the menstrual function of any woman in terms of a fraction, the numerator referring to the duration of the flow and the denominator to the length of the cycle from the beginning of one period to the beginning of the next. A normal cycle may, therefore, be represented by 4/28 **(Table 1)**.

General Disturbances Associated with Menstruation

A female has an average of 450 menses throughout her lifetime; therefore, it is important to understand the menstrual cycle and its physiology because of the various complications, consequences and distress that it may have for a female patient. There are various types of menstrual disorders, including dysmenorrhea, premenstrual symptoms, menorrhagia, polymenorrhea, abnormal vaginal bleeding, amenorrhea, oligomenorrhea and irregular menstruation, which may or may not require any active treatment.

Menstruation can also be accompanied by minor physical and nervous disturbances. It is estimated that only 20% of women are completely free from discomfort or upset and that only 3% of young nullipara do not experience premenstrual molimina of some kind. The degree of disturbance, however, depends to a large extent on the individual's outlook towards this physiological process and on her determination not to allow it to interfere with her normal life. Highly strung emotional women exaggerate the significance of menstruation while well-balanced individuals disregard it. About 50% of women <30 years of age experience an ache or pain in the lower abdomen, pelvis or back before or during menstruation.

Studies have shown that a large proportion of the female population of reproductive age suffers from menstruation-related health issues. Menstrual problems not only carry an economic burden but are also one of the most common causes of absenteeism and poor academic performance among young females. Stress can be a major contributor or cause of menstrual irregularities, and an association has been documented between stress and various menstrual irregularities including menorrhagia, oligomenorrhea, dysmenorrhea and premenstrual syndrome (PMS).

General manifestations mainly occur premenstrually and include a feeling of lethargy and tiredness, malaise, depression, excitability and irritability, headache, fullness and tenderness of the breasts, inability to concentrate and impairment of efficiency in both mental and physical activities **(Fig. 2)**. It is of interest to note that the majority of accidental and suicidal deaths among women occur during the luteal phase of the cycle. Oestrogen-associated migraine headaches can occur in relation to the menstrual cycle; headache should occur over a minimum of three menstrual cycles to make the diagnosis. These menstrual headaches occur in close temporal relationship to the onset of menstruation, starting from 2 days prior to 3 days after the first day of menses or withdrawal bleeding. These headaches do not occur outside of menses. The headaches can occur with or without an aura. Sometimes the combination of all these abovementioned symptoms related to menses is referred to as PMS where they experience a wide variety of cyclic and recurrent physical, emotional, behavioural and cognitive symptoms that begin in the luteal phase (second half) of the menstrual cycle and resolve shortly after the onset of menses. The core feature is the recurrent onset of symptoms during the end of the luteal phase of the menstrual cycle with a symptom-free period shortly after menses has begun, typically when the menstrual flow has ended. Moderate-to-severe PMS symptoms have been associated with reductions in health-related quality of life, as well as a decrease in work productivity, increase in work absenteeism and an increase in visits to ambulatory healthcare providers

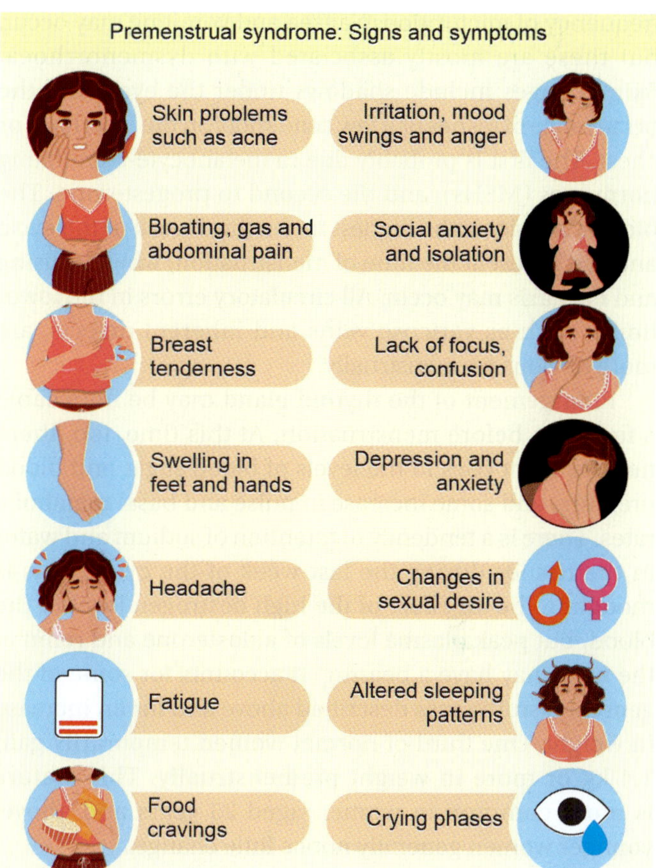

Fig. 2: Signs and symptoms of premenstrual syndrome.

Many women have a sensation of an impending period, which includes a feeling of weight in the pelvis, possibly related to congestion of the pelvic viscera. This is followed by a sensation of relief when the period is well-established. Changes in bowel function occur in 50% of women, the most common being a tendency to constipation (with abdominal distension) premenstrually and more frequent motions during menstruation. This is a result of a disturbance in the autonomic nervous system as may also be premenstrual frequency of micturition. Nausea and vomiting may occur, but these are mostly associated with dysmenorrhoea. Skin changes include shadows under the eyes, and the occurrence of rashes or a few acne spots on the face, back or chest. The first is probably due to melanocyte-stimulating hormones (MSHs), and the second to progesterone. The blood viscosity is the highest in the third week of the cycle and the lowest at the time of menstruation, when bruising and epistaxis may occur. All circulatory errors in the lower limbs, such as varicose veins and inherent defects, are more obvious premenstrually.

Enlargement of the thyroid gland may be noticeable a few days before menstruation. At this time, too, there may be slight rises in the levels of blood sugar and blood pressure, and some increase in pulse and basal metabolic rates. There is a tendency to retention of sodium and water in the tissues during the last week of the cycle. This is thought to be an effect of the high oestrogen level in the blood, but peak plasma levels of aldosterone and renin at the time may have a bearing. It accounts for some of the general disturbances described above and for an increase in weight. One third of normal women temporarily gain 1.4 kg or more in weight premenstrually. This feature is more common in women aged 25 years and above; younger women generally notice little change.

Management of Normal Menstruation

Menstruation is still a subject of taboo, superstition and folklore, and the handing on of these to young girls can be responsible for abnormal reactions to menstruation. One of the fallacies, which carries the support of religious practices, is that the menstruating woman is unclean. This idea alone is enough to instill feelings of shame, embarrassment and resentment. Again, it is commonly believed that girls are in a low physical state during menstruation, that they are especially vulnerable to all manner of ills, and that dire results will follow bathing or even washing their hair at this time. These beliefs are to be resisted and corrected. The menstrual function should be explained to girls truthfully, if simply, and they should be made to realise that it is not a method for excreting something which is noxious but rather a manifestation of womanhood. There is no need for them to stop playing games or for not undertaking anything to which they are accustomed. Indeed, they should be encouraged to live their usual life.

Many types of menstrual products absorb or collect blood during your period, including sanitary pads, tampons, menstrual cups, menstrual discs and period underwear can be used. In either case, regular and frequent changes are necessary if offensiveness and chafing are to be avoided.

Follow few instructions when you are using menstrual products, in addition to instructions that come with the product:

- Wash your hands before and after using the restroom and before using a menstrual product.
- *Discard used disposable menstrual products properly:* Wrap them with toilet paper, a tissue or other material and then toss them in a trash bin. Do not flush menstrual products down the toilet.
- *Sanitary pads:* Change sanitary pads every few hours, no matter how light the flow. Change them more frequently if your period is heavy.
- *Tampons:* Change tampons every 4–8 hours. Do not wear a single tampon for >8 hours at a time:
  - Use the lowest absorbency tampon needed. If you can wear one tampon for up to 8 hours without changing, the absorbency may be too high.
- *Menstrual cups:* Clean cups every day after use. Sanitise menstrual cups after your period is over by rinsing them thoroughly and then placing them in boiling water for 1–2 minutes.
- *Period underwear:* Most reusable period underwear is machine washable. Follow the product directions on the best way to clean.

Intravaginal tampons are comfortable, unobtrusive and convenient. It is said that they shorten the apparent duration of a period by 24 hours, because the last day of the flow ordinarily consists only of drainage from the vagina. Their disadvantages are as follows:

- They cannot be used unless the hymen is torn or stretched.
- One may be forgotten and left in the vagina for several weeks when it can cause pelvic infection. This should not happen to an intelligent woman, but it does, and a stinking tampon has sometimes to be removed in an outpatient clinic.
- They are inefficient if the flow is heavy.
- In general, the proper use of tampons does not lead to vaginitis, cervicitis, erosion or lowered fertility. In 1978, the toxic shock syndrome (TSS) was first described in children with acute infection due to *Staphylococcus aureus*. Subsequently, the syndrome was described in the United States in association with menstruation and the use of tampons. No particular type of tampon has

been implicated. One can reassure women that the risk of contracting TSS is very low and can be reduced by using tampons for part of the period only (using pads at night), and using only the standard size which are changed more frequently.

One possible contraindication to the use of tampons is the presence of an intrauterine contraceptive device, which has a tail lying in the cervical canal or vagina. This may become entangled with the result that the device is displaced on removal of the tampon.

A few hygiene practices can be followed to stay healthy and comfortable during menses:

- *Wear lightweight, breathable clothing:* Tight fabrics can trap moisture and heat, allowing germs to thrive
- *Change your menstrual products regularly:* Trapped moisture provides a breeding ground for bacteria and fungi. Wearing a pad or period underwear for too long can lead to a rash or an infection.
- *Keep your genital area clean:* Wash the outside of your vagina (vulva) and bottom every day. When you go to the bathroom, wipe from the front of your body towards the back, not the other way. Use only water to rinse your vulva. The vagina is a self-cleaning organ. Changing the natural pH balance of your vagina by washing or using chemicals to cleanse out the vagina can be harmful and may result in a yeast infection or bacterial vaginosis.
- *Use unscented toilet paper, tampons, or pads:* Scented hygiene products can irritate the skin and impact your natural pH balance.
- *Drink enough liquids:* This can help wash out your urinary tract and help prevent infections, such as vaginal candidiasis.
- *Track and monitor your period:* Your menstrual cycle is a valuable marker for your overall health. You can track your period on a calendar or with an app on your phone designed for this purpose.
- Visit a healthcare provider for your annual check-up. An annual well-woman examination is a full check-up that includes a pap smear, a pelvic exam and a breast exam. These exams are essential for good reproductive health as they can catch early signs of cancer or other health issues.

In some countries, young girls are taught to douche the vagina at the end of each menstrual period. This again is a relic of the old idea of uncleanliness. Vaginal douching as a hygienic measure at the end of a period, or at any other time, is unnecessary and is potentially harmful in that it washes away the natural protective discharges. The vagina can take care of itself and it is remarkable how it cleans itself of all menstrual debris in the course of a few hours. Girls and women should also be warned against the use of vulvar and vaginal deodorant powders and sprays. They are unnecessary and very liable to produce local reactions. Talc-containing deodorants have been implicated as an aetiological factor for ovarian cancer.

Although many married couples shun coitus during menstruation, its practice at such a time is probably more frequent than is generally realised. The menstrual phase is part of the safe period, and some women have a strong sexual desire at that time. Many women, however, react to menstruation with embarrassment and increased modesty (the taboo of uncleanliness) and resist coitus at that time. The Jewish law forbids coitus during the period (or for 5 days, whichever is the shorter) and for 7 days afterwards, making a total of 12 days in any one cycle. It is remarkable that this old code provided for abstinence during what is now recognised as a safe period and allowed resumption of marital relations at the optimum time for conception.

Medical arguments against the practice of coitus during menstruation are that sexual excitement may cause uterine congestion and increase the menstrual flow, that the more vascular and friable vaginal walls may be injured, and that the associated orgasm may encourage retrograde menstruation and the development of endometriosis. These are theoretical considerations of little practical significance. If there is a chronic or latent infection in the genital tract of either the male or the female, there is danger of causing salpingitis if coitus is practiced during menstruation, but in a healthy couple, there is no sound medical reason for advising against it. The only real objection is the obvious aesthetic one.

Artificial Deferment or Advancement of Menstruation

Some women, anticipating that a menstrual period will clash with an important business or social engagement, ask to have their onset changed. A dysmenorrhoeic student may fear that her period will commence on the day of a professional examination; the athlete is worried lest menstruation mar her performance; the prospective bride is embarrassed at the thought that her marriage is planned to coincide with the menses. In nearly all such cases, it is best to advise that no treatment be given, because a clash is not inevitable in that the date of the next menstrual period can never be calculated accurately, and the anticipation of the important occasion may itself make the period early or late; also, the hormone therapy necessary may be more upsetting than the period and may result in breakthrough bleeding.

If the circumstances appear to justify taking action, it is generally better to postpone than to advance the flow. This can be done by maintaining the ovarian hormone levels in the blood artificially at the time when their natural fall would lead to menstruation. For this purpose, oral therapy with one of the oestrogen-progestogen contraceptive preparations (one or two pills daily), or with a progestogen such as norethisterone, 5 mg TDS, is usually adequate. Treatment is commenced 3–6 days before the expected onset of the period and is continued until the crisis is over. The flow is to be expected 2 or 3 days after the treatment is suspended.

To bring on menstruation prematurely, it is necessary to start treatment early in the cycle and to suppress ovulation. This can be done by giving an oestrogen-progestogen oral contraceptive once daily. Treatment is commenced on the fifth day of the cycle and continued for 14 days. When it is suspended, menstruation (anovular) is likely to begin within 2 or 3 days, i.e. approximately 1 week before it would otherwise have occurred.

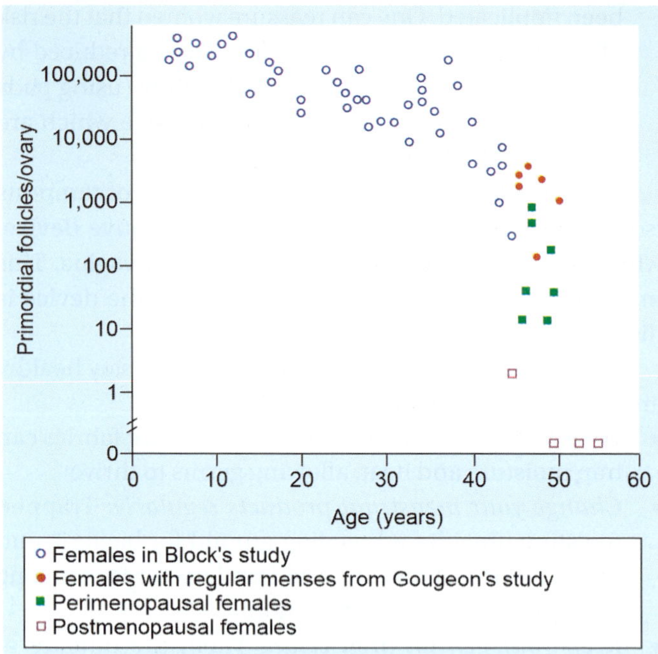

Fig. 3: A comparison of the relationship between age and primordial follicle number in Block's study of 44 females aged 7–44 years with that of Gougeon's study of females aged 45–55 years. Follicle depletion appears to accelerate in the decade preceding menopause.

Source: Block E. Quantitative morphological investigations of the follicular system in women; variations at different ages. Acta Anat. 1952;14:108.

Gougeon A. Caractères qualitatifs et quantitatifs de la population folliculaire dans lóvaire humain adulte. Contr Fert Sex. 1984;12:527.

THE MENOPAUSE AND THE CLIMACTERIC

Definition and Age

Definition

Menopause is defined as the permanent cessation of menses for 1 year and is physiologically correlated with the decline in oestrogen secretion resulting from the loss of follicular function. It occurs at a median age of 51.4 years and is a reflection of complete, or near complete, ovarian follicular depletion, with resulting hypoestrogenemia and high follicle-stimulating hormone (FSH) concentrations **(Fig. 3)**.

The terms menopause and climacteric are often used synonymously, but they refer to essentially different conditions. The climacteric is the counterpart of puberty and is a transitional phase lasting from 1 to 5 years during which the genital organs involute in response to the cessation of gonadal activity. The menopause is the counterpart of the menarche and refers only to cessation of menstruation; it is merely one manifestation of the climacteric (change of life) and precedes complete cessation of ovarian function by several months or years. The interval between the two may in part be explained by the secretion of oestrogen by the adrenal cortex or by the ovarian stroma. Hyperplasia of the stroma of the ovarian cortex is described as a frequent finding in women aged 40–60 years and is a postulated source of oestrogen, even after the menopause. The menopause and climacteric are peculiar to the human race; in lower animals, ovulation and fertility continue into old age. About 10% of men are also said to experience a climacteric (the andropause) but at a rather later age than women.

Age

The age of the menopause does not depend on the age of menarche, the type of menstrual cycle, the number of pregnancies which a woman has had, marriage, climate or environment. In the absence of general or pelvic disease, and with the possible exception of economic and social status, the only known factors governing it are familial and racial.

Black and Hispanic women have more frequent rates of premature and early menopause than White women. The incidence of premature menopause in black and Hispanic women is 1.4% versus 1% for White women. Similarly, the incidence of early menopause in Black and Hispanic women is 3.7–4.1% compared to 2.9% for white women. However, when confounding factors are considered, race does not seem to contribute to the differences in the timing of menopause for an individual patient. Yet, it may be a contributor when looking at the population level. Additionally, Black women consistently have more bothersome issues with vasomotor symptoms of menopause than other racial groups. 80% of Black women experience vasomotor symptoms, and the median duration is 10.1 years. Of White women, 65% experience vasomotor symptoms with a median duration of 6.5 years.

The menopause usually occurs between the ages of 45 and 52 years, but it is not uncommon to meet women of 53 or 54 years who are still menstruating regularly. The average age, which used to be 47 years in Britain and the United States, is now said to be 51 years. The mean has risen by 5 years in the last century, a change which probably reflects a general improvement in health and vigour of the community and a determination of women to stay young. In India, it is still estimated at 48 years.

Menstrual function may cease suddenly without warning, but the menopause is most often heralded by a gradual decrease in the amount and frequency of blood loss during several months or years. Excessive and prolonged bleeding is never a feature of the normal climacteric or approaching menopause. The menstrual cycle ceases, because the ovaries cease to react to the stimulus of the anterior pituitary gland. This is related to the disappearance of all the primary oocytes which is an ageing effect. The pituitary continues to pour out gonadotrophins and, indeed, being released from an inhibitive; influence produces them in very large amounts. Traditionally, menopause has been diagnosed retrospectively based on the lack of menstrual periods. With the advent of modern laboratory testing, menopause may now be more precisely defined as amenorrhoea, with signs of hypoestrogenaemia, and an elevated serum FSH level of >40 IU/L. Various symptoms such as hot flashes also point towards diagnosing menopause **(Table 2)**. Both early menopause and primary ovarian insufficiency have been associated with an excess risk of cardiovascular disease, bone loss and cognitive function concerns. Hot flashes and other acute symptoms associated with the perimenopausal period often become more intense near menopause when the levels of circulating oestrogen suddenly drop. These symptoms are especially intense in patients who experience premature ovarian failure or surgical menopause because of the peripheral conversion of both ovarian and adrenal androgens to oestrogen, the loss of ovarian function does not result in an absolute oestrogen deficiency. As a result, some women are less affected by oestrogen deficiency than others. The menopausal transition (or perimenopause) begins, on average, 4 years before the final menstrual period (FMP) and includes a number of physiologic changes that may affect a woman's quality of life. It is characterised by irregular menstrual cycles and marked hormonal fluctuations, often accompanied by hot flashes, sleep disturbances, mood symptoms and vaginal dryness. In addition, changes in lipids and bone loss begin to occur, both of which have implications for long-term health. Virtually all women experience the menstrual irregularity and hormonal fluctuations prior to clinical menopause; up to 80% develop hot flashes (the most common menopausal symptom), but only 20–30% seek medical attention for them.

Much of the available information about the endocrine and clinical manifestations of the menopausal transition comes from longitudinal cohort studies of mid-life women, the largest of which, the Study of Women's Health Across the Nation (SWAN), has followed a multiethnic, community-based cohort of over 3,000 women ages 42–52 years for 15 years. Based on data from these cohort studies, a staging system was developed that is now considered to be the gold standard for characterising reproductive aging from the reproductive years through menopause.

Physical Changes

Although in 50% of women, the effect is temporarily delayed by a trickle of oestrogen from the adrenal, the whole genital tract reacts to waning ovarian function by atrophy and inactivity. The breasts shrivel and become flat except in obese women in whom they may remain large and pendulous; this is because atrophy affects glandular tissue only. The anterior pituitary responds by histological as well as functional changes, and the workings of the thyroid and adrenal are also altered. Initially, thyroxine metabolism slows down, and there is a compensatory decrease in thyroxine secretion. Later, conversion of T4 to T3 decreases, and thyroid-stimulating hormone (TSH)

TABLE 2: The Stages of Reproductive Aging Workshop +10 staging system for reproductive aging in females.

Menarche							***FMP (0)***			
Stage	***−5***	***−4***	***−3b***	***−3a***	***−2***	***−1***	***+1a***	***+1b***	***+1c***	***+2***
Terminology	*Reproductive*				*Menopausal transition*		*Postmenopause*			
	Early	Peak	Late		Early	Late	Early			Late
					Perimenopause					
Duration	Variable				Variable	1–3 years	2 years (1+1)		3–6 years	Remaining lifespan
Principal criteria:										
Menstrual cycle	Variable to regular	Regular	Regular	Subtle changes in flow/strength	*Variable length:* Persistent ≥7-day difference in length of consecutive cycles	Interval of amenorrhea of ≥60 days				
Supportive criteria:										
Endocrine: • FSH • AMH • Inhibin B			Low Low Low	Variable* Low Low	↑ Variable* Low Low	↑ >25 IU/L¶ Low Low	↑ Variable Low Low		Stabilizes Very low Very low	
Antral follicle count			Low	Low	Low	*Low*	Very low		Very low	
Descriptive characteristics:										
Symptoms						Vasomotor symptoms likely	Vasomotor symptoms most likely			Increasing symptoms of urogenital atrophy

*Blood draw on cycle days 2–5.

¶Approximate expected level based on assays using the current international pituitary standard.

(AMH: anti-Müllerian hormone; Arrow: elevated; FMP: final menstrual period; FSH: follicle-stimulating hormone).

Source: Reproduced with permission from Harlow SD, Gass M, Hall JE, Lobo R, Maki P, Rebar RW, et al. Executive summary of the Stages of Reproductive Aging Workshop + 10: addressing the unfinished agenda of staging reproductive aging. J Clin Endocrinol Metab. 2012;97(4):1159-68.

levels increase (latent hypothyroidism). The incidence of hypothyroidism increases with age and is more common in women than in men. In a small proportion of women, overt hypothyroidism results.

As a result of the hormonal changes, the woman becomes coarser in build and appearance and develops features suggestive of a mild degree of acromegaly. The shoulders become fat, the waistline is lost, and there may be a slight growth of hair on the face **(Fig. 4)**. Axillary and pubic hair are not shed because these depend on the adrenal rather than the ovaries. Body hair becomes sparse only later in life, and this is part of a senile change affecting all organs.

The maximum and finite number of follicles in the ovary occurs in neonatal life. One million follicles are present at birth. At puberty, 250,000–400,000 follicles remain. In menopause, follicles age, and structures within the ovaries change. Ovarian aging involves not only a decrease in the number of follicles but also a decrease in the quality of oocytes. Changes are noted in the telomere, mitochondria

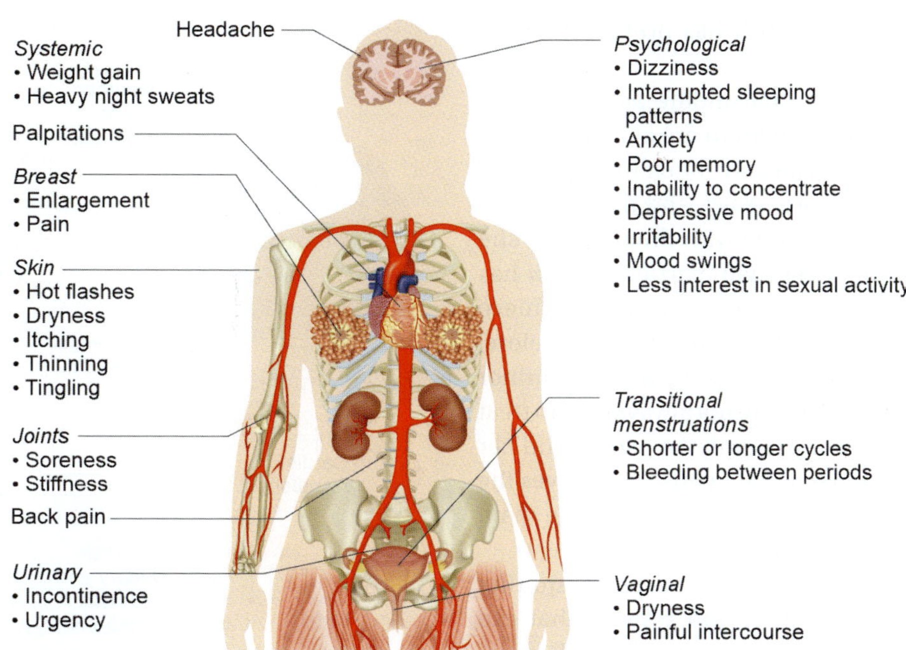

Fig. 4: Symptoms of menopause.

and other components of the ovary. Mechanisms involved in ovarian aging are still not thoroughly understood on a cellular level.

There is a significant change in the vulva and vagina during menopause due to decreasing levels of oestrogen. Inflammation of the mucosal surfaces occurs with resultant erythema and friability. An increase in vaginal pH and parabasal cells is noted. There is a narrowing of the introitus, labial thinning and decreased depth and width of the vagina.

Increase in weight is common in the climacteric but is not inevitable as is generally believed. When it does occur, it is often related to an increased appetite or eating in the face of emotional stress, as much as to an alteration in metabolism which lowers the nutritional requirements. The plasma and urinary levels of calcium and potassium tend to rise; this may have either a cause or an effect relationship to osteoporosis.

Psychological Changes

These vary considerably and depend largely on the makeup of an individual and on her previous outlook on the menopause and its significance. This, in turn, is influenced by whether the woman is single or married, and whether she is childless and grandchildless or surrounded by a happy family. In the well-adjusted and well-informed woman, psychological changes are few and insignificant, amounting to no more than a period of slight emotional instability. This is also true in the East where age brings with it an increase in social esteem.

Unfortunately, the menopause and the climacteric, such as other aspects of the menstrual function, are subjects about which there are many fallacious ideas. For this reason, many women approach the menopause with a dread which may have been with them for the previous 5–10 years. They fear insanity, loss of femininity, obesity and loss of their husband's affection. Some associate the menopause with the development of cancer. For many, it heralds the beginning of old age.

A fundamental reason for emotional upset is that the menopause represents the end of the reproductive era, and this means something to all women, even those who have as many children as they want. It inevitably means more to the barren and unmarried woman who had previously lived in hope. Married women are sometimes worried by the idea that the menopause means the end of sexual desire and physical love. In fact, unless the woman wills it otherwise, libido usually remains unchanged and marital relations continue after the menopause. It is reckoned that 75% of couples in Britain aged 60 years still practise coitus regularly. Sex life wanes only gradually as part of the ageing process in both partners. It is influenced more by culture and individual attitudes than by declining hormones. Sex urge in the woman may even be temporarily increased by the menopause, especially if it has previously been inhibited by fear of pregnancy.

One of the difficulties is that middle age is often a period of stress in the home. Children are at an age when they can cause parents much anxiety (often needless) and expense. Household duties are heavy, and the mother is no longer so physically fit to cope with them. Often, she is untrained for anything other than marriage, and it has become clear that her husband is never going to achieve the success at one time expected. It is no wonder, therefore, that many women in their 40s develop all manner of minor complaints and neuroses. These are not always easy to treat successfully, and it is tempting to both the patient and her doctor to attribute them to the menopause. This gives the menopause a bad name and is, in the long run, the main reason why so many women approach it with fear.

Perimenopausal women need access to quality health services and communities and systems that can support them. Unfortunately, both awareness and access to menopause-related information and services remain a significant challenge in most countries. Menopause is often not discussed within families, communities, workplaces or healthcare settings.

Women may not know that the symptoms they experience are related to menopause, or that there are counselling and treatment options that can help alleviate discomfort. Those experiencing menopausal symptoms may feel embarrassed or ashamed to draw attention to their experiences and ask for support.

Healthcare providers may not be trained to recognise perimenopausal and postmenopausal symptoms and counsel patients on treatment options and staying healthy after the menopausal transition. Menopause currently receives limited attention in the training curricula for many healthcare workers.

Many governments do not have health policies and financing for the inclusion of menopause-related diagnosis, counselling and treatment services as part of their routinely available services. Menopause-related services are a particular challenge in settings where there are often other urgent and competing priorities for health funding.

Climacteric (Menopausal) Symptoms

While the metabolic processes and the functions of other glands are becoming adapted to the cessation of ovarian function, a woman often experiences symptoms which are generally called menopausal but they are strictly climacteric **(Fig. 5)**. For this reason, they arise some months or years after the cessation of menstruation and never occur while menstruation remains regular. If there is enough oestrogen in circulation to produce a period, there is enough to prevent climacteric symptoms. The exception to this rule is the hot flush which is brought about by the relatively sudden change in hormone levels and is not seen in women who are chronically hypoestrogenic, e.g. Turner syndrome, or those subjected to bilateral oophorectomy in childhood. If this is recognised, then many women in their 40s will be spared the misery of being told that any discomforts they report are caused by the change of life.

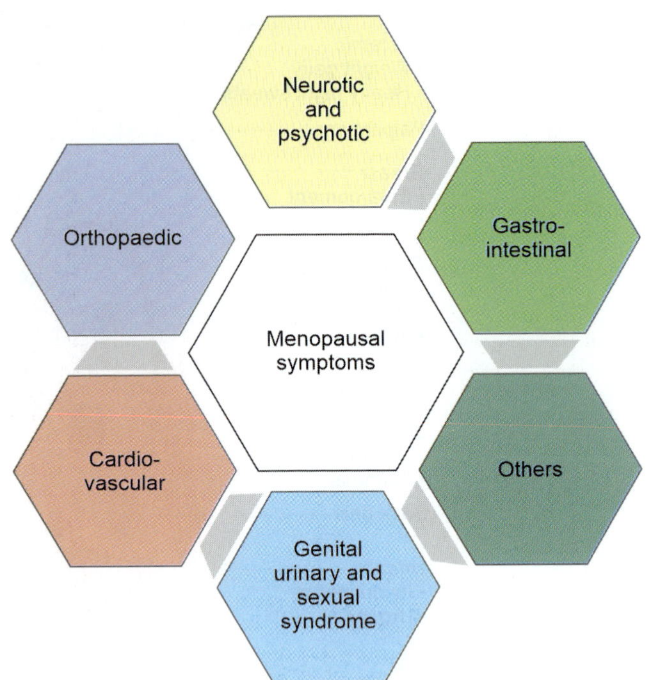

Fig. 5: Climacteric (menopausal) symptoms.

Just before the onset of the menopausal transition, serum inhibin B (a granulosa cell protein marker reflecting oocyte number) begins to decrease, allowing the rise in serum FSH while oestradiol levels are preserved. Luteal phase progesterone levels decrease as fertility potential begins to decline. Menstrual cycles are ovulatory, but the follicular phase begins to shorten. Women who are having difficulty conceiving often seek advice about their menopausal status during this stage. Although there is variability in age at any given stage of reproductive aging, women are typically in their 40s when cycles begin to shorten.

The immediate cause of climacteric symptoms is generally ascribed to oestrogen deficiency and the compensatory gonadotrophic overactivity of the hypothalamus and pituitary. The more irregular cycles are often accompanied by dramatic fluctuations in serum FSH and oestradiol concentrations. Consequently, a random serum sample may demonstrate high FSH and low oestradiol concentrations consistent with menopause, but soon thereafter, FSH and oestradiol may return to the normal premenopausal range. The mechanism is complex, because women who have never been exposed to ovarian hormones do not suffer from hot flushes even though their production of gonadotrophins is high. True climacteric symptoms certainly reflect an endocrine readjustment in which the adenohypophysis plays a part because they are not experienced by women with primary pituitary failure (e.g. Sheehan's syndrome), and their incidence is related to the level of gonadotrophins. The menopausal transition also includes a progressive decrease in serum inhibin B, as well as a decrease in anti-Müllerian hormone (AMH), another product of the ovary's granulosa cells. In addition, ovarian antral follicle count (AFC), defined as the remaining complement of follicles measuring 2–10 mm in diameter on transvaginal ultrasound, declines steadily across the reproductive years through postmenopause.

About 75% of women experience some disturbance at the time of the climacteric, but only 25% require to seek medical advice and not >5–10% need more than reassurance. The incidence, type and severity of climacteric symptoms depend on the physical, mental, emotional and social condition of the woman. Menopausal symptoms fall into several groups and can be broadly classified as shown in **Figure 5**.

Neurotic and Psychotic

These include depression, memory loss, nervousness, irritability and inability to concentrate. Headache is also common, and there may be insomnia, paraesthesia of the hands and feet, giddiness and head noises. These problems are seen frequently early after menopause, but their causal relationship with oestrogen is unclear. There is a significantly increased risk of new-onset depression as well in women during the menopausal transition compared with their premenopausal years. An 8-year longitudinal study determined risk factors for depressive disorders; a diagnosis of depression was 2.5 times more likely to occur in the menopausal transition compared with when the woman was premenopausal. This association is most marked for women with a prior history of depression or a mood problem. Postmenopausal women are prone to sleep disturbances. A distressing feature of hot flashes is that they are more common at night than during the day and are associated with arousal from sleep. However, peri- and postmenopausal women experience sleep disturbances even in the absence of hot flashes. Some women describe symptoms such as forgetfulness, difficulties with word retrieval, and 'brain fog', which requires attention as well.

Gastrointestinal

Appetite may be increased or decreased, and there may be various forms of dyspepsia, especially intestinal distension and constipation associated with colonic spasm.

Cardiovascular

Palpitations and precordial pains are not uncommon. The most important symptom, however, and the one, which is used as an index of the severity of climacteric upsets, is hot flushes.

There is considerable geographic variability in the prevalence of menopausal hot flashes. Among American and Japanese females, the prevalence of moderate to severe hot flashes is 35% and 15%, respectively. In a survey of menopausal females in five European countries, the overall prevalence of moderate to severe hot flashes was slightly higher than in the United States (40% vs. 35%), ranging from a low of 31% in France to a high of 52% in Italy. The reasons for the variation are unclear; smoking rates were similar in each country, and body mass indexes (BMIs) were not provided.

This is a manifestation of a vasomotor instability, which results in a tendency to flush or blush, especially around the face and neck. The flushes are brought on particularly by excitement, nervousness and a hot atmosphere, and they possibly correspond to the blushes of the adolescent. They vary in number from one or two in 24 hours to one every 15–30 minutes and are often associated with profuse sweating. They occur by night as well as by day, and sleep is disturbed by night sweats which leave the woman bathed in perspiration. Vasodilatation is followed by vasoconstriction, so after a flush comes a cold shiver. Synchronous with the onset of each flush is the release of a luteinizing hormone (LH) pulse. Each hot flush averages 2.7 minutes but is commonly 1–5 minutes in duration.

The incidence of coronary artery disease and myocardial infarction in women, which is about a fourth of that in men in the premenopausal years, rapidly increases in the postmenopausal years to approximately the same as in men. This has been attributed partly to alterations in lipid profile. The high-density lipoprotein (HDL) cholesterol level is about 10 mg/dL higher in both pre- and postmenopausal women than in men. However, total and low-density lipoprotein (LDL) cholesterol levels which are lower in premenopausal women rise rapidly after the menopause. Oestrogen may protect women through other mechanisms also which include the following: Direct inotropic effect on the heart; favourable impact on fibrinolysis; augmentation of vasodilating and antiplatelet aggregation factors, e.g. nitric oxide and prostacyclins; inhibition of smooth muscle growth which prevents intimal thickening; reduction of angiotensin-converting enzyme and renin levels and reduction of insulin and homocysteine levels.

Osteoporosis

Senile osteoporosis occurs in both sexes, but women lose more bone than men after the menopause. Osteoporotic fractures constitute a major public health problem. The main bone loss is in the vertebrae and the hip. About 50% of all fractures are vertebral. They may be asymptomatic, manifesting as a loss of height up to 2.5 cm or the dorsal kyphosis of the dowager's hump. Hip fractures at the femur neck lead to increased mortality and morbidity. Approximately 10% of these women die within 6 months due to surgical complications while a large number are unable to resume normal activities. The third most common site of fracture is at the distal end of the radius. Osteoporosis of the jawbone leads to tooth loss. The critical blood level of oestradiol required to maintain bone mass is 40–50 pg/mL (150–180 pmol/L). Oestrogen deficiency after menopause may also contribute to the development of osteoarthritis.

Genital Urinary and Sexual Syndrome

Genitourinary syndrome of menopause (GSM), formerly referred to as vulvovaginal atrophy, is defined as a collection of symptoms and signs caused by hypoestrogenic changes to the labia, clitoris, vagina, urethra and bladder that occur in menopausal women. Oestrogen deficiency leads to a decrease in blood flow to the vagina and vulva. This decrease is a major cause of decreased vaginal lubrication and sexual dysfunction in menopausal women. A pruritus vulva is never a symptom or result of the climacteric. Urethritis with dysuria, frequency and urgency occurs because of thinning of the mucosa of the urethra and bladder. The patients present with recurrent urinary tract infections and stress incontinence.

Others

All manner of other symptoms and signs are ascribed to the menopause. They include painful and tender breasts (fibrocystic disease), joint pains (menopausal arthropathy), fibrositis and myositis, pigmentation of the skin, the development of warts and naevi, keratoconjunctivitis sicca, menopausal hypertension and onset of Alzheimer's disease. Some of these conditions are age-related and some are directly related to waning ovarian function. Hypertension and arthritis, for example, are not prevented or reversed by oestrogens. Breast pain and tenderness are also common in the early menopausal transition but begin to diminish later on. Alzheimer's disease, on the other hand, has been shown to be linked with declining oestrogen levels and will hopefully be prevented by oestrogen replacement therapy. Osteoporosis associated with arthritis may be benefited from oestrogen therapy. Oestrogen deficiency is currently being linked to cancer of the colon, cataracts and retinal dysfunction. Treatment of keratoconjunctivitis sicca with oestradiol drops has shown a better response in the postmenopausal woman than artificial tear drops alone.

Management of the Menopause and Climacteric Symptoms

Whether to recommend hormone replacement therapy (HRT) to postmenopausal patients is a challenge facing many physicians. Equally difficult is an individual woman's decision to take or not to take HRT.

Controversies started with the publication of some of the literature. The findings of the Women's Health Initiative (WHI) study, a prospective, randomised trial of >16,000 healthy, postmenopausal women, published in July 2002, have thrown the use of HRT into question in both the medical and layman communities. Publications mention the increased risk of invasive breast cancer among women receiving the combined therapy, as well as heart attacks, stroke and clotting. These risks were not offset by the benefits: A decrease in colon cancer and hip fractures.

However, the average age of the women in the WHI was 63.2 years and does not reflect normal clinical practice where replacement is used mainly for symptoms including hot flashes, in women 10–30 years younger. Women in the WHI also had an average BMI of 28 kg/m^2, one third had hypertension and one half had a history of smoking. Thus, at the present time, the relative risk to benefit of using

HRT in younger, healthier women is largely unknown, and physicians cannot make all clinical decisions by the WHI study, as it appears to apply specifically to the population studied. Hormone replacement is still an important therapeutic modality for women for symptoms and quality of life issues which deserves further study and should be considered by physicians with their patients on an individual basis.

Evaluation

The basic details such as age, symptoms, onset and associated disorders and blood disorders are considered in the evaluation of a women in menopause.

As noted above, the Stages of Reproductive Aging Workshop (STRAW) staging system was developed based upon data from multiple longitudinal cohort studies. It is considered the gold standard for characterising reproductive aging from the reproductive years through menopause and includes criteria for the reproductive years, the menopausal transition, FMP, and postmenopause based upon bleeding patterns, endocrine findings and symptoms **(Flowchart 1)**. Although the STRAW system has been used primarily for women's health research, it may also be helpful in the clinical setting for patients and clinicians to assess fertility potential, contraceptive needs, and potential need for hormone therapy. We find the bleeding and symptom criteria of STRAW to be useful when counselling patients about what to anticipate in the coming years.

For women between 40 and 45 years who present with irregular menstrual cycles, with or without menopausal symptoms, possible diagnoses include early menopause or the menopausal transition. Evaluation would include laboratory tests such as:

- Pregnancy—serum hCG
- Hyperprolactinaemia—serum prolactin
- Hyper-/hypothyroidism—serum TSH
- Follicle-stimulating hormone

General

It is first necessary to exclude organic disease as a basis for whatever the complaints may be. Thereafter, it is essential to ensure that a woman understands that the menopause represents a change of life and not an end of life, and

Flowchart 1: Evaluation of suspected menopause in females >40 years.

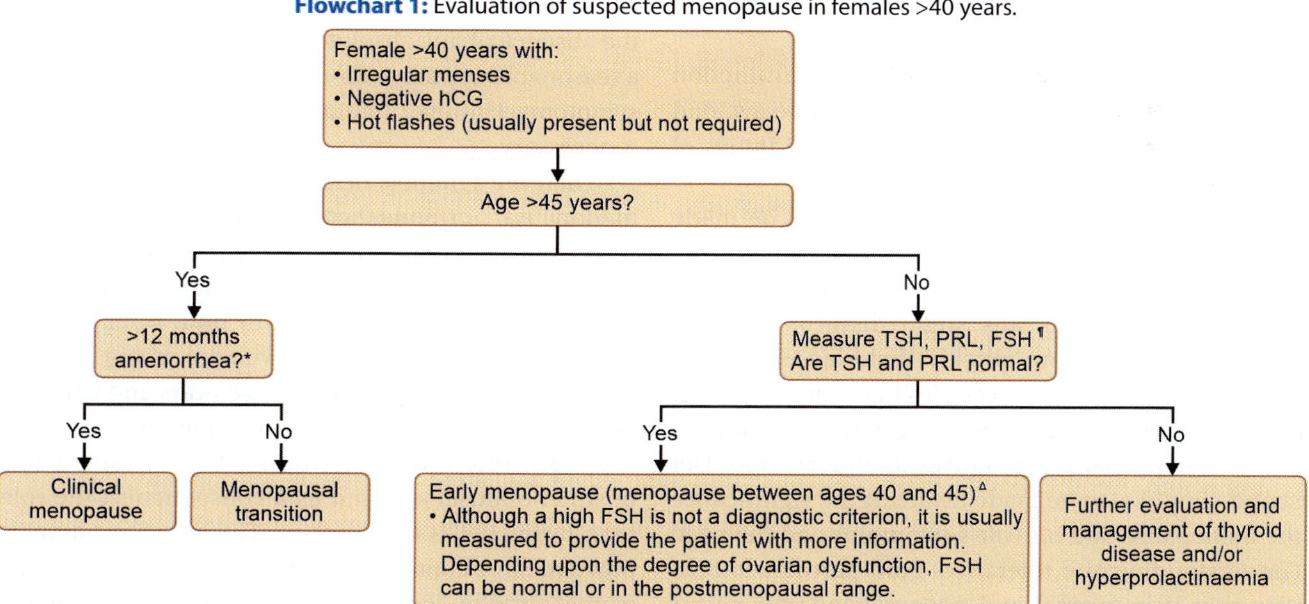

*The diagnosis of perimenopause/menopause in females over age 45 years is clinical and based upon the presence of irregular menses and/or menopausal symptoms. Laboratory evaluation is not necessary or suggested.

¶In females aged 40–45 years, the presence of irregular menses and hot flashes strongly suggests menopause. However, laboratory evaluation should be performed first to rule out other endocrine disorders.

ΔDiagnostic criteria for early menopause: Irregular menses, hot flashes and without another endocrine disorder (thyroid disease and hyperprolactinaemia).

(FSH: follicle-stimulating hormone; hCG: human chorionic gonadotrophin; PRL: prolactin; TSH: thyroid-stimulating hormone)

that, unless she allows it to do so, it will not result in her suddenly becoming aged and unattractive.

Middle-age spread can be prevented by reasonable restriction of diet and appropriate exercise. It is important for the woman to recognise the benefits of exercise and include a regular programme in her schedule for at least half an hour every day. Walking is the safest and easiest but does not have an impact on spinal bone density. Running, aerobics, weight lifting and climbing stairs are useful but should be done in consultation with the physician. Women who exercise three or more times a week have fewer menopausal symptoms, i.e. vasomotor symptoms, negative moods, loss of libido and memory loss. Relaxation exercises help to decrease hot flushes. Few studies have also shown that there were short-term improvements of psychological symptoms in menopausal women after yoga and meditation interventions. However, no evidence is being found for improvements regarding somatic, vasomotor, urogenital or total menopausal symptoms.

The diet should contain 1,000–1,500 mg of calcium. Milk, beans, broccoli, spinach and fish are good dietary sources of calcium but a supplement may be required. Phytoestrogens are present in soya beans, cereals and legumes and their adequate intake helps to prevent or relieve menopausal symptoms.

Cigarette smoking, high intake of salt and consumption of alcohol, coffee and aerated drinks should be avoided as these are associated with a higher incidence of osteoporosis.

The woman facing the climacteric should be made to see it as a physiological process, which calls for the adaptation of various body organs to new conditions. During this adaptation, any slight disturbances will correct themselves more quickly if she accepts them philosophically, and if she occupies her mind and body with interesting pursuits for which the new freedom of the postmenopausal era promises adequate time. Her husband should also be made aware of the significance of the menopause and his wife's symptoms and the need for understanding and tolerance. Both partners should realise that it is normal and advantageous for coitus to be continued regularly. Should dyspareunia occur, which is unlikely if the practice is regular; a water-soluble lubricant can be prescribed to overcome dryness of the vagina. If the woman is fearful of a menopausal pregnancy, the taking of one of the oral contraceptives may be indicated.

Medical

Those women who require more than explanation and encouragement but are reluctant to take hormone therapy sometimes find that small doses of sedatives help to control hot flushes.

Hypotensive agents such as clonidine hydrochloride are sometimes advised. By blocking the sympathetic nerves centrally, they can quieten vasomotor instability. But they are not without potentially serious adverse reactions, especially in women who are already hypertensive. When nervous symptoms predominate, tranquillisers may help.

Hormone Replacement Therapy

Since menopausal symptoms are directly related to the result of deprivation of oestrogen, the administration of this hormone should relieve them completely. The primary goal of hormonal therapy is to relieve hot flashes. Other symptoms associated with perimenopause and menopause that respond to oestrogen include sleep disturbances, mood lability/depression and, in some cases, joint aches and pains. It can, therefore, be used as a therapeutic test to make sure that disturbances in any case are climacteric. Short-term low-dose oestrogen, in the absence of any absolute contraindication to its use, is a reasonable approach for the relief of severe menopausal symptoms. However, frequent re-evaluation of the patient is necessary.

There are a number of factors to consider before starting menopausal hormone therapy (MHT) such as patient age, severity of symptoms and the patient's calculated risks for cardiovascular disease and breast cancer. The initiation of hormone therapy is found to be a safer option for healthy, symptomatic women who are within 10 years of menopause or younger than age 60 years and who do not have contraindications to hormone therapy.

About one third of a woman's life is spent in the postmenopausal era, and as a consequence, the role of long-term HRT is of relevance. The benefits, namely the prevention or control of vasomotor symptoms, insomnia, genital atrophy, coronary artery disease and osteoporosis, have to be balanced against the risks of iatrogenic disease as a consequence of medication. The greatest potential benefit of oestrogen therapy is the prevention of osteoporosis; oestrogen is considered by many authorities to prevent bone loss and osteoporosis if started before the disease is established and if maintained long enough.

Exercise may have a similar beneficial effect; in countries where female labour is common and in women who partake vigorous exercise, bone demineralisation and fractures seem to be avoided, regardless of endocrine status. The actual or potential hazards of prolonged oestrogen therapy include cancer of the endometrium and breast, gallbladder disease and thromboembolism. The association between unopposed oestrogen therapy, endometrial hyperplasia and endometrial carcinoma is well-established but can be countered by adequate progestogen therapy. The only real risk is that of breast cancer, the incidence of which is only marginally increased in current users up to 5 years (and may be up to 10 years) of therapy. Data for longer use are awaited.

Once the decision has been made to give oestrogen therapy, then the dose should be the lowest possible that gives symptomatic relief or has a bone-sparing effect. It is necessary to review the patient regularly whether the patient is receiving short- or long-term therapy. Regular reviews are important for all women, but particularly so in those who have a uterus.

Oestrogen: It acts at various levels on receptors all over the body. It also acts by inhibiting or reducing the output of gonadotrophins by the hypothalamic–pituitary system, though this is not consistent because of the loss of inhibin. If oestrogen is being prescribed for the relief of vasomotor symptoms, the effects can be judged by a daily hot flushes count. Natural oestrogens such as conjugated equine oestrogens can be used in a dose of 0.625 mg daily. If need be, the dose is gradually increased to achieve this effect. When the appropriate level is found, the same dose is maintained for 1 month and is then very gradually reduced over the course of 3 or 4 months. Gradual weaning is the secret of treatment, for if oestrogen is discontinued suddenly, symptoms return with renewed intensity. In order to mimic the natural cycle and to avoid continuous stimulation of the tissue, some authorities withhold treatment during 1 week out of every 4; however, even this regimen does not give the patient an actual oestrogen-free interval due to storage and release in adipose tissue.

A disadvantage of this form of treatment is that many women fail to obey instructions about reducing the dose and, once having experienced the relief which oestrogens provide, continue to take them haphazardly over the course of many years. In such circumstances, oestrogens are likely to cause uterine haemorrhage, endometrial hyperplasia and possibly carcinoma. Indeed, endometrial hyperplasia can develop in a young woman who has had radical intracavitary radium for a stage 1 carcinoma of the cervix!

The standard daily dose for providing osteo- and cardioprotection has been found to be 0.625 mg of conjugated equine oestrogen. Equivalent doses of other oestrogens have been worked out.

Low-dose progestins are also being considered in a few countries. Vaginal and oral micronised progestins are also sometimes considered, although they have side effects such as bloating, mood swings and cardiovascular diseases. Some clinicians choose off-label use of the lower dose levonorgestrel-releasing intrauterine device (IUD). Discussions about this approach are typically between the patient and their provider. Lower doses of levonorgestrel-releasing IUDs for use in menopausal women are available in many countries but are not labelled for this use in the United States.

Ethinyl oestradiol 10 μg has been used orally for vasomotor symptoms, but the dose-response effect on bone has not been sufficiently studied.

A transdermal oestradiol patch 50 μg twice weekly has a similar bone-sparing effect as 0.625 mg conjugated oestrogens. Its major advantage is that it avoids the hepatic first-pass effect; thus, it lowers triglycerides and can be administered to women with hypertriglyceridaemia. However, there is a high incidence of local skin reactions due to the presence of alcohol, especially in tropical countries during the summer months. This problem is reduced with the use of the thinner matrix patches.

Transdermal oestradiol gels have obviated this problem. Daily application of 1.5 mg oestradiol has an efficacy equivalent to that of oral oestrogen.

Oestradiol pellets (25–50 mg) can be implanted subcutaneously twice a year. These take several months to be absorbed but should never be used alone in women who still have a uterus. Once a depot is established, treatment is beyond control. The place for implants of oestrogen is especially in young women subjected to hysterectomy and bilateral oophorectomy. An oestrogen implant spares them with the effects of sudden deprivation of ovarian function. However, beneficial effects of transdermal oestrogens on lipoproteins may not occur because of the first-pass effect through the liver. Moreover, tachyphylaxis can occur over a period of time.

Oestrogens are well absorbed through the vaginal mucosa and while vaginal creams may be used to treat local genital atrophy, they are not the method of choice for long-term therapy. Some of the benefits gained by this treatment are related to the systemic rather than the local effect. All these approaches do not apply to women with primary ovarian insufficiency, who require a higher daily dose.

Newer delivery systems being developed include the continuous low-dose oestradiol-releasing vaginal silicon ring, which releases 5–10 μg oestradiol in 24 hours.

Oestrogens can be used alone only if the woman has already undergone hysterectomy. All women with an intact uterus, or even those who underwent hysterectomy for endometrial cancer (stage I), endometrioid ovarian tumours or endometriosis, or those with severe osteoporosis should receive combined oestrogen–progestogen therapy or be considered for the selective oestrogen receptor (ER) modulators (see further).

Combined oestrogen and progestogen preparations: With the possible exception of norethisterone, which is partly metabolised to an oestrogen, progestogens do not relieve climacteric symptoms. It is now generally accepted that progestogens should always be given if oestrogen therapy is to be continued for longer than 2–3 months in a woman with an intact uterus. The addition of progestogens is protective against endometrial cancer. Progestogens reduce oestrogen binding and are also capable of decreasing the amount of intracellular oestriol. They can be given cyclically or in the form of a continuous combined regimen. For the perimenopausal woman, one of the lower dose oral contraceptives may be appropriate, but these should be avoided in menopausal women as the amount of oestrogen is higher than that required. If an oestrogen preparation is used alone, it should be supplemented by progestogen for the last 10–12 days of treatment. Most treatment regimens are on a cyclical 3 weeks out of 4 basis; although the alternative of stopping treatment for the first 5–7 days of a calendar month is also popular. The advantage of having the oestrogen and progestogen preparations separate is that it allows the lowest possible dose of oestrogen to be determined for the individual patient. Medroxyprogesterone acetate 10 mg is administered daily for the last 10–12 days. Other options are dydrogesterone (10–20 mg), norethisterone (2.5 mg), desogestrel (150 mg) or micronised progesterone (200–300 mg). Of these, norethisterone has the potential for adverse effects on the lipid profile but may be advantageous in osteoporosis.

The majority of women with a uterus will have withdrawal bleeding in the intervals between treatment. This is generally accepted by those women who wish to avoid climacteric symptoms, genital atrophy and preserve a youthful appearance and outlook. However, most women prefer not to have withdrawal bleeding, and for them, the continuous combined regimen is recommended in which the daily dose of oestrogen is combined with 2.5–5.0 mg medroxyprogesterone acetate or 0.35 mg norethindrone. Combined oestrogen—progestogen patches containing 50 μg of oestradiol and 250 mg of norethisterone are also available in some countries. Vaginal rings which release 15–20 μg of ethinyl oestradiol and 1 mg norethindrone acetate per 24 hours are also being developed. Nearly half the women on combination therapy will experience breakthrough bleeding in the first 6 months of therapy. Bleeding which persists beyond this time requires evaluation preferably by transvaginal sonography (TVS), hysteroscopy and endometrial aspiration. Giving patients a planned withdrawal every 3–4 months may decrease the incidence of, and be more acceptable than, an unscheduled breakthrough bleeding.

In long cycle HRT, 0.625 mg of conjugated equine oestrogen or its equivalent is administered for 70 days, followed by 20 mg of medroxyprogesterone acetate for 15 days. Placebo tablets are administered for the next 5 days to complete the 90-day cycle while allowing withdrawal bleeding.

Regardless of the therapeutic regimen, patients receiving oestrogen and progestogen therapy must have regular examinations. These should include examination of the breasts and genital tract, blood pressure monitoring and appropriate blood tests to check for any potential adverse endocrine or metabolic effects, i.e. blood sugar, liver function tests and lipid profile. Dual-energy X-ray absorptiometry (DEXA) is the best index of bone mass but is not freely available in developing countries. Pap smear and TVS for evaluation of uterus, ovaries and endometrial thickness should be done annually and mammography performed every 2–3 years. Endometrial sampling may be required if there is persistent abnormal bleeding before or during HRT, or if the endometrium is markedly thickened on TVS. Combining the procedure with hysteroscopy improves the diagnostic sensitivity and specificity. Provided that proper medical supervision is maintained, the regular taking of a youth pill has benefits for appropriately selected postmenopausal women, especially those with early menopause.

Mixed oestrogen and androgenic preparations: Except possibly when massive and virilising doses are used, androgens do not inhibit hypothalamic-pituitary gonadotrophic function and by themselves are of no value in the treatment of climacteric symptoms. But preparations containing 3–4 mg methyltestosterone and 30–50 µg ethinyloestradiol were used, the recommended dose being one to two tablets daily. The oestrogen is said to prevent virilism while the androgen is alleged to inhibit oestrogenic stimulation of the uterus and breasts. Both are protein anabolics. Oestrogen depresses the output of gonadotrophin and androgen gives a sensation of well-being and raises morale. The claims that one hormone cancels out the ill-effects of the other have an insecure foundation; certainly, preparations of this kind can still cause uterine haemorrhage on the one hand, and hirsutism and voice changes on the other. If at all, they have a place, it may be in the treatment of depressed libido, where tibolone is either not available or not affordable.

Tibolone: It is a gonadomimetic synthetic steroid, similar to the 19-nortestosterone steroids. It is metabolised into isomers with three major metabolites, which have oestrogenic, progestogenic and androgenic effects, respectively. These metabolites vary in their effect, on different target tissues. In the endometrium, tibolone and its metabolites have a weak stimulatory effect because of a high progesterone receptor binding affinity. Thus, tibolone produces beneficial effects on bone, vasomotor symptoms, genital tract, libido and mood changes in the standard 2.5 mg dose, but in the endometrium, it generally induces atrophy. It has beneficial effects on coagulation factors, but not on lipoproteins. Total, HDL- and LDL-cholesterol are not altered; triglyceride levels decrease. It inhibits breast cell proliferation in vitro; in vivo, mammography pictures are more accurate, because it does not increase the breast density such as conventional HRT.

A major advantage of tibolone is its relatively low incidence of vaginal bleeding, seen mostly in small amounts within the first 4 months of therapy. It is also suitable for women with leiomyomas and endometriosis, in whom conventional HRT can cause an aggravation of the condition. The major side effects are weight gain and a bloated sensation. Some women complain of breast enlargement, tenderness and gastrointestinal symptoms. There have also been cases of breast cancer, endometrial hyperplasia and stroke following tibolone therapy. Lower doses of 1.25 mg have been tried which, while offering some bone protection and other benefits, may be associated with a higher incidence of breakthrough bleeding.

Selective oestrogen receptor modulators: Two ERs have been identified and are designated ER-α and ER-β. Binding of the same oestrogen to different receptors can produce variable, even opposite, effects, e.g. binding of oestradiol to ER-α can stimulate gene transcription whereas binding to ER-β will be inhibitory in some tissues and vice versa in others. The development of selective oestrogen receptor modulators (SERMs) has made use of this property to ensure that positive effects of HRT are affected on bone, lipids, brain, etc., while protecting from undesirable side effects by an inhibitory action on the endometrium and breast. Raloxifene and tamoxifen are being intensively studied in this regard. Raloxifene prevents osteoporosis and is an advantage in those patients unsuitable for, or reluctant to use, hormone therapy but is not a substitute for oestrogen. Apart from bone, it has favourable effects on lipoprotein-a, LDL-cholesterol, homocysteine level and fibrinogen but does not affect HDL levels, does not benefit atherosclerosis and may even increase hot flushes and leg cramps. Tamoxifen has side effects akin to oestrogen on bone mineral density and beneficial effects on coronary heart disease but has a stimulatory effect on the endometrium which precludes its use for this purpose. Other SERMs such as droloxifene, idoxifene and toremifene are under evaluation.

Problems with HRT and contraindications: In spite of its many benefits, overall compliance with HRT is poor, with dropout rates as high as 40–60% with conventional programmes. The main reasons for discontinuing HRT are vaginal bleeding, breast tenderness, nausea, vomiting, weight gain and the fear of breast cancer. Most of these symptoms settle after the first 2–3 months and may be less if therapy is initiated with a lower dose, especially in older women who are well into the menopause. Fear of cancer and the general belief that hormones are not good for the system are also important reasons for discontinuing or turning to alternate methods of HRT (see further).

Hormone replacement therapy is contraindicated in women with undiagnosed abnormal vaginal bleeding, breast lump, acute thrombosis, liver dysfunction, the acute phase of myocardial infarction and recently treated endometrial or breast cancer. Some relief of symptoms may be obtained in these women through lifestyle and dietary modifications and natural oestrogens.

Nonhormone Replacement Therapy Regimens

Osteoporosis can be corrected by non-HRT methods such as the bisphosphonates, which have a direct inhibitory action on osteoclasts. Alendronate is most commonly used; a 10-mg dose being administered in the fasting state for a period of 3–5 years. Other agents are etidronate, pamidronate and risedronate. Bisphosphonates are sometimes used in combination with HRT in severe cases of osteoporosis. Denosumab is a monoclonal antibody to the receptor activator of the nuclear factor kappa-B ligand, otherwise known as RANKL. It inhibits the osteoclasts and their activity, such that bone resorption decreases and bone density increases. In turn, it reduces the risk of fractures in menopausal women with osteoporosis. It is given as a subcutaneous injection on a biannual basis.

Selective serotonin reuptake inhibitors (SSRIs), serotonin–norepinephrine reuptake inhibitors (SNRIs) and gabapentin can be used for the treatment of vasomotor menopausal symptoms. SSRIs and SNRIs, such as paroxetine, escitalopram and venlafaxine, are antidepressants that treat vasomotor symptoms. Paroxetine, in particular, is the only Food and Drug Administration (FDA)-approved drug for this indication, and symptoms diminish within a week of initiating treatment. While not FDA-approved for the treatment of vasomotor symptoms, gabapentin has been shown to reduce hot flashes in menopausal women. High doses of gabapentin (900–2,400 mg/day) reduce hot flashes as much as oestrogen and at least up to two hot flashes per day.

Neurokinin B, acting through the neurokinin 3 receptors (NK3Rs) in the infundibular nucleus of the hypothalamus, has been recently implicated in the cause of hot flashes of menopause. The NK3R antagonists are showing encouraging treatment results and safety as nonhormonal therapy for vasomotor symptoms of menopause. Initial studies suggest that they may be more effective than SNRIs. Fezolinetant is now FDA-approved as an NK3R antagonist that is used for moderate-to-severe vasomotor symptoms. It is used as a single dose at 45 mg/day that does not need titration. Headache is the most common adverse effect. Oxybutynin 2.5 or 5 mg twice daily up to 15 mg extended-release daily may improve vasomotor symptoms of menopause in a dose-dependent fashion.

Salmon calcitonin has likewise been used when HRT is contraindicated (100 IU daily subcutaneously), but it is expensive and has the potential for immunologic reactions. It has the advantage of relieving the acute pain caused by subclinical vertebral fractures.

Slow-release sodium fluoride can be combined with calcium supplementation in a dose of 25 mg BD for a year, followed by a gap of 2 months, up to a maximum of 4 years. It is effective in reducing the fracture rate.

Alternative Therapy for the Menopause

Alternative therapy is increasing in popularity, and one of the largest segments of this industry is therapy for menopause. This includes the use of vitamin and mineral supplements according to specific nutritional recommendations in addition to dietary modifications; herbal therapies including traditional Ayurvedic and Chinese medicinal formulas as well as European herbs, homoeopathic formulas and mind–body medicine.

Nutraceuticals: Vitamin E is an antioxidant, which has been shown to decrease the risk of coronary artery disease by inhibiting the oxidation of LDL cholesterol and inhibiting platelet aggregation. A minimum daily intake of 400 IU for women under 50 years of age and 600 IU for those over 50 years is recommended. Vitamin E supplementation has been shown to decrease fatigue, nervousness, dizziness, headache, palpitations, joint pain and backache.

Supplementation of vitamins B6, B12 and folic acid facilitates conversion of methionine (derived from homocysteine) to the harmless amino acid cystathionine and protects against cardiovascular disease.

All vitamins or minerals which work synergistically need to be supplemented adequately, else negative effects can result, e.g. vitamin E without adequate vitamin C can have a pro-oxidant effect.

Natural oestrogens: Phytoestrogens are compounds derived from plants. They have a weak affinity for the ERs. Through this SERM-like action, they act as both oestrogen agonists and antagonists.

There are many classes of phytoestrogens, but the most important are the isoflavones which are found in legumes, especially soya beans and chickpeas, and the lignans which are found in many fibre-rich foods, wholegrain cereals and nuts.

In animal studies, the isoflavone genistein has been shown to be equivalent to conjugated equine oestrogens in maintaining bone mass by stimulating osteoblast number and function and by inhibiting osteoclast activity.

In women, 40 g of soya protein per day for a period of 6 months has been reported to increase the bone density by up to 2.2%, but the beneficial effect of phytoestrogen on bone density has still to be established. Ipriflavone is a synthetic isoflavone, which does not have oestrogenic effect but is used in the prevention and treatment of osteoporosis.

Phytoestrogens have been found to be useful in reducing hot flushes and may induce favourable changes in lipid metabolism and improve carbohydrate metabolism. High intake of phytoestrogens in the diet (>40 mg soya/day) has been correlated epidemiologically with a lower incidence of endometrial, breast and prostate cancers because of their SERM-like action.

Herbal therapies: Some herbs also contain oestrogen-like compounds, e.g. ginseng, red sage and dong quai, but there is not sufficient scientific data on these, and many herbal preparations contain high levels of harmful heavy metals such as lead. Several herbs are known for their antidepressant effects, e.g. gingko biloba and St. John's wort. Valerian, kava and chamomile have sedative properties. Liquorice and ginger are added to some herbal formulas to relieve gastrointestinal symptoms commonly associated with the menopause.

According to the Indian Menopause Society (2013), International Menopause Society (2016), and the North American Menopause Society (2012):

- MHT should begin within 10 years of menopause or <60 years of age.
- *Premature menopause:* MHT up to natural age of menopause 3–5 years
- Continuation of therapy should be decided at the discretion of the well-informed woman and her health professional.

ABNORMAL MENOPAUSE

Premature Menopause

It is rare for the menopause to occur before the age of 40 years, and the diagnosis of premature menopause should never be made until all other causes for amenorrhoea have been excluded. Nor should any symptoms ever be ascribed to the menopause unless they are accompanied by amenorrhoea. When the menopause does occur unusually early, there is often a history of a similar occurrence among other members of the family. Abnormal karyotype, hypothyroidism and autoimmune disorders including Addison's disease, pernicious anaemia and hypoparathyroidism have been linked with premature menopause.

No treatment is of any value, because the ovaries are refractory. They are without ova if the amenorrhoea is truly menopausal. Gonadotrophin levels are raised, and response to therapy is poor. Ovarian biopsy is not essential. HRT is recommended to prevent long-term sequelae. However, the role of oocyte donation in premature menopause for fertility needs to be considered.

Late Menopause

Regular menstruation up to the age of 53 years is not uncommon and is of little significance. Beyond that age, it should be regarded as unusual although not necessarily pathological; but if it continues beyond 55 years, then there is a clear indication for further investigation. The causes or associations of late menopause are constitutional (a familial or racial tendency), uterine leiomyomas, diabetes mellitus and an oestrogenic tumour of the ovary. The last causes irregular rather than cyclical bleeding.

Women who experience a late menopause are said to have an increased tendency to develop carcinoma of the body of the uterus later in life, and this is one reason why the condition should not be neglected. Unless there is a strong family history, a delayed menopause may be an indication for hysteroscopy, endometrial sampling and, occasionally, for hysterectomy.

Artificial Menopause and Climacteric

Surgical Menopause

This is caused by removal of the uterus, ovaries or both. If only the uterus is removed, and the blood supply of at least one ovary is not disturbed, ovarian function usually continues up to the normal age of the climacteric and no symptoms other than amenorrhoea develop. There are, however, reports of declining ovarian function after hysterectomy, even when both ovaries are conserved. In about 25–50% of women, ovarian function declines within 2–5 years after hysterectomy, especially in women who already have vasomotor symptoms. It is postulated that this may be caused by an interruption of blood supply from the uterine artery. This is one of the reasons why all efforts are made to conserve the uterus in young women even if further reproductive function is not desired.

Removal of both ovaries from a woman who is still menstruating causes climacteric symptoms in 75% of cases. The surgical climacteric is said to be more troublesome than the natural one, because the ovarian influence is withdrawn suddenly rather than gradually, though this is not always true. Symptoms continue for 4–24 months after operation, tending to have a higher incidence but persist for a shorter time in younger women. The rate of bone loss is greater in the first year after hysterectomy than it is in subsequent years or after a natural menopause.

Progesterone use in surgical menopause:

- After endometriosis surgery with hysterectomy to take care of residual tissue
- After supracervical hysterectomy
- After ablation technique on endometrium

Radiation Menopause

Ovarian function is suppressed by exposure to intense gamma radiation. Such treatment is likely to be followed by climacteric symptoms, which are as intense as those following bilateral oophorectomy. In a woman under 40 years of age, X-ray castration may not be permanent, the effect lasting only a few years. Thereafter, she may conceive, and there is a theoretical risk of the fertilised ovum being abnormal. Moreover, conception can occur before the woman has any warning by way of a return of menstruation. The menopause can also be induced by inserting radium and other isotopes into the uterus. These act not only by destroying the endometrium but also by depressing ovarian function. So, climacteric symptoms ensue, their frequency and intensity being midway between those which follow bilateral oophorectomy and those which occur at the natural climacteric.

Follicle-stimulating Hormone and Luteinizing Hormone in a Menopausal Woman

Follicle-stimulating Hormone

As the ovarian function declines in a woman, the FSH and LH increase. The most consistent finding in the menopausal transition is an elevation of serum FSH levels. In fertile menstruating women, FSH on cycle day 3 should be 5–10 IU/L with normally functioning ovaries. In fact, the quality of ovum is not very good when the basal levels of FSH are nearing 10 IU/L or when it is >10 IU/L. Elevated FSH levels (10–25 IU/L) suggest relative ovarian resistance consistent with the menopausal transition, even if oestradiol levels are in the normal range. Physiologically, this is believed to be the result of decreased inhibin production by the ovarian follicles during the last decade of menstrual function. However, levels of FSH >40 IU/L are consistent with complete cessation of ovarian function. Ovarian function can wax and wane over several years, and levels can fluctuate accordingly. Therefore, women with amenorrhoea and FSH >40 IU/L may resume menstruating for a short time in the future and occasionally may achieve pregnancy.

Luteinizing Hormone

In clinical practice, evaluation of LH levels appears to be of somewhat less value than other hormone assessments during the menopausal transition. In a normally menstruating woman, the LH is usually <10 IU/L, and it is elevated in a polycystic ovarian syndrome (PCOS) woman. Prior to menopause, LH levels are usually in the range of 5–20 IU/L. However, it is necessary to check both LH and FSH in women, especially young patients, with apparent loss of ovarian function.

OVULATION

Ovulation and the Menopause

It is generally asserted that menstruation is frequently anovular during 5–10 years before the menopause, and this is put forward as an explanation of lowered fertility after the age of 40 years. One of the few reported investigations into this matter showed that in women aged 40–45 years, 75% of cycles were ovular, and that in women aged >46 years, 60% of cycles were ovular. Ovulation certainly continues sporadically if not regularly up to the time of the menopause and sometimes afterwards. In England and Wales, prior to liberalisation of the abortion laws, 20–30 (1 in 28,000) births each year occurred amongst women aged 50 years and over; in the United States, 1 in 20,000 babies born had mothers aged 50 years or more. Most of the women who conceive late in life are still menstruating but there are reliable reports of conception occurring several months up to 11 years after the assumed menopause. In view of this, women should be advised not to discontinue contraceptive precautions until 2 years after the last menstrual period. After this time, the risk is so slight as to be negligible.

Spontaneous ovulation has been demonstrated, and pregnancies recorded, in women aged 52 years. The editor of the Guinness Book of Records was convinced of the authenticity of reports of babies being born to women aged 54 or 55 years (in Britain, 1956); and 57.5 years (in United States, 1956) [with assisted reproductive technology (ART), a woman aged 63 years has now given birth to a child].

Many women have the idea that there is an increased likelihood of conception at the change of life. This is not true; however, women may become careless about contraception as the menopause approaches.

Diagnosis of Ovulation

It is sometimes clinically important to be able to determine if and when a woman is ovulating and to distinguish between ovular and anovular menstruation. The following methods are available.

Analysis of Symptoms

Cyclical bleeding: The occurrence of regular normal menstrual losses is strong presumptive evidence of monthly ovulation.

Ovulation pain (mittelschmerz): Many women feel some discomfort in the hypogastrium, or in one or the other iliac fossa, for 12–24 hours just before or just after ovulation. An awareness of its significance allows them to determine the approximate time of their ovulation.

Ovulation bleeding or discharge (Mittelblüt): Some women experience a slight loss of blood or of mucus tinged with blood at the time of ovulation. This may be associated with ovulation pain, although each can occur independently. Those women who do not have obvious bleeding may notice an increase in the natural discharges. Occult ovulation bleeding, or the presence of glucose in the secretions (a postovulation phenomenon), can be detected if tampons or paper strips impregnated with appropriate chemicals are inserted into the vagina daily.

Premenstrual mastalgia: Premenstrual pain and tenderness in the breasts are in some way related to corpus luteum action, so its occurrence is fairly reliable evidence that ovulation has occurred during that particular cycle.

Temperature changes: The body temperature is raised by progesterone and is therefore higher during the luteal phase of the cycle and also during pregnancy. During the latter part of the menstrual flow and during the follicular phase, the temperature is relatively low. Ovulation is sometimes preceded by a low peak and is generally followed by a rise. However, a monophasic temperature chart does not always mean that ovulation has not occurred. The rise may occur suddenly within 24 hours or gradually over 4 days. After this, the temperature remains 0.2–0.5°C higher than in the follicular phase until the onset of the next period. This biphasic chart is evidence of ovular as opposed to anovular menstruation, and the thermal shift is a fairly accurate indication of the time of ovulation.

For this test to be of value, it is essential for the temperature to be recorded daily under standard conditions, before rising from bed in the morning and before eating or drinking. The drawbacks of this test are its poor correlation with hormone levels and the inconvenience to the patient.

Endometrial changes: The time of ovulation cannot be determined accurately by histological changes in the endometrium, but the fact that it has occurred previously can be deduced by recognising secretory activity in the glands during the week preceding, or at the onset of, menstruation **(Fig. 6)**. Such activity is highly reliable evidence of corpus luteum formation.

Endometrial biopsy or aspiration for this purpose can be carried out on the unanaesthetised patient without causing more than slight momentary discomfort. It is important that it is the surface endometrium and not the unresponsive basal layer which is examined.

Changes in cervical mucus: The different effects of oestrogen and progesterone on the physicochemical properties of cervical mucus are utilised in the fern test. Mucus is collected on cotton wool, spread thickly on a glass slide and allowed to dry. The fern pattern **(Fig. 7)** is seen under a low-power microscope from the 6th to 22nd days of the cycle, after which it is nonexistent. A failure to demonstrate ferning during the premenstrual week, after a positive finding earlier in the same cycle, denotes a dominant progesterone influence and suggests that ovulation has occurred. In performing this test, it is essential to prepare the glass slide by washing it in distilled water. The electrolytes in tap water prevent the crystallisation of mucus and so does contamination of the mucus with blood or semen.

Vaginal Smears

Provided that there is no complicating pathology to confuse the picture, the daily examination of vaginal smears from the lateral vaginal wall by an expert will pinpoint ovulation quite well. The superficial cells increase in number towards mid-cycle and the number of intermediate cells declines gradually. A single smear taken

Approximate relationship of useful morphological factors

Menses | Early proliferation | Mid proliferation | Late proliferation | Secretion

Gland mitoses
Indicate proliferation, they occur during menstruation because repair and breakdown are progressing simultaneously at that time

Pseudostratification of nuclei
This is characteristic of the proliferative phase but persists until active secretion begins. If is not resumed until the glands have involuted during menstruation

Basal vacuolation
This is the earliest morphological evidence of ovulation found in the endometrium. It begins approximately 36–48 hours following ovulation

Secretion
This curve represents visible secretion in the gland hymen, active secretion falls off more abruptly. In the later stages, the secretion becomes inspissated

Stromal oedema
This factor varies with the individual particularly the rise during proliferation which may be almost absent. The oedema which accompanies secretion is more constant

Pseudodecidual reaction
This is evident first around the arterioles and progresses until just before menstruation a superficial compact layer is formed

Stromal mitoses
These are most abundant during the proliferative phase, absent during active secretion but reappear during the stage of predecidual formation

Leucocytic infiltration
Throughout the cycle, there are always a few lymphocytes. Polymorphonuclear infiltration begins about 2 days before the onset of flow

Menses | Early proliferation | Mid proliferation | Late proliferation | Secretion

Fig. 6: Dating of the endometrium.
Source: Noyes RW, Hertig AW, Rock J. Dating the endometrial biopsy. Fertil Steril. 1950;1:3-25.

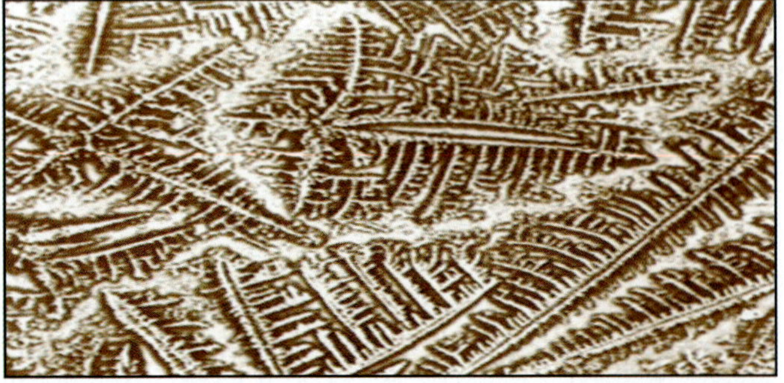

Fig. 7: The fern test. Crystallisation of cervical mucus on a glass slide to produce the pattern of a fern leaf (arborisation). This phenomenon reflects oestrogen influence and does not occur when progesterone is dominant.

in the second half of the cycle reliably shows whether a corpus luteum has formed. The intermediate cells now predominate. They have basophilic cytoplasm and large, pale and vesicular nuclei. The number of polymorphs increases. At menstruation, there is considerable debris with red and white blood cells and histiocytes.

Hormone Assays

Ovulation can be reliably confirmed by an estimation of the mid-luteal phase plasma progesterone level, i.e. 5–8 days after ovulation. A minimum of 6.5 ng/mL is taken to indicate ovulation.

Prediction of ovulation is possible by detection of the preovulatory LH surge, which precedes follicle rupture by 34–36 hours. Radioreceptor assays can estimate the levels of LH in plasma and urine within 2 hours of collecting the sample. Various kits utilise erythrocytes coated with anti-LH antibody; their different rates of sedimentation in the presence or absence of LH give an effective measure of the levels of LH, to enable the initiation of the surge to be detected rapidly. This demands repeated sampling to time the initial rise in LH, which is related to the follicle rupturing some 36 hours later. This information is helpful in relation to the timing of artificial insemination or the timing of oocyte collection. The study of daily oestrogen and progesterone levels is only likely to be undertaken in women in whom ovulation is being induced with gonadotrophins.

Ultrasound

The modern real-time ultrasonic apparatus has been used to describe ovarian and follicular characteristics throughout spontaneous and stimulated ovulatory cycles **(Fig. 8)**. It thus allows criteria to be set by which abnormal and possibly inadequate cycles may be identified prior to follicular rupture. This is helpful in the induction and confirmation of ovulation, artificial insemination and in vitro fertilisation (IVF). The wide range of follicular size of the dominant follicle still makes it impossible to predict the precise time of ovulation.

Once ovulation has occurred, the follicle appears as a smaller, irregular cyst, which progressively decreases in size over the next few days. Internal echoes are seen within the follicle. Occasionally, the follicle disappears completely. Sometimes, fluid is seen in the pouch of Douglas.

Direct Observation

Recent ovulation can be diagnosed by the finding of an active corpus luteum on inspecting the ovary during laparoscopy or laparotomy.

Ovarian Dysfunction

Ovarian dysfunction is classified into three main groups (WHO):

1. *Group I (10–15%):* Hypothalamic–pituitary failure, e.g. anorexia nervosa, Kallmann's syndrome and Sheehan's syndrome
2. *Group II (80–85%):* Hypothalamic–pituitary dysfunction, e.g. PCOS, congenital adrenal hyperplasia (CAH),

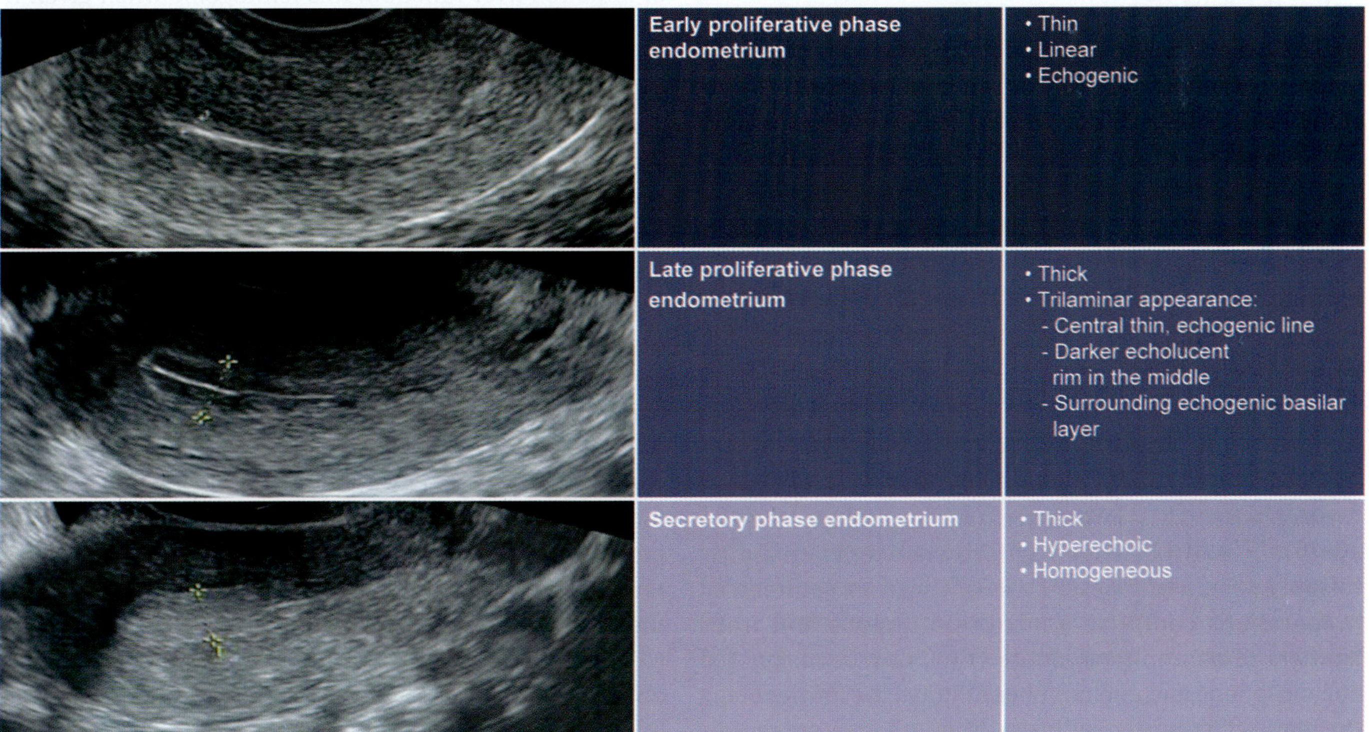

Fig. 8: Characteristic sonographic endometrial changes seen throughout the menstrual cycle.

adrenal tumours and androgen-producing ovarian tumours

3. *Group III (5%):* Ovarian failure, e.g. Turner syndrome, pure gonadal dysgenesis, Swyer's syndrome, autoimmune disorders, infection (e.g. mumps), radiotherapy or chemotherapy.

Treatment

The detailed treatment of all groups is discussed in the respective sections. Groups I and II are treated by induction of ovulation (see further) if they desire pregnancy. Group III patients will not respond to induction of ovulation but can be considered for oocyte donation.

Treatment of the cause: When general diseases such as diabetes, thyroid dysfunction, tuberculosis and anorexia nervosa are the basis of anovulation, treatment should be directed to cure these. Nevertheless, in resistant cases of anorexia nervosa, ovulation can be induced by gonadotrophin therapy.

The induction of ovulation: The induction of ovulation in clinical practice is only indicated when the object is to give a woman, infertile by reason of anovulation, a chance to conceive. It is not justified in the treatment of amenorrhoea alone. Moreover, no method can succeed unless the ovaries contain oocytes.

This means that it is pointless to attempt to induce ovulation in the postmenopausal woman or one suffering from streak gonads. Elevated serum gonadotrophin levels coupled with lack of withdrawal bleeding on progesterone challenge indicate ovarian failure.

Before treatment is planned, it is necessary not only to be reasonably certain that ova are available for stimulation but also to exclude the presence of all other possible bars to conception, male and female. This having been done, the methods whereby ovulation may be induced are as follows. Their results are always difficult to compute because of the possibility of ovulation occurring spontaneously irrespective of treatment.

Clomiphene: This substance is an analogue of the synthetic non-oestrogen chlorotrianisene, distantly related to diethylstilboestrol (DES). The usual commercial preparations comprise a mixture of the cis and trans isomers of clomiphene citrate (CC), now redesignated zuclomiphene and enclomiphene citrate, the former being the main active principle. Taken by mouth, they are rapidly absorbed and are metabolised in the liver. Although mildly oestrogenic in some animals, clomiphene acts mainly as an antioestrogen in human beings. It competes with natural oestrogens for receptors on the specific oestrogen-binding proteins and blocks their inhibitory action on the hypothalamic–pituitary system. The overall effect of clomiphene is therefore to bring about a release of gonadotrophins. An upsurge in the plasma level of FSH and LH is demonstrable after clomiphene administration. It is also suggested that clomiphene may potentiate ovarian sensitivity to gonadotrophins.

It follows that if clomiphene is to effect ovulation, the hypothalamic–pituitary system must be intact and capable of function. It is useless, e.g. in cases of Sheehan's syndrome. Some degree of ovarian activity also seems essential so, before clomiphene therapy is applied, it is necessary to establish, directly or indirectly, that the patient is producing a certain amount of endogenous gonadotrophins and oestrogens. The best results are seen when the level of the former is low and that of the latter is high. Some of the best indications for clomiphene therapy are the PCOS and the Chiari–Frommel syndrome, amenorrhoea and anovulation following the use of oral contraceptives, and infrequent ovulation and menstruation.

Clomiphene is a powerful drug and should not be given empirically. It is strongly contraindicated in the presence of impaired liver function. It is teratogenic when given in large doses to animals, so pregnancy should be excluded for certain before it is used.

The initial course of treatment consists of 50 mg clomiphene daily given orally for 5 days. This can be commenced at any time in the amenorrhoeic woman but, for the woman who has regular anovular menstruation, the starting point is usually the fifth day of the menstrual cycle (in IVF programmes, treatment is started from the second day to recruit more follicles). The treatment is monitored by daily charting of basal temperature and serum oestradiol levels or ultrasound for confirmation of ovulation, if practical. If it is successful, ovulation occurs 7–12 days after the last day of treatment, and coitus should be timed accordingly. If it fails, further courses of treatment can be related to the periods or at 30-day intervals in amenorrhoeic women if regular menses are not re-established. It is reasonable to increase the dose, if there is no evidence of ovulation or untoward reactions, to 100 mg or even 150 mg. If there are large cysts during observation of the follicular growth, then the persistence of the cyst should be evaluated on day 2 of menses since the next cycle of CC can be started only if there are no cysts.

In general, no >150 mg of clomiphene is given in 1 day. Moreover, if the ovaries do not respond to six courses of treatment, it is useless to give any more, and it may be dangerous to do so. Although the possible ill effects of long-term treatment are unknown, there are stray reports of an increased likelihood of ovarian cancer in women who had received ovulation induction with clomiphene for prolonged periods.

Women vary in their sensitivity to clomiphene and even small doses sometimes overstimulate the ovaries to make them the seat of pain, enlargement, cystic change, haemorrhage and multiple ovulations. Other side effects include hot flushes (which occur in 10% of cases and which coincide with peak releases of LH), nausea and vomiting, headache, visual disturbances, alopecia (rare) and galactorrhoea (rare). Such patients can often be successfully treated with 25 mg daily for 5 days or sometimes even for 3 days.

In well-selected cases, clomiphene induces ovulation in 70%, but conception does not always result. This may mean that the evidence for ovulation is not always reliable and may reflect pseudo-ovulation or luteinisation of an unruptured follicle due to clomiphene-induced inhibition of prostaglandin synthesis. Another possibility is that the antioestrogenic action of clomiphene makes the cervical mucus unreceptive to spermatozoa. Pregnancy occurs in 40–50% of women following treatment and, even though the dosage is carefully controlled, 5–10% of the conceptions are multiple.

Some patients with hyperinsulinaemia will not respond to clomiphene, and there is emerging evidence that correction of the hyperinsulinaemia with metformin 500 mg TDS will effect ovulation. If an ovulatory response is not seen in 3 months, clomiphene is restarted in addition, beginning at the lowest doses. Metformin should not be administered to women with compromised renal function.

Letrozole: Competitive nonsteroidal inhibitor of aromatase enzyme system and inhibits conversion of androgens to oestrogen. It blocks oestrogen production both in the periphery and brain. Mechanism inhibits peripheral oestrogen synthesis, which leads to increased gonadotrophin-releasing hormone (GnRH) pulsatility and consequent FSH and inhibin stimulation and secretion and stimulate ovarian follicle development, i.e. monofollicular growth. It is administered orally and metabolised in liver. Letrozole benefits in PCOS, clomiphene resistance/failure cases, unexplained infertility, in conditions where high oestradiol level would be contraindicated such as breast cancer. Effective in ovulation induction than CC. Dosage 2.5–5 mg/day for 5 days from day 3–7 of the period or a single dose of 20 mg on day 3 of the period. Side effects are well tolerated. No antioestrogenic effect on endocervix, endometrial growth and maturation and cervical mucus. No difference in overall rates of major and minor congenital malformations among newborns born in mothers who conceived after letrozole and no increased incidence of miscarriage and ectopic pregnancy.

Tamoxifen: This is a triphenylethylene compound which has antioestrogenic properties, probably because it competes with oestrogen for binding sites in target organs. It is an alternative to clomiphene and is used for the same type of case. The usual dose is 10 mg twice daily on the 2nd, 3rd, 4th, 5th and 6th days of the menstrual calendar. The dose may be increased, if there is no evidence of ovulation, to 20 mg twice daily and, if there is no response, up to a maximum of 40 mg twice daily. In women who are not menstruating, subsequent courses are recommended at 45-day intervals. If the patient responds with menstruation, the next course of treatment starts on the second day of the period.

It is often a matter of personal choice as to whether one uses tamoxifen or clomiphene. Since some women respond to one of these drugs and not the other, it is not unusual for the alternative preparation to be given after a 3–4-month gap following six unsuccessful courses (the maximum recommended). There appears to be a rebound phenomenon with each preparation, for some women conceive shortly after completing a course. Patients on tamoxifen should be monitored for clomiphene **(Fig. 9)**.

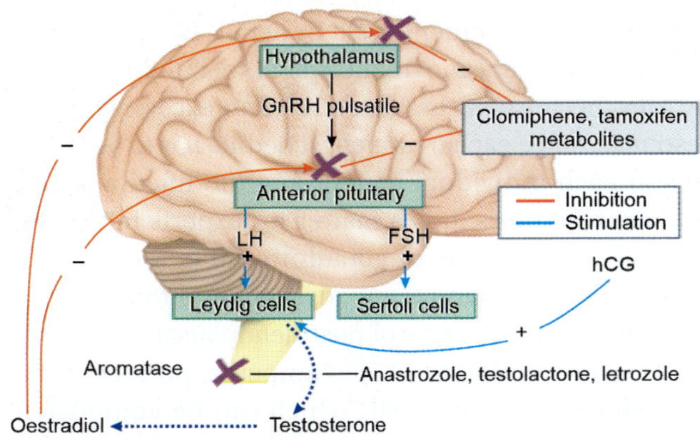

Fig. 9: Mechanism of ovulation tablets. (FSH: follicle-stimulating hormone; GnRH: gonadotrophin-releasing hormone; hCG: human chorionic gonadotrophin; LH: luteinizing hormone)

Corticosteroids: In CAH, regular treatment with small doses of cortisone or allied products usually corrects the ovarian function. The same is true for Addison's disease (adrenal cortical failure), the occult form of which is characterised by anovular, although often regular, menstruation. Without such clear indications for it, however, corticosteroid therapy is not of any value.

Dexamethasone has been added to clomiphene in women with hirsutism and high dehydroepiandrosterone sulphate (DHEAS) levels. Daily administration of 0.5 mg at bedtime blunts the adrenocorticotropic hormone (ACTH) peak.

Gonadotrophins: When ovulation is arrested because of a failure in the production of gonadotrophins by the hypothalamic-pituitary system, the logical treatment is to administer these hormones. They may also be tried when the simpler clomiphene therapy fails to produce ovulation. Indeed, except when pituitary failure is clearly established, the above methods should be applied before resorting to gonadotrophin therapy. Induction of ovulation with gonadotrophins has also been accomplished in hypophysectomised hypogonadotrophic women.

All patients considered for gonadotrophin therapy will have been screened to exclude causes of amenorrhoea and anovulation treatable by other means. It is important that, if gonadotrophin therapy is considered appropriate, both husband and wife appreciate what is involved and are aware that treatment is costly and dangerous, and that success cannot be guaranteed. In most centres, the number of treatments will be limited; we usually restrict it to six successful ovulations; ideally, these should be confirmed biochemically.

Gonadotrophin therapy should only be given in centres where appropriate facilities are available to monitor each treatment cycle in detail. Extreme caution is required when anovulation is associated with cystic ovaries, because of the high risk of an excessive ovarian response. Since each treatment schedule has to be tailored to suit each individual patient and modified according to daily responses, it is a matter for experts in the field. Several preparations of gonadotrophins are available. The oldest is human menopausal gonadotrophin (hMG) extracted from the urine of postmenopausal women with 75 IU each of FSH and LH per ampoule; purified urinary FSH and recombinant FSH which can be administered subcutaneously are also available. If day 3 LH levels are low, hMG is a better choice, whereas if LH is high, pure FSH is a better choice. Human chorionic gonadotrophin (hCG), recombinant hCG and recombinant LH are also available.

Follicle stimulation is achieved by daily administration of gonadotrophin for 7–14 days. It is customary to start with 75 IU (one ampoule) daily from day 2 and assess the response by ultrasound, preferably vaginal, to assess the number and size of the follicles. Circulating oestradiol is periodically assessed, if possible. On the 7th day, further dose assessment is done depending on the response, and the same dose is continued or it is stepped up. In the step-down method, the initial dose is higher (2–3 ampoules/day) and is reduced to one ampoule after the initial recruitment of follicles, thus mimicking the normal FSH changes.

Patients with polycystic ovaries are at greater risk of hyperstimulation and need earlier monitoring and lower doses.

Once the follicle has reached a size of 18–20 mm, the endometrium is showing the characteristic triple line and thickness of 9–10 mm, and the serum oestradiol level is 1,000–1,500 pg/mL, an ovulatory stimulus is given, either by 5,000–10,000 units of hCG or 0.1 mg of triptorelin. The former mimics the LH surge and the latter stimulates it. The patient is advised to have intercourse regularly on that day and the next 2 days. Even when the optimum dosage has been determined, stringent monitoring of every course of treatment is essential, because ovarian sensitivity varies from time to time, and the activity of the ampoules of the commercial hormone preparation is not constant. Moreover, ovulation sometimes occurs without hCG being given, this being explained by the fact that preparations of hMG contain variable amounts of LH.

The postovulation phase is also monitored since it helps to determine a subsequent dose of FSH. Ovulation results more frequently than conception; but overall, the PR should be at least 50% with good selection and has been reported to be as high as 90% in group I patients. The multiple PR is about 20%, with multiples over two forming 2–5%. Despite all precautions, there is clinical evidence of ovarian hyperstimulation in not less than 2–5% of treatment cycles.

Ovarian hyperstimulation syndrome: The OHSS is an iatrogenic condition. It has a varied spectrum but is usually manifested by ovarian pain, haemorrhage, enlargement and cystic change **(Fig. 10)**. Haemorrhage in particular can give rise to an acute abdomen and to unnecessary laparotomy. Any discomfort, with or without fainting, is most likely to commence 2–4 days after the administration

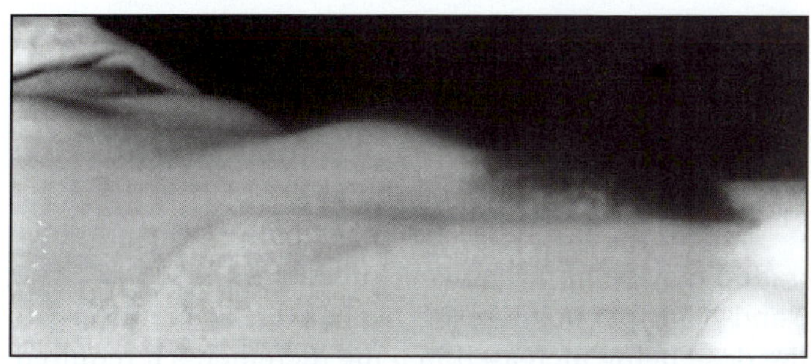

Fig. 10: Gross enlargement of the ovaries complicating treatment with human gonadotrophins and resulting in a tumour arising out of the pelvis and extending as high as the umbilicus. This developed 7 days after the giving of human chorionic gonadotrophin (hCG) preceded by follicle-stimulating hormone (FSH). The patient conceived during this cycle of treatment and the enlargement of the ovaries subsided only very gradually during the first 3–4 months of pregnancy.

of hCG; it increases for 7 days and wanes during the next 7 days. The patient should be warned accordingly. Another possible side effect is a painful reaction and swelling in the tissues at the injection sites.

When treatment has been less well controlled, there have been cases of serious complications and a few fatalities have been recorded. In these, and probably as a result of a high level of ovarian steroids in circulation affecting the vascular tree, electrolyte levels and renal function, there have developed hypovolaemia, renal failure, a shift of protein from the plasma to the peritoneal, pleural and rarely the pericardial cavities with consequent ascites and hydrothorax (pseudo-Meigs' syndrome) and venous thromboembolism. Massive intraperitoneal haemorrhage from the ovaries is also described. Acute respiratory distress syndrome (ARDS) is a rare but life-threatening complication, which can lead to cardiac arrest. Based on clinical, laboratory and ultrasonographic findings, OHSS is subdivided into mild, moderate and severe classes. If the ovaries are <8 cm in diameter and the patient complains of abdominal bloatedness, heaviness, tension or swelling with mild pain, the case is categorised as mild.

In moderate OHSS, the ovaries are 8–12 cm in diameter, ascites may be detected on ultrasound, and all symptoms are more severe and may be accompanied by nausea and vomiting.

In severe OHSS, the ovaries are >12 cm in diameter, and there are clinical ascites, sometimes hydrothorax. Laboratory assessment reveals haemoconcentration, hypoproteinaemia and electrolyte disturbance. There is hypovolaemic perfusion.

Management aims to provide symptomatic relief and prevent complications. In mild OHSS, outpatient management may suffice and the condition resolves with the onset of menstruation. Paracetamol and opiates are safe, but nonsteroidal anti-inflammatory drugs (NSAIDs) should be avoided as they interfere with the dispersion of the cumulus oophorus and ovum release. Antiemetics, adequate fluid intake orally or parenterally and discontinuation of hCG with changeover to progestogen are important ancillary measures. In moderate OHSS, the cysts take 2–4 weeks to resolve, but in conception cycles, they may take longer. Elastic stockings reduce the risk of thromboembolism.

The treatment of severe OHSS is to admit the patient and put her on bed rest with strict intake-output charting, frequent monitoring of vitals and daily weight record. The haematocrit, blood urea, serum creatinine, electrolytes, serum proteins with albumin-globulin ratio, coagulation studies and electrocardiogram are monitored serially. Plasma expanders, human albumin and electrolyte supplements are administered to restore the plasma volume and correct the electrolyte imbalance. Removal of the fluid from the pleural and peritoneal cavities may be required if life-threatening ARDS develops. Heparinisation is indicated in severely haemoconcentrated patients to prevent arterial and venous thromboses. Termination of pregnancy or surgery for haemorrhage or rupture of the cysts is rarely required.

The incidence of OHSS can be reduced by careful monitoring of serum oestradiol and serial ultrasonography. If serum oestradiol levels are high or there are a large number of maturing follicles, hCG is withheld and the cycle is cancelled; or, if facilities permit, the oocytes are collected for cryopreservation. These patients are asked to weigh themselves daily. If weight gain is >5 kg or any of the other symptoms develop, they must come to the hospital. Using GnRH agonists instead of hCG for ovulation, induction reduces the incidence of OHSS. All CC cycles must be monitored by sonography for response or hyperstimulation.

Clomiphene and gonadotrophins: When clomiphene alone fails to produce ovulation, it is supplemented with hCG 5,000–10,000 IU which mimics the LH surge.

The combination of clomiphene with FSH and LH decreases the requirement of gonadotrophins and therefore the cost of therapy. Clomiphene administration is begun on the second or third day of the cycle with 100 mg daily for 5 days, and then two ampoules of gonadotrophins are administered daily or on alternate days with monitoring. If the response is not seen with 100 mg CC, it is ideal to add gonadotrophins to CC for a few days (CC 100 mg day 2–6 plus add gonadotrophin 75 IU from day 7–10 for better response or give only gonadotrophin).

Bromocriptine: Although this drug does not specifically induce ovulation, it is the drug of choice for those women with amenorrhoea and/or infertility associated with hyperprolactinaemia. A raised level of prolactin is thought to cause anovulation by a central and/or peripheral effect at the hypothalamic level by inhibiting the release of GnRH and hence FSH and LH, and peripherally by antagonising the effects of LH and FSH on the gonadal ovulatory processes. The drug may also be used for those women who have normal prolactin levels but who have not ovulated with courses of clomiphene or tamoxifen, before considering using gonadotrophins for inducing ovulation. In most instances, irrespective of the final dosage, the optimum response with the minimum of side effects is best achieved by the gradual introduction of bromocriptine. It is recommended that the tablets should be taken with food, starting with one tablet (2.5 mg) at bedtime, increasing after 5–7 days to two tablets. The dose may then be increased by a further tablet 5–7 days later until a dose of 2.5 mg three times daily is reached. In infertile patients without an elevated serum prolactin level, the usual dosage is 2.5 mg twice daily. The lowest effective dose should be the objective of treatment in women with normal prolactin levels to avoid suppressing the prolactin level too much, since this would impair luteal function. Therefore, during the regular assessments, the prolactin levels should be checked, since the duration of treatment will usually last 6–9 months if pregnancy does not occur. Bromocriptine should be discontinued if pregnancy occurs, although there is no evidence of any teratogenic effects.

Hypothalamic-releasing Factors (Gonadotrophin-releasing Hormone)

When the anterior pituitary gland is intact and capable of function, e.g. when anovulation follows inhibition of the hypothalamus, it would appear appropriate to administer releasing factors instead of gonadotrophins. There are problems in administering GnRH because it has a very brief half-life and has to be given continuously in a pulsatile fashion by portable infusion pumps. This method is effective in women with hypothalamic amenorrhoea who do not have menstrual bleeding following a progestin challenge because of a deficiency of endogenous GnRH. It is also effective in women with hyperprolactinaemia who cannot tolerate bromocriptine.

The pump has to be worn constantly. Drug administration may be intravenous or subcutaneous, doses being 5 and 20 mg per bolus, respectively, every 90 minutes, with the dose being increased in 5 mg increments if required. Intravenous administration requires heparinisation.

After ovulation, the pump may be continued or alternatively hCG 2,000 IU is given intramuscularly every 3 days for luteal support.

The PR after six cycles is 80%; with polycystic ovaries, it is 30–40%. The incidence of multiple pregnancies is low. In spite of its physiological action and advantages, the pump has not been accepted well by patients and is not available in many countries.

Gonadotrophin-releasing Hormone Agonists and Gonadotrophin-releasing Hormone Antagonists

Women with elevated basal levels of LH, e.g. women with PCOS have a poorer response to hMG treatment and a higher rate of abortion. In such women, GnRH agonists are administered to convert these patients to a hypogonadotrophic state. GnRH agonists desensitise and downregulate pituitary GnRH receptors. Thus, endogenous hormone production is shut off. Removal of the premature LH release improves the PR, decreases the abortion rate and may even decrease the risk of ovarian hyperstimulation.

Administration of GnRH agonists causes an initial stimulatory response, the flare, which results in enlarged follicular cysts if the agonist is administered in the follicular phase or to anovulatory women. To obviate this problem, treatment is started in the mid-luteal phase of the previous cycle. The agonists are administered subcutaneously (e.g. leuprorelin 500 µg BD or 3.75 mg IM) or intranasally (e.g. nafarelin 200 µg BD). Complete downregulation takes 7–10 days if started in the mid-luteal phase and about 3 weeks if started in the follicular phase. At this time, patients develop menopausal-like symptoms, but these disappear once hMG is started.

Following downregulation, hMG administration is started **(Flowchart 2)**. Higher doses of gonadotrophins are usually required following GnRH therapy, which implies increased cost of therapy. The agonist is administered daily throughout the duration of gonadotrophin treatment

Flowchart 2: Long protocol of gonadotrophin-releasing hormone (GnRH) agonists.

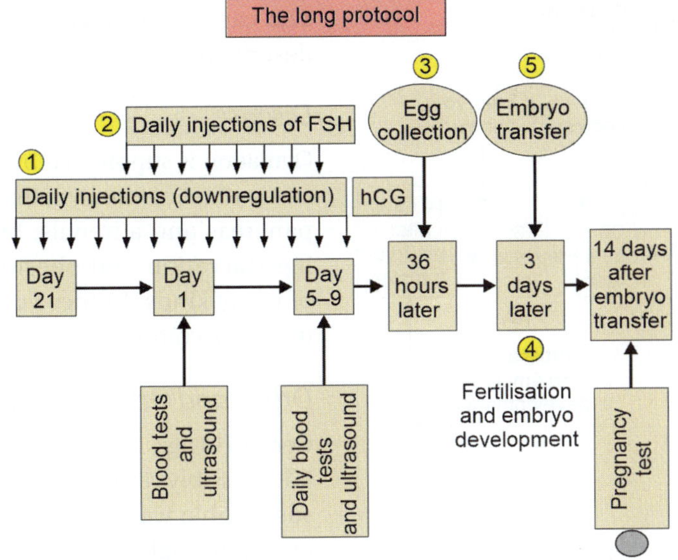

(FSH: follicle-stimulating hormone; hCG: human chorionic gonadotrophin)

until hCG is administered. Luteal support with hCG or progesterone is essential to compensate for the suppressed endogenous LH level. False-positive pregnancy tests can result from the luteal phase administration of hCG.

High LH levels have a negative role in IVF, so reduction in bioactive LH levels in the serum is desirable, particularly in the light of evidence associating raised LH levels in the follicular phase with adverse reproductive outcomes:

- Reduced fertilisation and PRs
- Increased spontaneous abortion rate. Most specialist infertility clinics attempt to minimise premature LH surges using pituitary downregulation. To achieve this, GnRH agonists (GnRH-a) were introduced into IVF superovulation regimens in the late 1980s and have become established as a component of standard regimens in most centres worldwide.

The inclusion of GnRH-a in ovarian stimulation protocols for ARTs has resulted in significant improvements in outcome:

- Cycle cancellation rates have decreased.
- Clinical PRs have increased. In fact, before GnRH-a became available, approximately 20% of stimulated cycles within an IVF programme were cancelled due to premature LH surges. By using the GnRH-a to prevent LH surges via gonadotrope GnRH receptor (GnRH-R) downregulation and desensitisation, this percentage decreased to about 2%, and concomitantly, the IVF and PRs per cycle initiated were increased.

Several treatment schedules currently are in use (long, short, or ultrashort protocol): The long protocol, in which the GnRH-a is begun in the luteal phase of the cycle preceding the treatment (stimulation) cycle and downregulation occurs before the start of the gonadotrophin-stimulation treatment phase, is generally the most effective regimen and is presently the most frequently used protocol. However, it has some disadvantages, such as hypoestrogenic side effects and an increase in the number of ampoules of FSH or hMG required for adequate stimulation.

Low doses of the native peptide delivered in a pulsatile manner to mimic that found in the hypothalamic portal vessels restore fertility in hypogonadal patients and are also effective in treating cryptorchidism and delayed puberty. Administration of high doses of GnRH or agonist analogues causes desensitisation of the gonadotrope gland with consequent decline in gonadal gametogenesis and steroid and peptide hormone synthesis. This phenomenon finds extensive therapeutic application in clinical medicine in a wide spectrum of diseases and in IVF to avoid LH increase. In addition, GnRH analogues could be used as new-generation male and female contraceptives in conjunction with steroid hormone replacement.

Gonadotrophin-releasing hormone-antagonists (GnRH-ants) inhibit the reproductive system through competition with endogenous GnRH for the receptor and, in view of their rapid effects, are being increasingly used

Flowchart 3: Protocol with antagonists.

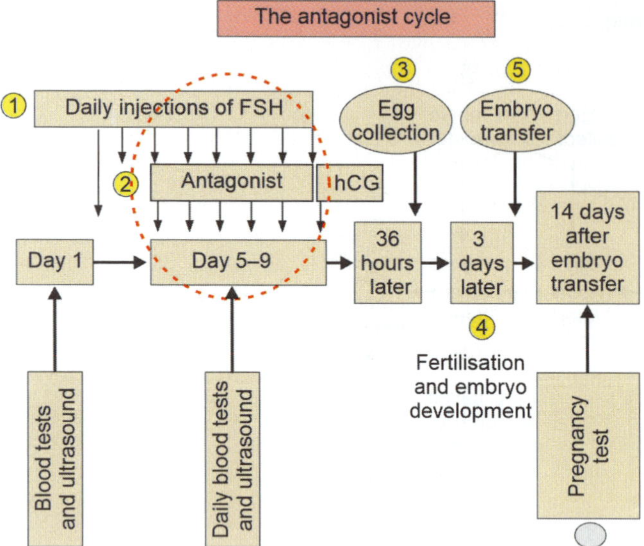

(FSH: follicle-stimulating hormone; hCG: human chorionic gonadotrophin)

for the abovementioned applications. GnRH antagonists are started mid-cycle to suppress LH. Hence, the doses of gonadotrophins are reduced. GnRH antagonists cause immediate suppression of LH **(Flowchart 3)**.

Surgical Procedures

Wedge resection of the ovaries was earlier practised in patients with polycystic ovaries who did not respond to medical induction of ovulation. Removal of stromal tissue resulted in decreased androgen and inhibin levels with a consequent rise in FSH levels and subsequent ovulation.

Most centres have now replaced wedge resection with laparoscopic procedures. The procedure is reserved for those women where an adequate trial of medical induction has been unsuccessful. The ovaries are drilled using cautery, diathermy or laser through the laparoscope. Multiple punctures are used, varying from 4 to 20 per ovary, following which there is spontaneous ovulation or at least an increased sensitivity to clomiphene. However, adhesions may develop in about 10–15% of cases. Severe haemorrhage may occur. Excessive tissue destruction has also been reported to result in premature ovarian failure, so current trials are evaluating the place of lesser punctures which may even be restricted to one ovary. The effect is temporary. Better results have been reported with cautery than with laser.

Suppression of Ovulation

The causes and means of suppression of ovulation are described here.

Disease

Ovulation is suppressed by psychoses and neuroses; by diseases affecting the hypothalamus, pituitary, ovary, thyroid, pancreas and adrenals; by metabolic disorders, including starvation and obesity and by debilitating diseases of many kinds. In these circumstances, ovarian failure is usually accompanied by amenorrhoea or oligomenorrhoea.

Drugs and Other Therapeutic Agents

Certain drugs, notably chlorpromazine and its derivatives, and possibly reserpine, can sometimes arrest ovulation in susceptible women. They probably act via the hypothalamus, through prolactin. Some chemotherapeutic drugs, notably mustard-type alkylating agents and busulfan, may cause permanent anovulation. Other drugs which have been implicated include the vinca alkaloids, bleomycin, cytosine arabinoside and hydroxyurea. Electroconvulsive therapy can have a similar effect.

Irradiation

It is possible to suppress ovulation temporarily or permanently by exposing the pituitary gland or the ovaries to ionising radiations.

Oestrogens and Progestogens

Ethinyloestradiol, 0.05–0.1 mg, administered daily from the 5th day of the cycle onwards, prevents ovulation by inhibiting the production of gonadotrophins. This is evidenced by the fact that it eliminates the normal mid-cycle upsurge of gonadotrophins in the plasma and urine. Progestogens given alone do not usually suppress ovulation. It is the oestrogen content of the combined oestrogen-progestogen oral contraceptives which mainly determines their antiovulatory effect.

Androgens

Any androgen given in a sufficient dose inhibits ovulation, mainly by direct inhibition of the ovarian follicles.

Danazol

This drug has antigonadotrophic effects that suppress the mid-cycle surge of gonadotrophins. Most women become amenorrhoeic within 6–8 weeks of treatment.

Analogues of Hypothalamic-releasing Factors

Ovulation can be inhibited by GnRH-a treatment.

SUGGESTED READING

1. American College of Obstetricians and Gynaecologists. ACOG Committee Opinion No. 651: menstruation in girls and adolescents: using the menstrual cycle as a vital sign. Obstet Gynecol. 2015;126:e143-6.
2. Burkard T, Moser M, Rauch M, Jick SS, Meier CR. Utilization pattern of hormone therapy in UK general practice between 1996 and 2015: a descriptive study. Menopause. 2019;26(7):741-9.
3. Ecochard R, Gougeon A. Side of ovulation and cycle characteristics in normally fertile women. Hum Reprod. 2000;15(4):752-5.
4. Ekpenyong CE, Davis KJ, Akpan UP, Daniel NE. Academic stress and menstrual disorders among female undergraduates in Uyo, South Eastern Nigeria—the need for health education. Niger J Physiol Sci. 2011;26:193-98.
5. Fortune JE. Ovarian follicular growth and development in mammals. Biol Reprod. 1994;50(2):225-32.
6. Freeman EW, Sammel MD, Lin H, Nelson DB. Associations of hormones and menopausal status with depressed mood in women with no history of depression. Arch Gen Psychiatry. 2006;63:375.
7. Menown SJ, Tello JA. Neurokinin 3 receptor antagonists compared with serotonin norepinephrine reuptake inhibitors for non-hormonal treatment of menopausal hot flushes: a systematic qualitative review. Adv Ther. 2021;38(10):5025-45.
8. Miro F, Parker SW, Aspinall LJ, Coley J, Perry PW, Ellis JE, et al. Origins and consequences of the elongation of the human menstrual cycle during the menopausal transition: the FREEDOM Study. J Clin Endocrinol Metab. 2004;89:4910.
9. Nappi RE, Kroll R, Siddiqui E, Stoykova B, Rea C, Gemmen E, et al. Global cross-sectional survey of women with vasomotor symptoms associated with menopause: prevalence and quality of life burden. Menopause. 2021;28:875.
10. Nappi RE, Siddiqui E, Todorova L, Rea C, Gemmen E, Schultz NM, et al. Prevalence and quality-of-life burden of vasomotor symptoms associated with menopause: a European cross-sectional survey. Maturitas. 2023;167: 66-74.
11. Neer RM, SWAN Investigators. Bone loss across the menopausal transition. Ann N Y Acad Sci. 2010;1192:66.
12. Santoro N, Brockwell S, Johnston J, Crawford SL, Gold EB, Harlow SD, et al. Helping midlife women predict the onset of the final menses: SWAN, the Study of Women's Health Across the Nation. Menopause. 2007;14:415.
13. Shifren JL. Genitourinary syndrome of menopause. Clin Obstet Gynecol. 2018;61(3):508-16.
14. Speroff L, Glass RH, Kase NG. Clinical Gynecologic Endocrinology and Infertility, 5th edition. Baltimore: Williams and Wilkins; 1994.
15. "The 2023 Nonhormone Therapy Position Statement of The North American Menopause Society" Advisory Panel. The 2023 nonhormone therapy position statement of The North American Menopause Society. Menopause. 2023;30(6):573-90.
16. Tsafriri A, Chun SY, Reich R. Follicular rupture and ovulation. In: Adashi EY, Leung PC (Eds). The Ovary, 1st edition. New York: Raven Press; 1993. p. 227.
17. Van der Merwe JV. Contemporary physiology of the menstrual cycle. Part II. The reproductive hormones, regulatory mechanisms and cyclical hormonal changes. S Afr Med J. 1981;59(23):834-8.
18. Van Look PF, Baird DT. Regulatory mechanisms during the menstrual cycle. Eur J Obstet Gynecol Reprod Biol. 1980;11(2):121-44.
19. Wang X, Wang L, Xiang W. Mechanisms of ovarian aging in women: a review. J Ovarian Res. 2023;16(1):67.
20. Williams M, Richard-Davis G, Weickert A, Christensen L, Ward E, Schrager S. A review of African American women's experiences in menopause. Menopause. 2022;29(11):1331-7.
21. Zhou M, Wege N, Gu H, Shang L, Li J, Siegrist J. Work and family stress is associated with menstrual disorders but not with fibrocystic changes: cross-sectional findings in Chinese working women. J Occup Health. 2010;52:361-6.

6

CHAPTER

Puberty and Adolescent Gynaecology

Roopa PS, Muralidhar V Pai

Chapter Outline

- Puberty and Adolescence
- Abnormalities of Puberty and Adolescence
- Prolactin
- Puberty Menorrhagia

PUBERTY AND ADOLESCENCE

Definition

Adolescence (Latin: *adolescere*—to grow) is the period of life during which the carefree child becomes the responsible adult. The period varies in duration from one individual to another and is difficult to define. A modern description of the adolescent is the *teenager*.

Puberty (Latin: *pubertas*—adulthood) is the state of becoming functionally capable of procreation. This is usually accepted as occurring at 12 years in girls and 14 years in boys, but total reproductive capacity is not usually attained until later. Puberty is characterised by physical and sexual differentiation and by the onset of activity of the sex organs **(Figs. 1 and 2 and Table 1)**.

Puberty is really the first part of adolescence, the remainder being concerned with the mental and emotional adaptation to sexual function and with the development of full maturity. The menarche (Greek: month + origin) is the onset of menstruation and is merely one manifestation of puberty.

Description

There is some activity of the hypothalamic-pituitary-ovarian (HPO) axis in infancy; however, its clinical relevance is unknown. There is a long period of inactivity followed by stimulation during growth and prepuberty. During childhood, the anterior pituitary is concerned mostly with physical growth. It is capable of gonadotrophic activity but is inhibited by the hypothalamus until the higher centres of the brain are more mature. At puberty, as a result of the increased secretion of releasing factors by the hypothalamus, and the increased responsiveness of the pituitary gland to these factors, all activities are increased. This is manifested by a sudden spurt in stature just before or after the menarche [growth hormone (GH) effect]; by enlargement of the thyroid [thyroid-stimulating hormone (TSH)]; by increased adrenal cortical activity [adrenocorticotrophic hormone (ACTH) effect]; by skin pigmentation [melanocyte-stimulating hormone (MSH) effect]; and by the onset of ovarian activity (gonadotrophin effect). The cyclical production of gonadotrophins and oestrogens in amounts approaching those found in the adult is often demonstrable by the age of 10 years. The secretion of oestrogen by the ovaries and of androgens by the adrenals induces epiphyseal closure, and skeletal growth then ceases.

Nevertheless, some sexual differentiation occurs in childhood. The nipples are rather more obvious in the female than the male by the age of 3 years, and there is a tendency to plumpness and roundness of the limbs at 6–8 years. The pelvis widens between the ages of 7 and 11 years. Definite signs of puberty are usually present by the age of 9 or 10 years when the breasts develop a 'bud' (thelarche, **Figs. 3A and B**), and soon afterwards, they become generally enlarged. By this time, hair begins to grow on the body, appearing first on the mons veneris (adrenarche). Meanwhile, body contours change by the deposition of fat, the growth spurt occurs and there is some evidence of skin pigmentation, notably on the vulva but sometimes around the eyes, mouth and nipples, and on the abdominal wall in the form of a linea nigra. Some development of the breasts and pubic hair usually precedes the onset of menstruation, the average interval being 2 years. Axillary hair appears later, often after the menarche. Hence, adolescence starts with thelarche (development

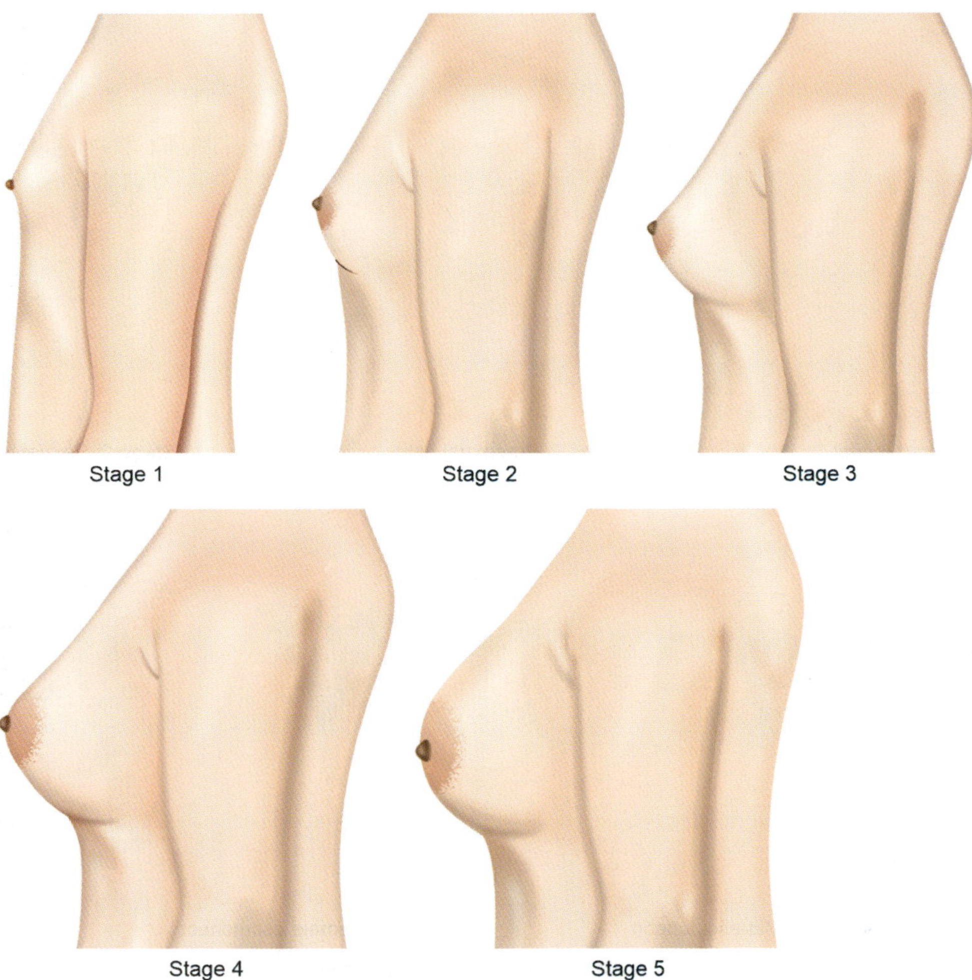

Fig. 1: Development of the female breast.

of breast buds), followed by pubarche (development of pubic hair), adrenarche (development of axillar hair) and menarche (the first menstruation) **(Flowchart 1)**.

Marshall and Tanner in 1969–1970 described the stages of normal pubertal development, which came to be known as 'Tanner stages.'

The first menstrual period usually occurs between the ages of 10 and 16 years, the average being 13.5 years in India, 13.0 years in Western Europe, and 12.5 years in North America. The age of the menarche varies to some extent with family, race, social class, family size, birth order, environment, diet and general health, but not with climate. Menstruation tends to occur earlier in the higher social classes and urban surroundings; this probably reflects general health. The age of the menarche and maturity in general is falling. Among Caucasian races at least, girls of 14–15 years are now as physically and sexually developed as their mothers were at the age of 16 years. In England and Wales, Western and Northern Europe and North America, the mean age of menarche dropped from 17 to 13 years during the 100 years up to 1960, decreasing at the rate of 4 months every 10 years. Similar trends were, and are being, seen in all countries and are variously credited to better nutrition, freedom from disease and increased outbreeding, which provides hybrid vigor. However, after 1965 (in girls born from 1946 onwards), the menarcheal age ceased to fall in Britain, North America and Western Europe and is now static at the levels indicated above. Whether this is a temporary or permanent stabilisation remains to be seen.

During the 2 years before the menarche, the development of the genital tract proceeds apace. The menstrual flow itself is often preceded by mucoid vaginal discharge and by periodic hypogastric pain caused possibly by uterine contractions. Rarely, ovulation and

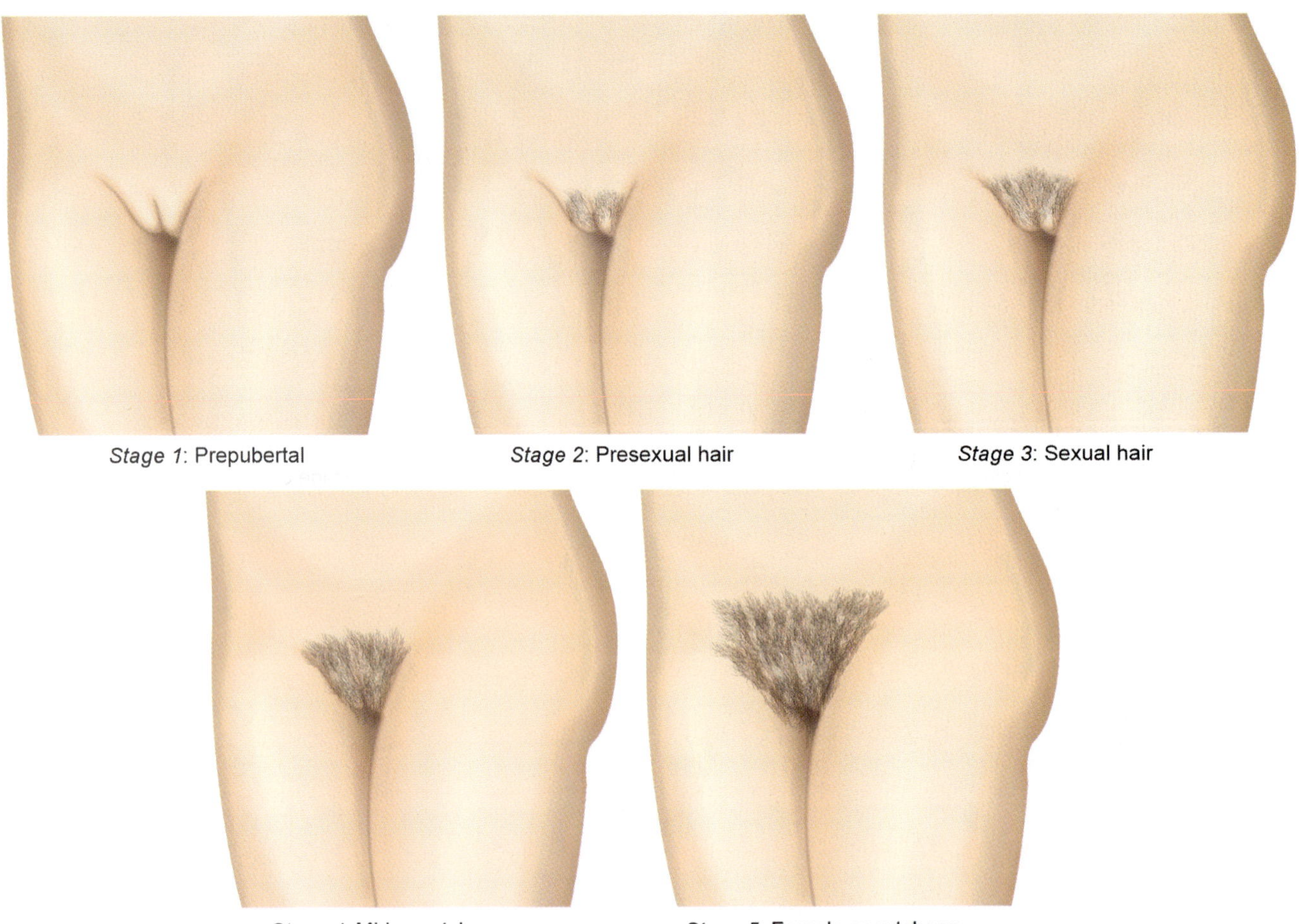

Stage 1: Prepubertal *Stage 2*: Presexual hair *Stage 3*: Sexual hair

Stage 4: Mid-escutcheon *Stage 5*: Female escutcheon

Fig. 2: Development of pubic hair.

even conception can precede the menarche. The phase of active physical growth makes the girl temporarily lanky and awkward in her movements. Thereafter, the figure becomes fuller and feminine, and the shrill voice of the child changes to the slightly deeper and more melodious tone of the adult. Girls reach peak height velocity early in puberty before menarche. As a consequence, they have limited growth potential after menarche whereas boys reach peak height velocity about 2 years later than girls. Boys grow an average of 28 cm during the growth spurt, in comparison to a mean of 25 cm for girls. The control of this is connected to the hormonal control of the pubertal growth spurt. GH, insulin-like growth factor 1 (IGF-1) and gonadal steroids play major roles. During puberty, the long bones in the body lengthen, and the epiphyses ultimately close. The bone or skeletal age of any individual can be estimated closely by comparing X-rays documenting the development of bones in the nondominant hand (most commonly), knee or elbow to standards of maturation for the normal population. Another practical clinical approach to predicting adult height uses midparental height. Several changes in body composition also occur during pubertal development. The changes in body contour in girls, with accumulation of fat at the thighs, hips and buttocks, occur during the pubertal growth spurt. Voice and other changes are also associated with the changes in body composition.

During puberty and adolescence, the psychological changes are profound. The happy-go-lucky tomboy changes into a self-conscious girl who is interested in her appearance, may be moody and secretive and is often imaginative and curious. She begins to feel that she has grown up, finds it more difficult to obey orders, and looks for independence. Her confidante becomes another girl rather than her mother. The sex urge becomes manifest and is often homosexual at first being evidenced by an unreasonable 'passion' for a particular older girl or woman. This phase is usually followed, sooner or later, by heterosexual impulses and activities.

TABLE 1: Tanner staging of development of secondary sex characteristics.

Stage	*Breast*	*Pubic hair*
1	Elevation of papilla	No pubic hair (prepubertal)
2	Elevation of breast and papilla as a small mound, increased areolar diameter (median age 9.8 years)	Sparse, long pigmented hair mainly along labia majora (median age 10.5 years)
3	Further enlargement without separation of breast and areola (median age 11.2 years)	Dark, coarse, curled hair sparsely spread over mons (median age 11.4 years)
4	Secondary mound of areola and papilla above breast (median age 12.1 years)	Adult-type, abundant hair, but limited to the mons (median age 12.0 years)
5	Recession of areola to contour of breast (median age 14.6 years)	Adult-type spread in quantity and distribution (median age 13.6 years)

Source: Speroff L, Glass RH, Kase NG. In: Mitchell C (Ed). Clinical Gynecologic Endocrinology and Infertility, 6th edition. Baltimore: Lippincott Williams & Wilkins; 1999.

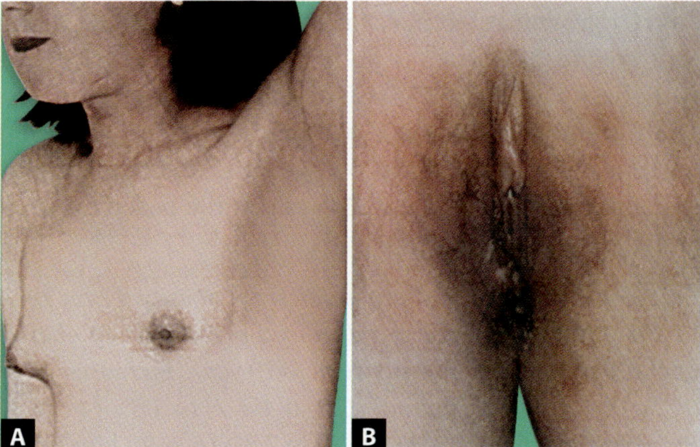

Figs. 3A and B: Delayed puberty. Girl, aged 17 years, complaining of primary amenorrhoea. (A) Breast development has commenced and is characterised by the areolar bud ordinarily seen in a girl aged 9–12 years. Axillary hair has not yet appeared; (B) The labia majora are poorly developed and pubic hair is scanty. Investigation, which did not include sex chromosome analysis, revealed no abnormality, and no treatment was given. Maturation proceeded spontaneously, and menstruation commenced 2 years later.

Flowchart 1: Phases of female development.

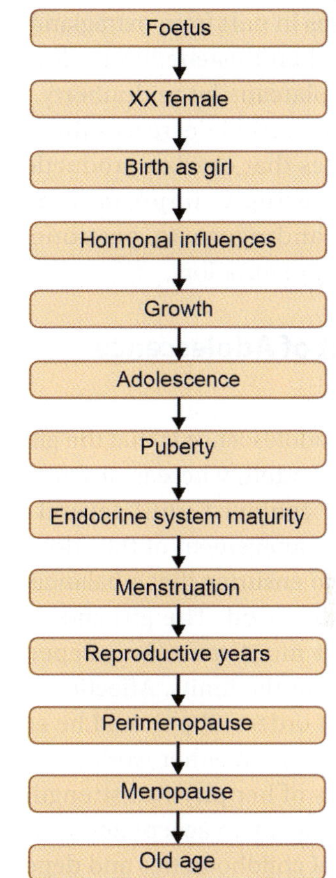

Temporary enlargement of the thyroid at puberty has already been mentioned. Acne of the face and back is often a nuisance for 1 or 2 years after the menarche; it is mainly the result of increased androgen secretion by the adrenal, which is also manifested by an increased excretion of 17-ketosteroids in the urine. Indeed, many of the manifestations of puberty (e.g. the growth of pubic and axillary hair) are the result of adrenal rather than of ovarian activity. Vasomotor instability is revealed by a tendency to blush at the slightest provocation.

Early in puberty, there is increased sensitivity of luteinising hormone (LH) to gonadotrophin-releasing hormone (GnRH). Gonadotrophins are always secreted in an episodic or pulsatile fashion; even before puberty, the pulsatile secretion of gonadotrophins is more easily documented as puberty progresses and basal levels increase. The appearance of the axillary and pubic hair is due to increased adrenal androgen secretion. A progressive increase in circulating levels of the major adrenal androgens, dehydroepiandrosterone (DHEA) and its sulphate (DHEA-S) accelerates at 7–8 years of age and continues until 13–15 years of age. The accelerated increases in adrenal androgens begin about 2 years before the increases in gonadotropin and gonadal sex steroid secretion. Oestrone, which is secreted in part by the ovaries and arises in part from extraglandular conversion of oestradiol and androstenedione, also increases early in puberty but plateaus by midpuberty. Thus, the ratio of oestrone to oestradiol decreases throughout puberty, and this indicates that ovarian production of oestradiol becomes increasingly important and peripheral conversion of androgens to oestrone becomes less important during maturation.

Management of Adolescence

Sex Education

The problem of adolescence is that the girl regards herself as grown up and adult, whereas physical and emotional maturity is not achieved until several years after the menarche. The management of the adolescent is difficult and is directed to ensuring that a balanced adult emerges from the testing period. The girl should not be teased or ridiculed but move towards independence, respect and control within the limits. Affection and trust should take the place of orders. She should be encouraged to be continually occupied in either work or healthy recreation within the limits of her physical strength. Above all, her parents must be ready to accept and even encourage the disappearance of childhood ties and dependence. Failure to do so means that their daughter will never adequately fulfil her intended roles as a wife and a mother. It should be recognised that some girls are extremely embarrassed by changes in figure, especially by the development of the breasts, which they may attempt to hide by adopting a round-shouldered posture. Such girls are sensitive to comment and are helped by the provision of loose-fitting upper garments.

On the other hand, there are many early 'teenagers' who worry because their breast development seems to them late or poor and who accept the menarche and its accompaniments with pride. These are the ones who have been well primed in what to expect. The onset of menstruation in a girl who is uninformed arouses emotions of fear and shame and can give her a psychological shock from which she never fully recovers. Failure of the adolescent to realise the implications and potential dangers of sex can lead to tragedy. Sex education should come naturally and piecemeal throughout childhood. Even infants are curious about their genitalia, and their curiosity should be satisfied. Children inevitably ask questions, and these should be answered simply but truthfully as they arise. Indeed, sex instruction should be merely part of the general education of the child, acquired from day to day in the course of family conversation and becoming more detailed with the passing of time.

In today's world, the very real risks of unwanted teenage pregnancy and sexually transmitted diseases cannot be ignored. The progressively decreasing age of menarche has resulted in the first and the increasing permissiveness of society in the second. Today's adolescent needs to be armed with sufficient information in order to be protected against the hazards of human immunodeficiency virus (HIV) infection, in addition to other reproductive tract infections, and to avoid the psychological and physical consequences of unwanted illegitimate pregnancy.

ABNORMALITIES OF PUBERTY AND ADOLESCENCE

Obesity

Obesity has become a major health concern and a global problem not only in adults but also in childhood and adolescence. It is associated with cardiometabolic and psychosocial comorbidity and premature mortality.

According to the 2007 World Health Organization (WHO) growth reference, for the age group 5–19 years, overweight is defined as body mass index (BMI) ≥1 SD and obesity as BMI ≥2 SD of the median for age and sex. The Centers for Disease Control and Prevention (CDC) for those aged 2–20 years, overweight as >85th to <95th percentile and obesity as ≥95th percentile based on CDC growth charts.

Prevalence of childhood and adolescent obesity: From 1975 to 2016, the global age-standardised prevalence of obesity in children and adolescents aged 5–19 years increased from 0·7% [95% credible interval (CrI) 0·4–1·2] to 5·6% (4·8–6·5) for girls and from 0·9% (0·5–1·3) to 7·8% (6·7–9·1) for boys.

Risk Factors and Implications of Childhood Obesity

Risk factors and implications of childhood obesity are shown in **Flowchart 2**.

The principles of management are (1) to reduce adiposity, (2) improve related physical and psychosocial complications, and (3) prevent the development of chronic diseases.

Multicomponent interventions include diet, physical activity, reducing screen time, behaviour

Flowchart 2: Risk factors and implications of childhood obesity.

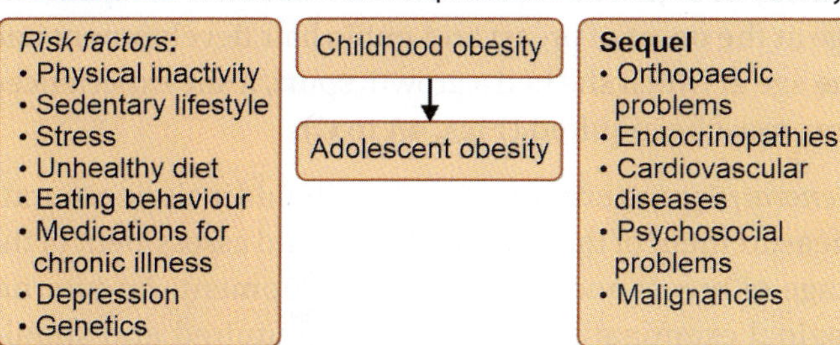

changes, adequate sleep, behavioural support activities, psychological interventions, antiobesity medications and metabolic and bariatric surgery as a last resort.

Adolescence is sometimes accompanied by a rapid increase in weight and the development of 'puppy fat.' This can be associated with the formation of striae on the breasts, flanks, buttocks and upper arms, which are reddish-purple at first but later fade to silver. The cause is a weakening of the elastic tissue by an increased production of adrenal corticoids together with stretching of the skin by subcutaneous fat.

Some of these girls may have an underlying problem, such as hypothyroidism or polycystic ovaries. Obesity in children and adolescents, irrespective of the underlying metabolic processes of the individual, is nearly always associated with overeating, or with eating predominantly carbohydrates. This is true no matter what the protesting parent may say. Adolescent obesity of a minor degree tends to disappear by the age of 20 years if the appetite is reasonably curbed. Obesity of a gross degree, however, requires strict dietetic control (1,000 kcal in 24 hours), lest it persist and progress to prejudice the girl's future menstrual and reproductive functions, as well as her health in general. There may be a variation in the age of menarche and the obesity of the girl. Typically, the age of menarche is earlier than average in children with moderate obesity (up to 30% above normal weight for age), whereas delayed menarche is common in those with severe malnutrition.

Menstrual Disorders

For details, refer to Chapter 39 (Amenorrhoea, Hypomenorrhoea, and Oligomenorrhoea) and Chapter 40 (Abnormal and Excessive Uterine Bleeding).

Delayed Puberty

Delayed puberty can be defined as the failure to begin sexual maturation at an age that is 2.5 standard deviations (SD) above the mean age of onset of puberty. Delayed puberty in girls can be described if there is no occurrence of breast development by the age of 13 years or no menarche by 3 years after breast development or by the age of 16 years. In boys, delayed puberty can be defined as no testicular enlargement by 14 years or a delay in development for 5 years or more after the onset of genitalia enlargement. In the US, the evaluation of delayed puberty is recommended at 13 years in girls and 14 years or older in boys who do not demonstrate any signs of sexual maturation. However, if other secondary sexual characteristics have developed normally in a girl with primary amenorrhoea, an expectant approach can be adopted until the age of 16 years, following which the girl must be investigated.

Aetiology

The main cause of delayed puberty is hypogonadism, which could be either hypogonadotropic hypogonadism (inactive hypothalamic-pituitary axis) or hypergonadotropic hypogonadism (primary gonadal failure) **(Table 2)**. In these cases, there is an absence of breast and pubic hair development. In cases of hypogonadotropic hypogonadism, there is an absent or reduced level of gonadotrophins. In hypergonadotropic hypogonadism, there is normal release of gonadotrophins, but there is no response from the gonads. As a result, there is no negative feedback to control gonadotrophin levels. Another important cause of delayed puberty is a constitutional delay of growth and puberty.

Constitutional growth delay: Constitutional growth delay is a temporary delay in skeletal growth and height of a child with no other physical abnormality causing the delay. This can be considered as one of the most important causes of delayed puberty and short stature. In cases of constitutional delay of puberty, normal prepubertal growth nadir is prolonged, and pulsatile GnRH secretion is slow to develop. Family history is often positive, with the siblings or parents also giving a history of delayed puberty. X-ray of the left hand and wrist demonstrates the bone age to be delayed. If the bone age reaches 13 years in girls or 14 years in boys without the evidence of puberty, the patient is more likely to have GnRH deficiency rather than constitutional delay of puberty. Also, in cases of constitutional delay of puberty, laboratory evaluation reveals prepubertal testosterone levels and low or normal gonadotrophin levels. In cases of constitutional delay of puberty, even though the puberty is delayed, it begins before the bone age of 13 years in girls or 14 years in boys.

TABLE 2: Various causes of delayed puberty.

Absence of breast and pubic hair development	
Hypogonadotropic hypogonadism	***Hypergonadotropic hypogonadism***
• Functional GnRH deficiency, reflecting a constitutional delay in the reactivation of the hypothalamic-gonadal axis • Normal variation, sometimes familial • Suppressive effects of chronic stress due to illness, malnutrition or excessive exercise • Systemic disease, e.g. malnutrition, cystic fibrosis, renal failure, heart disease, and malabsorption • Genetic defects (Kallman's syndrome) • Anatomic abnormalities (hypothalamic and pituitary tumours, e.g. craniopharyngioma) • Thyroid deficiency (hypothyroidism) • Hyperprolactinaemia • Pituitary failure • Androgen receptor defect, e.g. testicular feminisation (complete or partial defects) • Anorexia nervosa • Emotional deprivation • Excessive exercise	• Primary gonadal failure (primary testicular failure, e.g. Klinefelter's syndrome or primary ovarian failure, e.g. Turner's syndrome) • Previous treatment of malignancy (gonadectomy, chemotherapy, gonadal irradiation, etc.) • Galactosemia (in association with ovarian failure) • Autoimmune ovarian failure (may be associated with abnormalities such as Addison's disease, vitiligo and hypothyroidism) • Congenital adrenal hyperplasia (due to the deficiency of 17-α hydroxylase)
Normal breast and pubic hair development: Normal progression of puberty, but failure of menstruation	
• Anatomical abnormalities (e.g. Müllerian agenesis) • Imperforate hymen or transverse vaginal septum • Hyperprolactinaemia • Congenital adrenal hyperplasia (CAH)	
Normal breast development, but scanty or absent pubic hair	
Androgen insensitivity syndrome (failure of pubic hair development due to end-organ insensitivity to androgens)	

(GnRH: gonadotrophin-releasing hormone)

Height is often <5th percentile, but growth rate is normal for the skeletal age. The onset of adrenarche is delayed.

Diagnosis

Clinical presentation: A detailed history must be taken from the girl as well as her mother to determine if puberty itself is delayed or just the onset of menstruation is delayed. The age at the onset of breast and pubic hair development and the age at which she had a growth spurt, if she experienced any, must be inquired **(Figs. 4A to C)**.

General physical examination: This should include accurate measurement of the patient's height and assessment of the stage of breast and pubic hair development. An internal vaginal examination is usually not required and should be avoided in young girls. An inspection of the external genitalia usually proves to be sufficient.

Investigations

The investigations which are performed in cases of delayed puberty include the following:

- *Radiology:* An X-ray of the hand to assess bone age helps in revealing whether the child has reached a stage of physical maturation at which puberty should be occurring. Visible secondary sexual development usually begins when girls achieve a bone age of 10.5–11 years.
- *Gonadotrophin levels:* Measurement of gonadotrophin levels helps in revealing if the cause is due to the defect of the gonads (elevated gonadotrophin levels) or due to the deficiency of the sex steroids (reduced gonadotrophin levels).
- *Serum prolactin levels:* In cases of raised serum prolactin levels, imaging by magnetic resonance imaging (MRI) is indicated to rule out a pituitary lactotrophic adenoma, except in cases where hyperprolactinaemia can be attributed to secondary medications.
- *Measurement of serum TSH and free thyroxine levels:* Measurement of these can help in identifying the cases of primary and secondary hypothyroidism.
- *Measurement of serum DHEAS concentration:* Measurement of serum DHEAS levels is important to differentiate between constitutional growth delay and GnRH deficiency. Patients with congenital GnRH deficiency are likely to have normal adrenarche and therefore normal levels of DHEAS.
- *Karyotype analysis:* In cases of hypergonadotrophic hypogonadism, karyotype analysis must be performed, which helps in ruling out chromosomal abnormalities (especially Turner's syndrome and Klinefelter's syndrome). In a short female, chromosome analysis should be performed to rule out Turner's syndrome.
- *Serum testosterone levels:* High serum testosterone levels indicate androgen insensitivity (male

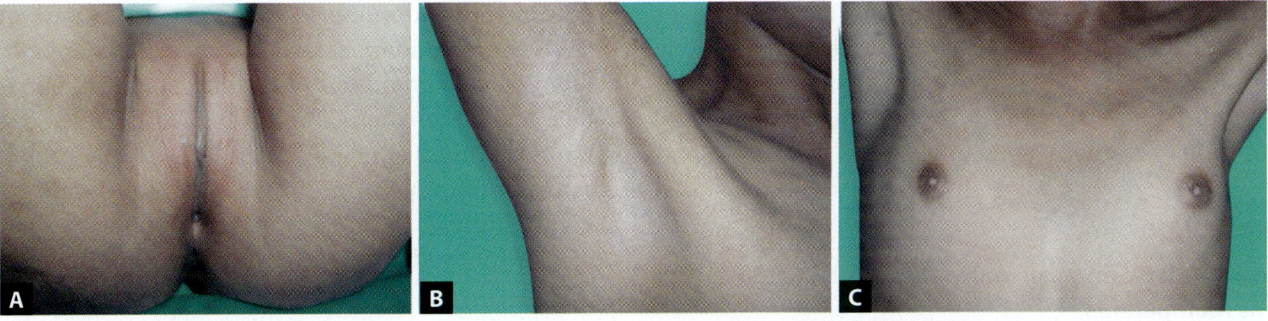

Figs. 4A to C: (A) Lack of pubic hair; (B) Lack of axillary hair; (C) Breasts are underdeveloped.

pseudohermaphroditism), which comprises a normal male karyotype (46, XY) with an abnormality in the androgen receptor. This results in unresponsiveness to androgens, which prevents masculinisation of male genitalia. As a result, there is the development of female external genitalia. The person is phenotypically a female with normal breasts, but absent pubic hair. There may be the presence of intra-abdominal testes.

- *Ultrasound examination:* This may be required to confirm the presence of uterus and ovaries **(Figs. 5 and 6)**.
- *Other tests:* Other tests, such as complete blood count (CBC), erythrocyte sedimentation rate (ESR) and liver function tests (LFTs), help in ruling out chronic illnesses.

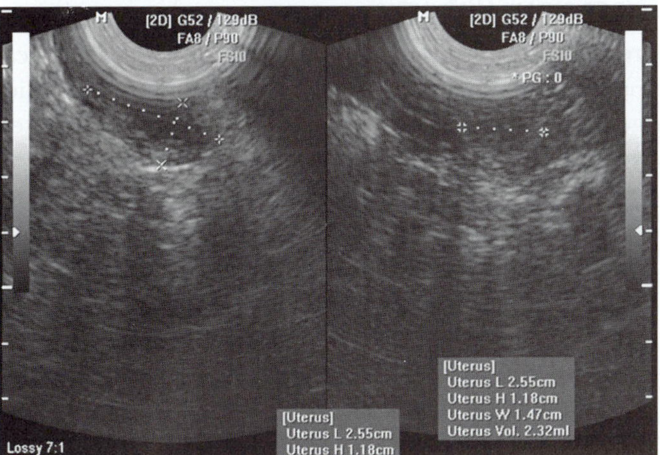

Fig. 5: Prepubertal uterus.

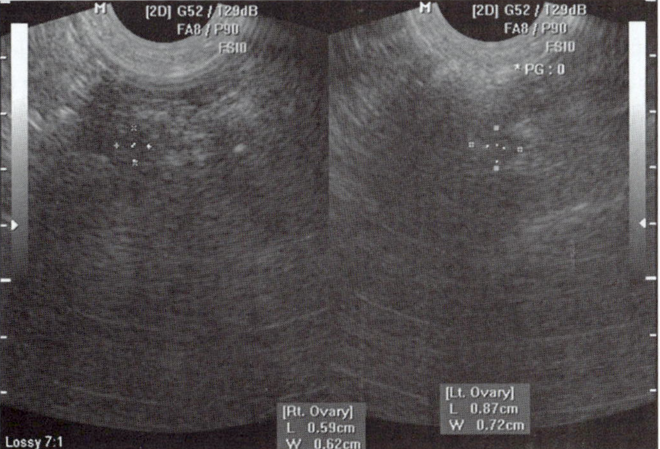

Fig. 6: Prepubertal ovaries.

Management

If no obvious cause of delayed puberty can be detected, reassurance and prediction of puberty based on bone age work in most cases. If, on radiological assessment, bone age is less than the chronological age, a wait-and-watch policy must be adopted. Most of these girls eventually develop secondary sexual characteristics and menarche over a period of time.

- *Therapy with sex hormones:* Pubertal delay due to gonadotrophin deficiency may be treated with testosterone replacement or human chorionic gonadotrophin (hCG). The treatment most commonly involves the administration of testosterone or related compounds to boys and oestrogens to girls in extreme cases. GH can also be sometimes prescribed. Treatment with pulsatile gonadotrophins has also been used. However, this treatment is difficult to sustain because subcutaneous injection attached to a portable pump may be required for several months. The more widely used approach involves the administration of low doses of ethinyl oestradiol in the dosage of 1–2 µg per day for 3–6 months.
- Hormone therapy can also be initiated in patients with congenital GnRH deficiency or constitutional delay of puberty over 12 years having no signs of spontaneous sexual maturation and causing significant distress or anxiety.

- *Treatment of the underlying cause:* This comprises treating the underlying cause, such as thyroid hormone replacement therapy (HRT) for hypothyroidism, therapy with dopamine agonists for hyperprolactinaemia and excision of craniopharyngioma.

Complications

Delayed puberty may cause anxiety or stress to the girls as well as their parents.

Precocious Puberty

Precocious puberty refers to the appearance of physical and hormonal signs of pubertal development at an earlier age than is considered normal. This can be characterised by the development of both breasts and pubic hair in girls and by the development of pubic hair and testicular enlargement in boys (testicular enlargement can be defined as an increase in the volume of >4 mL or a diameter of 2.5 cm).

Precocious puberty is defined as pubertal development occurring more than 2.5 SD earlier than the average age. If the average age of puberty was considered to be 10 years, the development of secondary sexual characteristics before 8 years in females **(Figs. 7A to C)** or the onset of menses before the age of 10 years (chronological age) would be defined as precocious puberty. The development of secondary sexual characteristics before 9 years in males is also considered precocious. A history of early puberty in a parent or sibling is relevant and decreases the likelihood that early puberty has an organic cause.

Aetiology

Precocious puberty can be of two types:

1. Central precocious puberty (CPP) (constitutional/true/complete precocious puberty), which is gonadotrophin dependent **(Figs. 8A and B)**
2. Precocious pseudopuberty, which is gonadotrophin-independent

The difference between CPP and precocious pseudopuberty is described in **Table 3**.

Diagnosis

Clinical presentation: The diagnosis is made with the help of a careful history and physical examination in conjunction with the use of radiologic and laboratory evaluations. The clinician must differentiate CPP from precocious pseudopuberty at the time of examination. In CPP, the secondary sexual characteristics appear in a chronological order, and eventually, regular menstrual cycles are established. Due to exposure to oestrogens, there is an initial spurt of height followed by premature closure of epiphysis due to which the ultimate height remains stunted. Future reproductive capacity is usually not compromised in cases of true precocious puberty.

Investigations

The following investigations are required in cases of precocious puberty:

Radiography: After taking a complete history and performing a physical examination, radiography of the hand and wrist must be performed in order to determine the bone age.

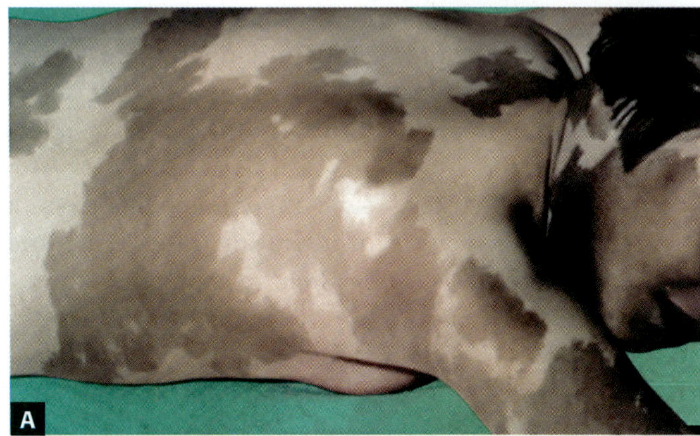

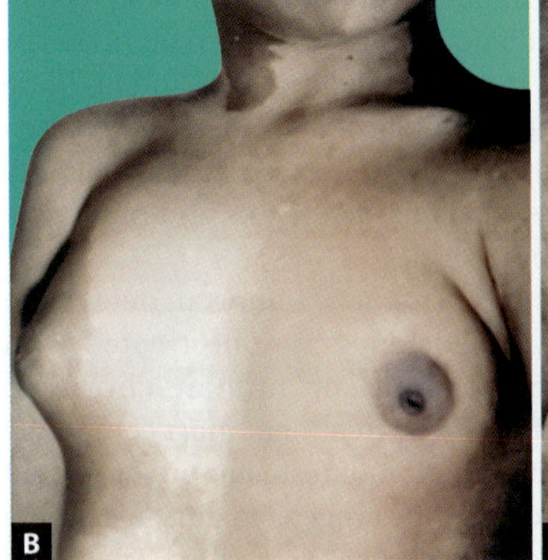

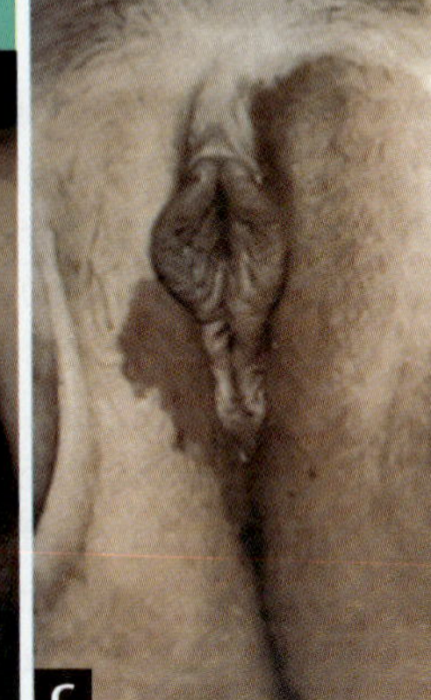

Figs. 7A to C: Precocious puberty as part of Albright syndrome. A girl, aged 7 years, with well-developed breasts and vulva who had been menstruating for 2 years. She had suffered many fractures, and both legs were in plaster at the time of photography. The patches shown in (A) are yellow-brown pigmentation; it is a typical feature.

The individuals who require further endocrine evaluation and imaging include the following:
- Children with advanced bone age
- Children with normal bone age accompanied by the development of both breasts and pubic hair
- Children with normal bone age associated with accelerated growth and breast or pubic hair development

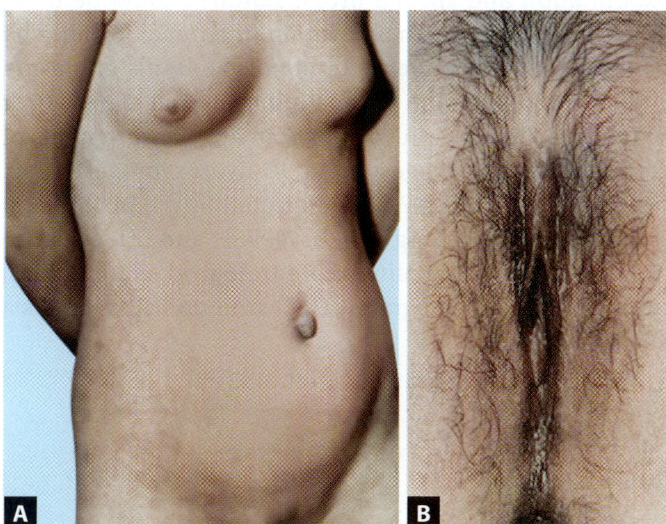

Figs. 8A and B: Precocious puberty. Child, aged 13 years 11 months, who had been menstruating for 18 months. The breasts, pubic hair, and the vulva are well developed. No abnormality was found on investigation, and the precocity was labelled 'constitutional,' but the after history of this case is unknown, so a lesion in the hypothalamic-pituitary system is not excluded.

Measurement of gonadotrophin levels: Measurement of GnRH-stimulated serum gonadotrophin levels helps in differentiating between the two types of precocious puberties. Measurement of the stimulated serum LH concentration can be considered the most useful diagnostic parameter. In case of gonadotrophin-dependent precocious puberty, there are elevated basal or stimulated serum LH levels. Other tests which may be required to evaluate the cause of CPP include the following:
- *Magnetic resonance imaging:* In cases of CPP, MRI of the head is indicated to exclude an intracranial lesion.
- *Thyroid function tests:* Thyroid function tests are not a routine requirement in the evaluation of precocious puberty. These may be required in case of clinical suspicion of thyroid dysfunction.

Evaluation of the causes of precocious pseudopuberty: In case of gonadotrophin-independent precocious puberty (as evidenced by normal basal and stimulated LH levels), other tests which need to be done include:

TABLE 3: Differences between gonadotrophin-dependent and gonadotrophin-independent precocious puberty.

Characteristics	***Gonadotrophin-dependent precocious puberty***	***Gonadotrophin-independent precocious puberty***
Alternative name	Also known as central precocious puberty or true precocious puberty	Also known as peripheral precocious puberty or pseudoprecocious puberty
Aetiology	It is characterised by early maturation and activation of the hypothalamic-pituitary-gonadal axis. However, the sequence of pubertal events is normal and proceeds at a normal pace	It is independent of GnRH and gonadotrophins. It usually results from exposure to sex-steroid hormones, which may be derived from the gonads, adrenals or the environment
Consistency of sexual characteristics with the child's gender	It is isosexual in nature, i.e., developing sexual characteristics are consistent with the child's gender	It could be either isosexual or contrasexual in nature, where sexual characteristics are inconsistent with the child's gender (e.g. virilisation in girls or feminisation in boys)
Levels of gonadotrophins	Levels of gonadotrophins, particularly FSH and LH, are increased	Levels of gonadotrophins are low
Causes	• Idiopathic (70–80%) • *CNS lesions:* Congenital such as hydrocephalus, acquired, such as postirradiation, infection, surgery, cysts or tumours (such as microscopic hamartomas, astrocytomas, ependymomas, pineal tumours and optic and hypothalamic gliomas) • Hypothyroidism	• McCune-Albright syndrome • Ovarian tumours (granulosa tumour, malignant teratoma or arrhenoblastoma of the ovary) • Adrenal cortical lesions (tumour or hyperplasia) • Testicular disorders (Leydig cell tumours) and administration of exogenous sex steroids

(CNS: central nervous system; GnRH: gonadotrophin-releasing hormone; FSH: follicle-stimulating hormone; hCG: human chorionic gonadotrophin; LH: luteinising hormone)

- Serum concentration of oestradiol, testosterone and hCG (for detection of functional ovarian cysts, tumours and functional adrenal tumours)
- Late afternoon cortisol levels (Cushing's syndrome)
- Dehydroepiandrosterone, DHEAS and premature adrenarche
- 17-hydroxyprogesterone (CAH)

Management

Approaches and laboratory findings related to precocious puberty are illustrated in **Flowchart 3** and **Table 4**.

Children presenting with vaginal bleeding before the age of 8 years should be examined for evidence of secondary sex characteristics. If these are not present, then the bleeding is probably not menstrual, and a local organic cause in the uterus or vagina should be looked for **(Figs. 9A and B)**.

If secondary sex characters are present, then examination and special investigations should be done to exclude an intracranial, ovarian or adrenal lesion. The demonstration of pubertal or abnormal levels of plasma gonadotrophins in the plasma indicates that the anterior pituitary is showing precocious activity. Measurements of serum oestradiol, progesterone, 17-hydroxyprogesterone, testosterone and DHEAS, as indicated by the history and physical findings, along with basal FSH and LH levels are helpful. Any abnormality on neurological examination, head computed tomography (CT) scan or MRI suggests a cerebral cause.

Flowchart 3: Approaches to precocious puberty.

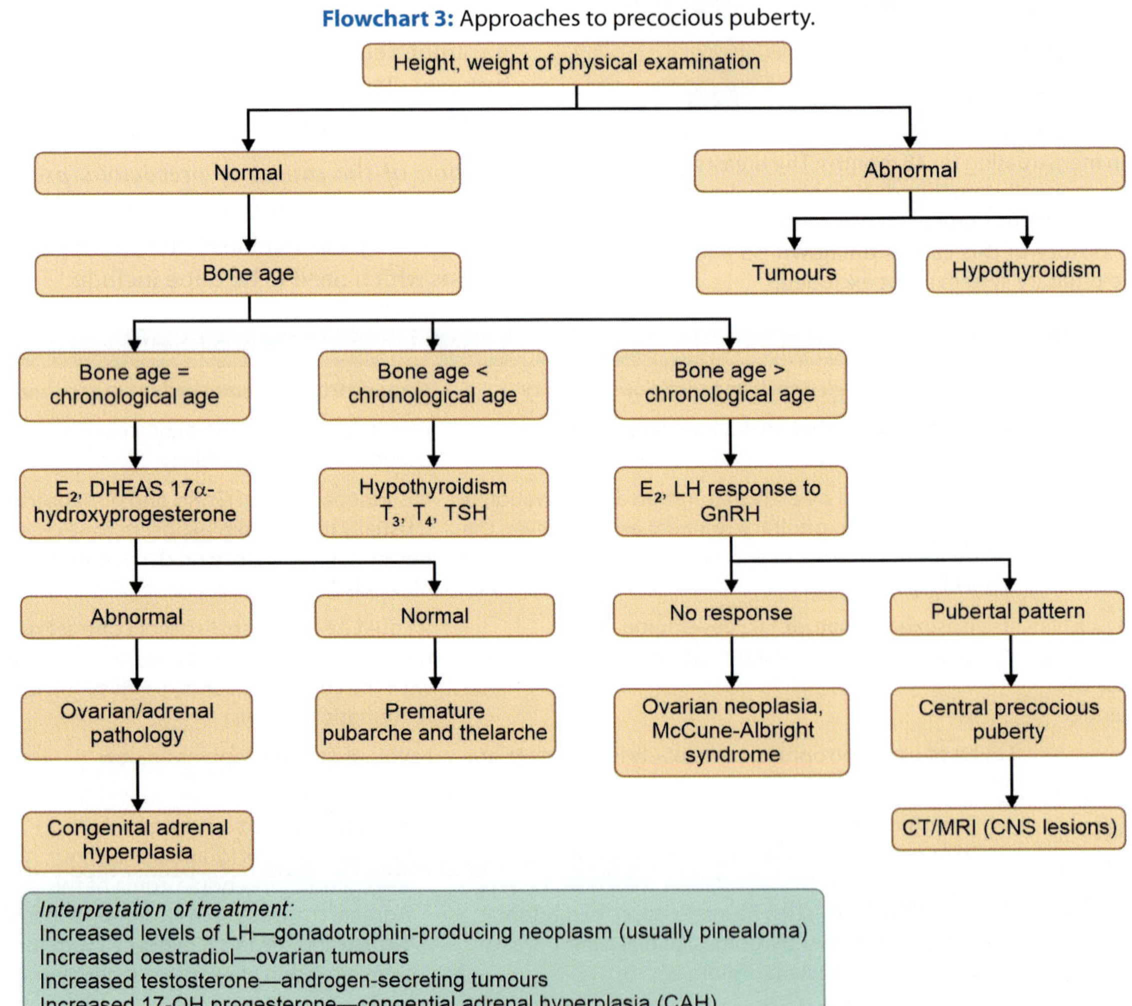

(CNS: central nervous system; CT: computed tomography; DHEA-S: dehydroepiandrosterone sulphate; GnRH: gonadotrophin-releasing hormone; LH: luteinising hormone; MRI: magnetic resonance imaging; TSH: thyroid-stimulating hormone)

TABLE 4: Laboratory findings in disorders producing precocious puberty.

	Gonadal size	*Basal FSH/LH*	*Oestradiol or testosterone*	*DHEAS*	*GnRH response*
Idiopathic	Increased	Increased	Increased	Increased	Pubertal
Cerebral cause	Increased	Increased	Increased	Increased	Pubertal
Gonadal cause	Unilaterally increased	Decreased	Increased	Increased	Flat
McAlbright syndrome	Increased	Decreased	Increased	Increased	Flat
Adrenal cause	Small	Decreased	Increased	Increased	Flat

(DHEAS: dehydroepiandrosterone sulphate; FSH: follicle-stimulating hormone; GnRH: gonadotrophin-releasing hormone; LH: luteinising hormone)

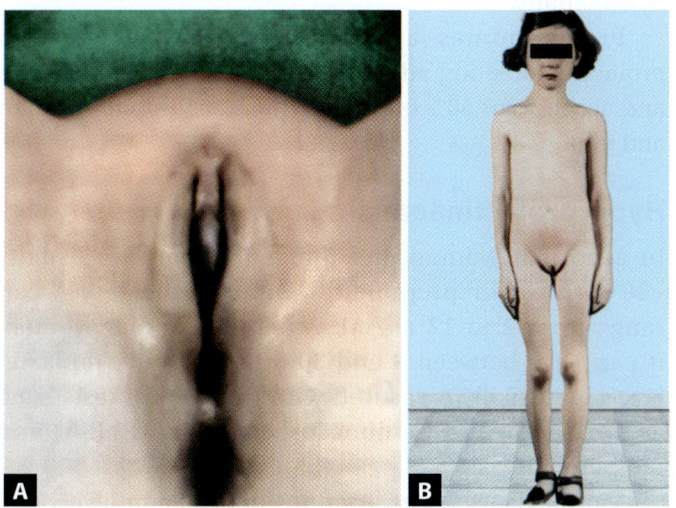

Figs. 9A and B: Alleged precocious puberty. A child, aged 7 years, who had bled vaginally on two occasions. There is no development of the breasts, pubic hair or vulva, and this indicates that the bleeding was not menstrual or the result of hormone stimulation. It was decided that it was caused by local interference of some kind, and it did not recur. A normal menstrual cycle, accompanied by physical maturation, began 6 years later. At a later stage in life, this patient was seen again and was then found to have a uterus didelphys and septate vagina. So, the bleeding in childhood was probably caused by injury to the lower border of the septum inflicted by the patient herself. The photograph of the vulva shows what looks like a prominent clitoris. This is usual in childhood and is explained by poor development of the labia.

The management depends on whether it is gonadotrophin dependent (in which case it is almost invariably of central origin) or gonadotrophin independent (of peripheral origin). The evaluation of precocious puberty is as follows:

- The first test should be the measurement of basal gonadotrophin levels.
- Thyroid function should also be evaluated to rule out primary hypothyroidism as the cause of precocious development.
- High levels of LH (which really may be hCG detected because of cross-reactivity with LH in immunoassays) suggest a gonadotrophin-producing neoplasm, most often a pinealoma (ectopic germinoma).
- Increased oestradiol levels suggest an oestrogen-secreting neoplasm, probably of ovarian origin.
- Increased testosterone levels suggest an androgen-producing neoplasm of the ovary or the adrenal gland. Such neoplasms may be palpable on abdominal or rectal examination. Increased 17α-hydroxyprogesterone levels are diagnostic of 21-hydroxylase deficiency (i.e., CAH). DHEAS levels are elevated in various forms of CAH as well.

Bone age should always be assessed in evaluating an individual with sexual precocity. Then management with GnRH agonist therapy initially increases circulating gonadotrophin and oestradiol concentrations for short periods of time. Chronic therapy is associated with the suppression of pulsatile gonadotrophin secretion and a blockade to the LH response of endogenous GnRH. Suppression is best monitored with GnRH challenge tests. Additionally, measurement of serum oestradiol (if elevated on prior analysis), height, bone age and assessment of secondary sexual characteristics may be helpful. Evaluation of ovarian morphology and uterine size by pelvic ultrasonography may, in some cases, provide additional evidence of such suppression. The various effects like cessation of menses, regression in physical pubertal signs (i.e., breast size and pubic hair) and a diminution of uterine and ovarian size usually occur within the first 6 months of therapy.

If these are normal, it is most likely to be idiopathic sexual precocity. If a feminising adrenal tumour is suspected (with elevated serum DHEAS and oestradiol and low gonadotrophins), abdominal and pelvic ultrasound or MRI can be done. Ovarian tumours are also associated with elevated oestradiol and low gonadotrophins and can be detected by imaging. Skeletal survey for bone age shows accelerated maturation (breast development with bone age 11 and menarche with bone age 13). Virilising ovarian tumours may result in elevated serum DHEAS or androstenedione levels. Ovarian and adrenal tumours should be surgically resected.

Precocious puberty with delayed bone age suggests primary hypothyroidism. Serum TSH is increased, serum T4 is low and galactorrhoea may be present along with increased serum prolactin. Serum gonadotrophins are in the pubertal range. The sella may be widened on imaging. All values return to normal with treatment.

Patients with Albright syndrome may have a very variable presentation, and sometimes a technetium-99 bone scan may be necessary to demonstrate areas of fibrous dysplasia in the bones.

The principles of management of true precocious puberty require (1) attention to maximising height, (2) arresting further maturation and (3) attenuating precocious features.

In the past, medroxyprogesterone acetate, cyproterone acetate and danazol were used with some success. The use of GnRH analogues has significantly improved the results of treatment. These can be administered subcutaneously or intranasally, daily or in long-acting depot forms. The last are obviously the most preferred. The goal of therapy is to maintain the serum oestradiol level <10 pg/mL. Treatment has to be continued till pubertal and chronological ages match. The final bone height is increased depending on how early treatment is instituted.

Prolonged observation is required to detect evidence of underlying disease in the pituitary, ovary or adrenal gland, which may appear later.

Parents should be warned to guard the precocious child from possible sexual assault.

Complications

- Rapid bone maturation can cause linear growth to cease too early and can result in an ultimately short adult stature.
- The early appearance of breasts or menses in girls and increased libido in boys can cause emotional distress for some children.
- Young girls with precocious puberty may be stressed, may become withdrawn, may exhibit behavioural problems (such as poor self-esteem and higher anxiety, irritability or withdrawal) and may have difficulty adjusting to wearing and changing pads.
- A precocious child should be guarded against possible sexual assault.

PROLACTIN

Prolactin is a peptide hormone, which is secreted in a pulsatile manner. Its function is mainly the preparation of mammary glands for the production of milk. Prolactin is present in the blood in two forms: (1) Monomeric and (2) polymeric. Secretion of prolactin is mainly controlled by dopamine.

Prolactinomas are the most common benign prolactin-secreting adenomas derived from lactotrophs and account for 50% of pituitary tumours in both women and men.

Hyperprolactinaemia

In a normal woman, the prolactin levels are usually <20 ng/mL. In prepubertal women, the levels can range from 2 to 12 ng/mL, whereas in adult women, it can vary between 3 and 30 ng/mL. Serum prolactin levels are usually measured with the help of tests such as enzyme-linked immunosorbent assay (ELISA) and radioimmunoassay.

Various causes for variations in prolactin levels and their management are discussed in **Table 5**.

TABLE 5: Variations in prolactin levels and their management.

Serum prolactin levels (ng/mL)	*Causes*	*Management*
<40	• Normal • Psychological • Stress • Drug induced	• No advice • Relieve stress • Stop drug
50–100	• Usually hypothalamic • Stalk compression • Polycystic ovarian syndrome	• Rule out thyroid • Complete evaluation • Repeat levels
>150	Probably tumours due to systemic disorders	Computed tomography/ magnetic resonance imaging (CT/MRI)
>200	Confirmed tumours	Medical or surgical advice

TABLE 6: Clinical features of hyperprolactinaemia.

Female	*Male*
• Galactorrhoea • Amenorrhoea • Oligomenorrhoea • Luteal phase defects • Follicular dysfunction • Infertility	• Sexual dysfunction • Azoospermia • Galactorrhoea

Clinical Features

Clinical features of hyperprolactinaemia for both males and females are shown in **Table 6**.

The causes of infertility due to hyperprolactinaemia are as follows:

- Disruption of normal follicular development
- Atresia of dominant follicle
- Premature destruction of corpus luteum.

Causes

- *Hormone disturbances:*
  - Primary hypothyroidism
  - Endogenous increased oestrogen
  - Use of oral contraceptive pills (OCPs)
  - Cushing's syndrome.
- *Use of dopamine receptor blocking agents:*
  - Phenothiazines
  - Haloperidol
  - Metoclopramide
  - Gonadotrophin analogues
- *Dopamine-depleting agents:*
  - Reserpine
  - α-methyl dopamine
  - Opiates
- *H_2 receptor antagonists:*
  - Ranitidine
- *Tumours:*
  - Pituitary adenomas
  - Craniopharyngiomas
- *Physiological:*
  - Stress
  - Exercise
  - Nipple stimulation
  - Sleep
  - Sex
- *Others:*
  - Renal failure (decreased clearance)
  - Cirrhosis of liver
- Idiopathic

Please note that drugs form an important and common cause of hyperprolactinaemia and should always be ruled out before going for higher investigations. Diligent history taking is of foremost importance.

Management

Management (both surgical and medical) has been discussed in **Flowchart 4**.

Medical management: Medical management of hyperprolactinaemia comprises the following medicines:

- *Bromocriptine:*
  - First used in the 1970s
  - Ergot derivative
  - Half-life 6–8 hours
  - Decreases tumour size and causes perivascular fibrosis. It is usually administered in the dosage of 1.25 mg HS and then increased based on the clinical parameters.
- *Cabergoline:* This is the preferred drug of choice presently.
  - Half-life 65 hours
  - Given in the dosage of 2.5 mg/week
  - Higher affinity for D2 receptors
- *Pergolide:*
  - Newer ergot derivative
  - Long acting
  - Used in bromocriptine resistance cases

Medical management is the first line of treatment in prolactinomas, and cabergoline is the drug of choice. Drugs should be started at a low dose and slowly increased to improve tolerability and compliance. A close watch on the adverse effects of the drugs should be advocated. Follow-up in 3–6 months is advised, which determines the effectiveness of treatment and helps in prognostication.

- Surgical management is offered for (1) spontaneous cerebrospinal fluid (CSF) rhinorrhoea; and (2) rapidly progressive vision loss due to a sellar mass effect or apoplexy; (3) intolerance or resistance to long-term dopamine agonist therapy; (4) young age in women could favour a choice of surgical treatment to avoid the need for dopamine agonist therapy over many decades; and (5) who desires pregnancy, as it reduces the risk of symptomatic mass enlargement during future pregnancy of the above-listed causes only the first one is a clear-cut indication for surgery, and the remaining indications need to be individualised.

Flowchart 4: Management of hyperprolactinaemia.

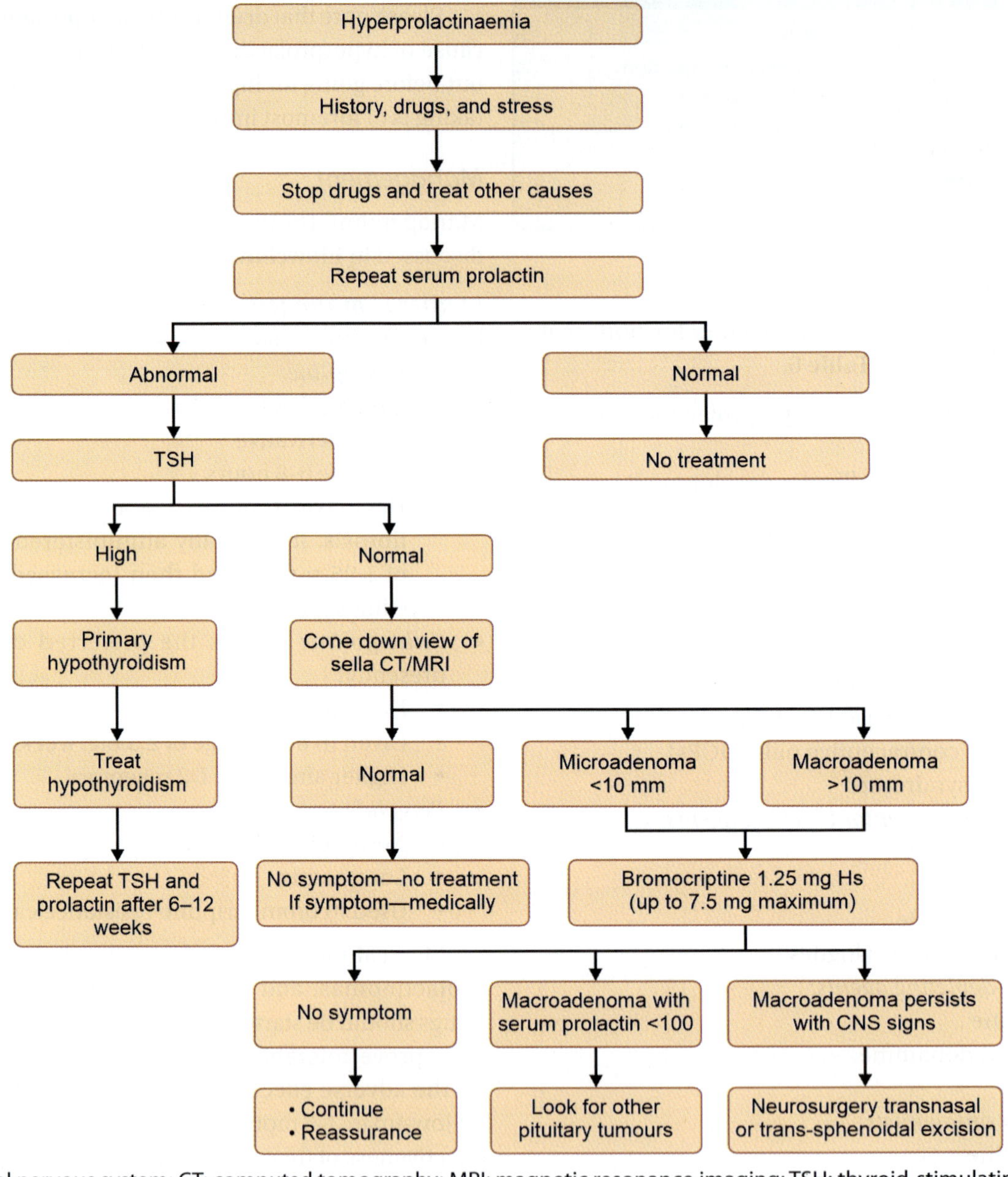

(CNS: central nervous system; CT: computed tomography; MRI: magnetic resonance imaging; TSH: thyroid-stimulating hormone)

Radiation therapy is the least used management approach for prolactinoma and is mainly offered when medical and surgical treatments have not been successful, usually in patients with size-progressing, aggressive prolactinoma or prolactin-secreting malignancies.

PUBERTY MENORRHAGIA

- Menarche usually occurs at the age of 12–14 years and coincides with Tanner stage 4 of breast or pubic hair.
- Menstrual problems are common in adolescence due to the slow maturation of the HPO axis, which is a mediator of the menstrual cycle.

Etiopathology

Adolescents lack a positive feedback mechanism to induce LH surge and subsequent ovulation despite increased oestrogen levels. The negative feedback mechanism is intact. So, there is pubertal anovulation.

TABLE 7: Causes of puberty menorrhagia.

Anovulation	*Blood dyscrasias*	*Others*
	• Coagulation defects. Idiopathic thrombocytopenic purpura (ITP) is the most common – Others—thalassemia and sickle cell – Platelet defects – Pernicious anaemia	• *Anatomic:* – Trauma – Foreign body – Sexual abuse – Polyps – Fibroids – Malignancies • *Hypothalamic:* – Stress – Eating disorders – Excessive exercise – Immunology – Ovarian antibodies – Follicle-stimulating hormone/luteinising hormone • *Infections:* – Pelvic inflammatory disease – Cervicitis • *Systemic disease:* – Thyroid – Adrenal – Diabetes mellitus – Renal • *Pregnancy related:* – Abortion – Ectopic • *Drugs:* – Oral contraceptive pills – Nonsteroidal anti-inflammatory drugs (NSAIDs) – Aspirin – Anticoagulants

Anovulation results in a state of unopposed oestrogen, leading to increased endometrial growth. This endometrium without the support of progesterone can break down spontaneously with random and excessive bleeding.

Elevated oestrogen by its negative feedback suppresses FSH, LH, GnRH and oestrogen itself, leading to vasoconstriction and collapse of hyperplastic endometrium and heavy prolonged bleeding. Heavy bleeding is also worsened by prostaglandin imbalance. There is an alteration in the ratio of PGF2α and PGE2.

- Heavy menstrual bleeding (HMB) in adolescence might be a sentinel for underlying blood disorders. A detailed medical and family history pertaining to bleeding disorders should be obtained.

An adolescent girl should be assessed for anaemia from blood loss, serum ferritin levels, the presence of endocrine disorders leading to anovulation and evaluation for the presence of bleeding disorders.

Causes of Puberty Menorrhagia

The causes of puberty menorrhagia are shown in **Table 7**.

Management of Puberty Menorrhagia

Management for the puberty of menorrhagia is shown in **Flowchart 5**.

Diet

- Vitamin A supplements 25,000 IU for 15 days
- Vitamin E supplements 100 IU alternate days for 3 months
- Vitamin C and flavonoids protect capillaries from damage
- *Others:*
  - Cinnamon
  - Periwinkle
  - Hazel
  - Oak

Flowchart 5: Management of puberty menorrhagia.

(APC: activated protein C; CBC: complete blood count; DUB: dysfunctional uterine bleeding; EUA: examination under anaesthesia; Hb: haemoglobin; IV: intravenous; MPA: medroxy-progesterone acetate; OCPs: oral contraceptive pills; PS: peripheral smear; USG: ultrasonography)

Hormones

- *Progesterone:* Inhibits the growth of the endometrium
- *Oestrogen depot:* Progynova 25 mg—arrests bleeding
- Cyclic OCPs
- *Desmopressin:* Analogous to DDAVP (1-deamino-8-D-arginine vasopressin); it is used as a nasal spray in the dose of 1.5 mg/mL in patients with inherited bleeding disorders.

Important points to be considered:

- Structural causes of acute abnormal uterine bleeding (AUB) in adolescents are rare, so imaging might not always be helpful and should be reserved based on clinical judgement.
- Depending on the presentations, individuals might require an acute management of bleeding with restoration of haemodynamic stability and simultaneous evaluation of the specific cause followed by management of the same.
- Medical management is the first line for management of all individuals.
- Majority of the anovulatory causes settle on the maturation of the HPO axis in 3–5 years of menarche.

SUGGESTED READING

1. ACOG Committee Opinion. (2019) Screening and management of bleeding disorders in adolescents with heavy menstrual bleeding. ACOG Committee Opinion Number 785. [online] Available from https://www.acog.org/clinical/clinical-guidance/committee-opinion/articles/2019/09/screening-and-management-of-bleeding-disorders-in-adolescents-with-heavy-menstrual-bleeding [Last accessed March, 2025].
2. Albanese A, Stanhope R. Investigation of delayed puberty. Clin Endocrinol (Oxf). 1995;43(1):105-10.
3. American Academy of Pediatrics. Sexuality education for children and Adolescents: Committee on Psychosocial Aspects of Child and Family Health and Committee on Adolescence. Pediatrics. 2001;108(2):498-502.
4. Bridges NA, Christopher JA, Hindmarsh PC, Brook CG. Sexual precocity: sex incidence and aetiology. Arch Dis Child. 1994;70(2):116-8.
5. Cesario SK, Hughes LA. Precocious puberty: a comprehensive review of literature. J Obstet Gynecol Neonatal Nurs. 2007;36(3):263-74.
6. Chalumeau M, Chemaitilly W, Trivin C, Adan L, Bréart G, Brauner R. Central precocious puberty in girls: an evidence-based diagnosis tree to predict central nervous system abnormalities. Pediatrics. 2002;109(1):61-7.
7. Crowne EC, Shalet SM, Wallace WH, Eminson DM, Price DA. Final height in girls with untreated constitutional delay in growth and puberty. Eur J Pediatr. 1991;150(10):708-12.
8. Harrington J, Palmert MR. Definition, etiology, and evaluation of precocious puberty. UpToDate. [online] Available from https://www.uptodate.com/contents/definition-etiology-and-evaluation-of-precocious-puberty [Last accessed March, 2025].
9. Jebeile H, Kelly AS, O'Malley G, Baur LA. Obesity in children and adolescents: epidemiology, causes, assessment, and management. Lancet Diabetes Endocrinol. 2022;10(5):351-65.
10. Jebeile H, Kelly AS, O'Malley G, Baur LA. Obesity in children and adolescents: epidemiology, causes, assessment,

and management. Lancet Diabetes Endocrinol. 2022;10(5):351-65.
11. Kaplowitz PB, Oberfield SE. Reexamination of the age limit for defining when puberty is precocious in girls in the United States: implications for evaluation and treatment. Drug and Therapeutics and Executive Committees of the Lawson Wilkins Pediatric Endocrine Society. Pediatrics. 1999;104(4 Pt 1):936-41.
12. Koliaki C, Dalamaga M, Liatis S. Update on the Obesity Epidemic: After the Sudden Rise, Is the Upward Trajectory Beginning to Flatten? Curr Obes Rep. 2023;12(4):514-27.
13. Lazar L, Padoa A, Phillip M. Growth pattern and final height after cessation of gonadotropin-suppressive therapy in girls with central sexual precocity. J Clin Endocrinol Metab. 2007;92(9):3483-9.
14. Ng SM, Kumar Y, Cody D, Smith CS, Didi M. Cranial MRI scans are indicated in all girls with central precocious puberty. Arch Dis Child. 2003;88(5):414-8.
15. Parent AS, Teilmann G, Juul A, Skakkebaek NE, Toppari J, Bourguignon JP. The timing of normal puberty and the age limits of sexual precocity: variations around the world, secular trends, and changes after migration. Endocr Rev. 2003;24(5):668-93.
16. Petersenn S, Fleseriu M, Casanueva FF, Giustina A, Biermasz N, Biller BMK, et al. Diagnosis and management of prolactin-secreting pituitary adenomas: a Pituitary Society international Consensus Statement. Nat Rev Endocrinol. 2023;19(12):722-40.
17. Trotman GE. Delayed puberty in the female patient. Curr Opin Obstet Gynecol. 2016;28(5):366-72.
18. Wei C, Crowne EC. Recent advances in the understanding and management of delayed puberty. Arch Dis Child. 2016;101(5):481-8.
19. Weihrauch-Blüher S, Wiegand S. Risk Factors and Implications of Childhood Obesity. Curr Obes Rep. 2018;7(4):254-9.

7

CHAPTER

Conception

Akhila Vasudeva, Muralidhar V Pai

Chapter Outline

- Process
- Early Development of the Ovum
- Formation of Foetus and Membranes
- Hormonal Control of Early Pregnancy

INTRODUCTION

By definition, conception is taken synonymous with fertilisation which is when the sperm meets the ovum, but to say the least, in humans, it is complicated from fertilisation to implantation to continuation of the viable embryo and development. We generally say that a woman has conceived when beta human chorionic gonadotrophin (β-hCG) is detected after missed periods in either blood or urine.

PROCESS

Conception starts with the sexual activity between male and female when semen is deposited in the vagina. Semen consists of sperm and seminal fluid. The opportunity for their meeting is provided by the deposition of semen in the upper vagina and on the external os during coitus. Even if spermatozoa are only deposited on the vulva, they can sometimes make their way up the vagina to the cervix. This explains the occasional pregnancy in apparent virgins and also failures of coitus interruptus as a method of contraception.

Once deposited in the vagina, spermatozoa find themselves in a hostile acid medium from which they must escape quickly if they are to survive. The seminal fluid itself is alkaline with a pH of 7.05–7.41, rising to 7.5–8.0 on standing in vitro. When mixed with vaginal secretion, the pH of the seminal pool is 6.2, and may be only 5.5 if the alkaline contributions from the cervix and Bartholin's glands are limited. All spermatozoa remaining in the vagina for 2 hours or longer are killed, and it is probable that only those which can enter the alkaline cervical canal within a few minutes retain their fertilising power. They enter the cervix under their own powers of propulsion, being directed by chemotaxis (acid repels and alkali attracts). They invade the mucus plug in the cervical canal which, at the time of ovulation, is arranged to form microchannels to allow easier penetration. Once through the cervix, spermatozoa ascend rapidly, so rapidly that it is believed that they are moved by contractions of the uterus and tubes in addition to their own power. These contractions may be stimulated by prostaglandins present in the semen. The chief function of its flagellum may be to allow the spermatozoon to penetrate the corona radiata and the capsule of the ovum.

The time taken for spermatozoa to travel from the vagina to the tubes may be as short as 5 minutes. Many are lost on the way, the semen being expelled from the introitus, the sperm digested by vaginal enzymes or phagocytised by the epithelial cells of the genital tract. Those that reach the tube travel against the cilial current, and some find their way into the peritoneal cavity. Of an average of 200–300 million spermatozoa deposited in the vagina, fewer than 200 finally reach the egg. Until they enter the female genital tract, spermatozoa do not possess the capacity to penetrate the zona pellucida and to fertilise the ovum. 'Capacitation' is only acquired after they have been in the cervix, uterus and tubes for 2–4 hours.

The seminal plasma factors coating the surface are removed, and the surface charge is modified when the capacitated sperm interacts with the follicular fluid, the sperm head undergoes the acrosome reaction, allowing the release of several enzymes including hyaluronidase, corona dispersing enzymes and acrosin. The sperm motility also increases remarkably. All these changes are critical for zona penetration.

An ovum leaves the ovary having already undergone the first maturation (reduction) division and is picked

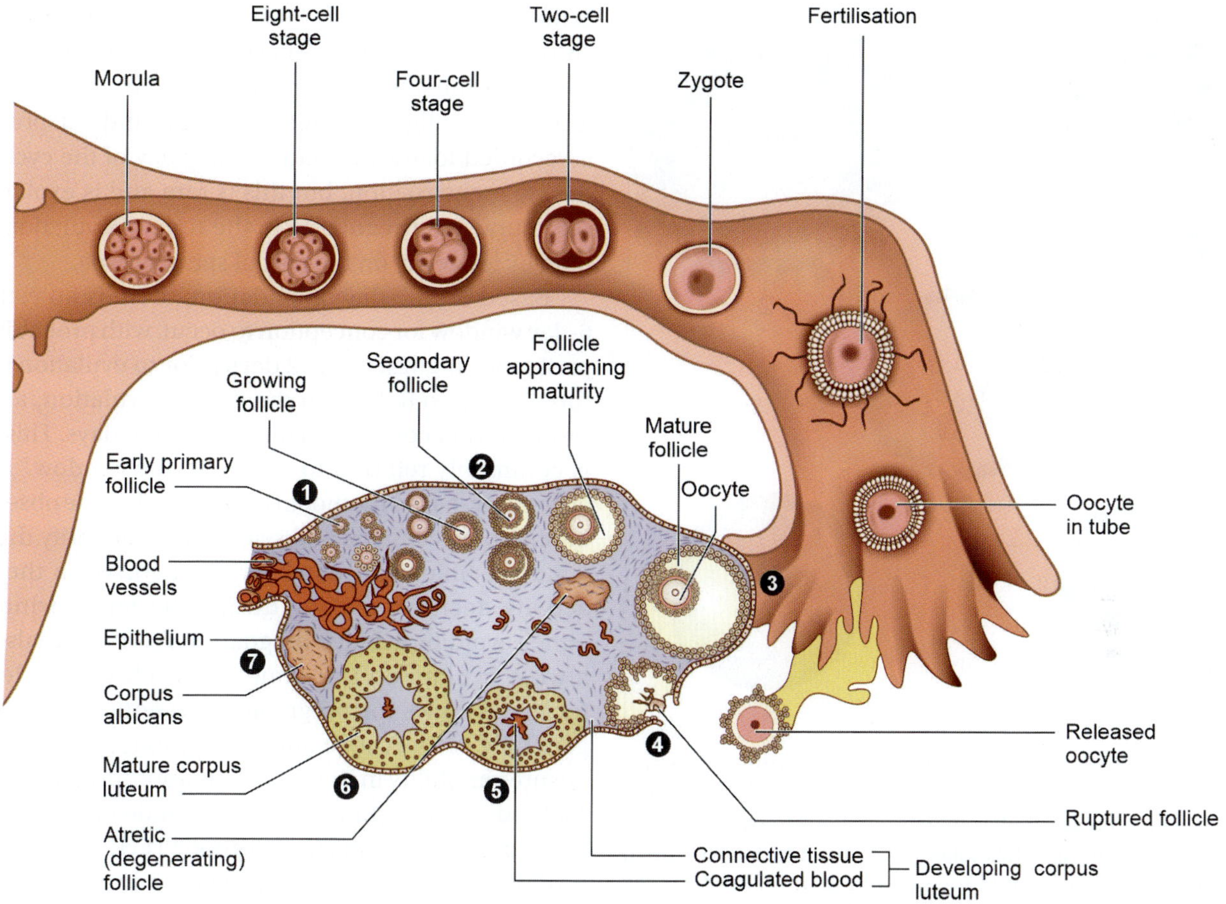

Fig. 1: Diagrammatic representation of ovulation, maturation of the ovum and fertilisation.

up by the fimbria of the fallopian tube **(Figs. 1 to 4)**. In the ampulla of the tube, the gamete, still enclosed by the corona radiata, is approached by numerous spermatozoa, some of which probably have the function of softening or preparing the envelope of the ovum by releasing hyaluronidase.

Ultimately, a single spermatozoon penetrates the ovum and then loses its tail and body. The pronucleus, contained in its head, does not actually fuse with the pronucleus of the ovum. As they complete their second maturation divisions, each gamete contributes its chromosomes to form a single nucleus containing 46 chromosomes. Thereafter, the fertilised ovum begins a series of cell divisions but, for the first 7 days, does not increase in the overall size.

Fertile Period

How long can human spermatozoa survive in the female genital tract? It is true that spermatozoa have been found to retain motility in the cervical canal and uterus for 5–7 days, and have been found in the tube 60 hours after

- Metaphase II (MII)
- No germinal vesicle
- The first polar body is present

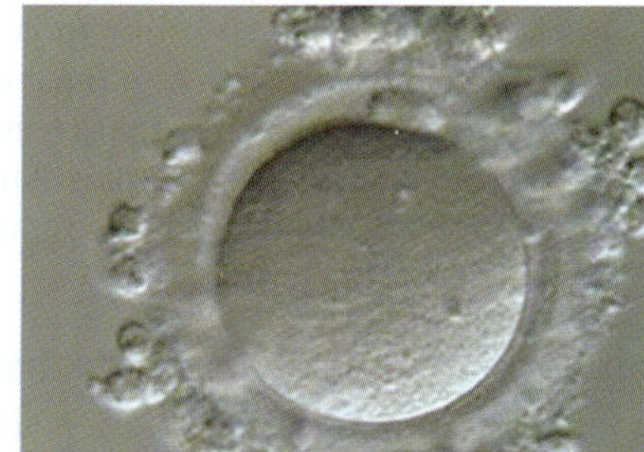

Fig. 2: Mature oocyte.

On fertilisation, second polar body, is extruded and the second meiotic division is completed.
Within a few hours, male and the female pronucleus is observed.

Nuclear membranes form around the decondensing sperm and oocyte chromatin and PN move closely in the centre of the oocyte within 3–6 hours of gamete fusion.

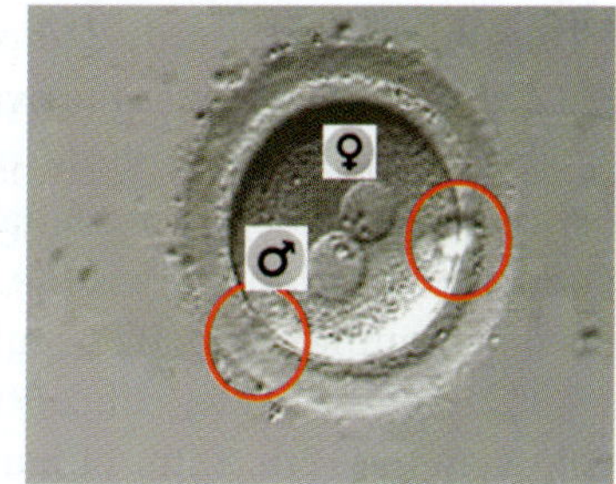

Fig. 3: Successful fertilisation process. (PN: pronuclei)

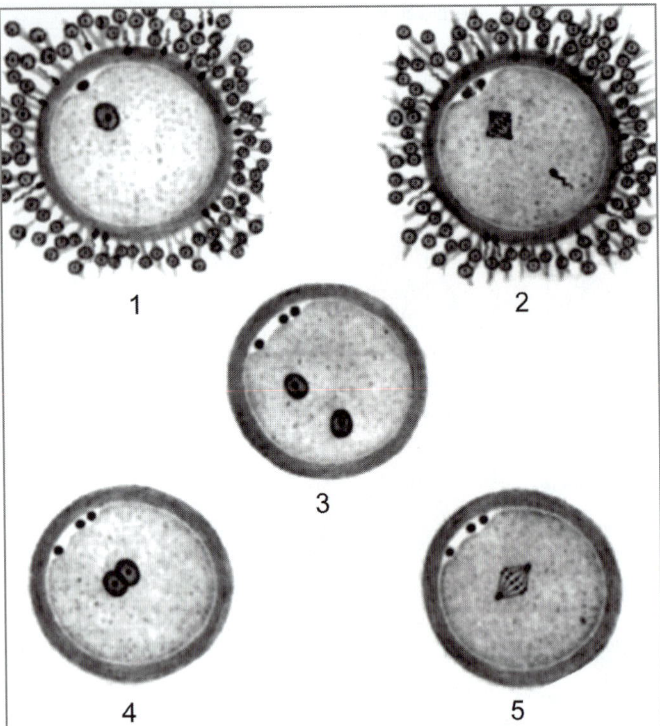

Fig. 4: Maturation and fertilisation of the ovum while still surrounded by the corona radiata. These events take place in the tube and are illustrated as follows: (1) Prior to ovulation, the first (reduction) division has taken place to give rise to a polar body, shown as a black dot to the side of the ovum itself; (2) The second division occurs, or is completed, after the spermatozoon penetrates the ovum; the polar body also divides, so that the ultimate result is three polar bodies; (3) The male and female pronuclei approach each other to contribute chromosomes which link together to form one nucleus; the pronucleus of the spermatozoon is smaller than that of the ovum but, for clarity, is here shown of similar size; (4) Fusion almost complete; (5) The first division after fertilisation to produce a two-cell ovum.

coitus, but this does not mean that they have the power to fertilise. Indeed, the evidence shows that spermatozoa do not retain this property for longer than 48 hours, and probably not for longer than 24 hours, after being implanted in the vagina. The ripe ovum can survive in a fertilisable form for only 24 hours and probably only for 8–12 hours after it leaves the ovary.

Conception is therefore extremely unlikely unless coitus takes place during 2 days before, or immediately after the ovulation. This is the basis for the fertile period of each monthly cycle. If ovulation always occurred on the 14th day of the cycle, conception could only result from coitus on the 12th, 13th, 14th and 15th days. In fact, there is some variability in the time of ovulation, so allowance is made for this and the fertile period in a woman with a 28-day cycle occupies 7–9 days. The other days in the cycle constitute the safe period but it should be recognised that it is relatively rather than absolutely safe. Indeed, pregnancy is recorded following coitus on any day of the cycle, even during menstruation, but this is rare and is explained by some unusual irregularity in the time of ovulation rather than by longevity on the part of spermatozoa.

Based on the day of ovulation, there is an estimated 6-day window for conception to occur, with probabilities of pregnancy highest in the 2 days prior to ovulation (~30%), then falling to 8–10% on the date of ovulation, and zero probability of conception on subsequent days. This period is commonly referred to as the 'fertile window.' Fertility awareness-based methods (FABMs) utilise the observation of physiological signs and symptoms to identify the fertile window, which subsequently can be used in the sexual activity decision-making during the fertile window, to either avoid or achieve pregnancy. As individuals do not always ovulate on the same day each cycle, identified fertile windows for pregnancy prevention purposes are generally conservative and usually longer than 6 days to ensure variability in the window is appropriately captured. Methods of predicting ovulation include urinary hormone measurement [luteinising hormone (LH) and oestrogen], FABMs (including tracking basal body temperatures, cervical mucus monitoring and calendar charting/tracking apps) and ultrasonography. The Cochrane Database of Systematic Review suggests that timed intercourse using urine ovulation tests probably improves live birth and pregnancy rates, compared to intercourse without ovulation prediction. As modern methods of contraception, each FABM has distinct perfect and typical use efficacy rates (a range of perfect-use pregnancy rates from 0.4 to 12.1, and a range of typical-use pregnancy rates from 1.8 to 33.6, depending on the method), though studies on efficacy and effectiveness for these methods have been more limited than other methods of contraception.

Tracking the ovulation is equally important for controlled ovarian stimulation and intrauterine insemination (COS/IUI) cycles for treatment of subfertility, wherein timing of insemination is usually done at 24 or 36 hours after hCG injection to suit the convenience of the clinic or care provider.

EARLY DEVELOPMENT OF THE OVUM

After fertilisation, the zona pellucida undergoes a striking change. From the moment of fusion of the gametes, the zona pellucida changes to become an impermeable membrane, separating the zygote physically and physiologically from the environment.

Cell Cleavage

As a result of fertilisation, cleavage is initiated. From this moment, the zygote will develop a number of daughter cells called blastomeres. A characteristic for this process is the fact that during cleavage, each new cell (blastomere) contains half the volume of the cytoplasm of the mother cell **(Figs. 5 and 6)**. This process will go on until a specific ratio is reached between the cell volume and the volume of the nucleus: the volumetric ratio between the nucleus and the cytoplasm has gained a value characteristic of the human organism in question. The amount of cytoplasm of the zygote is so large that this does not take place till the zygote reaches the 16-cell stage. This specific ratio is a necessity for the cell to have the bioactivity to continue, including protein synthesis. During the process of cleavage, the overall size of the zygote does not change.

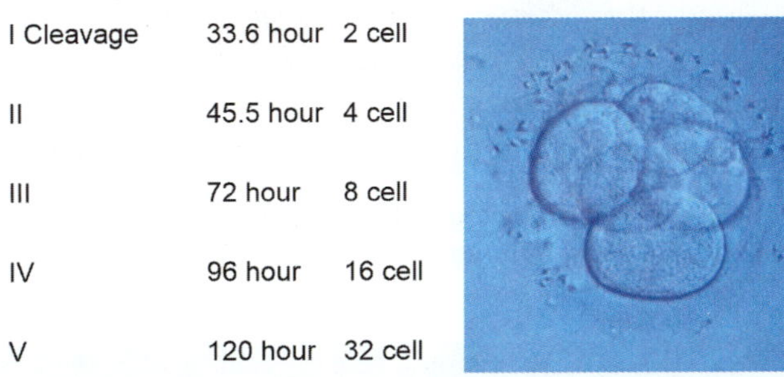

Fig. 5: Embryonic development rating (EDR).

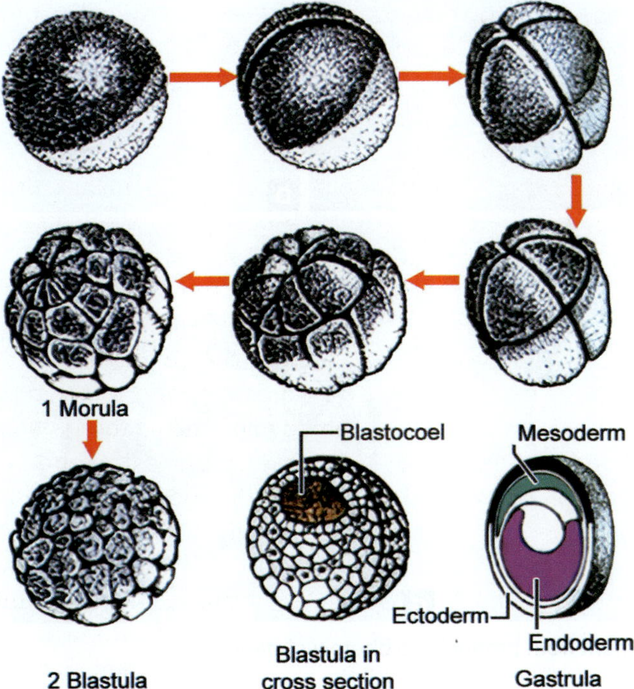

Fig. 6: The development of the fertilised ovum during the first 7 days. (1) Morula stage and (2) blastocyst stage. During this process, and to permit its transport along the tube, the ovum does not increase in size much. The diameter of the blastocyst is only 0.13 mm, that of the ovum immediately after fertilisation being 0.1 mm. The zona pellucida persists until the blastocyst embeds in the endometrium.

Compaction and Formation of Blastocyst

About 4 days after fertilisation, the formed cluster of blastomeres, now called the morula, undergoes the process of compaction. In compaction, the peripheral cells begin to stick together in a much closer contact than before, forming a denser structure. It is a process comparable to epithelialisation. These peripheral cells will give rise to the trophoblast. The inner cell mass will give rise to the embryo proper, and is therefore called the embryoblast.

The first division of the ovum into two cells occurs within 24–30 hours of fertilisation, and thereafter, each cell divides again and again to form a morula, a clump of cells 0.13 mm in diameter, by the third or fourth day. The morula, still covered by the zona pellucida, next becomes cystic as a result of fluid being either secreted by its own cells or absorbed from the genital tract. It is moved along the fallopian tube by the cilial current and by peristalsis, being nourished temporarily by the cells of the corona radiata and by the secretions of the endosalpinx. In approximately 4 days, it reaches the uterine cavity where it lies free for another 2 or 3 days during which it is supported by the secretions of progestational endometrium. Any factor affecting tubal peristalsis or cilial currents, such as chronic tubal disease due to pelvic inflammatory disease (PID) or progesterone-only contraceptives, can affect this process of embryo movement to the uterine cavity, thus predisposing to ectopic pregnancy. Rarely, transperitoneal migration of spermatozoa can also predispose to tubal ectopic pregnancy.

This blastocyst **(Figs. 7 and 8)**, present by the seventh day, consists of a single layer of cells surrounding the contained fluid, with a collection of cells forming a solid area on the inner aspect of the wall at one point. This is the inner cell mass from which the foetus is formed. The cyst wall of flattened cells is the trophoblast which soon becomes differentiated into two layers: an inner one of cuboidal cells—the cytotrophoblast and an outer one—the syncytiotrophoblast. The latter consists of irregular

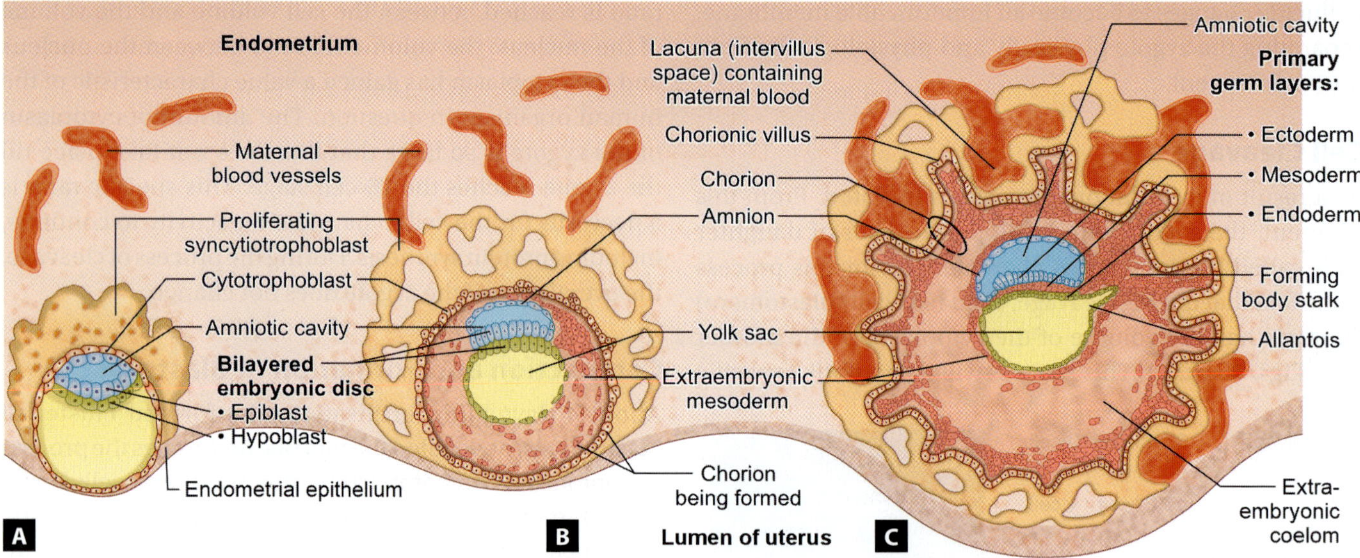

Figs. 7A to C: The stages of implantation with the formation of different layers in a developing embryo. (A) 7½-day implanting blastocyst; (B) 12-day implanted blastocyst; (C) 16-day embryo.

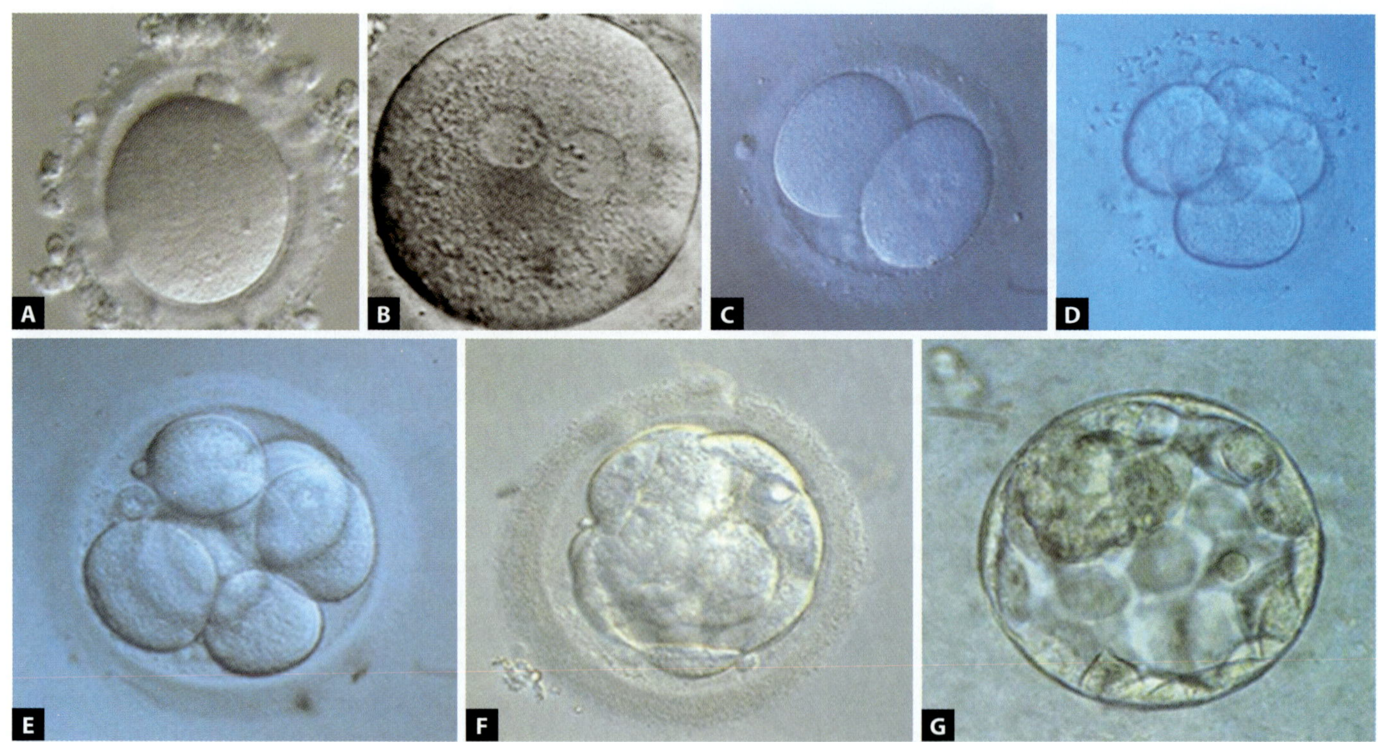

Figs. 8A to G: Different stages of early development from pronuclei to blastocyst stage.

masses of protoplasm with multiple nuclei and few cell walls. It is probably developed from the cytotrophoblast, and its formation from this source is continued throughout pregnancy. The function of the trophoblast is to attach the ovum to the wall of the uterus and thereafter to nourish it.

Implantation

About the seventh day, the blastocyst adheres itself to the wall of the uterus, normally in the upper part for which it has a special predilection, and then burrows into the endometrium (invasion). At this time, it loses its covering, the zona pellucida. The site of entry is quickly sealed. The invasive power is provided by enzymes of the syncytium and related proteins, e.g. implantation-initiating factor, fibronectin and blastokinin, and the endometrium, already sensitised by progesterone, reacts by a strong decidual change. A decidual reaction is also seen to a limited extent on the pelvic peritoneum and on the surface of the ovary.

So far as the uterus is concerned, the decidual reaction is protective in that it controls the degree of penetration by the chorion and prevents the erosion of large blood vessels. Nevertheless, fine capillaries of the endometrium are opened and the blood leaks out to form pools and lakes around the ovum. The trophoblastic epithelium acts as an intermediary or as a semipermeable membrane.

To facilitate the interchange of carbon dioxide during the early stages of the trophoblastic development, the endometrium is rich in carbonic anhydrase. This forms as a result of a progesterone influence and is probably vital to successful implantation.

The altered endometrium lying deep to the implanted ovum is the decidua basalis, and that which shields it from the uterine cavity is the decidua capsularis. The lining of the remainder of the uterus is the decidua vera. The decidua vera and decidua capsularis fuse by 12 weeks of gestation, obliterating the uterine cavity. Thus, there is no access to the tubes from the cervix after this time and no possibility of ascending infection.

One must remember that the foetus is a semiallograft, which escapes maternal immune rejection in a healthy pregnancy; hence, the immune system plays an important role in carrying on a successful implantation process. The uterine natural killer (uNK) cells are most prominent during early implantation, accounting for >70% of all leucocytes. Within the NK cell population, two primary subsets can be identified: CD56dimCD16þ cells, which constitute the majority (>90%) of the cells in peripheral blood, and the other main subset (10%), CD56brightCD16-, the uterine NK cells, whose main role is primarily immunological response regulation through cytokine production. Uterine NK cells are typically most abundant during the late secretory phase of the menstrual cycle and in the first trimester of pregnancy. Possibly, uNK cells play a role in implantation by secreting cytokines and angiogenic factors, such as transforming growth factor-b, angiopoietin 1 and 2, vascular endothelial growth factor, and placenta growth factor. They are involved in facilitating proper trophoblast invasion, vascularisation, and placentation.

It is theorised that an excessive number of uNK cells or overly cytotoxic uNK cell population could lead to increased peri-implantation blood flow and excessive oxidative stress to trophoblast cells, thereby increasing the risk of pregnancy loss. However, the evidence to support administration of any immunomodulator to women with recurrent pregnancy loss (RPL) to increase the live birth rate is not convincing at this moment.

FORMATION OF FOETUS AND MEMBRANES

As the cells of the inner cell mass proliferate, a fluid-filled space appears in their midst on the side adjacent to the trophoblast; this is the amniotic cavity and its lining cells become the amnion **(Figs. 7 to 9)**. A second cyst lined by a single layer of flattened cells appears on the other aspect of the inner cell mass: this is the yolk sac, a primitive structure in the human being. These two cavities are separated from each other by a double layer of cells. Between these two layers, the mesoderm develops (probably from the amniotic layer), and grows out to form the body stalk or umbilical cord. The amniotic cavity and the yolk sac are present by the seventh day. A reticulum of mesenchyme appears in the blastocyst and condenses to line the trophoblast on its inner aspect. There is now a flat plate between the amnion and the yolk sac comprising three layers—amniotic cells which become ectoderm; the intermediate mesoderm; and yolk sac cells or endoderm. It is from these primary layers that the whole foetus develops. The process of development is one in which the plate folds on itself in two dimensions so that ultimately a part of the yolk sac is included by engulfing mesoderm and ectoderm. The resulting tube-like structure stretching from end to end becomes the primitive gut and cloaca. This at first communicates with the remains of the yolk sac (vitelline duct) now lying in the body stalk. The allantois, also found in the body stalk, is a diverticulum from the primitive gut.

Migration

Just like cell division, compaction, migration is a very important part of development. During the last days of the second week, the connecting stalk 'migrates.' This 'migration' takes place during the enormous growth and differentiation of the germ disc that characterises the third week of development. The position of the amnion and definitive yolk sac including the germ disc changes rapidly in relation to the mesoderm lining the inner wall of

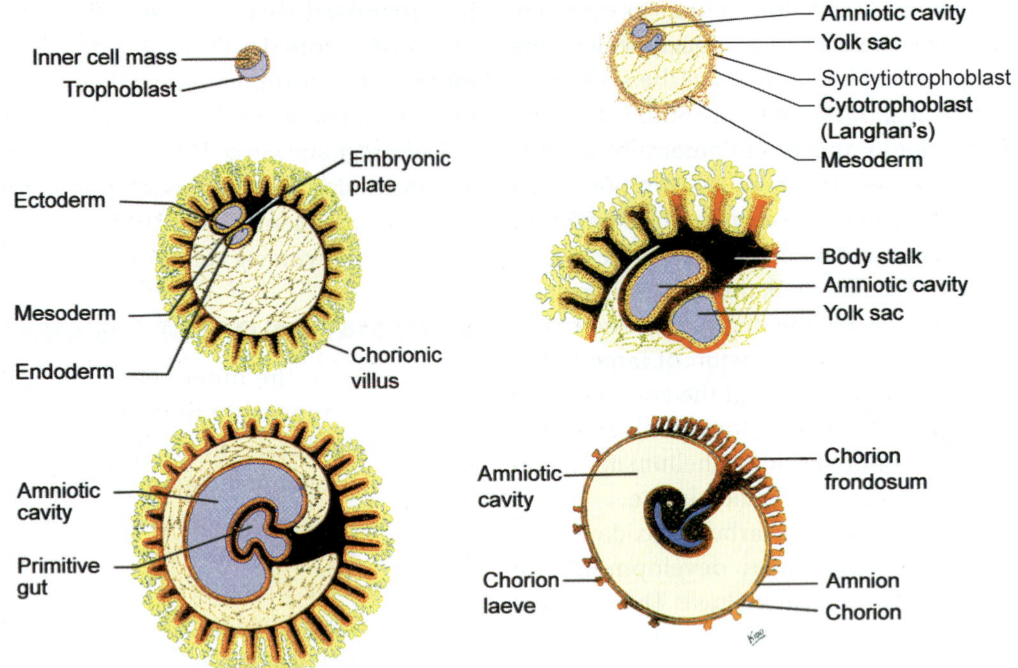

Fig. 9: The development of the early embryo and its membranes.

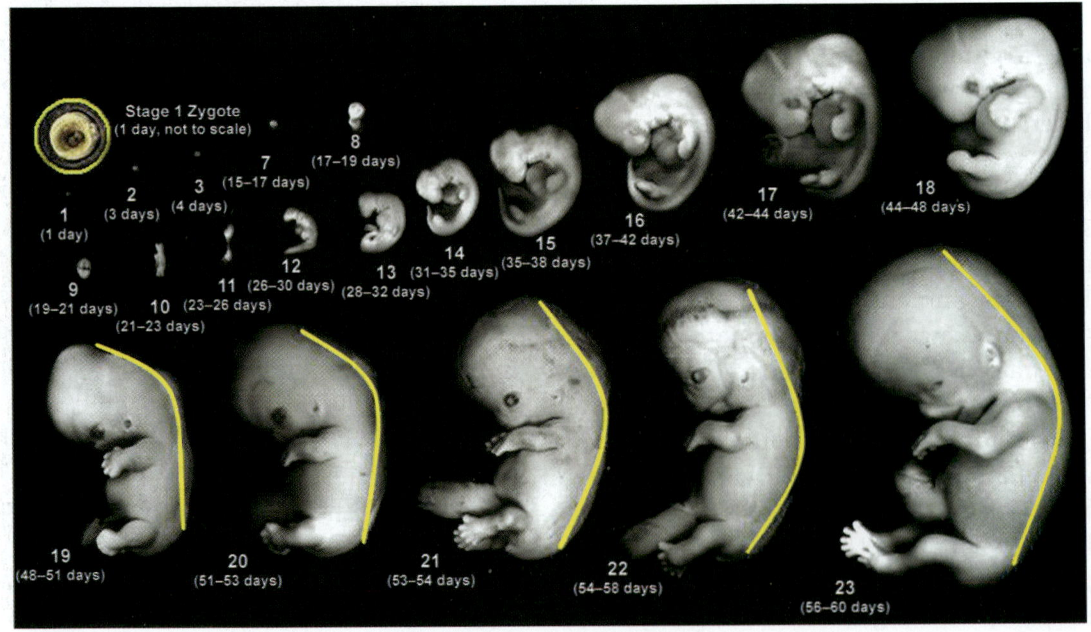

Fig. 10: Development of embryo.

the chorion. By the end of the third week, the connecting stalk is a mesodermal bridge between chorion and germ disc. It is attached to the embryoblast where amnion and definitive yolk sac come together. In later stages, it will emerge as the future caudal region of the embryonic body.

Stages of Development

The primitive streak develops in the dorsocaudal part of the epiblast in the midaxial region. From now on, the formation of the mesoderm and the notochord will occur with the invagination of epiblast cells through the primitive streak and primitive pit **(Figs. 7 and 10)**. The results of these new developments are the trilaminar germ disc, a central axis and bilateral symmetry of the embryo.

In the 17-day-old embryo, we can distinguish three directions: A dorsoventral direction (epiblast-hypoblast) and after development of the axial structures, a caudocranial direction and a left and right side **(Fig. 10)**. The germ disc now starts folding around a transversal axis in a cephalocaudal direction and around a longitudinal axis in a ventrolateral direction. An enormous expansion in all directions of the amnion takes place at the same time. During this process, the embryonic body will gradually become a separate structure freely floating in the amniotic fluid. The last connection with the environment will be the umbilical cord, which develops from the connecting stalk. The former 'open body form' will be changed into a cylinder-like 'closed bodily form.'

The body of a 17-day embryo has a median axial structure (primitive streak and notochordal cells) and is involved in the process of gastrulation, i.e. forming an inner cavity, an inner space. Both are highly specific processes of animal embryological development. The change from radial symmetry to bilateral symmetry and the differentiation of mesoderm support this interpretation. Mesoderm is a tissue that gives rise to muscles, bones, tendons and cartilage. These tissues are all precursors for structures, which are in some way connected with the ability of the organism to move. Morphologically, an 'inner world' develops between the ectoderm and endoderm.

The neural canal forms from an invagination of ectoderm; the mesoderm gives rise to the primitive muscles, blood vessels, bones and all structures intervening between the ectoderm and endoderm.

All the essential structures of the body are present in primitive but recognisable form by the sixth week.

Meanwhile, the trophoblast has developed villous projections on its outer aspect to give it the appearance of a fluffy ball. Mesenchyme invades each villus as a central core. When the trophoblast receives its inner layer of the mesoderm, it becomes known as chorion and its projections become chorionic villi. The situation can be thus summarised as: Cytotrophoblast + syncytiotrophoblast = trophoblast; trophoblast + mesoderm = chorion.

Chorionic villi are well formed by the 14th day. By the 21st day, blood vessels have developed from the mesoderm and are found in the foetus itself, in the body stalk, and in the core of each villus to form a continuous circulation. The chorionic villi are thus bathed in maternal blood and oxygen. Foodstuffs and foetal waste products are exchanged between this and the foetal blood in the vessels of each villus.

The villi are at first present on all aspects of the blastocyst. As the ovum grows, the decidua capsularis bulges into the uterine cavity and the chorionic villi within it atrophy on the side adjacent to the uterine cavity and persist on the side adjacent to the uterine wall. The part of the chorion still covered with villi is rough and shaggy—the chorion frondosum; the part devoid of villi is smooth—the chorion laeve. The villi of the chorion frondosum grow and invade the decidua basalis. With further development, the chorion frondosum becomes more and more clearly demarcated and restricted to one area, giving rise to the placenta. This is connected to the foetus by the umbilical cord, the umbilical vessels linking up those of the chorionic villi with those of the foetus.

While the foetus develops and the remains of the yolk sac shrivel, the amniotic cavity grows apace until it completely fills the original blastocyst. It comes into close contact with the chorion and adheres to it lightly; it covers the umbilical cord and is continuous with the skin of the foetus at the umbilicus. The foetus is suspended in amniotic fluid; around this are the membranes, which consist of an inner glistening thin but tough amnion and an outer thicker but more friable chorion.

When the ovum fills the uterine cavity, the decidua capsularis comes in contact and fuses with the decidua vera lining the opposite pole of the uterus. The arrangement of the membranes and the placental-foetal relationships then remain essentially unchanged until the end of pregnancy.

As the pregnancy progresses, trophoblastic cells continually break away and migrate into the decidua and myometrium; others enter the bloodstream from which they are sieved by the lungs. These are normal and harmless happenings but the decidual reaction to these 'wandering cells,' sometimes labelled syncytial endometritis, can be mistaken for choriocarcinoma by the histologist. Yet, others break away and collect at the internal os. Transcervical mucus plug aspiration prior to 12 weeks of gestation is a potential technique for first-trimester prenatal diagnosis of aneuploidies, trisomies, etc. which may be less invasive than chorion villus sampling which is done between 9 and 11 weeks for foetal chromosomal disorders but carries the risk of abortion, preterm labour, premature rupture of membranes and foetal limb reduction defects.

From the fourth and fifth week of human embryological development onwards, the folding process of the third week is partly unfolded to reach the typical human external bodily form: Upright posture. Unfolding creates a morphological movement opposite to flexion. This is superimposed on the folded bodily form of the early embryonic period **(Fig. 10)**.

Only human beings have a stable upright posture. The perfect rectangular relationship of the frontal, sagittal and horizontal planes in the human body is due to the persistence of the unfolding process of the vertebral column.

HORMONAL CONTROL OF EARLY PREGNANCY

The fertilised ovum is embedded in the endometrium on the 21st or 22nd day of the menstrual cycle, and by this time, it begins to secrete small amounts of hCG, which is luteinising and luteotrophic. This prevents the degeneration of the corpus luteum, which continues to maintain the progestational endometrium; amenorrhoea, and anovulation results.

Corpus Luteum of Pregnancy

The corpus luteum not only persists but also continues to enlarge slightly up to the 60th day of pregnancy when it may measure 3 cm in diameter. Individual cells are three to four times larger than those of the corpus luteum of menstruation. Soon after the 60th day, and presumably because of the dramatic fall in hCG production at about this time, the corpus luteum temporarily becomes cystic and its activity begins to wane by the 10th week. It shows evidence of colloidal degeneration by the 16th week but remains a recognisable structure throughout pregnancy. In the puerperium and after abortion, it occasionally undergoes calcification but is ultimately absorbed.

Placental Hormones, Enzymes and Proteins

The placenta produces a wide range of hormones in the syncytiotrophoblast, of which some are clinically different from the comparable maternal hormone. The steroid hormones, oestrogen and progestogen, cannot be produced by the placenta alone, because the necessary enzymes are absent. However, the foetal and maternal adrenals produce the precursors for the placental synthesis of the hormones. As a consequence of the shared biosynthesis of oestrogens by the foetal adrenal and the placenta, the concept of the foetoplacental unit was developed. The placenta transforms foetal adrenal dehydroepiandrosterone sulphate (DHEAS) to oestrogen using a placental sulphatase enzyme. The synthesis of DHEAS is regulated during early pregnancy by hCG and thereafter by foetal adrenocorticotropic hormone (ACTH). The placenta synthesises progesterone from maternal and foetal cholesterol throughout pregnancy, so that the maternal levels increase steadily during pregnancy.

Only the large protein hormones, hCG and human placental lactogen (hPL), will be discussed in this section, as the roles of the other hormones are largely unknown or speculative. Since the early 1970s, several new proteins of placental origin have been discovered in the maternal circulation and are called pregnancy associated plasma protein A (PAPP-A). Their concentration increases as pregnancy progresses; rather like hPL. So far, no definite physiological functions have been attributed to these proteins.

Human Chorionic Gonadotrophins

Chorionic gonadotrophins, although glycoproteins, differ chemically from pituitary gonadotrophins, but act similarly and have both a follicle-stimulating and luteinising action. The latter, however, is dominant. It is in the same family of glycoprotein heterodimers as thyroid-stimulating hormone (TSH), follicle-stimulating hormone and LH, which are produced by the pituitary gland. Each of these heterodimers shares a common α subunit but also has a unique β subunit. The β subunit is what confers biological specificity to each molecule. Interestingly, although the β subunit is unique to each molecule, there is a significant similarity between the β subunits of LH and hCG, which results in homology in their biological actions serving utility in assisted reproduction. However, the half-life of hCG is significantly longer than that of LH, with the former being approximately 37 hours and the latter 25–30 minutes.

As soon as the ovum is implanted in the endometrium, the production and excretion of hCG rises rapidly from approximately 100 IU/L in the maternal serum at the time of the expected menses to a maximum of approximately 100,000 IU/L at the 60th day of pregnancy; thereafter, they fall to a fairly constant low level **(Fig. 11)**. The purpose of hCG in circulation in early pregnancy is mainly concerned with maintaining the corpus luteum. Some of the suggested biological functions of hCG include stimulation of placental progesterone production, inhibition of maternal-foetal graft rejection, stimulation of the foetal adrenal and production of DHEAS and stimulation of the foetal gonads, in particular the production of testosterone by the testis.

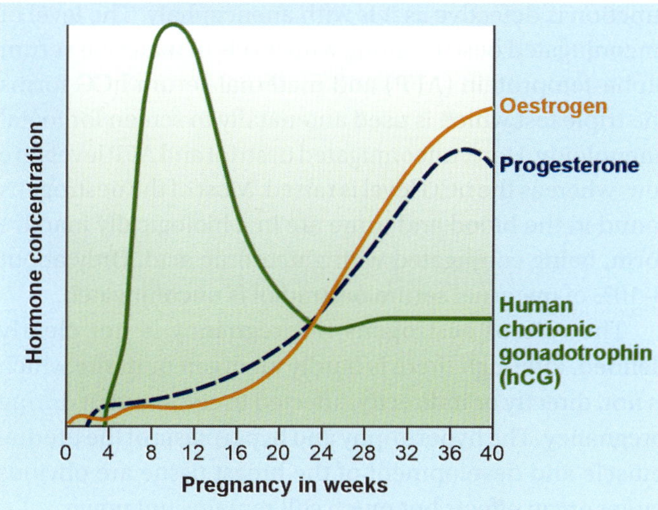

Fig. 11: Hormone levels during pregnancy.

Clinical Application of Human Chorionic Gonadotrophin

Testing for hCG is utilised in various settings including detection of pregnancy, aid in identifying normal versus abnormal early pregnancy, role in pregnancy of unknown location and diagnosis of ectopic pregnancy, malignancy monitoring (gestational trophoblastic neoplasia and germ cell tumours), and foetal aneuploidy screening. There is a 6–7-day window between fertilisation and implantation. In this early window, any pregnancy test will be negative because no hCG is being produced. Following this point in time, different pregnancy tests offer different sensitivity and specificity based on their timing. A urine pregnancy test detects hCG beginning at 20–50 mIU/mL, at approximately 32–35 days of amenorrhoea. In contrast, a serum pregnancy test typically detects hCG levels as low as 1–2 mIU/mL. The absence of intrauterine pregnancy in TVS with hCG levels beyond the discriminatory zone (15,000–2,000 IU/L) raises the suspicion of ectopic pregnancy.

The similarity between hCG and TSH has several implications in pregnancy including careful interpretation of thyroid function tests in the first trimester and symptoms of thyrotoxicosis in pathological conditions such as molar pregnancy.

Serum hCG levels are incorporated in aneuploidy screening programs, wherein the hCG level is typically elevated in Down syndrome and decreased in trisomy 18 and 13.

In the process of in vitro fertilisation (IVF), hCG is administered to help mature oocytes and simulate the LH surge before retrieval. This is possibly due to the homology between hCG and LH, which allows both to stimulate ovulation and support lutein cells. It is used to trigger ovulation in COS/IUI cycles as well.

Human Placental Lactogen

This hormone, also known as chorionic somatomammotrophin (hCS), is also secreted by the syncytiotrophoblast. It is demonstrable in the plasma by the sixth week of pregnancy and rises to a maximum in the third trimester of pregnancy to disappear quickly after delivery. It is a protein hormone with immunological and certain biological similarities to the growth hormone (GH). As its alternative name implies, it is growth-promoting, but is less than one twentieth as effective as GH, and is lactogenic, although this has only been proved in other animal species. Its action is weak compared with pituitary prolactin.

The hormone participates, directly or indirectly, in a number of metabolic processes. It has been suggested that it may function as a metabolic regulatory, albeit a fine one, in the mother to ensure that the nutritional requirements of the foetus are met. In the mother, hPL induces insulin resistance and carbohydrate intolerance. It mobilises lipids as free fatty acids. Thus, it ensures an adequate supply of fuels to the foetus between maternal meals. Alterations in the levels of hPL have been used in early pregnancy to assess viability in cases of threatened abortion, and in late pregnancy as an indication of placental function. However, biophysical techniques are more reliably predictive and sensitive for assessing foetal well-being.

Progesterone

The activity of the corpus luteum of pregnancy explains the slight rise in the level of progesterone in the blood during the first few days or weeks following conception. The placenta, however, soon takes over responsibility for producing progesterone in ever-increasing amounts until term or near term **(Fig. 11)**. The daily production of progesterone in late pregnancy is about 250 mg with blood levels of 100–200 ng/mL. Progesterone helps prepare and maintain the endometrium to permit implantation. It may have a role in suppressing maternal immunological response to foetal antigens, thus preventing maternal rejection. It reduces myometrial contractility. It also serves as the substrate for some of the foetal adrenal gland production of gluco- and mineralocorticoids.

The increased progesterone levels have an effect on the kidneys since progesterone competes with aldosterone for renal receptor sites. The sodium balance in pregnancy reflects, to some extent, the increased aldosterone and progesterone levels.

The secretion of progesterone by the human placenta explains why, in women, the corpus luteum is not important to the maintenance of pregnancy in contrast to other animals. Both ovaries, including the corpus luteum, can be removed in the first trimester without abortion taking place in 50% of the cases. There are reports of the human corpus luteum having been removed as early as on the 23rd day of the menstrual cycle (presumed to be the 9th day of pregnancy) without an untoward effect.

Nevertheless, if it is removed within the first 4 weeks (6 weeks' amenorrhoea), abortion usually occurs within 80 hours.

This is the basis for the use of the antiprogestogen, RU 486 (mifepristone) for medical induction of abortion in the early first trimester.

Although supplemental progesterone is commonly utilised for the treatment of luteal phase defect (LPD) and RPL, supporting data seems to be inconsistent. Dydrogesterone, an immunomodulator progestin, is often used in the first trimester for recurrent/threatened pregnancy loss or as luteal support in ART. Women with a history of miscarriage who present with bleeding in early pregnancy may benefit from the use of vaginal micronised progesterone 400 mg twice daily. Vaginal micronised progesterone is proven to be effective in reducing the risk of spontaneous preterm birth among those who have had an earlier spontaneous preterm birth and those with a short cervix at the midtrimester.

Oestrogens

These hormones are produced in ever-increasing quantities from the beginning to the end of pregnancy. The corpus luteum makes a contribution in the first few weeks but the main source, as described above, is the placenta. This secretes oestradiol, oestrone and oestriol. Oestrone and oestradiol levels increase to about 100 times the nonpregnant levels, but oestriol excretion is increased about 1,000 times **(Fig. 11)**. Although oestriol is a weak oestrogen, its high concentrations compensate and the biological effect is equivalent to oestradiol. If the foetus is removed and the placenta remains in situ, as in some cases of abdominal pregnancy, the level of oestriol falls considerably. This level is also low if the foetal adrenal function is defective as it is with anencephaly. The level of unconjugated oestriol along with levels of maternal serum alpha-fetoprotein (AFP) and maternal serum hCG forms the triple test which is used antenatally to screen for foetal aneuploidy. Here, unconjugated oestriol and AFP levels are low, whereas the hCG level is raised. Most of the oestrogens found in the blood and urine are in a biologically inactive form, being conjugated with glucuronic acid. Only about 8–10% of maternal serum oestradiol is unconjugated.

The role of oestrogens in pregnancy is not clearly defined, although there is hardly an organ or tissue which is not, directly or indirectly, affected to some extent during pregnancy. The hypertrophy and hyperplasia of the uterine muscle and development of the breast tissue are obvious target organ effects but much still remains unknown.

Low values and low growth rates of E2 (oestradiol) probably indicate bad pregnancy outcomes. However, unlike hCG estimation, serum oestradiol estimation has not found its place in clinical obstetrics, except in ART cycles. Serum E3 (oestriol) levels have been rarely used as low levels, which are associated with foetal aneuploidy (trisomy 21, 18), foetal genetic conditions (Smith-Lemli-Opitz syndrome, X-linked ichthyosis, aromatase deficiency and primary or secondary foetal adrenal insufficiency) and foetal demise. High levels have been associated with pending labour (PTL) and congenital adrenal hyperplasia.

Pregnancy-associated Plasma Protein A and Other Serum Biochemical Markers

The biological function of pregnancy-associated plasma protein A (PAPP-A) in human pregnancy is not completely understood, except that it plays a role in promoting optimal foetal growth. However, low levels of PAPP-A (<0.4 MoMs) in the first-trimester plasma are currently used as part of maternal screening programs for foetal chromosomal abnormalities, in particular Down syndrome, and for placental dysfunction disorders including preeclampsia (15–18). Additionally, foetuses with Cornelia de Lange syndrome, a rare condition involving incomplete foetal development and subsequent deformities, are associated variably with low levels of PAPP-A in the maternal circulation.

The identified pathophysiological mechanisms, including angiogenic imbalance, placental dysfunction and inflammatory responses, shed light on the intricate molecular landscape of preeclampsia and placental dysfunction disorders. In addition to low PAPP-A, low placental growth factor (PlGF) levels, low alkaline phosphatase (AP), higher sFlt-1 (soluble fms-like tyrosine kinase-1) levels, higher AFP levels and elevated levels of inflammatory markers such as free β-hGC, interferon-gamma (INF-γ) and tumour necrosis factor-α (TNF-α) may be associated with risks, including the onset of hypertensive disorders of pregnancy (HDP), foetal growth restriction (FGR) and delivery of SGA neonates. Comparatively, PAPP-A and PlGF appear to be the most important biochemical markers for the prediction of SGA and HDP. In addition, an sFlt-1:PlGF ratio of 38 or lower proves useful in predicting the short-term absence of preeclampsia in women where clinical suspicion exists. The therapeutic potential of PlGF and PAPP-A in preeclampsia is under rigorous investigation.

SUGGESTED READING

1. Collins LC, Gatta LA, Dotters-Katz SK, Kuller JA, Schust DJ. Luteal phase defects and progesterone supplementation. Obstet Gynecol Surv. 2024;79(2):122-8.
2. Conover CA, Oxvig C. The pregnancy-associated plasma protein-a (PAPP-A) story. Endocr Rev. 2023;44(6):1012-28.
3. Coomarasamy A, Devall AJ, Brosens JJ, Quenby S, Stephenson MD, Sierra S, et al. Micronized vaginal progesterone to prevent miscarriage: a critical evaluation of randomized evidence. Am J Obstet Gynecol. 2020;223(2):167-76.
4. da Fonseca EB, Damião R, Moreira DA. Preterm birth prevention. Best Pract Res Clin Obstet Gynaecol. 2020;69:40-9.
5. Fortune JE. Ovarian follicular growth and development in mammals. Biol Reprod. 1994;50(2):225-32.
6. Gibbons T, Reavey J, Georgiou EX, Becker CM. Timed intercourse for couples trying to conceive. Cochrane Database Syst Rev. 2023;9(9):CD011345.
7. Górczewski W, Górecka J, Massalska-Wolska M, Staśkiewicz M, Borowski D, Huras H, et al. Role of first trimester screening biochemical markers to predict hypertensive pregnancy disorders and SGA neonates-a narrative review. Healthcare (Basel). 2023;11(17):2454.
8. Herkert D, Meljen V, Muasher L, Price TM, Kuller JA, Dotters-Katz S. Human chorionic gonadotropin-a review of the literature. Obstet Gynecol Surv. 2022;77(9):539-46.
9. In: England MA (Ed). Life Before Birth, 2nd edition. St. Louis, MO: Mosby-Wolfe; 1996.
10. Ringler GE, Strauss JF. Recent advances in understanding the process of implantation. Curr Opin Obstet Gynecol. 1990;2(5):703-8.
11. Rogers PA. Current studies on human implantation: a brief overview. Reprod Fertil Dev. 1995;7(6):1395-99.
12. Simmons RG, Jennings V. Fertility awareness-based methods of family planning. Best Pract Res Clin Obstet Gynaecol. 2020;66:68-82.
13. Thakur AS, Tayade S, Patel D, Gupta A, Batra N. Unraveling the predictive power: placenta growth factor and pregnancy-associated plasma protein A in pre-eclampsia. Cureus. 2024;16(1):e52752.
14. Béquet YLBN, Lashley EELO, Goddijn M, van der Hoorn MP. The role of uterine natural killer cells in recurrent pregnancy loss and possible treatment options. Fertil Steril. 2023;120(5):945-47.

8

CHAPTER

Spontaneous Abortions (Including Recurrent Loss)

Akhila Vasudeva, Muralidhar V Pai

Chapter Outline

- Spontaneous Abortions
- Recurrent Early Pregnancy Loss

INTRODUCTION

Abortion is the termination of pregnancy by any means before the foetus is sufficiently developed to survive. In the United States, this definition is confined to the termination of pregnancy before 20 weeks based upon the date of the first day of the last normal menses. Another commonly used definition is the delivery of a foetus-neonate that weighs <500 g.

SPONTANEOUS ABORTIONS

When abortion occurs without medical or mechanical means to empty the uterus, it is referred to as spontaneous. Another widely used term is miscarriage. Although early pregnancy loss is often an emotionally difficult experience for patients, it is a very common event. Approximately 15–25% of clinically recognised pregnancies end in miscarriage, and when unrecognised early losses are included, the miscarriage rate may be as high as 30–60% of all pregnancies. It is estimated that 80% of pregnancy losses occur in the first trimester, while pregnancy losses between 12 and 20 weeks occur in just 1–5% of cases.

Pathology of Spontaneous Abortions

Haemorrhage into the decidua basalis and necrotic changes in the tissues adjacent to the bleeding usually accompany abortion. The ovum becomes detached and this stimulates uterine contractions that result in expulsion. When the sac is opened, fluid is commonly found surrounding a small, macerated foetus, or alternatively there may be no visible foetus in the sac, so-called blighted ovum (an embryonic gestational sac) **(Fig. 1)**.

A blood or carneous mole is an ovum that is surrounded by a capsule of clotted blood. The capsule is of varying thickness, with degenerated chorionic villi scattered through it. The small, fluid-containing cavity within appears compressed and distorted by the thick walls of old blood clot.

Chromosomal anomalies cause at least half of these early abortions, and their incidence likewise decreases thereafter.

Mechanism of Abortion

- *Up to 8 weeks:* The gestational sac tends to be expelled completely, and the decidua is shed thereafter.
- *From 8 to 12 weeks:* The decidua capsularis ruptures and the embryo is expelled either entire or after rupture of the amnion.
- *After 12 weeks:* The placenta is completely formed, and the process of abortion is like a miniature labour. It is more common for the foetus to be expelled but for the placenta to be retained due to firmer attachment to the uterine wall **(Figs. 2 and 3)**.

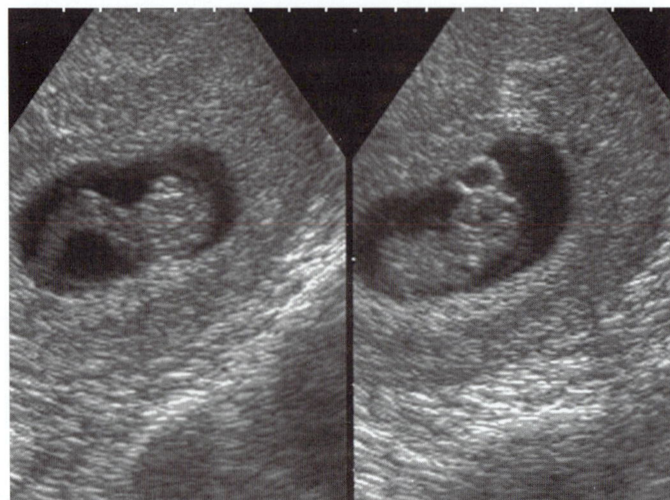

Fig. 1: Ultrasonographic picture of yolk sac and embryo.

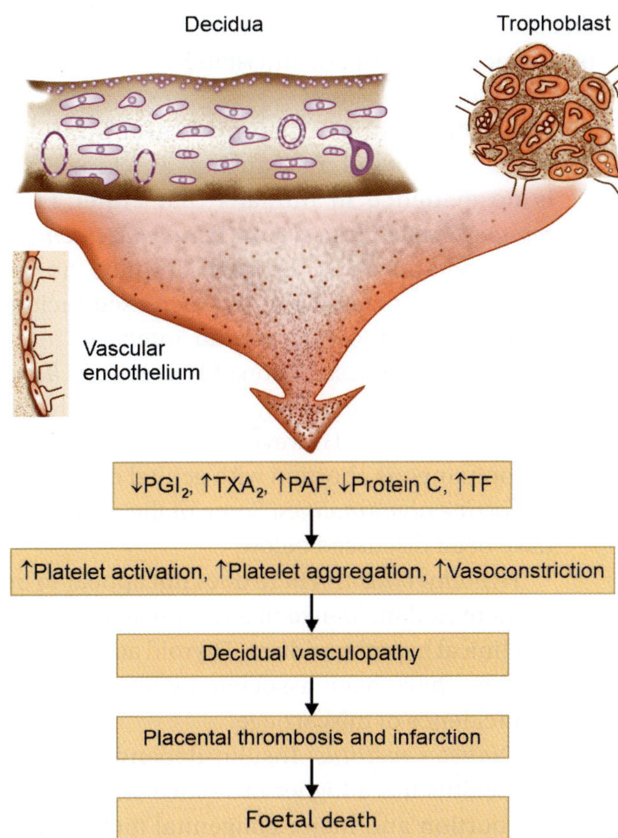

Fig. 2: Proposed mechanisms of foetal loss. (PAF: platelet-activating factor; PGI_2: prostacyclin; TF: tissue factor; TXA_2: thromboxane A2)

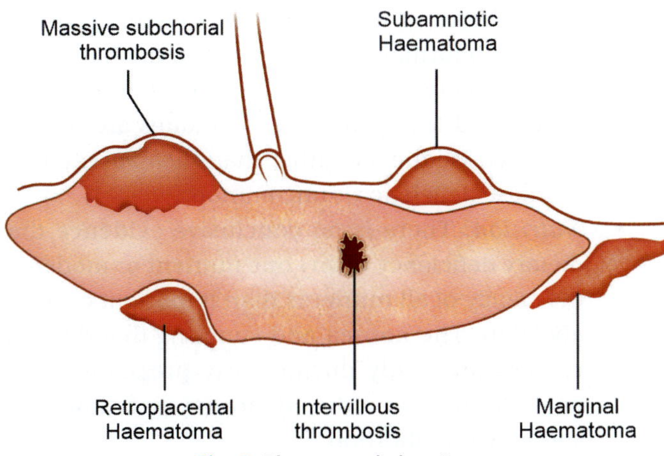

Fig. 3: Threatened abortion.

Causes of Spontaneous Abortion

The potential causes of spontaneous abortion are discussed here.

Genetic Factors (Aneuploid Abortions)

- Chromosomal abnormalities are diagnosed in over 50% of first-trimester miscarriages, becoming less prevalent in second- and third-trimester losses. On karyotyping, most chromosomal abnormalities are numerical (termed aneuploidy, usually because of chromosomal nondisjunction during meiosis), including autosomal trisomies (30–60%), triploidy (11–13%), monosomy X (10–15%) and tetraploidy (9%), whereas only a minority result from structural chromosome rearrangements (2–6%) and mosaicism (8%) (FertSterNov2023).
    - Autosomal trisomy is the most frequently identified chromosomal anomaly associated with first-trimester abortions. Trisomies can be the result of an isolated nondisjunction, a maternal or paternal balanced translocation, or a balanced chromosomal inversion. Balanced structural chromosomal rearrangements are present in 2–3% of couples with a history of recurrent abortions. Translocations may be identified in either parent. Balanced chromosomal inversions may also be identified in couples with recurrent abortions. Trisomies for all autosomes except chromosome number 1 have been identified in abortuses, but autosomes 13, 16, 18, 21, and 22 are the most common.
    - Monosomy X (454, X) is the next most common chromosomal abnormality and is compatible with live-born females (Turner syndrome).
    - Triploidy is often associated with hydropic placental degeneration. Incomplete hydatidiform moles may have foetal development, which is triploid or trisomic for chromosome number 16. Foetuses associated with these frequently abort early, and the few carried longer are all grossly malformed. Advanced maternal and paternal age are not associated with this abnormality. Tetraploid abortuses are rarely live-born and are most often aborted very early in gestation.
- Chromosomal structural abnormalities are unusual causes of abortion and have been identified only since the development of banding techniques. Some of these infants are live-born with balanced translocations and can be normal. Autosomal monosomy is extremely rare and is incompatible with life. Sex chromosomal polysomy (47, XXX or 47, XXY) is unusual in abortus material but is commonly seen in live births. In women

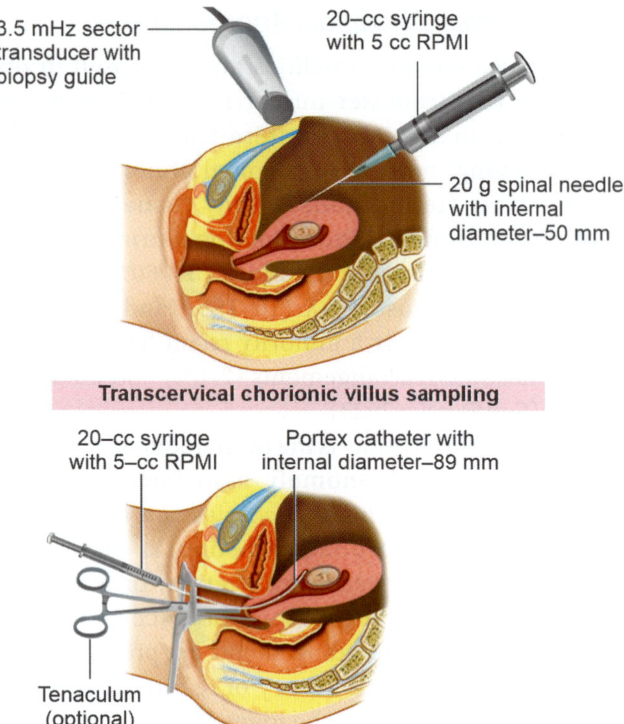

Fig. 4: Chorionic villi in spontaneous abortion.

with genetic problems can be offered chorionic villus sampling **(Fig. 4)**.

- Most chromosome anomalies in sporadic miscarriages appear to arise de novo.
- In addition to chromosome abnormalities, defects in genes involved in meiosis regulation, DNA repair and cell proliferation may impair gamete or embryonic development. Imprinting disorders arising during gametogenesis may be associated with miscarriage.
- As the number of successive pregnancy losses increases, factors other than embryonic genetic anomalies often lead to recurrent miscarriage.
- Parental chromosomal rearrangements are found in 2–5% of cases of recurrent miscarriage, increasing the risk of further pregnancy loss.

Euploid Abortion

Three-fourths of aneuploid abortions are before 8 weeks, while euploid abortions peaked at about 13 weeks.

The following causes are possibilities:

- A genetic abnormality such as an isolated mutation or polygenic factors.
- Approximately 0.5% of live births have chromosomal abnormalities, while at least 2% of live births have diseases associated with a single-gene mutation or a polygenic mechanism of inheritance.
- *Various maternal factors:*
  - *Infections:* Some chronic infections have been implicated in causing abortion. There is no evidence in humans that either *Listeria monocytogenes*, *Brucella* or *Chlamydia trachomatis* produce abortions. Herpes simplex, however, has been associated with an increased incidence of abortion following genital infection in early pregnancy. The association of *Mycoplasma hominis* and *Ureaplasma urealyticum* in abortion was suggested by few. However, there was no evidence of spontaneous abortion with genital mycoplasma.
  - *Endocrine abnormalities:* Some of the abnormalities have been discussed below.
    - *Hypothyroidism:* There does not appear to be an increased incidence of abortion associated with clinical hypothyroidism. Thyroid autoantibodies alone have been associated with an increased incidence of miscarriage.
    - *Diabetes mellitus:* Insulin-dependent diabetes mellitus has a higher incidence of spontaneous abortion and major congenital malformations. The risk is more related to the degree of metabolic control in early pregnancy.
    - *Progesterone deficiency:* Insufficient progesterone secretion by the corpus luteum or placenta has been associated with an increased incidence of abortion. It has been suggested that abnormal levels of one or more hormones might help to forecast abortion. Unfortunately, reduced levels of these hormones are usually the consequence rather than the cause. Luteal phase deficiency is uncommon.
  - *Nutrition:* There is no conclusive evidence that dietary deficiency of any one nutrient or moderate deficiency of all nutrients is an important cause of abortion. The nausea and vomiting that develop rather commonly during early pregnancy, and any inanition so induced, are rarely followed by spontaneous abortion.
  - *Drug use and environmental factors:* Different agents have been reported, but not confirmed, to be associated with an increased incidence of abortion. However, this is not proved.
    - *Smoking:* This has been associated with an increased risk for euploidic abortion.

- *Alcohol:* Both spontaneous abortion and foetal anomalies may result from frequent alcohol use during the first 8 weeks of pregnancy.
- *Caffeine:* Coffee consumption at greater than four cups per day appears to slightly increase the risk of abortion. This may be due to paraxanthine (a caffeine metabolite) levels of which are associated with a significant two-fold risk of spontaneous abortion. However, moderate consumption of caffeine is unlikely to be associated with spontaneous abortion.
- *Radiation:* In sufficient therapeutic doses, radiation is a recognised abortifacient. The exposure to less than 5 rads does not increase the risk of miscarriage.
- *Environmental toxins:* In most instances, there is little information to indicate any specific environmental agent; however, there is evidence that arsenic, lead, formaldehyde, benzene and ethylene oxide may cause abortion.
- *Parental age:* Female age is by far the strongest risk factor for miscarriage, with the probability of pregnancy loss being highest at the extremes of women's reproductive lives (i.e., <20 and >40 years, while an aging oocyte is likely to give rise to a chromosomally abnormal gamete).

- *Immunological factors:* Much attention has been focused on the immune system as important in recurrent pregnancy loss (RPL). Two primary pathophysiological models that have evolved are the autoimmune theory (immunity against self) and the alloimmune theory (immunity against another person).
  - *Autoimmune factors:* It has been determined from compiled studies that approximately 15% of over 1,000 RPL patients have recognised autoimmune factors. The most significant antibodies have specificity against negatively charged phospholipids and are most commonly detected by testing for lupus anticoagulant (LAC) and anticardiolipin antibody (ACA).

    The LAC is an immunoglobulin [immunoglobulin G (IgG), IgM or both] that interferes with one or more of the phospholipid-dependent tests of in vitro coagulation. The term is a misnomer because it is associated with clinically important increases in thromboembolic events. Importantly, the LAC is most often diagnosed in patients who do not meet the diagnostic criteria for lupus.

    Antiphospholipid antibodies are acquired antibodies targeted against a phospholipid. They can be of the IgG, IgA or IgM isotope. The mechanism of pregnancy loss in these women is thought to involve placental thrombosis and infarction.
  - *Alloimmune factors:* A number of women with RPL have been diagnosed as having an alloimmune cause. They have received a variety of therapies targeted at stimulating maternal immune tolerance of foetal material. Diagnosis of an alloimmune factor has centered on several tests:
    - Maternal and paternal human leucocyte antigen (HLA) comparison.
    - Assessment of maternal serum for the presence of cytotoxic antibodies to paternal leucocytes.
    - Maternal serum testing for blocking factors for maternal–paternal mixed lymphocyte reactions.

    In essence, those couples determined to have significant HLA-type homology, or in which the women were found to have minimal antipaternal antibodies, were judged to represent an alloimmune disorder. This view is doubtful.
- *Inherited thrombophilia:* There have been numerous reports of an association of spontaneous abortions and inherited thrombophilias. It has been found to have an increased incidence of activated protein C resistance and factor V Leiden mutation. Some reported that elevated serum homocysteine levels were also a risk factor.
- *Aging gametes:* Some researchers found an increased incidence of abortion relative to successful pregnancies when insemination occurred 4 days before or 3 days after the time of shift in basal body temperature. They concluded, therefore, that aging of the gametes within the female genital tract before fertilisation increased the chances of abortion.
- *Anatomical abnormalities:*
  - *Uterine fibroids:* Large and multiple uterine leiomyomas may cause abortion. More than the size, the location of myoma is more important,

especially the submucous variety which is not only responsible for infertility but also for spontaneous abortions. This is because of distortion or partial obliteration of the uterine cavity, decreased vascularity at the implantation site and uterine irritability.

- *Uterine synechiae (Asherman's syndrome):* It is caused by the destruction of large areas of endometrium by curettage. This, in turn, results in amenorrhoea and recurrent abortions believed to be due to insufficient endometrium to support implantation.
- *Development defects:* These defects are the consequence of abnormal Müllerian duct formation or fusion; some types, such as uterine septa or bicornuate may be associated with abortions, especially midtrimester. The causes are reduced intrauterine volume, reduced placental vascularity when implanted on the septum, increased uterine contractility and irritability.
- *Cervical insufficiency:* It is the inability of the uterine cervix to retain a pregnancy in the second trimester in the absence of clinical contractions, labour or both. It may occur in a single pregnancy or recur in consecutive pregnancies.
- It is characterised by painless cervical dilatation in the second trimester or perhaps early in the third trimester, with prolapse and ballooning of membranes into the vagina, followed by rupture of membranes and expulsion of an immature foetus. Unless effectively treated, this sequence tends to repeat in each pregnancy.
  - *Cause:* Previous trauma to the cervix such as dilation and curettage, conisation, cauterisation or amputation has been implicated but the cause still remains obscure.
  - *Diagnosis:*
    1. *Interconception period:* Numerous methods have been described in nonpregnant women to make the diagnosis, usually by documenting a more widely dilated internal cervical os than is normal.
    2. *Hystero-cervicography:* It shows a funnel-shaped shadow (premenstrual).

Pull-through techniques of inflated catheter balloons and acceptance without resistance at the internal or passage of specifically sized cervical dilators no. 6–8 beyond internal os without resistance and absence of internal os snap on its withdrawal.

During pregnancy, the following three types of diagnosis could be done:

1. *Obstetrical history-based diagnosis:* A classic history of greater than or equal to two consecutive prior second-trimester pregnancy losses/extremely preterm births (i.e., <28 weeks) associated with no or minimal mild symptoms. The presence of risk factors for structural cervical weakness supports the diagnosis. Most of these cases are pregnancy losses before 24 weeks.
2. *Ultrasound-based diagnosis:* Transvaginal ultrasound (TVS) has become the gold standard. In asymptomatic women with a past history of one second-trimester pregnancy loss/extremely preterm birth (i.e., <28 weeks) associated with no or minimal mild symptoms and those in whom a history-based diagnosis is uncertain, serial TVS examinations and diagnosis of cervical insufficiency are made when the cervical length is ≤25 mm before 24 weeks.

   The mean cervical length is 35–40 mm from 14 to 22 weeks and falls to approximately 35 mm between 24 and 28 weeks and 30 mm after 32 weeks. The cervical length from 22 to 32 weeks of gestation displays a normal bell-shaped distribution, with the 50th percentile approaching approximately 35 mm and the 10th and 90th percentiles at 25 and 45 mm, respectively. Hence, a cervix below 25 mm at midpregnancy is suggestive of a short cervix.

   Ultrasound images of the cervix in pregnancy have demonstrated that cervical effacement begins at the internal cervical os and proceeds distally through a process called funnelling. This process is usually established prior to dilatation of the external cervical os and can begin as early as 16–24 weeks in patients who eventually deliver preterm. Zilanti et al. described the appearance of cervical effacement as seen by TVS as the progression of the letters T, Y, V, and U to denote the relationship of the lower uterine segment to the axis of the cervical canal **(Fig. 5)**.
3. *Physical examination-based cervical insufficiency:* Diagnosis of physical examination-based cervical insufficiency in women 14 through 27 weeks of gestation with a dilated and effaced cervix on physical examination and no contractions or weak irregular contractions that appear inadequate to explain the

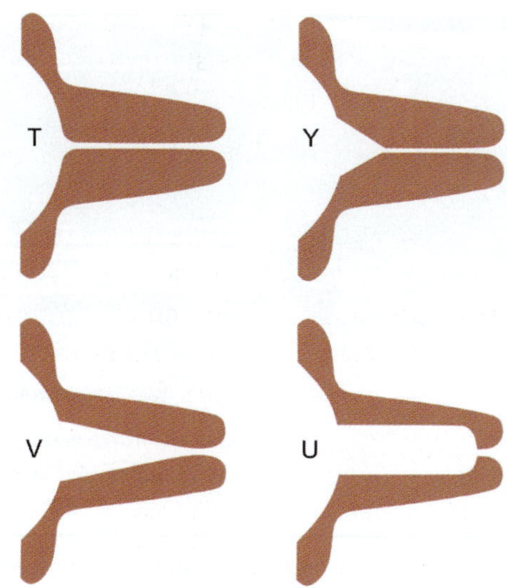

Fig. 5: Funnelling of cervix.

cervical dilation and effacement. The membranes may be prolapsed or ruptured.

Good evidence in the literature shows that a cervix <15 mm has a very high incidence of preterm labour. Insertion of a cervical suture may not substantially reduce the risk of prematurity. However, when diagnosed along with aggressive preterm tocolysis, antibiotics, etc., will help in a good number of those women who otherwise would have delivered preterm. Hence, TVS has a good positive predictive and negative predictive value for preterm labour and therefore could be used as a screening method in pregnancy.

- *Paternal factors:* Little is known about paternal factors in the genesis of spontaneous abortion. Certainly, chromosomal translocations in sperm can lead to abortion. DNA abnormalities may be contributory in these cases, and it may be worth assessing this.
- *Trauma:* External to the abdomen or during abdominal or pelvic operations.

Clinical Varieties of Spontaneous Abortions

Threatened Abortion

Clinical picture:

- Symptoms and signs of pregnancy coincide with its duration.
- Vaginal bleeding is slight or mild, bright red in colour originating from the choriodecidual interface.
- Pain is absent or slight.
- Cervix is closed.
- Pregnancy test is positive.
- Ultrasonography shows a living foetus.

Prognosis: If the foetus is normal in chromosomes with or without treatment, the chances of pregnancy continuation are 85%.

Treatment: Rest in bed for 1 week after the stoppage of bleeding. No intercourse as it may disturb pregnancy by the mechanical effect and the effect of semen prostaglandins on the uterus. Sedatives can be used if the patient is anxious. Progestogens and their role are controversial. However, a low plasma progesterone level is an indication of pregnancy failure. Progestogens may cause retention of the dead ovum, which leads to a missed abortion. Gonadotrophins [human chorionic gonadotrophin (hCG)] may be of benefit in cases of luteal phase deficiency, which is once again not proved.

Inevitable Abortion

Clinical picture:

- Symptoms and signs of pregnancy coincide with its duration. Vaginal bleeding is excessive and may be accompanied with clots.
- Pain is colicky, felt in the suprapubic region radiating to the back. The internal os of the cervix is dilated, and products of conception may be felt through it.
- Rupture of membranes between 12 and 28 weeks is a sign of the inevitability of abortion.

Treatment: Any attempt to maintain pregnancy is useless. Resuscitation and 0.5 mg of methyl ergometrine is given either intramuscular (IM) or Intravenous (IV) route to induce tetanic uterine contraction and stop bleeding.

- *If pregnancy is <12 weeks:* Termination is done by vaginal evacuation and curettage or suction evacuation under general anaesthesia.
- *If pregnancy is more than 12 weeks:*
  - Oxytocin is given by IV drip to expel the uterine contents.
  - If the placenta is retained, it is removed under general anaesthesia.

Cervical Abortion

It is a variety of inevitable abortion in which the products of conception (POC) have been separated from the uterine cavity but retained in the cervical canal causing its distension.

Clinical picture:
- The patient complains of considerable bleeding and severe lower abdominal pain referred to the back.
- On examination, the products of conception are felt through the dilated cervix.

Treatment: Under anaesthesia, the cervix is dilated, contents are removed, and the cavity is curetted to remove the decidua.

Incomplete Abortion

Retention of a part of the products of conception inside the uterus. It may be the whole or part of the placenta that is retained.

Clinical picture: The patient usually noticed the passage of a part of the conception products. Bleeding is continuous. On examination, the uterus is less than the period of amenorrhoea but still larger in size. The cervix is opened and retained contents may be felt through it.

Ultrasonography: It shows the retained contents.

Treatment: Complete the process by evacuation.

Complete Abortion

All products of conception have been expelled from the uterus.

Clinical picture:
- The bleeding is slight and gradually diminishes. Pain ceases.
- The cervix is closed. The uterus is slightly larger than normal.

Ultrasound: It shows an empty cavity.

Missed Abortion

Retention of dead products of conception for 4 weeks or more.

Carneous mole is a special variety of missed abortion in which the dead ovum in early pregnancy is surrounded by clotted blood.

Clinical picture:
Symptoms: Symptoms of threatened abortion may or may not be developed. Regression of pregnancy symptoms such as nausea, vomiting and breast symptoms. The abdomen does not increase and may even decrease in size. The foetal movements are not felt or cease if previously present. Milk secretion may start particularly in second-trimester abortion because of the decline in oestrogen secretion that was normally blocking the action of prolactin on the breasts. A dark brown vaginal discharge may occur (prune juice discharge).

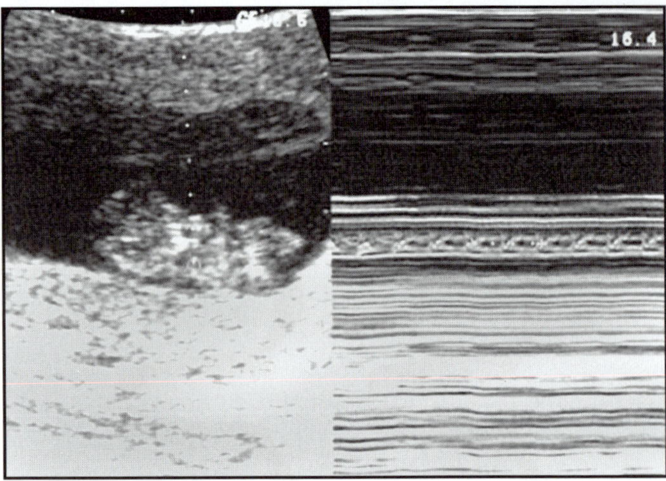

Fig. 6: *M-mode embryonic heart:* Embryonic and/or foetal cardiac activity must be documented.

Signs: The uterus fails to grow or even decreases in size and becomes firmer. The cervix is closed.

Investigations: A pregnancy test becomes negative within 2 weeks from the ovum death, but it may remain positive for a longer period due to persistent living chorionic villi. Ultrasound shows either a collapsed gestational sac, absent foetal heart movement or foetal movement **(Fig. 6)**.

Complications: Disseminated intravascular coagulation (DIC) may occur if the dead conceptus is retained for >4 weeks and superadded infection.

Treatment: The dead conceptus is expelled spontaneously in the majority of cases. *Evacuation of the uterus is indicated in the following conditions:* Spontaneous expulsion does not occur within 4 weeks. However, in clinical practice, one does not wait for too long, as there is an increased psychological feeling in the woman and her relatives. Hence, the same may be evacuated either medically or surgically, depending on the size of the uterus. The other indications to interfere are that when there is bleeding or infection or DIC.

Evacuation is carried out as follows: If the uterine size is <12 weeks' gestation; vaginal or suction evacuation is done. If the uterine size is >12 weeks' gestation, evacuation can be done by:
- *Prostaglandins:* Given intravaginally (PGE_2), intravenously, intra- or extra-amniotic ($PGF2\alpha$).

- Oxytocin infusion
- *Combination:* Starting with prostaglandin and completed with oxytocin
- *Hysterotomy:* It is not done in modern methods of evacuation.

Septic Abortion

It is any type of abortion, usually criminal abortion, complicated by infection.

Microbiology: Escherichia coli, bacteroides, anaerobic streptococci, clostridia, streptococci, and staphylococci are among the most causative organisms.

Clinical picture:

General examination: It includes:

- Pyrexia and tachycardia
- Rigors suggest bacteraemia
- A subnormal temperature with tachycardia is ominous and mostly seen with gas-forming organisms.
- Malaise, sweating, headache, and joint pain
- Jaundice and/or haematuria is an ominous sign, indicating haemolysis due to chemicals used in criminal abortion or haemolytic infection such as *Clostridium welchii.*

Abdominal examination:

- Suprapubic pain and tenderness
- Abdominal rigidity and distension indicate peritonitis.

Local examination:

Offensive vaginal discharge: Minimal inoffensive vaginal discharge is often associated with severe cases. Uterus is tender, products of conception may be felt, and local trauma may be detected. Fullness and tenderness of the Douglas pouch indicate a pelvic abscess which will be associated with diarrhoea.

Complications: Endotoxic (septic) shock may develop with its serious sequels such as acute renal failure and DIC.

Treatment:

- Isolate the patient. Bed rest.
- An IV line is established for therapy. In case of shock, a central venous pressure (CVP) line when needed to aid in the control of fluid and blood transfusion is added.
- *Observation for vital signs:* Pulse, temperature and blood pressure as well as fluid intake and urinary output. A cervicovaginal swab is taken for culture (aerobic and anaerobic) and sensitivity.
- *Antibiotic therapy:* Ampicillin or cephalosporin (as a broad spectrum) + gentamycin (for Gram-negative organisms) + metronidazole (for anaerobic infection) are given by IV route while awaiting the results of the bacteriological culture. Another regimen to cover the different causative organisms is clindamycin + gentamicin.
- *Fluid therapy:* For example, glucose 5%, normal saline and/or lactated ringer solutions can be given as long as there are no manifestations of acute renal failure, particularly if the urinary output is >30 mL/h.
- *Blood transfusion:* It is given if CVP is low (normal: 8–12 cm water). It is of importance also to correct anaemia, coagulation defects and infection.
- Antigas gangrene (in *C. welchii*) and antitetanic serum (in *C. tetani*)
- *Oxytocin infusion:* To control bleeding and enhance the expulsion of the retained products
- Surgical evacuation of the uterus can be done after 6 hours of commencing IV therapy but may be earlier in case of severe bleeding or deteriorating condition in spite of the previous therapy.
- Hysterectomy may be needed in endotoxic shock not responding to treatment, particularly due to gas gangrene (*C. welchii*).

RECURRENT EARLY PREGNANCY LOSS

Recurrent pregnancy (RM) loss affects somewhere between 1 and 5% of couples. There is a rising prevalence of RPL reported due to several reasons, including change in definition of RPL, changing reproductive epidemiology, early diagnosis of pregnancy, etc. Both the European Society of Human Reproduction and Embryology (ESHRE) and the American Society for Reproductive Medicine (ASRM) now recognise a more inclusive criteria for the diagnosis of RPL, which specifies the loss of two or more pregnancies. This shift from 3 to 2 pregnancy losses appears to have been prompted by evidence that there is minimal clinical significance in a reported history of two versus three early miscarriages. The ASRM describes "early" loss as occurring before 20 weeks gestational age or loss of a foetus weighing <500 g, although the ESHRE defines it as a loss before the point of viability, which is achieved at 24 weeks gestation. In addition, although previously the diagnosis specified the occurrence of consecutive pregnancy losses, it is currently acceptable to include nonconsecutive losses to meet diagnostic criteria.

TABLE 1: Suspected cause of recurrent pregnancy loss.

Cause	*Contribution to RPL (%)*	*Recommended screening*	*Supportive scientific evidence*	*Controversial scientific evidence*	*Not recommended*
Cytogenetic	2–5	Balanced reciprocal translocations			
aPL syndrome	8–42	Lupus anticoagulant, anticardiolipin IgG or IgM antibody, anti-β2 glycoprotein I	IgG and IgM antibodies, aPL testing for other phospholipids and β2 glycoprotein I	IgG or IgM anti-annexin A5, anti-factor XII, anti-prothrombin, IgA aPLs	ANA, antithyroid antibodies
Anatomic	1.8–37.6	Hysterosalpingography, sonohysterography	Congenital uterine abnormalities	Uterine fibroids, polyps	Cervical incompetence
Hormonal or metabolic		Prolactin, TSH, haemoglobin A1C	Uncontrolled diabetes or thyroid disease, prolactin	Polycystic ovary syndrome and insulin resistance, luteal phase progesterone	
Infectious		None		Bacterial vaginosis, endocervical infections	
Male factors		None		Abnormal sperm DNA	
Psychological		None		Psychological effect on uterine receptivity	
Alloimmune		None		Mucosal CD 16-NK cells, embryotoxic factors, cytokine profiles, blocking antibodies, HLA typing, antipaternal leucocyte antibodies and circulating CD16-NK cells	Circulating CD 16-NK cells
Environmental, occupational, or personal habits		History			Not related to recurrent pregnancy loss

(ANA: antinuclear antibodies; aPL: antiphospholipid; DNA: deoxyribonucleic acid; HLA: human leucocyte antigen; IgG: immunoglobulin G; IgM: immunoglobulin M; NK: natural killer; RPL: recurrent pregnancy loss; TSH: thyroid-stimulating hormone)

More than half of the RM cases following investigations are classified as idiopathic, that is, no identifiable cause in either partner; it is generally accepted that, within the idiopathic group, there is considerable heterogeneity and it is unlikely that one single pathological mechanism can be attributed to RM history **(Table 1)**.

Risk Factors for Recurrent Miscarriage (Fig. 7)

- *Epidemiological factors:* Number of previous miscarriages and advanced maternal age are two independent risk factors for RM. There is a decline in the number and quality of remaining oocytes with advancing age. The risk of miscarriage increases after each successive pregnancy loss, reaching 40% after three consecutive pregnancy losses and prognosis worsens with advancing maternal age. Advanced paternal age has also been identified as a risk factor. Among couples where the woman's age is >35 years and the man's age is >40 years, the risk of miscarriage is highest.

  Recent studies have suggested that obesity increases the risk of both sporadic and recurrent miscarriage.
- *Antiphospholipid syndrome (APS):* It is the most important treatable cause of RM.

  Revised Sapporo or Sidney criteria for classification of antiphospholipid antibody syndrome APS are present if one of the following clinical criteria and one of the laboratory criteria are met.

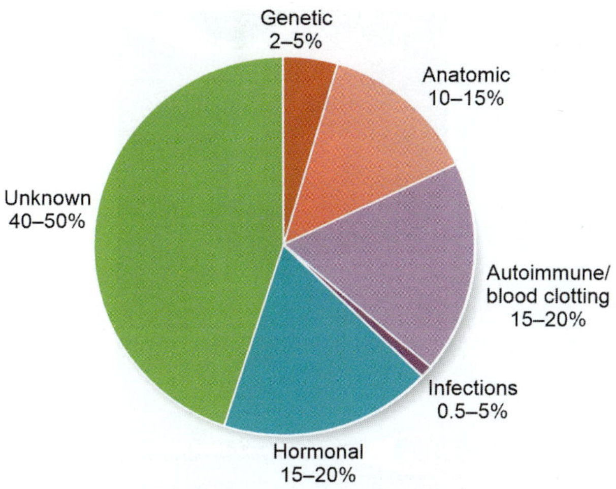

Fig. 7: Aetiology of recurrent pregnancy loss.

- *Clinical criteria:*
    - *Vascular thrombosis:* One or more episodes of venous, arterial or small vessel thrombosis, with unequivocal imaging or histologic evidence of thrombosis in any tissue or organ. Superficial venous thrombosis does not satisfy the criteria for thrombosis for APS.
    - *Pregnancy morbidity:* It includes:
        - One or more unexplained foetal deaths of morphologically normal foetuses after 10 weeks of gestation by ultrasound or direct examination of the foetus.
        - One or more premature births of a morphologically normal neonate before 34 weeks of gestation because of eclampsia or severe preeclampsia, or recognised placental insufficiency.
        - Three or more unexplained consecutive spontaneous abortions before 10 weeks with maternal anatomic or hormonal abnormalities and paternal and maternal chromosomal causes excluded.
- *Laboratory criteria:*
    - Lupus anticoagulant present in plasma on two or more occasions at least 12 weeks apart, or
    - Antocardiolipin antibody of IgG or IgM isotype in serum or plasma present in medium or high titre (>40 GPL or MPL or >99th percentile), on two or more occasions at least 12 weeks apart, or
    - Anti-β2-glycoprotein-1 antibody of IgG and/or IgM isotype in serum or plasma (in titre greater than 99th percentile), present on two occasions at least 12 weeks apart.

- *Genetic factors:*
    - *Parental chromosomal rearrangements:* One of the partners carries a balanced structural chromosomal anomaly, in approximately 2–5% of couples with RM. Most commonly a balanced reciprocal or Robertsonian translocation.
    - *Embryonic chromosomal abnormalities:* Chromosomal abnormalities of the embryo account for 30-57% of miscarriage. The risk increases with advancing maternal age **(Figs. 8A to G)**.
- *Anatomical factors:*
    - *Congenital uterine malformation:* Septate or arcuate uteri, unicornuate, didelphic, bicornuate. These congenital Müllerian tract anomalies are mostly associated with second-trimester pregnancy loss, along with other complications like preterm labour, foetal malpresentation and increased rates of caesarean delivery **(Figs. 9 to 11)**.
    - *Cervical insufficiency:* A recognised cause of recurrent second-trimester abortion. The diagnosis is based on a history of second-trimester abortion preceded by spontaneous rupture of membrane or painless cervical dilatation.
- *Endocrine factors:* Diabetes mellitus and thyroid disease have been associated with miscarriage. Women who have high haemoglobin A1c levels in the first trimester are at high risk of miscarriage and foetal malformations. In polycystic ovary syndrome (PCOS), increased risk of miscarriage is attributed to insulin resistance, hyperinsulinaemia and hyperandrogenaemia.
- *Immune factors:* Natural killer (NK) cells are found in peripheral blood and the uterine mucosa. There is no clear evidence that altered peripheral blood NK cells are related to recurrent miscarriage. Cytokines are immune molecules that control immune and other cells. In normal pregnancy, Th-2 cytokine response is predominant as compared to recurrent miscarriage, where Th-1 cytokine responses are mounted. But available data are not consistent with the association between cytokine polymorphisms and recurrent miscarriage.
- *Infective agents:* Sporadic miscarriage can be caused by any severe infections leading to bacteraemia or viremia. In recent literature, it has been described that infections may account for up to 15% of early miscarriages and up to 66% of late miscarriages. Among bacterial pathogens, syphilis, gonorrhoea, bacterial vaginosis, brucellosis, and listeriosis have

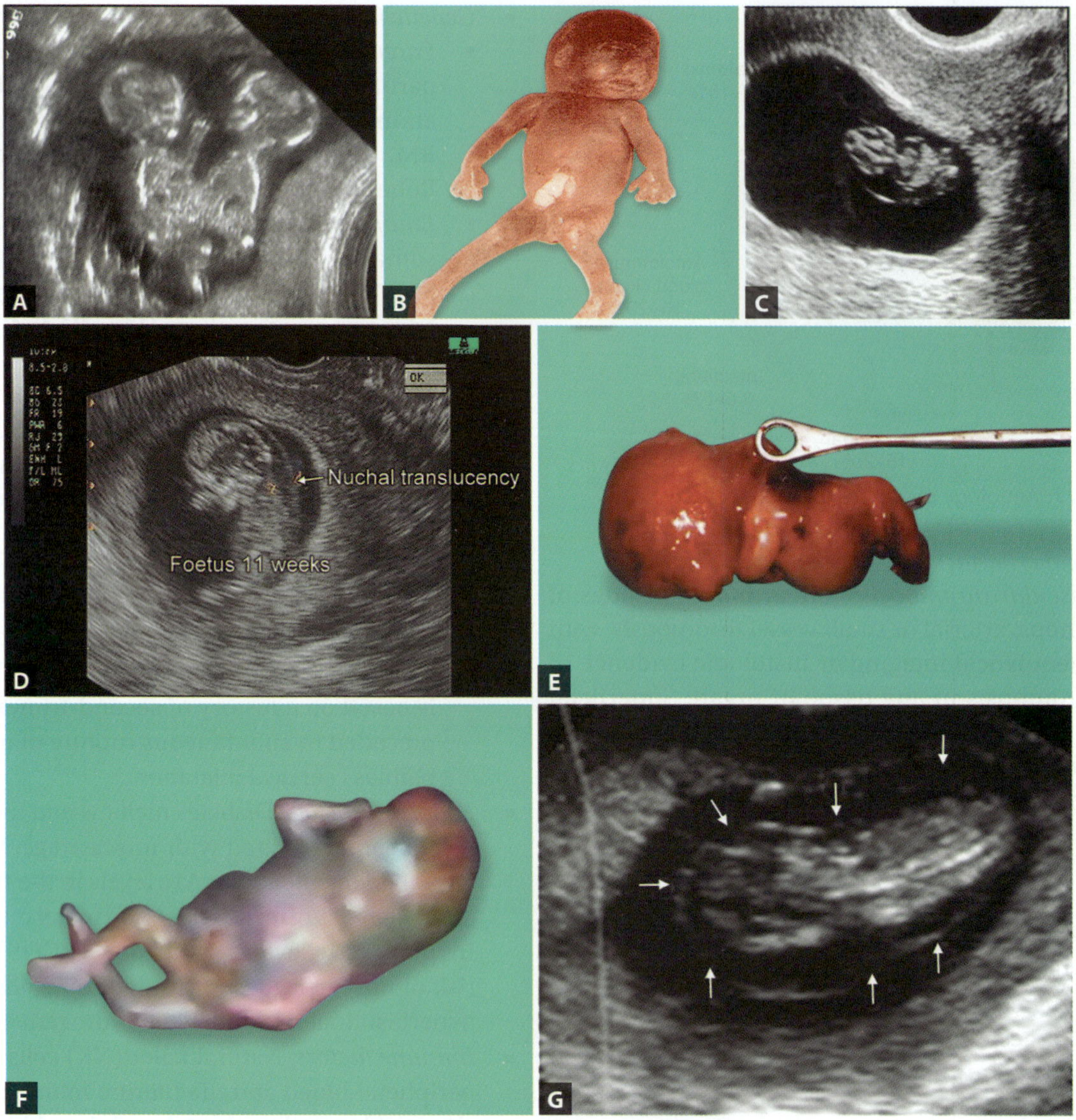

Figs. 8A to G: Genetic anomalies in the embryo.

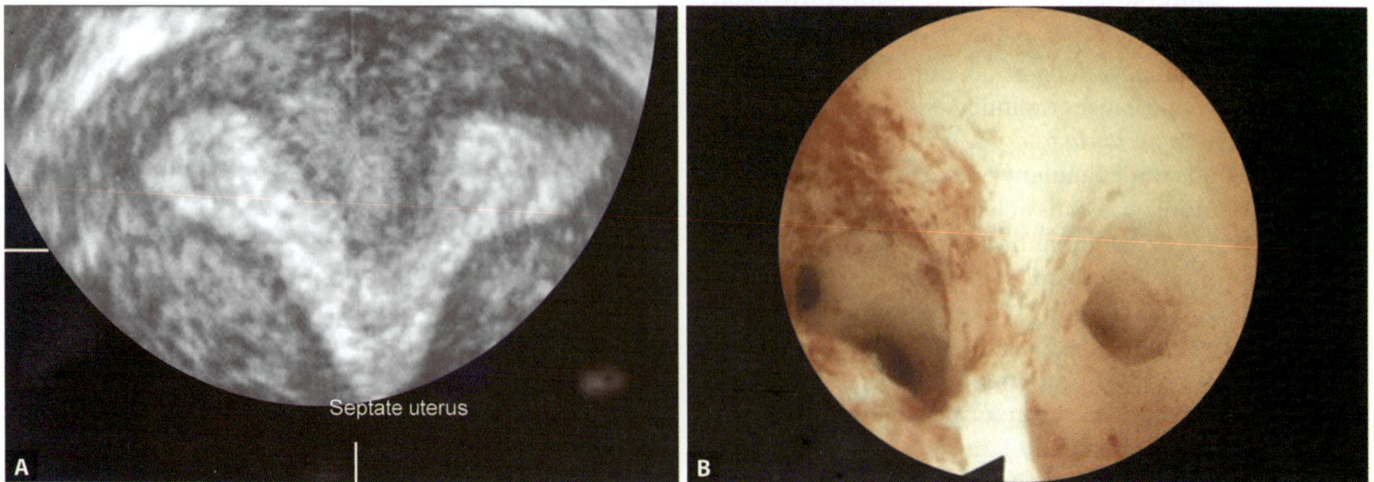

Figs. 9A and B: (A) Three-dimensional ultrasound septate; (B) Hysteroscopy showing septum.

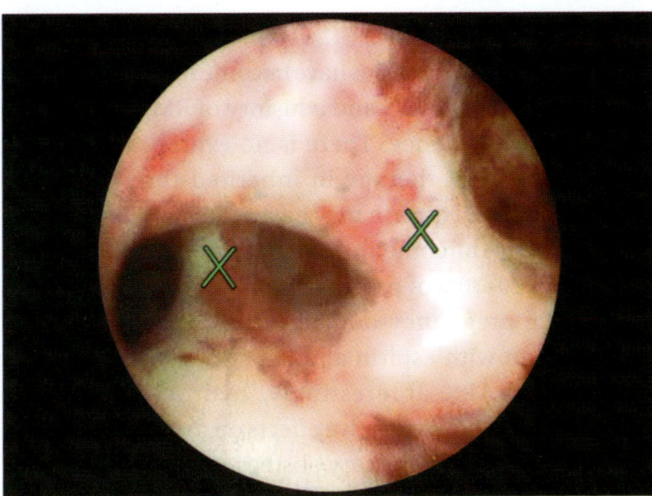

Fig. 10: Intrauterine adhesions.

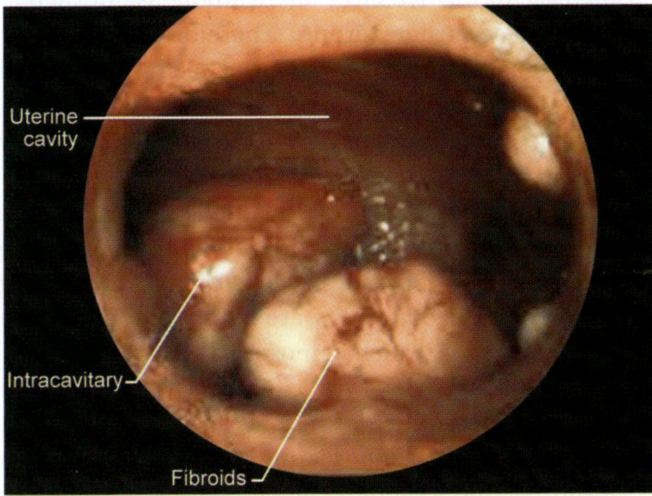

Fig. 11: Uterine submucosal fibroids.

been shown to consistently increase the chance of miscarriage. Rubella, human immunodeficiency virus (HIV), cytomegalovirus (CMV), herpes simplex virus (HSV), hepatitis B virus, Zika virus, dengue virus, and influenza viruses are associated with an increased risk of miscarriage. Among protozoa, malaria and toxoplasma have been associated with a higher risk of miscarriage. For repeated pregnancy loss, the infective agent to be implicated must be capable of persisting in the genital tract and avoiding detection or must cause insufficient symptoms to disturb the women. TORCH (toxoplasmosis, others, Rubella, cytomegalovirus, herpes) screening should be abandoned as they do not fulfil these criteria.

- *Inherited thrombophilic defects:* Inherited and acquired thrombophilias [activated protein C resistance (factor V Leiden mutation), deficiencies of protein C/S and antithrombin III, hyperhomocysteinaemia and prothrombin gene mutation] have been implicated as a possible cause in RPL and late pregnancy complications with the mechanism being thrombosis of uteroplacental circulations. Other coagulation abnormalities, including impaired fibrinolytic activity, factor XII deficiency and reduced activated partial thromboplastin time have also been reported to be associated with RM.

Investigations

- *Antiphospholipid syndrome:* Anticardiolipin antibodies (IgG and/or IgM); LAC to be done at least 12 weeks apart with medium or high titre.

  Dilute Russell's viper venom test with a platelet neutralisation procedure is more specific and sensitive than the activated partial thromboplastin time test or Kaolin clotting time test.
- *Genetic testing on the products of conception:* Cytogenetic analysis should be performed on products of conception of the third and subsequent consecutive miscarriage Royal College of Obstetricians and Gynaecologists (RCOG). In cases where testing of products of conceptions reports an unbalanced structural chromosomal abnormality, parental peripheral blood karyotyping of both partners must be performed. ESHRE and ASRM recommend this test only for explanatory purposes or to look for reasons for treatment failure. However, karyotyping has certain disadvantages, including inconclusive results in up to 20–40% of cases and possible false-negative results in up to 22–33% of samples. Chromosomal microarray (CMA) can diagnose submicroscopic chromosomal abnormalities. Compared with karyotyping, CMA offers several advantages, including improved resolution, detecting molecular gains or losses of DNA down to 10 kilobases within the genome. It is also less likely to yield inconclusive or false-negative results. Other advantages include avoidance of maternal cell contamination, no requirement for viable tissue and cell culture, a higher rate of results and more objective detection of genetic abnormalities. Using CMA can lead to a 13% increase in the detection rate of chromosome abnormalities in RPL, and thus the ESHRE recommends array comparative genomic hybridisation as the preferred method for cytogenetic testing of foetal tissue.

- *Parental genetic testing:* Parental chromosome rearrangements are involved in approximately 2–5% of recurrent miscarriage cases, of which most are balanced translocations. Where foetal cytogenetic testing renders inconclusive results or is impossible, parental karyotype is recommended. In addition, couples found to have a genetic abnormality should be referred for genetic counselling for discussion of the risks of future pregnancy and management options.
- Pelvic ultrasound (3D TVS ultrasound) hysteroscopy and laparoscopy in cases of suspected uterine anomalies.
- ASRM, ESHRE, and RCOG advise against routine testing of hereditary thrombophilia in patients with RPL as the association between hereditary thrombophilias and RPL is weak, and the clinical value of testing is minimal.
- Test for diabetes mellitus (Glyc Hb), hypo- or hyperthyroidism (TSH)
- *Other immunological factors:* ESHRE and RCOG suggest testing anti-thyroid peroxidase (TPO) antibodies (but not treating euthyroid antibody-positive women but to monitor their TSH during pregnancy). ESHRE recommends testing ANA (antinuclear antibodies) only for explanatory purposes as ANA positivity has been linked to a higher risk of RPL. However, various forms of immunotherapy and vitamin D supplementation have been studied to know their benefit in this context.

After a thorough evaluation following ASRM, ESHRE or RCOG diagnostic guidelines, over 50% of cases have no identifiable cause. This further contributes to parental stress and motivates patients and healthcare providers to pursue nonevidence-based therapy. Genetic testing of products of conception (POC) (using CMA) can reduce the proportion of this unexplained RPL. In a series of 378 cases of RPL, combination of ASRM workup and CMA analysis of POC revealed a definite or probable explanation for the loss in 91.8% of cases and decreased the rate of unexplained RPL from 57.1 to 8.3%. Authors claim that this improved diagnostic rate of RPL is potentially beneficial to patient wellbeing and reduced healthcare system costs. Based on this, although RCOG recommends genetic testing of POC from the third miscarriage onwards, CMA of POC can be considered from the second loss onwards, in addition to using the standard RPL work-up algorithm.

Management

- Aspirin and/or heparins have become routine treatment for women with APS and a history of RM, on the basis of limited evidence. There is no evidence to suggest benefit of this therapy in inherited thrombophilia. Empiric use of aspirin may have a deleterious effect on pregnancy outcome in women with RM and no APS. Around 20–30% of pregnant women with APS develop adverse pregnancy outcomes despite conventional treatment with aspirin and heparin, called refractory obstetric APS. Interestingly, hydroxychloroquine (HCQ) has shown positive effects on top of the standard of care in some refractory obstetric APS patients.
- For women with a history of one or more miscarriages experiencing vaginal bleeding, evidence shows an increase in the live birth rate with the use of vaginal micronised progesterone. Therefore, the current recommendation is to use 400 mg of micronised vaginal progesterone twice a day until 16 weeks' gestation in women presenting with vaginal bleeding and a history of one or more previous miscarriages.
- On the basis of the available evidence, levothyroxine treatment could be considered for women with subclinical hypothyroidism whose thyroid-stimulating hormone concentrations are above the laboratory reference range, which in most cases is approximately 4.0 mIU/L. Women with normal thyroid function who are positive for thyroid antibodies do not require levothyroxine treatment. Data is unclear on levothyroxine usage in women with mildly elevated thyroid-stimulating hormone concentrations (2.5–4.0 mIU/L) and positive for thyroid antibodies.
- Metformin may have a role in miscarriage prevention among women with PCOS. Metformin started preconceptionally and continued throughout the first trimester, has been shown to reduce miscarriage rates and improve pregnancy outcomes.
- The use of intravenous immunoglobulin (IVIG), anti-tumour necrosis factor (TNF), glucocorticoids or cellular therapies in order to prevent or reduce an excessive immune response remains controversial.
- Findings of an abnormal parental karyotype should prompt referral to a clinical geneticist. Preimplantation genetic screening has been advocated as a treatment option for women with recurrent miscarriage.
- In women with recurrent miscarriage and uterine septum, there is insufficient evidence to assess

the effect of septum resection to prevent further miscarriage.

- Cervical cerclage should be considered only in women who are likely to benefit due to hazards related to surgery and the risk of stimulating uterine contractions.
- In women with a singleton pregnancy and history of one second-trimester miscarriage attributable to cervical factors, with a cervical length of 25 mm or less detected by transvaginal scan before 24 weeks of gestation, cerclage should be offered.
- A small number of nonrandomised studies have reported that psychological support, that is, tender loving care (TLC) in early pregnancy, decreases miscarriage rates in women with unexplained RM.
- Regardless of whether or not a specific cause is obtained, patients should work to correct modifiable risk factors for RPL such as achieving normal body mass index (BMI). Lifestyle modifications known to prevent or reduce the risk of miscarriage, based on limited evidence are a balanced and varied diet, testing serum vitamin D levels followed by appropriate replacement, limiting caffeine intake to <150 mg/day, efforts to bring BMI within normal range, avoid smoking and alcohol intake, adequate sleep and reduce stress levels.
- *Male partner:* A systematic review found that paternal smoking of >10 cigarettes/day in the preconception period is associated with an increased risk of pregnancy loss, hence recommended smoking cessation in the preconceptional period. Moderation of alcohol consumption is also recommended.
- There are many strategies that need further research; for example, immunotherapy, prednisolone/ hydroxychloroquine for autoimmunity, preimplantation genetic testing, hCG administration, antibiotics for chronic endometritis and endometrial scratching. However, the body of evidence suggests no clear benefit for any of these interventions, and therefore they cannot be recommended routinely. However, in patients who are of advanced maternal age, the biological realities of aneuploidy and pregnancy loss should be addressed, and options such as preimplantation genetic testing for aneuploidy may be discussed.
- There is a lack of certainty regarding the correlation between uNK cell levels, cytotoxicity, RPL and potential treatments such as corticosteroids, and this is an area being studied intensively in ongoing trials.
- It is critical to offer adequate mental health support, acknowledgment and validation of their grief and provide the couple with information about their diagnosis as well as a path forwards.
- Delaying childbearing is increasingly common now. One may need to discuss with them the option of fertility preservation in the form of oocyte or embryo freezing, which may ultimately decrease their risk of experiencing RPL in future years when they are ready to build their family.

Lastly, a recent meta-analysis suggests that women who have had recurrent spontaneous abortions may have a higher prevalence of adverse pregnancy outcomes in their subsequent spontaneous conceptions, such as gestational diabetes, preeclampsia, antepartum haemorrhage, late miscarriage, preterm birth, caesarean section, perinatal death and neonatal intensive care unit (NICU) admissions [association with foetal growth restriction (FGR), foetal anomalies and postpartum haemorrhage (PPH) not clear]. Therefore, these are high-risk pregnancies that need vigilance.

SUGGESTED READING

1. Alberman ED, Creasy MR. Frequency of chromosomal abnormalities in miscarriages and perinatal deaths. J Med Genet. 1977;14(5):313-5.
2. Aleman A, Althabe F, Belizán J, Bergel E. Bed rest during pregnancy for preventing miscarriage. Cochrane Database Syst Rev. 2005;(2):CD003576.
3. Bagratee JS, Khullar V, Regan L, Moodley J, Kagoro H. A randomized controlled trial comparing medical and expectant management of first trimester miscarriage. Hum Reprod. 2004;19(2):266-71.
4. Benson J. Clinical management of abortion complications: a practical guide. WHO; 1994.
5. Blumenthal PD. Prospective comparison of Dilapan and Laminaria for pretreatment of cervix in second-trimester induction abortion. Obstet Gynecol. 1988;72(2):243-6.
6. Brunader R. Accuracy of prenatal sonography performed by family practice residents. Fam Med. 1996;28(6):407-10.
7. Bugalho A, Bique C, Almeida L, Bergström S. Application of vaginal misoprostol before cervical dilation to facilitate first-trimester pregnancy interruption. Obstet Gynecol. 1994;83(5 Pt 1):729-31.
8. Carbonell JL, Velazco A, Rodriguez Y, Tanda R, Sánchez C, Barambio S, et al. Oral versus vaginal misoprostol for cervical priming in first trimester abortion: a randomized trial. Eur J Contracept Reprod Health Care. 2001;6(3):134-40.
9. Castadot RG. Pregnancy termination: techniques, risks, and complications and their management. Fertil Steril. 1986;45(1):5-17.

10. Chen BA, Creinin MD. Contemporary management of early pregnancy failure. Clin Obstet Gynecol. 2007;50(1): 67-88.
11. Chen LH, Lai SF, Lee WH, Leong NK. Uterine perforation during elective first trimester abortions: a 13-year review. Singapore Med J. 1995;36(1):63-7.
12. Cleary-Goldman J, Malone FD, Vidaver J, Ball RH, Nyberg DA, Comstock CH, et al. Impact of maternal age on obstetric outcome. Obstet Gynecol. 2005;105(5 Pt 1):983-90.
13. Darney PD, Horbach NS, Korn AP. First-trimester elective abortion. Protocols for Office Gynecologic Surgery. Cambridge, MA: Blackwell Science; 1996. pp. 158-93.
14. Devaseelan P, Fogarty PP, Regan L. Human chorionic gonadotrophin for threatened miscarriage. Cochrane Database Syst Rev. 2010;(5):CD007422.
15. Donders GG, Van Bulck B, Caudron J, Londers L, Vereecken A, Spitz B, et al. Relationship of bacterial vaginosis and mycoplasmas to the risk of spontaneous abortion. Am J Obstet Gynecol. 2000;183(2):431-7.
16. Dresang LT, Rodney WM, Rodney KM. Prenatal ultrasound: a tale of two cities. J Natl Med Assoc. 2006;98(2):167-71.
17. Edwards JE, Darney PD, Paul M. Surgical abortion in the first trimester. In: Paul M, Lichtenberg ES, Borgatta L, (Eds). A Clinician's Guide to Medical and Surgical Abortion. New York: Churchill Livingstone; 1999. pp. 107-21.
18. Eliwa J, Papas RS, Kutteh WH. Expanding the role of chromosomal microarray analysis in the evaluation of recurrent pregnancy loss. J Reprod Immunol. 2024 Feb:161:104188.
19. ESHRE Recurrent Pregnancy Loss Guideline Development Group. Recurrent Pregnancy Loss. Guideline of European Society of Human Reproduction and Embryology; 2022, 2nd version 2:7-179.
20. Everett C. Incidence and outcome of bleeding before the 20th week of pregnancy: prospective study from general practice. BMJ. 1997;315(7099):32-4.
21. Everett CB, Preece E. Women with bleeding in the first 20 weeks of pregnancy: value of general practice ultrasound in detecting foetal heart movement. Br J Gen Pract. 1996;46(402):7-9.
22. Fielding WL, Lee SY, Borten M, Friedman EA. Continued pregnancy after failed first-trimester abortion. Obstet Gynecol. 1984;63:421.
23. Fierro JJ, Velásquez-Berrío M, Ospina A, Henning S, de Leeuw K, Cadavid JÁP. The effects of hydroxychloroquine and its promising use in refractory obstetric antiphospholipid syndrome. Rheumatol Int. 2024;44(2):223-34.
24. Forna F, Gülmezoglu AM. Surgical procedures to evacuate incomplete abortion. Cochrane Database Syst Rev. 2001;(1):CD001993.
25. Genovese HG, McQueen DB. The prevalence of sporadic and recurrent pregnancy loss. Fertil Steril. 2023;120(5):934-6.
26. Glick E. Surgical Abortion. Reno, Nevada: West End Women's Medical Group; 1998. pp. 17-22.
27. Gracia CR, Sammel MD, Chittams J, Hummel AC, Shaunik A, Barnhart KT, et al. Risk factors for spontaneous abortion in early symptomatic first trimester pregnancies. Obstet Gynecol. 2005;106(5 pt 1):993-9.
28. Grimes DA, Schulz KF, Cates WJ. Prevention of uterine perforation during curettage for abortion. JAMA. 1984;251:2108.
29. Grimes DA. Management of abortion in TeLinde's Operative Gynecology, 9th edition. Philadelphia: Lippincott Williams & Wilkins; 1997. p. 8.
30. Haas DM, Ramsey PS. Progestogen for preventing miscarriage. Cochrane Database Syst Rev. 2008;(2): CD003511.
31. Hallengren B, Lantz M, Andreasson B, Grennert L. Pregnant women on thyroxine substitution are often dysregulated in early pregnancy. Thyroid. 2009;19(4):391-4.
32. Hannafin B, Lovecchio F, Blackburn P. Do Rh-negative women with first trimester spontaneous abortions need Rh immune globulin? Am J Emerg Med. 2006;24(4):487-9.
33. Hasan R, Baird DD, Herring AH, Olshan AF, Jonsson Funk ML, Hartmann KE. Association between first-trimester vaginal bleeding and miscarriage. Obstet Gynecol. 2009;114(4):860-7.
34. Hasan R, Baird DD, Herring AH, Olshan AF, Jonsson Funk ML, Hartmann KE. Patterns and predictors of vaginal bleeding in the first trimester of pregnancy. Ann Epidemiol. 2010;20(7):524-31.
35. Henriksen TB, Hjollund NH, Jensen TK, Bonde JP, Andersson AM, Kolstad H. Alcohol consumption at the time of conception and spontaneous abortion. Am J Epidemiol. 2004;160(7):661-7.
36. Huggins GR, Cullins VE. Fertility after contraception or abortion. Fertil Steril. 1990;54(4):559-73.
37. Jia DM, Li X, Zhang BC, Zhang BR, Zhang QJ, Liu MW, et al. Adverse outcomes in subsequent pregnancies in women with history of recurrent spontaneous abortion: a meta-analysis. BMC Neurol. 2025;25(1):126.
38. Johns J, Jauniaux E. Threatened miscarriage as a predictor of obstetric outcome. Obstet Gynecol. 2006;107(4): 845-50.
39. Keder LM. Best practices in surgical abortion. Am J Obstet Gynecol. 2003;189(2):418-22.
40. Lede RL, Duley L. Uterine muscle relaxant drugs for threatened miscarriage. Cochrane Database Syst Rev. 2005;(3):CD002857.
41. Lichtenberg ES, Grimes DA, Paul M. Abortion complications: prevention and management. In: Paul M, Lichtenberg ES, Borgatta L, et al. (Eds). A Clinician's Guide to Medical and Surgical Abortion. New York: Churchill Livingstone; 1999. p. 197.
42. Li DK, Liu L, Odouli R. Exposure to non-steroidal anti-inflammatory drugs during pregnancy and risk of miscarriage: population based cohort study. BMJ. 2003;327(7411):368.

43. Luise C, Jermy K, May C, Costello G, Collins WP, Bourne TH. Outcome of expectant management of spontaneous first trimester miscarriage: observational study. BMJ. 2002;324(7342):873-5.
44. May W, Gülmezoglu AM, Ba-Thike K. Antibiotics for incomplete abortion. Cochrane Database Syst Rev. 2007;(4):CD001779.
45. Metwally M, Ong KJ, Ledger WL, Li TC. Does high body mass index increase the risk of miscarriage after spontaneous and assisted conception? A meta-analysis of the evidence. Fertil Steril. 2008;90(3):714-26.
46. Michels TC, Tiu AY. Second trimester pregnancy loss. Am Fam Physician. 2007;76:1341-6.
47. Molin A. Risk of damage to the cervix by dilation for first-trimester induced abortion by suction aspiration. Gynecol Obstet Invest. 1993;35:152.
48. Nakhai-Pour HR, Broy P, Bérard A. Use of antidepressants during pregnancy and the risk of spontaneous abortion. CMAJ. 2010;182(10):1031-7.
49. Nanda K, Peloggia A, Grimes D, Lopez L, Nanda G. Expectant care versus surgical treatment for miscarriage. Cochrane Database Syst Rev. 2006;(2):CD003518.
50. Neilson JP, Hickey M, Vazquez J. Medical treatment for early foetal death (less than 24 weeks). Cochrane Database Syst Rev. 2006;(3):CD002253.
51. Nelson DB, Grisso JA, Joffe MM, Brensinger C, Shaw L, Datner E. Does stress influence early pregnancy loss? Ann Epidemiol. 2003;13(4):223-9.
52. Ness RB, Grisso JA, Hirschinger N, Markovic N, Shaw LM, Day NL. Cocaine and tobacco use and the risk of spontaneous abortion. N Engl J Med. 1999;340(5):333-9.
53. Parazzini F, Chatenoud L, Tozzi L, Di Cintio E, Benzi G, Fedele L. Induced abortion in the first trimester of pregnancy and risk of miscarriage. Br J Obstet Gynaecol. 1998;105(4):418-21.
54. Paspulati RM, Bhatt S, Nour SG. Sonographic evaluation of first trimester bleeding. Radiol Clin North Am. 2004;42(2):297-314.
55. Paul M, Lackie E, Mitchell C, Rogers A, Fox M. Is pathology examination useful after early surgical abortion? Obstet Gynecol. 2002;99(4):567-71.
56. Pennes DR, Bowerman RA, Silver TM, Smith SJ. Failed first-trimester pregnancy termination: uterine anomaly as etiologic factor. J Clin Ultrasound. 1987;15:165.
57. Poulose T, Richardson R, Ewings P, Fox R. Probability of early pregnancy loss in women with vaginal bleeding and a singleton live fetus at ultrasound scan. J Obstet Gynaecol. 2006;26(8):782-4.
58. Practice Committee of the American Society for Reproductive Medicine. Definitions of inf and recurrent pregnancy loss: a committee opinion.Fertil Steril. 2020;113 (3):533-5.
59. Refary EL, Calder T, Wheatley DN, Templeton A. Cervical priming with prostaglandin analogues. Lancet. 1994;343:1207-9.
60. Royal College of Obstetricians and Gynaecologists. The Investigation and Treatment of Couples with Recurrent First Trimester and Second-Trimester Miscarriage. Green-top Guideline No. 17. London: RCOG; 2011.
61. Royal College of Obstetricians and Gynaecologists. The Investigation and Treatment of Couples with Recurrent Miscarriage. Guideline No. 17. London: RCOG; 2003.
62. Royal College of Obstetricians and Gynaecologists. The Management of Early Pregnancy Loss. Guideline No. 25. London: RCOG; 2006.
63. Royal College of Obstetricians and Gynaecologists. The Management of Gestational Trophoblastic Neoplasia. Guideline No. 38. London: RCOG; 2004.
64. Royal College of Obstetricians and Gynaecologists. The Management of Tubal Pregnancy. Guideline No. 21. London: RCOG; 2004.
65. Rumbold A, Middleton P, Crowther CA. Vitamin supplementation for preventing miscarriage. Cochrane Database Syst Rev. 2005;(2):CD004073.
66. Schauberger CW, Mathiason MA, Rooney BL. Ultrasound assessment of first-trimester bleeding. Obstet Gynecol. 2005;105(2):333-8.
67. Shirangi A, Fritschi L, Holman CD. Maternal occupational exposures and risk of spontaneous abortion in veterinary practice. Occup Environ Med. 2008;65(11):719-25.
68. Smith LF, Ewings PD, Quinlan C. Incidence of pregnancy after expectant, medical, or surgical management of spontaneous first trimester miscarriage: long term follow-up of miscarriage treatment (MIST) randomised controlled trial. BMJ. 2009;(339):b3827.
69. Sophie CM, Philippe B, Irving MS. Medical termination of pregnancy. N Engl J Med. 2000;342:946-55.
70. Stubblefield PG. Control of pain for women undergoing abortion. Int J Gynaecol Obstet Suppl. 1989;3:131.
71. Stubblefield PG. Surgical techniques of uterine evacuation in first- and second-trimester abortion. Clin Obstet Gynecol. 1986;13:53.
72. Suprato K, Reed S. Naproxen sodium for pain relief in first-trimester abortion. Am J Obstet Gynecol. 1984;150:1000-1.
73. Taylor HS, Pal L, Seli E. Recurrent early pregnancy loss. In: Speroff's clinical gynecologic endocrinology and infertility. 9th edition. Philadelphia: Wolters Kluwer; 2020:1174-204.
74. The Medical Termination of Pregnancy Act, 1971 (Act No 34 of 1971, 10th August 1971).
75. The Reproductive Health Access Project. First trimester bleeding algorithm. [online] Available from http://www.reproductiveaccess.org/mm/downloads/First_trimester_bleeding_algorithm.pdf [Last accessed March, 2025].
76. Tong S, Kaur A, Walker SP, Bryant V, Onwude JL, Permezel M. Miscarriage risk for asymptomatic women after a normal first-trimester prenatal visit. Obstet Gynecol. 2008;111(3):710-4.
77. Valle RF, Sabbagha RE. Management of first trimester pregnancy termination failures. Obstet Gynecol. 1980;55(5):625-9.

78. Wacholder S, Chen BE, Wilcox A, Macones G, Gonzalez P, Befano B, et al. Risk of miscarriage with bivalent vaccine against human papillomavirus (HPV) types 16 and 18: pooled analysis of two randomised controlled trials. BMJ. 2010;(340):c712.
79. Wahabi HA, Abed Althagafi NF, Elawad M. Progestogen for treating threatened miscarriage. Cochrane Database Syst Rev. 2007;(3):CD005943.
80. Wang X, Chen C, Wang L, Chen D, Guang W, French J. Conception, early pregnancy loss, and time to clinical pregnancy: a population-based prospective study. Fertil Steril. 2003;79(3):577-84.
81. Weeks A, Alia G, Blum J, Winikoff B, Ekwaru P, Durocher J. A randomized trial of misoprostol compared with manual vacuum aspiration for incomplete abortion. Obstet Gynecol. 2005;106(3):540-7.
82. Westfall JM, Sophocles A, Burggraf H, Ellis S. Manual vacuum aspiration for first-trimester abortion. Arch Fam Med. 1998;7(6):559-62.
83. Wieringa-de Waard M, Bonsel GJ, Ankum WM, Vos J, Bindels PJE. Threatened miscarriage in general practice: diagnostic value of history taking and physical examination. Br J Gen Pract. 2002;52(483):825-9.
84. Wieringa-De Waard M, Hartman EE, Ankum WM, Reitsma JB, Bindels PJE, Bonsel GJ. Expectant management versus surgical evacuation in first trimester miscarriage: health-related quality of life in randomized and non-randomized patients. Hum Reprod. 2002;17(6):1638-42.
85. Wilcox AJ, Wein CR, O'Connor JF, Baird DD, Schlatterer JP, Canfield RE,et al. Incidence of early loss of pregnancy. N Engl J Med. 1988;319:189-94.
86. Zhang J, Gilles JM, Barnhart K, Creinin MD, Westhoff C, Frederick MM. National Institute of Child Health Human Development (NICHD) Management of Early Pregnancy Failure Trial. A comparison of medical management with misoprostol and surgical management for early pregnancy failure. N Engl J Med. 2005;353(8): 761-9.

9

CHAPTER

Ectopic Pregnancy and Pregnancy of Unknown Location

Shripad Hebbar, Kavisha Bhat, Muralidhar V Pai

Chapter Outline

Ectopic Pregnancy
- Frequency of Ectopic Pregnancy
- Sites of Ectopic Pregnancy
- Aetiology of Ectopic Pregnancy
- Ectopic Pregnancy in Fallopian Tubes
- Management and Treatment Options of Ectopic Pregnancy
- Expectant Management
- Medical Management
- Surgical Management
- Complications of Ectopic Pregnancy
- Ovarian Pregnancy
- Cornual Pregnancy
- Cervical Pregnancy
- Caesarean Scar Pregnancy
- Abdominal Pregnancy
- Interstitial Pregnancy
- Intraligamentary Pregnancy

Pregnancy of Unknown Location
- Outcome of Ectopic Pregnancy
- Diagnosis
- Management of Pregnancy of Unknown Location

ECTOPIC PREGNANCY

INTRODUCTION

An ectopic pregnancy is one in which the fertilised ovum becomes implanted in a site other than the normal uterine cavity. Although extrauterine pregnancy is often used as a synonymous term, it is different in that it does not include certain rare types, such as pregnancy in the rudimentary horn of a bicornuate uterus. Ectopic pregnancy is the consequence of an abnormal implantation of the blastocyst.

FREQUENCY OF ECTOPIC PREGNANCY

Ectopic pregnancy is seen in about 2% of all pregnancies in the United States, with a 3–4% of worldwide incidence. In some studies, the incidence of ectopic pregnancies reported is as high as 20.7 per 1,000 pregnancies.

Ectopic pregnancy is the leading cause of first-trimester maternal mortality, accounting for 4% of maternal deaths even after advanced medical care being available. After one ectopic pregnancy, the risk of a subsequent ectopic pregnancy increases by 7-13-fold. The chance that a subsequent pregnancy will be intrauterine is 50–80%, and that of tubal pregnancy will be 10–25%; the remaining patients will be infertile.

SITES OF ECTOPIC PREGNANCY

Any pregnancy occurring outside the uterine cavity is labelled as ectopic pregnancy. The possible sites can be classified according to the above downwards and according to frequency.

Above Downwards

- Abdominal cavity
- Ovary
- Fallopian tubes
- Broad ligament
- Rudimentary horn of the uterus
- Cervix

Frequency

- Fallopian tubes: 95–98%
- Uterine cornu: 2–2.5%
- Ovary, cervix and abdominal cavity: <1%
- Caesarean scar pregnancy (CSP) <1%
- Heterotopic pregnancy 1–3%

Ectopic pregnancy is more common on the right side. The possible risk factors of ectopic pregnancy are described in **Box 1**.

BOX 1: Risk factors.

- Pelvic inflammatory diseases (sixfold increased risk)
- Use of intrauterine contraceptive devices (IUCDs) (3–5% increased risks)
- Smoking (2.5% increased risk)
- Assisted reproductive technology (ART) pregnancies (3–5% increased risk)
- Tubal damage (surgical occlusions or cilia damage)
- Tubal surgery (5.8% increased risk)
- Salpingitis isthmica nodosa (3.5% increased risk)
- Prior ectopic pregnancy (10-fold increased risk)
- The age risk of ectopic pregnancy is threefold greater in women of 35–44 years compared to 18–24 years
- Non-white race (1.5-fold increased risk)
- Endometriosis (1.5-fold increased risk)
- Developmental errors
- Overdevelopment of the ovum and external migration

AETIOLOGY OF ECTOPIC PREGNANCY

The cause of ectopic pregnancy is tubal damage or altered motility that results in the blastocyst being improperly transported and abnormally implanted. Tubal damage accounts for one-third of ectopic cases. The most common cause is acute salpingitis in almost 50% of cases. In almost 40% of cases, no risk factor is apparent.

Pelvic Inflammatory Disease

Infection of the tubes is seen as the most common cause preceding ectopic pregnancy, and histopathological evidence of salpingitis is identified in almost 50% of tubes harbouring ectopic pregnancy **(Box 1)**.

Salpingitis causes peritubal adhesions, partial tubal lumen occlusion, intratubal adhesions, diverticula and disturbed tubal functions. Salpingitis [pelvic inflammatory disease (PID)] may be due to *Chlamydia*, gonococcal infection, tuberculosis, postabortal, puerperal or secondary to pelvic peritonitis infection and the source could also be extragenital, such as appendicitis (20% cases may give history of previous surgery, usually appendicectomy). Since tubal disease is nearly always bilateral, there is a strong tendency for ectopic pregnancy to occur first on one side and then at a later date on the other. In a woman who has already had one tubal pregnancy, the risk of a second is 7–13 times greater than the overall risk. The aetiological influence of faulty tubes is also shown by the fact that ectopic pregnancy is often preceded by several years of infertility. The incidence of ectopic pregnancy in women previously investigated for infertility is two-and-a-half times the normal.

Use of Intrauterine Contraceptive Devices

Tubal pregnancy is more likely in women using intrauterine contraceptive devices (IUCDs). IUCDs prevent intrauterine pregnancy (IUP), hence the ratio of ectopic to IUPs appears to be higher. Women using IUCDs have a 53% chance of having an ectopic pregnancy. Ectopic pregnancy is more likely with progesterone IUCDs rather than copper IUCDs. Copper has a phagocytic and a toxic effect on sperm, oocytes and embryos. Progesterone devices may alter tubal motility and polarity and hence lead to abnormal implantation.

Smoking

Cigarette smokers who smoke >20 cigarettes/day may have a relative risk of 2.5 times compared to nonsmokers, while those who smoke 1–10 cigarettes have a relative risk of 1.3. Nicotine is thought to alter tubal motility, ciliary activity and blastocyst implantation.

Assisted Reproductive Techniques

There is a higher incidence of ectopic pregnancy after in vitro fertilisation (IVF). These may be the result of direct injection of embryos into the fallopian tube, retrograde propulsion by uterine contraction, and pre-existing tubal damage. The position of the catheter in the uterine cavity and the volume of transfer medium may also be risk factors. Cauterisation of the cornual ends of the tubes was practised earlier to decrease this risk. However, this does not eliminate the possibility of an interstitial pregnancy.

Surgical Obstruction (Tubal Damage)

The fertilised ovum sometimes implants on the stump of a tube after partial salpingectomy. Tubal pregnancy is also recorded after tubal ligation, and after hysterectomy with conservation of the tube, when the operation is performed within 48 hours of coitus. In such a case, the surgeon unwittingly imprisons the ovum. Tubal pregnancy is also more likely in cases of sterilisation failures, these being the most common within 2 years of sterilisation and more often with cauterisation procedures than with conventional minilaparotomy.

Abnormalities of the two agents which normally propel the ovum into the uterus represent developmental anomalies or the results of previous infection.

Tubal Surgery

Ectopic pregnancy is seen following surgery for blocked tubes and reversal of sterilisation. The risk depends on the method and site of ligation, residual tube length and adhesions, and is also higher following cauterisation procedures.

Salpingitis Isthmica Nodosa

This is a condition seen in chronic infections such as tuberculosis, and in this, the tubal epithelium extends into the myometrium and forms a true diverticulum where the blastocyst is likely to implant.

Prior Ectopic Pregnancy

Women who have had one ectopic pregnancy have a 10% risk of having an ectopic pregnancy again, even after a surgical removal of the tube has been done in the first instance. This risk is due to the fact that PID and salpingitis are bilateral diseases and the risk factor will be the same for the other side, even after ectopic pregnancy on one side.

Age: It has been observed that older age group women (35–44 years) are at a threefold increased risk of an ectopic pregnancy compared to younger women (18–24 years). This may be due to the fact that the older the age, the more the likelihood of a chromosomally abnormal blastocyst and the more the likelihood of this abnormal embryo implanting at an abnormal site.

Non-white race: Asians, blacks and other non-white races have a slightly higher risk of having an ectopic pregnancy.

Endometriosis: Endometriosis of the fallopian tubes leads to a patchy differentiation of endosalpinx into endometrium, and this may provide a site for implantation. Adhesions and faulty transport within the tube may also be a reason.

Developmental Errors of the Tube

Rarely, the fallopian tube may show developmental errors such as hypoplasia, undue tortuosity, undue length, diverticula, and accessory lumen. These may trap the travelling embryo and impede its progress, leading to a faulty implantation.

Overdevelopment of the Ovum—External Migration of the Ovum

An ovum discharged from one ovary can be fertilised in the peritoneal cavity and cross the pelvis by a process of external migration to enter the tube on the opposite side. Meanwhile, its early development has proceeded to such an extent that it may be too big to pass the isthmic portion of the tube or, more importantly, it has acquired its trophoblast, which encourages its implantation before it reaches the uterus. The phenomenon is not rare and is evidenced by the finding of the corpus luteum in the ovary on the side opposite to that of the tubal pregnancy. External migration is assumed in such cases but bearing in mind how rare is conception in the woman with only one tube and only one ovary, those being on opposite sides, Professor Jeffcoate often wonder that whether the migration is sometimes internal rather than external, that is, from one tube to the other across the uterine cavity. That this can occur is reliably reported.

ECTOPIC PREGNANCY IN FALLOPIAN TUBES

Sites

Excluding tubal 'stump pregnancy', the ovum implants in one of five main positions **(Figs. 1A to D)**.

1. *Fimbriated opening:* A primary implantation at this site is unusual (17%) **(Fig. 2)**
2. *Ampulla:* This is the most common and the least dangerous site (70%)**(Fig. 3)**
3. *Isthmus:* This is less common but is more dangerous because of the likelihood of tubal rupture (25%)
4. *Interstitial:* This is probably rare, although some cases may be missed because the pregnancy can be discharged through the uterus; it is said to be the site in 3% of all tubal pregnancies
5. Diverticulum of the fallopian tube **(Fig. 4)**.

Reactions of the Tube

The ovum burrows into the tube as it does into the uterus and, in doing so, induces a decidual reaction in the cells of the endosalpinx **(Figs. 5A and B)**. This reaction is patchy, feeble and relatively ineffective in controlling the invasion of the trophoblast into the tube wall and blood vessels. The muscle undergoes only limited hypertrophy, so, for one or both reasons, there is a high risk of choriodecidual haemorrhage and of erosion or rupture of the tube wall.

Reactions of the Uterus

The uterus itself is under the influence of the hormones of the corpus luteum and of the trophoblast, so it responds by generalised enlargement, increased vascularity, hypertrophy of all tissues and decidual reaction in the endometrium.

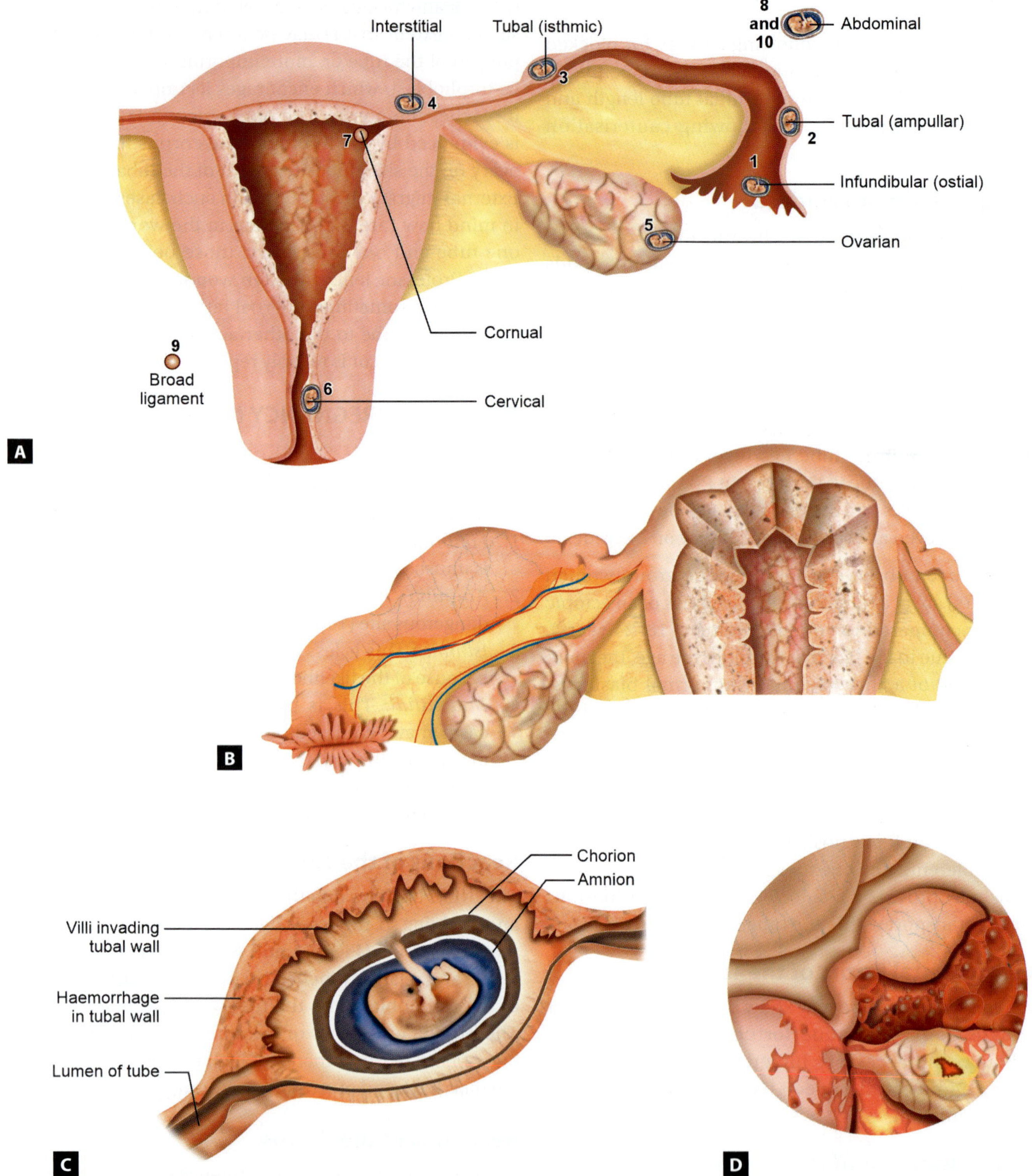

Figs. 1A to D: (A) The sites of ectopic pregnancy. (1) Fimbrial, (2) Ampullary, (3) Isthmic, (4) Interstitial, (5) Ovarian, (6) Cervical, (7) Cornual- rudimentary horn, (8) Secondary abdominal, (9) Broad ligament, (10) Primary abdominal—a disputed site, but see the text; (B) Unruptured tubal pregnancy; (C) Section through tubal pregnancy; (D) Culdoscopic view.

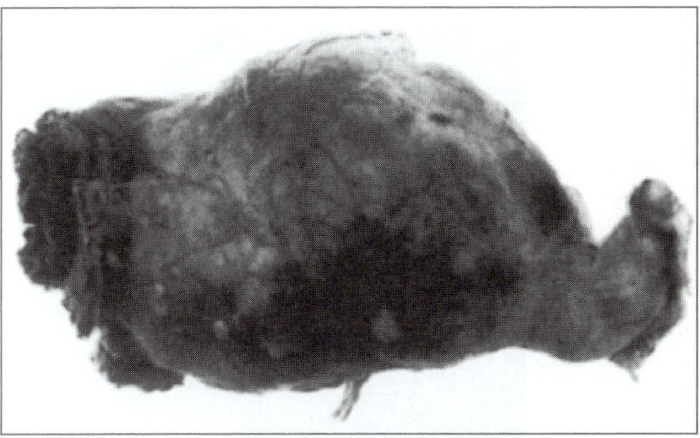

Fig. 2: An unruptured tubal pregnancy situated near the fimbriated extremity.

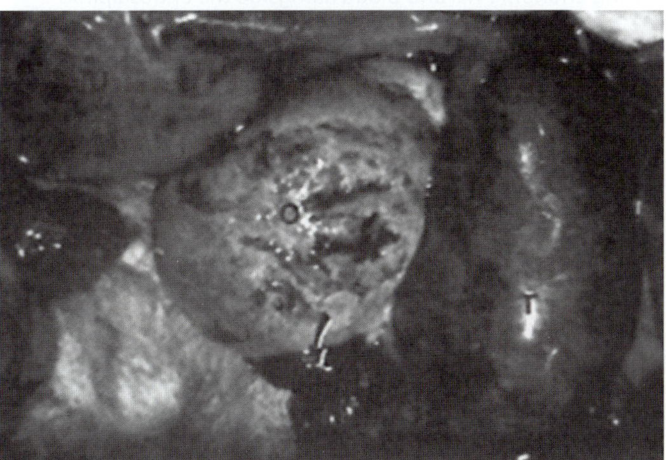

Fig. 3: Ampullary ectopic pregnancy.

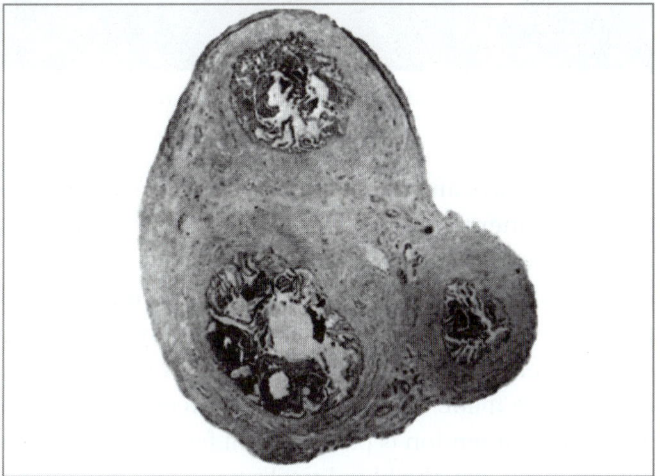

Fig. 4: An early ectopic pregnancy in a diverticulum of the fallopian tube. The cross-section of the tube shows the normal lumen at the top with accessory lumina below. Of the latter, the left one contains blood and chorionic villi. Both diverticula had blind ends, as was established by serial sections.

A special appearance of the endometrial glands (the Arias-Stella reaction) is seen in 10–15% of cases. This is characterised by a mixed pattern of atypical proliferative and secretory activity, the epithelial cells being enlarged and having hyperchromatic and gigantic bizarre-shaped nuclei, which are sometimes polypoidal. Their cytoplasm can be vacuolated and foamy. These histological features, which, except for the secretory activity, are rather suggestive of malignant change, represent an unusual response to steroid hormones and are not, as was once thought, peculiar to ectopic pregnancy. They can sometimes be found in association with normal early IUP, abortion, hydatidiform mole, choriocarcinoma, endometriosis and after prolonged intake of oestrogens and progestogens.

The decidua is maintained until some accident overtakes the pregnancy, when it separates and is discharged from the uterus, either as a whole cast or in fragments **(Figs. 6 and 7)**. Decidual separation is accompanied by slight continuous uterine bleeding, the mechanism, so far as the vascular apparatus is concerned, being the same as in menstruation. Prior to this, and while the pregnancy is alive, the patient is amenorrhoeic.

General Reactions

The woman responds to pregnancy in the usual way and may experience nausea, vomiting, changes in appetite, and pain and tenderness in the breasts.

Clinical Features

Tubal pregnancy presents as a chronic or acute illness, or as an acute-on-chronic illness. The first is much more common, but the acute picture is so dramatic that it tends to receive more attention.

Symptoms and Signs

- Normal symptoms and signs of pregnancy (amenorrhoea and uterine softening)
- Acute abdominal pain (dull, crampy or colicky pain)
- Evidence of haemodynamic instability (hypotension, collapse, signs and symptoms of shock)
- Adnexal mass (with or without tenderness)
- Vaginal bleeding
- Signs of peritoneal irritation
- Absence of gestational sac on ultrasound with a β-human chorionic gonadotrophin (β-hCG) of ≥2,500 mIU/mL
- Abdominal pregnancy

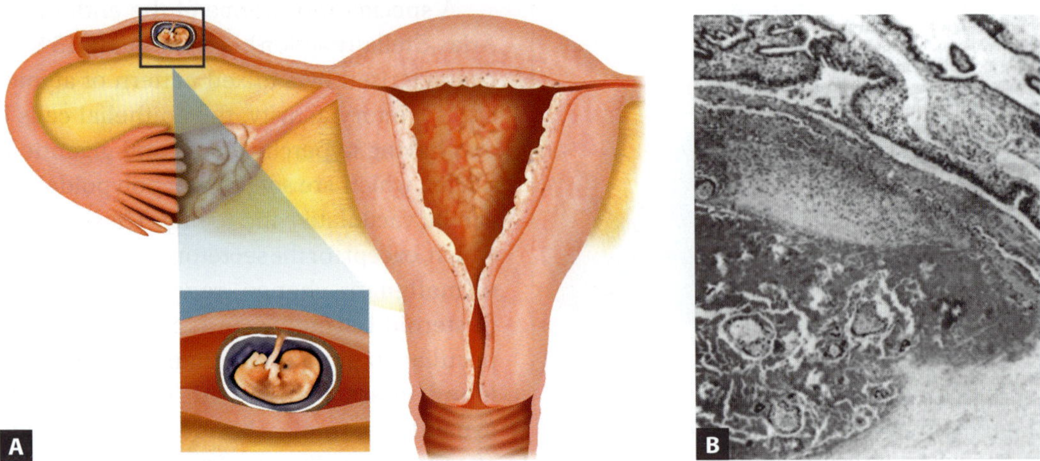

Figs. 5A and B: (A) Tubal pregnancy; (B) A photomicrograph showing chorionic villi and blood alongside the endosalpinx.

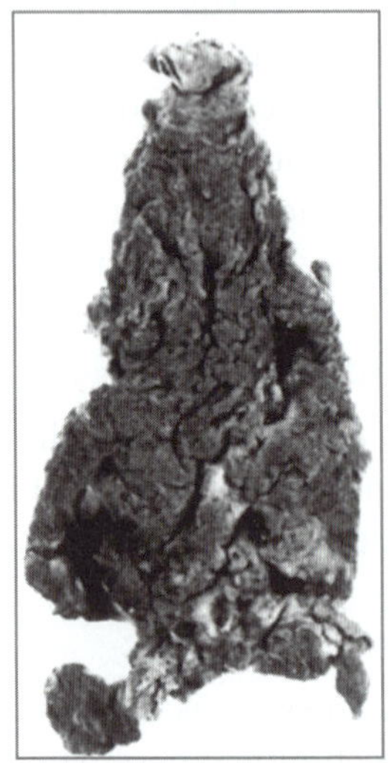

Fig. 6: Decidual cast from a case of ectopic pregnancy.

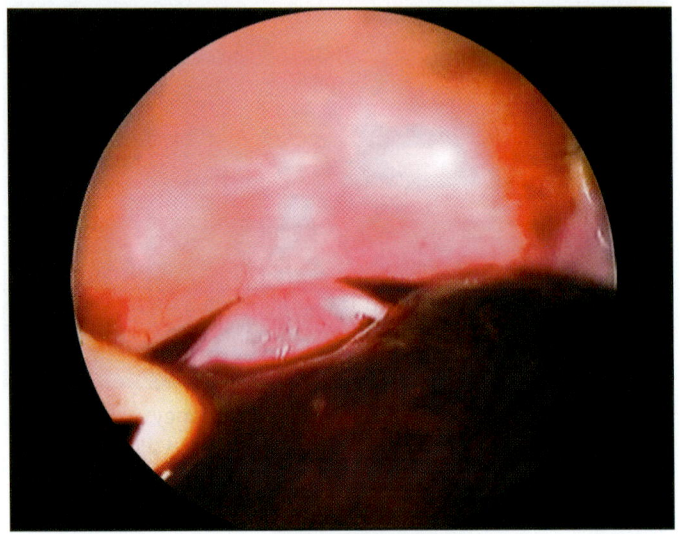

Fig. 7: Ruptured ectopic with haemoperitoneum.

Clinical Picture in Chronic Ectopic Pregnancy

This is seen when intraperitoneal bleeding from the tube is small in amount but recurrent, as in tubal abortion and tubal mole. The patient has a short period of amenorrhoea and sometimes notices other symptoms of early pregnancy, such as nausea and breast pain. When a menstrual period is overdue by a few days (i.e. when the pregnancy is only 2–3 weeks old), distension or contractions of the tube may cause aching in one or other iliac fossa. This is not so noticeable, however, as are attacks of sharp stabbing pain caused by choriodecidual haemorrhages or by the escape of blood into the peritoneal cavity. The severity of pain depends on the amount of blood lost, and there is nearly always an associated syncope. The latter varies from a momentary feeling of faintness to collapse and unconsciousness, but a combination of pain and syncope is the most constant and characteristic symptom of ectopic pregnancy. Many published analyses of symptoms put syncope relatively low on the list, but this is because the analyses are made retrospectively on incomplete records in which no attention is paid to slight faintness. When the patient lies down, the blood tracks to the diaphragm, and this is manifested by shoulder tip pain, or by epigastric pain, which is worse on inspiration.

Slight vaginal bleeding follows lower abdominal pain, and this is easily mistaken for the late onset of a menstrual period. It is uterine in origin and indicates separation of the decidua, although some authorities consider that, in part at least, it comes from the affected tube. Once this bleeding has begun, it tends to continue (if only as a brown discharge) without intermission; this is a diagnostic feature. A decidual cast may be recognised in the discharge **(Fig. 6)**. A large pelvic haematocele **(Fig. 7)** can cause acute retention of urine as a leading symptom. The collection of blood in the pouch of Douglas can also mean that the patient finds it difficult to sit on a hard chair without some ill-defined discomfort.

Examination may or may not reveal early pregnancy changes in the breasts. Tenderness and muscle guarding over the lower abdomen, especially on the affected side, is a striking feature. The amount of blood in the peritoneal cavity is unlikely to be sufficient to give rise to signs of free fluid, but some degree of intestinal distension is a common and important diagnostic sign. Haemoperitoneum of 2 or 3 weeks' standing can cause the appearance of bruising around the umbilicus (Cullen's sign). It is rarely seen nowadays in ectopic pregnancy, but Sir Norman Jeffcoate has found it to be the clue to the diagnosis of haemoperitoneum due to other lesions.

The possible findings on vaginal examination include arterial pulsation in the fornix on the affected side, an irregular and tender enlargement of the adnexum on the affected side, and an ill-defined tender semisolid swelling in the pouch of Douglas, indicative of pelvic haematoma. Tenderness in the pelvis is the most constant sign.

The patient looks pale, and the pulse rate is likely to be raised, especially after an attack of pain. It is also not uncommon to find slight intermittent pyrexia—the effect of absorption of products of degenerated blood. The bilirubin content of the blood is increased, and the patient may ultimately become jaundiced. In the ordinary case, there is a slight rise in the leucocyte count and in the erythrocyte sedimentation rate. A long-standing haemoperitoneum, however, can cause a high leucocyte count; this, in association with a low haemoglobin level, is a diagnostic point.

Acute Clinical Picture

This is seen when there is a sudden massive intraperitoneal haemorrhage **(Fig. 7)** and is typical of tubal rupture rather than tubal abortion. It may supervene on a previously chronic picture.

After a short period of amenorrhoea, and sometimes none, the patient is seized with a severe lancinating pain in one iliac fossa or in the hypogastrium. This is immediately followed by profound collapse marked by pallor, low blood pressure, subnormal temperature and a weak, rapid pulse. Death may ensue in a very short time. Usually, however, the haemorrhage is temporarily arrested and the general condition improves within a few hours. Pain persists, however, and is referred to the epigastrium or the shoulder.

Examination reveals obvious signs of shock and anaemia. The lower abdomen (and sometimes the upper as well) is usually acutely tender. The presence of free blood in the peritoneal cavity may be indicated by dullness in the flanks and intestinal distension in front. Vaginal examination should not ordinarily be carried out for fear of precipitating more bleeding but if it is (and it should be very gentle), some enlargement of one adnexum may be detected. This sign is not easy to elicit because of tenderness. Again, acute tenderness and the production of pain by movement of the cervix are the leading signs.

Classical Triad

A patient with amenorrhoea, pain and vaginal bleeding should always be suspected to have an ectopic pregnancy. The dictum to early diagnosis and successful management is to 'think ectopic' but also not to 'overthink ectopic'.

Outcome of Ectopic Pregnancy

The tube is capable of only limited distension and is also unable to provide secure placentation due to the unsatisfactory environment. 80% of these embryos are malformed, and >99% of these pregnancies do not progress beyond 6 weeks. The course of pregnancy is illustrated in **Flowchart 1** and **Figures 8A to D**. Usually, this condition will lead to a disaster in one of the following ways:

- *Tubal abortion:*
  - Complete absorption
  - Complete abortion
  - Incomplete abortion
  - Missed abortion (tubal mole)
- Tubal rupture
- Chronic ectopic adnexal mass
- Foetal survival to term

Tubal Abortion

This implies discharge of the gestational sac into the lumen of the tube. If the discharged sac reaches the fimbrial end, it may separate from its attachment to the tube and its trophoblastic shell. This could lead to complete

Flowchart 1: Course of ectopic pregnancy.

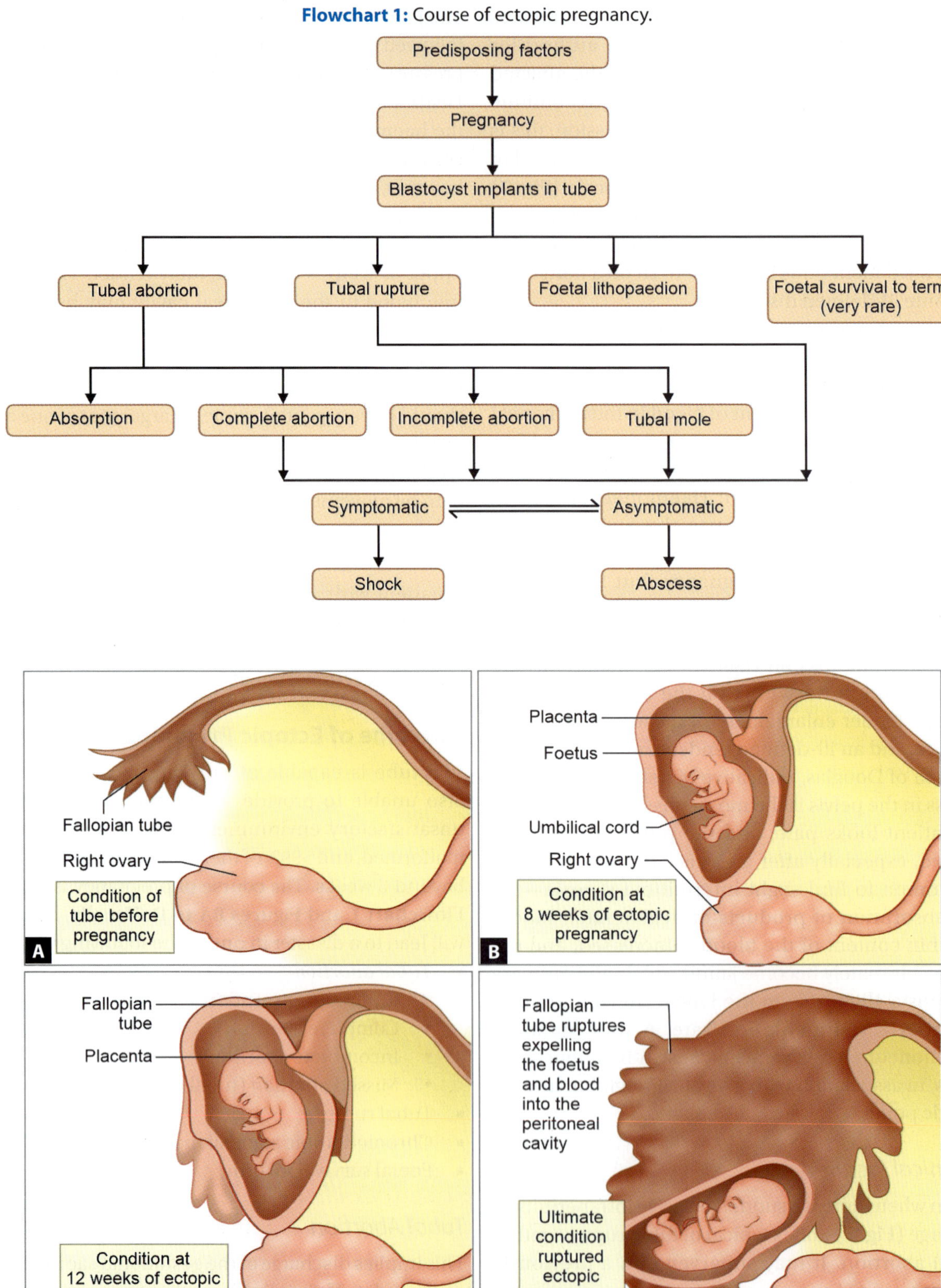

Figs. 8A to D: Course of ectopic pregnancy with the increasing gestational age.

absorption, complete abortion, incomplete abortion or missed abortion (tubal mole).

Complete absorption: It is difficult to prove as a very small embryo may abort in the peritoneal cavity and get absorbed without any signs and symptoms.

Complete abortion: The embryo is expelled out of the fimbrial end by tubal contractions into the peritoneal cavity. This may occur with only slight bleeding (asymptomatic or mild symptoms) and may later be absorbed. Complete abortion may also lead to continuous bleeding and haemoperitoneum and shock-like symptoms.

Incomplete abortion: Some of the products of conception one expelled out of the fimbrial end. Usually, bleeding continues, and the condition is symptomatic.

Missed abortion (tubal mole): The embryo dies due to a faulty environment and faulty implantation and is converted into a carneous mole. Usually, it will get partially absorbed and liquefied and give rise to a symptomless haematosalpinx, or the process may progress, leading to haematosalpinx, peritubal haematocele and even pelvic haematocele.

The haematocele, if asymptomatic and not treated, will form a pseudocapsule around the organised blood and lymph. Later, it will lead to adhesions to omentum, bowel uterus, pelvic peritoneum, and ultimately it will get infected and form pelvic abscess.

Tubal Rupture

The fallopian tube may rupture due to its thin lumen at the isthmus and ampulla. The lumen is incapable of distension due to the blastocyst burrowing and eroding the tubal wall. Rupture of tubes usually causes severe bleeding and complete or partial extrusion of chorionic villi, leading to a haemodynamic unstable patient presenting with shock-like features. The rupture is usually intraperitoneal, leading to pelvic and peritoneal haematocele. Rarely rupture may be extraperitoneal, if rupture is at the broad ligament attachment, such a condition will present as broad ligament haematoma or pelvic haematoma. Ultimately, the broad ligament haematoma will either rupture intraperitoneal or form an abscess.

Chronic Ectopic Adnexal Mass

Sometimes the products of conception are partially extruded through the fimbria or through a partial rupture. After a slight or mild-to-moderate bleeding, the haemorrhage may get arrested and result in an adnexal mass involving the tube, ovaries, and clots. This may present as chronic pelvic pain in many women.

Foetal Survival to Term

The foetus usually does not develop beyond 6 weeks in the fallopian tubes; however, in rare conditions, pregnancy may progress and foetal death occurs later with formation of calcified lithopaedion which may even be detected many years later as expulsion of foetal bones through rectum, bladder, and pouch of Douglas or in abdominal cavity.

Very rarely, pregnancies have been known and reported to have survived up to term in the abdominal cavity (secondary abdominal pregnancies). The chorionic villi and placenta have been reported to be implanted in the broad ligament, bowel, omentum, liver surface and even the diaphragm. Such pregnancies have a poor foetal outcome (80% do not survive) and also have a 20% chance of maternal mortality due to haemorrhage.

Differential Diagnosis

All women in the reproductive age group complaining of the classical triad or any one of the three symptoms should raise the suspicion of ectopic pregnancy, even though the patient is on effective contraception or has had a tubal occlusion operation.

The picture of ectopic pregnancy is extremely variable and can mimic any intra-abdominal disease.

It should be kept in mind here that:

- 85–90% of patients have abdominal pain
- 80–85% of patients have amenorrhoea
- 80–85% of patients have vaginal bleeding.

In ectopic pregnancy, the clinical diagnosis is more on symptoms rather than signs (negative physical signs should not be allowed to overrule symptoms). The following conditions are most likely to be confused with ectopic pregnancy. These may be pelvic diseases or nongynaecological nonobstetric diseases.

Obstetric Diseases

- Abortion of an early IUP
- Abortion followed by salpingitis
- Early pregnancy with pelvic tumours
- Retroverted gravid uterus (threatened abortion)
- Septic abortion

Gynaecological Diseases

- Degenerating fibroid
- Dysfunctional uterine bleeding
- Endometriosis
- Ovulation (Mittelschmerz)
- Ruptured corpus luteum
- Torsion of adnexal mass
- Acute or subacute salpingitis (including tuberculosis)
- Dysmenorrhoea

Nongynaecological Conditions

- Appendicitis
- Gastroenteritis
- Mesenteric thrombosis
- Perforated peptic ulcer
- Renal colic
- Intraperitoneal haemorrhage from any source (rupture of splenetic aneurysm or tumours).

Diagnosis

Mostly the diagnosis is based on the classical clinical triad of pelvic pain, vaginal spotting and amenorrhoea (5–9 weeks). Other classical symptoms are dizziness, pregnancy symptoms and vaginal passage of clot/tissue. The most common classical finding is adnexal tenderness and adnexal mass.

Ruptured ectopic may present as shock (tachycardia with hypotension). Shoulder pain due to diaphragmatic irritation is a late sign of haemoperitoneum.

Investigations

The following investigations must be done in the suspected cases of ectopic pregnancy:

Blood Group Typing (ABO and Rh Type)

Blood typing [ABO and Rhesus (Rh)] and antibody screening should be done in all pregnant patients with bleeding to identify Rh-negative pregnant patients in whom bleeding would be associated with an increased risk of Rh isoimmunisation. Such patients require to be injected with 50 μg (280 IU) of anti-D immunoglobulins (Rhogam) to prevent the occurrence of haemolytic disease of the newborn. Blood must be typed and cross-matched in order to ensure the availability of blood products in case of excessive blood loss.

Complete blood count (CBC) and estimation of haemoglobin and/or haematocrit must be done in these patients for evaluation of maternal anaemia. In cases of tubal rupture with severe intra-abdominal bleeding, measurement of platelet count and/or coagulation tests is also indicated. If administration of methotrexate (MTX) is considered in cases of unruptured ectopic gestation, a CBC must be done as part of the pretreatment laboratory evaluation.

Urine or Serum β-Human Chorionic Gonadotrophin Levels

In the emergency department, pregnancy is diagnosed by determining the levels of β-hCG in the urine or serum. This hormone may be detected in the urine and blood as early as 1 week before an expected menstrual period. While urine testing may detect levels up to 20–50 IU/L, serum testing may detect levels as low as 5 IU/L. In most cases of suspected ectopic pregnancy, screening is initially done with a urine pregnancy test. Determination of serum β-hCG levels is a time-consuming procedure and may not be a practical option at the time of emergency. However, if pregnancy is strongly suspected, even when the urine pregnancy test has a negative result, serum testing becomes necessary. The quantitative level of β-hCG found in ectopic pregnancy varies. In a normal pregnancy, the β-hCG levels double every 48–72 hours until they reach 10,000–20,000 mIU/mL. Normal IUPs are associated with a doubling time of 1.4–2.1 days. According to the American College of Obstetricians and Gynecologists (ACOG) recommendations (2008), an increase in serum hCG of <53% in 48 hours confirms an abnormal pregnancy. The increase in hCG concentration is at a much slower rate in most, but not all cases of ectopic and nonviable IUPs. A falling, slow-rising or plateauing hCG concentration is most consistent with a failed pregnancy (e.g. anembryonic pregnancy, tubal abortion, spontaneously resolving ectopic pregnancy, complete or incomplete abortion, etc.). A single serum measurement of the β–hCG concentration, however, cannot definitely identify the presence of an intrauterine gestational sac. Although women with an ectopic pregnancy tend to have lower β-hCG levels than those with an IUP, there is considerable overlap. Therefore, serial β-hCG measurement is often used for women with first-trimester bleeding or pain, or both. However, similar to a single measurement, serial measurement of β-hCG levels also cannot confirm the intrauterine location of the gestational sac. In a patient with a subnormal increase in β-hCG concentration, nonviability is assumed, and more invasive investigations must be used for differentiating between miscarriage and ectopic pregnancy. Though the falling β-hCG levels confirm nonviability, at the same time, they do not rule out ectopic pregnancy. The lack of an IUP when the β-hCG level is above the discriminatory zone represents an ectopic pregnancy or a recent abortion.

Discriminatory zone of β-hCG: The discriminatory zone of β-hCG is the level above which a normal IUP is reliably visualised in nearly 100% cases. Ectopic pregnancy is suspected if transvaginal ultrasonography (TVS) does not show an intrauterine gestational sac and the patient's β-hCG level is 1,000 mIU/mL (1,000 IU/L) or greater. A negative ultrasound examination at hCG levels below the discriminatory zone is suggestive of an early viable IUP or an ectopic pregnancy, or a nonviable IUP. Such cases where the location of the gestational sac (whether intrauterine or extrauterine) cannot be identified on ultrasound examination are termed 'pregnancy of unknown location (PUL)'.

The level of the discriminatory zone may vary depending upon the patient's clinical scenario. These levels are dependent upon the parameters such as quality of the ultrasound equipment, the experience of the sonographer, prior knowledge of the woman's risks, symptoms and the presence of physical factors such as uterine fibroids and multiple pregnancies. A discriminatory zone of 1,000 IU/L can be used for specialised units performing high-resolution vaginal ultrasound, having prior knowledge about the woman's symptoms and serum β-hCG levels. Units where a diagnostic TVS is offered without prior knowledge about the patient's clinical or biochemical parameters, a discriminatory zone of 1,500 IU/L or 2,000 IU/L is acceptable.

Serum hCG levels above the discriminatory zone: Visualisation of an intrauterine gestational sac at the serum hCG levels above the discriminatory zone almost always excludes the presence of an ectopic pregnancy. However, there may be some exceptions to this rule, such as heterotopic pregnancy or the pregnancy in a rudimentary uterine horn or cornual pregnancy. Diagnosis of an extrauterine pregnancy is almost certain if there is the absence of an intrauterine gestational sac and presence of a complex adnexal mass at hCG concentrations above the discriminatory zone. Presence of embryonic cardiac activity or a definite yolk sac in this adnexal mass is certain evidence of an ectopic gestation. In these cases, treatment of ectopic pregnancy should be started. The diagnosis is less certain if there is the absence of a complex adnexal mass or an intrauterine gestational sac on ultrasound examination with serum hCG levels >1,500 IU/L. Absence of intrauterine gestational sac in the presence of serum β-hCG levels above the discriminatory zone may sometimes be indicative of multiple gestations, since there is no proven discriminatory level for multiple gestations. Therefore, in these cases, TVS examination and serum β-hCG concentration must be repeated again after 2 days. If an IUP is still not observed on TVS, then the pregnancy is abnormal. In these cases, serial follow-up with serum β-hCG levels is required:

- If the serum hCG concentration is observed to be increasing or has plateaued, treatment for ectopic pregnancy can be instituted.
- If the serum hCG concentration is observed to be decreasing, this is most consistent with a failed pregnancy (e.g. miscarriage, blighted ovum, and tubal abortion).

The rate of fall is slower with an ectopic pregnancy than with a complete abortion. Weekly hCG concentrations should be monitored in these cases until the serum hCG levels become undetectable.

Serum hCG levels below the discriminatory zone: In case the serum β–hCG levels are below the discriminatory zone, evaluation of serum hCG levels must be repeated after 3 days in order to observe the trend. As previously mentioned, in normal viable intrauterine gestation, serum hCG concentration usually doubles every 1.4–2 days until 10 weeks of gestation when it peaks. After that, it either declines or plateaus. A normally rising hCG concentration should be evaluated with TVS examination when the serum hCG levels reach the discriminatory zone. At that time, an IUP or an ectopic pregnancy can be diagnosed. If the hCG concentration does not double over 72 hours, then the pregnancy is most likely abnormal (an ectopic gestation or IUP that is destined to abort). The clinician can be reasonably certain that a normal IUP is not present in these cases. A falling hCG concentration is also most consistent with a failed pregnancy.

Imaging Studies

Ultrasonography, especially TVS or endovaginal ultrasonography, should be the initial investigation of choice for symptomatic women in their first trimester.

TVS can be performed either in the outpatient clinic or the emergency department to diagnose IUP. TVS has been reported to have a sensitivity of 90%, specificity of 99.8%, with positive and negative predictive values of 93% and 99.8%, respectively. Not only is this highly accurate in identifying ectopic pregnancy, but it also helps in determining the health and viability of the patient's IUP.

Signs of an intrauterine pregnancy on TVS: The presence of a gestational sac with a sonolucent centre (>5 mm in diameter) is indicative of an IUP. The gestational sac is surrounded by a thick, concentric, echogenic ring located within the endometrium and contains a foetal pole, yolk sac, or both. A normal gestational sac, an ovoid collection of fluid adjacent to the endometrial stripe, can be visualised by means of the transvaginal probe at a gestational age of about 5 weeks. It can often be seen when it is 2 mm or 3 mm in diameter and should be consistently seen at 5 mm. Since a pseudogestational sac is often associated with an ectopic pregnancy, the presence of a sac alone cannot confirm IUP. The earliest embryonic landmark, the yolk sac, appears when the sac is 8 mm or more in diameter, usually during the 5th week of gestation. Cardiac activity can be observed with endovaginal scanning when the embryo reaches 4–5 mm in diameter, at a gestational age of 6–6.5 weeks.

Probably abnormal intrauterine pregnancy: The IUP visualised on TVS is probably abnormal if the gestational sac is >10 mm in diameter without a foetal pole or with a definite foetal pole but without cardiac activity. In these cases, the gestational sac frequently has an irregular or crenate border.

Definite ectopic pregnancy: Signs of a definite ectopic pregnancy on TVS examination are as follows:

- *Presence of an extrauterine echogenic ring*: A thick, bright echogenic, ring-like structure, which is located outside the uterus, having a gestational sac containing an obvious foetal pole, yolk sac or both. This usually appears as an intact, well-defined tubal ring (Doughnut's or Bagel's sign, **Fig. 9**). Though this finding confirms the diagnosis of ectopic pregnancy, it may not always be present.
- *An empty uterus or presence of a pseudogestational sac* ***(Figs. 10A and B):*** Pseudogestational sac is typically formed due to endometrial changes and fluid collection in the endometrial cavity occurring with implantation of extrauterine pregnancy.

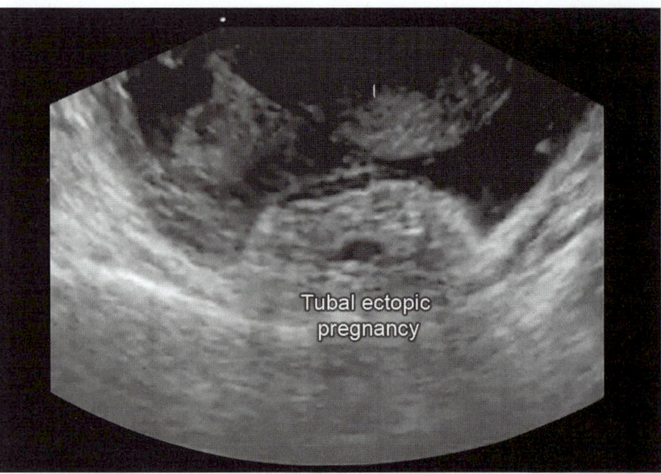

Fig. 9: Ultrasound examination showing the Bagel's sign, which can be defined as the thickened fallopian tube due to the presence of a gestational sac inside it.

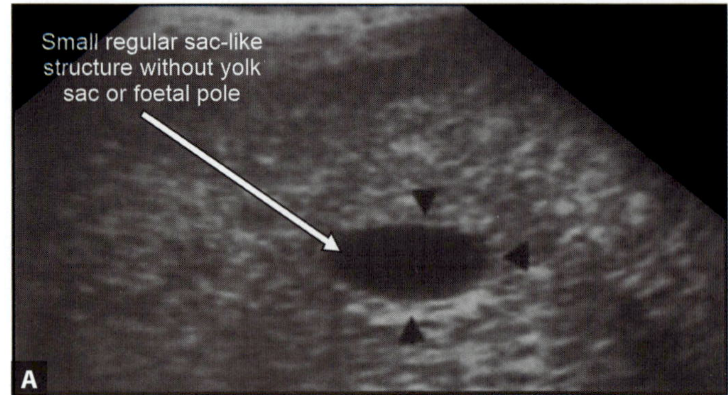

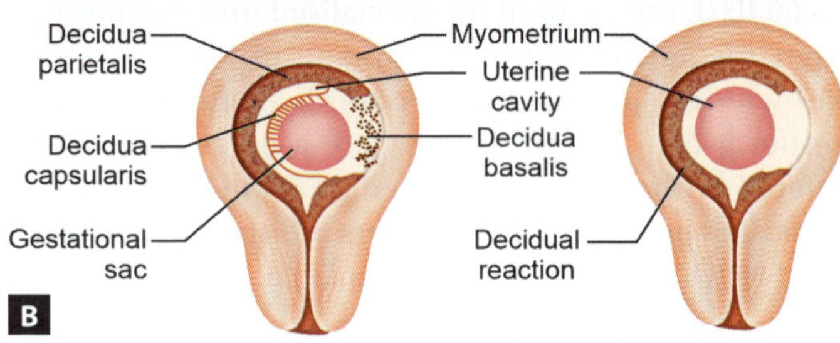

Figs. 10A and B: Uterine findings of pseudosac.

The gestational sac of a normal IUP is placed eccentrically, whereas a pseudogestational sac is centrally placed. An empty uterus on TVS images in patients with a serum β-hCG level greater than the discriminatory cut-off value is considered to be an ectopic pregnancy until proven otherwise. An empty uterus also may represent a recent abortion. However, in that case, serum β-hCG levels would not be greater than the discriminatory cut-off value.

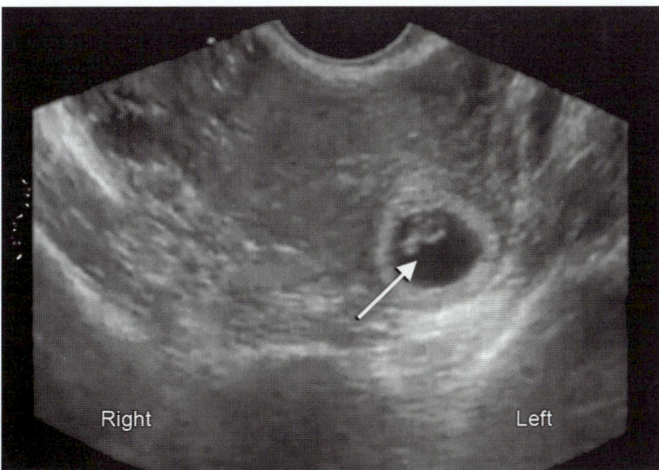

Fig. 11: Cornual ectopic pregnancy (indicated by arrow) shows the presence of a gestational sac in the left horn of the bicornuate uterus. A gestational sac with a sonolucent centre can be identified.

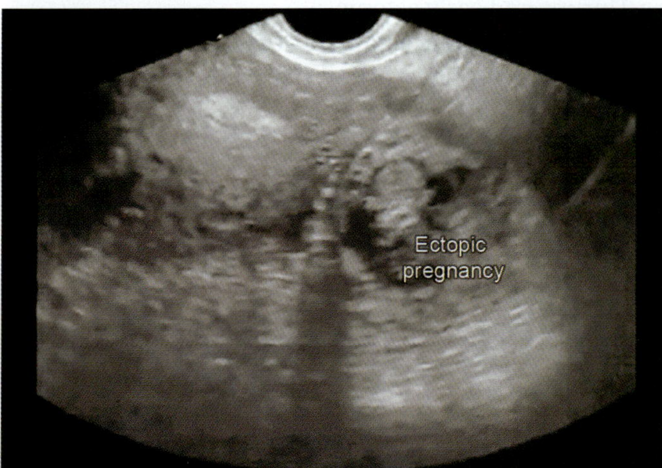

Fig. 12: Left-sided ectopic pregnancy.

- *Adnexal mass:* Cystic or solid adnexal or tubal masses (including the tubal-ring sign, representing a tubal gestational sac) **(Figs. 11 and 12)** and severe adnexal tenderness with probe palpation are also suggestive of ectopic pregnancy.
- *Haematosalpinx:* There may be haematosalpinx (presence of free fluid or blood in the fallopian tubes) and echogenic or sonolucent cul-de-sac fluid.
- *Ruptured ectopic pregnancy:* In case of a ruptured ectopic pregnancy, the ultrasonographic findings include the presence of free fluid or clotted blood in the cul-de-sac or in the intraperitoneal gutters (Morison's pouch).

TABLE 1: The criteria for transvaginal ultrasonography (TVS) diagnosis of ectopic pregnancy.

Stages	***TVS finding***
Type 1A	Well-defined tubal ring displaying foetal heart
Type 1B	Well-defined tubal ring displaying no foetal heart
Type 2	Ill-defined tubal mass
Type 3	Free pelvic fluid, empty uterus, displaying no adnexal mass

The criteria for TVS diagnosis of ectopic pregnancy, given by Rottem et al., are described in **Table 1**. If a low-risk patient's ultrasonography is negative for IUP, she is haemodynamically stable and has a β-hCG level <1,000 mIU/mL, the physician should take another β-hCG measurement after 48 hours. Patients with a nondiagnostic TVS result and a β-hCG level of 1,000 mIU/mL or greater are at an increased risk for ectopic pregnancy and may require a surgical consultation and must remain under vigilance. Serial measurement of β-hCG and progesterone concentrations may also be useful when the diagnosis remains unclear.

Other Tests

Serum Progesterone Levels

Serum progesterone levels have been used by some in the assessment of an ectopic pregnancy. While a value of 25 ng/mL is associated with normal pregnancies in 98% of cases, a value of <5 ng/mL identifies a nonviable pregnancy without regards of the location of pregnancy. Most women with an ectopic pregnancy would show serum progesterone levels somewhere in between these two values, limiting the clinical usefulness of progesterone in diagnosing an ectopic pregnancy. Measurement of the serum concentration of progesterone has been investigated as a potentially useful adjunct to serum β-hCG measurement, since progesterone levels are stable and independent of gestational age in the first trimester. Rapid progesterone analysis can identify two important subgroups of patients in the emergency department with symptomatic first-trimester bleeding or pain, or both: (1) stable patients with progesterone levels above 22 ng/mL, who have a high (but not certain) likelihood of viable IUP; and (2) patients with levels of 5 ng/mL or less, who almost certainly have a nonviable pregnancy. Invasive diagnostic testing (e.g. dilatation and curettage) could be offered to the latter, as treatment with

MTX could be offered to the latter group, without fear of interrupting a potentially viable IUP. Serum progesterone levels can detect pregnancy failure and identify patients at risk for ectopic pregnancy, but they are not diagnostic of ectopic pregnancy. Sensitivity for the diagnosis of ectopic pregnancy is very low (15%); therefore, 85% of patients with ectopic pregnancy will have normal serum progesterone levels. Therefore, serum progesterone levels are not routinely measured, because the results of this test merely confirm the provisional diagnosis, which had already been established by hCG measurements and TVS.

Colour Flow Doppler Examination

Blood flow in the arteries of the fallopian tube, which contains an ectopic pregnancy, is approximately 20–45% higher in comparison to the opposite tube. As a result, the Doppler waveforms in the tube containing an ectopic pregnancy show low impedance flow. Colour Doppler may also demonstrate a 'ring of fire' appearance due to an increased blood flow in the tubal mass **(Figs. 13A and B)**. However, investigations such as TVS and serum hCG measurements are usually sufficient for establishing the diagnosis in the usual clinical practice, and routine Doppler ultrasound examination is not normally required.

Magnetic Resonance Imaging

Though magnetic resonance imaging (MRI) can be used for diagnosing ectopic pregnancy, it is not usually used due to the high costs involved.

Diagnostic Procedures

Laparoscopic examination: Sometimes, in case of doubt, laparoscopic examination may be performed to diagnose an ectopic pregnancy. In case the diagnosis of ectopic pregnancy is confirmed on laparoscopic examination, definitive treatment (salpingectomy or salpingostomy) may be carried out.

MANAGEMENT AND TREATMENT OPTIONS OF ECTOPIC PREGNANCY

In all cases of suspected ectopic pregnancy, the patient should be admitted to the hospital. Shock must be treated before she is moved.

For treatment options, the management will depend on:

- Condition of patient (haemodynamic stability)
- Acute ruptured ectopic
- Chronic ectopic
- Unruptured early ectopic
- Unruptured dying ectopic
- Ectopic in places other than the fallopian tubes (cervical, abdominal, ovarian, interstitial, and uterine scar).

Surgical or medical management will depend on the aforementioned factors.

Emergency Management

In case of a collapsed patient with suspected ectopic pregnancy, the following needs to be done as described next.

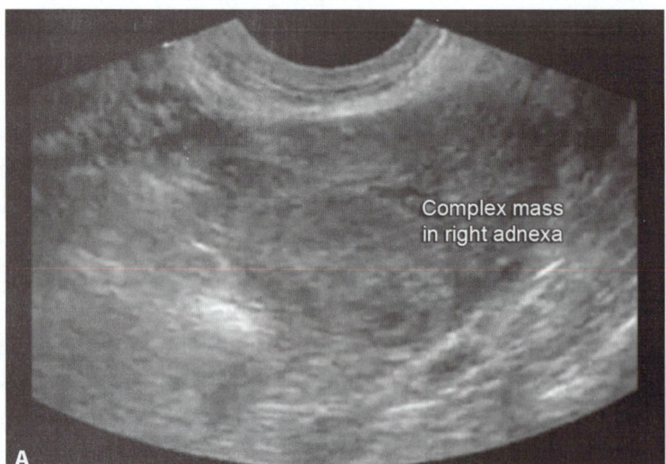

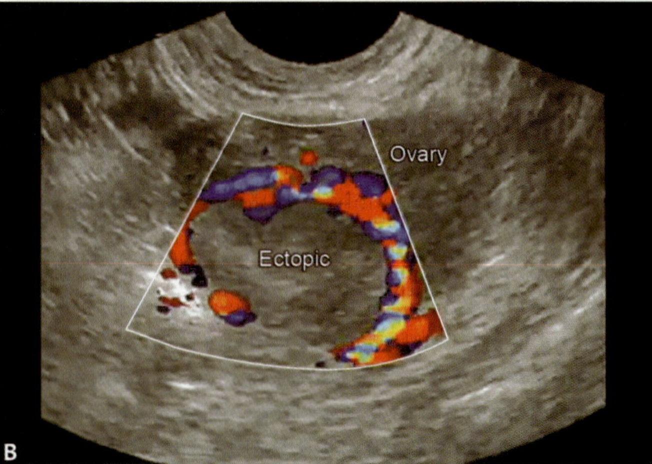

Figs. 13A and B: (A) Complex right echogenic adnexal mass in this figure represents haematosalpinx (presence of free fluid or blood in the fallopian tubes); (B) Doppler ultrasound in the same case showing a 'ring of fire' appearance due to increased vascularity of the surrounding fallopian tube.

Flowchart 2: Treatment plan for patients with ectopic pregnancy.

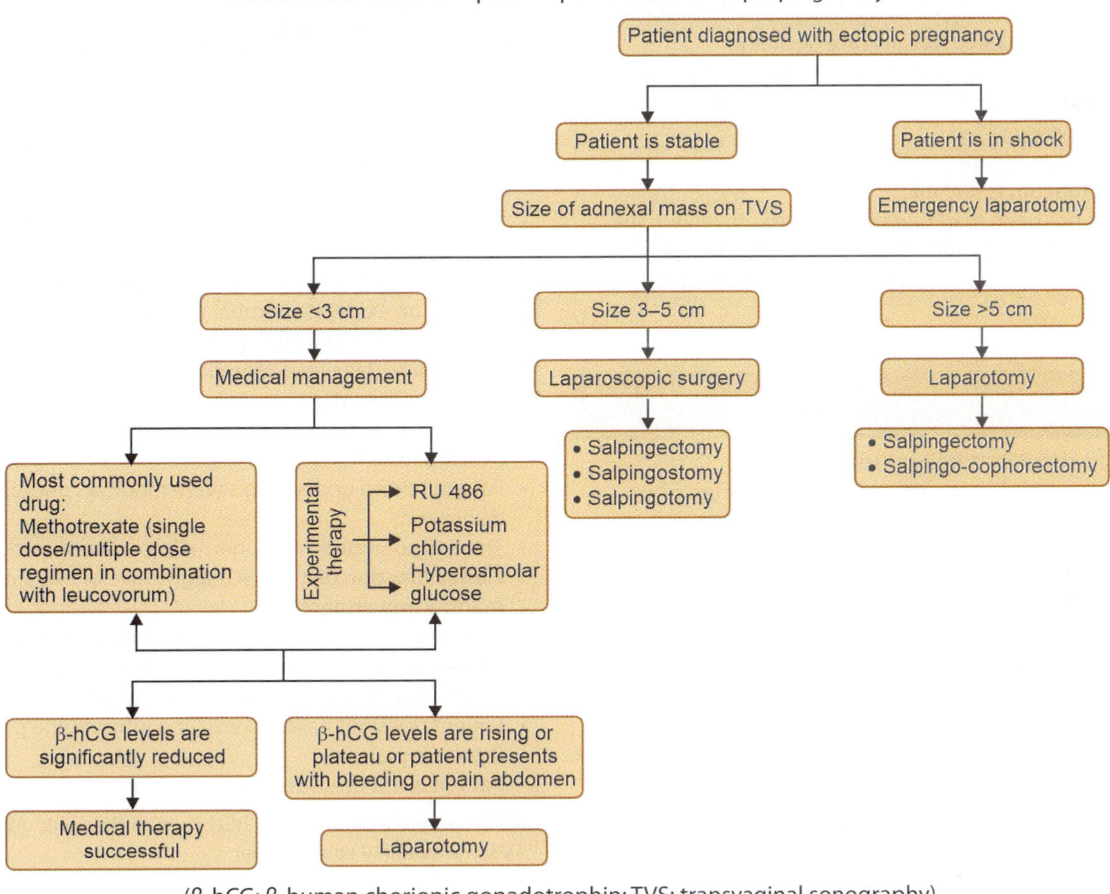

(β-hCG: β-human chorionic gonadotrophin; TVS: transvaginal sonography)

Hospital Admission

Whenever tubal pregnancy is diagnosed or suspected, the patient should be admitted to the hospital immediately, provided that she is not in a state of shock. Shock must be treated before she is moved.

Treatment of Shock

Lay the patient flat, keep her still and quiet, and give morphine or pethidine. With these simple measures alone, and so long as no vaginal examination is made to confirm the diagnosis and to cause more haemorrhage, the general condition usually improves. Transfusion with blood, plasma or substitutes should be arranged as soon as possible, if need be, in the patient's home.

Management Plan for Established Ectopic Pregnancy

Management plan of patients with suspected diagnosis of ectopic pregnancy and various treatment options for cases of ectopic pregnancy, including expectant management, medical management and surgical treatment, are described in **Flowchart 2**. The particular management option must be tailored according to the patient's clinical condition and her requirements for future fertility. Surgical treatment in the form of open surgery (laparotomy) or minimally invasive surgery (laparoscopy) is the most commonly used treatment option. The procedures which can be performed at the time of both laparotomy and laparoscopy include salpingectomy or salpingotomy.

EXPECTANT MANAGEMENT

Expectant management is an option for women with minimal symptoms who are clinically stable with a PUL or in cases of clinically stable asymptomatic women with an ultrasound diagnosis of ectopic pregnancy, showing declining serum hCG levels, initially <1,000 IU/L **(Box 2)**. Contraindications for expectant management of ectopic pregnancy are listed in **Box 3**. Women who are being managed expectantly should be followed twice weekly

BOX 2: Criteria for expectant management of ectopic pregnancy.

- Serum hCG levels ≤1,000 IU/L and are declining
- Ectopic pregnancy is suspected, but TVS fails to reveal any gestational sac or an extrauterine mass suspicious for an ectopic pregnancy
- Size of ectopic pregnancy is <3.5 cm
- Haemoperitoneum is <50 mL
- The patient has been made aware of the risks involved; she accepts the risks and is able to comply with follow-up
- The patient should be within easy access to the hospital in question

BOX 3: Contraindications for expectant management of ectopic pregnancy.

- Patient is haemodynamically unstable
- Presence of signs of impending or ongoing rupture of ectopic mass
- Serum hCG levels ≥1,000 IU/L, is increasing, or is not declining
- Noncompliant patient, who is unwilling or unable to follow up with monitoring
- The patient does not have timely access to a medical institution

(hCG: human chorionic gonadotrophin)

with serial hCG measurements to ensure that the hCG levels are rapidly decreasing. Ideally, the hCG levels must become <50% of their initial level within 7 days. These women must also be followed weekly by transvaginal examinations to ensure that there is a reduction in the size of the adnexal mass by 7 days. Measurement of weekly hCG levels and TVS examinations are advised thereafter until serum hCG levels become <20 IU/L. Recent studies have suggested that expectant management is as safe and efficacious as MTX treatment in selected patients.

MEDICAL MANAGEMENT

Medical therapy should be offered to suitable women who fulfil the criteria mentioned in **Box 4**. Contraindications for MTX therapy are listed in **Box 5**. The hospital units dispensing medical treatment should have appropriate protocols for treatment and follow-up. Presently, the most widely used medical treatment option is the administration of intramuscular MTX in the form of a single dose, calculated from the patient's body surface area (50 mg/m^2). For women with an average body mass index (BMI), this dose varies between 75 and 90 mg. Following the administration of this dose of MTX, serum hCG levels are checked on days 4 and 7. A further dose of MTX is given if hCG levels have failed to fall by more than 15% between days 4 and 7. **Box 5** describes the protocol for single-dose MTX. One of the most important advantages of outpatient medical therapy is that it is likely to result in considerable savings in the cost of treatment.

BOX 4: Prerequisites for starting medical treatment of ectopic pregnancy.

- Patient is haemodynamically stable and does not have pelvic pain
- Patient desires future fertility
- Patient appears to be reliable and compliant, and will return for post-treatment follow-up care
- Ectopic pregnancy <4 cm in diameter and no foetal heart activity on TVS, or <3.5 cm with presence of cardiac activity and absence of any free fluid in the pouch of Douglas
- There is no evidence of tubal rupture
- Serum hCG is <5,000 IU/L, with minimal symptoms
- Availability of facilities for follow-up care following the use of methotrexate (MTX)
- Patient agrees to use reliable contraception for 3–4 months post-treatment
- Patient has no underlying severe medical condition or disorder
- There is no underlying abnormality of liver function test, kidney function test or CBC, suggestive of liver, renal or bone marrow impairment
- Patient does not have any known contraindications to MTX
- Patient is not currently taking nonsteroidal anti-inflammatory drugs, diuretics, penicillin and tetracycline group of drugs
- Patient does not have a coexisting intrauterine pregnancy (heterotopic)
- Patient is not breastfeeding

(CBC: complete blood count; hCG: human chorionic gonadotrophin; TVS: transvaginal sonography)

SURGICAL MANAGEMENT

The option of surgical treatment must be considered if an adnexal mass suggestive of ectopic pregnancy can be observed on TVS examination or there are clear signs demonstrating the presence of an ectopic pregnancy on ultrasound examination. If no abnormality is observed on the ultrasound examination, there is a high probability that an ectopic pregnancy would not be visualised at the time of surgery. Surgical treatment in the form of open surgery (laparotomy) or minimally invasive surgery (laparoscopy) is the most commonly used treatment option. Some indications for surgical therapy are described in **Box 6**. The procedures, which can be performed at the time of both laparotomy and laparoscopy, include salpingectomy

BOX 5: Contraindications to methotrexate therapy.

- *Absolute contraindications:*
- Patient is haemodynamically unstable
- Presence of signs of impending ectopic mass rupture (i.e. severe or persistent abdominal pain or >300 mL of free peritoneal fluid outside the pelvic cavity)
- Pregnant and lactating mother
- Hepatic, renal, or haematological dysfunction, e.g. liver disease with a transaminase level two times greater than normal, renal disease with a creatinine level >1.5 mg/dL (133 µmol/L)
- Overt or laboratory evidence of immunodeficiency with a WBC count <1,500/mm^3 (1.5 × 10^9/L)
- Active pulmonary disease
- Peptic ulcer disease
- Alcoholism, alcoholic liver disease or other chronic liver disease
- Pre-existing blood dyscrasias, such as bone marrow hypoplasia, leucopaenia, thrombocytopenia [platelet count <100,000/ mm^3 (100 × 10^9/L)] or significant anaemia
- Known sensitivity to methotrexate
- Coexistent viable intrauterine pregnancy
- Patient is unwilling to be compliant with post-therapeutic monitoring, or there is a lack of timely access to a medical institution
- Relative contraindications:
- Large ectopic size (≥3.5 cm)
- Presence of embryonic cardiac activity
- High hCG concentration (>5,000 mIU/mL)
- Presence of foetal cardiac activity
- Presence of fluid in the peritoneal cavity
- *Other relative contraindications requiring further research:* Sonographic evidence of a yolk sac; isthmic location of ectopic mass rather than ampullary; high pretreatment levels of folic acid, etc.

(hCG: human chorionic gonadotrophin; WBC: white blood cell)

BOX 6: Indications for surgical therapy.

- Candidate not suitable for medical therapy (not willing to comply with post-treatment medical therapy follow-up or contraindications to the use of methotrexate)
- Failed medical therapy
- Heterotopic pregnancy with a viable intrauterine pregnancy
- Patient is haemodynamically unstable and requires immediate treatment
- Impending or ongoing rupture of the ectopic mass
- Absence of timely access to a medical institution for managing tubal rupture
- Patient desires a permanent method of contraception

(tube removal) or the tube-conserving procedures (salpingotomy or salpingostomy). Salpingotomy is the procedure involving surgical incision of the fallopian tube, so that the contents of ectopic pregnancy can be removed or flushed out, following which the incision is closed. Salpingostomy is a similar tube-conserving procedure where a surgical incision is made over the fallopian tube to remove the ectopic pregnancy. However, unlike salpingotomy, where the incision is closed, in salpingostomy, the incision is not closed and is left to heal itself by secondary intent. Salpingectomy, on the other hand, is the surgical excision of the fallopian tube. In case of ruptured ectopic pregnancy, salpingectomy is invariably performed. No benefit has been shown to closing the incision through suturing (a salpingotomy) beyond that which is needed to obtain haemostasis. Salpingotomy is an obsolete procedure now, no longer practised.

Management of tubal pregnancy in the presence of haemodynamic instability should be by the most expedient and rapid method. In most cases, this will be laparotomy. While in a haemodynamically stable patient, a laparoscopic approach is usually preferred over laparotomy, in cases of haemodynamic instability, laparotomy is the most preferred option.

Failure to conceive again after a tubal pregnancy is sometimes voluntary but is also to some extent explained by the abnormality of the other tube. Professor Jeffcoate postulated that unilateral salpingectomy reduces the chances of pregnancy by approximately one-half. When an ovum is produced by the ovary on the side from which the tube has been removed, and this is likely on average during half the cycles, it can be fertilised and implanted only if it undergoes external migration. This phenomenon, if it ever occurs, would add to the risk of an ectopic pregnancy on the other side. If unilateral salpingo-oophorectomy is carried out, the chances of subsequent pregnancy are doubled, because ovulation must then always take place from the ovary, which still has its oviduct. It follows that in a woman who is particularly anxious about future fertility, it may be better to sacrifice than to save the ovary on the affected side **(Figs. 14A and B)**.

Salpingostomy versus Salpingectomy

The choice between salpingostomy and salpingectomy for the treatment of ectopic pregnancy presently remains controversial. Both procedures are associated with similar rates of operative morbidity. The main disadvantage of salpingostomy is the potential risk of persistent trophoblast and/or recurrent ectopic pregnancy. Salpingostomy is, therefore, performed in those women

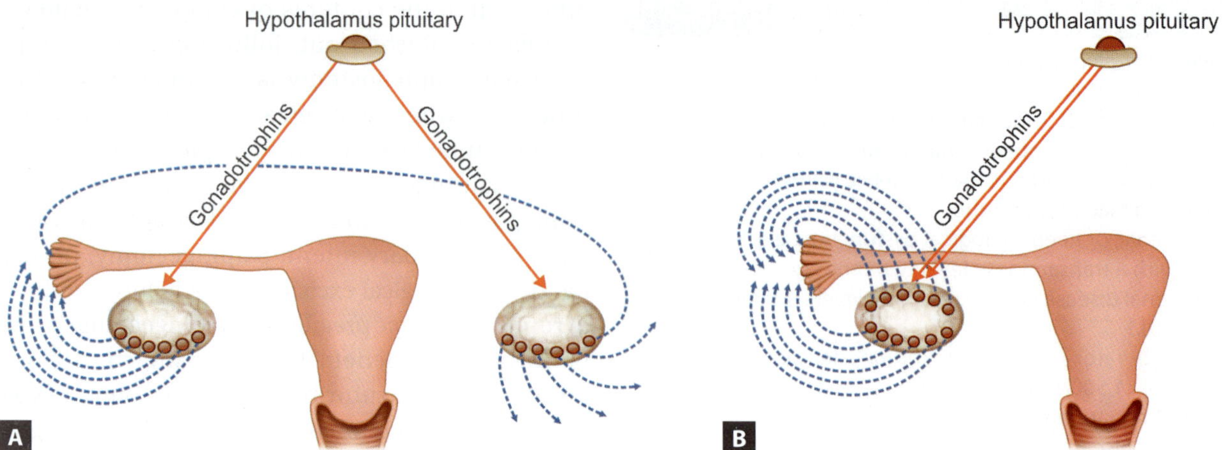

Figs. 14A and B: Jeffcoate's theory of the different effects of salpingectomy and salpingo-oophorectomy on subsequent fertility (see text). (A) After salpingectomy, approximately half the ova shed are from the ovary without an oviduct and, unless they migrate across the pelvis, are lost; (B) After salpingo-oophorectomy, all the ova are produced by the remaining ovary and are available for fertilisation and passage down the tube into the uterus.

BOX 7: Indications for performing salpingectomy instead of salpingostomy.

- Uncontrolled bleeding from the implantation site/ruptured ectopic
- Recurrent ectopic pregnancy in the same tube
- Severely damaged tube
- Large tubal pregnancy (i.e. >5 cm)
- Women who have completed their childbearing
- Women who may be treated with IVF in future
- Sterilisation failure resulting in ectopic pregnancy

who are haemodynamically stable and with a reasonable probability of future normal tubal function in the affected tube. If the woman does not conceive in the first 12–18 months following surgical therapy for ectopic pregnancy or her contralateral tube is damaged or absent, the clinician must resort to the option of IVF. Salpingectomy, instead of salpingostomy, is performed in the situations listed in **Box 7**.

According to two recent randomised trials, ESEP (European Surgery in Ectopic Pregnancy) study and DEMETER (Greek goddess of fertility) study, presently, there is no clear evidence regarding the use of salpingotomy in preference to salpingectomy in patients with a healthy contralateral tube. There are four cohort studies suggesting that salpingotomy may be associated with a higher rate of subsequent IUP. However, the magnitude of this benefit is likely to be small. The use of conservative surgical techniques is likely to expose the women to a small risk of tubal bleeding in the immediate postoperative period. There may be a potential requirement for further treatment of persistent trophoblast tissue. Therefore, if the option of salpingotomy is being considered, the surgeon must discuss both these risks and the possibility of further ectopic pregnancies in the conserved tube with the patient before undertaking such surgery.

Laparoscopic salpingostomy should be considered as the major treatment option for patient with ectopic pregnancy who desires future fertility, in the presence of contralateral tubal disease. It is likely to be associated with a higher rate of subsequent IUP in comparison with laparoscopic salpingectomy in women with contralateral tubal disease **(Figs. 15A to F)**. Due to a higher risk of persistent ectopic pregnancy, a follow-up of hCG levels is mandatory after a salpingostomy. Incidence of persistent EP after conservative tube-preserving surgery ranges from 5% to 29%.

Moreover, in women with a damaged or absent contralateral tube, the procedure of IVF is likely to be required for future pregnancy if salpingectomy is performed. Due to the requirement for postoperative follow-up and the treatment of persistent trophoblast, the short-term costs of salpingotomy are greater than those of salpingectomy. However, in the long term, due to the requirement of assisted conception for future pregnancies with salpingectomy, salpingostomy may be considered as a more cost-effective option in comparison to salpingectomy. Therefore, in the presence of contralateral tubal disease, the use of salpingotomy appears to be more appropriate.

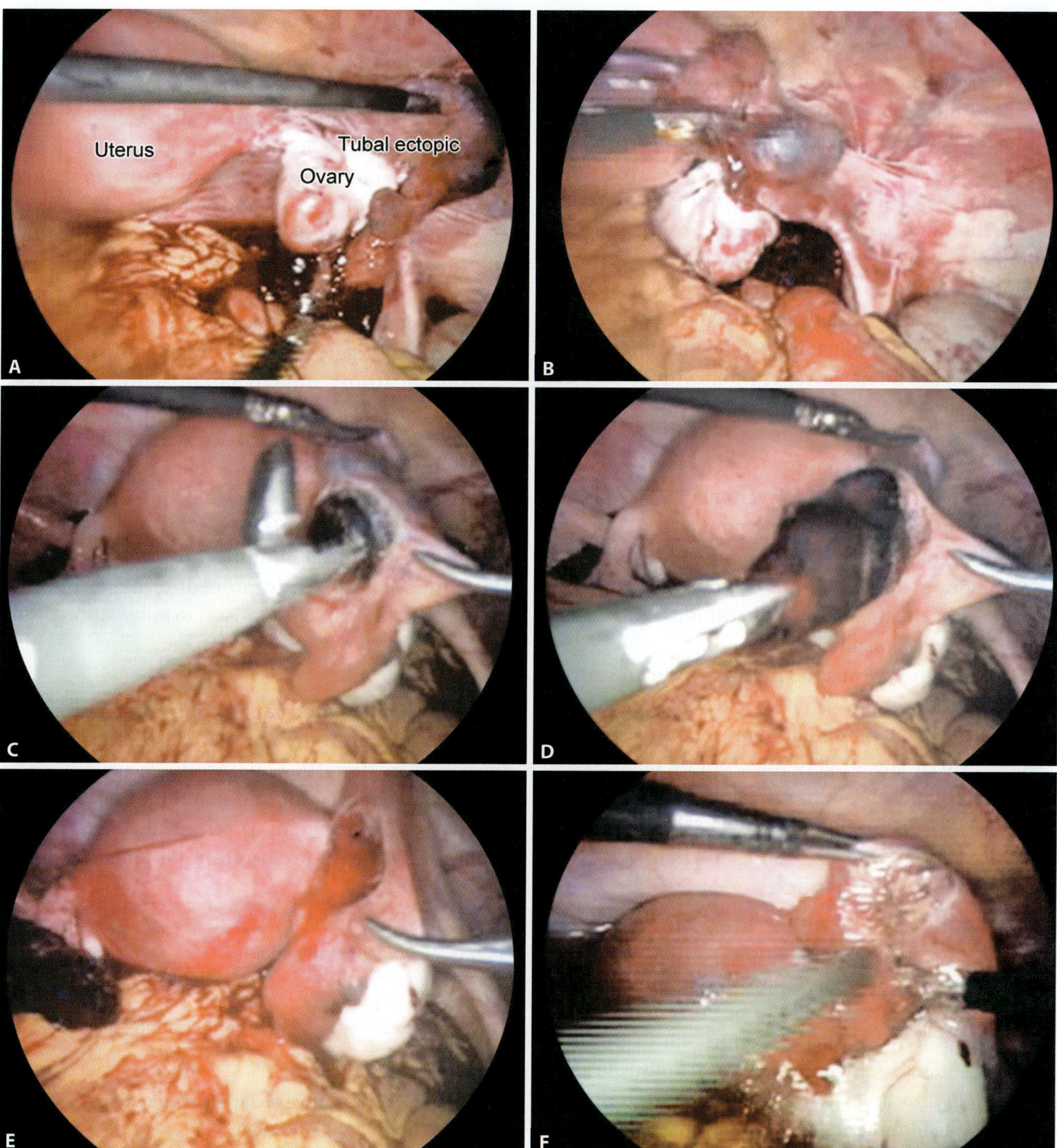

Figs. 15A to F: Laparoscopic salpingotomy: (A) Laparoscopic view showing the uterus, adnexa and the tubal ectopic pregnancy; (B) Grasping the tube containing ectopic pregnancy, before giving the incision; (C) A small 1 cm incision is given over the tubal ectopic; (D) Tubal contents being removed out of the tube; (E) The entire salpingotomy incision is left unstitched, only the bleeding vessels on the incision site are coagulated; (F) Irrigation of the area of incision with normal saline before closing the abdomen.

Surgical treatment is associated with reduced requirement of time for resolution of the ectopic pregnancy and avoidance of the requirement for prolonged monitoring. Some prerequisites which must be taken into consideration before deciding surgical treatment include the following:

- Treatment needs to be explained to the woman and her partner, and written informed consent must be obtained.
- Patient's blood sample needs to be typed and cross-matched (ABO and Rh) and blood needs to be arranged. Anti-D immunoglobulins need to be administered to women who are Rh negative. The following steps need to be taken for women who are haemodynamically unstable:
  - Immediate resuscitation
  - Securing immediate intravenous (IV) access by inserting large-bore venous cannula
  - Sending blood for CBC and cross-matching and arranging at least four units of blood
  - Informing the theatre staff, anaesthetist and on-call gynaecology consultant
  - Foley's catheter must be inserted prior to starting the procedure.
  - The urgency of the situation must be stressed to all concerned. The surgery must not be delayed and should be performed even before blood and fluid losses have been completely replaced.

Types of Surgical Approach

Surgical therapy may be either in the form of open laparotomy or via the laparoscopic route. Nowadays, the trend is towards using a laparoscopic approach for surgery. Numerous factors need to be considered before deciding on the type of surgical approach to be used. Some of these factors include history of multiple prior surgeries, pelvic adhesions, skill of the surgeon and surgical staff, availability of the equipment, condition of the patient and size and location of ectopic pregnancy. As previously described, a laparoscopic approach to the surgical management of tubal pregnancy must be used in haemodynamically stable patients. On the other hand, management of tubal pregnancy in the presence of haemodynamic instability should be by laparotomy. There is no role for medical management in the treatment of tubal pregnancy or suspected tubal pregnancy when a patient is showing signs of hypovolaemic shock.

Laparoscopic Surgery

A laparoscopic approach to the surgical management of tubal pregnancy, in the haemodynamically stable patient is preferable to an open approach. Laparoscopic management is associated with considerably reduced postoperative morbidity, shorter operative times, reduced intraoperative blood loss, shorter duration of hospital stay, lower analgesic requirements, lower complication rate and time duration of return to normal activity level. Most cases of ruptured as well as unruptured tubal pregnancy can be treated laparoscopically. The main advantages of laparoscopic surgery are enumerated in **Box 8**.

Complications due to laparoscopic management of ectopic pregnancy: In experienced hands, there is no specific complication directly related to the laparoscopic procedure, but if the surgeon is not trained enough in laparoscopy, then there is the chance of complications as described in **Box 9**. However, in experienced hands, the chances of these complications are extremely rare. Altogether, laparoscopic procedure has a much lower complication rate in comparison to conventional surgery.

Laparotomy

There are times when laparotomy is favoured over the laparoscopic approach. Some of these indications are described in **Box 10**. Laparotomy is usually preferred in cases of haemodynamic instability or when ectopic pregnancy is cervical, interstitial, abdominal, etc. Laparotomy is also preferred in patients having a large

BOX 8: Advantages of laparoscopic surgery.

- Reduced postoperative pain
- Faster recovery
- Short hospital stay
- Lower rate of postoperative complications such as wound infection
- Cost-effectiveness
- Reduced postoperative analgesic requirement
- Reduced adhesion formation

BOX 9: Complications due to laparoscopic surgery.

- Missed diagnosis
- Bleeding
- Incomplete removal of ectopic pregnancy
- Visceral injury
- Leakage of purulent exudates
- Intra-abdominal abscess
- Hernia

BOX 10: Indications for laparotomy.

- Patient is haemodynamically unstable
- Cervical, interstitial or abdominal ectopic pregnancy
- Patients having a large haematoma due to a large ruptured ectopic pregnancy
- Presence of more than 1,500 cc haemoperitoneum
- Patients with underlying cardiac diseases and chronic obstructive pulmonary disease
- History of abdominal surgery in the past
- Patients at increased risk of complications with general anaesthesia

haematoma due to a large ruptured ectopic pregnancy or in case of the presence of >1,500 cc haemoperitoneum. Patients with cardiac diseases and chronic obstructive pulmonary disease may not be good candidates for laparoscopic management. Laparoscopic management of ectopic pregnancy may also be more difficult in patients who have had previous lower abdominal surgery or those who may also be at an increased risk for complications with general anaesthesia combined with pneumoperitoneum, e.g. the elderly patients.

Surgical Procedures at the Time of Laparotomy

Salpingectomy: The surgical procedure performed during laparotomy is usually salpingectomy. Salpingectomy involves the removal of the ectopic pregnancy along with the fallopian tube of the affected side. Milking of pregnancy through abdominal ostium (transfimbrial extraction) had been advocated in the past if the haemorrhage was easy to control and pregnancy was fimbrial. However, the risk of recurrent ectopic pregnancy in these cases is twice as high. Therefore, this procedure is no longer recommended. Regardless of the route of approach (whether laparotomy or laparoscopy), salpingectomy is indicated in the situations enumerated in **Box 11**. The clinician has the option of choosing between partial and total salpingectomy. The choice for partial versus total salpingectomy is based on the patient's age and her desire to conceive in future. Partial salpingectomy is usually done in cases where the patient might opt for tubal anastomosis at a future date. Total salpingectomy is usually performed in those cases where IVF appears to be the likely treatment option.

Procedure of salpingectomy: The procedure of salpingectomy involves the following steps:

- The tube between the uterus and the ectopic pregnancy is clamped using a clamp. The pedicle is then cut and ligated.

BOX 11: Indications for salpingectomy.

- The tube is severely damaged
- There is uncontrolled bleeding
- There is a recurrent ectopic pregnancy in the same tube
- There is a large tubal pregnancy of size >5 cm
- The ectopic pregnancy has ruptured
- The woman has completed her family, and future fertility is not desired
- Ectopic pregnancy has resulted due to sterilisation failure
- Ectopic pregnancy has occurred in a previously reconstructed tube
- Patient requests sterilisation
- Haemorrhage continues to occur even after salpingotomy
- Cases of chronic tubal pregnancy

- The tubo-ovarian artery is also clamped, cut and ligated, while preserving the utero-ovarian artery and ligament.
- The mesosalpinx must be continued to be clamped, cut and ligated until the tube is free and can be removed.
- Following the excision and removal of the tube, the pedicles are ligated using a 2-0 or 3-0 synthetic absorbable suture.

Partial salpingectomy: It may be sometimes performed instead of complete salpingectomy if the pregnancy is in the midportion of the tube, none of the indications for salpingectomy are present, and the patient appears to be a candidate for tubal reanastomosis in future. In these cases, a clamp is placed through an avascular area in the mesosalpinx under the ectopic pregnancy. This creates spaces through which two free ties are placed, which are tied around the tube on each side of the ectopic pregnancy. The isolated portion of the tube containing the ectopic pregnancy is then cut and removed.

Follow-up: All patients who have not had the entire ectopic pregnancy removed by salpingectomy need to have their weekly hCG levels observed until these levels return to nonpregnant values. If, during this time span, the hCG level either plateaus or rises, the patient must be treated with MTX. Patients should be advised to use some form of effective contraception until their hCG levels have returned to nonpregnant levels.

Salpingotomy: Tube-sparing salpingostomy or salpingotomy is a procedure in which the gestational sac is removed, without the removal of the tube, through a 1-cm long incision on the tubal wall. This surgery is preferred over salpingectomy, because not only is salpingotomy less invasive, but also associated with comparable rates of subsequent fertility and ectopic pregnancy. Laparoscopic salpingotomy should especially be considered as the primary modality of treatment if the woman has contralateral tube disease and desires future fertility. When salpingotomy is used for the management of tubal pregnancy, follow-up protocols (weekly serum β-hCG levels) are necessary for the identification and treatment of women with persistent trophoblastic disease. Persistent trophoblast is detected by the failure of serum hCG levels to fall as expected after initial treatment.

Procedure: After infiltrating the mesosalpinx with vasopressin (20 IU in 50 mL normal saline), a 1–2 cm incision is made on the antimesenteric side of the tube. A syringe filled with saline is inserted deep into the incision, and the fluid is injected forcefully in such a way as to dislodge the ectopic pregnancy and clot. The contents of the ectopic pregnancy and clots are then aspirated out. Following this, the bed of the ectopic pregnancy must be irrigated well. In case some trophoblastic tissue remains, prior injection of vasopressin may lead to anoxia and death of the trophoblasts, preventing postoperative growth. Bleeding may be controlled by applying pressure with blunt tissue forceps for 5 minutes.

Postoperative follow-up: Regular follow-up must be done following surgery in order to ensure that the patient's hCG levels have returned to zero. This may take several weeks. Elevated hCG levels could mean that some ectopic trophoblastic tissue, which was missed at the time of removal, is still remaining inside. This tissue may have to be removed using MTX or additional surgery.

- The patient must be instructed to visit the clinician after 1 week for removal of sutures.
- The patient must be counselled that she may experience mild bleeding or pain during the 1st postoperative week. In case of mild pain, she can use simple analgesic drugs available over the counter. In case of pain or bleeding of severe intensity, she must be instructed to report to the clinician immediately.

COMPLICATIONS OF ECTOPIC PREGNANCY

Ruptured ectopic pregnancy can result in life-threatening haemorrhage, hypovolaemic shock and/or disseminated intravascular coagulation (DIC), which may even prove fatal. In the past few decades, ruptured ectopic pregnancy was amongst the leading causes of maternal mortality. Presently, with the improvement in imaging and minimally invasive procedures in cases of ectopic pregnancy, the mortality rate has considerably reduced. Nowadays, the trend is towards the use of minimally invasive surgery in cases of ectopic pregnancy. Although operative laparoscopy is associated with its own inherent complications, in experienced hands, there are usually minimal complications related to the laparoscopic procedure. However, if the surgeon is not trained enough in laparoscopy, then there is a chance of complications as described in **Box 9**. In experienced hands, the chances of these complications are extremely rare. Altogether laparoscopic procedure has a much lower complication rate in comparison to the conventional surgery. Conventional surgery can also be associated with complications such as bleeding, infection and damage to the surrounding viscera such as bowel, bladder, ureters and other major vessels. Ectopic pregnancy can be associated with significant psychological distress to the parents because most mothers may perceive ectopic pregnancy as the loss of their pregnancy. A patient with a history of ectopic pregnancy is associated with an approximately 10% risk of developing ectopic pregnancy in the future. Conceiving a future IUP is not a problem even if one of the tubes is removed. About 65% of the women are likely to achieve a successful pregnancy in future within 18 months of having an ectopic pregnancy. Occasionally, fertility treatment such as IVF may be required.

OVARIAN PREGNANCY

Ovarian pregnancy is very rare, with many apparent examples being explained by an extruded tubal pregnancy becoming adherent to the surface of the ovary. Incidence ranges from 1% to 3% of ectopic pregnancy. In true ovarian pregnancy, the ovum is fertilised while it is in the abdominal cavity, in the Graafian follicle or in the process of leaving the follicle. The pregnancy then develops within a capsule of ovarian tissue with the corpus luteum immediately alongside it **(Fig. 16)**.

Endometriosis on the surface of an ovary is said to favour implantation of an ovum fertilised in the peritoneal cavity.

The criteria for a diagnosis of ovarian pregnancy are—the tube and its fimbriae are normal and separate from the pregnancy sac; the pregnancy sac is in the position of the ovary; the pregnancy sac is attached to the uterus by the ovarian ligament; ovarian tissue is histologically recognisable in several areas of the wall around the pregnancy. These criteria are generally attributed to Spiegelberg **(Box 12)**.

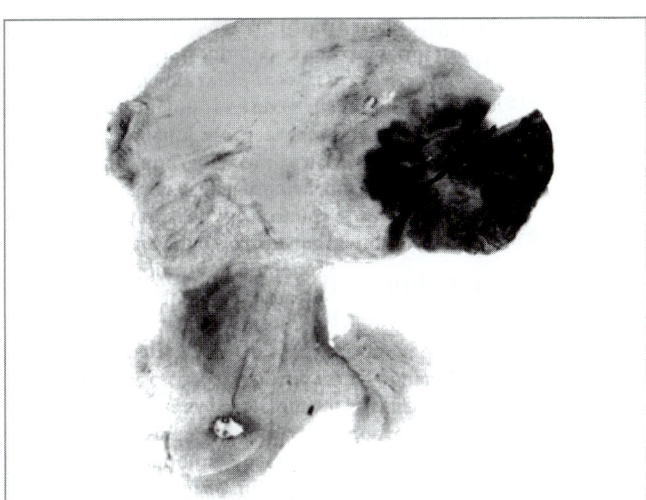

Fig. 16: Ovarian pregnancy with the outer end of a normal fallopian tube above.

BOX 12: Spiegelberg criteria for ovarian pregnancy diagnosis.

- The fallopian tube on the affected side must be intact
- The foetal sac must occupy the position of the ovary
- The ovary must be connected to the uterus by the ovarian ligament
- Ovarian tissue must be located on the sac wall

Source: Spiegelberg O. Casusistik der ovarialschwangerschaft. Arch Gynaecol. 1878;13:73.

Pathology

The general and local reactions of the body are the same as in tubal pregnancy. Decidual reaction occurs in the endometrium and, to a limited extent, in the stroma of the ovary. The ovary can only accommodate the pregnancy for a very short period; within 2–3 weeks, the capsule bursts or is eroded and is the source of intra-abdominal haemorrhage.

Clinical Features and Differential Diagnosis

These are the same as for tubal pregnancy, and an ovarian site for the pregnancy is usually unsuspected before laparotomy. At operation, the conditions likely to be confused are—haemorrhage from the corpus luteum of menstruation or of pregnancy; ovulation haemorrhage; and haemorrhagic cysts of all kinds. These are often only distinguished by histological examination of removed tissues.

Treatment

The principles of treatment are the same as for tubal pregnancy. At operation, the affected ovary usually has to be sacrificed.

CORNUAL PREGNANCY

In this rare form of ectopic pregnancy, implantation occurs in the cavity of a rudimentary horn of the uterus. The horn does not always communicate with the rest of the uterine cavity, in which case it must be assumed that spermatozoa ascend through the other horn and tube and fertilise an ovum in the peritoneal cavity. This then enters the tube of the rudimentary horn.

Pathology

The general and local reactions are the same as for tubal pregnancy. An important feature of cornual pregnancy, however, is that the sac is surrounded by myometrium and, even though this is poorly developed, it can contain the pregnancy for a longer time than can the tube or ovary. Rupture of the horn, therefore, does not usually take place until the 12th–20th week but when it does, there is nearly always severe bleeding, which makes the condition extremely dangerous.

In some respects, cornual pregnancy resembles the interstitial type of tubal pregnancy, and they can be confused at operation. A distinguishing feature is *the insertion of the round ligament, which is always lateral to a cornual pregnancy*. In both cases, it is possible for the pregnancy to be discharged into the main cavity of the uterus.

Clinical Features and Differential Diagnosis

These are similar to those of tubal gestation except that dramatic symptoms occur late. Before the occurrence of rupture, the condition most likely to be confused is a painful leiomyoma complicating pregnancy. The pregnant horn differs from a myoma in that it can be felt to contract.

Asymmetrical enlargement of the uterus, real or apparent, is a feature of normal early pregnancy. If exaggerated, an implantation of the conceptus into the cornu of a normal uterus is sometimes postulated, and the condition is called an angular pregnancy. The asymmetry disappears by the 12th week but, meanwhile, might be confused with a cornual pregnancy.

Treatment

This is governed by the principles described under tubal pregnancy, the affected horn together with the pregnancy being usually removed.

CERVICAL PREGNANCY

This rare form of ectopic pregnancy is one in which the ovum becomes implanted in the cervical canal and distends it as it grows. The major risk factors include in vitro fertilisation, endometrial injury caused by PID or postsurgical trauma such as caesarean section or uterine curettage, history of abortions, intrauterine device use and structural uterine anomalies.

Clinical criteria for diagnosis of cervical pregnancy are: The uterus above the distended cervix is smaller; the internal os is closed; no placental tissue is obtained on endometrial curettage; and the external os opens earlier than in spontaneous abortion.

Ultrasound criteria have been described to differentiate a true cervical pregnancy from a spontaneous abortion. These include empty uterine cavity or a false gestation sac; hour-glass uterine shape; ballooned cervical canal containing the gestation sac and placental tissue; and closed internal os. MRI has also been used to establish the diagnosis **(Box 13)**.

The condition can be mistaken for an incomplete abortion of a normally sited pregnancy, placenta praevia or, if the external os is not dilated, for a cervical leiomyoma or cervical carcinoma.

The cervical pregnancy may be mistaken for CSP. The differentiating feature is that cervical pregnancy is located below the internal os, while scar pregnancy is located above, at the level of the caesarean scar incision. It may also be misdiagnosed as an ongoing abortion. The two situations are best distinguished by the sliding sign, which means that when gentle pressure is applied on the cervix with the ultrasound probe, the implanted cervical pregnancy does not slide, whereas the gestational sac of the abortion slides.

BOX 13: Ultrasound criteria for cervical pregnancy.

- Echo-free uterine cavity or the presence of a false gestational sac only
- Decidual transformation of the endometrium with dense echo structure
- Diffuse uterine wall structure
- Hour-glass uterine shape
- Ballooned cervical canal
- Gestational sac in the endocervix
- Placental tissue in the cervical canal
- Closed internal os

Source: Hofmann HM, Urdl W, Höfler H, Hönigl W, Tamussino K. Cervical pregnancy: case reports and current concepts in diagnosis and treatment. Arch Gynecol Obstet. 1987;241:63-9.

Abortion usually takes place sooner or later and when it does, bleeding from the nonretractile cervix can be so severe as to necessitate hysterectomy **(Fig. 17)**. Continuance of the pregnancy to produce a viable child has been described.

CAESAREAN SCAR PREGNANCY

It is the implantation of the gestational sac over the previous caesarean scar. Recently, there has been an increase in the incidence of CSP due to the increased rate of caesarean delivery. CSP account for about 4.2% of ectopic pregnancies. Caesarean scar ectopic pregnancies may increase the risk of severe morbidity, such as life-threatening haemorrhage, placenta accreta spectrum, uterine rupture and hysterectomy with subsequent loss of fertility, and higher chances of maternal mortality.

Transvaginal ultrasound-based diagnostic criteria for CSP:

- Empty uterine cavity
- Empty cervical canal
- Anterior part of the uterine isthmus showing presence of a gestational sac with or without foetal cardiac activity
- Absence or thinning of the myometrium at the level of the bladder

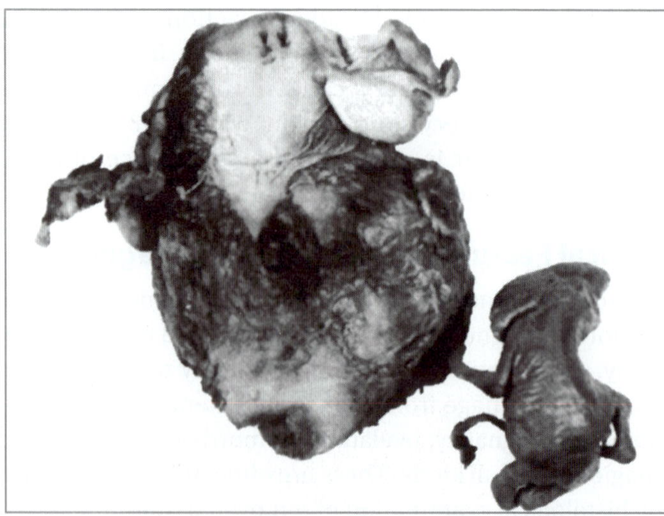

Fig. 17: A cervical pregnancy with a small misshapen foetus still attached to its placenta within the pregnancy sac. The latter is in the supravaginal cervix and bulging out into the right broad ligament. The external os is visible at the lower pole. As is usual, the bleeding in this case was so severe and uncontrollable that hysterectomy was necessary.

- Peritrophoblastic or periplacental flow surrounding the caesarean scar ectopic pregnancy appearing on Doppler flow ultrasonogram.

Treatment options include systemic or local MTX therapy, needle aspiration followed by local MTX, uterine curettage, hysteroscopy, resection of CSP through a transvaginal approach, uterine artery embolisation, laparoscopy and high-intensity focused ultrasound with hysteroscopic dilation and curettage (D and C).

ABDOMINAL PREGNANCY

Some authorities doubt whether a primary abdominal pregnancy, that is, one in which a fertilised ovum implants itself initially on some abdominal organ, ever occurs. Well-documented cases, in which both tubes and ovaries were normal and separate from the pregnancy sac, are reported. However, most cases of abdominal pregnancy are secondary in that the pregnancy is first implanted in the tube, ovary or uterus. In the case of the last it escapes by way of rupture of a scar **(Fig. 18)**. The criteria for diagnosis of primary abdominal pregnancy are—normal tubes and ovaries with no evidence of recent or past pregnancy; no evidence of uteroplacental fistula; pregnancy related to the peritoneal surface and early enough to eliminate the possibility of secondary implantation **(Box 14)**.

Pathology

The usual sequence of events is for the foetus and chorion to commence their development in the tube. After a few weeks, the foetus is extruded through the abdominal ostium or through a break in the wall of the tube, but does not die, because its chorionic attachment and amniotic sac remain intact. When the amnion is intact, the amount of liquor amnii is always small, probably because the normal contribution from the decidua, via the membranes, is missing. The chorion grows through the rent and forms attachments to the pelvic peritoneum, broad ligament, uterus, omentum and intestine. These structures react by developing large blood vessels to serve the placenta, and their anatomy becomes grossly disturbed. The foetus develops in the peritoneal cavity, its amniotic sac becoming supported by an outer coat of organising lymph and blood exudate.

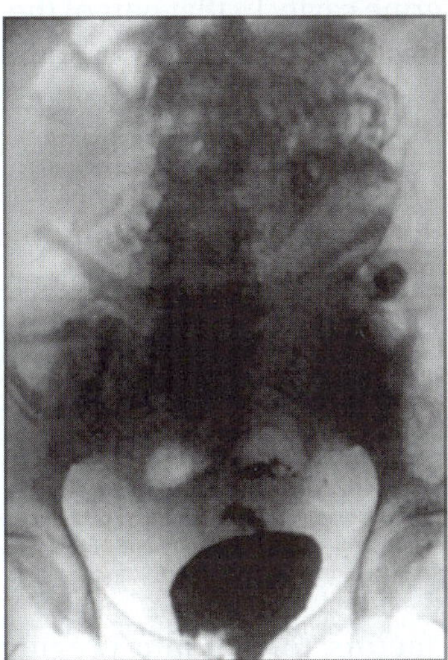

Fig. 18: Secondary abdominal pregnancy, the empty uterine cavity being demonstrated by hysterography.

The placental attachment is so insecure and the local decidual reaction so weak that retroplacental and intra-abdominal haemorrhage is likely at any time. Nevertheless, some abdominal pregnancies proceed to term when spurious labour ensues. The uterus then contracts painfully and rhythmically, and there is some dilatation of the cervix with a discharge of blood and decidua. The foetus dies but remains in the abdominal cavity where it undergoes maceration **(Fig. 19)**.

Clinical Features

If closely questioned, the patient usually gives a history suggestive of tubal implantation in the early weeks. The pregnancy then proceeds apparently normally, except it is unusually uncomfortable; intestinal distension, periodic abdominal pain, and occasional slight uterine bleeding are common. The foetus usually takes up an abnormal attitude and position. Contrary to what might be expected, the foetus is not especially easy to feel—the whole tumour is asymmetrical but difficult to define, and the abdomen is tender in one or other area. The uterus may be felt as a tumour separate from the pregnancy sac and is mistaken for a leiomyoma or cyst, the distinguishing feature being that it contracts from time to time. The pregnancy mass, on the other hand, does not contract. On vaginal examination,

BOX 14: Studdiford's criteria for diagnosis of primary abdominal pregnancy.

- Presence of normal tubes and ovaries with no evidence of recent or past pregnancy
- No evidence of uteroplacental fistula
- The presence of pregnancy, related exclusive to the peritoneal surface and early enough to eliminate the possibility of secondary implantation after primary tubal nidation

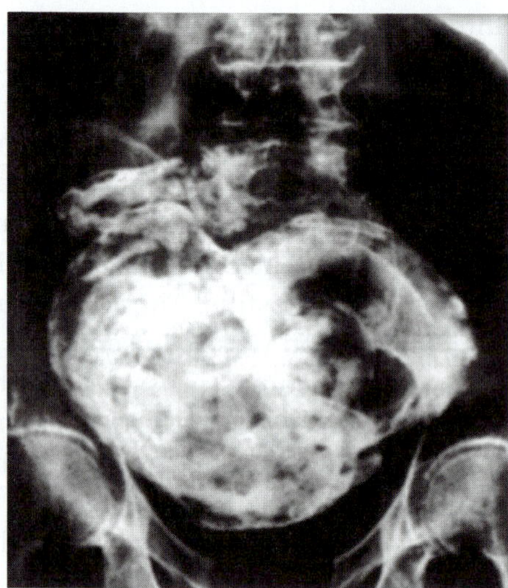

Fig. 19: A lithopaedion in the abdomen of a woman aged 84 years. It was left untreated (Mr CH Walsh's case).

the cervix is nearly always found displaced, often upwards and forwards with foetal parts lying below and behind it.

Diagnosis

This can be surprisingly difficult. Earlier diagnosis was difficult, and many cases were missed until late in pregnancy before the more routine use of ultrasound. Sometimes the diagnosis is suspected only when repeated attempts at induction of abortion or labour are unsuccessful. Pregnancy in one horn of a uterus didelphys can be difficult to exclude. Radiological examination is particularly helpful for it not only reveals an unusual foetal attitude and position but also gas shadows of coils of intestine superimposed on the foetal skeleton. Lateral radiographs of the standing woman may also show some part of the foetal skeleton on a plane posterior to the anterior border of the maternal spine. Hysterography confirms the diagnosis but cannot be employed so long as there is any chance of the pregnancy being within the uterus **(Fig. 18)**. Experience of rare conditions takes time to accumulate, but the ultrasonic findings are in essence similar to those described above, and the empty uterus is more easily identified.

Treatment

Laparotomy should generally be undertaken as soon as the diagnosis of abdominal pregnancy is made. The operation is dangerous because the anatomical relations are likely to be disturbed, and great skill and gentleness are necessary if serious haemorrhage is to be avoided. The difficulty is to control the sinuses of the placental site when it involves the intestines and the peritoneum. If the site is such that the maternal vessels leading to it are easily ligated, the foetus and placenta are removed. If the placenta is implanted dangerously, it is often better to remove the foetus without disturbing its sac. The umbilical cord is cut short, and the placenta and membranes are left to be absorbed during the next 1 or 2 years. Only rarely do they have to be removed later, and then usually because of abscess formation. In such cases, the hCG and plasma progesterone levels fall only gradually during the course of 8–12 weeks. MTX has been used to manage the residual placenta, but it can accelerate tissue necrosis and cause severe infection. Laparoscopic treatment must be considered for early abdominal pregnancy.

There may be circumstances, when it offers the patient her only chance of a live child, for example, in which it is justifiable to delay operating until the foetus is viable. This course is only to be followed after considering the serious maternal risk involved, and in the knowledge that the child is likely to be misshapen, albeit not permanently, and that the neonatal death rate is 50%.

If the foetus dies in the abdomen, it is sometimes wiser to defer operation to allow the placental sinuses to become thrombosed. In such cases, the maternal coagulation profile needs to be monitored.

INTERSTITIAL PREGNANCY

Interstitial or intramural ectopic pregnancy can be defined as the most common type of ectopic pregnancy, located outside the uterine cavity in that part of the fallopian tube, which penetrates the muscular layer of the uterus. It also refers to the presence of a pregnancy located within the cavity in one of the two upper 'horns' of a bicornuate uterus. Since it occurs within the interstitial portion of the fallopian tube, it has the potential to grow to a larger in size in comparison to the standard tubal ectopic pregnancies by the time of its presentation. It accounts for nearly 2–4% of all tubal pregnancies. This can be estimated as 1 in every 2,500–5,000 live births. The incidence of interstitial pregnancies is rising further due to the growing use of IVF.

Risk Factors

Various risk factors for ectopic pregnancy include a previous history of tubal ectopic pregnancy, tubal infection, tubal surgery and/or IVF.

Clinical Presentation

Typical symptoms of interstitial pregnancy are similar to the classical signs of ectopic pregnancy and include amenorrhoea, abdominal pain and vaginal bleeding. 25% of the patients may present with haemorrhagic shock. On an average, gestational age at the time of presentation is 7–8 weeks. When undiagnosed, they present late in the second trimester, associated with rupture and catastrophic bleeding, with a mortality rate of 2–2.5%.

Diagnosis

Imaging Modalities

Features suggestive of an interstitial pregnancy on TVS include the following:

- *Interstitial line sign:* This is represented by an echogenic line extending from the edge of the mass to the endometrial echo complex. This is associated with a sensitivity of about 80% and a specificity of 98%.
- *Empty uterine cavity:* Gestational sac is present, separate from the uterine cavity.
- *Presence of an eccentric gestational sac:* An eccentric intrauterine gestational sac may be visualised, or there may be decidual reaction located high in the fundus. There is a paucity of myometrium around the gestational sac, with <5 mm of surrounding myometrium in all planes. This is often termed as the 'myometrial mantle'. Moreover, there may be the absence of myometrium in some of the planes.

Three-dimensional ultrasound and MRI examination may be helpful for delineating the location of the gestational sac.

β-Human Chorionic Gonadotrophin Assay

Quantitative β-hCG assay may also be useful in these cases.

Management

Management is largely dependent on the clinical situation. Emergency laparotomy is required in cases of ruptured ectopic pregnancy. Surgical procedures comprise cornual evacuation, cornuostomy (incision of cornua and removal of ectopic pregnancy), cornual resection or corneal wedge resection. Cornuectomy or hysterectomy may be used as an emergency procedure in cases of life-threatening haemorrhage. Due to increased vascularity of the interstitial region, there may be excessive blood loss at the time of surgery.

Conservative Management

Conservative management can be undertaken in asymptomatic patients who are haemodynamically stable. Conservative management of an interstitial ectopic includes the use of one of the following:

- Methotrexate (either systemic or local)
- Potassium chloride (KCl) injection
- Conservative laparoscopic surgery
- Uterine artery embolisation

In patients with conservative surgical therapy, there is a high risk of persistent ectopic pregnancy due to the presence of deeply embedded surviving trophoblastic tissues. These patients thus require regular monitoring of the β-hCG levels until they become undetectable.

Complications

Interstitial pregnancies, on an average, have a higher risk of uterine rupture and haemorrhage, and overall mortality in comparison to usual tubal ectopic pregnancies. Uterine myometrial rupture usually tends to occur by the second trimester of pregnancy.

Patients with interstitial pregnancy who were surgically managed must be monitored using TVS in their subsequent pregnancies in order to ensure its proper location and to assess the intactness of the surgically repaired area. Caesarean section is recommended during subsequent pregnancies to avoid uterine rupture during labour.

INTRALIGAMENTARY PREGNANCY

Intraligamentary pregnancy is similar to secondary abdominal pregnancy in that it arises secondarily to tubal implantation, the tube rupturing extraperitoneally and discharging the foetus between the layers of the broad ligament. If the chorionic attachment remains undisturbed and the foetus lives, the further progress, clinical features, complications and treatment are similar to those of abdominal pregnancy.

PREGNANCY OF UNKNOWN LOCATION

INTRODUCTION

Pregnancy of unknown location can be defined as 'pregnancy with a positive pregnancy test (β-hCG) but with no signs of either intrauterine or extrauterine pregnancy or retained products of conception on TVS or even laparoscopy'. Incidence of PUL has been found to vary between 10% and 31%.

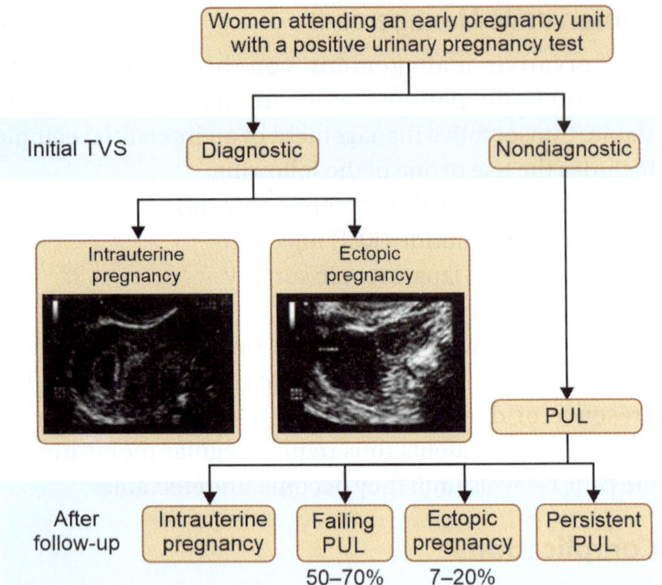

Fig. 20: Diagrammatic representation of the outcome of PUL. (PUL: pregnancy of unknown location; TVS: transvaginal sonography)

The risk of being ectopic (outside the uterus) in location is low in the majority of PUL. It is necessary to correctly diagnose an ectopic pregnancy. This is due to the reason that even if at least 15% of ectopic pregnancies resolve spontaneously, there is no other method of distinguishing these from those that would eventually rupture and put the woman's life in danger, i.e. high-risk group of becoming ectopic in future. In patients with a PUL, 30% may end up having a normal IUP.

The four possible outcomes of PUL are as follows **(Fig. 20)**:

1. Disappearance of results from failing to resolve pregnancy (44–69%) and the spontaneous decrease in levels of hCG to <5 IU/L.
2. Progression to confirmation of a normal IUP, where up to 75% of PUL develops in viable IUPs.
3. The frequency of ectopic pregnancy in the case of PUL ranges from 8.1% to 42.8%.
4. Ultimately, 2% of cases account for persisting PULs, which are defined as those where there is no decrease in the levels of hCG, show no signs of trophoblastic disease and the position of the pregnancy cannot be recognised. Such cases can be managed with the administration of MTX.

The majority of PULs are nonaggressive. They represent either failing intrauterine or ectopic pregnancies, which are never visualised utilising TVS (failing PULs or IUPs that are too early to be detected on TVS).

Easy access to urine pregnancy tests, improved availability of ultrasound scans and increased anxiety among women to confirm a pregnancy after missing the next normal menstrual cycle (even before missing a period!) are a few causes of the increasing frequency of PULs.

The detection of ectopic pregnancies within the PUL group is the main challenge. Also, ectopic pregnancies within this PUL population pose the highest risk, because they are the predominant cause of maternal mortality in early pregnancies.

OUTCOME OF ECTOPIC PREGNANCY

Failing Pregnancies of Unknown Location

In PUL, the contribution of failing pregnancies is 50–70%, and it resolves spontaneously with expectant management. Failing pregnancies could be intrauterine or extrauterine. In these cases, the levels of serum progesterone will be <20 nmol/L and at 0 and 48 hours, the serum hCG levels continue to fall by more than 15%. Till the concentration is <5 IU/L, the weekly monitoring hCG levels is essential. However, the follow-up with TVS is not mandatory.

Intrauterine Pregnancy

Approximately 30–37% of PUL occurs due to IUPs and 75% of these women show viable IUP on follow-up. At 2 days, the increase in levels of serum hCG is >66%, whereas the serum progesterone will be >60 nmol/L. To confirm IUP by scan, weekly serial hCG estimation is done till the level is >1,000 IU/L.

Ectopic Pregnancy

In a nonspecialised scan centre, approximately 8.1–42.8% is the average prevalence of early ectopic pregnancy in the PUL population, whereas in a specialised scan centre, it ranges from 8.1% to 14%. The diagnostic accuracy in specialised centres is about 87–93%, and only some portion of PULs shows high-risk ectopic pregnancy.

Serum hCG or serum progesterone levels are used in the diagnosis of ectopic pregnancy, where there is suboptimal increase or decrease in serum hCG, and the serum progesterone varies between 20 and 60 nmol/L. On repeated scan, instead of the absence of an intrauterine sac on TVS, it may indicate a complex adnexal mass or echogenic fluid. With TVS, when the levels are above 1,000–1,500 IU/L, an ectopic pregnancy will usually be visualised. However, there is a lack of methods which will be useful for predicting whether ectopic pregnancies are likely to be self-limiting or are dangerous.

Persisting Pregnancy of Unknown Locations

When serum hCG level does not decline but is <500 IU/L, it is diagnosed as persisting PULs with unidentifiable normal or abnormal pregnancy, either by scan or laparoscopy. In this group of women, the treatment option may be the medical management with MTX.

DIAGNOSIS

Serum Inhibin A and Activin A Levels

Prediction of pregnancy loss and failing PULs in women can be made by examining maternal serum inhibin A levels, whereas levels of activin A correlate weakly with the pregnancy outcome. Ectopic pregnancy can be best predicted when the inhibin A level decreases over 48 hours. For PUL outcome, activin A levels are not a good predictor, and their levels may increase in failing PULs compared with IUPs.

The foetoplacental unit secretes both glycoproteins inhibin A and activin A. For accurate prediction of all three possible final outcomes of PULs, neither single nor serial measurements of inhibin A or activin A can be used. Identification of a universal marker of PUL outcome, which combined accuracy, reproducibility and simplicity, is the major challenge that still exists. In order to increase sensitivity and specificity for several outcomes, however, an amalgamation of markers may be required. Until such a marker is identified, the value of serum hCG levels at 0 and 48 hours is the ideal way for predicting PUL outcome.

MANAGEMENT OF PREGNANCY OF UNKNOWN LOCATION

Management options in cases of PULs are:

- Expectant
- Medical
- Surgical

Expectant Management

This management is carried out where hCG levels are below the discriminatory zone. Conservative management of asymptomatic cases should be done. Until pregnancy is located or intervention becomes necessary, follow-up must be continued with serial hCG and TVS. In selective cases of symptomatic women (having abdominal pain and vaginal bleeding), who are clinically and haemodynamically stable with normal ultrasound, expectant treatment can be done.

Though expectant management is considered to be safe and is not associated with any serious adverse outcome and reduces unnecessary surgical intervention, but for the final diagnosis, multiple visits are required.

Medical Management

Methotrexate indications are persisting PUL and ectopic gestation.

Methotrexate and Pregnancy of Unknown Location

An antimetabolite drug, MTX, which is a folic acid antagonist, inhibits the enzyme dihydrofolate reductase and thereby prevents reduction of folic acid to folinic acid. The crucial metabolic processes required for DNA and RNA synthesis are impaired due to the interaction of these agents with intracellular enzymes. For medical management of ectopic gestation and persistent PUL, MTX is the drug of choice and is also chiefly used for treatment of persistent gestational trophoblastic disease and germ cell tumours. It should be remembered that in PUL population, the high-risk factors for ectopic pregnancy should be considered **(Table 2)**.

TABLE 2: High-risk factors for ectopic pregnancy.

Risk factors	***Risk***
High risk	
• Tubal corrective surgery	21.0
• Tubal sterilisation	9.3
• Previous ectopic pregnancy	8.3
• In utero DES exposure	5.6
• Intrauterine device	4.5–45
• Documented tubal pathology	3.8–21
Moderate risk	
• Infertility	2.5–21
• Previous genital infection	2.5–3.7
• Multiple partners	2.1
Slight risk	
• Previous pelvic/abdominal surgery	0.93–3.8
• Smoking	2.3–2.5
• Douching	1.1–3.1
• Intercourse <18 years	1.6

(DES: diethylstilbestrol)

Indications for use of methotrexate:

- A patient with normal haemogram, liver and renal function should be haemodynamically stable. They are also likely to keep follow-up appointments.
- Unruptured tubal pregnancy
- Absence of evidence related to IUP
- Ectopic mass <3.5 cm
- Levels of hCG with <15,000 IU/L
- Absence of foetal heart tones
- <6 weeks of gestation.

For treatment of ectopic pregnancy and persistent PUL, generally single-dose protocol of MTX therapy is used **(Tables 3 and 4)**.

Various contraindications for the use of methotrexate are:

- Active intra-abdominal haemorrhage
- >4 cm of ectopic mass
- Breastfeeding
- Immunodeficiency
- Liver or kidney disease
- Blood dyscrasias
- Peptic ulcer

TABLE 3: Single-dose protocol of methotrexate.

Regimen	*Follow-up*
Methotrexate (50 mg/m^2 IM)	The levels of β-hCG are measured on days 4 and 7: • If difference is ≥15%, repeat weekly until <15 mIU/mL • If difference is <15%, repeat the methotrexate dose and begin a new day 1 • On day 7, if foetal cardiac activity is present, repeat methotrexate dose, begin new day 1 • If levels of β-hCG are not decreasing or foetal cardiac activity persists after three doses of methotrexate, surgical treatment is done

(β-hCG: β-human chorionic gonadotrophin; IM: intramuscular)

TABLE 4: Different failure rates of single-dose methotrexate.

hCG level (IU/L)	*Failure (%)*
<1,000	2
1,000–1,999	7
2,000–4,999	8
5,000–9,999	13
10,000–14,999	18
>15,000	32

(hCG: human chorionic gonadotrophin).

Emergency surgery, such as laparoscopy or laparotomy, is required in 5% of cases where tubal rupture can occur. Vaginal bleeding, abdominal and pelvic pain, weakness, dizziness or syncope are few signs and symptoms of tubal rupture that must be observed properly and sonography must be done in case of urgent examination. If serum β-hCG is not detected, then sexual intercourse is prohibited. Multivitamins with folic acid must be prohibited. Treatment success rate with single-dose MTX is 87%, tubal patency 81%, subsequent uterine pregnancy 61% and subsequent ectopic pregnancy is 13%.

Surgical Management

Indications are as follows:

- Persisting PUL attributed to IUP or ectopic pregnancy
- Transvaginal scan with suspicious findings of ectopic pregnancy, which cannot be concluded
- Ectopic gestation
- Pregnancy of unknown location in clinically and haemodynamically unstable women.

Surgical Procedure

For a surgical procedure, in case of persisting PUL (IUP or ectopic pregnancy), curettage or laparoscopy is indicated in a few circumstances. The differentiation between IUP and ectopic pregnancy can be done by finding the chorionic villi with the help of the vacuum aspiration or curettage technique. For prediction of an abnormal IUP, thereby excluding an ectopic pregnancy, there should be a decrease in hCG levels by ≥50 within 24 hours after manual vacuum aspiration or curettage. Persisting IUP is expected to be present if there is a decrease in hCG levels, and on histopathological examination of curettings, chorionic villi are revealed. Weekly follow-up is necessary in these cases and is continued till the normal value of hCG levels is attained.

In contrast, persistent PUL due to ectopic pregnancy is suspected if hCG levels do not decrease and there is the absence of chorionic villi as revealed by curettings. Diagnostic laparoscopy is carried out in cases where an ectopic sac is visualised or where it is not. MTX is given if the ectopic sac is not visualised, and management by MTX or laparoscopic surgery is done when the ectopic sac is visualised.

Some of the other indications for laparoscopy, where TVS is not conclusive in suspected cases of ectopic pregnancy, are as follows:

Flowchart 3: Management of pregnancy of unknown location.

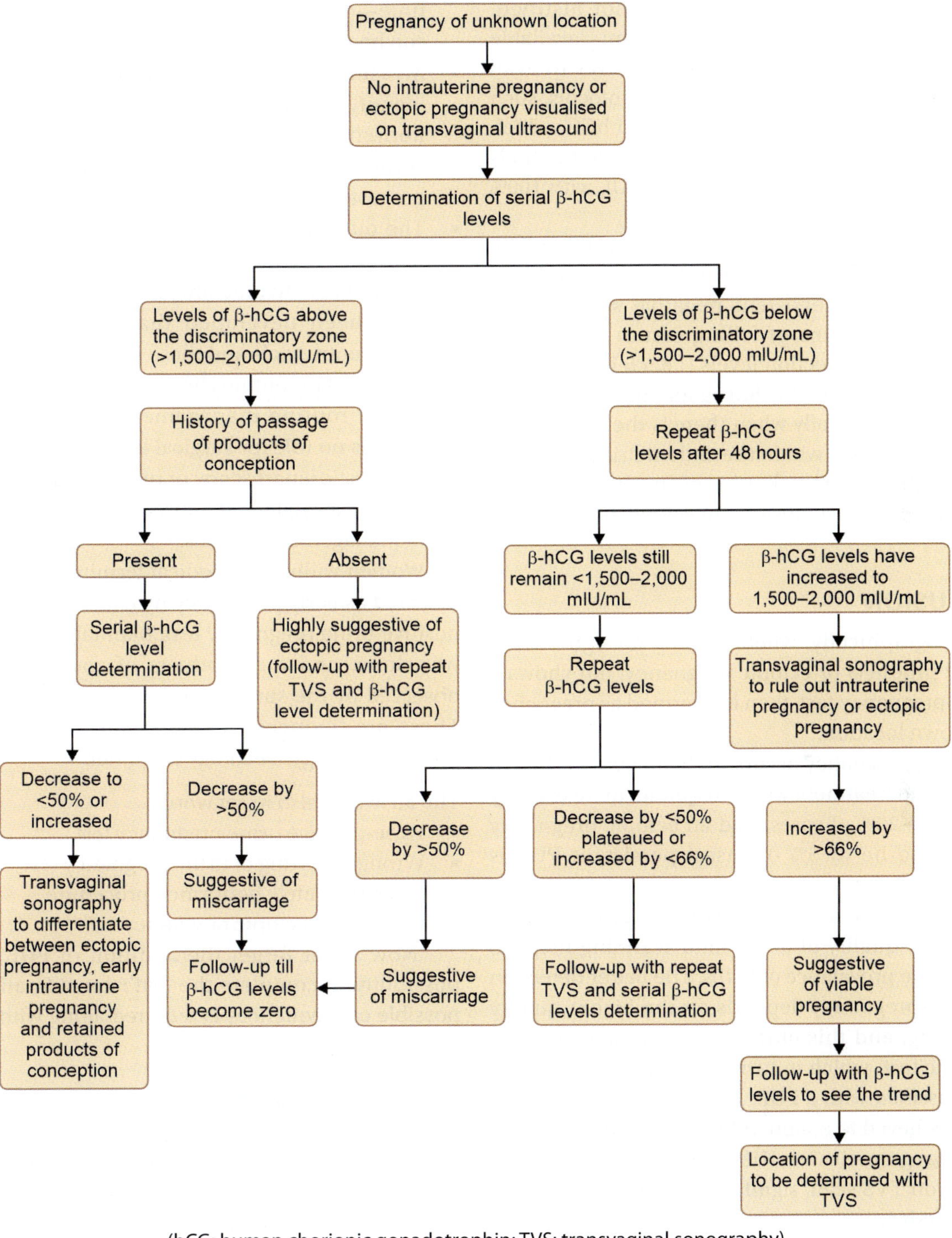

(hCG: human chorionic gonadotrophin; TVS: transvaginal sonography)

- Adnexal mass, which is associated with PUL
- Little free fluid in the pouch of Douglas
- Prevention of proper visualisation by TVS due to a fibroid uterus
- Symptomatic PUL with TVS findings indicating ectopic pregnancy and PUL with hCG levels above the discriminating zone

All the following factors should be considered, while a uniform, straightforward approach is not justified, depending on the type of clinical presentation—available resources, attitude of women and her relatives to avail resources. Though there are the following protocols, such as combining TVS, serum progesterone and hCG, which may be considered to be useful but there are no methods which can predict the clinical outcome of PUL with 100% accuracy **(Flowchart 3)**.

Until a final diagnosis is made, a failing PUL, an IUP or an ectopic pregnancy, careful follow-up should be done. If there were persistent negative sonographic findings in the presence of failing serum hCG levels ultimately reaching detection levels (i.e. <5 U/L), then it is confirmed as failing PUL. During follow-up, an IUP is confirmed sonographically when there is the presence of a gestational sac placed within the endometrial cavity. On the basis of the positive visualisation of an adnexal mass or a gestational sac, the diagnosis of an ectopic pregnancy is carried out.

CONCLUSION

- Ultrasonographically, when there is no sign of IUP, retained products or ectopic pregnancy, but shows a positive pregnancy test, then it is termed as pregnancy of unknown location.
- A resolving pregnancy occurs in the majority (70%) of cases, and no treatment will be required; there is a very early IUP in 25% of cases, and an ectopic pregnancy turns out to be in 5% of cases; persistent PUL is extremely rare.
- The range of PUL in different studies varies from 8% to 31%. The quality of ultrasound scanning helps to ascertain the prevalence of PULs. The better detection of ectopic pregnancy depends on the higher quality of scanning, and this ultrasound is used as a single diagnostic test, which in turn results in fewer women being classified with a PUL. Most modern units using TVS are believed to maintain PUL rate below 10%.
- Failing pregnancies or IUPs, that are too early to visualise on TVS scan, signify PULs, which are mostly nonaggressive.
- Expectant management should be performed in clinically stable woman with PULs and for expectant management there must be no signs of haemoperitoneum on ultrasound scan.
- The prognosis of pregnancy outcome does not depend on initial levels of serum hCG.
- To predict the failing PULs, change in serum hCG over time—doubling, hCG ratio and progesterone levels can be used.
- Measurements of serum progesterone can help to identify women at risk for ectopic pregnancy, but are nonreliable in diagnosing ectopic pregnancy with certainty due to the discriminative capacity of serum progesterone.
- The outcome of PUL cannot be predicted by serum markers—activin A and inhibin A.
- To predict PUL outcome, many mathematical models have been developed that need to be tested in multicentre trials and these models do not prove to be beneficial in routine clinical approach.
- In the routine management of women with PUL, there is no role for surgical intervention in the form of diagnostic laparoscopy or uterine curettage.
- To have a single visit approach is improper in the case of management of PULs.

Women willing for medical termination of pregnancy, detected as early pregnancy by clinical evaluation with a positive urine pregnancy test. Manual vacuum aspiration was done, and the products of conception were not observed by the surgeon. What can be the possibilities? These are frequently asked favourite questions of the obstetrics and gynaecology examiner.

The answer is also in set words:

- False-positive urine pregnancy test
- Wrong reporting of urine pregnancy test
- Inappropriately performed procedure
- Chances of ectopic pregnancy

'Now never forget the addition of PUL as the fifth possibility to complete the list!'; consideration of all its possible consequences is required along with meticulous follow-up.

SUGGESTED READING

1. American College of Obstetricians and Gynecologists (ACOG). ACOG practice bulletin no. 193: tubal ectopic pregnancy. Obstet Gynaecol. 2018;131:e91-103.
2. American College of Obstetricians and Gynecologists (ACOG). ACOG Practice Bulletin No. 94: medical management of ectopic pregnancy. Obstet Gynecol. 2008;111(6):1479-85.
3. Ankum WM, Hajenius PJ, Schrevel LS, Van der Veen F. Management of suspected ectopic pregnancy. Impact of new diagnostic tools in 686 consecutive cases. J Reprod Med. 1996;41(10):724-8.

4. Bangsgaard N, Lund C, Ottesen B, Nilas L. Improved fertility following conservative surgical treatment of ectopic pregnancy. BJOG. 2003;110(8):765-70.
5. Berg CJ, Callaghan WM, Syverson C, Henderson Z. Pregnancy related mortality in the United States, 1998 to 2005. Obstet Gynecol. 2010;116:1302.
6. Bignardi T, Condous G, Alhamdan D, Kirk E, Van Calster B, Van Huffel S, et al. The hCG ratio can predict the ultimate viability of the intrauterine pregnancies of uncertain viability in the pregnancy of unknown location population. Hum Reprod. 2008;23:1964-7.
7. Birch Petersen K, Hoffmann E, Rifbjerg Larsen C, Svarre Nielsen H. Cesarean scar pregnancy: a systematic review of treatment studies. Fertil Steril. 2016;105(4):958-67.
8. Cacciatore B, Stenman U, Ylöstolalo P. Diagnosis of ectopic pregnancy by vaginal ultrasonography in combination with a discriminatory serum hCG level of 1000 IU/L (IRP). BJOG. 1990;97(10):904-8.
9. Callen PW. Ultrasonography in Obstetrics and Gynecology, 4th edition. Philadelphia: WB Saunders Co; 2000.
10. Casikar I, Reid S, Condous G. Ectopic pregnancy: ultrasound diagnosis in modern management. Clin Obstet Gynecol. 2012;55(2):402-9.
11. Colombo GE, Leonardi M, Armour M, Di Somma H, Dinh T, da Silva Costa F, et al. Efficacy and safety of expectant management in the treatment of tubal ectopic pregnancy: a systematic review and meta-analysis. Hum Reprod Open. 2020;2020(4):hoaa044.
12. Comstock C, Huston K, Lee W. The ultrasonographic appearance of ovarian ectopic pregnancies. Obstet Gynecol. 2005;105:42-5.
13. Condons G, Kirk E, Lu C, Van Huffel S, Gevaert O, De Moor B, et al. Diagnostic accuracy of varying discriminatory zones for the prediction of ectopic pregnancy in women with a pregnancy of unknown location. Ultrasound Obstet Gynecol. 2005;26:770-5.
14. Condous G, Kirk E, Syed A, Van Calster B, Van Huffel S, Timmerman D, et al. Do levels of serum cancer antigen 125 and creatine kinase predict the outcome in pregnancies of unknown location? Hum Reprod. 2005;20:3348-54.
15. Creanga AA, Shapiro-Mendoza CK, Bish CL, Zane S, Berg CJ, Callaghan WM. Trends in ectopic pregnancy mortality in the United States; 1980-2007. Obstet Gynecol. 2011;117:837-47.
16. Durston WE, Carl ML, Guerra W, Eaton A, Ackerson LM. Ultrasound availability in the evaluation of ectopic pregnancy in the ED: comparison of quality and cost-effectiveness with different approaches. Am J Emerg Med. 2000;18(4):408-17.
17. Elsherbiny M, Lim ET, Ma K. Interstitial Ectopic Pregnancy: Laparoscopic Cornuostomy. J Minim Invasive Gynecol. 2023;30(6):439-40.
18. Farquhar CM. Ectopic pregnancy. Lancet. 2005;366(9485): 583-91.
19. Fernandez H, Capmas P, Lucot JP, Resch B, Panel P, Bouyer J. Fertility after ectopic pregnancy: the DEMETER randomized trial. Hum Reprod. 2013;28(5):1247-53.
20. Flanagan HC, Duncan WC, Lin CJ, Spears N, Horne AW. Recent advances in the understanding of tubal ectopic pregnancy. Fac Rev. 2023;12:26.
21. Fujishita A, Masuzaki H, Khan KN, Kitajima M, Hiraki K, Ishimaru T. Laparoscopic salpingotomy for tubal pregnancy: comparison of linear salpingotomy with and without suturing. Hum Reprod. 2004;19:1195-200.
22. Fylstra DL. Ectopic pregnancy within a cesarean scar: a review. Obstet Gynecol Surv. 2002;57:537-43.
23. Gray DT, Thorburn J, Lundorff P, Strandell A, Lindblom B. A cost-effectiveness study of a randomised trial of laparoscopy versus laparotomy for ectopic pregnancy. Lancet. 1995;345(8958):1139-43.
24. Health Encyclopedia. University of Rochester Medical Center. HCG (blood). [online] Available from https://www.urmc.rochester.edu/encyclopedia/content?contenttypeid=167&contentid=hcg_serum [Last accessed May, 2025].
25. Hillard T. Yearbook of Obstetrics and Gynaecology. London: RCOG Press; 2008. pp. 22-6.
26. Hochner-Celnikier D, Ron M, Goshen R, Zacut D, Amir G, Yagel S. Rupture of ectopic pregnancy following disappearance of serum beta subunit of hCG. Obstet Gynecol. 1992;79(5):826-7.
27. Houser M, Kandalaft N, Khati NJ. Ectopic pregnancy: a resident's guide to imaging findings and diagnostic pitfalls. Emerg Radiol 2022; 29(1): 161-172.
28. Job-Spira N, Bouyer J, Pouly JL, Germain E, Coste J, Aublet-Cuvelier B, et al. Fertility after ectopic pregnancy: first results of a population-based cohort study in France. Hum Reprod. 1996;11(1):99-104.
29. Jurkovic D, Gruboeck K, Campbell S. Ultrasound features of normal early pregnancy development. Curr Opin Obstet Gynecol. 1995;7:493-504.
30. Jurkovic D, Hillaby K, Woelfer B, Lawrence A, Salim R, Elson CJ. First-trimester diagnosis and management of pregnancies implanted into the lower uterine segment cesarean section scar. Ultrasound Obstet Gynecol. 2003;21:220-7.
31. Kaakaji Y, Nghiem HV, Nodell C, Winter TC. Sonography of obstetric and gynecologic emergencies: Part I, Obstetric emergencies. AJR Am J Roentgenol. 2000;174(3): 641-9.
32. Kadar N, DeVore G, Romero R. Discriminatory hCG zone: its use in the sonographic evaluation for ectopic pregnancy. Obstet Gynecol. 1981;58(2):156-61.
33. Kelley RW, Martin SA, Strickler RC. Delayed hemorrhage in conservative surgery for ectopic pregnancy. Am J Obstet Gynecol. 1979;133(2):225-6.
34. Kirk E. Ultrasound in the diagnosis of ectopic pregnancy. Clin Obstet Gynecol. 2012;55(2):395-401.

35. Lin EP, Bhatt S, Dogra VS. Diagnostic clues to ectopic pregnancy. Radiographics. 2008;28(6):1661-71.
36. Lipscomb GH, McCord ML, Stovali TG, Huff G, Portera SG, Ling FW. Predictors of success of methotrexate treatment in women with tubal ectopic pregnancies. N Engl J Med. 1999;341:1974-8.
37. Lund CO, Nilas L, Bangsgaard N, Ottesen B. Persistent ectopic pregnancy after linear salpingotomy: a non-predictable complication to conservative surgery for tubal gestation. Acta Obstet Gynecol Scand. 2002;81:1053-9.
38. Lundorff P, Thorburn J, Hahlin M, Källfelt B, Lindblom B. Laparoscopic surgery in ectopic pregnancy: a randomized trial versus laparoscopy. Acta Obstet Gynecol Scand. 1991;70(4-5):343-8.
39. Lundorff P, Thorburn J, Lindblom B. Fertility outcome after conservative surgical treatment of ectopic pregnancy evaluated in a randomized trial. Fertil Steril. 1992;57(5):998-1002.
40. Mateer JR, Valley VT, Aiman EJ, Phelan MB, Thoma ME, Kefer MP. Outcome analysis of a protocol including bedside endovaginal sonography in patients at risk for ectopic pregnancy. Ann Emerg Med. 1996;27(3):283-9.
41. Miller R, Timor-Tritsch IE, Gyamfi-Bannerman C. Society for maternal-fetal medicine (SMFM) consult series #49: cesarean scar pregnancy. Am J Obstet Gynecol. 2020;222:B2–14.
42. Mol BW, Matthijsse HC, Tinga DJ, Huynh T, Hajenius PJ, Ankum WM, et al. Fertility after conservative and radical surgery for tubal pregnancy. Hum Reprod. 1998;13(7):1804-9.
43. Mol F, van Mello NM, Strandell A, Strandell K, Jurkovic D, Ross J, et al. Salpingotomy versus salpingectomy in women with tubal pregnancy (ESEP study): an open-label, multicentre, randomised controlled trial. Lancet. 2014;383(9927):1483-9.
44. Murphy AA, Nager CW, Wujek JJ, Kettel LM, Torp VA, Chin HG. Operative laparoscopy versus laparotomy for the management of ectopic pregnancy. Fertil Steril. 1992;57(6):1180-5.
45. Muttukrishna S, Jauniaux E, Greenwold N, McGarrigle H, Jivraj S, Carter S, et al. Circulating levels of inhibin A, activin A and follistatin in missed and recurrent miscarriages. Hum Reprod. 2002;17:3072-8.
46. Naveed AK, Anjum MU, Hassan A, Mahmood SN. Methotrexate versus expectant management in ectopic pregnancy: a meta-analysis. Arch Gynecol Obstet. 2022;305(3):547-53.
47. Panelli DM, Phillips CH, Brady PC. Incidence, diagnosis and management of tubal and nontubal ectopic pregnancies: a review. Fertil Res Pract. 2015;1:15.
48. Rastogi R, Gl M, Rastogi N, Rastogi V. Interstitial ectopic pregnancy: A rare and difficult clinicosonographic diagnosis. J Hum Reprod Sci. 2008;1(2):81-2.
49. Rottem S, Thaler I, Timor-Tritch E. Classification of tubal gestations by transvaginal sonography. Ultrasound Obstet Gynecol. 1991;1(3):197-201.
50. Royal College of Obstetricians and Gynaecologists (RCOG). The management of tubal ectopic pregnancy. Guideline No. 21. London: RCOG Press; 2010.
51. Royal College of Obstetricians and Gynaecologists. The management of early pregnancy loss. Green-top Guideline No. 25. London: RCOG; 2006.
52. Rulin MC. Is salpingostomy the surgical treatment of choice for unruptured tubal pregnancy? Obstet Gynecol. 1995;86(6):1010-3.
53. Saraj AJ, Wilcox JG, Najmabadi S, Stein SM, Johnson MB, Paulson RJ. Resolution of hormonal markers of ectopic gestation: a randomized trial comparing single-dose intramuscular methotrexate with salpingostomy. Obstet Gynecol. 1998;92(6):989-94.
54. Seifer DB, Lambert-Messerlian GM, Canick JA, Frishman GN, Schneyer AL. Serum inhibin levels are lower in ectopic than intrauterine spontaneously conceived pregnancies. Fertil Steril. 1996;65:667-9.
55. Sgili H, Mohamed K. Pregnancy of unknown location: an evidence based approach to management. Obstet Gynaecol. 2008;10:224-30.
56. Silva PD, Schaper AM, Rooney B. Reproductive outcome after 143 laparoscopic procedures for ectopic pregnancy. Obstet Gynecol. 1993;81(5 Pt 1):710-5.
57. Sowter M, Frappell J. The role of laparoscopy in the management of ectopic pregnancy. Rev Gynaecol Practice. 2002;2:73-82.
58. Sowter MC, Farquhar C, Petrie KJ, Gudex G. A randomized trial comparing single dose systemic methotrexate and laparoscopic surgery for the treatment of unruptured tubal pregnancy. BJOG. 2001;108(2):192-203.
59. Stabile G, Mangino FP, Romano F, Zinicola G, Ricci G.. Ectopic cervical pregnancy: treatment route. Medicina. 2020;56:1-11.
60. Timor-Tritsch IE, Monteagudo A, Cali G, D'Antonio F, Kaelin Agten A. Cesarean scar pregnancy: diagnosis and pathogenesis. Obstet Gynecol Clin North Am. 2019;46:797-811.
61. Timor-Tritsch IE, Monteagudo A, Santos R, Tsymbal T, Pineda G, Arslan AA. The diagnosis, treatment, and follow-up of cesarean scar pregnancy. Am J Obstet Gynecol. 2012;207:44.e1-13.
62. Van Den Eeden SK, Shan J, Bruce C, Glasser M. Ectopic pregnancy rate and treatment utilization in a large managed care organization. Obstet Gynecol. 2005;105:1052
63. Vermesh M, Silva PD, Rosen GF, Stein AL, Fossum GT, Sauer MV. Management of unruptured ectopic gestation by linear salpingostomy: a prospective, randomized clinical trial of laparoscopy versus laparotomy. Obstet Gynecol. 1989;73(3 Pt 1):400-4.

64. Vial Y, Petignat P, Hohlfeld P. Pregnancy in a cesarean scar. Ultrasound Obstet Gynecol. 2000;16:592-3.
65. Vora PH, Jassawalla MJ, Bhalerao S, Nadkarni T. Cervical ectopic pregnancy: a clinician's dilemma. J Obstet Gynaecol India. 2016;66:617-9.
66. Xie RH, Guo X, Li M, Liao Y, Gaudet L, Walker M, et al. Risk factors and consequences of undiagnosed cesarean scar pregnancy: a cohort study in China. BMC Pregnancy Childbirth. 2019;19:383.
67. Zhang C, Zhang Y, He J, Zhang L. Outcomes of subsequent pregnancies in patients following treatment of cesarean scar pregnancy with high intensity focused ultrasound followed by ultrasound-guided dilation and curettage. Int J Hyperthermia. 2019;36(1):926-31.

10
CHAPTER

Gestational Trophoblastic Disease

Priya Ballal K, Suprajna Shetty

Chapter Outline

- Types of Tumours
- Aetiology
- Pathology
- Clinical Features
- Evaluation and Treatment
- Postmolar Surveillance
- Persistent Trophoblastic Disease
- Classification and Staging of Gestational Trophoblastic Disease
- Treatment of Gestational Trophoblastic Tumours
- Management of Metastasis
- Postchemotherapy Surveillance for High-risk Gestational Trophoblastic Tumours

INTRODUCTION

Gestational trophoblastic disease (GTD) is a group of disorders that arise from trophoblastic tissue. GTD does not include benign disorders of the trophoblast but only the malignant or those with malignant potential. Incidence is varied throughout the globe, having ethnic, racial and geographic propensity to the Hispanic population, African, Asian, Southeast Asian countries, Indonesia, Philippines, Japan, etc., with very low incidence in Europe and America. Global incidence is 0.5–2.5 per 1,000 pregnancies. Complete and partial moles, although benign, have a malignant potential, with the incidence of persistent trophoblastic disease ranging from 3% to 25%. Among which 77% are invasive mole, 10–30% choriocarcinoma and 6–25% have the risk of being metastatic disease. Diagnosis and evaluation are based on serum beta human chorionic gonadotrophin (hCG) values. Gestational trophoblastic neoplasia (GTN) most often has a good prognosis with chemotherapy and almost 100% cure rates. Surgical treatment and hysterectomy as well as radiation are used for select situations.

TYPES OF TUMOURS

The World Health Organization (WHO) classification distinguishes GTD into complete mole, partial mole and GTN, also called as gestational trophoblastic tumours (GTTs) **(Table 1)**. While complete and partial moles may be considered as those with malignant potential or premalignant, the GTTs are either locally invasive or metastatic and aggressive. Benign trophoblastic tumours, such as exaggerated placental site or placental site nodule, are not included among the GTD. GTTs are invasive mole, placental site trophoblastic disease and choriocarcinoma. A rare variant called epithelioid trophoblastic tumour is a highly aggressive type of GTT. GTT can be triggered from a molar pregnancy or arise de novo from any gestational event, including term pregnancy, spontaneous abortion or MTP or even an ectopic pregnancy.

TABLE 1: Classification of gestational trophoblastic disease.

Gestational trophoblastic disease	• Complete mole • Partial mole • Gestational trophoblastic tumours: – Choriocarcinoma – Placental site trophoblastic tumour – Invasive mole – Epithelioid trophoblastic tumour

Choriocarcinoma are nature's first cancer and man's first cure. It is one of the earliest cancers to be completely cured by chemotherapy. One need not have representative tissues from the uterus or metastases in order to start treatment; an elevated titre of hCG in the appropriate clinical situation is all that is required to initiate treatment. Although the prognosis may be affected to a certain degree by the type of tumour, histologically it is impossible to reliably assess the malignant potential of a given tumour. In practice, the biological activity and clinical behaviour of the tumour are better indices of prognosis.

AETIOLOGY

Normal trophoblasts behave in many ways, such as malignant growth. It locally invades maternal tissues, and fragments of it enter the bloodstream to lodge in the lungs. These properties, however, are normally controlled by certain maternal factors (immunological) or other nonfactors so that invasion of the uterine wall is limited and any extrauterine deposits are destroyed. In this respect, it must be recognised that the trophoblast is made up of tissues, which are only 50% maternal. The paternal contribution is presumably foreign to the host, so there must normally also be some mechanism whereby its rejection is prevented. The occurrence of a trophoblastic tumour can be regarded as the result of a breakdown in what must be a complicated and delicate host-invader balance.

The idea of an underlying breakdown in normal host resistance could explain why choriocarcinoma often appears months and even years after the causal pregnancy. This suggests that the woman is able to resist fragments of trophoblast and to keep them dormant until a time comes when her powers of resistance fail for some reason. In those cases, in which spontaneous regression of metastatic deposits occurs, it can also be supposed that the woman has in some way recovered from a temporary failure in normal host response. Thus, the lack of ability to control trophoblastic activity has two possible bases: An inherent or immunological one, and one which results from malnutrition and debility.

Age-related risk of GTD is higher in teenage pregnancies as well as in women older than 40 years of age (10-fold increase). Previous history of molar pregnancy in the past increases the risk of GTD 25–40 times that of the general population. Women who experience recurrent miscarriages have a higher risk of GTD, proportionate to the number of pregnancy losses, probably again attributable to genetic/immunological factors. There is no strong evidence to implicate consanguinity or family history.

Gestational trophoblastic disease has been found more among high-parity women, those with malnutrition, debilitating disease; however, evidence is inconclusive on implicating nutrition as an aetiological factor. High carotene content in diet has been inversely related to the incidence of GTD.

Trophoblastic tumours have a striking geographical distribution. In Europe and North America, they are rare; they are more common in the Middle East, and occur most frequently in South-East Asia, Malaysia, Singapore, Hong Kong, Indonesia, Philippines and China.

BOX 1: Aetiology.

- Immunological
- Genetic/blood group, human leukocyte antigen (HLA) type, paternal chromosomes
- Racial
- Geographic
- Dietary
- Environmental
- Age related
- Antecedent pregnancy
- Parity

The incidence is also relatively high in Central Africa. Asia has an incidence of molar pregnancy 10 times higher than Europe and North America. The incidence varies in different parts of India as well, to the extent of neighbouring states having significant differences of GTN.

Higher incidence of GTD has been noted among women with AB or A blood type compared to the others. Women with recurrent GTD were found to be of blood type B. Cytogenetic studies indicate a higher incidence of balanced translocations in women with GTD (4.6%) compared to (0.6%) in normal unaffected population. Those with balanced translocations have higher chance of abnormal events during meiosis and inducing empty/inactive eggs.

Other genetic factors **(Box 1)** include:

- Expression of tumour suppressor genes and receptors such as DOC-2lbDAb2, TNF-alpha and partially derived H19.
- Oncoproteins-p53, p21, Rb and mbm 2, with considerable overlap among variants of GTD.
- Increased circulating soluble interleukins-2 receptors (SIL-2R) and decreased serum interleukin-2 levels.

Increased risk of GTD has been noted among smokers; those women using OC pills have a relative risk of 2.6 with more than 4 years of use, and increases proportionately with increasing years of use. A sixfold increase in choriocarcinoma has been reported with more than 5 years of OC pills. However, this is not significant enough to implement changes in OC pill recommendation.

PATHOLOGY (TABLE 2)

Complete Mole (Molar Pregnancy)

Complete mole has abnormal excessive proliferation of only trophoblastic tissue, with dilated and oedematous chorionic villi—hydropic degeneration, giving a characteristic appearance of grape-like vesicles filling the cavity of the uterus and absent foetal tissue **(Figs. 1 and 2)**.

TABLE 2: Comparison between complete and partial hydatidiform mole.

Features	*Complete mole*	*Partial mole*
Hydropic changes	Diffuse and placenta not present	Focal
Hyperplasia of trophoblasts	Marked	Mild to moderate
Foetal tissue	Absence of foetus	Present, malformed or FGR
Foetal vessels	Absent	Present
Karyotype	46XX mostly and paternally derived	69XXY
Malignant potential	15–20%	Rare
Beta hCG	Very high	Comparatively low

(FGR: foetal growth restriction; hCG: human chorionic gonadotrophin)

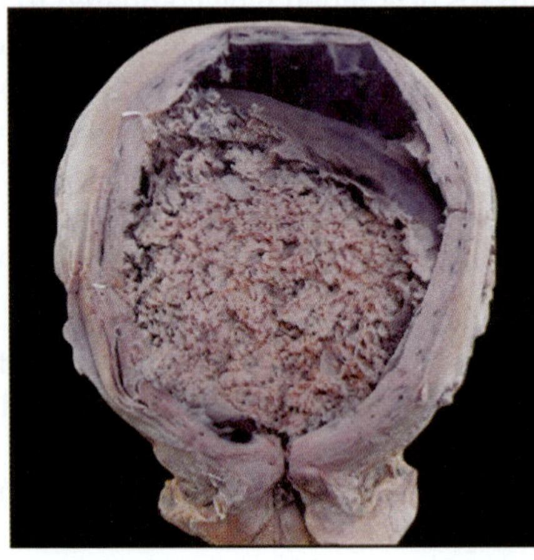

Fig. 1: Complete mole.
Courtesy: Department of Pathology, KMC, Mangalore.

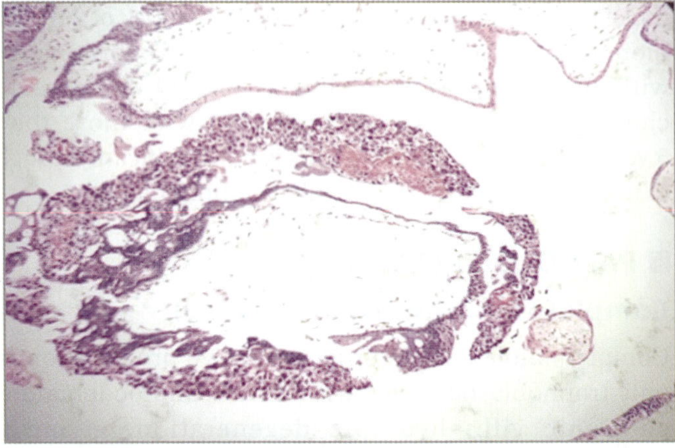

Fig. 2: Microscopic picture of complete mole.
Courtesy: Department of Pathology, KMC, Mangalore.

Microscopically, villi contain fluid-filled cisterns having a vesicular pattern, and the translucent and thin-walled nature earns the name—vesicular mole or hydatidiform mole. Prior to 8 weeks, characteristic features are not seen and hence difficult to differentiate from an abortus. Absence of proliferation on microscopy and immunohistochemistry [p57 (kip2)] helps to differentiate the two. The presence of foetal tissue is possible in twin pregnancy with one molar and the other normal foetus, which has to be differentiated from partial mole.

Partial Mole

The partial mole has a few enlarged villi alongside normal trophoblastic tissue. Presence of foetal tissue, which could sometimes be malformed, is pathognomonic of partial mole **(Fig. 3)**. Microscopy reveals two types of villi—large, oedematous with central cisterns and small with stromal fibrosis. Focal circumferential fibrosis gives a scalloped outline to the villi (Fjord-like) **(Fig. 4)** with identifiable foetal tissue and red blood cells (RBCs).

Ploidy studies play an important role in differentiating partial and complete moles. Complete moles are 46XX. They arise either by diandric diploidy (94%)—an empty pronucleus fertilised by haploid sperm undergoing duplication, or diandric dispermy (4%)—two sperms fertilise an empty egg **(Figs. 5A and B)**. A biparental complete mole can arise in women who are carriers for the mutation NLRP7 or KHDC3L. Partial moles are triploid in nature with 69 chromosomes—diandric triploidy—two sperms fertilise an oocyte **(Figs. 5A and B)**.

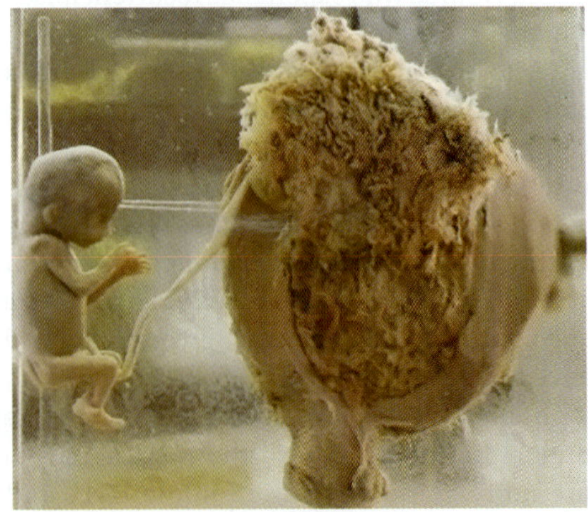

Fig. 3: Partial mole.
Courtesy: Department of Pathology, KMC, Mangalore.

Invasive mole (older terminology—chorioadenoma destruens, malignant mole, villous choriocarcinoma): When a molar pregnancy invades the myometrium or causes metastasis to distant organs, it is called an invasive mole. Grossly, a mass is seen protruding into the myometrium, and sometimes, there may be perforation. Microscopically, trophoblastic villi are seen within the myometrium or at distant sites. The clue is persistently elevated levels of serum hCG. It can be confused with choriocarcinoma. Invasive mole is more common than choriocarcinoma and can be distinguished based on microscopy.

Nonmolar Lesions

Choriocarcinoma: Choriocarcinomas arise from any antecedent pregnancy event, most commonly from molar pregnancy **(Table 3)**.

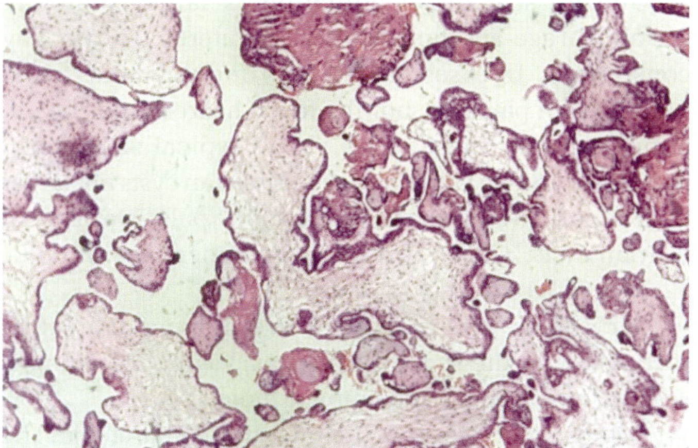

Fig. 4: Microscopic picture of partial mole.
Courtesy: Department of Pathology, KMC, Mangalore.

The tumour appears haemorrhagic **(Fig. 6)**. Microscopically, the absence of chorionic villi with cluster spread of syncytiotrophoblasts and cytotrophoblasts is pathognomonic. Nuclear pleomorphism with or without atypia is seen **(Fig. 7)**. Choriocarcinomas are highly metastatic, but extremely chemosensitive, resulting in high cure rates even if there is metastasis.

Differential diagnosis includes early gestational trophoblasts, exaggerated placental site, placental site trophoblastic tumour (PSTT), molar pregnancy or endometrial cancer.

Placental Site Trophoblastic Tumour

Placental site trophoblastic tumour is rare, arising from intermediate cytotrophoblasts or syncytiotrophoblasts. Grossly, it is a well-circumscribed solid tumour invading myometrium or protruding into the cavity, with haemorrhage and necrosis. Microscopically, cells resemble intermediary trophoblasts of the implantation site with mononuclear, abundant cytoplasm infiltrating and splaying smooth muscles and the vessel wall. Immunohistochemistry shows no hCG expression, although human placental lactogen (HPL) and inhibin are noted. Distant metastasis is rare.

Epithelioid Trophoblastic Tumours

Epithelioid trophoblastic tumours are rare tumours arising from the intermediate trophoblast of chorionic variety, following an antecedent normal pregnancy. They arise as a mass in the myometrium or cervix. They lack myometrial infiltration of PSTT. They stain with inhibin and cytokeratin 18 on immunohistochemistry.

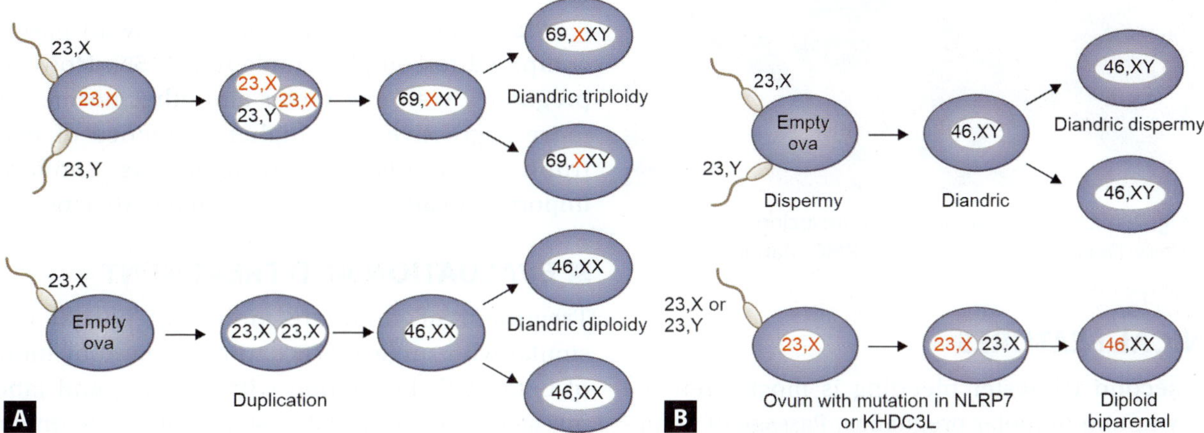

Figs. 5A and B: Aetiopathogenesis of molar pregnancy.

TABLE 3: Incidence of choriocarcinoma in relation to antecedent pregnancy.

Antecedent gestational event	*Incidence of choriocarcinoma*
Molar gestation	50%
Spontaneous abortion	25%
Normal pregnancy	22.5%
Ectopic pregnancy	2.5%

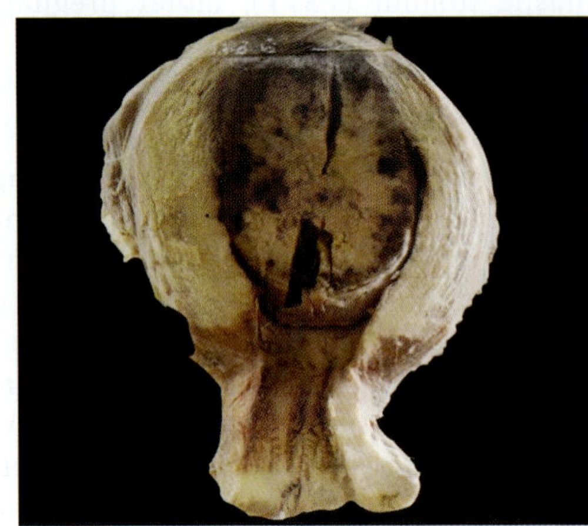

Fig. 6: Choriocarcinoma.
Courtesy: Department of Pathology, KMC, Mangalore.

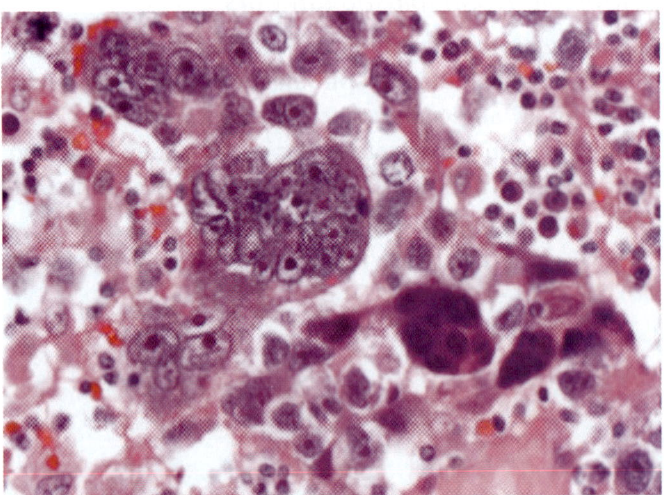

Fig. 7: Microscopic picture of choriocarcinoma.
Courtesy: Department of Pathology, KMC, Mangalore.

CLINICAL FEATURES

First or second trimester bleeding is most often the earliest symptom of molar pregnancy. Passage of grape-like vesicles is a late symptom heralding expulsion. These patients most often suffer from hyperemesis gravidarum. Features of hyperthyroidism are a possibility with molar pregnancy, either due to excessive hCG production mimicking thyroid-stimulating hormone (TSH) or TSH synthesised by trophoblastic tissue. Values of beta hCG can be as high as >1 × 10^5 mIU/mL. With current practices of antenatal care, a molar pregnancy is diagnosed during the dating scan, even before the symptoms present.

BOX 2: Complications of molar pregnancy.

- Early-onset pre-eclampsia
- Anaemia
- Uterine perforation
- Torsion/rupture of theca lutein cyst
- Respiratory distress
- Thyroid storm
- Persistent trophoblastic disease
- Malignant transformation (5%)

Uterine size on examination is larger than the gestational age-appropriate size of the uterus, with doughy consistency. In cases of second-trimester mole, foetal parts are not palpable, nor the foetal heart sounds heard. Sonography in these cases shows typical snowstorm appearance along with thin-walled ovarian cysts not larger than 10 cm; 25–50% of cases present with palpable bilateral ovarian cysts. The cysts resolve spontaneously within 8–12 weeks after molar evacuation.

Partial mole presents with fewer symptoms, most often recognised in the second trimester. Vaginal bleeding is seen in fewer cases than complete mole.

Sonographic features include cystic changes in the placenta and a possible nonviable or malformed foetus.

Patients may also present with features of complications due to molar pregnancy other than thyrotoxicosis, as mentioned in **Box 2**.

Malignant transformation is rare with partial mole compared to complete mole that is 5%. However, twin pregnancy with one molar and other normal twin are more aggressive with higher incidence of persistent trophoblastic disease and metastasis. Similarly, it is important to differentiate these from partial mole.

EVALUATION AND TREATMENT

Treatment of complete mole and partial mole are similar with surgical evacuation followed by monitoring of beta hCG. Evaluation with imaging and laboratory investigations along with histopathology are important in diagnosis, prognostication and staging of GTD along with identifying complications. Stepwise evaluation has been described in **Box 3**.

The procedure for evacuation of a mole has been described in **Table 4**.

Preevacuation preparation of the cervix with prostaglandin E2 (PGE2) is safe for use as recommended by the Royal College of Obstetricians and Gynaecologists (RCOG) despite the theoretical risk of embolisation. Use of mifepristone or misoprostol is currently not recommended in molar pregnancy.

BOX 3: Evaluation.

- Human chorionic gonadotrophin (hCG)
- Ultrasound
- Complete blood count
- Thyroid-stimulating hormone
- Liver function test
- Renal function test
- Electrolytes
- Chest X-ray

TABLE 4: Evacuation technique.

Preoperative preparation	• Address medical complications • Stabilise the patients' haemodynamics • Large-bore intravenous (IV) access • Adequate cross-matched blood to be reserved • Keep prepared for laparotomy • Prostaglandin E1 (PGE1) for priming of the cervix
Procedure	• Position in dorsal lithotomy after appropriate anaesthesia • Visualise and grasp cervix with atraumatic vulsellum or sponge holder • Do not sound the uterus • Cervix dilated by mechanical dilatation to accommodate a 12–14 mm suction cannula • Introduce the cannula gently to place the tip at the lower portion of the uterine cavity • It is now time to start an oxytocin infusion • Place the left hand on the fundus of the uterus to identify involution and reduce the risk of perforation • Cannula may be rotated • Following palpable involution (decreasing height of fundus) cannula may be advanced to scrape the uterine cavity and complete evacuation • Pitocin may be continued postevacuation • Anti-D administration required only in case of a partial mole with Rh-negative blood group

Hysterectomy is a procedure reserved for older women with no requirement of fertility preservation in an effort to reduce the risk of malignant transformation to 3.5% in comparison to uterine evacuation.

POSTMOLAR SURVEILLANCE

Regular follow-up is the key to the diagnosis of persistent trophoblastic disease and preventing complications. Enough emphasis is to be laid on this when counselling patients with GTD. Patients are advised to avoid conception for the initial 6 months of surveillance.

Regular estimation of beta hCG levels in the blood is mentioned in **Table 5**.

It is good practice to examine the patient at least monthly, with additional imaging whenever required. To rule out metastasis especially vaginal and lung metastasis with rising beta hCG titres.

Prophylactic chemotherapy is used in women who are at an increased risk of developing postmolar GTT **(Flowchart 1)**. However, considering recent evidence of developing drug resistance to methotrexate as well as the toxicity and complications of chemotherapy and considering the fact that prophylactic chemotherapy does not eliminate the risk of GTT completely, its routine use has fallen out of favour. Given the efficacy of treating postmolar GTD, most centres have given up prophylactic chemotherapy.

PERSISTENT TROPHOBLASTIC DISEASE

Persistent trophoblastic disease (PTD) complicates 3–25% of cases following molar pregnancy, of which 7–90% are likely to develop invasive mole, and only 10–30% have the propensity to develop choriocarcinoma. Metastatic disease, however, varies between 6% and 25%. Diagnosis is made with rising or plateauing levels or persistent high levels of beta hCG showing no signs of decline on postmolar surveillance or following ectopic pregnancy. Abnormal uterine bleeding after a term pregnancy also

TABLE 5: Beta human chorionic gonadotrophin (hCG) evaluation.

Frequency	*Duration*
48 hours postevacuation	
Weekly	Until 3 normal values
Once in 15 days	Up to 3 months
Monthly	Up to 6 months

Flowchart 1: Protocol for diagnosis and evaluation of low-risk gestational trophoblastic disease.

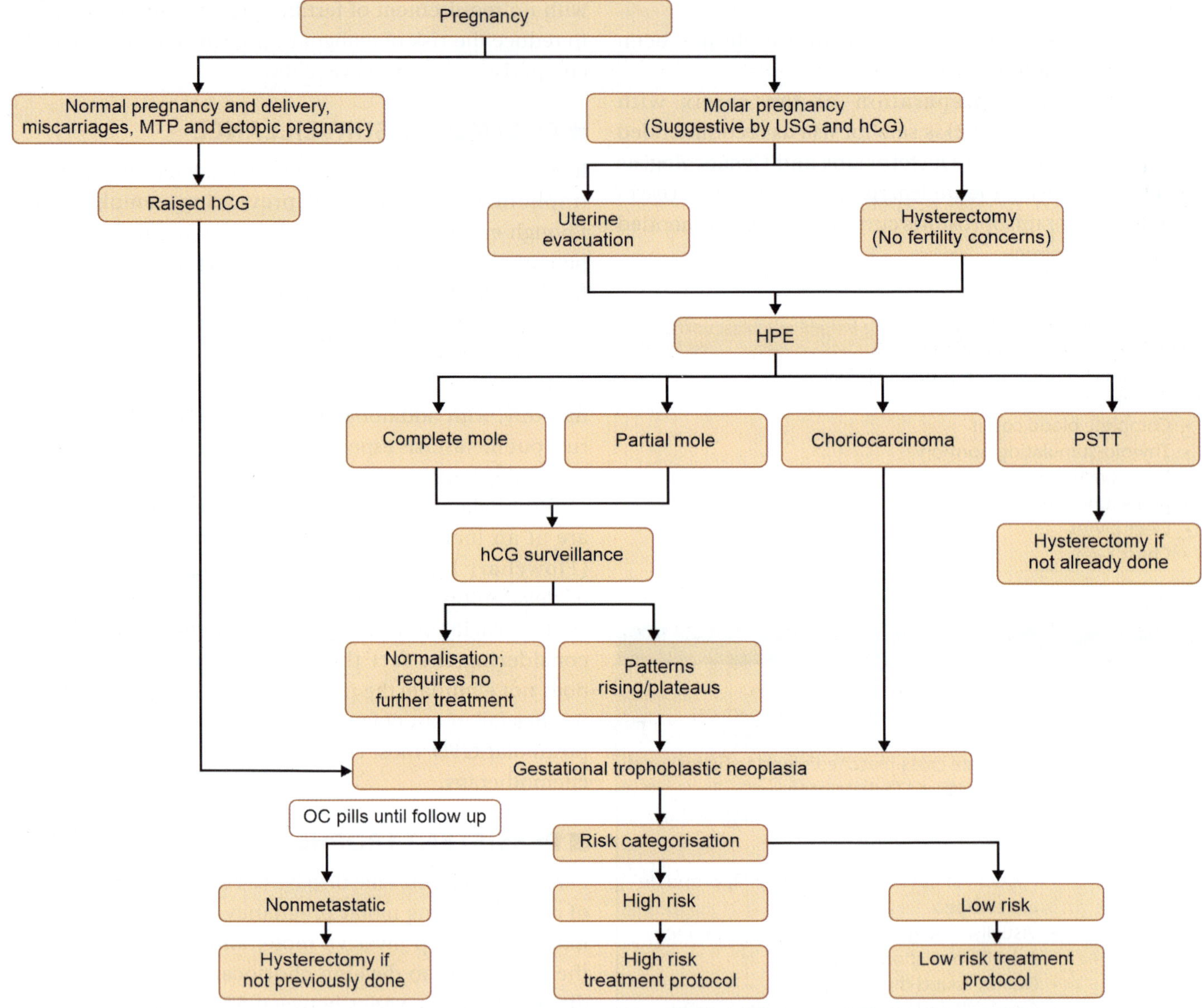

(hCG: human chorionic gonadotrophin; HPE: histopathological examination; MTP: medical termination of pregnancy; OC: oral contraceptive; PSTT: placental site trophoblastic tumour)

warrants beta hCG estimation to rule out PTD among other causes. PTD can also be diagnosed based on histopathological examination showing choriocarcinoma, PSTT or metastatic disease.

Parameters reflecting trophoblastic proliferation are mentioned in **Box 4**.

Chemotherapy should be started in all such cases of elevated beta hCG or vaginal bleeding. Suction evacuation for histopathological diagnosis is discouraged in view of complications such as uterine perforation and haemorrhage. Invasive trophoblastic antigen (ITA) has

BOX 4: Parameters that reflect trophoblastic proliferation.

- Uterine size is larger than period of gestation
- Bilateral theca lutein cyst
- Beta human chorionic gonadotrophin (hCG) >100,000 mIU/mL
- Hyperthyroidism
- Postevacuation haemorrhage, respiratory distress and subinvolution

100% sensitivity and specificity in diagnosing invasive mole. *Quiescent gestational trophoblastic disease* is a term used when persistently low (<50 mIU/L) levels are noted for a long period of time. Here, patients require surveillance without chemotherapy until beta hCG rises or ITA is positive.

Women with slightly higher (200–300 mIU/L) persistent levels of beta hCG may be a result of false-positive beta hCG assay caused by nonspecific heterophile antibodies termed as 'phantom hCG'. A case not responding to chemotherapy with persistent postchemotherapy values should be evaluated for this condition before subjecting them to second-line chemotherapy.

Other than being locally invasive PTD can present as metastatic disease with venous spread to vaginal plexus resulting in bluish suburethral vaginal nodule, which can lead to torrential haemorrhage. Mainstay of treatment is chemotherapy, however, vaginal packing followed by embolisation can be emergency management. Disease can also spread to distant sites such as lung, liver, brain, GI tract and kidneys. Lymphatic spread is rare. Methods used to evaluate PTD are mentioned in **Box 5**.

CLASSIFICATION AND STAGING OF GESTATIONAL TROPHOBLASTIC DISEASE

Many classification systems have evolved over the years, taking into consideration risk factors affecting prognosis, anatomical spread of disease, as well as resistance to single-agent chemotherapy.

Described in **Table 6** is the International Federation of Gynaecology and Obstetrics (FIGO) staging with the WHO prognostic scoring system adapted by FIGO. It is expressed by stage in Roman numerals separated by the sum of risk factor scores in Arabic numerals, separated by a colon, e.g. Stage II:6. A consolidated score of <6 is considered to be low risk.

BOX 5: Evaluation of persistent trophoblastic disease (PTD).

- Chest X-ray
- USG pelvis—to rule out pregnancy/tumours
- CT thorax, abdomen and pelvis
- MRI brain

TABLE 6: FIGO staging with WHO prognostic scoring system.

FIGO anatomical staging	*Stages* I. Disease confined to the uterus II. GTN spreads outside the uterus, limited to genital structures III. Lung metastases with or without genital tract involvement IV. Other metastases			
Modified WHO Prognostic Scoring System as Adapted by FIGO				
Scores	*0*	*1*	*2*	*4*
Age	<40 years	≥40 years	-	-
Antecedent pregnancy	Mole	Abortion	Term	-
Interval months from index pregnancy	<4	4–6	7–12	>12
Pretreatment serum hCG (IU/L)	$<10^3$	$10^3–10^4$	$10^4–10^5$	$>10^5$
Largest tumour size (including uterus)	<3 cm	3–4 cm	≥5 cm	-
Site of metastases	Lung	Spleen, kidney	Gastrointestinal	Liver, brain
Number of metastases	-	1–4	5–8	>8
Previous failed chemotherapy	-	-	Single drug	≥2 drugs
	Risk status • Low • High		Total score ≤6 ≥7	

(hCG: human chorionic gonadotrophin; FIGO: International Federation of Gynaecology and Obstetrics; GTN: gestational trophoblastic neoplasia; WHO: World Health Organization)

TREATMENT OF GESTATIONAL TROPHOBLASTIC TUMOURS

Chemotherapy is the mainstay in the treatment of GTN. Surgical management as well as radiation is also included in individual cases based on the recurrence, risk factors as well and to deal with complications. Low-risk patients, including those with metastatic disease, require less aggressive or single-dose chemotherapy **(Table 7)**. PSTT are considered high risk, and hysterectomy should be performed in these women. Choriocarcinoma, also termed high risk, requires chemotherapy as well as individual management of the metastasis **(Box 6)**. 100% cure rates are possible among low-risk patients. Failure of first-line chemotherapy warrants second-line course, and even such patients can expect 100% cure rates. Drugs used in low-risk cases include methotrexate, etoposide, actinomycin D and 5-fluorouracil. Regimens are described in **Table 8**. Multidrug regimens are reserved for patients who fail despite second-line chemotherapy. Monitoring is done by serial beta hCG measurements, and remission is achieved when three consecutive values have normalised. Chemotherapy is continued for one more cycle beyond remission.

Postchemotherapy surveillance includes beta hCG estimation as in **Table 9**. Contraception is suggested during the year of surveillance. A 10% increase in beta hCG on serial monitoring or appearance of metastasis indicates resistance to treatment. Recurrence ranges from 2.5% to 3.5% in low-risk GTT.

High-risk Gestational Trophoblastic Tumours

High-risk GTT requires multidrug chemotherapy. EMACO is the most commonly used combination with a success rate of 80–82% and hence the treatment of choice; however, several modifications, including cisplatin and others, have been used. Nausea, vomiting and alopecia are the most common side effects; neutropenia, thrombocytopenia and the development of secondary malignancies such as colon, breast cancers as well as myeloid leukaemia are possible toxaemias related to EMACO.

Relapse of high-risk GTN occur in 15–30% of patients requiring second-line chemotherapy and surgical resection of persistent disease/metastatic sites. The EMA-EP regime with overall success rate of 85%, is the combination of choice. VIP (cisplatin, vincristine and ifosfamide) combination are also used.

Those refractory to EMA-EP are found to benefit from taxane-based regimens. These multidrug regimens are required to be given for 2–3 cycles after normalisation of

TABLE 7: Low-risk gestational trophoblastic tumour.

Clinical classification	***Low-risk metastatic disease***
FIGO	Stage III or less
WHO	<6
Charing cross	<8

BOX 6: Indications for hysterectomy.

- Molar pregnancy in patients not desirous of fertility and advanced maternal age
- Placental site trophoblastic tumour (PSTT)
- Nonmetastatic gestational trophoblastic tumours

TABLE 8: chemotherapy options for low-risk malignant GTN.

Methotrexate	• 20–25 mg (0.4 mg/kg) IM Q day × 5 days (repeat in 7–14 days) • 30–50 mg/m^2 IM (repeat weekly)
Methotrexate and folinic acid	• Methotrexate 1 mg/kg IM/PO days 1, 3, 5, 7 alternating with folinic acid 0.1 mg/kg IM/PO days 2, 4, 6, 8 (repeat every 14 days) • Methotrexate 300–500 mg/m^2 IV followed by folinic acid 15 mg PO Q 6°× 4 doses (repeat every 14 days)
Actinomycin D	• 9–13 µg/kg IV Q day × 5 days (repeat every 14 days) • 1.25 mg/m^2 IV bolus (repeat every 14 days)
Methotrexate and actinomycin D	Methotrexate 20–25 mg (0.4 mg/kg) IM Q day × 5 days in week 1 alternating with actinomycin D 9–13 µg/kg IV Q day × 5 days in week 2 (repeat every 14 days)
5-FU	28–30 mg/kg/day (continuous 10-day infusion)
Etoposide	200 mg/m^2 for 5 days orally (repeat every 2 weeks)

(5-FU: 5-fluorouracil; GTN: gestational trophoblastic neoplasia; IM: intramuscular; IV: intravenous)

TABLE 9: Post-therapy beta hCG evaluation.

Frequency	***Duration***
Once in 2 weeks	3 months
Once a month	3 months
Once in 2 months	6 months

beta hCG. Peripheral stem cell therapy may also be tried in such patients.

MANAGEMENT OF METASTASIS

Lung metastasis: Identified by multiple pulmonary nodules on X-ray, not resolved after treatment. Lung resection is an option for those with residual disease.

Hepatic metastasis indicates a poor prognosis, with fatal hepatic haemorrhage being the complication. Radiation to the liver, hepatic artery embolisation or partial hepatectomy are therapeutic options.

Brain metastasis (10–15%) seen on frontal and parietal lobes presents with symptoms of raised intracranial pressure. Whole brain irradiation in combination with multidrug chemotherapy is the treatment. Intrathecal administration of the drug can also be used. Craniotomy and tumour resection are reserved for individual cases. Resection and anastomosis of the bowel is opted for when GI metastasis is identified. Vaginal nodules may require resection if they are the only site of metastasis. Radiation or embolisation may be used to control haemorrhage in these sites.

POSTCHEMOTHERAPY SURVEILLANCE FOR HIGH-RISK GESTATIONAL TROPHOBLASTIC TUMOURS

Postchemotherapy surveillance for high-risk GTT is for a period of 2 years after remission with serial beta hCG monitoring. Follow-up continues for 5 years after therapy. Pregnancy to be discouraged for 1 year after completion of treatment. Prognosis for high-risk GTT is 86% 5-year survival after treatment.

SUGGESTED READING

1. Alteri A, Franceshchi S, Ferlay J, Smith J, La Vecchia C. Epidemiology and aetiology of gestational trophoblastic diseases. Lancet Oncol. 2003;4(11):670-8.
2. American College of Obstetricians and Gynecologists (ACOG). Diagnosis and treatment of gestational trophoblastic disease. Washington (DC): American College of Obstetricians and Gynecologists (ACOG); 2004. p. 13. (ACOG practice bulletin; no. 53).
3. Azab M, Droz JP, Theodore C, Wolff JP, Amiel JL. Cisplatin, vinblastine, and bleomycin combination in the treatment of resistant high risk gestational trophoblastic tumors. Cancer. 1989;64(9):1829-32.
4. Bagshawe KD. Treatment of high risk choriocarcinoma. J Reprod Med. 1984;29:813-20
5. Ballal PK, Kushtagi P, Shetty N, Polnaya R. Variation in prevalence of gestational trophoblastic disease in India. Indian J Gynecol Oncol. 2016;14:41.
6. Benson CB, Genest DR, Bernstein MR, Soto-Wright V, Goldstein DP, Berkowitz RS. Sonographic appearance of first trimester complete hydatidiform moles. J Ultrasound Obstet Gynecol. 2000;16(2):188-91.
7. Berkowitz RS, Cramer DW, Bernstein MR, Cassells S, Driscoll SG, Goldstein DP. Risk factors for complete molar pregnancy, case control study. Am J Obstet Gynecol. 1985; 152:1016-20.
8. Bower M, Newlands ES, Holden L, Short D, Brock C, Rustin GJ, et al. EMA/CO for high risk gestational trophoblastic tumors: results from a cohort of 272 patients. J Clin Oncol. 1997;15:2636-43.
9. Costa HL, Doyle P. Influence of oral contraceptives in the development of post molar trophoblastic neoplasia: a systematic review. Gynecol Oncol. 2006;100(3):579-85.
10. Deng L, Yan X, Zhang J, Wu T. Combination chemotherapy for high-risk gestational trophoblastic tumour. Cochrane Database Syst Rev. 2009;2:CD005196.
11. DuBeshter B, Berkowitz RS, Goldstein DP, Bernstein MR. Vinblastine, cisplatin and bleomycin as salvage therapy for refractory high-risk metastatic gestational trophoblastic disease. J Reprod Med. 1989;34:189-92.
12. FIGO Oncology Committee. FIGO staging for gestational trophoblastic neoplasia 2000. Int J Gynecol Obstet. 2002;77:285-7.
13. Fowler DJ, Lindsay I, Seckl MJ, Sebire NJ. Routine pre-evacuation ultrasound diagnosis of hydatidiform mole: experience of more than 1000 cases from a regional referral center. Ultrasound Obstet Gynecol. 2006;27:56-60.
14. Gestational Trophoblastic Disease (Green-top guideline NO. 38). RCOG; 2010.
15. Gestational trophoblastic diseases: Report of a WHO scientific group. WHO Tech Rep Ser. 1983;692:51.
16. Gestational Trophoblastic Neoplasia. Union for International Cancer Control 2014. Review of Cancer Medicines on the WHO List of Essential Medicines.
17. Gordon AN, Kavanagh JJ, Gerhenson DM, Saul PB, Copeland LJ, Stringer CA. Cisplatin, vinblastine, and bleomycin combination therapy in resistant gestational trophoblastic disease. Cancer. 1986;58:1407-10.
18. Hammond CB, Borchert LG, Tyrey L, Creasman WT, Parker RT. Treatment of metastatic trophoblastic disease: good and poor prognosis. Am J Obstet Gynecol. 1973;115: 451-7.
19. Johns J, Greenwold N, Buckley S, Jauniaux E. A prospective study of ultrasound screening for molar pregnancies in missed miscarriages. Ultrasound Obstet Gynaecol. 2005;25:493-7.
20. Lorigan PC, Sharma S, Bright N, Coleman RE, Hancock BW. Characteristics of women with recurrent molar pregnancies. Gynecol Oncol. 2000;78:288-92.

21. Lurain JR, Brewer JI, Torok EE, Halpern B. Natural history of hydatidiform mole after primary evacuation. Am J Obstet Gynecol. 1983;145:591-5.
22. Lurain JR, Sand PK, Carson SA, Brewer JI. Pregnancy outcome subsequent to consecutive hydatidiform moles. Am J Obstet Gynecol. 1982;142:1060.
23. Ma Y, Xiang Y, Wan XR, Chen Y, Feng FZ, Lei CZ, et al. The prognostic analysis of 123 postpartum choriocarcinoma cases. Int J Gynecol Cancer. 2008;18(5):1097-101.
24. Newlands ES, Bagshawe KD, Begent RH, Rustin GJ, Holden L, Dent J. Developments in chemotherapy for medium and high risk patients with gestational trophoblastic tumors. (1979–1984). Br J Obstet Gynaecol. 1986;93: 63-9.
25. Newlands ES, Bagshawe KD, Begent RH, Rustin GJ, Holden L. Results with EMA/CO (etoposide, methotrexate, actinomycin D, cyclophosphamide, vincristine) regimen in high risk gestational trophoblastic tumors, 1979 to 1989. Br J Obstet Gynaecol. 1991;98:550-57.
26. Newlands ES, Mulholland PJ, Holden L, Seckl MJ, Rustin GJ. Etoposide and cisplatin/etoposide, methotrexate, and actinomycin D (EMA) chemotherapy for patients with high-risk gestational trophoblastic tumors refractory to EMA/Cyclophosapmide and vincristine chemotherapy and patients presenting with metastatic placental site trophoblastic tumors. J Clin Oncol. 2000;18:854-9.
27. Newlands ES, Paradinas FJ, Fisher RA. Recent advances in gestational trophoblastic diseases. Hematol Oncol Clin North Am. 1999;13:225-42.
28. Ngan HYS, Seckl MJ, Berkowitz RS, Xiang Y, Golfier F, Sekharan PK, et al. Update on the diagnosis and management of gestational trophoblastic disease. Int J Gynaecol Obstet. 2018;143 Suppl 2:79-85.
29. Palmer JR. Advances in the epidemiology of gestational trophoblastic disease. J Reprod. Med. 1994;39:155.
30. Royal College of Obstetricians and Gynaecologists. The management of gestational trophoblastic neoplasia. Green-top Guideline No. 38. London: RCOG; 2010. Available from: https://www.rcog.org.uk/files/rcog-corp/GT38ManagementGestational0210.pdf [Accessed April 2025].
31. Rustin GJ, Newlands ES, Lutz JM, Holden L, Bagshawe KD, Hiscox JG, et al. Combination but not single agent methotrexate chemotherapy for gestational trophoblastic tumors increases the incidence of second tumors. J Clin Oncol. 1996;14:2769-73.
32. Sebire NJ, Seckl MJ. Gestational trophoblastic disease: Current management of hydatidiform mole. BMJ. 2008;337:453-58.
33. Secakl MJ, Sebire NJ, Fisher RA, Golfier F, Massuger L, Sessa C, et al. Gestational trophoblastic disease: ESMO clinical practice guidelines for diagnosis, treatment and follow up. Annals Oncol. 2013;24(6):vi39-50.
34. Seckl MJ, Rustin GJ. Late toxicity after therapy for gestational trophoblastic tumours. In: Hancock BW, Newlands ES, Berkowitz RS, Cole LA (Eds). Gestational Trophoblastic Disease, 3rd edition. London: International Society for the Study of Trophoblastic Disease; 2003. pp. 470-84.
35. Sekharan PK. The management of gestational trophoblastic neoplasia FOGSI – ICOG consensus statement. SOGC Practice Guidelines. Gestational Trophoblastic Disease. J Obstet Gynaecol Can. 2002;24(5):434-9.
36. Soper JT, Evans AC, Conaway MR, Clarke-Pearson DL, Berchuck A, Hammond CB. Evaluation of prognostic factors and staging in gestational trophoblastic tumor. Obstet Gynecol. 1994;84:969-73.
37. Soper JT, Lewis JL, Hammond CB. Gestational trophoblastic disease. In: Hoskins WJ, Perez CA, Young RC (Eds). Principles and Practice of Gynecologic Oncology, 2nd edition. Philadelphia: Lippincott-Raven; 1996. pp 1039-77.
38. Soper JT. Trophoblastic disease update. In: Hawkins JL, editor. Obstetric anesthesia. Clin Obstet Gynecol. 2003;46(3).
39. Takeuchi S. Incidence of gestational trophoblastic disease by regional registration in Japan. Hum Reprod. 1987;2:729.
40. Tidy JA, Rustin GJ, Newlands ES, Foskett M, Fuller S, Short D, et al. The presentation and management of women with choriocarcinoma after non molar pregnancy. Br J Obstet Gynaecol. 1995;102(9):715-9.

11

CHAPTER

Breast Function and its Disorders

Shripad Hebbar, Rajani Upadhyaya, Muralidhar V Pai

Chapter Outline

- Breast Development
- Developmental Anomalies of the Breast
- Breastfeeding and Lactation
- Endocrine Disorders (Galactorrhoea and Breast Atrophy)
- Benign Breast Condition
- Screening for Breast Diseases
- Benign Breast Disease
- Breast Cancer
- Epidemiology

BREAST DEVELOPMENT

The female breasts (mammary glands) develop rapidly between the age groups of 10 and 20 years. The adolescent breast development takes place according to sexual maturity rating, and the breast bud development is the first sign of puberty in girls at around 8 years of age.

Embryologically, the breasts (mammary glands) develop on the mammary line/ridge, which is a thickened ectoderm from the axilla to the inguinal region.

On this mammary line, the ectoderm thickens as a mass of epidermal cells and projects into the dermis in the pectoral region and this forms the mammary glands on both sides. About 15–20 outgrowths arise from this thickened epidermal mass and grow into the dermis to get surrounded by fat and vascular and connective tissue. The distal part of these outgrowths forms secretory elements and the proximal part cannulates to form lactiferous ducts. All the ducts open into a pit which becomes elevated to form a nipple. The breast lobes develop at puberty in response to endocrine stimulation **(Figs. 1 and 2)**.

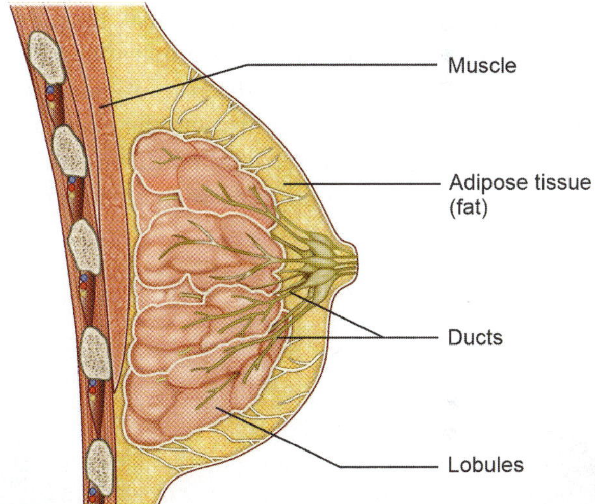

Fig. 1: Side view of breast.

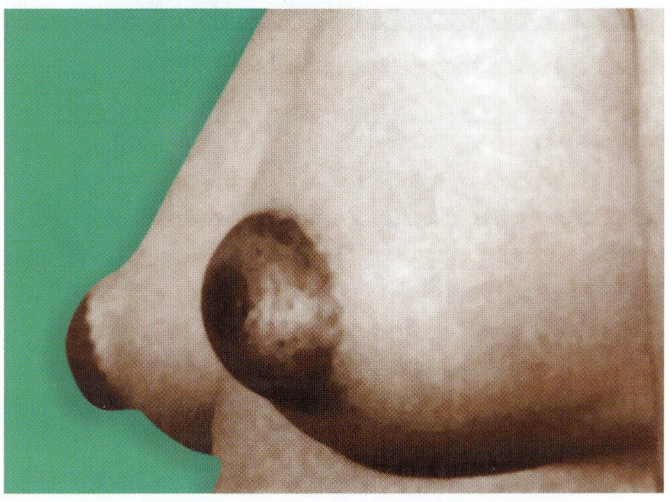

Fig. 2: Areolar bud (Patient on oestrogen therapy).

Stages of Breast Development at Puberty

The embryological origins of breast tissue date back to the fifth week of gestation, with the formation of the mammary ridge. Recent studies emphasise the role of mesodermal-ectodermal interactions in forming the glandular and stromal components. Anomalies during this stage can lead to clinical conditions such as polymastia or polythelia.

At birth, the breast is a simple system of ducts without alveoli. By 9–10 years, female breasts begin to enlarge, but, first, the area around the nipples enlarges.

- The ducts and acini develop in the next 3–4 years.
- By menarche, there is fat deposition and breasts become prominent and round.
- Further enlargement of breasts occurs till 18 years of age.
- Prepubertal development is mainly due to oestrogens from the ovary and also due to growth hormone and adrenal corticoids.
- The hormones that are required by a nonlactating breast to grow are oestrogens, progesterone, growth hormone, insulin, cortisol, thyroxine and prolactin (PRL) **(Fig. 3)**.
- The receptors in mammary glands (cytoplasm of mammary epithelium) depend on PRL, and these receptors respond to oestrogen. Adequate fat deposition is also needed for normal breast development, and this adipose tissue provides a loose matrix for glandular and ductal expansion under hormonal stimulation.
- Recent studies emphasise the role of mesodermal–ectodermal interactions in forming the glandular and stromal components. Anomalies during this stage can lead to clinical conditions such as polymastia or polythelia.

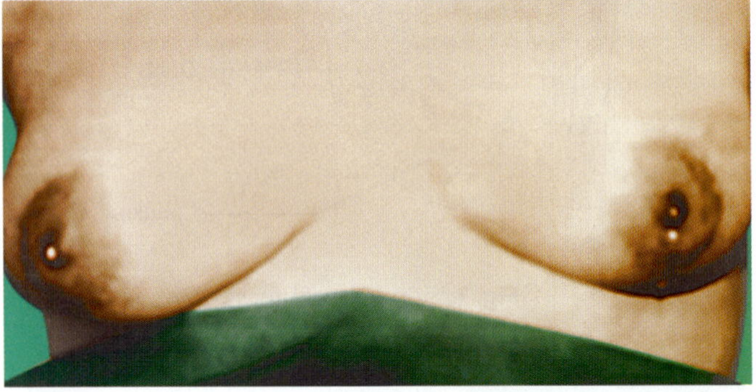

Fig. 3: Chiari–Frommel syndrome.

- The morphological changes in breasts at puberty are described by Tanner in five stages (P1–P5) **(Fig. 4)**.

Tanner's Staging (Fig. 5)

- *P1:* Prepubertal (Breast bud only)
- *P2:* Early development of subareolar bud, widening of areolae, small amount of labial or axillary hairs
- *P3:* Increase in the size of palpable breast tissue and areolae. Increased dark pubic hair on mons veneris and axillary hair and characteristic body odour
- *P4:* Further increase in breast size and areola that protrudes above breast level. Adult sexual hair but limited to pubes. Acne and menarche may occur.
- *P5:* Adult breast and areolae. Adult amount and distribution of pubic hair with extension to upper thigh. Menarche occurs.

Endocrine Control of Female Breast

The mature breasts undergo a cycle that corresponds to the ovarian cycle. Oestrogen will stimulate ductal elements, whereas oestrogen and progesterone stimulate glandular elements and increase in water content of the breast. In the luteal phase, there is an increased epithelial activity (slight secretion) in the ducts and acini; this regresses during menstruation. The breast as a whole increases in size during a week before menstruation, and this is mainly due to congestion and oedema of the connective tissue between lobules. This is manifested as premenstrual heaviness, pain and tenderness in the breasts **(Table 1)**.

During pregnancy, there is an active development of both ducts and acini (many acini are formed for the first time). The breast enlarges and its vascularity increases. The acini secrete a small amount of glairy fluid (colostrum). The development of the breast during pregnancy is endocrine

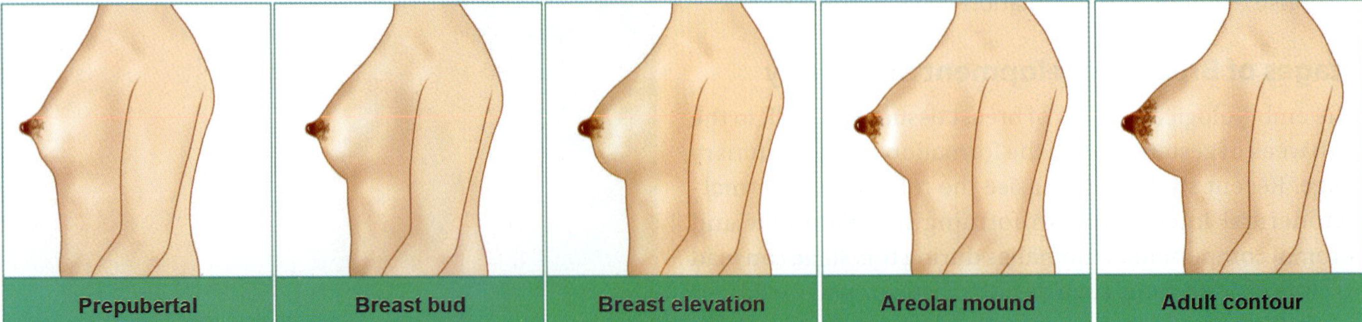

Fig. 4: Morphological changes in the breast at puberty.

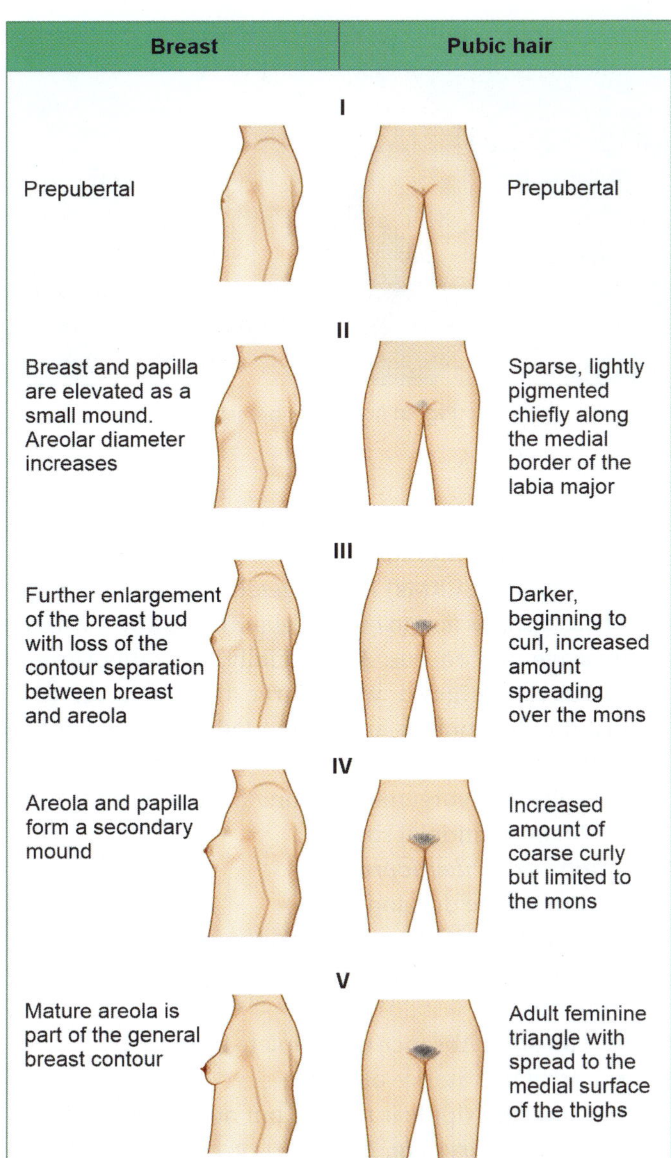

Fig. 5: Tanner's staging.

hormone (oestrogen + progesterone) dependent for full preparation for lactation and is also dependent on an adequate diet, corticosteroids and PRL (placental or pituitary) **(Fig. 6)**.

At menopause, as the level of sex steroid hormones decreases, the breast tissue, both glandular and stromal, undergoes atrophy. The breast size will decrease, and this may also contribute to psychological disturbance during menopause. The breast is also an important secondary sexual organ, and it is an erogenous zone, the stimulation of which aids in orgasm. Breasts give women a female identity; hence, changes in breast size and problems with breast cause a lot of psychological upset and trauma.

Recent insights into receptor-mediated pathways reveal the intricate balance of oestrogen and progesterone, not only in glandular development but also in influencing breast cancer risk. Emerging research on HER2 (human epidermal growth factor receptor 2) and ER (oestrogen receptor) receptors provides promising therapeutic avenues.

DEVELOPMENTAL ANOMALIES OF THE BREAST

The breast development may show various anomalies, which are seen during the adolescent growth period and cause a lot of psychological trauma. The breast anomalies are classified as follows:

- *Congenital anomalies* ***(Figs. 7 to 9):***
  - Absence
  - Supernumerary
  - Ectopic position (accessory breast/nipple)
  - Midline webbing
  - Retracted nipples

TABLE 1: Endocrine control of female breast development and function from prepubertal stage to pregnancy.

Stage	***Duct system***	***Major hormones***	***Permissive hormones***
Prepubertal		None	Unknown
Adult		Oestrogen (Progesterone)	
Pregnancy		• Progesterone • Prolactin • Human placental lactogen	• Insulin • Thyroxine • Glucocorticoids • Growth hormone

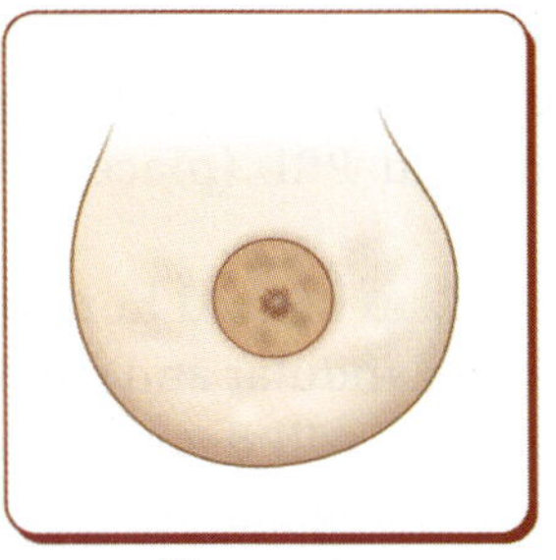

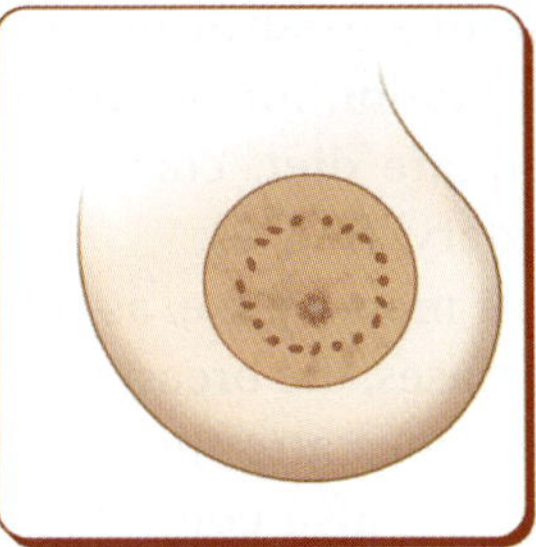

Fig. 6: Breast enlargement in pregnancy and lactation.

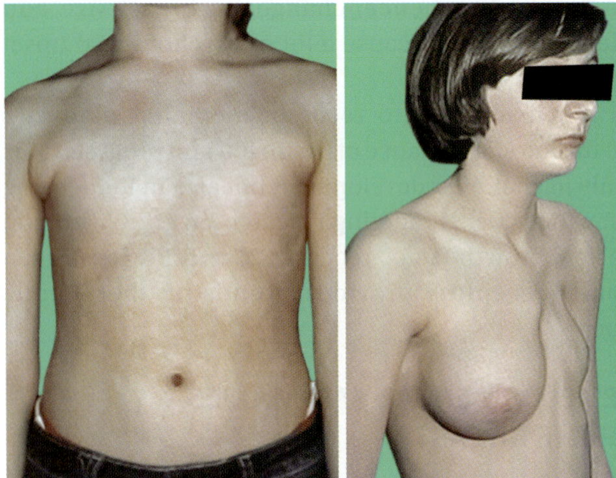

Fig. 7: Bilateral athelia and unilateral amazia.

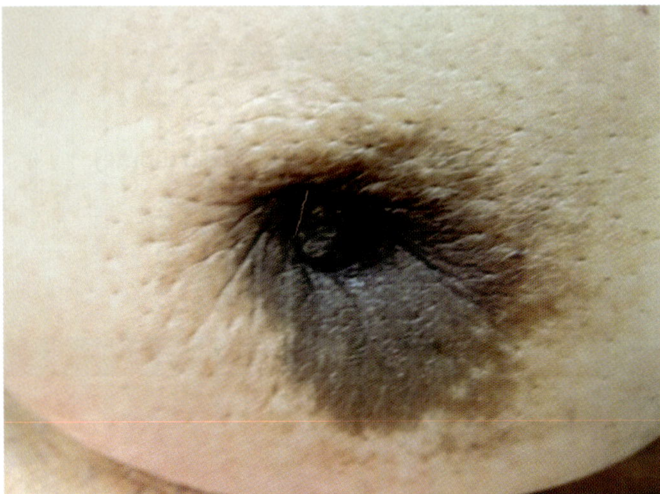

Fig. 8: Retracted nipple.

- *Modification of physiological response:*
  - Hypoplasia or aplasia
  - Asymmetry
  - Hypertrophy

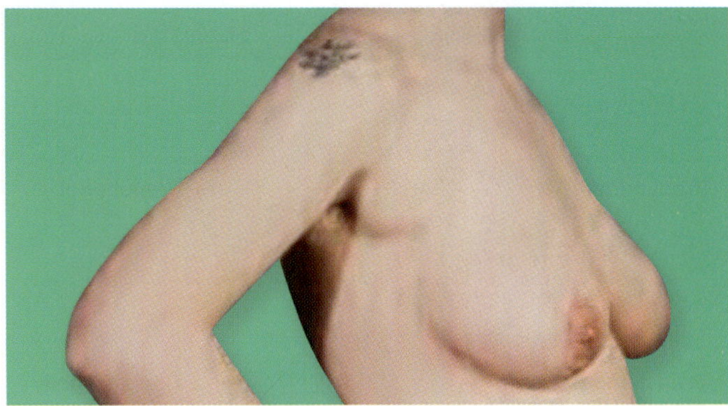

Fig. 9: Accessory breast.

New therapeutic approaches for managing hypertrophy include selective oestrogen receptor modulators (SERMs) and targeted endocrine therapy. These options aim to control glandular growth without invasive procedures. Additionally, wearable support systems designed with three-dimensional (3D) printing technology are being trialled for nonsurgical symptom management.

  - Painful engorgement (neonatal or pubertal)
  - Malformation of shape
- *Faulty sexual development:*
  - Premature development
  - Delayed or failure of development
  - Changes in pregnancy and lactation
- *Absence:*
  - *Amastia:* Absence of complete breast
  - *Athelia:* Absence of nipple
  - *Amazia:* Nipple is formed but not breast tissue
- *Supernumerary **(Fig. 10)**:*
  - *Polymastia:* Multiple breast
  - *Polythelia:* Multiple nipples
  - *Polythelia areolaris:* Only multiple areolas
  - Only glandular tissue
- Ectopic position of nipple or breast (accessory breast and nipples)
- *Symmastia:* Midline webbing between breasts

Congenital breast anomalies should be identified early, and mostly reassurance and counselling are needed for corrective surgery in most of the cases. Recent advancements have identified the role of maternal hormones in the development of congenital anomalies, including polythelia and polymastia.

Imaging techniques like high-resolution ultrasound and MRI are increasingly being used to diagnose accessory

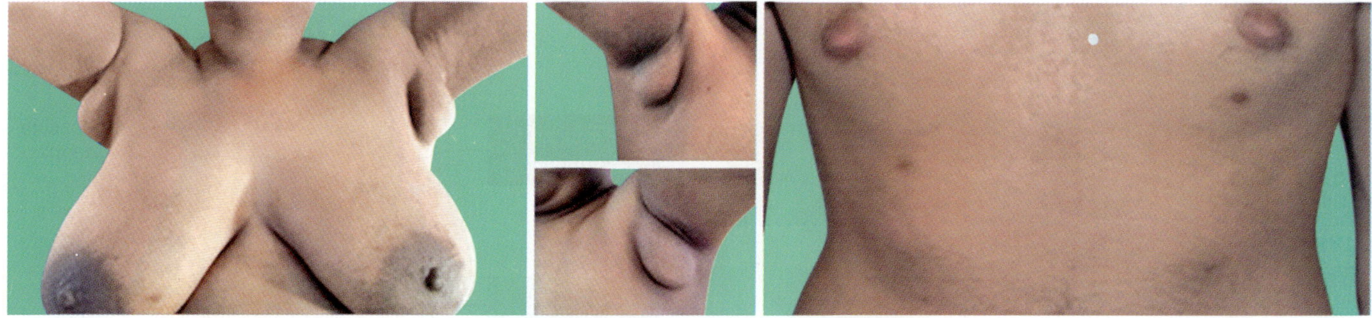

Fig. 10: Polythelia versus polymastia.

breast tissue, providing more precise surgical planning for corrective procedures. The surgeries done for such anomalies are augmentation mammoplasty, surgical removal of supernumerary breast or nipples, mammary prosthesis or glandular flap for unequal breasts.

Modification of Physiological Response

Aplasia or Hypoplasia

Varying degrees of underdeveloped breasts are seen in young women and are usually due to fat and glandular tissue. The treatment for hypoplasia ranges from good diet, exercises of pectoral muscles, massage, oestrogen therapy in cases of low ovarian oestrogens and plastic surgery.

Fat grafting for hypoplasia has seen improvements with the addition of platelet-rich plasma, enhancing graft survival rates and promoting vascularisation. Long-term studies are currently evaluating the efficacy of combining stem-cell enriched grafts with minimally invasive surgical techniques.

True hypertrophy (not adiposity) is uncommon. The cause is not yet known and it affects glandular tissue and not nipples. It is usually bilateral and is seen at puberty. These breasts may weigh as much as 6–13 kg. These breasts will further develop hypertrophy during pregnancy and lactation, but they do not lactate. Treatment is support or surgical reduction (subtotal mastectomy). Bromocriptine may be of some benefit during pregnancy.

Asymmetry

Like other paired organs, the breast will show some inequality in size. However, in 7% of cases, the disparity in size disappears as woman grows. Breast measurement is done with a centimetre tape from 3 o'clock to 9 o'clock and then from 12 o'clock to 6 o'clock over the nipples. The two measurements are multiplied, and the figure is called 'breast unit'. The right breast normally tends to be slightly larger than the left breast **(Table 2)**. The fault of asymmetry of breasts is always an inherent fault in target tissue; hence, endocrine treatment is of no value. If the asymmetry is too much, then surgery is the only answer (usually reduction of the larger breast and sometimes enlargement of the smaller).

TABLE 2: Breast unit.

Age (years)	Right breast		Left breast	
	Measure (cm)	Unit	Measure (cm)	Unit
14	19 × 13	247	18 × 14	252
15	21 × 17	357	17 × 20	340
16	22 × 18	396	18 × 21	378

Painful Engorgement (Mastitis) (Neonatal or Adolescent)

Breasts of male or female babies sometimes become enlarged and hard for 3–4 days after birth. This is due to congestion related to the withdrawal of the influence of maternal oestrogens. A discharge may also occur from the nipple, known as 'witch's milk'. No treatment is required. Adolescent mastitis is a nodular, painful enlargement of the breasts in both boys and girls. It is due to an upsurge of pituitary hormones. No treatment is required. Reassurance and sometimes analgesics might be required for symptom relief. A well-fitting brassiere may be used for breast support.

Malformation of Shape

Usually, the malformation involving the inferior quadrant will be present with various degrees of severity. Minor malformations are high submammary sulcus, hypoplasia of the inferior quadrant. Major malformations are flatness of the whole inferior quadrant, leading to 'funnel breast' or

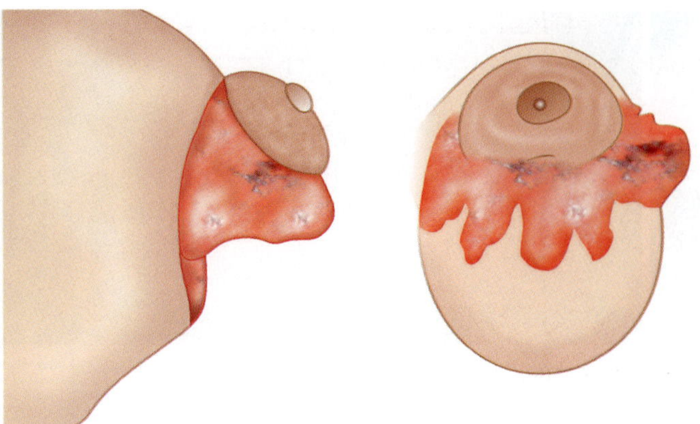

Fig. 11: Tubular breast: Excision of glandular tissue.

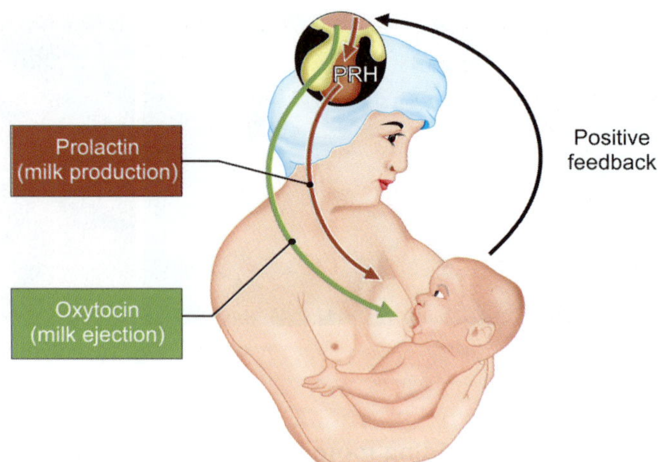

Fig. 12: Physiological changes. (PRH: prolactin-releasing hormone)

'tubular breasts,' also known as 'nipple' breast or 'snoopy' breasts. Surgical correction is the only treatment **(Fig. 11)**.

Faulty Sexual Development

Premature Development

Where breast growth starts before the age of 8 years (premature thelarche), it is due to increased organ sensitivity. This is usually self-limiting. If breast growth is associated with other secondary sexual characters and menstruation, then it is known as 'precocious puberty.'

Delayed or Failure of Development of the Breast

Absence of breast growth by the age of 14 years is regarded as abnormal. If menses is normal, then it is hypoplasia due to the target organ receptor. If amenorrhoea is there, then the causes could be gonadal dysgenesis, pituitary-hypothalamic lesion or androgen-producing tumours. Complete endocrine and genetic investigations with CT skull may be required.

Delayed breast development can now be analysed with advanced endocrine profiling and genetic sequencing, allowing early interventions with customised therapies. This includes targeted hormone replacement for individuals diagnosed with receptor insensitivity or hormonal pathway deficiencies.

Changes in Pregnancy and Lactation

The mature breast is a collection of sweat glands modified during evolution to produce milk. Developed breast (mammary gland) has stroma and glands, which consist of fat, connective tissue, ducts and lobuloalveolar system. Breasts undergo mammogenesis during pregnancy.

Anatomic Changes

- General enlargement up to two to three times
- Increased vascularity and engorgement of superficial veins
- Brown pigmentation of the areola
- *Raised areas of areola:* Montogomery's tubercle
- Formation of secondary areola
- Increased erectility of breasts
- Nodularity of breasts
- Secretion of a glairy fluid (colostrum)
- Pain and tenderness

Anatomic changes are more pronounced in primigravida rather than multigravida.

Physiological Changes ***(Fig. 12)***

- Mammogenesis
- Lactogenesis
- Galactokinesis
- Galactopoiesis

The preparation of breasts (mammogenesis) begins during pregnancy. Synthesis and secretion of milk (lactogenesis) occur due to high PRL and a fall in oestrogen and progesterone after delivery of the placenta. The understanding of lactogenesis has evolved with the identification of key molecular signals like signal transducer and activator of transcription 5 (STAT5) and mammalian target of rapamycin (mTOR) pathways, which regulate milk production. Innovative lactation aids, such as wearable biosensors, are also emerging to help monitor milk flow and prevent lactation-related complications.

The hormones responsible for mammogenesis or lactogenesis are cortisol, growth hormone, thyroxine and insulin. Galactokinesis is a centrally mediated reflex of milk letdown. Galactopoiesis is the maintenance of lactation and depends on frequent suckling of the breast by the infant.

BREASTFEEDING AND LACTATION

Breast milk is universally recognised as the preferred nutrition for infants. Exclusive breastfeeding is promoted internationally as optimum feet up to 4–6 months. Breast milk is nutritionally and immunologically superior to any substitute. The advantages of breastfeeding to the infant are nutrition, fat demand of the baby, lactose content, protein content, vitamins and minerals and protective role against infections [due to immunoglobulin A (IgA), lactoferrin, bifidus factor, unsaturated fatty acids, antibodies, lactoperoxidase, interferons and chemotactic factor]. Breastfeeding also has benefits for the mother:

- Breastfeeding women return to the prepartum state faster
- Lower risk of premenopausal breast cancer
- Inhibits ovulation, hence contraceptive value

Other advantages include:

- Economic
- Benefits to the community and the country
- Ecologic benefits
- Psychological advantages
- *Other benefits to baby:* Minerals, protective role, lactoferrin, bifidus factor, unsaturated fatty acids, antibodies and nonspecific factors against viruses, other cellular components and development of brain and central nervous system (CNS).

The benefits of breastfeeding also extend to the mother and these include:

- Faster return to prepartum state
- Low risk of long-term osteoporosis
- Lower risk of premenopausal breast cancers
- Exclusive breastfeeding, inhibits ovulation and hence delays the return of fertility (contraceptive benefits).

The role of healthcare professionals is very important in initiating breastfeeding in women during the first few days of hospital stay. The World Health Organization (WHO) and the United Nations Children's Fund (UNICEF) have also launched the Baby-Friendly Hospital Initiative (BFHI) in India as a part of a global effort to protect, promote and support breastfeeding.

Recent studies have highlighted the importance of exclusive breastfeeding for up to 6 months, with evidence showing long-term benefits in preventing childhood obesity and reducing maternal risk of type 2 diabetes. New guidelines emphasise the role of lactation consultants in supporting mothers during the early postnatal period.

Special Conditions

Breastfeeding can be reliably continued in various maternal health problems, except in heart failure, severe lung and kidney diseases and severe psychosis or postnatal depression. Mastitis and breast abscess do not contraindicate breastfeeding. In mothers suffering from open tuberculosis, breastfeeding can be continued, and the infant should be given prophylactic isoniazid. Breast milk is a primary form of immunisation for the infant; hence, in human immunodeficiency virus (HIV) and hepatitis B-infected mothers, the benefits overweight the risk of transmission. Maternal malnutrition does not affect breast milk; however, extreme prematurity and bilateral cleft palate may be a contraindication.

In HIV-positive mothers, antiretroviral therapy during lactation has been shown to significantly reduce the risk of vertical transmission without compromising the nutritional benefits of breast milk. For mothers with mastitis, recent data suggest that probiotics may aid in faster recovery alongside conventional treatments.

Breast Diseases in Lactation

The most common problems during lactation are mastitis and abscess formation. The mother may develop tender, painful masses of galactoceles, which can be diagnosed and cured by aspiration. Fibroadenomas may enlarge and become painful due to infarction. Breast cancer diagnosis becomes delayed if it occurs during lactation.

Advanced imaging techniques, such as high-resolution ultrasound, are now recommended for the early diagnosis of galactoceles and mastitis. Additionally, new minimally invasive procedures, like ultrasound-guided aspiration, have shown high success rates in managing breast abscesses.

Failure of Lactation

Lactation fails if not initiated by early suckling. In 70% of the cases, lactation can be restored by counselling, good nutrition, rest and frequent suckling. If there is

TABLE 3: Ratio of drug distribution in milk/plasma.

Drug type	*M:P ratio*
Lipid soluble	+1
Water soluble (with molecular weight 200)	+1
Weak acids	≤1
Weak bases	≥1
Actively transported drugs	>1

complete failure (agalactia) or very less breast milk, then a galactagogue may be tried (chlorpromazine or metoclopramide). Also, it is possible to induce breast milk in nonpuerperal mothers.

Emerging therapies for agalactia include the use of domperidone, a safer alternative to metoclopramide, and nonpharmacological interventions like acupuncture. Early initiation of breastfeeding within the first hour of birth remains the most effective strategy for preventing lactation failure.

Suppression of Lactation

In some conditions, breast milk needs to be suppressed up to 60–70%. This can be achieved by no suckling and breast support. Drugs used for suppression are oestrogen and progesterone and androgen combination. This combination can reduce engorgement and discomfort, but there is a risk of thromboembolism and rebound engorgement. Pyridoxine is a cheap and effective drug for lactation suppression. Bromocriptine is effective but has side effects. Cabergoline in a single 1 g dose is very effective.

Drugs and Lactation

Safety of prescribing any drug during lactation is questioned and a thorough knowledge of pharmacokinetics excretion in breast milk and probable hazards to the infant should be kept in mind. Drug therapy beneficial to mother and not detrimental to infant is the ultimate goal. **Tables 3 to 6** and **Boxes 1 and 2** include safe and unsafe drugs.

The updated list of contraindicated drugs now includes newer antiretrovirals and immunosuppressants, which may enter breast milk and pose risks to infants. Real-time lactation pharmacology databases are becoming indispensable tools for healthcare providers in prescribing safe medications during lactation.

TABLE 4: Drugs with limited safety in lactation.

Anthraquinones	*Nalidixic acid*
Barbiturates (safe in low doses)	Oral contraceptives (safe in low doses)
Cimetidine	Phenylbutazone
Indomethacin	Reserpine
Isoniazid	Sulphonamides
Methyldopa	Tetracycline
Metronidazole	Thiazide diuretics

TABLE 5: Probable safe drugs in lactation.

Alcohol	*Erythromycin*	*Nitrofurantoin*
Ampicillin	Folic acid	Paracetamol
Antihistamines	Frusemide	Penicillin
Caffeine	Gentamycin	Pentazocine
Carbamazepine	Guanethidine	Pethidine
Carbenicillin	Heparin	Phenothiazines
Cephaloridine	Heroin	Potassium iodide
	Imipramine	Propantheline
Chlordiazepoxide	Iron	Quinine
Chloroquine	Kanamycin	Salicylates
Chlorpromazine	Lincomycin	Sodium fusidate
Codeine	Mefenamic acid	Streptomycin
Desipramine	Methylergometrine	Thyroxine
Dichloralphenazone	Morphine	Tolbutamide
Digoxin	Nitrazepam	Warfarin

ENDOCRINE DISORDERS (GALACTORRHOEA AND BREAST ATROPHY)

Galactorrhoea

About 5–10% of normally menstruating women and 22% of infertile women have a milky discharge from breast nipples known as galactorrhoea. Milk discharge from nipples can be scanty or abundant expressed or spontaneous, intermittent or persistent and unilateral or bilateral. Galactorrhoea needs to be evaluated in nulliparous women and in women who have stopped breastfeeding for a year. Nipple discharge can be confirmed as milk by examining on a slide with coverslip under a microscope to see for fat droplets.

TABLE 6: Analgesics and anti-inflammatory drugs.

Drugs	*Quantity in milk*	*MP ratio*	*Adverse effects (infant)*	*Comments*
Aspirin	Trace	<1	Platelet	Cautious use
Mefenamic acid	Negligible	–	NS	Compatible
Indomethacin*	Excreted	0.37	Seizures and may be nephrotoxic	Compatible
Morphine	Trace	–	Neonatal addition in high doses	Compatible
Phenylbutazone	Trace	0.13	NS	Compatible
Pentazocine	Not excreted	None	NS	Compatible

(NS: not significant)
*Case report.

BOX 1: Factors affecting drug transfer into milk.

Maternal pharmacology:
- Drug dose, frequency and route of administration
- Clearance rate
- Plasma protein binding
- Metabolite profile

Breast:
- Blood flow and pH
- Yield capacity
- Ion and other transport mechanisms

Milk:
- Composition (fat, protein, water)

Infant:
- Suckling time and amount/feed
- Feeding intervals

Drug:
- PKa
- Solubility characteristics in fat
- Protein binding characteristics, molecular weight

BOX 2: Drugs contraindicated in lactation.

- Antineoplastic
- Diazepam
- Lithium
- Phenindione
- Radiochemicals
- Amiodarone

Recent findings suggest a connection between galactorrhoea and increased stress hormone levels, which may indirectly affect PRL secretion. Mind-body interventions, such as yoga and meditation, are being explored as complementary therapies.

Prolactin is a polypeptide secreted from the anterior pituitary gland and also by chorion, endometrium and decidua. Normal midmorning fasting levels of PRL are 0–20 ng/mL. PRL release is in pulses every 1–1.5 hours more in night time (circadian rhythm). Secretion is highest from midnight to 6 AM. PRL secretion is affected by eating, stress (physical or mental) exercise and sexual intercourse (but rarely >30 ng/mL).

In pregnancy, levels may increase up to 100–200 ng/mL, i.e. 5–10 times from the 10th week onwards, and during postpartum, levels may go up by 15 times, i.e. up to 300–600 ng/mL. **Figure 13** shows how PRL hormone is regulated.

Pathophysiology of Galactorrhoea (Fig. 14)

The final pathway for milk discharge from breast is an oestrogen-primed breast and hyperprolactinaemia. All the cases of hyperprolactinaemia may not have galactorrhoea (28%). Idiopathic galactorrhoea may occur without a PRL rise, and one-third of these women may menstruate normally.

Causes of Galactorrhoea (Table 7)

The most common cause is due to pituitary tumours (seen in 40% of the cases) and due to drugs.

Clinical Features

- Oligomenorrhoea
- Amenorrhoea
- Dysfunctional uterine bleeding
- Luteal phase defects
- Infertility
- Hirsutism
- Osteoporosis

Galactorrhoea can cause a spectrum of physical and emotional challenges, including fatigue and anxiety

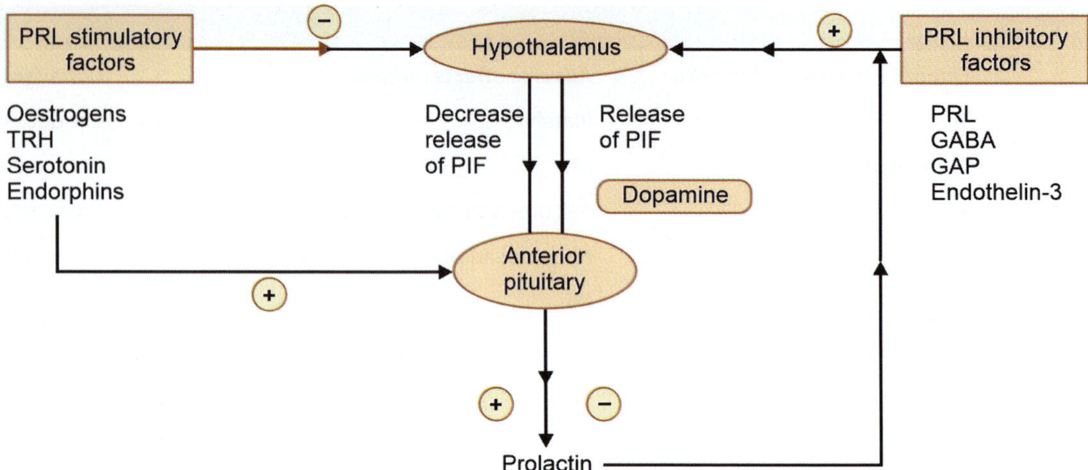

Fig. 13: Control of prolactin secretion. (GABA: gamma aminobutyric acid; GAP: GnRH-associated protein; PIF: prolactin-inhibiting factor; PRL: prolactin; TRH: thyrotropin-releasing hormone)

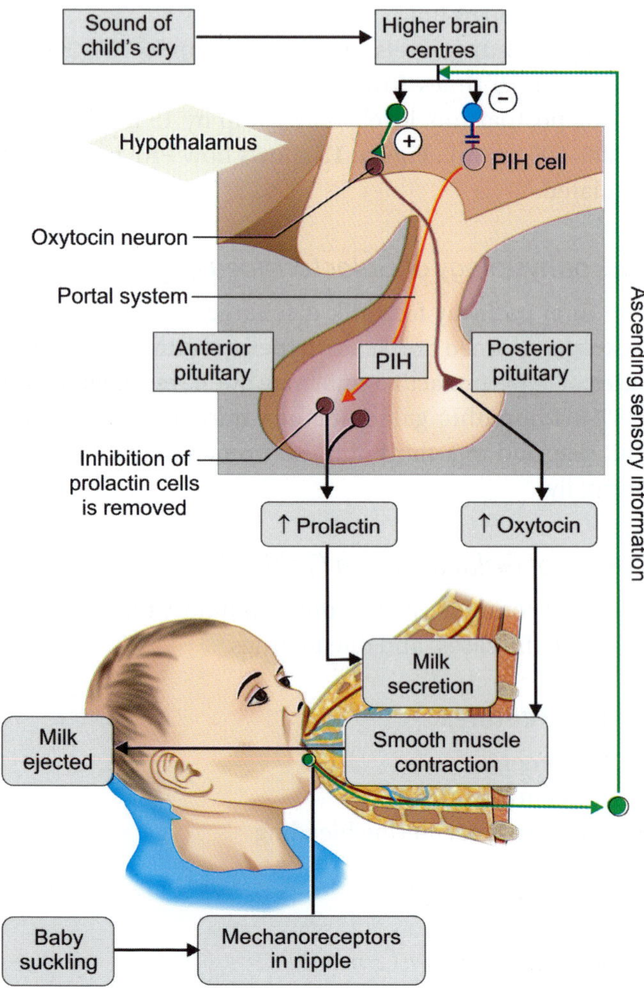

Fig. 14: Galactopoiesis reflex. (PIH: pregnancy-induced hypertension)

linked to underlying hormonal imbalances. Addressing these symptoms holistically is gaining traction in clinical practice.

Diagnosis

All the preliminary routine mandatory investigations include serum PRL, thyroid and renal function tests. A serum PRL should be done on two occasions as a mid-morning fasted, nonstressed, no drugs and in the follicular phase of the menstrual cycle **(Table 8)**.

The introduction of serum PRL bioassays has enabled the differentiation between biologically active and inactive PRL forms, improving diagnostic precision and reducing unnecessary interventions.

Table of Levels

Screening for pituitary tumours is done by imaging sella turcica using the various imaging modalities, as shown in **Table 9**.

Endocrinal tests to discriminate hypothalamic and pituitary causes include **(Table 9)**:

- Gonadotrophin-releasing hormone (GnRH) stimulation
- Thyrotropin-releasing hormone (TRH) stimulation

Endocrine tests do not give any additional value than a coned-down view of the sella turcica. Visual field examination is not useful as these may be altered only in very large tumours, which are evident by radiological examination.

TABLE 7: Causes of galactorrhoea.

Cause		***Mechanism***
I	Pharmacological	Certain drugs
II	Persistent breast stimulation	Neurogenic reflexes from chest and nipples to CNS decrease PIF and release oxytocin
III	*Chest lesions:* • Thoracotomy scars • Herpes zoster, cervical spinal lesions	
IV	• Hypothalamic dysfunction • Chiari–Frommel syndrome (Galactorrhoea persists after delivery) • Del–Castillo syndrome (Galactorrhoea without antecedent delivery)	Psychogenic disturbance alters brain transmitters that decrease PIF
V	Forbes–Albright syndrome (it signifies an organic brain lesion):	
	A. *Pituitary tumour:* Prolactinomas (micro and macro), mixed growth hormone/PRL secreting (acromegaly), mixed ACTH/PRL secreting (Cushing's disease)	Hypersecretion of prolactin
	B. *Nonpituitary lesions:* Craniopharyngioma, empty sella syndrome, other tumours (pinealoma, meningioma, astrocytoma metastasis, neurofibromatosis head trauma, encephalitis)	Pituitary stalk compression
VI	Primary hypothyroidism	TRH stimulates PRL release
VII	Renal disease	Decreased excretion of PRL
VIII	*Ectopic prolactin-secreting tumours:* Bronchogenic carcinoma, hypernephroma leiomyoma	Ectopic prolactin secretion
IX	Idiopathic	

(ACTH: adrenocorticotrophic hormone; CNS: central nervous system; PIF: prolactin inhibiting factor; PRL: prolactin; TRH: thyrotropin-releasing hormone)

Treatment

Treatment depends on aetiology, stopping aggravating drugs and treating hypothyroidism, chest lesions and renal disease. If a pituitary tumour is diagnosed, there are three options: Medical, radiation or surgery.

In cases of microadenoma, only close surveillance in noninfertile parous women is the treatment option.

TABLE 8: Correlation of PRL levels in nonpregnant, nonlactating women.

Prolactin levels (ng/mL × 43.86 = Pmol/mL)	***Probable diagnosis***
≤20 ng/mL	Normal
20–100 ng/mL	Functional or tumour
100–200 ng/mL	Very suggestive of a tumour
200–300 ng/mL	Tumour present in 90% of cases
>300 ng/mL	Tumour is invariable
>34–386 ng/mL	Pregnant women

(PRL: prolactin)

Breast Atrophy

Breasts are a symbol of femininity, maternal and sexuality. Having not well-formed breasts and small atrophic breasts after puberty have a psychological feeling of disfigurement, loss of womanhood, social rejection or isolation. Breast atrophy or deformity is the most emotionally and devastating feature of physical deformities in women.

Classification

- *Developmental breast hypoplasia (micromastia):*
  - Congenital
  - Iatrogenic
- *Late-onset breast atrophy:*
  - Postpartum
  - Postmenopausal
  - Secondary breast atrophy
  - Idiopathic

Innovative therapies, such as bioidentical hormone replacement and laser-based collagen stimulation, are now being tested for their efficacy in reversing early stages of breast atrophy with minimal side effects.

Aetiology

Causes of small breasts are shown in **Table 10**.

Clinical Features and Evaluation

- Age (adolescent, postpregnancy, postmenopausal)
- History (weight loss or gain)

TABLE 9: Imaging techniques of sella turcica.

Lateral coned-down view of sella turcica	*Computer axial tomographic scan in coronal plane with intravenous contrast (enhancement CT scan)*	*Magnetic resonance imaging (MRI)*
Detects macroadenoma and craniopharyngioma	Uses 1 mm slices of the pituitary gland and hypothalamus. It visualises pituitary tissue and surrounding soft tissue. Therefore, it can diagnose microadenoma, suprasellar extension and empty sella syndrome	Best imaging technique for sella turcica: It gives a resolution of 1 mm, is more sensitive than a CT scan, and gives better accuracy in assessing extrasellar extension and empty sella syndrome. It has no biological hazard
Advantages: Cheap and easily available		
Disadvantages: • It is not very sensitive for small tumours as interpretation is dependent upon bony changes occurring in sella turcica secondary to tumour enlargement • In large tumours, it cannot detect suprasellar extension	*Disadvantages:* • *High cost:* They typical radiation exposure during CT scan results in 3 rads dosage delivery to pituitary and 7 rads to eye lens. Repeated exposures may result in cataract formation and multiple CT scans should be avoided	*Disadvantages:* • Very expensive • Requires a lengthy period of time to obtain images

TABLE 10: Causes of small breasts.

Clinical type	*Causes*
Developmental breast hypoplasia	• Congenital • *Iatrogenic in prepubertal age:* – Trauma – Infections – Incision – Radiation therapy
• *Late-onset breast atrophy:* – Postpartum atrophy – Postmenopausal atrophy – Secondary atrophy	Hormonal
	Oestrogen deficiency • *Endogenous factors:* – Neoplasms – Adrenal and ovarian tumours – Non-neoplastic conditions – CAH – Late-onset CAH – Cushing's syndrome – PCOD
	• *Exogenous-drug induced:* – Androgens and anabolic steroids – Danazol, Dilantin – Minoxidil, diazoxide – Oral contraceptives
Idiopathic	Unknown viral

(CAH: congenital adrenal hyperplasia; PCOD: polycystic ovarian disease)

- Development (puberty/pregnancy/lactation)
- Endocrine (secondary sex characters)
- Breast masses
- Family history of breast cancer
- Psychological
- Medical diseases

In secondary breast atrophy:

- Virilism
- Congenital adrenal hyperplasia (CAH) or Cushing's disease
- Ovarian tumours

Laboratory Tests

- 17 ketosteroids and hydroxyketosteroids in urine
- Plasma testosterone and free testosterone
- Plasma androstenedione, luteinising hormone (LH), follicle-stimulating hormone (FSH) and PRL
- Adrenal and ovarian vein studies
- CAT scan and MRI
- Ultrasound
- Laparoscopy

Management

Look for underlying causes in the adolescent group and treat them to increase breast size. Mammary augmentation surgery is required **(Flowchart 1)**.

Flowchart 1: Management of breast atrophy.

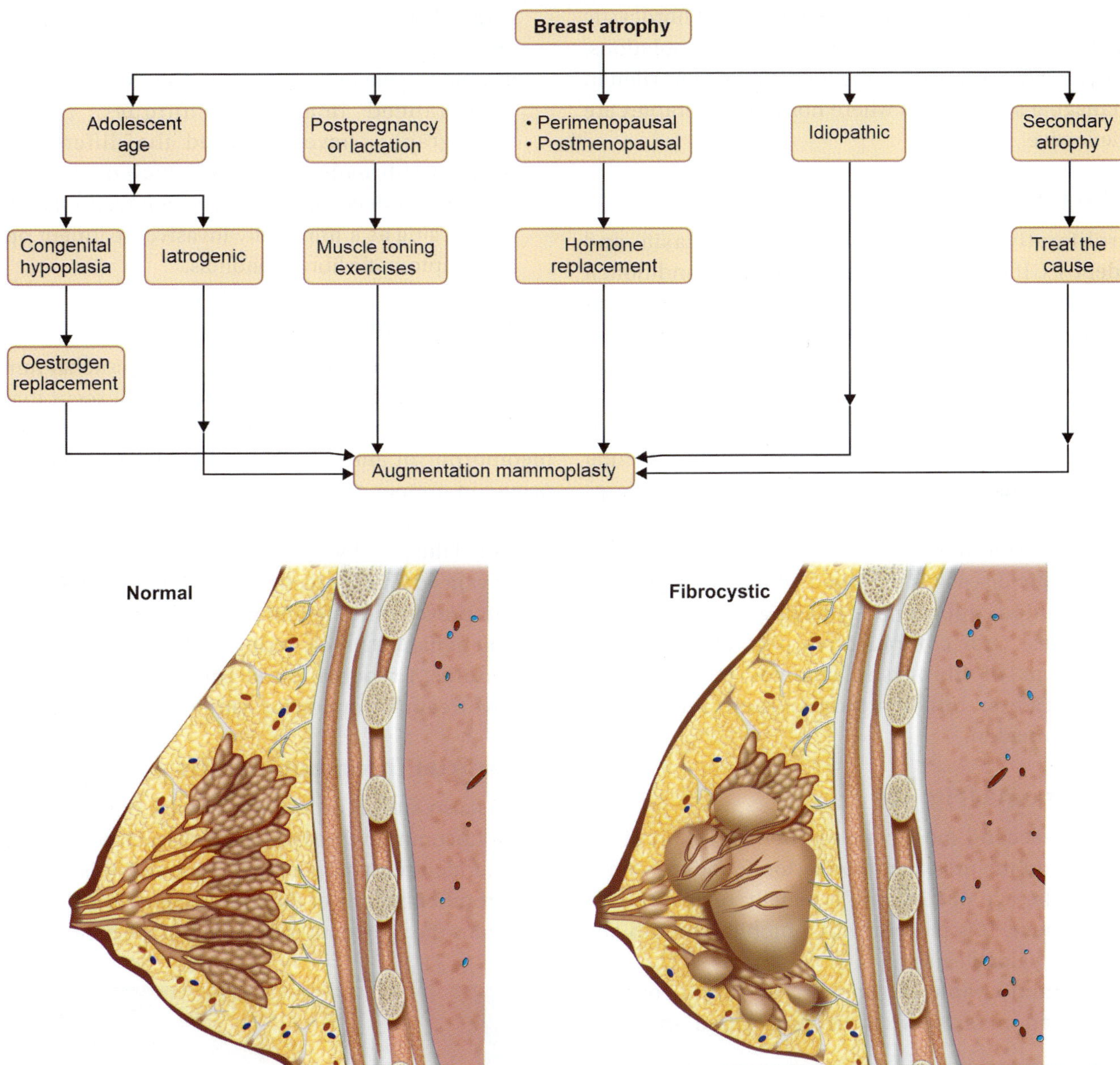

Fig. 15: Fibrocystic changes.

BENIGN BREAST CONDITION

Fibrocystic Changes (Fig. 15)

- It is the most common benign breast condition in women. It is because of the fluctuating hormone levels and is commonly found in premenopausal women between 20 and 56 years. It is usually bilateral and associated with pain and tenderness, especially during the premenstrual phase of the cycle.
- Fibrocystic change is not a precancerous condition in majority of the women.
- Two histological changes are noted with fibrocystic changes—proliferative and nonproliferative.

- Recent studies highlight the role of iodine supplementation in reducing symptoms of fibrocystic changes, particularly in iodine-deficient populations. Research has also shown the potential of tamoxifen in managing severe cases where hormonal therapies are ineffective.

Proliferative Changes

- Proliferative changes include hyperplasia and adenosis. If atypia is associated with this condition, it has a fivefold increase in breast cancer risk. Adenosis is caused by changes in the active distal mammary nobble. Sclerosing adenosis may present as a palpable mass in women.
- Ductal proliferation can lead to papilloma, which is a papillary lesion with a branching of fibrovascular cone present with serosanguineous nipple discharge in 25–50% of the patients and a small palpable mass adjacent to the areola 90% of the time.
- Fibrocystic disease is managed with regular physical examination, appropriate imaging and supportive measures. Oral contraceptive pills also suppress symptoms of fibrocystic changes in 70–90% of the patients, but symptoms often recur after discontinuation.

Fibroadenoma (Fig. 16)

- It is the second most common benign lesion of the breast and the most common lesion found in women under the age of 25 years. It usually regresses after menopause. It is present with a mobile, smooth and painless palpable mass.
- On mammography, it appears as round, oval or lobulated masses with circumscribed margins; fibroadenoma rarely converts to carcinoma. It requires surgical treatment if it continues to enlarge; fine-needle aspiration (FNA) or core biopsy is inconclusive or yields atypia or the patient desires for excision.

Advanced imaging techniques, including elastography, have improved the differentiation between fibroadenomas and malignant masses, reducing the need for invasive procedures. Cryoablation is emerging as a minimally invasive treatment option for symptomatic fibroadenomas.

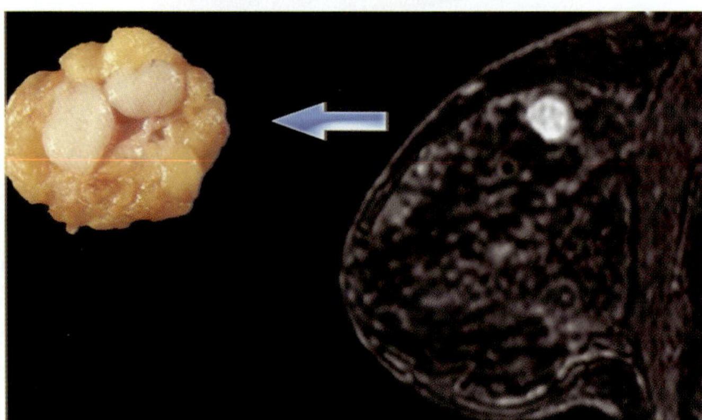

Fig. 16: Fibroadenoma.

Phyllodes Tumour

It is an uncommon, slow-growing fibroepithelial tumour. It is very much similar to fibroadenoma, except that the stromal component is hypercellular with increased pleomorphism and mitotic activity. It more commonly occurs in premenopausal women. Malignant conversion is rare. Treatment is by total surgical exclusion with a wide margin of the healthy tissue **(Fig. 17)**.

Advanced imaging techniques, including elastography, have improved the differentiation between fibroadenomas and malignant masses, reducing the need for invasive procedures. Cryoablation is emerging as a minimally invasive treatment option for symptomatic fibroadenomas.

Superficial Thrombophlebitis

- It is also known as Mondor disease of the breast. It is an uncommon disease, usually associated with breast trauma, breast surgery or pregnancy. It is because of thrombophlebitis of the thoracoepigastric vein, which drains the upper outer quadrant of the breast.

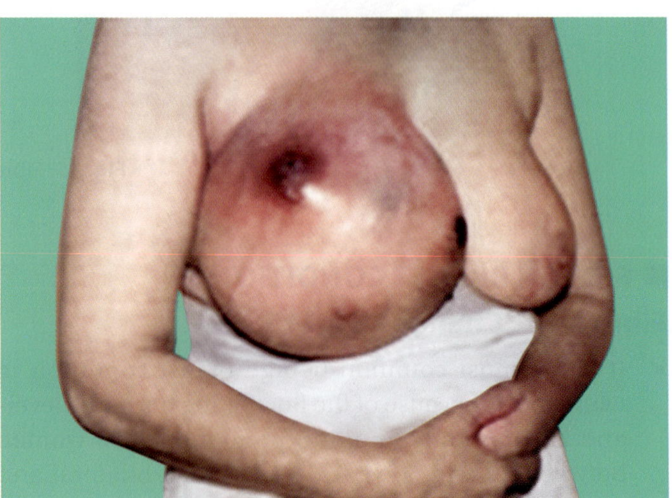

Fig. 17: Phyllodes tumour.

- Analgesics and application of heat are the treatment options.

  Recent advancements suggest that topical heparin and nonsteroidal anti-inflammatory drugs can significantly alleviate symptoms of Mondor disease. Ultrasonography is increasingly used to confirm the diagnosis and rule out deeper vein involvement.

Mastitis (Fig. 18)

It is because of the skin-organising *Staphylococcus aureus* and *Streptococcus* causing infection of nipple and breast ducts. It usually occurs during lactation because milk is an excellent medium for infection.

Probiotic therapy has shown promise in reducing the recurrence of mastitis by promoting a healthy microbiome. Ultrasonographic guidance is now recommended for the drainage of abscesses to minimise surgical interventions.

- The treatment is with antibiotics. If antibiotics fail, mastitis may progress to breast abscess formation, which requires incision and drainage of pus. Probiotic therapy has shown promise in reducing the recurrence of mastitis by promoting a healthy microbiome. Ultrasonographic guidance is now recommended for the drainage of abscesses to minimize surgical interventions.

Duct Ectasia (Fig. 19)

This usually occurs in premenopausal or postmenopausal women. Patients usually present with a hard, tender mass adjacent to the areola with a thick greenish-black discharge. This may be present in some cases.

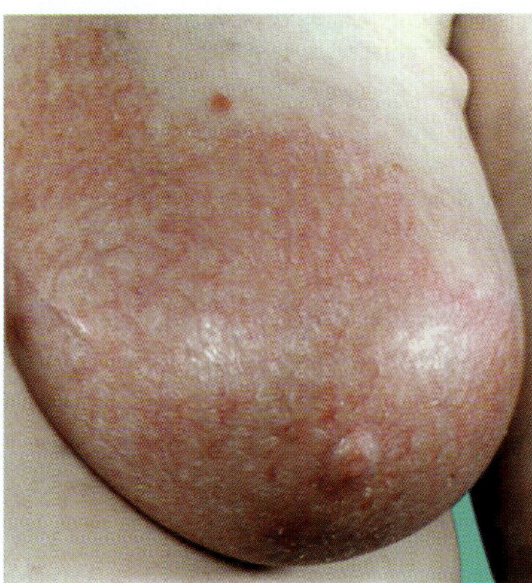

Fig. 18: Mastitis.

The role of chronic inflammation in duct ectasia is being actively researched, with anti-inflammatory therapies emerging as potential treatments. MRI is proving valuable in distinguishing duct ectasia from malignancies.

Fat Necrosis (Figs. 20 and 21)

It is an uncommon benign condition caused due to breast trauma. Mass can mimic a carcinoma. On mammography, multiple calcifications are seen. It does not increase the risk of carcinoma but has to be differentiated from it.

High-resolution mammography combined with digital breast tomosynthesis (DBT) is enhancing the differentiation of fat necrosis from malignant lesions, reducing unnecessary biopsies. Autologous fat transfer

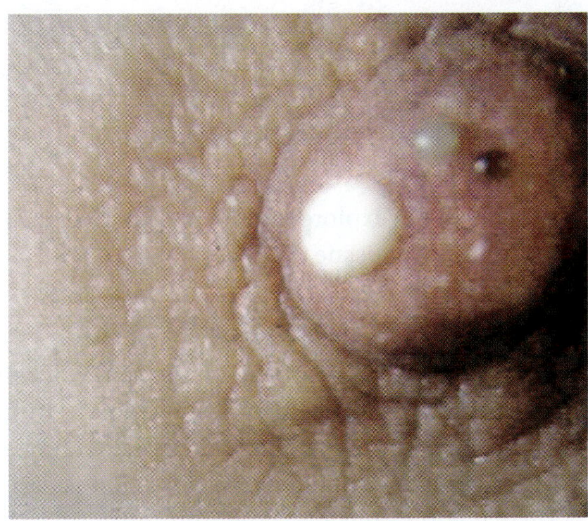

Fig. 19: Duct ectasia.

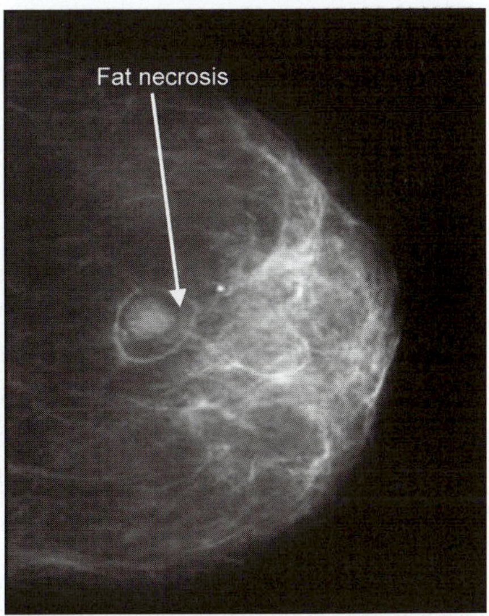

Fig. 20: Fat necrosis.

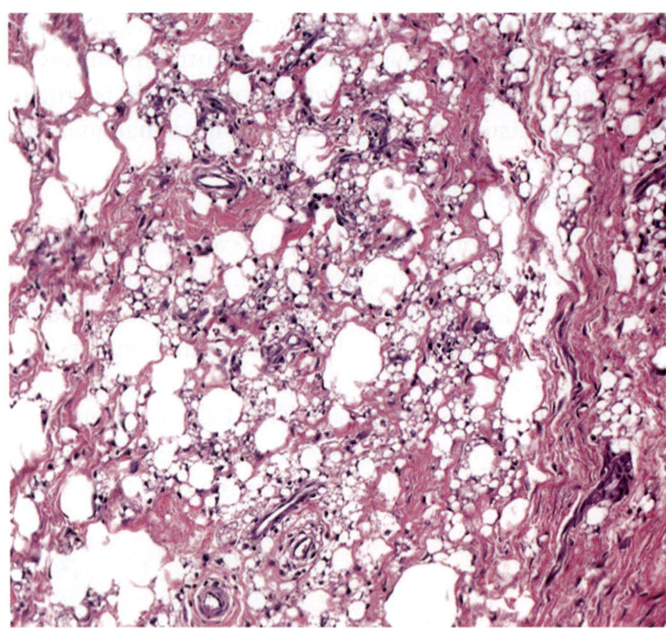

Fig. 21: Histology of fat neurosis.

techniques are being explored for reconstructive purposes in cases of significant tissue damage.

SCREENING FOR BREAST DISEASES

In the western countries, breast cancer is the foremost killer. The incidence is as high as 1 in 9 women. In India, breast cancer is second to cervical cancer in incidence and mortality. To reduce mortality, early detection is essential and statistics show that by screening mortality can be reduced by 25% **(Table 11)**.

TABLE 11: Breast cancer screening methods.

Age (years)	*Methods*	*Comments*
Starting 20s	*Breast self-exam:* The technique should be reviewed by a health professional during a physical examination	Women may find a breast lump by chance or be aware of what is abnormal (lump, swelling, skin irritation, dimpling, nipple pain or retraction). Women may feel stressed by trying to perform the self-exam technique correctly
20s–30s	Clinical breast exam by a health professional at least every 3 years	Provides an opportunity for women and health professionals to discuss any changes in their breasts, early detection testing and risk factors
40s and older	Per ACS, mammogram every year and continue as long as in good health. The USPSTF recommends biennial screening mammography for women aged 50–74 years	Very effective and valuable method to detect breast cancer; however, a mammogram will miss some cancers and sometimes give false-positives
High-risk women	MRI and mammogram every year for women having a lifetime risk of breast cancer ≥20%; BRCA1 or BRCA2 gene mutation (or first-degree relative); radiation therapy to the chest between ages 10 and 30 years; or certain genetic syndromes*	MRI is not recommended for women with a lifetime risk of breast cancer <15%. MRI can detect cancer better than a mammogram, but it can miss some cancers that a mammogram can detect

*Li-Fraumeni syndrome, Cowden syndrome, Bannayan–Riley–Ruvalcaba syndrome, or first-degree relatives with one of the syndromes.
(ACS: American Cancer Society; BRCA: breast cancer susceptibility gene; USPSTF: US Preventive Services Task Force)

Risk Factors

Age

At the age of 70 years, a woman has 10 times more risk than a 40-year-old. Screening will benefit women aged 50–69 years most as there will be a 29% reduction in mortality. Recommended screening is 2-yearly mammography (National Cancer Institute). As the incidence of breast cancer is <10% before 40 years, these women benefit maximum by screening. 20% of women in the 30–54 years age group and 29% of women aged 55–84 years are at risk. Every woman is assumed at risk and must be screened.

Genetics (Familial)

Almost 5–10% of breast cancer cases are seen to have a familial pattern over many generations. The relative risk is 1.5–2 with one first-degree relative and 4–6 with two first-degree relatives. *BRCA-1* gene on the long arm of chromosome 17, *BRCA-2* on chromosome 13, *p53* mutation and the tumour suppressor gene are implicated.

Reproductive Factor

Early menarche is a weak risk factor, relative risk of 1.2 for women with a menarche before 12 years, as compared to 14 years. Chinese women have a five times less risk of breast cancer as compared to American women, as the menarche is 17 years. Incidence is doubled in women with natural menopause occurring after 55 years. Nulliparity and delay of first child birth are also risk factors, increasing the risk by 3.5. Lactation is a weak-to-moderate protector.

Recent studies highlight that lifestyle modifications, such as regular exercise and a balanced diet, can significantly reduce breast cancer risk in high-risk populations. Additionally, advances in genetic testing now allow for better risk stratification and targeted preventive strategies.

Recent meta-analyses indicate that high levels of chronic stress may correlate with increased breast cancer susceptibility, emphasising the importance of psychological well-being in prevention strategies.

Environmental exposures, such as prolonged contact with endocrine-disrupting chemicals (EDCs), are being investigated for their potential role in increasing breast cancer risk. Reducing exposure through lifestyle adjustments is now part of preventive recommendations.

BENIGN BREAST DISEASE

Women with a history of benign breast disease contribute to 5% of breast cancer cases.

Diet/Obesity/Alcohol

High fat contents in the diet might influence, though obesity is not a major risk factor. Alcohol consumption of even one drink per day is a moderate risk factor.

Hormones and Breast Cancers

Oestrogen and very long-term use of oral pills appear to increase risk, but the risk drops as soon as the drug is stopped.

Ionising Radiation

There is no increase of risk in low-dose exposure as low-dose screening mammography. Risks increase from atomic blast exposure (Japanese women), radiation exposure for postpartum mastitis and tubercular patients undergoing multiple fluoroscopy.

Screening Strategy

Screening is basically done by:

- Breast self-examination (BSE) (every month)
- Clinical examination by physician (annually)
- Screening mammography (every 2 years)

Artificial intelligence (AI)-based tools are being increasingly used to improve the accuracy of mammogram interpretations, reducing false positives and negatives. AI-assisted diagnostic models are particularly beneficial in dense breast tissues.

Thermography, though still under evaluation, is being explored as a radiation-free adjunct to traditional mammography. It shows potential in early detection, especially in women with dense breast tissue.

Recent innovations in optical imaging techniques, including diffuse optical tomography, are showing potential as complementary tools for breast cancer screening, particularly in resource-limited settings.

Breast Self-examination

It should be done every month after the menstrual period when breasts are soft **(Figs. 22A to F)**. The woman is asked to unclothe to the waist and sit in front of the mirror:

- Hands by the side
- Hands pressed against the hips
- Hands above the head
- Stooping forwards

The woman is taught to look for changes in size, contour, nipple retraction, elevation, visible lumps and skin changes like erythema, dimpling and ecchymosis. The breast should fall forwards on stooping. The woman should palpate after inspection in both the sitting and supine positions. Palpate the right breast with the left hand and vice versa. Teach the woman to palpate using the palmar surface and the areola is compressed to demonstrate nipple discharge, and then feel the supraclavicular area.

Mobile health applications are emerging as effective tools to teach and remind women about regular BSEs. These apps provide step-by-step guidance, improving adherence to screening practices.

Training programs led by healthcare professionals have demonstrated a significant increase in the accuracy and effectiveness of BSEs, highlighting the role of education in preventive care.

Community-based awareness campaigns have proven effective in increasing the uptake of regular BSEs, particularly in rural and underserved populations.

Clinical Examination by Physician

A complete and thorough history, assessment of reproductive history, counselling, handing out pamphlets

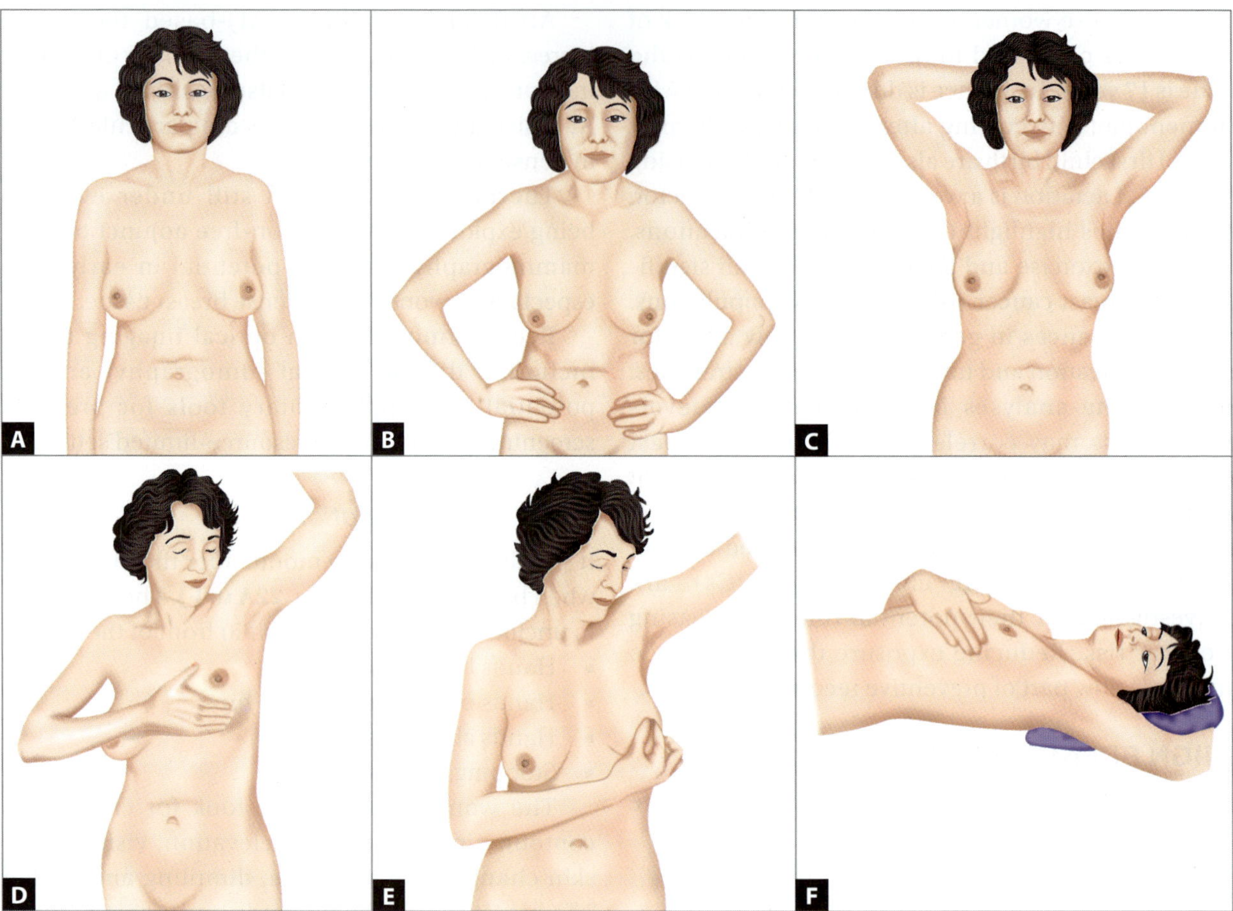

Figs. 22A to F: *Routine breast self-examination:* (A) Inspect breasts in the mirror hands by the side; (B) Hands on the hip; (C) Hands above the head inspect breast tissue leading to axilla; (D) Palpate breast tissue concentrically; (E) Compress areola to demonstrate nipple discharge; (F) Palpate axilla and top of clavicle.

and reteaching BSE are examined by the physician. The clinical examination is the same as BSE but is done by the physician **(Figs. 23A to D)**.

Screening Mammography

The breast imaging can be done by ultrasound (high-resolution probes) or radiologically by mammography (film-screen mammography or xeromammography). For screening purposes, breast mammography should be done every 2 years. Breast ultrasound is done by a 5–7.5 MHz transducer. The entire quadrant is scanned in sagittal and transverse planes. Both film screen and xeromammography are sensitive techniques in evaluating breast diseases.

Film screen mammography has a sensitivity of 90%. It is the only method that allows reproducible and reliable detection of a prognostically relevant nonpalpable carcinoma **(Tables 12 and 13)**. Xeromammography provides good penetration, especially in dense breasts **(Fig. 24)**. The procedure is dry, quick and does not need a darkroom, but only 5% of mammograms are performed with xeromammography due to the high dose of radiation and some technical disadvantages.

Digital breast tomosynthesis is becoming the standard for mammographic screening, offering better sensitivity and specificity compared to traditional 2D mammography. It is especially useful in detecting lesions in dense breasts. Recent guidelines recommend initiating mammographic screening earlier for women with significant family history or genetic predispositions, ensuring timely detection and improved prognosis.

Contrast-enhanced spectral mammography (CESM) is gaining attention for its ability to detect tumours with high sensitivity, particularly in patients with inconclusive ultrasound or standard mammography findings.

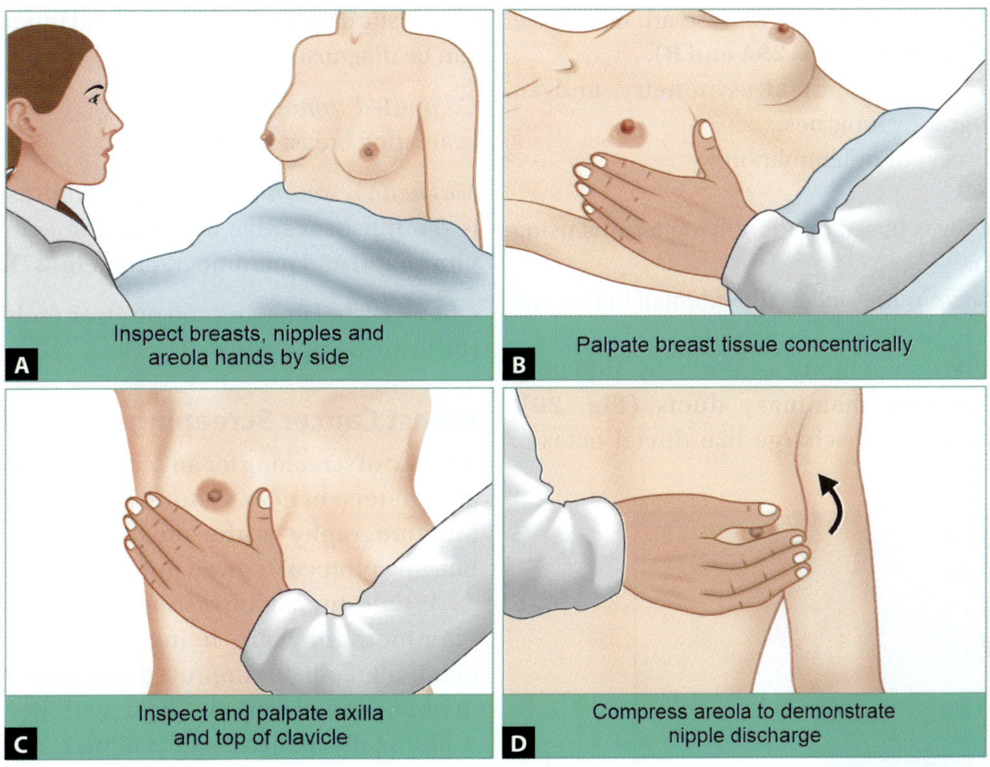

Figs. 23A to D: Breast examination by a physician.

TABLE 12: Screening guidelines for women under age 40 years.

Condition	*Timing of annual mammography*
Lobular cancer in situ or breast cancer diagnosis	At the time of diagnosis
First-degree relative with premenopausal breast cancer	10 years earlier than the relative's age at diagnosis, but not younger than 25 years
Mantle irradiation for Hodgkin's disease	8 years after completion of radiation therapy
BRCA1 or BRCA2 mutation	Age 25–35 years; specific age chosen based on adequacy of mammography imaging in the first study and patient choice

Source: American College of Obstetricians and Gynecologists. Primary and Preventive Care: Periodic Assessments. ACOG Committee Opinion No. 246. Washington, DC; 2000.

Today, high-resolution *ultrasound* with high-frequency probes and the newest introduction of elastography (still under trial as screening for breast cancer) have revolutionised breast imaging, and the ultrasound is becoming indispensable after a clinical examination. Ultrasound is quick, reliable, cheap and reproducible with patient comfort. Also, almost all the interventional

TABLE 13: American College of Radiology (BI-RADS) assessment categories.

(BI-RADS) Category	*Assessment*
0	Need additional imaging evaluation; assessment is incomplete
1	Negative
2	Benign finding(s)
3	Probably benign finding; initial short interval, follow-up suggested
4a	Low suspicion for malignancy
4b	Moderate suspicion for malignancy
4c	High suspicion for malignancy
5	Highly suggestive of malignancy, appropriate action should be taken
6	Known biopsy; proven malignancy; appropriate action should be taken

(BI-RADS) Breast Imaging Reporting and Data System

Note: By subdividing category 4 into 4a, 4b, and 4c, it is encouraged that relevant probabilities for malignancy be indicated within this category so that the patient and her physician can make an informed decision on the ultimate course of action.

Source: American College of Radiology, Illustrated Breast Imaging Reporting and Data System (BIRADS), 4th edition. Reston, VA; 2003. Reprinted with permission of the American College of Radiology. No other representation of this material is authorised without expressed, written permission from the American College of Radiology.

procedures for diagnosis in breast disease are now done under ultrasound guidance **(Figs. 25A and B)**.

Thermography shows thermal asymmetry, and an abnormal thermography indicates:

- A localised abscess or inflammation
- Alveolar lesions

Diaphanography is based on identifying lesions using transillumination.

Pneumocystography may tell us the extent of intracystic tumour.

Ductography/galactography is done by injecting radiographic dye into mammary ducts **(Fig. 26)**. Abnormalities of nipple discharge like ductal ectasia, fibrocystic changes, papillomas and intraductal carcinoma can be diagnosed.

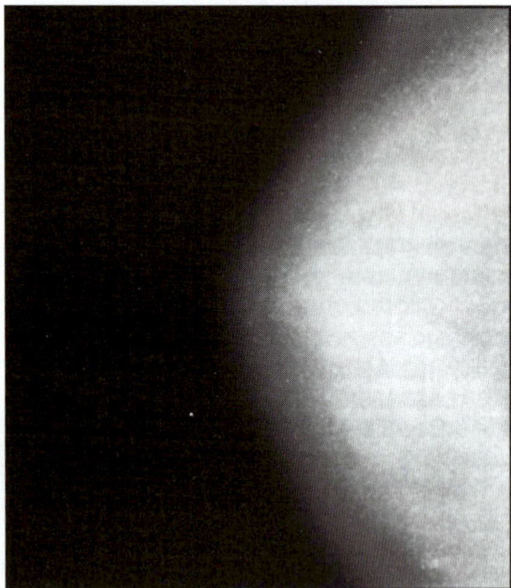

Fig. 24: Benign breast disease—mammogram shows diffuse increased density with no evidence of calcification.

Computed tomography scan: A CT scan is of no use in evaluating breast lesions.

Magnetic resonance imaging: A contrast-enhanced MRI is the most sensitive additional imaging modality after ultrasound and mammography **(Fig. 27)**.

Others: Digital imaging and positron emission tomography (PET) are being evaluated.

Breast Cancer Screening

The aim of screening for any cancer is to decrease mortality and detect cancer before it becomes symptomatic. Mammography is the most sensitive method. Feig's imaging protocol is given in **Table 14**.

Whole-breast ultrasound and contrast-enhanced mammography are being evaluated as adjuncts to mammography for improved detection rates, particularly in younger women and those with dense breast tissue. Additionally, genetic counselling is now recommended alongside imaging for high-risk women.

Liquid biopsy, using circulating tumour DNA (ctDNA) and other biomarkers, is emerging as a promising noninvasive tool for early breast cancer detection and monitoring, complementing traditional imaging methods.

Advanced genomic profiling is being integrated into screening protocols to identify women at higher genetic risk, allowing for more personalised and frequent monitoring strategies.

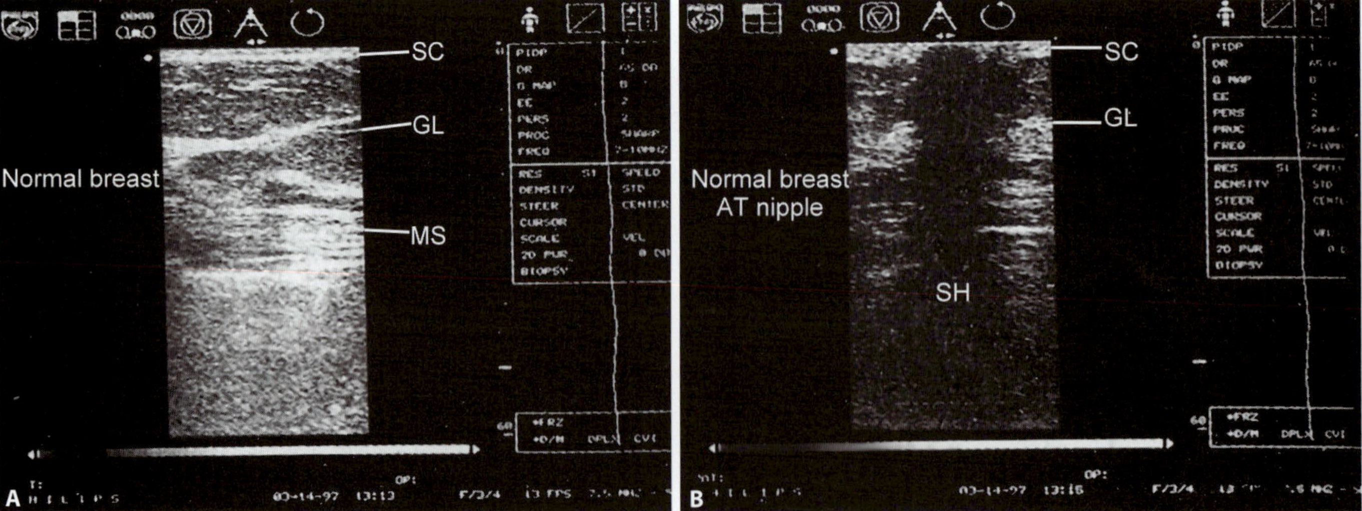

Figs. 25A and B: Ultrasound shows normal anatomy of breast disease.

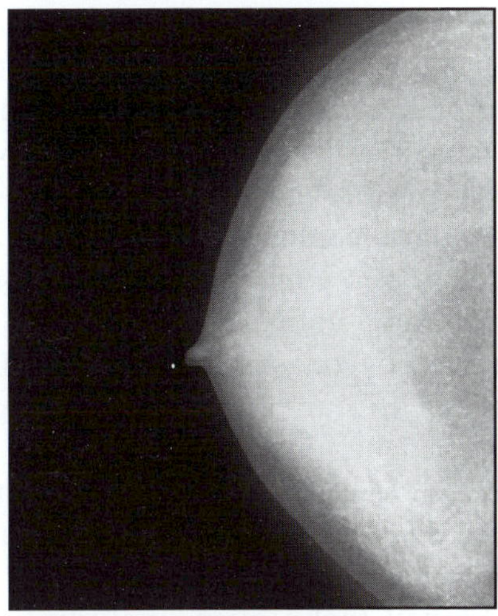

Fig. 26: Galactography shows normal and dilated ducts in otherwise normal mammography but history of nipple discharge.

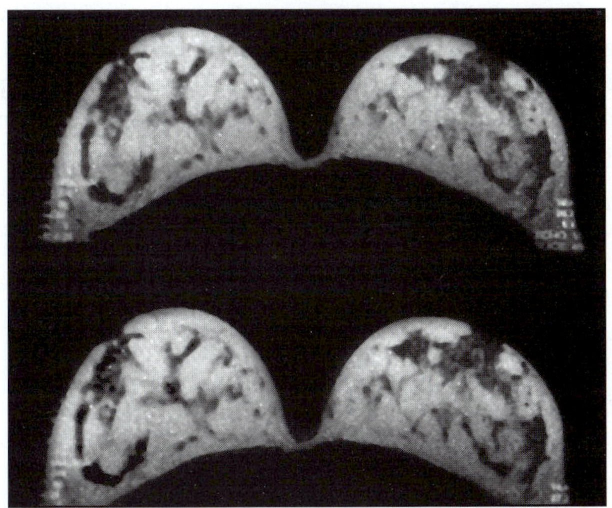

Fig. 27: MRI shows normal breast, T_1- and T_2-weighted images.

TABLE 14: Feig's imaging protocol.

Patient age in years	*Imaging*
<20	Sonography alone
20–30	Sonography + mammography
30–35	Sonography + mammography
>35	Bilateral views per breast mammography, then sonography and magnetic resonance imaging

BREAST CANCER (FIG. 28)

Breast carcinoma is the most common cancer in women in Europe, the USA and Australia and in India, it is the second most common after cancer of the cervix.

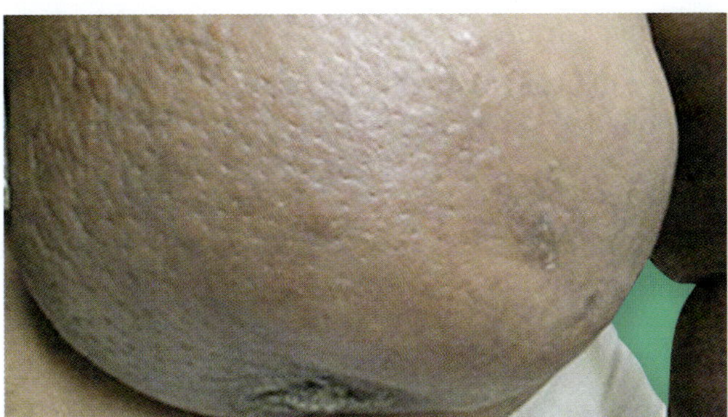

Fig. 28: Breast carcinoma.

BOX 3: Risk factors for breast carcinoma.

- Early menarche
- Late menopause
- Obesity
- Nulliparity
- Late age of first birth
- Never breastfed
- Nipple discharge
- Radiation exposure
- High dietary fat intake
- Oestrogen replacement therapy
- First-degree relative with a breast
- Carcinoma in the other breast
- Previous carcinoma endometrial
- *BRR 1* and *BRR 2* mutation

EPIDEMIOLOGY

According to the American Cancer Society, 1,82,460 women in the USA are diagnosed with breast cancer annually. The incidence of breast cancer appears to have a sigmoid function in women <55 years. The incidence is about 6.6% in <40 years, 2.4% in <35 years and 1% in <30 years of age. Most commonly, it originates in the upper-outer quadrant (38.5%), central area (29%), upper-inner quadrant (14.2%), lower-outer quadrant (8.8%) and lower-inner quadrant (5%) **(Box 3)**.

Prognostic Factors

Axillary Lymph Node Status

It is the most important prognostic factor. The number of lymph nodes involved and also presence of metastasis correlate with distant metastasis.

Tumour Size

It is important even in the absence of lymph node involvement. Size <1 cm and good histologic types have a good prognosis.

Histologic Grade

Poorly differentiated tumours have more aggressive behaviour and poor prognosis.

Oestrogen and Progesterone Receptors

Positive hormone receptors correlate with response to antihormonal agents and also better prognosis.

HER 2/neu

Overexpression or amplification of this oncogene has been correlated with poor prognosis.

P-53

Accumulation of this tumour superior gene correlates with reduced survival.

Recent advancements include the identification of molecular subtypes of breast cancer, such as luminal A, luminal B, HER2-enriched and triple-negative, which are now integral to prognosis and treatment planning.

Recent findings highlight the prognostic significance of Ki-67 proliferation index, which is now widely used to stratify patients and tailor adjuvant therapy choices. This marker has become essential in managing aggressive breast cancer subtypes.

Clinical Features

It usually presents as an ill-defined lump in the breast associated with the indrawing of the nipple.

Stage I: Discrete palpable lump of 2 cm or less

Stage II: Discrete lump <5 cm with palpable ipsilateral mobile axillary lymph node

Stage III: Large lump with local extension:

- Skin ulcer
- Peau d'orange
- Satellite skin nodules
- Fixed chest wall
- Fixed ipsilateral lymph nodes

Stage IV: All the above features plus:

- Supraclavicular lymph node
- Liver enlargement
- Krukenberg tumour
- Ascites
- Pleural effusion
- Bone pains and swelling
- Headache and epileptic episodes
- Chronic cough and recurrent haemoptysis
- Emerging data suggest that inflammatory breast cancer, though rare, requires heightened awareness due to its aggressive nature and rapid progression. Early diagnosis through imaging and biopsy is critical for improving outcomes.
- Lymphoedema, a common complication of breast cancer, is now being managed with advanced techniques like decongestive therapy and microsurgical lymphaticovenular anastomosis, significantly improving patients' quality of life.

Diagnosis is based on clinical examination, and a thorough search should be made with all investigative modalities for extension and secondaries.

Liquid biopsy techniques, including circulating tumour DNA (ctDNA) analysis, are being integrated into diagnostic protocols for their potential to detect minimal residual disease and guide personalised treatment strategies. Advanced imaging technologies, such as molecular breast imaging (MBI), are emerging as valuable tools for detecting cancers missed by traditional mammography, especially in dense breast tissue.

Staging: TNM staging and classification **(Table 15)**. Investigations are aimed to:

- Confirm diagnosis
- Assess the extent of the disease
- Predict response

Modalities and Tests

- Ultrasound
- Mammography
- Fine needle aspiration cytology (FNAC)
- Doppler studies
- Bone scan
- CAT and MRI scans
- Hormone receptor studies

Management of breast cancers depends on the staging **(Tables 16 to 19)**.

Treatment of Breast Cancer (Table 15)

Mastectomy

- Radical mastectomy includes removal of the breast and axillary contents but preservation of the pectoral muscle and more skin.
- Extended radical mastectomy includes embolic removal of the internal mammary chain at the time of radical mastectomy.

TABLE 15: TNM system of classification and staging.	
Breast: Left right	
Tumour size ______ cm × ___ cm × ___ cm	
Lymph nodes total number with metastasis	
Definitions:	
Primary tumour (T)	
TX	The primary tumour cannot be assessed
T0	No evidence of primary tumour
Tis	*Carcinoma in situ:* Tis (DCIS) Intraductal carcinoma, Tis (LCIS) lobular carcinoma in situ or Tis (Paget's) Paget's disease of the nipple with no tumour
T1	Tumour 2 cm or less in greatest dimension
T1mi	Tumour ≤1 mm in greatest diameter
T1a	Tumour >1 but ≤0.5 mm or less in greatest dimension
T1b	>0.5 cm, but not >1 cm in greatest dimension
T1c	>1 cm but not >2 cm in greatest dimension
T2	Tumour >2 cm but not >5 cm in greatest dimension
T3	Tumour >5 cm in greatest dimension
T4	Tumour of any site with direct extension to the chest wall or skin
T4a	Extension to the chest wall
T4b	Oedema (including peau d'orange) or ulceration of the skin of the breast or satellite skin nodules confirmed on the same breast
T4c	Both T4a and T4b
T4d	Inflammatory carcinoma
Regional lymph nodes (N):	
NX	Regional lymph nodes cannot be assessed (e.g. previously removed or removed for pathologic study)
N0	No regional lymph node metastasis
N1	Metastasis to movable ipsilateral axillary lymph node(s)
N2	Metastasis to ipsilateral level 1,2 auxiliary lymph nodes that are clinically fixed or matted or in a clinically detected ipsilateral internal mammary node in the absence of clinically evident axillary lymph node metastasis
N2a	Metastasis in ipsilateral level 1, 2 axillary lymph nodes fixed to one another (matted) or to other structures
N2b	Metastasis only in clinically detected ipsilateral internal mammary nodes and in the absence of clinically evident 1, 2 axillary lymph node metastasis
N3	Metastasis to ipsilateral infraclavicular (level 3 axillary) lymph node(s), with or without level 1, 2 axillary node involvement or in clinically detected ipsilateral internal mammary lymph node(s) and in the presence of clinically evident 1, 2 axillary lymph node metastasis: or metastasis in ipsilateral supraclavicular lymph node(s), with or without axillary or internal mammary lymph node involvement
N3a	Metastasis to ipsilateral infraclavicular lymph node
N3b	Metastasis to the ipsilateral internal mammary lymph node and the axillary lymph node
N3c	N3c metastasis to ipsilateral supraclavicular lymph node
Distant metastasis (M):	
MX	Presence of distant metastasis cannot be assessed
cM0(i+)	No clinical or radiographic evidence of distant metastases, but deposits of molecularly or microscopically detected tumour cells in circulating blood, bone marrow or other nonregional nodal tissue that are no >0.2 mm in a patient without symptoms or signs of metastases
M1	Distant detectable metastasis as determined by classic clinical and radiographic means and/or histologically proven >0.2 mm

TABLE 16: Anatomic stage/prognostic group.

Stage	***T***	***N***	***M***
0	Tis	N0	M0
IA	T1	N0	M0
IB	T0	N1mi	M0
	T1	N1mi	M0
IIA	T0	N1	M0
	T1	N1	M0
	T2	N0	M0
IIB	T2	N1	M0
	T3	N0	M0
IIIA	T0	N2	M0
	T1	N2	M0
	T2	N2	M0
	T3	N1	M0
	T3	N2	M0
IIIB	T4	N0	M0
	T4	N1	M0
	T4	N2	M0
IIIC	Any T	N3	M0
	Any T	Any N	M1

TABLE 17: Histological grade.

GX	Grade cannot be assessed
G1	Low combined histological grade (favourable)
G2	Intermediate combined histological grade (moderately favourable)
G3	High combined histologic grade (unfavourable)

Breast Conservation Therapy

- In this surgery, a wide local excision with excision of a 1–2 cm rim of normal tissue is performed. It is commonly known as lumpectomy or tumourectomy.
- In quadrantectomy, resection of the tumour with the overlying skin and the involved quadrant of the breast is performed.
- Local recurrence is reported to be 18–40% with lumpectomy and only 2–14% with lumpectomy and radiation. So, radiation therapy is an important component of breast conservation.

Management of the Axilla

- Axillary lymph nodes are divided relative to the pectoralis minor into three levels:
  - *Level I:* Lateral to the lateral border of the pectoralis minor muscle
  - *Level II:* Behind the pectoral is minor muscle
  - *Level III:* Medial to medial border of pectoralis minor
- Lymph node metastasis occurs in a step-wise manner; complete Level I and Level II dissection provides good local control with reduced recurrence to <1%.

Sentinel Lymph Node Biopsy

- This modality minimises the morbidity associated with axillary lymph node dissection, still providing important staging information.
- Blue dye and isotope when used in combination approaches 100% positive predictive value and 95% negative productive value.
- Sentinel lymph node biopsy is widely employed in invasive breast cancer. But in some cases, standard axillary dissection should be considered like:
  - Palpable suspicious lymph node
  - Large lesions
  - Prior radiation, large excisional cavity close to the axilla, or disruption of lymphatics

Systemic Treatment

- Randomised studies demonstrated that addition of chemotherapy improves the survival of breast cancer patients. But the use of adjuvant chemotherapy or hormonal therapy depends on factors like size of the primary tumour, lymph node status, the presence or absence of metastasis and expression or lack of expression of oestrogen and progesterone receptors.
- For patients with positive nodes or large tumours, the combination of cyclophosphamide, methotrexate and 5-fluorouracil (CMF) has been used. 5-fluorouracil, adriamycin, cyclophosphamide (FAC) is used in patients with a high risk of recurrence. Paclitaxel has also been used in these cases. FAC is more toxic than CMF, but trials showed superiority with this regimen.

Metastatic Disease

Palliative therapy is the goal, as cure is unlikely. Tamoxifen or aromatase inhibitors like letrozole or anastrozole are the first-line agents. On failure of these agents, chemotherapy can be used.

In metastatic settings, antibody-drug conjugates like trastuzumab deruxtecan show promising results in

TABLE 18: Pathological grade (pN).

pNX	Regional lymph nodes cannot be assessed
pNO	No regional lymph node metastasis was identified histologically
pNOi–	No regional lymph node metastasis histologically, negative IHC (immunohistochemistry)
pNOi+	Malignant cells in regional lymph node(s) ≤0.2 mm [detected by haematoxylin-eosin (H & E) stain or IHC, including ITC]
pNOmol–	No regional lymph node metastasis histologically, negative molecular findings (reverse transcriptase polymerase chain reaction (RT-PCR)
pNOmol+	Positive molecular findings (RT-PCR) but no regional lymph node metastases detected by histology or IHC
pN1	Micrometastases, or metastases in 1–3 axillary lymph nodes and/or in internal mammary nodes, with metastases detected by sentinel lymph node biopsy but not clinically detected
pN1mi	Micrometastases (>0.2 mm and/or >200 cells, but none >2 mm)
pN1a	Metastases in 1–3 axillary lymph nodes (at least 1 metastasis >2 mm)
pN1b	Metastases in internal mammary nodes, with micrometastases or macrometastases detected by sentinel lymph node biopsy but not clinically detected
pN1c	Metastases in 1–3 axillary lymph nodes and in the internal mammary lymph node, with micrometastases or macrometastases detected by sentinel lymph node biopsy but not clinically detected
pN2	Metastases in 4–9 axillary lymph nodes or in clinically detected internal mammary lymph nodes in the absence of axillary lymph node metastases
pN2a	Metastases in 4–9 axillary lymph nodes (at least 1 tumour deposit >2 mm)
pN2b	Metastases in clinically detected internal mammary lymph nodes in the absence of axillary lymph node metastases
pN3	Metastases in ≥10 axillary lymph nodes; or in infraclavicular (level 3 axillary) lymph nodes; or in clinically detected ipsilateral internal mammary lymph in the presence of ≥1 positive level 1,2 axillary lymph node; or in >3 axillary lymph nodes and in internal mammary lymph nodes, with micrometastases or macrometastases detected by sentinel lymph node biopsy but not clinically detected or in ipsilateral supraclavicular lymph nodes
pN3a	Metastases in ≥10 axillary lymph nodes (at least 1 tumour deposit >2 mm; or metastases to the infraclavicular (level 3 axillary lymph) nodes
pN3b	Metastases in clinically detected internal mammary lymph nodes in the presence of ≥1 positive axillary lymph node, or in >3 axillary lymph nodes and in internal mammary lymph nodes, with micrometastases or macrometastases detected by sentinel lymph node biopsy but not clinically detected
pN3c	Metastases and ipsilateral supraclavicular lymph nodes

Notes: ITCs (isolated tumour cell clusters) are defined as small clusters of cells ≤0.2 mm, or a single tumour cell, or a cluster of <200 cells in a single histologic cross-section; ITCs may be detected by routine histology or by immunohistochemistry (IHC) methods.
Classification is based on axillary lymph node dissection, with or without sentinel lymph node biopsy. Classification is based solely on sentinel lymph node biopsy without subsequent axillary lymph node dissection, designated (sn) for 'sentinel node,' for example, pN0 (sn).
'Not clinically detected' is defined as not detected by imaging studies (excluding lymphoscintigraphy) or not detected by clinical examination.
'Clinically detected' is defined by imaging studies (excluding lymphoscintigraphy) or by clinical examination and having characteristics highly suspicious for malignancy or presumed pathologic macrometastases on the basis of fine needle aspiration (FNA) biopsy with cytological examination.

HER2-positive breast cancer, even in heavily pretreated patients. Immunotherapy, particularly with programmed cell death protein 1 (PD-1)/programmed death-ligand 1 (PD-L1) inhibitors, is being actively investigated for triple-negative breast cancer.

Patients with brain metastases are benefiting from newer targeted agents like tucatinib, which have demonstrated the ability to penetrate the blood-brain barrier effectively. These therapies are expanding options for patients with advanced disease.

- *Targeted therapies,* such as poly(ADP-ribose) polymerase (PARP) inhibitors for *BRCA*-mutated cancers, and immunotherapies, like checkpoint inhibitors, are revolutionising the management of advanced breast cancer. These modalities are being increasingly included in treatment guidelines.

TABLE 19: Management depending on the stage of carcinoma.

Stage	*In all cases*	*Special staging tests*
IA IB	• CBC, urinalysis, LFT, KFT, X-ray chest, EKG • Mammogram, USG abdomen	Bone scan, CT/MRI only if indicated
IIA	Do	Do
IIB	Do	Bone scan selective vs. universal
IIIA	do	Bone scan in all cases CT/MRI if indicated
IIIB IIIC	Do Mammogram	Do
IV	Do Mammogram	Bone scan in all cases CT/MRI in all cases

(CBC: complete blood count; CT: computed tomography; EKG: electrocardiogram; LFT: liver function test; KFT: kidney function test; MRI: magnetic resonance imaging; USG: ultrasonography)

- *Neoadjuvant therapies*, including dual HER2-targeted therapies (e.g. trastuzumab and pertuzumab), have shown remarkable success in downstaging tumours, making breast-conserving surgery a viable option for more patients.

Radiation Therapy

- It is used in conjunction with lumpectomy for patients opting for breast conservation. The dose is 1.8–2.0 Gy/day for a total of 45–50 Gy with 10–15 Gy boost to the lumpectomy bed.
- Patients with large tumours and more than four positive lymph nodes are given chest wall radiation in a dose of 50 Gy over 5 weeks with a 10 Gy boost to the mastectomy scar.
- Radiation therapy can be used for metastatic lesions to the bone or brain for palliative treatment.
- *Hypofractionated radiation schedules,* delivering higher doses over fewer sessions, are now standard for many patients, offering comparable outcomes with improved convenience and reduced toxicity. Proton beam therapy is also gaining traction for its precision in treating complex cases.
- *Adaptive radiation therapy,* guided by advanced imaging techniques, is optimising treatment delivery by accounting for changes in tumour size and position during the course of therapy. This approach is improving outcomes and reducing complications.

SUGGESTED READING

1. American College of Radiology: Breast Imaging Reporting and Data System (BI-RADS), 2nd edition. Reston, VA, American College of Radiology; 1995.
2. Baines CJ, To T. Changes in breast self-examination behavior achieved by 89,835 participants in the Canadian National Breast Screening Study. Cancer. 1990;66:570-6.
3. Barnes AB. Diagnosis and treatment of abnormal breast secretions. N Engl J Med. 1966;275:1184-7.
4. Bassett LW, Kimme-Smith C. Breast sonography. Am J Roentgenol. 1991;156:449.
5. Bassett LW, Liu TH, Giuliano AE, Gold RH. The prevalence of carcinoma in palpable vs impalpable mammographically detected lesions. Am J Roentgenol. 1991;157:21-4.
6. Bernstein JL, Thompson WD, Risch N, Holford TR. The genetic epidemiology of second primary breast cancer. Am J Epidemiol. 1992;136:937-48.
7. Cady B, Steele GD Jr, Morrow M, Gardner B, Smith BL, Lee NC, et al. Evaluation of common breast problems: guidance for primary care providers. CA Cancer J Clin. 1998;48(1):49-63.
8. Ciatto S, Cariaggi P, Bulgaresi P. The value of routine cytologic examination of breast cyst fluids. Acta Cytol. 1987;31:301-4.
9. Clare S, Morrow M. Management of the palpable breast mass. In: Harris JR, Lippman ME, Morrow M, Osborne CK (Eds). Diseases of the Breast, 3rd edition. Philadelphia: Lippincott Williams & Wilkins; 2000:38.
10. Costa MJ, Tadros T, Hilton G, Birdsong G. Breast fine needle aspiration cytology: utility as a screening tool for clinically palpable lesions. Acta Cytol. 1993;37:461-71.
11. Costanza ME. Breast cancer screening in older women: synopsis of a forum. Cancer. 1992;69(7):1925-31.
12. Dawes LG, Bowen C, Venta LA, Morrow M. Ductography for nipple discharge: no replacement for ductal excision. Surgery. 1998;21:685- 91.
13. Diercks DB, Cady B. Lawsuits for failure to diagnose breast cancer: tumor biology in causation and risk management strategies. Surg Oncol Clin N Am. 1994;3:125-39.
14. Donegan WL. Evaluation of a palpable breast mass. N Engl J Med. 1992;327:937-42.
15. Edeiken S. Mammography and palpable cancer of the breast. Cancer. 1988;61:263-5.
16. Ernster VL, Goodson WH, Hunt TK, Petrakis NL, Sickles EA, Miike R. Vitamin E and benign breast "disease": a double-blind, randomized clinical trial. Surgery. 1985;97:490-4.
17. Fletcher SW, Black W, Harris R, Rimer BK, Shapiro S. Report of the International Workshop on Screening for Breast Cancer. J Natl Cancer Inst. 1993;85:1644-56.
18. Gateley CA, Miers M, Mansel RE, Hughes LE. Drug treatments for mastalgia: 17 year's experience in the Cardiff Mastalgia Clinic. JR Soc Med. 1992;85:12-5.

19. George H. Sakorafas. Breast cancer surgery—historical evolution, current status and future perspectives. Acta Oncol. 2001;40(1):5.
20. Haas JS, Kaplan CP, Brawarsky P, Kerlikowske K. Evaluation and outcomes of women with a breast lump and a normal mammogram result. J Gen Intern Med. 2005;20(8):692.
21. Hammond S, Keyhani-Rofagha S, O'Toole RV. Statistical analysis of fine needle aspiration cytology of the breast: a review of 678 cases plus 4,265 cases from the literature. Acta Cytol. 1987;31:276-80.
22. Hankey BF, Miller B, Curtis R, Kosary C. Trends in breast cancer in younger women in contrast to older women. J Natl Cancer Inst Monogr. 1994:7-14.
23. Harris VJ, Jackson VP. Indications for breast imaging in women under age 35 years. Radiology. 1989;172:445-8.
24. Kaufman Z, Shpitz B, Shapiro M, Rona R, Lew S, Dinbar A. Triple approach in the diagnosis of dominant breast masses: combined physical examination, mammography, and fine-needle aspiration. J Surg Oncol. 1994;56:254-7.
25. Kelsey JL. Breast cancer epidemiology: summary and future directions. Epidemiol Rev. 1993;15:256-63.
26. Kleinberg DL, Noel GL, Frantz AG. Galactorrhea: a study of 235 cases, including 48 with pituitary tumors. N Engl J Med. 1977;296:589-600.
27. Kline TS, Joshi LP, Neal HS. Fine-needle aspiration of the breast: diagnoses and pitfalls: a review of 3545 cases. Cancer. 1979;44:458-64.
28. Manchon P, Borràs JM, Ferro T, Espinàs JA. Breast cancer OncoGuia. Clin Transl Oncol. 2010;12(2)113.
29. Morrow M, Wong S, Venta L. The evaluation of breast masses in women younger than forty years of age. Surgery. 1998;124:634-40.
30. Morrow M. Management of common breast disorders: breast pain. In: Harris JR (Ed). Breast diseases, 2nd edition. Philadelphia: Lippincott; 1991. pp. 63-71.
31. Morrow M. The evaluation of common breast problems. Am Fam Physician 2000; 61:2371.
32. Nekhlyudov L, Nicola M, Jung I, Buechler E. Clinicians' knowledge and attitudes about breast symptom management: is there a use for clinical guidelines? J Women's Health. 2008;17(1):57.
33. Newcomb PA, Weiss NS, Storer BE, Scholes D, Young BE, Voigt LF. Breast self-examination in relation to the occurrence of breast cancer. J Natl Cancer Inst. 1991;83:260-5.
34. Preece PE, Baum M, Mansel RE, Webster DJ, Fortt RW, Gravelle IH, et al. Importance of mastalgia in operable breast cancer. Br Med J (Clin Res). 1982;284:1299-300.
35. Pruthi S. Detection and evaluation of a palpable breast mass. Mayo Clinic Proc. 2001;76(6):641.
36. Recht A, Houlihan MJ. Conservative surgery without radiotherapy in the treatment of patients with early-stage invasive breast cancer: a review. Ann Surg. 1995;222:9-18.
37. Richardson LC, Royalty J, Howe W, Helsel W, Kammerer W, Benard VB. Timeliness of breast cancer diagnosis and initiation of treatment in the National Breast and Cervical Cancer Early Detection Program, 1996–2005. Am J Pub Health. 2010;100(9):1769.
38. Rodden AM. Common breast concerns. Prim Care. 2009;36(1):103.
39. Seltzer MH. Breast complaints, biopsies, and cancer correlated with age in 10,000 consecutive new surgical referrals. Breast J. 2004;10(2):111.
40. Smart CR, Hendrick RE, Rutledge JH 3rd, Smith RA. Benefit of mammography screening in women ages 40 to 49 years: current evidence from randomized controlled trials. Cancer. 1995;75:1619-26.
41. Takahashi PY, Okhravi HR, Lim LS, Kasten MJ. Preventive health care in the elderly population: a guide for practicing physicians. Mayo Clinic Proc. 2004;79(3):416.
42. Urban JA. Non-lactational nipple discharge. CA Cancer J Clin. 1978;28:130-40.
43. Wujcik D, Fair AM. Barriers to diagnostic resolution after abnormal mammography. Cancer Nurs. 2008;31(5):E16.

12

CHAPTER

Development of the Urogenital System

Latha Kharka, Muralidhar V Pai

Chapter Outline

- Gonad
- Wolffian System
- Müllerian Ducts
- Mesenteries and Ligaments
- Development of the Vagina, Bladder and Urethra
- Development of the Vulva

INTRODUCTION

The development of the three primary layers of the foetus is described in Chapter 7: Conception. By the 21st day or during the third week of development, the embryo properly acquires the form of a three-layered disc, called the embryonic disc, made of three layers—ectoderm (outer), primitive gut or endoderm (inner) and mesoderm (middle). With the formation of head and tail folds and the subsequent development of the primitive gut by endoderm, the primitive gut has acquired a dorsal mesentery, which attaches it to the posterior wall of the body cavity (coelom). The lining of the latter develops from mesenchyme; between it and the ectoderm is the mesoderm **(Figs. 1A to D)**. On either side of the root of the

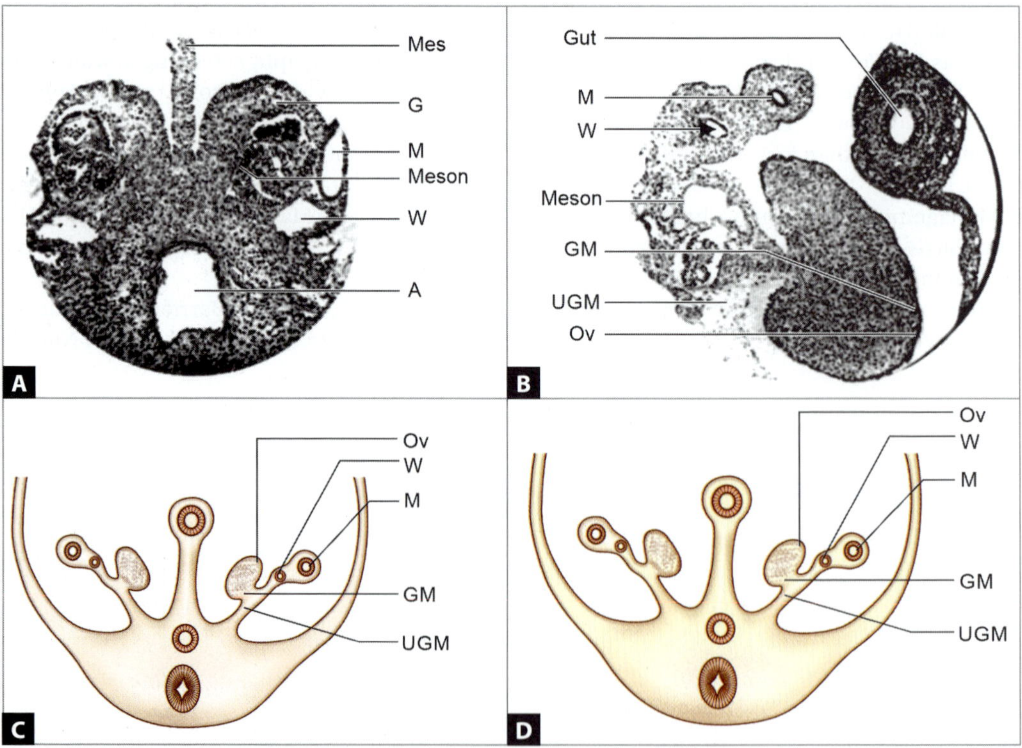

Figs. 1A to D: (A) Cross-section through the trunk of a 4–5-week-old embryo, showing the posterior coelomic wall with the root of the mesentery and the urogenital ridge on either side; (B) Similar cross-section through a slightly older embryo showing the left urogenital ridge and the mesentery of the gut; (C) Diagrammatic representation of (A); (D) Diagrammatic representation of (B) the right side being jittered. (A: aorta; G: gonad; GM: genital mesentery; M: Müllerian duct; Mes: mesentery of gut; Meson: mesonephric tubules; Ov: ovary; UGM: urogenital mesentery; W: Wolffian duct).

mesentery is the intermediate cell mass of mesoderm, and one part of this proliferates to form the urogenital ridge or nephrogenic cord, surface of it covered by the coelomic epithelium. This extends from the cervical to the caudal region of the embryo. The medial part of the urogenital ridge is the genital ridge, which forms the genital system, and the lateral part of the nephrogenic cord forms the urinary system.

With the exception of the vulva, lower vagina, bladder and urethra, all the organs of the genital and urinary systems develop in these ridges. Urinary and genital systems are interconnected in their formation, topography and function. Developmentally, they are complementary to each other as one induces the other. Among the two systems, the urinary system is formed first.

GONAD

Gonads appear at first as a pair of longitudinal ridges called the genital ridge. They are formed by the proliferation of coelomic epithelium on the medial aspect of the intermediate cell mass and the underlying mesodermal cells. This is seen in the cervical and thoracic regions of the 4–5-week-old embryo.

The coelomic cells form the germinal (surface) epithelium and hence the cortex of the ovary; the underlying mesoderm gives rise to the medulla. Germ cells do not appear in the genital ridges until the sixth week of development. Primordial germ cells differentiate into oogonia which are formed at a very early stage from cells of the dorsal part of the hindgut (originally yolk sac). During the fourth week, they migrate by amoeboid movement along the dorsal mesentery of the hindgut to reach the gonad.

Before and during the arrival of primordial germ cells, at an early stage, the cells from the surface germinal epithelium proliferate as mesenchymal downgrowths that grow into the underlying mesoderm. These are the connective tissue cords or septa that develop into primitive sex cords or medullary cords. The cords break up into clumps (cell clusters) and eventually collect around the primordial ova to form primitive follicles. Secondary downgrowths (Pflüger's tubules) occur later and also contribute to pregranulosa cells. So, although the ovarian stroma is derived from basal mesoderm, all the granulosa and theca elements develop from coelomic epithelium. It is suggested that the differentiation of the mesenchyme cells into granulosa and theca cells is dependent on the presence of ova, each one of which acts as an organiser of the cells around it to form a primordial follicle. Oogonia become encapsulated with pre-granulosa or granulosa cells by about the 16th–20th week; these cells are essential to their survival (refer to **Fig. 3,** Chapter 3: Ovarian Functions).

In males, the primary sex cords subsequently differentiate to form seminiferous tubules. The sex cords are separated from the surface epithelium by the development of the connective tissue from the mesenchymal cells, which is called the tunica albuginea. Meanwhile, the primordial germ cells migrate to the region of the developing testis and get incorporated into the seminiferous tubules. The interstitial cells are partly derived from sex cords and also from the surrounding mesenchyme. The tunica albuginea completely separates the sex cords from the germinal epithelium, and thereafter, this epithelium can make no further contribution to testicular tissue. In females, the tunica albuginea does not appear at this stage, and as no tunica albuginea is formed, the germinal epithelium may contribute to the ovary even in postnatal period.

Originally a limited number, the oogonia divide rapidly to produce, according to one estimate, 600,000 oocytes at 8 weeks, and 7 million at 22 weeks. Thereafter, cell division ceases and, coincident with a proliferation of stroma, many, and particularly those which have not acquired a covering of pregranulosa cells, are destroyed. Hence, the number of primary oocytes present in the ovaries at birth is not >2 million, and these are in the dictyate stage of meiotic division.

The ovary descends from the lumbar region, where it is first formed, to the true pelvis. A gubernaculum forms, as in the male and extends from the ovary to the labium majus, it becomes attached to the developing uterus at its junction with the uterine tube, the part of the gubernaculum that persists between the ovary and the uterus becomes the ligament of the ovary, the part between the uterus and the labium majus becomes the round ligament of uterus.

WOLFFIAN SYSTEM

Three slightly overlapping kidney systems are formed in a cranial to caudal sequence during intrauterine life in humans, the pronephros, mesonephros and metanephros. The first of these systems is rudimentary and nonfunctional, the second may function for a short time during the early foetal period and the third forms the permanent kidney.

By the 22nd or 23rd day, small tubules develop in the cervical portion of each urogenital ridge, lateral to the future site of the gonad **(Figs. 1 to 3)**. These constitute

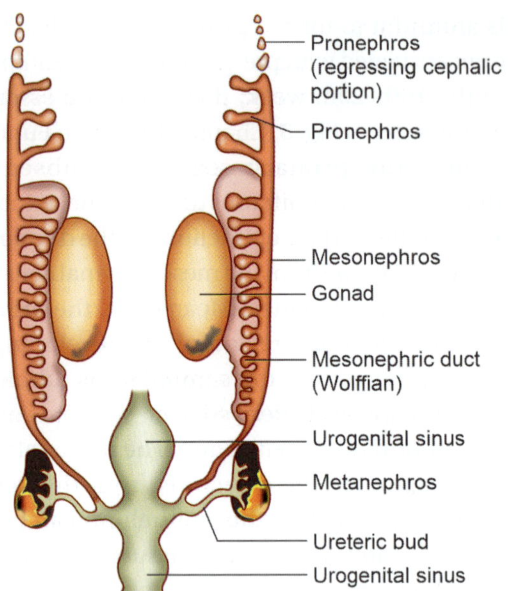

Fig. 2: Diagrammatic representation of the urogenital system in a 6-week-old embryo as seen from the front. The Müllerian duct is not shown.

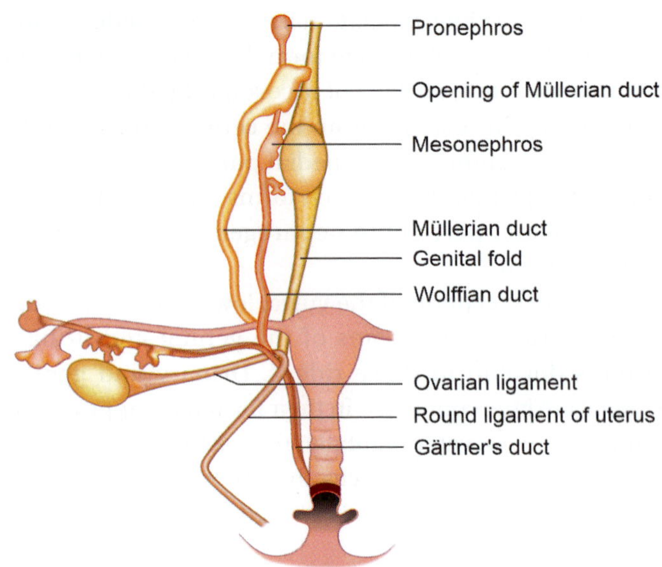

Fig. 4: The ultimate fate of the ducts and ligaments before and after descent of the ovary and its associated structures. H-hydatid of Morgagni; E-epoophoron; P-paroophoron.

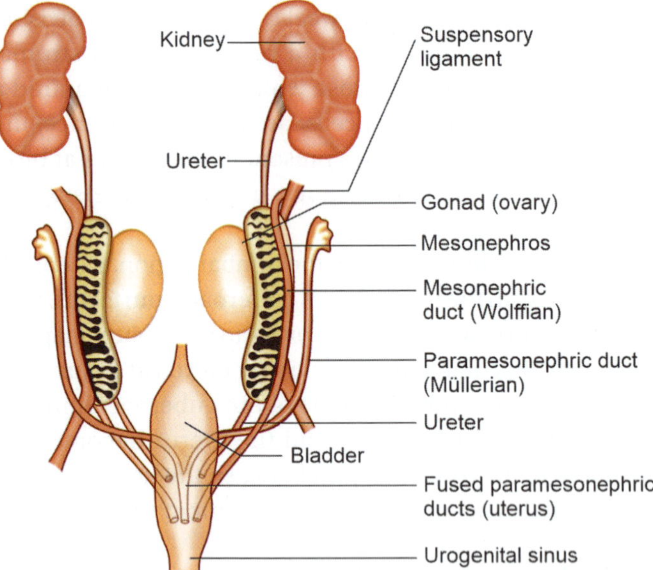

Fig. 3: The developing urogenital system as seen from the side.

the pronephros, and they acquire a duct that extends down to meet the cloaca, which is the caudal extremity of the primitive gut. The pronephros is non-functional and disappears soon after its formation, however, the pronephric (Wolffian) duct persists to serve the mesonephros, and the only remains of the pronephric duct in the adult female are the hydatid of Morgagni and possibly Kobelt tubules **(Fig. 4)**.

The pronephros is succeeded by a second system of tubules mesonephros, which appear in the thoracic region on the 29th or 30th day, and the mesonephric duct drains the excretory tubules of mesonephros. The mesonephros also quickly degenerates, disappearing almost completely by the seventh week. A few caudal tubules persist as the functional vasa efferentia and rete of the testis in the male, and as the vestigial paroophoron, epoophoron (organ of Rosenmüller) in the female **(Figs. 1 to 6)**.

In the male, the Wolffian duct persists as the vas deferens and epididymis, and is connected to the testis by the vasa efferentia and rete testis, which are of mesonephric origin. The seminal vesicle is an outgrowth from the Wolffian duct. But, in the female, the Wolffian duct proper begins to degenerate at the eighth to ninth week and only remains in the adult as the rudimentary Gartner's duct (refer to **Fig. 4 and Fig. 16** of Chapter 2: Anatomy).

In both sexes, the ureteric bud forms the ureter, the pelvis and calyces of the kidney and, by its contribution to the wall of the urogenital sinus, part of the base of the bladder and the urethra.

It will be noted that the kidney is at first situated at a low level in the foetal trunk. Its subsequent ascent is more apparent than real, being mainly explained by the disproportionate growth of the caudal end of the foetus.

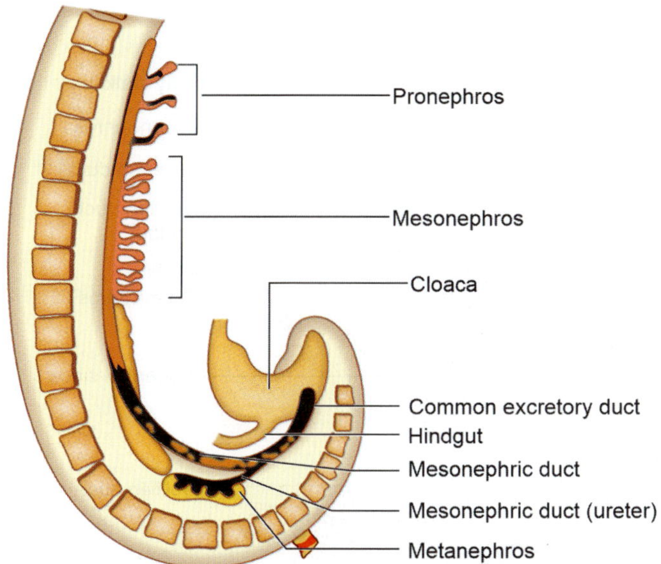

Fig. 5: Diagrammatic representation of a later stage in the development of the Wolffian and Müllerian ducts.

MÜLLERIAN DUCTS

The Müllerian (paramesonephric) ducts appear between the fifth and sixth week in the intermediate mesoderm **(Fig. 1)** and are formed as buds by invagination of coelomic epithelium. They lie lateral to the mesonephric ducts in the cranial part of the nephrogenic cord, and each one grows down lateral to the corresponding Wolffian duct until it reaches a low level. There it turns inwards and, crossing anterior to the Wolffian duct, joins its fellow from the opposite side at the back of the urogenital sinus **(Fig. 5)** and fuse in the midline to form the uterovaginal canal, the caudal end of this canal comes in contact with the dorsal wall of the definitive urogenital sinus **(Fig. 7)**. In the female, this part of the sinus gives rise to the vestibule. The paramesonephric ducts give origin to the uterine tubes, the uterus, and part of the vagina.

In the male, the action of a specific Müllerian-inhibiting substance, liberated by the foetal testes, causes regression of the paramesonephric (Müllerian) duct system and is the likely signal for differentiation of Leydig cells from the surrounding mesenchyme. Testosterone produced by the Leydig cells is responsible for the evolution of the mesonephric (Wolffian) duct into male genital system.

In the female, the Müllerian ducts persist, and their lower ends fuse to form the uterus while their separated upper parts with open ends become the fallopian tubes and the abdominal ostia. They also give off solid downgrowths to form the upper vagina. The epithelium of the uterus thus develops from the fused paramesonephric duct, and the myometrium is derived from surrounding mesoderm. As the thickness of the myometrium increases, the Müllerian ducts fuse from below upwards, their adjacent walls breaking down to form a single cavity. The unfused horizontal parts of the two paramesonephric ducts come to be partially embedded within its substance and help to form the fundus of the uterus.

Fusion begins at the seventh or eighth week but is not complete until the 12th week of intrauterine life. The top of the uterus is at first flat, the domed fundus being a later postnatal development. Differentiation of the cervix from the body of the uterus is recognisable by the 10th week but the cervix is not clearly separated from the vagina until the 20th week. Primitive endometrial glands are present by the 16th week and cervical glands by the 28th week. These later come under the influence of placental hormones, so at birth, they show evidence of some proliferation and even secretory activity, which subsides during the early days of extrauterine life.

Various types of Müllerian anomalies occur due to malformations at various levels during the development stages. They have been classified by the American Fertility Society Society (refered to Chapter 13: Malformations and Maldevelopments of the Genital Tract).

MESENTERIES AND LIGAMENTS

As the gonad and Wolffian systems develop, they project into the coelom until ultimately, they are attached to its posterior wall by the urogenital mesentery **(Figs. 1B and D)**; this is destined to become the broad ligament. The gonad then develops its own genital mesentery, which is ultimately the mesovarium. The part of the urogenital mesentery lying outside or above the attachment of the genital mesentery contains the Müllerian duct, Wolffian (Gartner's) duct and the remains of the pronephros and the mesonephros; it is thus recognisable as the mesosalpinx.

Below the gonad, the genital ridge is continued down the posterior coelomic wall and turns forward to what will become the lower abdominal wall. It is called the genital ligament or gubernaculum and plays an important part in the ultimate descent of the gonad, especially in the male. In the female, the genital ligament is caught up by the Müllerian ducts, where they come together and are thus divided into two parts. The lower part becomes the round ligament running from the cornu of the uterus to the abdominal wall. The upper part is the ovarian ligament

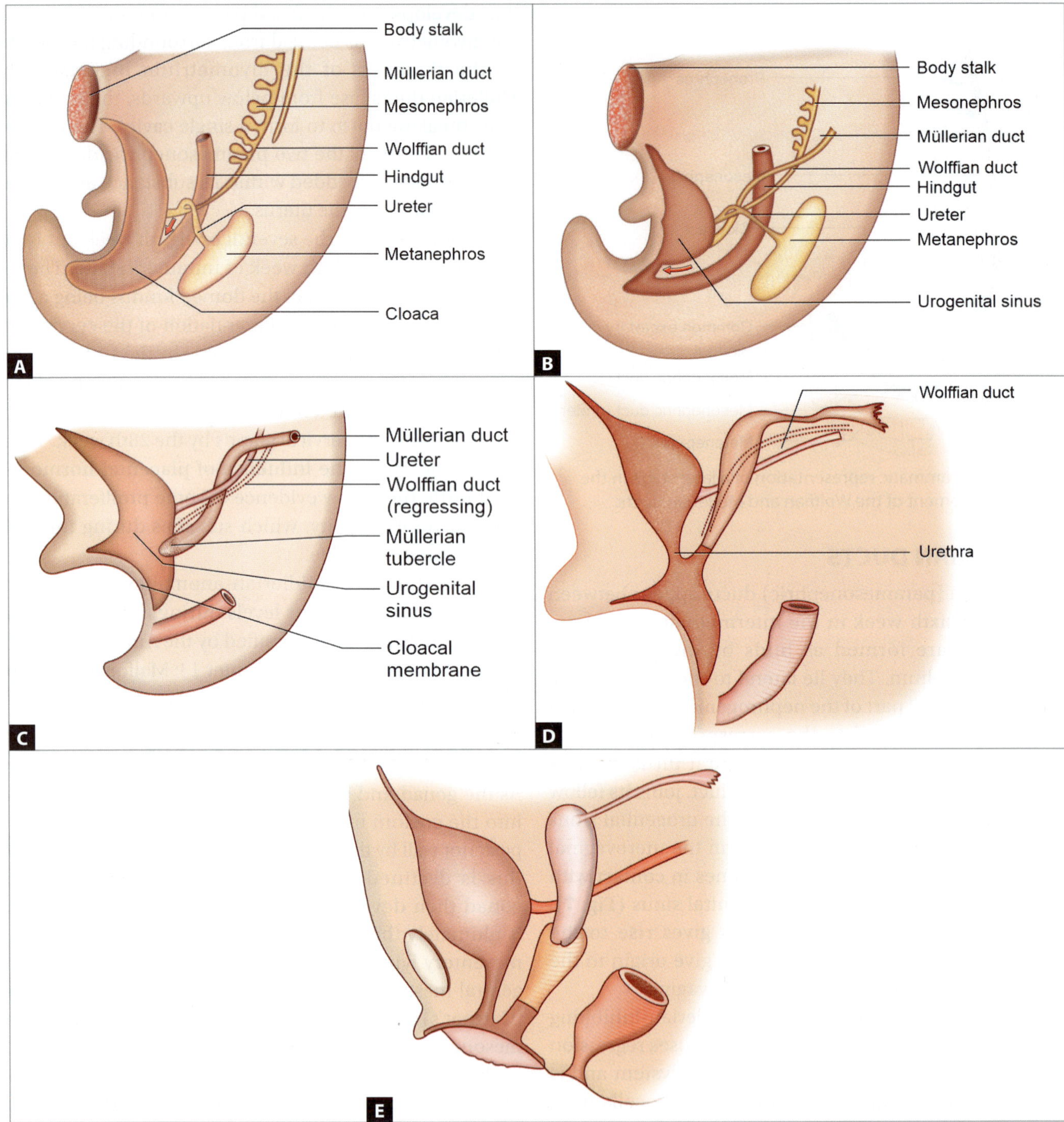

Figs. 6A to E: *Diagrammatic explanation of the partition of the cloaca and the development of the vagina:* (A) The early situation, hindgut and cloaca developing from endoderm. The arrow indicates a mesodermal downgrowth; (B) The urogenital sinus is forming as the urorectal septum of mesoderm (arrowed) divides the cloaca and separates the hindgut; (C) The Müllerian ducts impinge on the urogenital sinus and form the Müllerian tubercle. The sinovaginal bulbs develop at this site. The ureter now opens separately into the urogenital sinus; (D) The urogenital sinus above the Müllerian tubercle narrows to form the urethra. The lower vagina forms from the urogenital sinus; (E) The cloacal membrane breaks down to expose the opened-up lower part of the urogenital sinus, which is the vulva. The posterior part of the cloacal membrane opens to form the anus.

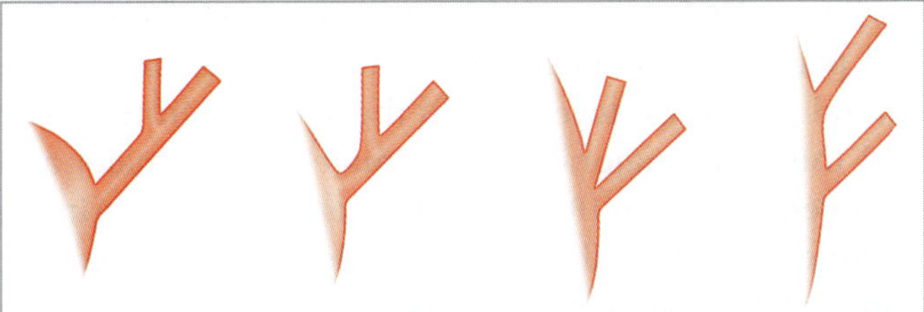

Fig. 7: The stages whereby the lower parts of the mesonephric (Wolffian) duct are opened out to form part of the wall of the urogenital sinus. By this process, the duct and its ureteric bud come to have separate openings into the sinus.

attaching the ovary to the cornu of the uterus **(Fig. 4)**. As their foetal development proceeds, the unfused portions of the Müllerian ducts and the adjacent gonads descend towards the pelvis; this accounts for the fallopian tubes lying at right angles to the uterus and for the change in direction of the urogenital mesenteries to become the broad ligaments.

DEVELOPMENT OF THE VAGINA, BLADDER AND URETHRA

The cloaca is the lower end of the included yolk sac (endoderm) and, at an early stage of development, is divided into the hindgut and urogenital sinus by a downgrowth of mesoderm, which forms the urorectal septum and ultimately the perineal body **(Fig. 6)**. With the formation of the urorectal septum, the cloacal membrane becomes subdivided into a ventral urogenital membrane, and a caudal anal membrane.

The lower ends of the fused Müllerian ducts lie in close association with the posterior part of the urogenital sinus and give rise to a solid downgrowth of tissue, which invaginate the urogenital sinus to produce a prominence called the Müllerian tubercle **(Fig. 6)**. There is a proliferation of endodermal cells of urogenital sinus tissue such as solid evaginations to form the bilateral sinovaginal bulbs.

The upper three-quarters of the vagina is formed from the Müllerian downgrowths, which become canalised. The lower part of the vagina develops by canalisation of the sinovaginal bulbs, a process, which is not complete until the 21st week. Thus, the vagina has dual origin, upper part derived from uterine canal (mesoderm) and lower part derived from urogenital sinus (endoderm). Incomplete breakdown of the junction between the bulbs and the urogenital sinus proper leaves the hymenal membrane.

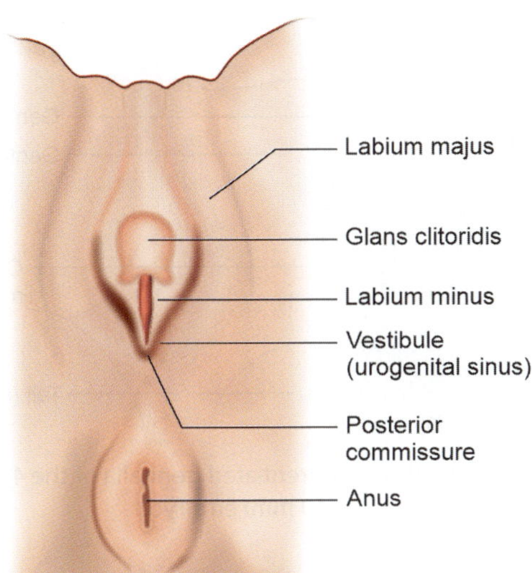

Fig. 8: The external genitalia of the 10–12-week-old female embryo. The cloacal membrane has broken down to expose the urogenital sinus (vestibule).

The urogenital membrane becomes elongated in a craniocaudal direction, and the mesoderm on either side of it is soon heaped up to form two longitudinal elevations called the primitive urethral folds. The urogenital membrane breaks down in its centre at the sixth week to expose the lower parts of the urogenital sinus, which are destined to become the vestibule, urethra and lower vagina **(Figs. 6 and 8)**. The primitive urethral folds now form the labia minora. It will be obvious that they are lined on the outside by the ectoderm, and on the inside by the endoderm. The vaginal fornices are of paramesonephric origin differentiated by the 20th week.

The part of the urogenital sinus immediately above the Müllerian tubercle becomes narrowed to produce the urethra; the part below opens out to become the vestibule of the vulva with the urethra and vagina opening into it **(Fig. 6D)**.

The bladder itself is the upper part of the urogenital sinus and at first has a diverticulum (allantois) into the body stalk. This later retrogresses, its remains being the urachus running from the fundus of the bladder to the umbilicus.

DEVELOPMENT OF THE VULVA

The external genitalia develop in the area bounded in front and above by the body stalk, and below and behind by the tail of the embryo **(Fig. 9)**. It is not easy to recognise the sex of the external genitalia until the 11th or 12th week (50 mm CR embryo). By the fourth or

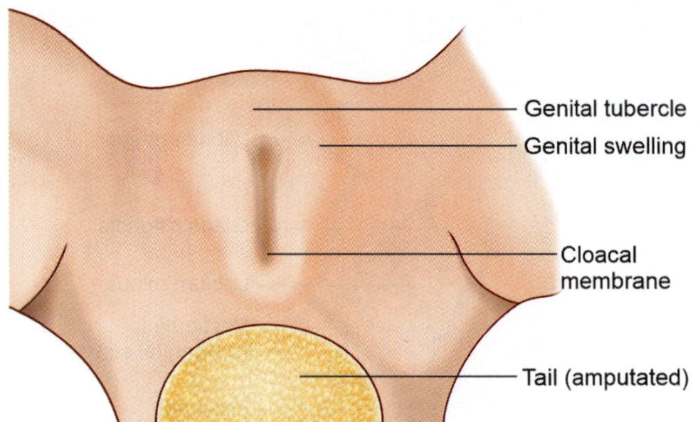

Fig. 9: The sexually undifferentiated genitalia of the 4–5-week-old (10 mm) embryo.

fifth week, the genital tubercle is formed in front by the fusion of two mesodermal thickenings. From this, the genital swellings sweep backwards one on either side towards the tail; between them is the cloacal membrane, which is two-layered, ectoderm without and endoderm within. The urorectal septum of mesoderm, which grows down to separate the urogenital sinus from the hindgut, divides this membrane into urogenital and anal parts, and forms the perineal body.

The genital tubercle ultimately becomes the phallus (the penis in the male and the clitoris in the female); the genital swellings develop into the scrotum in the male and the labia majora in the female. In the male, and commencing at the 10th week, the genital folds fuse in the midline to form the floor of the penile urethra. In females, they remain separate as the labia minora.

Bartholin's glands and Skene's tubules are developed from outgrowths of the urogenital sinus, the former being homologous to Cowper's (bulbourethral) glands, and the latter to the prostate, in the male. The female urethra is homologous to the upper part of the prostatic portion of the male urethra.

SUGGESTED READING

1. Schoenwolf GC, SB Bleyl, Brauer PR, Francis-West PH. Larsen's Human Embryology, 5th edition. Elsevier; 2025.
2. Roly ZY, Backhouse B, Cutting A, Tan TY, Sinclair AH, Ayers KL, et al. The cell biology and molecular genetics of Müllerian duct development. Wiley Interdiscip Rev Dev Biol. 2018;7(3):e310.
3. Sadler TW (Eds). Langman's Medical Embryology, 12th edition. Philadelphia: Wolters Kluwer Health/Lippincott Williams & Wilkins; 2012.

13

CHAPTER

Malformations and Maldevelopments of the Genital Tract

Priyankur Roy, Muralidhar V Pai

Chapter Outline

- Causes of Malformations
- Cytogenetics
- Uterine Anomalies
- Ovary
- Fallopian Tube
- Uterus
- Conical Cervix and Pinhole Ostium
- Vagina
- Vulva
- Errors Arising in Connection with the Cloaca
- Malformations of the Urinary Tract

INTRODUCTION

Congenital malformations of the female genital tract are defined as deviations from normal anatomy resulting from embryological maldevelopment of the Müllerian or paramesonephric ducts. An understanding of congenital anomalies as they are encountered in clinical practice is greatly enhanced by not only knowledge of normal embryology and the mechanism of formation of normal infants but also an insight into the processes that result in the development of anomalies. An awareness of malformations and a systematic examination and appraisal of every neonate will greatly increase the number of such anomalies found. In some instances, e.g. congenital adrenal hyperplasia, imperforate anus, diaphragmatic hernia and oesophageal atresia, early detection and prompt intervention may be lifesaving.

Congenital malformations of the female genital tract represent a rather common benign condition with a prevalence of 4–7%. Moreover, depending on the type and degree of anatomical distortion, they are associated with health and reproductive problems. In adults, amenorrhoea is an important clue and may suggest an imperforate hymen, vaginal septum or absence of the uterus. The finding of one anomaly should stimulate a careful gynaecologist to carry out a complete study to detect renal and ureteral anomalies, particularly the solitary pelvic kidney, which might be removed as a *pelvic mass*. Many anomalies occur infrequently, so only physicians in large medical centres may see them frequently enough to be aware of the possible anomalies and their causation, prognosis and, in some cases, correction. The identification and interpretation of such abnormalities constitute a real challenge to the clinician. The knowledge of the problems and pitfalls in the management of these defects will benefit both the obstetrician and the gynaecologic surgeon.

CAUSES OF MALFORMATIONS

The causes of congenital malformations or abnormalities present at birth may be either environmental or genetic (chromosomal abnormalities). It is not always easy to separate the two factors; both may be at work in the same embryo or foetus. Rapidly growing embryonic organs are the most sensitive to environmental influences. Millen has classified the mechanisms of anomaly production as follows:

- Developmental arrest—cessation of development before completion
- Agenesis or aplasia—failure of normal development
- Hyperplasia or local overgrowth
- Aberrant development
- Failure of normal resorption (either too much or too little) or resorption in the wrong locations
- Secondary degeneration of normally developed structures.

Millen also emphasises *that the period when environmental agents may affect the development of an embryo* is *very short, being nearly over by the end of the 8th week of pregnancy*. Organogenesis occurs from day 13 to day 60; teratogenic (G. teras, monster) agents are most dangerous during this period. There is a time relationship between specific organ systems and sensitivity to environmental factors as well as a relationship between

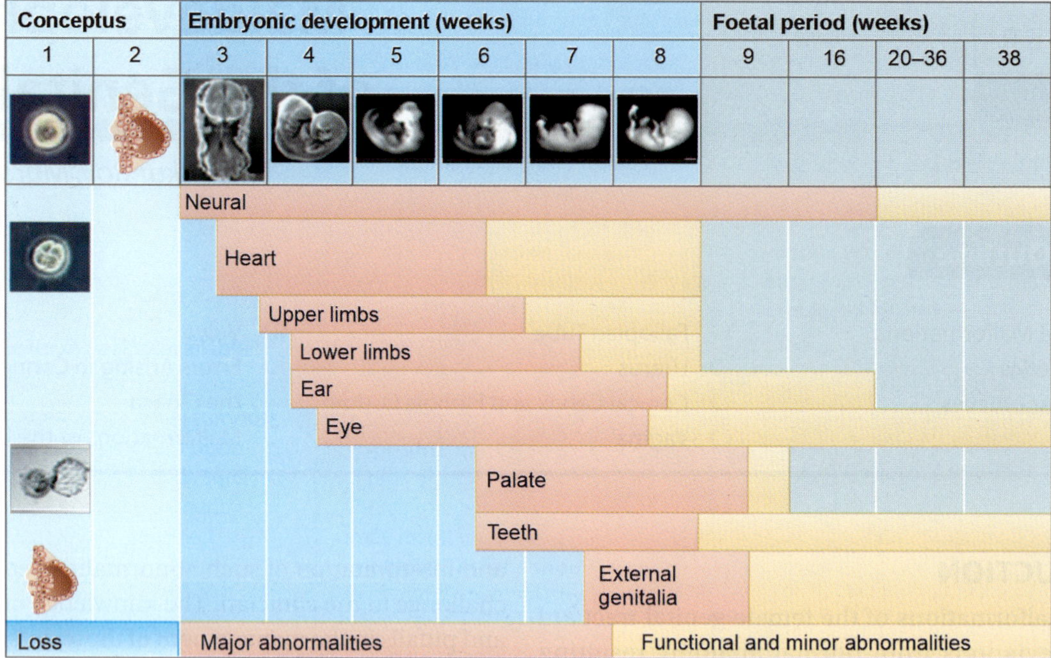

Fig. 1: Major, functional and minor abnormalities.

specific teratogens and specific organ systems. Examples are rubella infections occurring in the first trimester, with a high incidence of cataracts, deafness and cardiac malformations, and use of thalidomide, with varied malformations of arms and legs **(Fig. 1)**.

Nugent has evaluated in detail the mechanisms of action of various environmental teratogenic factors. These include the following:

- Ionising radiation
- Vital disease and related infections
- Chemical factors
- Immunologic disturbances
- Hormones
- Nutritional factors

Ionising radiation is probably one of the best known damaging factors. Infections such as rubella virus, cytomegalovirus, and *Toxoplasma gondii* can cause severe damage to the eyes and central nervous system **(Fig. 2)**. Chemicals include aminopterin (causing skeletal defects and nervous system damage), methotrexate and thalidomide. Immunologic disturbances include Rhesus incompatibilities. Hormone damage is particularly interesting; the administration of exogenous testosterone, synthetic progestogens and similar preparations can cause iatrogenic deformities of the female genitalia. Pathologic hyperandrogenaemia, as seen in luteomas of pregnancy, can result in virilisation in the female newborn. Environmental factors, such as exposure to diesel fumes, have also been associated with virilisation due to inhibition of aromatase and accumulation of excess testosterone. Nutritional factors apparently have little direct teratogenic effect on the foetus. The timetable of development of the female genetic tract is discussed in **Table 1**.

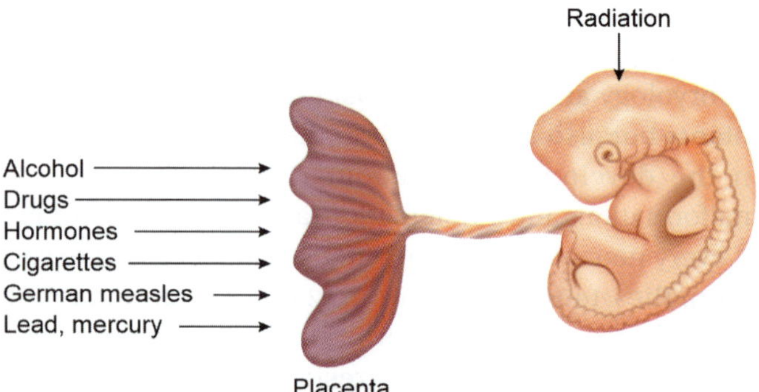

Fig. 2: Mechanism of action of various environmental teratogenic factors.

CYTOGENETICS

In 1923, Painter reported that there were 48 chromosomes in the normal human cell. The correct number of 46 was established in 1956 by Tjio and Levan. In 1956, Down syndrome, Turner syndrome, and Klinefelter syndrome

TABLE 1: Timetable of development of the female genital tract **(Fig. 3)**.

Size (mm)	*Age (weeks)**	
0.08	7.5 days	Bilaminar disc embryo
0.21	13 days	Yolk sac forming hindgut and foregut
0.36	20 days	Allantois formed
1.5	2+	• Gonocytes are located in yolk sac endoderm • Urogenital ridge begins to form
2	3	• Wolffian duct appears as coalescence of pronephric ducts • Allantois well formed, joins hindgut at cloaca • Cloacal membrane forms as cloaca contacts hind-end ectoderm
4	4	Wolffian ducts open into urogenital sinus (cloaca)
5		Primordium of gonad appears
6	4+	Primordial germ cells in mesenchyme
7	1 month+	Indifferent gonad developing
	5	• Wolffian ducts open to urogenital sinus • Ureteric buds • External genital tubercle forming
8		• Sex cords budding from coelomic epithelium • Anlage of adrenal cortex forms • Urorectal septum starts partition of cloaca
10		Free ends of sex cords form rete testis
11	5.5	• Müllerian funnel and duct begin to form • Primary bifurcation of ureteric bud • *Sex difference in external genitalia:* Urethral groove shorter in female • Urethral folds develop lateral to central groove
15	5¾	• Differentiation of gonad into testis in male • Ureter opens separately from Wolffian duct into urogenital sinus
16	6	• Cloaca subdividing; urorectal septum completed • Phallus forming from genital tubercle
18		• Secondary bifurcation of ureteric bud • Urethral membrane (and cloacal membrane) perforates
20	7	Gonad recognizable as ovary; cortex forming Labioscrotal folds developed (lateral genital swellings)
23	8	
25		• Coronary sulcus of phallus appears • Female phallus shows caudal curvature
30		Interstitial cells recognisable
32	9	• Müllerian ducts reach urogenital sinus • Müllerian tubercle formed
42		Lower Müllerian ducts fused
45	10	• Wolffian ducts begin to regress in female • Coronary sulcus of phallus forms a groove (easily recognised)
50		• Posterior commissure formed • Great increase of Leydig cells from mesenchyme • Prostatic buds first appear in male

Contd...

Contd...

Size (mm)	**Age (weeks)***	
56	11	• Sex differences in external genitals first noticeable • Uterovaginal canal formed, fusion of Müllerian ducts with sinovaginal bulbs
65		• Wolffian ducts begin to disappear • Longitudinal folds in urogenital sinus • Sinovaginal bulbs formed, obliterate Müllerian tubercle
70	12	Beginning solidification of uterovaginal canal by proliferation of both Müllerian and sinovaginal epithelium
94		Sinus upgrowth along vaginal plate
100	16	• Wolffian ducts have disappeared by this stage • External genitalia of male fully formed
125		Foetal ovarian stroma differentiates
150		• Primordial follicles in central part of ovary • Vagina canalises from urogenital sinus forward • Maximum development of Leydig cells
175	20	Beginning shrinkage and degeneration of Leydig cells
180		Vagina fully canalised; glycogenated epithelium
187		Seminiferous tubules coiled; lumina
200	24	
240	7 months (early)	Testes descend into scrotum
250	28	During cortical differentiation, medullary cords crowded centrally; some medullary tubules provided with germ cells persist in hilum
286	32	Reduction in Leydig cells (male)
		Disappearance of medullary cords in ovary (female)

*Except as otherwise noted.
Source: Dougherty CM, Spencer R. Female Sex Anomalies. Hagerstown, MD: Harper & Row; 1972.

were shown to be the result of chromosomal anomalies. Porter pointed out that we can now distinguish every individual chromosome and different regions of each chromosome. Normal variants can be defined reliably, extra chromosomes involved in abnormalities can be identified accurately, small defects previously missed can now be recognised, and structural defects can be mapped accurately by tracing exchange segments of chromosomes. A clear cytogenetic diagnosis can serve as a guide to a rational plan of management, to counselling with regard to prognosis and genetic problems and in the monitoring of pregnancies in people with an increased risk of having children with defects.

There are hundreds of chromosomal abnormalities; most involve visible morphologic defects, which should alert the clinician to the possibility of chromosomal anomalies. Disorders of gonadal development such as Klinefelter syndrome (47,XXY) and Turner syndrome (45,X) have been described with sex chromosome aneuploidy. Even deletions within regions of the X or Y chromosome can be deleterious to normal development. Gene deletions in the distal arms of the X chromosome (Xp22.3) cause short stature, mental retardation, X-linked ichthyosis and Kallmann syndrome. The distal region of the Y chromosome contains the sex-determining region Y (SRY) chromosome that encodes the gene for testis-determining factor (TDF). Deletions in this region cause gonadal dysgenesis and streak gonads. Transfer of this region to the X chromosome causes an XX male. Another region of interest within the Y chromosome is the azoospermia factor (AZF) region that is related to spermatogenesis. It has been discovered that one subset of gene rearrangements on the Y chromosome, *microdeletions*, is a major cause of male infertility in some populations. With refined cytogenetic mapping, we will be able to better correlate phenotype with genotype.

The complexity of the rapidly changing field of cytogenetics is not only startling but also a fascinating promise of new knowledge, new discoveries and new clinical tools. With these new tools, challenges emerge for the obstetrician/gynaecologist, reproductive endocrinologist, and paediatrician. Genetic analysis may become routine for every embryo, foetus, or neonate. Embryos can be biopsied, and a single cell screened for aneuploidy prior to implantation. This technique has the potential to improve pregnancy outcomes and decrease miscarriage rates, especially in couples with multiple foetal losses. The public health implications are startling, and indications for testing are increasing.

The cumbersome terms *mesonephric* (Wolffian) and *paramesonephric* (Müllerian) have always been difficult to keep clearly differentiated **(Fig. 4)**. Mesonephric means *middle kidney* (pronephric elements are not a factor in human development). The eponym *M*üllerian duct is deeply ingrained in the literature as relating to uterus, tubes and vagina, while the term *paramesonephric*, meaning *alongside the middle kidney system*, is less difficult to remember. The concept of the paramesonephric (Müllerian) duct system as a double-barrelled organ (suggesting a shotgun) is useful in understanding developmental anomalies, since various growth arrests and failures of development at this stage explain many of the anomalies encountered.

UTERINE ANOMALIES

The most frequent uterine anomalies are those resulting from varying degrees of failure of fusion of the Müllerian ducts. This variability makes classification difficult and determination of the true incidence uncertain. Many of these malformations are detected by radiologic or sonographic studies. Estimates of incidence vary from 0.13% to 4.0%. The incidence of Müllerian anomalies in patients with infertility has been reported to be as high as 4–6%.

There are two systems for classification of female genital tract malformations **(Table 2 and Fig. 5)**:

1. The American Society for Reproductive Medicine [formerly American Fertility Society (AFS)] classification of Müllerian duct anomalies 1998
2. European Society of Human Reproduction and Embryology (ESHR) and European Society of Gynaecological Endoscopy (ESGE) 2013

Type and classes of uterus are shown in **Box 1** and **Figures 6A to F**.

Pregnancy occurs in many women despite these anomalies. The complication rates with pregnancy are considerably increased; complications include abortion, prematurity, postpartum haemorrhage, retained placenta, and breech presentation. Not surprisingly, the rate of caesarean delivery is markedly higher.

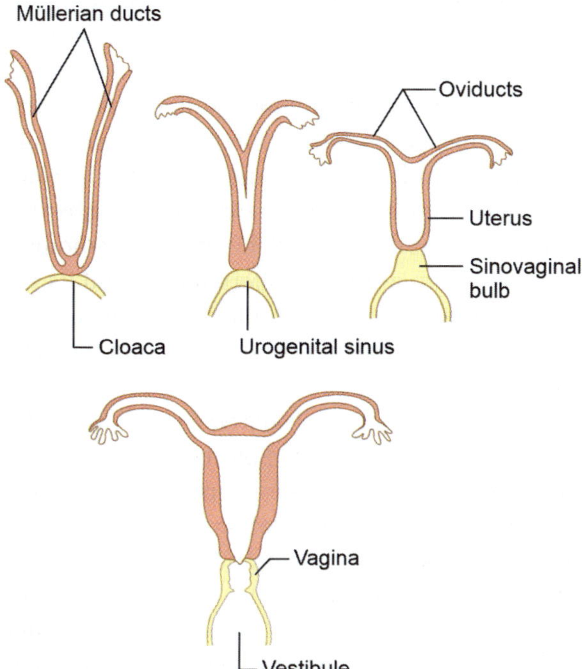

Fig. 3: Embryonic formation of the female reproductive system.

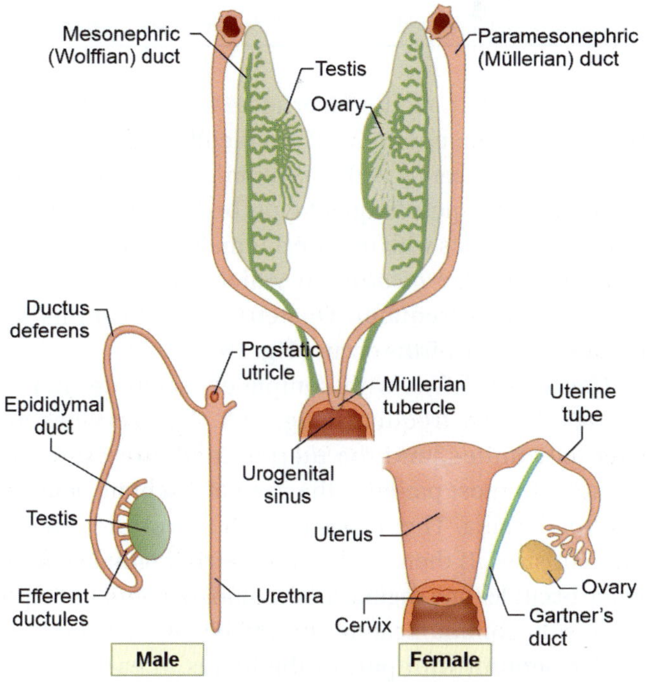

Fig. 4: Mesonephric and paramesonephric.

TABLE 2: Classification and complications of female genital tract malformations.

Female genital tract malformations	***Complications***
Segmental Müllerian hypoplasia or agenesis:	
• Vaginal • Cervical • Uterine fundus • Tubal • Combined anomalies	9.4% infertile population have a hypoplastic uterus
Unicornuate uterus:	
• Communicating rudimentary horn • Non-communicating horn • No endometrial cavity • No rudimentary horn	• 6% infertile women • 2.3% recurrent miscarriages
Uterine didelphys	• 2.9% infertile women • 0.8% recurrent miscarriages
Bicornuate uterus:	
• Complete (division to internal ostium) • Partial	• 10% infertile women • 5.3% recurrent miscarriages
Septate uterus:	
• Complete (division to internal ostium) • Partial	• 46% infertile women • 26.5% recurrent miscarriages
Arcuate	24% infertile women
Diethylstilbestrol related	65% recurrent miscarriage

Uterus duplex, or the bicornuate uterus, is the most frequent uterine anomaly. The unicollis type in which there is a single cervix with a septum that does not reach the cervix is the most frequent type, occurring in over one third of all patients with uterine anomalies **(Fig. 7A)**.

Uterus duplex bicollis, in which two cervices are present, is less frequent. Obstetric complications are frequent, but live births occur **(Fig. 7B)**.

Uterus didelphys, with completely separate uterine cavities, is also frequent **(Fig. 7C)**. The cervices are externally united, and the uterine fundi are externally separate. In most patients, the vagina is septate, causing a double vagina. The halves of such uterus are often of different sizes. If there is an asymmetric vaginal septum, which occludes one vagina, mucocolpos or haematocolpos may result. Communicating uteri, involving an incomplete uterine septum with part of the foetus in each uterine cavity, occasionally occur.

Uterus septus is an essentially normal uterus with a septum reaching to the cervix **(Fig. 7D)**.

Uterus subseptus involves a partial septum that does not reach the cervix. Twins apparently occur approximately three times more often in women with this condition than in women with normal uteri; the cause is not clear **(Fig. 7E)**.

Uterus arcuatus is a normal uterus without a septum. The fundus, however, is notched or flattened. There is usually no interference with normal pregnancy **(Fig. 7F)**.

Uterus unicornis is a uterus with a single horn. A normal vagina and a single normal tube are usually present. The other half of the uterus is usually absent or rudimentary. In most patients, the kidney is missing on the side of the missing uterus. Successful pregnancy can occur **(Fig. 7G)**.

Separate hemiuteri with separate vaginas is a rare condition that is usually associated with duplications of urethra and bladder or of the colon and anus. Pregnancy in each of the two hemiuteri in the same woman at different times has been reported.

These anomalies result from failure of fusion of the paired Müllerian ducts, but in some instances, there is a true duplication of the ducts on one or both sides. Such duplications result from splitting of the Müllerian duct during the 7th week of development. Accessory tubes or ovaries may be present.

Semmens extensively reviewed the literature on genital tract anomalies and evaluated 56 personal patients as well as 500 cases from the literature. He employed a simplified classification, based entirely on the functional capacity of the uterine cavity, which divided genital tract anomalies into two groups: group I—hemiuterus of single Müllerian origin, paired and group II—uterus of dual Müllerian origin, associated with varying degrees of absorption. He concluded that if the entire functional component has been derived from a single Müllerian duct and its vaginal outlet is a cervical canal of similar origin, its capacity is smaller than that of the uterus resulting from the fusion of bilateral ducts.

In contrast, if the uterus is derived from two Müllerian ducts, its capacity is larger. Semmens concluded that the space available for the developing foetus as well as the variations in uterine circulation had a direct effect on the length of gestation, onset and behaviour of labour and overall foetal salvage. The diagnosis of uterine anomalies during pregnancy is always difficult. The most important factor is awareness of their existence and frequency and of the problems that frequently develop.

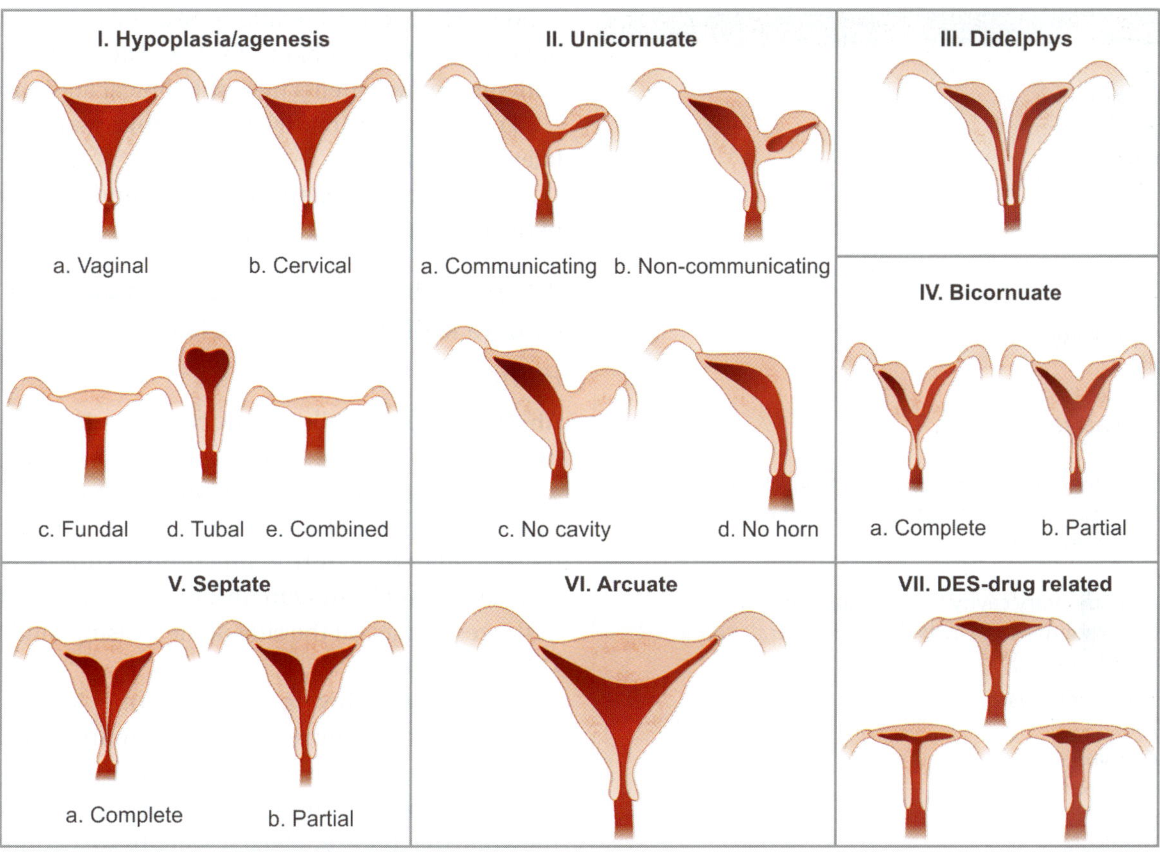

Fig. 5: Female genital tract malformations.

Findings such as a floating head at term without apparent cause, notching and broadening of the uterine fundus, abnormal lie, recurrent breech presentations, prolonged third stage of labour, and trapped or retained placenta indicate the possibility of an anomaly. In abnormal uteri, triangular spasm and cornual pocketing of the placenta may occur and necessitate manual removal of the placenta. The administration of oxytocin under these circumstances usually increases the degree of pocketing in an abnormal uterus. Among antepartum patients, pyelitis (often associated with a urologic anomaly), passage of a decidual cast, haemorrhage and premature rupture of the membranes are the most common complications. Intrapartum complications include septal dystocia, incarcerated non-gravid horn, uterine inertia and retained placenta. Foetal dystocia is considerably increased. Postpartum complications are few and include haemorrhage, retained placenta and failure of uterine involution. Most complications of uterine anomalies in the pregnant woman can be anticipated and managed successfully if the clinician is alert to the possibility of anomalies and if the nature of the anomaly is known. The finding of an asymmetrically located cervix in the vaginal fornix, an excessively large cervix whether or not a septum is present, or a duplicated cervix suggests uterine abnormality. Abnormal configurations of the fundus of the uterus in the third trimester should suggest abnormalities to the clinician, as should abnormal presentations and failure of the presenting part to engage without apparent reason. An obstetric history of successive abortions, recurrent breech presentations or recurrent pyelitis should alert the obstetrician to the possibility of anomalies and, in non-pregnant women, to the need for hysterosalpingogram, saline sonography, magnetic resonance imaging (MRI) and renal imaging.

Clinical Aspects

Patients usually present between 15 and 18 years of age with primary amenorrhea. Growth and secondary sexual characteristics are normal.

Although findings on local examination are usually as described above, some patients may have a small vaginal

BOX 1: Types of uterus.

Uterus
- Normal uterus
- *Dimorphic uterus:*
  - T-shaped
  - Infantilis
  - Others
- *Septate uterus:*
  - Partial
  - Complete
- *Bicorporeal uterus:*
  - Partial
  - Complete
  - Bicorporeal septate
- *Hemiuterus:*
  - With rudimentary cavity (communicating or not horn)
  - Without rudimentary cavity (bi- or unilateral uterine remnants/aplasia)
- *Aplastic:*
  - With rudimentary cavity (bi- or unilateral horn)
  - Without rudimentary cavity (bi- or unilateral uterine remnants/aplasia)

Unclassified malformation

Cervix (C):
- Normal cervix
- Septate cervix
- Double cervix
- *Unilateral cervix:*
  - Cervical aplasia

Vagina (V):
- Normal vagina
- Longitudinal non-obstructing vaginal septum
- Longitudinal obstructing vaginal septum
- Transverse vaginal septum
- Vaginal aplasia

pouch developed as a result of repeated attempts at intercourse. On rectoabdominal examination, the uterus cannot be palpated.

Ultrasound confirms the absence of the uterus and demonstrates the ovaries. Occasionally, the rudimentary uterine horns can be seen. If ultrasound is inconclusive, MRI or laparoscopy is required. MRI is the ideal method for demonstrating uterine malformations.

Chromosomal analysis is not usually required in these patients; however, some patients who present before puberty may require a karyotype to distinguish the condition from one of the forms of male pseudohermaphroditism.

Renal anomalies are the most common associated features seen in 40% of cases, ranging from complete agenesis to malposition (usually a pelvic kidney), to subtle architectural alterations. Skeletal abnormalities can involve the spine, limbs or ribs. These are seen in 10–15% of patients. Some patients have subclinical auditory defects.

Treatment is primarily by vaginoplasty and is discussed later in the chapter.

The clinical aspects are discussed under malformations of the tubes, uterus and vagina.

Absence or Incomplete Development of One Müllerian Duct (Class II)

Pathology

Absence of one Müllerian duct results in a unicornuate uterus with only one fallopian tube (class II). The cervix and vagina may be normal in appearance and function, but they represent strictly only one half of the fully developed organs. A true unicornuate uterus is rare and is usually associated with absence or gross malformation of the renal tract on the side of the missing Müllerian duct **(Figs. 2 and 4)**.

Incomplete development of one Müllerian duct gives rise to the more common apparent unicornuate malformation; this is distinguished by the finding of a fallopian tube and round ligament, rudimentary though they may be, on the affected side. In this condition, two kidneys are usually present, although, occasionally, the one on the affected side may also be hypoplastic and not show on intravenous pyelography **(Figs. 8A and B)**.

Symptoms

A unicornuate uterus causes few symptoms and is usually only discovered by chance or as a result of pregnancy complications. If it happens that the patient has dysmenorrhoea, the pain is limited to the side on which the horn is present. The condition does not, as a rule, lower fertility significantly, but it favours abortion and premature labour, breech presentation of the foetus and fundal insertion of the placenta. The uterus usually contracts efficiently in all stages of labour.

Diagnostic Signs

The uterus which leans well to one side of the pelvis and which cannot easily be straightened should always be suspected as being unicornuate, but the diagnosis can only be made for certain by inspection of the pelvic organs. Hysterosalpingographs are helpful but do not always distinguish between true and apparent unicornuate deformity **(Figs. 6 and 8)**.

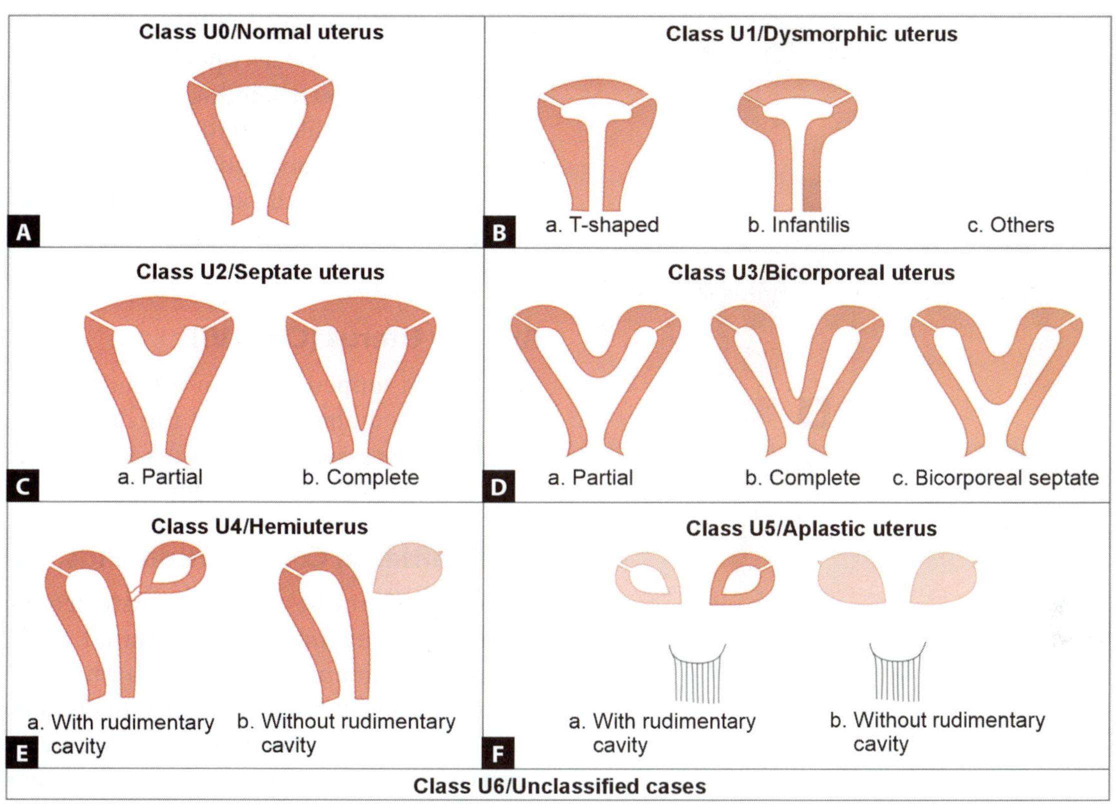

Figs. 6A to F: Classes of uterus.

Treatment

No treatment is indicated for the true unicornuate uterus. The rudimentary horn of an apparent unicornuate uterus may have to be excised if it causes symptoms (see below).

Imperfect Fusion of the Müllerian Ducts

Pathology

Failure of fusion of the Müllerian ducts occurs in varying degrees **(Figs. 6A to F)**. If minor degrees involving uterine shape are included, this type of malformation is extremely common and can be demonstrated in 10–15% of fertile women. The different nomenclatures and classifications of the resulting deformities are confusing. Sometimes, the external and internal shapes of the uterus are both affected, and sometimes only one. From the standpoint of obstetrical complications, the shape of the cavity is more important.

Uterus Didelphys (Class III)

If the two Müllerian ducts remain separate, the two halves of the uterus remain distinct and each has its own cervix **(Figs. 2, 5, and 6F)**. Some distinguish between uterus didelphys and uterus pseudodidelphys according to the degree of separation of the two ducts, and they believe that even the vulva should be duplicated in a true didelphys uterus. However, this view is not widely held. Occasionally, and especially if they are rudimentary, the horns are very widely separated and rarely may be found in the sacs of inguinal hernias.

Bicornuate Uterus (Class IV)

In this condition, only the lower parts of the ducts fuse, leaving the cornua separate **(Figs. 6, 9E to 11)**. The cervix and vagina may be single or double.

Septate and Subseptate Uterus (Class V)

The uterus is outwardly normal but contains a complete or incomplete septum, which reflects a failure in breakdown of the walls between the two ducts **(Figs. 6 and 9D)**. The cervical canal may be single or double, and the vagina whole or septate.

Septate and Subseptate Vagina

A sagittal septum with a crescentic lower edge may be present in the upper vagina or throughout its length **(Figs. 12A to F)**. It can occur alone or in conjunction with

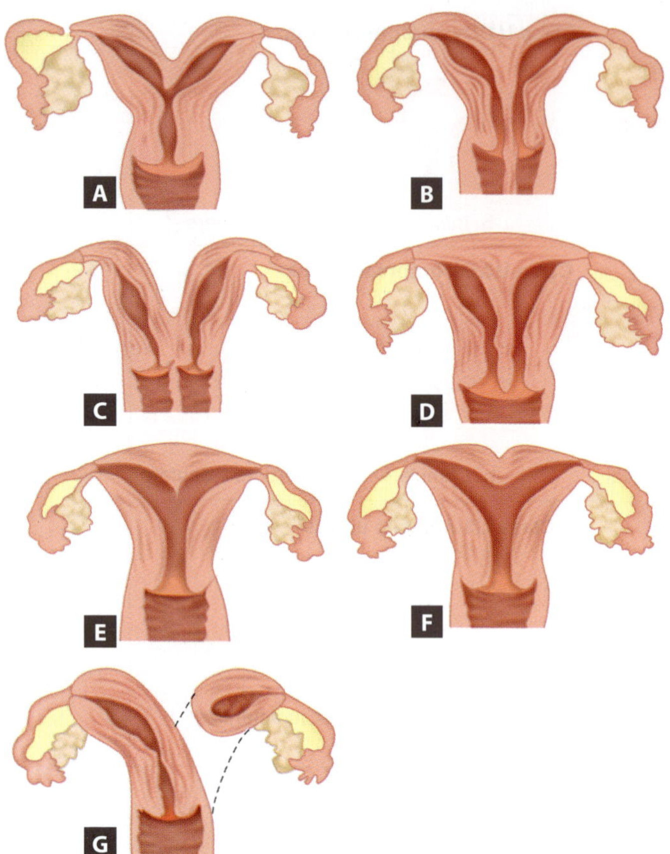

Figs. 7A to G: Uterine anomalies. (A) Uterus duplex unicollis; (B) Uterus duplex with double vagina; (C) Uterus didelphys; (D) Uterus septus with single vagina; (E) Uterus subseptus; (F) Uterus arcuatus; (G) Uterus unicornis with rudimentary contralateral hemiuterus.

a septate or bicornuate condition of the uterus and may have one or two cervices opening into it. This condition arises either because late fusion of the Müllerian ducts gives rise to two Müllerian tubercles or because of failure of proper canalization of the two sinovaginal bulbs. Very rarely, the septum is disposed from side to side, and this is supposed to be explained by rotation of the Müllerian ducts on each other.

Arcuate Uterus (Class VI)

This is a flat-topped uterus in which the fundal bulge has not developed after fusion of the ducts **(Figs. 2 and 9)**. If only the exterior of the uterus is affected, the fundal myometrium is abnormally thin.

Deformities in Combination (Figs. 6 and 13)

The above deformities occur in all manner of combinations. Moreover, they may be associated with atresia or underdevelopment of one or both Müllerian ducts. For example, one half of a uterus didelphys may communicate with the vagina and the other may not. Again, one or both horns of a bicornuate uterus may be rudimentary.

Diethylstilbestrol-related Anomalies (Class VII)

Several characteristic anomalies have been described in women who were exposed to diethylstilbestrol (DES) in utero. Benign vaginal adenosis and cervical hoods, septate, collars and cockscombs are seen in a large

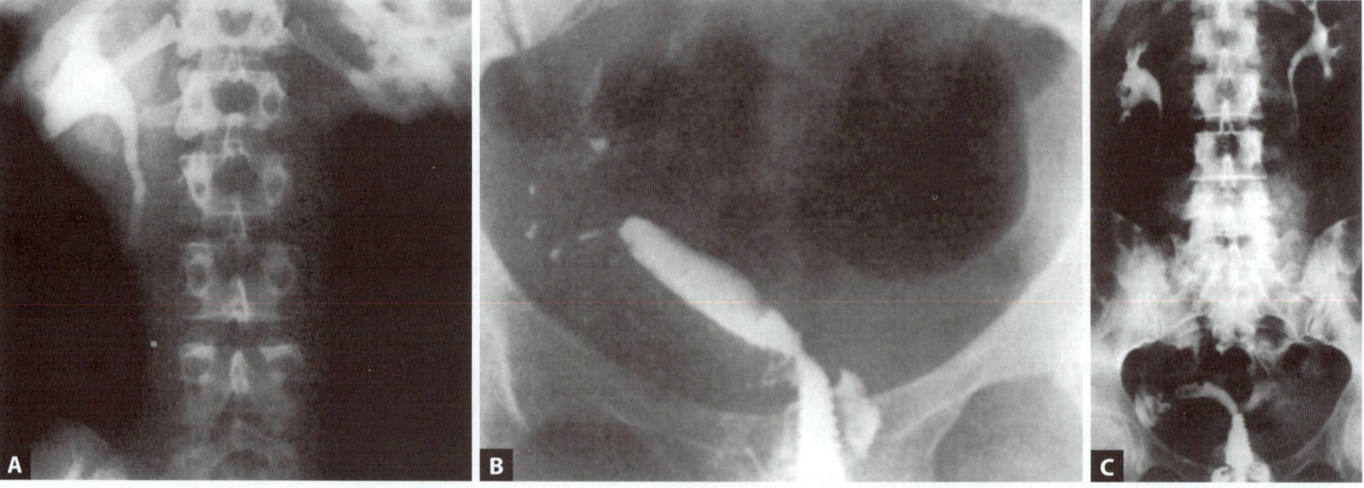

Figs. 8A to C: (A and B) Hysterosalpingogram and intravenous pyelogram in the same woman, illustrating congenital absence of the left Müllerian duct and Wolffian system. A true unicornuate uterus is, thus, associated with absence of the kidney on the opposite side; (C) A hysterogram showing an apparent right-sided unicornuate uterus, but the presence of kidneys, indicated by the pyelogram on the same woman, proves that the uterus must be bicornuate with a hypoplastic horn on the left side not communicating with the cavity of the uterus. This was proved at laparotomy.

number of cases. T-shaped uteri, wide lower segments and constriction bands have also been described. There is a high incidence of perifimbrial paratubal cysts. Vaginal clear cell adenocarcinoma is very rare. Unlike all other congenital uterine malformations, the DES uterus is not associated with an increase in renal anomalies.

Aetiology

The Müllerian ducts are ordinarily pulled together by subperitoneal fibromuscular tissue, and it is suggested that a defect in this process is a cause of these malformations.

The causes of Müllerian anomalies have yet to be fully clarified. The karyotypes are normal (46,XX) in 92% of the women with Müllerian anomalies and abnormal (sex chromosome mosaicism) in 8% of these women. The majority of these developmental abnormalities are infrequent and sporadic and are thus attributed to polygenic and multifactorial causes. A recent study attributed persistence of the intrauterine septum to a deficiency in the antiapoptotic protein Bcl-2, which is responsible for the process of apoptosis and absorption of the septum.

Events such as hypoxia that occurs during pregnancy, use of medications such as methotrexate or DES, ionising radiation and viral infections may also contribute towards the occurrence of Müllerian malformations. Among the

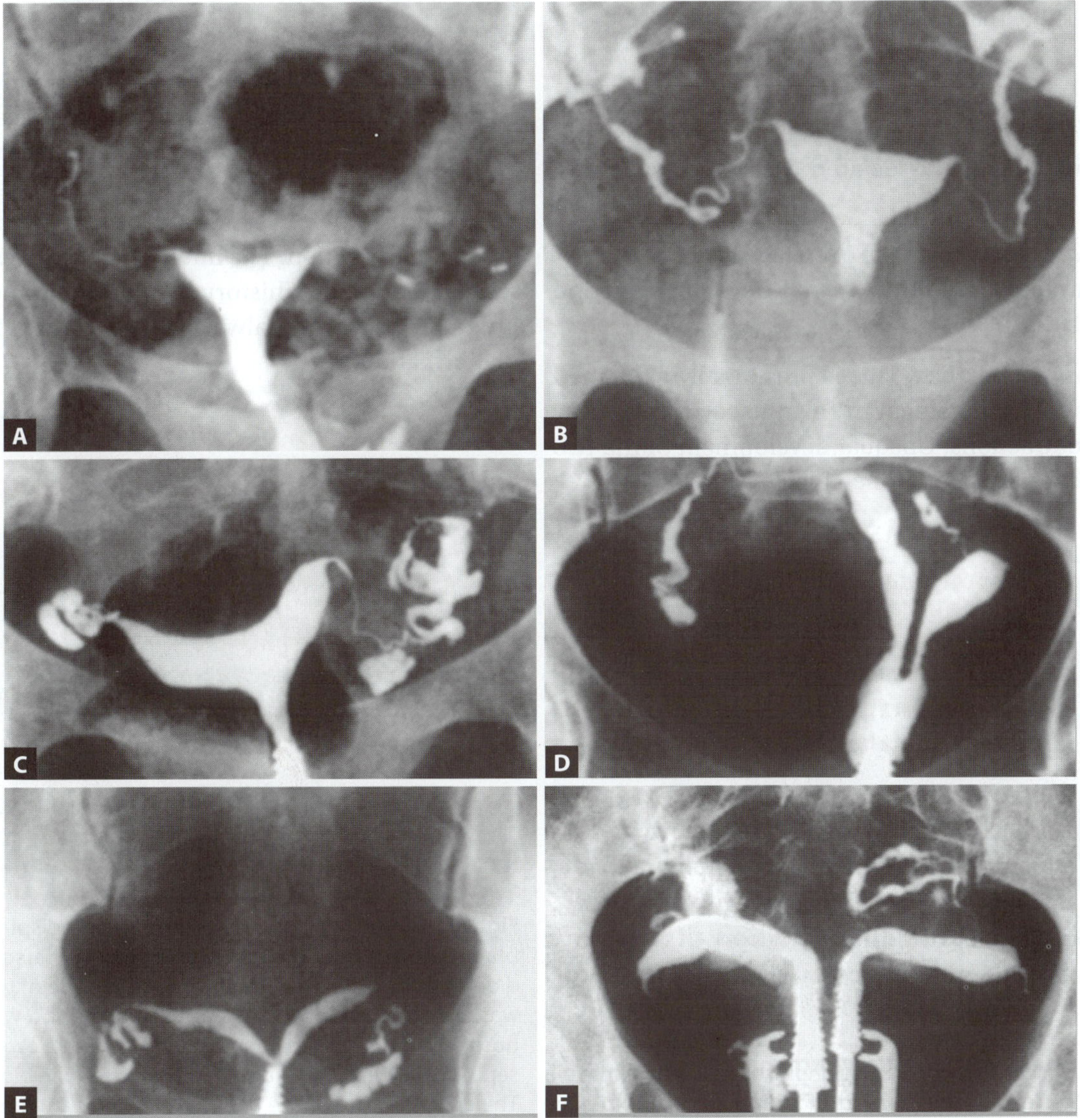

Figs. 9A to F: Certain types of Müllerian duct malfusion deformity revealed by hysterosalpingography. (A and B) Degrees of arcuate deformity; (C) A minor degree of bicornuate malformation; this type of radiograph is difficult to interpret because a similar picture can be produced by a fundal leiomyoma; (D) Septate uterus; (E) Uterus bicornis unicollis; (F) Uterus didelphys with a cannula in each cervix.

drugs that induce Müllerian malformations, thalidomide and DES lead to malformations of the uterine cavity.

The uterus didelphys and bicornuate uterus often have unusually thick and strong round ligaments, and a tough vesicorectal fold running between each horn; it may be that these prevent the Müllerian ducts from coming together.

Symptoms

These abnormalities are relatively common, but they pass unnoticed because they are often symptomless. The majority is first recognised during pregnancy or as a result of a pregnancy mishap; this only goes to show that, excepting the condition of septate vagina, they do not as a rule lower fertility materially.

Menstrual

The menstrual cycle is usually normal. Menstrual abnormalities that are associated with these cases are given in the following text.

Menorrhagia: Menorrhagia can occur because of the larger bleeding surface offered by two well-developed uterine horns **(Fig. 10)**.

Spasmodic dysmenorrhea: This is presumably explained by the unusual arrangement of the musculature and by abnormal contractions. Unequal development of the two horns can be manifested by one-sided dysmenorrhoea.

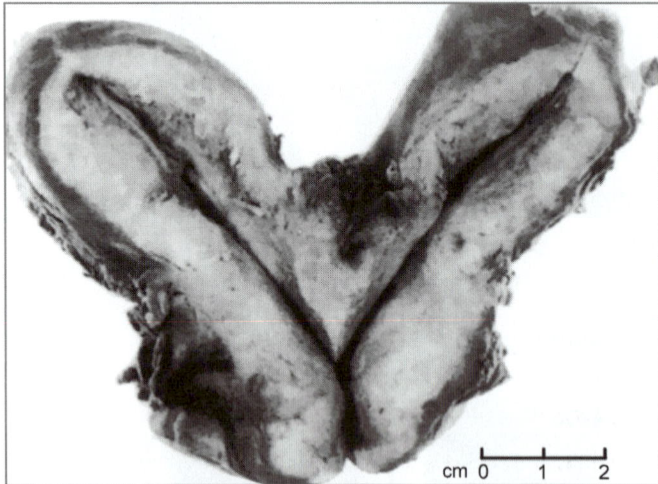

Fig. 10: Uterus bicornis unicollis. Both horns are equally and well developed; the resulting increased bleeding surface explains why the patient concerned always had very heavy periods, which ultimately necessitated hysterectomy.

Failure to contain flow: Failure to control the menstrual outflow by means of a single intravaginal tampon can give a clear lead to the diagnosis of a septate vagina and uterus didelphys.

Coital

Dyspareunia: A vaginal septum may cause difficulty in coitus, but this is often overcome without the couple realising the abnormality. One half of the vagina is then usually dilated, and the septum is pushed to the side.

Bleeding: Attempts at coitus or at the insertion of a tampon sometimes cause bleeding from a vessel in the lower edge of the septum **(Fig. 11)**.

Obstetric Symptoms

Malpresentation: Malpresentation of the foetus and the related fundal or cornual insertion of the placenta are often explained by an abnormality in the shape of the uterus. A subseptate or bicornuate deformity favours a transverse lie; a uterus didelphys or a unicornuate uterus favours a breech presentation. The finding of a transverse lie, which resists version, or a history of malpresentation in several pregnancies, should always raise a suspicion of uterine malformation.

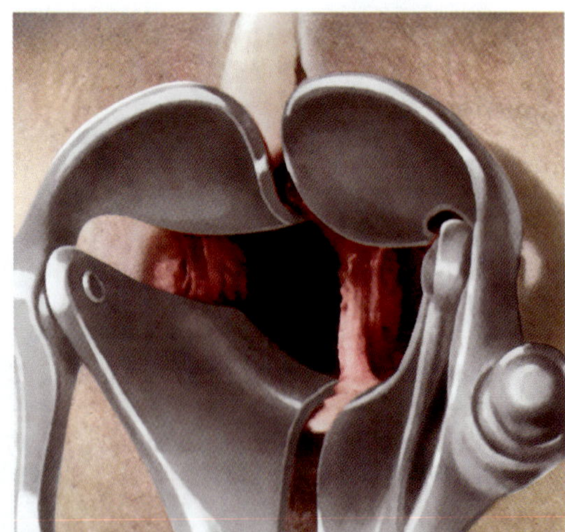

Fig. 11: Septate vagina, the septum being displayed by a four-bladed speculum. The patient concerned also had a uterus didelphys with a cervix opening on either side of the septum. She was an unmarried woman, aged 31 years, who was admitted to hospital suffering from haemorrhage from the lower border of the septum and was so exsanguinated as to require blood transfusion. The alleged cause of the haemorrhage was an attempt to insert a menstrual vaginal tampon for the first time; it may, however, have been an attempt at coitus.

Abnormal uterine action: This is not often seen in the first and second stages of labour but is common in the third stage. Manual removal of the placenta may be necessary in cases of bicornuate, septate and subseptate uterus, and the incidence of postpartum haemorrhage is increased. If the horns are completely separate, however, expulsive action is generally good. A high vaginal septum can prevent the cervix from dilating.

Obstructed labour: The non-pregnant horn of a uterus didelphys enlarges during pregnancy, being subjected to the same hormone influences as the pregnant horn. Sometimes, it remains low in the pelvis and then constitutes a tumour, which obstructs the delivery of the foetus. Labour may also be obstructed by a vaginal septum, a classical situation arising when the breech presents astride the septum.

Infertility

The only form of malfusion deformity which may lower fertility significantly is a fully septate vagina. In such circumstances, coitus may take place in the half, which does not communicate with the cervix or with the better developed cervix and uterus. Even if coitus is practiced sometimes on one side and sometimes on the other side of the septum, there is always a 50% chance that semen is deposited in the Müllerian duct, which does not serve the ovary that has ovulated in that particular cycle.

Cornual Pregnancy

Site of the conceptus: In successive pregnancies, this is not necessarily the same cavity of the *double* uterus. If both horns are well developed, either may be used.

Sacculation of the uterus: This presents as either an organic or a functional abnormality during pregnancy. When the saccule is sited on the line of junction of the Müllerian ducts, it may be a manifestation of a fusion defect.

Abortion and Premature Labour

These are common when the uterus is malformed because of abnormal contractions, inadequate stretching and hypertrophy to accommodate the pregnancy, poor implantation, or placentation on a septum **(Figs. 12A to F)**. Uterine malformation tends to cause late, rather than early, abortion because of an associated incompetent ostium.

Diagnostic Signs

A septate vagina and two cervices may be obvious on vaginal examination, and either finding should immediately raise the possibility of a fusion defect in the uterus. On bimanual examination, it may be possible to feel the two separate uterine horns or a depression in the fundus; failing that, a very suggestive sign is an impression that the uterus is unusually wide from side to side. A septate uterus cannot be diagnosed on bimanual examination but may be recognised by passing a sound, as may the more extreme malformations. Apart from laparotomy or laparoscopy (which may fail to reveal a septate uterus), the diagnosis of uterine malfusion defects is best made by hysteroscopy or hysterosalpingography **(Figs. 9A to F)**.

Magnetic resonance imaging is an excellent modality for accurate diagnosis, but it is more expensive and not universally available.

The clinical diagnosis of septate vagina and of uterus didelphys can be extraordinarily elusive, particularly if there is unequal development of the two sides and if a septum is displaced. At times, the other cervix and uterus are not recognised, leading to clinical situations such as doing procedure on wrong uterus. This will lead to persistence of symptoms and many a times, the diagnosis is missed.

During pregnancy, most of these anomalies go unnoticed diagnosed during pregnancy or during caesarean section. Abnormal contour of fundus, recurrent malpresentations and history of preterm labour should raise the suspicion, and evaluation may be done with sonography or during caesarean section. Ultrasonography should be done to rule out associated urinary system anomalies. A diagnosis of uterus bicornis or didelphys is made by feeling the non-pregnant horn lying to one side and a little in front of or behind the main tumour **(Fig. 14)**. Whenever a placenta has to be removed manually or curettage carried out to complete an abortion, the cavity of the uterus should carefully be explored by hand, finger, sound or curette to exclude a septum or bicornuate deformity.

Treatment

The treatment depends on the severity present and on the menstrual, sexual and reproductive symptoms produced. Each case requires separate consideration. Many go unnoticed and if asymptomatic are best left untreated. Vaginal septa are removed unless they are symptomless,

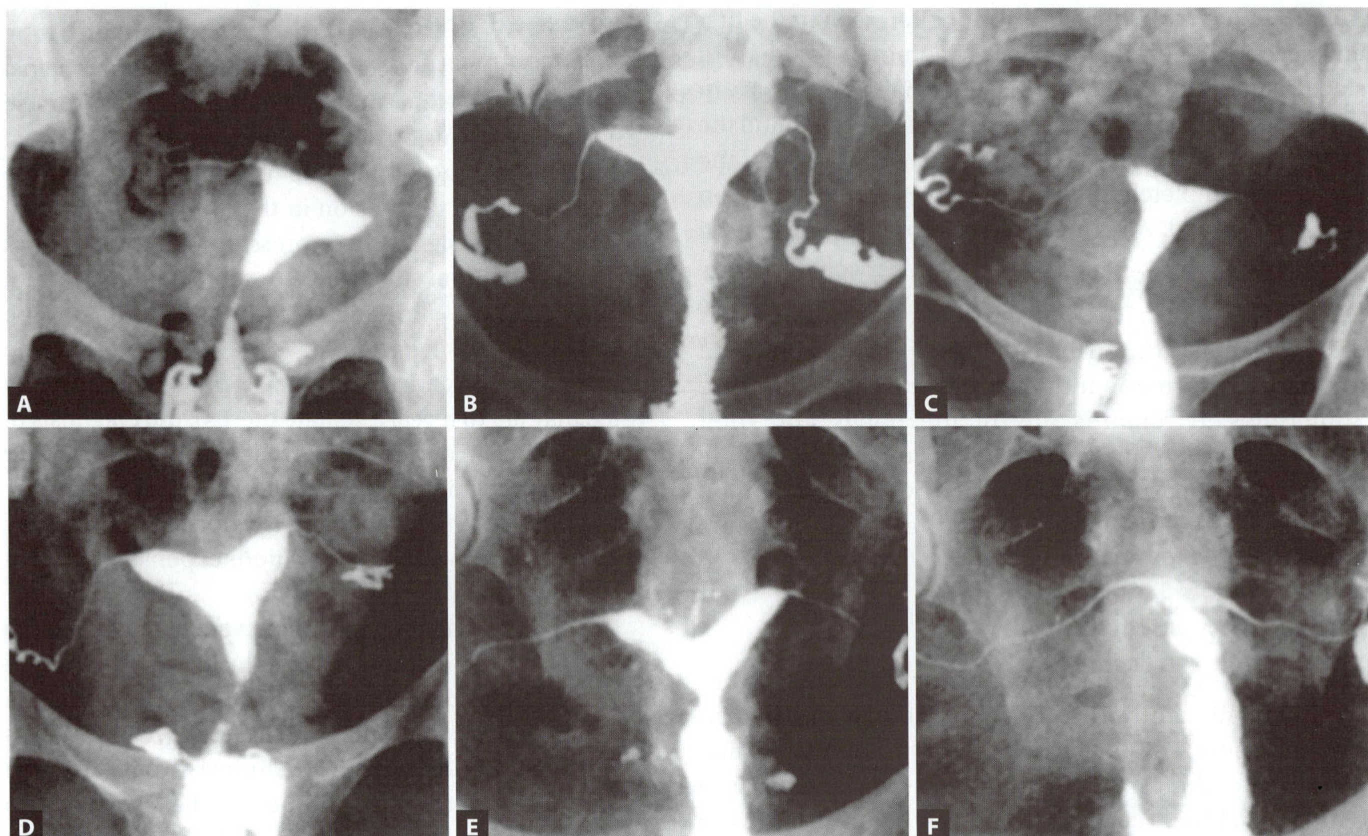

Figs. 12A to F: Hysterograms illustrating uterine causes of abortion. (A) A normal uterus for comparison with the other hysterograms. Note the well-shaped fundus and constriction at the level of the isthmus and internal os; (B) A normal fundus but a defective internal os (*funnel cervix*) in a woman who had repeated abortions and premature labours; (C) A funnel cervix and a minor degree of bicornuate deformity in the uterus of a woman who had a series of premature labours; (D) A competent cervix but a bicornuate malformation in a woman who had one abortion and one premature labour; (E) A bicornuate uterus in a patient with a history of four successive pregnancies ending in mid-trimester abortion or premature labour and stillbirth; (F) The same case as (E) after metroplasty. After this, radiograph was obtained, the woman conceived again and the pregnancy progressed well until 37th week when bleeding from a placenta praevia prompted a caesarean section; a live healthy baby resulted.

and there is no prospect of marriage and childbearing. Noncommunicating rudimentary uterine horns are painful and may cause complications and should be treated with excision.

When a bicornuate or septate uterus has caused not less than three miscarriages and no pregnancy has resulted in a viable child, surgery may be indicated. Prior to surgery, a thorough work-up is mandatory to exclude all other causes of recurrent abortion. In the case of bicornuate uterus, an incision is made over the uterus and the two horns are sutured together to form a single cavity. The results depend on a careful choice of cases according to the exact anatomy as shown by hysterography. In such cases, there is a place for elective caesarean section. These surgeries are well done these days with laparoscopy.

Surgeries such as Jones metroplasty, Tompkins procedure, Strassman metroplasty, and transcervical lysis of uterine septum all have now only historic importance. Operative hysteroscopy has replaced all of above by a simple procedure wherein the septum is cut hysteroscopically by scissors, resectoscope or laser (argon, KTP or neodymium-doped yttrium-aluminium-garnet) after inducing endometrial atrophy by administering gonadotrophin-releasing hormone (GnRH) analogue for 2 months. Laparoscopic guidance is required to confirm that the uterus is indeed septate and not bicornuate and to determine the end point of resection—the myometrial fibres can be seen hysteroscopically and the light can be seen transmitted through the fundus uniformly. Healing of the septal areas occurs in 2 months, and they are covered by

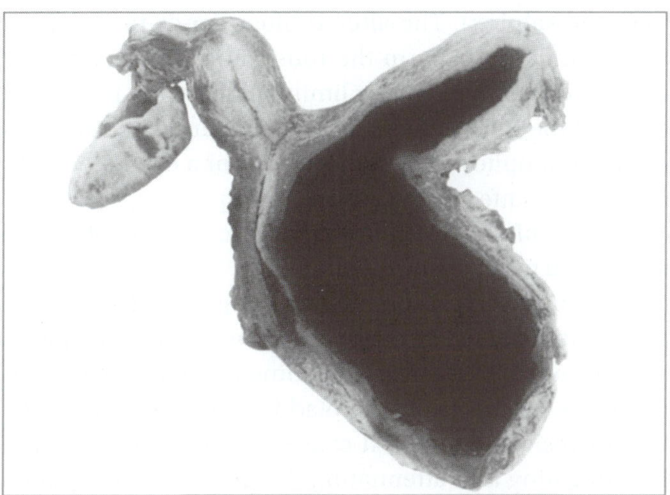

Fig. 13: Uterus didelphys with one half of a septate vagina imperforate. This has resulted in unilateral haematocolpos and haematometra, the diagnosis of which in life might have been missed because the patient concerned menstruated normally from the other side.

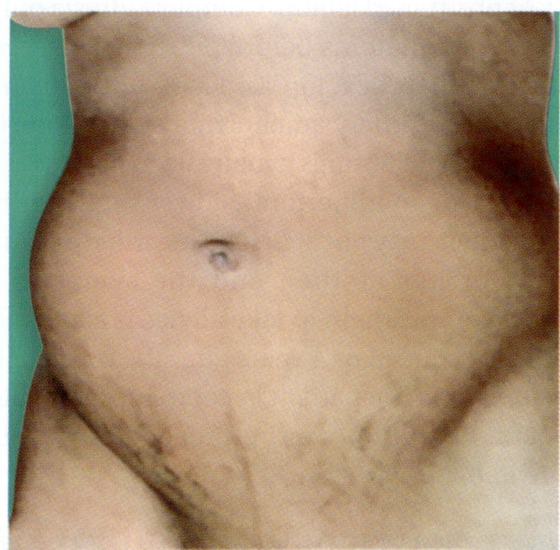

Fig. 14: A bicornuate uterus containing a pregnancy of 32 weeks' duration. The broad-topped uterus with a depression between the horns is clearly visible. This condition may cause a transverse lie, but, in this case, the patient delivered normally at term.

endometrium. Evidence suggests that prophylaxis against intrauterine adhesion formation by the use of oestrogens, intrauterine Foley balloon catheters or intrauterine contraceptive devices (IUCDs) is not required.

Duplication and Diverticula of Müllerian Ducts

If the Müllerian ducts are duplicated, a true double uterus with four fallopian tubes can result, but this is a condition of extreme rarity. More common are diverticula of the ducts which give rise to accessory abdominal ostia of the tube, accessory tubes, diverticula of the tube, or a uterine diverticulum or accessory horn. In the last condition, which is sometimes called a Mülleroma and is very rare, the third horn is not supplied with a fallopian tube or round ligament. If functional, it can cause severe dysmenorrhoea.

Incomplete Canalization of Müllerian Ducts: Congenital Gynatresia

The Müllerian buds have solid tips behind which canalisation takes place progressively. The Müllerian and sinovaginal bulb tissues, which form the vagina, are also lumenless at first. Failure to canalise results in either solid organs or membranes of varying thicknesses obstructing the genital canal. Thus, a rudimentary uterus sometimes lacks a cavity, and the vagina may be represented by an uncanalised column of tissue. Atresia may affect only one Müllerian duct so that one horn of a bicornuate uterus may fail to communicate with the cervical canal or one half of a septate vagina may be a closed cavity **(Fig. 13)**. Unilateral haematocolpos, mucocolpos and pyocolpos are not common. They can give rise to difficulty in diagnosis because the retained secretions create a tumour lying beside an apparently anatomically and functionally normal genital tract.

Sites

Cervical Atresia

Congenital atresia of the cervix of an otherwise normal uterus or of a bicornuate uterus is rare. When it occurs, a reasonably normal vagina is invariably present. It is more common to encounter apparent cervical atresia in association with absence of the lower vagina **(Figs. 7A to G)**.

Vaginal Atresia

This occurs in various degrees and forms. The whole vagina may be represented by a solid strand of tissue, which is difficult if not impossible to recognise. Whether or not this is present, the condition is labelled congenital absence of the vagina. Next, the upper (46%), middle (40%) or lower (14%) zones of the vagina may be imperforate over an area 0.5–6.0 cm in depth. More frequently, the vagina is obstructed by a thinner membrane situated low in the vagina, just above the hymen. It represents a failure in breakdown of the partition between the Müllerian and sinovaginal bulb contributions to the vagina.

This condition of imperforate vagina is frequently misdiagnosed as much less common imperforate hymen. However, the distinction between the two is largely academic because their effects and treatments are identical.

An obstructing membrane situated across the upper vagina, just below the cervix, may be complete but usually has a laterally placed tiny opening through which menstrual discharge escapes. This condition is sometimes called phimosis of the cervix. A minor degree of this deformity, amounting to no more than an annular constriction of the upper vagina, is more common.

Pathology

Atresia of the lower genital tract has no serious ill effects if the uterus is absent or functionless. If the uterus is present, it is unusual to see any harm arise in childhood, although a collection of mucus, sometimes bloodstained, in the uterus or upper vagina (mucocolpos) is possible. This may even be present at or soon after birth, the secretions of the uterus and cervix having been stimulated by placental hormones **(Figs. 15A to C)**.

When the uterus begins to menstruate, the fact is not recognised because the blood remains hidden behind the obstruction, a condition of cryptomenorrhoea. With each monthly discharge, the vagina fills with blood which remains fluid. Some of its water content is continually being absorbed, so the material becomes inspissated. Nevertheless, the amount gradually increases and in the course of months or years distends first the vagina (haematocolpos), then the cervix and uterus (haematocervix and haematometra), and finally the tube (haematosalpinx). The altered blood tends to set up an aseptic inflammation in the tubes, and this closes their outer ends and prevents or limits spill into the peritoneal cavity. If the tubes remain open, pelvic endometriosis is a possible complication. A mucocolpos or a haematocolpos can become infected to cause a pyocolpos.

Atresia of the cervix has similar results, but only the uterus and tubes are affected.

The vagina can accommodate a large quantity of blood and, as it distends, forms a tumour, which fills the pelvis and extends into the lower abdomen. The pelvic tumour displaces the fundus of the bladder upwards but not the urethrovesical junction. It causes retention of urine, not by elongating and attenuating the urethra, as is so often stated, but by interfering with the opening of the internal urethral sphincter.

Clinical Features

An incomplete vaginal membrane may cause dyspareunia, infertility or obstructed labour. Complete atresia only occasionally causes symptoms before puberty. The secondary sex characters then develop as usual, but menstruation does not appear. Primary amenorrhoea, therefore, is often the complaint, which brings gynatresia to light.

In the case of an imperforate lower vagina or hymen, the amenorrhoea may not at first be regarded as significant by the girl or her mother, and the symptom which sometimes prompts them to take advice is acute retention of urine. This occurs 3 or 4 years after the onset of hidden menstruation, and the patient is, therefore, generally aged 15–18 years. Retention can be preceded by a phase of bladder irritability.

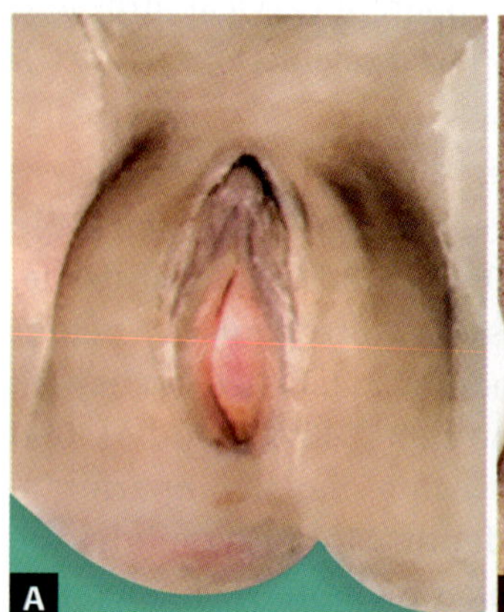

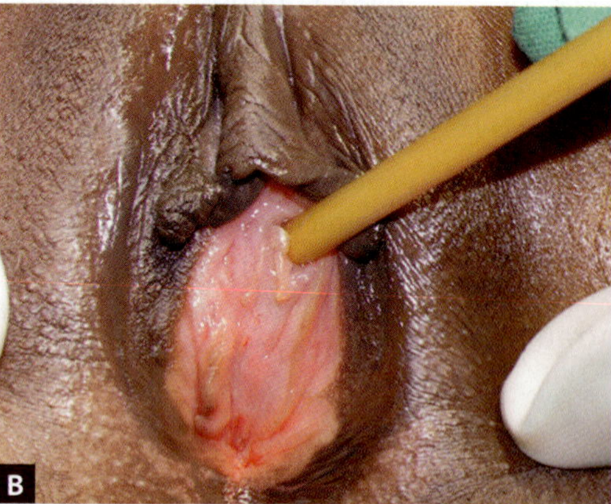

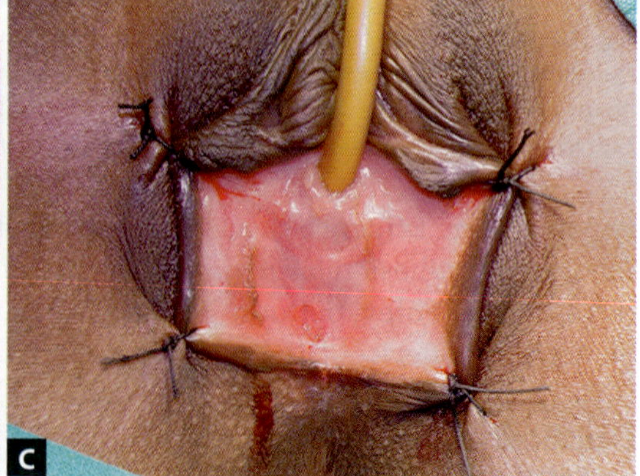

Figs. 15A to C: A mucocolpos in a newborn baby with the imperforate lower vaginal membrane bulging. This was incised when the baby was 3 days and 500 mL of mucoid fluid escaped.
Courtesy: Francis HH.

Often, there is a history of monthly attacks of lower abdominal pain or backache with menstrual molimina. Pelvic discomfort and rectal pain are also noticed by some patients.

On examination, a tumour, dull to percussion, is found in the lower abdomen. This is caused partly by an overfull bladder with hypertrophied walls. When a catheter has been passed, however, a tumour may still extend to the level of the umbilicus or higher, and this consists of the distended vagina with the uterus perched on top **(Figs. 16A and B)**. Even in babies, a mucocolpos can result in a large abdominal tumour. If the obstructing membrane is thin and situated low in the vagina, it can be seen bulging at the introitus; the underlying blood gives it a bluish colour. Rectal examination is all important to the diagnosis.

With atresia of the upper vagina or cervix, the patient is more likely to present with attacks of severe abdominal pain occurring at monthly intervals. The tumour then consists of a distended uterus, cervix or upper vaginal compartment, or combinations of these **(Figs. 7A to C)**. It is not likely to be as large as in the case of a classical haematocolpos because the severe pain forces the patient to seek advice at an earlier stage. If the lower vagina is absent, the swelling is usually only palpable on rectal examination.

Differential Diagnosis

Conditions most likely to be confused are pregnancy and tuberculous peritonitis, both of which cause amenorrhoea and a lower abdominal swelling; acute or subacute appendicitis—attacks of pain; all causes of true amenorrhoea; ovarian cyst and pelvic kidney; this is common when the vagina is absent and may be mistaken for a haematometra. Ultrasound helps in the diagnosis.

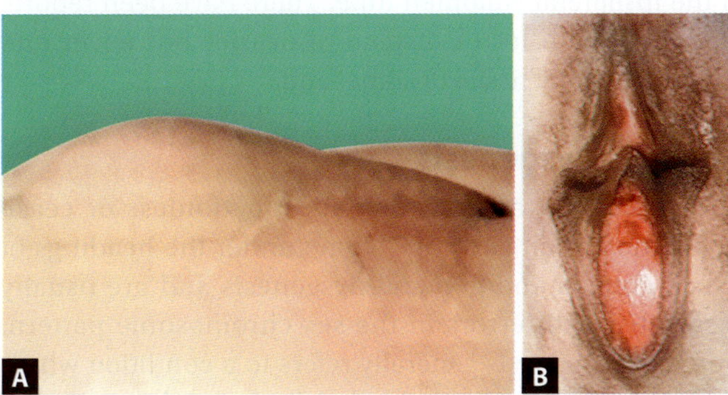

Figs. 16A and B: (A) Haematocolpos resulting from an imperforate vagina producing, in a girl aged 15 years, a tumour, which extends from the pelvis to the umbilicus; (B) The bulging membrane at the introitus, made dark by the underlying tarry blood.

Treatment

Once the diagnosis of cryptomenorrhoea is made, surgical treatment is urgently required since every menstrual episode further dilates the genital tract and threatens permanent impairment of reproductive function.

Obstruction at the level of the cervix is least often encountered but is the most controversial. The conservative approach is uterovaginoplasty, while the radical method is to perform a hysterectomy. The decision is based on the clinical features, psychological status, approach and experience of the surgeon and, not the least, the wishes of the patient and her family.

When the vagina is well developed and the uterus is well formed and functional, uterovaginoplasty can be attempted by a combined abdominovaginal approach. This is a technically difficult operation in which the uterus and vagina are opened, the collected menstrual blood is drained from the uterus, and the posterior wall of the vagina is sutured to that of the uterus. A Foley catheter is inserted through the vagina into the uterus and anchored there. The uterine body is then reconstructed and sutured to the anterior vaginal wall. The Foley catheter remains as a stent for 8–12 weeks to permit epithelialisation of the new tract.

In patients with cervical atresia, restenosis may occur in 50%, and hysterectomy is then required. In some of these patients, severe sepsis may result, and even the occasional fatality has been reported. All these patients have severe morbidity from the incapacitating pain. These features prompt many gynaecologists to recommend a hysterectomy to patients with cervical atresia. However, since these are young women, the psychological sequelae of such radical steps are tremendous; hence, most surgeons nowadays attempt reconstructive surgery at least once.

Pregnancy has occurred in some cases after creation of a neocervix, and this fact further encourages surgeons towards the conservative approach.

When the outflow of menstrual blood is prevented by a thick vaginal membrane at any level, incision of the latter alone is inadequate. The raw area in the vagina always seals over rapidly within days if not hours. It is, therefore, essential to cover any deficiency with vaginal epithelium; this is best done by dissecting free the upper vaginal walls and *advancing* them downwards to be sutured to the margins of the vagina around the lower limit of the

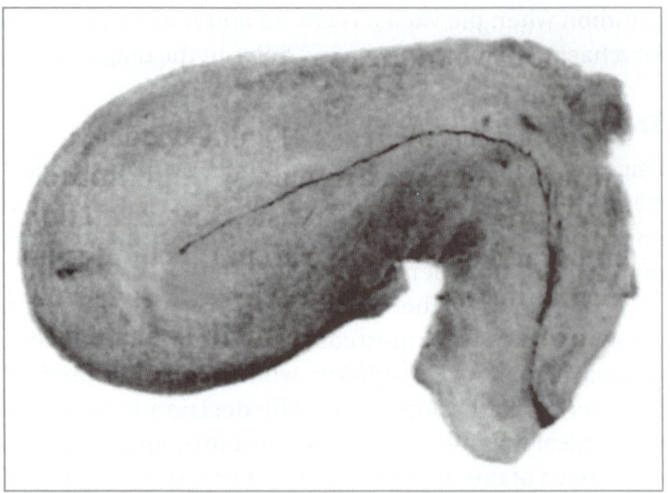

Fig. 17: Acute anteflexion of the cervix (cochleate uterus).

obstruction **(Fig. 17)**. Alternatively, the raw area can be covered with a skin graft, as for the creation of an artificial vagina, but this is usually unnecessary. Pregnancy following such procedures is not very rare and is often best terminated by elective caesarean section.

The treatment of the more common and typical cases of haematocolpos, when the obstructing membrane is thin and low down, is simple. The membrane is merely excised (not incised) and the edges subsequently heal rapidly. However, this apparently minor operation demands great care over asepsis, as the more complicated ones mentioned above. The vagina has been closed throughout life, so it is without protecting lactobacilli, its epithelium is poorly formed, and its reaction is alkaline or weakly acid. There is, therefore, a little natural resistance to bacteria entering from below; indeed, the degenerated blood and debris offer a favourable medium for their growth. Postoperative salpingitis and peritonitis are, therefore, real hazards and, in the past, were sometimes fatal. Bilateral hydrosalpinges occur as late sequelae.

The fluid which escapes after removal of the obstruction resembles liquid chocolate. It is devoid of fibrinogen and prothrombin and contains mucin (from the cervix), lactic acid (from the blood), calcium and altered blood pigments. Its amount varies from 200 mL to 2 L or more, and it may take several days to run away. Its escape should not be hurried by the insertion of a drainage tube or by intermittent pressure over the lower abdomen because such procedures encourage the entry of organisms. For the same reason, vaginal examination should be avoided, and the state of the uterus and tubes is left in doubt for 1–2 months. Meanwhile, the vulva is kept covered with a sterile pad and the patient is discouraged from sitting in a bath.

At the end of the prescribed time, vaginal examination is carried out to see if there is any remaining evidence of haematometra or haematosalpinx. Fortunately, the uterus and tubes show enormous power of recovery, so radical treatment such as salpingectomy and hysterectomy is rarely necessary. A high percentage of girls treated for haematocolpos later prove to be fertile.

Incomplete atresia such as stricture of the upper vagina is treated by dilatation or by incision and suture on the principles of plastic surgery. Occasionally, excision of fibrous tissue and coverage of the raw area by freeing the adjacent vaginal wall are necessary.

OVARY

The sex of each human is determined at the time of union of spermatozoon and ovum, but no morphologic sex differentiation in the ovaries can be demonstrated until the 7th week. The primordial germ cells are first found on the 24th day near the allantois. The germ cells proliferate and migrate to reach the genital ridge, which by the 5th week becomes elevated and thickened. Sex differentiation becomes visible early in the 8th week. Proliferation of oogonia (germ cells) by mitosis continues until approximately the 15th week. By the 4th month, primary follicles appear. In the meantime, the ovary has become recognisable as a discrete organ, which *descend*s to the level of the pelvic brim and undergoes lateral rotation.

Malformations may affect one or both ovaries.

Absence or Underdevelopment

Absence of the gonads is extremely rare and betokens a fundamental error in the formation of the urogenital ridge. It is usually associated with renal agenesis and absence of the ipsilateral Fallopian tube. There have been reports of women with testes instead of ovaries but never one without gonadal tissue of some kind.

Gonadal Dysgenesis

Rudimentary ovaries, which are functionless or cease to function at an early age, come under the headings of streak gonads and gonadal dysgenesis and are usually associated with errors in the sex chromosome pattern. Gonadal dysgenesis generally refers to a condition where gonadal development is abnormal, often only presenting streaks of connective tissue that are often called *streak gonads*. Streak ovaries extend from the lateral pelvic wall to the attachment of the utero-ovarian ligaments. They vary considerably in size but are usually approximately

4 cm in length and 2–3 mm in width. Dysgenetic ovaries are characterised by the absence of follicular structures and oocytes. In women, the most common cause of gonadal dysgenesis is Turner syndrome, 45X. Phenotypic females with streak gonads can also have XX gonadal dysgenesis, XY gonadal dysgenesis or mixed gonadal dysgenesis. In phenotypic females with a Y chromosome, there is a high risk of the development of a gonadoblastoma, and removal of the gonads is usually indicated.

Accessory and Supernumerary Ovaries

True ovarian duplication is rarely reported; it occurs in conjunction with duplication of genital ridge and a duplicated Müllerian duct. An accessory ovary on one or both sides is not uncommon, but the condition as a rule is one in which a single ovary is divided into two portions which are attached to each other by fibrous tissue.

Nevertheless, true supernumerary ovaries or portions of ovarian tissue have been found in the broad ligament and elsewhere; they probably account for the occasional reports of menstruation continuing, and of pregnancy occurring, after the removal of both ovaries.

Failure of Descent

The ovary may remain at the level of the pelvic brim or even near the lower pole of the kidney. Sometimes, it is found in a hernial sac.

FALLOPIAN TUBE

The Fallopian tubes are formed from the most cephalic portions of the Müllerian ducts. Late in the 6th week (crown–rump length, 11 mm), a shallow depression can be observed near the mesonephric duct. Commencing as a groove, a tube forms, a lumen develops and the paramesonephric ducts grow caudal, lying lateral to the Wolffian ducts. The ostia at the cephalic ends remain open. Anomalies of the oviducts are not prominent and frequently pass unnoticed. Malformations of the tube are described under Müllerian duct anomalies. They include absence in whole or part, underdevelopment, congenital atresia, excessive length, duplication, accessory tubes, diverticula and accessory ostia.

Absence of one or both tubes may occur and is almost always associated with absence of the uterus as well as with other anomalies. Localised factors may result in an incomplete tube. Rudimentary tubes occur as fibromuscular cords without lumens. If the tube is a long, thin hypoplastic structure and responds to appropriate endocrine therapy, it is classified as infantile. Occasionally, ostia are duplicated or an accessory tube may be present. Most anomalies as such do not require treatment.

UTERUS

Absence

Complete absence of the uterus results when the Müllerian ducts fail to develop and are often associated with an error in the sex chromosome makeup. The uterine agenesis–hypoplasia spectrum accounts for ~10–15% of all Müllerian duct anomalies. The upper vagina is inevitably absent as well. If the Fallopian tubes or their fimbriated extremities are present, they taper inwards to a transverse fold—the plica transversalis.

Hypoplasia

Types

Hypoplasia of the uterus occurs in varying degrees as the result of an error in either antenatal or postnatal development. Sometimes, the organ consists of nothing more than a small nodule of solid or hollow functionless tissue, a condition often mistaken for absence of the uterus. The uterus may, however, be essentially normal in shape and structure yet have reduced dimensions. Persistence of the infantile proportions in which the cervix is long in relation to the corpus is another feature.

Causes

- An inherent error in Müllerian duct tissues, often associated with sex chromosome abnormality, resulting in a uterus which is incompletely formed or which is incapable of responding to the normal postnatal growth stimulus of oestrogen
- Failure of the ovaries and adrenals to supply the oestrogen stimulus to a basically normal uterus at the time of puberty
- Some disease or circumstance which destroys oestrogen or nullifies its effect on the uterus

Clinical Features

The traditional symptoms of uterine hypoplasia are primary amenorrhoea, late menarche, infrequent menstruation and infertility. All except the first are more likely to be manifestations of an underlying ovarian inactivity than of the uterine abnormality. There is no reason why smallness of the uterus per se should prevent conception or alter the ovarian cycle. Scanty menstruation (hypomenorrhoea) may be a symptom but is often found with normal-sized uteri. Some believe that the first pregnancy is more likely to abort if the uterus is hypoplastic, but the evidence for this is insecure.

On examination, the uterus is found to be small in overall length and width, although the cervix may be relatively long. The endometrium is thin.

When the complaint is secondary amenorrhoea, the finding of a small uterus means atrophy rather than hypoplasia; it is sometimes difficult, if not impossible, to distinguish between these two states.

Diagnosis

The diagnosis of uterine hypoplasia is made all too frequently on a mere impression that the uterus feels small on bimanual examination. Indeed, uterine hypoplasia is more often a convenient label than a proven state, especially in cases of infertility where the cause is unknown. The essential criteria of uterine hypoplasia are a subnormal menstrual cycle, a uterine cavity measurement of 6 cm or less and an endometrium which appears unstimulated on microscopy. All must be present.

Treatment

Treatment needs to be directed at the cause. The results of treatment with exogenous oestrogens are unsatisfactory for the following reasons:

- If hypoplasia is the result of the uterus being unresponsive to the ovaries, oestrogens have no effect on it.
- If hypoplasia is the result of an inadequate ovarian stimulus, then oestrogens will promote full development of the uterus, but the effect is temporary and, unless ovarian function becomes normal in the meantime, the uterus returns to its former state when treatment is suspended.

In practice, therefore, the administration of oestrogen is of more value as a diagnostic than as a therapeutic procedure. It may be added that, when the complaint is infertility, attention should be directed to establishing normal ovarian function rather than correcting the consequential uterine hypoplasia.

Cochleate Uterus

Pathology

In young nulliparous women, it is not uncommon to find a uterus which is cochleate or C-shaped when viewed from the side. The position of the body of the uterus is normal and the deformity arises because the cervix is angled forwards. The condition is, therefore, also called acute anteflexion of the cervix **(Fig. 17)**. A similar malformation in reverse can occur when the body of the uterus is directed backwards and is a common feature of congenital retroflexion of the uterus. In these states, the cervix is usually longer, narrower and more conical than normal, the corpus being well developed.

Menarche is at a normal age and menstruation is free and regular. A cochleate uterus should, therefore, be regarded as being maldeveloped rather than underdeveloped, the site of the trouble being at the level of the internal os. The deformity nearly always disappears after pregnancy.

Clinical Features

A cochleate uterus rarely gives rise to symptoms, and its rinding is incidental. There is a greater likelihood of spasmodic dysmenorrhoea, possibly because of disturbed uterine polarity. When both the body of the uterus and the cervix can be defined, the acute angle between them can be demonstrated by being able to feel each lying in close contact with opposite sides of one finger **(Fig. 18)**.

Treatment

Treatment is directed to the symptoms, if any.

CONICAL CERVIX AND PINHOLE OSTIUM

The normal cervix varies in shape and size but occasionally it is so conical or its external ostium appears so small as

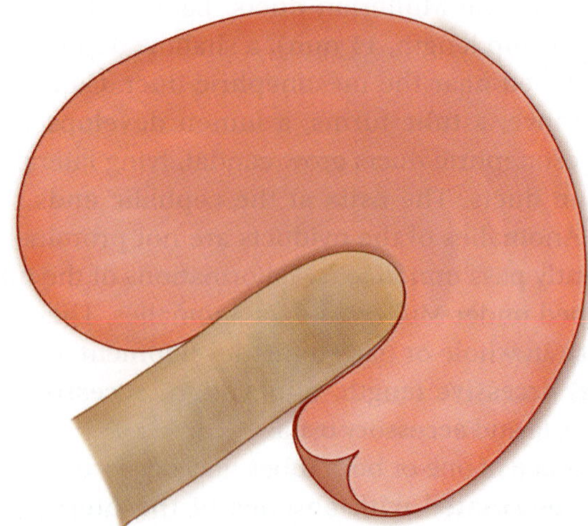

Fig. 18: Acute anteflexion of the cervix determined clinically by apposition of the body of the uterus and of the cervix to the sides of one finger.

to warrant these descriptions. Conical cervix and pinhole ostium often go together and the cervix as a whole tends to be long and narrow. These diagnoses are largely a matter of fashion and personal opinion; at present, they are out of fashion.

Congenital Hypertrophy of Cervix

This condition is developmental rather than congenital and a malformation rather than hypertrophy. Congenital hypertrophy of the cervix is, in fact, merely a name for an unusually long cervix. The elongation affects the vaginal rather than the supravaginal cervix, and the diagnosis is only made in nulliparous women. The condition is usually symptomless. Sometimes, the cervix is so long that the patient is conscious of it during straining and during coitus; this is particularly true if the vagina happens to be short.

VAGINA

As the paramesonephric (Müllerian) ducts grow caudal, they reach the urogenital sinus by approximately the 9th week (32 mm) and fuse with it to form an elevation known as the Müllerian tubercle, with the openings of the paramesonephric ducts on either side of it. A ribbon of epithelium replaces the uterovaginal canal and is the precursor of the vagina. The vagina is formed between the 16th and 20th weeks by the development of lacunas; complete canalisation later occurs to form the vaginal lumen. The principal congenital anomalies of the vagina include the following:

- Longitudinal septum
- Transverse septum
- Vaginal agenesis
- Mesonephric remnants

Absence/Agenesis of Vagina

Pathology

The vagina may be completely absent **(Fig. 5)** or, more often, the Müllerian duct portion is absent and the urogenital sinus part is present as a depression of variable depth. The condition can be associated with intersexuality, but in otherwise apparently normal women the sex chromosomes are usually XX. Agenesis of the vagina may only be detected on pelvic examination for amenorrhoea. Absence of a vagina is always associated with absence of a hymen. Since agenesis of the vagina is usually misdiagnosed as imperforate hymen, this is of diagnostic importance. In nearly every case of vaginal agenesis, there is an absent or very rudimentary uterus; ovarian agenesis may be present. Nearly all patients without a vagina have associated anomalies of the urinary tract, including renal agenesis, ectopic pelvic kidney, and ureteral anomalies. The mechanism of these vaginal anomalies is not entirely clear; they may result from failure of development of the epithelial vaginal mass or from failure of development of the urogenital sinus.

Clinical Features

If the uterus is present and functional, an upper compartment of the vagina is invariably present, and deep-seated haematocolpos and haematocervix develop after puberty. These cause monthly attacks of pain associated with apparent amenorrhoea. If the uterus is functionless, the complaints are primary amenorrhoea and dyspareunia or apareunia. In fact, absence of the vagina is usually diagnosed during the investigation of amenorrhoea before marriage.

Treatment

If cryptomenorrhoea is present, a plastic operation can be carried out to connect the upper vagina and uterus to the lower vagina and introitus **(Figs. 19A to C)**. In neglected cases, hysterectomy may be necessary.

If the aim is merely to permit coitus, then it is usually advised that treatment should be deferred until 6–9 months before marriage and that a plastic operation should only be carried out with the knowledge and consent of the partner. This attitude rarely deserves modification, even though there are young women who consider it unfair to encourage a proposal of marriage until their physical handicap has been corrected as far as possible. Several lines of treatment are available.

If the lower vagina is present as a depression or pouch, then continued or repeated pressure with an obturator (or repeated attempts at coitus) over the course of several months will often stretch the vagina sufficiently to allow reasonably normal coitus. Success or failure with this method depends very much on the outlook and determination of the patient. In this respect, the patient should always be told that the vaginalis underdeveloped rather than absent; this encourages in her the idea that it is capable of being stretched. The same holds good if it becomes necessary to create an artificial vagina by one of the following methods:

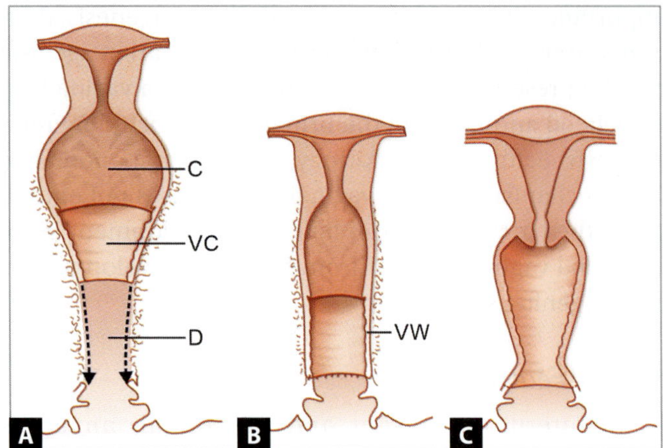

Figs. 19A to C: Advancement of the upper compartment of the vagina in dealing with all except minor degrees of lower vaginal aplasia or atresia causing a haematocervix. In the past, such vaginal deficiencies were often dealt with by creating and skin grafting a lower vagina, but the results are not always good, and a stricture tends to form at the junction of the artificial vagina and true vaginal compartment above. Once the diagnosis is made, there is no need even for laparotomy. Careful dissection from below leads to the collection of blood above and after this has been released, the upper vagina and cervix are mobilised so freely that they can be brought down to be sutured to the introitus. (A) A path through the obstruction is dissected (D) and the vaginal compartment and the cervix containing the menstrual blood. Vaginal compartment and cervix are freed to be advanced to a lower level as indicated by the arrows; (B) The operation is completed, VW being the vaginal wall; (C) This shows the final result; the cervix returns to its normal shape and what was an upper compartment of vagina adapts to produce a vagina of good length.

- A space is dissected between the bladder and rectum and lined with a skin graft carried on a mould made of light plastic material or foam. Even after the graft has been taken, the patient has to wear an obturator or mould for at least 6 months afterwards to prevent contracture and may have to use it indefinitely unless coitus is practised regularly. The danger of the operation is injury to the bladder and rectum with fistula formation. Contracture of the artificial vagina is common, but if the patient is determined to get coitus established, the result can be very satisfactory **(Figs. 20A and B)**. A rare late sequel to this type of operation is enterocoele formation.
- A more recent development has been the use of an amnion graft instead of a skin graft. The dissection is as above, but the mould is covered with amnion (obtained under sterile conditions at a caesarean section delivery and kept in sterile solution until used). The mould is sutured in situ and removed after 7 days. The vagina is washed out. A new mould with amnion may be inserted for further 5–7 days. The epithelium of the lower part of the vagina appears to grow over or into the amnion and, therefore, gives a more satisfactory end result than a skin graft in my opinion.
- A pouch, superficial to the vestibule and opening anteriorly, is created by suturing together a linear U-shaped incision in the hairless aspects of the labia majora (Williams' operation). This is a simple and

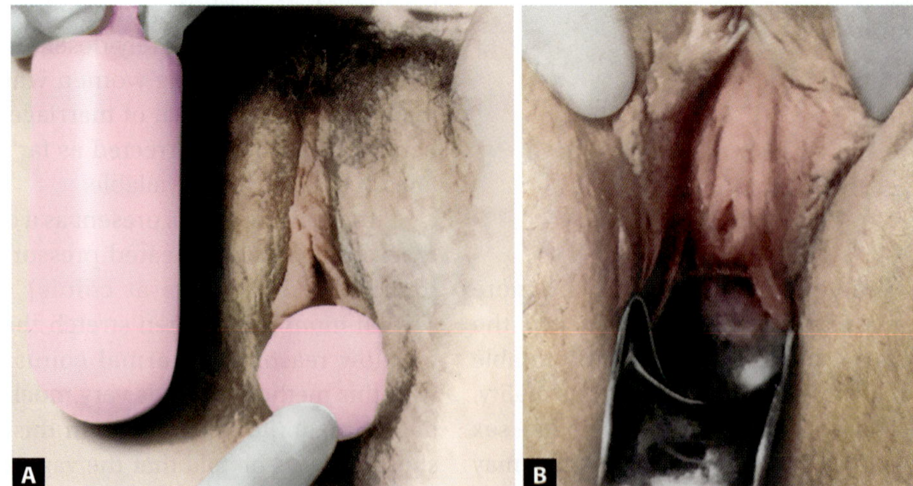

Figs. 20A and B: Artificial vaginas created surgically by dissection and skin grafting of a space between the bladder and rectum. Photographs were taken 1 year after the operations. (A) The vulva looks normal and the vagina accommodates a good-sized obturator. This is one type of light plastic obturator which the woman inserts and wears regularly to prevent contracture; (B) A second case with the artificial vagina demonstrated by means of a Sims' speculum.

safe procedure. Once coitus is established, it permits a gradual indentation of the vestibule to lengthen the available canal. However, the angle of the neovagina is not physiological. Also, if the pouch is too close to the urethra, urine can collect in it. This method is sometimes used for patients with a pelvic kidney or following radical surgery.

- Muscle and skin flaps have also been used for reconstruction of the vagina following radical surgery. The gracilis myocutaneous flap has a high failure rate due to vascular problems. Neurovascular pudendal-thigh flaps (the Singapore flap) are reported to have better blood supply and innervation.
- The labia majora and minora have been used to create a satisfactory vagina, but this distorts the vulvar anatomy. Labiovaginal flaps created by tissue expansion techniques have been used to overcome this problem.
- Operations involving the transplantation of an isolated loop of colon into a space dissected between the bladder and rectum are described. They are unjustified for congenital absence of the vagina but may be used following radical cancer surgery (pelvic exenteration).
- Laparoscopic techniques using an olive device, which exerts traction on the pseudohymen through the abdominal wall, have been used (Vecchietti method), but the device has not been approved by the Food and Drug Administration (FDA).

Before any of these operations is undertaken, the presence of associated kidney malformations and impairment of renal function should be excluded.

Nonsurgical approach (Frank procedure): The Frank technique was initially described in 1938. The goal was to increase the depth and calibre of the vagina with the use of graduated dilators, thus avoiding the need for surgical intervention. The Ingram *bicycle seat* represented a dramatic improvement in the Frank procedure. The major advantage of this racing-type bicycle seat is that it is positioned between the buttocks and is therefore, in better contact with the perineum, providing direct pressure from the graduated dilator on the incompletely developed vagina.

In the Frank's non-surgical method first, the patient is instructed to use a mirror to examine her genitalia at home, identifying the external structures and introital dimple. Dilators of graduated sizes are used to create pressure on the vaginal dimple, beginning with a dilator approximately 1.5 cm in diameter and 2–3 cm in length. The same is used for 20–30 minutes three to four times daily. She should be seen monthly, not only for physical evaluation but also for continued encouragement and motivation; she should be made aware that consistent use of this technique will enable her to avoid surgery and will eliminate the risk of postoperative scarring and the need for painful, potentially disfiguring skin grafting. Steady progress should be readily apparent on periodic pelvic examination. Adequate vaginal calibre and depth can usually be demonstrated in 14–16 weeks.

On occasion, the position may be difficult to manage because of the shallowness of the vaginal dimple. In these cases, the patient can begin with the lithotomy position, applying manual pressure to hold the dilator firmly in contact with the vaginal dimple until there is sufficient invagination to accommodate the bicycle technique comfortably. Some women can pedal a stationary bicycle during dilatation after several weeks of non-surgical treatment, but this should be discontinued if there is any chafing or discomfort. The Ingram technique is successful in approximately 90% of cases, and Ingram himself contended that surgery should not be considered until the patient had undergone a sufficient trial of this approach.

The Frank and Ingram techniques are successful in a fair number of girls and can be considered until the patient has undergone a sufficient trial of this approach.

Vaginal Hypoplasia

Vaginal hypoplasia is evidenced by shortness, narrowness, shallow fornices and by thin and inactive epithelium. It is caused either by an inherent fault in the Müllerian ducts or by absence of the oestrogen stimulus from the ovary. In the latter case, it is always associated with uterine hypoplasia and can be overcome by oestrogen therapy.

This treatment is worthwhile if the complaint is dyspareunia because, once the vagina is well formed, it does not contract back to its former state so long as coitus is continued regularly.

Congenital Atresia and Stricture

See page 273.

Septate and Subseptate Vagina

See page 267.

Double Vagina (Duplication)

This is extremely rare, occurring in association with double vulva, double uterus, double bladder and urethra, and sometimes with supernumerary lower limbs **(Fig. 21)**. The condition really represents an included twin. In most cases labelled *double vagina*, the vagina is single but septate.

VULVA

Absence, Gross Underdevelopment and Duplication

These curiosities are usually only found with other malformations incompatible with life **(Fig. 21)**.

Hypoplasia

This is seen in association with hypoplasia of the rest of the genital tract in states of hypo-oestrogenism (e.g. infantilism, streak gonads). The secondary sex characters are poorly developed as well.

Bifid Clitoris (Diphallus)

The genital tubercle is formed from two mesodermal bands which grow round from the dorsal aspect of the foetus in the third week. These also provide for the musculature of the abdominal wall, musculature of the anterior walls of the bladder and urethra, and symphysis pubis. Failure of these bands to develop properly or to fuse results in a bifid clitoris (bifid or double penis in the male), ectopia vesicae, epispadias, a muscular defect of the lower abdominal wall, divarication of the foreparts of the labia majora, absence of the hair-bearing skin of the pubes and a split pelvis **(Figs. 22 and 23)**.

The vulvar deformity is often associated with shortness of the vagina and stricture of the introitus, and there is a strong predisposition to uterine prolapse.

For this condition, the primary object of treatment is to close the bladder wall anteriorly, but it is often necessary

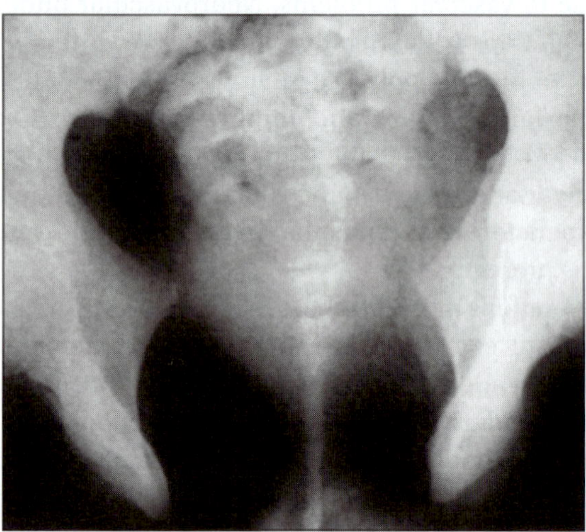

Fig. 22: Split pelvis in a woman aged 21 years suffering from ectopia vesicae and bifid clitoris. Her urinary incontinence was controlled by transplantation of the ureters into the pelvic colon at the age of 10 years. There was normal renal function and electrolyte balance 11 years later.

Fig. 21: Duplication of the vulva in a baby which died from multiple malformations 7 weeks after birth. There was a single anus and rectum but two bladders, a uterus didelphys and a *double* vagina. There were only two kidneys, one grossly hydronephrotic.

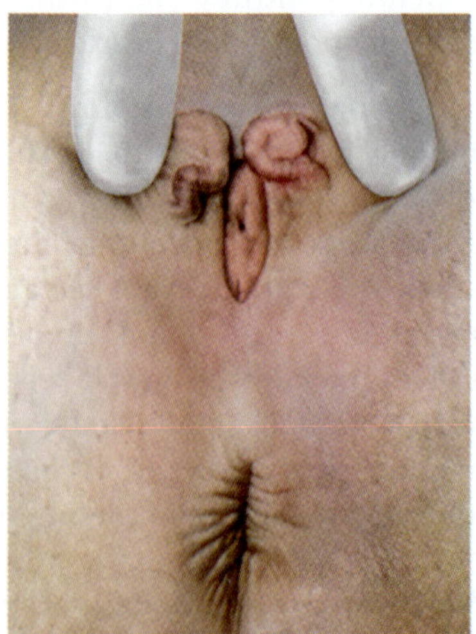

Fig. 23: Bifid clitoris and divarication of the labia associated with a defect of the lower abdominal wall, ectopia vesicae and split pelvis.

to divert the urinary stream to ensure some sort of continence. I know of three cases in which the ureters were transplanted to the colon in childhood and in which the women remained healthy 15–20 years later. One of these women had two normal pregnancies followed by easy vaginal deliveries.

Hypertrophy of the Clitoris

See Chapter 14.

Abnormalities of the Hymen

The hymen may be absent, imperforate or tough. The last cause apareunia.

Atresia of the Labia Minora

In a young female embryo, the genital folds may fuse as they do in the male. The introitus then becomes enclosed by a membrane which represents the two labia minora, with an exit for urine anteriorly. This is a feature of congenital adrenal hyperplasia and can be caused by any virilising agent acting on the foetus before vulvar development is complete.

In most cases of fused nymphae seen in children aged 1–3 years, the abnormality is the result of adhesions forming after acute vulvitis of infancy rather than an error in development.

Hypertrophy of the Labia Minora (Spaniel Ear Nymphae)

Pathology

Hypertrophy may affect one or both labia minora and does not ordinarily become obvious until puberty. It is sometimes stated that bilateral hypertrophy of the labia minora is the result of masturbation. There is no doubt that manipulation and stretching of the labia as practised by some primitive tribes can lead to their permanent gross enlargement. Nevertheless, the hypertrophy seen in civilised communities is rarely attributable to anything more than a developmental peculiarity **(Fig. 24)**.

Symptoms

Usually, there are no symptoms, but the patient may complain of a *tumour* or of *something hanging* from the vulva. If the labia are very long, they can become chafed, oedematous and ulcerated during exercise. Such symptoms are mostly seen during adolescence when there is a tendency for leucorrhoea and uncleanliness.

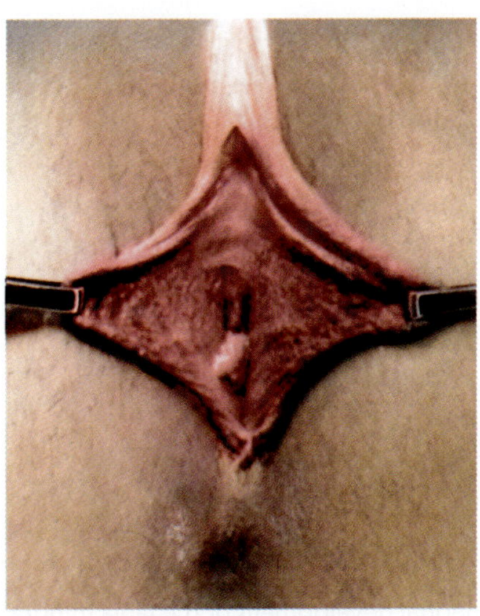

Fig. 24: Bilateral hypertrophy of the labia minora in a virgin aged 14 years. She complained of recurrent discomfort caused by abrasion, so the labia were trimmed down to size by a simple plastic procedure.

Treatment

No treatment other than reassurance and attention to hygiene is usually necessary. Talcum powder should be avoided because it cakes in the crevices. A barrier cream or zinc and castor oil cream can be applied before exercise. If these conservative measures fail, the size of the labia can be reduced by a simple plastic operation which gives excellent results.

Asymmetry of the Labia Minora

Like all paired organs, the labia minora are often unequal in size. One may be unusually large or small **(Fig. 25)**. The condition is rarely more than of interest; often, the patient is unaware of the inequality.

No treatment is necessary unless the larger labium causes chafing, when its size can be reduced surgically.

ERRORS ARISING IN CONNECTION WITH THE CLOACA

Defects in the proper partition of the cloaca into the hindgut and urogenital sinus result in a persistent cloaca with a common opening for the bladder, vagina and bowel (this is extremely rare); a fistula between the rectum or anus and the vagina; a perineal, vestibular or vaginal anus **(Fig. 26)**; or an imperforate anus.

A perineal or vaginal anus is not too uncommon and is characterised by a deficiency in the perineal body and

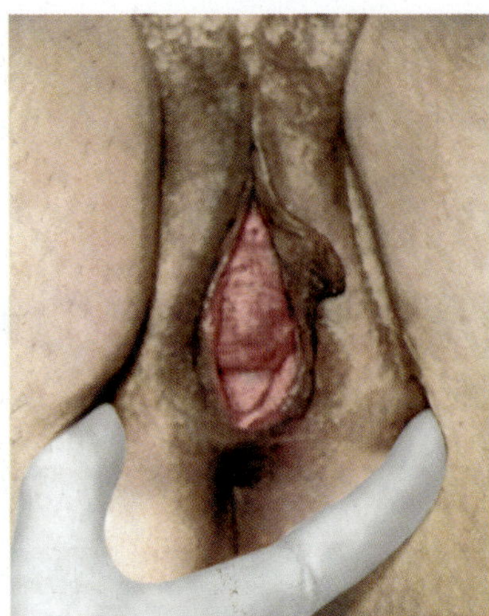

Fig. 25: Unequal development of the labia minora, which is a common finding. Vaginal prolapse is also present in this case.

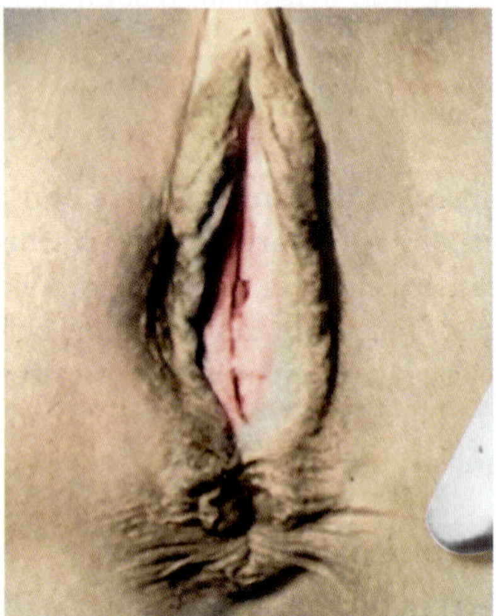

Fig. 26: Perineal anus. The anus is just outside the fourchette; sometimes, it opens nearer to or just within the vagina.

by the lower bowel opening low down on the posterior vaginal wall or at the fourchette. A vaginal anus is usually recognised in the newborn and is distinguished from imperforate anus by the escape of meconium from the vagina. Nevertheless, it is the subject of much unnecessary and harmful surgery in children. Rarely, the anus is so narrow as to obstruct the passage of meconium. In that case, a simple *cutback* operation is indicated and does not generally result in faecal incontinence in later life. Usually, the opening is sufficiently large not to obstruct the bowel and, in that case, should be left alone. The baby, as it grows, develops quite good sphincter control. In adult life, the individual suffers little or no inconvenience but, if the opening is high and the vagina gets badly contaminated, a reconstruction operation may be necessary before marriage. A high vaginal anus is exceptional and is usually associated with a failure in development of the lower rectum, pelvic floor and sacrum. As a rule, however, no surgery is necessary at any age.

A perineal anus is only a problem during childbirth when the thin rectovaginal septum is vulnerable to trauma in the second stage of labour. A rectovaginal fistula with faecal incontinence is not an inevitable result, but the risk is sufficient to justify elective caesarean section in many of these cases.

If it does become necessary to transplant a vaginal or perineal anus backwards, one of the difficulties is to provide it with a sphincter. The operation may have to be preceded by temporary colostomy.

An imperforate anus results when the cloacal membrane over the hindgut fails to breakdown or when the division of the cloaca leaves a blind lower end of the bowel. The latter can be some distance away from the ectoderm in which case surgical correction of the error can be difficult. All babies should be examined at birth to see if the anus is perforate; if it is not, operative treatment is urgent.

MALFORMATIONS OF THE URINARY TRACT

Some of these come within the remit of the gynaecologist and some have already been mentioned. They often occur in association with abnormalities of the uterus, vagina and vulva.

Epispadias and Ectopia Vesicae

See page 282.

Urethral Diverticula

See Chapter 26.

Accessory and Aberrant Ureter (and Kidney)

Duplication of the renal pelvis and ureter is common and arises as a result of an accessory ureteric bud from the Wolffian duct **(Figs. 27A and B)**. The accessory ureter always links with the upper pole of the kidney and crosses posterior to the main ureter. Its importance is that it may be injured during pelvic operations because the surgeon is usually unaware of its existence.

Sometimes, the ureter, but more often an accessory ureter, opens into the anterolateral wall of the uterus,

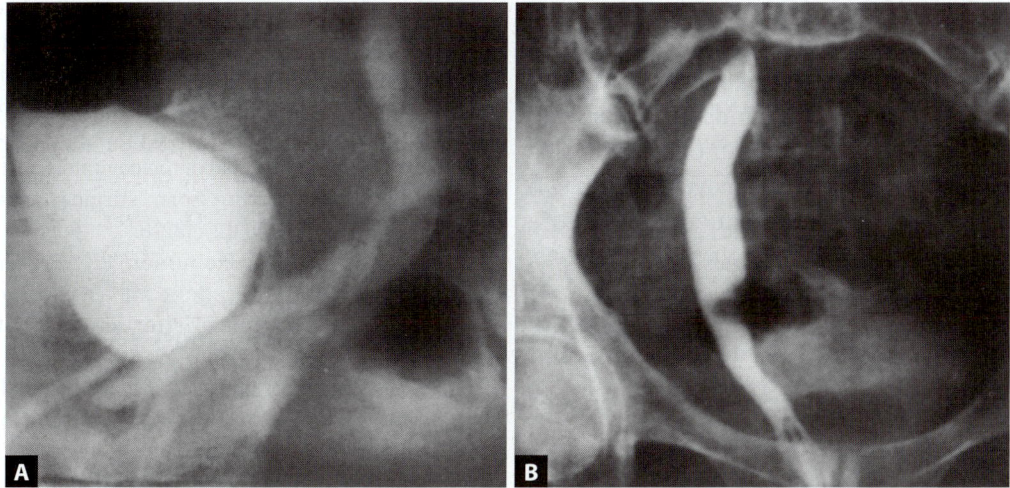

Figs. 27A and B: Bilateral aberrant ureters. In this case, a girl, when aged 12 years, had bilateral aberrant kidneys and the upper parts of their ureters had removed. She remained symptom free until her first pregnancy at the age of 22 years when she developed what was first thought to be stress incontinence of urine. Investigation then showed that the pelvic parts of the aberrant ureters were still present; the left one entered the bladder just above the internal urethral meatus and caused no trouble. The right one opened into the urethra at a low level and is here shown as the dilated structure lying behind the bladder and upper urethra. It was removed successfully. (A) Lateral urethrocystogram with the aberrant right ureter filled from below with radio-opaque medium; (B) Anteroposterior exposure of the lower part of the right aberrant ureter.

vagina, vestibule or urethra; the most common site is the vestibule. It then causes incontinence of urine, which is frequently mistaken for enuresis in childhood. The amount of urine which escapes can be small and intermittent, so bearing in mind that micturition is otherwise normal, the leakage may be regarded as vaginal discharge. An aberrant ureter may become infected.

The diagnosis of an accessory ureter can be extremely difficult and sometimes eludes the expert for years. That part of the kidney served often has poor function, so neither it nor the ureter may be revealed by intravenous pyelography. Moreover, the opening on the vestibule or elsewhere is usually tiny and difficult to locate unless a bead of urine happens to escape at the time of examination.

Treatment is by excision of the aberrant structure and of the kidney tissue, which it drains.

Absence of One Kidney and Ureter

This is commonly associated with absence of the Müllerian duct on the same side or with gross malfusion deformities of the uterus (***see* Figs. 8A to C**).

Fusion of the Kidneys—Horseshoe Kidney

Pelvic Kidney

Failure of the kidney to ascend results in a pelvic kidney which lies extraperitoneally, sometimes at the pelvic brim but more often below the brim in front of the sacroiliac joint (**Fig. 28**). It is more likely than a normal kidney to develop hydronephrosis and pyonephrosis. It may

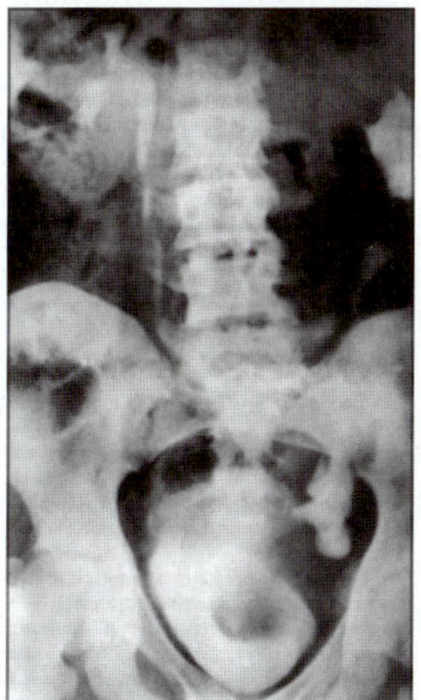

Fig. 28: An intravenous pyelogram showing three separate kidneys, a normal one on the right, a hydronephrotic one on the left, and one in the left side of the pelvis. The site of the last is typical for a pelvic kidney. This situation was discovered during the investigation of a girl aged 16 years complaining of primary amenorrhoea and who had the stigmata of Turner syndrome, including stunted growth and webbing of the neck. She was nevertheless chromatin positive and later menstruated normally so she did not have streak gonads. The sex chromosome pattern was not determined but was almost certainly abnormal.

present merely as a pelvic tumour, palpated during vaginal examination, or obstructing labour. It is usually mistaken for an ovarian tumour, and this sort of error can only be avoided by keeping the condition in mind and by carrying out pyelography in the case of any tumour of the right size and position which is more fixed than an ovarian cyst.

A pelvic kidney, or a single horseshoe kidney in the pelvis, is not uncommon in cases of vaginal agenesis. It can be mistaken for a haematometra.

SUGGESTED READING

1. Acien P, Acien M, Sanchez-Ferrer M. Complex malformations of the female genital tract. New types and revision of classification. Hum Reprod. 2004;19(10):2377-84.
2. Acien P, Acien MI. The history of female genital tract malformation classifications and proposal of an updated system. Hum Reprod Update. 2011;17(5):693-705.
3. Aittomaki K, Eroila H, Kajanoja P. A population-based study of the incidence of mullerian aplasia in Finland. Fertil Steril. 2001;76(3):624-5.
4. The AFS classification of adnexal adhesions, distal tubal occlusion, tubal occlusion secondary to tubal ligation, tubal pregnancies, mullerian anomalies and intrauterine adhesions. Fertil Steril. 1988;49:944-55.
5. Brucker SY, Rall K, Campo R, Oppelt P, Isaacson K. Treatment of congenital malformations. Semin Reprod Med. 2011;29(2):101-12.
6. Buttram VC, Gibbons WE. Mullerian anomalies: a proposed classification (an analysis of 144 cases). Fertil Steril. 1979;32(1):40-6.
7. Chan YY, Jayarpakasan K, Tan A, Thornton JG, Coomarasamy A, Raine-Fenning NJ, et al. Reproductive outcomes in women with congenital uterine anomalies: a systematic review. Ultrasound Obstet Gynecol. 2011;38(4):371-82.
8. Fedele L, Bianchi S, Zanconato G, Berlanda N, Bergamini V. Laparoscopic removal of the cavitated non-communicating rudimentary uterine horn: surgical aspects in 10 cases. Fertil Steril. 2005;83(2):432-6.
9. Joki-Erkkila MM, Heinonen PK. Presenting and long-term clinical implications and fecundity in females with obstructing vaginal malformations. J Pediatr Adolesc Gynecol. 2003;16(5):307-12.
10. Pena-Alonso R, Nieto K, Alvarez R, Palma I, Nájera N, Eraña L, et al. Distribution of Y-chromosome-bearing cells in gonadoblastoma and dysgenetic testis in 45,X/46,XY infants. Mod Pathol. 2005;18(3):439-45.
11. Rock JA, Carpenter SE, Wheeless CR, Jones HW. The clinical management of maldevelopment of the uterine cervix. J Pelvic Surg. 1995;1:129-33.
12. Tomazevic T, Ban-Frangez H, Ribic-Pucelj M, Premru-Srsen T, Verdenik I. Small uterine septum is an important risk variable for preterm birth. Eur J Obstet Gynecol Reprod Biol. 2007;135(2):154-7.
13. Troiano RN, McCarthy SM. Mullerian duct anomalies: imaging and clinical issues. Radiology. 2004;233(1):19-34.
14. Noordegraaf AV, Huirne JAF, Brölmann HAM, van Mechelen W, Anema JR. Multidisciplinary convalescence recommendations after gynaecological surgery: a modified Delphi method among experts. BJOG. 2011;118(13):1557-67.

14

CHAPTER

Disorders of Sex Differentiation

Rajeshwari G Bhat, Muralidhar V Pai

Chapter Outline

- Factors Responsible for Normal Sexual Patterns
- Turner Syndrome 45, XO
- Triple X Syndrome (47, XXX) (From Old Jeffcoate's)
- Klinefelter Syndrome (47, XXY) (From Old Jeffcoate's)
- YY Syndrome
- Disorders of Sex Development with Normal Sex Chromosomes
- Approach to a Neonate with Atypical Genitalia
- Intersex Developing after Birth

INTRODUCTION

The normal sex of an individual is determined by the following factors:

- Chromosomal sex (genetic sex)
- Gonadal sex
- Secondary sex characteristics
- Internal anatomical sex
- Sex of rearing
- Gender role (societal role)

FACTORS RESPONSIBLE FOR NORMAL SEXUAL PATTERNS

Chromosomal Factors

Sex is primarily determined when the ovum is fertilised by the type of sex chromosome supplied by the spermatozoon. The nucleus of every cell of the human body normally carries 46 chromosomes arranged in 23 pairs. One of these pairs, the sex chromosomes, is mainly concerned with sex; the remaining 22 pairs are designated autosomes **(Fig. 1)**. In females, the two sex chromosomes are similar, the upper arms of the X being much shorter than the lower. In males, they are dissimilar-XY, Y being a much smaller structure than X and having very short upper arms **(Fig. 1)**. The reduction division of the mature ovum results in 22 separate autosomes and 1 X sex chromosome. Mature spermatozoa, however, carry either an X or a Y chromosome and are, therefore, of two types. If the X chromosome fertilises the ovum, it results in a female zygote whose karyotype is expressed as 46, XX; if the other is operative, the outcome is a male with the karyotype of 46, XY **(Flowchart 1)**.

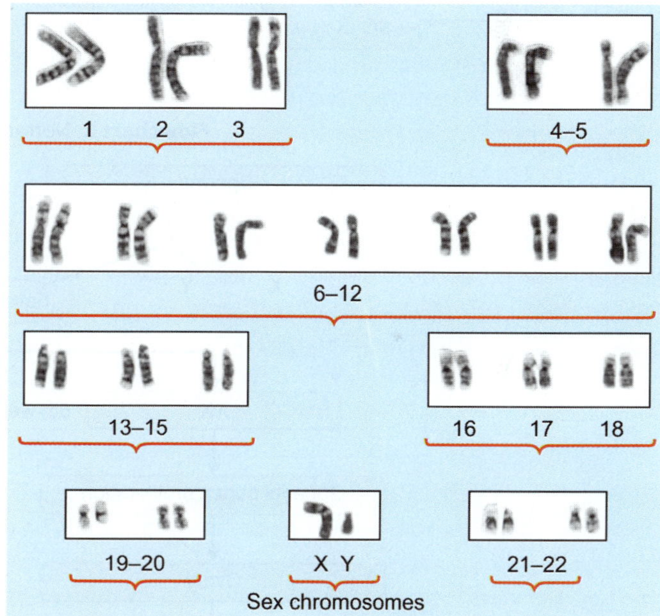

Fig. 1: The 23 pairs of chromosomes in the normal human male, numbered according to an internationally agreed system. The chromosomes are obtained from cultures of lymphocytes or fibroblasts and identified from a metaphase spread using special stains (in this case G banding using Giemsa stain plus trypsin).

To begin with, every embryo possesses bipotent gonads, which can become either testis or ovary. Gonads have internal duct systems of both sexes, one of which normally differentiates and the other regresses, and the embryo also has undifferentiated, potentially bisexual external genitalia **(Flowchart 2)**.

Flowchart 1: The normal distribution of autosomes (A) and sex chromosomes (SC) before and after reduction division of the ovum and spermatozoon and after fertilisation.

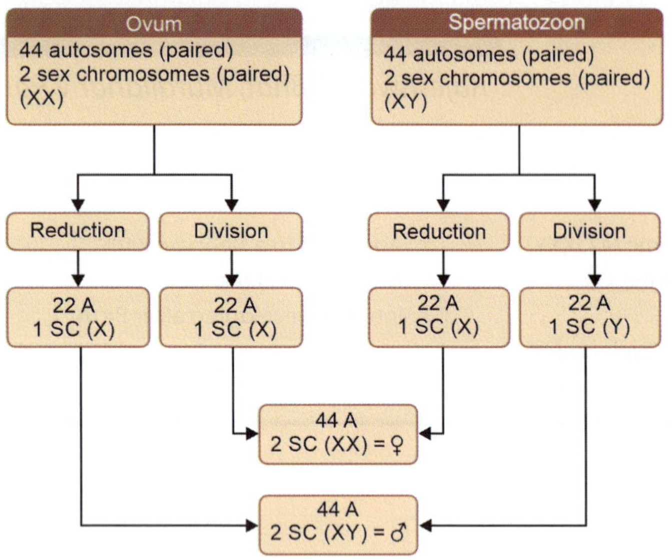

Gonadal Differentiation

Primordial germ cells originate in the endoderm of the yolk sac and migrate through dorsal mesentery during the 4th and 5th weeks of intrauterine life to reach the primitive gonad. The undifferentiated gonad arises from the coelomic epithelium on the urogenital ridge, overlying some mesenchymal tissues. It is situated on either side of the midline on the dorsal aspect of the embryo. There are many genes (*WT1*, *SF1/NR5A1*) involved in the development of the bipotential gonad and the testis [sex-determining region Y (*SRY*), *SOX9*, *GATA4*]. The ovarian development is not passive in the absence of the *SRY* gene as thought earlier; several genes are crucial for the normal development of ovaries (*DAX1*, *RSPO1*, *FOXL2*, *WNT4*) **(Fig. 2)**. At approximately 40 days of gestation, divergent gonadal differentiation becomes evident under the influence of the *SRY* gene on the Y chromosome. *SRY* is the testis-determining factor (TDF). It is situated on the

Flowchart 2: Normal sexual development.

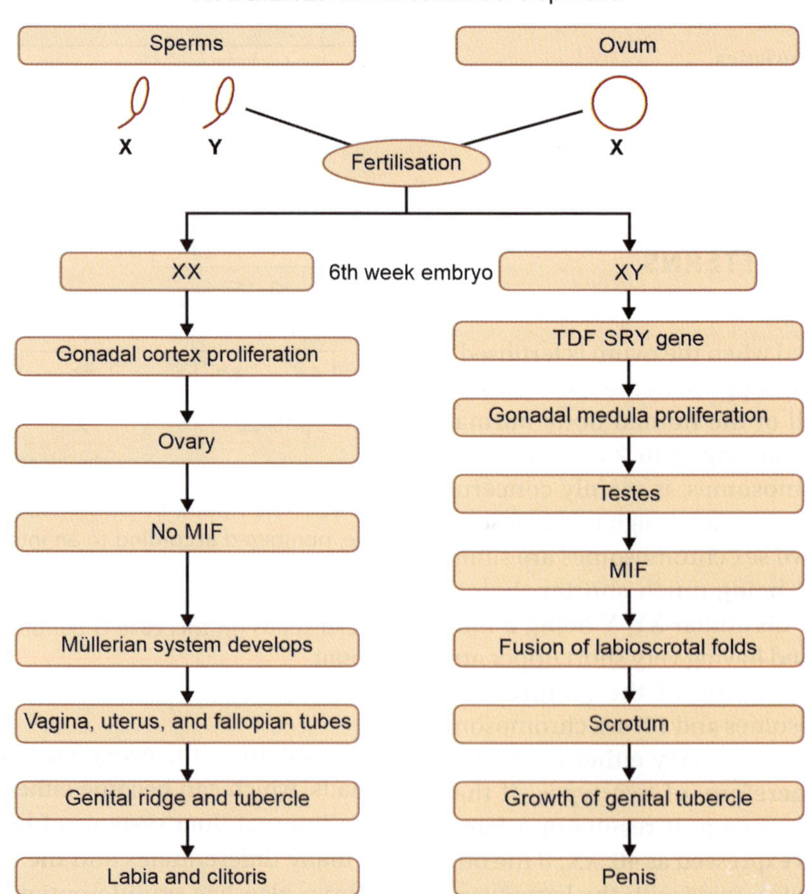

(MIF: Müllerian-inhibitory factor; SRY: sex-determining region Y; TDF: testis-determining factor)

short arm of the Y chromosome near the pseudoautosomal region. The expression of SRY in the gonad directs cells of the gonadal primordium to differentiate as Sertoli cells, which aggregate to form spermatogenic cords and then seminiferous tubules. Leydig cells are formed a week later.

The bipotent gonad develops into an ovary about 2 weeks later than testicular development in a XX individual, as there is no Y chromosome. The cortical zone develops and contains germ cells, and the medullary portion regresses. Normal ovarian differentiation requires the presence of germ cells and complete 46 XX chromosomal components.

Duct System Differentiation

The Wolffian (mesonephric) ducts and the Mullerian (paramesonephric) ducts coexist in all embryos for up to 8 weeks. One type of duct system normally persists, giving rise to special ducts and glands, whereas the other disappears during the 3rd month. In males, Sertoli cells secrete anti-Müllerian hormone (AMH), also called Müllerian-inhibiting substance or Müllerian-inhibiting factor. AMH causes regression of the Müllerian ducts on the ipsilateral side, which is completed in 8 weeks **(Flowchart 3)**. Leydig cells produce testosterone at 8 weeks; peak concentration is reached at approximately 16 weeks. Local testosterone produced by the foetal testis promotes ipsilateral Wolffian duct maturation into the epididymis, vas deferens and seminal vesicle. This effect requires a high local concentration of testosterone because Wolffian differentiation is not induced by systemic androgenic administration. In female embryos, in the absence of the Y chromosome, testosterone and AMH, the Wolffian system regresses and the Müllerian system (paramesonephric ducts) develops into fallopian tubes, uterus and upper vagina.

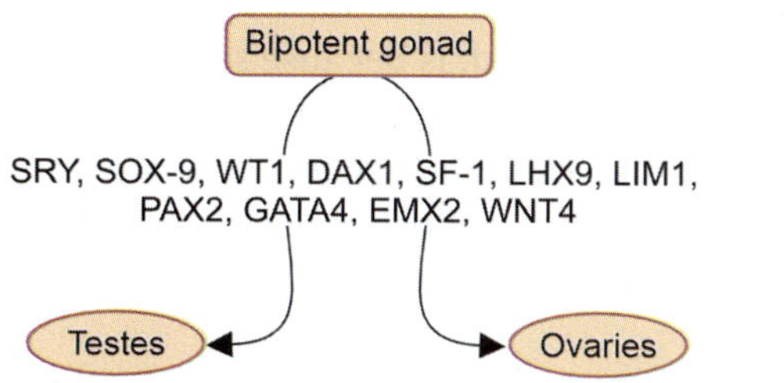

Fig. 2: *Various genes involved in the development of differentiated gonads.*
Source: García-Acero M, Moreno O, Suárez F, Rojas A. Disorders of Sexual Development: Current Status and Progress in the Diagnostic Approach. Curr Urol. 2020;13(4):169-78.

External Genitalia Differentiation

Like gonads, the external genitalia are initially identical in all foetuses regardless of genetic sex. Bipotential external genitalia develops in the male line under the influence of dihydrotestosterone (DTH). The enzyme 5α reductase converts testosterone into DHT in the skin fibroblasts of external genitalia, which causes elongation of genital tubercle, becomes the penis; urethral folds fuse to become

Flowchart 3: Development of male external genitalia and internal genital organs.

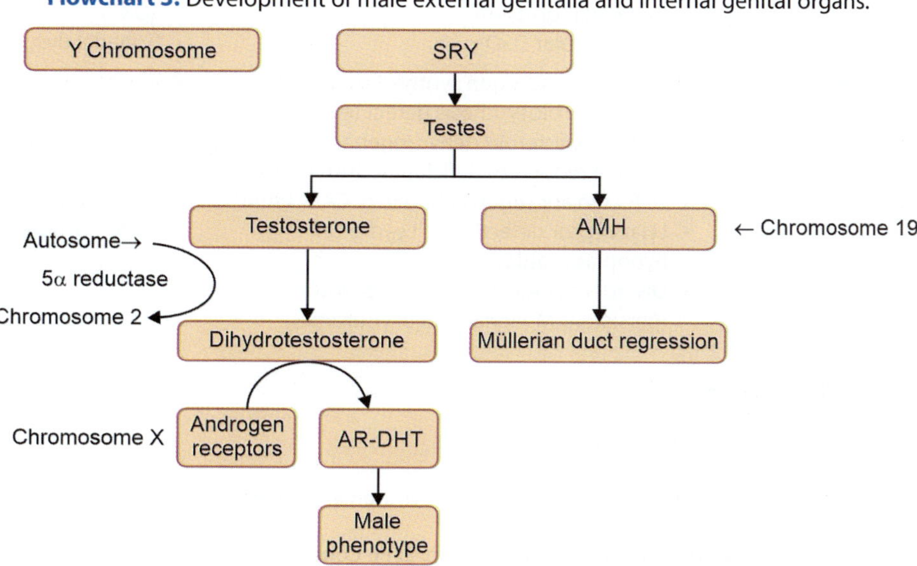

(AMH: anti-Müllerian hormone; SRY: sex-determining region Y)

the floor of the penile urethra and the corpus spongiosum that encloses the penile urethra **(Flowchart 3)**. Labioscrotal swellings fuse in the midline to become the scrotum. In the female, as there is no DTH, the genital tubercle becomes the clitoris, and the urethral folds and labioscrotal swellings do not fuse becoming labia minora and labia majora, respectively.

Money et al. introduced the concept of psychosexual development to the above sequence. Gender identity is defined as the self-representation of a person as male, female or even neither. Gender role (sex typical behaviour) describes behaviour, attitudes and traits that a society identifies as masculine or feminine. Sexual orientation denotes the individual responsiveness to sexual stimuli, which includes behaviour, fantasies and attractions (hetero/bi/homosexual).

Disorders of sex development (*DSD*) is a new terminology for congenital conditions in which there is a discrepancy in chromosomal, gonadal or anatomic sex. DSDs are classified based on the sex chromosome composition into three categories: (1) 46, XX DSDs, (2) 46, XY DSDs and (3) sex chromosomal DSDs **(Table 1)**.

Mechanism of Abnormal Chromosomal Formation (Jeffcoate's)

- *Errors in sex chromosome division and distribution:* During the cell division, the chromosomes normally split *longitudinally, one-half of each going to each of two daughter* cells. When cleavage does not take place, the phenomenon is termed nondisjunction; this is not uncommon, especially during the first meiotic (reduction) division leading to the formation of a mature ovum or spermatozoon. The result is an oocyte, which may contain either two X chromosomes or no sex chromosome at all, and a spermatozoon with either XY or no sex chromosomes. When fertilisation takes place, the outcomes that are possible are zygotes whose chromosome makeup is 45, XO; 45, YO; 47, XXX; and 47, XXY **(Flowchart 4)**. An embryo with a chromosome pattern of 45, YO has never been found. This, it is assumed, is because such an arrangement is incompatible with the life of a cell or an early embryo.
- During the mitotic division of the fertilised ovum, errors in the distribution of the chromosomes, even if their original complement is normal, can still occur.

TABLE 1: Classification of disorders of sex development (DSD).

Sex chromosome DSD	***46, XY DSD***	***46, XX DSD***
45, XO (Turner syndrome and variants)	Disorders of gonadal (testicular) development: • Complete gonadal dysgenesis (Swyer syndrome) • Partial gonadal dysgenesis • Gonadal regression • Ovotesticular DSD	Disorders of gonadal (ovarian) development: • Ovotesticular DSD • Testicular DSD (e.g. SRY+, duplicate SOX9) • Gonadal dysgenesis
47, XXY (Klinefelter syndrome and variants)	Disorders in androgen synthesis or action: • Androgen biosynthesis defect (e.g. 17-hydroxysteroid dehydrogenase deficiency, 5-alpha reductase deficiency, StAR mutations • Defect in androgen action (e.g. CAIS, PAIS) • LH receptor defects (e.g. Leydig cell hypoplasia, aplasia) • Disorders of AMH and AMH receptor (persistent Müllerian duct syndrome)	Androgen excess: • Foetal (e.g. 21-hydroxylase deficiency, 11-hydroxylase deficiency • Foetoplacental (aromatase deficiency, POR) • Maternal (luteoma, exogenous, etc.)
45, XO/46, XY (mixed gonadal dysgenesis, ovotesticular DSD)		
46, XX/46, XY (chimeric, ovotesticular DSD)		

(AMH: anti-Müllerian hormone; CAIS: complete androgen insensitivity syndrome; PAIS: partial androgen insensitivity syndrome; SRY: sex-determining gene Y)

Source: Hughes IA, Houk C, Ahmed SF, Lee PA, LWPES Consensus Group. ESPE Consensus Group. Consensus statement on management of intersex disorders. Arch Dis Child. 2006;91(7):554-63.

Flowchart 4: Errors in sex chromosome division and distribution.

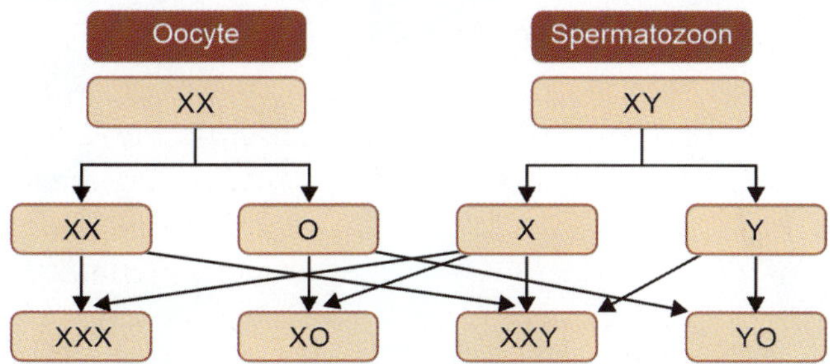

Nondisjunction is again possible or, if cleavage takes place, all the resulting products can pass to one daughter nucleus to give it a 48, XXXX or 48, XXYY complement. This is known as duplication.

- Sometimes during cell division, all or part of a chromosome may be lost (by anaphase lag, depletion or fragmentation). One or two of the arms of an X, for example, may disappear or, on the other hand, become displaced and link with an autosome (translocation). Even the translocation of part of a Y to an X chromosome, the so-called X–Y interchange, is described. Another possibility is for chromosomes to divide across their centrosomes instead of longitudinally producing isochromosomes **(Fig. 3)**. For example, long-armed X and short-armed X isochromosomes.
- Errors of these kinds, affecting only one or two cells at a very early stage of segmentation of the ovum, are reproduced in their offspring, and the outcome is two or more cell lines in the foetus. These can be found throughout the whole body or each may be localised or dominant in particular tissues. This phenomenon is called mosaicism, and the affected individual is a mosaic. How far mosaicism is present in all men and women is unknown, but, in minor degrees, it may be universal. Mosaicism of a gross degree is not uncommonly found in men and women suffering from aberrations in sex differentiation and reproductive function. The possible combinations are endless. A few examples are 46, XX/45, XO; 46, XY/45, XO; 46, XX/46, XY; 46, XX/45, Xf (f meaning a fragment); and 46, XY/47, XXY. The effects on the genital apparatus and phenotype depend on the relative numbers of the different types of cells, i.e. on which cell line is dominant and on their tissue distribution. Thus, if the primitive gonad is predominantly 45, XO, it is not likely to develop or function even though most other tissues in the body are 46, XX; if it is 46, XY, it will

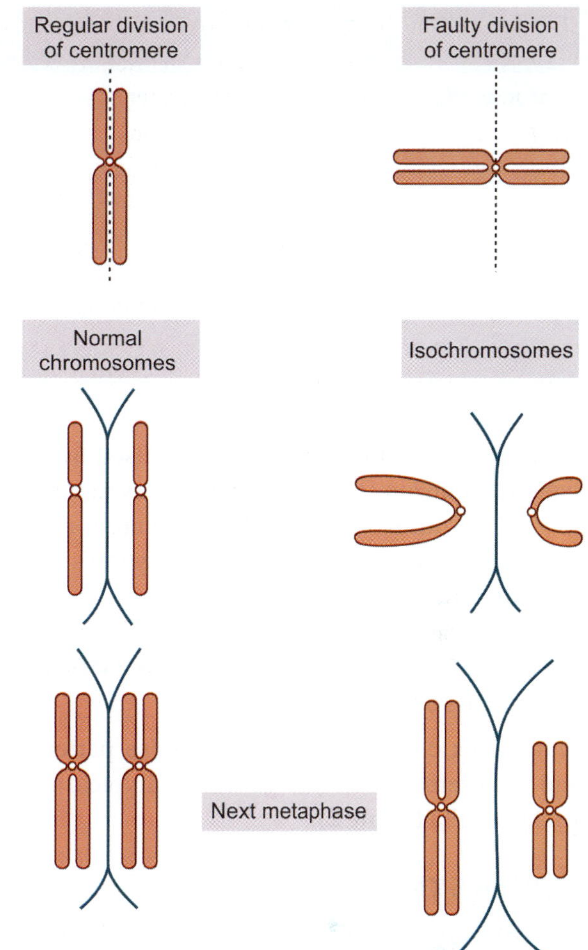

Fig. 3: The abnormal division of chromosomes, across their centrosomes instead of longitudinally, producing isochromosomes.

become a testis even though elsewhere the dominant cell line is 45, XO. The earlier in embryogenesis that any of the abnormalities in the sex chromosome pattern arise, the more widespread and serious their effect. Three to four per 1,000 live babies are born with clearly recognisable sex chromosome aberrations. This, however, understates the incidence since many affected foetuses, especially those with XO patterns, are aborted (likely >99%) (UpToDate).

- *Chimerism and dispermy:* The one type of mosaicism that is difficult to understand is the rare combination of XY/XX. This is said to arise under two circumstances. If binovular twins of different sexes have placentas with vascular connections, their blood intermingles to result in each having leucocytes, some of which are XY and some XX. This is the condition of chimerism. When a singleton foetus shows XY/XX mosaicism, the

TABLE 2: Abnormal chromosomal pattern and external genitalia.

External genitalia	*Chromosome complement*
Female	• 45, XO (Turner syndrome) • 47, XXX (superfemale)
Atypical	• 45, XO/46, XY • 46, XX/46, XY • Triploidy 69, XXY
Male	• 47, XXY (Klinefelter syndrome) • 47, XYY • 46, XX male

probability is that the ovum was fertilised by at least two spermatozoa (dispermy), one carrying an X and one a Y chromosome. Double fertilisation of a two-nucleated ovum and fusion of two zygotes are also postulated happenings.

Abnormal Sex Differentiation with Abnormal Sex Chromosome Component

It is called sex chromosomal DSD. These patients can present with female external genitalia, atypical or male external genitalia **(Table 2)**.

TURNER SYNDROME 45, XO

Turner syndrome was first described in 1957 by Henry Turner. This is the classical syndrome associated with streak gonads, and the underlying error is a karyotype of 45, XO or a mosaic containing this cell line. In this case, the nondisjunction of the sex chromosomes, the single X chromosome, is of maternal origin in 75–79% of cases. Many of 45, XO embryos are aborted but those that are not malformed and, in addition to having streak gonads, present the features of Turner syndrome at and after birth. Being without a Y chromosome, all affected individuals appear female, and their incidence is 0.2 per 1,000 live girl babies. The diagnosis can often be made in infancy, being prompted by somatic defects.

Clinical Presentation

The presentation of Turner syndrome varies throughout a patient's life.

The diagnosis should be considered in:
- Female foetus with hydrops
- Increased nuchal translucency
- Cystic hygroma or lymphoedema

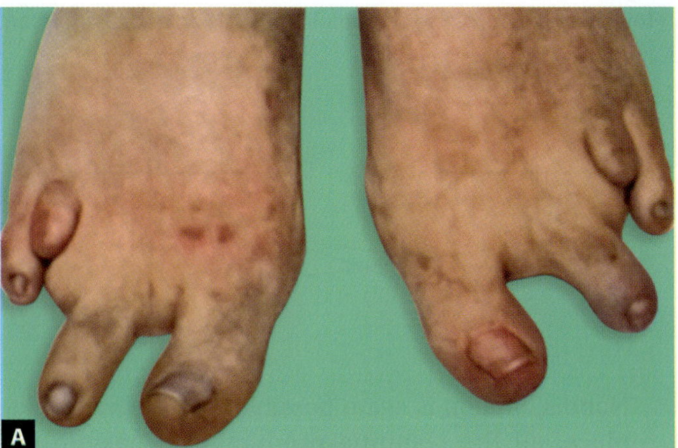

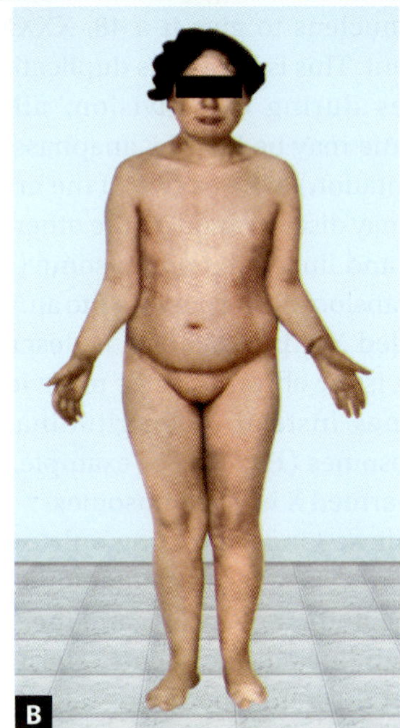

Figs. 4A and B: Turner syndrome with presumed streak gonads. The patient, aged 17 years, complained of primary amenorrhoea. Height 130 cm. Note the short wide neck, barrel-shaped trunk, increased carrying angle, deformities of the toes, and the absence of secondary sex characteristics.

- Characteristic facial features can be subtle **(Figs. 4 and 5)** and include:
  - Short stature
  - A webbed neck
  - A low posterior hairline
  - Misshapen or rotated ears
  - A narrow palate with crowded teeth
  - A broad chest with widely spaced nipples
  - Cubitus valgus
  - Hyperconvex nails
  - Multipigmented nevi

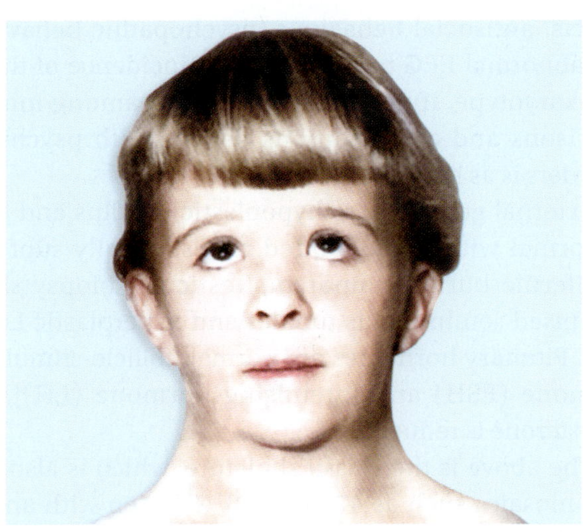

Fig. 5: Turner syndrome. Girl aged 7 years showing webbing of the neck and exaggerated epicanthic folds. She also had a congenital abnormality of the heart. Sex chromosomes 45, XO.

Other important systems involved are given as follows:

- *Cardiac malformation:* Patients with Turner syndrome are at risk of congenital heart defects (e.g. coarctation of aorta, bicuspid aortic valve) and may have progressive aortic root dilatation or dissection.
- *Bone deformity:* Kyphosis and scoliosis in 20% of patients
- Increased upper limb to lower limb ratio (UpToDate)
- Renal malformation (e.g. horseshoe kidney, duplicated or cleft renal pelvis)
- Sensorineural hearing loss, ocular abnormalities, including colour blindness, and skin lesions (pigmented nevi, pilomatrixoma)
- Osteoporosis, obesity, diabetes, atherogenic lipid profile, autoimmune thyroiditis and coeliac disease
- Liver enzymes are mildly elevated in approximately 35–45% of adult patients (UpToDate).

Patients usually have normal intelligence but may have problems with nonverbal, social and psychomotor skills.

At puberty, girls present with a lack of breast development and amenorrhoea, with elevated follicle-stimulating hormone levels by 14 years of age and infertility in women.

The homeobox gene, short stature homeobox-containing gene on the X chromosome (*SHOX*), is associated with short stature in Turner syndrome. For gonadal insufficiency, a gene for bone morphogenetic protein 15 (BMP15) on the short arm of the X chromosome (Xp), as well as two genes encoding fragile X messenger ribonucleoprotein or FMRP (*FMR1* and *FMR2*), on the long arm (Xq) has been implicated.

The ovaries in Turner syndrome characteristically consist of small amounts of connective tissue without follicles or only a few atretic follicles ('streak gonads'). However, the degree of ovarian dysfunction is variable, ranging (at the extremes) from no ovarian function to completely normal function with normal menarche and normal reproductive function for at least a few years after menarche. Because of the broad range of gonadal function, it is not easy to predict which girls will have an absence of breast development versus those girls who will have spontaneous thelarche or even menarche. The gonadal failure is caused by accelerated apoptosis rather than abnormal germ cell formation. The underlying mechanisms for this increased rate of loss of oocytes could be due to haploinsufficiency of genes on the X chromosome [i.e. two copies of these gene(s) are necessary for normal oocyte survival]. Evidence suggests that measurement of AMH is a sensitive marker of prepubertal follicular development and will be helpful in the ovarian assessment of Turner syndrome throughout childhood (UpToDate).

Overall mortality rates in patients with Turner syndrome are increased approximately threefold when compared with the general population, with excess risk occurring at all ages and for most major causes of death (UpToDate).

Streak and dysgenetic gonads have a high potential for neoplasia if the karyotype contains a Y chromosome. In such cases, the risk of a tumour, such as a dysgerminoma or gonadoblastoma, developing in later life is put at 20–30%. Unless a Y chromosome is in the background, however, streak gonads carry a negligible risk in this respect (from old Jeffcoate's).

TRIPLE X SYNDROME (47, XXX) (FROM OLD JEFFCOATE'S)

One per 1,000–1,200 women have a 47, XXX chromosome makeup; this being mostly the result of nondisjunction during oogenesis **(Flowchart 4)**, i.e. X sperm fertilising XX ovum. These were originally described as superfemales, which they are not, for they are, likely to suffer from oligomenorrhoea, secondary amenorrhoea, infertility, genital tract hypoplasia and premature menopause. Other features of the triple X syndrome are low intelligence, sometimes gross mental deficiency or psychosis, and often abnormal electroencephalography (EEG) patterns and the presence of two Barr bodies. But majority of women with a 47, XXX karyotype appear to be normal in every way and are fertile. Moreover, the taint is not transmitted to their offspring, the extra X being lost during oogenesis, even though there is a theoretical risk of XXX or XXY.

KLINEFELTER SYNDROME (47, XXY) (FROM OLD JEFFCOATE'S)

Klinefelter syndrome is also known as primary microorchidism. The 47, XXY karyotype is found only with a male phenotype, its incidence being 1.5–2.0 per 1,000 men. It is correctly known as 'seminiferous tubule dysgenesis.' It usually results from nondisjunction, the additional X chromosome being maternal in 60% of cases **(Flowchart 4)**. The typical effect is Klinefelter syndrome, which combines a tall eunuchoid figure with testicular and genital hypoplasia **(Figs. 6A and B)**. Slender male with female distribution of fat. The testes are very small and may or may not be descended. Their embryological history is rather like that of the streak gonad. Germ cells are present in the genital ridge in the embryo but disappear early in foetal life. After birth, the tubules are aplastic and functionless, so sterility is the rule. The secretion of gonadotrophins is sometimes increased. Gynaecomastia develops in adults in 15% of cases, and there is a much increased risk of carcinoma of the breast in later life. Klinefelter syndrome is also characterised by mental defects, antisocial behaviour (psychopathic behaviour) and abnormal EEG patterns. So, the incidence of the 47, XXY karyotype, if not of the syndrome, among inmates of prisons and of institutions dealing with psychiatric disorders is as high as 1–10%.

External genitalia are hypoplastic, phallus and small or normal with undescended testes, usually subfertile or infertile but not impotent. Testicular biopsy shows hyalinised seminiferous tubules and hyperplastic Leydig cells. Pituitary hormones are normal [follicle-stimulating hormone (FSH) and luteinising hormone (LH)], and testosterone is reduced.

The above is the classical picture, which is also seen with mosaics such as 47, XXY/46, XY. Men with an XXY complement in their chromosome makeup can be completely normal, physically and mentally, and may even have superior intelligence and drive. Moreover, they can be fertile and produce normal 46, XY and 46, XX offspring, the additional X being lost during the maturation of spermatozoa.

YY SYNDROME

As a result of errors in the nuclear division, such as duplication in the zygote, there are men with two or more Y chromosomes and with karyotypes such as 47, XYY, 48, XYYY, 48, XXYY and mosaic patterns containing these. Such men often suffer from the 'YY' syndrome, which

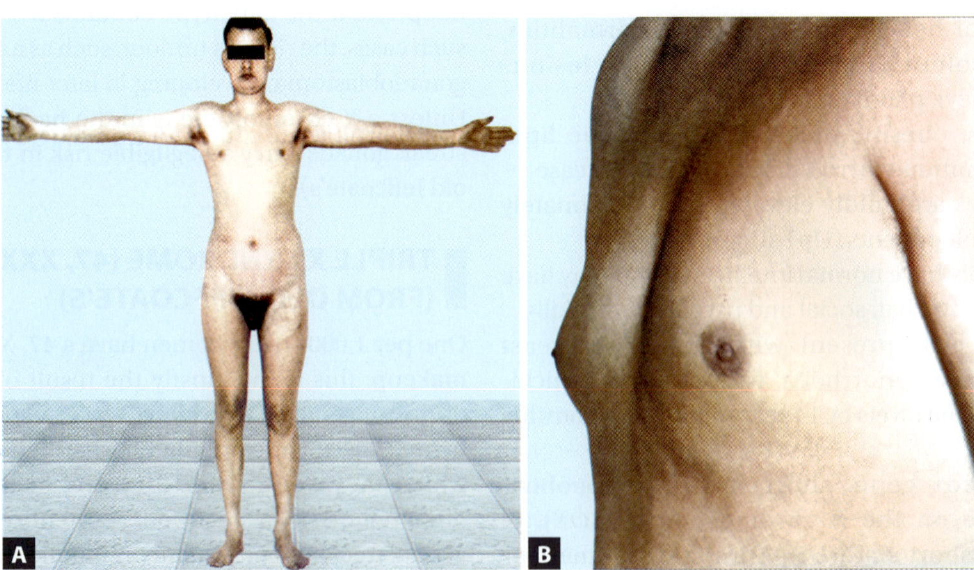

Figs. 6A and B: Klinefelter syndrome. Man aged 28 years, married but infertile and complaining of gynaecomastia. Chromosomes 47, XXY (Professor Sir Cyril Clarke's case). (A) An apparently normal male but tall. The scrotum is small and contains very hypoplastic testes; (B) Slight enlargement of the breasts.

is characterised by excessive tallness, aggressive and antisocial behaviour, and criminal tendencies with or without mental subnormality. Their genital development and fertility are usually normal. The possible aberrations of sex chromosome numbers and types and their combinations in mosaics are endless, but their effects are always in line with the principles stated above (Old Jeffcoate's).

DISORDERS OF SEX DEVELOPMENT WITH NORMAL SEX CHROMOSOMES

46, XX Disorders of Sex Development

The steroid hormones cross the placenta, and the large amounts of oestrogen and progesterone in circulation during pregnancy do not influence sex differentiation in the foetus. Elevated androgens cause virilisation of female foetus.

- Congenital adrenal hyperplasia:
  - 21-Hydroxylase deficiency
  - 11β-Hydroxylase deficiency
  - 3β-Hydroxysteroid dehydrogenase deficiency
- Elevated androgen in maternal circulation
- Drug intake
- Maternal androgen-producing tumours
- Foetal aromatase deficiency
- Tumours of the ovary (e.g. luteoma, androblastoma, mucinous cystadenoma or Krukenberg tumours) and adrenal (e.g. adenoma)

The degree and type of virilisation depend on the timing and strength of the hormone influence, but, since there is no Müllerian inhibitor, the tubes, uterus and vagina develop normally. The effects are seen only in the external genitalia and consist of enlargement of the clitoris, with or without fusion of the labia minora. To produce gross deformity, the androgenic impulse must be applied before the 14th week.

Congenital Adrenal Hyperplasia (Old Terminology—Adrenogenital Syndrome)

This condition is responsible for approximately one half of atypical (ambiguous) genitalia. This is an autosomal recessive disorder and results from a deficiency of one of the enzymes required for the adrenal synthesis of cortisol. The hypothalamic–pituitary axis reacts to the low level of cortisol by elevated adrenocorticotropic hormone (ACTH) secretion resulting in a hyperplastic adrenal cortex that produces androgens as well as corticoid precursors in abnormal quantities up to the enzymatic block in the steps of the biosynthetic pathway.

The clinical picture results from inadequate production of cortisol, aldosterone, excess accumulation of precursors and excessive androgens (refer to **Flowchart 5**). Excess androgens cause masculinisation of genetic female and excessive masculinisation of genetic male. The extent of masculinisation of female foetus depends on the time of onset, quantity available and duration of exposure of the foetus to androgen. The presence of excessive androgens is manifested by varying degrees of fusion of the labioscrotal folds, clitoral enlargement and anatomic changes of the urethra and vagina. High androgen levels earlier than the 10th week of foetal age cause fusion of labia and variable closure of urethra along the phallus, but after the 10th week, vagina and urethra are separated, and excess androgen can cause only clitoral hypertrophy **(Fig. 7)**. As gonads are ovaries, there is no AMH; hence, fallopian tubes and uterus develop normally. Wolffian duct development requires a high local concentration of testosterone secreted by the testis; excessive circulating androgen produced by adrenal glands cannot induce

Flowchart 5: Pathway for steroid biosynthesis.

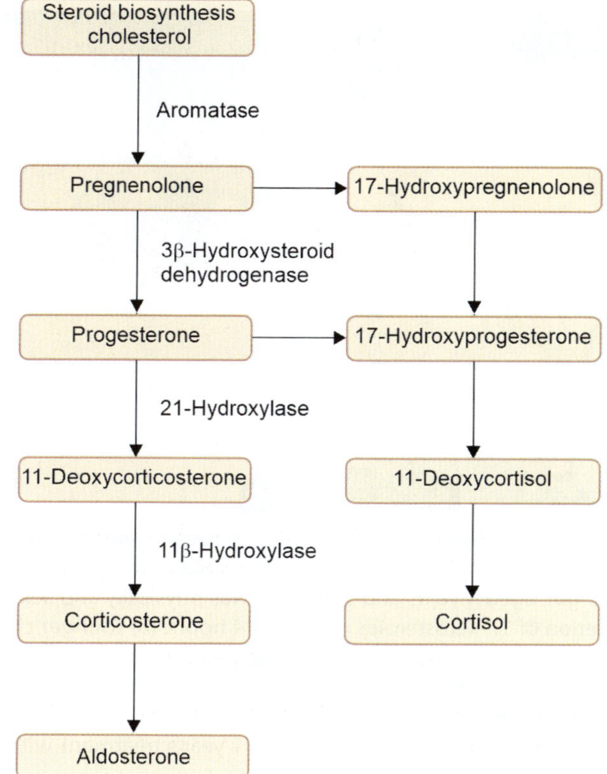

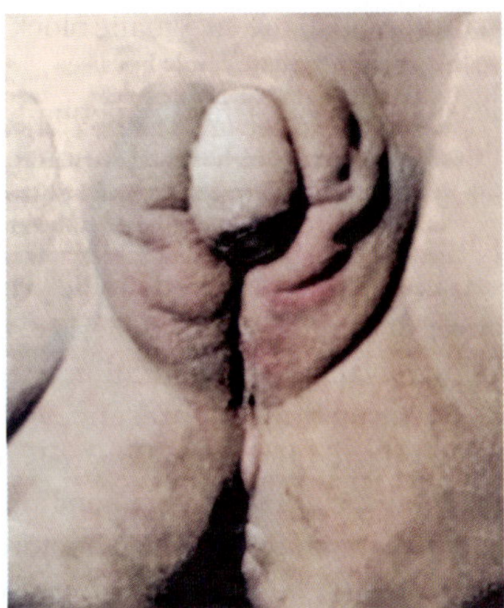

Fig. 7: The virilised external genitalia of a newborn female suffering from congenital adrenal hyperplasia. This condition was diagnosed before birth because the mother, known to be at special risk of having such a child, was subjected to amniocentesis. Examination of the liquor showed it to contain unusually large amounts of pregnanetriol and of 17-ketosteroids (the latter being less significant). These substances were contributed by the foetal urine. This was the first case in which the diagnosis of any form of foetal metabolic error was made before birth, the possibility having come to mind when it was realised that, since the foetus normally urinates in utero, its urine can be examined (via the liquor) before birth. It was this case that led to all subsequent developments in this field.

Wolffian duct development. If untreated, the female with adrenal hyperplasia will develop signs of progressive virilisation postnatally. In addition to sexual changes, patients can present with metabolic disorders such as electrolyte imbalance and hypertension. An electrolyte imbalance of the salt-losing type is due to inadequate aldosterone production **(Figs. 8A to F)**.

21-Hydroxylase Deficiency

This is the most common form of CAH. This condition may be of varied spectrum from partial to almost complete absence of the enzyme. The incidence is 1 in 14,000 newborns worldwide. Three different clinical forms are recognised representing the spectrum of severity given as follows:

1. Salt losing
2. Simple virilising (adequate aldosterone)
3. Nonclassic (late onset, acquired adrenal hyperplasia).

Salt losing and simple virilising forms are associated with masculinisation of foetus, salt losing accounts for 66% of reported cases, and simple virilising 32%.

The classic presentation of 21-hydroxylase deficiency (salt losing) is that of hyponatraemic dehydration, hyperkalaemic acidosis and vascular collapse. Nonclassic

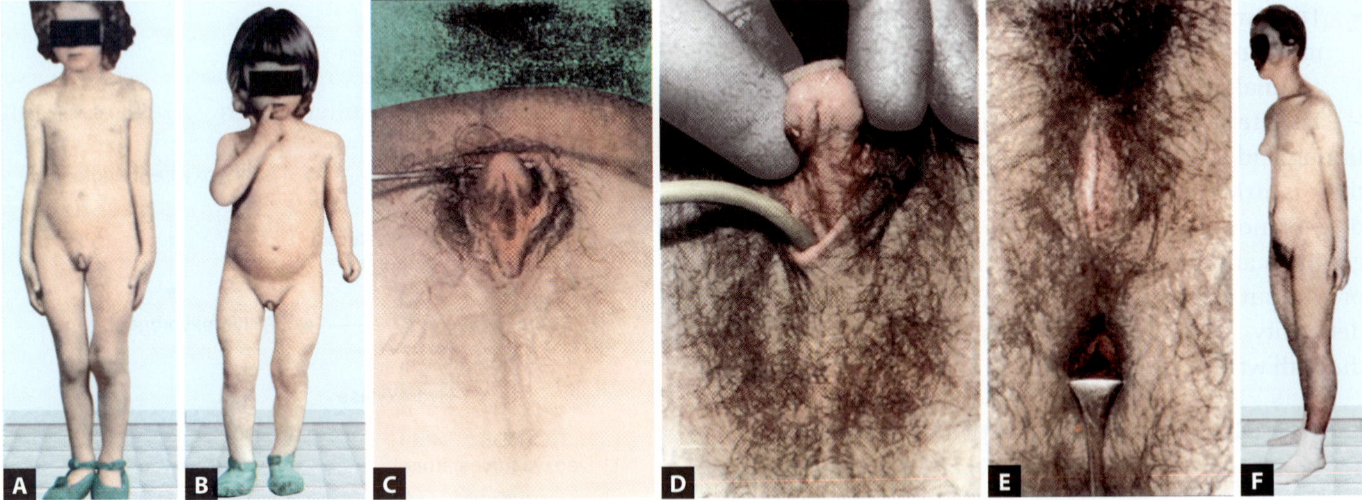

Figs. 8A to F: Sisters each exhibiting congenital adrenal hyperplasia. Another child of the same parents had been born earlier and registered as a male. It died when 6-week-old from "wasting"; so, it was probably affected and died from electrolyte imbalance. (A) The older girl, aged 4 years and 6 months, was physically and sexually precocious. Axillary and pubic hair is present and voice is breaking. Excretion of 17-ketosteroids = 25 mg/24 hours; (B) Younger child aged 2 years and 6 months and precocious. 17-ketosteroid excretion = 15 mg/24 hours; (C) The external genitalia were identical in appearance, and this shows the finding in the child aged 2 years and 6 months. The uterus, tubes, and ovaries were normal in both; (D) The external genitalia at the age of 10 years; the catheter is inserted for the purpose of a vaginogram; (E) The external genitalia 3 months after a reconstruction operation at the age of 10 years; (F) Breast development, previously absent, after 1 year's treatment with prednisolone. Regular menstruation also resulted from this treatment. Both girls responded equally well.

individuals may have completely normal genitalia in the newborn period and become apparent at adolescence or beyond and present with hirsutism, menstrual irregularities and infertility.

Blockage of 21-hydroxylase activity impairs the conversion of progesterone and 17-OH progesterone to deoxycorticosterone and 11-deoxycortisol, respectively, resulting in the accumulation of progesterone and 17-OH progesterone.

11β-Hydroxylase Deficiency

Deoxycortisol and deoxycorticosterone are not converted into cortisol and corticosterone, respectively. However, elevated 11β-deoxycorticosteroid causes salt retention and hypertension in contrast to 21-hydroxylase deficiency. Excess androgen synthesis causes masculinisation. 5.8% of cases of CAH are due to 11β-hydroxylase deficiency.

3β-Hydroxysteroid Dehydrogenase Deficiency

Deficiency of this enzyme results in impaired conversion of pregnenolone and 17-OH pregnenolone to progesterone and 17-OH pregnenolone, respectively. In addition, the conversion of dehydroepiandrosterone to testosterone is impaired. Therefore, there is decreased synthesis of glucocorticoids, mineralocorticoids, androgens and oestrogen. The infants are severely ill at birth and rarely survive. Partial deficiency of enzyme results in masculinisation of the genetic female and incomplete masculinisation of the genetic male resulting in atypical genitalia. Milder, nonclassic cases may be seen.

Masculinisation Due to Elevated Androgens in the Maternal Circulation

Elevated androgens in the maternal circulation can be due to either androgen-secreting maternal tumour or intake of exogenous androgenic substances such as progestin and danazol by the mother. Virilisation is not progressive as there is no inborn error of metabolism; therefore, no hormonal therapy is needed. Surgical correction of abnormalities in the external genitalia is the only treatment required.

46, XY Disorders of Sex Development

These individuals have 46, XY; therefore, genetic sex is male, gonads are testes, but external genitalia are not normally of male.

Causes

- Androgen synthesis defects
- Defective responses in androgen-dependent tissues—androgen insensitivity syndromes
- 5-α reductase deficiency
- Leydig cell agenesis or hypoplasia [testicular unresponsiveness to human chorionic gonadotrophin (hCG) and LH, gonadotrophin-resistant testes]
- Defects in synthesis, secretion or response to AMH

Inborn Errors of Testosterone Biosynthesis

Cholesterol side chain cleavage, 3β-OH steroid dehydrogenase, 17α-hydroxylase, 17, 20-desmolase and 17β-OH dehydrogenase deficiencies all cause incomplete masculinisation of the genetic male. 3β-hydroxysteroid dehydrogenase is most likely to result in atypical genitalia; other lesions usually result in highly feminised individuals. Genetic sex is male (46, XY), possesses testicles, internal genitalia are incompletely developed, and no Müllerian structures as AMH is present, with atypical or female genitalia **(Flowchart 6)**.

Complete Androgen Insensitivity Syndrome

Individual has male karyotype but is phenotypically female. It is transmitted by X-linked recessive gene. There is congenital insensitivity to androgens. Testes are normally developed but abnormally positioned. Wolffian ducts do not develop. Mullerian structures are absent. External genitalia is of female type with blind vagina **(Figs. 9A to C)**.

- They may present with an inguinal hernia or palpable inguinal mass in early childhood.
- At puberty, there is breast development (may be the result of the action of oestrogen uninhibited by androgen).
- Pubic and axillary hair are absent and present with primary amenorrhoea.

Differential diagnoses for primary amenorrhoea are Mayer–Rokitansky–Kuster–Hauser syndrome (uterus absent) and Turner syndrome (uterus is present but gonads fail to produce oestrogen).

Partial Androgen Insensitivity Syndrome

This condition is less common than complete androgen insensitivity and is X-linked recessive. Clinical presentation ranges from almost complete failure of virilisation to

Flowchart 6: Testosterone biosynthesis.

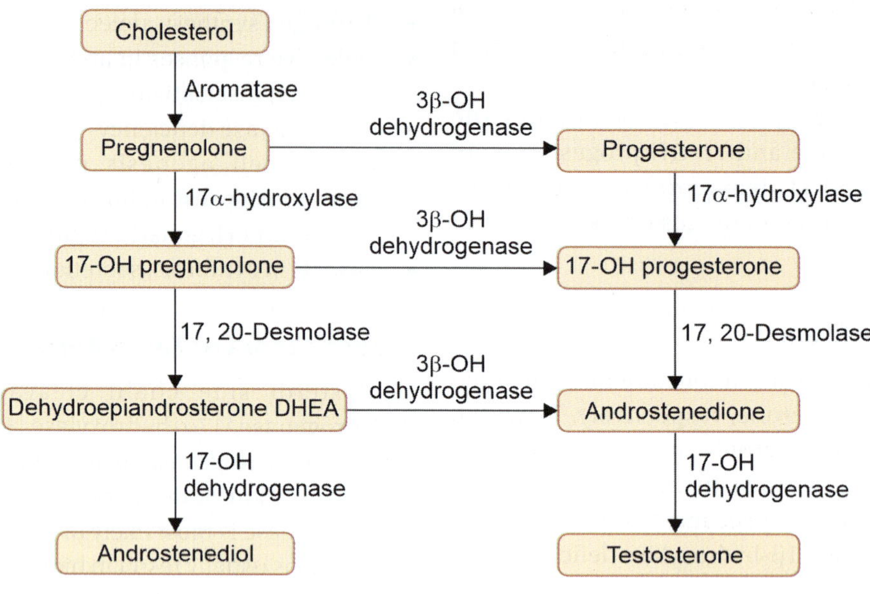

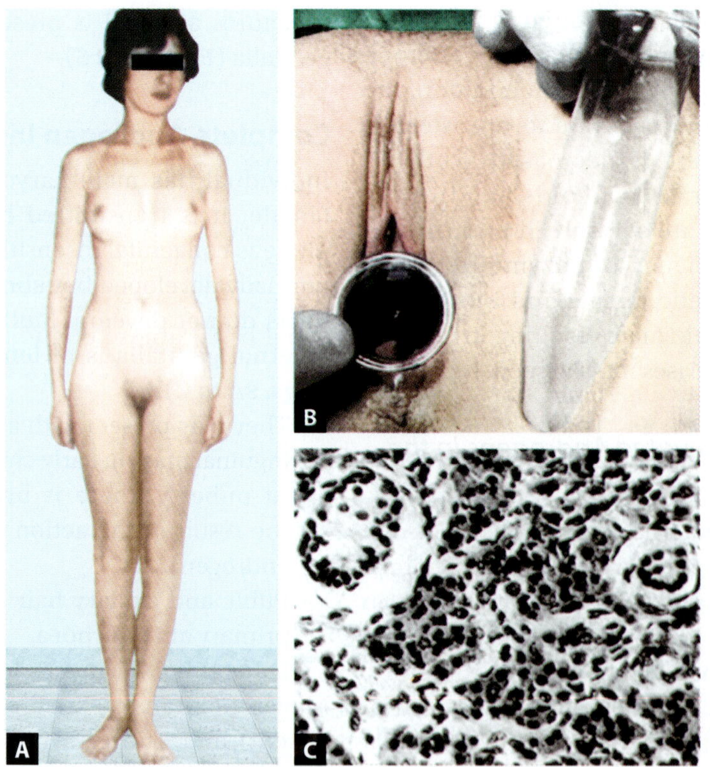

Figs. 9A to C: Complete androgen insensitivity syndrome (testicular feminisation syndrome). A girl aged 18 years complaining of primary amenorrhoea, although her breasts had developed well since she was 12 years old. Interests and outlook feminine; chromosome pattern 46, XY. Undescended testes were removed, and there was no sign of tubes or uterus at operation. She married 1 year later and had normal heterosexual libido and coitus. (A) A very attractive female figure with a well-developed bust and smooth hairless skin; (B) Feminine external genitalia although the pubes and vulva are characteristically almost devoid of hair. The vagina is of good length, although it must represent a urogenital sinus component only; (C) Section of one of the gonads, showing inactive seminiferous tubules and large islands of interstitial (Leydig) cells.

complete male phenotype, with atypical genitalia in between. All intermediate forms are termed Reifenstein syndrome. Forty percent of men with infertility due to azoospermia or severe oligospermia have incomplete androgen insensitivity. Usually, there is inadequate virilisation at puberty and they can have gynaecomastia. These individuals are infertile. Some men with partial androgen insensitivity may respond to androgen treatment with enhanced virilisation.

The endocrine profile of complete and partial androgen insensitivity includes:

- Normal to elevated FSH
- Mildly elevated LH
- ↑ Testosterone and oestradiol

Defects in Testosterone Metabolism: 5α-Reductase Deficiency

It is an autosomal recessive condition with deficiency or reduced activity of enzyme 5α-reductase, which converts testosterone to DHT. The condition is characterised by severe perineal hypospadias and separate urethral and vaginal openings and was known as pseudovaginal perineoscrotal hypospadias. Genetic sex is male (46, XY), testes are present, and testosterone-dependent structures such as Wolffian ducts differentiate normally, whereas DHT-dependent structures such as external genitalia, urethra and prostate do not develop along male lines. Affected individuals have less body hair and temporal recession of hair. Spermatogenesis, muscle mass, male libido and deepening of voice are normally present. DHT presence is required only in foetal life. Early correction of cryptorchidism and hypospadias can preserve fertility and allow male life. If the sex assignment is female, early gonadectomy is necessary to prevent virilisation at puberty.

Diagnosis can be established by demonstrating an elevated blood T/DHT ratio, especially after hCG stimulation and diminished 5α/5β urinary steroid ratios.

Gonadotrophin-resistant Testis

There is either agenesis or abnormal differentiation of Leydig cells, which have reduced responsiveness to LH/hCG characterised by atypical genitalia and cryptorchidism. There may be varying degrees of masculinisation reflecting some amount of Leydig cell function.

Abnormal Anti-Müllerian Hormone (Hernia Uterine Inguinale, Uterine Hernia Syndrome and Persistent Müllerian Duct Syndrome)

These individuals appear to be normal males but have relatively well-differentiated Müllerian duct structures. Usually, the uterus and tubes are found in the inguinal sac, with undescended testes. There is a failure of AMH function either because of failure of Sertoli cell secretion or because of inability of the Müllerian ducts to respond to AMH. Fertility is rare, which may be due to cryptorchidism or aplasia of the epididymis and upper part of vas deferens.

Ovotesticular Disorders of Sex Development

Patients with ovotesticular DSD have both ovarian and testicular tissue. There may be ovarian and testicular tissue within the same gonad (ovotestis) or in opposite gonads. They are further classified into unilateral, if there is ovotestis on one side and either ovary or testes on the other side, and bilateral, if ovotestis is present on both sides.

Approximately 60% of patients have 46, XX karyotypes, followed by 46, XX/46, XY and 46, XY karyotypes. Proposed mechanisms include mosaicism, chimerism or translocation of Y chromosomal material to an autosome or to the X chromosome.

External genitalia are often atypical, and the majority are reared as males because of the size of the phallus. Gonads may be either intra-abdominal, in the inguinal canal or in labioscrotal fold. Internal ducts correspond to the ipsilateral gonad **(Fig. 10)**. The uterus is usually present. Spermatogenesis is deficient. Breast development and menstruation/cyclical haematuria occur at puberty. Occasionally, ovulation may occur; individuals may become pregnant and deliver normal offspring.

Clinical Presentation

Infancy:

- Atypical (ambiguous genitalia):
  - Congenital adrenal hyperplasia
  - Incomplete androgen insensitivity syndrome
  - Testosterone synthesis defect
  - Ovotesticular DSD
  - 5α-reductase deficiency
- Metabolic derangements and electrolyte imbalance: Congenital adrenal hyperplasia
- Inguinal hernia:
  - Complete androgen insensitivity

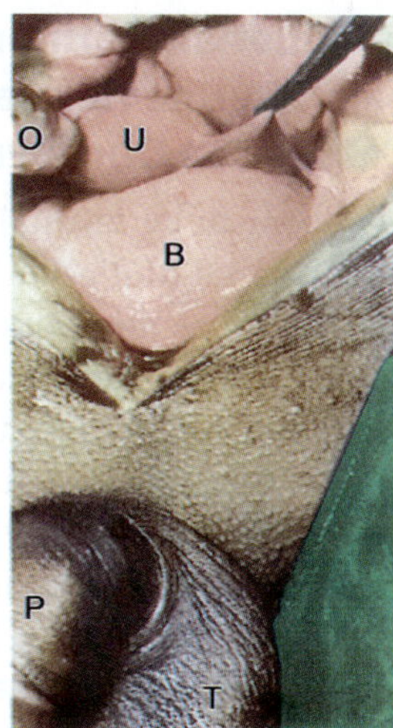

Fig. 10: Influence of the gonad on development of the genital ducts. An adult African man with a normal phallus (P) and scrotum but only the left testis (T) descended. Within the abdomen and behind the bladder (B) is a right-sided unicornuate uterus (U) with a tube and ovary (O). The ovary contains a recent corpus luteum. It is the absence of a testis on the right side that explains the persistence of the Müllerian duct on that side. The buccal smears were chromatin positive, but the chromosomal pattern was not determined. It might have been 46, XX/46, XY.

- Leydig cell agenesis
- Hernia uteri inguinale
- Ovotesticular DSD

  Every female baby with a hernia should be approached with disorders of sex development in mind.

- Hypospadias, cryptorchidism, micropenis and mass in labia

  Any degree of hypospadias associated with any degree of bilateral or unilateral gonadal undescended requires evaluation.

Puberty:

- *Female phenotype:*
  - Primary amenorrhoea: Turner syndrome
    - Complete androgen insensitivity syndrome (CAIS)
  - Infertility and oligomenorrhoea
    - Congenital adrenal hyperplasia
    - Turner mosaic
    - Ovotesticular DSD
  - Virilisation:
    - Congenital adrenal hyperplasia
    - Testicular biosynthesis defect
    - Partial androgen insensitivity syndrome (PAIS)
    - Ovotesticular DSD
- *Male phenotype:*
  - Gynaecomastia:
    - Incomplete androgen insensitivity syndrome
    - Testicular biosynthesis defect
    - Ovotesticular DSD
  - No virilisation
  - Infertility

APPROACH TO A NEONATE WITH ATYPICAL GENITALIA

Definition of atypical genitalia warranting diagnostic evaluation in a neonate is given as follows:

- Penis and a bilaterally nonpalpable testis (cryptorchidism)
- Unilateral cryptorchidism with hypospadias
- Severe penoscrotal, scrotal or perineal hypospadias, with or without microphallus, even if the testes are descended
- Apparently female appearance with enlarged clitoris (clitoromegaly >8 mm) and/or inguinal hernia(s) or palpable gonad(s)
- Asymmetry in size, pigmentation or rugation of labioscrotal folds

This is a social and medical emergency. It is very important to rule out life-threatening salt-losing variety of congenital adrenal hyperplasia in a newborn with atypical genitalia because most infants with atypical genitalia are masculinised females, and the most common cause for that is congenital adrenal hyperplasia. Diagnosis may be difficult in certain situations, and a period of delay is better than reversal of the sex assignment later.

Teamwork is important, and a team of experts in endocrinology, genetics, neonatology, gynaecology, psychology, surgery, urology, specialist nurse, social worker and medical ethicist may be necessary. Parents must be informed about potential adverse sequelae, life-threatening metabolic complications, risk of malignancy, impact of inadequate genitalia, psychological impact of the diagnosis on the child and risk of further children having similar problems.

History

History of previously affected relative, neonatal death of sibling (strongly suggests congenital adrenal hyperplasia) and history of maternal exposure to drugs should be elicited.

Physical Examination

General Examination

The presence of hyperpigmentation, dehydration and hypo-/hypertension suggests congenital adrenal hyperplasia. Turner syndrome is associated with somatic features.

Examination of external genitalia: Careful examination of external genitalia may help to differentiate enlarged clitoris from small penis and fused labia from bifid scrotum. The penis has a midline ventral frenulum, and the clitoris has two folds that extend from the lateral aspects of the clitoris to the labia minora. A male with hypospadias always has a chordee. The ratio of the distance from the anus to the edge of the vagina divided by the distance from the anus to the base of the clitoris/glans is <0.5 in normal males; a ratio >0.5 indicates some degree of fusion. The presence of midline raphe is a male feature.

Palpation for gonads in the inguinal region or labioscrotal fold is important. Gonads in the inguinal region or in the scrotal folds are almost certainly testes. Ovaries are not found in scrotal folds or in the inguinal region. Testicles may be intra-abdominal. If gonads are not palpable, the infant should be considered to have congenital adrenal hyperplasia until proven otherwise.

Rectal examination: Gentle rectal examination may be done to palpate the uterus.

Investigations

- Imaging
- Hormonal assay
- Karyotyping and fluorescence in situ hybridisation (FISH)

Imaging to detect the uterus, ovaries, or undescended testes:

- Pelvic ultrasound
- MRI
- Retrograde injection of dye into the urogenital orifice to outline the urethra and/or vaginal anatomy **(Figs. 11A and B)**.

Hormonal assay: Gonadotrophins—FSH and LH

17-OHP (17-hydroxyprogesterone) 11-Deoxycorticosterone 17-OH pregnenolone 11-Deoxycortisol	Resting and after ACTH stimulation
Androgens: Androstenedione Dehydroepiandrosterone Dehydroepiandrosterone sulphate	Resting and after hCG stimulation

- Assay of AMH to detect the presence of functioning testicular tissue
- Testosterone:DHT ratio
- Testosterone:Androstenedione ratio

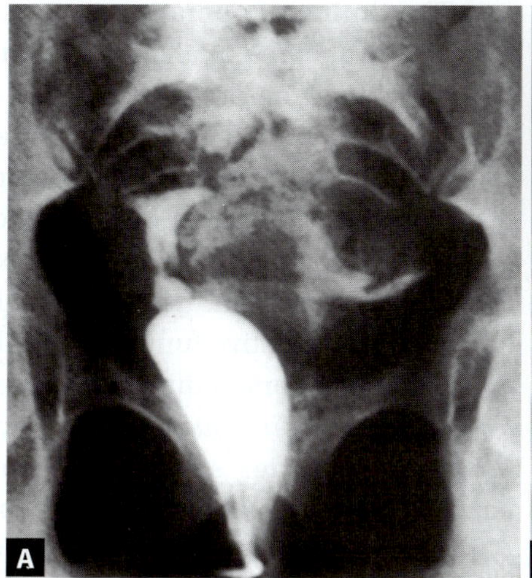

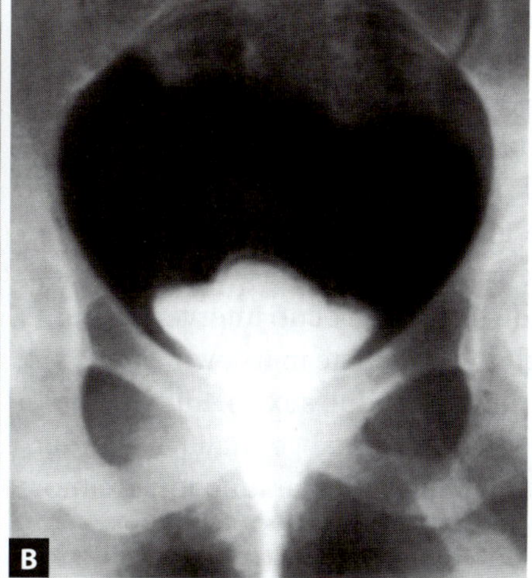

Figs. 11A and B: Congenital adrenal hyperplasia. Vaginograms were obtained by running radiopaque fluid through a catheter inserted. As shown in Figure 7D, the head of the patient being slightly lowered. (A) In this case, the fluid not only filled the obscured vagina but ran into the uterus and even into the peritoneal cavity. Girl aged 11 years. (B) Here, the fluid entered both the urethra and vagina to produce a cystogram superimposed on a vaginogram. Girl aged 8 years (Jeffcoate's).

- Laparoscopy if needed for the detection of Müllerian structures and gonadal biopsy for the diagnosis of ovotesticular DSD and gonadal dysgenesis
- Genetic testing, including screening of androgen receptor gene for mutations, molecular testing for 5-alpha reductase-2 gene mutations, androgen receptor expression and androgen-binding study in genital skin fibroblasts.

Management

Accurate diagnosis, using all the available diagnostic tests, is important. A multidisciplinary team is required for gender assignment and follow-up of these children and during their transition to adulthood. The patients and their families should be involved in decision making. Each individual with DSD is unique and management should be tailored.

Gender Assignment

Gender is how a person views himself as a man or woman and how that person is viewed by others. If there is a problem with the correct sex assignment, it is better to delay than to reverse it later.

Principles: The principles of treatment are as follows:

- Sex of rearing should not be changed if possible
- Careful counselling
- It is easier to remove a small penis or enlarged clitoris and convert it to female genitalia
- Abnormal gonads have a 4% risk of malignancy, so they should be removed
- Supportive hormone therapy
- Counselling for sexual activity and fertility

While dealing with parents, terms such as hermaphrodite and ambiguous genitalia should be avoided. Parents are given the opportunity to make an informed and educated choice regarding gender selection. Options should include the choice of no intervention until the child is old enough to participate in its own care.

Though genetic and gonadal sex is important in selecting the sex of rearing, external genitalia, secondary sexual characteristics and future sexual function are more important.

Therefore, gender assignment will depend on:

- The projected appearance of genitalia after puberty, e.g. penile adequacy for coital function
- Future fertility:
  - Future fertility is unaffected in:
    - All masculinised females; therefore, should be reared as females
    - 5α-reductase deficiency reared as males
    - Turner mosaics may ovulate and conceive
    - Fertility in genetic males with atypical genitalia may be possible in case of isolated hypospadias and repaired isolated cryptorchidism
  - All other patients with atypical genitalia are sterile.

Medical

This is a very important form of treatment in the case of salt-losing type of congenital adrenal hyperplasia as it is lifesaving. It also halts the further masculinisation of a female child.

Hormone replacement: Oestrogen initially and later oestrogen and progesterone are required in Turner syndrome; growth hormone has also been used to increase height. Oestrogen replacement is required for all genetic males who are reared as females.

Testosterone replacement is indicated in those individuals who are reared as males but have no properly functioning testes, e.g. testicular biosynthesis defect.

Surgical reconstruction: Feminity is neutral and masculinity is superimposed. Technically, the construction of female genitalia is easier, and it is difficult to reconstruct a functional male phallus. Therefore, the female sex is usually chosen **(Figs. 12A to F)**.

The timing of operative treatment is also important. The removal of the phallus from a 'girl' should, if possible, be performed before she is aware of its presence. This means before the age of 5 years, and some would say 2 years. Testes are best excised before the age of 14 years. Once an individual is conditioned to live as a member of one sex, it is better not to revert to sex at a later date unless, with a new sex, the individual is capable of normal married life and reproductive function or if the individual opts for reversal by understanding his/her genetic sex (change).

Reconstructive surgeries include feminine reconstructive surgeries such as clitoroplasty, vaginoplasty and labioplasty. Masculine reconstruction consists of the reconstruction of the phallus with vascularised pedicle flaps, correction of chordee, scrotoplasty and testicular prosthesis. The advantage of early separation of urethra and vagina is that the presence of oestrogen in early infancy has beneficial effects on wound healing.

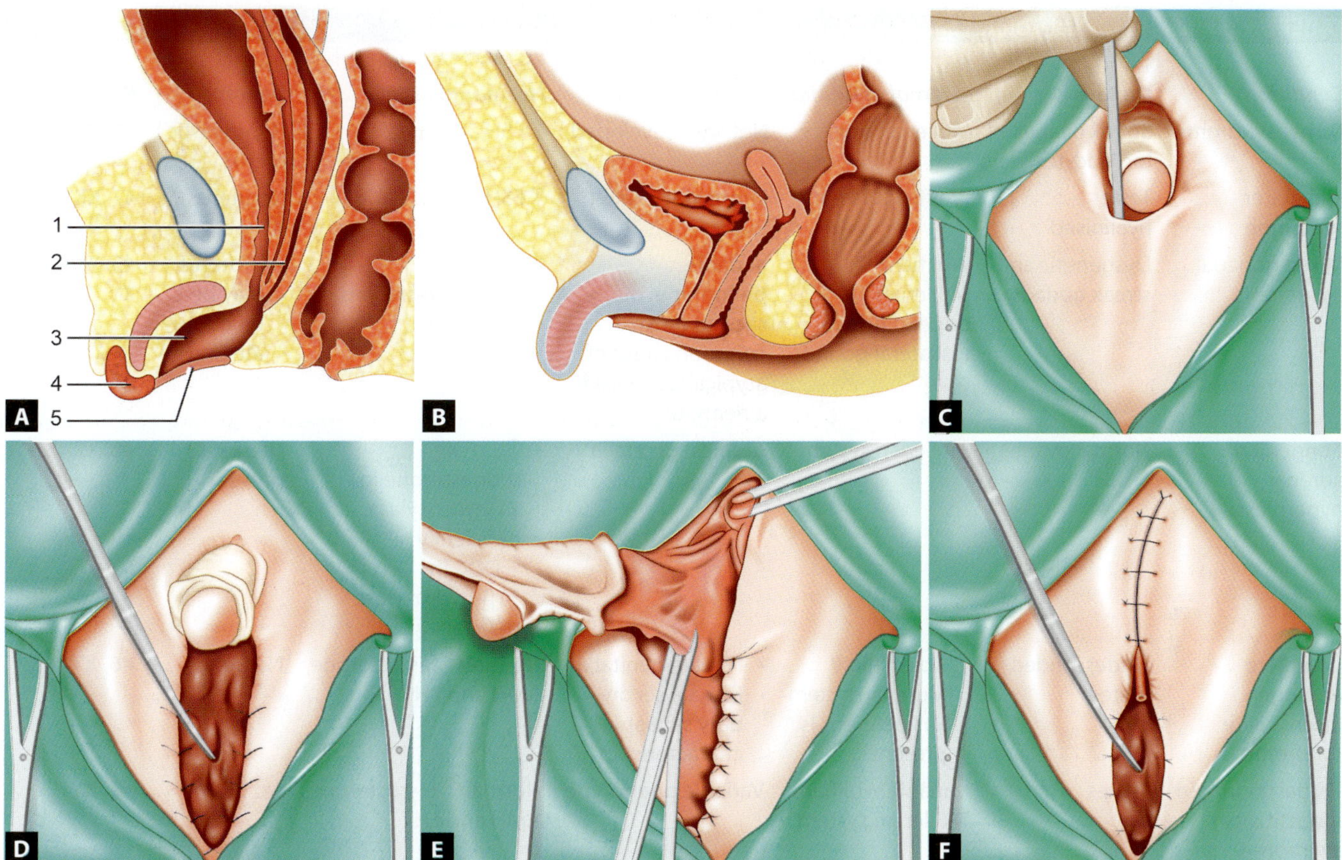

Figs. 12A to F: Correction of the deformity of the external genitalia in congenital adrenal hyperplasia. (A) The normal development of the vulva, vagina, and urethra at the 4th month (after Hamilton, Boyd, and Mossman). (1) Urethra, (2) vagina, (3) vestibule forming from the urogenital sinus, (4) clitoris, and (5) site of cloacal (urogenital) membrane; (B) The deformity in the adrenogenital syndrome represents essentially a fusion of the genital folds to form a perineal membrane that obscures the introitus and vagina; (C) The occluding membrane demonstrated; (D) Incision of the membrane reveals the urethra and vagina; (E) Removal of the enlarged clitoris; (F) The ultimate result; compare with **Figure 7E**.

The chance of postoperative stricture formation is thought to be less. Vaginal dilatation is required at puberty.

Gonadectomy (orchidectomy) may be indicated to prevent malignancy or to prevent unwanted endocrine changes during puberty. It is important to remove any testicular tissue in patients raised as females (androgen insensitivity syndrome, testosterone synthesis defects, mixed gonadal dysgenesis, testicular DSD). Even when male gender assignment is made, the streak gonad is always removed. If histological tests are not dysgenetic and if it has or can be made to have a scrotal position, it can be retained.

It is better to avoid gonadectomy (unless indicated for cancer risk) too early. In the case of male gender assignment, orchidopexy for undescended testes should be performed by the first year of life to preserve testicular function. Hypospadias repair and correction of chordee are best performed early in childhood.

A summary of the clinical features and investigations of DSDs and the management of DSDs are mentioned in **Tables 3 and 4**, respectively.

INTERSEX DEVELOPING AFTER BIRTH

Sex differentiation after birth is controlled by hypothalamic–pituitary, thyroid, adrenal and gonadal hormones as well as by inherent genetic forces. Any disturbances in the functions of these glands, due to a genetic taint or acquired disease, can modify the sexual apparatus and behaviour of the otherwise normal male and female. The development of feminine traits in the male is *called feminism* and that of masculine traits in the female is called *virilism*.

TABLE 3: Summary of clinical features and investigations of DSDs.

Condition	Gonads	Internal genitalia	Secondary sexual characteristics	Hormonal assay	Imaging	Karyotyping
Turner syndrome	Streak ovaries (no oocytes)	Müllerian ducts	Not well developed	↑ FSH and LH	Hypoplastic uterus	45, XO
Klinefelter syndrome	Testes—hyalinised	Wolffian system	Eunuchoid male	↑ FSH than LH	No uterus	47, XXY
Mixed gonadal dysgenesis	Dysgenetic and streak gonads	Wolffian/ Müllerian depending on ipsilateral gonad	Variable phenotype, the second most common cause of atypical genitalia in a neonate	• ↑ FSH/LH • Variable testosterone and AMH	• ± Uterus • May be unicornuate	45, XO/46, XY
Congenital adrenal hyperplasia	Normal ovaries	Müllerian system	Atypical genitalia	• ↑ 17-OH progesterone in 21-hydroxylase deficiency • ↑ DOC in 11β-hydroxylase deficiency	Uterus is present	46, XX
Complete androgen insensitivity syndrome	Undescended testes	• No Wolffian/ Müllerian system • Vas deferens is present	• Female genitalia • Female secondary sexual characteristics	Normal/↑ testosterone, AMH and LH	No uterus	46, XY
Partial androgen insensitivity syndrome	Testes	Variable Wolffian/ Müllerian system	Variable phenotype	Normal/↑ testosterone, AMH and LH	No uterus	46, XY
Testosterone biosynthesis defect	Normal testes	Underdeveloped Wolffian system	Atypical genitalia, under masculinised male	Absence of ↑ in FSH and LH after hCG stimulation	Uterus present	46, XY
5α-reductase deficiency	Testes	Wolffian system	Atypical genitalia with undervirilised male	• Normal testosterone and AMH • T/DHT ratio is >30	No uterus	46, XY

(AMH: anti-Müllerian hormone; DSD: disorders of sex development; DHT: dihydrotestosterone; DOC: deoxycorticosteroid; FSH: follicle-stimulating hormone; hCG: human chorionic gonadotrophin; LH: luteinising hormone; T: testosterone)

Feminism

Manifestations

Sex organs: Feminine features appearing after birth include failure of the testes to descend or develop, hypoplasia of the phallus and gynaecomastia. Galactorrhoea can, but usually does not, accompany gynaecomastia. Gynaecomastia can occur without genital aberrations and may be unilateral or bilateral **(Fig. 13)**.

Secondary Sex Characters

Feminism is indicated by a feminine figure with poor muscular development, broad hips and narrow shoulders, a characteristic gait, a high-pitched voice and smooth skin with a weak growth of hair on the trunk and face.

Libido: Heterosexual impulses may be weak or absent, and the man may be impotent. Homosexuality and transsexuality are extreme examples of abnormal libido.

Causes

Physiological: Slight gynaecomastia (often familial) is common in pubertal and adolescent boys but disappears in 1.5 years. It is caused either by increased hypothalamic–pituitary activity or by temporary hyperoestrogenism resulting from disturbed metabolism of androgens.

Genetic and constitutional: An inborn weakness of masculinising genes explains some disorders of behaviour

TABLE 4: Summary of management.

Condition	Most suitable gender	Medical therapy	Surgical reconstruction	Gonadectomy
Turner syndrome	Female	Growth hormone, oestrogen, progesterone	Not required	If Y chromosome is present
Klinefelter syndrome	Male	Testosterone	Not required	Not defined yet
46, XY gonadal dysgenesis	Female	Oestrogen replacement therapy	Vaginoplasty	Gonadectomy
Congenital adrenal hyperplasia	Female	Glucocorticoids with or without mineralocorticoids	Cliteroplasty and separation of labioscrotal fold, vaginal reconstruction	No
Complete androgen insensitivity syndrome	Female	Oestrogen replacement therapy	Vaginoplasty	Gonadectomy after puberty
Partial androgen insensitivity syndrome	Female/male	According to gender selected	Surgery accordingly	If female gender is assigned/ after molecular tests
Testosterone biosynthesis defect	Female/male	According to the gender selected	Surgery accordingly	If female gender is assigned/if male follow-up is required
5α-reductase deficiency	Male	Not required	Reconstruction	Not to be done if reared as male

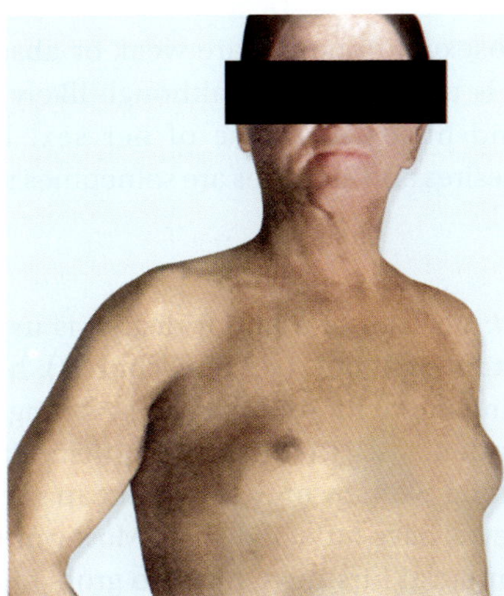

Fig. 13: Gynaecomastia which developed rapidly in a man aged 50 years. The cause proved to be the application of an oestrogenic ointment for pruritus ani; only two tubes were used to produce this effect.

and personality. It can also account for a weak beard, high-pitched voice and failure of the phallus to develop at puberty. This is because the sensitivity of target organs to sex hormones is determined genetically.

Androgen deficiency: Hypoplasia, injury, disease and removal of either the adrenals or testes can cause feminism. If the testes are removed before puberty, the resulting eunuch has a tall feminine figure, soft hairless skin, a high-pitched voice and weak or absent heterosexual interests. The effect of removal of testes later in life is less obvious, but gynaecomastia is recorded as a sequel.

The undescended testis or the one damaged by orchitis usually preserves its endocrine function even though it does not produce spermatozoa.

Oestrogenism: Excessive production of oestrogen is a possible explanation of the rare cases of feminism associated with adrenal cortical tumours and hyperplasia. The administration of oestrogens to the male inhibits testicular activity, suppresses sex drive and causes gynaecomastia. Feminism is also sometimes seen when the liver is damaged by disease or by malnutrition; this is because the liver is no longer able to inactivate oestrogen normally secreted by the adrenal. Gynaecomastia in association with raised blood oestrogen levels is described as a complication of refeeding after starvation, pulmonary tuberculosis, chronic renal failure, renal dialysis, psoriasis, eczema and bronchogenic carcinoma. In the case of the last, the tumour itself can secrete oestrogens and sometimes other hormones, including gonadotrophins.

Diseases of the pituitary, hypothalamus and midbrain (hyperthyroidism): They cause feminism by suppressing androgen production of the adrenals and testes or by increasing the oestrogen secretion of the adrenals.

Drugs

Testosterone and other androgens, by being metabolised to oestrogens, can cause gynaecomastia in young boys. This condition is also seen following the administration of gonadotrophins for cryptorchidism and of drugs such as reserpine and phenothiazine derivatives, which act on the hypothalamus. Digitalis and methyldopa are also reported causes.

Treatment

This varies with the cause of feminism and its manifestation. Oestrogenic tumours can be removed, and cryptorchidism and gynaecomastia may require surgery. An androgen deficiency can be made good by giving testosterone, but this hormone is of little value when the cause of feminism is constitutional, psychological or a genetically determined insensitivity of the target organs.

Virilism

Manifestations

Because of variations in the sensitivity of target organs, these can occur singly or in various combinations. This sensitivity may depend on the high or low capacity of the local tissues to convert testosterone to its active end product, which mediates cell response.

Sex organs: Hypertrophy of the clitoris and hypoplasia or atrophy of the breasts and the genital tract are the main evidence of acquired anatomical virilism. Functional virilism includes amenorrhoea, infertility and failure to lactate.

Secondary sex Characters

Virilism is indicated by coarse features, acne, a heavy angular build, well-developed muscles, broad shoulders and narrow hips with a striding gait. Exceptional athletic skill, especially in those sports that involve throwing, can betoken masculinity. Many international women athletes have been virilised females or congenital DSDs, and some have been disqualified on this account. Other signs of virilism are a prominent larynx (Adam's apple) and a deep voice.

Hair: Growth of hair over the triangle between the pubes and the umbilicus is said to be a masculine trait but occurs in approximately one third of all women. It carries no special significance. Similarly, a slight down on the upper lip and on the arms and legs is as much a female as a male characteristic. The first is found in 25% of young normal women and in 40% of those aged >40 years. Seventeen percent of normal women aged 18–25 years have hair on the chest and breasts.

The more important signs of virilism are hirsutism affecting the beard area and back, a heavy growth of hair on the arms and legs, eyebrows that extend over the bridge of the nose, hair in the nostrils and ears and on the dorsal aspects of the toes, and baldness of the scalp. Significant hirsutism is accompanied by thickening of the affected skin whose collagen content is increased (male features). The sweat gland response is also masculine. So, hirsutism is sometimes called cutaneous virilism.

Personality and outlook: Under this heading come a forceful manner, a weak maternal instinct, disregard for appearance and dress and an assumption of male attire and habits.

Libido: Heterosexual impulses are weak or absent. The virile woman is usually asexual although likely to have platonic friendships with those of her sex. Frankly, homosexual desires and activities are sometimes regarded as virilism.

Causes:

Constitutional: Virilism of a minor degree is usually an inherent constitutional trait (*see* **Flowchart 4**); hirsutism and a masculine build, for example, show strong familial and racial tendencies. Hirsutism by British standards is general among women of Mediterranean races. The Chinese, however, have little body hair. Most women who seek advice for facial hirsutism have no gross endocrine disturbance; their only trouble is that they have hairy parents or parents with hairy brothers and sisters. They generally have good menstrual and reproductive functions, and assessment of ovarian and adrenal function proves normal. Their problem is the undue sensitivity of hair follicles to normal amounts of androgen.

If the onset of hirsutism is acute or associated with masculinisation, the androgen excess might be due to a functional tumour of the ovary or adrenal glands as described later.

Psychological: Masculine trends in outlook and behaviour are often of psychological origin. For one reason or another, there is a conscious or subconscious determination to suppress or deny the female sex, and this sometimes amounts to overt transvestism and trans-sexuality.

Oestrogen deficiency: Failure of the ovaries to function, or removal of the ovaries, results in genital hypoplasia or atrophy but does not lead to positive virilism.

Excessive androgen stimulus

Administration of androgens: Testosterone and danazol therapy in women, unless carefully controlled, causes facial hirsutism, amenorrhoea, atrophy of the breasts and uterus and deepening of the voice. The last is permanent, hirsutism may persist, but the others disappear when treatment is suspended.

Adrenal: Androgenic tumours of the adrenal cortex, which may be benign or malignant, cause a postnatal adrenogenital syndrome that is biochemically different from the congenital one. The manifestations are also different in that the genital organs are normally formed before being exposed to an excessive androgen stimulus. However, the clitoris enlarges, menstruation and follicular ripening are suppressed, the breasts and uterus remain infantile or undergo atrophy, and there are usual manifestations of virilism, including personality changes **(Figs. 14A to D)**. The types of tests used in the diagnosis of virilism are to measure the concentration of some or all the following: Dehydroepiandrosterone (DHEA), DHEA sulphate (DHEAS), testosterone (free preferable to total) and androstenedione by radioimmunoassay techniques in the peripheral circulation. Adrenal tumours generally produce elevated plasma DHEAS levels, which are not suppressed with high doses of dexamethasone. Methods such as ultrasonography and computed tomography (CT) scan may demonstrate these tumours.

After puberty, however, it may be due to nonclassical congenital adrenal hyperplasia. It does not usually suppress menstruation completely; it results in excretion levels of 17-ketosteroids (usually <50 mg/24 h), and this level can be raised by giving ACTH and lowered by dexamethasone. Because of the adrenal response, severe burns and other stress sometimes initiate hirsutism.

In Cushing syndrome, hirsutism and oligomenorrhoea are associated with a rapid increase in weight, striae formation, hypertension, polycythaemia and hyperglycaemia. These reflect a disturbance in the output of sex hormones and corticosteroids by the adrenal. The urinary excretion of 17-ketosteroids is moderately raised and that of 17-hydroxycorticoids grossly raised. Plasma cortisol levels are assayed in the late evening and after single-dose overnight dexamethasone suppression (1 mg at 11 PM). If plasma cortisol is <5 µg/dL, it is normal, whereas if it is >10 µg/dL, it is diagnostic of adrenal hyperfunction.

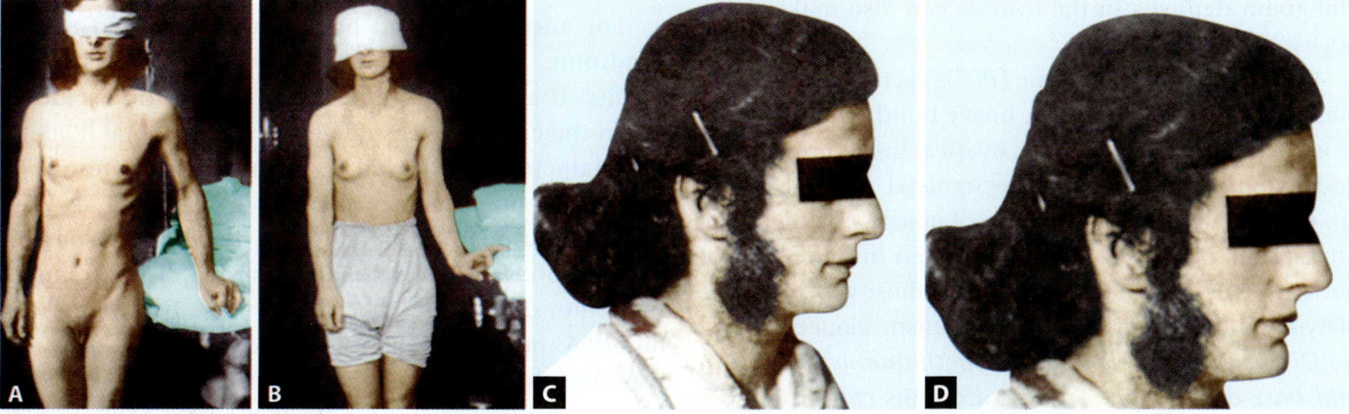

Figs. 14A to D: Postnatal adrenogenital syndrome caused by an adrenal tumour. Woman aged 31 years complaining of primary amenorrhoea and hirsutism. Genitalia are infantile except for enlargement of the clitoris. An adrenal cortical adenoma was found and removed; thereafter, menstruation became established spontaneously in 3 months. (A) Before operation (abdomen and pubes shaved). Note the masculine figure and enlargement of the clitoris; (B) Three months after operation and without hormone therapy. The breasts are now well formed, and increased modesty is indicated by the patient's refusal to be photographed nude; (C) Before operation, showing the growth of hair on the face; the hair on the chin and upper lip had been removed with a razor; (D) Facial appearance 1 year after operation. The growth of hair on the face ceased only very slowly and, at the time of photography, this woman still had to shave, although infrequently.

An abnormal result can be confirmed by the 2-day low-dose dexamethasone suppression (0.5 mg 6-hourly) test. Twenty-four hours of urinary 17-hydroxysteroids and free cortisol can be assayed together. The cause is often a primary adrenal disorder. A malignant or benign tumour may be present, but sometimes there appears to be nothing more than an oversensitivity of the gland to normal amounts of ACTH.

The anterior pituitary may show a predominance of basophil cells (pituitary basophilism), but this is probably the result rather than the cause of the adrenal upset. Occasionally, however, the syndrome is caused by a primary hypothalamic or pituitary lesion.

A true Cushing syndrome is quite rare. Many suspected cases prove to be nothing more than fat and slightly hairy women with oligomenorrhoea but without a demonstrable gross endocrine disturbance. This picture is sometimes labelled 'Cushingoid.' Other conditions associated with this presentation include alcoholism, response to stress, anorexia and bulimia nervosa.

Ovary: Certain rare tumours of the ovary such as the androblastoma and the hilus cell tumour are androgenic. They usually occur in young adults and cause enlargement of the clitoris, suppression of menstruation, hirsutism, acne and voice change. These features are not associated with an increase in the output of 17-ketosteroids but if the serum testosterone level is above 1.5 ng/mL, the possibility of an ovarian tumour should be considered. Secondary malignant deposits in the ovaries can also make these organs androgenic.

Polycystic ovary syndrome (PCOS) is characterised by oligomenorrhoea, infertility, heavy build and hirsutism in association with polycystic ovaries. Insulin resistance and hyperinsulinaemia are recognised correlates and are exacerbated in the presence of obesity. Using pelvic ultrasound, polycystic ovaries are seen in up to 20% of normal women and higher numbers in those with evidence of hyperandrogenism, e.g. acne, hirsutism, alopecia.

Diseases of the pituitary, hypothalamus, midbrain and base of the skull: These conditions can produce a measure of virilism by way of their effect on the adrenal or gonad. Acromegaly, for example, is characterised by angular masculine features, heavy build, amenorrhoea, voice change, loss of libido and atrophy of the breasts and uterus. It is not infrequently mistaken for the adrenogenital syndrome. Prolactin-secreting tumours can have the same effect.

Drugs

Apart from androgens, other hormones and drugs such as ACTH, progestogens, corticosteroids and anabolic agents can sometimes cause virilism.

Diagnosis

Successful treatment depends on finding the cause of the virilism. This can sometimes be determined by clinical methods. Vaginal examination, for example, may reveal a palpable ovarian tumour. Generally, special investigations are necessary: Hormone assays—measurement of serum testosterone, sex hormone-binding globulin (SHBG), FSH, LH, androstenedione, DHEAS and 17-OHP; studies of the effects of giving adrenal cortical stimulators and depressants; electrolyte and metabolic studies and radiographs of the sella turcica; CT scanning and ultrasonography of the pelvis; and IVP and laparoscopy.

Treatment

Surgical: Removal of androgenic tumours of the adrenal and ovary results in the reversal of all signs of masculinity except deepening of the voice. The effect is not always as dramatic as might be expected in that the hirsutism subsides only slowly over the course of many months or years; the clitoris may also never revert completely to normal. Both ovarian and adrenal androgenic tumours may be malignant, so the ultimate result is not always good from the standpoint of life and health.

For adrenal cortical hyperplasia and for Cushing syndrome, partial adrenalectomy gives unsatisfactory results. If a primary pituitary lesion can be excluded, and if the condition is sufficiently serious, total bilateral adrenalectomy followed by substitution therapy is sometimes practised. In the case of polycystic ovaries, treatment depends on whether the patient desires conception or not. For those desirous of procreation, induction of ovulation should be tried. In women who do not want conception at the time of presentation, oral contraceptive pills are the treatment of choice. Laparoscopic ovarian drilling is done only if medical induction of ovulation fails. Its effects are usually temporary.

Medical: If drugs are the cause of virilism, they are discontinued. Mild acne requires only regular washing with soap and water or with lotions containing chlorhexidine. If it does not respond, local nightly application of preparations containing benzoyl peroxide and retinoic acid is advised. For severe acne, antibiotics for at least 3 months (or longer, if necessary) are advised.

Hormonal:

Oestrogen: Although it is the 'female sex hormone', oestrogen never completely overrides an androgen effect. It is used alone or in combination with progestogens and is effective in decreasing adrenal and ovarian steroid production and reducing hair growth in two thirds of hirsute patients. Combined oral contraceptive pills containing ethinyl oestradiol with desogestrel or gestodene have been found to be useful in mild hirsutism.

Medroxyprogesterone acetate: It decreases gonadotrophin-releasing hormone (GnRH) production, and gonadotrophin release and therapy decrease testosterone and oestrogen levels. It can be administered orally (20–40 mg daily in divided doses) or intramuscularly (150 mg of the depot form every 6–12 weeks) with excellent results in decreasing hair growth.

GnRH agonists: Leuprolide acetate intramuscularly every 4 weeks decreases hair growth and diameter in idiopathic hirsutism and in hirsutism with PCOS. Add-back therapy with oral contraceptives or conjugated oestrogen prevents bone loss, vasomotor symptoms and genital atrophy.

Corticosteroids: Dexamethasone can be tried in cases of postpubertal adrenal cortical hyperplasia and PCOS. The rationale is an attempt to depress the output of ACTH by the pituitary. Low doses of 0.25 mg daily improve hirsutism and acne. Serum cortisol should be monitored.

Antiandrogens:

Cyproterone acetate: A synthetic antiandrogen drug such as cyproterone acetate, which has progestational as well as antiandrogenic and antigonadotrophic properties, can be used. It is widely used but is not always effective, and hirsutism may recur after the therapy is stopped. For mild androgenic states, e.g. acne, it is given in a dose of 2 mg/day combined with ethinyl oestradiol. This serves the dual purpose of regularising the menstrual cycle as well as preventing conception during therapy as it is teratogenic. In severe cases of hirsutism with PCOS, it is given in a dose of 50–100 mg from day 5 through 16; ethinyl oestradiol is given from day 5 through 26 in a dose of 30–50 μg. The maximum dose of cyproterone acetate is 300 mg/day.

Spironolactone: This mineralocorticoid antagonist has a beneficial effect on hirsutism without serious side effects but is ineffective for the other signs of virilism. It acts by competitive inhibition of DHT at the intracellular receptor level, suppression of testosterone biosynthesis and increase in testosterone catabolism. It improves hirsutism when taken in a dose of 100 mg for 6 months, but side effects include menstrual irregularity, nausea, fatigue, scalp hair loss, mastodynia and urticaria. A contraceptive must be used because of the possible risk of feminising a male foetus. Its use for the treatment of hirsutism has not been approved in the United States and United Kingdom.

Finasteride: This is a follicular 5α-reductase inhibitor. It is administered in a dose 1–5 mg daily. Finasteride can cross the placenta.

Flutamide: This is a nonsteroidal antiandrogen, which is a weak inhibitor of testosterone biosynthesis. It is not used now because of hepatotoxicity.

Cosmetic: This is indicated mainly in cases of hirsutism without a definite organic cause, and these comprise the majority. It is also often a necessary supplement to more definitive treatment. If the hair growth is slight, nothing more than bleaching may be required. Otherwise, the superfluous hair is best removed by means of a depilatory wax, a razor or a pumice stone. After centuries of experience, men know that shaving is the most efficient method, but women are prejudiced against it, often because they have heard tell that it encourages a stronger growth of beard; this is not true. Electrolysis is painful and leaves scars. Thermolysis and laser epilation give better cosmetic results. The new chemical depilatories (destroyers of hair) are, unlike the older ones, relatively harmless to the skin and can be useful. In the form of pastes or creams, they commonly contain mercaptans as the active principle as these act in the presence of an alkaline material.

SUGGESTED READING

1. Ahmed SF, Cheng A, Dovey L, Hawkins JR, Martin H, Rowland J, et al. Phenotypic features, androgen receptor binding, and mutational analysis in 278 clinical cases reported as androgen insensitivity syndrome. J Clin Endocrinol Metab. 2000;85(2):658-65.
2. Ahmed SF, Tucker P, Mayo A, Wallace AM, Hughes IA. Randomized, crossover comparison study of the short-term effect of oral testosterone undecanoate and intramuscular testosterone depot on linear growth and serum bone alkaline phosphatase. J Pediatr Endocrinol Metab. 2004;17(7):941-50.
3. Alizai NK, Thomas DF, Lilford RJ, Batchelor AG, Johnson N. Feminizing genitoplasty for CAH: what happens at puberty? J Urol. 1999;161(5):1588-91.

4. Rangecroft L; British Association of Paediatric Surgeons Working Party on the Surgical Management of Children Born With Ambiguous Genitalia. Surgical management of ambiguous genitalia. Arch Dis Child. 2003;88(9):799-801.
5. Brown J, Warne G. Practical management of the intersex infant. J Pediatr Endocrinol Metab. 2005;18(1):3-23.
6. Callens N, van der Zwan YG, Drop SL, Cools M, Beerendonk CM, Wolffenbuttel KP, et al. Do surgical interventions influence psychosexual and cosmetic outcomes in women with disorders of sex development? ISRN Endocrinol. 2012;2012:276742.
7. Clayton PE, Miller WL, Oberfield SE, Ritzen EM, Speisser PW, ESPE/LWPES CAH Working Group. Consensus statement on 21-hydroxylase deficiency from the Lawson Wilkins Pediatric Endocrine Society and the European Society for Paediatric Endocrinology. Horm Res. 2002;58(4):188-95.
8. Conn J, Gillam L, Conway G. Revealing the diagnosis of androgen insensitivity syndrome in adulthood. BMJ. 2005;331(7517):628-30.
9. Cools M, van Aerde K, Kersemaekers AM, Boter M, Drop SL, Wolffenbuttel KP, et al. Morphological and immunohistochemical differences between gonadal maturation delay and early germ cell neoplasia in patients with undervirilization syndromes. J Clin Endocrinol Metab. 2005;90(9):5295-303.
10. Creighton S, Minto C. Managing intersex. BMJ. 2001;323(7324):1264-5.
11. Creighton SM, Minto CL, Steele SJ. Objective cosmetic and anatomical outcomes at adolescence of feminising surgery for ambiguous genitalia done in childhood. Lancet. 2001;358(9276):124-5.
12. Creighton SM. Long-term outcome of feminization surgery: the London experience. BJU Int. 2004;93(Suppl 3):44-6.
13. Crouch NS, Minto CL, Laio LM, Woodhouse CR, Creighton SM. Genital sensation after feminizing genitoplasty for congenital adrenal hyperplasia: a pilot study. BJU Int. 2004;93(1):135-8.
14. Dreger AD, Chase C, Sousa A, Gruppuso PA, Frader J. Changing the nomenclature/taxonomy for intersex: a scientific and clinical rationale. J Pediatr Endocrinol Metab. 2005;18(8):729-33.
15. El-Mansoury M, Berntorp K, Bryman I, Hanson C, Innala E, Karlsson A, et al. Elevated liver enzymes in Turner syndrome during a 5-year follow-up study. Clin Endocrinol (Oxf). 2008;68(3):485.
16. García-Acero M, Moreno O, Suárez F, Rojas A. Disorders of sexual development: current status and progress in the diagnostic approach. Curr Urol. 2020;13:169-78.
17. Gastaud F, Bouvattier C, Duranteau L, Brauner R, Thibaud E, Kutten F, et al. Impaired sexual and reproductive outcomes in women with classical forms of congenital adrenal hyperplasia. J Clin Endocrinol Metab. 2007;92(4):1391-6.
18. Grumbach MM, Hughes IA, Conte FA. Disorders of sex differentiation. In: Larsen PR, Kronenberg HM, Melmed S, Polonsky KM (Eds). Williams Textbook of Endocrinology, 10th edition. Philadelphia: WB Saunders; 2003. pp. 842-1002.
19. Hannema SE, Scott IS, Rajpert-De Meyts E, Skakkebaek NE, Coleman N, Hughes IA. Testicular development in the complete androgen insensitivity syndrome. J Pathol. 2006; 208(4):518-27.
20. Houk CP, Hughes IA, Ahmed SF, Lee PA. Writing Committee for the International Intersex Consensus Conference Participants. Summary of consensus statement on intersex disorders and their management. International Intersex Consensus Conference. Pediatrics. 2006;118(2):753-7.
21. Hughes IA, Houk C, Ahmed SF, Lee PA, LWPES Consensus Group. ESPE Consensus Group. Consensus statement on management of intersex disorders. Arch Dis Child. 2006;91(7):554-63.
22. Ismail-Pratt IS, Bikoo M, Liao LM, Conway GS, Creighton SM. Normalization of the vagina by dilator treatment alone in complete androgen insensitivity syndrome and Mayer-Rokitansky-Kuster-Hauser syndrome. Hum Reprod. 2007;22(7):2020-4.
23. Köhler B, Kleinemeier E, Lux A, Hiort O, Grüters A, Thyen U. Satisfaction with genital surgery and sexual life of adults with XY disorders of sex development: results from the German clinical evaluation study. J Clin Endocrinol Metab. 2012;97(2):577-88.
24. Lee PA, Witchel SF. Genital surgery among females with congenital adrenal hyperplasias: changes over the past five decades. J Pediatr Endocrinol Metab. 2002;15(9):1473-7.
25. Marx JS, Pagadala M, Carney J, Gerlach E, Swiatek P, Zabinsky JA, et al. A retrospective review at a pediatric tertiary care medical center. J Pediatr Orthop. 2023;43(5):299.
26. Mayo A, Macintyre H, Wallace AM, Ahmed SF. Transdermal testosterone application: pharmacokinetics and effects on pubertal status, short-term growth, and bone turnover. J Clin Endocrinol Metab. 2004;89(2):681-7.
27. Mazur T. Gender dysphoria and gender change in androgen insensitivity or micropenis. Arch Sex Behav. 2005;34(4):411-21.
28. Migeon CJ, Wisniewski AB, Gearhart JP, Meyer-Bahlburg HF, Rock JA, Brown TR, et al. Ambiguous genitalia with perineoscrotal hypospadias in 46, XY individuals: long-term medical, surgical, and psychosexual outcome. Pediatrics. 2002;110(3):e31.
29. Money J, Hampson JG, Hampson JL. An examination of some basic sexual concepts: the evidence of human hermaphroditism. Bull Johns Hopkins Hosp. 1955;97:301-19.
30. Morel Y, Rey R, Teinturier C, Nicolino M, Michel-Calemard L, Mowszowicz I, et al. Aetiological diagnosis of male sex ambiguity: a collaborative study. Eur J Pediatr. 2002;161(1):49-59.
31. Morgan T. Turner syndrome: diagnosis and management. Am Fam Physician. 2007;76(3):405-10.

32. Newman K, Randolph J, Parson S. Functional results in young women having clitoral reconstruction as infants. J Pediatr Surg. 1992;27(2):180-3.
33. Ogilvy-Stuart AL, Brain CE. Early assessment of ambiguous genitalia. Arch Dis Child. 2004;89(5):401-7.
34. Priyadarshini S. Sharma R. Disorders of sex development in office practice. Indian J Pediatr. 2023;90:1030-7.
35. Ramani P, Yeung CK, Habeebu SS. Testicular intratubular germ cell neoplasia in children and adults with intersex. Am J Surg Pathol. 1993;17(11):1124-33.
36. Randolph J, Hung W, Rathlev MC. Clitoroplasty for females born with ambiguous genitalia: a long-term study of 37 patients. J Pediatr Surg. 1981;16(6):882-7.
37. Robson S, Oliver GD. Management of vaginal agenesis: review of 10 years practice at a tertiary referral centre. Aust NZ J Obstet Gynaecol. 2000;40(4):430-3.
38. Rogol AD. New facets of androgen replacement therapy during childhood and adolescence. Expert Opin Pharmacother. 2005;6(8):1319-36.
39. Rørth M, Rajpert-De Meyts E, Andersson L, Dieckmann KP, Fosså SD, Grigor KM, et al. Carcinoma in situ in testis. Scand J Urol Nephrol Suppl. 2000;205:166-86.
40. Sarma VP. A review of the essential concepts in diagnosis, therapy, and gender assignment in disorders of sexual development. Ann Pediatr Surg. 2022;18:13.
41. Steiner E, Woernie F, Kuhn W, Beckmann K, Schmidt M, Pilch H, et al. Carcinoma of the neovagina: case report and review of the literature. Gynecol Oncol. 2002;84(1):171-5.
42. Toniolo D, Rizzolio F. X chromosome and ovarian failure. Semin Reprod Med. 2007;25(4):264-71.
43. Warne G, Grover S, Hutson J, Sinclair A, Metcalfe S, Northam E, et al. A long-term outcome study of the intersex conditions. J Pediatr Endocrinol Metab. 2005;18(6):555-67.
44. Warne G. Support groups for CAH and AIS. Endocrinologist. 2003;13:175-8.
45. Warne GL, Grover S, Zajac JD. Hormonal therapies for individuals with intersex conditions: protocol for use. Treat Endocrinol. 2005;4(1):19-29.
46. Weidemann W, Peters B, Romalo G, Spindler KD, Schweikert HU. Response to androgen treatment in a patient with partial androgen insensitivity and a mutation in the deoxyribonucleic acid binding domain of the androgen receptor. J Clin Endocrinol Metab. 1998;83(4):1173-6.

15

CHAPTER

Injuries

Kavitha D Nayak, Muralidhar V Pai

Chapter Outline

- Different Types of Injuries

INTRODUCTION

Female genital tract injuries are often ignored, and they usually present late with complications. Female genital tract injuries involve direct trauma to vulva and vagina, foreign body in the genital tract, vaginal burns and obstetric complications such as laceration of cervix, perineal tear, rupture of uterus, broad ligament haematoma, genital tract fistula and its sequelae. Female genital organs and external genitalia have a rich blood supply, and injuries to the female genital tract can bleed torrentially at times. It can lead to haemodynamic instability. Hence, timely diagnosis and management become crucial in saving the life of women. In addition, certain conditions such as complete perineal tear, rectovaginal fistula, can make women's life miserable, and most of the time she suffers in silence. Therefore, it is important we learn, understand, and aim for primary management of these conditions to prevent their consequences.

DIFFERENT TYPES OF INJURIES

Direct Trauma to Vulva and Vagina

There is often a history of road traffic accident with fracture to the pelvis or history of fall or history of coitus. It can occur in difficult delivery, instrumental delivery. Patients can present with bleeding or in shock. The first thing is to explore and examine the vulva and vagina for tears with the help of good light. If required, the patient has to be taken to the operating theatre (OT) for examination. Sometimes childbirth trauma leads to the formation of vulvovaginal haematoma. It is due to inadequate suturing of tears.

Tips and tricks: When examining for vaginal tears, it is good practice to do per rectal examination and rectovaginal examination to check integrity of rectovaginal septum. Always identify the apex of any vaginal tear and ensure it is sutured. It is usually seen in deep-seated tears that the apex is left unsutured and the patient ends up in shock.

If a woman is unable to pass urine postdelivery, suspect vaginal haematoma. Also, when bleeding is not much but the patient is in shock, look for a haematoma.

Clinical/surgical tips: Vulvar haematoma presents with painful, tender swelling. Vaginal haematoma presents with a swelling deeper inside. If a haematoma develops above the pelvic diaphragm, it can spread retroperitoneal. Management includes resuscitation, to estimate blood loss, correct hypovolaemia with aggressive fluid management, and blood transfusion. Tears or haematomas have to be explored with good antibiotic cover. Haematoma requires surgical exploration, primary closure, and compression for 12–24 hours **(Flowchart 1)**. In case of direct trauma, bleeding vessel to be identified and ligated and vaginal pack can be kept.

Foreign Body and Its Effects

A foreign body can be present in vagina or inside the uterine cavity [e.g. intrauterine contraceptive device (IUCD)]. It is mostly retrieved from small girls or mentally retarded women. Various substances have been recovered from vagina such as hair pins, toys, fruit seeds and abortion sticks. In reproductive women, there can be forgotten tampons or condoms. Sometimes, there can be left vaginal

Flowchart 1: Management of haematomas based on size.

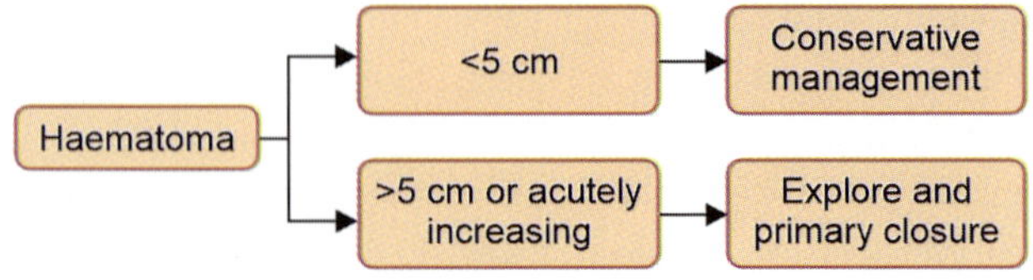

packs or swabs used for delivery. In older women with prolapse, women often fail to come for the 3-monthly follow-up of the pessary. This can cause the formation of tissue over the pessary, and the pessary is forgotten.

Tips and tricks: Any woman presenting with offensive vaginal discharge needs to be examined thoroughly and symptom should not be ignored. Sometimes, examination of anaesthesia will be needed. Foreign body to be removed.

Clinical/surgical tips: In case of an IUCD, per speculum examination is to be done, and the thread is to be visualised. With the help of per vaginal examination, the thread can be felt. X-ray/transvaginal ultrasound will help to confirm the presence of an IUCD inside the uterine cavity.

Hysteroscopy can also be used. Hysteroscopic removal of IUCD is nowadays the preferred procedure for removal, especially when an IUCD is displaced higher, and the thread is not seen. Laparoscopy is combined in cases of suspected perforation. Also, to rule out bowel injuries.

Vaginal Burns

These are not commonly seen. It can be due to chemical injury by hot vaginal douches. It can be radiotherapy-induced burns. Sometimes, it is accidental burns of vagina with cautery at surgery [e.g. during loop electrosurgical excision procedure (LEEP)].

Clinical tips: Minor burns can cause a burning sensation and can be managed with local creams. Large areas can cause fibrosis and lead to dyspareunia and haematometra. This requires adhesiolysis.

Rupture and Perforation of Uterus

In gynaecology, perforation of the uterus can occur during dilatation of the cervix, hysteroscopic septal resection, hysteroscopic adhesiolysis or insertion of an IUCD.

Tips and tricks: Be vigilant in cases where perforation can occur, such as menopausal uterus, pyometra, postpartum and endometrial cancer cases.

Clinical tip/surgical tip: During hysteroscopy, suspect perforation when there is loss of resistance of uterine sound, loss of vision and drop in vitals. The first step is to stop the procedure.

Management depends on size of perforation, type of instrument, associated bowel injuries and haemodynamic instability. The patient has to be adequately resuscitated. If the perforation is small, no bleeding, patient is stable, then observation can be done. Even for perforation by a small instrument, such as a sound or dilator can be observed.

If perforation occurs with a suction cannula or hysteroscope, laparoscopy must be done, and the concurrent status of bowel and omentum to be checked. If the perforation is small, it can be sutured laparoscopically. If perforation is bleeding involving uterine artery or a large perforation, or there is bowel injury, it requires laparotomy and management. Sometimes, total abdominal hysterectomy +/– bilateral salpingo-oophorectomy (BSO) may be needed. Bowel injuries will need help of a gastroenterologist and resection and anastomosis/primary closure, depending on size of bowel perforation, perforation is through and through (involving mucosa) and site of injury and bowel preparation.

Perineal Tear

Perineal tears are classified based on Royal College of Obstetricians and Gynaecologists (RCOG, 2015) into the following, as described in **Table 1**.

Tip and tricks: To identify risk factors for perineal tears early, such as gestational diabetes with a big baby, shoulder dystocia, occipitoposterior position, instrumental delivery and elderly primigravida (rigid perineum). We can reduce perineal tears by using liberal episiotomy in the above cases. Proper perineal support is a crucial step towards the prevention of perineal tears. Controlled delivery of the head by Ritgen manoeuvre also helps in preventing perineal tears.

Clinical/surgical tip: Third- and fourth-degree perineal tear is called OASIS (obstetric anal sphincter injuries). All perineal tears need to be sutured. It requires good analgesia, good light and good suturing techniques. Third-degree tear can be sutured by end-to-end or overlap technique. End-to-end suturing technique is preferred.

TABLE 1: Classification of perineal tears.

Grade of tear	*Involved structures*
First degree	Vaginal epithelium or perineal skin only
Second degree	Perineal muscles
Third degree: • Grade 3a • Grade 3b • Grade 3c	Anal sphincters • <50% thickness of external sphincter • >50% thickness of external sphincter • Internal sphincter
Fourth degree	Anal epithelium

Flowchart 2: Types of fistulas.

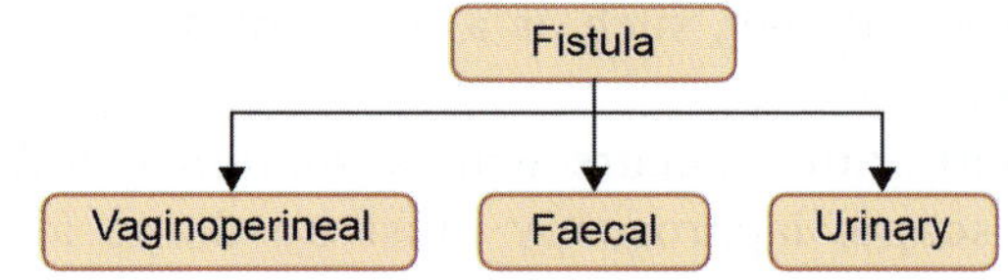

Flowchart 3: Types of faecal fistula.

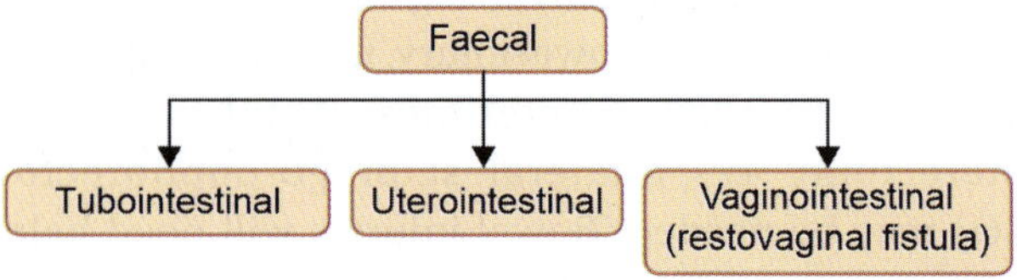

Different types of fistulas are depicted in **Flowchart 2**.

Genital Fistula

Usually, vaginoperineal results from incomplete healing of the obstetrical perineal tear. If symptomatic, requires sinogram and complete excision.

Faecal Fistula (Flowchart 3)

Tips and tricks: Faecal fistula often presents with incontinence of faeces and flatus. Mostly, they result due to obstructed labour causing ischaemic necrosis, instrumental delivery. It can result due to unidentified rectal injury during gynaecological surgery. In India, tuberculosis is an important cause. It can also occur due to radiotherapy, pelvic abscess, diverticulitis or carcinoma colon.

Surgical tip: Rectovaginal fistula (RVF) is more commonly seen in clinical practice. It can be low RVF when opening is in distal third of vagina. It is mid-RVF when opening is in middle third of vagina (above fourchette). It is a high RVF near the cervix and opens into the sigmoid colon. Identification can be done with rectovaginal examination, rectal probe test, proctoscopy, dye test and CT scan. Endoanal ultrasound helps to identify associated sphincter defects. A low rectovaginal fistula can be converted to a complete perineal tear and stitched layer-wise. For the transvaginal approach, repair of the fistula involves incision around the fistula. Vaginal mucosa is widely mobilised from rectum. The rectum defect is then sutured with 3-0 Vicryl in two layers. Vaginal mucosa is then sutured with 2-0 Vicryl in two layers. If the fistula is higher then it requires an abdominal approach and repair.

Broad Ligament Haematoma

It occurs due to trauma (lacerations/tears) to the cervix, upper vagina or uterus that extends into uterine or vaginal vessels or vessels of the broad ligament. It can occur following operative delivery, trauma or surgery or after spontaneous vaginal delivery or dilation and curettage (D and C).

Tips and tricks: Suspect broad ligament haematoma in cases of unexplained shock when bleeding is not much. The definitive treatment of broad ligament haematoma is variable according to size, location and severity of patient. However, a strong clinical suspicion, prompt diagnosis and timely intervention are the important factors for successful treatment.

Clinical/surgical tip: Clinically, patient can have excess perineal pain, urinary retention, rectal tenesmus, unexplained pyrexia and signs of hypovolaemia. On examination, uterus deviated upwards and laterally to opposite side from broad ligament haematoma. Diagnosis is done with the help of ultrasound, CT and MRI for location, size, and extent.

Broad ligament haematoma may be treated either conservatively with blood transfusion, fluid resuscitation and observation or with surgical exploration and evacuation. Conservative management in the form of broad-spectrum antibiotics and continuous monitoring can be done if the haematoma is <5 cm and not expanding. However, in case of larger and expanding haematoma or patient becomes hemodynamically unstable then emergency exploration should be done. Surgical intervention can be in the form of haematoma evacuation, ligation of the internal iliac artery, uterine artery embolisation (UAE) or even hysterectomy.

Differential diagnoses (DD): DD include pelvic mass, abscess and intra-abdominal bleeding.

Laceration of Cervix

Cervical laceration can occur during instrumental delivery, precipitate labour or delivery through an incompletely dilated cervix. It can occur during gynaecology procedures such as D and C, and with vulsellum too.

Cervical tears are commonly seen on the left side than right side. It can be multiple tears causing a stellate appearance of external os. Cervical tear can extend deep into fornix and can cause broad ligament haematoma or incomplete rupture of uterus.

Tip and trick: Always do cervical exploration in case of instrumental delivery. Cervical exploration requires two sponge-holding forceps, and the method is called as 'walking over the cervix'. First, apply a sponge-holding forceps at 12 o'clock position. Then apply another sponge-holding forceps at 3 o'clock position and inspect the area between them. Now release the sponge holder at 12 o'clock position and apply it over 6 o'clock position and continue all around the cervix.

Clinical/surgical tip: Only deep cervical tears >1 cm and/or bleeding actively have to be sutured. Cervical repair needs good analgesia, good lighting and adequate exposure. Always identify the apex, and suturing is started 1 cm above the apex. Interrupted sutures are used, and the tear is approximated.

Urinary Fistula (Flowchart 4)

Causes include pelvic surgery, cancer +/- radiotherapy, obstetrical trauma.

Clinical/surgical tip: Obstetric fistula occurs due to prolonged, obstructed labour due to cephalopelvic disproportion (CPD)/malposition, resulting in ischaemic necrosis of the bladder between foetal head and pubic symphysis. Usually, fistula develops 7–10 days later postdelivery and usually involves trigone of bladder. During LSCS, bladder base may be torn, and involved suture can cause a fistula later. Also, in extension of uterine angles, the ureter is at risk while suturing.

Gynaecological causes of fistula are a result of pelvic surgery. In cases of hysterectomy, ureter can be injured at IP ligament ligation, at pelvic brim, at adnexal masses dissection, at base of broad ligament, floor of pelvis. This results in ureterovaginal fistula. Vesicovaginal fistula results during vaginal vault closure and in carcinoma cervix, radiotherapy.

Conservative management: Usually, vesicovaginal fistula (VVF) heals in 3 weeks to 3 months with continuous bladder drainage. If it fails, surgery is planned after 3–4 months after the initial injury/previous attempt to repair. This allows tissue reaction to subside.

Small VVF (<3 mm) can be managed with superficial bladder fulguration using electrocautery/laser. Postirradiation fistula takes 6 months to 2 years to be ready for repair. Early repair for small, uncomplicated fistula within 1–8 weeks can be attempted.

Flowchart 4: Types of urinary fistula.

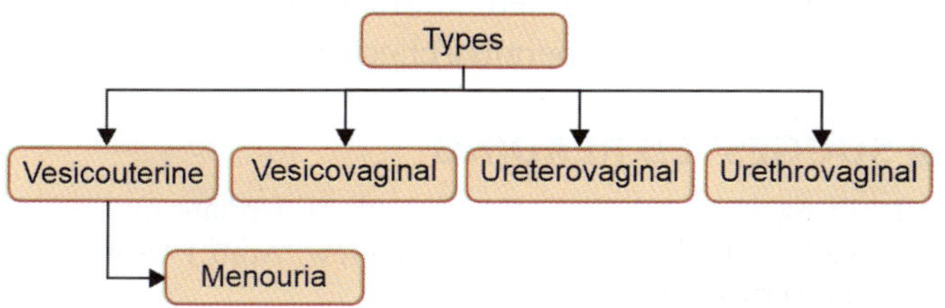

Surgical management:
- *Ureteric fistula:* Treatment includes transplantation of ureter into bladder or Boari operation or ileal conduit or ureteric diversion into colon.
- *Uterovesical fistula:* Hysterectomy if fistula is large. Otherwise, identify the fistulous tract, suture the uterine and bladder defects in layers, and interpose vesical peritoneum.
- *Vesicovaginal fistula:* First is to perform cystoscopy to know size, location of fistula and distance to ureteric orifice and then the repair is planned. Better to do ureteric stent in case fistula is close to ureter.

Vaginal approach of repair is preferred than transvesical approach. It includes adequate dissection and mobilisation of tissues, excision of the fistula tract and all scar tissue. Suturing is done with 3-0 Vicryl. The first row of sutures is placed in bladder. This is tested with methylene blue, reinforced, if necessary, by a second covering in muscularis. The vagina is closed without tension (least tension is in transverse direction).

In cases of posthysterectomy VVF can be closed vaginally by Latzko's partial colpocleisis after ureteral catheterisation.

- *The transperitoneal transvesical approach is used:* If fistula is close to ureteric orifice, an omental flap is used, ureteroneocystostomy is needed, or an ileal/cecum conduit is needed. If tissue loss is excessive, Martius graft is used in vaginal approach, omental flap abdominally. Other grafts are the gracilis muscle flap, rectus abdominis flap and peritoneal flap.

  These days laparoscopic approach is preferred in abdominal repair. Post-repair requires continuous bladder drainage for 2–3 weeks, and input and output chart has to be maintained.
- *Urethrovaginal fistula:* The easiest and most successful technique involves dissection of the floor of urethra from the external meatus up to and including the fistula. The vagina is the freed from urethra. Closure of urethra from above downwards. During

closure, lumen is protected by a small polythene tube. The vagina wall is closed, and a catheter is placed in urethra for continuous drainage for 14 days.

- *Surgery for complicated fistula:* Complicated fistula includes fistula that are extensive, postirradiation, postmalignancy fistula, combined fistula and those with intestinal fistula. For a fistula with gross loss of tissue, ureteroileocolostomy is preferred. For active malignancy, exenteration may be indicated. For a combined fistula, a large radiation one involving bladder and rectum is managed by colpocleisis. It is so planned that the contents flow from bladder to rectum and not the other way around.
- *Pregnancy after cure of fistula or complete perineal tear:* If a woman is cured after urinary or faecal fistula communicating with vagina, elective classical caesarean section is preferred.
- Similarly, in case of complete perineal tear in previous pregnancy who are symptomatic or who have abnormal endoanal ultrasonography and/or manometry should be delivered by elective lower segment caesarean section (LSCS).

Prevention of fistula: For obstetric fistula, improvement in obstetric care, early recognition of CPD, preventing prolonged and obstructed labour and timely LSCS are the key factors.

In gynaecology, sharp dissection of bladder and pushing the bladder down to be followed. Use of DJ stenting preoperatively in cases of endometriosis to recognise ureter. Early recognition and management of bladder and ureteric injury intraoperatively. One step is to instill methylene blue into bladder and look for spillage intraoperatively. Postoperatively, suspect bladder injury if haematuria occurs/abdominal pain/distension/paralytic ileus. Ureteric injury typically will have flank pain.

Old Complete Perineal Tear

This occurs due to unsutured/unhealed third- or fourth-degree perineal tear and occurs 3 months postdelivery.

Tip and trick: They present with incontinence to flatus and faeces. This incontinence of faeces occurs during loose motion. This is because these women develop better levator ani tone and use it as a sphincter. So, they become incontinent only during loose motion. However, if sphincter is completely damaged, they can have incontinence of solid stools as well.

Usually, on inspection, diagnosis becomes evident. There will be no perineum and red shinning mucus membrane of anal canal and pinkish vaginal wall is seen. There will be two dimples seen at 3 o'clock and 9 o'clock representing the cut ends of external anal sphincter. There will be radial folds seen only on posterior half and absent on anterior half.

Important differential diagnoses will be rectovaginal fistula, which also presents with faecal incontinence. Hence, a speculum examination and rectovaginal examination must be performed to rule out this condition.

Surgical tip: The treatment of choice for a complete perineal tear is surgery. It is to be performed either within 24 hours of delivery or after 3 months. After 3 months as it helps in tissue inflammation to heal. Delaying beyond 6 months can cause dense scar tissue, and surgery becomes difficult. Important points to be remembered before surgery are good bowel preparation, treatment of infection and vaginal douching.

The surgical procedure is a layered method of repair under anaesthesia in lithotomy position. First is to give transverse incision at vaginal and rectal mucosa. Then incision extended midline in posterior vaginal wall. Some also follow inverted V incision over posterior vaginal wall called 'Warrens flap' method. Then the vaginal mucosa and rectal mucosa are separated. The anal mucosa is closed with continuous 3-0 Vicryl. Then the internal sphincter is closed over the anal mucosa with 3-0 Vicryl. Next the ends of external anal sphincter are identified and closed either by end-to-end or by overlap technique. Afterwards, the levator ani is brought together and sutured with interrupted sutures. Perineorrhaphy is done. Then the vaginal mucosa is closed with 2-0 Vicryl. Finally, the perineal skin is closed with subcuticular or interrupted sutures.

Postoperative care involves antibiotics, stool softener, intravenous (IV) fluids, followed by a liquid diet, then a soft diet. Patient is advised contraception and to review after 6 weeks for postoperative checkup.

SUGGESTED READING

1. El-Azab AS, Abolella HA, Farouk M. Update on vesicovaginal fistula: a systematic review. Arab J Urol. 2019; 17(1):61-8.

2. Korde-Nayak V, Biniwale P. Broad ligament haematoma. In: Sharma A (Ed). Labour Room Emergencies. Singapore: Springer; 2020. pp. 395-402.
3. Rafi J, Khalil H. Maternal morbidity and mortality associated with retroperitoneal haematomas in pregnancy. JRSM open. 2018;9(1):2054270417746059.
4. RCOG. (2015). The management of third- and fourth-degree perineal tears. RCOG green top guidelines no. 29. Available from https://www.rcog.org.uk/guidance/browse-all-guidance/green-top-guidelines/third-and-fourth-degree-perineal-tears-management-green-top-guideline-no-29/ [Last accessed April, 2025].
5. Wilson AN, Homer CS. Third-and fourth-degree tears: a review of the current evidence for prevention and management. Aust N Z J Obstet Gynaecol. 2020;60(2): 175-82.

16

CHAPTER

Female Genital Mutilation

Rajeshwari G Bhat, Muralidhar V Pai

Chapter Outline

- Classification of Female Genital Mutilation
- Prevalence of Female Genital Mutilation
- Indications
- Complications
- Diagnosis
- Management in Obstetric and Gynaecological Practice
- Management of Short-term Complications
- Management during the Antenatal Period
- Management during the Intrapartum Period
- Postnatal Care
- Eradication

INTRODUCTION

Female genital mutilation (FGM), also known as 'female genital cutting,' or 'cutting,' or 'female circumcision' refers to 'all procedures involving partial or total removal of the external female genitalia or causing injury to the female genital organs for nonmedical reasons.' In December 2012, the United Nations General Assembly adopted a historic resolution on the elimination of FGM across the globe, urging states to pursue a comprehensive, culturally sensitive, systematic approach that incorporates a social perspective and is based on human rights and gender equality principles. The February 6 of each year has been recognised as the International Day of Zero Tolerance to FGM. The United Nations strives to eradicate the practice by 2030, with its inclusion as target 5.3 in the Sustainable Development Goal (SDG).

Female genital mutilation has been practiced since early 450 BC and was widely performed throughout ancient Egypt in many other societies and cultures. In the early 1800s to the mid-1950s, surgeries such as clitoridectomy, hysterectomy and oophorectomy were commonly performed in the United States and Great Britain for the treatment of various disorders such as masturbation, lesbianism, falling of the womb, floating womb, emaciation, debility, nymphomania, seizures, and hysteria.

The procedure of FGM is usually performed by traditional practitioners, who have received no formal medical training. As a result, the procedure is performed without the use of anaesthetics, using crude instruments such as knives, scissors or razor blades. However, there has been a global trend towards the medicalisation of FGM. In some countries, a significant number of FGM procedures are performed by health professionals. These include countries such as Egypt, Sudan and Kenya. FGM is likely to occur among all socioeconomic groups. However, daughters of urban and educated women are less likely to undergo FGM in comparison to the daughters of rural and less educated women.

Female genital mutilation is almost always carried out on girls between infancy and the age of 15 years. However, the age at which the procedure is performed significantly varies between countries. It is estimated that in over half of the countries practicing FGM, the procedure is performed under the age of 5 years. In some communities, reinfibulation (defibulation) may be performed in an adult woman following childbirth.

CLASSIFICATION OF FEMALE GENITAL MUTILATION

The widely accepted classification of FGM was developed by the World Health Organization (WHO) in 1995, and the updated version of the WHO handbook 2018 is shown in **Table 1** and **Figures 1A to D**.

PREVALENCE OF FEMALE GENITAL MUTILATION

As per the estimates by the United Nations Children's Fund (UNICEF), over 200 million women and girls have undergone FGM worldwide. There are more than

TABLE 1: World Health Organisation's classification of female genital mutilation.

Type I	Partial or total excision of the clitoris and/or the prepuce • *Type Ia:* Removal of the prepuce/clitoral hood (circumcision) • *Type Ib:* Removal of the clitoral glans with the prepuce (clitoridectomy)
Type II	Partial or total removal of the clitoris and the labia minora, with or without excision of the labia majora • *Type IIa:* Removal of the labia minora only • *Type IIb:* Partial or total removal of the clitoral glans and the labia minora (prepuce may be affected) • *Type IIc:* Partial or total removal of the clitoral glans, the labia minora and the labia majora (prepuce may be affected)
Type III	Infibulation or narrowing of the vaginal orifice by cutting and appositioning the labia minora and/or the labia majora, with or without excision of the clitoris • *Type IIIa:* Only appositioning of the labia minora • *Type IIIb:* Appositioning of the labia majora also
Type IV	Any other procedure which is performed for nonmedical reasons and causes injuries to the female genital organs such as pricking, piercing or incision of the clitoris and/or labia; stretching of the clitoris and/or labia; cauterisation by burning of the clitoris and surrounding tissues; scraping of tissue surrounding the vaginal orifice; introduction of corrosive substances or herbs into the vagina for the purpose of tightening or narrowing it, etc.

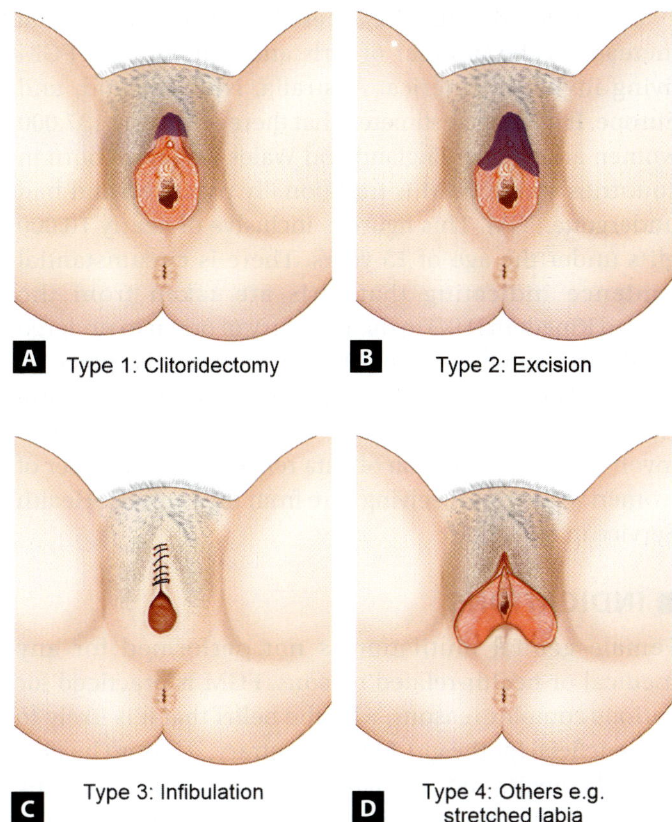

Figs. 1A to D: World Health Organisation's classification of female genital mutilation.

three million girls at risk each year. It is considered a traditional cultural practice in several African countries. The prevalence of FGM in various African countries is demonstrated in **Figure 2**. Outside Africa, FGM is also practiced in Yemen, Iraqi Kurdistan and parts of Indonesia and Malaysia. Though FGM has been culturally restricted in countries where it presently occurs, these laws are poorly enforced.

The type of FGM varies between countries. Type 3 FGM is practiced almost entirely in Africa, with the highest prevalence in North-Eastern Africa, including Somalia, Sudan, Ethiopia, Eritrea, and Djibouti. Prevalence of FGM is also likely to vary within a particular country, where it may be associated with ethnic groups.

Female genital mutilation is a cultural rather than a religious practice. There is no mention of alteration of the female genitalia in any officially adopted text of any religion.

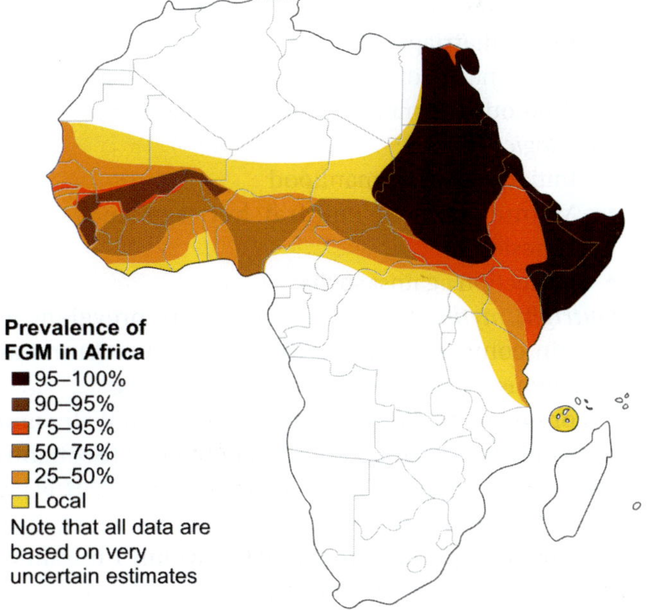

Fig. 2: Map of Africa showing the prevalence of female genital mutilation in the country. (FGM: female genital mutilation)

As a result of migration, there has been a substantial increase in the number of girls and women with FGM living in North America, Australia, New Zealand, and Europe. It has been estimated that there are nearly 137,000 women and girls in England and Wales who were born in countries where FGM is traditionally practiced and had undergone FGM. This figure is inclusive of nearly 10,000 girls under the age of 15 years. There is circumstantial evidence indicating that girls are taken from the United Kingdom (UK) to their country of origin to undergo FGM, and some cases of FGM may also take place in the UK. The Health and Social Care Information Centre (HSCIC), implemented by the Department of Health, is involved in the collection of data related to the number of women with FGM receiving care from the National Health Service in England.

INDICATIONS

Female genital mutilation is not performed for any medical or health-related reasons. FGM is practiced for various complex reasons, with the belief that it is likely to be beneficial for the girl. On the contrary, it has no health-related benefits and may harm girls and women in many ways. FGM is a practice that violates human rights and is a form of child abuse. It can be considered a severe form of violence against women and girls.

The likely reasons given for FGM include the following:

- *Psychosexual causes:*
  - Maintenance of a woman's chastity and virginity before marriage
  - Maintenance of her fidelity during marriage
  - Promotion of morally appropriate fertility
- *Sociological causes:*
  - Initiation into womanhood
  - Maintenance of cultural heritage and social cohesion
  - Protection against spells
- *Outright myths:* Bizarre traditions are prevalent in certain communities, which consider the clitoris as dangerous and can cause damage to a penis.

According to the FGM Act 2003 in England, Wales and Northern Ireland, and the Prohibition of FGM (Scotland) Act 2005 in Scotland, FGM is illegal in the UK. If FGM is confirmed in a girl under the age of 18 years, it is compulsory to report this to the police within 1 month of its confirmation.

Female genital cosmetic surgery is also barred in the UK unless it is essential for the maintenance of the patient's physical or mental health. Surgeons undertaking such surgery must take appropriate measures to ensure compliance with the FGM Acts. Reinfibulation refers to the resuturing (usually after childbirth) of the incised scar tissue in a woman with FGM type 2 or 3. Previously, there was uncertainty as to whether reinfibulation was covered by the FGM Acts. However, it is now accepted that reinfibulation is illegal and should not be performed under any circumstances. Reinfibulation is an illegal procedure. There is no clinical justification for this procedure, and it should not be undertaken under any circumstances.

The UN resolution 67/146 in December 2012, took a resolution for 'intensifying global efforts for the elimination of female genital mutilations'. Female genital mutilation is a degrading practice that does serious harm to women's physical and moral integrity. Today, more than 100 million women and young girls are the victims of a practice that is justified under false cultural and religious pretenses and remains a taboo subject that is misunderstood and misinterpreted in numerous societies. Resolution 67/146, which was just adopted, is not just a strong political message engaging the entire international community, but also a message of hope for millions of girls and women who, each year, risk suffering that odious and discriminatory practice in the name of tradition and, falsely, of religion. Moreover, it allows us to further mobilise all stakeholders, in particular States, international organisations and civil society, to engage more effectively in the struggle to eliminate female genital mutilation by fully implementing and putting into practice the existing national, regional and international measures.

COMPLICATIONS

Short-term Complications

The most common short-term complications related to FGM include haemorrhage, urinary retention, genital swelling, infection, fever, etc. Haemorrhage is the most common and life-threatening complication of FGM. If the clitoral dorsal artery or labial branches of the pudendal artery are cut, haemorrhage has been documented in the range of 4–19%. Active haemorrhage, subsequent hypotension, hypovolemic shock and death may occur in these cases.

Long-term Complications

Reported long-term complications of FGM are as follows:

- *Genital scarring:* Female genital mutilation can result in unsightly and painful genital scarring. Keloid scarring has been reported in up to 3% of women. There may be a formation of epidermoid inclusion cysts and sebaceous cysts, which may require surgical excision. Infibulation cysts and neuromas can also occur.

- *Urinary tract complications:* Complications of the lower urinary tract are particularly more common in women with type 2 or type 3 FGM. Various urinary tract complications can occur, such as poor flow of urine beneath the infibulation scar, which may result in symptoms of urinary obstruction. Stasis of urine due to obstruction may result in recurrent urinary tract infections and urinary or vaginal calculi. The recommended treatment in these cases of urinary obstruction is deinfibulation. Damage to the urethra during FGM of any type may result in the development of a urinary stricture or fistulae. These may require assessment by a urologist or urogynaecologist.
- *Impaired sexual function:* Female genital mutilation may be associated with several consequences related to sexual health, including dyspareunia, apareunia, impaired sexual functioning, etc. Dyspareunia may occur as a result of vaginal narrowing and formation of painful scar tissue. Sometimes, a complete inability to perform sexual intercourse or apareunia and vulvovaginal lacerations may also result. The removal of sexually sensitive tissue of the clitoris and labia minora may reduce sexual sensation. This may be associated with numerous sexual consequences such as a reduction in sexual desire and arousal, reduced frequency of orgasm or anorgasmia, decreased lubrication and poor sexual satisfaction.
- *Psychological sequelae:* Female genital mutilation is likely to have several psychological effects, such as panic attacks, anxiety and post-traumatic stress disorder. FGM has been linked to an increased incidence of domestic violence in Africa. Health professionals need to be aware of the psychological consequences of FGM and the different factors influencing FGM perception. Indeed, a feeling of 'Being abnormal' can be awakened among patients because of health professionals' incorrect behaviours.
- *Menstrual difficulties:* Female genital mutilation is likely to result in haematocolpos. Dysmenorrhoea has also been reported among women with FGM. However, the underlying mechanisms behind this presently remain unclear.
- *Genital infection and pelvic inflammatory disease:* Female genital mutilation has been associated with an increased risk of genital infections such as bacterial vaginosis and herpes simplex (especially type 2). However, currently, there is no conclusive evidence to show that FGM is associated with an increased risk of pelvic inflammatory disease.
- *Infertility:* Female genital mutilation is likely to cause infertility by causing complications such as apareunia, dyspareunia, impaired sexual function and ascending infections. However, presently, there is limited evidence to indicate that FGM might result in infertility. While any randomised trials have demonstrated no such link, one case-control study has shown a positive association between primary infertility and FGM.
- *Human immunodeficiency virus (HIV) and hepatitis B infections:* Although it is believed that FGM may increase the risk of transmission of viruses, such as hepatitis B, hepatitis C and HIV, probably due to the sharing of nonsterile instruments when FGM is performed in groups, there is presently no definite epidemiological evidence to support this.
- *Obstetric complications:* Various obstetric complications are likely to occur with various types of FGM. However, the risk is greater with greater tissue damage. A meta-analysis by Berg et al. reviewed maternal outcomes in women with FGM. Though this meta-analysis included some studies from the US and Europe, most were from Africa. The meta-analysis also reported an increased risk of complications such as prolonged labour, postpartum haemorrhage (PPH) and perineal trauma in association with FGM. A large prospective study by the WHO, which investigated both maternal and perinatal outcomes among 28,000 women belonging to six African countries, has shown an increased risk of caesarean delivery, low birth weight, an increased requirement for neonatal resuscitation and risk of stillbirths and early neonatal deaths.
- Other obstetric consequences that have been described with FGM include fear of childbirth, difficulty in the performance of simple obstetric procedures such as application of foetal scalp electrodes and foetal blood sampling, difficulty in catheterisation during labour, wound infection and retention of lochia. FGM is also likely to increase the risk of the development of subsequent obstetric fistulae in the future because of obstructed labour.
- *Complications in the male partner:* A history of FGM in the female can result in the following complications in

the male partner—difficulty in penetration, wounds and infections on the penis and psychological problems.

DIAGNOSIS

Clinical Presentation

- *Antenatal examination:* All women, especially those coming from communities where FGM is traditionally practiced, should be asked for a history of FGM at their booking antenatal visit so that this can be identified early in the pregnancy. This should be documented in the woman's maternity case notes.
- *Gynaecological examination:* Sometimes women with FGM may present with symptoms directly associated with FGM or with coexisting gynaecological morbidity, e.g. dyspareunia and menstrual abnormalities. The vulva should be inspected to determine the type of FGM. The external examination would also help in determining if deinfibulation is indicated, to enable vaginal examination and carrying out gynaecological tests (e.g. Pap smear, genital infection screening, etc.). The external examination would also be useful in identifying any other FGM-related morbidity, e.g. epidermoid inclusion cysts.
- *Psychological referral:* All women who have undergone FGM in the past should be referred for psychological and/or psychosexual assessment and treatment.

Investigations

- *Screening for blood-transmitted infections:* These women should be tested for infections such as HIV and hepatitis B and C.
- *Sexual health screening:* Screening for sexually transmitted infections should be done.

MANAGEMENT IN OBSTETRIC AND GYNAECOLOGICAL PRACTICE

- All acute trusts or health boards should appoint a selected consultant obstetricians and midwives responsible for the care of women with FGM.
- All gynaecologists, obstetricians and midwives should receive mandatory training on FGM and its management, including the technique of deinfibulation. They should complete the programme of FGM e-modules developed by Health Education, England. Healthcare professionals should be cautious regarding the clinical signs and symptoms of recent FGM, such as pain, haemorrhage, infection and urinary retention.
- Most specialist FGM services in the UK are available in the major cities. They are usually located in a hospital or community clinic (e.g. GP surgery or sexual health clinics). Consultant obstetrician and/or gynaecologist must lead the specialist multidisciplinary FGM services, which may offer the following services—information and advice about FGM; risk assessment tools for safeguarding children; gynaecological assessment; deinfibulation; access to other services, etc. Healthcare professionals must adopt a sensitive and nonjudgemental approach towards such patients and consult with them in a safe and private environment. In case the healthcare professional is unable to understand the woman's language, professional interpreters must be used; family members should not be used as interpreters.
- Specialist FGM services should offer access to services such as psychological assessment and treatment, psychosexual services, screening and treatment of sexual health-related diseases and services pertaining to gynaecological subspecialties such as urogynaecology and infertility.
- Specialist FGM services should work in collaboration with other healthcare providers, including general physicians (GPs) and acute trusts, voluntary sector organisations, the police, social services and schools.
- When providing care for FGM survivors, healthcare providers and forensic practitioners must abstain from making assumptions, or expressing negative opinions, reactions and anger towards FGM.

Instead, it is essential to develop a trusting relationship and provide holistic care in a culturally sensitive and nonjudgmental manner. An accurate record of the findings at the time of clinical examination should be maintained in the patient's clinical records. This could be supported by a photographic record of the lesions where appropriate. All women and girls with acute or recent FGM must be referred to the police and social services.

MANAGEMENT OF SHORT-TERM COMPLICATIONS

- Management of pain—analgesics and sedatives
- *Haemorrhage:* If bleeding is minimal, the area is cleaned with an antiseptic solution and pressure is applied. If the bleeding is heavy and the girl/lady is in haemorrhagic shock, she should be managed according to the protocol at the higher centre.
- Injection of tetanus toxoid and antibiotics

- *Urinary retention:* It may be due to inflammation and swelling, pain or injury to the urethra.
    - Nonsteroidal anti-inflammatory drugs
    - Encourage the girl to pass urine
    - Foley's catheterisation
    - Referral if urethral injury is suspected.

To reverse infibulation, a multidisciplinary approach is required. This includes evaluation of psychological/social needs, which is as important as taking care of the physical effects of FGM. A team of plastic and gynaecological surgeons to correct the aesthetic features and functionality of the vulva. A combination of regenerative and surgical procedures may be performed to restore sexual function, normal voiding, menstruation and to facilitate vaginal examinations, cervical screening and intrapartum care.

MANAGEMENT DURING THE ANTENATAL PERIOD

- The woman should be referred for psychological assessment and treatment. Clinicians should be aware of the psychological sequelae and other complications associated with various types of FGM.
- Besides routine antenatal screening tests such as hepatitis B, HIV and syphilis, screening for hepatitis C should also be offered.
- The appropriate plan of care must be discussed and recorded by the midwife or obstetrician.
- *Requirement for deinfibulation:* Deinfibulation is the surgical procedure that aims at the division of the scarred tissue sealing the vaginal introitus in type 3 FGM. This helps in opening up the closed vaginal introitus **(Figs. 3A to D)**. Deinfibulation has been shown to improve maternal and obstetric outcomes, reducing the risk of caesarean section, postpartum haemorrhage, infection and urinary retention. This is an elective procedure that must be performed by an appropriately trained midwife or an obstetrician. During the antenatal visit, the vulva must be inspected to determine the type of FGM and to assess if there is any requirement for deinfibulation. If the introitus is sufficiently open to permit vaginal examination and the urethral meatus is visible, deinfibulation may not be required. However, adequate vaginal assessment during labour may be impossible for women with type 3 FGM. In these cases, deinfibulation is recommended during the antenatal period, typically at around 20 weeks of gestation.
- If there is a requirement for deinfibulation, it may be performed antenatally, in the first stage of labour, at the time of delivery or perioperatively after caesarean section. It is usually performed under local anaesthetic in a delivery suite. The procedures of deinfibulation (when the introitus is narrowed) and selective episiotomy (based on assessment at the time of delivery) may help in improving the clinical outcomes in these women.
- Women should be informed that reinfibulation would not be undertaken under any circumstances.

MANAGEMENT DURING THE INTRAPARTUM PERIOD

- Women with FGM should preferably be delivered in units having immediate access to emergency obstetric care.
- Intravenous access must be established in labour, and a blood sample should be taken for complete blood count (CBC), blood group and save.

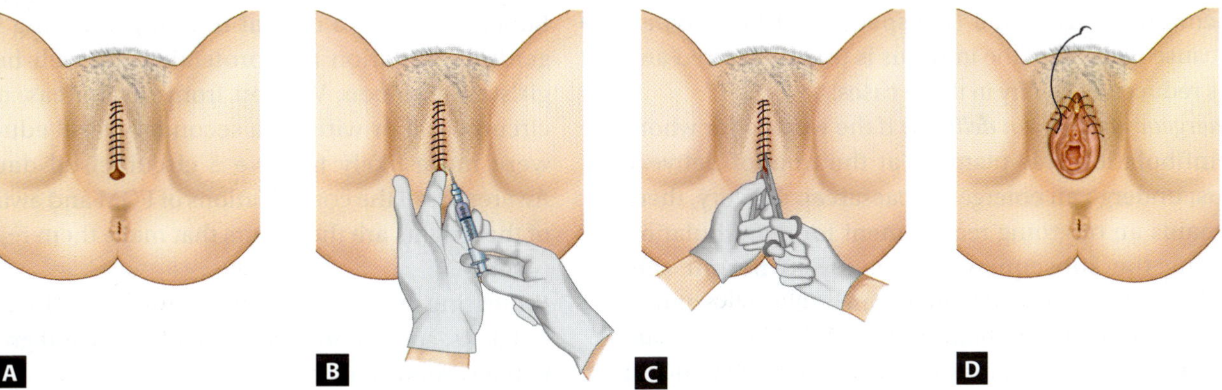

Figs. 3A to D: Technique of deinfibulation: (A) Infibulation of the vaginal introitus, resulting in the formation of midline scarred tissue; (B) Infiltration of midline scar with local anaesthetic agent; (C) Incision of midline scar until the external urethral meatus is visible; (D) Suturing of cut edges with absorbable sutures.

- Most cases of FGM should be provided care by a consultant obstetrician.
- The impact of FGM on labour and delivery should be sensitively discussed with the patient, and a plan of care must be agreed upon.
- *Deinfibulation in the intrapartum period:* If during the intrapartum period, vaginal examination is not possible or it is not possible to perform various intrapartum procedures such as urinary catheterisation, then deinfibulation is recommended during the first stage of labour. This is usually performed after administration of an epidural, which covers not only the procedure but also subsequent vaginal examinations and delivery. If vaginal access is adequate during the intrapartum period, then deinfibulation can be performed at the time of delivery under local anaesthetic. Deinfibulation is sometimes described as the reversal of FGM. However, this is not completely correct, because this procedure does not replace genital tissue, nor does it restore the normal genital anatomy and function.

  The technique and principle of deinfibulation at the time of delivery are similar to deinfibulation performed during the antenatal or postpartum period. However, when deinfibulation is performed prepregnancy, during the antenatal period or during the first stage of labour, either a scalpel or scissors may be used to make the incision. In contrast, when deinfibulation is performed at the time of delivery, the incision should preferably be made with scissors (rather than a scalpel) just before the crowning of the foetal head. Local anaesthesia in the form of local infiltration with lidocaine without adrenaline should be used. Once the procedure has been performed, the requirement for episiotomy may be assessed. Nevertheless, episiotomy is commonly required (irrespective of FGM type), because the skin of the introitus is usually scarred and has reduced elasticity in these cases.
- *Emergency caesarean delivery:* If the woman for whom deinfibulation was planned at the time of delivery must undergo an emergency caesarean delivery, there remains an on-going requirement for deinfibulation during the subsequent pregnancy to permit safe vaginal delivery. Such a woman can be given the option of undergoing perioperative deinfibulation after safe caesarean delivery of the baby, once the maternal and neonatal well-being has been confirmed. This option should be discussed with the mother before she is transferred to the operation theatre.
- Labial tears in women with FGM should be managed like those in women without FGM. Repairs should be performed where clinically indicated, after discussion with the woman. Appropriate materials and techniques should be used for suturing.
- *Role of clitoral reconstruction:* Reconstructive clitoral surgery is believed to restore clitoral function. However, according to the available evidence, clitoral reconstruction should not be performed, because it is associated with unacceptable complications without any conclusive evidence of benefit. Surgery is unlikely to replace clitoral tissue removed at the time of FGM. Moreover, surgical exploration of the clitoral area may result in further damage to the clitoral nerves and vasculature, resulting in the loss of sensation.

Also, the existing studies are retrospective with poor follow-up. There is no standardised method for the assessment of sexual function. Presently, there is a requirement for well-designed clinical trials in the future to investigate the safety and effectiveness of this procedure.

POSTNATAL CARE

If a planned deinfibulation cannot be performed due to delivery by an emergency caesarean section, the woman should be followed up in the gynaecology out-patient department or FGM clinic, so that deinfibulation can be offered to her before a subsequent pregnancy.

- Before the patient is discharged, all documentation must be complete, and all legal and regulatory processes must have been adhered.

ERADICATION

- Education plays a crucial role in preventing female genital mutilation and protecting the well-being of girls and women. Women from rural areas, already circumcised or without a secondary level education, were more likely to have a circumcised daughter. Awareness of the complications of FGM and awareness of their rights are the factors that make them reject the practice.
- Educating boys and men, as well as educational, religious, social and community figures and groups, is equally important.
- Active participation of fathers in the decision-making process could free mothers from the social pressure and responsibility of carrying on traditions, creating a more

favourable environment for FGM/C abandonment. Training and awareness are required for healthcare staff and paramedics in identifying patients at risk, how to approach the subject, and where to refer patients for further care and support.

SUGGESTED READING

1. Almroth L, Almroth-Berggren V, Hassanein OM, Al-Said SS, Hasan SS, Lithell UB, et al. Male complications of female genital mutilation. Soc Sci Med. 2001;53(11):1455-60.
2. Almroth L, Elmusharaf S, El Hadi N, Obeid A, El Sheikh MA, Elfadil SM, et al. Primary infertility after genital mutilation in girlhood in Sudan: a case-control study. Lancet. 2005; 366(9483):385-91.
3. Alsibiani SA, Rouzi AA. Sexual function in women with female genital mutilation. Fertil Steril. 2010;93(3):722-4.
4. Andersson SH, Rymer J, Joyce DW, Momoh C, Gayle CM. Sexual quality of life in women who have undergone female genital mutilation: a case–control study. BJOG. 2012; 119(13):1606-11.
5. Balogun OO, Hirayama F, Wariki WM, Koyanagi A, Mori R. Interventions for improving outcomes for pregnant women who have experienced genital cutting. Cochrane Database Syst Rev. 2013;(2):CD009872.
6. Banks E, Meirik O, Farley T, Akande O, Bathija H, et al.; WHO study group on female genital mutilation and obstetric outcome. Female genital mutilation and obstetric outcome: WHO collaborative prospective study in six African countries. Lancet. 2006;367(9525):1835-41.
7. Barstow DG. Female genital mutilation: the penultimate gender abuse. Child Abuse Neglect. 1999;23(5):501-10.
8. Bazi T. Female genital mutilation: the role of medical professional organization. Int Urogynecol J. 2017;28(4): 537-41.
9. Beeson S, Vincent H, Frankland J. Combating female genital mutilation. Br J Midwifery. 2024;32(1):46-9.
10. Behrendt A, Moritz S. Post-traumatic stress disorder and memory problems after female genital mutilation. Am J Psychiatry. 2005;162(5):1000-2.
11. Berg RC, Denison E. Does female genital mutilation/cutting (FGM/C) affect women's sexual functioning? A systematic review of the sexual consequences of FGM/C. Sex Res Soc Policy. 2012;9(1):41-56.
12. Berg RC, Odgaard-Jensen J, Fretheim A, Underland V, Vist G. An updated systematic review and meta-analysis of the obstetric consequences of female genital mutilation/ cutting. Obstet Gynecol Int. 2014;2014:542859.
13. Berg RC, Underland V, Odgaard-Jensen J, Fretheim A, Vist GE. Effects of female genital cutting on physical health outcomes: a systematic review and meta-analysis. BMJ Open. 2014;4(11):e006316.
14. Blatant World. (2010). Map showing approximate prevalence of FGM across Africa. [online] Available from www.flickr.com/ photos/ blatantworld/5052042739/in/set-72157622910728412. [Accessed March, 2025].
15. Browning A, Allsworth JE, Wall LL. The relationship between female genital cutting and obstetric fistulae. Obstet Gynecol. 2010;115(3):578-83.
16. Byard RW, Behnia-Willison F. Female genital mutilation—an overview for forensic practitioners. J Forensic Leg Med. 2024;101:102624.
17. Care of Women and girls living with female genital mutilation: a clinical handbook. Geneva: World Health Organization; 2018.
18. Cook RJ, Dickens BM, Fathalla MF. Female genital cutting (mutilation/circumcision): ethical and legal dimensions. Intl J Gynecol Obstet. 2002;79(3):281-7.
19. Elmusharaf S, Elkhidir I, Hoffmann S, Almroth L. A case-control study on the association between female genital mutilation and sexually transmitted infections in Sudan. BJOG. 2006;113(4):469-74.
20. Female Genital Mutilation in England and Wales. Updated statistical estimates of the numbers of affected women living in England and Wales and girls at risk: Interim report on provisional estimates. London: City University London; 2014.
21. Foldès P, Cuzin B, Andro A. Reconstructive surgery after female genital mutilation: a prospective cohort study. Lancet. 2012;380(9837):134-41.
22. Gissler M, Alexander S, Macfarlane A, Small R, Stray-Pedersen B, Zeitlin J, et al. Stillbirths and infant deaths among migrants in industrialized countries. Acta Obstet Gynecol Scand. 2009;88(2):134-48.
23. Gombau-Giménez L, Almansa-Martínez P, Suarez-Cortés M, Molina-Rodríguez A, Leal-Costa C, Jiménez-Ruiz I. Obstetric complications in women from Sub-Saharan Africa—a cross-sectional study. Int J Environ Res Public Health. 2022;19(16):10101.
24. Gupta S, Latthe P. Female genital mutilation deinfibulation: antenatal or intrapartum? Obstet Gynaecol Reprod Med. 2018;28(3):92-4.
25. Health and Social Care Information Centre (HSCIC). Female Genital Mutilation (FGM) Enhanced Dataset. Requirements Specification. Leeds: HSCIC; 2015.
26. Libretti A, Bianco G, Corsini C, Remorgida V. Female genital mutilation/cutting: going beyond urogynecologic complications and obstetric outcomes. Arch Gynecol Obstet. 2023;308.
27. Morison L, Scherf C, Ekpo G, Paine K, West B, Coleman R, et al. The long-term reproductive health consequences of female genital cutting in rural Gambia: a community-based survey. Trop Med Int Health. 2001;6(8):643-53.
28. Morris JG, Donohoe M. The history of hysteria. Pharos Alpha Omega Alpha Honor Med Soc. 2004;67(2):40-3.
29. Peltzer K, Pengpid S. Female genital mutilation and intimate partner violence in the Ivory Coast. BMC Women's Health. 2014;14:13.

30. Peterman A, Johnson K. Incontinence and trauma: sexual violence, female genital cutting and proxy measures of gynecological fistula. Soc Sci Med. 2009;68(5):971-9.
31. Phonsombat S, Master VA, McAninch JW. Penetrating external genital trauma: a 30-year single institution experience. J Urol. 2008;180(1):192-6.
32. Reman T, Balligand V, Schoefs B, Feipel V, Bertuit J. Psychological consequences of female genital mutilation: A mixed-method systematic review. S Afr J Physiother. 2023;79(1):1877.
33. Royal College of Midwives (RCM), Royal College of Nursing, Royal College of Obstetricians and Gynaecologists (RCOG), Equality Now, Unite. Tackling FGM in the UK: Intercollegiate recommendations for identifying, recording and reporting. London: RCM; 2013.
34. Royal College of Obstetricians and Gynaecologists (RCOG). Female Genital Mutilation and its Management. Green-top Guideline No. 53. London: RCOG Press; 2015.
35. Salihu HM, August EM, Salemi JL, Weldeselasse H, Sarro YS, Alio AP. The association between female genital mutilation and intimate partner violence. BJOG. 2012;119(13):1597-605.
36. Small R, Gagnon A, Gissler M, Zeitlin J, Bennis M, Glazier R, et al. Somali women and their pregnancy outcomes postmigration: data from six receiving countries. BJOG. 2008;115(13):1630-40.
37. United Nations Children's Fund. Female Genital Mutilation/Cutting: A statistical overview and exploration of the dynamics of change. New York: UNICEF; 2013.
38. United Nations General Assembly. Resolution adopted by the General Assembly on 20 December 2012: 67/146. Intensifying global efforts for the elimination of female genital mutilations. New York: United Nations; 2012. [online] Available from https://documents.un.org/doc/undoc/gen/n12/487/36/pdf/n1248736.pdf [Last accessed April, 2025].
39. United Nations. Goal 5: Achieve gender equality and empower all women and girls. [online] Available from https://www.un.org/sustainabledevelopment/gender-equality/. [Last accessed March, 2025].
40. Van Eekert N, Barrett H, Kimani S, Hidayana I, Leye E. Rethinking the definition of medicalized female genital mutilation/cutting. Arch Sex Behav. 2024;53(2):441-53.
41. World Health Organization (WHO). Eliminating female genital mutilation: an interagency statement. Geneva: WHO; 2008.
42. World Health Organization (WHO). Female genital mutilation: A joint WHO/UNICEF/UNFPA statement. Geneva: WHO; 1997.
43. World Health Organization. (2023). Female genital mutilation (Fact sheet). [online] Available from https://www.who.int/news-room/fact-sheets/detail/female-genital-mutilation. [Last accessed March, 2025].
44. Yusuf L, Negash S. Vaginal calculus following severe form of female genital mutilation: a case report. Ethiop Med J. 2008;46(2):185-8.
45. Zou Q, Fu Q. Diagnosis and treatment of acute urogenital and genitalia tract traumas: 10-year clinical experience. Pak J Med Sci. 2015;31(4):925-9.

Pelvic Organ Prolapse

Rajeshwari G Bhat, Muralidhar V Pai

Chapter Outline

- Uterine and Vaginal Prolapse
- Prolapse of the Ovaries

Pelvic organ prolapse refers to protrusion of the pelvic organs into or out of the vaginal canal.

UTERINE AND VAGINAL PROLAPSE

Prolapse, procidentia (from the Latin *procider*, to fall) or downwards descent of the vagina and uterus is a common and disabling condition. Vaginal prolapse can occur without uterine prolapse, but the uterus cannot descend without carrying the upper vagina with it.

Pericervical ring: Collar of connective tissue encircling supravaginal cervix. Its function is cervical stabilisation.

Supports of Uterus (Figs. 1A and B and Table 1)

Apart from the normal position—anteverted and anteflexed, there is a three-tier system consisting of the following:

1. Upper
2. Middle (the strongest and important)
3. Lower

Upper Tier

- Weak
- Mostly by maintaining the uterus in anteverted position
- Endopelvic fascia
- Round ligaments
- Broad ligaments with intervening pelvic cellular tissues.

Middle Tier

- The strongest support of uterus
- Cervicovaginal junction
- Pelvic cellular tissue

Lower Tier

- Indirect support to the uterus
- Principally given by the musculofascial tone of the hollow vagina, which is amply supported by the fascial condensation at the vault and by the pelvic floor at the lower end.

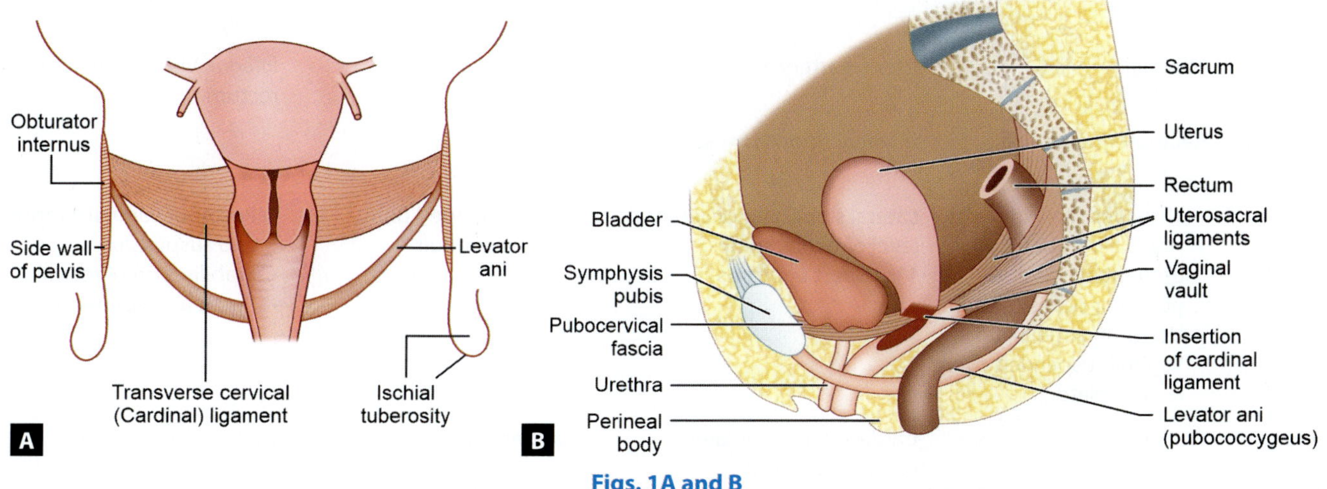

Figs. 1A and B

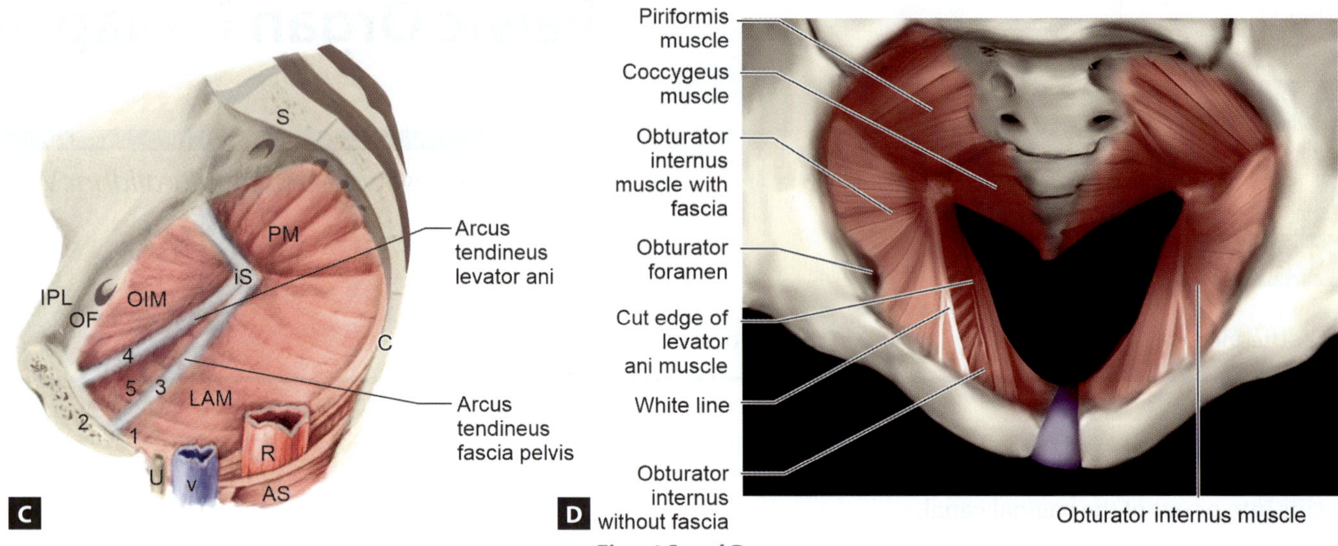

Figs. 1C and D

Figs. 1A to D: (A and B) Different supports of uterus; (C and D) Arcus tendineus fascia pelvis.

TABLE 1: Components and functions of major support of uterus.

	Uterosacral ligament	***Mackenrodt's ligament***	***Pubocervical ligament***	***Rectovaginal septum***
Origin	Periosteum of sacral vertebra 2, 3 and 4	Hypogastric roots with fibrous connective tissue to lateral abdomen and pelvic walls	Inner surface of superior pubic ramus medially	Trapezoid shape with fibroelastic and connective tissue and smooth muscle
Insertion	Posterior and lateral supravaginal cervix at 5 and 7 o' clock	Lateral supravaginal cervix at 3 and 9 o'clock forms part of pericervical ring	11 and 1 o'clock	*Boundaries:* • *Distal:* Perineal body • *Lateral:* Distal-half vagina levator ani
Neurology content	Uterosacral plexus of autonomic nerves	Portion of uterosacral plexus	Artery and veins of bladder pillar	• *Proximal:* Uterosacrals and pericervical rings • *Superior:* Epithelium of vagina
Vascular content	Minimal	Uterine artery and veins		*Inferior:* Visceral fascia of rectum
Muscular content	Rectouterine muscle	Minimal smooth muscle		
Function	• 1° suspensory elements • Holds cervix behind urogenital hiatus in posterior pelvis • Uterus in anteflexion • Vaginal suspended over levator plate	Lateral stabilising of cervix at level of ischial spines. 1° support of uterus	Least developed only vascular conduit	• Posterior vaginal support and suspension • Stabilisation of rectum • Perineal suspension
Synonym	Rectal pillar	Cardinal ligament lateral cervical ligament	Bladder pillar	Denonvilliers' fascia

Supports of Vagina

Delancey divided the supports of vagina into three levels: (1) Proximal, (2) midvaginal and (3) distal.

Proximal

- Mostly attributed to uterosacral and cardinal ligaments
- Damage results in uterovaginal prolapse, posthysterectomy, vault prolapse and enterocele.

Midvaginal

- Mostly by the lateral attachment of the pubocervical fascia to the arcus tendineus fascia pelvis (ATFP) (white line). It is a thickening of the parietal fascia of the belly of the iliococcygeus that extends from the ischial spine to pubic ramus. It lies inferior to the arcus tendineus levator ani and provides midvaginal lateral support **(Figs. 1C and D)**.
- Damage results in paravaginal and pararectal defects.

Distal

- Attributed to the fusion of the deep endopelvic fascia to the urogenital diaphragm and rectovaginal septa.
- Damage results in urinary incontinence anteriorly and perineal body deficit posteriorly.

Types

Uterine (Uterovaginal) Prolapse

The pelvis may be said to consist of three compartments: (1) Anterior, (2) middle and (3) posterior. Descent of the anterior compartment results in cystocele and urethrocele, that of the middle compartment in descent of the uterine vault and enterocele, and that of the posterior compartment in rectocele. In order to descend, the uterus becomes slightly retroverted to lie in the axis of the vagina. When the prolapse is reduced, however, the uterus is often found to be anteverted. Normally, external os of the cervix is at the level of ischial spines. The imperfection of the grading systems is evident from the number of systems that have been developed over the years. Various classifications have been described. According to one scheme, three degrees of uterine descent are recognised **(Fig. 2A)**.

1. *First degree:* Descent of the uterus but the cervix remains within the introitus.
2. *Second degree:* Descent to the extent that the cervix projects through the vulva when the woman is straining or standing **(Fig. 2B)**.

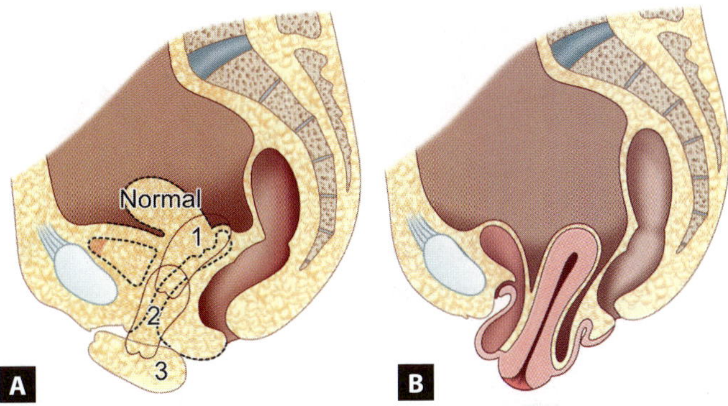

Figs. 2A and B: (A) Degrees of uterine prolapse; (B) The anatomy of second-degree uterine prolapse associated with cystocele and enterocele. A rectocele is not present. The supravaginal cervix is elongated.

3. *A third degree, i.e. complete procidentia or general prolapse:* The entire uterus prolapses outside the vulva. The whole vagina, or at least the whole of its anterior wall, is everted.

In Shaw's classification **(Fig. 3A)**, descent is classified into four degrees: (1) The first degree remains the same as above, (2) the second degree is one where the cervix descends to the level of the introitus, (3) the third degree when it projects through the vulva (4) and the fourth degree is complete procidentia.

Palpation is done to differentiate between third-degree prolapse and procidentia. The thumb is kept anteriorly on the most proximal part of the prolapse with the other four fingers on the posterior proximal part. In procidentia, as the uterine fundus has prolapsed below the introitus, one can easily approximate fingers from both sides **(Fig. 3B)**.

Baden's system of grading is similar to Shaw's but uses the hymen as a reference point. Each component is graded from 0 to 4 with the patient straining. The aim of the Baden-Walker system was to restore the vaginal support to its original anatomic location.

Baden–Walker Halfway System

Extent of prolapse is recorded using numbers 0–4 at each of six defined sites of vagina **(Fig. 4)**.

- Six numbers are recorded as a measure of descent.
- Zero indicates—(N) anatomical position.
- Four represents maximum prolapse.
  - Normal
  - Descent to halfway to hymen
  - Progression to hymen
  - Progression halfway through hymen
  - Maximal progression through hymen

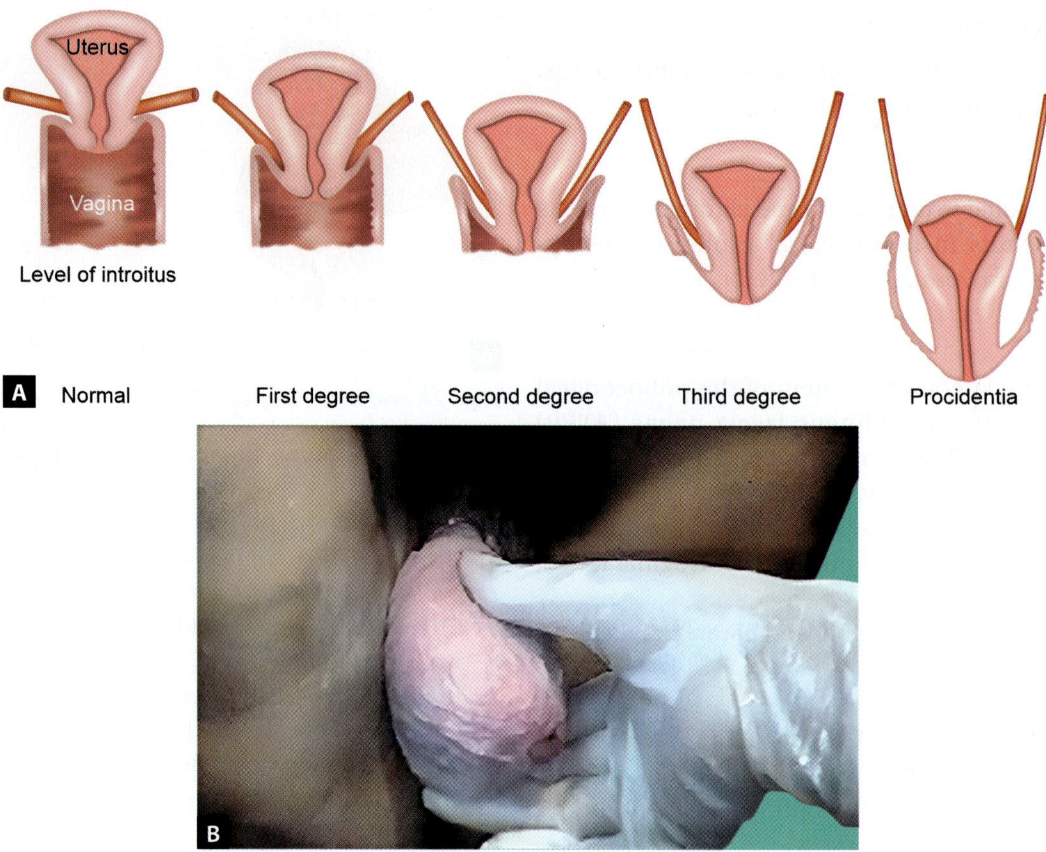

Figs. 3A and B: (A) Shaw's classification; (B) Differentiating third-degree prolapse from procidentia.

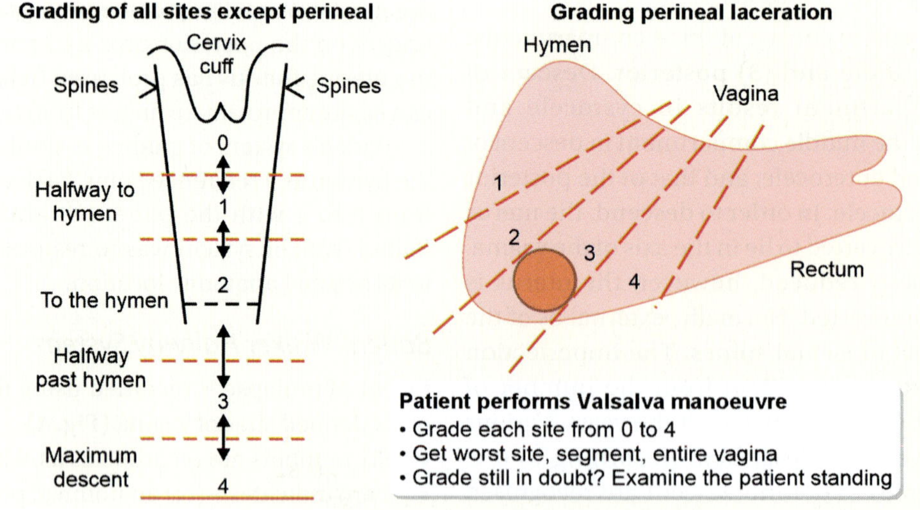

Fig. 4: Baden–Walker halfway system.

Enterocele

0. Normal (maximum of 2 cm of cul-de-sac between posterior cervix and rectum)
1. Herniation of cul-de-sac to one-fourth of distance to hymen
2. Herniation to two-fourths of distance towards hymen

3. Herniation to three-fourths of distance towards hymen
4. Herniation to hymen.

Chronic Perineal Laceration

0. Normal (no more than hymenal laceration)
1. Involvement of anterior half of perineal body
2. Involvement of perineal body but not anal sphincter
3. Involvement including anal sphincter
4. Involvement including anal mucosa.

However, these systems do not provide accurate quantification for scientific comparison, lack reproducibility and specificity, and may not accurately describe the structures associated with the sites of prolapse. To address these problems, the International Continence Society has, therefore, approved a new system, the Pelvic Organ Prolapse Quantification (POP-Q) staging system, which measures (in centimetres) the positions of nine sites on the vagina and perineal body in relation to the hymen **(Figs. 5A and B)**. These nine sites are given as follows:

1. Aa—located 3 cm proximal to the urethral meatus on the anterior vaginal wall
2. Ba—the most distal position of the upper anterior vaginal wall
3. C—the most distal edge of the cervix or vaginal cuff
4. D—the location of the posterior vaginal fornix
5. Ap—located 3 cm proximal to the hymen on the posterior vaginal wall
6. Bp—the most distal position of the upper portion of the posterior vaginal wall
7. gh—the diameter of the genital hiatus
8. pb—width of the perineal body
9. tvl—the total vaginal length.

Last three sites (gh, pb and tvl) are measured and recorded on a grid form **(Fig. 5B)**. A final prolapse stage from 0 to 4 can be assigned according to the severity of the greatest degree of prolapse.

Stages of Pelvic Organ Prolapse (POP-Q Staging System)

- *Stage 0:* No prolapse is demonstrated.
- *Stage 1:* The most distal portion of the prolapse is >1 cm above the level of hymen.
- *Stage 2:* The most distal portion of the prolapse extends from <1 cm above and 1 cm below the level of hymen.
- *Stage 3:* The most distal portion of the prolapse is >1 cm below the level of hymen but protrudes no further than 2 cm less than the total vaginal length (tvl).
- *Stage 4:* Complete eversion of vagina, i.e. distal portion of the prolapse protrudes to greater than or equal to 2 (tvl ≥2) cm **(Fig. 6)**.

It is important to recognise that these measurements can change according to the position of the patient, e.g. standing or lithotomy, and by insertion of a speculum. It is also important to mention whether the patient was straining or whether traction was applied. Measurements at points gh and pb are completed first. A speculum is then placed in the vagina to allow introduction of a spatula and measurement of tvl. Points C and D are next measured during maximal Valsalva effort. Lastly, points Aa, Ba, Ap and Bp are measured. Complete procidentia is not

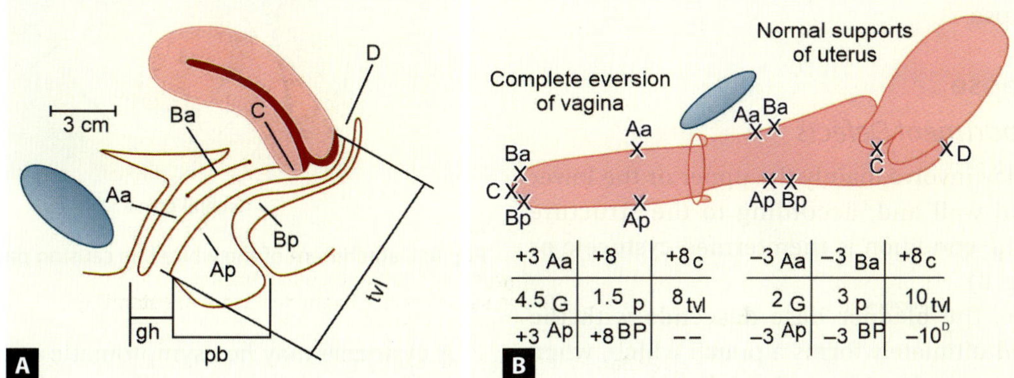

Figs. 5A and B: (A) Graphic representation of points used to quantify prolapse (see *text*). (B) Line diagram showing contrasting measurements of normal supports (a) and posthysterectomy vaginal eversion (b) International Continence Society Standardisation of Terminology of Female Pelvic Organ Prolapse and Pelvic Floor Dysfunction.

Source: Bump RC, Mattiasson A, Bø K, Brubaker LP, DeLancey JO, Klarskov P, et al. The standardization of terminology of female pelvic organ prolapse and pelvic floor dysfunction. Am J Obstet Gynecol. 1996;175:12-4.

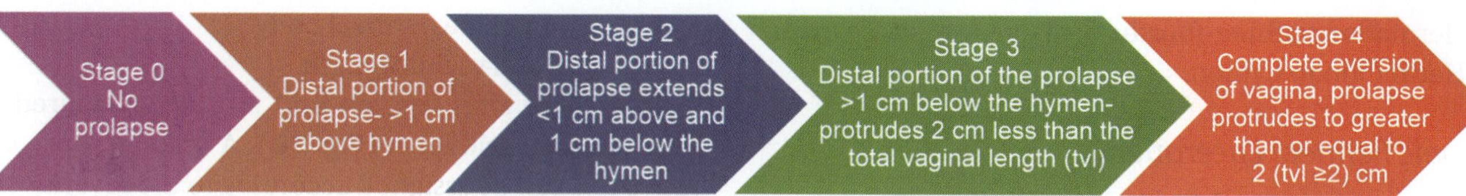

Fig. 6: Pelvic Organ Prolapse Quantification staging system.

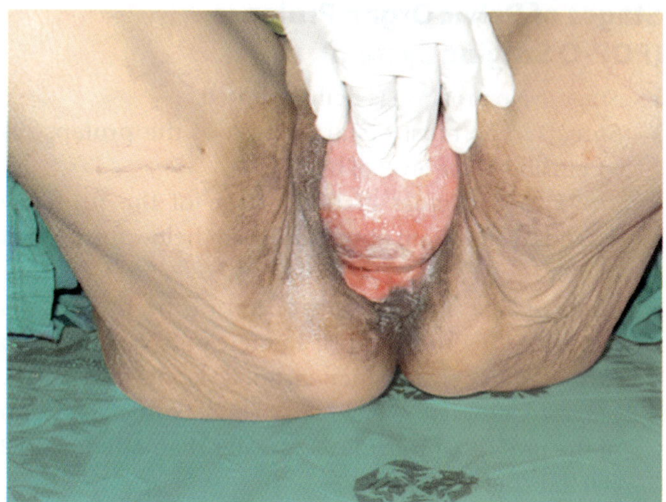

Fig. 7: Uterovaginal prolapse with decubitus ulcer.

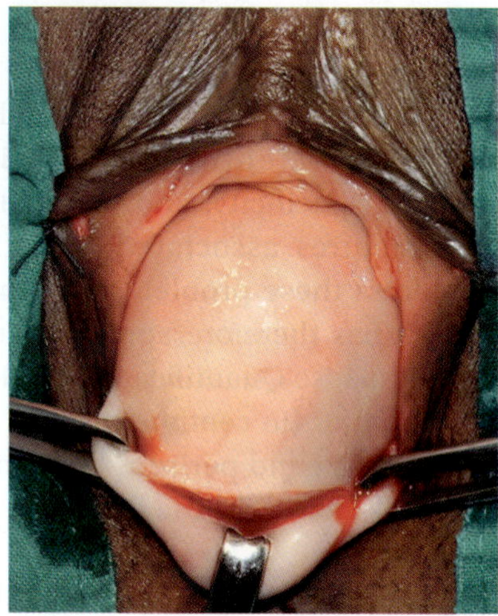

Fig. 8: Cystocele.

common, and many cases so diagnosed are real examples of severe second-degree prolapse. The mistake is made because elongation, hypertrophy, congestion and oedema of the cervix account for such a large protrusion of tissue as to make it appear that the whole uterus must be outside the vulva **(Fig. 7)**. In fact, the uterus cannot escape from the introitus unless it remains small; when it does, a failure in all the genital supports is implied—a condition of total or general prolapse.

Vaginal Prolapse

Anterior Compartment Defects

The prolapse may involve mainly the upper or the lower anterior vaginal wall and, according to the structure underlying it, the condition is then termed cystocele or urethrocele **(Fig. 8)**.

In cystocele, the bladder base descends with the vaginal wall and ultimately forms a pouch which, when the patient strains, reaches a lower level than the internal urethral meatus. Cystocele can be central when the defect is in midline or lateral when there is a paravaginal defect. A paravaginal defect results when the pubocervical fascia is detached from the white line **(Fig. 9)**.

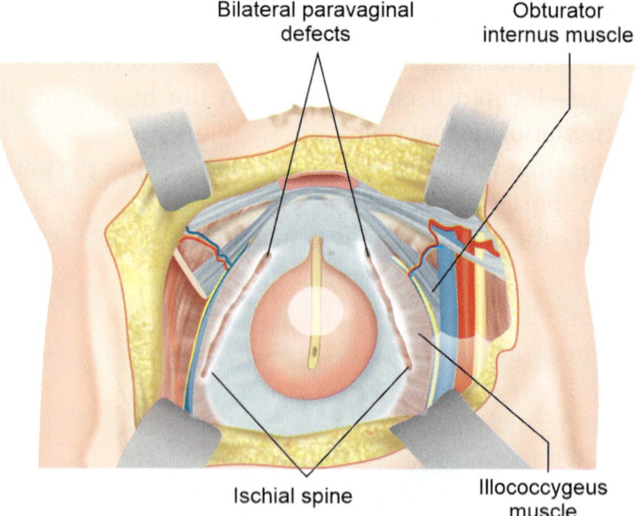

Fig. 9: Detachment of the white line causing paravaginal defect.

A cystocele may be asymptomatic or may be noticed protruding through the vaginal introitus. If it is very large, it leads to difficult or incomplete emptying of the bladder.

In urethrocele, the urethra is dislocated from the subpubic angle and is displaced backwards and downwards on straining. This lesion means damage to

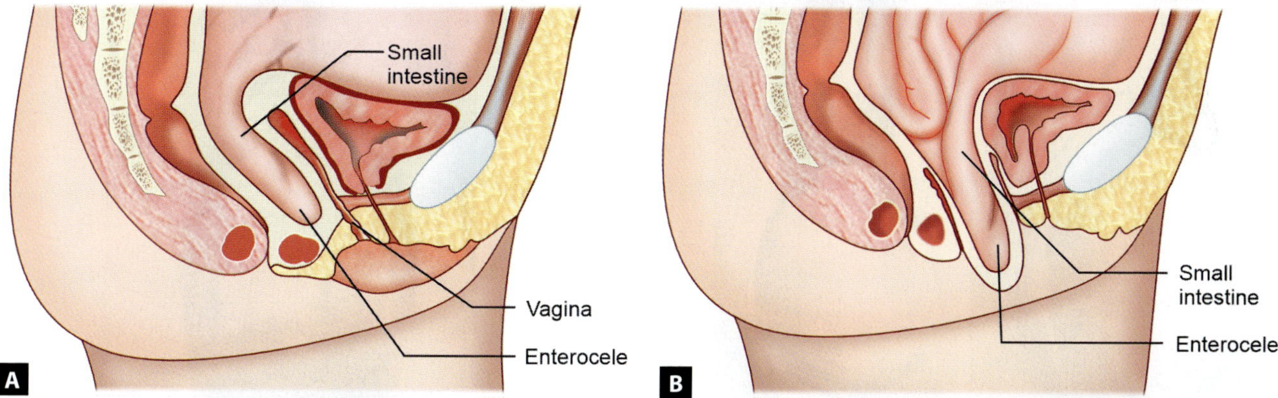

Figs. 10A and B: Uterine prolapse with an enterocele bulging behind a congested and oedematous cervix.

the triangular ligament, which ordinarily fixes the urethra forwards; the urethra itself is not dilated. Radiologically, there is a resultant loss of the urethrovesical angle.

Middle Compartment Defects

This includes enterocele and massive eversion of the vagina. The enterocele **(Figs. 2 and 10)** is a herniation of the pouch of Douglas, which contains loops of small bowel, as the name suggests, or omentum. This is an important condition, because if its correction is overlooked at the time of surgery, the patient may present with a recurrence of the prolapse.

Three types of enterocele are identified:

1. *Pulsion enterocele:* The vaginal vault is pushed outwards by conditions, which increase intra-abdominal pressure, e.g. chronic respiratory problems and lifting of heavy weights.
2. *Traction enterocele:* A pre-existing weakness in the anterior compartment and uterine descent pull down the vault.
3. *Iatrogenic enterocele:* This follows a vault suspension procedure or procedures such as Burch or Marshall–Marchetti-Krantz, which produces a change in the vaginal axis and subjects the vault to abnormal pressures.

Massive eversion of the vagina or vault prolapse may or may not exist with cystocele, rectocele and enterocele.

Patients with enterocele and vault prolapse present with backache, pelvic heaviness and pressure or a *bearing down* sensation.

Posterior Compartment Defects

Rectocele and perineal body descent are the main components of the posterior compartment defects. The importance of perineal body descent has been recognised as an additional component in the New York modification of the POP-Q staging system.

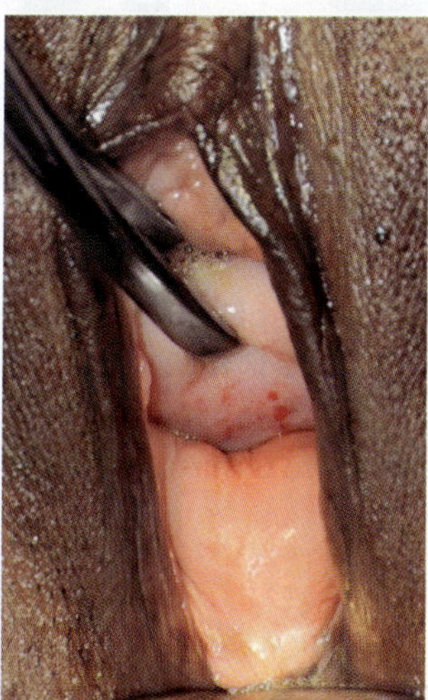

Fig. 11: A small rectocele.

Rectocele **(Figs. 11 and 12)** is caused by the weakening of the fibres of the rectovaginal fascia (Denonvilliers' fascia). As with anterior compartment defects, it is important to assess the condition by rectovaginal examination and in the erect position, if necessary, the exact location and type of defect, i.e. upper, mid or lower third of the vagina; linear or transverse.

Assessment of the levator plate by palpation between the two fingers inside the vagina and thumb outside on the perineum is also an essential part of the assessment. Integrity of this plate is vital to maintaining the vagina in its correct position. Adequacy of vaginal length, so that its apex is well above the levator plate, is essential for preventing recurrence of the prolapse. The only exception

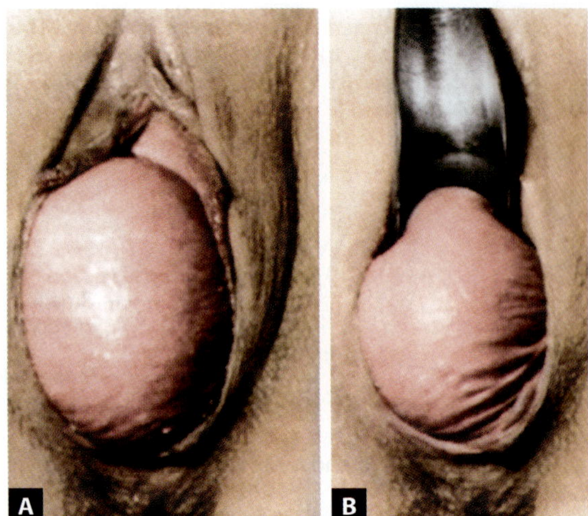

Figs. 12A and B: (A) Gross prolapse of the vaginal wall and, without further investigation, it is impossible to say whether it is a cystocele or rectocele; (B) Insertion of a speculum to hold back the anterior vaginal wall shows that the lesion is a rectocele.

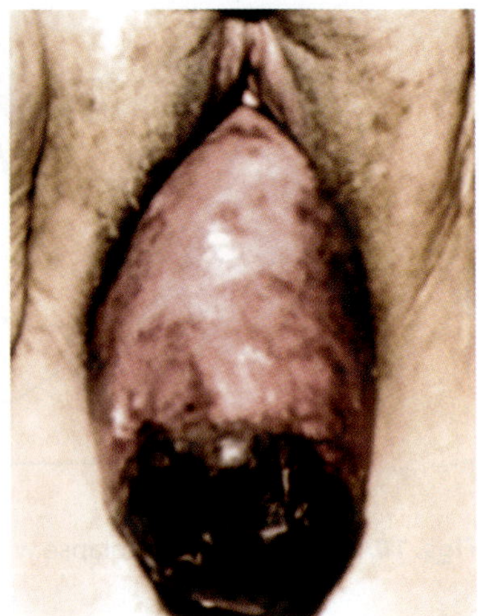

Fig. 13: Uterovaginal prolapse with decubital ulceration of the cervix. Without further investigation, it is impossible to say whether this represents prolapse or complete procidentia.

to this rule is in the case of radical surgery where, despite a short vagina, prolapse is never seen. This is because of the extensive scarring, which occurs around the vagina consequent to extensive tissue dissection.

Complications

- *Keratinisation of the vagina:* The epithelium of the prolapsed vaginal walls and of the portio vaginalis, being constantly exposed to the air and possibly to trauma, becomes thickened, corrugated and white with keratin **(Fig. 7)**.
- *Decubitus ulcer:* Ulceration of the prolapsed tissue is often said to be caused by friction with the thighs and clothing. Although this may be partly true, it is notable that the ulcer is nearly always on the most dependent part of the cervix or vagina and not at the sides where friction is greatest **(Figs. 7 and 13)**. It is to be regarded, therefore, more as the result of circulatory and tissue anoxia due to venous stasis and as being aetiologically similar to a varicose ulcer of the leg.

Hypertrophy of the Cervix

Elongation of the Supravaginal Cervix (Fig. 2B)

If the lower cervix and vaginal vault descend while the upper cervix remains well supported, the supravaginal cervix becomes elongated. In this way, the total length of the uterus can become considerably increased, and a cavity measurement of 12–15 cm is by no means uncommon. This change does not occur in total prolapse where all the supports of the uterus fail.

Congestion and Oedema (Fig. 10)

The downwards displacement of the uterus puts tension on the descending vascular connections of the cervix, interfering with the venous and lymphatic drainage.

Glandular Hypertrophy (Adenomatous Change)

The state of chronic congestion sometimes leads to actual hypertrophy or hyperplasia of the glandular and connective tissue elements in the cervix.

Obstructive Lesions of the Urinary Tract

A large cystocele, with angulation of the urethra during straining, causes difficulty in emptying the bladder; this results in hypertrophy of the bladder wall and trabeculation. The downwards movement also involves the lower ends of the ureters, so they become attenuated and constricted in the ureteric canals at the sides of the uterus. Back pressure from the bladder and obstruction of the lower ureter ultimately lead to hydroureter and hydronephrosis **(Fig. 14)**.

Infection of the Urinary Tract: Renal Failure

If the pouch of a cystocele is low, it may not be emptied during micturition. In such circumstances and if the

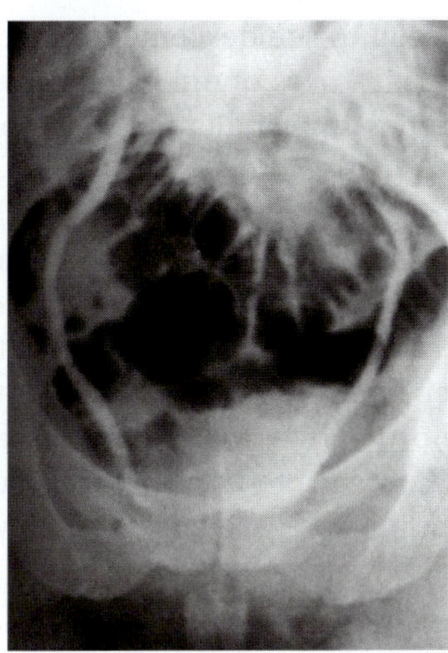

Fig. 14: Dilated and displaced ureters associated with uterovaginal prolapse, demonstrated by intravenous pyelography.

cystocele is chronically unreduced, a calculus can form in the pouch **(Fig. 14)**. The residual urine favours the growth of organisms, so *cystitis* complicates cystocele sooner or later. There may also be pyelitis and pyelonephritis, especially if the upper urinary tract is dilated. The final outcome may be renal failure.

Incarceration of the Prolapse

The extruded cervix and adjacent vaginal walls sometimes become so congested and oedematous that the patient finds the prolapse irreducible. If true incarceration occurs, it is first treated by catheterising the bladder and applying glycerine magnesium sulphate dressing to the congested tissues.

Carcinoma of the Cervix or Vagina

It is a remarkable fact that, irrespective of chronic irritation and ulceration, cancer of the cervix or vagina is rarely seen in untreated cases of prolapse. When it is, the symptoms of prolapse often disappear as the tissues become fixed.

Genital Prolapse and Pregnancy

If the woman suffering from genital prolapse conceives, no special problems usually arise. In the first trimester, increased uterine weight associated with relaxation and congestion of pelvic tissues tends to accentuate the prolapse. Later, however, when the uterus and its contents rest on the pelvic brim, the prolapse is often less troublesome. Nevertheless, the uterus sometimes remains low in late pregnancy, and delivery at term through a cervix lying outside the vulva is described.

Aetiology

The occurrence of prolapse implies failure of one or more of the supports of the uterus and vagina, which are described in Chapter 2: Anatomy.

In 95% of cases of prolapse, the patient is multiparous, and the implication is that childbearing is an important causal factor. Nevertheless, it should be recognised that the majority (probably not <80%) of middle-aged women are parous, and that those who develop prolapse might have done so even if they had remained childless. The part played by childbirth should not, therefore, be overestimated.

Predisposing Factors

Congenital or Developmental Weakness of the Supports

This is the most important of all factors, and it operates in multiparous as well as nulliparous prolapse. It may explain why prolapse often follows easy rather than difficult labour, the inherent weakness of the fibromuscular tissues allowing rapid dilatation of the birth canal as well as subsequent prolapse. Sometimes, during the examination of a young nulliparous woman, it will be noted that the vaginal wall is atonic, and that the uterine supports are weak; it is then possible to foretell that, if she ever has a baby, she will inevitably develop prolapse. Syndromes such as the Ehlers-Danlos syndrome are characterised by fascial and connective tissue weaknesses. These women have a high incidence of urinary incontinence, and most authors believe that the incidence of pelvic organ prolapse is also increased in this group. Congenital weakness of pelvic floor ligaments and fascia may also be found with spina bifida or bladder exstrophy.

Other developmental features, which favour prolapse, are shortness of the vagina, deep uterovesical and uterorectal peritoneal pouches and, possibly, uterine retroversion, but this is not as important as was formerly believed.

The part played by an inherent defect in the supporting tissues is also evidenced by the fact that prolapse, both nulliparous and multiparous, has a strong familial incidence **(Figs. 15A and B)**.

True *congenital prolapse* is rare, but cases are described in which the uterus is displaced outside the vulva at birth. When the baby is, otherwise, normal, this happening may

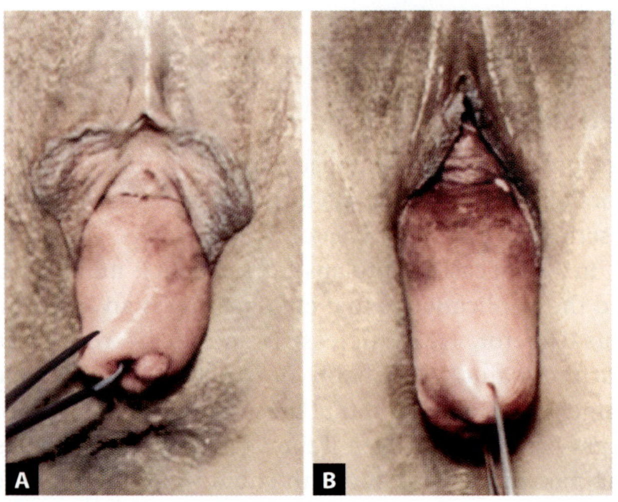

Figs. 15A and B: Nulliparous uterovaginal prolapse occurring in sisters. (A) Virgin aged 50 years; (B) Virgin aged 45 years. A third sister had one child and was operated on for prolapse 5 years previously.

be related to prolonged pressure of the birth canal on the foetal abdomen during breech delivery. In such a case, immediate replacement of the uterus is said to be followed by *permanent* cure; it is difficult to believe that the prolapse does not recur in adult life.

Injury Sustained During Childbirth

The delivery of a child inevitably disturbs stretches and sometimes tears the supports of the pelvic viscera; if these are already weak, they subsequently fail. The exact injury and the mechanism whereby it is sustained are unknown. One possibility is premature bearing down or fundal pressure before full dilatation of the cervix. Traction on the presenting part before the cervix is fully dilated could damage the cardinal ligaments, so vacuum extractor should not be used during the first stage of labour. Denervation changes have been documented in the pelvic floor and anal sphincter following vaginal delivery. These are thought to lead to temporary and sometimes permanent, urinary and faecal incontinence. Use of positions other than squatting for delivery may increase the incidence of prolapse.

Perineal and vaginal tears, even if they become infected, do not cause prolapse, although they are alleged to do so. Indeed, it will often be noted that a scarred area of the vagina is the only part, which does not prolapse, and that the uterus sometimes depends for its support on a deep laceration in the cervix and vaginal vault. Moreover, it is a well-accepted clinical observation that it is very uncommon to see descent of either the uterus or the vaginal walls in cases of unhealed complete perineal tear. Good puerperal rehabilitation by proper exercises is important in preventing prolapse.

To summarise, the evidence so far available suggests that overstretching or prolonged distension of the vagina with disruption of its fascial envelope is more conducive to vaginal prolapse than obvious tearing, and that a perineal laceration or episiotomy, which allows a quicker second stage, may be protective, although there are some who doubt this. With regard to uterine prolapse, little can be said except that it is rarely seen in women who have only been delivered by caesarean section!

Surgical Injury

Contrary to what is often stated, hysterectomy is not a cause of subsequent vaginal or vault prolapse. This operation, however, sometimes reveals a preexisting weakness. Thus, a very large or well-supported uterus may hold up a vagina whose own supports are weak, and this defect may become apparent when hysterectomy is carried out.

Vault prolapse is more likely to occur after subtotal than after total hysterectomy, despite the fact that the latter involves division of more elements of the transverse cervical ligaments. But it leaves more fibrosis, and the scar tissue might have a supporting role. If the cervix is not removed, it may act like the apex of an intussusception and encourage the vault to evert.

Vaginal hysterectomy is alleged to be more commonly followed by vault prolapse than abdominal hysterectomy. But this is because many gynaecologists only adopt the vaginal approach when there is some degree of prolapse already present. If they fail to strengthen the vaginal supports and to excise any enterocele while removing the uterus, subsequent vault prolapse is almost inevitable. Other things being equal; vaginal hysterectomy is no more likely to be followed by vaginal prolapse than abdominal hysterectomy; it should be less likely, because it offers the surgeon an opportunity to correct any weakness already present.

Vaginal or uterovaginal prolapse is sometimes seen following abdominoperineal excision of the rectum and is said to be a late complication of 4% of such operations.

Atrophy of Supporting Tissues at the Climacteric

Congenital or developmental weakness of the pelvic supports, and obstetrical injuries to them, often does not become manifest until after menopause. Until that time, the supports remain adequate, but the atrophy, which follows cessation of ovarian function, is the *final straw* and is followed by prolapse within a few years. Prolapse sometimes suddenly appears 3 or 4 weeks after delivery, whereupon the woman rests for a few days and then often has no more trouble until menopause. Nulliparous prolapse is mostly seen in unmarried girls in their late teens.

Role of Oestrogen in Pelvic Support

Oestrogen has a profound effect on the pelvic collagen synthesis. Collagen forms a major component of connective tissue. Type I collagen is present in organised fibres and ligamentous tissue, while type III collagen is present in loose areolar tissue. Oestrogen can increase type I collagen expression and deform type III collagen expression. Thus, oestrogen plays a vital role in maintaining the strength of the pelvic connective tissue.

Activating Factors

If a weakness is present, the circumstances likely to precipitate the onset of prolapse are given as follows:

- Increased intra-abdominal pressure caused by a chronic cough, chronic constipation, ascites, tumour formation, lifting heavy weights, doing extra work (e.g. nursing a sick friend or relative) and straining at stool.
- Increased weight of the uterus resulting from subinvolution, myohyperplasia or a small tumour. A uterine tumour, which is so large that it rests on the pelvic brim, prevents prolapse.
- Traction on the uterus by vaginal prolapse or by a large cervical polyp. In other words, descent of the vagina can precede and possibly cause uterine prolapse. The rough surgeon can precipitate prolapse by pulling strongly on the cervix during an operation.
- Diabetes mellitus due to its neuropathy and associated obesity contribute to the tendency of prolapse.
- Smoking in addition to chronic cough has antioestrogenic properties.
- Corticosteroid therapy for any chronic disease has a weakening effect on connective tissues.
- Any connective tissue disorder such as Ehlers–Danos syndrome increases the risk of prolapse.

Conditions that May Reduce the Chance of Prolapse

- Pelvic inflammatory disease
- Endometriosis
- Puerperal and postabortal infections.

Symptoms

The amount of discomfort and inconvenience experienced by the patient is extremely variable. Some women suffer complete procidentia for many years without being seriously incapacitated and without having to restrict their activities. On the other hand, other women complain bitterly when they suffer only a moderate degree of uterine or vaginal descent; the difference may in part be explained on the basis of resistance offered by the supporting ligaments. Little resistance, as in gross uterovaginal prolapse, means little discomfort. As a rule, only a few of the following possible symptoms are seen in any one case. The characteristic of nearly all symptoms is that they are immediately and completely relieved by lying down.

Sensation of Swelling or Fullness in the Vagina

This or a complaint of *something coming down outside* is common. The swelling or *something* may be the cervix, cystocele, rectocele or all three.

Dragging Discomfort in the Lower Abdomen and Pelvis

This sort of symptom is also described as a *bearing down sensation,* because the swelling in the vagina gives the woman a desire to evacuate it.

Urinary Symptoms

Urinary symptoms depend on descent of the anterior vaginal wall and displacement of the bladder and urethra.

Frequency

This at first is only diurnal and is due to mechanical irritation of the trigone on incomplete voiding. When the frequency becomes nocturnal as well as diurnal and is accompanied by scalding, it means that the situation is complicated by cystitis. Urgency may also occur, but it is important to exclude other causes such as detrusor instability.

Difficulty in Emptying the Bladder

The patient finds it difficult to empty the pool of urine in a large cystocele, and the more she strains, the greater the difficulty. Thus, when she relaxes at what she believes is the completion of the act, she has a desire to pass urine again immediately. In severe uterovaginal prolapse, the urethra may become so acutely angled that retention results. The intelligent woman gets over these difficulties by digitally holding up the prolapse during micturition.

Stress Urinary Incontinence

Although traditionally regarded as a symptom of prolapse, stress incontinence of urine occurs frequently in women without, as in those with, genital prolapse. In both groups, the incidence is 40%. Urethral incompetence is neither related to the type or severity of the displacement of the uterus and anterior vaginal wall nor to the position of the bladder and urethra in the pelvis. The cure for stress incontinence is not dependent on the anatomical success of an operation for prolapse. For these and other reasons, urethral incompetence is best dissociated from prolapse.

Difficulty in Emptying the Rectum

This is a common symptom of rectocele, although many women are too embarrassed to mention it spontaneously. Faeces collect in the forwards bulge of the bowel and cannot be evacuated unless the rectocele is held back digitally. Symptoms are sometimes disproportionate to the degree of defect.

Backache

This is in the midline at the lumbosacral or sacral level and is diffuse, deep seated and unaccompanied by local tenderness.

It is completely and immediately relieved by rest and is never experienced in bed or on rising in the morning; it comes on gradually during the day. Contrary to what was formerly believed, prolapse is a rare cause of backache; when this symptom is cured by an operation for prolapse, it is most often because the operation provides the patient with a period of enforced rest. Vaginal prolapse certainly does not cause backache; if uterine prolapse does, it is because of traction on the uterosacral and cardinal ligaments.

Discharge

A purulent and sometimes bloodstained vaginal discharge is a manifestation of decubitus ulcer. Leucorrhoea can be caused by increased activity of the cervical glands associated with congestion.

Physical Signs

The presence, type and extent of prolapse and presence of stress incontinence, if any, can usually be determined by asking the patient to bear down or to cough during examination. Minor degrees of uterine prolapse may only be recognised by feeling descent of the cervix while the patient is straining. Rectal examination is useful to demonstrate rectocele and to distinguish it from enterocele.

Sometimes, fairly severe degrees of prolapse are not evident at the time of examination, because the woman is not straining hard for fear of causing an escape of flatus or faeces; she may have been resting immediately prior to examination; if she has been wearing a pessary for a long time, it may be several days or weeks before the prolapse becomes obvious again.

If there is doubt, the patient should be asked to stand or walk for some time before examination. Occasionally, it is necessary to test for uterine descent by pulling on the cervix with a vulsellum.

Differential Diagnosis

From the standpoint of symptoms and signs, prolapse has to be distinguished from the following:

- A vulvar tumour or any polypoid tumour, which projects through the vulva on straining. A cervical polyp **(Fig. 16)** and a urethral caruncle are the most frequent causes of confusion. Metastases from uterine tumours, e.g. adenocarcinoma or choriocarcinoma, may be seen.
- Hypertrophy and elongation of the cervix.

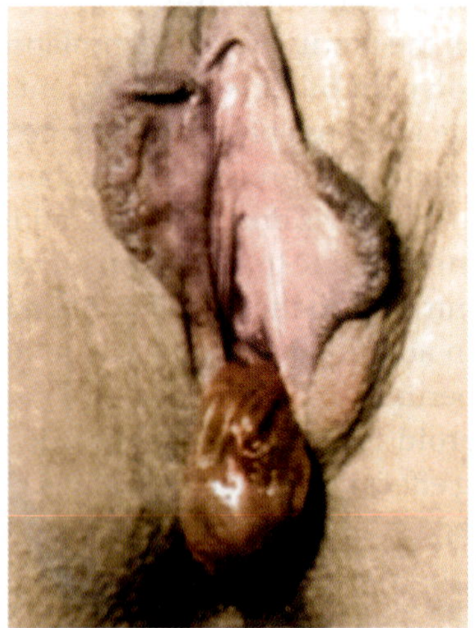

Fig. 16: A cervical polyp simulating prolapse. The woman in this case, aged 55 years, had a repair operation for prolapse several years previously. Her complaint was a 'recurrence of the prolapse.' The tumour, however, proved to be a cystic adenoma arising from the cervical stump (cervix previously amputated) of a well-supported uterus.

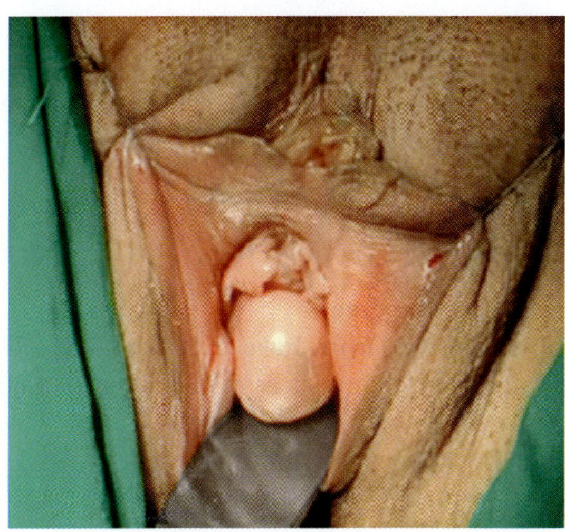

Fig. 17: Vaginal cyst simulating prolapse.

- Vaginal or periurethral cysts. These may be congenital, e.g. Gartner's cyst or inclusion dermoid cysts following trauma or surgery. They simulate cystocele or rectocele but are different in that they cannot be reduced **(Fig. 17)**. If there is doubt, a rectal examination or the passage of a sound into the bladder indicates the anatomy of the swelling.
- A diverticulum or prolapse of the urethra. This can be mistaken for urethrocele or cystocele.
- Inversion of the uterus.
- Inversion of the bladder.
- Varicose veins of the vulva or vagina, haemorrhoids and rectal prolapse.
- All other causes of low backache.
- All other causes of bladder symptoms.

Although prolapse can usually be recognised easily, it may be difficult to say whether it is responsible for the patient's particular symptoms, especially if the prolapse is not severe and the complaint is an ache or a pain. If there is doubt, a pessary test should be applied. Only if the discomfort is relieved by a ring, and if it returns when the ring is removed; it can be credited to the prolapse with reasonable certainty.

Prevention

During Labour and the Puerperium

- Avoid attempts at delivery, by the patient as well as by the attendant, before the cervix is fully dilated.
- Avoid an unnecessarily long second stage by episiotomy and, if need be, by low forceps or vacuum extraction.
- Repair all tears and incisions accurately in layers.
- If possible, use delayed absorbable sutures for the repair of the muscle layer.
- Do not express the uterus when attempting to deliver the placenta.
- Deliver the placenta by controlled cord traction.
- Encourage pelvic floor and other postnatal exercises. These favour involution of all the pelvic tissues. Early ambulation is more likely to prevent than to cause prolapse.
- Treat puerperal constipation in order to avoid strong bearing down efforts while supporting ligaments are slack.
- The correction of puerperal retroversion, once advocated strongly, is of no value.

At Hysterectomy

Many suggest that the chance of subsequent vaginal prolapse can be reduced if, during abdominal hysterectomy, the stumps of the uterosacral and cardinal ligaments are stitched to the vaginal vault. A deep cul-de-sac should be obliterated by Moskowitz sutures. Sacropexy can be done in high-risk situations, e.g. collagen disorders.

During vaginal hysterectomy, excision of redundant peritoneum, tightening of the cardinal and uterosacral ligaments and their inclusion in the vaginal vault are important prophylactic steps.

The increasing acceptability of oestrogen replacement therapy in postmenopausal women may decrease the incidence and severity of prolapse.

Treatment

Physiotherapy

When there is only a minor degree of prolapse and especially during 6 months following delivery, Kegel's pelvic floor exercises carried out regularly are of some value. Their effect is limited, however, because they only influence the voluntary muscles, i.e. the bulbocavernosus, superficial and deep transverse perineal and levator ani muscles and not the main fascial supporting tissues.

Vaginal cones of increasing weight have been tried by some with limited success.

Pessary Treatment

Palliative treatment consists of preventing the descent of the uterus and vaginal wall by means of a supporting pessary of which there are many types. Those most commonly employed are 'rings.'

The insertion of a pessary may be indicated in the following circumstances:

- During pregnancy
- Immediately after pregnancy and during lactation
- When further childbearing is intended in the near future
- This is a debatable indication
- Medical disorders, which make operation unsafe
- Refusal of operation on the part of the patient
- As a therapeutic test to determine if symptoms are due to prolapse
- Hippocrates—inserted half pomegranate soaked in wine into vagina
- 16th century—brass and waxed cork pessaries
- Primary indication of fitting a pessary is the non-surgical relief of symptoms associated with pelvic organ prolapse. Also used for alleviation of stress incontinence
- *Types:*
    - Supportive
    - Derived by a spring mechanism and thought to be supported by symphysis pubis (Ring, Gehrung, lever type)
    - Space filling:
        - Supported by creation of suction between pessary and vaginal walls or by providing a diameter larger than genital hiatus (Donut, Inflatoball, Shaatz)

Ring:
- Hinged spring circumference
- Silicone coated for ease of insertion
- Inserted behind pubic symphysis
- Self-removal and insertion
- May be worn during coitus

Donut:
- Supported by levator muscles
- Fills the vagina completely
- Insertion through introitus is in vertical plane, and pessary is turned to horizontal plane when inserted beyond levator ani muscle
- Coitus is not possible
- Difficult to be removed by patient herself

Inflatoball
- Made of latex rubber
- Can be easily inserted and removed when deflated
- Inflated using manual pump
- Sits above levator plate
- As made of latex absorbs secretion and odour

Gellhorn
- Used in severe degree
- Support derives from base that sits above levator plate and stem that rests as distal posterior vagina of perineum
- Cannot be inserted or removed by patient
- Coitus is difficult

Shaatz
- Has no stem
- Similar to Gellhorn
- Coitus possible
- Self-management is possible

Gehrung
- Arc-shaped with pliable metal frame
- Keels of pessary rest on lateral aspects of posterior vagina.

Incontinence Pessaries

Usually involve the addition of a knob that is positioned under the urethra at level of bladder neck to help prevent descent and facilitate temporary compression of urethra.

Complications

- Discharge and odour
- Mucosal erosion and abrasion
- Infections
- Fistulas
- Herniation and incarceration of cervix.

A pessary does not cure prolapse; it merely holds up the tissues. Sometimes, however, if a slight prolapse is controlled for some months, the supports recover tone, and the patient may then be able to manage without the pessary for some time. This is particularly true in the puerperium. However, without concomitant exercises, the symptoms gradually worsen, and the size of pessary required may increase with time.

Operative Treatment

Indications

Some sort of surgical procedure is nearly always the best treatment for established prolapse but is only necessary if the condition is causing symptoms or interfering with the woman's normal activities. If the prolapse is an incidental finding, and if it is not certain that a patient's symptoms are attributable to it, operation is best deferred. Nothing is lost by waiting and, even if the condition becomes worse in the meantime, the subsequent operation is not technically more difficult; indeed, it may be easier.

Youth and the intention to have more children in the future are not contraindications to operation, although they may modify surgical techniques (see further). Even if the prolapse recurs after further pregnancies, and this is not inevitable if the management is good, the original operation is not to be regarded as a waste of time. It is unreasonable to advise the young and potentially active mother and wife to persevere with makeshift measures until she is too old and inactive to enjoy the comfort which surgery can give.

Equally, old age and ill health are not necessarily contraindications, for the operation involves little risk if care is taken over anaesthesia. It is easily performed under regional anaesthesia in old women.

Preoperative Management

In assessing and correcting the general health of the patient before operation, particular attention should be paid to the urinary system. Urinalysis and blood urea estimations are essential in all cases; abdominal sonography should be done to look for hydronephrosis in long-standing cases. Urinary tract infection should be eliminated lest it shows an exacerbation postoperatively.

If the vaginal walls are senile and atrophic, oestrogen cream may be administered vaginally daily, 1–2 weeks before operation. The objective is to improve the healing power of the tissues.

Although some say it is unnecessary, decubitus ulcer should be treated before operation. The ulcer is always secondarily infected, and its presence means that the tissues have a low healing capacity. To cure it, admit the patient to hospital and keep her lying flat in bed as much as possible. The prolapsed organs are replaced and are packed in position by a gauze tampon soaked in antiseptic solution, which is changed every day. By this method, fairly large ulcers heal in 5–7 days. If the ulcer still shows no signs of healing, a biopsy is warranted.

Types of Operation

The aim of surgery is to restore the normal anatomy. A normal vaginal length should be maintained with its axis directed towards S3–S4. Hysterectomy is not essential, but it facilitates the repair of an enterocele. In the postmenopausal woman, it allows the removal of an organ, which may harbour unsuspected disease or be a focus for such a problem in the future. Most importantly, the strength of various supporting structures should be assessed and surgery planned accordingly, supplementing ligamentous and fascial repair with synthetic materials attached to alternate supports, e.g. the sacrospinous ligament and sacral promontory, if required.

Anterior Colporrhaphy

This is designed to cure cystocele and urethrocele. The vaginal wall is dissected free from the fascia, bladder and urethra, and its redundant part is excised. The excised portion is usually elliptical or triangular with its base at the cervix and its apex near the urethral orifice **(Figs. 18A to D)**. If there is a transverse ridge about 1 cm above the urethral orifice, it is best not disturbed because it marks an intact triangular ligament and compressor urethrae. The bladder is well separated from the uterus and displaced upwards; the pubovesicocervical fascia and the pubourethral ligaments are then stitched together in the midline to support the bladder, and the vaginal wall is closed. It is important to avoid overcorrection of the posterior cystocele to prevent a run-off type of urinary incontinence. The surgical management of stress incontinence is often done at the same time. It is also important to use delayed absorbable sutures in all cases. In fact, some go so far as to advise the use of a first layer of nonabsorbable sutures for fascial support, covered over with a second row of delayed absorbable sutures. Paravaginal defects can be repaired through an abdominal retropubic approach, through a vaginal retropubic incision, or laparoscopically, all of which aim to reattach the pubocervical fascia to the ATFP and to the fascia overlying the obturator internus muscle.

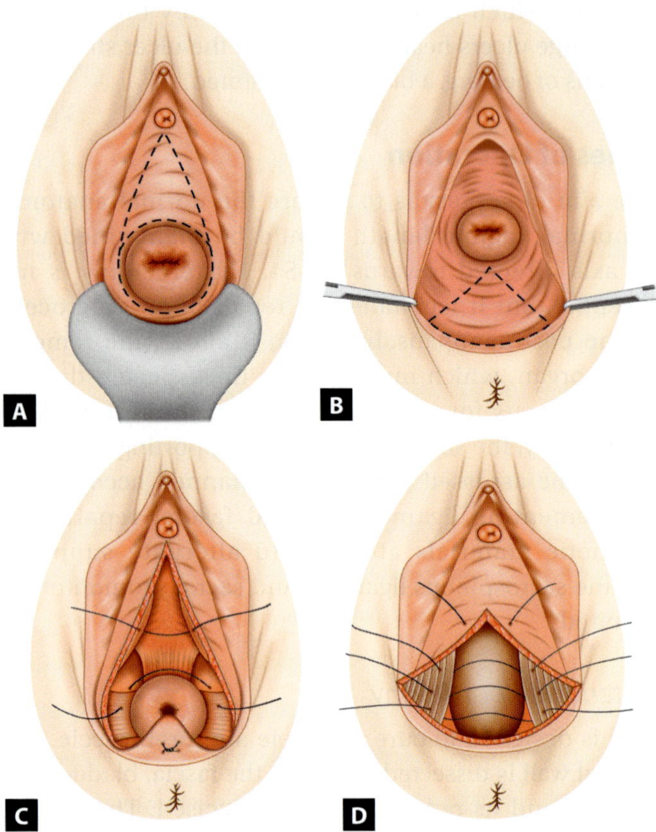

Figs. 18A to D: The principles of the Manchester operation for uterovaginal prolapse. (A) Incisions for anterior colporrhaphy and for amputation of the cervix; (B) Incisions for posterior colporrhaphy, a procedure included in the classical operation but unnecessary unless a rectocele is present; (C) Suturing of the bases of the cardinal ligaments in front of the cervix before completing the covering of the cervical stump with vaginal epithelium. Suturing the pubocervical fascia before closing the vaginal wall from above downwards; (D) Sutures placed in the edges of the levator ani before closure of the vaginal wall and perineum. Not shown here, but essential in every repair of this kind, is the opening of the pouch of Douglas behind the cervix immediately after the amputation. All redundant peritoneum is then excised, and a culdoplasty is done.

Steps of anterior colporrhaphy:

Principles:

- To excise a portion of the relaxed anterior vaginal wall
- To mobilise the bladder and push it upwards after cutting the vesicocervical ligament
- Bladder is permanently supported by tightening the pubocervical fascia.

Operative Steps (Figs. 19A to H)

- Triangular vaginal flaps, including the fascia, separated from endopelvic fascia
- Line of cleavage vesicovaginal space
- Pubocervical ligament is divided
- Bladder is pushed upwards
- Pubocervical fascia is plicated with interrupted Vicryl sutures
- Thus, closing the hiatus through which bladder herniates
- Redundant portion of the vaginal mucosa is cut on either sides
- Cut margins of the vagina apposed.

Anterior Prolapse Repair with Grafts

An anterior prolapse can be repaired by using grafts to strengthen the support. However, its use remains controversial. Different types of graft materials can be used that include synthetic absorbable materials such as polyglactin 910 mesh and synthetic permanent materials such as polypropylene or biologic grafts.

Complications associated with the use of graft may vary from pelvic pain, groin pain, dyspareunia to erosion and extrusion of the mesh.

Therefore, the use of grafts should be reserved for high-risk individuals, recurrent anterior prolapse or comorbid medical conditions.

Some surgeons perform a bladder neck plication along with the anterior prolapse repair to treat or prevent stress urinary incontinence.

Enterocele Repair

At vaginal hysterectomy, an enterocele sac should always be looked for and excised after dissection from above downwards. A high ligature of the peritoneum can be done by a purse-string ligature, which incorporates the uterosacral ligaments as well. The third important step is colporrhaphy to shorten the cardinal-uterosacral complex support of the vaginal cuff. When the uterosacral ligaments are long and strong, a McCall type of culdoplasty is indicated. If, on the other hand, the strength of the cardinal-uterosacral ligaments is doubtful, it is safer to anchor the vaginal vault to the sacrospinous ligament as a primary procedure.

The enterocele can be corrected abdominally by obliterating the pouch of Douglas by the Moskowitz or Halban technique.

Posterior Colpoperineorrhaphy

This is a similar type of operation for rectocele and a deficient perineum. Ordinarily, a rough triangular portion

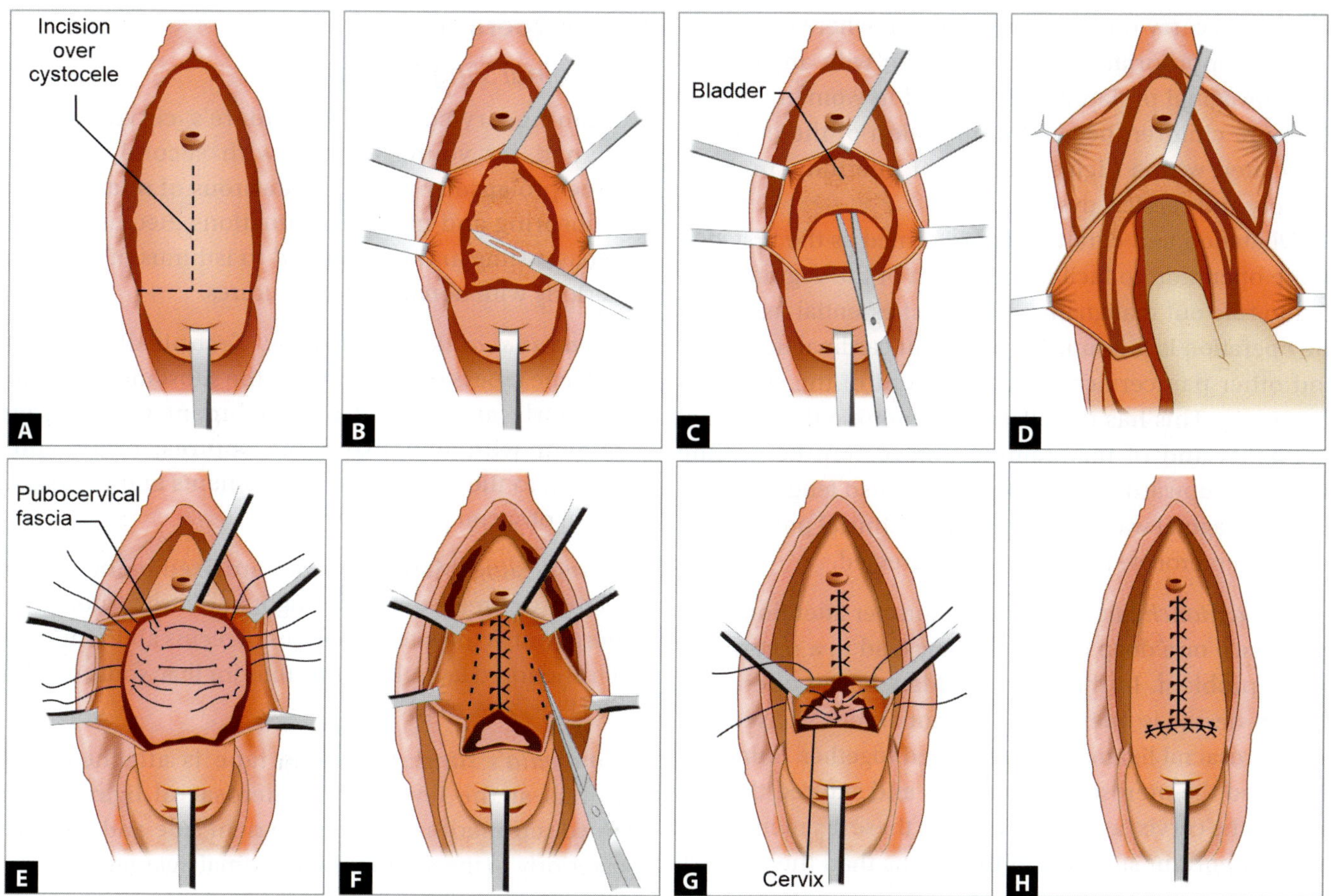

Figs. 19A to H: Steps of anterior colporrhaphy.

of the posterior vaginal wall is excised, the base of the triangle being at the introitus and the apex just above the level of the rectocele. In case of a high rectocele, dissection right up to the cervix and excision of redundant peritoneum of the pouch of Douglas are necessary. The underlying rectovaginal fascia is sutured, and the edges of the levator ani are brought together in the midline. The vaginal wall is then sutured and finally the superficial perineal muscles and skin. The operation has the effect of lengthening the perineum and tightening the introitus. The goal is a normal vaginal axis and a depth of about 10 cm, which can take the vault above the levator plate and prevent later development of enterocele.

Postmenopausal women who have undergone repair operations should be advised to continue local oestrogen application lifelong.

The traditional routine performance of posterior colpoperineorrhaphy as a part of all operations for genital prolapse has a historical rather than a sound anatomical basis. Repair of the posterior vaginal wall and perineum is not necessary for at least 50% of operations for prolapse and then only for the cure of undoubted rectocele (which is the least common form of prolapse).

The advantages of avoiding perineorrhaphy in association with other procedures for repair of cystocele and uterine prolapse are that the patient hardly ever has postoperative retention as they are free from postoperative local discomfort and is unlikely to suffer anatomical dyspareunia subsequently. Here, it must be emphasised, however, that adequate preoperative examination is essential; otherwise, a weakness in the posterior wall left uncorrected may set the stage for recurrence of prolapse.

Fothergill or Manchester operation ***(Figs. 18A to D)***: This operation variously credited to Donald and to Fothergill, both from Manchester, combines anterior colporrhaphy, amputation of the cervix and posterior colpoperineorrhaphy in one procedure. Fothergill did not always carry out a posterior repair, whereas Donald did. It is appropriate in young women with any degree of uterovaginal prolapse. It is avoided in women anxious for more children because amputation of the cervix is associated with a high incidence of infertility, preterm delivery and cervical dystocia.

Dilatation and curettage is performed as the first step of the operation to facilitate creation of the vaginal flaps and to rule out malignancy. The most essential feature of the operation is the suturing of the cut cardinal ligaments and other paracervical tissues in front of the stump of the cervix. This has the effect of tightening the cardinal ligaments and of maintaining anteversion by pulling the cervix upwards and backwards; it also lengthens the anterior vaginal wall—an important technical point.

If an enterocele is present, it is corrected.

Extended Manchester operation: Improper attention to an enterocele or a deep cul-de-sac may lead to a recurrence of the problem. In the extended Manchester operation, the cul-de-sac is opened, the peritoneum is excised and the uterosacral ligaments are plicated together. Shirodkar dissected the uterosacral ligaments and sutured them in front of the cervix, as he believed that these ligaments were more important supports of the uterus than the cardinal ligaments. Further, in his operation, amputation of the cervix was avoided, thus offering a better alternative for women who desired further childbearing.

Vaginal Hysterectomy with Anterior Colporrhaphy and Posterior Colpoperineorrhaphy

Vaginal hysterectomy is preferred in premenopausal patients when prolapse is complicated by abnormal uterine bleeding or disease, when some condition such as diabetes or obesity indicates a higher than average risk of the subsequent development of uterine cancer, or when the patient is over 40 years of age. In postmenopausal patients, both tubes and ovaries may be removed vaginally at the same time.

Vaginal hysterectomy by itself does not cure prolapse. For this purpose, it remains essential, after the uterus is removed, to excise any redundant peritoneum, to strengthen the vaginal vault by approximating the uterosacral and broad ligament pedicle, and to tighten the pubocervical fascia. If proper attention is paid to these matters, it is not necessary to add posterior colpoperineorrhaphy unless a rectocele is present.

Other Operations

Abdominal Sling Operations

Abdominocervicopexy (Purandare's cervicopexy) is designed for young women with second- or third-degree prolapse and who are desirous of retaining their childbearing and menstrual functions. Rectus sheath is used as a sling and is anchored to isthmus of the uterus anteriorly with nonabsorbable sutures.

Shirodkar's abdominal sling: Technically difficult. Mersilene tape is passed through the substance of isthmus posteriorly at the level of attachment of uterosacral ligament with nonabsorbable sutures; other end is attached to the anterior sacral ligaments and periosteum in front of sacral promontory.

Khanna's sling: Mersilene tapes are fixed to the isthmus, and the two free ends are brought out retroperitoneally to emerge out at the lateral margins of rectus abdominus and then anchored laterally to the anterior iliac spine on either side **(Figs. 20A to C)**.

Soonawala's sling: Mersilene tape is attached to the isthmus at the level of the uterosacral ligament and passed retroperitoneally on the right side and then fixed posteriorly to the anterior longitudinal ligament.

Virkud sling: Mersilene tape is fixed to the anterior longitudinal ligament and then passed retroperitoneally to emerge at the isthmus where it is fixed and then continues on to the left side between the broad ligament to be brought anteriorly and fixed to the rectus compartment.

Partial obliteration of the vaginal lumen by creating a septum between the anterior and posterior vaginal walls *(Le Fort's operation)* is sometimes advocated for severe prolapse in old women and for vaginal eversion after hysterectomy. The Le Fort's operation, however, is just as safe, and the results are better, especially if the surgeon is prepared to sacrifice coital function by making a *pencil vagina*. Moreover, the drag of the septum, created in Le Fort's operation, is liable to open the internal urethral sphincter to cause stress incontinence. The Le Fort's operation can be done under local anaesthesia, and this may be of value in some old women with severe medical problems.

Operations for Vaginal Prolapse after Hysterectomy

Eversion of the vagina following hysterectomy in an older and more sedentary patient is best treated by a

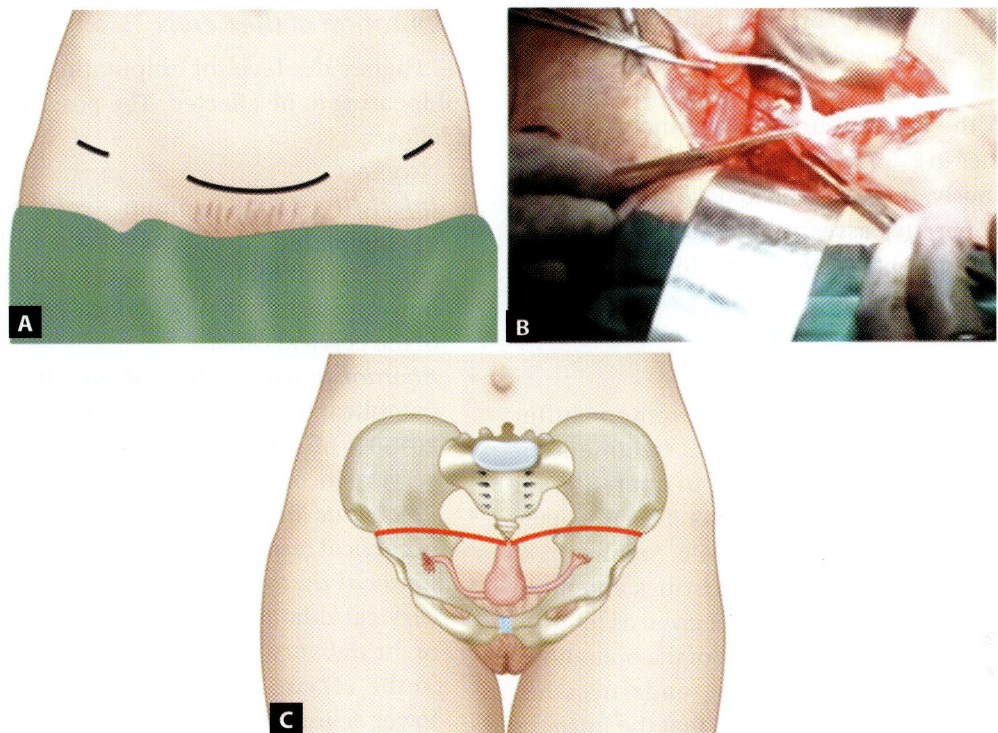

Figs. 20A to C: Khanna's abdominal sling operation. (A) Incisions given for Khanna's sling operation; (B) Attachment of the Mersilene tape to the uterine isthmus posteriorly; (C) Diagrammatic representation of the completed Khanna's sling surgery.

transvaginal vault suspension with anterior colporrhaphy and posterior colpoperineorrhaphy. This method is also suitable for women with a previous abdominal hernia repair with a mesh in situ or with a history of intestinal obstruction or adhesive disease. Sacrospinous ligament fixation is a suitable method in these patients. Injury to the pudendal vessels and nerves can occur. It is important to identify and correct an enterocele and narrow the vagina, if necessary.

Abdominal sacral colpopexy provides the surest and strongest correction for vaginal vault prolapse and is preferred in younger patients with more strenuous physical activity or those with associated diseases that increase intra-abdominal pressure chronically, e.g. asthma, chronic obstructive pulmonary disease and chronic constipation. It is also the preferred operation in patients with previous failed repairs and a shortened, scarred vagina. Mersilene or Teflon mesh is used to attach the vault to the anterior longitudinal ligament of the first sacral vertebra. The mesh is peritonealised to avoid bowel entrapment. The venous plexus in front of, and the pelvic nerves lateral to, this ligament can be injured. A culdoplasty by the Halban or Moskowitz technique is done as an essential part of the procedure. The vaginal vault can also be attached to the anterior abdominal wall by Mersilene mesh. Strips of fascia from the anterior rectus sheath have been used, but these have poorer long-term results, and occasionally the patient develops a hernia. Stress incontinence may occur or be aggravated in 10–25% of cases if there is excessive tension on the anterior vaginal vault, for which reason some would also recommend performing a Burch colposuspension routinely.

Laparoscopic sacrocolpopexy has been undertaken, but long-term results are awaited.

Results of Operations

The results of operations for prolapse depend very much on the skill of the surgeon and on selection of operation according to the case- and site-specific defect. In general, the anatomical results are good, being permanently satisfactory in at least 90% of cases. Symptomatic results are also good except in respect of the following.

Stress Incontinence

If the woman treated for prolapse happens also to suffer from urinary stress incontinence, this symptom is not always cured by anterior colporrhaphy alone even though the anatomical result of anterior colporrhaphy is satisfactory. Moreover, anterior colporrhaphy, by interfering with the internal urethral sphincter, causes stress incontinence in 2–3% of women who do not have this complaint previously. It is essential to have adequate and appropriate preoperative assessment of all women with urinary symptoms and prolapse and perform additional procedures accordingly.

Dyspareunia

It is not always realised how often women suffer dyspareunia and apareunia after surgical treatment for prolapse. About 25% of women coming to operation for prolapse have already discontinued coitus. This is usually because of waning libido in husband or wife. Another 25%, however, find that the cure of prolapse brings an end to marital relations. The reasons for this are given as follows:

- Fear that coitus will impair the result of the operation.
- An early attempt at coitus, before tenderness has subsided and without the realisation that the introitus is narrower, causes pain. This, together with fear of injury, causes vaginismus.
- Often, the operation is done at an age when senile atrophy is to be expected. Coitus is discontinued for several months and, when it is attempted again, contracture has taken place.
- Narrowing and shortening of the vagina and introitus are the most important causes. Much of the trouble arises over unnecessary perineorrhaphy. The introitus should be about two fingers loose at the end of surgery.

Posterior colpoperineorrhaphy is to be avoided unless it is clearly indicated; the assessment being made before the woman is anaesthetised. It is also important preoperatively to ask every woman, no matter how old she may be, whether she still practises coitus. If she does, a careful operative technique should be followed by explanation and guidance about the subsequent resumption of the practise.

Postoperative vaginal oestrogen therapy is of benefit in improving the results of operation by improving the tone of the tissues and also reducing symptoms of atrophy.

Pregnancy after Repair Operations

The effects of operations for prolapse on subsequent pregnancies vary with the technique employed. Some are related to amputation of the cervix and some to colporrhaphy.

Amputation of the Cervix

The Higher the level of amputation, the more likely is childbearing to be affected. The possible effects are given as follows:

- No effect
- *Infertility:* Many women avoid conception after operation, but 75–90% of women with opportunity to conceive fail to do so after cervical amputation. This may be due to a loss of cervical mucus and distortion of the cervical canal.
- *Abortion and premature labour:* The incidence of these complications is decidedly increased. They occur in 20–50% of subsequent pregnancies and are due to cervical incompetence.
- *Precipitate labour:* This occurs because of the absence of cervical resistance.
- *Cervical dystocia:* Excessive fibrosis interferes with cervical dilatation and results in obstructed labour or in delivery at the expense of a deep laceration in the cervix. The injury may extend to involve the lower segment. Cervical dystocia calls for caesarean section.
- Traumatic intrapartum and postpartum haemorrhage: This occurs from tearing of rigid tissues in the cervical stump.

Women in whom the cervix has been amputated should be delivered only in a fully equipped hospital because of the risks to both mother and baby.

Colporrhaphy

The possible effects of this procedure on childbearing are as follows:

- No effect
- Dyspareunia, apareunia and, therefore, infertility
- Delay in the second stage of labour. This is due to failure of scar tissue in the vagina and perineum to stretch. The delivery may ultimately be achieved at the expense of extensive perineal tear.
- *Recurrent prolapse:* The chance of prolapse recurring after a subsequent labour is difficult to compute; it varies with the type of operation. After a Manchester operation, there is little risk of pregnancy and labour causing a return of prolapse. If, however, anterior colporrhaphy and posterior colpoperineorrhaphy are carried out without amputation of the cervix, as is often the case in young women, there is a high recurrence rate after labour. If the operation has consisted only of perineorrhaphy, vaginal delivery does not usually

cause a return of trouble, providing episiotomy is carried out.

- Stress incontinence of urine cured by urethropexy and anterior colporrhaphy frequently relapses with a subsequent pregnancy or labour.

Previous colporrhaphy always calls for delivery in a fully equipped hospital. Caesarean section is indicated not <20% of all cases and should be made the rule for women cured of urinary stress incontinence. When the vaginal route is chosen for delivery, episiotomy should be carried out as a routine to shorten the second stage and to minimise stretching and tearing of the paravaginal supports.

PROLAPSE OF THE OVARIES

This is a relatively unimportant example of prolapse. The ovaries can be very mobile, but they are not often significantly low in the pouch of Douglas unless they are the seat of a tumour or unless there is an associated retrodisplacement of the uterus. The only symptom likely to be produced is occasional sharp deep-seated sickening pain when one or other ovary is touched during coitus. This sensation is reproduced by pressure on the ovary during bimanual examination. In fact, deep-seated dyspareunia attributed to prolapsed ovaries is mostly caused by pressure on the associated retroverted uterus.

Symptomatic treatment is preferable; dyspareunia, for example, can nearly always be avoided by modifying coital posture. If an operation is carried out, usually for some other reason, the ovary is usually suspended from the cornu of the uterus by shortening the ovarian ligament, with or without an associated ventrosuspension of the uterus.

SUGGESTED READING

1. Antosh DD, Dieter AA, Balk EM, Kanter G, Kim-Fine S, Meriwether KV, et al. Sexual function after pelvic organ prolapse surgery: a systematic review comparing different approaches to pelvic floor repair. Am J Obstet Gynecol. 2021;225:475.e1-19.
2. Baggish MS, Karram MM. Anatomy of the support of the anterior and posterior vaginal walls. In: Baggish MS, Karram MM (Eds). Atlas of Pelvic Anatomy and Gynecologic Surgery, 5th edition. Philadelphia: Elsevier; 2021.
3. Bump RC, Mattiasson A, Bø K, Brubaker LP, DeLancey JO, Klarskov P, et al. The standardization of terminology of female pelvic organ prolapse and pelvic floor function. Am J Obstet Gynecol. 1996;175(1):10-7.
4. Cheung RYK, Lee JHS, Lee LL, Chung TKH, Chan SSC. Vaginal pessary in women with symptomatic pelvic organ prolapse. Obstet Gynecol. 2016;128(1):73-80.
5. DeLancey JO. Anatomic aspects of vaginal eversion after hysterectomy. Am J Obstet Gynecol. 1992;166(6 Pt 1): 1717-24.
6. DeLancey JO. Anatomy and biomechanics of genital prolapse. Clin Obstet Gynecol. 1993;36(4):897-909.
7. Handa VL, Harris TA, Ostergard DR. Protecting the pelvic floor: obstetric management to prevent incontinence and pelvic organ prolapse. Obstet Gynecol. 1996; 88(3):470-8.
8. Hefni M, El-Toucky T. Uterine prolapse in young women. Best Pract Res Clin Obstet Gynaecol. 2011;25:157-65.
9. Kowalski JT, Barber MD, Klerkx WM, Grzybowska ME, Toozs-Hobson P, Rogers RG, et al. International urogynecological consultation chapter 4.1: definition of outcomes for pelvic organ prolapse surgery. Int Urogynecol J. 2023;34(11):2689-99.
10. Kudish BI, Iglesia CB. Posterior wall prolapse and repair. Clin Obstet Gynecol. 2010;53(1):59-71.
11. Lentz GM. Anatomic defects of the abdominal wall and pelvic floor: abdominal and inguinal hernias, cystocele, urethrocele, enterocele, rectocele, uterine and vaginal prolapse and rectal incontinence: diagnosis and management. In: Katz VL, Lentz GM, Lobo RA, Gershenson DM (Eds). Katz: Comprehensive Gynecology, 5th edition. Philadelphia: Mosby Elsevier; 2007.
12. Maggiore ULR, Alessandri F, Remorgida V, Venturini PL, Ferrero S. Vaginal sacrospinous colpopexy using the Capio suture-capturing device versus traditional technique: feasibility and outcome. Arch Gynecol Obstet. 2012;287(2): 267-74.
13. Maher C, Yeung E, Haya N, Christmann-Schmid C, Mowat A, Chen Z, et al. Surgery for women with apical vaginal prolapse. Cochrane Database Syst Rev. 2023;7(7):CD012376.
14. Nappi RE, Cucinella L. Sexuality, pelvic floor/vaginal health and contraception at menopause. Best Pract Res Clin Obstet Gynaecol. 2022;81:85-97.
15. Oktem M, Isik G, Guner H. The effectiveness of prophylactic sacrospinous ligament fixation after vaginal hysterectomy. J Minim Invas Gynecol. 2016;23(7):S251-2.
16. Practice Bulletin No. 185: pelvic organ prolapse. Obstet Gynecol. 2017;130:e234-50.
17. Schulten SF, Claas-Quax MJ, Weemhoff M, van Eijndhoven HW, van Leijsen SA, Vergeldt TF, et al. Risk factors for primary pelvic organ prolapse and prolapse recurrence: an updated systematic review and meta-analysis. Am J Obstet Gynecol. 2022;227:192-208.
18. Siff LN, Barber MD. Native tissue prolapse repairs. Obstet Gynecol Clin North Am. 2016;43(1):69-81.
19. van Le L, Handa VL. Surgery for pelvic floor disorders. In: Van Le L, Handa VL (Eds). Te Linde's Operative Gynecology, 12th edition. Philadelphia: Lippincott Williams & Wilkins; 2019.
20. Ward RM, Velez Edwards DR, Edwards T, Giri A, Jerome RN, WU JM. Genetic epidemiology of pelvic organ prolapse: a systematic review. Am J Obstet Gynecol. 2014;211(4):326-35.

18

CHAPTER

Other Displacements of the Uterus

Jyothi Shetty, Muralidhar V Pai

Chapter Outline

- Upward Displacement of the Uterus
- Lateral Displacement of the Uterus
- Forward Displacement of the Uterus
- Backward Displacement of the Uterus
- Retroverted Gravid Uterus
- Inversion of the Uterus
- Chronic Inversion

INTRODUCTION

The uterus normally has a limited range of movement, so its position in the pelvis is affected by filling of the bladder and rectum, by increasing the intra-abdominal pressure through coughing, laughing, and bearing down effort and by alterations in posture. The uterus is lower when the woman is standing than when she is lying and lowest when she is squatting. Nevertheless, the supravaginal cervix is relatively fixed, and movement or displacement of the uterus often consists of rotation of the organ around this axis or of bending of the corpus on the cervix.

UPWARD DISPLACEMENT OF THE UTERUS

The uterus can be lifted upwards to become an abdominal organ, and the external os may be above the level of the upper border of the symphysis pubis and out of reach of the vaginal examining fingers.

Causes

- A vaginal or paravaginal tumour
- Haematocolpos
- A broad ligament tumour and especially a low cervical leiomyoma
- Any tumour impacted in the pouch of Douglas
- A collection of pus or blood in the pelvis.

Treatment

Treatment is directed to the cause, the displacement itself being of no consequence.

LATERAL DISPLACEMENT OF THE UTERUS

There may be lateral deviation of the uterus as a whole, or lateral tilting with the corpus directed to one side and the cervix to the other. Except as a sign of the lesion causing it, a displacement of this type is of no significance.

Causes

- A unilateral tumour, inflammatory exudate or collection of fluid, especially if situated in the broad ligament, pushes the uterus to the opposite side.
- Adhesions can pull the uterus to one side. Malkani described the deviation of the uterus and cervix to one side of the pelvis as a sign of genital tuberculosis, wherein postinfection scarring results in contractures and pulls the uterus to the affected side.
- Operative removal of one adnexum often leaves the uterus leaning towards the side of the operation site.
- Unicornuate or bicornuate deformity.
- *Idiopathic:* It is common for the uterus to lie or lean to one side without there being an abnormality **(Fig. 1)**. In this case, the uterus is mobile and can be manipulated temporarily to a normal position.

Treatment

No treatment other than that of the cause is necessary.

FORWARD DISPLACEMENT OF THE UTERUS

Forward displacement of the uterus as a whole is usually the result of a tumour or a collection of fluid in the pouch

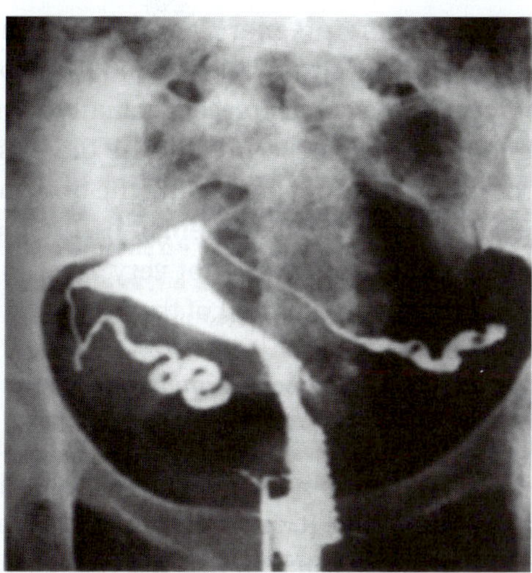

Fig. 1: Lateral deviation of the uterus, which is common and not significantly abnormal.

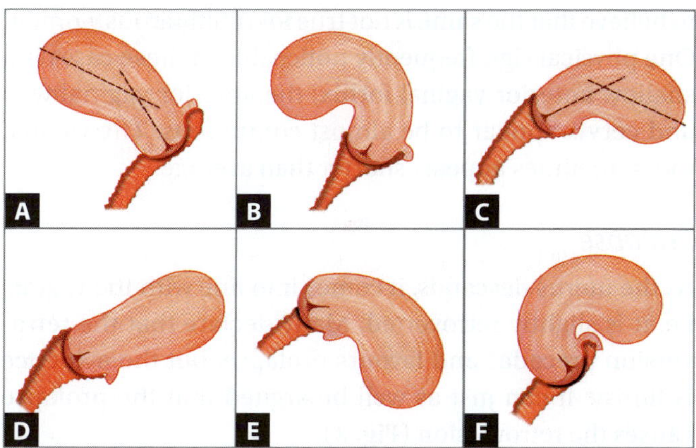

Figs. 2A to F: Uterine version and flexion. (A) Normal anteflexion and version; (B) Cochleate uterus or acute anteflexion of the cervix. The axis of the cervix indicates retroversion but the angle of anteflexion is increased, so that the corpus is in a normal position in the pelvis; (C) Retroversion and retroflexion; (D) Retroversion; (E) Extreme retroflexion and retroversion; (F) Cochleate type of uterus in reverse; an essentially anteverted uterus (from the direction of the cervix) is sharply retroflexed.

of Douglas and is then associated with upward displacement. It can also be explained by a previous ventrofixation operation. Acute anteflexion of the uterus (or forward displacement of the corpus) is not to be confused with acute anteflexion of the cervix (cochleate uterus). It is a normal finding in early pregnancy when the fundus is heavy and the supravaginal cervix is soft and atonic. A fundal leiomyoma or an ovarian tumour can push the corpus downwards.

These displacements have no importance in themselves. This was not recognised in bygone centuries, and it is of interest to recall that one of the early uses of mechanical pessaries was to correct anteversion, even normal anteversion, rather than retroversion.

BACKWARD DISPLACEMENT OF THE UTERUS

Backward displacement of the uterus as a whole (*retropronation* or *retroposition*) is the normal reaction to a full bladder and can be caused by any tumour occupying the front compartment of the pelvis. It also occurs as a developmental peculiarity in certain women. In no circumstances, it is of any significance. More important are the states of *retroversion* and *retroflexion* with which the remainder of this section is concerned **(Figs. 2A to F)**.

Definitions

Retroversion

In this condition, the axis of the *cervix* is directed upwards and backwards in relation to a line drawn through the long axis of the trunk **(Figs. 2C to E)**.

Retroflexion

In this condition, the long axis of the corpus is bent backwards on the axis of the cervix **(Figs. 2C, E and F)**.

According to these definitions, it is theoretically possible to have retroflexion in an anteverted uterus and anteflexion in a retroverted uterus; such states are described, although they are of academic interest only. In practice, retroversion and retroflexion usually occur together, and they are often both loosely called retroversion or retrodisplacement. No attempt is made to separate them here, although it may be noted that, of the two, retroflexion is more likely than retroversion to cause symptoms.

Degrees of retroversion and retroflexion are also described but are of no practical value.

Frequency

Retrodisplacement of the uterus is found in approximately 15% of women.

Causes

Developmental (Congenital)

Retrodisplacement of the uterus is most often a developmental anomaly. It is not a congenital malformation because the uterus is without version and flexion at birth. Nearly, all cases of retroversion and retroflexion in nulliparous women are of this type, and there is no reason to believe that the same is not true for multiparous women. One physical sign frequently noticeable in these cases is a shallow anterior vaginal fornix; the anterior vaginal wall and cervix appear to be almost continuous. The vagina, too, sometimes appears shorter than average.

Prolapse

As the uterus descends, it comes into line with the vagina, i.e. it is slightly retroverted. Many declare that the retroversion precedes and favours prolapse, but the evidence is flimsy; it can just as well be argued that the prolapse causes the retroversion **(Fig. 3)**.

Tumours and Adhesions

A tumour lying in front of the uterus pushes it backwards; adhesions behind may pull it backwards. Endometriosis of the uterosacral ligaments and pouch of Douglas is very commonly found in association with retroversion and is a cause of displacement of a previously anteverted uterus.

Puerperal

Retrodisplacement is often found to be present when the uterus involutes after pregnancy because, it was once said, it falls backwards while its controlling ligaments are slack and subinvoluted. The uterus is certainly unusually mobile during the weeks after delivery and I have often noticed that a uterus, which is retroverted 3–6 weeks after delivery, becomes anteverted within the following months and vice versa.

When the uterus remains *permanently* retroverted after pregnancy, it is generally safe to conclude that it was in a similar position before pregnancy and that it has merely returned to its normal state. This explains why puerperal retrodisplacement, even if treated, usually recurs after each pregnancy. It also accounts for the old observation that if retroversion does not occur after the first pregnancy, it is unlikely to do so after subsequent ones. Pregnancy and faulty involution are, therefore, not very common causes of permanent retrodisplacement of the uterus.

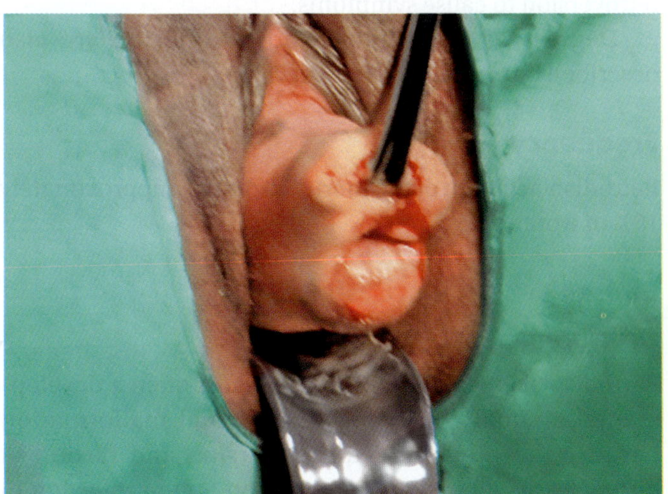

Fig. 3: Second-degree prolapse.

Symptoms

It cannot be emphasised too strongly or too often that a mobile retrodisplacement of the uterus is nearly always symptomless, and that it can be regarded as a normal physical trait of many women. Its only real disadvantage is that it favours perforation of the uterus when a sound or other instrument is inserted, in or out of pregnancy.

If, however, the uterus is fixed backwards, symptoms are usually present, these being caused by the lesion fixing the uterus rather than by the retrodisplacement itself. These are considered elsewhere.

The possible clinical manifestations of a mobile retrodisplacement and their mechanisms are described here.

Spasmodic Dysmenorrhoea

Developmental retrodisplacement does not affect menstruation but, if the uterus is cochleate in type, spasmodic dysmenorrhoea can be associated. The symptomatology and treatment are the same as for acute anteflexion of the cervix; the retroflexion is incidental and does not need correction.

Pelvic Congestion Syndrome

When the uterus assumes or resumes a position of retroversion and retroflexion after pregnancy, involution may be slightly retarded or so it is said. In explanation, it is postulated that the torsion of the broad ligament interferes with the venous and lymphatic return, leaving the pelvic organs congested and oedematous.

Persistence of such a circulatory error might later lead to congestive dysmenorrhoea, menorrhagia, polymenorrhagia, premenstrual low back pain, diffuse suprapubic pain, dyspareunia and leucorrhoea. This is an entirely theoretical concept, and it is extremely doubtful whether such symptoms, which are features of the 'pelvic congestion' syndrome, are ever attributable to uterine retrodisplacement. They certainly cannot be if the displacement is developmental in origin because the circulation will be adapted to this. Some of these patients have psychosomatic and psychiatric complaints as well.

Low Backache and Pelvic Pain

Despite statements to the contrary, a mobile retroversion probably never causes these symptoms.

Rectal Symptoms

Uterine retrodisplacement alone never produces pressure on the rectum or symptoms referred to the lower bowel.

Dyspareunia

This is one of the few genuine symptoms of retrodisplacement but is present in only a minority of cases, depending possibly on the length of the vagina. The pain is deep seated and is caused by direct pressure on the uterus itself rather than on an associated prolapsed ovary. It is position dependent, and a change of coital position may avoid or reduce discomfort. Some of these patients may have endometriosis.

Infertility

Although women with retroversion ordinarily conceive readily, a few find it difficult, and it is postulated that this is because the cervix is directed forwards away from the seminal pool, and the ejaculation of semen directly into the external os is less likely. Moreover, the external os tends to be closed by the anterior vaginal wall when coitus is complete **(Fig. 2E)**. More importantly, however, some of these women may have associated pelvic pathology such as endometriosis or pelvic inflammatory disease, which is the cause of both the retroversion and infertility.

Abortion

Contrary to former belief, retrodisplacement of the uterus is not an important cause of abortion, unless the uterus is impacted in the pouch of Douglas, and there is a disturbance in the uterine vascularity. In such cases, it may be a factor in a few cases, operating between the 10th and 14th weeks.

Physical Signs

Inspection of the cervix through a vaginal speculum is often enough to make a provisional diagnosis of retroversion. It is characteristic that the cervix comes into view unusually easily and that the external os points forwards. On bimanual examination, the position and direction of the cervix are again valuable signs, especially if it is difficult to define the corpus.

To be certain of the diagnosis, the body of the uterus should be felt in the pouch of Douglas and recognised by its size, shape and continuity with the cervix. Tenderness is a striking, although unexplained feature of the retroflexed uterus, even when there is no associated disease (hence the dyspareunia).

In the past, when more importance was attached to retroversion, the uterine position was often confirmed by passing a sound. This is now rarely done except as a precaution preliminary to the insertion of an instrument or an intrauterine contraceptive device.

Differential Diagnosis

Uterine retroversion and retroflexion have to be distinguished from the following:

- Acute anteflexion of the cervix, confusion arising because of the forward direction of the cervix.
- A tubal or ovarian swelling prolapsed in the pouch of Douglas or adherent to the back of the uterus.
- Faeces or other mass in the lower bowel
- A tumour such as endometriosis in the pouch of Douglas or the rectovaginal septum, pelvic haematocele and an abscess.
- A leiomyoma or other tumour in the posterior wall of the uterus.

Management and Treatment

When retroversion or retroflexion of the uterus is diagnosed, it becomes necessary to determine whether the uterus is fixed or mobile. This is done by attempting to replace it by moving the cervix backwards and by pushing the fundus upwards. Only very rarely is examination under anaesthesia necessary to ascertain mobility.

When the uterus is fixed, treatment should be directed primarily to the disease causing the fixation and the symptoms. If the patient has other symptoms and limited mobility of the uterus, a laparoscopy may help to establish the correct diagnosis.

If the uterus is found to be mobile, the general conclusion should be that it is not causing symptoms and that no treatment is required. In most of these cases, the patient should not even be informed of the presence of the retroversion or, if she is, she should be assured that it is a normal feature of her development.

The possible lines of treatment for uterine retrodisplacement are discussed here.

Prevention

Preventive measures used to be suggested during the weeks immediately after abortion or labour, and they consisted of the following:

- Regular emptying of the bladder to avoid overdistension
- Pelvic floor exercises
- Early ambulation
- *Posture:* The puerperal woman used to be advised to lie face downwards for 30 minutes—1 hour once or twice daily with the idea of encouraging anteversion. If this treatment had any value, the most important time for it was between the 10th and 28th days after labour; before then, the uterus was so large that the sacral promontory prevented retroversion.
- Pessary treatment.

The above is in line with tradition and, since a puerperal retroversion usually represents merely a return to a prepregnancy state, it does not require treatment of any kind. So, as a rule, the finding should be made without comment, or at most, the patient told to report within the first 3 months of her next pregnancy.

Replacement of the Uterus and Insertion of a Pessary

Principles of Treatment

A supporting pessary inserted into the upper vagina will hold the uterus in a normal position temporarily, but it cannot cure a retrodisplacement except possibly in the puerperium. The most efficient instrument for this purpose is the Hodge-type pessary. The pessary achieves its objective by putting tension on the posterior vaginal fornix and the overlying uterosacral ligaments, and this, in turn, holds the cervix backwards. The pessary does not press on the body of the uterus; this stays forward merely because its backward rotation is prevented by fixation of the cervix **(Fig. 4)**. A pessary, therefore, only exerts its effect after the uterine position has been corrected.

Indications for Insertion of a Pessary

A fixed retroversion cannot be replaced, and a pessary is, therefore, of no value in its treatment. A mobile retroversion may be treated with a pessary under the following circumstances.

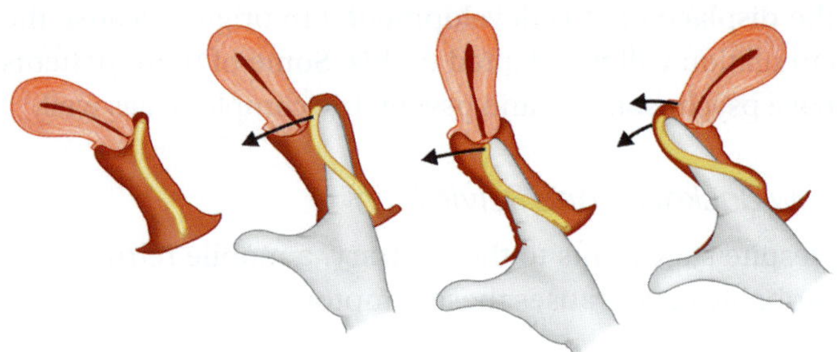

Fig. 4: Correction of retroversion by means of a Hodge pessary.

Pessary Test

When there is reasonable doubt whether the symptoms are caused by the displacement, a therapeutic test can be applied. It has to be kept in mind that the insertion of a pessary can have a good effect psychologically on an overanxious patient with vague complaints, and this possibility has to be excluded. The pessary is put in place, and the woman is asked to report the effect on her symptoms at the end of 1 month. No indication is given to her as to whether relief is expected or not. If the symptoms are not improved, the retroversion is blameless and requires no further consideration. If they are improved, the pessary treatment is continued for 2–3 months in all, and the device is then removed. At that time, the patient is assured that the malposition is corrected and that nothing more is required. In fact, the retroversion recurs immediately, but the patient is unaware of this, so if she returns promptly with a recurrence of symptoms, it may be concluded that her observation is without prejudice and that treatment is indicated. Automatically rotates the fundus forwards until it can be caught by the abdominal hand and manoeuvred into the final position.

During Pregnancy

Pessary treatment is rarely required but may be used if the uterus does not correct its own position by the 10th–12th weeks (see further).

Technique of Replacement of the Uterus

- Bimanual manipulation of the uterus is one method, the secret of success being to move the cervix backwards. This automatically rotates the fundus forwards until it can be caught by the abdominal hand and manoeuvred.
- The easiest and best method is to use the pessary as a lever for replacement of the uterus. This gives the

patient very little discomfort; often, she does not realise that the uterus is being repositioned. The pessary is inserted while the uterus is still retroverted; its upper rim then lies in front of the cervix. Finger pressure on the upper part of the pessary then forces the cervix backwards, and the fundus begins to rotate forwards **(Fig. 4)**. As the cervix moves backwards, the rim of the pessary slips past and comes to lie in its proper place, the posterior fornix. If anteversion is not then complete, the pessary can be used to pull the cervix further backwards by 'stroking' the upper posterior vaginal wall. An advantage of this method is that there is no opportunity for the retroversion to recur between the replacement manoeuvre and the insertion of the pessary.

- A finger inserted into the rectum may help to push the corpus forwards.

In a difficult case, the knee-chest position can be of help. Rarely, general anaesthesia is necessary to allow the manipulation. If the pessary itself is used to lever the uterus into position, anaesthesia is hardly ever required.

Size of Pessary

The size of a pessary is determined by introducing two fingers into the vagina and guiding them to the posterior fornix. The thumb of the same hand is placed to measure the distance to the posterior edge of the symphysis pubis. This distance from the tip of the finger is measured and that becomes the size of the pessary. Once the pessary is fitted in place one should be able to pass a finger between it and the anterior vaginal wall. If not, then an immediately smaller number pessary is used.

Management of Pessary

Taking care of the pessary is easy and can be done every 6 months. The pessary is removed every 6 months, washed thoroughly with water, and placed in an antiseptic solution for 24 hours and then reintroduced.

Operative Treatment for Retrodisplacement

Indications

Operative treatment is rarely necessary and is only indicated in the following circumstances:

- When the displacement has been proved to be causing symptoms by an adequately controlled pessary test.
- When a retroflexion is causing severe dyspareunia. This is a definite indication but, even so, an operation can often be avoided by instructing the couple to change coital posture so that the woman's back is towards the man (coitus *a tergo*).
- As part of an operation for an associated condition such as pelvic infection, endometriosis and leiomyoma.
- In a few cases of infertility and habitual abortion, when all other causes have been eliminated.

Techniques

There are >200 operations described for the retroversion of uterus.

Surgical Methods for Correction

More than 200 operations for retrodisplacement have been described, and these include the following:

- Various methods of intraperitoneal looping and shortening of the round ligaments and uterosacral ligaments. In the *Baldy-Webster operation,* round ligament loops are passed through the anterior and posterior leaves of the broad ligament, stitched together behind the uterus, creating a hammock-like effect.
- Bringing a loop of each round ligament out through the internal abdominal ring and suturing it to the back of the rectus sheath (modified *Gilliam's operation*) using a permanent suture. This again has the effect of shortening the round ligaments. Provided the loops are kept extraperitoneal, it is the method that I favour. It has no ill effect on subsequent pregnancy and childbirth.
- Laparoscopic ventrosuspension is favoured by some operators.
- Shortening of the uterosacral ligaments may be attempted at laparotomy and is useful when combined with a modified Gilliam suspension, but care must be taken to avoid excessive tucking, which can result in kinking or ligature of the ureter and also cause dyspareunia.

RETROVERTED GRAVID UTERUS

The uterus is retroverted during the early weeks in 15% of all pregnancies.

Outcome and Effects

Spontaneous Correction of the Position of Uterus

This occurs by the 10th week of pregnancy in nearly all cases. Since many women do not take medical advice before this time, the previous presence of the displacement is often not known. The capacity of the uterus to correct its position is remarkable. It succeeds even in the presence of adhesions, presumably because they soften and stretch in pregnancy, as evidenced by the following.

Two patients attended a clinic for infertility for years. Both had widespread endometriosis in the pelvis and ultimately, laparotomy was carried out. Tarry cysts were dissected from the ovaries, but the uterus was fixed backwards by adhesions, which were so dense that it was impossible to separate them without injury to the bowel. The uterorectal pouch was obliterated. Both women had ovulation suppressed for 9 months with a combined oestrogen and progestogen pill. In both cases, the uterus was retroverted and limited in mobility prior to conception. Subsequently, both women became pregnant, and the uterus in each patient was, of course, still retroverted when seen at the 8th and 10th weeks, respectively. By the 12th and 14th weeks, respectively, each uterus was inclined forwards and out of the pelvis. The pregnancy in each case progressed uneventfully.

Impaction of the Uterus

Pathology

Very, very occasionally, the fundus of the uterus fails to clear the promontory of the sacrum and becomes impacted in the pelvis at the 12th–14th weeks. The uterus then fills the pelvis and displaces the fundus of the bladder upwards and the base of the bladder forwards. The first symptom may therefore be bladder irritability, but the one which usually brings the patient for advice is acute retention of urine. The latter is caused by the tumour interfering with the opening of the internal urethral sphincter posteriorly, not by lengthening and attenuation of the urethra as is so often stated. Acute retention of urine is often precipitated by an episode of excessive drinking, or by a circumstance interfering with the woman emptying her bladder when she first feels the urge. That is, it is brought on by over-distension of the bladder.

Impaction of the pregnant uterus is most likely to occur when the pelvis is small and has an overhanging sacral promontory. The fact that pelvic contraction of a severe degree is disappearing probably explains why this complication, once comparatively common, is now comparatively rare. A leiomyoma in the posterior wall of a pregnant uterus sometimes determines impaction.

Diagnosis

The diagnosis can be made with reasonable certainty whenever a woman of reproductive age complains of acute retention of urine associated with 3–4 months of amenorrhoea. On examination, a soft tender tumour is found arising from the pelvis and may be mistaken for the uterus. It is, in fact, the distended bladder **(Fig. 5)**. Vaginally, it is difficult to find the cervix, which is drawn high up in the anterior fornix; behind and filling the pelvis is the tense but soft uterus.

The condition has to be distinguished from all others causing retention of urine and from other tumours, which may occupy the pouch of Douglas—particularly a large haematocele associated with ectopic pregnancy. Confusion with ectopic pregnancy is a very real possibility because the presence of some uterine bleeding may be wrongly attributed to threatened abortion associated with the retroversion.

Treatment

The immediate treatment is to catheterise the patient, and this can be done easily because the urethra itself is not compressed. Care is necessary since the rapid release of the contents of an over-distended bladder can cause collapse of the patient. Sudden decompression is also said to precipitate rupture of the rapidly refilling blood vessels of the bladder wall, but this theory is no longer acceptable.

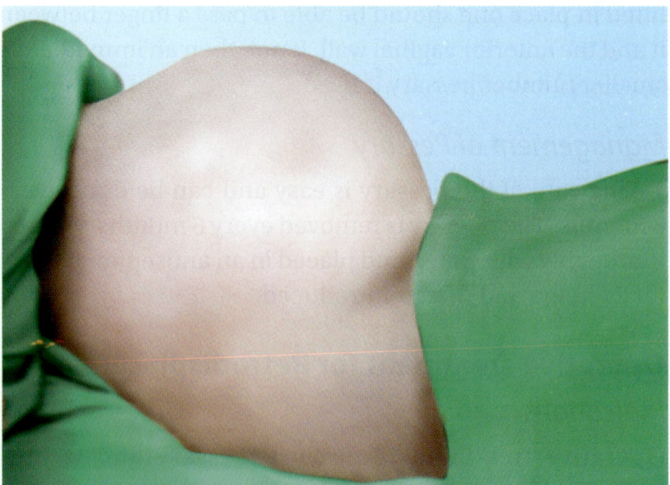

Fig. 5: Retention of urine associated with an impacted retroverted gravid uterus. A multiparous woman with 15 weeks' amenorrhoea complained of an inability to void. The uterus was entirely in the pelvis, and the abdominal 'tumour,' which reached well above the umbilicus, was the distended bladder.

Haematuria, when it occurs, is evidence of severe cystitis, which can even progress to gangrene.

Slow emptying of the bladder, the patient meanwhile being kept prone or in an exaggerated Sims' position, often results in correction of the retroversion. Some authorities say that spontaneous cure always occurs if the catheterisation is properly managed, but this is an overstatement. If correction does not occur, the bladder is kept empty by continuous drainage, and a large-sized pessary is inserted into the vagina. This exerts continuous slight pressure in the posterior fornix and backward traction on the cervix and usually restores the position of the uterus to normal within a few days. Failing this, the uterus may be manipulated by one of the methods described previously, with or without general anaesthesia. It is said that, as a last resort, laparotomy may have to be carried out. I have never encountered a case in which this proved to be necessary, even when the uterus was known to be bound down by adhesions.

Sacculation of the Uterus

A very rare outcome is for the fundus to remain beneath the sacral promontory, the pregnancy continuing to grow by expanding the anterior wall of the uterus. This ultimately produces a saccule or diverticulum of the uterus. If this condition goes unrecognised, the main body of the uterus remains in the pelvis throughout pregnancy and acts as a tumour, which obstructs the delivery of the foetus from the sacculation. The only safe treatment for this exceptional state of affairs is by caesarean section.

Management of the Uncomplicated Retroverted Gravid Uterus

A practical problem is the management of symptomless retroversion found during routine examinations early in pregnancy. Bearing in mind that the uterus is almost certain to correct itself, many take the view that no treatment is necessary. The only advice necessary is to tell the patient to make sure that she does not allow her bladder to get too full. This is not usually a problem as frequency is often the case in early pregnancy. However, if, for example, in hot weather, the patient has a lot of fluid to drink, she should be advised to empty her bladder frequently.

INVERSION OF THE UTERUS

Inversion is a condition in which the uterus turns inside out, the fundus prolapsing through the cervix. It is rare and interesting but dangerous. Inversion varies in degree from a mere dimpling of the fundus to involvement of the whole uterus and cervix **(Figs. 6A to C)**. It is seen in acute and chronic forms.

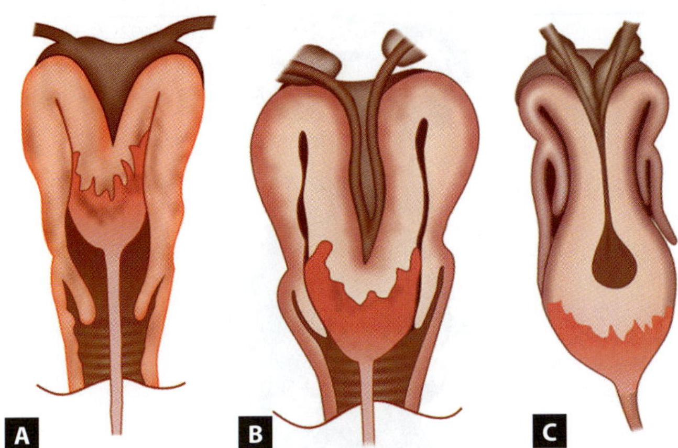

Figs. 6A to C: Degrees of inversion. (A) First degree; (B) Second degree; (C) Third degree.

Acute Inversion

This occurs during, or immediately after, the third stage of labour. The cervix is then open and atonic, and the fundus passes through it because of mismanagement of the third stage of labour, pressure on the fundus by the attendant, traction on the umbilical cord of an unseparated placenta or if insufficient time has been allowed for syntometrine to work effectively in the active management of the third stage. If the degree of inversion is gross, the fundus (with or without the placenta attached) appears outside the vulva.

Otherwise, it remains inside the vagina or the lower part of the uterus, and the diagnosis may then only be made by exploring the vagina and uterine cavity with a hand.

Even if it does not cause postpartum haemorrhage, acute inversion nearly always produces a severe degree of shock, which can be quickly fatal. It was said that shock is produced by pressure on the ovaries, which, together with the fallopian tubes, are drawn inside the inverted fundus **(Fig. 7)**. In fact, examination of specimens shows that the ovaries are usually clear of the ring. So, the shock is due to cervical distension and traction on the peritoneum and peritoneal ligaments. It may even come from stimuli arising in the uterine wall itself.

It might be thought that an alteration in the height and shape of the fundus would be obvious on abdominal examination immediately after delivery, and thus make

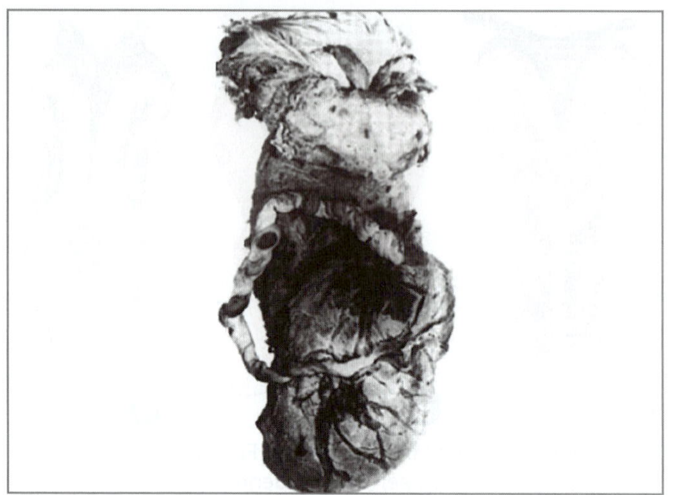

Fig. 7: Acute puerperal inversion of the uterus in a woman who died from the resulting shock during the third stage of labour. The autopsy specimen shows the fundus of the uterus completely inverted with the tubes and ovaries dipping into the ring at the top. The placenta is still attached to the inverted fundus.

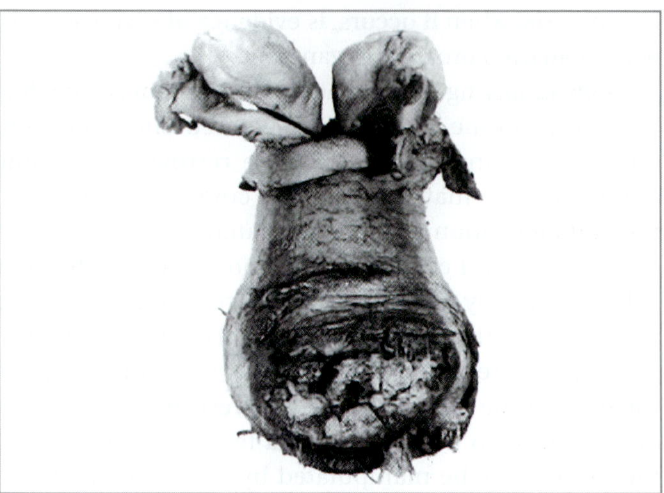

Fig. 8: Chronic puerperal inversion with ulceration and infection of the inverted fundus of the uterus. The patient from whom the specimen was obtained was aged 44 years and was treated by hysterectomy when the condition was discovered 3 months after labour. The endometrial surface is invariably infected and ulcerated.

the diagnosis easy. This, however, is not the case; the uterine mass generally feels reasonably normal.

Acute inversion is an obstetrical problem, and it suffices to say here that the most important part of treatment is to remove the cause of the shock, that is, to anaesthetise the patient and to replace the fundus. This is usually done manually or by hydrostatic pressure obtained by filling the vagina with fluid. Traction on the round ligaments at laparotomy is only occasionally necessary. The transfusion of blood and other fluids should be carried out simultaneously, but by itself is not likely to cure the shock. If attempts to replace the uterus are deferred in the hope that the general condition will improve, they are likely to be forestalled by the patient's death.

Replacement of the uterine fundus under general anaesthesia takes precedence over resuscitation.

CHRONIC INVERSION

Puerperal

Pathology

Occasionally, the uterus undergoes incomplete inversion at the time of delivery without producing much shock; or perhaps shock is ascribed to postpartum haemorrhage or other causes, the partial inversion being overlooked. It is also possible that the process of inversion can occur gradually during the puerperium. At any rate, there are cases in which the inversion is 'chronic' in the sense that it is only discovered a few weeks or months after delivery. By that time, the exposed endometrial surface is invariably infected and ulcerated **(Fig. 8)**.

Clinical Features

The complaint is vaginal discharge and irregular bleeding dating from confinement, and there may be a history of postpartum haemorrhage or obstetric shock. Other symptoms are low backache and chronic pelvic pain.

On examination, an infected haemorrhagic mass is found in the vagina and is likely to be confused with a sloughing polyp, a retained portion of the placenta, an ulcerated prolapsed cervix and even a malignant neoplasm. The diagnosis is made by recognising that the mass is coming through the cervix and by demonstrating the shortness of the uterine cavity with a sound.

Treatment

The first objective is to clear up the infection by keeping the patient lying flat in bed, by douching and by antiseptic packing of the vagina. Occasionally, this treatment results in *spontaneous cure of the inversion.* When inversion persists and the prolapsed fundus is clean, a special repositor (Aveling's repositor or its modification), consisting of a cup on a metal stem, can be placed over the inverted fundus.

Continuous pressure is applied by bracing it to the patient's waist and shoulders. Tight vaginal packing around the cup keeps it in place, and the woman's discomfort is relieved by analgesics. This treatment is generally successful within a few days. One of the secrets of replacing either an acute or chronic inversion is to lift the uterus high in the pelvis. This puts traction on the round ligaments, which in turn pull the fundus out of the inversion cup. This view, put to Professor Jeffcoate by Dr AB Johnson of New York, would explain why filling the vagina with saline solution (O'Sullivan's method), and the repositor, achieve their effect; it would also account for spontaneous cures with posture and vaginal packing.

More commonly, however, the uterine fundus can often be lifted into place by traction on the round ligaments at laparotomy. This procedure is also applicable to acute inversion.

In longstanding and resistant cases, replacement may require incision of the constricting ring of the cervix. This can be done abdominally (Haultain's operation) or vaginally (Spinelli's operation). The former is more common.

Hysterectomy, vaginal or abdominal, may be indicated, especially if further childbearing is not important to the patient.

Senile Inversion

Spontaneous inversion of the uterus is sometimes seen in old age, especially if the cervix has previously been amputated at a high level **(Fig. 9)**. The inversion is probably due to cervical atony and incompetence. The symptoms and signs are the same as those of chronic inversion. The condition is usually mistaken for an ulcerated prolapse. Hysterectomy is the best treatment.

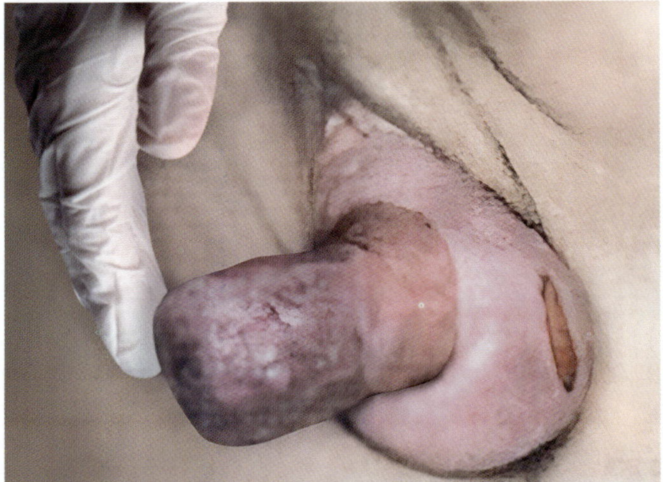

Fig. 9: Spontaneous inversion of the uterus associated with recurrent prolapse. The patient concerned was senile and had a Manchester operation several years previously. The factors causing the inversion are probably high amputation of the cervix and senile change in the tissues.

Inversion due to Pedunculated Tumour

When a tumour (usually a myoma) arises from a stalk attached to the interior of the uterus, it tends to be expelled into the vagina. If the pedicle is stout and reluctant to stretch, the traction produces a dimple in the uterine wall and ultimately quite a severe degree of inversion **(Figs. 10A and B)**. The patient's symptoms are those of the polyp, and the associated inversion may be missed unless the possibility is kept in mind. If it is overlooked, the result can be disastrous because, in dividing what is regarded as the pedicle of the polyp **(Fig. 11)**, the surgeon cuts across the fundus of the uterus and opens into the peritoneal

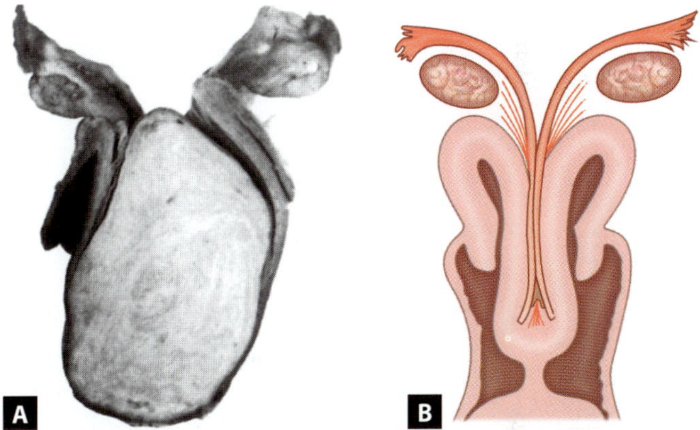

Figs. 10A and B: Inversion of the uterus caused by tumours. (A) A fundal leiomyoma is the cause in this case; the specimen is unusual because the tumour is not polypoidal; (B) A diagrammatic representation of the more common type of leiomyoma causing inversion.

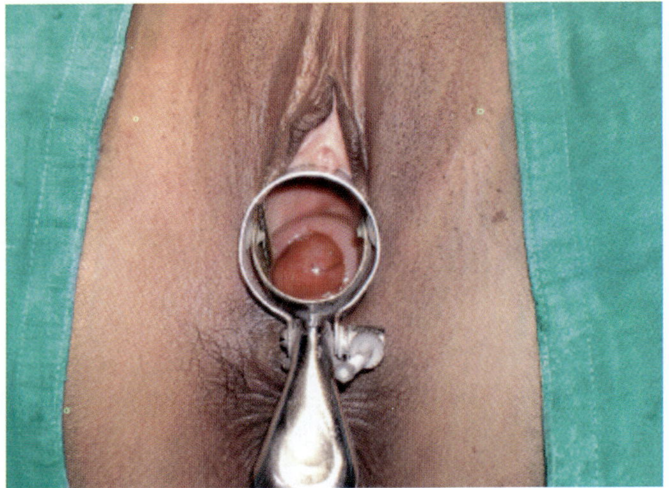

Fig. 11: A polyp projecting from the os.

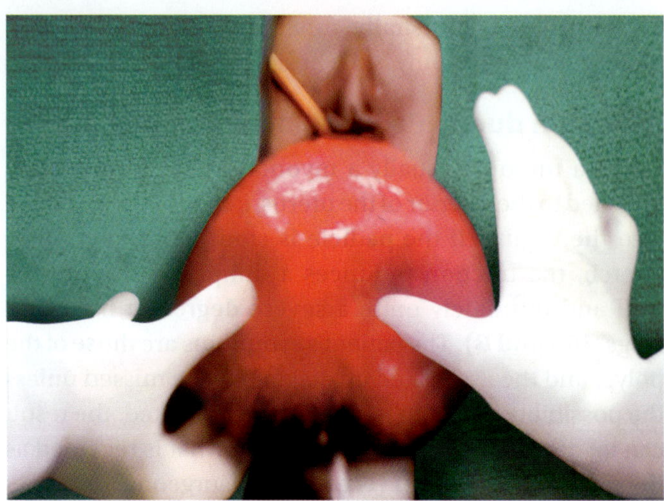

Fig. 12: A prolapsed gravid uterus, which is replaced and kept in place by a pessary.

cavity. Before any such polyp is removed, the length of the uterine cavity should always be tested by sound. Moreover, if there is any possibility of an inversion being present, the tumour should be removed by shelling it from its capsule rather than by dividing its pedicle. Rarely, gravid uterus may prolapse completely, and these have to be pushed back and treated conservatively till delivery, by the use of a pessary **(Fig. 12)**.

SUGGESTED READING

1. Alvarez Moro FJ, Molino Trinidad C, Junyent Parés MP, Calvo Mateo MA. Comparative study of ureteral displacements. Arch Esp Urol. 1978;31(2):167-86.
2. Johnston HW. The treatment of displacements of the uterus. Can Med Assoc J. 1932;27(5):513-4.
3. Tew WP. Displacements of the uterus. Am J Surg. 1930;8(6):1250-5.

19

CHAPTER

Torsion of Pelvic Organs

Latha V Khakra, Muralidhar V Pai

Chapter Outline

- Torsion in Normal and Abnormal Uterus
- Aetiology
- Differential Diagnosis
- Treatment

INTRODUCTION

Torsion is an uncommon but notable complication that can occur in many free-floating abdominal and pelvic organs. The sudden onset of pain caused by twisting of anchoring structures such as peritoneum and ligaments leads to restricted blood flow, resulting in ischaemia and potentially progressing to gangrene. Timely intervention is crucial to prevent further tissue damage and complications.

TORSION IN NORMAL AND ABNORMAL UTERUS

A minor degree of rotation of the uterus around its long axis is common and insignificant **(Fig. 1)**. This is particularly observed during pregnancy, where the uterus typically rotates to the right (dextrorotatory).

Torsion occurs when the rotation of the uterus is >45° around its long axis. In about two-thirds of diagnosed cases, torsion that is severe enough to impair blood flow usually does not occur in a healthy, normal uterus.

Symptomatic significant uterine torsion, whether in a pregnant or nonpregnant state, typically occurs only when the uterus is asymmetrical because of a tumour, Müllerian duct fusion deformity, or when it is twisted by an adjacent lesion. Torsion most often happens at the level of the supravaginal cervix, leading to obstruction of the uterine blood vessels. As a result, the uterus becomes congested, fills with blood and can eventually progress to gangrene.

Though uterine torsion is most commonly observed during pregnancy, it typically occurs in the third trimester and can result in significant maternal and perinatal complications.

In rare instances, it may be present in young girls due to congenital uterine abnormalities. Torsion of the pedicle of a subserosal pedunculated leiomyoma is also a relatively frequent occurrence.

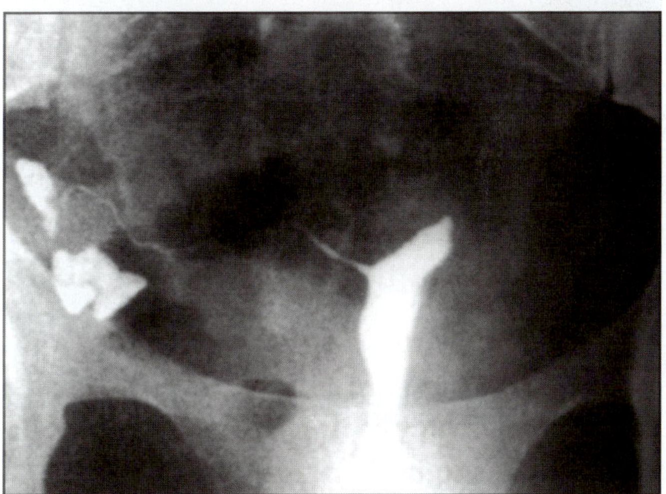

Fig. 1: Rotation of the normal uterus as revealed by hysterography. The degree of twist is not of significance, but radiographs showing this sort of picture are often misinterpreted as showing a uterine malformation.

Tube and Ovary

Torsion of the normal ovary alone is exceptional, but torsion of the normal fallopian tube with or without the ovary is not uncommon. This occurs when the fallopian tube rotates around its own axis, and sometimes only the free, outer end of the tube is involved **(Fig. 2)**. The torsion may be partial and self-resolving, but it often recurs. In more severe cases, the tube can undergo multiple complete twists. Initially, the venous return is obstructed, leading to significant congestion and blood extravasation. Eventually, the arterial supply is compromised, causing the tissue distal to the twist to become gangrenous.

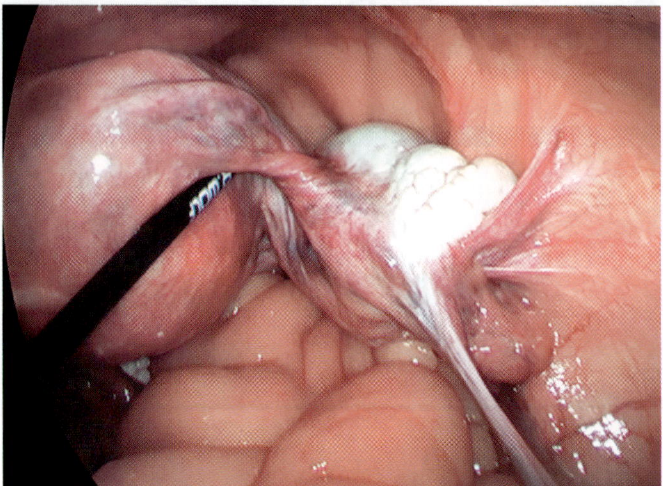

Fig. 2: Torsion of normal tube and ovary.

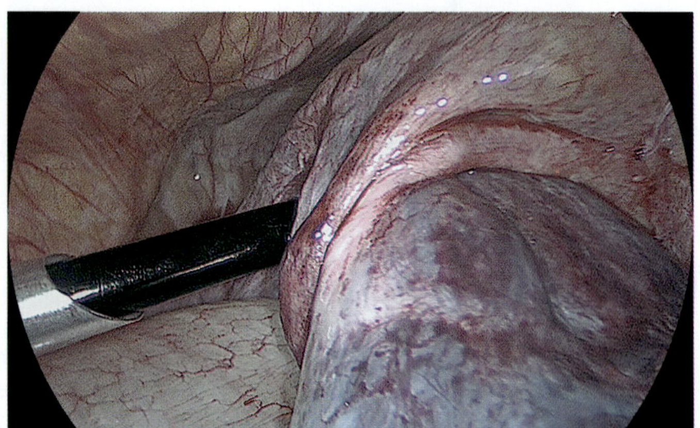

Fig. 4: Torsion of left adnexa.

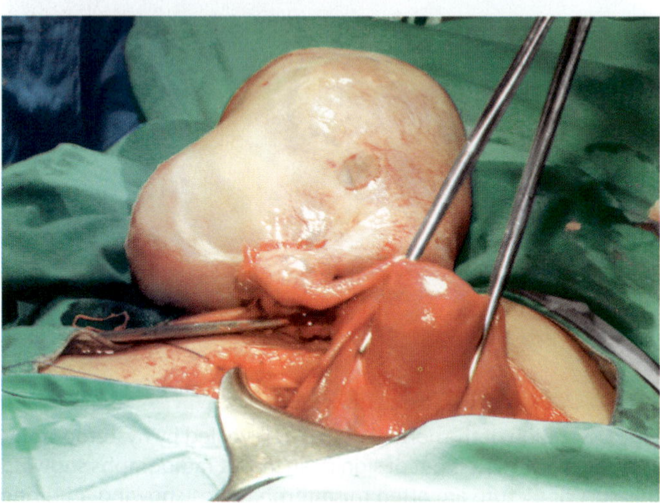

Fig. 3: Torsion of solid ovarian tumour.

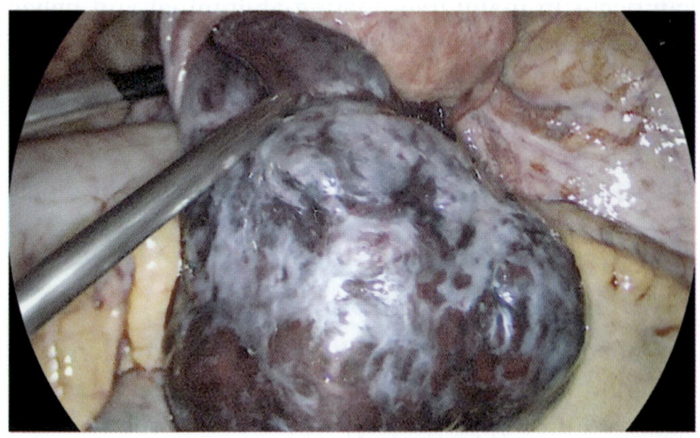

Fig. 5: Torsion leading to extreme congestion and extravasation leading to gangrene.

Torsion of Ovaries

Ovarian tumours are commonly complicated by torsion of their pedicle and in some cases, the fallopian tube may also be affected **(Figs. 3 and 4)**. Involvement of the ovary in torsion of a hydrosalpinx or fimbrial cyst depends on the exact site at which the twist occurs in relation to the mesovarium.

In ovarian torsion, the ovarian vascular pedicle undergoes partial or complete rotation, leading to an obstruction of blood flow. When the torsion exceeds 360°, the risk of necrosis and gangrene increases **(Fig. 5)**.

The patient is usually a child or adolescent who experiences a sudden onset of severe pain in the lower abdomen, often localised to one side of the midline. This may be intermittent with a previous history of a similar pain. It can cause vomiting and sometimes bladder and bowel irritability. Shock is rarely present; the temperature remains normal at first, but the pulse rate may be raised. Mild uterine bleeding often occurs within a few hours. Muscle guarding or rigidity over the lower abdomen is usual. Since the patient is nearly always young and virginal, pelvic examination is difficult. Rectal examination may reveal tenderness on one side of the uterus, although adnexal swelling is usually too small to be detected.

Misdiagnosis can result in ovarian ischaemia, necessitating prompt surgical intervention to prevent gonadal dysfunction. Diagnosis is extremely challenging due to nonspecific clinical presentation. Normal-appearing ovaries on ultrasound may delay diagnosis. Doppler imaging can aid in identifying ovarian torsion. Ultrasound is also a useful tool; however, if the ovary is not enlarged, its effectiveness is reduced. Computed tomography (CT) is another reliable diagnostic method.

Laparoscopic detorsion is the recommended treatment option. However, the increased use of this procedure may lead to retorsion. Preventative measures, such as oophoropexy, which involves fixing the ovaries to the pelvic wall, can help reduce the incidence of retorsion. Ovarian torsion can also occur in premenopausal and postmenopausal women.

Torsion of Tube

Torsion of tube most frequently occurs during the reproductive years. Due to nonspecific clinical symptoms, preoperative diagnosis is challenging. As a result, it is rarely diagnosed before surgery, which is often performed too late. Spontaneous torsion of the fallopian tubes can lead to primary infertility even in the absence of any prior medical conditions.

The lesion of the tube preceding torsion is mostly a hydrosalpinx **(Fig. 6)**. The interference in blood supply converts this to a haematosalpinx **(Fig. 7)**. The clinical features are the same as for torsion of the normal tube except that a tumour is more likely to be found on examination. During surgery, it is often difficult to say whether the tube was previously normal or the seat of a hydrosalpinx.

Torsion of the tube can occur with the rare carcinoma of the fallopian tube. Torsion of the tube also inevitably occurs when there is torsion of a paraovarian (fimbrial) cyst, because the tube is tightly stretched over the wall of the cyst.

Salpingectomy is the most commonly performed procedure for isolated fallopian tube torsion due to necrosis, although more conservative treatment options such as detorsion may be performed.

AETIOLOGY

The factors determining the axial rotation of organs and tumours are discussed here.

Unusual Mobility of Organs

Physiological mobility of organs in childhood and adolescence explains why torsion of a normal tube and ovary is mostly seen at these ages. Instability of the outer end of the tube, caused by resection of the middle portion for purposes of sterilisation, can also result in its torsion. For similar mechanical reasons, it is the small rather than the large tumour, with a long pedicle, which is most likely to be affected by this complication.

Pregnancy and the Puerperium

Torsion of tumours is more often seen during pregnancy or in the puerperium when abdominal wall tension and intra-abdominal space are altering rapidly. Changes in the size of the uterus also act as rotating forces **(Figs. 8 and 9)**.

Movement of the Trunk

Torsion can be started by certain movements and often appears to follow turning over in bed.

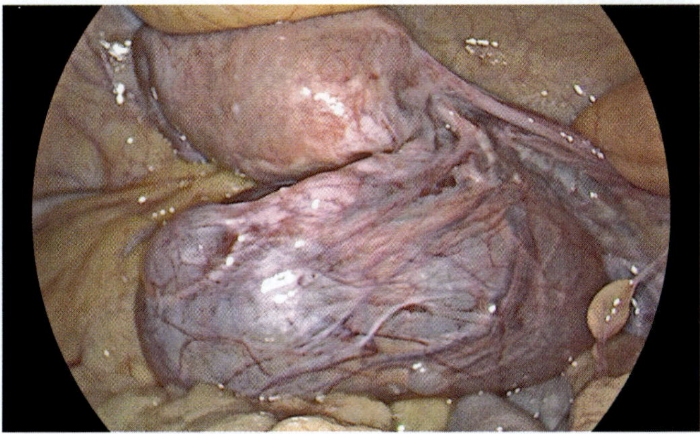

Fig. 6: Hydrosalpinx of right fallopian tube prone to torsion.

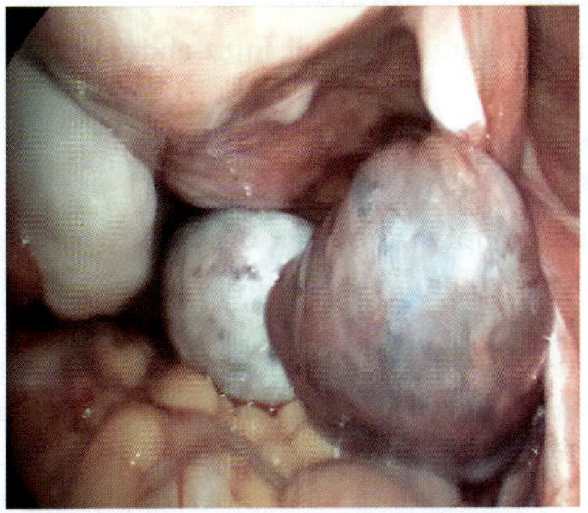

Fig. 7: Torsion of right fallopian tube with haematosalpinx.

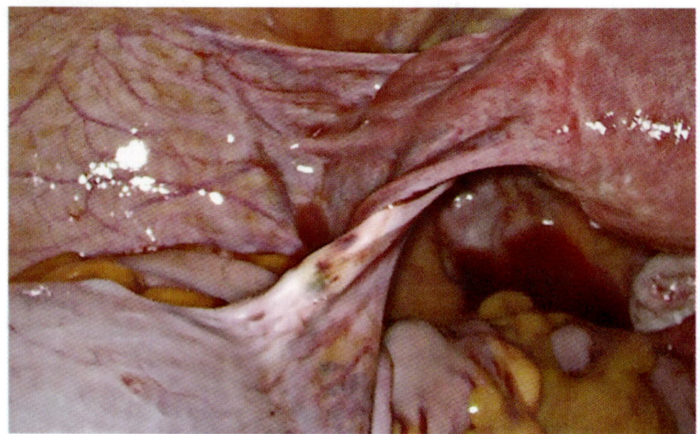

Fig. 8: Torsion of left adnexa in 12 weeks of pregnancy.

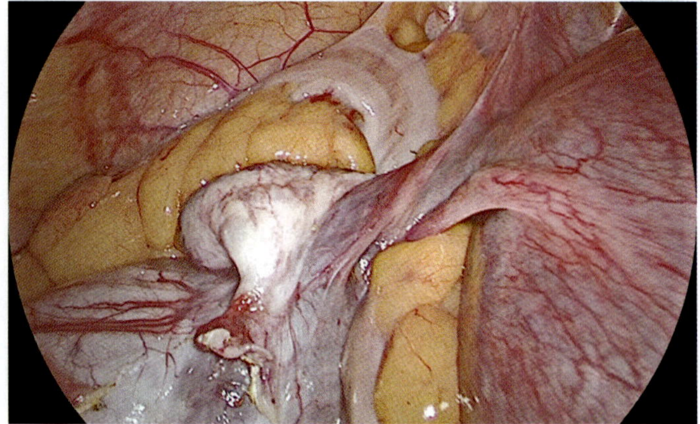

Fig. 9: Torsion of left tube and ovary in 18 weeks of pregnancy.

Flowchart 1: Torsion of pelvic organs.

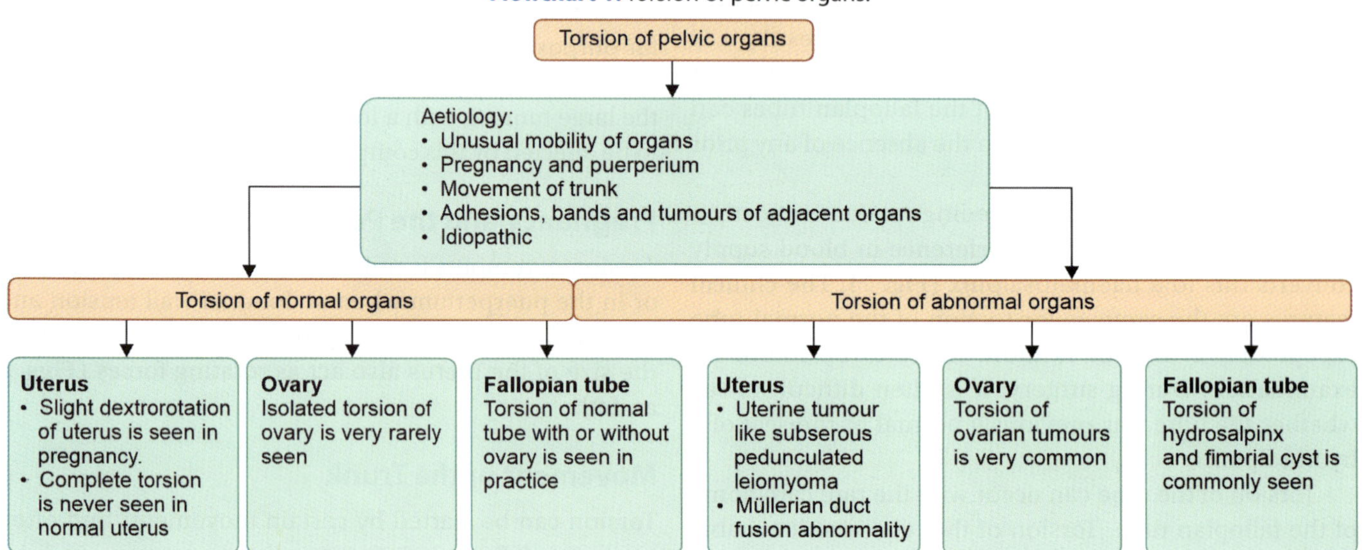

Defecation and Micturition

These can operate by altering intra-abdominal relations.

Adhesions, Bands, and Tumours in Adjacent Organs

A normal fallopian tube can become twisted around a ventrofixation band. This sort of accident is described after various operations for uterine retroversion.

Whatever be the force which commences the rotation of the pedicle or mesentery, it is widely believed that the further twisting is brought about by haemodynamics—possibly by pulsation in the vessels supplying the tumour or organ.

Idiopathic

In many cases, there is no obvious cause.

DIFFERENTIAL DIAGNOSIS

Torsion of a pelvic organ or tumour has to be distinguished from acute salpingitis, ruptured cyst, ectopic pregnancy, all causes of intraperitoneal haemorrhage, acute appendicitis and diverticulitis, rupture of an endometriotic cyst, ovulation pain, degeneration in a leiomyoma, retroplacental haemorrhage during pregnancy, intestinal obstruction and renal colic.

Before operation, it may be impossible to say which organ or tumour has undergone torsion, although guides are offered by the age, previous history and menstrual function of the patient, and by the position of a tumour.

TREATMENT

If torsion is suspected or diagnosed, immediate laparoscopy or laparotomy is required; the surgical procedure then depends on the exact nature of the finding.

If the torsion is incomplete or recent, the tissues may still be viable; it is then possible to conserve them and to stabilise them by suture. Hence, detorsion is recommended where vascularity is maintained along with oophoropexy to prevent repeat torsion. Risk of embolism is low.

Ovarian cystectomy, as distinct from removal of the whole ovary with its tumour, is sometimes a reasonable procedure. If the organ has undergone more than three twists, blood supply is occluded beyond correction. When the tissues are gangrenous beyond recovery, they have to be removed. With recent advancements and technological development and the expertise available, almost all cases of torsion can be managed laparoscopically, if not possible laparotomy should be done.

Flowchart 1 summarises the torsion of pelvic organs.

SUGGESTED READING

1. Cook KE, Jenkins SM. Pathologic uterine torsion associated with placental abruption, maternal shock, and intrauterine fetal demise. Am J Obstet Gynecol. 2005;192(6):2082-3.
2. Guié P, Adjobi R, N'guessan E. Uterine torsion with maternal death: our experience and literature review. Clin Exp Obstet Gynecol. 2005;32(4):245-6.
3. Sikora-Szczęśniak D, Szczęśniak G, Łegowik T, Sikora W. Torsion of the uterus with myomas in a postmenopausal woman—case study and review of the literature. Prz Menopauzalny. 2014;13(2):145-9.
4. Sparić R, Pervulov M, Stefanović A, Tadić J, Gojnić M, Milićević S, et al. Uterine torsion in term pregnancy. Srp Arh Celok Lek. 2007;135(9):572-5.

20

CHAPTER

Infections Including Sexually Transmitted Diseases

Jayaraman Nambiar M, Muralidhar V Pai

Chapter Outline

- Natural Defences of the Genital Tract
- Variations in the Efficiency of Defence Mechanisms
- Types of Infecting Organisms
- Sexually Transmitted Diseases
- Genital Tuberculosis
- Sarcoidosis
- Actinomycosis
- Schistosomiasis (Bilharzia)
- Amoebiasis

NATURAL DEFENCES OF THE GENITAL TRACT

The genital tract forms a continuous open pathway from the exterior to the peritoneal cavity, and a natural defence system against ascending infection is therefore necessary. This is all the more important in view of the proximity of the urethra and anus to the vaginal orifice.

Defence Mechanisms

Vulva

The vulva and perineum of the mature woman have a remarkable inherent resistance to infection; so, incisions and tears, even if contaminated, heal well if sutured with care over haemostasis. Additionally, the secretion of the apocrine glands is said to be rich in undecylenic acid, which is fungicidal. These properties, as well as closure of the introitus by apposition of the labia, protect the genital tract above.

Vagina

- Closure by apposition of its anterior and posterior walls
- A well-developed stratified squamous epithelium, unbroken by entrances to glands
- Vaginal acidity
- *Vaginal flora:* All manners of organisms ordinarily inhabit the vagina, but the gram-positive anaerobic lactobacillus is normally predominant and it is this which, by its production of lactic acid, keeps the others in check. The efficiency of the vaginal defence is directly proportional to the relative number of lactobacilli present. Organisms that do not attach to the underlying tissue are swept away by the mucus stream and do not produce tissue damage or local inflammatory response. Glycoprotein and carbohydrate seem to be the factors responsible for adherence.
- The mucosal immune response—antibodies are present although titres are low. Phagocytic cells and cytokines have also been identified.

Cervix

Functional closure of the cervix is affected by mucus, which is also said to be bacteriolytic.

Uterus

Periodic shedding of surface endometrium during menstruation tends to eliminate any infection, which may try to gain a hold. The cavity of the uterus was formerly regarded as being sterile, but it is now known that it often harbours nonpathogenic anaerobic streptococci, especially after abortion and labour. These may well play a beneficial scavenger role in clearing away debris after menstruation and pregnancy.

VARIATIONS IN THE EFFICIENCY OF DEFENCE MECHANISMS

With Age

The defences are imperfect during childhood and after the menopause when the vagina has a thin and vulnerable epithelium, when its content of glycogen and lactobacilli is low, and when its pH approaches 7. The endometrium is also poorly developed or atrophied at these ages and does not undergo cyclical shedding and reformation.

With Menstruation

During menstruation, the cervical plug is absent and vaginal acidity is lowered by the alkaline menstrual discharge. Gonococcal infection is therefore more virulent if contracted during menstruation and is more likely to ascend to the uterus and tubes at that time. Similarly, Trichomonas vaginitis tends to occur or relapse during menstruation.

During the Puerperium

In the adult woman, the genital tract defences are the weakest during and immediately after abortion or labour because: There is a raw placental site; there are often breaks in the epithelial linings of the cervix and vagina; the tissues are bruised and devitalised; the vulva, vagina, and cervix are wide open; the discharge of liquor and lochia (both alkaline) reduces vaginal acidity; degenerating blood clots and fragments of decidua offer a nidus for infection; and the patient's general resistance is lowered by the strain of pregnancy and possibly by anaemia and malnutrition.

These circumstances are the basis of what was, in the past, the scourge of midwifery—puerperal sepsis—and which, with the development of antibiotic resistance by organisms, is again becoming a threat **(Figs. 1 and 2)**.

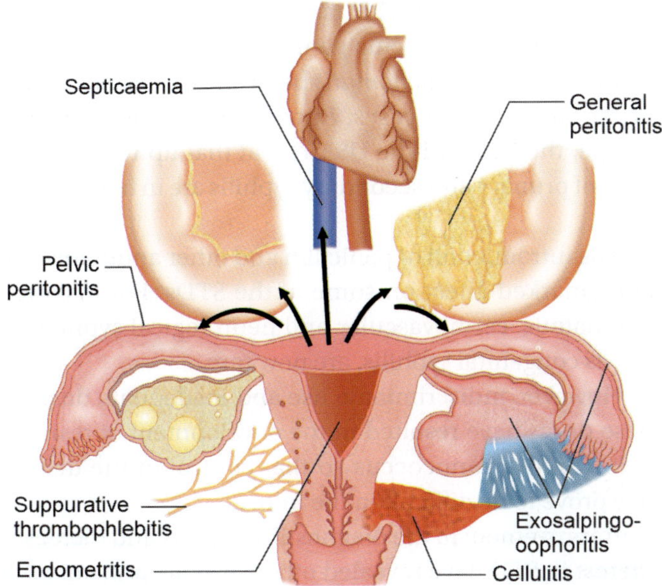

Fig. 1: Diagrammatic representation of the mode of spread and lesions produced in puerperal (including postabortal) infection.

TYPES OF INFECTING ORGANISMS

The organisms commonly causing infection of the genital tract are *Treponema pallidum, Neisseria gonorrhoeae, Gardnerella vaginalis, Haemophilus ducreyi, Prevotella* spp., *Bacteroides, Peptostreptococcus, Calymmatobacterium granulomatis, Chlamydia trachomatis, Mycobacterium tuberculosis (MTB)*, the parasite *Trichomonas vaginalis, Candida albicans*, the viruses herpes simplex virus (HSV) types 1 and 2, human papillomavirus (HPV), and the greatest scourge of recent times—the human immunodeficiency virus (HIV).

Almost all the pathogenic organisms known, however, can be responsible at times and those worthy of mention are: *Streptococcus* (aerobic and anaerobic, haemolytic and non-haemolytic species), *Staphylococcus, Pneumococcus, Escherichia coli, Clostridium tetani, Clostridium welchii, Salmonella typhi* and *S. paratyphi*, the *Actinomycetes* and other *Streptothrix* organisms, the filarial worms, *Schistosoma haematobium*, and amoebae.

Many of the above organisms, even *C. welchii*, are frequently found in the vagina without being pathogenic. Their presence may represent either a normal or a carrier state.

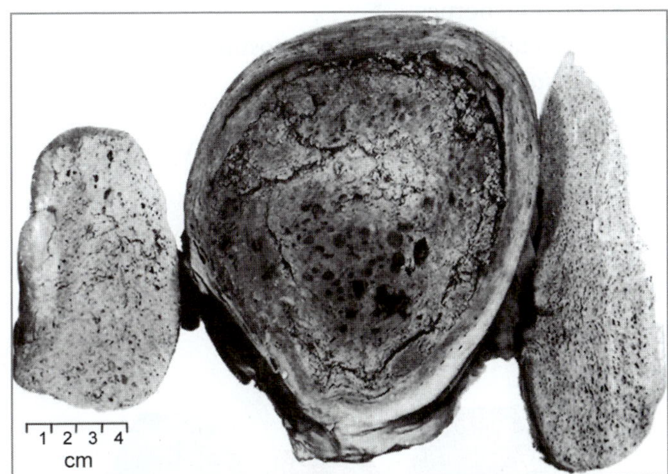

Fig. 2: Puerperal infection caused by *Clostridium welchii*. A primigravida aged 20 years was found to be suffering from hydatid form mole, and bougies were inserted into the uterus in an attempt to induce labour. The patient died 4 days later with signs of an overwhelming infection. This was in the days prior to the discovery of sulphonamides and antibiotics. The specimens obtained at autopsy are, from left to right, a portion of the spleen, the uterus with the products of conception still retained and a slice of liver. All the tissues are riddled with gas-containing spaces.

SEXUALLY TRANSMITTED DISEASES

Sexually transmitted diseases (STDs), also called venereal diseases, after Venus, the Greek goddess of love, are infections acquired during heterosexual or homosexual intercourse with an infected partner.

Various Types of Sexually Transmitted Diseases

Historically, they comprised only three common bacterial infections:

1. Gonorrhoea
2. Syphilis
3. Chancroid

Other Sexually Transmitted Infections

Many other infections of the female genital tract can be acquired by intercourse with an infected partner but can also arise in other ways; in some cases, the latter are the more important. The following infections can, or possibly can, be transmitted during the close bodily contact involved in coitus **(Fig. 3)**.

- *Viral:*
  - HIV infection and acquired immunodeficiency syndrome (AIDS)
  - Genital HPV
  - Genital herpes
  - Genital molluscum contagiosum
- *Bacterial:*
  - *C. trachomatis* infections
  - Lymphogranuloma venereum (LGV)
  - Genital mycoplasmas
  - Granuloma inguinale

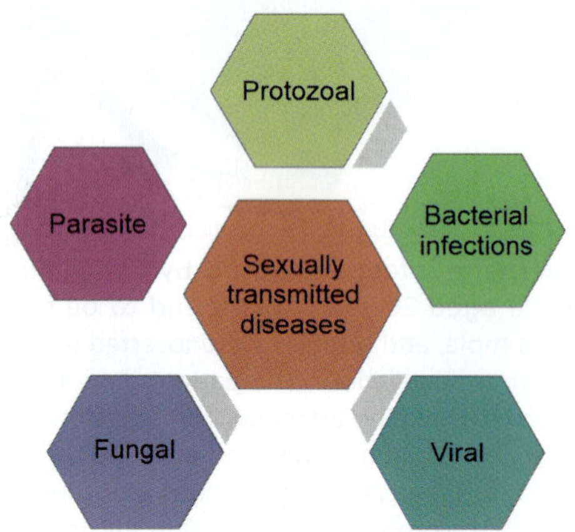

Fig. 3: Sexually transmitted infections.

- *Protozoal:*
  - Trichomoniasis
- *Fungal:*
  - Vulvovaginal candidiasis
- *Parasite:*
  - Pediculosis pubis
  - Genital scabies

Bearing in mind its relationship to the previous practice of coitus and infection with HPV, some would now include carcinoma of the cervix occurring in later life as a STD.

Hepatitis B virus is a major cause of acute and chronic liver disease including primary liver cancer. The detection of the virus in saliva suggests that sexual transmission may be involved, and there is good evidence for infection resulting from both heterosexual and homosexual contacts. Direct transmission from the mother to the foetus or a neonate is also of importance in areas where the carrier rate is high. The development of an effective vaccine offers hope of controlling the spread of the virus.

The true incidence of STDs is difficult to determine, and all figures are an underestimate, as 80–90% of cases are treated privately and not reported. Throughout the world, increasing numbers of cases of syphilis and gonorrhoea are being reported annually along with other STDs. One important factor is that worldwide, there are more people at risk each year. The expectation of life has increased, especially for women, so that the lowering of the age of puberty combined with a longer span of healthy life provides a much greater period for acquiring STD.

The incidence of STD is rising. The most common condition is a nonspecific genital infection (urethritis in the male), with *C. trachomatis* being probably responsible for 40–50% of these cases. Reports from major cities in Europe, the UK, and the USA reveal that up to 70% of all cases of primary and secondary syphilis are in homosexual males.

The introduction of penicillin and other antibiotics has had a marked effect on some of the STDs. For instance, gummatous, cardiovascular and neurological syphilis, as well as congenital syphilis, are now rare.

However, indiscriminate use and inadequate doses of these drugs have resulted in the development of resistant strains of the gonococcus so that control of the disease may prove to be difficult in the future.

Improvement in the diagnostic methods and increased interest in STD have revealed other sexually transmissible agents, several of which are viral. The manifestations of this group of diseases vary from local discomfort to chronic disability, infertility, ectopic gestation, stillbirth, and neonatal death. Cases of urethritis and cervicitis due to *Chlamydia*, *Gardnerella*, and other agents greatly outnumber new cases of gonorrhoea and are increasing rapidly.

Many patients with STD are between 18 and 24 years, and in recent years, there has been a marked increase in the number of girls aged between 16 and 17 years. The radical changes in attitudes to sex and in sexual behaviour during the past 25 years have resulted in a marked increase in STD. This is the price that girls and women everywhere are paying for their sexual liberation.

The reasons for the world crisis in STD are as follows:

- *Promiscuity:* This, the weakening of family life and the fact that modern conditions of life provide more opportunity for promiscuous behaviour are the most important factors. With so many individuals in any community having asymptomatic infections, it requires relatively few partners before an infected one is encountered.
  - Modern methods of contraception, such as the oral contraceptive pill and intrauterine contraceptive devices (IUCDs), do not offer protection as did the older barrier methods, and at the same time they may encourage casual intercourse.
  - Development of antibiotic-resistant organisms
  - Shifts in the population and overseas travel
  - Increase in world population and life expectancy
- *Ignorance of the risk of becoming infected:* The youth of today, especially in urban areas, is generally better informed on all matters pertaining to sex. But many refuse to accept that STD is anything more serious than the common cold and believe that it is readily cured without leaving any permanent ill effect. They adopt toward it an attitude of indifference if not contempt.
  - Multiple sexual partners, heterosexual partners, men who have sex with men (MSM), HIV positive patients and patients with tuberculosis (TB) are at a high risk of contracting sexually transmitted infections (STIs) **(Box 1)**.

BOX 1: Genital discharge causative organisms.

- Gonorrhoea
- Chlamydia
- *Candida*
- *Trichomonas*
- Bacterial vaginosis

Syphilis

Aetiology

Syphilis is caused by a spirochaete, *T. pallidum*, and this organism is to be found in all lesions—primary, secondary and tertiary. This disease is sometimes congenital (transplacental, from 9th week of gestation) but is usually acquired by direct contact with another person who has an open primary or secondary syphilitic lesion. One thirds of people having sexual intercourse with an infected person will develop syphilis. It may be spread by heterosexual or homosexual contact. It can also occur in drug abusers and through blood transfusion. The site of infection may be on the hands as a consequence of touching a syphilitic lesion, a risk to which doctors and nurses are especially exposed if there is a break in their skin or mucous membrane.

Here, we are mainly concerned with syphilitic lesions of the female genital tract acquired as a result of sexual intercourse. Patients with syphilis may have coexisting HIV infection. There are approximately 18 million prevalent cases of syphilis worldwide [World Health Organization (WHO) 2016].

Clinical Features

Primary stage: The primary lesion or chancre **(Fig. 4)** is found most commonly on the labium majus, labium minus, fourchette, clitoris, urethral orifice or cervix, but it may be anywhere on the lower genital tract, even the vaginal wall. In 10% of cases, more than one primary lesion is present. The chancre usually appears 10–20 days after exposure, but the incubation period may be as long as

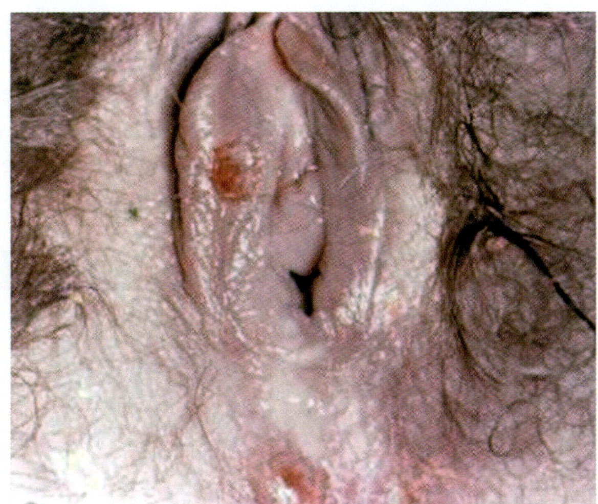

Fig. 4: Syphilis chancre.

90 days. The first manifestation is a small papule, which quickly breaks down to form an ulcer, the classical features of which are a sharply defined serpiginous outline and a brownish red colour. In practice, however, the lesion is often so slight that it passes unnoticed, and it rarely has the characters of the typical chancre with a hard base as seen in the male. Indeed, any sort of discrete relatively *painless* ulceration on the vulva may be a primary syphilitic lesion. An inflammatory reaction in the surrounding tissues is unusual but oedema can be present.

On the cervix, a chancre commences as a grey or purple nodule but, when it ulcerates, can resemble an erosion and may be mistaken for one. Sometimes, it presents as a diffuse induration of the cervix. Primary chancre usually heals in 3–8 weeks.

The inguinal glands enlarge when the primary chancre is on the vulva or lower vagina. They are hard and shotty but painless and do not suppurate.

Secondary stage: The primary chancre heals spontaneously in 3–8 weeks and soon afterward the secondary stage of syphilis, which results from entry of the spirochaetes into the bloodstream, is manifested by general systemic upset with lassitude, anorexia, headaches, and pyrexia, which is usually less severe than in the male; macular, papular, or pustular skin rashes, which are typically nonirritant, pleomorphic, bilaterally symmetrical in distribution and copper coloured; occasional loss of scalp hair; white mucous patches in, or ulceration of, the mouth and pharynx; generalised adenitis—symmetrical enlargement of the epitrochlear glands is said to be diagnostic; iritis; and condylomata lata on the vulva and around the anus—these differ from the common multiple warts (condylomata acuminata) **(Box 2)** in that they are coarse, flat-topped, moist and necrotic **(Fig. 5)**.

Sometimes, secondary manifestations occur before the primary heals, or they may not occur at all. The first and second stages can last up to 2 years, during which time the woman is a source of infection. Secondary syphilis may also cause hepatitis, glomerulonephritis (mediated by antibody treponeme complex deposition) and splenomegaly. A small percentage of patients may develop meningitis or eye manifestations during secondary syphilis.

Tertiary stage: In untreated syphilis, this stage occupies many years during which the spirochaetes attack bones, joints, eyes, blood vessels, heart and central nervous system (CNS). Tertiary syphilis is also characterised by the formation of localised granulomas (gummas) in any part of the body. Gummas of critical organs such as heart, brain and liver can be fatal. Gummas of the genital tract are rare, but when they do occur, they are most often found on the vulva where they break down to form ulcers with a serpiginous outline and surrounding oedema. They are not painful unless secondarily infected. These late forms are rarely seen nowadays.

Latent syphilis: After infection with *T. pallidum*, there are periods when the patient is seroreactive but shows no evidence of disease. They should all be evaluated for signs of tertiary disease.

Syphilis in Pregnancy

Syphilis can be transmitted transplacentally in any stage in pregnancy. It can present as miscarriage, preterm labour, foetal distress, intrauterine device (IUD), hydrops, polyhydramnios and congenital syphilis. Maternal HIV coinfection can increase the risk of syphilis transmission. It is recommended to screen all antenatal women for

BOX 2: Differential diagnosis of anogenital warts.

- Condyloma acuminata—human papillomavirus (HPV)
- Molluscum contagiosum
- Skin tags
- Seborrhoeic keratosis
- Secondary syphilis
- Other sexually transmitted infections (STIs)
- Intraepithelial neoplasia
- Malignancy

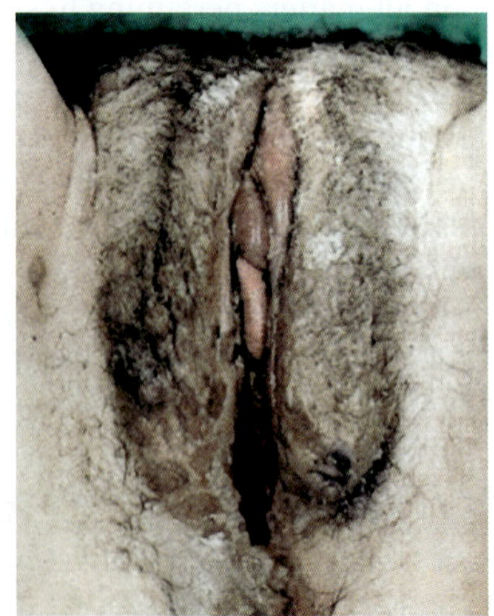

Fig. 5: Secondary syphilitic lesions on the vulva. These consist of brownish, slightly raised plaques and a few flat-topped, coarse condylomas.

syphilis at the first visit. In case of high-risk women, the test should be repeated in the third trimester.

Congenital syphilis can be early (with 2 years) or late (after 2 years). Manifestations of early syphilis include rash, haemorrhagic rhinitis, generalised lymphadenopathy, hepatosplenomegaly and skeletal abnormalities. Involvement of bone, kidney and CNS may occur. Late congenital syphilis can cause keratitis, Clutton's joints, Hutchison's incisors, high palatial arch, perioral fissures, deafness, bossing, short maxilla, saddle nose and intellectual disability.

Infants born to mother with syphilis: They should undergo serological test on infant blood (not cord blood) and should be examined for signs of congenital syphilis.

Diagnosis

The diagnosis during the primary stage is made by examining serum from the base of the primary chancre for the presence of *T. pallidum*, using dark-ground illumination microscopy. Treponemas can also be seen in fluid from most lesions of secondary syphilis. Routine culture of the organism is not yet possible. Polymerase chain reaction (PCR) test can also be used in secretions to diagnose syphilis.

Serological tests are positive in all but the earliest stage of primary syphilis (they are negative until about 2 weeks after the appearance of the chancre, i.e. about 3–5 weeks after infection) and sometimes in very late syphilis. In suspected congenital syphilis or when the infection has progressed beyond the second stage, the diagnosis can only be determined by serological tests. The serological tests for syphilis may be grouped into those which are nonspecific or nontreponemal and those which are specific or treponemal. Most laboratories carry out a test of each type. The nonspecific tests are complement fixation or flocculation tests. The Wassermann reaction (WR) test was the prototype of complement fixation tests and in its various modified forms remains the mainstay of this type of test. A flocculation type of test for a non-specific antibody, regain, namely the venereal disease research laboratory (VDRL) slide test, is the most commonly used nonspecific test for screening purposes. The VDRL test may be positive in the absence of specific tests, i.e. a biological false-positive reaction. This can occur in pregnancy, during or shortly after any infective illness such as infectious mononucleosis, measles, chickenpox, mumps, HSV, herpes zoster or viral pneumonia, or following recent immunisation. The false-positive reactions are of a temporary nature but may persist in certain chronic diseases such as leprosy, TB, and autoimmune diseases (lupus erythematosus, haemolytic anaemia, thyroiditis, and rheumatoid arthritis). Antibody to cardiolipin is also measured by the rapid plasma regain (RPR) test. Although this is an autoantibody (hence the term *non-treponemal antibody*), it provides a useful marker of activity of disease and is helpful in follow-up, especially where only a few samples are being run at a time.

Specific antibody tests include: Treponemal enzyme immunoassay (EIA) or treponemal chemiluminescence immunoassay (CLIA); *Treponema pallidum* haemagglutination assay (TPHA); *Treponema pallidum* particle agglutination assay (TPPA), fluorescent treponemal antibody absorption test (FTA-abs), *Treponema pallidum* immunoblot, and *T. pallidum*-specific immunoglobulin M (IgM) antibody tests: Antitreponemal IgM EIA and immunoblot.

Tests should be repeated after 2 or 3 weeks to ensure that no test has become positive during that time, as can occur in early syphilis. In high-risk situations, repeating the test in the third trimester of pregnancy is recommended. Once positive, the VDRL may remain positive for life. A quantitative RPR/VDRL test is recommended for monitoring the serological response to treatment.

Interpretation of the serological tests may be difficult if there is a past history of other treponemal infections, particularly the non-venereal tropical disease yaws, which is endemic in the West Indies. The causative organism of yaws, *Treponema pertenue*, is morphologically identical to *T. pallidum* and gives indistinguishable serological results. As well as giving positive serological tests, this disease also has three stages—(1) primary granulomas or papules, (2) desquamation, and (3) ulceration—and can cause visceral and periostotic lesions. The skin lesions are commonly seen on the vulva, breasts and legs. In the absence of a satisfactory history of treatment for yaws, the patient should be regarded as having a treponemal disease, which might be syphilis and treated accordingly.

Treatment

The treatment of syphilis is a matter for the specialist venereologist. Screening for other STDs should be done. Sexual contact with an infected person should be refrained until the lesions of early syphilis are completely cured or first follow-up of serology shows cure.

Local treatment is useless because the spirochaetes invade deeply and spread by vascular channels at an early stage. The best medication for early syphilis is penicillin to which the treponemes have not so far developed a resistance. A single dose of 2.4 million units (MU) of benzathine penicillin intramuscularly (IM) appears to cure primary or secondary syphilis. If there is any doubt about the duration of disease or where it is known to have been present for longer than a year, 3 weekly doses of 2.4 MU are recommended. Intramuscular injection of 600,000 units of aqueous procaine penicillin daily for 10–14 days is equally efficient. The treponemes usually disappear from active lesions within 24 hours, and serological tests become negative in weeks or months. Observation for 2 years following treatment is desirable.

For patients sensitive to penicillin, doxycycline (100 mg twice daily for 14 days), ceftriaxone (1 g IM daily for 10–14 days), oxytetracycline (500 mg 6 hourly for 14 days) or erythromycin (500 mg 6 hourly for 30 days) may be substituted. However, both erythromycin and tetracyclines are less effective in treating syphilis compared to penicillin. Late syphilis is also treated with penicillin, but the schemes of dosage and number of courses vary with its manifestations. Treatment should be preceded by radiological examination of the heart and aorta and by tests on the cerebrospinal fluid (CSF).

The rare Jarisch–Herxheimer reaction is a minor acute febrile reaction of this type accompanied by headache, myalgia and other symptoms, which occurs in 50% of patients after the first administration of any therapy for syphilis, and warning of this should be given. It is seen particularly when there are lesions in the larynx, meninges, heart and aorta, but can be seen in one third of patients of primary syphilis and two thirds of secondary syphilis. Therapy need not be discontinued. Most cases can be managed by reassurance of the patient and administration of ibuprofen or aspirin. Prednisolone is not usually necessary.

In pregnancy, the treatment is the same as above. The woman who is allergic to penicillin should be treated with ceftriaxone. Erythromycin does not reliably cure the foetus. Doxycycline should not be used in pregnancy.

The baby should be assessed at birth, and at 6 weeks and 3 months after birth. Penicillin treatment is indicated in infants with suspected congenital syphilis, or whose mothers were treated inadequately, documentation is missing, treated <4 weeks prior to delivery and treated with non-penicillin regimens.

Gonorrhoea

Gonorrhoea is the second most common bacterial STI.

Pathology and Clinical Features

Gonorrhoea is an infection caused by a gram-negative diplococcus—*N. gonorrhoeae* (the gonococcus)—and, in the adult woman, is contracted by sexual contact with an infected male. Transfer by other means is little more than a theoretical possibility except in babies, who can be infected during their passage through the birth canal, the most serious result being ophthalmia neonatorum. There is usually an interval of 2–5 days between the exposure and the development of symptoms, but this interval varies from 1 to 10 days. However, an asymptomatic carrier state can persist for weeks or even months, and throughout this time infection can be transmitted. The bacteria attack first those tissues of the lower genital tract which are not covered by stratified squamous epithelium—the endocervix, the urethra (including the paraurethral tubules) and the ducts and acini of Bartholin's glands **(Fig. 6)**. Gonococci also commonly spread to the anorectum; they may sometimes be implanted there during anal coitus. Infection can also occur in conjunctiva.

The initial complaints of the patient are a purulent vaginal discharge, dysuria and frequency. This discharge

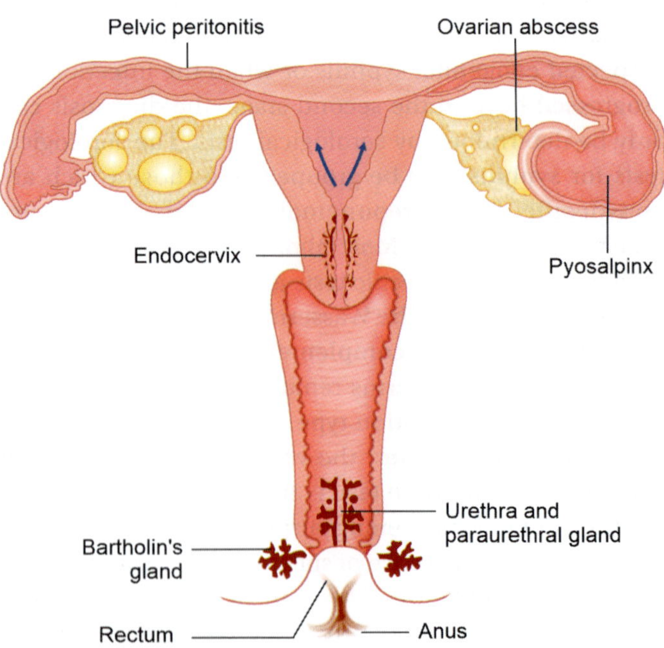

Fig. 6: Diagrammatic representation of the mode of spread and the sites of infection in gonorrhoea.

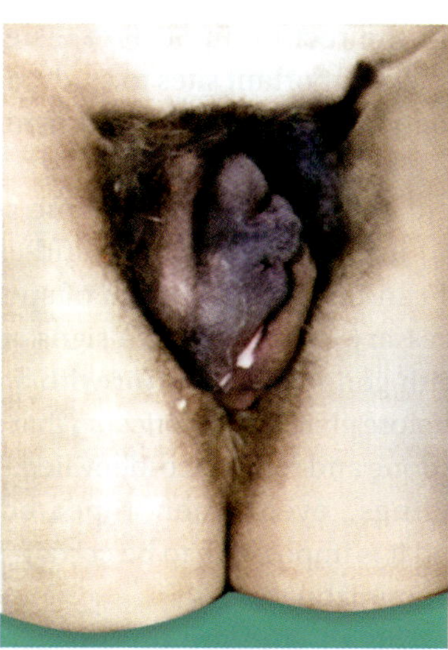

Fig. 7: Acute gonorrhoea with right-sided bartholinitis and associated oedema of the labia. The purulent discharge can be seen escaping from the vagina.

causes soreness but not pruritus unless there is an associated *Trichomonas* infection. In severe cases, the whole vulva becomes reddened and swollen **(Fig. 7)**.

When the vulvar reaction is acute, inguinal adenitis is the rule and some constitutional upset is likely. Cystitis and proctitis can develop. In exceptional cases, gonococcal septicaemia is described and may be manifested by pyrexia and even a vesicular or pustular dermatitis. Gonococcal tonsillitis or pharyngitis occurs as the result of genito-oral contact. Lesions involving joints, tendons and ligaments, once regarded as gonococcal, are usually explained by an associated nongonococcal infection (see Reiter's disease) but gonococcal arthropathy does occur, and the organisms can be cultured from the joint effusion.

Generally, the infection remains limited to the lower genital tract but, in 10% cases of proven gonorrhoea, it spreads upwards to cause salpingo-oophoritis of varying degrees. The organisms ascend through the uterus to the tubes, producing a fleeting acute endometritis on the way. The last is not clinically evident, being overshadowed by the symptoms of salpingitis. Both tubes are always involved, and the essential lesion is an endosalpingitis. The organisms pass through the abdominal ostia to produce pelvic peritonitis and oophoritis. Generalised peritonitis is rare. It has long been the belief of gynaecologists that gonococcal salpingitis is a self-limiting disease in that the bacteria in the tubes die within 3–4 weeks. Nevertheless, positive cultures are sometimes obtained as long as 6 months after the original infection.

Moreover, even if the gonococci die out, a pyosalpinx is often secondarily infected. The above is the classical clinical picture of gonorrhoea with some of its rare and even bizarre variations. It must be emphasised that it is not often encountered. Most women, even in the acute and subacute stages of the primary infection, notice nothing more than slight frequency, dysuria and slight discharge that they pay little attention to. Indeed, 60–70% of women from whom gonococci can be cultured from the lower genital tract are free from symptoms and obvious physical signs of the disease. It is they who are responsible for the spread of infection, and they can only be found and treated by an efficient system of *contact tracing*. Routine mass screening using meticulous bacteriological techniques is, according to most reports, of little value.

Even salpingitis can develop without producing an acute picture and in a subclinical degree is probably quite common. No matter whether it has a dramatic or quiet onset, gonorrhoea persists as a chronic but contagious disease for many years. The organisms linger in the endocervix, Bartholin's glands, periurethral tubules and rectum but give rise to no symptoms or, at most, to a slight chronic mucopurulent vaginal discharge.

The most important and tragic sequel to gonorrhoea is tubal damage and closure, which threaten future reproduction. Unlike the situation in the male, urethral stricture following gonococcal urethritis is almost unknown in the female. Disseminated gonococcal infection is a rare complication in <3% of cases. These patients may also present with endocarditis and meningitis. Rarely infection can spread to joints and can cause arthralgia and tenosynovitis.

Diagnosis

In the classical case, the diagnosis of gonorrhoea is usually suggested by the history of exposure, the acuteness of the onset of a purulent discharge, the associated urethritis, and the appearance of zones of congestion (maculae) around the orifices of Bartholin's ducts. In practice, it is the occurrence of urethritis in the patient's consort which often brings the woman to investigation, she herself having no symptoms.

Sixty percent of women with proven gonorrhoea also suffer from *T. vaginalis* and/or *C. trachomatis. C. albicans*, HSV, etc. are also associated. So, the disease should be suspected whenever there is a complaint of vaginal discharge.

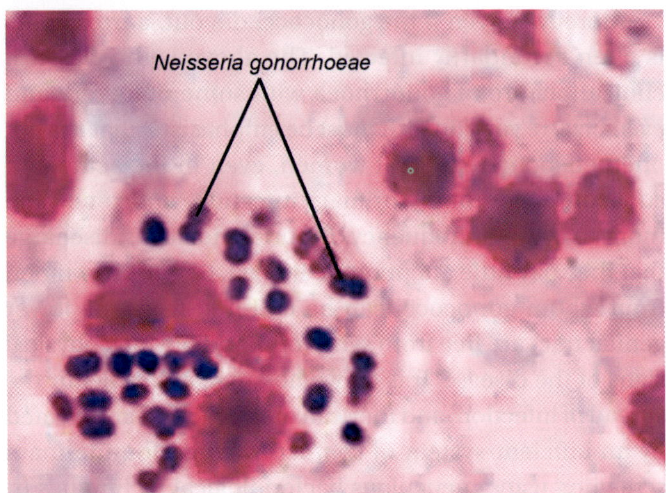

Fig. 8: Gonorrhoea diplococci.

The diagnosis can only be proved by the demonstration of gonococci in the genital tract secretions or in the lower rectum. In the female, it is rare to find typical gram-negative intracellular diplococci in direct smears of vaginal discharge **(Fig. 8)**, unless a very acute infection is present. Smear has a low sensitivity. Hence, nucleic acid amplification test (NAAT) or culture is a better method of diagnosis. The setting up of cultures is therefore mandatory, and material for these is obtained from the endocervical canal. Cultures of the urethra, anal canal and pharynx are recommended but produce only a slight increase in the yield. When gonococcal septicaemia, pharyngitis or arthritis is suspected, it is necessary also to prepare cultures from the blood, throat swabs and synovial fluid. Gonococci will survive on ordinary swabs for approximately 2 hours. A longer interval than this between the collection of specimens and their arrival in the laboratory means the use of transport media such as Stuart's agar and crystal violet, or one of the proprietary preparations in the market. Alternatively, plates of warmed chocolate agar or of Thayer-Martin medium can be inoculated directly by the patient's bedside. Sensitivity also should be tested at the time of culture.

The woman should not have passed urine or used a douche before examination. Having wiped its orifice clean, the urethra is milked to obtain discharge from the paraurethral glands. Further material is obtained by milking Bartholin's glands and their ducts. Swabs are next taken from the endocervix and finally from the anal canal and rectum. In proven cases of gonorrhoea, the organisms are found in Bartholin's ducts in 30%, in the endocervix in 90%, and in the rectum in 50–60%. The last two are therefore the most important sites to study, and it is stated that a combination of their findings provides an almost 100% accurate diagnostic test.

Nucleic acid amplification test is more sensitive than culture (>96%) in both symptomatic and asymptomatic infection and can test a wider range of specimen types. Culture is necessary in patients with signs and symptoms compatible with gonorrhoea and/or with a confirmatory NAAT result, before giving antibiotics, so that susceptibility testing can be done and resistance identified. Nevertheless, negative findings, even when repeated, are never conclusive, and it is impossible to be certain that a woman does not have gonorrhoea.

Similarly, tests of cure are unsatisfactory although negative bacteriological findings on three occasions are the accepted criteria. The best time to perform these is immediately after menstruation. Enzyme-linked immunosorbent assay (ELISA) tests have been developed, which offer greater reliability.

Whenever gonorrhoea is diagnosed or suspected, it is essential to entertain the possibility of the patient having contracted syphilis at the same time. The case must therefore also be investigated from this standpoint and, meanwhile, no treatment given which might mask, without curing, this disease.

Antibiotic sensitivity of the organism is becoming important because of the resistant or less-sensitive strains. The detection of penicillinase-producing strains of *N. gonorrhoeae,* which are totally resistant to penicillin and relatively insensitive to several other antibiotics is important as these strains are spreading throughout the world.

Treatment

Treatment is indicated in microscopy, culture and NAAT positive for *N. gonorrhoeae* from any site, recent partner of confirmed cases of gonococcal infection and following sexual assault. Patients should be advised to refrain from unprotected sexual intercourse (UPSI) for a week and should be screened for other STIs. NAATs are more sensitive than culture (>96%) in both symptomatic and asymptomatic infection and can test a wider range of specimen types. Culture is necessary in patients with signs and symptoms compatible with gonorrhoea and/or with a confirmatory NAAT result, before giving antibiotics so that susceptibility testing can be done and resistance identified.

If there is a severe systemic reaction, or if acute salpingitis is present, the patient should be put completely at rest in hospital and given intensive antibiotic therapy in divided doses. Otherwise, she can remain ambulant but should be warned against coitus until pronounced cured. Except for the drainage of an abscess, local treatment should be avoided lest it encourages the spread of infection.

The British Association for Sexual Health and HIV recommends the following antibiotic regimen: Ceftriaxone 1 g IM as a single dose or Ciprofloxacillin 500 mg orally as a single dose. Cefixime 400 mg orally as a single dose plus azithromycin 2 g orally may be recommended to patients who do not want to take injections.

Sex partners should be notified, tested and treated, especially those exposed within 2 weeks prior to onset of symptoms or 4 weeks prior to diagnosis in an asymptomatic patient. Repeat cultures for test of cure are no longer recommended for all patients as cure rates of currently used regimens approach 90%. They may be indicated if there is a doubt of patient compliance.

Chancroid (Soft Sore) (Fig. 9)

Chancroid is becoming increasingly rare everywhere but is still an important STD in some areas in developing countries. It is much more common in men than women. In north India, it still accounts for 24% of genitourinary ulcer disease.

Pathology and Clinical Features

The infection is caused by a gram-negative streptobacillus—*H. ducreyi*. The disease appears 2–5 days after coitus and takes the form of multiple small papules or vesicles which quickly break down to leave acutely painful shallow ulcers that discharge offensive pus. These are usually multiple, but can be single, and are distributed on the labia majora and minora and sometimes within the introitus and around the anus. Each ulcer is ringed with a bright red zone of congestion and surrounded by oedema. The ulcers bleed easily on gentle cleaning. Oedema is a striking physical sign. Autoinoculation from primary lesion on opposing skin leads to *kissing ulcers*.

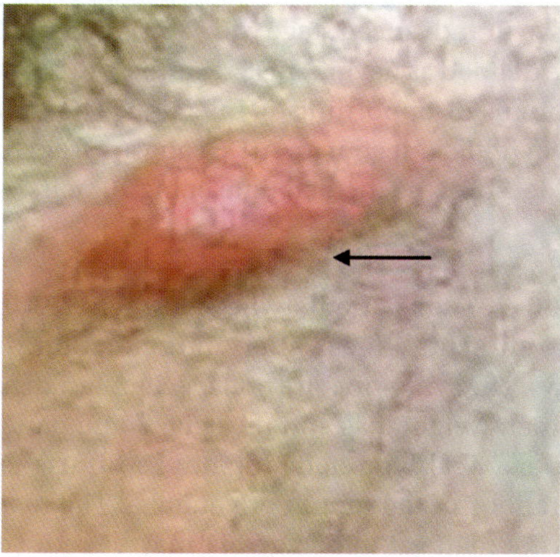

Fig. 9: Chancroid (soft sore).

The draining lymph nodes are usually unilateral and inguinal. They are painful and tender and become *matted* together in a unilocular abscess (bubo formation)—a distinguishing feature from syphilitic adenitis. Secondary infection is common and can produce much tissue destruction. Untreated, the inguinal abscess bursts onto the skin, forming a sinus. The infection does not spread and, although it can cause malaise and pyrexia, has no serious systemic effects.

Diagnosis

The clinical features may be suggestive, but the diagnosis can only be made by the demonstration of *H. ducreyi* in the discharge from the ulcers or in pus obtained by aspiration of an inguinal node or by PCR. Culture medium for growing *H. ducreyi* is not easily available. Chancroid lesions can be confused with those of Behçet's syndrome, the type and sites of the genital ulcers being identical **(Box 3)**.

Treatment

Differential clinical diagnosis is often unreliable. Hence, one should either do combined testing to rule out other genital ulcer diseases (GUDs) like syphilis and HSV-2 or use syndrome in treatment to cover all possible treatable causes. Patients should refrain from any sexual contact till completion of treatment.

BOX 3: Differential diagnosis of genital ulcer.

- *Painful:*
  - Herpes simplex viruses 1 and 2
  - Chancroid
  - Systemic conditions—Behçet's syndrome
- *Painless:*
  - Syphilis
  - Human papillomavirus (HPV)
  - Granuloma inguinale
  - Lymphogranuloma venereum (LGV)

Experience is now so limited that it is difficult to judge the best antibacterial agent to use *H. ducreyi* that were initially susceptible to sulphonamides, trimethoprim, tetracycline, streptomycin and chloramphenicol. Presently, azithromycin (1 g orally single dose), erythromycin (500 mg 6 hourly for 7 days) or ceftriaxone (250 mg IM single dose) are the recommended drugs. Erythromycin or ceftriaxone should be used in pregnancy, lactation and children. No adverse effect of chancroid on foetus and pregnancy has been noted.

Along with antibiotics, the patient is advised to rest during the acute stage of ulceration and her pain can be relieved with analgesics. If the inguinal nodes suppurate, the abscesses are aspirated from adjacent healthy skin. Healing usually occurs within 2 weeks.

Test of cure is not recommended. Sexual partners of last 10 days should be examined and treated even in absence of symptoms as asymptomatic carriage can occur. Screening is not recommended.

Human Immunodeficiency Virus Infection and Acquired Immunodeficiency Syndrome

Acquired immunodeficiency syndrome is a disease of the immune system caused by a retrovirus, the HIV that results in the development of either life-threatening opportunistic infections or the development of unusual malignant lesions or both. Although AIDS is classified as an infectious disease, its transmission requires sexual contact or direct entry of virus-infected blood or blood products into the circulation. There is little evidence that AIDS is transmitted by any nonsexual form of person-to-person contact.

The first recognised cases of AIDS occurred in male homosexuals, and such individuals constitute the main risk group (about three quarters of reported cases occur in homosexual or *bisexual* males). Drug users who share infected needles constitute another high-risk group. AIDS has been diagnosed in female sexual partners of affected males, and this is the predominant mode of transmission today, although this has always been the case in Africa. Vertical transmission occurs from mother to foetus. In Asia, the infection is now moving into the low-risk general population and is likely to move from the urban to the rural areas. Occupational transmission of HIV from patients to health care and laboratory workers is a small but definite risk. While the converse is theoretically possible, it is very rare.

Human immunodeficiency virus has been isolated from the blood, semen and saliva of affected individuals. Some individuals who have been exposed to, or are infected by, the virus do not show any evidence of such disease. This suggests either a long incubation period or the operation of other factors during the incubation period which, together with the HIV, precipitate the loss of cell-mediated immunity. It is estimated that 36 million people are infected with HIV, with approximately two thirds in Africa and one fourth in Asia. Explosive patterns of the disease are being seen in India and Thailand. In the 21st century, it is expected that the magnitude of the epidemic in these regions will exceed that in sub-Saharan Africa.

Pathology

The human immunodeficiency viruses, HIV-1 and HIV-2, belong to the family of human retroviruses and the subfamily of lentiviruses. HIV-1 is the most common cause of HIV disease throughout the world, but different subtypes are prevalent in different areas. HIV-2 was originally seen in West Africa, but it has now been identified in Europe and America as well. Infections with HIV-2 tend to be less severe than HIV-1. Some individuals may have infection with both HIV-1 and HIV-2.

Human immunodeficiency virus infection results in a progressive decline in the number and function of helper T lymphocytes, e.g. the CD4 cells and monocytes. This results in the development of a profound immunodeficiency state with clinical manifestations in virtually all systems of the body.

CD4 counts >800 cells/mm^3 are considered normal. In the early stage of disease, the count is >500 cells mm^3 and in the intermediate stage 200–500 cells mm^3. HIV-positive patients in the advanced stage with CD4 counts < 200 cells/mm^3 are defined as having AIDS regardless of the presence of symptoms or opportunistic infection. The duration of time from initial infection to AIDS can vary from 3 years to several decades, the median time being 10 years.

Clinical Features

About 30–70% of patients who contract HIV infection develop an acute illness after an incubation period of 7–10 days. The symptoms are nonspecific, i.e. fatigue, fever, sore throat, weight loss and myalgia. Some patients may develop cervical lymphadenopathy, a diffuse skin rash or ulcerations of the mouth or genitalia. The diagnosis is usually not made at this stage but may be retrospectively diagnosed later in the course of the illness.

In the stage of clinical latency, patients may remain entirely asymptomatic. As CD4 counts decline, the appearance of an opportunistic infection may be the first manifestation of HIV disease. Persistent generalised lymphadenopathy is also a feature of early symptomatic disease.

Oral manifestations develop in almost all patients at some point in the course of their disease depending on the type, frequency and severity of disease. Various manifestations seen in the early stage include oral hairy leucoplakia, candidiasis, HSV infection, aphthous ulcers and gingivitis. Impaired skin immunity leads to cutaneous manifestations: Molluscum contagiosum, herpes zoster, HSV infection, seborrhoeic dermatitis, scabies and folliculitis. Thrombocytopenia manifests as bleeding gums, petechiae and easy bruisability. Peripheral neuropathy can occur at all stages of the disease. Aseptic meningitis occurs in all but the very late stages. Later in the course of the disease, HIV-infected individuals present with oesophagitis, diarrhoea, malabsorption and weight loss. There is a 10-fold increase in the incidence of pneumonia. *Pneumocystis carinii* pneumonia (PCP) is pathognomonic of AIDS and is generally seen when CD4 count is <200 cells/mm^3. Similarly, TB is also generally seen with CD4 counts of <200 cells/mm^3. While pulmonary TB in early-stage HIV has a presentation similar to that in non-HIV patients, AIDS patients have an atypical presentation characterised by diffuse pulmonary infiltrates.

Other secondary infections include infection with *Toxoplasma gondii, Cryptosporidiidae, Cryptococcus, Cytomegalovirus, T. pallidum, Histoplasma*, and *Bartonella*. Kaposi's sarcoma is another presentation virtually pathognomonic of AIDS.

Ocular manifestations are seen, the most serious being cytomegalovirus retinitis. Endocrine disorders in these patients may be consequent to general debility. These include adrenal insufficiency and hypogonadism. HIV-associated nephropathy, myocarditis or dilated cardiomyopathy has also been described. Infection of the CNS results in an AIDS-dementia complex in the majority of patients late in the course of the illness. Seizures occur frequently and may be caused by neoplasms, opportunistic infections or HIV encephalopathy.

Mother-to-infant transmission occurs in about 25% of cases. The risk is increased in advanced stages of the disease and higher levels of viral replication, and now with highly affective retroviral therapy (HAART) the infection of foetus can be prevented.

The incidence of pelvic inflammatory disease (PID) and preinvasive lesions of cervix and carcinoma cervix is more common in women with HIV, and regular screening for carcinoma cervix is warranted. These infected women are more prone to developing *Candidiasis*.

The WHO clinical staging for HIV/AIDS for adults and adolescents, 2006 divides patients into four stages depending on the severity of symptoms as given in **Table 1**.

Diagnosis

The diagnosis of HIV infection requires the demonstration of antibodies to HIV or its direct detection. Three rapid tests are done and if all three are positive, a diagnosis of HIV is made. If the results are indeterminate, the Western blot test is done and is considered positive if it contains bands to at least two of the following gene products: *p24*, *gp41*, and *gp120/160*. If the Western blot test is indeterminate, it is repeated after 1 month.

A PCR test can also be done and is the most specific. Deoxyribonucleic acid (DNA) and ribonucleic acid (RNA) PCR are both possible. The high cost of PCR and the problem of false-positive results due to contamination have resulted in it being used only when standard serologic tests fail to provide a definite answer.

Human immunodeficiency (HIV-1) disease markers such as CD4 cell count and plasma HIV-1 RNA levels are important indicators of disease stage and are used in laboratory monitoring of patients.

Treatment

Counselling of the patient regarding the natural history of the disease, transmission, nature and goals of therapy should be done in all cases. Support systems with qualified personnel are essential. Before starting, a thorough assessment of the patient should be done and any opportunistic infections like TB must be identified. All baseline investigations must be done.

Minimum baseline investigations:

- Haemogram/complete blood count (CBC)
- Urine for routine and microscopic examination
- Fasting blood sugar
- Blood urea and serum creatinine
- Serum bilirubin, alanine aminotransferase (ALT), serum glutamic-pyruvic transaminase (SGPT)
- VDRL

TABLE 1: WHO staging for HIV/AIDS for adults and adolescents, 2006.

Adults and adolescents	***Children***
Clinical stage 1	
• Asymptomatic • Persistent generalised lymphadenopathy (PGL)	• Asymptomatic • PGL
Clinical stage 2	
• Moderate unexplained weight loss (<10% of presumed or measured body weight) • Recurrent respiratory tract infections (sinusitis, tonsillitis, otitis media, pharyngitis) • Herpes zoster • Angular cheilitis • Recurrent oral ulceration • Papular pruritic eruption • Fungal nail infections • Seborrhoeic dermatitis	• Unexplained persistent hepatosplenomegaly • Recurrent or chronic upper respiratory tract infections (otitis media, otorrhoea, sinusitis, tonsillitis) • Herpes zoster • Lineal gingival erythema • Recurrent oral ulceration • Papular pruritic eruption • Fungal nail infections • Extensive wart virus infection • Extensive molluscum contagiosum • Unexplained persistent parotid enlargement
Clinical stage 3	
• Unexplained severe weight loss (>10% of the presumed or measured body weight) • Unexplained chronic diarrhoea for >1 month • Unexplained persistent fever (intermittent or constant for longer than 1 month) • Persistent oral candidiasis • Oral hairy leucoplakia • Pulmonary tuberculosis • Severe bacterial infections (such as pneumonia, empyema, pyomyositis, bone or joint infection, meningitis, and bacteraemia) • Acute necrotising ulcerative stomatitis, gingivitis or periodontitis • Unexplained anaemia (<8 g/dL), neutropenia ($<0.5 \times 10^9$/L) and/or chronic thrombocytopaenia ($<50 \times 10^9$/L)	• Unexplained moderate malnutrition not adequately responding to standard therapy • Unexplained persistent diarrhoea (14 days or more) • Unexplained persistent fever (above 37.5°C, intermittent or constant, for longer than 1 month) • Persistent oral candidiasis (after the first 6 weeks of life) • Oral hairy leucoplakia • Lymph node tuberculosis • Pulmonary tuberculosis • Severe recurrent bacterial pneumonia • Acute necrotising ulcerative gingivitis or periodontitis • Unexplained anaemia (<8 g/dL), neutropenia ($<0.5 \times 10^9$/L) or chronic thrombocytopaenia (50,000/L) • Symptomatic lymphoid interstitial pneumonitis • Chronic HIV-associated lung disease, including bronchiectasis
Clinical stage 4	
• HIV wasting syndrome • Pneumocystis (jirovecii) pneumonia • Recurrent severe bacterial pneumonia • Chronic herpes simplex infection (orolabial, genital or anorectal of >1 month duration or visceral at any site) • Oesophageal candidiasis (or candidiasis of trachea, bronchi or lungs) • Extrapulmonary tuberculosis • Kaposi's sarcoma • Cytomegalovirus infection (retinitis or infection of other organs) • *Central nervous system:* Toxoplasmosis • HIV encephalopathy • Extrapulmonary cryptococcosis, including meningitis • Disseminated nontuberculous mycobacterial infection (NTM) • Progressive multifocal leucoencephalopathy (PML) • Chronic cryptosporidiosis • Chronic isosporiasis • Disseminated mycosis (extrapulmonary histoplasmosis, and coccidioidomycosis) • Lymphoma (cerebral or B-cell non-Hodgkin's) • Symptomatic HIV-associated nephropathy or cardiomyopathy	• Unexplained severe wasting, stunting or severe malnutrition not responding to standard therapy • Pneumocystis (jirovecii) pneumonia • Recurrent severe bacterial infections (such as empyema, pyomyositis, bone or joint infection, meningitis, but excluding pneumonia) • Chronic herpes simplex infection (orolabial or cutaneous of >1 month duration or visceral at any site) • Oesophageal candidiasis (or candidiasis of trachea, bronchi or lungs) • Extrapulmonary tuberculosis • Kaposi's sarcoma • Cytomegalovirus infection (retinitis or infection of other organs with onset at age >1 month) • *Central nervous system:* Toxoplasmosis (after the neonatal period) • HIV encephalopathy • Extrapulmonary cryptococcosis, including meningitis • Disseminated NTM • PML

(AIDS: acquired immunodeficiency syndrome; HIV: human immunodeficiency virus; WHO: World Health Organization)

- CD4 count
- Chest X-ray posteroanterior (PA) view.

Antiretroviral therapy (ART) is the cornerstone of treatment. Zidovudine (ZDV) was the first drug used. It is a nucleoside analogue which functions as a reverse transcriptase inhibitor. Its major side effect is bone marrow suppression. Proximal myopathy is also commonly seen. Emergence of strains, which are resistant to ZDV, has limited its use as a long-term monotherapy **(Table 2)**.

There has been a rapid decline in HIV-related mortality and morbidity due to the wider availability of affordable, more efficacious and less toxic antiretroviral (ARV) drugs over the last two decades. ART uses a combination of three different classes of drugs to suppress viral load. Continued suppression of viral load improves immune functions and prolongs survival. HIV infection now is a chronically manageable disease. ART cannot cure HIV infection. However, it suppresses the viral load and improves immune functions.

All patients with HIV must be started on ART medication, irrespective of clinical stage or CD4 count. They need lifelong treatment and should be counselled about the need for taking medications lifelong. A combination of tenofovir (TDF 300 mg) + lamivudine (3TC 300 mg) + dolutegravir (DTG 50 mg) regimen is taken as a fixed-drug combination as a single pill. Patients with severe diabetes and hypertension should be monitored more closely for TDF toxicity. Patients on DTG must be monitored for weight gain and development of diabetes. Viral load declines to <1,000 copies/mL when on treatment. If the viral copies remain >1,000 copies/mL, they should be referred to an ART specialist for further treatment.

Prophylaxis for *P. carinii* pneumonia is started in all patients with clinical stages 3 and 4 and those with CD4 <350 cells/mm^3.

The management of opportunistic infections is a very important aspect of care of the AIDS patient. Treatment regimens for all opportunistic infections have been clearly defined.

Prevention of HIV infection requires education of all adolescents and adults regarding the method of spread of disease, safe sexual practices, use of disposables and testing of blood products.

Regular use of condoms can prevent HIV infection in a large number of cases. The addition of nonoxynol-9 improves the protection as it is toxic to HIV. It also improves the contraceptive efficacy. Partners of HIV-positive patients must be instructed in the use of condom protection even if they are using other contraceptive methods. Physicians and surgeons must observe universal precautions at all times as 90% of HIV-infected individuals are asymptomatic. Screening for cervical cancer is important in patients with HIV. If three annual smears are negative, patients should go for 3-year pap smear.

Genital Human Papillomavirus

Papillomaviruses are a group of small DNA viruses that produce epithelial cell proliferation (papillomas). More than 30 HPV types infect the genital tract. These have been grouped into high- and low-risk types, based on the malignant potential.

Pathology and Clinical Features

Human papilloma viruses are epitheliotropic, and their replication depends on the presence of differentiating

TABLE 2: Classes of drugs available.

Nucleoside reverse transcriptase inhibitor (NRTI)	*Nonnucleoside reverse transcriptase inhibitor (NNRTI)*	*Protease inhibitor*	*Nucleotide reverse transcriptase inhibitors (NtRTI)*	*Fusion inhibitor*	*Integrase inhibitor*	*Ccr5 entry inhibitor*	*Post-attachment maturation inhibitor*
Zidovudine	Nevirapine	Saquinavir	Tenofovir	Enfuvirtide	Dolutegravir	Maraviroc	Ibalizumab
Stavudine	Efavirenz	Ritonavir			Raltegravir		
Lamivudine	Delavirdine	Nelfinavir			Elvitegravir		
Didanosine		Amprenavir			Bictegravir		
Zalcitabine		Indinavir			Cabotegravir		
Abacavir		Ritonavir					
		Tipranavir					

squamous epithelium. HPV-infected epithelium characteristically has a hyperplastic prickle cell layer (acanthosis). The stratum corneum consists of one to two layers of parakeratosis. There are deep dermal papillae and a sharp border with the dermis. Koilocytes have been considered a marker for HPV infection. They are mature squamous cells with a large, clear perinuclear zone. The nuclei are enlarged and hyperchromatic; double nuclei may be present. Koilocytes may be scattered throughout the outer cell layers. Koilocytic changes may, however, be mimicked by other cellular changes or may be subtle.

Human papillomaviruses infection is most common in young, sexually active women and is seen in 20–25% of women in the third decade. Not all of these women will become symptomatic. Very often, the infection disappears spontaneously after 1–2 years. Women over the age of 30 years with persistent HPV infection are most likely to manifest disease.

Two major manifestations of genital HPV are Genital warts, which can be seen by the naked eye (usually caused by type 6 or 11), and squamous intraepithelial lesions (SILs) of the cervix, which are detected by cytology and colposcopy (usually caused by type 16 or 18). Although SILs are seen in the vulva, vagina and penis also, the clinical significance of these is unclear.

The four morphological types of genital warts are: (1) Condylomata acuminata, which have a cauliflower appearance **(Fig. 10)**; (2) papular warts, which are flesh-coloured, dome-shaped, 1–4 mm in diameter; (3) keratotic warts, which have a thick, crusty layer, resembling common skin warts; and (4) flat-topped macular warts.

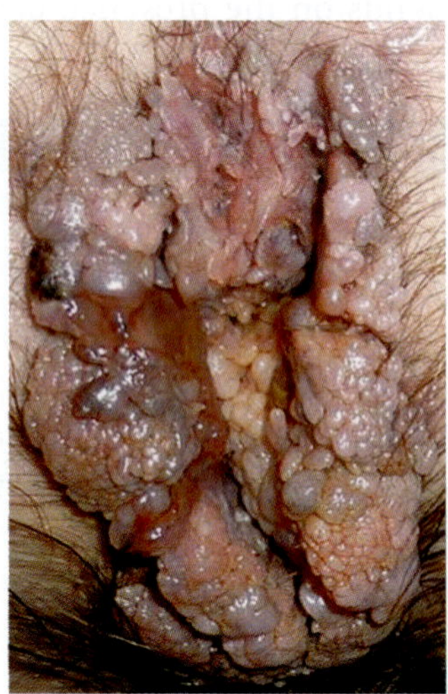

Fig. 10: Condyloma acuminata.

Generally, condylomata occur on moist, partially keratinised epithelium, keratotic and papular warts on fully keratinised epithelium, and macular warts on either partially or fully keratinised epithelium.

Condyloma may resolve on its own. Otherwise, surgical or laser excision can be done. Local application of 3.75% imiquimod cream is also an effective method of treatment.

Chlamydia trachomatis Infections

Chlamydia trachomatis is being increasingly recognised as the pathogen responsible for a variety of conditions, many of which resemble gonococcal infections. However, many chlamydial infections produce few or no symptoms in women and escape detection. Moreover, lack of adequate laboratory facilities for testing has led to the high prevalence of these infections in several parts of the world. It is most common in women <25 years of age.

Prevalence ranges from 3 to 5% in asymptomatic women to over 20% in those attending STD clinics. In industrialised countries, this is now recognised as the most common cause of PID and the most common STI.

Pathology

Chlamydia trachomatis is one of four species within the genus *Chlamydia*. The chlamydia have a unique growth cycle. They are obligate intracellular parasites and cannot be cultivated on artificial media because they depend on their host for adenosine triphosphate (ATP) and nutrient supplies. They survive by a replicative cycle that results in death of the infected host cells. Thus, they can never be part of the normal flora of the genital tract and are always pathogenic when present.

Virtually, all chlamydial infections are sexually transmitted. Infants may acquire the infection by passage through an infected birth canal and develop ophthalmia neonatorum. It infects the epithelium of cervical glands and can present as mucopurulent discharge. It can also affect the urethra.

Many serotypes have been identified based on an immunofluorescent antibody typing system of which L1, L2 and L3 are associated with LGV, and D, E, F, G, H, I, J and K have been associated with nongonococcal urethritis, cervicitis, salpingitis, proctitis, epididymitis, and inclusion of conjunctivitis and pneumonia of newborns. Extensive subepithelial inflammation, epithelial ulceration, and scarring are the end result.

Clinical Features

Infections caused by *C. trachomatis* are very similar to those caused by *N. gonorrhoeae* in terms of the pattern of infection and sequelae. However, chlamydial infections are more insidious in onset and generally produce very mild or no symptoms at all.

Patients may present with mucopurulent discharge from the endocervical canal and hypertrophic ectopy of the cervix, which bleeds on touch. On colposcopy, they may be seen to have immature squamous metaplasia. Dysuria and frequency of micturition with bacteriuria $<10^5$ organisms/mL of urine is pathognomonic of chlamydial infection in young, sexually active women. Clinical evidence of bartholinitis may be due to chlamydial infection alone or in combination with gonococcal infection. Menorrhagia and metrorrhagia, often seen in association with salpingitis, may be the manifestations of concomitant endometritis. *Silent* salpingitis is the hallmark of chlamydial infection, which results in tubal scarring and infertility, or ectopic pregnancies.

The Fitz-Hugh–Curtis syndrome of perihepatitis with salpingitis, long considered a complication of gonococcal infection, has now been recognised as being more common with chlamydial infection. Patients present with right upper quadrant abdominal pain, fever, nausea or vomiting. While salpingitis may not be diagnosed clinically, laparoscopy shows extensive tubal scarring, adhesions and inflammation. Periappendicitis may also occur.

Among men, it is estimated that 35–50% of cases of nongonococcal urethritis are caused by *C. trachomatis*. Reiter's syndrome has also been linked to *C. trachomatis*. This is a combination of nonspecific urethritis, polyarthritis and conjunctivitis, sometimes with uveitis and skin lesions. The sexually transmitted variety is almost always confined to young adult men.

Diagnosis

The first cultures of *C. trachomatis* were done on hen's egg yolk sacs. Cell culture plates are expensive; hence nonculture diagnostic tests, which detect the antigen, are used that are equally reliable, e.g. direct fluorescent antibody (DFA) and ELISA. Samples are taken with cotton-tipped swabs, which after mopping should pick up columnar epithelial cells from the exudate. DFA is the reference standard; ELISA can be done in larger numbers than DFA but is less reliable (40–70% sensitive). PCR is used in developed countries even as a screening modality, but widespread use of these methods is still not available in developing countries. NAATs are more sensitive and specific than ELISA (90–95%).

Treatment

Unprotected sexual intercourse should be avoided for 1 week. Explain long-term implications. Screen for other STIs. Uncomplicated infection is not an indication for removal of IUD.

Tetracyclines administered in a dose of 100 mg twice daily for 7 days eradicate *C. trachomatis.* Azithromycin 1 g may be given as a single dose. All neonates should receive topical ocular prophylaxis for the prevention of gonococcal and *Chlamydia* ophthalmia neonatorum. After 3 months of treatment, ideally patients should be tested for cure. Treatment of partner is also advised.

Lymphogranuloma Venereum

This disease is mostly seen in tropical countries. Elsewhere it is rare but is sometimes found in immigrants and prostitutes in seaports where it is introduced by sailors. It occurs most commonly among the African races, notably those in the West Indies and in India, and parts of South-East Asia and South America. It more often affects men than women, and personal uncleanliness appears to be a predisposing factor.

It is usually, but not always, contracted by sexual intercourse. It is caused by *C. trachomatis* serotypes L1, L2 and L3.

Clinical Features

The incubation period is 7–14 days. The disease has three stages: A papule initially followed by painful lymphadenopathy and fibrosis. The initial lesion is a painless papule, pustule or ulcer on the vulva and may quickly disappear. The infection persists in the lymphatics and spreads (mainly by lymphatics) to involve not only the tissues of the vulva but also those around and within the vagina and anus. Between 3 and 4 weeks, the inguinal and femoral lymph nodes (groove sign) are involved. These painful swellings may be the first sign of the disease. The double genitocrural fold is a sign typical of LGV which is seen in approximately 20% of cases, caused by the formation of a groove between groups of inflamed inguinal lymph nodes. The nodes tend to undergo necrosis and to form abscesses which release an offensive discharge, leaving

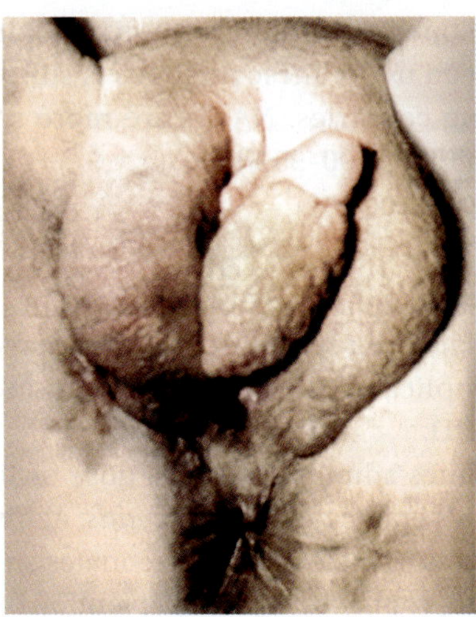

Fig. 11: False elephantiasis resulting from healed lymphogranuloma venereum. There are also residual scars on the perineum and around the anus. The patient concerned gave a history of ulceration which persisted for 2 years.

chronic deep sinuses and much surrounding fibrosis. If the ulceration of the vulva and perianal region is extensive, it also heals with scarring and contracture. Fenestration is a characteristic end result. Chronic lymphatic obstruction and induration can result in vulvar elephantiasis and make the vaginal walls feel rigid or rubbery inconsistency **(Fig. 11)**. Destruction or stricture of the urethra can occur. Rectal strictures and fistulas are not uncommon and can give rise to erroneous diagnoses of malignant disease. When the rectum is involved, there is diarrhoea and the passage of blood and pus per anus. Constitutional upset and pyrexia accompany the active stages of the disease. Rarely, perihepatitis (Fitz-Hugh-Curtis syndrome) may occur.

Diagnosis

This is suggested by clinical features and laboratory findings. The Frei test is no longer used.

The diagnosis can be made by isolating the organism if facilities for culturing *Chlamydia* are available. The organism may be obtained either from a smear of material from lesions or from a lymph node abscess, rectal swabs and urethral swabs. NAAT is a reliable mode of testing. Antibody against LGV serotypes can be detected by a microimmunofluorescent technique. A test for anti-*Chlamydia* antibody is available: The LGV complement fixation test. If the antibody titre exceeds 1 in 64, it is most likely to be due to LGV rather than other chlamydial infections. PCR is highly sensitive and specific to demonstrate *Chlamydia* in infected secretions or tissues.

Treatment

The Centers for Disease Control and Prevention (CDC) recommends doxycycline 100 mg twice daily for 21 days. Erythromycin is an alternative treatment. The end results of tissue destruction and fibrosis sometimes require reconstructive surgery on the vulva, urethra and vagina.

Screen for other possible causes of genital ulcerative diseases. Biopsy of lymph node may be required to exclude neoplasia.

Genital *Mycoplasmas*

Mycoplasma hominis and *Ureaplasma urealyticum* are the most common *Mycoplasmas* to be isolated from the genital tract. They can be acquired during passage through the birth canal or later, after puberty, usually as a result of sexual contact.

Pathology and Clinical Features

Mycoplasmas belong to the class *Mollicutes* and has developed from anaerobic bacteria by the process of gene deletion. Of the 16 *Mycoplasmas* detected in human beings, 6 are known to inhabit primarily the genitourinary tract. Some of these may be found in the oropharynx because of orogenital contact.

Genital *Mycoplasmas* have been implicated in a wide variety of clinical conditions. They were initially implicated in the aetiology of nongonococcal urethritis, but this has not been supported. *U. urealyticum* appears to play an important role in the aetiology of *Chlamydia*-negative nongonococcal urethritis, although these varieties of inflammatory response diminish with repeated inoculations.

Mycoplasma hominis may have a role in PIDs; here ureaplasmas do not seem to have any significance. *M. genitalium* has not been shown to be involved in bacterial vaginosis (BV), but the role of *Mycoplasmas* in BV needs further understanding. *M. hominis* can produce postabortal and postpartum fever. Ureaplasmas may also be causative in postpartum pyrexia. *Mycoplasma* group of organisms has been implicated in urethritis, cervicitis and PID.

The genital *Mycoplasmas* have a more important impact on disorders of reproduction. Treatment of ureaplasma infection has been shown to improve sperm motility and quantity in patients with infertility, although the conception rates have not been shown to increase. Most importantly, a significant association has been shown between mycoplasmal infection and recurrent spontaneous abortion, preterm delivery, preterm premature rupture of membranes and chorioamnionitis. *Ureaplasma* infection has been associated with low-birth-weight infants.

Diagnosis

Specialised media have been used to culture *M. hominis*, but several *Mycoplasmas* are fastidious and difficult to culture. Nonculture procedures (PCR) are important in this latter group. Serological tests have been popular in this regard (antibody titre). NAAT is also available in some nations.

Treatment

Azithromycin 1 g orally is more effective than doxycycline. In resistant cases, moxifloxacin 400 mg twice daily for 7–14 days is used.

Granuloma Inguinale (Donovanosis) (Fig. 12)

Donovanosis was first described from India and is now mostly seen in some developing countries. Whilst there is much confusion between this disease and the rather more common LGV, the regional lymph nodes are not involved in the early stages of this disease.

Pathology

The infecting organism is a gram-negative bacillus, *C. granulomatis*, with large capsules which can be seen within mononuclear cells when stained by the Giemsa method. The disease usually manifests itself 10–50 days after coitus with an infected partner. The initial lesion is nearly always on the vulva and presents as a papule which breaks down to form a chronic red ulcer with rolled edges, features that simulate those of cancer or a chancre. The ulcer spreads directly, rather than by lymphatics, to involve the whole vulva and sometimes the vagina, cervix, anus and the skin of the groins (the esthiomene stage). The condition is not particularly painful and ultimately heals to leave fibrosis, distortion of the tissues, and false elephantiasis or hypertrophy of the vulva. Sections of affected tissues often disclose epithelial unrest. Indeed, cancer can supervene. In pregnancy, the disease has a more aggressive course.

In the active stage of the disease, the inguinal nodes are enlarged but do not suppurate; this is a distinguishing feature from LGV.

Diagnosis

The diagnosis of granuloma inguinale is proved by finding Donovan bodies **(Fig. 13)** within mononuclear cells in material obtained from the ulcer. These are encapsulated diplobacilli, which show up with Giemsa and Leishman stains. It is common not to find these bodies, and this leaves the diagnosis in doubt. No serological tests are currently in use. However, the clinical picture is characteristic.

Treatment

Treatment recommended by the CDC (2015) is azithromycin 1 g once weekly for at least 3 weeks and until lesions are completely healed. Resolution may take weeks.

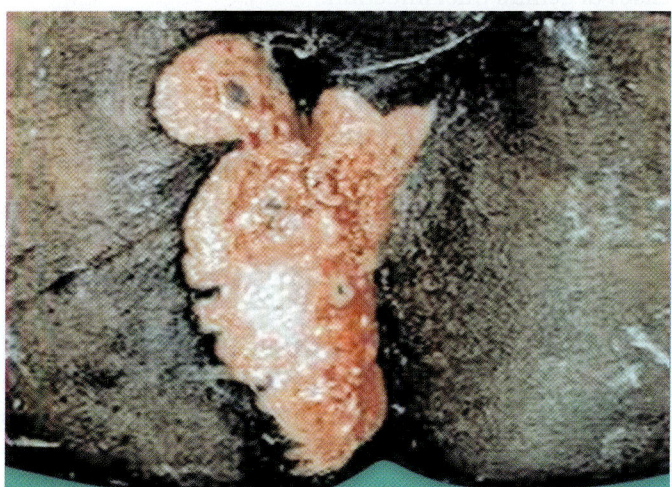

Fig. 12: Granuloma inguinale.

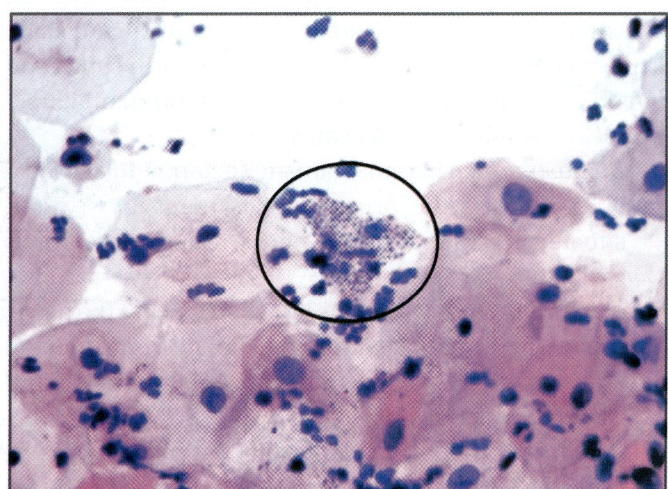

Fig. 13: Donovan bodies.

The end results of the destructive process may ultimately require plastic surgery or excision of the vulva in whole or in part.

GENITAL TUBERCULOSIS

The incidence of female genital tuberculosis (FGTB) varies in different countries from 1% in infertility clinics of USA, 6.15–21.1% in South Africa, and 1–19% in various parts of India. In infertility patients, the incidence of FGTB varies from 3 to 26% in India. Similarly, the incidence of FGTB is also very high in women seeking ART 24.5% overall but as high as 48.5% with tubal factor infertility. There has been a fivefold increase in the overall incidence of TB in countries with high prevalence of HIV. It is an important cause of chronic pelvic pain, infertility, dyspareunia and menstrual disturbances. FGTB is increased with women with diabetes, chronic renal disease or HIV coinfection.

Aetiology

Tuberculosis of the female genital tract is common among all communities where pulmonary or other forms of extragenital TB are prevalent, and this despite early recognition and effective treatment of such lesions. Those who take a contrary view do not conduct a proper search for it sufficiently often. It follows that genital TB is nearly always secondary to a focus elsewhere in the body, but the spread takes place at a very early stage of the disease—usually in adolescence or early maturity. Thus, by the time the genital lesion is found, which can be at any age, the primary lesion has often healed and is inconspicuous. Nevertheless, 50% of affected women give a past history of an extragenital infection, and a further number can recall, if questioned closely, contact with the disease in childhood or adolescence. The tubercle bacilli reach the genital tract by one of the following mechanisms:

- *Bloodstream:* This mechanism accounts for at least 90% of cases, the primary focus being most often situated in the lungs, lymph nodes, urinary tract, bones and joints—in that order.
- *Descending:* In this type, the infection reaches the pelvic organs by direct or lymphatic spread from infected adjacent organs such as the peritoneum, bowel and mesenteries nodes **(Fig. 14)**.
- *Ascending:* There is a theoretical possibility that a few cases of TB of the vulva and vagina, and of primary TB of the cervix, are explained by children sitting unclothed where others have spat or coughed, and in adults having coitus with a male suffering from urogenital TB. It can spread through sexual intercourse though rare.

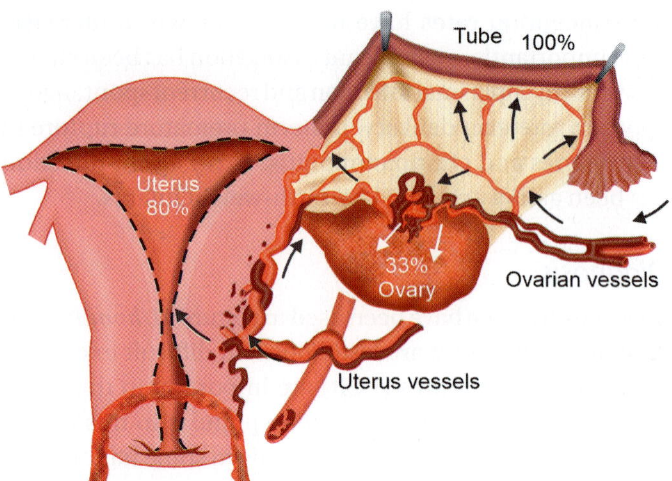

Fig. 14: Mode of transmission of tuberculous pelvic infection. Tubercle bacillus invades pelvic organs by way of the bloodstream from distant focus in the lung or other organ.

Pathology and Bacteriology

When the pelvic disease is secondary to tuberculous peritonitis, or when the primary focus is in the lymph nodes or bowel, the bovine bacillus *(MTB bovis)* is likely to be involved. In all other cases, it is generally the human bacillus *(MTB)* which is found. So, in those countries where cattle or their milk are relatively free from the tubercle bacilli, the human bacillus is found in 95% of cases of genital tract infection.

Any part of the genital tract can be affected but the common sites are the Fallopian tubes and the endometrium. The tubes are involved in at least 90% of cases and, following bloodstream spread, the genital disease probably starts there. It begins in the submucosa at their outer ends and gradually progresses inward, bombarding the endometrium with bacilli. The finding of endometrial TB almost always means that the tubes are infected, but tuberculous salpingitis can exist without associated endometritis.

The genital infection can be an acute and rapidly extending disease but is mostly indolent. There are several cases reported in which the disease appeared to commence, or to become violently active, immediately after pregnancy. In such circumstances, fatal miliary spread is not uncommon.

Vulva and Vagina

Tuberculosis of the vulva and vagina usually takes the form of shallow, superficial, indolent ulcers with undermined edges. The ulceration tends to spread slowly, healing in some areas with the formation of scar tissue. A vulvar hypertrophic lesion is less common and mostly represents inflammatory induration and oedema resulting from fibrosis and lymphatic obstruction.

Cervix

Clinically recognisable TB of the cervix can be ulcerative but more often appears as a bright-red papillary erosion, which bleeds easily. It can be confused with carcinoma. As a histological finding, cervical TB is not uncommon in cases of endometrial TB.

Uterus

The uterus usually looks normal to the naked eye, although a typical tuberculous ulcer may rarely be seen in the endometrium. Extensive involvement can result in collections of caseous material to form a type of pyometra or to cause abscesses in the myometrium **(Fig. 15)**. Adhesions and partial obliteration of the cavity are also described. Ordinarily, however, tuberculous endometritis is only recognised by histological and bacteriological examinations of the tissues.

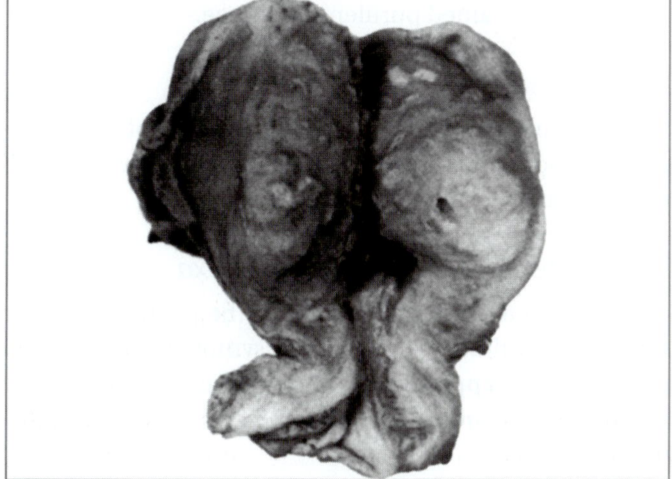

Fig. 15: Multiple tuberculous abscesses in a chronically thickened myometrium. This is a rare manifestation of tuberculosis and the appearance of the lesion might be mistaken for that of adenomyosis.

Fallopian Tubes

The appearance of tuberculous tubes varies widely and depends to some extent on whether the infection is bloodborne or spreads directly from the peritoneum or bowel. In one case, the disease is primarily an endosalpingitis, and in the other an exosalpingitis with the possibilities of tubercles on the surface and of dense surrounding adhesions.

Sometimes, the tubes look completely normal; more often they appear red, oedematous and swollen when the infection is active and fibrosed when it is chronic. They do not always have tubercles on their surface. *Tubercles* when seen on tubes and the peritoneum at laparoscopy or laparotomy are not always caused by TB. They may be an end result of any chronic inflammation, whether infectious or noninfectious, e.g. talc or starch granulomas, or peritoneal deciduosis. The tubal lumina are closed in only 50% of cases in which there is bacteriological and histological evidence of endometrial disease. In this respect, however, it seems likely that many examples of tubal obstruction of uncertain aetiology represent completely inactivated, and unprovable, old tuberculous lesions. In TB, the obstructions are typically multiple, and the tube wall is thickened and shotty. Sometimes, a localised closure at the outer end results in the formation of a hydrosalpinx or a pyosalpinx with thick fibrous walls which can become calcified or even ossified **(Figs. 16 and 17)**. A tuberculous pyosalpinx is often remarkably free from adhesions and may be so large that the patient's complaint is the presence of an abdominal tumour **(Figs. 16 and 18)**.

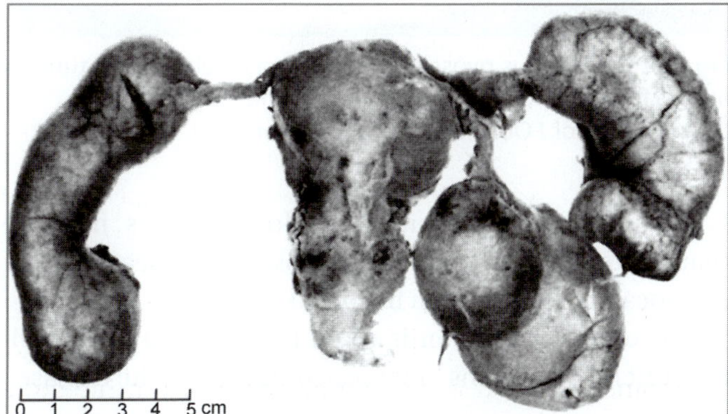

Fig. 16: Tuberculous pyosalpinges are relatively free from adhesions, as they commonly are. There is also a small cyst in the right ovary. This specimen was removed from a nulliparous woman aged 40 years whose only complaint was the presence of a lower abdominal tumour.

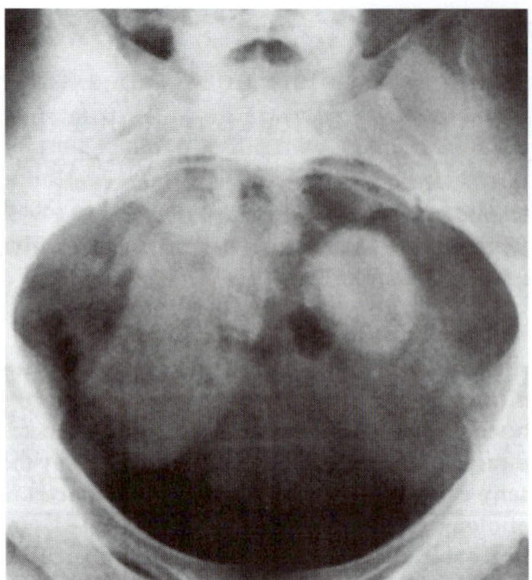

Fig. 17: Direct radiograph of the lower abdomen and pelvis. The pyosalpinges are visible because of slight calcification in their walls. This appearance permitted a preoperative diagnosis of tuberculosis.

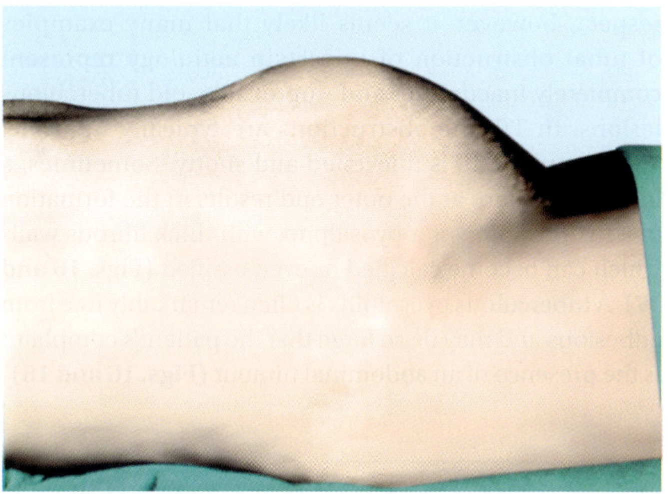

Fig. 18: Tuberculous pyosalpinges causing an abdominal tumour arising from the pelvis and extending to the umbilicus.
Source: Editor of J Obstet Gynaecol Br Commonw.

A hypertrophic form of endosalpingitis has the macroscopic and sometimes microscopic appearances of adenocarcinoma and can be mistaken for such.

Secondary infection is often present and may itself account for symptoms or for exacerbations of the disease.

Ovaries

The ovaries are infected in at least 30% of cases of tuberculous salpingitis, but ovarian TB without tubal involvement is rare. The disease can manifest by way of surface tubercles, adhesions and thickening of the capsule, and retention cysts and sometimes by caseating abscess cavities in the substance of the ovary **(Fig. 19)**. Often, however, the ovaries have a normal macroscopic appearance, and the diagnosis is only revealed by laboratory studies of excised tissue.

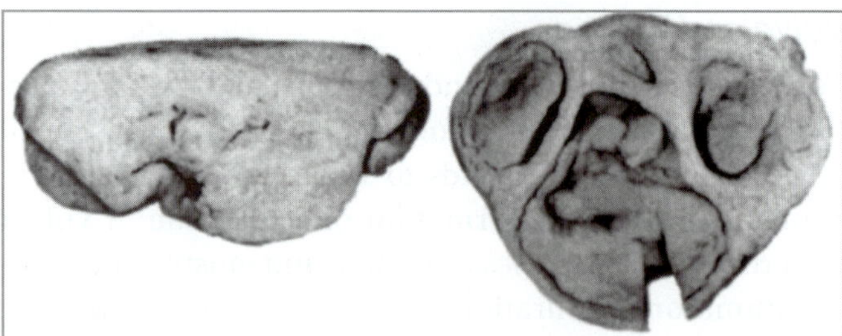

Fig. 19: Tuberculosis of the ovaries. There are typical multiple caseating abscesses in one and diffuse fibrosis and enlargement of the other.

Fistulas and Sinuses

Tuberculous fistulas and sinuses involving the abdominal wall, tubes, uterus, vagina, bladder and bowel can arise spontaneously **(Figs. 20A and B)**, but are mostly the result of inadequate or injudicious surgery.

Clinical Features

Tuberculosis of the Vulva and Vagina

Vulvar lesions are usually painful and tender; vaginal ulcers, unless sited at the introitus, are painless. Both often cause a bloodstained purulent discharge.

Overt Tuberculosis of the Cervix

This is painless but causes the same type of discharge and also postcoital bleeding. A cauliflower growth, which closely mimics malignancy, is often seen.

Tuberculosis of the Uterus and Adnexa

This is often a silent disease. It may be present for 20 or more years without producing any symptoms, the woman remaining in apparently excellent health. The pelvic organs also feel normal on bimanual examination in 50% of proven cases.

The presence of pelvic TB is most often revealed by the investigation of childlessness and therefore is usually discovered in women aged 20–40 years. In developed countries, tuberculous infection of the uterus and tubes is

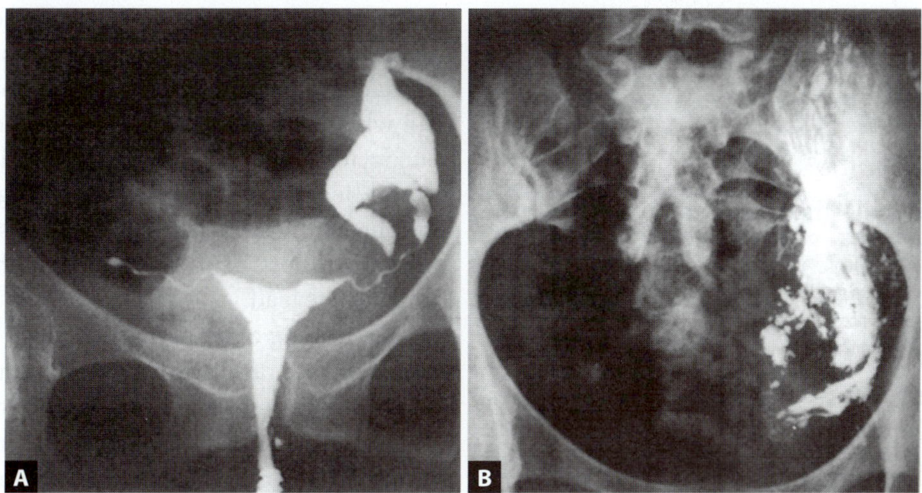

Figs. 20A and B: A tuboretroperitoneal fistula resulting from tuberculous salpingitis. A woman aged 27 years complained of infertility and was first subjected to tubal insufflation and curettage. The insufflation was positive (misleadingly so as was subsequently shown) and the endometrium was histologically and bacteriologically negative for tuberculosis. (A) A salpingogram showing the right tube closed at its outer end. From the distal end of the left tube, which is dilated, there is a small track through which the medium passed; (B) A straight radiograph taken 24 hours later shows that the medium escaped not into the peritoneal cavity but extraperitoneally. Laparotomy confirmed that the outer end of the left tube communicated by way of a caseating abscess with the extraperitoneal tissues on the side wall of the pelvis.

now demonstrable in <1% of all cases of infertility studied, varying with the prevalence of pulmonary TB in any community 15–20 years previously.

The frequency with which it is found in both symptomless and complaining women, however, depends on the care taken to look for it. Moreover, the symptoms credited to it, and their statistical importance, depend on the types of cases in which tests for TB are made. Thus, if the search is limited to all women complaining of infertility, one picture of associated symptomatology appears; if it is extended to all women complaining of amenorrhoea or to women with menorrhagia or postmenopausal bleeding, different pictures emerge.

It should be routine practice to look for bacteriological and histological evidence of endometrial TB in all cases of infertility and of amenorrhoea, and otherwise only when there are grounds for clinical suspicion. The special symptoms are as follows.

Infertility

Although 10% of women with proven endometrial infection have had babies or abortions, the most common symptom of pelvic TB is primary infertility. This is a feature of 70% of cases and occurs even though the Fallopian tubes are open. It then reflects abnormal tubal and endometrial function. TB causes damage to tubes, destruction of endometrium and damage to ovaries. All these can lead to infertility. TB by damaging the endometrium can cause recurrent implantation failure.

Ectopic Pregnancy

Every woman who has, or has had, a tubal pregnancy should also be suspected of having tubal TB, active or healed, apart from the more obvious causes nowadays, including chlamydial infection. Indeed, tubes removed for this condition should still be examined bacteriologically from this standpoint.

Menstrual Disturbance

In approximately 50% of cases, the menstrual function is normal. In the others, it is generally held that the change is mostly in the direction of menorrhagia and polymenorrhoea. In my experience, however, and unlike other infections, TB more often causes amenorrhoea or oligomenorrhoea. This is sometimes explained by suppression of ovarian function; in such cases, compensatory overactivity of the anterior pituitary can result in a raised excretion of gonadotropins. In other cases, however, there is evidence that ovulation continues; the amenorrhoea is then attributable to the endometrial damage.

Menopausal and postmenopausal bleeding can have endometrial TB as a basis. Dysmenorrhoea rarely, if ever, occurs.

Intermenstrual Discharge

This can be bloodstained if there is ulceration of either the cervix or the endometrium.

Pain

An intermittent chronic ache in the lower abdomen, often of longstanding nature, is noted in 20–30% of cases. Indeed, 20% of sufferers from pelvic TB have previously had a normal appendix removed. Unusual activity of the infection occasionally causes symptoms and signs of acute or subacute peritonitis. Exacerbations of this kind are sometimes precipitated by tubal patency tests.

General Disturbances

Conditions such as malaise, loss of weight, night sweats, and pyrexia are only seen during an unusually active phase of the disease.

Signs

There may not be any obvious signs. Pallor may be present. It is important to look for any lymphadenopathy. There may be an abdominal mass, and ascites sometimes may be present. There may be a lesion on vagina or cervix. Abnormal discharge per vagina can occur. If there is pyometra, the uterus may be enlarged. There may be adnexal tenderness or mass. Rarely TB can result in fistula within the genital tract.

Diagnosis

The clue to the diagnosis of pelvic TB is to have the condition in mind, although the incidence of TB is falling in many countries, immigration may bring problems. The only difficulty arises over those cases, and there must be many, where infection in adolescence has become quiescent leaving no active organisms, merely residual damage and clinical suspicion. Some of the guidelines are as follows.

Tuberculosis should be suspected and excluded in every woman whose infertility or amenorrhoea is not explained by other causes. Any virgin having symptoms and signs of chronic pelvic infection should be assumed to have TB until it is proved to the contrary. Any pelvic infection, which is slow to respond to the ordinary methods of treatment, is suspected, and so is one which shows an exacerbation after curettage or tubal patency tests, or one which is not accompanied by polymorphonuclear leucocytosis. Sometimes, a previous history of peritonitis, appendicectomy with slow healing, pleurisy, and a prolonged illness in childhood, or a history of TB affecting other members of the family and childhood contacts, provides the lead.

The finding of an active or healed extragenital lesion should always raise suspicions, as should the radiological demonstration of calcification in the tube or ovary or the classical appearance of isthmica nodosa on a hysterosalpingogram performed before the diagnosis is suspected or made.

If TB is suspected and the lesion is accessible (as in the case of the cervix and vulva or of the tube at laparotomy), the diagnosis is made by examining biopsy material both bacteriologically and histologically. Otherwise, advantage is taken of the fact that the endometrium is nearly always involved and can be obtained for examination by endometrial biopsy or aspiration. Specimens should preferably be taken from the cornual regions. The most likely time in the cycle to find evidence of endometrial TB is during the week preceding menstruation. This is because the tubercles and bacteria are mostly found in the surface layers, which are shed during menstruation and which have to be reformed and reinfected from the tubes downward.

Endometrial Aspirate or Biopsy

- *Acid-fast bacilli (AFB) microscopy:* Ziehl–Neelsen (ZN) staining is a rapid and cost-effective method to detect AFB, but this method lacks sensitivity. Fluorescent dyes (auramine and rhodamine) with light emitting diode (LED) microscopy have better sensitivity.
- *AFB culture* is gold standard in the diagnosis of TB. Various methods of culture include: (1) Conventional egg-based solid media like Lowenstein–Jensen (LJ) medium and agar-based 7H10 or 7H11 broth, which takes 6 weeks to get the result; (2) BACTEC-MGIT 960 (Mycobacterium Growth Indicator Tube) which takes 2 weeks to grow but results are reported at 6 weeks and (3) Versa TREK which is liquid-based culture and has good sensitivity.
- *NAAT* is WHO-accredited real-time PCR (RT-PCR) that has high specificity and can detect drug resistance.

- *PCR* has high sensitivity but cannot be used to treat TB. Further testing such as laparoscopy and biopsy is needed.
- *Loop-mediated isothermal amplification (LAMP):* It is a faster and economical test, which can give result in just 40 minutes. It cannot detect drug resistance.
- *Histopathology* detection of granuloma

Endoscopic Techniques

Diagnostic laparoscopy can detect tubercules, and encysted lesions can be biopsied. A real problem is to diagnose tubal TB in the absence of endometrial involvement. Here, laparoscopy has a place providing tuberculous peritonitis, and adhesion formation can be excluded with reasonable certainty. Biopsies and washings from the cul-de-sac can be subjected to the same tests described above. Salpingography sometimes reveals characteristic tubal patterns but is unreliable and is so dangerous from the standpoint of causing an exacerbation that it should never be carried out if there is a real possibility of the disease being present. Despite meticulous investigation, it is sometimes difficult to clinch the diagnosis and repeated tests may be necessary. I know of several patients with normal pelvic organs who had to have endometrial sampling carried out three or four times over a few years before tubercle bacilli were found. It is also my practice, when carrying out tubal surgery for infertility, to send material for bacteriological culture for TB as well as for routine histological analysis **(Box 4)**.

As no test is 100% sensitive, multiple tests may need to be done to confirm the diagnosis of TB.

BOX 4: Investigations for genital tuberculosis (TB).

- *Blood test:* Anaemia, leucocytosis with lymphocytosis, and raised erythrocyte sedimentation rate (ESR)
- Nonspecific serological tests like enzyme-linked immunosorbent assay (ELISA) (not very sensitive and specific)
- Moderate rise in level of CA-125
- Mantoux test and interferon gamma assays; poor sensitivity and specificity
- Chest X-ray for pulmonary TB
- *Imaging methods:* Ultrasonography, CT scan, and MRI are useful for tubo-ovarian masses
- *Positron emission tomography (PET) scan:* Tubo-ovarian masses
- *Hystero/sonosalpingography:* Synechiae formation, distorted, obliterated or T-shaped cavity, and venous and lymphatic intravasation
- Endometrial biopsy, curettage or aspirate
- *Histopathology:* Demonstration of epithelioid granuloma
- Mycobacterial smear and culture
- PCR and NAAT

(NAAT: nucleic acid amplification test; PCR: polymerase chain reaction)

Treatment

The choice of treatment depends to some extent on whether genital TB is found in association with an active lesion elsewhere and must therefore be preceded by a full investigation from this standpoint. Radiological examination of the chest and an examination of the urine for tubercle bacilli are especially important.

General

It is important to improve the patient's natural resistance to the disease by attention to diet and general well-being. Women frequently ask whether there is any chance of their husbands contracting urogenital TB during coitus. This risk cannot be denied, although it is small and can be obviated by the use of a condom until the infection is under control.

Medical Treatment

Female genital TB is treated like pulmonary TB for a total duration of 6 months. Four drugs—rifampicin (R), isoniazid (H), pyrazinamide (Z), and ethambutol (E)—are given orally daily for 2 months in the intensive phase followed by three drugs—rifampicin, ethambutol, and isoniazid orally daily for the remining 4 months (continuation phase). This is recommended by the WHO. Pyridoxine is used to prevent side effects.

Patients with TB resistant to first-line drugs are treated with second-line drugs. These have a lower degree of efficacy and a higher degree of toxicity, so these patients should ideally be referred to a specialised unit. Second-line drugs include kanamycin, amikacin and capreomycin, which are injectable preparations, and ethionamide, cycloserine, para-aminosalicylic acid (PAS), ofloxacin, sparfloxacin, clofazimine, thiacetazone and amoxycillin/clavulanic acid, which can be administered orally. Rifabutin is a long-acting rifamycin derivative under evaluation for cases resistant to rifampicin which may be effective in a once-weekly dose.

Directly-observed Treatment Short-course Strategy Treatment

Directly-observed treatment short-course strategy (DOTS) of FGTB is favoured and recommended by the WHO.

Daily treatment is given under direct supervision of a treatment supporter. Four drugs isoniazid (H), rifampicin (R), pyrazinamide (Z), and ethambutol (E) are given for 2 months (HRZE), followed by H, R, and E (HRE) daily for 4 months. Thrice-weekly regimen is no longer used. Drug resistance is ruled out before starting DOTS by NAAT and line-probe assays.

A standard regimen recommends a daily dosing schedule using combination tablets in patients who can adhere to treatment. DOTS is favoured by the WHO to prevent multidrug resistance (MDR) and for better results.

Treatment of Chronic Cases, Drug-resistant and Multidrug-resistant Female Genital Tuberculosis

It is the same as for pulmonary MDR with second-line drugs and is needed for long duration (18–24 months).

During treatment, patients should be monitored for drug toxicity. The most important and most common of these is hepatitis (every monthly liver function).

Patients on rifampicin should be warned that their urine, saliva and other body secretions will be coloured orange-red, but this should not be confused with the dark urine of hepatitis which is accompanied by loss of appetite. If there is marked derangement of hepatic function, drugs should be stopped and reintroduced once at a time after recovery. Other complications include optic neuritis with ethambutol, eighth nerve damage with streptomycin, and autoimmune thrombocytopenia with rifampicin; the development of these warrants discontinuation of these drugs. Hyperuricaemia and arthralgia may develop with pyrazinamide, but the drug is discontinued only if the patient develops gouty arthritis. Minor problems such as gastrointestinal symptoms and pruritus are treated symptomatically without alteration of therapy.

Tuberculosis of the vulva, vagina and cervix is often cured quite dramatically by antibiotics. In the case of endometrial TB, the patient is subjected to endometrial aspiration after 6 months for a test of cure. The results in the case of endometrial and tubal disease are more difficult to evaluate but experience suggests the following. By itself, antibiotic therapy is usually inadequate when chronic caseating abscesses are present.

In the more favourable cases, with only microscopic foci, the infection is eradicated in the majority of cases. Sometimes, after an initial apparent cure, positive endometrial cultures are obtained again 12 or more months later. This may happen in 5–10% of cases.

Cure to the extent of restoring the patient's fertility is not common, the total salvage being not more than 2 live babies for every 100 women treated.

If the tubes are closed at the outset, permanent sterility is likely and attempts at salpingostomy following suppression of the active infection may be followed by reclosure.

If the tubes are open, pregnancy is possible but, because of residual infection or of scarring and distortion of the endosalpinx, tubal implantation is likely. Indeed, ectopic pregnancy following antibiotic therapy for pelvic TB is now a recognised clinical syndrome. Abortion of intrauterine pregnancies is also common.

Reported experience and our own indicates that of all women treated, only 8% conceive. Of the pregnancies, 50% are tubal and 20–30% end in abortion, leaving only 20–30% resulting in live births. The subsequent obstetrical history of one patient was abortion, live baby, and ectopic pregnancy.

It is not always possible to relate subsequent fertility to treatment because spontaneous cure of the disease can happen and because conception occasionally occurs despite the presence of active TB.

In vitro fertilisation (IVF) is now one possible alternative. If after antituberculosis treatment (ATT) their tubes are still damaged but their endometrium is receptive (no adhesions or mild adhesions which can be hysteroscopically resected), IVF–embryo transfer (ET) is recommended. However, if they have endometrial TB causing damage to the endometrium with a shrunken small uterine cavity with Asherman's syndrome, adoption or gestational surrogacy is advised.

Surgery

When TB is localised to any site in the body, there is usually a place for excision of the affected area; this is true for genital TB where the disease can be remarkably localised and accessible. A hypertrophic lesion of the vulva, which fails to respond to antibiotics, may require excision.

Removal of the uterus and adnexa for tuberculous salpingitis and endometritis is often decried on the grounds that it is a dangerous operation and likely to result in a fistula or chronic sinus. If, however, the cases are well chosen, this risk is small even without antibiotic cover.

Now that surgery is covered by antibiotics, it is even less dangerous.

Indications for Surgery

Tuberculosis responds well to treatment. The only indication for surgery is drainage of abscess that does not respond to therapy.

Contraindication to Surgery

Active TB is a contraindication to surgery.

SARCOIDOSIS

Although not an infection, sarcoidosis is included here for comparison with genital TB. Sarcoidosis is mainly seen in people living in temperate climates—in Europe and North America. It is a granulomatous disease of the reticuloendothelial system with a wide distribution throughout the body. It occurs as a rarity in the uterus, tubes and ovaries, often symptomless but sometimes giving rise to a complaint of infertility. The diagnosis is a histological one, the lesions having microscopical appearances similar to those of TB with follicles consisting of an aggregation of epithelioid cells and a variable number of giant cells surrounded by a narrow zone of lymphocytes. Complete absence of caseation and a relative scarcity of lymphocytes distinguish it from the TB follicle **(Fig. 21)**.

Active sarcoidosis appears to be the result of an exaggerated cellular immune response to antigens, self or nonself, which stimulate predominantly or helper-induced T-cell response.

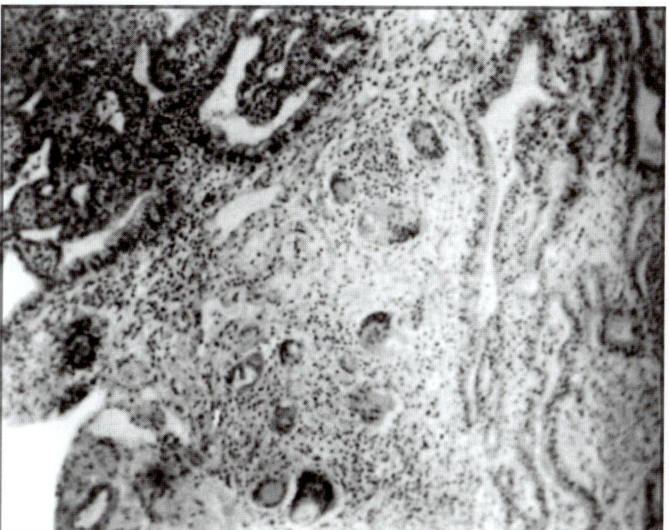

Fig. 21: Sarcoidosis of the tube.

Sarcoidosis is self-curative in 50% of cases but resolution can leave permanent tissue damage—in the Fallopian tubes. Nevertheless, it is best left untreated or attention paid only to relief of symptoms. The lesions disappear when corticosteroids are administered but return as soon as treatment is suspended.

ACTINOMYCOSIS

Actinomycetes, most often *Actinomyces israelii*, are occasionally found to be the cause of pelvic infection. Since the majority of infections reported in the past involved the right ovary and tube it was considered that the source of infection originated in the caecum or appendix or occurred as a result of bloodstream spread.

Presently, an association between the use of an IUCD and this infection is recognised, and it is postulated that the vagina is the portal of entry. Actinomycetes have been noted in cervical smears taken from asymptomatic IUCD wearers. The disease usually develops after at least 2 years of IUCD use. The organisms may persist in the genital tract for some time after the removal of the IUCD. Other possible routes of entry may be by orogenital sex, ascent from the rectum or spread from the appendix.

The clinical manifestations of PID caused by actinomycetes in association with an IUCD are more likely to be chronic rather than acute: Fever, weight loss, abdominal pain, and abnormal vaginal bleeding discharge. Endometritis may progress to the formation of an adnexal mass or a tubo-ovarian abscess. A delay in diagnosis can lead to a frozen pelvis; which has to be differentiated from endometriosis or disseminated malignancy.

Pseudomycelial-like clumps of organisms are seen in the Pap smear along with positive staining for fluorescein isothiocyanate-labelled antisera against *A. israelii.* Diagnosis is made by culture and PCR to identify the organism. Histopathological examination specimen also aids in the diagnosis. For women who are symptomatic but do not have an adnexal swelling, the IUCD should be removed and sent for culture. Diagnosis is made by prolonged courses of penicillin for 6–12 months are recommended. Ceftriaxone, macrolides (e.g. erythromycin), lincosamides (e.g. clindamycin) and tetracyclines (e.g. doxycycline) can be used if the patient has hypersensitivity to penicillin. If patients with pelvic masses do not respond to antibiotics, surgical excision of the masses may be required in addition. Asymptomatic patients are not treated.

SCHISTOSOMIASIS (BILHARZIA)

Genital schistosomiasis is seen in all tropical and subtropical countries, notably Egypt, other countries such as Africa, India, Malaysia, Indo-China, and Central and Southern America, where the causal worm and its immediate host—a water snail—are prevalent. The worm, *Schistosoma haematobium* having entered the skin from infested water, spreads by the bloodstream to invade the tissues where it deposits ova which cause local inflammatory reactions. Adult *S. haematobium* worms live in the genitourinary veins. The lesions are predominantly in hollow viscera, especially the bladder and rectum, but any part of the genital tract from the vulva to the ovaries can be involved. The most common genital site is the cervix; vulvar lesions are mostly seen in children. The infestation is chronic and can persist for a lifetime, the carrier continually excreting ova which contaminate the environment.

The inflammatory reaction is a severe one with each ovum being surrounded by a giant cell, epithelial cells, lymphocytes and eosinophils. In some respects, the microscopic appearances resemble those of TB.

Bladder and bowel symptoms predominate and the discomfort referred to the reproductive organs varies with the site infected. Schistosomiasis of the vagina and cervix can cause discharge, bleeding and dyspareunia; it also favours infertility in that antibodies to the disease are spermatotoxic.

To the naked eye, the disease appears in the form of nodules, plaques, ulcers or papillomas with surrounding induration. On the cervix, the disease can simulate erosion and leucoplakia. In any site, it can be mistaken for cancer.

It is suggested that schistosomiasis occasionally favours the development of cancer. Praziquantel is effective against all human schistosomes, and the dose is 40 mg/kg as a single oral dose. The organophosphorus compound metrifonate is only effective against *S. haematobium* infections and is given orally. The prognosis is good for treatment in the early stage but poor in the late stages of the disease.

AMOEBIASIS

Amoebiasis of the genital tract occurs at any age wherever intestinal infection is common that is among the less privileged communities living in warm climates. The parasite (*Entamoeba histolytica*) spreads from the lower bowel when standards of hygiene are poor. It causes ulcerative lesions in the vagina, cervix and endometrium, and these can be mistaken for cancer on naked-eye examination.

Apart from any bowel symptoms, the patient complains of a bloodstained purulent vaginal discharge. The diagnosis is made by the microscopic demonstration of the parasites in stools, vaginal discharge and tissue sections; the finding of the organism incidentally during cervical cytology is also described. A negative gel diffusion precipitation test, or amoebic latex agglutination test, carried out on serum, excludes active disease but a positive finding may only mean a previous infection.

The treatment of choice is metronidazole in large doses, 400–750 mg three times daily for 5–10 days. Metronidazole is relatively ineffective in chronic asymptomatic intestinal amoebiasis in which only cysts are present in the stool. In these cases, diloxanide furoate is the drug of choice.

SUGGESTED READING

1. BASHH. British Association for Sexual Health and HIV (BASHH) guidelines. [online] Available from www.bashh.org/resources/guidelines/ [Last accessed April, 2025].
2. Centers for Disease Control and Prevention (CDC). (2021). Sexually Transmitted Infections Treatment Guidelines, 2021. [online] Available from www.cdc.gov/std/treatment-guidelines/default.htm [Last accessed April, 2025].
3. NACO. (2021). National AIDS Control Organization (NACO) guidelines for HIV care and treatment. [online] Available from https://naco.gov.in [Last accessed April, 2025].
4. Sharma JB, Sharma E, Sharma S, Dharmendra S. Recent advances in diagnosis and management of female genital tuberculosis. J Obstet Gynaecol India. 2021;71(5):476-87.

21

CHAPTER

Infections as They Affect Individual Organs

Jayaraman Nambiar M, Muralidhar V Pai

Chapter Outline

- Vulvitis
- Bartholinitis
- Vaginitis
- Cervicitis
- Endometritis
- Metritis
- Salpingo-oophoritis
- Oophoritis
- Pelvic Peritonitis
- Pelvic Cellulitis
- Chronic Cellulitis
- Pelvic Inflammatory Disease
- Suppurative Thrombophlebitis of the Pelvic Veins

VULVITIS

Pyogenic Infections

Infection of Abrasions and Wounds

Local injuries or abrasions resulting from sanitary towels and tight under clothing—often impregnated with irritant detergents left from washing—are common sources of vulvar dermatitis. Excoriation of the skin can also be caused by vaginal discharge and by ammonia liberated by urea-splitting organisms when the vulva is exposed to constant leakage of urine. All these lesions can become secondarily infected to cause local pain and tenderness. Treatment consists of rest, warm baths and removal of the cause.

Intertrigo: Smegma concretions: Lack of cleanliness leads to a collection of irritating sebum and other secretions in the skin folds, and secondary infection follows. The only treatment required is care over hygiene.

Inattention to the skin in the area of the clitoris can result in the collection of a concretion of smegma resembling a small stone under the prepuce. This may have to be removed **(Figs. 1A and B)**.

Furunculosis: Infection of vulvar hair follicles leads to boils and carbuncles which are sometimes recurrent. Glycosuria must be excluded in such cases. Otherwise, recurrent boils mean that pathogenic staphylococci are being harboured in a carrier site (e.g. the nose or axilla) of the patient or a close associate. These have to be found and eliminated. For the vulvar skin, the remedies are scrupulous attention to cleanliness, swabbing with an antiseptic solution and regular applications of topical antibiotics. During a phase of active furunculosis, a full course of treatment with penicillin, or of other antibiotic appropriate to the infecting organism, should be given *systemically*, not locally.

Infection of Sebaceous and Apocrine Glands

Single abscesses, often representing secondary infection of a retention cyst of an apocrine or sebaceous gland, have the clinical characteristics of a boil and are treated in the same way. If they recur in the same site, the underlying cyst has to be excised when free from inflammatory reaction.

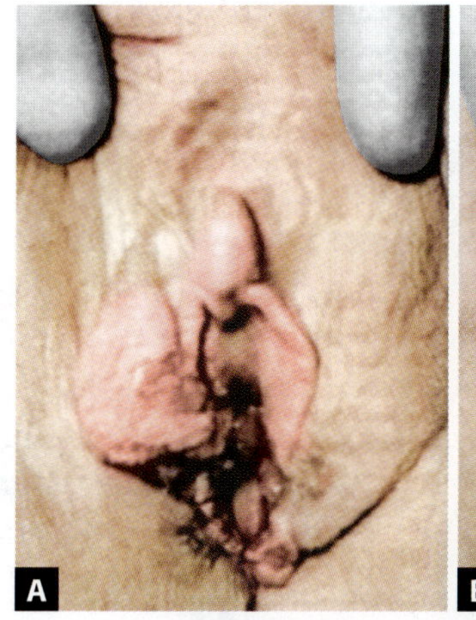

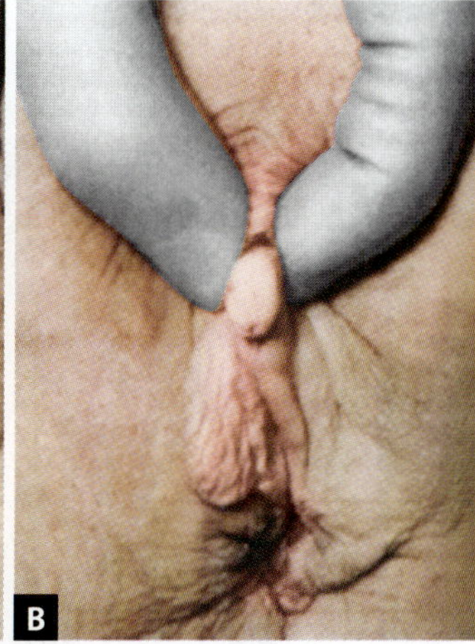

Figs. 1A and B: A smegma concretion beneath the prepuce of the clitoris. Patient aged 70 years with a carcinoma of the fourchette extending onto the perineum. (A) The hidden concretion gives the appearance of a tumour or hypertrophy of the clitoris; (B) The concretion being expressed; in this case, a small incision was necessary to provide an exit.

Hidradenitis suppurativa, which is rare and more likely to be seen in hot climates, is a condition of chronic bacterial infection of many apocrine glands which shows periodic exacerbations. It occurs in the axilla and the vulva, but only after puberty when the glands become active. On the vulva, the disease presents as a series of tender nodules which suppurate and coalesce to form abscesses. Sinuses develop, and these extend deeply and widely.

Radical and repeated incisions to lay open all abscesses and tracts, combined with antibiotics, are the treatment. Diffuse hidradenitis, however, is very refractory and in healing leaves extensive scarring and distortion.

Infantile and senile vulvitis: When the vulvar epithelium is thin and inactive, as in childhood and old age, any of the organisms to which it is normally resistant can set up a simple vulvitis. This sometimes leads to labial adhesions. This type of vulvitis is often associated with vaginitis.

Acute Simple Ulcers (Figs. 2A to C)

Herpes Genitalis

Changing sexual habits in the last few decades have been associated with an increased incidence of genital herpes. Indeed, genital herpes simplex infections now have a higher incidence than syphilis and are the most common cause of genital ulceration in industrialised nations. Genital herpes is important not only because of its increasing incidence but also because of the physical and psychological trauma it can induce. The risk of serious complications includes a link with cervical cancer and the risk of transfer of maternal infection to neonates. Disseminated herpes in the newborn is certainly one of the most severe manifestations of herpes infection. Prematurity and spontaneous abortion have also been associated with active maternal genital herpes.

Herpes genitalis is most often caused by infection with herpes simplex virus (HSV) type 2 (85%), which has usually been sexually transmitted by an infected partner, but may possibly be transmitted by orogenital contact. HSV type 1 infection accounts for about 15% of cases. Infection is transmitted by secretions containing the virus and not by fomites or aerosolisation, as the virus is readily inactivated at room temperature or by drying.

Genital diseases caused by either of these viral types are clinically indistinguishable. As with other herpes infections, the virus replicates in the epithelium giving rise to painful symptoms and signs. These typically, but not invariably, follow a course which commences with redness and inflammation, leading to the formation of vesicles which progress to pustules. These pustules then erode

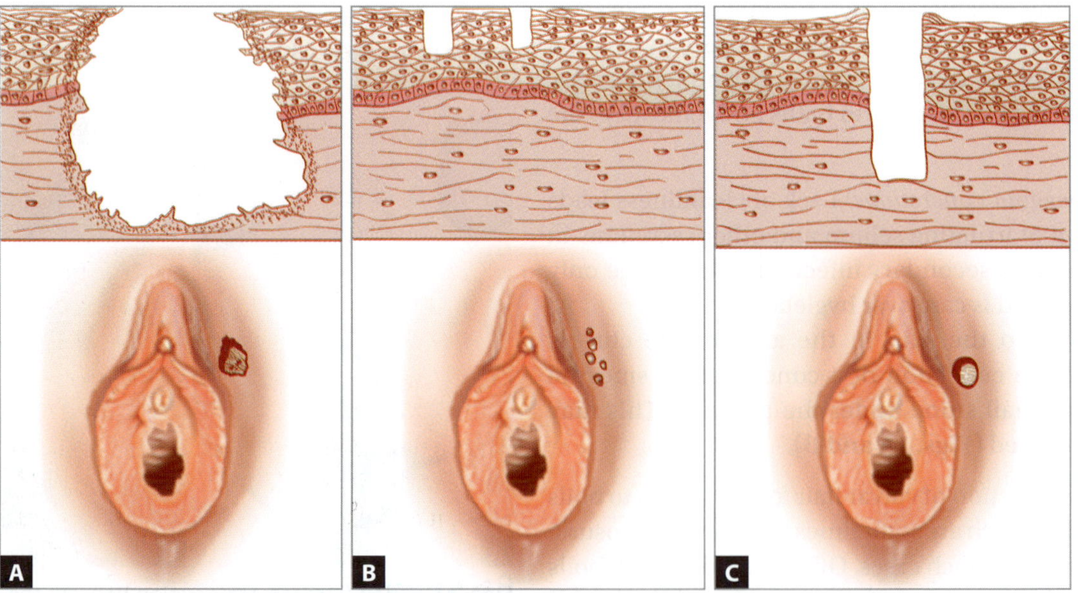

Figs. 2A to C: Appearance of the ulcers of (A) chancroid, (B) herpes and (C) syphilis. The ulcer of chancroid has irregular margins and is deep with undermined edges. The syphilis ulcer has a smooth, indurated border and a smooth base. The genital herpes ulcer is superficial and inflamed.

Source: Modified from Schmid GP, Shcalla WO, DeWitt WE. Chancroid. In: Morse SA, Moreland AA, Thompson SE (Eds). Atlas of Sexually Transmitted Diseases. Philadelphia, PA: JB Lippincott; 1990.

to form multiple, small and shallow ulcers found on the labia and around the introitus. Lesions may also be found in the urethra and vagina, on the cervix and, occasionally, on the thighs and buttocks. These coalesce to form larger ulcers and resolve with crusting and healing. This cycle may take up to 3 weeks in a primary infection. Herpetic lesions may also occur in cervix, vagina or rectum. After a primary infection, the virus remains quiescent in the sacral ganglia and can re-emerge to cause recurrences at a later time. The symptoms of recurrent genital herpes tend to be milder and of shorter duration and are often preceded by a prodromal phase consisting of cutaneous itching or burning and redness in the affected region. The frequency of recurrence can vary from days to years. Rarely, herpes genitalis can also cause meningitis, encephalitis and hepatitis.

Diagnosis and management: The presence of multiple painful ulcers is suggestive of the diagnosis, but other causes of multiple painful ulcers such as Behçet's disease, chancroid, Stevens–Johnson syndrome and vulvitis should be excluded. In all instances, a search should be made for extragenital lesions.

When genital herpes is suspected, it is important to confirm the diagnosis with laboratory culture, if possible, which also permits subtyping of the virus and can be done within 1–4 days of the infection. HSV antigen detection by enzyme immunoassay (EIA) or fluorescent antibody (FA) and HSV DNA detection by polymerase chain reaction (PCR) are also possible. Seroconversion and serodiagnosis are useful in documenting first-episode infection, but in recurrent infection, there may be no rise. Once the diagnosis is made, a sympathetic explanation should be given to the patient, who may be very upset. The natural history of the disease should be explained, and advice should be given on genital hygiene. It is obviously important to trace sexual partners, and it would be wise to inform the obstetrician if the patient is pregnant. In view of the possible link with cervical cancer, a cervical smear once a year would be a sensible precaution.

Acyclovir (ACV) is the therapy of choice in primary herpes simplex genitalis and severe recurrent attacks. It is an acyclic nucleoside analogue that is a substrate for HSV-specific thymidine kinase. In primary genital HSV infection, oral ACV (400 mg three times daily for 10–14 days) is given. ACV does not cure the disease but decreases its severity.

Concomitant urethral, cervical and oral infections are common in first-episode infection, so oral therapy is preferable to topical. Symptoms are reduced within 48 hours. The duration of viral shedding is also decreased with antiviral therapy. ACV has a very low toxicity to cells which are not infected with herpes simplex.

In very severe attacks, for patients in the hospital or patients with serious complications, intravenous ACV may be appropriate.

In recurrent disease, oral ACV, famciclovir and valacyclovir have all been shown to help in reducing the duration of the episode. Treatment should be initiated by the patient herself as soon as she notices the first sign or symptom of recurrence. If the patient is immunocompetent, therapy may not always be required as the episodes are self-limiting. Measures such as local application of calamine lotion may provide relief. The topical preparation in aqueous base may provide better relief than the polyethylene glycol base. For recurrent disease, ACV 400 mg three times daily for 5 days is given.

Suppressive therapy with long-term ACV therapy (400 mg bd) has been used in some women having 4–12 episodes per year and who are emotionally disturbed or in severe physical discomfort. No serious side effects have been reported. Treatment should be interrupted every 12 months to reassess the need for continued therapy.

If secondary infection is present, it should be treated. Patients should be advised to have regular cervical smears to avoid intercourse when lesions are present and to inform their medical attendants of a past history of herpes when pregnant.

Syphilis (chancroid) is the next common cause of sexually transmitted genital ulcers **(Figs. 2A to C)**. Diagnosis is made, based on history and clinical and serological tests for syphilis. A painless, minimally tender ulcer without lymphadenopathy is likely to be a syphilitic ulcer. It may also present as vesicles mixed with small ulcers. Chancroid is usually one or two extremely painful ulcer with tender lymphadenopathy. Also, inguinal bubo with ulcer is likely to be chancroid, and without ulcer, it is likely to be lymphogranuloma venereum (LGV).

Recurrent Genital (Buccal) Ulceration

This is not an uncommon condition, and the ulcers, identical in appearance with those described above, may be on the vulva alone, in the mouth alone or simultaneously in both sites. When it is associated with conjunctivitis, it becomes part of Behçet's disease. It is not sexually transmitted.

Lymphogranuloma Venereum and Granuloma Inguinale (Figs. 3 and 4)

Lymphogranuloma venereum and granuloma inguinale (donovanosis) are rare sexually genital diseases. These are associated with an increased risk for human immunodeficiency virus (HIV) infections.

Acute necrosis or gangrene of the tissues of the vulva is often associated with a fusospirochetal infection. This is a term covering two microorganisms living in symbiosis—(1) *Fusobacterium* and (2) *Spirochaeta*. Both live anaerobically and can exist in a nonpathogenic form in the mouth and on the vulva. When found on ulcers, they are considered by some to be secondary invaders rather than causal agents. It can arise as a complication of acute infectious fever in debilitated children but is now rare in outside tropical countries. In these, it is still seen in destitute malnourished children and adults. Because of the underlying debilitation of the patient, the condition can be fatal.

Diabetic Vulvitis

Glycosuria, whether it be due to diabetes mellitus or not, causes a diffuse inflammation which gives the vulvar skin a typical purplish-red appearance. The symptom is intense pruritus. Although chemical changes in the epithelial cells may play a part, the vulvitis is mainly the result of infection with *Candida albicans* (this organism thrives in the presence of carbohydrates with which the vulva is contaminated). Treatment consists of controlling the glycosuria and instructing the patient to wash the vulva free from all urine (and sugar) immediately after micturition. Sponging with a 1% sodium bicarbonate solution gives temporary relief from pruritus, but the specific remedies for the infection are local applications of ointments or powders containing one of the fungicides. An ointment combining a fungicide with hydrocortisone is especially helpful.

Candidiasis

Candida infection of the vulva also occurs without glycosuria and may or may not be associated with a similar infection of the vagina, perianal skin, hands and feet. It not infrequently follows the use of antibiotics which interfere with the normal flora of the vagina and bowel.

The appearance of the vulva varies from a diffuse erythema to pallor and oedema and is sometimes similar to that seen in diabetic vulvitis.

Candidiasis typically causes pruritus vulvae. Its diagnosis and treatment is described below in this chapter under candidiasis.

Tinea Cruris (Ringworm)

Fungal infection of the vulva is rare in women or at least is difficult to prove. Nevertheless, irritating vulvar skin changes are not uncommon in women suffering from some sort of fungal infection of the feet and hands.

Pediculosis Pubis

This affects the pubis rather than the vulva. The 'crab louse', *Pthirus pubis*, infects the hair-bearing area of

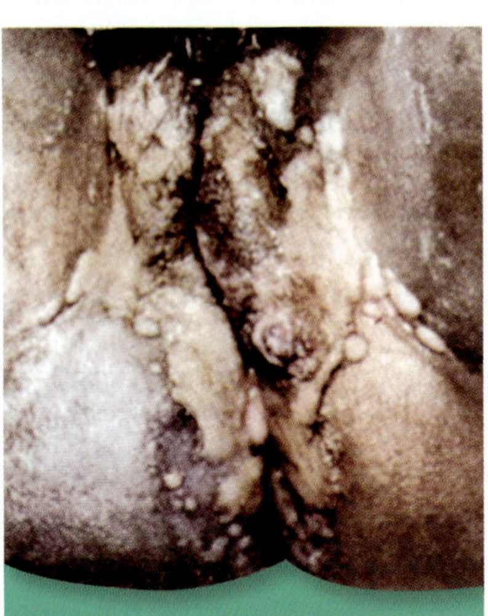

Fig. 3: Granuloma inguinale.

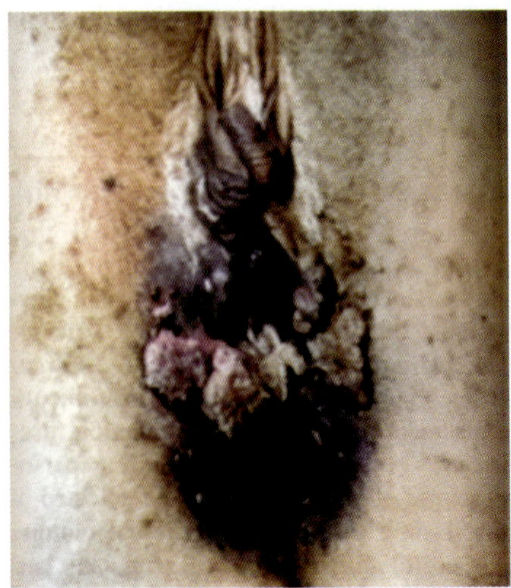

Fig. 4: Condyloma acuminatum of the vulva.

the mons, and the parasites or their eggs can be seen clinging to the hairs. The infection is transferred from one individual to another by contaminated clothing or by close bodily contact, including intercourse. The underlying cause is uncleanliness, and the symptom is pruritus. Treatment consists of shaving the vulva, frequent washing and applications of malathion lotion, shampoo or other pediculocides. Clothing has to be decontaminated.

Elephantiasis

This is a condition of chronic lymphatic oedema with associated thickening and hypertrophy of the epithelial tissues of the vulva. The skin is rough, warty and weeping. True elephantiasis is caused by infestation with the filarial worm *Wuchereria bancrofti*, but this is rare in temperate zones, where a more common cause of lymphatic obstruction is any chronic infection which heals by fibrosis. So, it is seen as an end result of healed tuberculosis, LGV, granuloma inguinale and possibly syphilis, and is then called false elephantiasis. Occasionally, the cause is obscure.

If the condition is severe enough to cause discomfort or dyspareunia, the affected tissue has to be excised. Even then, it may recur despite the discovery and treatment of the underlying infection.

Other Infections

All types of infection can involve the vulva on occasion. Those worthy of mention are diphtheria, actinomycosis, psoriasis **(Fig. 5)** and tetanus.

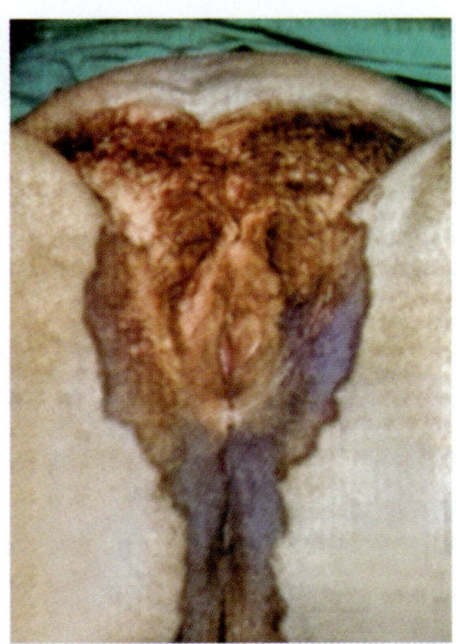

Fig. 5: Psoriasis of the vulva. Note the extent of the lesion extending laterally to the inner thighs and posteriorly to involve the perianal skin and cleft.

BARTHOLINITIS

Aetiology

The occurrence of bartholinitis always raises the suspicion of a gonococcal infection, but the disease can be caused by *Escherichia coli*, *Staphylococcus*, *Streptococcus faecalis*, *Streptococcus pneumoniae*, *Haemophilus* spp., *Trichomonas vaginalis* and, indeed, by any pyogenic organisms. Chlamydial infection may be present alone or in combination with the gonococcus. The role of bacterial vaginosis (BV) is unclear.

Pathology

Both duct and gland are involved and show the usual inflammatory reactions. The lining of the duct becomes swollen, and its orifice can be seen as a small red macula of congestion. Acute bartholinitis may resolve completely, but frequently an abscess forms and ultimately discharges through the lower vaginal wall. The infection sometimes persists in the chronic form with periodic exacerbations and abscess formation. The gland then becomes permanently enlarged and fibrotic, so that it can be felt between the fingers like a small hard pea. The duct often heals by fibrosis with closure of the orifice; this leads to cyst formation. Many Bartholin 'abscesses' are secondarily infected cysts. **Table 1** differentiates between a Bartholin cyst and abscess.

Clinical Features

The complaint is one of local discomfort which becomes very severe when an abscess forms. An acutely tender swelling appears beneath the posterior part of the labium majus extending inwards to the base of the labium minus. The overlying skin is reddened, and the surrounding tissues are indurated and oedematous. The position of the swelling at the junction of the anterior two thirds and posterior one third of the labia majora is diagnostic **(Fig. 6)**. The differential diagnosis is from adenoma and hamartomas, and in older women, from carcinoma.

Treatment

This consists primarily of rest in bed, the administration of antibiotics to cover gonococcal and chlamydial infections, as well as anaerobic bacteria and the relief of

TABLE 1: Differentiation between Bartholin abscess and Bartholin cyst.

Bartholin abscess	***Bartholin cyst***
Enlarged gland	Enlarged gland
Erythema is present in the skin overlying and surrounding the gland	Erythema absent
Skin overlying the gland is typically warm to the touch	No increase in temperature
Fever present, especially with tachycardia	Fever absent
Advancing cellulites can be present	Cellulites absent
WBC count elevated	WBC count not elevated
Bacteria and WBCs are present in the fluid (pus) contained within Bartholin gland	No bacteria or WBCs present in (serous) fluid contained within the cyst

(WBC: white blood cell)
Source: Faro S. Vulvovaginal infections. In: Bieber EJ, Sanfilippo JS, Horowitz IR, Shafi MI (Eds). Clinical Gynecology. Pennsylvania: Churchill Livingstone Elsevier; 2006. pp. 249-58.

pain with analgesics and warm baths. Since the infection is polymicrobial, good coverage is selected, and suitable single-agent oral outpatient therapy includes, among others, trimethoprim-sulfamethoxazole, amoxicillin-clavulanate or second-generation cephalosporins. Depending on patient risks, nucleic acid amplification tests (NAATs) for *Neisseria gonorrhoeae* and *Chlamydia trachomatis* and screening for other sexually transmitted diseases (STDs) may be done. When it is certain that an abscess has formed, free drainage is established by an incision placed outside the introitus; this is better than allowing the abscess to burst spontaneously. The operation of choice, however, is to marsupialise the edges of the abscess cavity to the skin of the introitus. By providing permanent drainage, this reduces the chance of subsequent cyst or abscess formation. The operator should wear protective goggles.

Excision of the gland and duct cannot be carried out while active infection is present, but it is indicated in the intervals between recurrent abscess formation when the gland remains palpable. This operation is more difficult than it sounds.

Technique of Marsupialisation

This technique preserves the secretory function of the gland for lubrication by avoiding the excision of the gland. It can be performed under local, regional or general anaesthesia. A wedged-shaped, vertical incision is made in the centre of vaginal mucosa just outside the hymenal ring as wide as possible to maintain the postoperative patency of the stoma-cyst wall is opened and the contents drained. Then, the lining of the cyst is exerted and approximated to the vaginal mucosa with 3-0 delayed absorbable interrupted suture. Recurrence rate is 10–15%.

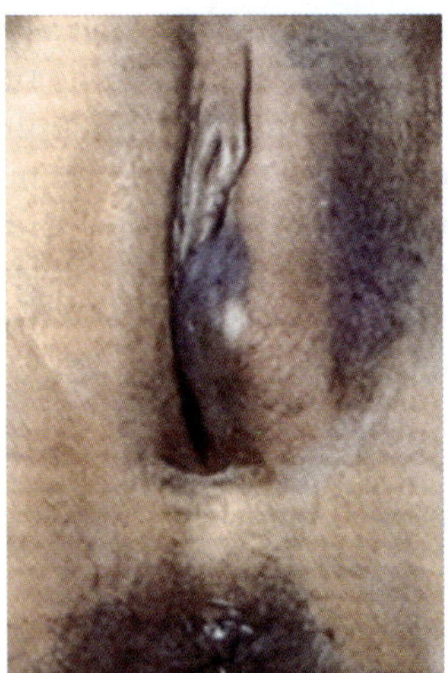

Fig. 6: A small left-sided Bartholin abscess which is distorting the vulva and pointing just within the introitus.

Technique of Excision

An elliptical incision in vaginal wall is made as close as possible to the size of gland origin. Blunt-pointed Mayo scissors allow dissection of the cyst from its bed. Cyst can further be mobilised with the handle of the scalpel. Complete cyst with adherent gland tissue is essential because residual glandular tissue can form a tender nodule or recurrent cyst; to ensure haemostasis, the entire cavity must be obliterated by approximating the walls with fine delayed absorbable suture material after excision of the cyst.

VAGINITIS

Vaginitis (Vulvovaginitis) in Infancy

Aetiology and Pathology

Although local infection in infancy is essentially one of vaginitis, the urethra and vulva are usually involved as well. The common age is 1–5 years. The infection arises because vaginal resistance has not been developed, and the organisms are transmitted from adults or another child by hands, clothing or utensils. The most serious form of infection is gonococcal, but this is now rare, and other organisms such as *C. albicans*, *Streptococcus*, *Staphylococcus*, *E. coli*, *Pneumococcus* and even *T. vaginalis* are more likely to be found. Threadworms (*Enterobius vermicularis*) can infest the infantile vagina as well as the lower bowel.

Occasionally, the basis of the infection is a foreign body inserted into the vagina by the child. The accidental entry of sand or shreds of clothing, especially from woollen pants, is another possibility.

Clinical Features

The main symptom is a purulent discharge, but the child may also complain of pain and soreness of the vulva. These interfere with walking and cause dysuria. In a young child, often, the parent notices her crying during urination or scratching herself. The vulva is reddened, sometimes oedematous or excoriated, and bathed in discharge. If the discharge is bloodstained, the presence of a foreign body, or some other condition such as a cervical polyp (even the rare sarcoma botryoides), should be suspected and excluded.

Diagnosis

The diagnosis of infantile vulvovaginitis is usually obvious, but the causal organism can only be determined by examining (including culturing) the discharge obtained by a swab or fine pipette inserted through the hymenal opening. This also excludes the possibility of leucorrhoea of infancy exaggerated by a fussy mother. Digital vaginal examination is not possible, but if a small girl is laid on her side, it is surprising how much of the vagina can be visualised. Rectal examination may enable a foreign body to be felt by counter-pressure against the symphysis pubis or against a hand placed on the abdomen. Ordinarily, however, the presence of a foreign body is excluded by sonography, examination under anaesthesia, and inspection of the upper vagina through an aural or nasal speculum, a baby's laryngoscope, a hysteroscope (vaginoscopy) or by radiography.

Treatment

Any foreign body must be removed; for this purpose, aural forceps can be useful. Otherwise, treatment consists of administering antibiotics or fungicides, modifying the dose to suit the age of the patient. Treatment for pinworms is instituted where required.

If the vulva is sore and excoriated, the child should be kept at rest, and the vulva sponged regularly. Adhesions of the labia can be prevented by the application of oestrogen cream locally.

It is necessary to take steps to prevent the spread of infection to the conjunctiva and other children. It is also important to avoid the young child becoming morbidly interested in her genital organs, which she quickly does—especially if the mother is overanxious.

Senile Vaginitis (Atrophic Vaginitis)

Aetiology and Pathology

This is caused by any of the common pyogenic organisms invading tissues, which have lost their resistance. Senile endometritis or vulvitis is sometimes present as well. The vaginitis is often granular, i.e. it appears as small multiple reddened areas, which are mostly seen in the vault and around the urethral orifice. Patchy ulceration can result in adhesions forming between the anterior and posterior walls to produce partial closure of the vagina—*adhesive vaginitis*.

Clinical Features and Diagnosis

The main complaint is postmenopausal yellowish discharge, sometimes bloodstained, which causes excoriation and soreness of the vulva. Dysuria (from urethral involvement) and a sensation of fullness in the vagina are also common.

The diagnosis can only be made by excluding other possible causes of postmenopausal discharge—senile endometritis or cancer of some part of the genital tract. Examinations under anaesthesia, diagnostic curettage and cervical cytology or biopsy are, therefore, essential in all cases before vaginitis is assumed to be the cause of symptoms. Even if vaginitis is present, the patient may still have carcinoma of the uterus as well.

Senile vaginitis should not be diagnosed merely on the finding of a speckled red vagina; for this, it can be a normal climacteric change. A discharge must also be present.

Treatment

The vaginal resistance is quickly restored by giving any of the oestrogen preparations in full dosage for 3 weeks, followed by an interval of 1 week and then repeated if necessary. Oestrogens can also be given locally in the form of a cream to be inserted into the vagina each night. By any route, they may induce uterine bleeding, and the patient should be warned of this. Any uterine bleeding must be reported; however, further investigation is then justified to exclude any more serious cause of postmenopausal bleeding. Local treatment with antiseptics or antibiotics is usually unnecessary.

When hormone therapy is suspended, the vagina atrophies again, but, if the infection has been eradicated, the disease should not relapse.

Trichomonas Vaginitis and Urethritis (Trichomoniasis)

Aetiology

This is the most common form of vaginitis and is found in approximately 50% of women complaining of vaginal discharge and in 60% of those with proven gonorrhoea. It occurs at any age from birth onwards but most often in the young adult.

The *Trichomonas* group of organisms is a large one, and certain members are commonly, if not normally, found in the mouth, bladder and large bowel. *T. vaginalis*, which is responsible for vaginitis, has morphological characteristics slightly different from the others. It is an ovoid motile flagellated parasite 15–20 μm in length and 8–10 μm in width, although smaller forms are described. It has four anterior flagella and an axostyle which traverse its body to end in a spike **(Fig. 7)**. It is a highly transmissible flagellated protozoan.

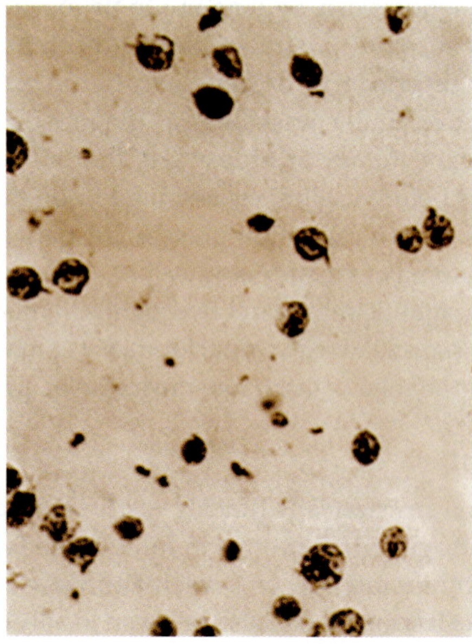

Fig. 7: *Trichomonas vaginalis* organisms, as seen in a preparation made from cultures of vaginal discharge.

In the vagina, the parasite is invariably accompanied by staphylococci, streptococci, enterococci or coliform organisms, but it is the trichomonads and not these which cause the vaginitis.

The infection is often contracted during intercourse with a male harbouring the organisms in the prepuce, urethra or prostate; the incubation period is 3–28 days. The partner of a man with proven *Trichomonas* infection can nearly always be shown to carry the organisms. Some say that trichomonads can be found in the urethra of 2% of all men and 10% after prostatic massage. Estimates of their frequency in cases of male nonspecific urethritis vary from 5% to 70%, depending possibly on the efficiency of the tests. Nevertheless, the male carrier is generally symptom free, and it has clearly been shown that a man can transfer the organisms from one woman to another without himself developing any signs of the disease.

This does not mean that *Trichomonas vaginitis* is always venereal in origin. It is not uncommon in virgins, children and old women. Transfer of the organism from one individual to another by indirect contact certainly happens. Contaminated domestic towels, bed linen and personal clothing, improperly sterilised surgical instruments such as specula, bath tubs and possibly swimming pools are likely media for transfer. Patients sometimes date the onset of symptoms to a stay in hospital where they may be exposed not only to infection by certain of the above means but to diseases and treatments which convert a carrier to an infected state. 20% of asymptomatic pregnant and nonpregnant women harbour the parasites in the vagina so, if debilitating illness lowers their resistance, or if they are given antibiotics which alter the vaginal flora, the disease can become manifested.

The effect of lowered local resistance is well illustrated by the fact that *Trichomonas vaginitis* often first manifests itself immediately after a menstrual period—during which the vaginal pH is raised. The optimum pH for the trichomonads is 5.5–6.5, and this or a slightly higher level is usually found in the vagina when the disease is present.

Trichomoniasis increases the chances of HIV infection if not treated. In women with HIV, trichomoniasis infection increases the chance of developing HIV infection.

Pathology

The infection is essentially of the vaginal epithelium, and the parasites shelter between the rugae. It is possible that they may penetrate between the surface cells but no deeper, and they induce the usual tissue inflammatory reaction. In 70–80% of cases, the trichomonads can also be cultured from the urethra, where they cause acute or chronic urethritis. Bartholin's glands and Skene's tubules are sometimes infected.

Trichomonas endocervicitis is also postulated, but it is doubtful whether it exists as a clinical entity. There are reliable reports of the organisms having been found in the cervix, the body of the uterus, the fallopian tubes and even in the bloodstream, but their significance in these sites is questionable.

Clinical Features

The first symptom is usually a sudden onset of purulent vaginal discharge, often dating from menstruation. It is said to be cream-colored and frothy, but its physical characteristics vary widely. The discharge is thin/thick, green, yellow or white, frothy and odorous in trichomoniasis. It may be profuse or scanty, and the most constant feature is that it causes pruritus, the itching being felt around and within the introitus. At the outset, dysuria and frequency of urine are also common complaints. Vaginal tenderness and congestion result in dyspareunia.

In the acute stage, the labia minora and introitus are sometimes oedematous. The vagina may be diffusely fiery red in colour but often presents a strawberry appearance which, on the cervix, can be confused with erosion. The external urethral meatus is congested and pouting. Later, when the reactions are less severe, the disease is manifested by a 'granular' vaginitis, which is most obvious in the fornices, on the portio vaginalis and around the urethral orifice.

The infection can become very chronic with pruritus more prominent than discharge and is subject to periodic exacerbations over the course of many years. The same is true of the urethritis; so 'recurrent cystitis' in women is very often explained by flare-ups of a persistent *Trichomonas urethritis*. This sort of chronic infection is also the main if not only cause of the pseudocaruncle or granulomatous caruncle of the urethra which is so often mistaken for a true caruncle.

Diagnosis

The diagnosis should be suspected in all cases where discharge causes pruritus but is made certain by demonstrating the presence of *T. vaginalis* organisms. Not infrequently, they are discovered incidentally during routine cervical cytology. Ordinarily, however, they are looked for in the vaginal discharge or, in cases of suspected urethritis, in swabs taken from within the urethra. A single negative test is never conclusive, and several studies may have to be done before the parasites are found.

In the office, wet smear preparation can be made. Specimens, uncontaminated by lubricant, are taken from the vagina or urethra by a swab or pipette and can be examined immediately microscopically. For this purpose, the material is mixed with saline solution on a warm slide, covered with a glass slip and left unstained. The trichomonads are recognised by their shape (larger than a pus cell but less than half the size of a vaginal squame) and by their motile flagella and rotatory movements. The sensitivity of wet mount secretion is low (51–60%).

However, this 'bedside' examination is very unreliable. Culture methods were considered gold standard until the advent of molecular methods of diagnosis (e.g. NAAT). The specimen of discharge, or preferably the whole cotton tip of the swab, is added immediately to a small tube of Kupferberg or Feinberg–Whittington medium. The latter is a proteolysed liver and inactivated horse serum preparation with streptomycin and penicillin added. It eliminates all organisms except *Trichomonas* and *C. albicans*; these thrive. Incubation preferably at 34°C rather than at 37°C is followed by examination of drops of the fluid for organisms at 24 and 48 hours and, if need be, later. Providing care is taken to make sure the culture medium is satisfactory; this method reveals *T. vaginalis* in twice as many female patients as does direct microscopic examination of discharge. It is the only means of reliably testing the male. NAAT is highly sensitive for the detection of *T. vaginalis*.

The finding of *Trichomonas vaginitis* indicates a need to exclude gonorrhoea as well. *Candida* and *Trichomonas* infestations also commonly coexist, but the dual nature of infection is not always evident until the dominant organism (*Trichomonas*) has been eliminated. The persistence of symptoms after treatment with trichomonacides, therefore, calls for repeated cultures for both *Candida* and gonococci.

Treatment

Systemic therapy is superior to topical therapy because *T. vaginalis* often infects the urethra and periurethral glands. These organisms can result in subsequent reinfection. The recommended regimen is metronidazole,

2 g in a single oral dose, for both partners. An alternative regimen in case of single-dose failure is one tablet of 500 mg given twice daily by mouth for 1 week. Tinidazole can be given as a 2-g single dose.

Whilst under treatment, the patient should be told of the need for care in the disposal of her underclothing and to keep her own bath towel to minimise the chance of her infecting other female members of the family. She should also be warned against coitus. The physical effect is irritant to inflamed tissue, and the male partner may become infected.

As many as 60% of the husbands of women suffering from *Trichomonas vaginitis* can be shown to harbour the parasite in the urethra and its associated glands or beneath the prepuce. Unless, during the period of abstinence, the organisms disappear spontaneously from the male urogenital tract, resumption of coitus when the wife's treatment is complete results in her being reinfected. Because of this, it is important to treat the consort of every woman suffering from *Trichomonas vaginitis*. He is given metronidazole simultaneously and in the same dosage. The couple should abstain from sex until treatment is completed.

It is generally stated that metronidazole administered orally is excreted in only small amounts through the vaginal wall; so its efficacy is difficult to understand. The fact that the treatment is generally efficient after total hysterectomy rather rules out the possibility of a significant secretion by the endometrial and cervical glands. It has been suggested that the real nidus of infection is in the bladder and urethra, and it is this which is eradicated by a renal excretion of the drug.

Oral medication with metronidazole is curative in 85–90% of cases, and the figure rises to 95% if the patient's consort is treated simultaneously. Tinidazole or metronidazole 2 g as a single oral dose is also effective and has lesser side effects. Chronic trichomoniasis in old women sometimes proves resistant, and, in such cases, treatment with the oral trichomonacide can with advantage be preceded by or combined with oestrogen therapy as for senile vaginitis.

Patients taking metronidazole or any of these drugs should be warned of the possible disulfiram (Antabuse)-like effect of these drugs in association with alcohol. Unless patients are warned, they quite logically give up the tablets rather than the alcohol. Metronidazole crosses the placenta but in very small amount. Treatment with metronidazole can be started after first trimester of pregnancy. Local metronidazole is not very effective in treating infection. Nonoxynol-9 and povidone–iodine are also trichomonacidal, but these are not recommended for use in pregnancy.

Nearly one in five women get reinfected within 3 months after treatment. So, follow-up and contact tracing and treatment are imperative. Recurrent YOU CAN BUY MEN infections are treated with metronidazole or tinidazole 2 g daily orally for 7 days.

Candida Vaginitis

Aetiology

This condition, also called vaginal thrush, is caused by the yeast-like organism *C. albicans*, a small gram-positive fungus which develops pseudomycelial threads with septate divisions and clusters of blastospores **(Fig. 8)**. It thrives on carbohydrate and likes an acidic medium (pH 4.0–5.5). This explains why the patient's symptoms are temporarily relieved by bathing or douching with a 1% sodium bicarbonate solution and during menstruation.

Candida albicans has a wide distribution in the body but is ordinarily nonpathogenic, being kept in check by the normal flora bacteria. It can be demonstrated in the mouths of 25% of all women, on the perianal skins of 8% and in the vaginas of 20–25%. Most vaginal (as well as alimentary and systemic) infections probably represent a change from the carrier state determined by circumstances which favour the growth of the fungus at the expense of other organisms. *Candida vaginitis* is often determined by glycosuria because of the availability of carbohydrate. It occurs frequently during pregnancy, because the vagina

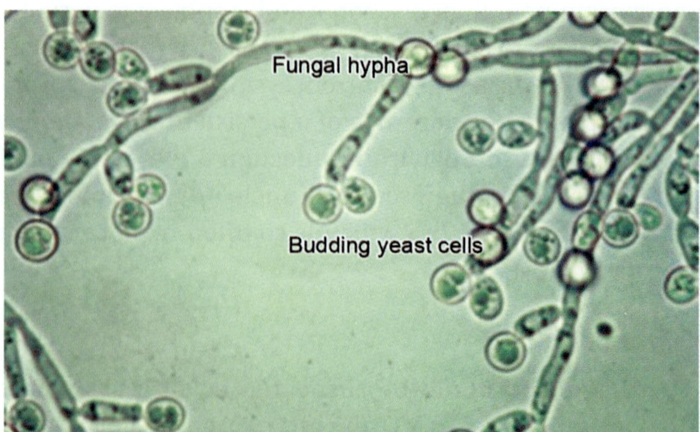

Fig. 8: *Candida albicans* showing hyphae and spores. This preparation was made from cultures of vaginal discharge.

then contains much glycogen, glycosuria is common and the high vaginal acidity tends to destroy other bacteria. The use of oral contraceptives favours the disease, but, in nonpregnant women, the most common cause is the taking of antibiotics, especially those covering a broad spectrum of bacteria. These, administered for incidental illnesses, alter the vaginal flora in favour of *Candida*. Indeed, the irresponsible use of these is responsible for the present widespread manifestations of candidiasis in both sexes throughout all communities. Almost 75% of women will have at least one episode of *Candida* infection in their lifetime.

Vaginal infection can be associated with lesions elsewhere in the body—the alimentary tract, hands, feet and perianal skin—of the patient or her consort. It can also be contracted during coitus with a man suffering from urethritis and balanitis or it is said so. In fact, these conditions are so uncomfortable as to prohibit intercourse; it is the asymptomatic male carrier who is more likely to be responsible.

A combination of *Candida vaginitis* and *Trichomonas vaginitis* is quite common, the dual infection again being possibly sexually transmitted **(Fig. 9)**.

Pathology and Clinical Features

The main symptoms are vaginal discharge associated with vaginal and vulvar pruritus, the latter often being out of all proportions to the amount of discharge. Local soreness causes dyspareunia. The discharge is typically thick, white and cheesy, tending to form plaques, which are lightly adherent to the vaginal wall **(Fig. 10A)**. They pull away to leave multiple haemorrhagic spots. In fact, the discharge is often atypical and may be watery or purulent, while the vaginal walls and introitus can appear diffusely reddened, oedematous or reasonably normal.

A very rare complication of *Candida* vaginitis is wide dissemination of the parasites to produce a dangerous systemic infection.

Transfer of Infection

One of the features of vaginal candidiasis is that the husband may also complain of burning or itching of the external genitalia for a few days following each act of coitus. The only causes of this symptom are *Candida* infection, *Trichomonas* infection and allergy to the rubber or chemical constituents of contraceptives. This is a valuable point in diagnosis. The woman who harbours the organisms in the vagina in late pregnancy may also infect the baby during its birth. This may be the origin of candidal stomatitis (thrush) in the newborn.

Diagnosis

The diagnosis of pruritus with discharge nearly always means either *Candida* or *Trichomonas* infection. A wet mount or saline preparation of the vaginal discharge should routinely be done, which can identify the presence of mycelia and yeast cells and also exclude clue cells and trichomonads. A 10% potassium hydroxide preparation is even more sensitive, as it dissolves the red and white blood cells (WBCs) and improves visualisation. If on direct

Fig. 9: *Trichomonas vaginalis*. The protozoa are seen only in a wet film and are of varying shapes. They may be adherent to a squamous cell or they may be attached to pus cells.

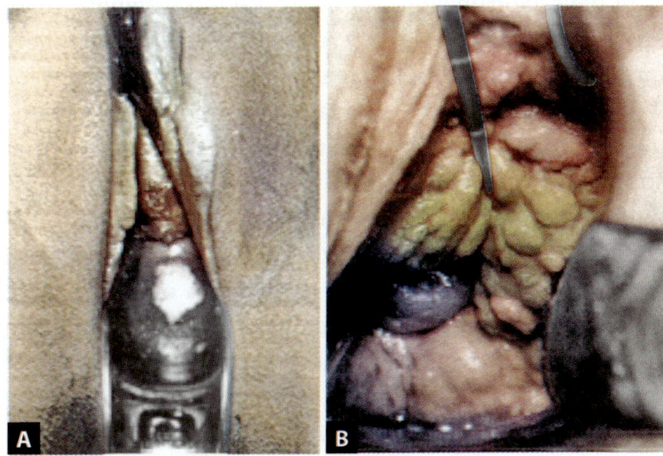

Figs. 10A and B: Two types of vaginitis. (A) *Candida* infection showing the classical patch of vaginal thrush; (B) Vaginitis emphysematosa occurring in midpregnancy.

microscopy, a large number of white cells are seen and the pH is >4.5, mixed infection should be suspected. If WBCs are absent and the pH is <4.5, antifungal treatment can be instituted. If direct microscopy does not show yeast cells or any other specific features, the vaginal swabs must be kept moistened with warm normal saline solution transported to the laboratory and cultures using Sabouraud broth or Nickerson medium prepared for reliable results. Better still is the inoculation of a tube of Feinberg–Whittington medium beside the patient. This permits the detection of both *Candida* and *Trichomonas* in one specimen. Antifungal treatment can be started after submitting the cultures. PCR test is also available for the diagnosis of *Candida* infection.

Treatment

Treatment with fungicides needs to be accompanied by controlling glycosuria, discontinuing oral contraceptives temporarily and eliminating any other aetiological factor. The one that cannot be removed is pregnancy, and it can be difficult to eradicate *Candida* completely from the vagina until after delivery. The pregnant as well as the nonpregnant woman, and their consorts, if necessary, are treated by local applications of one of the many fungicides available.

Of these, the traditional gentian violet solution, used in the past, is now outmoded. Although effective, it is messy and can cause severe local reactions with exfoliation of the superficial layers of the epithelium.

Recommended treatment for *Candida* infection includes clotrimazole 1% cream 5 g intravaginally daily for 7–14 days, clotrimazole 2% cream 5 g intravaginally daily for 3 days, miconazole 2% cream 5 g intravaginally daily for 7 days, miconazole 4% cream 5 g intravaginally daily for 3 days, miconazole 100 mg vaginal suppository one suppository daily for 7 days, miconazole 1,200 mg vaginal suppository one suppository for 1 day, tioconazole 6.5% ointment 5 g intravaginally in a single application, butoconazole 2% cream (single-dose bioadhesive product) 5 g intravaginally in a single application or terconazole 0.4% cream 5 g intravaginally daily for 7 days. Fluconazole 150 mg may be given as a single dose.

For recurrent infections, oral fluconazole 150 mg orally every 3 days for a total of three doses is recommended. Oral fluconazole (i.e. a 100-, 150- or 200-mg dose) weekly for 6 months is the indicated maintenance regimen.

Bacterial Vaginosis

Bacterial vaginosis is the most common cause of vaginal discharge in the reproductive age group.

Pathology

In BV, a polymicrobial infection with anaerobic bacteria displaces the normal flora of *Lactobacillus* spp. causing clinical symptoms.

Gardnerella vaginalis is the organism most commonly associated with BV. It is a small pleomorphic coccobacillus that may be Gram variable when stained and is found attached to epithelial 'clue cells' in smears of vaginal exudate or discharge. It is considered to be sexually transmitted. It is associated with multiple male partners. Male circumcision reduces the chance of BV. Usually, BV results from ascending infections **(Fig. 11)**.

Other microorganisms isolated from vaginal culture in BV include genital *Mycoplasma* and anaerobic bacteria such as *Peptostreptococci*, *Bacteroides* spp., *Prevotella* spp. and *Mobiluncus* spp. Lactobacilli are decreased or absent. The microbial ecosystem of the vagina is, thus, altered. Amines produced by the microbial flora, possibly by microbial decarboxylases, result in the characteristic fishy odour on mixing vaginal fluid with 10% KOH (whiff test).

It is often associated with other STDs. BV also increases the chances of acquisition of HIV infection.

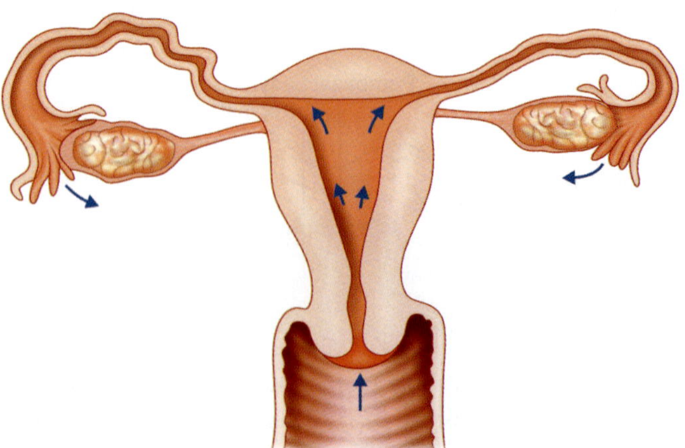

Fig. 11: Microorganisms originating in the endocervix ascend into the endometrium, fallopian tubes and peritoneum, causing pelvic inflammatory disease (endometritis, salpingitis and peritonitis). *Source:* Soper DE. Upper genital tract infections. In: Copeland LJ (Ed). Textbook of Gynecology. Philadelphia, PA: WB Saunders; 1993.

Clinical Features

The patients characteristically present with a homogeneous, white, nonviscous, malodorous, uniformly adherent, vaginal discharge. The discharge may be profuse enough to be seen at the labia. When other infections such as *Trichomonas* and *Candida* are associated, as they may be in 25% of cases, the picture may be modified. Some patients may be asymptomatic. Intrauterine contraceptive device (IUCD) use predisposes to BV.

Bacterial vaginosis has been implicated in postpartum endometritis, in posthysterectomy vaginal cuff cellulitis and in postabortion pelvic inflammatory disease (PID).

Diagnosis

Amsel's criteria:

1. Characteristic homogeneous thin, yellow, white adherent discharge
2. *Presence of clue cells on microscopy*
3. Vaginal fluid pH >4.5
4. Release fishy odour on adding 10% KOH.

Amsel's criteria are considered positive if any three of four criteria are positive.

The presence of clue cells is the most important criterion for diagnosis. A wet mount examination shows squamous epithelial cells covered with multiple bacteria, which gives the cells a stippled look with obscured borders **(Figs. 12A and B)**. Vaginal cultures are not as useful as *G. vaginalis* may be isolated even in the absence of BV. For the same reason, vaginal cultures cannot be used as a test of cure.

Nucleic acid amplification test is also available to diagnose BV infection.

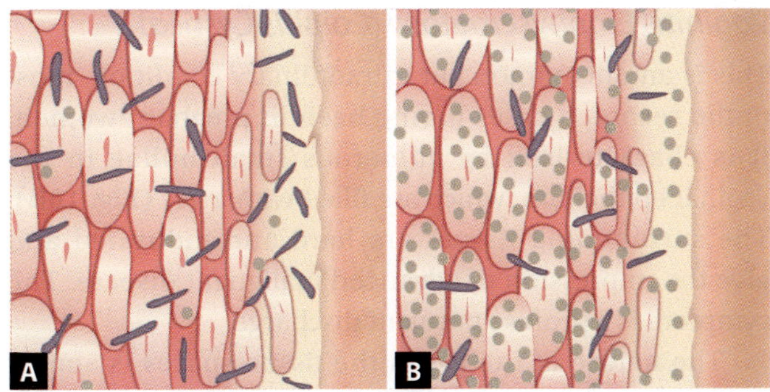

Figs. 12A and B: (A) Normal mature vaginal cells. The bacterial flora is dominated by lactobacteria (rod-shaped); (B) The field is dominated by 'clue cells'. Few lactobacilli are also seen.

TABLE 2: CDC-recommended regimen (2015).

Drug	*Dose*	*Duration (days)*
Metronidazole	500 mg oral, twice daily	7
Metronidazole gel 0.75%	One applicator (5 g), intravaginally, once daily	5
Clindamycin cream 2%	One applicator (5 g), intravaginally at bedtime	7

(CDC: Centers for Disease Control and Prevention)

TABLE 3: Alternative regimens.

Drug	*Dose*	*Duration (days)*
Tinidazole	2 g orally, once daily	2
Tinidazole	1 g orally, once daily	5
Clindamycin	300 mg orally, twice daily	7
Clindamycin	100 mg vaginally, once at bedtime	3

Treatment

Metronidazole 500 mg twice daily for 7 days results in 80% cure rates. Intravaginal metronidazole has fewer side effects but lowers the cure rates. Metronidazole gel 0.75% is used vaginally for 5 days. Oral clindamycin 300 mg twice daily for 7 days is as effective as oral metronidazole and is preferred in pregnancy. Clindamycin cream 2% can be given at bedtime for 7 days. Tinidazole 2 g orally for 2 days is another effective treatment for BV. Treatment of the male partner does not improve the clinical outcome. Vaginal acidifiers may suppress but do not kill anaerobic organisms, and alternative treatments such as *Lactobacillus*, yoghurt and disinfection have limited use in the treatment of BV **(Tables 2 and 3)**.

Oral probiotic therapy with Lactobacillus: It has been seen that lactobacilli taken orally will pass through the gastrointestinal (GI) tract and are seen to colonise the vagina via migration over the perineum.

Treatment of bacterial vaginosis is described in **Tables 2 and 3**.

Other Vaginal Infections

Some rare causes of vaginitis are the gonococcus and pneumococcus, which are seen mainly in children. Infections due to diphtheria, *Salmonella typhi* and *S. paratyphi* are also very rarely seen. The term puerperal vaginitis is sometimes used to cover infection of vaginal lacerations sustained during childbirth.

Vaginitis Emphysematosa (Colpitis Cystica)

This is an uncommon but extraordinary condition, most of the recorded cases having been in pregnant women. It is characterised by numerous small bullae in the vaginal epithelium, which are filled with a gas **(Fig. 10B)**. The surrounding tissues are hard and indurated and give the impression of advanced malignant disease. The symptom is a profuse purulent discharge.

The nature of the gas in the tissue spaces is almost certainly carbon dioxide. The cause of vaginitis emphysematosa is disputed, but, in the great majority of cases, trichomonads can be found in the vagina. These parasites, possibly by unusually deep penetration of the vaginal wall, are the most likely agents. *G. vaginalis* is also blamed.

The disease can cure itself spontaneously within a few weeks or months, often before the pregnancy is over. On the evidence, it should respond to treatment with metronidazole; although prior to the introduction of the drug, the cysts often regressed spontaneously.

Noninfective Vaginitis

Traumatic: Infection and ulceration can be the result of foreign bodies placed in the vagina and can complicate the anatomical and vascular changes which accompany uterovaginal prolapse. Occasionally, severe and recurrent vaginitis with ulceration is caused by self-inflicted trauma, prompted possibly by sexual perversion or other psychological upsets. This cause can be difficult to prove.

Allergy and drug sensitivity: A local reaction to chemicals is not uncommon, and the patient presents with discharge, pruritus and a fiery-red vagina. Antiseptics such as arsenic, mercury, iodine, picric acid, phenol preparations and gentian violet are used to be common causes. Presently, toilet preparations such as soaps, deodorants and bath salts; contraceptives such as rubber or materials used in the preparation of synthetic devices, the powder in which they are packed and chemical spermicides and nylon underwear are the common causes.

The diagnosis is made by careful enquiry about the onset of symptoms, bearing in mind the possibility of skin sensitivity. The treatment consists of removing the cause and arranging for saline douches and warm baths. Antihistamines by mouth and local applications of hydrocortisone may also relieve symptoms. The reaction not uncommonly includes cystitis and urethritis.

Idiopathic: There are some isolated cases of troublesome, chronic and resistant vaginal ulceration, sometimes multifocal, the causes of which are never discovered. These have been treated empirically by vitamins, antihistamines, antiseptics, various fungicides and trichomonacides and, in the case of postmenopausal women, with oestrogens.

CERVICITIS

Infection of the stratified squamous covering of the vaginal cervix as part of vaginitis is not usually regarded as cervicitis; this is a term reserved for inflammatory lesions in the endocervix, including the glands and deeper tissues.

Acute Cervicitis

This is mainly gonococcal, chlamydial or puerperal in origin, and the lesion is relatively unimportant in itself, the symptoms and physical signs being overshadowed by those caused by simultaneous infection of other tissues. Organisms gain entry through the gland openings in the endocervix and through obstetrical and surgical injuries.

The cervix is congested and enlarged with a swollen mucous membrane pouting at the external os. It is tender when touched or moved, and a profuse purulent discharge exudes from the cervical canal.

Acute cervicitis may resolve completely or progress to a state of chronic cervicitis. Its treatment is that of the more widespread infection of which it is merely a part.

Chronic Cervicitis

Aetiology

Chronic cervicitis is variously estimated to be present in some degree in 35–85% of women. It can probably arise as a result of vaginal organisms becoming pathogenic; it occasionally follows chronic and repeated injury from pessaries, tampons and unsatisfactory contraceptive devices; it may be gonococcal but is usually the end result of puerperal cervicitis. The puerperal type is often associated with laceration of the cervix and with chronic cellulitis.

Pathology

Although organisms can linger in the glands of the endocervix for many years, the condition of chronic cervicitis does not usually represent an active inflammatory state. It is the end result of injury and inflammation.

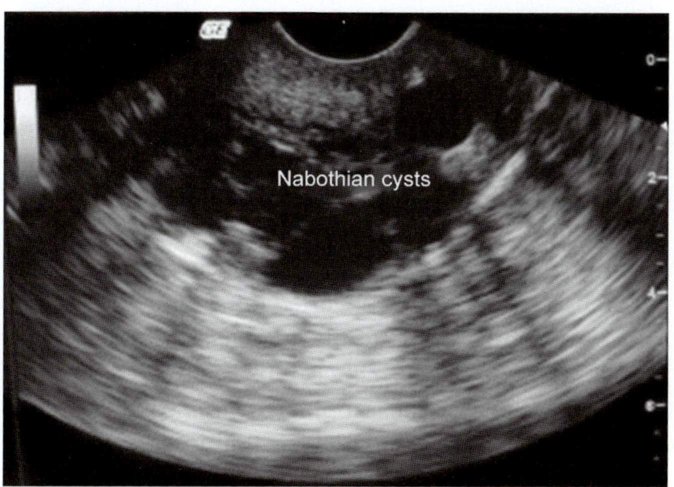

Fig. 13: Retention cysts (Nabothian follicles) in the cervix.

The mucosa and deeper tissues are fibrosed, congested and infiltrated with leucocytes and plasma cells. There may also be hypertrophy of glandular tissue to produce what was previously described as an *adenomatous cervix*. The ducts of certain glands become obstructed by plugs of epithelial cells and inspissated mucus, or by fibrosis, to cause retention cysts—*Nabothian follicles*. These are often visible to the naked eye and can become quite large **(Fig. 13)**.

A relationship between chronic cervicitis and the development of cervical cancer, once postulated, is no longer acceptable, and chronic cervicitis is not a cause of erosion as was once believed and still is in some quarters.

Clinical Features

Chronic cervicitis is usually a histological diagnosis without clinical significance. Some evidence of it is found in nearly all multiparous, and many nulliparous, cervices submitted to histological examination. Only when the injury and reaction are very severe, they cause symptoms, and all these, with the exception of discharge, mostly derive from an associated cellulitis. They tend to be worse premenstrually and include mucopurulent discharge—the mucus is due to overactivity of the glands themselves; low backache which is only partly relieved by rest; aching in the lower abdomen and pelvis; deep-seated dyspareunia; contact bleeding; menorrhagia and congestive dysmenorrhoea possibly from associated endometritis and infertility, alleged to result from changes in the physical characters of the cervical plug, from a decreased pH of the cervical canal and from an increased pH of the vagina—a profuse discharge can raise the vaginal pH to 5–7.5. The last symptom is questionable, and certainly many women with gross chronic cervicitis conceive without difficulty.

All manner of other conditions and symptoms have been ascribed to chronic cervicitis—arthritis, dyspepsia, pain on defaecation and bladder irritability. Indeed, cauterisation or other treatment of an allegedly infected cervix has been claimed to cure nearly all the ills to which the woman is subjected. It should, therefore, be emphasised that the only symptom clearly attributable to cervicitis *per se* is discharge, and this usually dates from an attack of infection, from abortion or from labour.

Diagnosis

The physical signs in the cervix which may lead to the diagnosis are enlargement and congestion, ectropion, cystic glands, pouting and florid endocervix, fixation, tenderness to the touch and pain when the cervix is moved or pierced with a vulsellum. It can be difficult to distinguish chronic cervicitis from carcinoma, and this may be impossible sometimes without biopsy. Vaginal cytology and colposcopy aid the diagnosis of malignancy. The exclusion of malignancy is especially important before using ablative methods of therapy.

Treatment

Antiseptics: Since any infection is always deep-seated, the superficial application of antiseptics by means of pessaries or paints is useless. Douching has only the merit of removing discharge and odour temporarily, but it may introduce the discharge into the upper genital tract and is no longer recommended.

Antibiotics: Antibiotics are useful only in case of active infection, e.g. gonorrhoea or chlamydia.

Cauterisation, cryotherapy or laser ablation: Chemical caustics employed in the past are of little value and have been replaced by electric or diathermy cauterisation, or cryotherapy, to destroy diseased areas.

By cautery, cystic glands are punctured, ectropion is corrected by deep linear burns and any coincidental erosion is coagulated. The cervical canal is treated only with caution or left alone.

Cryotherapy is preferable to cautery. It is done using the probe which best fits the lesion, and the entire lesion is frozen.

Laser ablation, e.g. with the CO_2 laser, has the advantage of cure rates similar to cryotherapy but with the transformation zone maintained in its normal position. Following cryotherapy, it usually recedes into the endocervical canal and is not visible for further evaluation if required.

These forms of treatment are office or outpatient procedures; general or even local anaesthesia is seldom required.

Following treatment, a slough separates in approximately 10 days. This is attended by an increase in discharge and often by frank bleeding. Following cryotherapy and laser, the discharge is extremely profuse, and the patient should be advised replacement of electrolytes to avoid feeling very weak. Thereafter, the discharge slowly subsides in 4–6 weeks, which is the time taken for squamous epithelium to grow over the raw area.

The late sequelae of overenthusiastic cauterisation are obstruction of the ducts to cause more cystic glands and cervical stenosis.

Trachelorrhaphy: The edges of lacerations can be excised, and the cervix is reconstituted by a plastic operation.

Hysterectomy: If the condition of cervicitis is so severe that it cannot be treated satisfactorily with diathermy, cryotherapy or cone excision, and if future fertility is not desired, hysterectomy is sometimes indicated.

Special Forms of Cervicitis

Tuberculosis, syphilis, schistosomiasis, amoebiasis and other special infections and ulcers of the cervix have already been described along with vaginitis in Chapter 20: Infections Including Sexually Transmitted Diseases.

ENDOMETRITIS

Acute Endometritis

Apart from infections introduced at operations and by instrumentation, acute endometritis is either gonococcal or puerperal in type.

Chronic Endometritis

Aetiology

In theory, every case of acute endometritis might go on to chronic endometritis. In fact, the regrowth of new surface endometrium during each menstrual cycle prevents the persistence of any infection which is not deep-seated. Chronic endometritis is, therefore, a rare disease between the menarche and the menopause and only occurs when the uterus is permanently injured or when there is opportunity for it to be continually reinfected. Its causes are foreign bodies within the uterus, malignant disease of the uterus, infected polyps and retained products of conception, with inflammatory cells, including altered macrophages known as 'foam cells'. Its lining epithelium becomes destroyed and converted into granulation tissue. This exudes pus, which tends to collect in the uterus to form a *pyometra* because the cervix is narrowed by senile change and because the atrophied myometrium is unable to expel it. The uterus enlarges by thinning its walls, and spontaneous rupture followed by peritonitis is described as a rare complication. Sometimes, in response to pyometra, the endometrial epithelium undergoes metaplasia into a stratified squamous type. Senile endometritis is a condition associated with cancer. The ultimate growth is usually an adenocarcinoma but can contain squamous cell elements.

Clinical Features

A purulent and very offensive postmenopausal discharge, sometimes bloodstained, is the main complaint. When a pyometra forms, the discharge occurs intermittently, ceasing for a few days or weeks and then returning immediately after colicky lower abdominal pain. The uterus generally feels small and atrophic but, in the case of pyometra, may be enlarged, soft and cystic.

Diagnosis

The clinical features are identical to those of carcinoma of the body of the uterus, so the diagnosis of senile endometritis can only be made by curettage. If a pyometra is present, pus escapes as the cervix is dilated, and conventional curettage then involves the risk of spreading the infection to cause cellulitis and peritonitis. To avoid this, curettage may have to be deferred for 1 or 2 weeks but must be carried out sooner or later if carcinoma is to be excluded. When it is done, a cover of antibiotics is desirable. Some form of suction curettage or endometrial lavage is less hazardous.

Treatment

The drainage of the uterus afforded by dilatation of the cervix is enough to cure some cases. There is, however, much to be said for hysterectomy in all cases of senile endometritis if the patient is reasonably fit. This not only makes for a certain cure; it circumvents the difficulty of excluding the presence of an underlying carcinoma and removes a potentially malignant organ.

Pyometra (Pyohaematometra)

The collection of pus, or of a mixture of pus and blood, within the uterus is described in this and other chapters. It is convenient here to summarise the possible causes which are:

- Congenital atresia of the vagina or cervix
- Stenosis of the cervix or vagina following operations, burns and radiotherapy
- Puerperal endometritis with retention of the lochia
- Tuberculous endometritis
- Endometritis
- Carcinoma of the cervix
- Carcinoma corporis.

The most common of these are malignant states of the uterus, acting alone or in association with radiotherapy; after these, senile endometritis. Benign tumours of the uterus, even infected polyps, rarely if ever cause pyometra because they do not obstruct the cervix.

METRITIS

Aetiology

The myometrium may be involved as part of a widespread pelvic infection, but metritis is rarely an entity in itself. Some degree of acute metritis is present in all cases of spreading puerperal endometritis. In prolonged labour with devitalisation of the lower segment and certain cases of abortion complicated by *Clostridium welchii* infection or induced by the injection of chemical irritants, the uterine wall becomes gangrenous **(Fig. 14)**. Curettage in the presence of endometrial infection can also cause metritis.

Pathology

The myometrium shows the usual reaction to infection—congestion and inflammatory cell infiltration in its early stages and possibly fibrosis ultimately. There may even be abscess formation.

Clinical Features

These are obscured by those of other inflammatory lesions which are always present. An abscess causes intermittent pyrexia and possibly pyaemia.

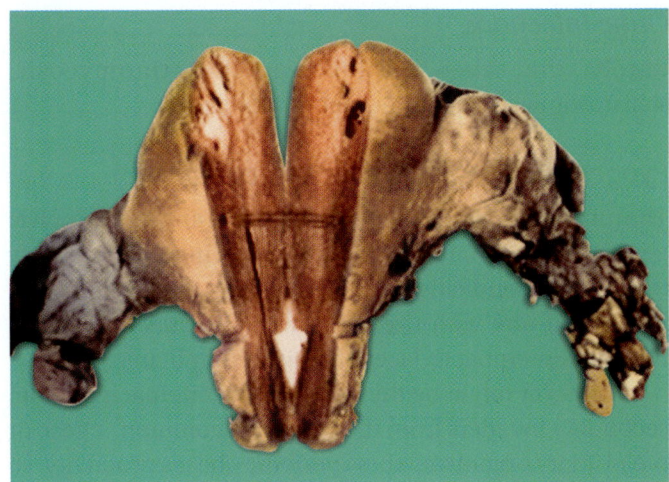

Fig. 14: Chronic abscesses in the uterine wall associated with chronic salpingo-oophoritis and pelvic cellulitis. This condition arose as a result of puerperal infection and caused death of the patient from pyaemia several weeks after delivery.

SALPINGO-OOPHORITIS

When the fallopian tubes are infected, the ovaries are usually affected as well, although often to a minor extent. The term salpingitis should, therefore, generally be taken as meaning salpingo-oophoritis. Salpingo-oophoritis is nearly always bilateral (unless one adnexum has been removed) and is essentially a disease of the young adult.

Aetiology

Ascending Infection

Acute salpingitis is a polymicrobial infection. In gonorrhoea and chlamydial infection, the organisms ascend through the uterus and along the tube to produce an endosalpingitis. Other organisms such as *G. vaginalis*, *Bacteroides* spp., especially *B. fragilis*, peptostreptococci, *Proteus* and *Klebsiella* spp. may also originate from the vagina.

Puerperal and Postabortal

The organisms concerned in puerperal infections are usually streptococci, staphylococci, *E. coli*, the genital mycoplasmas and *C. trachomatis*. They spread from the uterus by lymphatics and veins to the peritoneum to cause pelvic peritonitis. The adnexa are only involved as part of the pelvic peritonitis, and this explains why the old term for this condition was perimetritis. Although intraluminal spread of infection occurs to a limited extent, the tube is attacked mainly from the outside.

Other Infections

Rarely, the tubes are involved in actinomycosis, schistosomiasis and other special infections.

Pyogenic Infection of Pelvic Peritoneum

The tubes and ovaries become involved in any state of pelvic peritonitis. Often, the primary cause is in the alimentary tract (e.g. appendicitis and diverticulitis), and the infection is a mixed one with the coliform organisms and gram-negative Enterobacteriaceae being predominant.

Whatever might be the nature of the original infection, secondary invaders from the bowel are common. These or the primary organisms show periodic phases of activity, so salpingo-oophoritis tends to be a recurrent disease. In the case of gonorrhoea, however, repeated attacks probably always represent reinfection.

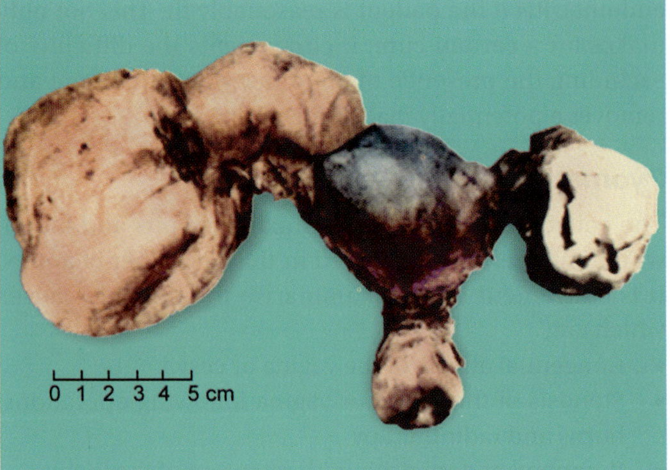

Fig. 15: Bilateral tubo-ovarian abscesses, probably gonococcal in origin.

Pathology

Ordinarily, the endosalpinx is affected along its whole length, but the gonococcus shows a predilection for the outer part to leave permanent damage of a characteristic type. In the acute phase of any infection, the tissues become reddened and oedematous showing, on microscopic examination, the usual inflammatory responses. Thereafter, the following developments are possible.

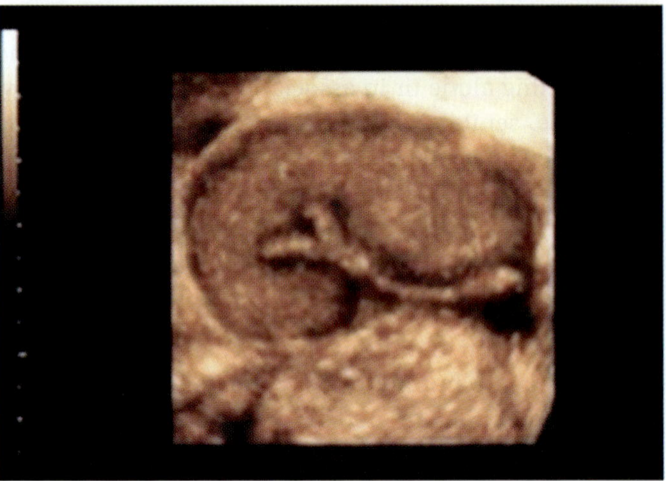

Fig. 16: Pyosalpinx 3D ultrasound.

Resolution

The tubes and ovaries can return to normal structure and function if the infection does not cause appreciable tissue destruction.

Abscess Formation

If the endosalpinx is destroyed in part or whole and converted into granulation tissue, pus is formed. This can escape into the peritoneal cavity or be retained within the tube depending on whether and when the abdominal ostium becomes closed. So, it may collect in the tube to result in a pyosalpinx, in the ovary to form an ovarian abscess, in both to produce a tubo-ovarian abscess **(Fig. 15)**, or in the pouch of Douglas to cause a pelvic abscess. The walls of a chronic pyosalpinx **(Fig. 16)** can ultimately become calcified, although such a happening generally betokens a tuberculous basis.

Healing by Fibrosis

When this happens, the tube wall thickens in part or whole; the plicae adhere together to obstruct or distort the lumen, and the tube and ovary become adherent to adjacent organs, to the broad ligament and to the uterorectal pouch. The parts of the tube most likely to be obstructed are the abdominal ostium and the narrow isthmus. In the latter site, chronic infection causes beading and thickening which give rise to the name *salpingitis isthmica nodosa*. This old term describes nodular lesions felt in the tube and of uncertain cause. Some use the term for tuberculous infection, although the nodules may be caused by either an endosalpingitis or a perisalpingitis.

Hydrosalpinx

When the inflammation subsides to leave the fimbrial end sealed, but the tubal epithelium elsewhere intact, the natural secretions cannot escape, and the tube gradually distends with watery fluid to become a hydrosalpinx. This is a retort-shaped swelling, which only exceeds the size of an orange in exceptional cases **(Fig. 17)**. An extraordinary feature of a hydrosalpinx is that the inner end of the tube is nearly always open, and yet the fluid does not drain into the uterus. Perhaps, the tubal muscle is so damaged or stretched that it cannot expel the fluid; perhaps, the tube normally drains into the peritoneal cavity rather than into the uterus. Examination of specimens suggests that the phenomenon is not explained by a valve mechanism at the uterine end. This feature is fortunate in that it enables the diagnosis to be made by hysterosalpingography **(Figs. 18A and B)**. An uncomplicated hydrosalpinx is usually too soft and flaccid to be palpable on bimanual examination. With high-resolution transvaginal ultrasound and three-dimensional (3D), the diagnosis of hydrosalpinx can also be made. Classical ultrasound findings are elongated cystic mass with incomplete septations **(Fig. 19)**.

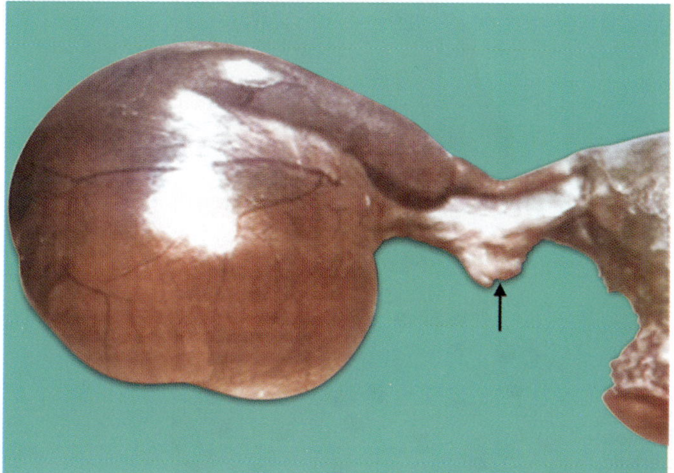

Fig. 17: Hydrosalpinx. The retort-shaped enlargement of tube with closure of the outer end. Disappearance of the fimbria and absence of adhesions are typical and suggest a previous gonococcal infection. The ovary (indicated by an arrow) is separate from the tumour.

The pathogenesis of hydrosalpinx is not agreed. It has been suggested that it represents the end result of pyosalpinx—the pus having liquefied. Bearing in mind the comparatively thick walls of a pyosalpinx and the destruction of the endosalpinx which goes with it, it is difficult to believe that the thin-walled hydrosalpinx is lined by normal, although compressed endosalpinx can ever be its offspring. The outlook as far as fertility is concerned is unfavourable, although the endothelium is able to secrete it is functionally impaired. Moreover, when a hydrosalpinx is found, there is usually no history of a severe previous infection; often, there is no history of salpingitis sufficient to cause symptoms. Nevertheless, the most likely cause of this condition is a gonococcal infection whose after-effects are limited to the ampullary area of the tube, one which produced few or no clinical manifestations when it happened. The apparent absence of fimbriae strongly supports this concept.

Other possible backgrounds, when there is no history of previous disease, are previously unrecognised subclinical infections related to *Chlamydia* and other organisms,

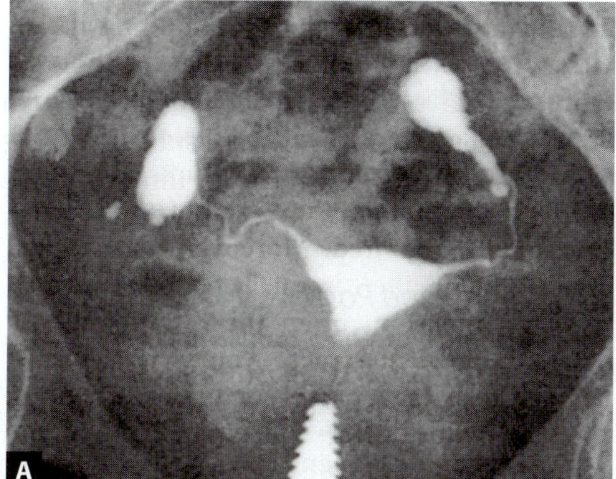

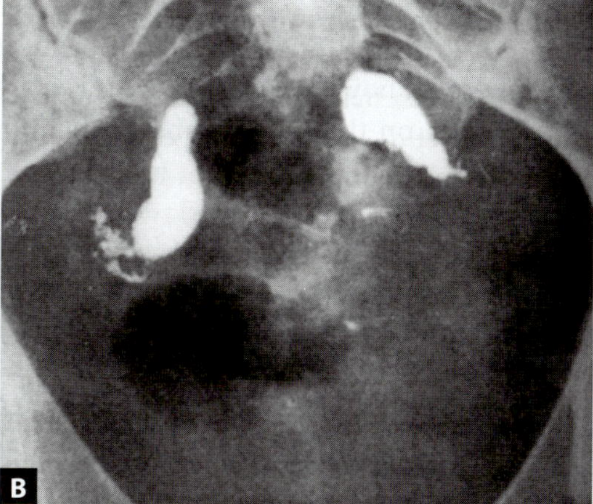

Figs. 18A and B: Bilateral hydrosalpinges, revealed by salpingography, in a woman aged 24 years who complained of infertility. She gave a history of gonorrhoea and of one abortion prior to marriage, but this condition is much more likely to be the result of gonococcal salpingitis than of postabortal infection. (A) Radiograph taken immediately after the injection of an oily radio-opaque material. The appearance of the globules in the dilated outer end of the left tube represents a failure of the oil to mix with the watery contents of the tube; (B) 24 hours later, the medium remains loculated in the hydrosalpinges.

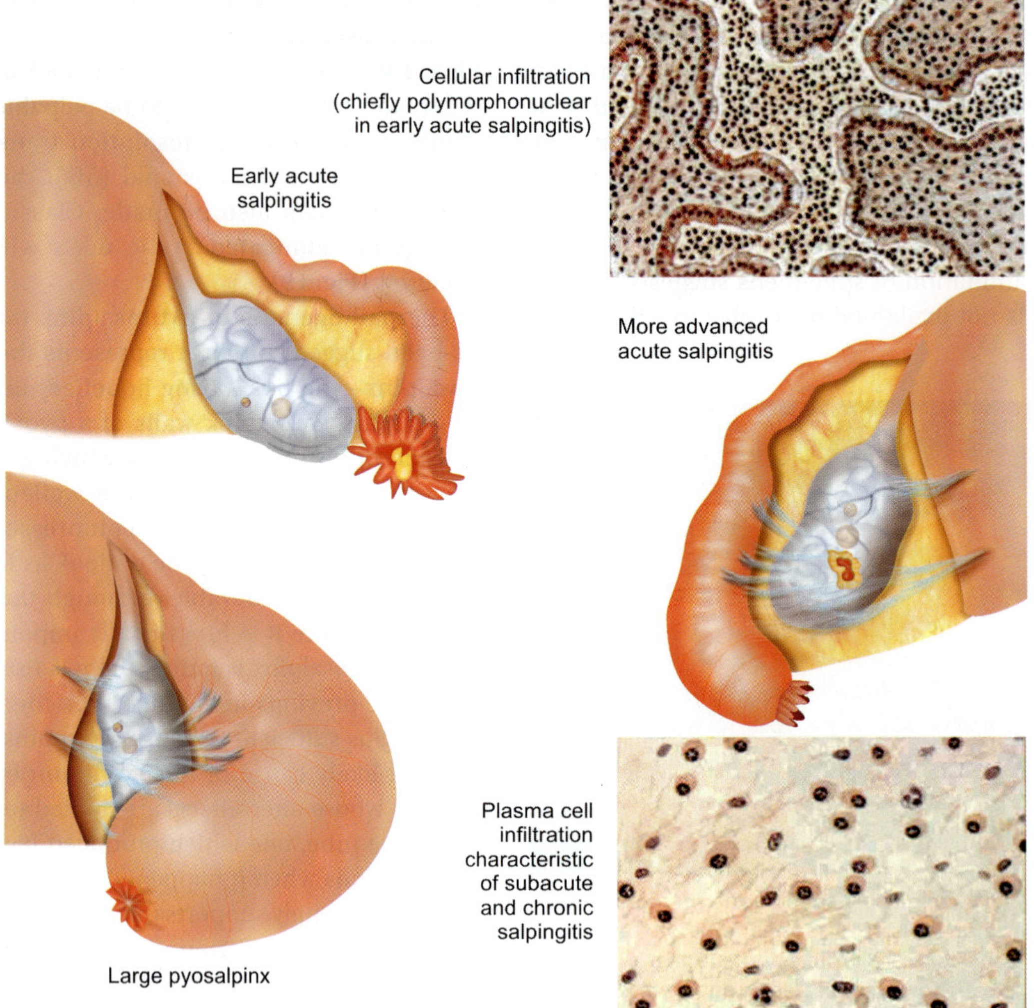

Fig. 19: Hydrosalpinx and pyosalpinx.

perhaps even including gonococcal or tubercular infections. In tuberculosis, however, the appearances are very variable depending on the site and mechanism of infection.

Tubo-ovarian Mass

When a hydrosalpinx is adherent to an ovary containing one or more follicular cysts, the two conditions give the appearance of a single multilocular structure. Sometimes, the dividing wall breaks down, but, even if it does not, the lesion is called a tubo-ovarian mass. In Western countries, tubo-ovarian masses rarely exceed the size of a foetal head. In the Far East, however, they commonly develop to the size of a pregnancy at term and are difficult to distinguish from large ovarian neoplasms.

Peritoneal Cysts and Pseudocysts

These are not uncommonly result from adhesions following perimetritis. When such a cyst lies outside the ovary and has a wall formed by intestines and omentum, it is sometimes called a pseudocyst.

Puerperal and Postabortal Infection

This, being essentially an exosalpingitis, results in peritubal and periovarian adhesions with thickening of the tube wall and ovarian capsule. Pyosalpinx and hydrosalpinx are not common, and, when the adhesions are separated, the fimbriae are found in a reasonably healthy state; even the tube lumen may be patent and lined by normal epithelium. Infections arising from the alimentary tract also have a similar effect.

Clinical Features

Acute Salpingo-oophoritis

This is a disease seen mainly in sexually active women of the reproductive age group. The clinical features mainly reflect pelvic peritonitis. The illness begins with acute lower abdominal pain, pyrexia, tachycardia, malaise and sometimes vomiting. The pain is situated diffusely across the lower abdomen or in both iliac fossae. A menstrual period may be delayed in onset by a few days or be precipitated early, and it is often heavy and prolonged. There may be symptoms of urethritis as well. There is often a history of recent confinement or abortion, of a discharge suggesting gonorrhoea, of exposure to risk of infection, or of previous attacks of salpingitis. Symptom-producing salpingitis hardly ever occurs during pregnancy. After the first 12 weeks, the decidua vera and decidua capsularis fuse, and a new infection cannot ascend through the uterus, while a pre-existing chronic infection may have caused tubal damage. Cases of acute salpingo-oophoritis in pregnancy are rare, except when secondary to acute appendicitis. Similarly, it is rarely seen in premenarchal girls or postmenopausal women. Women on oral contraceptive pills are also at a lesser risk possibly because of the thickening of the cervical mucus plug.

The patient looks flushed and toxic and has a dirty mouth. The lower abdomen is tender with some muscle guarding. There may be obvious signs of lower genital tract infection, but, on bimanual examination, it is often impossible to define either the uterus or the adnexa because of generalised tenderness. In any case, the adnexa are not usually enlarged at this stage. A valuable test is to rock the cervix gently from side to side. This puts tension on the broad ligaments and adnexa and produces pain if salpingitis is present. There is a brisk polymorphonuclear leucocytosis and a raised erythrocyte sedimentation rate.

With spreading peritonitis, intestinal distension and constipation are likely; a pelvic abscess causes a swinging temperature, diarrhoea, pain on defaecation and sometimes retention of urine. A very serious complication is rupture of a pyosalpinx which causes an 'acute abdomen' and sometimes extreme shock. Bacteraemic shock in its severest form may complicate gonococcal salpingitis.

Acute salpingo-oophoritis has to be distinguished from the following:

- *Acute appendicitis:* In this, the pain commences higher in the abdomen and becomes unilateral; anorexia and vomiting are more likely; muscle rigidity is localised and more obvious; menstrual disturbance and discharge are absent.
- *Ectopic pregnancy:* Here, the pain is mainly unilateral and causes collapse or fainting. There is little, if any, pyrexia, and the leucocyte count is only slightly increased.
- Torsion of the pedicle of a leiomyoma or ovarian cyst
- Rupture of an ovarian cyst
- Rupture of an endometriotic cyst
- Ovulation pain and corpus luteum haematoma
- Diverticulitis
- Intestinal obstruction
- Pyelitis and cystitis
- Other causes of an 'acute abdomen'

Subacute Salpingo-oophoritis

The onset of salpingo-oophoritis does not always produce the dramatic picture painted above. More often, the disease is subacute from the beginning and can persist in this form for several weeks. The symptoms and signs are then less striking, and the patient may be only moderately incapacitated, with less discomfort, less pyrexia and less pelvic tenderness. The clinical features in general are intermediate between those described above and those below.

Chronic Salpingo-oophoritis

Chronic salpingo-oophoritis may follow an acute or subacute stage, but, in the case of certain causal organisms, the disease is chronic from the outset. Also, a previous acute infection may have been subclinical and have passed unnoticed. Chronic salpingo-oophoritis is mostly asymptomatic and often is only discovered by the finding of obstructed tubes during the investigation of infertility or during surgery for ectopic pregnancy.

Otherwise, the symptoms are chronic aching in the lower abdomen or in both iliac fossae and sometimes in the lumbosacral region. The pain tends to be worse during the week preceding menstruation and to ease gradually as congestion subsides during menstruation. Ovarian involvement results in more frequent periods and uterine congestion to increased loss; so, the complaint is of heavy and frequent periods. Except when the infection is tuberculous in type, amenorrhoea never occurs, even when there are bilateral ovarian abscesses. There is often a mucoid or mucopurulent vaginal discharge intermenstrually. Deep-seated dyspareunia and involuntary infertility are other common complaints; rectal discomfort and bladder irritability are seen occasionally. General health is affected by way of malaise, anorexia, lethargy, increased irritability and sometimes loss of weight.

Examination may disclose no abnormality. On the other hand, bimanual palpation may reveal generalised tenderness and fixation of the pelvic organs. According to their pathology, the adnexa may be palpably enlarged. Often, they feel nodular and hard. A fixed retroversion of the uterus and some degree of cellulitis in the uterosacral or broad ligaments are common findings.

Chronic salpingo-oophoritis has to be distinguished from the following:

- Ectopic pregnancy
- Appendicitis, diverticulitis and other diseases of the bowel, especially if adhesions have occurred.
- Ovarian tumours, especially bilateral ones
- Pelvic endometriosis
- Congestive dysmenorrhoea and premenstrual syndrome
- Colonic and rectal spasm—irritable bowel and distended caecum syndromes

Treatment of Acute Salpingo-oophoritis

The treatment of acute salpingo-oophoritis is always conservative in the first place; hence, the importance of distinguishing this disease from abdominal conditions requires emergency surgery. Treatment should be preceded by taking cervical, rectal and urethral swabs to determine the nature of the infection.

General

Admission to hospital may be required. It ensures adequate rest, constant observation and efficient treatment. Once the diagnosis is made, all local interference such as pelvic examination should be avoided. Even if she is not kept in bed continually, the patient's physical activity should be severely restricted until her temperature and pulse rate have been normal for at least 5 days.

Relief of Pain

Warmth to the lower abdomen is soothing, and, once the diagnosis is reasonably sure, pain should be relieved by analgesics, anti-inflammatory agents or even opiates.

Antibiotics

These are given in full dosage for gonorrhoea, *Chlamydia* or postabortal infection.

Surgical Treatment

This is only indicated in the following circumstances: When there is evidence of spreading peritonitis despite adequate medical treatment, rupture of a pyosalpinx or ovarian abscess, intestinal obstruction resulting from adhesions, pelvic abscess formation, if the diagnosis is in reasonable doubt and if it is difficult to be sure that the condition is not one of acute appendicitis or other lesion requiring urgent surgery. Laparoscopy is sometimes suggested in the acute phase if the diagnosis is uncertain, but if there is any real possibility of peritonitis and adhesion formation, laparotomy may be safer. In cases of salpingitis, laparoscopy will reveal tubal hyperaemia and oedema, sticky exudates on the tubal surface and/or pus pouring out of the tubal ostia. It is generally wise to leave the pelvic organs untouched, except for taking a swab from any pus for bacteriological analysis or if laparotomy has been performed to close the abdomen without drainage. It is amazing how apparently hopeless tubes can recover to the extent of being functional.

When there are large pyosalpinges, they are sometimes best removed—even in the acute phase.

Treatment of Subacute and Chronic Salpingo-oophoritis

Before initiating treatment, it is again important to investigate bacteriologically for the source of infection. When the disease is chronic, however, and excepting tuberculosis or other rare special infections, it is unlikely that a significant organism will be found. Tests may need to be repeated several times before the organism is isolated.

Conservative Treatment

An important part of treatment is a period of physical rest. Appropriate antibiotic therapy is indicated for the subacute disease but rarely helps if the salpingitis is truly chronic and consists of little more than residual damage resulting from previous infection. Pelvic heat applied by means of hot water bottles 4 hourly, or by shortwave therapy, is comforting and sometimes appears to assist resolution of a subacute inflammatory reaction.

As swelling and fixation of the adnexa subside, as the uterus becomes more mobile, and when the temperature and pulse rate have remained normal for several days, the patient is allowed to resume activity gradually. Coitus should be forbidden until it is reasonably certain that the inflammatory process is completely inactive.

Surgical Treatment

Indications:

- For persistence of symptoms despite trial of conservative measures
- For recurrent attacks or exacerbations of the disease
- For persistence of gross enlargement of the adnexa
- Sometimes for infertility

Surgery is only really safe and likely to give the best results if it is carried out during a quiet phase, i.e. when the temperature has been normal for at least 2 weeks, there is no rise in pulse rate or temperature after a test vaginal examination, the white cell count is normal and the erythrocyte sedimentation rate is normal.

Nature of operation: This necessarily depends on the findings at laparoscopy or laparotomy. For infertility, the objective is to try to restore tubal function by *salpingolysis, salpingostomy* or *reimplantation of the tube* into the uterus. Even if reproductive function has to be sacrificed, menstrual function should be preserved, if possible, in young women; ovarian function, in particular, should be preserved because of the possibility of in vitro fertilisation at a later date. The disadvantages are that sometimes the ovaries later become cystic, and the patient may be left with menorrhagia for which hysterectomy ultimately becomes necessary.

In the case of salpingectomy with conservation of the uterus, it is important to excise the cornu of the uterus which contains the intramural portion of the tube. This may be infected, and, if it is not removed, it can be the source of further symptoms.

For widespread chronic pelvic infection with disorganisation of both adnexa, total hysterectomy with removal of both tubes (and sometimes both ovaries) is often the best treatment. Indeed, this is often the eventual outcome after previous conservative surgery.

OOPHORITIS

Oophoritis without salpingitis is rare and only occurs as a result of blood or lymph-borne infection from elsewhere.

Aetiology

Oophoritis occurs as a complication of septicaemia, typhoid and paratyphoid fevers, pneumonia and viral diseases such as mumps and influenza. Of these, the most common is mumps, the oophoritis being the equivalent of the orchitis complicating parotitis in the male.

Tuberculosis, sarcoidosis, syphilis and actinomycosis are very occasional causes.

Pathology

The acute inflammatory reaction nearly always subsides completely without permanent ill effect. However, abscess formation or healing with fibrosis and fibrocystic change are recorded. Mumps rarely has a sterilising or other ill effect in female, because the capsule of the ovary is more elastic than that of the testis; so, ischaemic injury to the Graafian follicles is not likely. Even if some follicles are destroyed, enough remain for full reproductive function.

Clinical Features

The only evidence of oophoritis as a rule is the occurrence of lower abdominal pain for a few days during an acute infective illness. A single menstrual period may be disturbed in its onset, but it is difficult to know whether this is the effect of the oophoritis or the general systemic upset. If an abscess forms or if the condition becomes chronic, the clinical features are those described under salpingo-oophoritis.

Treatment

In the acute phase, no treatment other than that of the causal illness is required. If an abscess forms, the treatment is as described for salpingo-oophoritis.

PELVIC PERITONITIS

Aetiology

- Any infection of the genital tract
- *Infection from the alimentary tract:* Appendicitis and diverticulitis
- *As part of general peritonitis:* Pneumococcal and tuberculous infections
- *Foreign bodies:* These reach the peritoneum via the bowel, uterus or the posterior vaginal fornix or are left at operations
- Rupture or perforation of an infected uterus

- *Following pelvic haematocele*: Infection of blood clot is seen in ectopic pregnancy and also following pelvic operations—postoperative pelvic peritonitis
- *Chemical*: This includes a variety of possible irritants—urine, bile, vernix caseosa, meconium (spilled at the time of caesarean section), radio-opaque media used in salpingography, talc from gloves or drapes used at operations and the contents of ruptured cysts. The fluid from endometriotic cysts is irritant, but the worst in this respect is the sebaceous fluid from dermoid cysts. This, like vernix caseosa, can produce the most violent reaction which ultimately leads to very dense adhesions.

Irritant fluids used for the purpose of douching, and especially those used by women themselves with the idea of inducing abortion, may pass through the uterus and tubes to produce pelvic or general peritonitis. Abortifacient pastes are another cause.

Pathology

The initial acute inflammatory reaction may subside or be followed by exudation and pus formation. Although complete resolution is possible, pelvic adhesions are left in most cases. Pus can collect to form a pelvic abscess, and the causes of this condition are all those stated above. If neglected, the abscess ultimately bursts into the rectum or bladder but very rarely into the vagina whose investing fascia is strong.

Clinical Features

These are the same as for acute salpingo-oophoritis and, in the case of residual pelvic adhesions, as for chronic salpingo-oophoritis. The leading symptom of acute pelvic peritonitis, with or without abscess formation, is often diarrhoea.

Treatment

In the acute stage, the treatment is the same as for salpingo-oophoritis, except that any cause such as a foreign body or ruptured cyst must be removed. A pelvic abscess or a collection of infected blood requires drainage; this is usually best established through the posterior vaginal fornix, not the rectum. Sometimes, abdominal drainage is more efficient.

Residual pelvic adhesions only require surgery if they cause symptoms.

PELVIC CELLULITIS

Pelvic cellulitis is a condition of inflammation affecting any of the loose cellular tissue lying above the levator ani. It occurs most obviously in the bases of the broad ligaments (parametritis) and the uterosacral ligaments (posterior parametritis).

Acute and Subacute Cellulitis

Aetiology

Organisms travel to the cellular tissue from infected adjacent pelvic organs by way of lymphatic channels, but they can also gain direct access through perforations and tears, surgical or obstetrical, in the vaginal fornix, cervix, uterus, rectum and bladder.

Adjacent infections:

- Cervicitis and endometritis, including secondary infection complicating neoplasms and foreign bodies. Cellulitis associated with cancer of the cervix makes it difficult to define the extent of the growth.
- *Salpingo-oophoritis:* Some degree of parametritis invariably accompanies severe salpingo-oophoritis. It accounts in large measure for the fixation of the pelvic organs in this disease.
- Diverticulitis, carcinoma of the rectum and other conditions of the large bowel can lead to cellulitis of the uterosacral ligaments.
- Carcinoma of the bladder and cystitis, if extensive, can cause cellulitis in the uterovesical space.

Pelvic operations:

- Dilatation and curettage, especially if carried out in the presence of endometritis
- Ablative procedures on an infected cervix
- *Hysterectomy:* Some degree of cellulitis of the tissues at the vaginal vault is common after total abdominal or vaginal hysterectomy but is usually preceded by haematoma formation.
- *Lower segment caesarean section:* In this case, the cellulitis is anterior rather than lateral and often represents secondary infection of a haematoma.
- Other obstetrical operations
- The insertion of intrauterine contraceptive devices or of instruments to terminate pregnancy.

Radiotherapy: Radiotherapy in the presence of infection can cause cellulitis. This risk is mostly seen in the case of malignant disease, but cellulitis following the insertion of radioisotopes occurs.

A special form of noninfective ischaemic 'cellulitis' is seen as a late complication of radiotherapy.

Pathology

Anaerobic streptococci, staphylococci and *E. coli* are the most likely pathogens. The loose connective tissue reacts by inflammatory infiltration and oedema; an indurated mass results. The possible further developments are complete resolution, abscess formation, the pus tracking according to the distribution of the cellular tissue and its connections and healing by fibrosis and scar formation. One complication is suppurative thrombophlebitis of the veins of the broad ligament, and the clinical features of this can obscure those of cellulitis.

Cellulitis of the broad ligament and paracolpos is nearly always *unilateral* and, in puerperal infection, is most often left-sided, as are cervical lacerations. Puerperal cellulitis is also more extensive and obvious because the amount of cellular tissue is increased, and the vascular channels are dilated by pregnancy. Cellulitis of the uterosacral ligaments is usually bilateral and appears as a horseshoe-shaped swelling with the two arms passing back beside the rectum.

Clinical Features

Symptoms and signs do not usually make their appearance until 7–14 days after the original infection. The typical picture is presented by puerperal cellulitis. This ordinarily becomes manifested around the 10th day when the patient experiences a rise in temperature and pulse rate accompanied by malaise. On reviewing the case, it may be noted that slight evening pyrexia has been present for some days previously for no apparent cause. The patient does not appear to be seriously ill but may complain of discomfort in the lower abdomen or pelvis on the affected side. The pain is not severe, and muscular rigidity is absent because the lesion is extraperitoneal. Other possible complaints are frequency of micturition, dysuria, diarrhoea and painful defaecation. The formation of an abscess brings further general systemic disturbance with a high swinging temperature and rigours.

The physical signs are very striking. The cellulitis gives the impression of a hard mass, continuous with the uterus and extending towards the wall of the pelvis. It may be so large as to be palpable abdominally; otherwise, it is detected on pelvic examination. Induration of the uterosacral ligaments is often felt more easily per rectum. If the broad ligament is involved, the swelling is unilateral and pushes the uterus to the opposite side. The mass is tender, woody in consistency and fixes all organs in its vicinity, especially the uterus.

An abscess may point into the rectum; into the bladder; into the vagina; on the lower anterior abdominal wall, especially above the inguinal ligaments; over the femoral canal; in the thigh via the obturator foramen or in the buttock via the sacrosciatic notch.

Diagnosis

The diagnosis is usually easy, but confusion may arise over the following:

- *Acute salpingo-oophoritis and pelvic peritonitis:* In this condition, the pain is *bilateral* and more intense, abdominal rigidity is present and the temperature is usually higher. Diarrhoea is more likely. Any swelling is separate from the uterus.
- *Malignant disease:* Extension of growth from the cervix, corpus or ovary into the broad or uterosacral ligaments
- Diverticulitis and carcinoma of the lower bowel
- Ectopic pregnancy, especially if it is intraligamentary
- Broad ligament haematoma

Treatment

Medical and general: As for acute salpingo-oophoritis.

Surgical: An abscess which is pointing and easily accessible should be drained; otherwise, surgery is to be avoided. The ideal drainage route is through the posterior vaginal fornix, but the site of incision is determined to a large extent by where the abscess points. An extraperitoneal inguinal approach is best in certain cases.

Prognosis

Except in old and debilitated women, the prognosis is good, and the cellulitis usually resolves completely. It sometimes heals by fibrosis (see further). Unlike salpingo-oophoritis and because the endosalpinx is not affected, cellulitis does not lower fertility. Moreover, future pregnancies do not involve any special risk of reawakening the infection.

CHRONIC CELLULITIS

Aetiology and Pathology

Chronic cellulitis is a condition of fibrosis, or of long persisting inflammatory exudation, in the broad and uterosacral ligaments. It usually represents the quiescent end result of acute cellulitis but can be a response to a chronic low-grade infection in an adjacent organ such as the cervix and rectum, e.g. an infected cancer.

Clinical Features

The symptoms are chronic aching pain in the pelvis, often one-sided; deep-seated dyspareunia; sacral backache, especially if the uterosacral ligaments are involved and menorrhagia and discharge if there is an associated congestion of the uterus and cervix. On vaginal examination, a scar in the cervix and vaginal vault, with underlying induration in the broad ligament, is easily detected. When the uterosacral ligaments are implicated, they feel prominent, hard and tender. The uterus is fixed on the affected aspect; attempts to move it reproduce the patient's pain.

Diagnosis

The diagnosis of chronic cellulitis should not be made a cover for all one-sided pelvic pains for which another cause cannot be found. Clear evidence of previous infection or associated disease should be present. Posterior parametritis has to be distinguished from endometriosis of the uterosacral ligaments and rectovaginal septum.

Treatment

Medical and General

This is the same as for chronic salpingo-oophoritis.

Nerve Block

Injection in the ilioinguinal region with long-lasting anaesthetic solutions may relieve pain and tenderness and can usefully be combined with treatment of associated cervical lesions.

Surgery

Trachelorrhaphy, freeing of cervical and vaginal scars and treatment of associated chronic cervicitis may give relief, especially if the complaint is dyspareunia.

PELVIC INFLAMMATORY DISEASE

Pelvic inflammatory disease comprises a spectrum of inflammatory disorders of the upper female genital tract, including any combination of endometritis, salpingitis, tubo-ovarian abscess and pelvic peritonitis. In the foregoing sections, the infections, as they affect individual organs, have been discussed. What follows here is a summary to present the condition as usually encountered in clinical practice.

Aetiology

While most cases of PID are caused by *N. gonorrhoeae* and *C. trachomatis*, other organisms can be encountered less frequently: *G. vaginalis*, *Prevotella*, *Peptostreptococcus*, streptococci, *Haemophilus influenzae* and pneumococci.

Clinical Features and Diagnosis

Some patients may be asymptomatic or have subtle nonspecific complaints.

The classic triad, however, is given as follows:

- Lower abdominal pain
- Cervical excitation pain
- Adnexal tenderness, often in the presence of fever.

In severe cases, abdominal rebound tenderness may be present; vaginal discharge may be seen. Some women may have associated menorrhagia, metrorrhagia and urinary symptoms.

One or more of the below additional findings may increase the detection and specificity of the diagnosis of PID:

- Oral temperature of >101°F (>38.3°C)
- Mucopurulent cervical discharge/friable cervix
- Presence of increased WBCs in vaginal discharge
- Elevated erythrocyte sedimentation rate
- Elevated C-reactive protein
- Laboratory documentation of cervical infection with *N. gonorrhoeae* or *C. trachomatis.*

The most specific criteria for gonorrhoea, *Chlamydia* or other organisms may be positive, and an endometrial diagnosis of PID includes:

- Endometrial biopsy, if performed, may show with histopathological evidence of endometritis.
- Transvaginal sonography or magnetic resonance imaging showing thickened, fluid-filled tubes with or without free fluid in the pelvis or tubo-ovarian complex or Doppler studies suggestive of pelvic infection (hyperaemia)
- Laparoscopic findings are consistent with PID.

Sequelae

The most important long-term sequelae of PID are chronic pelvic pain, ectopic pregnancy and infertility.

Treatment

Treatment should be initiated as soon as a presumptive diagnosis of PID is made, because early effective treatment is crucial to prevent long-term sequelae. The Centers for Disease Control and Prevention (CDC) guidelines (2021) for outpatient treatment of PID are shown in **Boxes 1 and 2**.

Cefoxitin [2 g intramuscular (IM) single dose plus 1 g probenecid orally] or ceftriaxone (500 mg IM) or equivalent third-generation cephalosporin (e.g. ceftizoxime or cefotaxime) along with doxycycline (100 mg orally twice daily for 14 days and metronidazole 500 mg orally twice daily for 14 days). Alternative regimen consists of levofloxacin 500 mg orally once daily in combination with metronidazole 500 mg orally 2 times/day for 14 days or moxifloxacin 400 mg orally once daily for 14 days. Hospitalisation is recommended in cases of severe disease, suspected pelvic abscess, cases where the diagnosis is uncertain, adolescent patients and where there is failure of or noncompliance with outpatient therapy **(Box 1)**.

Inpatient regimens have been explained in **Box 3**. Once clinical improvements occur, oral regimen is started. The oral regimen is described in **Box 3**.

Patients are discharged when the temperature is normal for 24 hours, and other signs decrease or disappear. The treatment of sexual partners is important.

Indications for surgery include failed antibiotic therapy, ruptured abscess and suspected sepsis. Surgery may be image-guided drainage under ultrasound, laparoscopy or laparotomy. Surgery usually involves removal of abscess cavity wall and drainage of pus.

BOX 1: Criteria for hospitalisation of patients with acute pelvic inflammatory disease.

The following criteria for hospitalisation are suggested:
- Surgical emergencies (such as appendicitis) cannot be excluded
- The patient is pregnant
- The patient does not respond clinically to oral antimicrobial therapy
- The patient is unable to follow or tolerate an outpatient oral regimen
- The patient has severe illness, nausea and vomiting or high fever
- The patient has a tubo-ovarian abscess

BOX 2: Centers for Disease Control and Prevention (CDC)-recommended treatment regimens for oral therapy of acute pelvic inflammatory disease (PID).

Oral therapy can be considered for women with mild-to-moderately severe acute PID, as the clinical outcomes among these women are similar to those treated with inpatient therapy. The following regimens provide coverage against the frequent aetiologic agents of PID. Patients who do not respond to oral therapy within 72 hours should be re-evaluated to confirm the diagnosis and should be administered parenteral therapy on either an outpatient or inpatient basis.
- *Regimen A:* Ceftriaxone 500 mg IM in a single dose plus doxycycline 100 mg orally 2 times/day for 14 days with metronidazole 500 mg orally 2 times/day for 14 days
- *Regimen B:* Cefoxitin 2 g IM in a single dose and probenecid 1 g orally administered concurrently in a single dose plus doxycycline 100 mg orally twice a day for 14 days *with* metronidazole 500 mg orally twice a day for 14 days
- *Regimen C: Other parenteral third-generation cephalosporin (e.g. ceftizoxime or cefotaxime) plus doxycycline 100 mg orally 2 times/day for 14 days with metronidazole 500 mg orally 2 times/day for 14 days*

The optimal choice of a cephalosporin for regimen B is unclear; although cefoxitin has better anaerobic coverage, ceftriaxone has better coverage against *Neisseria gonorrhoeae*.
Clinical trials have demonstrated that a single dose of cefoxitin is effective in obtaining short-term clinical response in women who have PID. However, the theoretical limitations in its coverage of anaerobes may require the addition of metronidazole to the treatment regimen. Metronidazole will also effectively treat BV, which is frequently associated with PID. No data have been published regarding the use of oral cephalosporins for the treatment of PID. Limited data suggest that a combination of oral metronidazole plus doxycycline after primary parenteral therapy is safe and effective.
- *Alternative oral regimens:* Levofloxacin 500 mg orally once daily in combination with metronidazole 500 mg orally 2 times/day for 14 days or moxifloxacin 400 mg orally once daily for 14 days

(BV: bacterial vaginosis; IM: intramuscular)

SUPPURATIVE THROMBOPHLEBITIS OF THE PELVIC VEINS

Definition

Suppurative thrombophlebitis is a condition in which the veins of the broad ligament become thrombosed as a result of infection within their lumen. It is to be distinguished from *phlebothrombosis* in which the vessel wall and the clot are not infected.

Aetiology and Pathology

Suppurative pelvic thrombophlebitis is nearly always the result of puerperal or postabortal infection with anaerobic streptococci or staphylococci. The thrombi in the uterine sinuses become infected, and the processes of thrombosis

BOX 3: Centers for Disease Control and Prevention (CDC)-recommended treatment regimens for parenteral therapy of acute pelvic inflammatory disease.

- Ceftriaxone 1 g IV every 24 hours plus doxycycline 100 mg orally or IV every 12 hours plus metronidazole 500 mg orally or IV every 12 hours
- Cefotetan 2 g IV every 12 hours plus doxycycline 100 mg orally or IV every 12 hours
- Cefoxitin 2 g IV every 6 hours plus doxycycline 100 mg orally or IV every 12 hours
- After clinical improvement with parenteral therapy, transition to oral therapy with doxycycline 100 mg 2 times/day and metronidazole 500 mg 2 times/day is recommended to complete 14 days of antimicrobial therapy
- Clindamycin (900 mg IV 8 hourly) along with gentamicin (loading dose 2 mg/kg body weight IM or IV, followed by 1.5 mg/kg 8 hourly). When using the clindamycin and gentamicin alternative parenteral regimen, women with clinical improvement after 24–48 hours can be transitioned to clindamycin (450 mg orally 4 times/day) or doxycycline (100 mg orally 2 times/day) to complete the 14-day therapy. However, when tubo-ovarian abscess is present, clindamycin (450 mg orally 4 times/day) or metronidazole (500 mg orally 2 times/day) should be used to complete 14 days of therapy with oral doxycycline to provide more effective anaerobic coverage

(IM: intramuscular; IV: intravenous)

and infection spread to the venous plexuses in the broad ligament and ultimately to the ovarian and uterine veins. The ovarian veins are more often affected. Portions of the infected clot break away to cause pyaemia with repeated embolism. Some degree of parametritis is nearly always present but is not usually obvious. Neither is the primary uterine infection, although gangrene and abscesses of the uterus are rare concomitants **(Fig. 14)**.

Clinical Features

Since the original uterine infection is generally low grade and gives little evidence of its presence, the disease usually only becomes clinically manifested approximately 10 days (with a range of 2–30 days) after abortion or labour. The onset can then be dramatic with a sudden rise of temperature (39–40.5°C) accompanied by a rigour. This denotes a breaking off of an infected clot into the bloodstream. There may be typical symptoms and signs of pulmonary embolism (or a 'fainting attack'). The pulse rate rises, the patient feels ill and leucocytosis is present, but localising symptoms, such as lower abdominal pain, are exceptional. Thereafter, the temperature fluctuates, and there may be recurrent pulmonary infarction. The fully established picture is one of pyaemia with the formation of embolic abscesses.

The physical signs in the pelvis are not remarkable unless there is associated cellulitis. The most that is found is a suggestion of thickening and tenderness in one broad ligament; the veins themselves may be palpable, but it requires an expert observer to detect this. Swelling of one or both legs gives evidence that the thrombosis has spread to the common iliac vein or to the inferior vena cava.

Treatment

General and Medical

This is the same as for postabortal infection, although massive doses of antibiotics may be required. The mainstay of treatment is antibiotics and heparin. Fever usually subsides within 48 hours of treatment. Treatment is usually continued for 7–10 days. Serious complications include extension of thrombus or pulmonary embolism.

Surgery

Ligature of the main vein proximal to the thrombosis is indicated only when recurrent embolism threatens life and cannot be controlled by other means. The ovarian and common iliac veins, and even the inferior vena cava, have been ligated with success in these circumstances. The need for such desperate measures is exceptional. It only arises mainly among poorly nourished women living in squalor and in whom septic abortion (probably criminal) has been neglected.

SUGGESTED READING

1. BASHH guidelines https://www.bashh.org/guidelines
2. CDC guidelines on pelvic infections available at cdc.gov
3. Gershenson DM, Valea FA, Lentz GM, Lobo RA (Eds). Comprehensive Gynecology, 8th edition. Elsevier; 2021.

22

CHAPTER

Genital Tuberculosis

Pesona Grace Lucksom, Latha V Kharka, Muralidhar V Pai

Chapter Outline

- Clinical Profile
- Classification
- Diagnosis
- Management
- Pathology of Pelvic Organs

INTRODUCTION

Tuberculosis (TB), a highly morbid yet preventable and usually curable disease, was the world's second leading cause of death in 2022, after the coronavirus infection (COVID-19). According to the Global tuberculosis report in 2022, 30 high TB burden countries were responsible for 87% of the world's TB cases, of which India accounted for 27%, which is the highest. TB affects more than 10 million people every year, due to which all Member States of the United Nations (UN) and the World Health Organization (WHO) set a goal to end the global TB epidemic by 2035. Globally, the net reduction of TB from 2015 to 2022 was 8.7%, far from the WHO End TB Strategy milestone of a 50% reduction by 2025.

Female genital TB (FGTB) is a variant of extrapulmonary TB **(Fig. 1)**, which usually occurs secondary to TB in other sites (mainly the lungs). The spread to the genital organs usually occurs through haematogenous (90%) or lymphatic routes. Direct inoculation of tubercle bacilli can also take place over vulva, vagina or cervix during sexual intercourse with a partner suffering from tuberculous lesions of genitalia. The fallopian tubes are affected in almost 100% of the cases followed by the endometrium in 50%, ovaries in 20%, cervix in 5% and vagina and vulva in <1%. Few reports have found the endometrium to be the most commonly involved site. The incidence of FGTB is underestimated as the majority of women with the disease are asymptomatic and may be diagnosed only during evaluation for infertility. Incidence of FGTB at infertility clinics varies significantly at various regions, ranging from <1% in the US to 3–26% in India. Although most of the affected females belong to the reproductive age group, the disease has also been reported in postmenopausal females. Drug therapy for FGTB is similar to the standard drug regimens used for pulmonary TB.

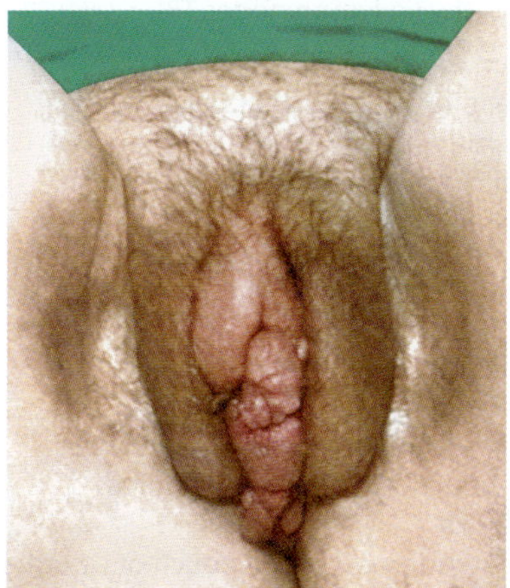

Fig. 1: Hypertrophic tuberculosis of vulva. Note considerable oedema of the labia majora and elephantiasis-like appearance of the labia minora.

Source: McLeod J, Read G. Gynaecology. London: Churchill Livingstone.

CLINICAL PROFILE

The majority of women suffering from FGTB are asymptomatic, however, some women may complain of chronic lower abdominal or pelvic pain. Women may also give symptoms of amenorrhoea or other menstrual disturbances or abnormal vaginal discharge. The antigonadotrophic effect of *Mycobacterium tuberculosis* may be responsible for menstrual irregularities that take place in cases of active pulmonary tuberculosis having no demonstrable lesions in the genital tract. The spectrum of infection outcomes by *M. tuberculosis* is described in **Figure 2**.

Genital TB should be suspected when a woman attends a clinic with a history of infertility (primary or secondary), especially in regions where the prevalence of TB is very high. FGTB may be detected in 2–30% of women having infertility, while infertility is seen in 60–80% of women with FGTB. Infertility may occur due to distortion or obstruction of the fallopian tubes, endometrial destruction and intrauterine adhesions, causing inadequate endometrial receptivity, or destruction of ovarian tissue leading to decreased ovarian reserve. Entry of harmful cytokines into the decidua, decreased subendometrial vascularity and vascular microthrombus formation following the tubercular infection of the endometrium leads to implantation failure and miscarriage. The incidence of ectopic pregnancies is also higher in women with FGTB due to tubal involvement by the disease and its distortion.

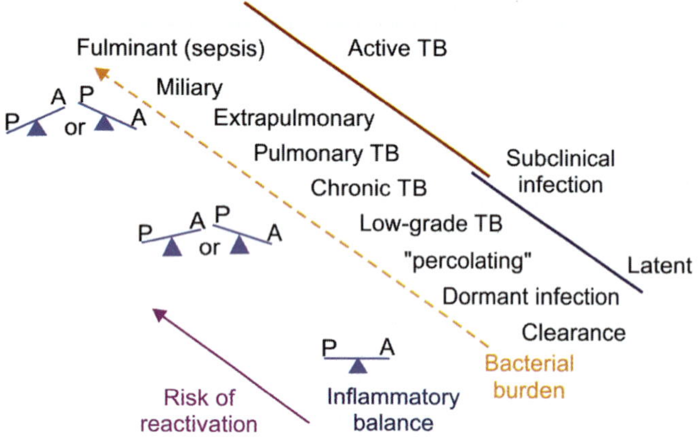

Fig. 2: Spectrum of *Mycobacterium tuberculosis* infection outcomes. (TB: tuberculosis)

In postmenopausal women, FGTB may present with postmenopausal bleeding, heavy white discharge and pyometra.

Women suffering from genital TB may have constitutional symptoms of TB (low-grade fever, weight loss, etc.) that may indicate concurrent infection elsewhere. Symptoms related to extra-genital TB (abdominal, CNS, bone and lymph nodes, etc.) may also be found in the affected individuals. Pelvic examination may show cervical growth, adnexal tenderness and tubo-ovarian mass.

Clinical Signs and Symptoms of Female Genital Tuberculosis

Clinical signs and symptoms of female genital tuberculosis are shown in **Table 1**.

CLASSIFICATION

Two types of tuberculosis infections in humans are as follows:

- *Latent TB*: Exposure to tuberculosis, but the organism is dormant or inactive. Only 5–10% of latent TB will progress to active disease in one's lifetime.

TABLE 1: Signs and symptoms of female genital tuberculosis.

Symptoms	***Signs***
Asymptomatic (10%)	No sign (10%)
General systemic symptoms	Raised temperature
• Pyrexia, anorexia, weight loss, feeling unwell, malaise and cough	Lymphadenopathy (in lymph nodes TB)
Menstrual symptoms: • Puberty menorrhagia • Heavy menstrual bleeding (in early stage) • Postmenopausal bleeding • Amenorrhoea and oligomenorrhoea • Hypomenorrhoea • Dysmenorrhoea (primary and secondary)	*Abdominal examination:* • Vague or definite abdominal or pelvic lump • Ascites • Doughy feel of the abdomen
Infertility (primary and secondary)	Crackles on chest auscultation (PTB)
Urinary incontinence or faecal incontinence Abdominal or pelvic mass Abdominal and pelvic pain	*Vaginal examination:* • Soft, tender and enlarged uterus (pyometra) • Tenderness and induration in the fornices • Lump in adnexa • Fullness and tenderness in the pouch of Douglas
Vaginal discharge	• Solid lesions on the external genitalia • Ulcers on external genitalia • Genital fistula

(PTB: pulmonary tuberculosis)

TABLE 2: Difference between active and latent tuberculosis infections in humans.

Active	*Latent*
• A big pellet of mycobacteria enters the body to surpass one's immunity or • Dormant bacteria in the body start multiplying due to lowered immunity to start active disease damaging the cells and tissues	• TB bacteria enter humans and stimulate the immune system to stimulate cell-mediated immunity, after which it remains dormant as bacteria or its DNA or antibodies

- *Active TB*: Occurs by active multiplication of the bacteria to cause disease and tissue destruction in the body **(Table 2)**.

DIAGNOSIS

The diagnosis of the disease is difficult. Apart from varied clinical presentation, a past history of tuberculosis or a history of contact may not be forthcoming, and evidence of tuberculous lesions elsewhere may be lacking. The abdominal and vaginal examinations may be normal. The key to the diagnosis is a high index of suspicion.

- A high erythrocyte sedimentation rate and a positive Mantoux test. These tests are nonspecific.
- The *chest radiograph* is normal in most cases. A pelvic ultrasound and hysterosalpingography examinations may be of some help.
- *Abdominal and pelvic USG (TVS):* Uterus, adnexa and pelvis to be evaluated preferably by transvaginal scan and the endometrial cavity and vascularity to be looked carefully with colour Doppler—cogwheel appearance of tubes; uterine cavity may show thin diffuse endometrium with irregular borders.
- *Computed tomography (CT)/Magnetic resonance imaging (MRI):* These can be used for evaluation of tubo-ovarian masses.
- *Endometrial sampling or biopsy* with Pipelle device or Karman cannula (4 mm) for microbiological and histopathological examination needs to be done to detect endometrial TB.
- *Endoscopy:* Hysteroscopy can be done to look for tubercles, pale endometrium and endometrial adhesions, and laparoscopy to evaluate uterus, adnexa and other pelvic organs, which may show tubercle-like lesions on the uterus, tubes and other pelvic organs, including peritoneum, and caseous nodules. An endoscopic-guided biopsy from the peritoneum or abdominal/pelvic lesions can be done, and the specimen subjected to microbiological and histopathological examination. Histopathological evidence in biopsy or demonstration of tubercle bacilli in culture of menstrual blood or endometrial curettage can only provide a certain diagnosis of the disease. Histopathological examination (HPE) of the specimens shows typical features of TB infection in the form of granulomatous caseous lesions. The demonstration of typical caseous granulomas with giant epithelioid cells is suggestive of TB; however, these lesions also appear in fungal infections, syphilis, leprosy, rheumatoid arthritis, systemic lupus erythematosus, pneumoconiosis and sarcoidosis. The best time for examining the endometrium is a few days before the expected menses, when the tubercles reach their maximum growth. The portion of the endometrium most likely to show tubercles is the cornual region, where spread from the tube first occurs.
- *Menstrual blood:* The success of identifying tuberculosis is less with menstrual blood. Menstrual blood should not be used for nucleic acid amplification tests (NAATs).
- *Hysterosalpingography:* It may show calcification, irregular calcified adnexa, blocked fallopian tubes (usually cornual), a rigid pipe stem appearance and beaded appearance, hydrosalpinx, which is usually moderate or slight with a club-like appearance to the ampulla (tobacco pouch appearance), multiple constrictions, filling defect in the uterine cavity (Asherman syndrome) **(Figs. 3 to 44)**. Hysterosalpingography must be avoided in acute phase.
- *Polymerase chain reaction (PCR):* PCR positivity is not taken as the 'Gold standard' for diagnosis of extrapulmonary TB since they are capable of detecting nonviable bacilli and hence may not reflect active disease.
- *Bacterial culture and staining:* Traditionally, the laboratory diagnosis of TB depends on demonstration of the causative organism, *Mycobacterium tuberculosis,* by acid-fast staining and/or growth of the organism on Löwenstein-Jensen (LJ) medium. Microscopic examination of acid-fast bacilli (AFB) requires the presence of at least 10,000 organisms/mL in the sample, while culture is more sensitive, requiring as little as 100 organisms/mL. However, *M. tuberculosis* may take up to 8 weeks to grow in LJ medium.

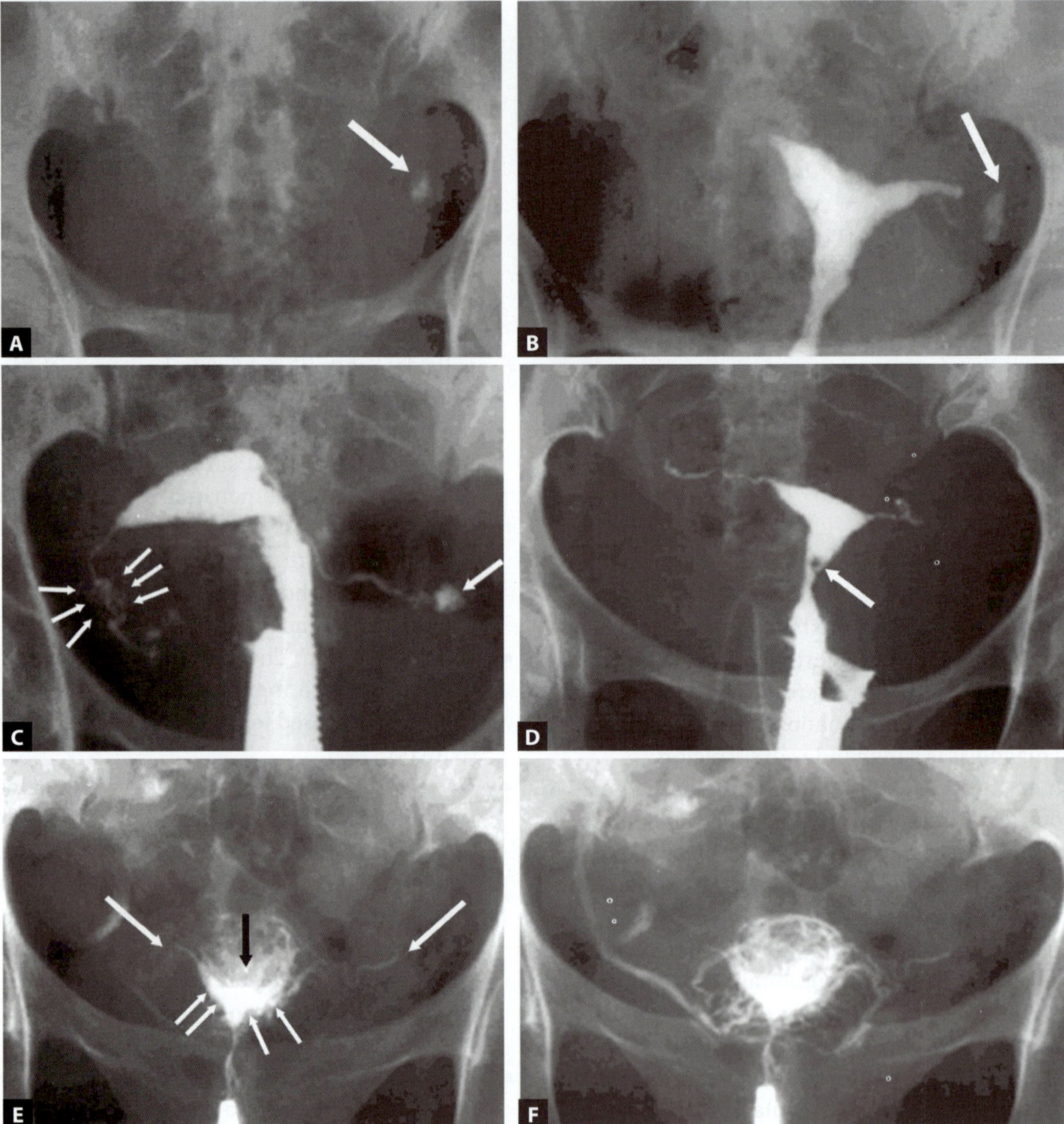

Figs. 3A to F: (A) Plain film of the pelvis frontal projection shows 1066 mm calcific density (arrow) on the left side; (B) Hysterosalpingogram frontal projection shows isthmic obstruction of the left fallopian tube just proximal to the calcification. There is an obstruction in the interstitial part of the tube on the right side. The endometrial cavity shows irregularity; (C) Hysterosalpingogram frontal projection shows occlusion of both fallopian tubes. The tubes appear rigid, 'pipestem', and are beaded. There is a lucent filling defect in the lower uterine segment suggestive of adhesion (arrow); (D) Hysterosalpingogram showing lead pipe rigidity and filling defect suggestive of intrauterine adhesions near the lower end; (E and F) Hysterosalpingogram shows isthmic obstruction of both the tubes (large arrows). The uterine cavity is deformed and shows 'T' shaped configuration (small arrows). Also note the intravasation of the contrast medium. There is a fundal impression on the uterine cavity (black arrow).

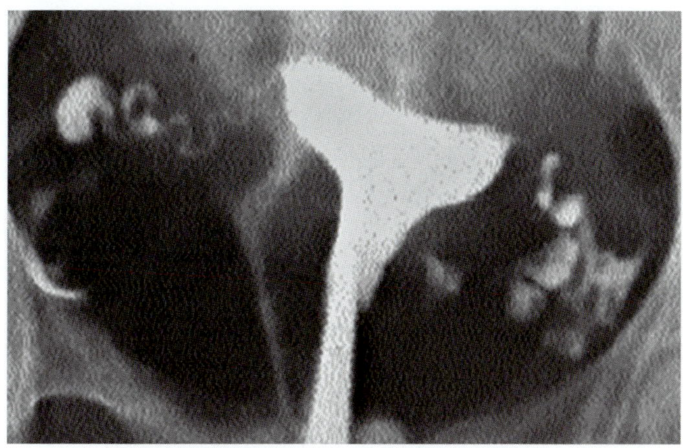

Fig. 4: Normal look of tubes at hysterosalpingography. Note the wavy outline of tubes that spill on both sides.

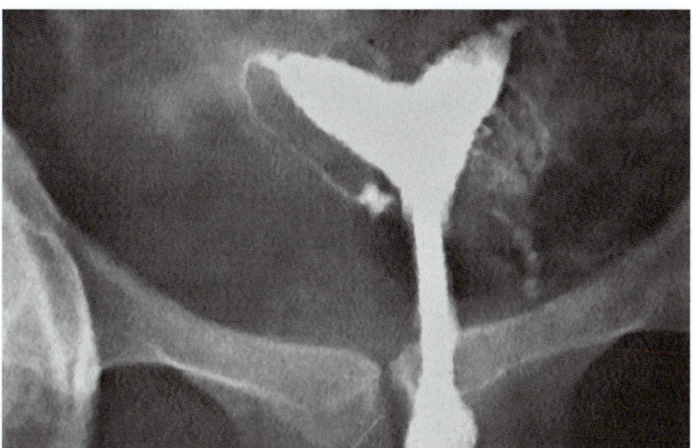

Fig. 7: Right tube lead pipe with left side intravasation.

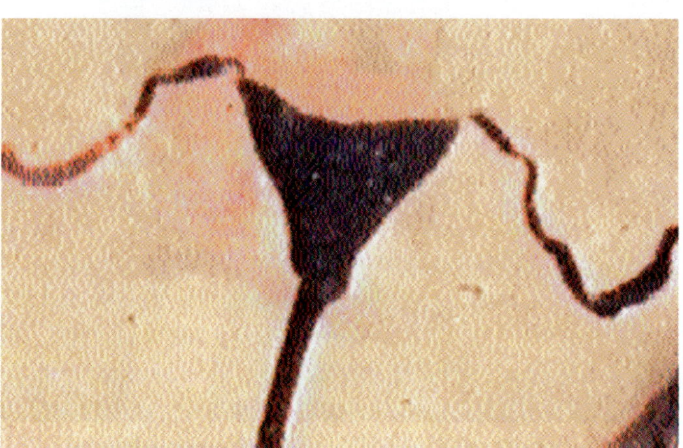

Fig. 5: Rigid pipeline tubes of proven Koch.

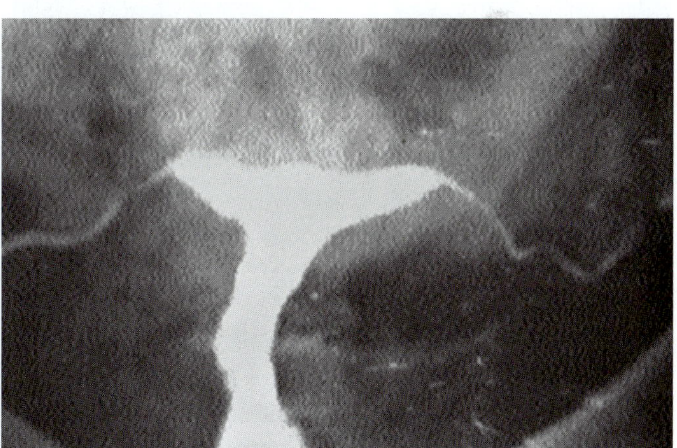

Fig. 8: Both tubes are lead pipe type.

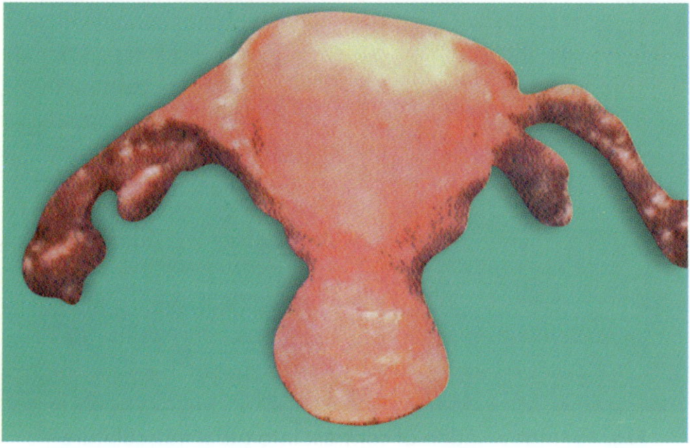

Fig. 6: The specimen after hysterectomy.

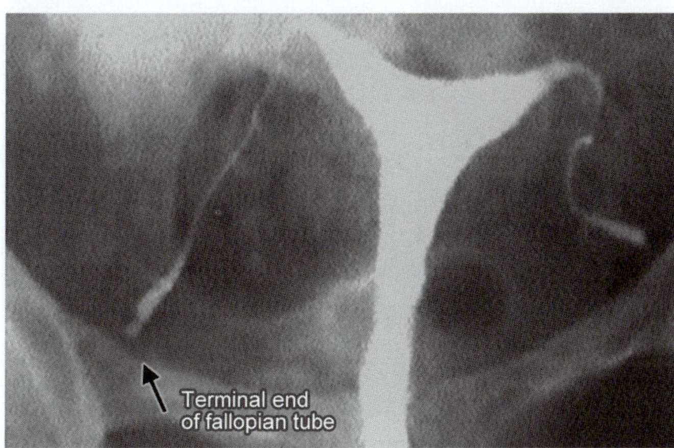

Fig. 9: Tubes straight + Typical terminal ends looking like sperm head.

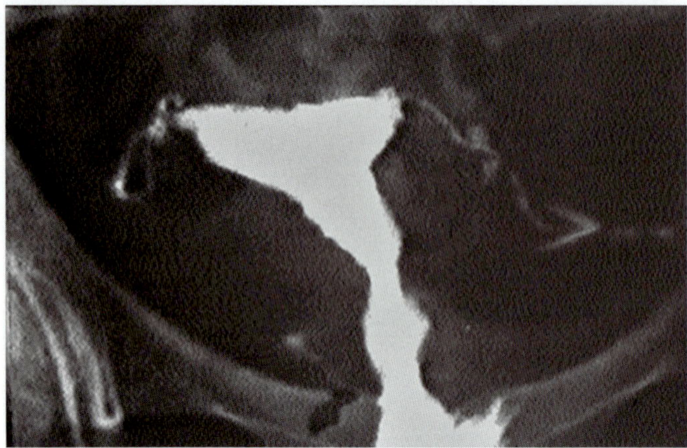

Fig. 10: Both tubes are eroded-looking. Inner lining of the uterine cavity (moth-eaten appearance).

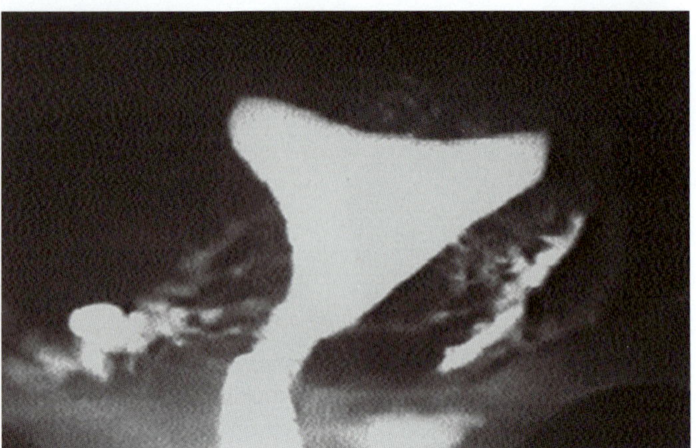

Fig. 13: Bilateral cornual block and intravasation.

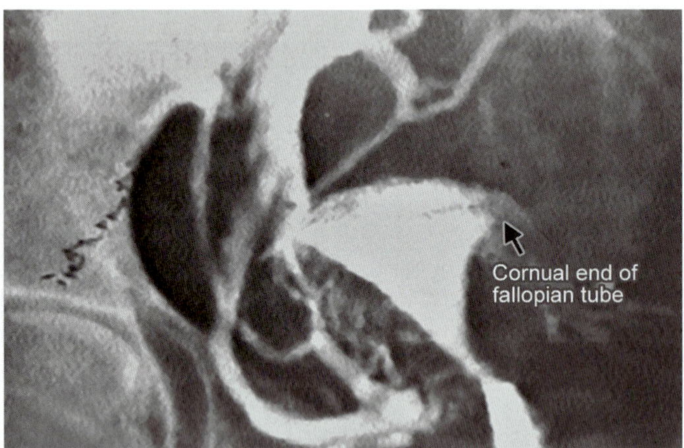

Fig. 11: Bilateral cornual block and intravasation of dye into vessels and lymphatics.

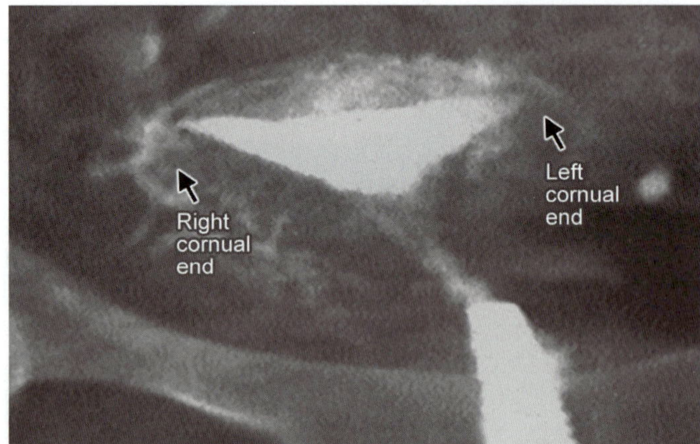

Fig. 14: Bilateral cornual block with intramyometrial intravasation.

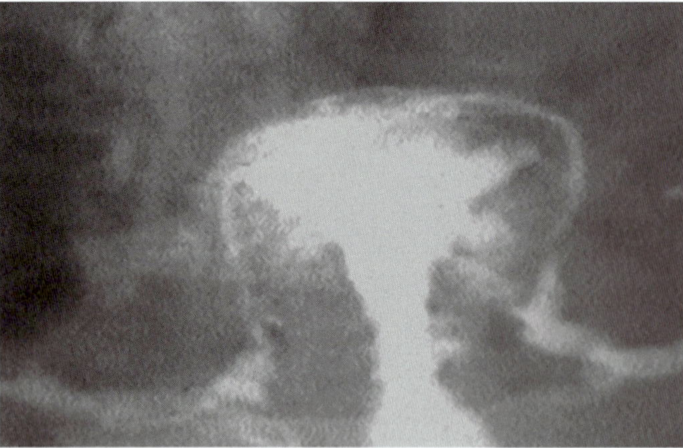

Fig. 12: Bilateral rigid pipeline tubes with intravasation of contrast.

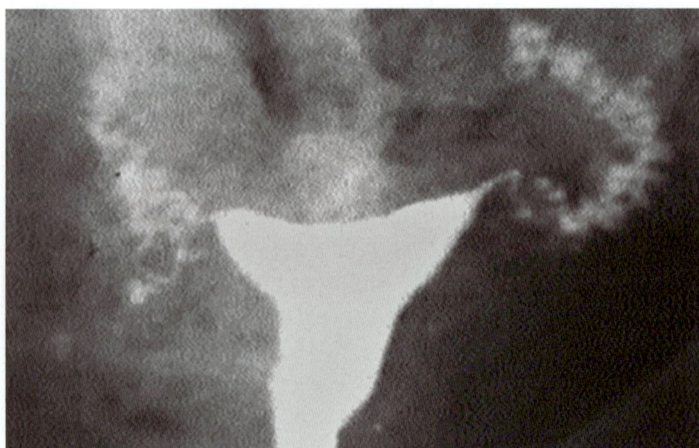

Fig. 15: Intravasation of contrast into tubal musculature—salpingitis isthmica nodosa.

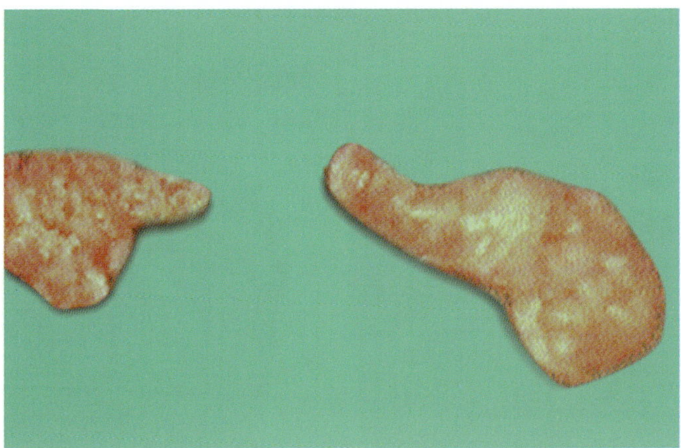

Fig. 16: Same tubes after removal.

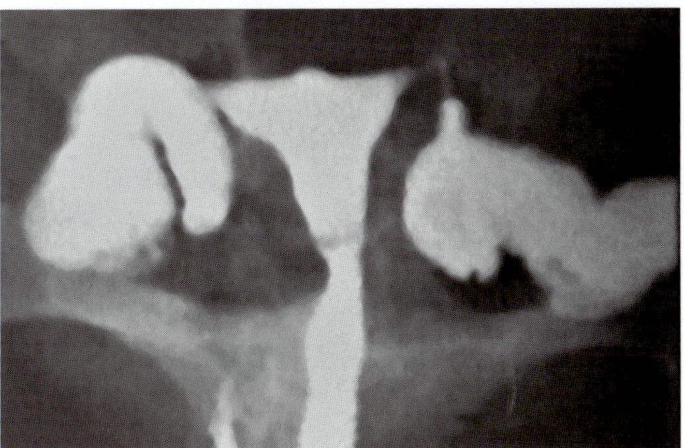

Fig. 19: Bilateral masses, even after antitubercular therapy (ATT) for 1 year, had repeated attacks of intestinal obstruction.

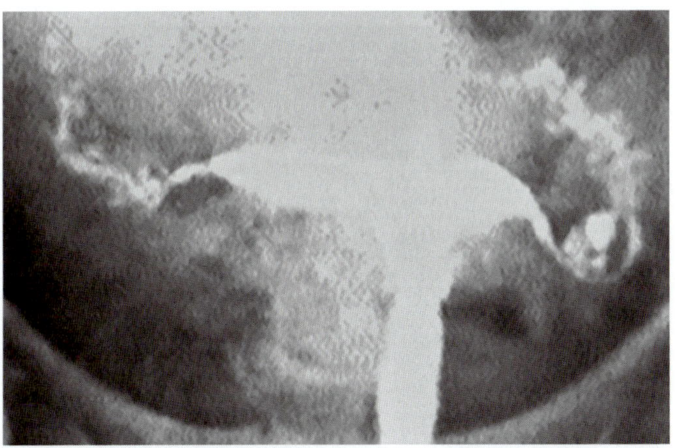

Fig. 17: Severe form of salpingitis isthmica nodosa.

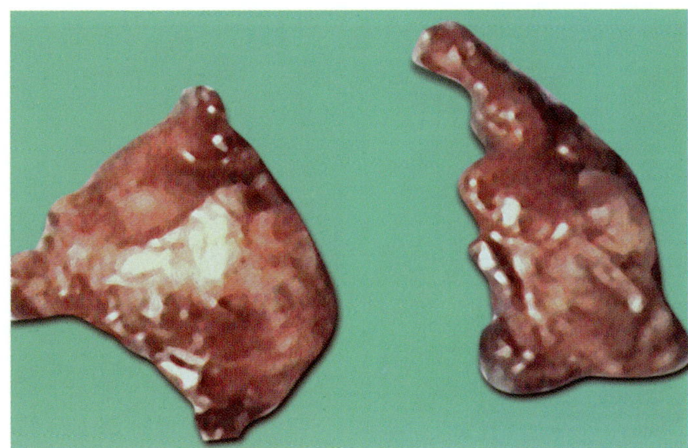

Fig. 20: Hence, bilateral salpingo-oophorectomy done.

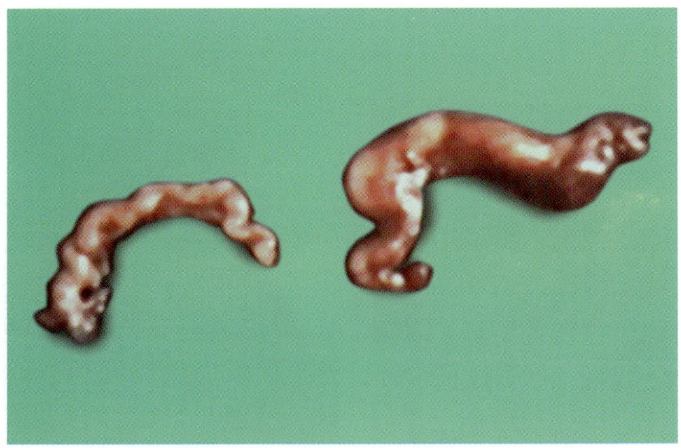

Fig. 18: Same tubes after removal of nodosa.

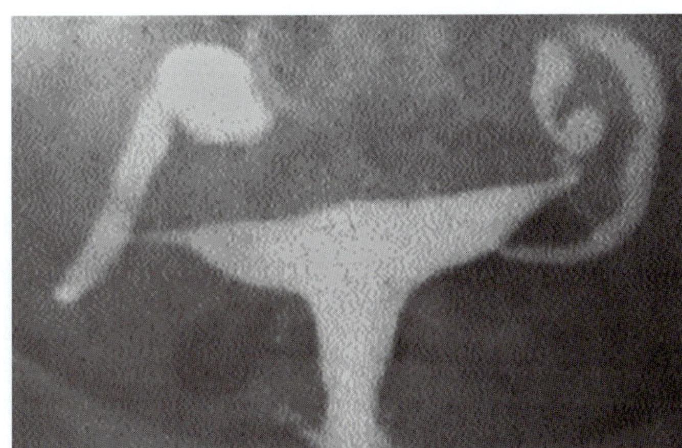

Fig. 21: Bilateral hydrosalpinx. Antitubercular therapy given for 2 years.

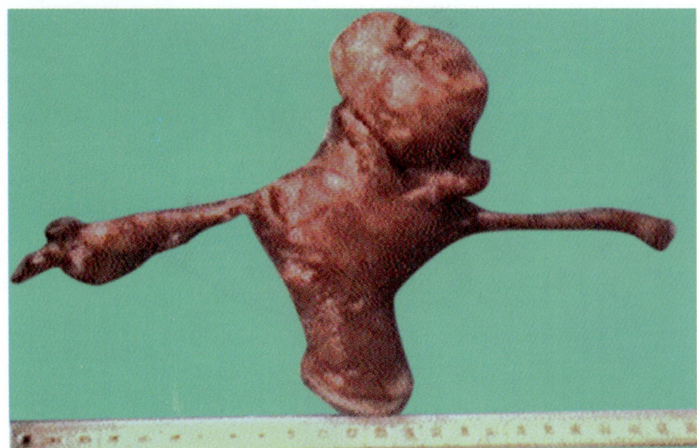

Fig. 22: Same patient developed a fibroid and hence underwent hysterectomy.

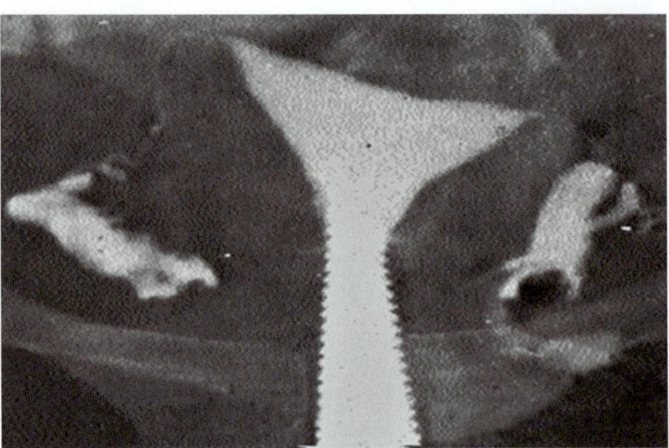

Fig. 25: Bilateral tobacco pouch appearance as described by Greenberg.

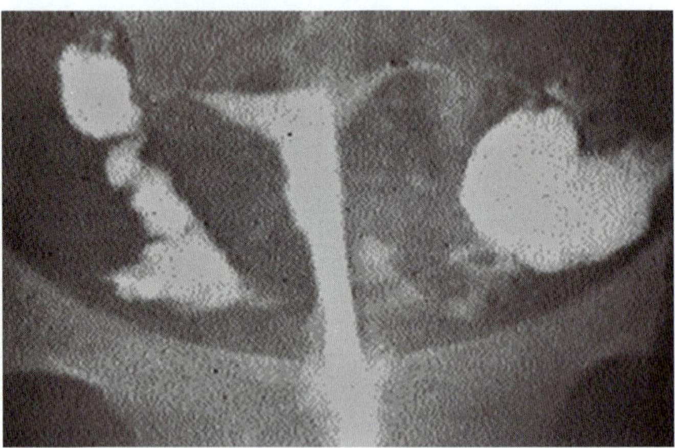

Fig. 23: Bilateral terminal hydrosalpinx typical of genital Koch's.

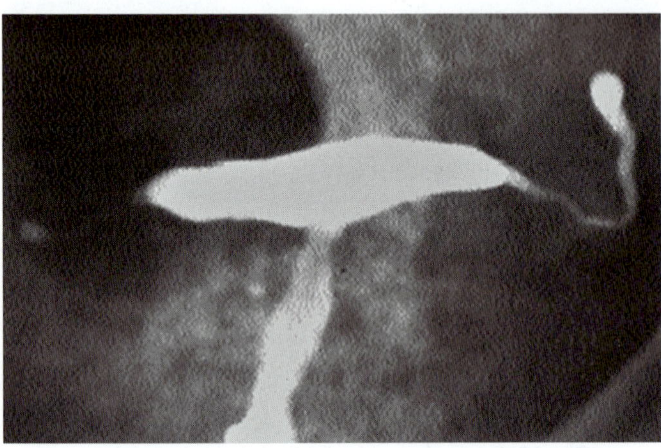

Fig. 26: The left tube appears as if a tubectomy has been done. The look of a sperm head.

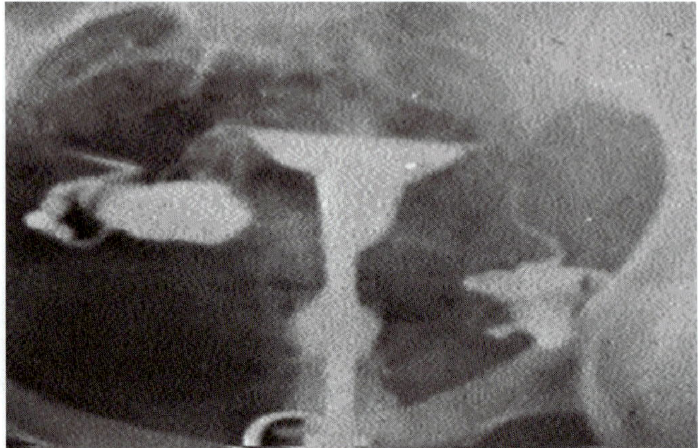

Fig. 24: Bilateral hydrosalpinx—tobacco pouch appearance of genital Koch's.

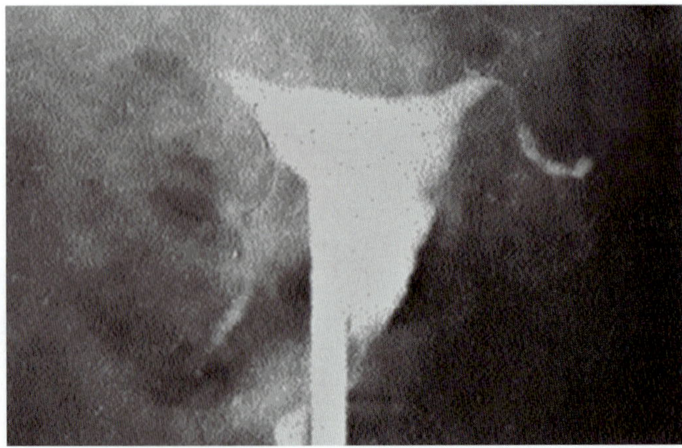

Fig. 27: Left tubes as if tubectomy is done, beaded appearance at hysterosalpingography (HSG) typical of Koch's.

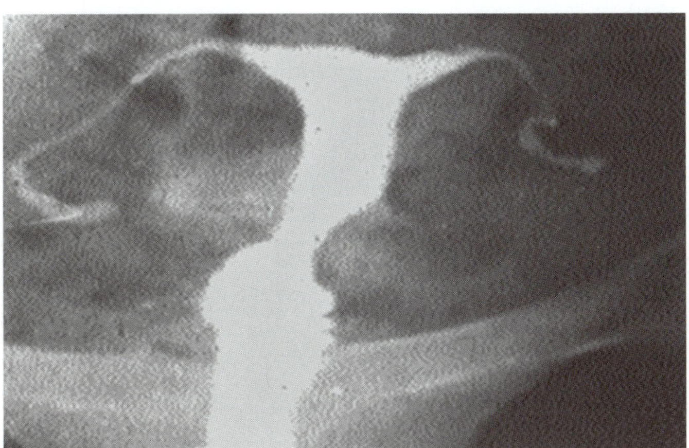

Fig. 28: Appearance similar to bilateral tubal ligation. Elongation and dilatation of cervical canal.

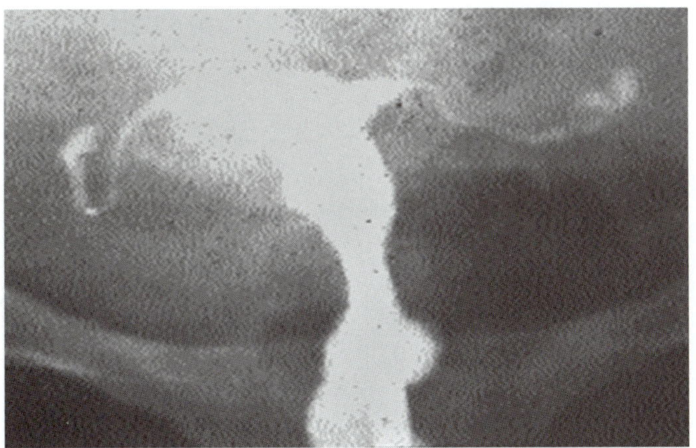

Fig. 29: Appearance as if bilateral tubal ligation has been done. Elongation and dilatation of cervical canal.

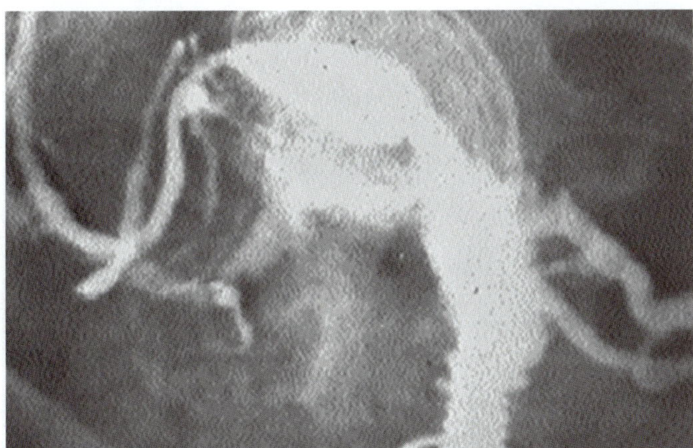

Fig. 30: Previous figures on injecting more dye intravasation into the myometrium and lymphatics.

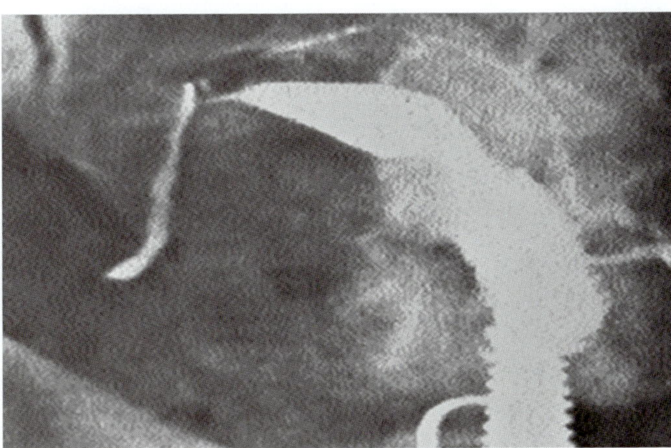

Fig. 31: Unicornuate uterus. Sperm head appears at the terminal end of the tube. Dilated cervical canal.

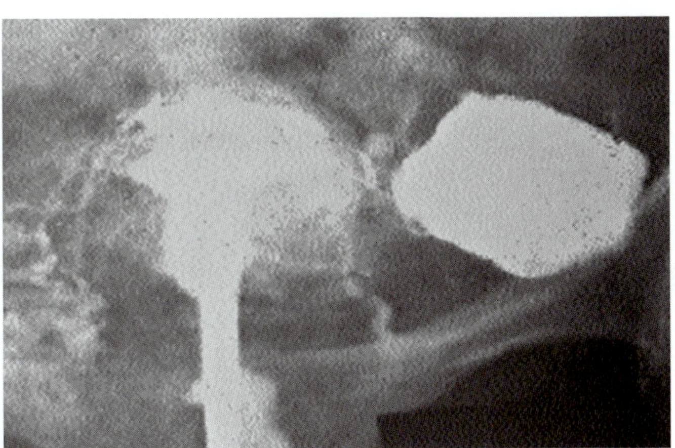

Fig. 32: Intravasation of dye into myometrium and lymphatics and left terminal hydrosalpingography.

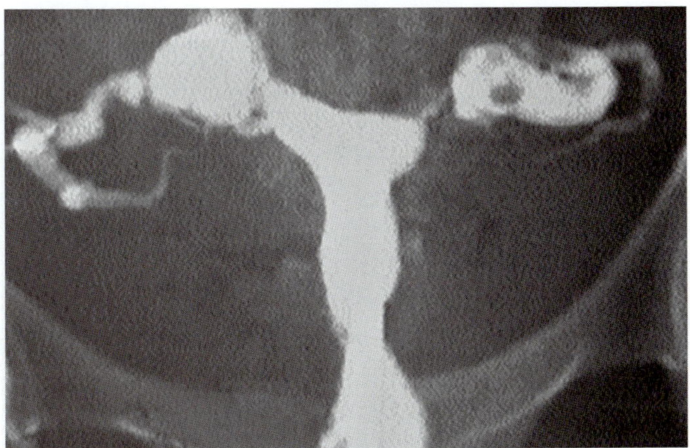

Fig. 33: Bilateral terminal hydrosalpingography. Right tube shows nodularity.

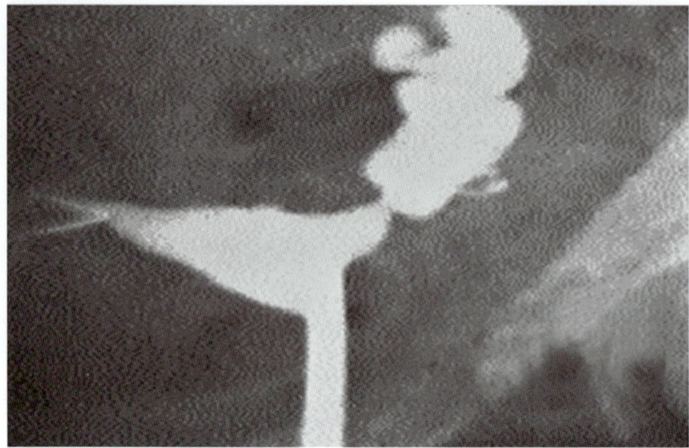

Fig. 34: Left terminal hydrosalpingography and right cornual block.

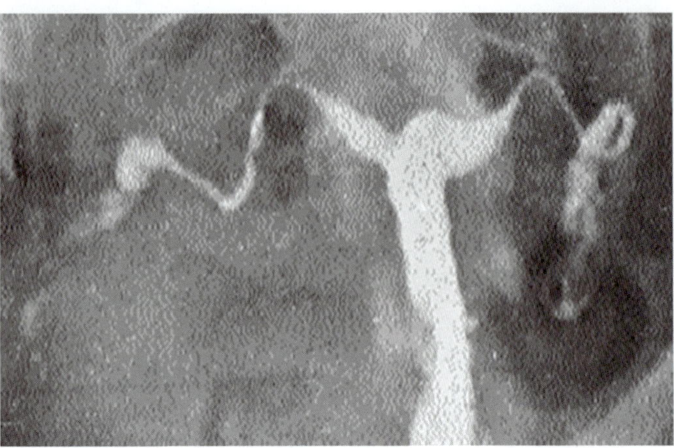

Fig. 37: Dilated fimbrial ends of bilateral fallopian tubes.

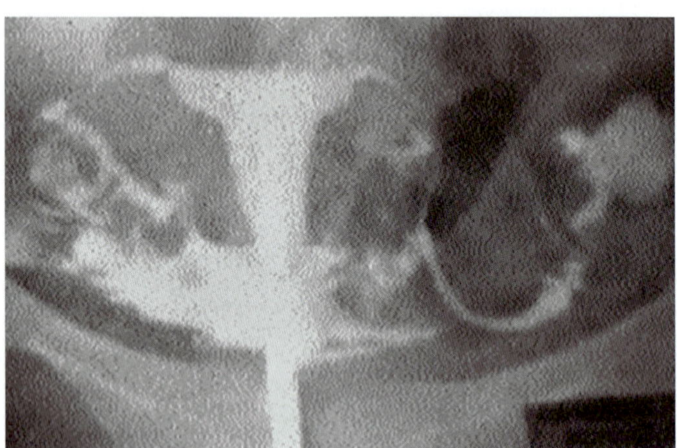

Fig. 35: Left terminal hydrosalpingography filling defect in left tube, right tube thick but patent.

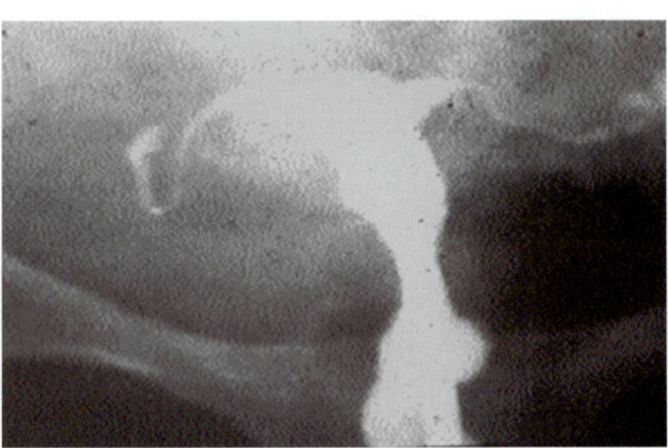

Fig. 38: Both terminal ends of the tubes are dilated.

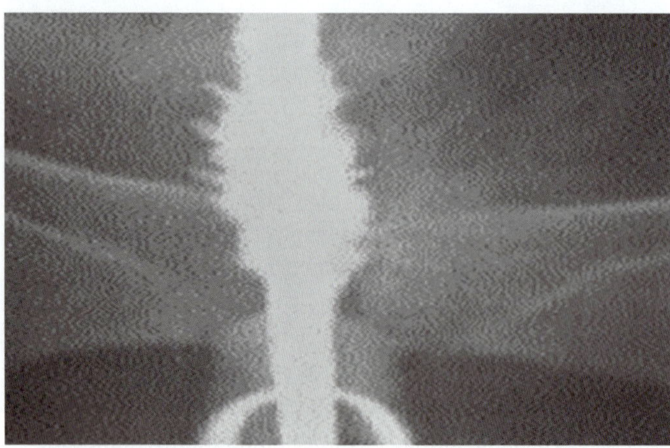

Fig. 36: Elongation and crypts in cervical canal.

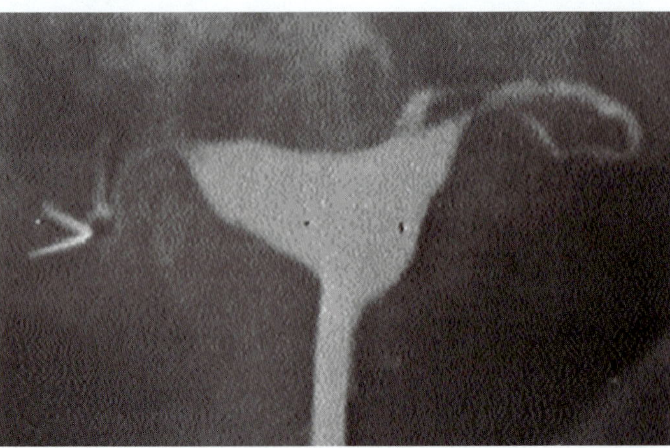

Fig. 39: Beaded appearance.

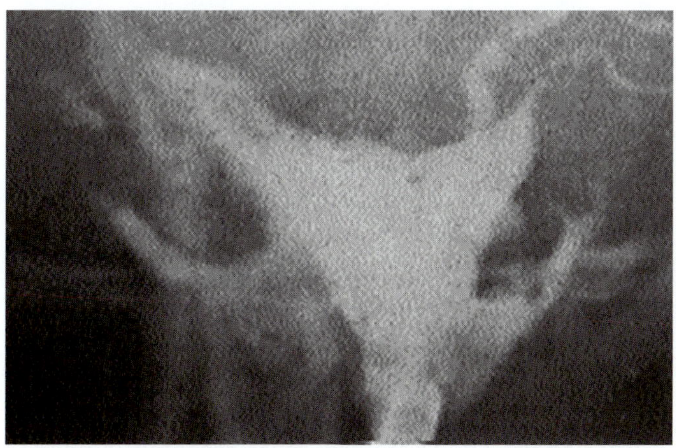
Fig. 40: Beaded appearance is more on the left side.

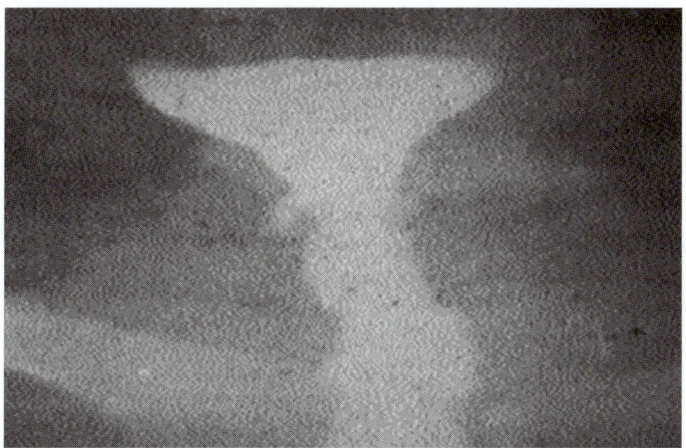
Fig. 41: Bilateral cornual block, cervical dilatation.

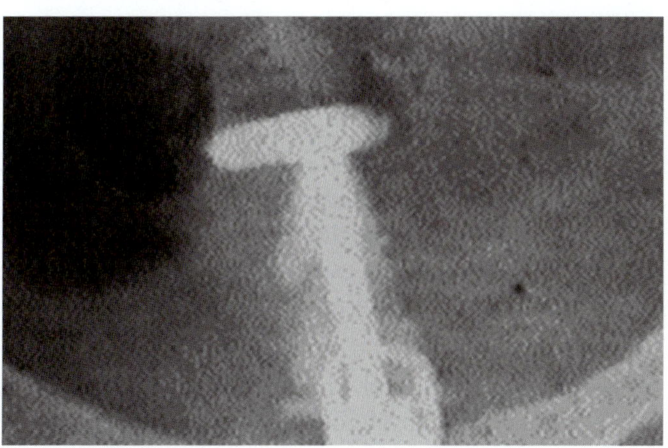
Fig. 42: Dwarfed uterine bilateral cornual block.

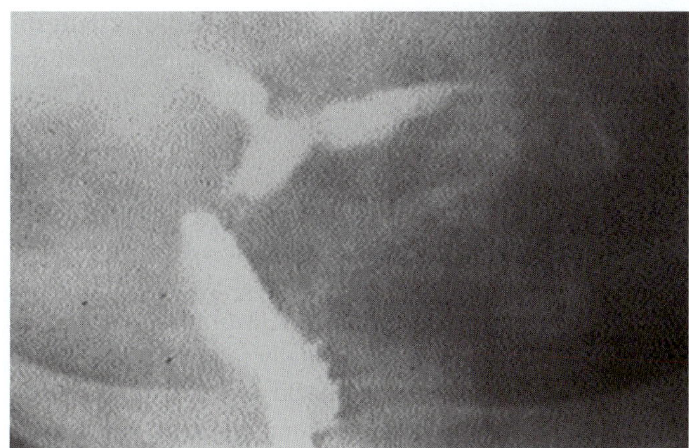
Fig. 43: Deformed uterus. It is not a bicornuate uterus.

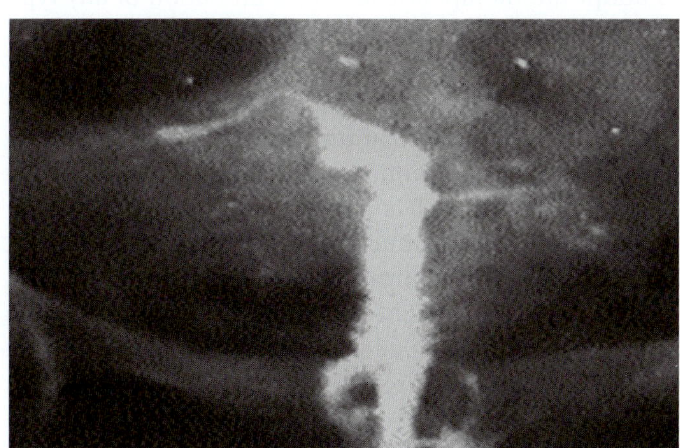
Fig. 44: Expansion and elongation of the cervix.

Besides technical drawbacks in demonstrating *M. tuberculosis* in the laboratory, a substantial number of TB lesions of the genital tract are bacteriologically mute.

- Mycobacterial culture is more sensitive compared to AFB microscopy, requiring as little as 10–100 organisms/mL. BACTEC radiometric culture is based on the measurement of carbon dioxide released by bacteria during growth in liquid medium. This new method has decreased the time for diagnosis to 2–3 weeks. BACTEC has a sensitivity of 80–90%, whereas LJ medium has only 30–40%.
- *Truenat*^{TM}, an indigenous molecular test, has been validated for TB, multidrug-resistant tuberculosis (MDR-TB),

extrapulmonary TB (EPTB) and paediatric pulmonary TB (PPTB) and is currently being used under the National TB Elimination Programme in India. The test has also been recommended by the WHO for the detection of TB and MDR-TB.

MANAGEMENT

Female genital tuberculosis is treated using a multidrug antitubercular regimen using rifampicin, isoniazid, pyrazinamide and ethambutol daily for 2 months, which is followed by rifampicin, isoniazid and ethambutol daily for the next 4 months. In women detected with drug resistance, treatment is given for 18–24 months using the second-line drugs.

In view of the problems of making a definitive diagnosis of genital TB in females, many physicians tend to adopt the therapeutic test for elimination of any type of TB, including the genital type, by prompt execution of antitubercular therapy (ATT) for the requested period of time. But a prescription error or poor compliance can delay the response to treatment, leading to failure, thereby resulting in continued morbidity despite the fact that good quality ATT is available. However, rifampicin has been known to induce menstrual disturbances in a few cases, which got normalised on further continuation of their ATT. Rifampicin-induced increased enzymatic catabolism of oestrogens is believed to affect the luteinising hormone surge, resulting in anovulatory cycles and causing minimal peeling of the functional layer in proliferative endometrium, which manifests in the form of oligomenorrhoea or amenorrhoea. Reversal of these disturbances is thought to take place due to the transitory nature of the effect or lowered threshold for the pituitary stimulus.

Surgery is avoided in active cases of TB. Surgery is done when there is persistence of pelvic mass, positive endometrial culture or histology and recurrence of pain or bleeding after 9 months of treatment. Surgery should be performed at least 6 weeks after initiation of anti-TB therapy, because antimicrobial treatment facilitates the surgical procedure and reduces the risk of perioperative complications.

Continuing search is needed for finding simpler and practicable methods for making definitive diagnosis in respect of female genital TB, and the use of therapeutic tests should be avoided. Prompt ATT and appropriate surgical intervention have improved the results in terms of cure from disease, restoration of female reproductive function and reduction of procedural and postoperative complications. The chances of pregnancy in females suffering from genital TB have so far been poor (5%) even after the completion of treatment. But results have been reported in difficult cases managed timely with combined medical treatment and surgical intervention.

In vitro fertilisation has also provided a ray of hope to the desperate infertile women in recent times. Further research may help further improve the fertility rate after the cure of genital TB. It may be mentioned that research is considerably hampered due to the non-availability of clear criteria for monitoring the treatment efficacy, unlike in pulmonary TB. Therefore, more research is needed so that the delivery of therapy can become more certain and therapeutic effects can be better defined in terms of the normalisation of the pathological process and the desirable reproductive function.

Flowchart 1 briefly describes the infection and management of tuberculosis.

Female Genital Tuberculosis Stepwise Decision

Clinical history:

- General physical and pelvic examination
- Pelvic ultrasound
- As indicated in infertility hysterosalpingography (HSG)

Definite FGTB needing ATT if any of the following tests are positive:

- Acid-fast bacilli microscopy positive
- Acid-fast bacilli culture positive
- Gene Xpert or other NAAT +ve
- Histopathological demonstration of epithelioid granuloma

Probable FGTB needing ATT if any of the following are positive:

- Clinical findings/suspicion of TB with tubo-ovarian masses on imaging studies
- Clinical findings/suspicion of TB with laparoscopic findings of beaded tubes, caseous nodules, tubercles, adhesions, hydrosalpinx and pyosalpinx, etc.
- Clinical findings/suspicion of TB with hysteroscopic findings of tubercles, caseous nodules, pale endometrium, intrauterine adhesions, etc.

Negative FGTB: No ATT:

- No microbiological, histological, radiological, laparoscopic and hysteroscopic evidence of FGTB

Menstrual blood should not be used for NAAT.

Flowchart 1: Tuberculosis.

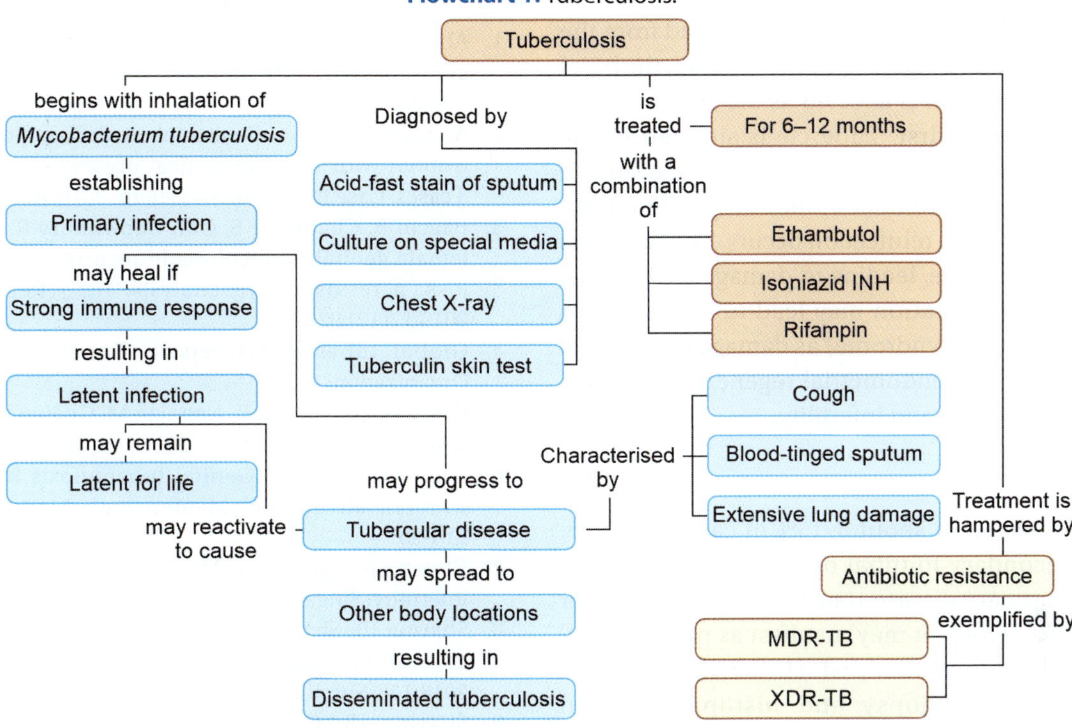

(INH: isoniazid; MDR-TB: multidrug-resistant tuberculosis; XDR-TB: extensively drug-resistant tuberculosis)

PATHOLOGY OF PELVIC ORGANS

Fallopian Tubes

Fallopian tubes are affected in 95–100% of genital TB. The ampullary region of the fallopian tubes shows the earliest changes, and the fimbrial processes become swollen later. The ampullary end is the most commonly affected site due to its rich blood supply from the uterine and ovarian arteries, as tubes are commonly affected through the haematogenous route from a primary site (primarily, the lung). The tubal site of infection is the submucosal layer (interstitial salpingitis) **(Fig. 45)**. Infection spreads medially causing destruction of muscles, which are replaced by fibrous tissues. Walls get thickened. Salpingitis isthmica nodosa is nodular thickening of the tube due to proliferation of tubal epithelium within hypertrophied myosalpinx. Fimbriae are everted. Elongated and distended distal tube with patent abdominal Ostia gives the appearance of a *tobacco pouch*. Tubercles burst, pouring caseous material into the lumen, producing tubercular pyosalpinx **(Fig. 46)**. Infection may spread outwards, producing perisalpingitis, causing adhesion.

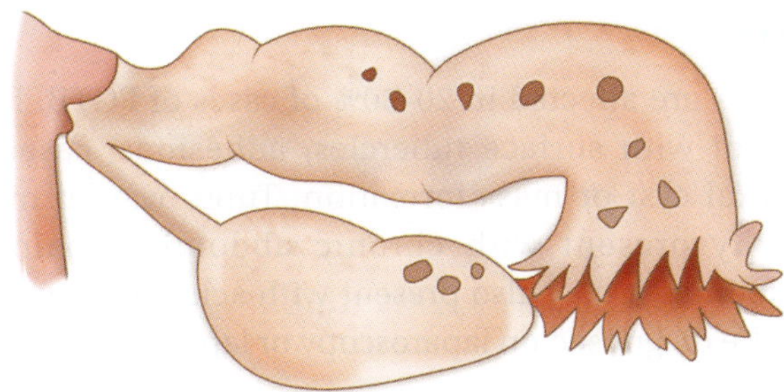

Fig. 45: Tubercular salpingitis.

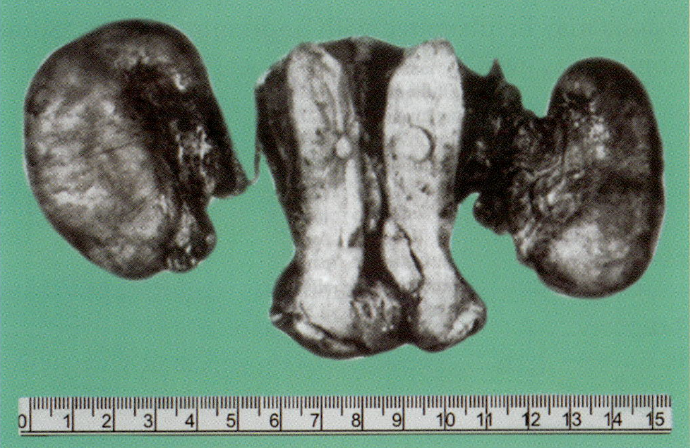

Fig. 46: Bilateral tuberculous pyosalpinx. Note the retort-shaped tubes, absence of surface tubercles and adhesions.

Uterus

Endometrium may be affected in 50–60% of FGTB either from direct spread from the fallopian tubes or by lymphatics or haematogenous spread. Cornual ends are commonly affected when there is a direct spread from the fallopian tubes. During a haematogenous spread, the basal layer of the endometrium is affected as the spiral arteries supply the basal layer first. Tubercle is situated in the basal layer of endometrium and only comes to the surface premenstrual when there is endometrial proliferation. After each menstruation, reinfection occurs. The tubercles may enlarge and ulcerate, leading to damage to the basal layer. Endometrial ulceration may lead to adhesions or synechiae (Asherman's syndrome) as damage to the basal layer leads to failure of endometrial regeneration, which may cause amenorrhoea and infertility.

Cervix

The cervix is affected in about 5–15% of cases of FGTB. It is usually secondary to tubal or endometrial TB, but may rarely be primary disease transmitted by the partner through infected semen. It may manifest as proliferative/nodular growth or ulceration, which may be mistaken for cervical cancer. Biopsy and histopathological demonstration of granulomatous inflammation are thus necessary to differentiate it from malignancy.

Ovary

Ovaries are affected in 20–30% of cases of FGTB. It may present with surface tubercles, adhesions, caseation, adnexal cyst or mass formation. Tubo-ovarian masses usually present with chronic abdominal pain, but sometimes it may also present with acute abdomen and may be diagnosed on laparoscopy or laparotomy.

Vulva and Vagina

Vulva and vagina are rare sites to be involved (1%). Affected lesions may be ulcerated with undermined edges. Some women may even present with perineal fistulas.

SUGGESTED READING

1. Abbara A, Davidson RN. Etiology and management of genitourinary tuberculosis. Nat Rev Urol. 2011;8(12): 678-88.
2. Arora A, Sadath SA. Genital tuberculosis in postmenopausal women with variable clinical presentations: a report of 3 cases. Case Rep Womens Health. 2018;18:e00059.
3. Bagchi B, Chatterjee S, Gon Chowdhury R. Role of latent female genital tuberculosis in recurrent early pregnancy loss: a retrospective analysis. Int J Reprod Biomed. 2019;17(12):929-34.
4. Global tuberculosis report. Geneva: World Health Organization; 2023.
5. Grace G, Devaleenal B, Natrajan M. Genital tuberculosis in females. Indian J Med Res. 2017;145(4):425-36.
6. Ishrat S, Fatima P. Genital tuberculosis in the infertile women: an update. Mymensingh Med J. 2015;24(1): 215-20.
7. Khanna A, Agrawal A. Markers of genital tuberculosis in infertility. Singapore Med J. 2011;52:864-7.
8. Sharma JB, Sharma E, Sharma S, Dharmendra S. Female genital tuberculosis: revisited. Indian J Med Res. 2018;148(Suppl):S71-83.
9. Sharma JB. Current diagnosis and management of female genital tuberculosis. J Obstet Gynaecol India. 2015;65(6):362-71.
10. Standard Treatment Workflows of India. Special Edition on Paediatric and Extrapulmonary Tuberculosis. New Delhi: Indian Council of Medical Research; 2022.
11. Tal R, Simoni M, Pal L. Latent and genital tuberculosis in the infertile population in US—experience at an academic fertility center in the north east underscores a need for vigilance. Fertil Steril. 2017;108:E117-8.
12. WHO. (2015). The End TB Strategy WHO. Global strategy and targets for tuberculosis prevention, care and control after 2015. [online] Available on https://www.who.int/publications/m/item/the-end-tb-strategy-brochure. [Last accessed April, 2025].
13. Yadav S, Singh P, Hemal A, Kumar R. Genital tuberculosis: current status of diagnosis and management. Transl Androl Urol. 2017;6(2): 222-33.

23

CHAPTER

Endometriosis and Chronic Pelvic Pain

Anjali Mundkur, Muralidhar V Pai

Chapter Outline

Endometriosis and Allied States
- Endometriosis and Adenomyosis
- Adenomyosis
- Endosalpingiosis
- Cervical Endometriosis
- Causes in The Genital Tract
- Extragenital Causes
- Management and Treatment

Chronic Pelvic Pain
- General Considerations
- Step-wise Evaluation of Chronic Pelvic Pain
- Examination
- Diagnostic Investigations
- Management

ENDOMETRIOSIS AND ALLIED STATES

ENDOMETRIOSIS AND ADENOMYOSIS

General Considerations

Endometriosis is a benign disease of the female reproductive system, which induces chronic inflammatory reactions. Endometriosis is defined as the presence of functioning uterine glands and stroma in any site outside the uterus. The condition is one of unusual interest and, although it gives rise to tumour formation (i.e. swelling), it is not a neoplasm. This does not mean that ectopic endometrium cannot occasionally be the site for the development of malignant growth, although this is uncommon (see further).

The disease occurs in two forms: (1) In extrauterine organs and tissues and (2) in the uterine wall.

Extrauterine Endometriosis

In extrauterine endometriosis, ectopic endometrium is found, usually in other pelvic organs but sometimes in more remote sites (see further). Although the true nature of the lesions was recognised towards the end of the 19th century, it is only during the last 50 years that proper attention has been paid to the condition. Previously, pelvic endometriosis was mistaken for an inflammatory reaction because of the commonly associated adhesions. Now that it is recognised by the surgeon, it is realised that it is so common that evidence of present or past external endometriosis is found in 10–20% of laparotomies carried out by a gynaecologist on White patients. It was thought to be comparatively rare in African and Asiatic women. However, it is recognised with increasing frequency in these populations and also with the increasing use of laparoscopy and other diagnostic modalities.

Adenomyosis

In adenomyosis, the myometrium is invaded by endometrial glands from within. A minor degree of microscopic invasion of the muscle by the basal endometrium is normal, and this can be somewhat exaggerated when the endometrium is hyperplastic. These facts explain the misleading statements to the effect that adenomyosis is found in 50% of all uteri removed. The penetration has to be at least one high-power field from the basal endometrium for it to justify the label of adenomyosis **(Fig. 1)**. If this criterion is accepted, adenomyosis is not particularly common, not nearly as frequent as uterine leiomyomas, although all three conditions may coexist.

General Pathological Considerations

An endometriotic lesion has the typical histological appearance of an endometrium **(Figs. 2 to 5)**. Both glands and stroma must be present to justify the designation, although the relative amounts of each vary. It is said that the glands appear first and act as organisers for the stroma. The lesion promotes a fibrous or fibromuscular tissue reaction in the host. This reaction is a diffuse one

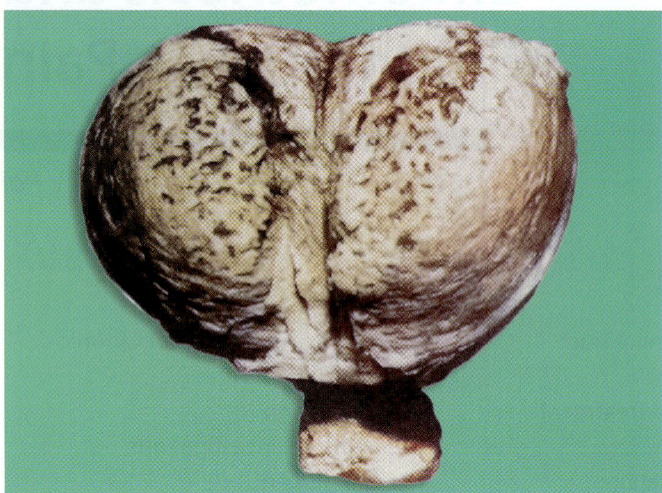

Fig. 1: A uterus bisected to show adenomyosis infiltrating its walls. In this case, there are some small menstrual blood cysts although this condition is not very hormone responsive. This specimen came from a woman aged 32 years complaining of infertility and menorrhagia.

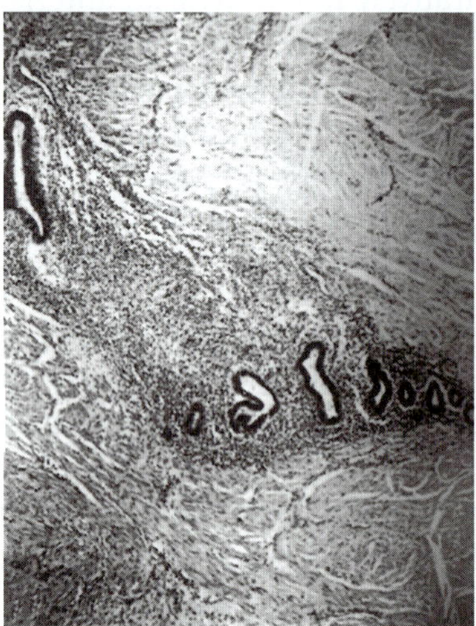

Fig. 2: Adenomyosis uteri.

and, except sometimes in the ovary, does not lead to encapsulation of the endometrioma.

Ectopic endometrium also resembles the uterine mucosa, in that, it is subservient to ovarian hormones. It therefore typically only proliferates when the ovaries are active and atrophies after the menopause. Ordinarily, an islet of endometriosis shows the cyclical changes characteristic of menstruation and, during pregnancy, its stromal cells exhibit a decidual reaction. However, there is no outlet for its menstrual discharge so blood and debris collect within the tissues to form a cyst. With each menstrual episode, the collection increases in size, but continual

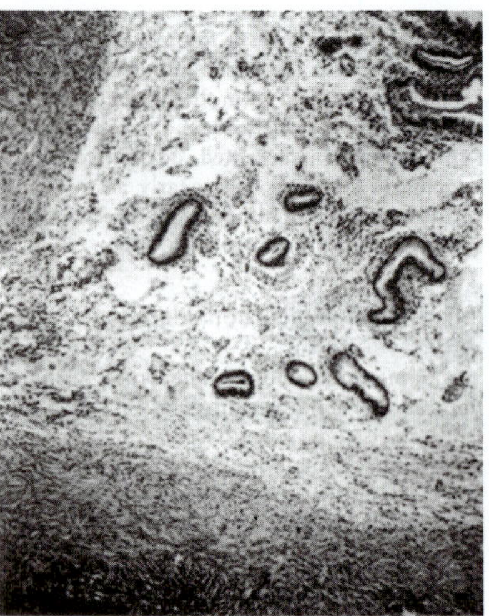

Fig. 3: Endometriosis of the ovary.

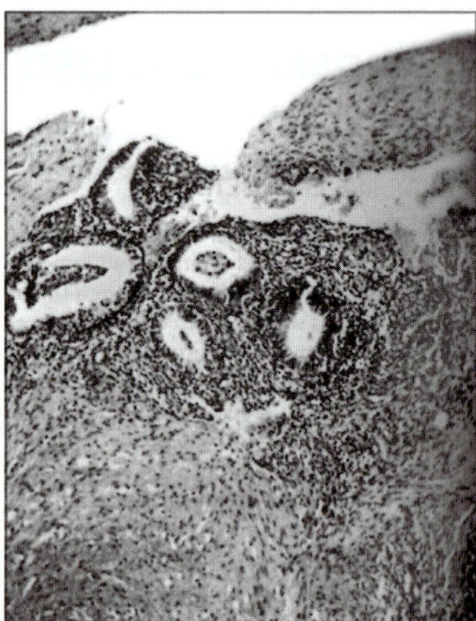

Fig. 4: Endometriosis of the surface of the ovary.

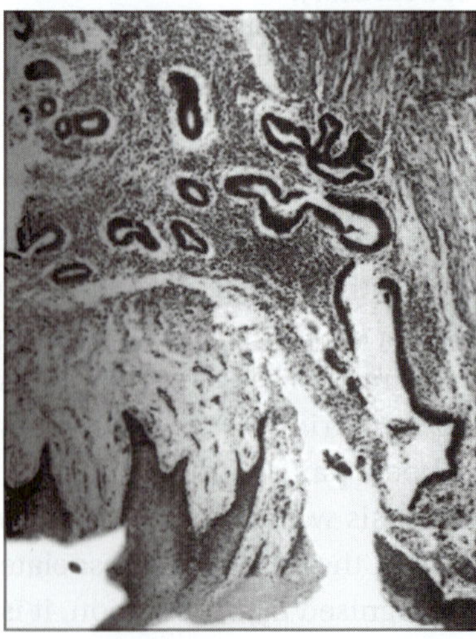

Fig. 5: Endometriosis of the vulva. The squamous epithelium of the skin lies immediately below the lesion.

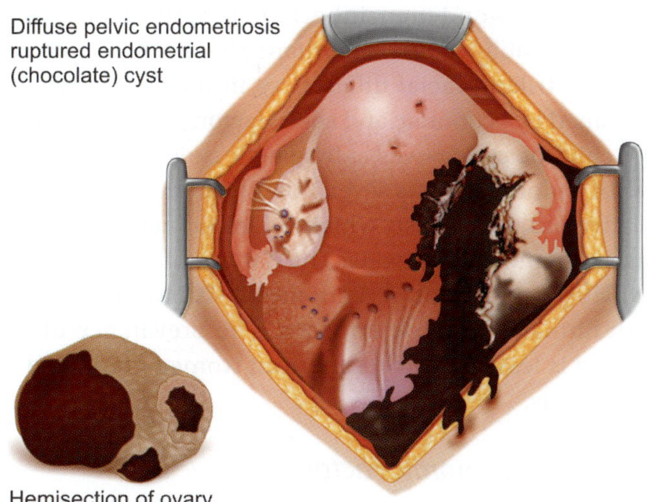

Fig. 6: Pathological lesions in endometriosis.

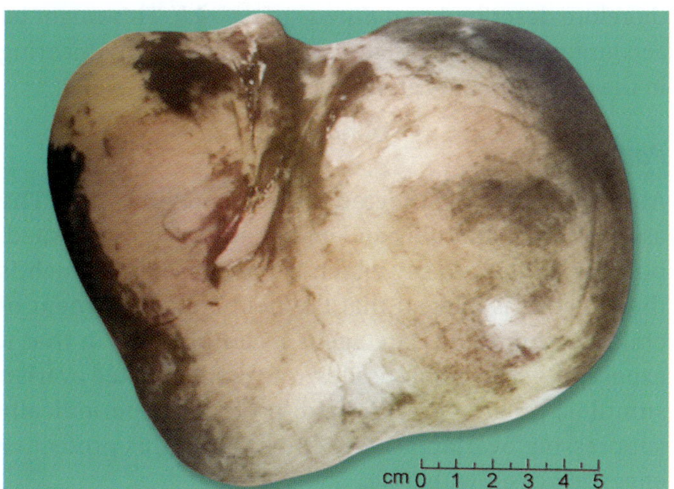

Fig. 7: An unusually large endometriotic cyst of the ovary, with tarry fluid leaking onto its surface.

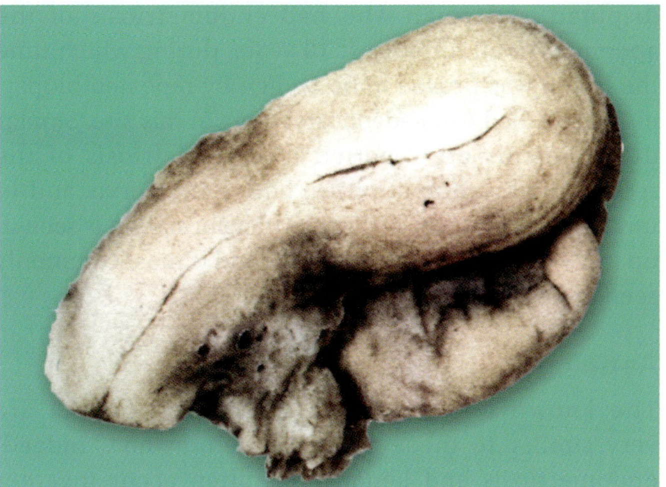

Fig. 8: Endometriosis of the uterosacral ligaments and the rectovaginal septum. The dark areas are tiny chocolate cysts. The uterus is retroverted, and the ovary is adherent to the back of it and to the mass of endometriosis.

absorption of some of the fluid elements causes the blood to become inspissated and dark coloured to produce a *tarry* or *chocolate* cyst **(Figs. 6 and 7)**. As the cyst grows, its endometrial lining is thinned and ultimately destroyed. So larger tarry cysts, such as are seen in the ovary, are lined by granulation tissue or by pseudoxanthoma cells rich in haemosiderin and their real nature may not be recognised. For this reason, the operative diagnosis of extrauterine endometriosis is not confirmed histologically in >50% of cases. This figure rises if the pathologist consults with the surgeon when selecting tissues for section and is prepared to examine many blocks. On the other hand, any ovarian cyst into which there has been haemorrhage may be diagnosed incorrectly as endometriosis if the presence of a tarry content and pigment-laden lining cells are accepted as the only criteria.

Rupture of endometriotic cysts, even small ones, is common; scatter of their contents, which include endometrial cells, can lead to the development of further areas of endometriosis. The peritoneum reacts sharply to the cyst material, and this causes dense adhesions to seal the hole. Adhesion and fixation are also encouraged by the fact that endometriosis infiltrates adjacent issues **(Fig. 8)**. No matter how extensive the adhesions are; however, it is characteristic of endometriosis that the fallopian tubes are almost invariably patent. This observation is of great importance from the standpoint of the retrograde menstruation theory of the origin of the disease.

Although it is generally recognised that the condition almost always becomes quiescent with the cessation of ovarian function, it is not always realised that it often does so before the climacteric. Indeed, the lesion appears sometimes to have a very limited phase of activity, after which it becomes burnt out to leave merely adhesions and a few old blood cysts. This situation is not infrequently encountered unexpectedly at laparotomy. One of the conditions which favour retrogression is pregnancy. Generally speaking, however, the disease continues to progress and is known to progress and recur after therapy, with recurrence rates reaching 40% in 5 years.

The possibility of adenocarcinoma or other malignant disease arising in an island of endometriosis is no longer disputed. A woman who had endometriosis of the abdominal wall for at least 10 years, during which time the lesion was proved to be benign by repeated biopsy, ultimately died from adenocarcinoma at this site. Similar developments are reported in endometriosis of the rectovaginal septum, ovaries, bowel and cervix and in uterine adenomyosis. Malignant transformation is seen in up to 1% of cases of endometriosis and is most commonly seen in the ovary.

Aetiology

The known and supposed aetiological factors are very similar to those of uterine leiomyoma; indeed, endometriosis and leiomyomas often occur together **(Fig. 9)**.

Age

Active endometriosis is seen most commonly between the ages of 25–35 years. It can, however, occur at any time between menarche and menopause, even before the age of 20 years. Most cases of endometriosis in women under the age of 17 years are seen with Müllerian outflow tract anomalies and obstruction.

Race and Family

Endometriosis has a family history in many. The risk of endometriosis is seven times greater if a first-degree relative has been affected by endometriosis. Because no specific Mendelian inheritance pattern has been identified, multifactorial inheritance has been postulated.

The striking racial differences in incidence may be explained by economic and social factors, age of marriage and child-bearing as well as by genetic considerations. The risk of endometriosis is seven times higher if a first-degree relative has the disease, which is further increased in the case of homozygotic twins. The pattern of inheritance is probably multifactorial. Endometriosis has been linked with human leucocyte antigens. The prevalence of the disease is less in African American women compared to Caucasians.

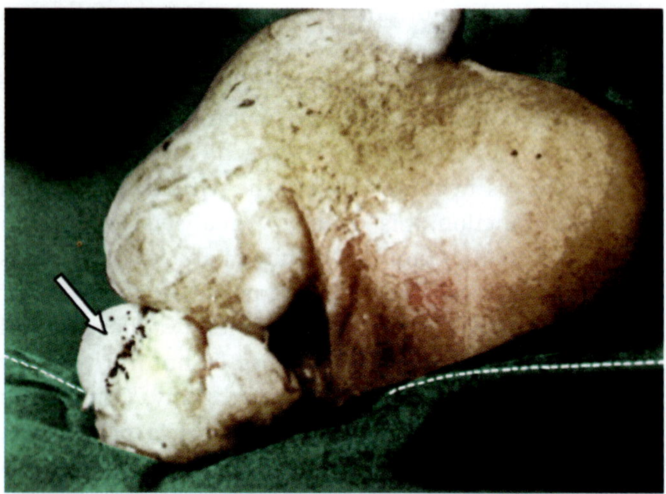

Fig. 9: Surface endometriosis of the ovary (arrow) shown by the dark puckered areas and the ends of broken adhesions. As is so often the case, the lesion is associated with multiple leiomyomas in the uterus.

Social and Economic Factors

Endometriosis is more common among highly civilised communities and their well-to-do members. It is four times as frequent in private as in hospital practice and is therefore described as *a disease of the rich*. This might be accounted for in part by late marriage and late childbearing in the higher income groups.

Parity

About 30–40% of affected women are infertile. The association of infertility and endometriosis is established, but it is difficult to say which is the cause and which is the effect. It is alleged that the deliberate deferment of childbearing until a late age is a causal factor in that it exposes the susceptible tissues to an uninterrupted ovarian stimulus; pregnancy, it is said, protects by periodically suppressing ovarian activity **(Box 1)**, but this protective effect decreases with time.

Luteinised Unruptured Follicle

The association of endometriosis with the luteinisation of an unruptured follicle (LUF) has been noted and it has

BOX 1: Risk factors.

- Late marriages
- Late child bearing
- Genital tract obstruction
- Frequent and prolonged menstrual cycles
- Nulliparity
- Early menarche
- Prenatal exposure to DES
- Low body mass index
- Heavy consumption of alcoholism and caffeine

(DES: diethylstilbestrol)

been suggested that, as a consequence of the reduced output of hormones, endometrial fragments might be able to take root and develop on the ovarian surface or pelvic peritoneum. Although the evidence is limited, it does appear that some women suffer from recurrent luteinisation of unruptured follicles, which might account for some women having both endometriosis and infertility problems.

Retroversion

Extrauterine endometriosis is often found with retroversion and it may be that the displacement is an aetiological factor in that it favours retrograde menstruation (see further).

Substantial evidence suggests that endometriosis is associated with a state of subclinical peritoneal inflammation, marked by an increased peritoneal fluid volume, increased peritoneal fluid white blood cell concentration (especially macrophages with increased activation status), and increased inflammatory cytokines, growth factors and angiogenesis-promoting substances.

Sites of Endometriosis

Endometriosis can occur anywhere in the body and is described even in the tissues of the arm, leg, pleura, lungs, diaphragm and kidney. Usually, however, it is confined to the organs and tissues of the abdomen and pelvis, at or below the level of the umbilicus. These include the omentum. Visceral lesions are often multiple.

Ovary

The ovary is the most common site and is involved in 30–40% of cases. The lesion is nearly always bilateral. It sometimes takes the form of multiple *burnt match head* spots on the surface of the ovary **(Figs. 9 to 11)**, sometimes as the typical tarry cysts in a disorganised organ surrounded by dense adhesions **(Fig. 12)**. It should be noted, however, that not all *tarry cysts* in the ovaries are endometriotic. Any cyst containing old blood can present a similar naked-eye appearance.

An endometriotic cyst can reach the size of a foetal head but is rarely larger. It is usually impossible to remove it intact from its adhesions, because the presence of these is a sign that the cyst wall has already been breached.

Pelvic Peritoneum Including the Uterovesical Pouch and the Pouch of Douglas

The peritoneum of the pouch of Douglas is the second most common site and a lesion there is often associated with one in the ovaries. It may represent secondary seeding from the ovarian condition. The tarry cysts seen on the pelvic peritoneum are rarely bigger than a pea; the lesions are manifested more by puckering and thickening of peritoneum and by adhesions. The last often occludes the uterorectal space, fixing the uterus in retroversion **(Fig. 8)**.

Outer Coat of Uterus

Endometriosis of the ovary, pelvic peritoneum and associated ligaments, when adherent to the uterus, often

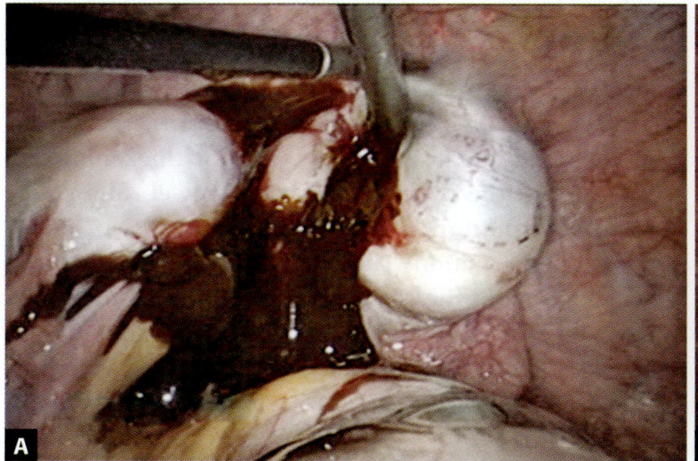

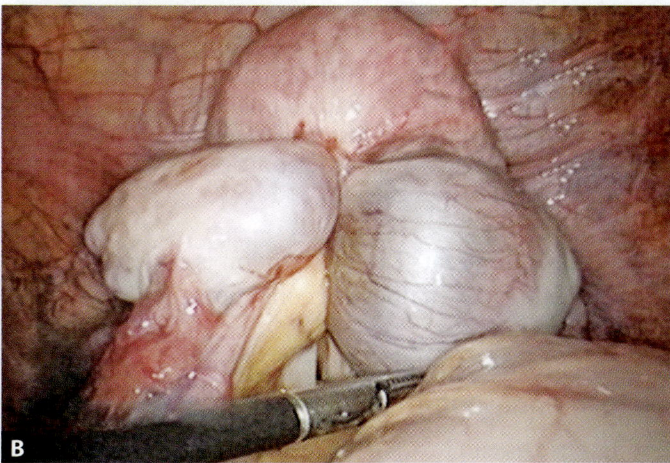

Figs. 10A and B: (A) Ovarian endometrioma; (B) Kissing ovaries.
Courtesy: Dr Sanjay Patel, Mayflower Hospital, Ahmedabad.

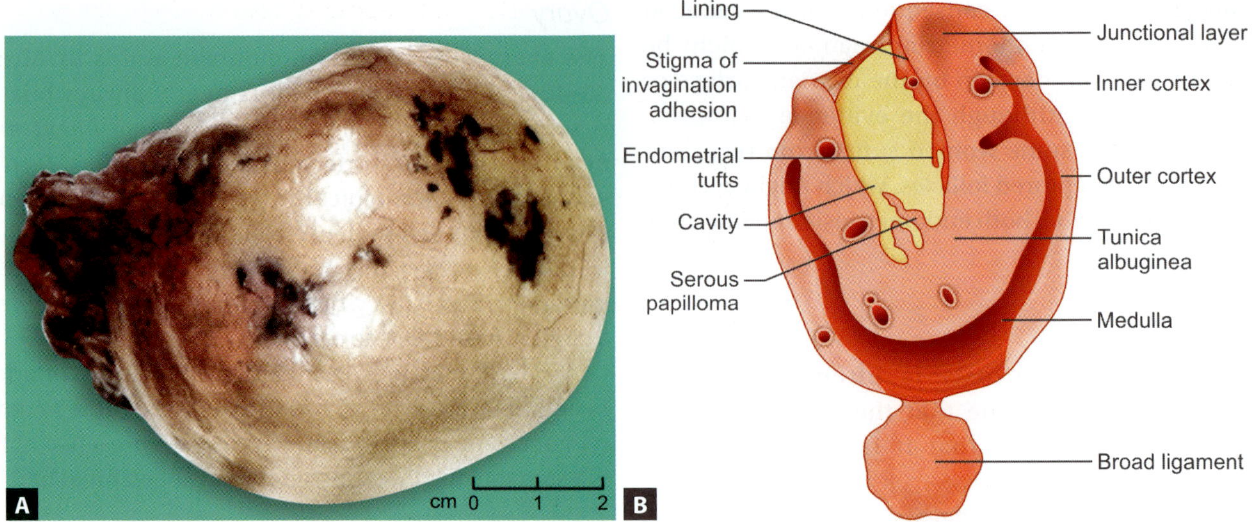

Figs. 11A and B: (A) A serous cystadenoma of the ovary with multiple areas of menstruating endometriosis on its surface. This is a fortuitous combination but the appearance of the lesions is typical of pelvic endometriosis; (B) Endometriotic burrowing through ovarian tissue.

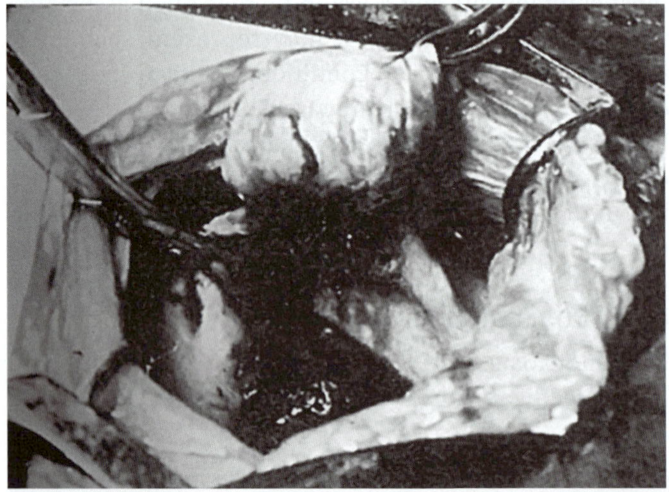

Fig. 12: Pelvic endometriosis. The right ovary, the seat of an endometriotic cyst, has been lifted from a mass of adhesions in the pelvis. Tarry fluid is seen escaping from the cyst and lying in the pelvis. The patient in this case was young and the ovary was conserved after resection of the affected areas. A similar procedure can be carried out laparoscopically.

invades its outer coat. The penetration is superficial and of little significance: It does not constitute adenomyosis.

Round Ligament, Uterosacral Ligament and Rectovaginal Septum

Endometriosis can involve the round ligament in either its pelvic or inguinal canal portion. In the latter case, it forms an abdominal wall tumour. The uterosacral ligaments are much more commonly affected and a lesion there tends to spread into the rectovaginal connective tissue. Endometriosis of the uterosacral ligaments can occur with or without involvement of the peritoneum of the pouch of Douglas.

Fallopian Tube

Endometriosis of the outer surface of the fallopian tube occurs as part of peritoneal endometriosis **(Fig. 13)**.

Intestine

The rectum and pelvic colon can be implicated by invasion from peritoneal and ovarian deposits or by seeding. The ileum, caecum and appendix are also possible sites. No matter how extensive it may appear, the lesion rarely penetrates the mucosa, so rectal haemorrhage and the visualisation of blood cysts on sigmoidoscopy are unlikely. The main pathological change is fibrotic thickening and puckering of the outer coats of the bowel, often with stricture formation and adhesions which can cause intestinal obstruction. The condition is easily mistaken for carcinoma of the rectum or pelvic colon, and many unexpected surgical cures of apparent malignant disease in these sites can be accounted for on this basis.

Bladder and Ureter

Endometriosis of these organs is usually explained by invasion from an adjacent site **(Figs. 14A and B)**.

Vagina and Vulva

Islets of endometriosis are sometimes found in surgical or obstetrical scars in the vagina and perineum but the most common site for vaginal endometriosis is the posterior fornix which becomes infiltrated from the pouch of Douglas or the rectovaginal septum. The lesion appears as multiple small blue-domed cysts in an indurated area of the vaginal vault **(Figs. 15 and 16)** and, when it becomes ulcerated, can be mistaken for carcinoma.

Abdominal Wall

Endometriosis occurs spontaneously in the umbilicus and the inguinal canal, usually without any associated intrapelvic endometriotic lesion. It causes a swelling which becomes bigger and more painful about the time of menstruation. It may appear blue from an underlying blood cyst and sometimes it discharges menstrual blood. The tumour is not encapsulated and the surrounding tissue is indurated. A lesion with similar characteristics sometimes occurs in abdominal wall scars following operations on the uterus or tubes (scar endometriosis). The operations most likely to be followed by this complication are hysterectomy, classical caesarean section, myomectomy, ventrofixation, removal of pelvic endometriosis and operations involving a section of the fallopian tube. It is also seen in episiotomy scars. All offer the possibility of a spill of Müllerian epithelium into the incision **(Fig. 17)**.

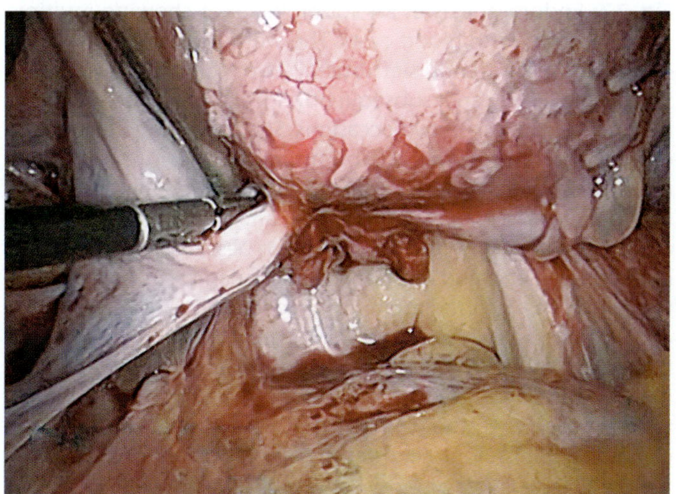

Fig. 13: Kissing fallopian tubes.
Courtesy: Dr Sanjay Patel, Mayflower Hospital, Ahmedabad.

Lungs and Pleura

The pleura is more often affected than the lungs and, even there, endometriosis is extremely rare. The characteristic effect is the cyclical development of pleuritic pain, and haemothorax (right-sided) or haemoptysis, with each menstrual period.

The cyclical occurrence of haemoptysis or haemothorax is suggestive but not conclusive evidence of an endometriotic lesion in the lungs or pleura.

Mechanism of Origin

Many theories have been put forward to account for the development of external endometriosis but none explains all aspects of this disease **(Table 1)**.

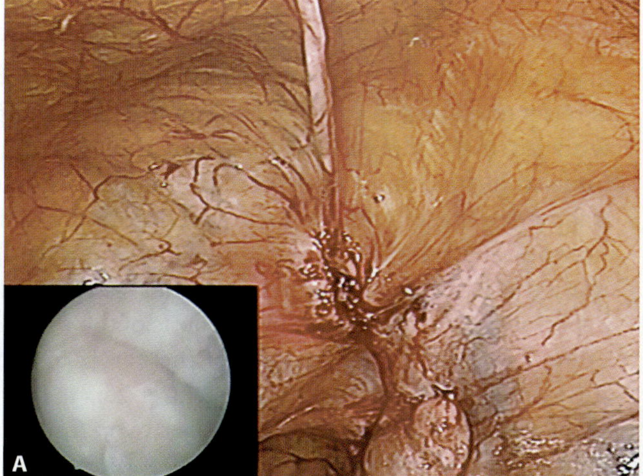

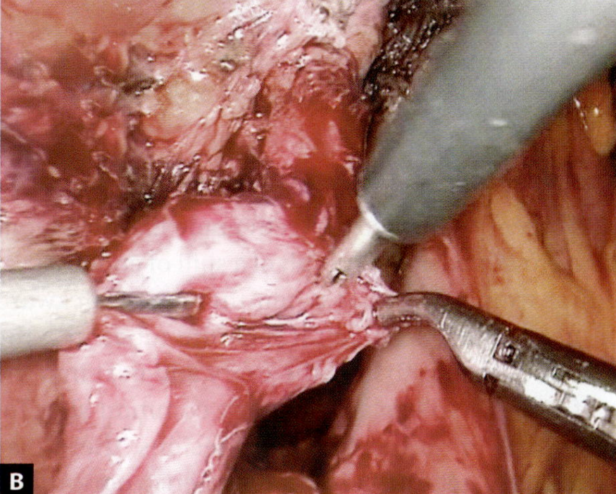

Figs. 14A and B: (A) Bladder endometriosis; (B) Ureteric endometriosis.
Courtesy: Dr Sanjay Patel, Mayflower Hospital, Ahmedabad.

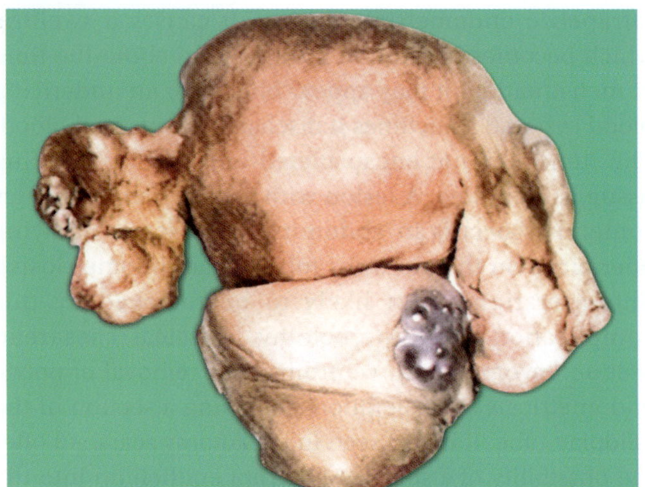

Fig. 15: Endometriotic cysts in the vaginal vault. The cuff of the vagina, removed at the time of total hysterectomy, has been turned back to show the posterior fornix with the *blue-domed* cysts of menstrual blood lying subepithelially.

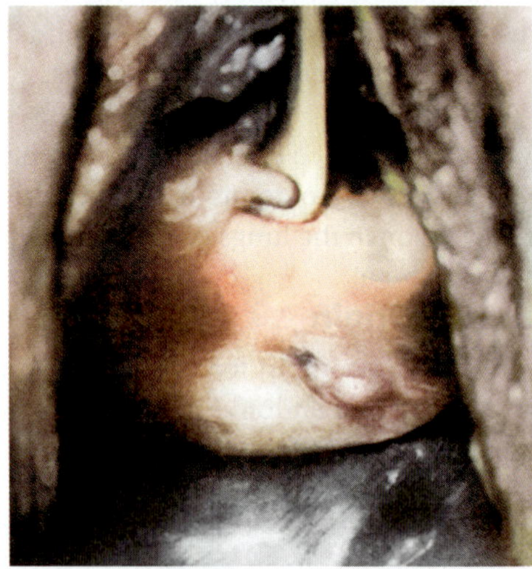

Fig. 16: Endometriotic cysts in the posterior vaginal fornix, the cervix being pulled forward by a vulsellum on its posterior lip.

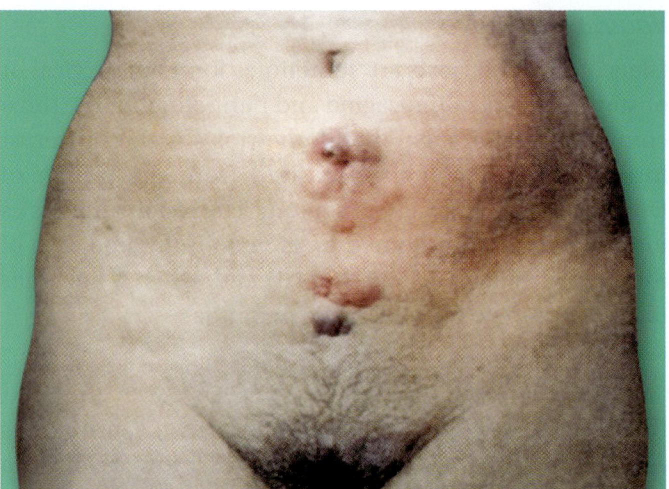

Fig. 17: Endometriosis of an abdominal scar showing multiple small tumours with blood cysts. The woman affected was aged 49 years and had endometriotic cysts of the ovaries removed 5 years previously and, subsequently, local removal of cysts from the abdominal wall on two occasions. She complained of swelling of, and bleeding from, the abdominal wall lesions with each menstrual period. The endometriosis extended deeply and widely in the muscle of the abdominal wall and it did not respond to continuous high-dose treatment with an oestrogen–progestogen preparation. So, it, and any remaining ovarian tissue in the pelvis, was exposed to X-irradiation. This reduced the size of the mass and permitted its wide, although still incomplete, surgical excision. Four years later, the disease was as troublesome as ever and the masses were large. They again failed to respond to progestogen therapy and, when the woman was 55 years of age it was clear, clinically and histologically, that the lesion was malignant. During the previous 7–8 years, biopsy had been carried out on at least five occasions and always the microscopic appearances were those of endometriosis with no evidence of malignancy. There is no doubt that, in this case, a benign endometriotic condition ultimately changed to an adenocarcinoma and killed the patient.

Endometrial Spill

Sampson's theory (the theory of retrograde menstruation) is that the growth arises as a result of a spill of endometrial epithelium from the uterus when there is a backward flow of menstrual discharge through the tubes into the peritoneum. This falls first on the ovary and next into the pouch of Douglas to explain the most common sites for endometriosis. From these primary lesions, there may be a secondary scatter. Retrograde menstruation is a common phenomenon as can be seen during laparoscopy or laparotomy in 90% of women. It is said to be more likely when the uterus is the seat of leiomyomas, when it is retroverted and in cases of endometriosis as compared with normal women. It is now established that the menstrual discharge does contain viable endometrial fragments; these have been recovered from the dialysate in women undergoing peritoneal dialysis during the menstrual period. Endometriosis has been produced experimentally in monkeys by implants of their menstrual efflux or surgical transposition of the cervix to produce intra-abdominal menstruation. Moreover, it has been shown that artificially produced retroversion in these animals favours the development of the condition.

The endometrial spill theory adequately explains endometriosis in scars in the abdominal wall, vagina and

TABLE 1: Theories of sites of endometriosis.

Site	***Theory***
Pelvic tissues	Retrograde menstruation
Pelvic peritoneum	Coelomic metaplasia
• Abdominal viscera • Rectovaginal septum umbilicus	Coelomic metaplasia
• Abdominal scar • Episiotomy scar • Vagina and cervix	Direct implantation
Lymph nodes	Lymphatic spread
Others (lungs, pleura and skin)	Vascular, genetic and immunologic

perineum following pelvic operations or childbirth; and accounts for the common finding of multiple pinhead-sized areas of endometriosis on the ovarian surface and pelvic peritoneum in adolescent girls suffering from cryptomenorrhoea. In these, however, the disease does not persist or cause trouble once the obstruction to the outflow of menstrual blood is removed.

Though the retrograde endometrial spill explains the physical displacement of endometrial cells to the peritoneal cavity, further predisposing factors are essential for the development of endometriosis. These include genetic and epigenetic factors, altered hormonal milieu and immunological factors. The spill theory fails to account for a primary lesion in the umbilicus and endometriosis in remote areas such as the kidney and limbs.

Coelomic Metaplasia

This theory is associated with the names of Ivanoff and Meyer and is based on the fact that the uterus develops from coelomic cells which form the Müllerian ducts. It postulates that embryonic cells capable of differentiating into Müllerian tissue remain in and around the peritoneum of the pelvis and the surface epithelium of the ovary, or that adult cells in these sites retain the potential to differentiate into endometrium and myometrium.

This concept offers an explanation for the common finding of fibromuscular tissue alongside ectopic endometrium. It can also account for lesions in all sites except those outside the abdomen and pelvis, and possibly those in the perineum. But even the last might have this basis because, during development, a tongue of coelom accompanies the down growth of the mesodermal urorectal septum which goes to form the rectovaginal septum and perineum. It is said that even limb buds receive a contribution from coelom. However, this theory is not well-supported by clinical data.

The induction theory is an extension of the theory of coelomic metaplasia and proposes that some biochemical factors such as hormonal or immunological agents may be responsible for the transformation of undifferentiated peritoneal cells to endometrial glands and stroma.

Lymphatic and Vascular Embolism

There is a body of evidence to show that tiny fragments of uterine endometrium frequently, and presumably normally, break off and enter the lymph or bloodstreams. They can be found in routine sections of lungs taken at autopsies, for example. Moreover, microscopic islands of endometrium are demonstrable in the pelvic lymph nodes in a high proportion of cases of endometriosis. Cell embolism which, incidentally, was also postulated by Sampson, is becoming more and more acceptable in the explanation of certain endometriotic lesions, especially those remote from the pelvis.

It may be concluded that, although endometriosis probably is usually a result of cellular spill, the present evidence suggests that it can arise by any of the above mechanisms. They are all, however, only potential causes of the disease for they are operating in all women. Once endometrial cells are shifted from their normal site, they still require other factors to make them survive and proliferate: One of the most important of these is a good supply of oestrogen from the ovary.

Immunological

It has been proposed that certain immunologic factors may explain why all women who have retrograde menstruation do not develop endometriosis. However, there are no consistent reports regarding decreased natural killer cell activity or decreased autologous cell-mediated cytotoxicity in endometriosis. Increased secretion of tumour necrosis factor (TNF), epidermal growth factor, macrophage-derived growth factor from macrophages and adhesion molecules such as integrins may promote pelvic implantation of endometrial tissue. T and B lymphocytes can be recruited by activated macrophages. These lymphocytes may then synthesise antibodies which may play a role in the propagation of endometriosis.

Immune Factors

- Impaired cellular immune response to autologous endometrial antigen allows translocated endometrial cells to implant at ectopic sites.
- Cytokines serve as immunomodulators, angiogenic factors or agents promoting endometrial cell growth.
- Interleukin-6 (IL-6) is a T-cell-derived cytokine. Its secretion is increased by peritoneal macrophages in endometriosis and by stromal cells of ectopic endometrium.
- IL-8 facilitates the attachment of endometrial cells to peritoneal surfaces, invasion of extracellular matrix, local angiogenesis and endometrial proliferation.
- TNF-α is secreted by activated macrophages and has potent inflammatory properties.

Altered Hormonal Milieu

There is an altered hormonal milieu with oestrogen dependence and progesterone resistance. The endometriotic tissue shows increased expression of aromatase and decreased expression of 17-hydroxy steroid dehydrogenase resulting in increases in locally available oestrogen. Also, there is decreased progesterone receptor expression resulting in progesterone resistance. Also, there is increased Cox-2 activity leading to high local production of prostaglandin (PG): PGE2 and PGF2 alpha. It also causes vasoconstriction, myometrial contractions and pain. The current literature suggests that stem cells, dysfunctional immune response, genetic predisposition and aberrant peritoneal environment may all be involved in the establishment and propagation of endometriotic lesions.

Epigenetic Changes

Epigenetic changes in endometriotic tissue led to increased local oestrogen production via increased activity of SF1. There is also upregulation of oestrogen receptor beta (ER-β) and downregulation of progesterone receptors in endometrial tissue.

Other current theories suggest that stem cells, dysfunctional immune response, genetic predisposition and aberrant peritoneal environment may all be involved in the establishment and propagation of endometriotic lesions.

Symptoms (Fig. 18)

Surprisingly, there may be no symptoms, even when the endometriosis is widespread and advanced. There are six *Ds*: Dysmenorrhoea, disorders of menstruation, dyspareunia, dyschezia, dull ache of abdomen and delay in conception (infertility). Delay infertility is a major problem with endometriosis.

Dysmenorrhoea is progressive which is characteristic of endometriosis. Postmenstrual dysmenorrhoea is the maximum compared to premenstrual and menstrual as the ectopic endometrium bleeds a little later than the endometrium. The symptoms and signs do not correlate with the findings as with small lesions there may be maximum symptoms; maximum symptoms with minimal lesions.

Dysmenorrhoea

The classical symptom of extrauterine endometriosis is secondary dysmenorrhoea, commencing after the age of 30 years and gradually getting worse. In fact, it is present in only approximately 50% of cases. The explanations for this are by the time the lesion is found it may have been inactive for several years. The pain comes on gradually for a few days before the period, when the endometriosis is becoming congested, but is more severe during menstruation when there is bleeding into a closed space. It can reach a maximum at the end of menstruation. Thereafter, the pain subsides slowly but may not disappear completely between periods. The severity of symptoms does not correlate with the severity of the disease except in deeply infiltrating endometriosis (DIE).

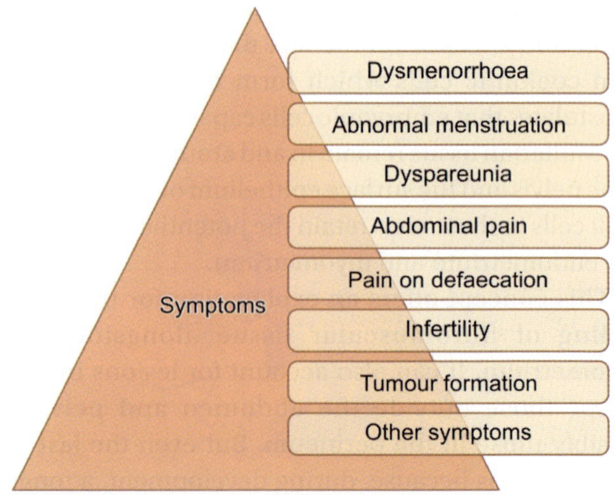

Fig. 18: Symptoms pyramid.

The site of the pain depends on the site of the lesion. With multiple pelvic deposits, it is deep-seated in the lower abdomen, pelvis, rectum and lower back. The pain of endometriosis on the body surface is localised to the tumour itself.

Dyspareunia

Deep-seated pain on coitus is particularly likely when the pouch of Douglas and rectovaginal septum is affected, and when there is an associated fixed retroversion.

Pain on Defaecation

This symptom is often only elicited by a leading question. It occurs when the endometriosis involves or is close to the rectum and is more noticeable at the time of menstruation when the tumour is larger and tenderer.

Tumour Formation

The patient may notice a swelling, especially in the case of a lesion of the abdominal wall or perineum. This exhibits cyclical enlargement and tenderness with menstruation and, if superficial, may discharge blood.

Abdominal Pain

Mechanisms for pain in endometriosis:

- Production of substances such as cytokines and growth factors by activated macrophages associated with endometric implants.
- Effect of bleeding from ectopic implants causing peritoneal irritation and fibrosis.
- Invasion of pelvic nerves by endometriosis implants.

Dyspareunia is attributed to the presence of endometriotic lesions over the uterosacrals and also due to the presence of dense adhesions in cul-de-sac making uterus, retroverted with restricted mobility.

Chronic: Endometriosis forming cysts and adhesions among the pelvic organs causes a chronic aching discomfort in the lower abdomen and pelvis sometimes referred to the groins, hips and thighs. This undergoes menstrual exacerbations.

Acute: A sudden and severe pain, with all the accompanying symptoms and signs of an acute abdomen, is experienced when a blood cyst ruptures. Such an accident is most likely about the time of menstruation and this coincidence, together with careful analysis of other symptoms and signs, helps to avoid the common error of diagnosing acute appendicitis. I have even seen such a case opened as a case of ectopic pregnancy.

Abnormal Menstruation

Excessive bleeding is present in approximately 60% of cases of pelvic endometriosis. Menorrhagia, polymenorrhoea and polymenorrhagia are all seen. A change in the cycle usually means ovarian involvement. Because of residual adhesions and vascular upset, abnormal bleeding can continue even when the disease is quiescent.

Infertility

The investigation of infertility, especially since the introduction of the laparoscope, has led to an increase in the diagnosis of endometriosis. Several possible mechanisms have been suggested for this association. The tubes are invariably open, but there may be pelvic adhesions, distorted anatomy and altered tubal motility which result in impaired ovum pick-up; the alterations in PGs, macrophages and cytokines mentioned above may lead to enhanced phagocytosis of sperm; hormonal dysfunction may lead to anovulation, the luteinised unruptured follicle and luteal phase deficiency; and there may be early pregnancy losses. We still do not fully understand how endometriosis causes infertility or how infertility causes endometriosis **(Flowchart 1)**.

Other Symptoms

General ill-health and malaise are not uncommon with pelvic endometriosis. Intermittent pyrexia, especially at the time of menstruation, is present in at least 10% of cases and is caused by absorption of the degenerated products of the retained blood. Frequency, strangury and sometimes haematuria at the time of menstruation are features of urinary tract endometriosis. Other possibilities include symptoms of intestinal and ureteric obstruction.

Physical Signs

Small multiple lesions may not give any sign of their presence during physical examination. The vulva, vagina and cervix should be inspected first with a speculum to rule out any deposits, though these are rare. Larger or easily accessible deposits are palpable as fixed, tender and nodular swellings with surrounding induration. Even if a definite tumour is not palpable, some or all of the pelvic organs are fixed and any attempt to move them reproduces the patient's pain. A fixed retroversion is a common

Flowchart 1: Altered immune response.

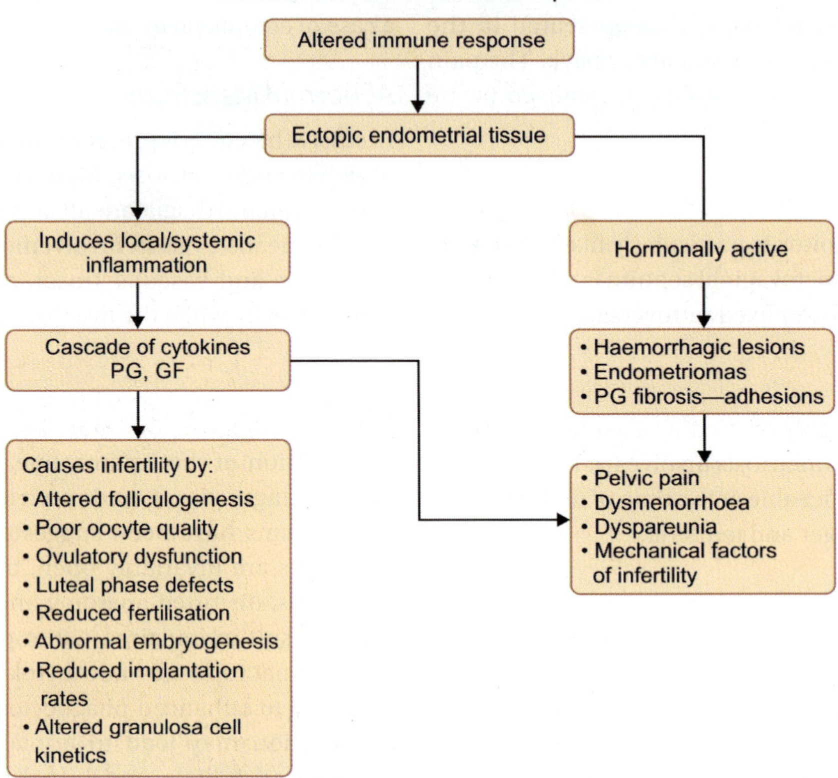

(GF: growth factor: PGs: prostaglandins)

finding. Involvement of the uterosacral ligaments and rectovaginal septum gives rise to a characteristic tender shotty thickening (*cobblestones*) above and behind the posterior fornix, which may be better appreciated during the menses.

Diagnosis

It must first be emphasised that symptom-producing endometriosis which is active, and sometimes when it is inactive, can usually be diagnosed before the operation. The diagnosis merely requires proper attention to the details of symptoms and physical signs. It is possible even when the lesion is too small to feel or is masked by large myomas. Nevertheless, tiny islets are often only revealed by laparoscopy carried out during the investigation of infertility or other complaints. Typical laparoscopic findings are the *powder-burn* lesions on the peritoneal surface.

However, apart from these dark-brown or bluish nodules or cysts, there may be subtle lesions, which include red implants, white plaques, scarring, serous or clear vesicles, pseudocysts and yellowish-brown colour of the peritoneum, and adhesions on the under surface of the ovaries. Therefore, a meticulous examination of the pelvic and abdominal cavity is required to map the extent of the disease. Larger cysts including endometriomas may be seen, which are usually <12 cm in diameter. Histological confirmation should be sought wherever possible.

Ultrasound **(Fig. 14A)**, transvaginal ultrasound (TVS), has 90% sensitivity and almost 100% specificity for the detection of endometriomas. CT scan or magnetic resonance imaging (MRI) can be used only as additional diagnostic modalities. Pelvic ultrasound helps to detect endometriomas which appear as ovarian cysts with irregular walls, low-level echoes within and occasional high-level echogenic areas which are blood clots. Peritoneal deposits cannot be delineated. CT scan and MRI do not offer any additional advantage and are more expensive. CA-125, a marker for ovarian cancer, is found to be raised in endometriosis although the levels are lower than they are in cancer. The levels have also been seen to correlate with the severity of the disease, but since there is a wide range and a wide variety of conditions in which the levels are elevated, its greatest use may be in monitoring a patient serially for recurrence. In about 30% of cases, the disease is steadily progressive, while in the rest, it remains stable. Spontaneous resolution has been reported. Endometriosis has to be distinguished from the following:

- *Chronic salpingo-oophoritis:* Menstrual irregularities and menorrhagia, dysmenorrhoea, infertility, dyspareunia, bilateral fixed tender adnexal masses, fixation of pelvic organs, general malaise and pelvic ache, and even pyrexia are common to both. In endometriosis, the dysmenorrhoea is intra- or postmenstrual, there is no history of infection and the tubes are patent, although they may be distorted by adhesions.
- Corpus luteum cysts or neoplastic cysts
- Uterine leiomyomas
- Malignant disease of the ovary or metastases on the pelvic peritoneum
- Carcinoma of the cervix and vagina. The difficulty here arises mostly in relation to endometriosis of the rectovaginal septum and vaginal vault.
- Carcinoma of rectum and colon, and diverticulitis
- All causes of an acute abdomen, in the case of rupture of a tarry cyst
- All causes of intestinal obstruction
- All tumours of the umbilicus
- Hernia and other swellings in the inguinal canal
- All causes of haematuria. In endometriosis, haematuria is limited to the time of menstruation.

Classification: Various classification systems have been proposed and these help to compare trials of therapeutic methods, but they correlate poorly with the degree of symptoms experienced by the patient **(Table 2)**.

TABLE 2: The American Society for Reproductive Medicine revised classification of endometriosis.

Stage I (minimal)	1–5			
Stage II (mild)	6–15			
Stage III (moderate)	16–40			
Stage IV (severe)	>40			
Total	Prognosis			
Ovary peritoneum	Endometriosis	<1 cm	1–3 cm	>3 cm
	Superficial	1	2	4
	Deep	2	4	6
	R superficial	1	2	4
	Deep	4	16	20
	L superficial	1	2	4
	Deep	4	16	20
Tube ovary	Posterior cul-de-sac obliteration adhesions	Partial	Complete	
		4		40
		<1/3 enclosure	1/3–2/3 enclosure	>2/3 enclosure
	R filmy	1	2	4
	Dense	4	8	16
	L filmy	2	4	4
	Dense	4*	8*	16
	R filmy	1	2	4
	Dense	4*	8*	16
	L filmy	1	2	4

**If the fimbriated end of the fallopian tube is completely enclosed, change the point assignment to 16.*

Source: Revised American Society for Reproductive Medicine classification of endometriosis: 1996. Fertil Steril. 1997;67(5):817-21.

Laparoscopic Findings

Laparoscopy with the histological examination is the gold standard for the diagnosis of endometriosis. Laparoscopy is the standard technique for visualising pelvis and establishing a definitive diagnosis **(Fig. 19A)**.

- During diagnosis laparoscopy, complete inspection in a clockwise or counterclockwise fashion with a blunt probe, of the bowel, bladder, uterus, tubes, ovaries, cul-de-sac and broad ligament should be included.
- Characteristic findings indeed typical *powder burn* or gunshot lesions on the peritoneal serosal surfaces which are black, dark-brown, bluish nodules or small cysts containing old haemorrhage surrounded by variable degree of fibrosis. These lesions should be confirmed histologically for diagnosis of endometriosis. However, the majority of implants are typical and may be red and vascular.
- DIE may have the appearance of minimal disease resulting in an underestimation of the disease severity. Careful inspection of all sides of both ovaries is essential for diagnosis of ovarian endometriosis. Large ovarian endometriotic cysts are usually located on anterior surface of the ovary and contain a thick, vicious dark-brown fluid (chocolate fluid).
- Biopsy and removal of ovarian cyst for histologic confirmation is essential for diagnosis in revised endometriosis classification. Ovarian endometriotic cyst has the following diagnostic features:
  - Cyst diameters of <12 cm
  - Adhesions to pelvic sidewall or broad ligament
  - Endometriosis on the surface of the ovary
  - Tarry, chocolate-coloured fluid content

Treatment

Expectant

The treatment of endometriosis varies with its extent, site and symptoms and also with the age of the patient. If the lesions are small and multiple and are producing few symptoms, it may be best to leave them alone; they sometimes become inactive after a period of time. Expectant management may also be indicated in women approaching menopause.

If a woman known to have endometriosis becomes pregnant, there need be little fear about the outcome. Rupture of chocolate cysts during pregnancy does occur but is rare; a fixed retroversion corrects itself; even large masses in the pelvis rarely obstruct labour, they disappear as pregnancy advances.

The following explanations are put forward to account for the disappearance or inactivation of endometriosis during pregnancy: The absence of follicular activity and ovulation; the suppression of menstruation and therefore of recurrent retrograde spill of endometrium; the conversion of ectopic endometrium to decidua, a change which favours its necrosis and absorption of the glands. This in fact is what happens when a state of pseudopregnancy is induced with progestogens **(Fig. 20)**.

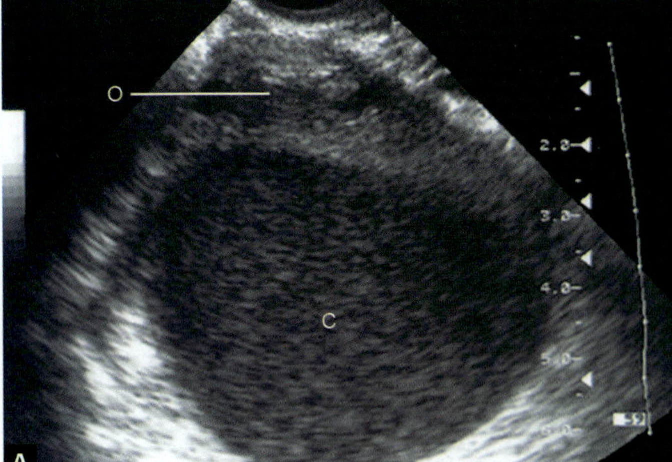

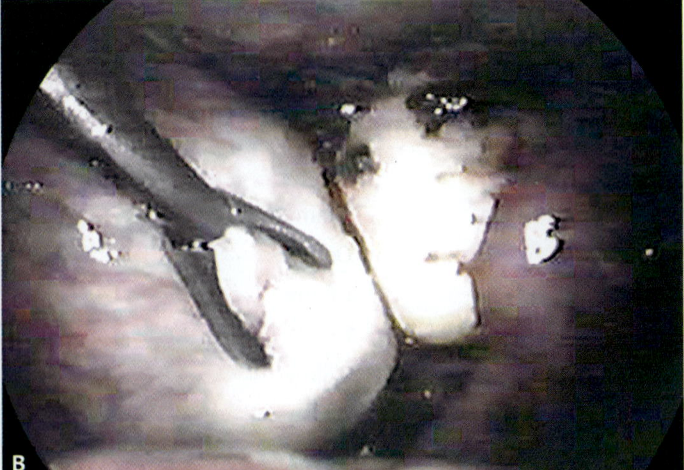

Figs. 19A and B: (A) Ultrasound pictures of endometriotic cyst which shows fine stippling inside ovary (ground glass appearance); (B) Laparoscopy findings of endometrioma.

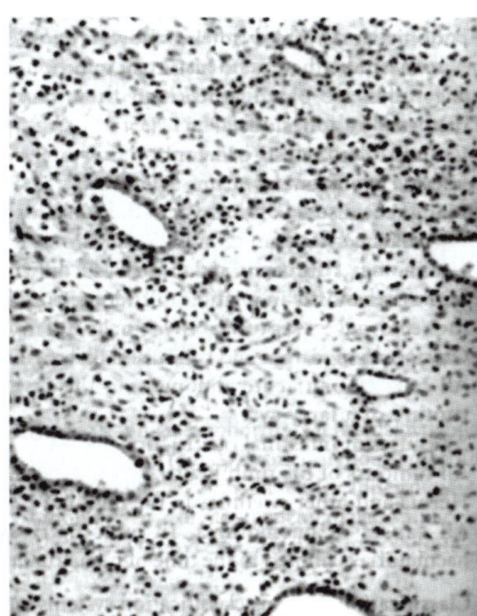

Fig. 20: The effect of oestrogen–progestogen antiovulatory preparations on endometriosis. Continuous administration in large doses causes proliferation and decidual reaction of the stroma—a progestogen effect. The glandular elements undergo *exhaustion* atrophy and appear small and inactive.

Medical Treatment

There is no evidence of medical management in the treatment of infertility; however, the medical therapy is effective in relieving the pain in endometriosis. On the medical line of management, the woman has amenorrhoea for 6–9 months as it is not effective and more over the woman becomes older and has fecundity lowered. In order to get amenorrhoea, medications are given to manipulate the endogenous hormonal milieu, and this is the basis for the medical management of endometriosis. Progestins may exert an antiendometriotic effect by causing initial decidualisation of endometrial tissue followed by atrophy. They can be considered as the first choice for the treatment of endometriosis, because they are as effective as danazol or gonadotrophin-releasing hormone (GnRH) analogues and have a lower cost and a lower incidence of side effects than these agents. In most studies, the effect of treatment has been evaluated after 3–6 months of therapy. Medroxyprogesterone acetate (MPA) has been the most studied agent. It is effective in relieving pain starting at a dose of 30 mg/day and increasing the dose based on the clinical response and bleeding patterns. However, a recent randomised placebo-controlled study reported a significant reduction in stages and scores of endometriosis in both the placebo group and the group treated with MPA, 50 mg/day, and placebo at laparoscopy within 3 months after cessation of therapy. These findings raise questions about the need for medical therapy.

TABLE 3: Medical treatment of endometriosis-associated pain: Effective regimens (usual duration: 6 months).

	Administration	***Dose***	***Frequency***
OCP			
Progestogens			
Medroxyprogesterone acetate	PO	30 mg	Daily
Megestrol acetate	PO	40 mg	Daily
Lynoestrenol	PO	10 mg	Daily
Dydrogesterone	PO	20–30 mg	Daily
Dienogest	PO	2 mg	Daily for 3 months
Antiprogestins			
Gestrinone	PO	1.25 or 2.5 mg	Twice weekly
Danazol	PO	400 mg	Daily
Gonadotrophin-releasing hormone			
Leuprolide	SC IM	500 mg 3.75 mg	Daily Monthly
Goserelin	SC	3.6 mg	Monthly
Buserelin	IN SC	300 µg 200 µg	Daily
Nafarelin	IN	200 µg	Daily
Triptorelin	IM	3.75 mg	Monthly
Intrauterine devices			
Levonorgestrel	Intrauterine	20 µg/day	Up to 5 years

(IM: intramuscular; IN: intranasal; OCP: oral contraceptive pill; PO: oral; SC: subcutaneous).

Hormone Therapy

Medical treatment of endometriosis-associated pain: Effective regimens are discussed in **Table 3**.

Oestrogens and Progestogens

Treatment with a combination of these hormones was introduced to mimic the conditions occurring during pregnancy, which has long been known to have a beneficial effect. Large doses given continuously suppress ovulation and menstruation and often quickly bring about clinical improvement in the condition with relief of the patient's symptoms. In the endometriotic lesions, they produce a widespread decidual change in the stroma, and this in turn brings about glandular atrophy and quiet **(Fig. 20)**. If this effect is maintained for a sufficiently long time, the glands may be destroyed and the endometriosis permanently cured. Generally, however, the result is only temporary and reawakening of the endometriosis can occur as long as 2 years after apparent cure.

Oestrogen–progestogen therapy is less effective for adenomyosis than for extrauterine endometriosis, because the endometrium in the former is relatively insensitive to hormones. Hormone therapy also generally gives unsatisfactory results when extrauterine endometriosis takes the form of large tumour masses and chocolate cysts. Its place is in the treatment of endometriosis-associated dysmenorrhoea, dyspareunia and chronic pelvic pain (CPP). In these circumstances, a good or satisfactory response is seen in 80% of cases, and 50% of patients with opportunity to subsequently conceive.

Any of the low-dose oestrogen–progestogen oral contraceptive preparations can be used. It is usual to administer it continuously and increase it if required, to suppress menstruation. Once the adequate level of dosage is reached, it is continued daily for 6–9 months. The advantage of this regime is the low cost.

The difficulties and disadvantages of this treatment are as follows:

- Nausea, vomiting and malaise at the outset
- Slight breakthrough bleeding often occurs, but this is of little consequence and can be controlled by stepping up the dose.
- It can cause gross hypertrophy of the uterus and enlargement of any leiomyomas, which may be present. With this treatment, uterine leiomyomas may increase considerably in size. The explanation is probably oedema and degeneration, rather than hyperplasia and hypertrophy of the tumours.
- During the treatment phase, the patient is inevitably infertile. If pregnancy occurs, there may be a risk to the foetus.
- Long-term benefits are questionable.

Progestogens

Mainly because of the last disadvantage listed above, treatment with progestogens alone, continuously or intermittently, is now advocated. Again, any of several agents can be used but popular ones are MPA, dydrogesterone and megestrol acetate. Injections of depot medroxyprogesterone acetate (DMPA) can also be effective.

By any technique, treatment for 6–9 months is necessary. During this time, ovulation may or may not be suppressed, even if menstruation is, so conception is possible.

Progestogens are often used as a first line of medical management, because they produce symptomatic relief and their side effects and cost are less. MPA is started at a dose of 30 mg/day, megestrol acetate at 40 mg/day and dydrogesterone at 20–30 mg/day. The dose is increased as required. DMPA is administered in a dose of 150 mg at intervals of 6–12 weeks.

The disadvantages of this regimen are as follows:

- Nausea, weight gain and fluid retention
- *Breakthrough bleeding:* This may require short-term oestrogen administration for about a week.
- Mood changes, depression
- DMPA should be avoided if fertility is desired as return of ovulation as well as menstruation is variable.

The levonorgestrel (LNG)-releasing intrauterine device (IUD) can be used for women with deep infiltrating rectovaginal endometriosis.

Medroxyprogesterone acetate (150 mg) given intramuscularly every 3 months is also effective for the treatment of pain associated with endometriosis, but it is not indicated in infertile women, because it induces profound amenorrhoea and anovulation, and a varying length of time is required for ovulation to resume after discontinuation of therapy. Megestrol acetate has been administered in a dose of 40 mg/day with good results. Other treatment strategies have included dydrogesterone (20–30 mg/day, either continuously or on days 5–25) and lynestrenol (10 mg/day). The effectiveness of natural progesterone has not been evaluated.

Side effects of progestins include nausea, weight gain, fluid retention and breakthrough bleeding due to hypoestrogenaemia. Breakthrough bleeding, although common, is usually corrected by short-term (7 days) administration of oestrogen. Depression and other mood disorders are a significant problem in about 1% of women taking these medications.

Local progesterone treatment of endometriosis-associated dysmenorrhoea with an LNG-releasing intrauterine system (IUS) for 12 months has resulted in a significant reduction in dysmenorrhoea, pelvic pain and dyspareunia; a high degree of patient satisfaction and a significant reduction in the volume of rectovaginal endometriotic nodules. Although the results are promising, none of these pilot studies included a control group. Further randomised evidence is needed to determine whether intrauterine progesterone treatment is effective in the suppression of endometriosis.

Dienogest

Dienogest is an oral progesterone, which has been used for the treatment of endometriosis; it does not have undesirable androgenic side effects. It causes decidualisation of endometrium followed by atrophy of endometriotic tissue. The recommended dosage is 2 mg/day for the period of 12 weeks.

Antiprogestins

Danazol

Danazol is a synthetic 2,3-isoxazol derivative of 17-α-ethinyl testosterone, an orally active 19-norsteroid with minimal androgenic activity. It appears to have multiple actions at various levels of the reproductive system, including direct inhibition of GnRH and/or gonadotrophin secretion, interaction with intracellular androgen and progesterone receptors, direct inhibition of multiple enzymes of steroidogenesis and alteration of endogenous steroid metabolism. It also reverses some of the immunological changes known to occur in endometriosis (see further). The net result of danazol administration is a pseudomenopause state. There is no stimulant phase comparable to that seen in the pseudopregnancy state with oestrogen and progestogen preparations but primary atrophy of the ectopic endometrium occurs. This leads to more rapid symptomatic relief, usually in 2–4 weeks with danazol, compared with 12–16 weeks for pseudopregnancy regimens. The complex pharmacological actions of danazol make it an effective agent for the medical treatment of endometriosis, but it is expensive and associated with significant androgenic and hypo-oestrogenic side effects. It is not the first-choice therapeutic agent. The dosage regimens vary from 400 to 800 mg but the lowest dose to produce relief of symptoms is the most appropriate.

The drawbacks of this treatment are as follows:

- Nausea, weight gain and fluid retention
- *Androgenic side effects*: Acne, oily skin, hirsutism and reduced breast size
- Hot flushes, atrophic vaginitis, emotional instability and reduced libido
- Fatigue, muscle cramps
- Irreversible deepening of voice
- Liver dysfunction
- Androgenic effects on the foetus if conception occurs.

Gestrinone

Gestrinone is a synthetic trienic 19-norsteroid, which has antiprogestogenic mild androgenic and antigonadotrophic effect. It binds to the progesterone and androgen receptors but not to ERs, thus resulting in progressive endometrial atrophy. The basal gonadotrophin levels are maintained but the mid-cycle surge is inhibited, ovarian steroidogenesis is diminished and the sex hormone-binding globulin (SHBG) levels are reduced. Symptomatic relief is seen in 80–90% of patients within 2 months.

The dosage is 2.5–5.0 mg orally twice weekly for 6–9 months. Side effects include weight gain, reduced breast size, muscle cramps and breakthrough bleeding but frank androgenic effects such as hirsutism and voice change are less common. Although it is not yet widely available, it is poised to replace danazol in the treatment of endometriosis.

Gonadotrophin-releasing Hormone Agonists

Gonadotrophin-releasing hormone agonist's initially stimulate the synthesis and release of follicle-stimulating hormone (FSH) and luteinising hormone (LH) by binding to pituitary GnRH receptors, eventually leading to a loss of pituitary receptors and downregulation of GnRH activity. FSH and LH levels decline leading to an inhibition of the production of ovarian steroids. Thus, this is another method of inducing a pseudomenopause. Presently, several GnRH agonists are available: Buserelin, nafarelin, goserelin, leuprorelin and triptorelin. The earliest ones were administered by intranasal spray up to five times daily. Depot formulations are now available for intramuscular and subcutaneous use. The intramuscular preparation can be administered once every 4 weeks and has greater patient acceptability. Doses vary with the agent used, e.g. buserelin 300–400 μg intranasally tds; nafarelin 200 μg intranasally bd; goserelin 3.6 mg subcutaneously monthly; and leuprorelin 3.75 mg intramuscularly monthly (refer to Chapter 43: Hormone Therapy in Gynaecology).

Results with GnRH agonists are similar to those with danazol or progestogens. Side effects are related to oestrogen deprivation. Hot flushes occur but these disappear rapidly after cessation of treatment, as do other atrophic symptoms. Significant bone loss occurs: 3–5%

in vertebral bone. Reversibility of bone loss is equivocal, especially if serum oestradiol levels are lower than 30–45 pg/mL. Add-back regimens have been proposed to compensate for this and to treat vasomotor symptoms while maintaining the efficacy of treatment: This is based on the threshold theory by which lower oestrogen levels are needed to protect the bones and prevent menopausal symptoms than to activate endometriotic tissue. Conjugated equine oestrogens along with MPA, norethisterone alone or tibolone.

Progesterone Antagonists

Progesterone antagonists and progesterone receptor modulators may suppress endometriosis based on their antiproliferative effects on the endometrium, without the risk for hypo-oestrogenism or bone loss that occurs with GnRH treatment. Mifepristone and ulipristal are two selective progesterone receptor modulator (SPRM), which have been approved for the treatment of endometriosis.

Mifepristone (RU-486) is a potent antiprogestogen with a direct inhibitory effect on human endometrial cells and, in high doses, an antiglucocorticoid action. The recommended dose for endometriosis is 25–100 g/day. In uncontrolled studies, mifepristone, 50–100 mg/day, reduced pelvic pain and induced 55% regression of the lesions without significant side effects. In an uncontrolled pilot study, mifepristone, 5 mg/day, resulted in pain improvement, but there was no change in endometriosis lesions, suggesting that this dosage is probably too low.

Aromatase Inhibitors

Aromatase inhibitors surpass oestrogen production leading to a decrease in endometriosis. However, due to severe antioestrogenic side effects (vaginal dryness, hot flushes, and bone depletion), they should only be used when other treatment strategies have failed. The European Society of Human Reproduction and Embryology (ESHRE) recommends AI be used in combination with oral contraceptive pill (OCP), progesterone or GnRH analogues only in refractory cases to prevent these side effects. Treatment of severe postmenopausal endometriosis with an AI, anastrozole, 1 mg/day, and elemental calcium, 1.5 g/day for 9 months, resulted in hypo-oestrogenism, pain relief after 2 months, and after 9 months a 10-fold reduction in the 30-mm diameter size of red, polypoid vaginal lesions, along with remodelling to grey tissue. No other data are available, except this case report.

Nonsteroidal Anti-inflammatory Drugs

Nonsteroidal anti-inflammatory drugs (NSAIDs) have been widely used as a first line of treatment for pain due to endometriosis. However, they may be associated with side effects such as inhibition of ovulation, gastric ulceration.

Investigational Nonhormonal Therapies

Emerging therapies that selectively target cell survival and proliferation pathways are currently under investigation for treating endometriosis.

Antiangiogenic Drugs

Endometriosis progression relies heavily on angiogenesis. Bevacizumab, a recombinant humanised monoclonal antibody against vascular endothelial growth factor (VEGF), resulted in a larger regression of endometriotic lesions. Dopamine agonists, including cabergoline, have been shown to enhance pain relief in addition to reducing VEGF receptor 1 and being well tolerated with no major side effects.

Immunomodulatory Drugs

Immunomodulators have the potential to suppress endometriotic activity by controlling inflammatory cytokines such as TNF-α, nuclear factor kappa B (NF-κB) and ILs.

Antioxidants

Oxidative stress plays a key role in stimulating the synthesis of inflammatory mediators in endometriotic implants. Metabolites from the lipoxygenase pathway and omega-3 polyunsaturated fatty acids suppress the growth of new endometriotic implants and significantly reduce the size of endometriotic lesions.

Surgery

In most women with endometriosis, preservation of reproductive function is desirable. Therefore, the least invasive and least expensive approach that is effective should be used. The goal of surgery is to excise or coagulate all visible endometriotic lesions and associated adhesions—peritoneal lesions, ovarian cysts, deep rectovaginal endometriosis—and to restore normal anatomy.

Surgical management of minimal and mild endometriosis: The association between infertility and minimal to mild endometriosis is controversial and poorly understood.

The clinical pregnancy rate (PR) per cycle after controlled ovarian hyperstimulation (COH) with or without intrauterine insemination (IUI) is reportedly lower in women with surgically untreated minimal to mild endometriosis than in women with unexplained infertility. It is possible that prior laparoscopic removal of minimal/mild endometriosis has a positive effect on the clinical PR after COH and IUI. However, it has been estimated that laparoscopies need to be performed to gain one additional pregnancy.

Surgical management of grade III/IV endometriosis: In women with stage III/IV disease who have other significant infertility factors, conservative surgical treatment with laparoscopy improves fertility.

Tumours on the body surface are best excised. Deep-seated lesions call for surgery when symptoms are acute, when the diagnosis is in doubt, when tumour masses are large and when hormone therapy fails or is ruled out.

In general, it can be said that laparoscopic surgery is now the method of choice in most women who require conservative surgery. It is less invasive, less expensive, has less morbidity and better postoperative results than laparotomy. Endometriotic lesions and adhesions are excised or coagulated using bipolar coagulation or CO_2 laser. The cyst wall of an endometrioma is removed and the remnants, if any, are fulgurated by bipolar electrocoagulation or laser. If the cyst is very small, it should be vaporised. It is important to remove the cyst wall if recurrence is to be prevented. At the same time, adhesiolysis and preservation of normal ovarian tissue are essential in a woman who desires fertility. In general, bipolar electrocoagulation results in less adhesion formation than the laser, but recurrence rates are the same with both procedures.

Where laparoscopic facilities are not available, the same conservative surgery can be performed at laparotomy too. Limited and incomplete excision of endometriosis is followed by surprisingly good results, even when ovarian function is not sacrificed. In young women, the subsequent PR is at least 30%, even when hormones are not administered postoperatively.

Ovarian endometriosis superficial ovarian lesions can be vaporised. Small ovarian endometrioma (<3 cm in diameter) **(Fig. 21)** can be aspirated, irrigated and inspected with ovarian cystoscopy for intracystic lesions; their interior wall can be vaporised to destroy the mucosal lining of the cyst. Large (>3 cm in diameter) ovarian endometrioma should be aspirated **(Fig. 22)**, followed by incision and removal of the cyst wall from the ovarian cortex. To prevent recurrence, the cyst wall of the endometrioma must be removed, and normal ovarian tissue must be preserved.

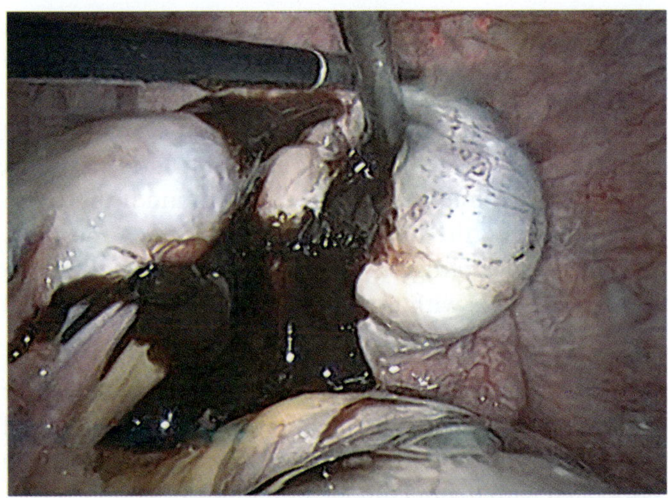

Fig. 21: Ovarian endometrioma.
Courtesy: Dr Sanjay Patel, Mayflower Hospital, Ahmedabad.

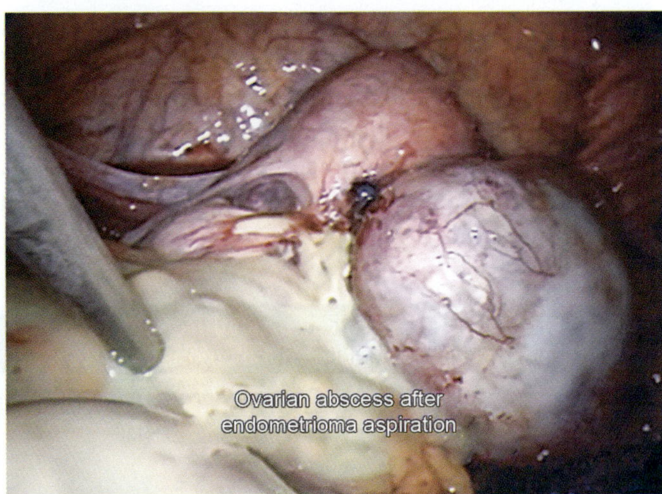

Fig. 22: Ovarian abscess endometrium aspiration.
Courtesy: Dr Sanjay Patel, Mayflower Hospital, Ahmedabad.

There is increasing concern that ovarian cystectomy with concomitant removal or destruction of primordial follicles may reduce ovarian volume and reserve and diminish fertility. However, it was found that there was a higher incidence of recurrences of cysts when the cyst was not excised. Therefore, based on the current evidence, ovarian cystectomy appears to be the method of choice. There is a 2.4% risk of ovarian failure after bilateral removal of ovarian endometrioma.

Laparotomy is usually considered for patients with advanced-stage disease, over the age of 40 years, where fertility is no longer required. In such cases, it is often best to remove the uterus and both ovaries. While it is important to remove as much endometriotic tissue as possible, small fragments can be left behind if there is a risk of injury to the bowel because of dense adhesions, and will usually retrogress of their own accord. If there are dense adhesions with the bowel and bladder, a subtotal hysterectomy may be a safer option.

Deep rectovaginal and rectosigmoidal endometriosis: The surgical excision of deep rectovaginal and rectosigmoidal endometriosis is difficult and can be associated with major complications. Postoperative bowel perforations with peritonitis have been reported in 2–3% of cases **(Table 4)**.

Oophorectomy and hysterectomy: Radical procedures such as oophorectomy or total hysterectomy are indicated only in severe situations and can be performed either laparoscopically or by laparotomy.

The exact procedure must vary from case to case. Rarely, in the case of obstruction, it is necessary to even resect the intestine.

TABLE 4: Suggested surgical procedure according to classification of deeply infiltrating endometriosis (DIE).

DIE classification	*Operative procedure*
A: Anterior DIE *Al:* Bladder	Laparoscopic partial cystectomy
P: Posterior DIE *P1:* Uterosacral ligament *P2:* Vagina	• Laparoscopic resection of USL • Laparoscopically assisted vaginal resection of DIE infiltrating the posterior fornix
P3: Intestine solely intestinal location without vaginal infiltration (V–) with vaginal infiltration (V+)	• Intestinal resection by laparoscopy or by laparotomy • Laparoscopically assisted vaginal intestinal resection or exeresis by laparotomy
Multiple intestinal location	Intestinal resection by laparotomy

(DIE: deeply infiltrating endometriosis; USL: uterosacral ligament)
Source: Chapron C, Fauconnier A, Vieira M, Barakat H, Dousset B, Pansini V, et al. Anatomical distribution of deeply infiltrating endometriosis: surgical implications and proposition for a classification. Hum Reprod. 2003;18:157-61.

Combined Medical and Surgical Therapy (Flowcharts 2A and B)

The medical treatment has not much of place preoperatively but more postoperatively to deal with residual macro- or microscopic disease. In women who desire fertility, it is a matter of speculation whether patients should be subjected to further suppression or induction of ovulation. In general, it is agreed that if adequate surgery has been possible, the sooner the patient is allowed to conceive the better, as the best outcome for fertility is immediately after surgery. Compared with surgery alone or surgery plus placebo, postoperative hormonal treatment has no effect on PRs. Postoperative medical therapy may be required in patients with incomplete surgical resection and persistent pain.

Based on several retrospective studies, several investigators have suggested that the PR after in vitro fertilisation (IVF) may be lower in women with endometriosis than in women without the disease.

Treatment of Recurrent Endometriosis

Therapeutic options and decisions remain the same in recurrent endometriosis, but before planning repeated conservative surgery in a patient with severe symptoms, it may be in her best interests to discuss the benefits of a radical surgical approach.

Selective Oestrogen Receptor Modulators

Raloxifene: In animal models, raloxifene therapy resulted in regression of endometriosis. The effect was seen in both a surgically prepared, rat uterine explant model and in rhesus macaques diagnosed with spontaneous endometriosis before exposure.

Mechanism of Action of Aromatase Inhibitors

Aromatase, a cytochrome p450-dependent enzyme, acts as final step in the synthesis of oestrogen, catalysing conversion of androgen to oestrogen. AIs act as competitive inhibitors **(Flowchart 3)**.

Assisted Reproduction and Endometriosis

The treatment of endometriosis-related infertility is dependent on the age of the woman, the duration of infertility, the stage of endometriosis, the involvement of ovaries, tubes, or both in the endometriosis process, previous therapy, associated pain symptoms and the

Flowcharts 2A and B: Algorithm for treatment of endometriosis-associated pain (A) and infertility (B). Where multiple pathways are shown, the path is guided by medical judgement and patient preference. In the infertility pathway, some practitioners dispense with the operative laparoscopy and recommend assisted reproductive technologies directly.

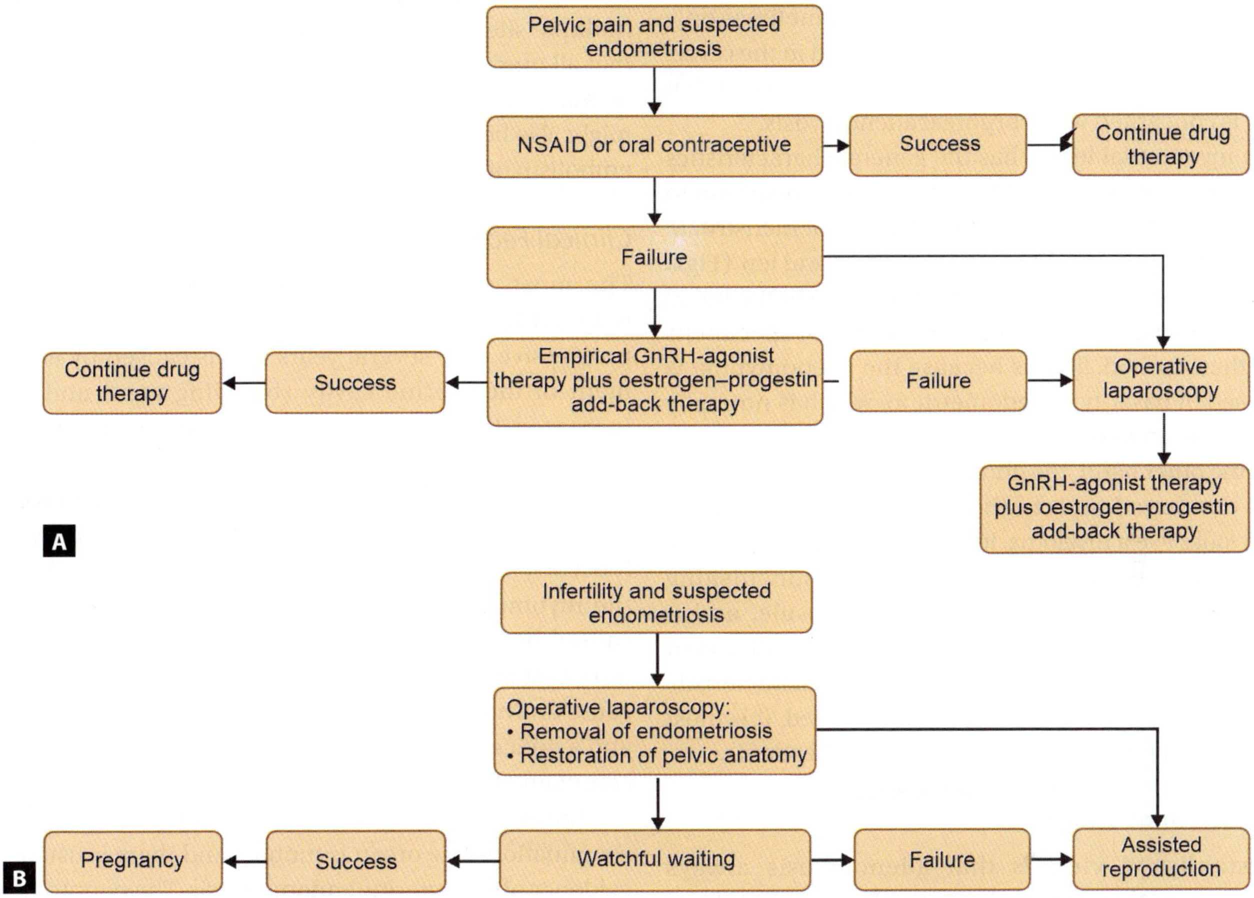

Pelvic pain and suspected endometriosis
NSAID or oral contraceptive
Success
Continue drug therapy
Failure
Empirical GnRH-agonist therapy plus oestrogen–progestin add-back therapy
Success
Continue drug therapy
Failure
Operative laparoscopy
GnRH-agonist therapy plus oestrogen–progestin add-back therapy
A
Infertility and suspected endometriosis
Operative laparoscopy:
• Removal of endometriosis
• Restoration of pelvic anatomy
Watchful waiting
Success
Pregnancy
Failure
Assisted reproduction
B

(GnRH: gonadotrophin-releasing hormone; NSAIDs: nonsteroidal anti-inflammatory drugs)
Source: Olive DL, Pritts EA. Treatment of endometriosis. N Engl J Med. 2001;345:267.

Flowchart 3: Mechanism of action of aromatase inhibitors.

Pregnenolone
17-OH-pregnenolone
DHEA
17α-OH
Androstenedione
Aromatase*
Aromatase*
Oestrone
Testosterone
Oestradiol

* Action of aromatase inhibitors

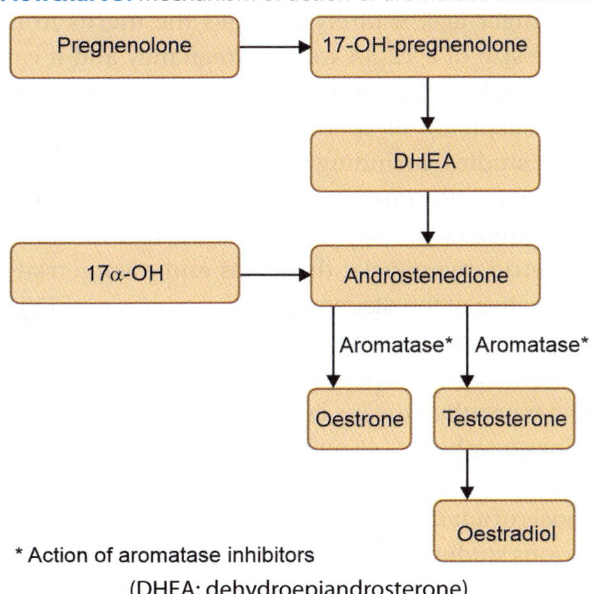

(DHEA: dehydroepiandrosterone)

priorities of the patient, taking into account her attitude towards the disease, the cost of treatment, her financial means and the expected results. Assisted reproduction, including COH with IUI, IVF and gamete intrafallopian transfer, may be options for infertility treatment in addition to surgical reconstruction and expectant management. IVF is the method of choice when distortion of the tubo-ovarian anatomy contraindicates the use of superovulation with IUI or gamete intrafallopian transfer.

- Super ovulation with IUI is indicated in women with minimal to mild endometriosis, especially after surgical correction of the disease.
- IVF-embryo transfer (ET) is indicated for women with moderate to severe endometriosis who fail to conceive after initial conservative surgery.
- GnRH agonists given for a period of 3–6 months prior to IVF in women with endometriosis increase the PRs.

ADENOMYOSIS

Pathology

Adenomyosis usually involves the corpus, sometimes only one of its walls or a part of it. Rarely, it is found in the cervix **(Fig. 23)**. Cervical endometriosis has special facets. What follows is concerned with corporeal adenomyosis.

The myometrial lesion has the general characteristics of endometriosis. Its special feature is that its response to ovarian hormones is limited; often it does not menstruate at all, and tarry cysts when present are small and few **(Figs. 2 and 3)**. Secretory activity in the glands during the luteal phase of the cycle is found in only 10–30% of specimens and is then limited. This is because the adenomyoma is composed of basal-type endometrium, which is normally insensitive to an endocrine stimulus.

On the other hand, the fibromyomatous tissue reaction is well developed and, to the naked eye, the resulting tumour looks like a myeloma, its cut surface having a similar striated and whorled appearance. The distinguishing features are that adenomyosis has no capsule, and it usually produces a diffuse enlargement of the uterus in contrast to the well-circumscribed nodules characteristic of leiomyomas. When adenomyosis is localised, it is most likely to be situated in the posterior wall of the uterus.

Mechanism of Origin

The established view is that adenomyosis always represents a down growth from the basal layer of the endometrium. No matter how deeply it may be situated, a gland, it is said, can always be shown by serial sections to communicate with the uterine cavity. It is sometimes suggested, however, that adenomyosis arises de novo in the myometrium and that the change may commence in multiple sites. This is not unreasonable, bearing in mind that all uterine tissues have a common origin. The finding of adenomyosis unconnected with the endometrium might also be explained on the basis of venous or lymphatic embolism of endometrial elements.

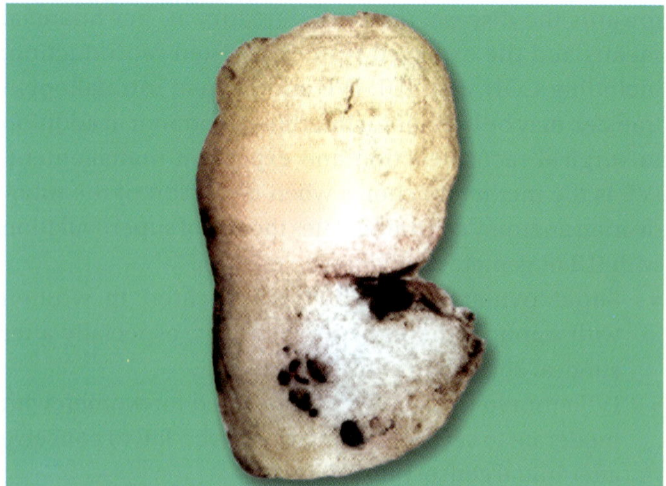

Fig. 23: Endometriosis of the cervix with multiple small tarry cysts.

Clinical Features and Diagnosis

The most common symptom is menorrhagia, which is found in approximately 75% of cases. It is gradually progressive over several years and is caused by enlargement of the uterine cavity (bleeding area) and by an increased blood supply. Other theoretical causes for the menorrhagia are impaired contractility of the myometrium and associated endometrial hyperplasia. Dysmenorrhoea is noted by only 30% of patients and, when it occurs, is mainly intramenstrual. It is more likely when the myometrium is deeply penetrated and is probably caused by disturbed uterine contractions rather than by tarry cyst formation. The increased size of the uterus can cause diurnal frequency, a sensation of weight in the pelvis and a noticeable abdominal tumour. The patient may also complain of infertility.

The enlargement of the uterus is detected on bimanual examination. The organ is mobile, and there is usually no evidence of extrauterine endometriosis. The symptoms and signs are so similar that it may be impossible to distinguish clinically between adenomyosis and leiomyoma. Pointers in favour of adenomyosis are as follows: It tends to occur at a younger age, it rarely enlarges the uterus to more than the size of a 12–14 weeks' pregnancy and it causes a regular rather than a nodular uterine enlargement. A clinical suspicion of adenomyosis can be suggested by imaging studies, including transvaginal ultrasonography (TVUS) and MRI. *Blurring* of endomyometrial interface, subendometrial linear striations, echogenic nodules, asymmetric myometrial thickness and myometrial cyst are indicative of the diagnosis of adenomyosis by TVUS.

The deep penetration of the glands is said to give rise to a characteristic hysterographic appearance, but this finding more often means endometrial hyperplasia. Gland openings may be visible on hysteroscopy.

The junctional zone thickness value specific to the diagnosis of adenomyosis has been debated and evaluated by various studies.

Transvaginal sonography has several advantages over MRI. It is widely available, and relatively inexpensive compared to MRI. It is well tolerated by most patients and generates high-quality images not limited by patient size or uterine position. However, it has its limitations. It is operator dependent and may not be reproducible in patients on follow-up. The presence of intramural fibroids can hinder assessment of the adjacent myometrium. MRI, on the other hand, is less operator dependent.

Treatment

Surgical Treatment

If symptoms are present, the primary line of treatment is by operation. This is the only means of making the diagnosis certain. Unfortunately, the tumour cannot be removed easily, because it has no capsule. Hysterectomy is therefore usually necessary; although in young women desirous of having children, resection of the main portion of the diseased uterine wall has rarely been carried out **(Fig. 24)**. In such cases, some of the adenomyosis was often left behind, but this was not necessarily incompatible with a good result. Indeed, pregnancy has been reported subsequently, and this is without any special postoperative therapy.

Palliative and Medical

Medical treatments: With the establishment of diagnostic criteria for imaging studies, it is now possible to offer women options for nonsurgical treatments. These range from local treatments such as IUDs to systemic preparations of GnRH analogues.

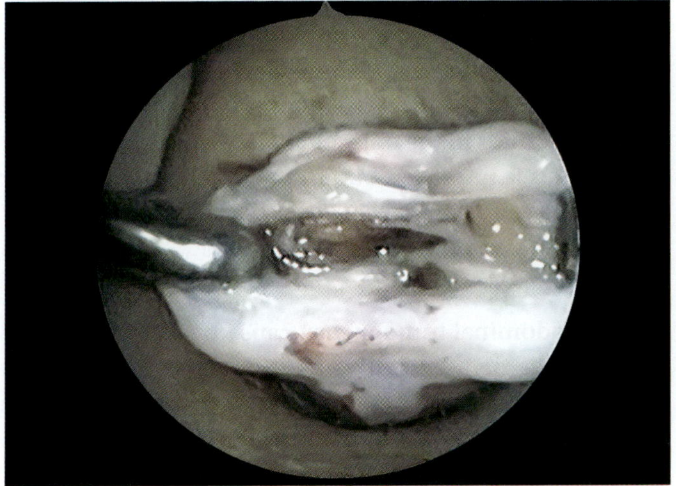

Fig. 24: Port site endometriosis.
Courtesy: Dr Sanjay Patel, Mayflower Hospital, Ahmedabad.

Levonorgestrel intrauterine system: Although the IUD was originally designed as a method of contraception, the addition of progesterone to the device means that it can now be used for managing menstrual disorders. Although the majority of the studies have been in women with heavy menstrual bleeding, LNG-IUS also has the potential to be used in women with endometriosis and adenomyosis. The LNG-IUS releases 20 mg LNG per day and has been shown to result in a profound reduction in menstrual blood loss in women with heavy menstrual bleeding; 20% of the women using the LNG-IUS are amenorrhoeic after 1 year of treatment. The LNG-IUS, which has contraceptive efficacy for 5 years, has also been reported to improve dysmenorrhoea. It is likely that some of the women with dysmenorrhoea may also have undiagnosed adenomyosis. A major disadvantage of the device is frequent and variable intermenstrual bleeding and spotting during the first few months of use. There are several mechanisms that could explain the role of the LNG-IUS in adenomyosis. Use of the LNG-IUS is associated with decidualisation of the endometrium followed by atrophic changes. As a result, there is a marked reduction in menstrual blood loss. LNG also acts directly on the adenomyotic deposits. Downregulation of ERs, which are present in both glandular and stromal endometrial tissues, occurs shortly after placement of the device and persists for at least the first year of use. Local LNG levels following uterine placement of the LNG-IUS result in very high endometrial levels of LNG compared to those in serum.

ENDOSALPINGIOSIS

Tubal epithelium has the same origin as endometrium and has similar potentialities. Certain cases of ovarian endometriosis are thought by some authorities to be endosalpingiosis. This is because the lesions do not menstruate and because, on section, they show a tubal type of epithelium without typical endometrial stroma.

Endosalpingiosis of the tube causes no symptoms other than infertility and, as a rule, is only diagnosed by microscopic examination of the excised tissue. In the ovary, too, it is only a histological diagnosis.

CERVICAL ENDOMETRIOSIS

In cervical endometriosis, the ectopic glands are truly endometrial and menstruate to some extent **(Fig. 17)**.

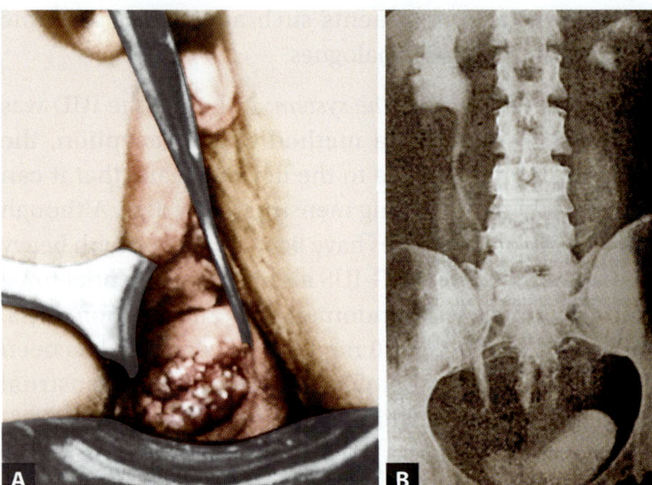

Figs. 25A and B: Endometriosis of the cervix in a woman aged 30 years and complaining of a bloodstained vaginal discharge for 18 months in addition to infertility: (A) A polypoid mass of endometriotic tissue protruding through the external os. The lesion was primarily in the posterior wall of the cervix but fungated into the cervical canal and also caused an opening into the posterior fornix. Extension into the right broad ligament produced physical signs similar to those of stage II or III cancer of the cervix; (B) Pyelography reveals obstruction of the lower end of the right ureter by the extension of the endometriosis into the broad ligament on that side. The patient was ultimately treated by total hysterectomy and bilateral salpingo-oophorectomy because of the threat to renal function.

Their presence is explained by direct implantation, embolism or metaplasia of the Müllerian duct tissue. The condition is not uncommonly seen after operations which involve simultaneous injury to the cervix and spill of endometrium, e.g. curettage with amputation of the cervix. Endometriosis of the posterior cervix may represent a spread from a lesion in the rectovaginal septum. Sometimes, however, the disease begins spontaneously in the substance of the cervix and then extends in the same manner as cervical cancer—to the endocervix to produce polypoid masses, to the posterior fornix to produce cysts and sinuses and to the bases of the broad ligaments to surround and obstruct the ureters **(Figs. 25A and B)**.

The lesions vary. They may be merely superficial tiny blood cysts on the portio; they may be deep-seated to cause distortion and fibrosis of the cervix with adhesions to the bladder base. Sometimes the cervix is grossly enlarged, completely fixed and ulcerated, the physical signs being similar to those of cancer except for the absence of friability.

Cervical endometriosis may cause no symptoms. Otherwise, the complaints are irregular bleeding and discharge, contact bleeding, dyspareunia and bladder irritability.

If surgical treatment becomes necessary because of failure to respond to drug therapy, extracervical adhesions and spread can create great technical difficulties. It is usually impossible to dissect broad ligament endometriosis from around the ureters, and renal function is sometimes only saved by resecting the ureter or by sacrificing both ovaries. In one case, it proved necessary to form an ileal conduit because of ureteric obstruction.

CAUSES IN THE GENITAL TRACT

Any backache caused by a gynaecological lesion is always diffuse. It is situated in the midline or has a bilateral distribution. Its level is sacral or lumbosacral and never higher than the fourth lumbar vertebra. Any backache which can be indicated with a finger point, or which is associated with local tenderness, is not due to an intrapelvic lesion.

Gynaecological conditions which may cause backache are the following.

Prolapse and Retroversion

Vaginal prolapse never causes backache; uterine prolapse and retroversion may on rare occasions do so by dragging on the uterosacral and cardinal ligaments. Backache caused by uterine prolapse is immediately relieved by lying down, a crucial point in diagnosis.

Chronic Cervicitis

This is a debatable cause of backache. It probably only operates when there is associated gross scarring and chronic cellulitis in the adjacent ligaments. Backache with such a basis is improved but is not completely relieved by rest. Cervical erosion never causes backache.

Tumours

A large abdominal tumour may cause backache, because the muscles of the trunk have to support the added burden, as well as maintain the lordosis necessary for the patient's balance. A tumour impacted in the pelvis can cause a sacral ache associated with deep pelvic discomfort. Sacrococcygeal teratomas, large fibroids or an ovarian cyst may present with low backache.

TABLE 5: Differential diagnosis of acute pelvic pain.

Pregnancy	• Ectopic • Abortion
Adnexa	• Haemorrhagic functional ovarian cyst • Torsion of adnexa • Rupture of ovarian cyst
Gastrointestinal tract	• Gastroenteritis • Appendicitis • Bowel obstruction • Inflammatory bowel disease
Musculoskeletal	• Abdominal wall haematoma • Hernia
Infection	• Acute endometritis • Acute pelvic inflammatory disease • Tubo-ovarian abscess
Genitourinary	• Cystitis • Pyelonephritis

Pelvic Congestion, Pelvic Varicocele and Premenstrual Syndrome

Slight discomfort low in the back is so common premenstrually that it is regarded as one of the normal menstrual molimina; it becomes exaggerated with pelvic congestion and in the premenstrual syndrome.

Uterine Contractions

Expulsive uterine contractions, or cervical resistance to them, can cause pain over the area of the sacrum. This can occur, e.g. during labour, abortion and attempts to expel polypoid growths, pus and blood from the uterine cavity. It is also a feature of spasmodic dysmenorrhoea. Nevertheless, this type of discomfort is subsidiary to the accompanying abdominal pain and does not come under the heading of what is usually meant by *low backache* **(Tables 5 and 6)**.

Gynaecological Operations

Gynaecological operations not infrequently cause sacroiliac strain or other forms of low backache. These complaints follow the use of the lithotomy position or prolonged lying on a flat table with relaxed muscles. To avoid injuries in the first position, it is important to raise and lower both legs at the same time; in the second position, the lumbar curve should be maintained by a special pillow.

Postoperatively, lying in a sagging bed can result in backache of muscular or ligamentary origin. The conclusion is that, contrary to what was formerly believed, and still is in some quarters, pelvic lesions are rare and unimportant direct causes of low backache in women, accounting for only 0.2% of such complaints. The fact that operative treatment for pelvic conditions is sometimes followed by the relief of backache does not establish a cause-and-effect relationship (see further). Indeed, the only reasonable certain gynaecological causes of low backache are malignant, inflammatory and endometriotic infiltration of pelvic cellular tissue and uterosacral ligaments, together with spinal metastases from pelvic cancer.

The woman who complains of backache nearly always has something wrong with her back.

TABLE 6: Differential diagnosis of chronic pelvic pain.

Noncyclic pain	***Cyclic pain***
Adhesion	Primary dysmenorrhoea
Endometriosis	Mittelschmerz
Salpingo-oophoritis	Secondary dysmenorrhoea
Retained ovary syndrome	Uterine or vaginal anomalies with obstruction to outflow
Pelvic congestion	Intrauterine device (IUD)
Ovarian neoplasms	• Endometrial polyp • Adenomyosis • Pelvic congestion syndrome • Fibroids

EXTRAGENITAL CAUSES

Muscular and Ligamentary Lesions

The possibilities under this heading are numerous, but many are merely names without proven pathology. Those deserving mention are lumbago, fibrositis, myositis, acute or chronic strains of the attachments of muscles and ligaments, rheumatic conditions and sacroiliac strain. In all cases, the pain tends to be localised and accompanied by tenderness; sometimes it is one-sided and often it extends higher than the lumbosacral region. It is worse premenstrually and during pregnancy and shows a definite relationship to exercise, rest, position and movement of the trunk. Sacroiliac strain and *fibrositis* are often worse in bed; the former is related especially to lying flat on the back and to rotatory movements of the trunk.

Sometimes there is a history of injury or strain but often there is not. Minor repeated trauma is commonly

Flowchart 4: Stepwise assessment.

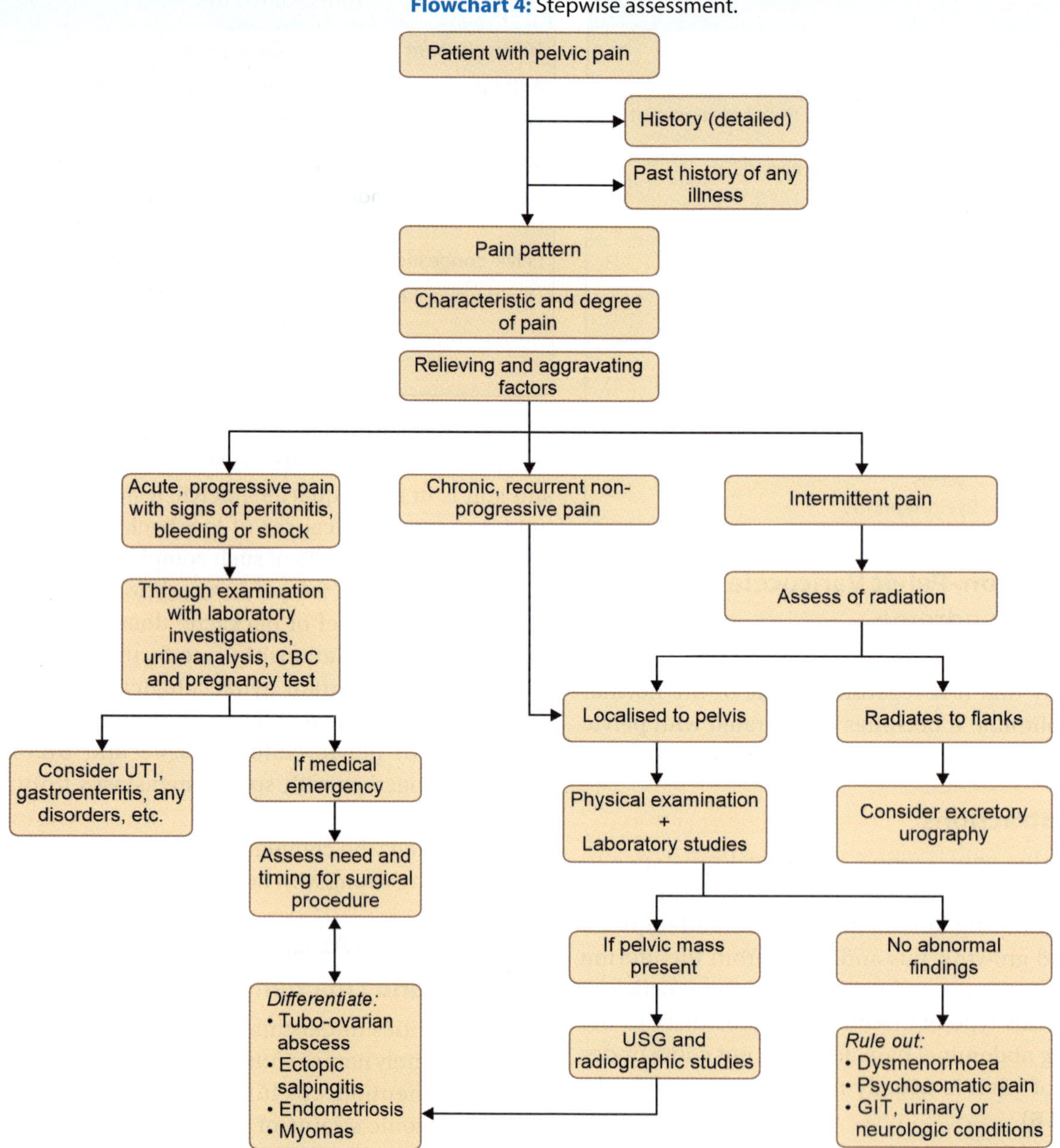

(CBC: complete blood count; GIT: gastrointestinal tract; USG: ultrasonography; UTI: urinary tract infection)

accounted for by obesity, bending and lifting, poor posture, pendulous abdomen, visceroptosis, flat feet, badly designed shoes with high heels (which increase the already relatively high angle of inclination of the pelvis) and long hours at the wheel of a car or an office desk.

Many of the above conditions are characterised by spasm of muscles, or groups of muscles, and it is suggested that the spasm may be the cause rather than the effect. This is one of the justifications for treatment by the injection of local anaesthetics at the site of the pain.

Lumbago and other pains are sometimes caused by disc prolapse rather than by a disorder of the muscles and ligaments.

Bone and Joint Lesions

Deep-seated causes of backache include arthritic conditions of the spine, disc lesions, tuberculosis of bones and joints, primary and metastatic growths, ankylosing spondylitis, osteitis deformans, bone injuries, spondylolisthesis, spondylitis, sacralisation of the fifth lumbar vertebra, scoliosis, kyphosis and degenerative changes associated with ageing. Many of these lesions involve nerve roots and cause pain referred down the back of the leg. Otherwise, pain and tenderness tend to be localised and often they are worse immediately after rest, easing as the joint works loose with movement.

Diseases of the Kidney and the Ureter

Renal pain is usually unilateral, and its characteristic site and distribution make it comparatively easy to identify.

Diseases of the Rectum

Carcinoma or any condition of the rectum producing spasm can cause sacral discomfort or a sensation which the patient calls backache.

Psychological Factors

In the majority of cases of low backache in women, a gross lesion is not found and an obvious cause is not demonstrated. Patients tend, therefore, to be handed from physician to gynaecologist to orthopaedic surgeon, and back again. No one is willing or anxious to take responsibility for the case and, sooner or later, the complaint is ascribed to anxiety neurosis or other psychological disturbance. It is undoubtedly true that many of the sufferers from chronic backache are of over anxious and complaining disposition. Nevertheless, even in these, there is likely to be an organic basis for the localisation of their complaint.

MANAGEMENT AND TREATMENT

The essential step in the management of low backache is to determine its cause by meticulous enquiry into the features of the pain **(Flowchart 4)**. These include its mode and date of onset, its exact site and spread, and its relation to rest, lifting, bending and other movements of the trunk. The discovery of local tenderness over a joint or muscle attachment during examination is also significant.

Apart from pelvic examination, radiography of the spine and pelvis is required in all cases, with the object of excluding major diseases of bone rather than providing the diagnosis. In most cases, sometimes even when there is a disc lesion, the radiological findings are negative. MRI is useful in evaluating such cases.

The treatment depends on the cause but, when a definite lesion is not found, the main requirements are reassurance and understanding, correction of posture, a well-fitting corset, abdominal and spinal exercises, appropriate footwear and advice about organising life to provide interest and periods of rest. In the more serious cases, an orthopaedic surgeon may decide to give local injections of anaesthetic solutions, manipulate joints or give other forms of treatment.

The response to treatment in any case can easily lead to false conclusions. For example, a woman may be treated surgically for prolapse or for an erosion of the cervix and thereafter be cured of her backache—for some time at least. It is then tempting to conclude that the backache was caused by the pelvic condition. More careful observations will, however, often make it clear that the operation cured only because it ensured that the woman had a period of prolonged rest, care, sympathy and relief from domestic duties.

CHRONIC PELVIC PAIN

Chronic pelvic pain is defined as the pain that occurs anywhere in the area between the umbilicus and the hips, which lasts for >6 months and is severe enough to cause functional disability.

The type of pain is usually vague and cannot be pinpointed. It may be intermittent or a steady dull ache, it varies in intensity from mild to severe, and it can be a feeling of heaviness or pressure deep in the pelvis. The pain may be associated with functions such as sitting or standing for prolonged intervals or voiding of bowel or bladder or with sexual intercourse.

GENERAL CONSIDERATIONS

The incidence of CPP is 2–24% of the female population worldwide. It affects one in six of the adult female population mainly in the reproductive age group of 25–35 years.

About 10–15% of women have CPP with or without backache. Patients with CPP are frequently anxious and depressed. Anywhere from 20 to 80% of patients undergoing laparoscopy for CPP have no intraperitoneal pathology or have tissue distortion that does not correlate with the pain, certain types of prevalent intraperitoneal pathology, such as endometriosis, adhesions or venous congestion. Nongynaecologic causes of pain, such as irritable bowel syndrome, interstitial cystitis, abdominal wall or pelvic floor myofascial syndrome or nerve entrapment, are frequently overlooked but common causes of CPP.

Red flag findings that may indicate systemic disease include postcoital bleeding, postmenopausal bleeding or onset of pain, unexplained weight loss, pelvic mass and haematuria.

STEP-WISE EVALUATION OF CHRONIC PELVIC PAIN

History: A thorough history is one of the most important tools in the evaluation of patients with CPP. The COLDERR acronym may be used to gain a general understanding of the patient's history of present illness.

Character: What does the pain feel like? (sharp, dull and crampy)

Onset: Does the pain come on suddenly or gradually? Is it cyclic or constant?

Location: Is the pain localised or diffuse?

Duration: How long has the pain been present and how has it changed over time?

Exacerbation: What activities or movements make it worse?

Relief: What medication, activities and positions make it better?

Radiation: Does the pain radiate anywhere (back, groin and flank)?

The patient should be questioned about symptoms associated with pain to have an idea of the organ system involved:

- Genital (abnormal vaginal bleeding, discharge, dysmenorrhoea, dyspareunia and infertility)
- Enterocolic (constipation, diarrhoea, flatulence, haematochezia and relationship of pain to bowel movements)
- Musculoskeletal (trauma, exacerbation with exercise or postural changes)
- Urologic (urgency, frequency, nocturia, dysuria, incontinence and haematuria)

EXAMINATION

A complete physical examination should be performed, with particular attention directed to the abdominal, lumbosacral, external genital, vaginal, bimanual and rectovaginal examination.

Carnett test can help in differentiating visceral pain from abdominal pain. The patient is laid supine and the rectus abdominis muscles are contracted by the head or leg rising. The examiner places the finger on the painful abdominal site to determine whether the pain increases during the manoeuvre. The assumption is that it potentially increases myofascial pain such as entrapped nerve, hernia or myositis, whereas true visceral sources of pain may be less tender when the abdominal muscles are tensed.

DIAGNOSTIC INVESTIGATIONS

Laboratory Testing

Complete blood count, an erythrocyte sedimentation rate (ESR), urine analysis and testing for sexually transmitted diseases can be done to rule out chronic infection.

Hormone analysis such as thyroid-stimulating hormone (TSH) to rule out hypothyroidism, especially in patients with depression and FSH and oestradiol levels in ovarian remnant syndrome may be helpful.

Radiology

Investigations needed may be ultrasound, Doppler ultrasound for pelvic congestion, radiography of joints and intravenous pyelogram (IVP) in accordance with history and examination. A CT scan or an MRI can be done or a detailed study of the identified pathology.

If ultrasound is not showing any abnormality, then a diagnostic laparoscopy is recommended in severe pain if other somatic causes are ruled out, and the results of the psychological evaluation are negative.

MANAGEMENT

The goal of the treatment is to involve the patient in self-management and improve the quality of life and functional disability. Pain is a complex and subjective symptom; hence, its management requires a comprehensive approach, including physical, behavioural, psychological and sexual components **(Flowchart 5)**.

Treat the cause when it is identified. A multidisciplinary therapy by gynaecologist, psychologist and an anaesthetist is usually preferable in patients with no obvious pathology. Guidelines by the European Association of Urology provide greater detail regarding the treatment of CPP.

Drug Therapy

The drug therapy consists of the following options:

- *NSAIDs*: Evidence shows benefit in dysmenorrhoea but not endometriosis

Flowchart 5: Management.

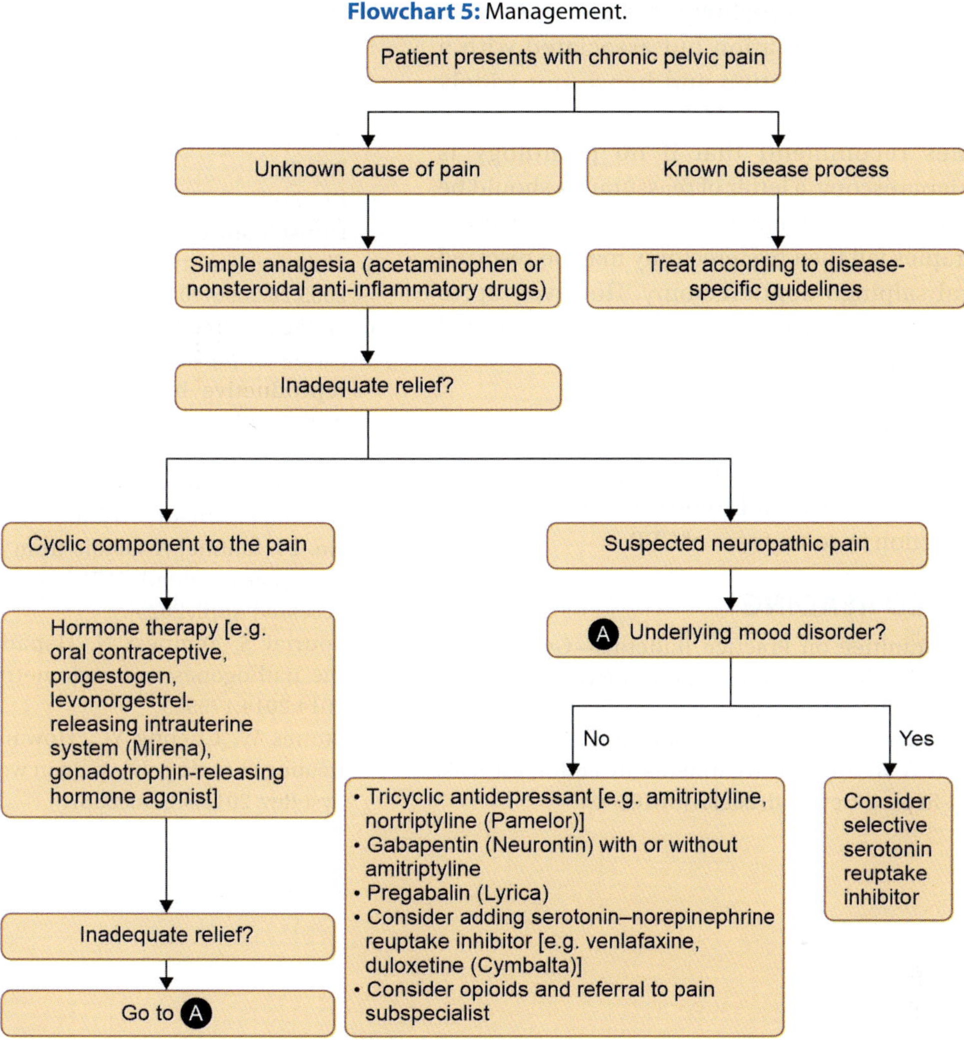

- *Acetaminophen*: Works best in arthritic pain
- *Opioids*: Good analgesia but questionable for long-term use
- *Gabapentin and pregabalin*: Can be used in neuropathic pain
- *Tricyclic antidepressants and selective serotonin reuptake inhibitors*: Benefit the depression component
- The overall effect seems to be good with a low dose of a tricyclic antidepressant, which is combined with behavioural therapy directed towards reducing reliance on pain medication. Psychotherapy is indicated for women who have pronounced depression, sexual difficulties or indications of past-trauma.

Hormones as oral contraceptives suppress ovulation, so pain due to endometriosis is reduced. MPA can be given for 9–12 months. Micronised progesterone is a natural progesterone available as oral and vaginal tablets. GnRH agonist can be tried similarly in severe cases. Antioestrogens can reduce the pelvic blood flow and congestion. Another drug under trial is diethyl ergotamine, which has been shown to reduce the severity of pelvic pain within 48 hours of IV injection. Both American and UK guidelines encourage an empirical trial of GnRH agonists for women suspected of endometriosis who do not desire a definitive diagnosis or wish to defer invasive surgical investigation.

Surgical Management

Laparoscopic removal of cysts, masses and fulguration of endometriotic lesions are effective in reducing pain. However, division of intraperitoneal adhesions is of unclear benefit. Interruption of nerve plexus have been tried in a few cases. Presacral neurectomy was more effective than uterosacral nerve ablation but associated with a high incidence of constipation and hence not widely practised.

Guidelines recommend that if no pathology is identified at laparoscopy, a letter of reassurance should be offered and the women contacted a year later for review.

If all therapies fail then hysterectomy may be resorted with bilateral salpingo-oopherectomy. However, up to 40% will have persistent pain and in 5% the pain will worsen after the surgery.

Other Treatment Modalities

Pelvic floor physical therapy and behavioural modifications have helped reduce stress and improve pain experience and motor function in some cases of CPP.

SUGGESTED READING

1. ACOG Committee on Practice Bulletins—Gynecology. ACOG Practice Bulletin No. 51. Chronic pelvic pain. Obstet Gynecol. 2004;103(3):589-605.
2. Bahi E, Maya G, Emily C Y, Catherine A, Paul J Y, Mohamed A B. Medical treatments of endometriosis: A review. Reprod Dev Med. 2023;7(3):166-79.
3. Daniels JP, Middleton L, Xiong T, Champaneria R, Johnson NP, Lichten EM, et al. Individual patient data meta-analysis of randomised evidence to assess the effectiveness of laparoscopic uterosacral nerve ablation in chronic pelvic pain. Hum Reprod Update. 2010;16(6): 568-76.
4. Kennedy S, Bergqvist A, Chapron C, D'Hooghe T, Dunselman G, Greb R, et al. ESHRE guideline for the diagnosis and treatment of endometriosis. Hum Reprod. 2005;20:2698-704.
5. Latthe P, Latthe M, Say L, Gülmezoglu AM. WHO systematic review of prevalence of chronic pelvic pain: a neglected reproductive health morbidity. BMC Public Health. 2006;6:177.
6. Royal College of Obstetricians and Gynaecologists Guidelines and Audit Committee. (2006). The investigation and management of endometriosis. Green-top Guideline No. 24. [online] Available from https://poliklinika-harni.hr/images/uploads/171/rcog-endometrioza.pdf. [Last accessed April, 2025].
7. Sourial S, Tempest N, Hapangama DK. Theories on the pathogenesis of endometriosis. Int J Reprod Med. 2014;2014:179515.
8. Stones W, Cheong YC, Howard FM. Interventions for treating chronic pelvic pain in women. Cochrane Database Syst Rev. 2015;3:CD000387.

24

CHAPTER

Polycystic Ovary Syndrome

Meghna A Nayak

Chapter Outline

- Oligomenorrhoea and Anovulation: Definition
- Hyperandrogenism (Clinical and/ or Biochemical)
- Polycystic Ovaries on Ultrasound or Elevated Serum Anti-Müllerian Hormone
- Pathophysiology
- Ovarian and Other Endocrine Aspects of Polycystic Ovary Syndrome
- Metabolic Component of Polycystic Ovary Syndrome
- Pathology
- Clinical, Biochemical and Metabolic Features of Polycystic Ovary Syndrome
- Ultrasonographic Examination
- Puberty and Polycystic Ovary Syndrome
- Management
- Infertility
- Weight Loss

INTRODUCTION

Polycystic ovary syndrome (PCOS) is a multifaceted enigmatic disease. It has significant endocrine, reproductive, dermatological, metabolic, cardiovascular and mental health implications in those individuals affected by it. It is by far the most common cause of anovulatory subfertility affecting 10% of reproductive-aged women worldwide. Approximately 75% of anovulatory women of any cause have polycystic ovaries and 20–25% of women with normal ovulation demonstrate ultrasound findings typical of polycystic ovaries **(Fig. 1)**.

Since there are so many clinical and biochemical features in PCOS, the exact definition of PCOS can be confusing. The diagnostic criteria for PCOS are as per the revised consensus Rotterdam criteria **(Fig. 2)**.

In adults, the presence of two of the three following criteria is required to diagnose PCOS:

1. Ovulatory dysfunction
2. Clinical/biochemical hyperandrogenism

Fig. 1: Normal and polycystic ovaries.

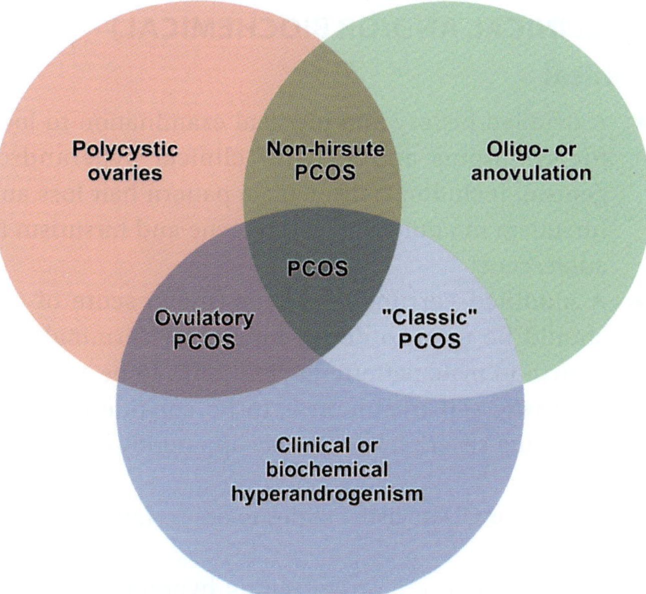

Fig. 2: Venn diagram illustrating the Rotterdam criteria for polycystic ovary syndrome (PCOS).

3. Polycystic ovaries on ultrasound or elevated anti-Müllerian hormone (AMH) levels, after other causes of these features are excluded.

Where irregular menstrual cycles and hyperandrogenism are present, ultrasound or AMH is not required for diagnosis.

In adolescents, both hyperandrogenism and ovulatory dysfunction are required, with ultrasound and AMH not recommended.

OLIGOMENORRHOEA AND ANOVULATION: DEFINITION

- Irregular cycles are normal and expected for the first year post menarche when the hypothalamopituitary axis is maturing.
- Up to 3 years post this period, 21–45 day cycles are normal.
- More than 3 years postmenarche to perimenopause, 21–35 day cycles are normal, <21 days or >35 days are irregular and likely anovulatory or less than eight cycles in a year
- 1 year postmenarche any cycle >90 days
- Occasionally, women with PCOS may have regular cycles that may be anovulatory which can be assessed by serum progesterone levels on day 21 to check for ovulation.

HYPERANDROGENISM (CLINICAL AND/OR BIOCHEMICAL)

Clinical

- A detailed history and physical examination to look for symptoms and signs of clinical hyperandrogenism, including acne, female pattern hair loss and hirsutism in adults and severe acne and hirsutism in adolescents
- A modified Ferriman–Gallwey (mFG) score of 4–6 should be used to detect hirsutism. Terminal hair growth in male pattern distribution is to be assessed. Cosmetic self-treatment is to be considered while assessing severity, as this may apparently reduce the score.
- Ludwig or Olsen visual scales to assess female pattern hair loss
- New-onset severe or worsening hyperandrogenism, including hirsutism, needs to rule out androgen-secreting tumours and ovarian hyperthecosis.

Biochemical

Biochemical evaluation is to be done when clinical features are minimal or missing:

- Total and free testosterone to be used to assess biochemical hyperandrogenism in the diagnosis of PCOS
- Dehydroepiandrosterone sulphate (DHEAS) and androstenedione are less specific.
- If levels of androgens are markedly elevated, check for differentials such as ovarian and adrenal neoplastic growths, congenital adrenal hyperplasia, Cushing syndrome, ovarian hyperthecosis (after menopause), iatrogenic causes and syndromes of severe insulin resistance.

POLYCYSTIC OVARIES ON ULTRASOUND OR ELEVATED SERUM ANTI-MÜLLERIAN HORMONE

- Follicle number per ovary (FNPO) ≥20, or follicle per cross-section (FPCS) ≥10, or ovarian volume >10 mL in at least one ovary is the detection criterion for PCOS morphology in adults.
- Ultrasound diagnosis is not recommended in adolescents.
- Serum AMH may be used in adults to diagnose PCOS but not in adolescents.

PATHOPHYSIOLOGY

Hypothalamopituitary Level (Flowchart 1)

The hypothalamic–pituitary compartment participates in aspects critical to the development of PCOS.

There is an elevated pulsatile release of gonadotropin-releasing hormone (GnRH) by the hypothalamus in PCOS. This elevation is due to reduction in hypothalamic opioid inhibition due to the chronic absence of progesterone resulting from persistent anovulation.

An elevated GnRH pulse favours the release of luteinising hormone (LH) more than follicle-Stimulating hormone (FSH). This results in an elevated LH:FSH ratio >2 or 3 to 1 characteristically found in approximately 60% of these patients.

Follicle stimulating hormone is not increased with LH, probably because of the synergistic negative feedback of chronically elevated oestrogen levels and normal follicular inhibin B.

Flowchart 1: Hypothalamic–pituitary compartment in polycystic ovary syndrome (PCOS).

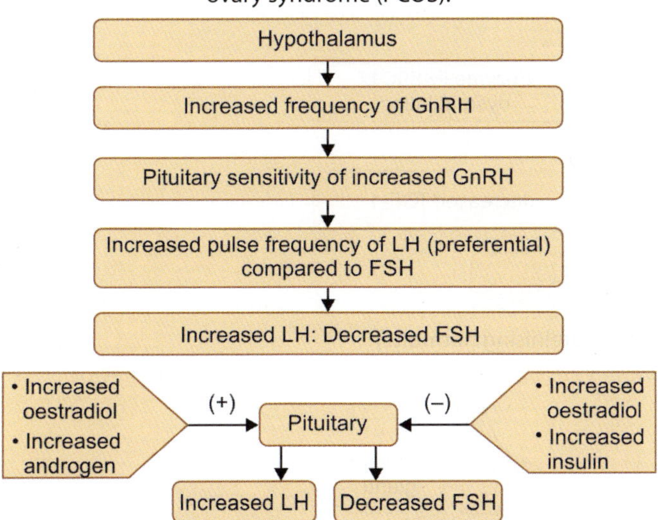

(FSH: follicle stimulating hormone; GnRH: gonadotrophin-releasing hormone; LH: luteinising hormone)

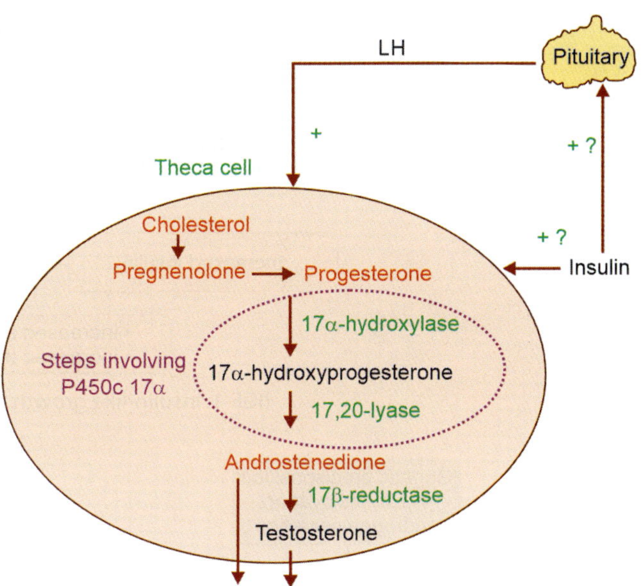

Fig. 3: Steps of P450c17 alpha enhancing the conversion of progesterone to testosterone due to increased luteinising hormone (LH) and insulin.

There is an increase in LH pulse amplitude and frequency but mainly amplitude. There is also an increased level of LH bioactivity; this is correlated with the levels of circulating oestrogen.

This altered state is also associated with a change in the circadian patterns with the highest LH values occurring in late afternoon rather than at night.

The increased pituitary and hypothalamic sensitivity can be attributed to the increased free oestrone levels, resulting from 50% reduction in sex hormone-binding hormone concentration due to increased testosterone and in patients with hyperinsulinaemia, due to a direct insulin effect on the liver.

About 25% of patients with PCOS exhibit elevated prolactin levels (generally <40 ng/mL). Hyperprolactinaemia may result from abnormal oestrogen feedback to the pituitary gland. In some patients with PCOS, bromocriptine has reduced LH levels and restored ovulatory function.

OVARIAN AND OTHER ENDOCRINE ASPECTS OF POLYCYSTIC OVARY SYNDROME

The hyperandrogenism and anovulation that accompany PCOS may be caused by abnormalities in four endocrinologically active compartments: (1) Ovaries, (2) adrenal glands, (3) periphery (fat) and (4) hypothalamus-pituitary compartment **(Flowchart 1)**.

There is allegedly an associated enzymatic dysregulation specifically of P450c17, the enzyme responsible for both 17α-hydroxylase and 17,20-lyase activities **(Fig. 3)**. This may account for the altered steroidogenesis in both ovaries and adrenal glands. The intermediates from 17α-hydroxypregnenolone and androstenedione hyper-respond, and testosterone rises slightly yet significantly and oestrone and oestradiol marginally. The 3 hydroxy intermediate pregnenolone, 17-hydroxyprogesterone and DHEA rise only slightly. This coupled with hyper-responsiveness of DHEAS to adrenocorticotropic hormone (ACTH) in the adrenals completes the background for the formation of PCOS. There is growing evidence that hyperinsulinaemia may stimulate P450c17 enzyme, resulting in hyperandrogenism.

Ovaries

In patients with PCOS, the ovarian compartment is the most consistent contributor of androgens. The ovarian stroma, theca and granulosa contribute to ovarian hyperandrogenism and are stimulated by LH. This hormone relates to ovarian androgenic activity in PCOS in a number of ways **(Flowchart 2)**, and they are given as follows:

- Total and free testosterone levels correlate directly with LH levels.

Flowchart 2: Excess of androgen.

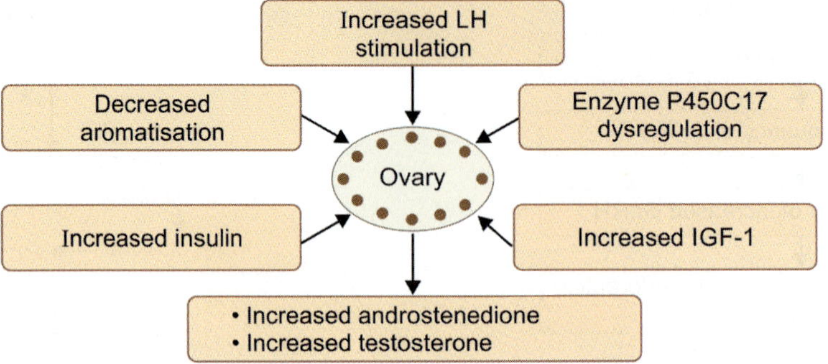

(IGF-1: insulin-like growth factor 1; LH: luteinising hormone)

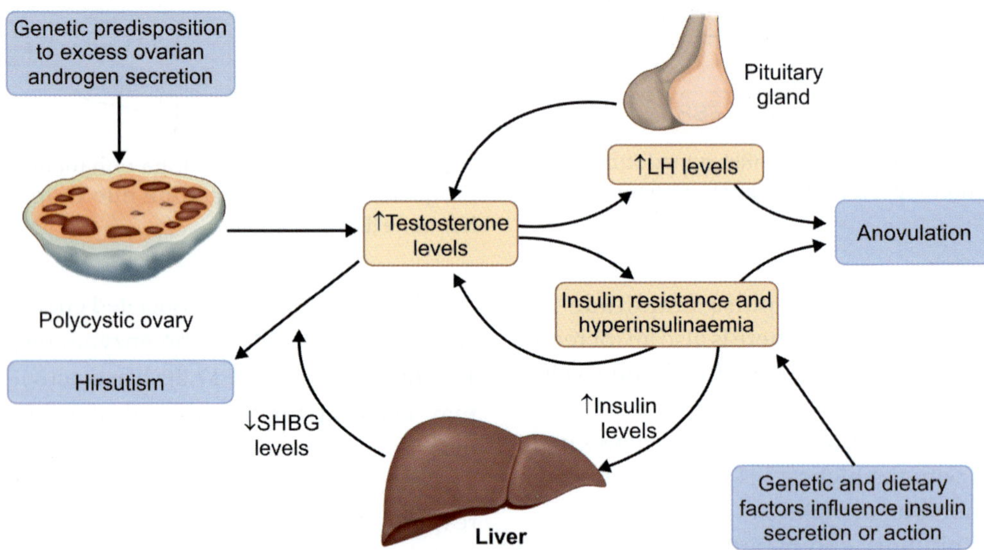

Fig. 4: Summary of clinical, biochemical and metabolic features of polycystic ovary syndrome (PCOS). (LH: luteinising hormone; SHBG: sex hormone-binding globulin)

- The ovaries are more sensitive to gonadotropic stimulation, possibly as a result of CYP17 dysregulation.
- Treatment with a GnRH agonist effectively suppresses serum testosterone and androstenedione levels.
- Larger doses of a GnRH agonist are required for androgen suppression than for oestrogen suppression.

The serum total testosterone levels are usually no more than twice the upper normal range (20–80 ng/dL). However, in ovarian hyperthecosis, values may reach 200 ng/dL or more. High intraovarian androgen concentrations inhibit follicular maturation. Although ovarian theca cells are hyperactive, the retarded follicular maturation results in inactive granulosa cells with minimal aromatase activity for conversion to oestrogens.

Since the FSH levels are not totally depressed, new follicular growth is continuously stimulated, but not to the point of full maturation and ovulation, in the form of multiple follicles measuring 2–10 mm in diameter. These follicles are surrounded by hyperplastic theca cells, often luteinised in response to high LH levels. The accumulation of follicular tissue in various stages of development allows an increased and relatively constant production of steroids in response to gonadotropic stimulation. This process is self-sustaining. As various follicles undergo atresia, they are immediately replaced by new follicles of similar limited growth potential. The elevated androgen levels compound the problem through the process of extraglandular conversion as well as suppression of sex hormone-binding globulin (SHBG) synthesis, resulting in elevated oestrogen levels and associated increase in free testosterone **(Fig. 4)**. This prevents normal follicular development and induces premature atresia.

Approximately 70–80% of women with PCOS demonstrate frank elevations in circulating androgens,

Flowchart 3: Obesity and insulin resistance.

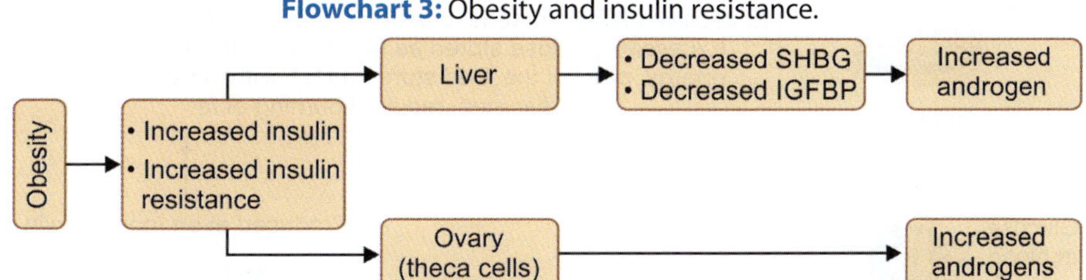

(IGFBP: insulin-like growth factor binding protein; SHBG: sex hormone-binding globulin)

particularly free testosterone. The ovaries of about 70% of patients with PCOS usually contain intermediate and atretic follicles measuring 2–8 mm in diameter, resulting in a *polycystic appearance* at sonography.

Adrenal

The adrenal compartment also plays a role in the development of PCOS. About 25–50% will have elevated levels of the adrenal androgen metabolite, DHEAS. Although the hyperfunctioning CYP17 androgen-forming enzyme coexists in both the ovaries and the adrenal glands, DHEAS is increased in only about 50% of patients with PCOS. The hyper-responsiveness of DHEAS to stimulation with ACTH at the onset of symptoms around puberty and the observation that 17,20-lyase activation (one of the two CYP17 enzymes) is a key event in adrenarche have led to the concept of PCOS as an exaggerated adrenarche.

Peripheral

The peripheral compartment, defined as the skin and the adipose tissue, manifests its contribution to the development of PCOS in several ways:

- The presence and activity of 5α-reductase in the skin largely determines the presence or absence of hirsutism.
- Aromatase and 17β-hydroxysteroid dehydrogenase activities are increased in fat cells, and peripheral aromatisation is increased with body weight.
- The metabolism of oestrogens, by way of reduced 2-hydroxylation and 17α-oxidation, is decreased. Genetic association and linkage analysis studies presently underway suggest an oligogenic origin for PCOS.

METABOLIC COMPONENT OF POLYCYSTIC OVARY SYNDROME

While not part of the diagnostic criterion, many women with PCOS appear to be uniquely insulinresistant.

Flowchart 4: Pathophysiology.

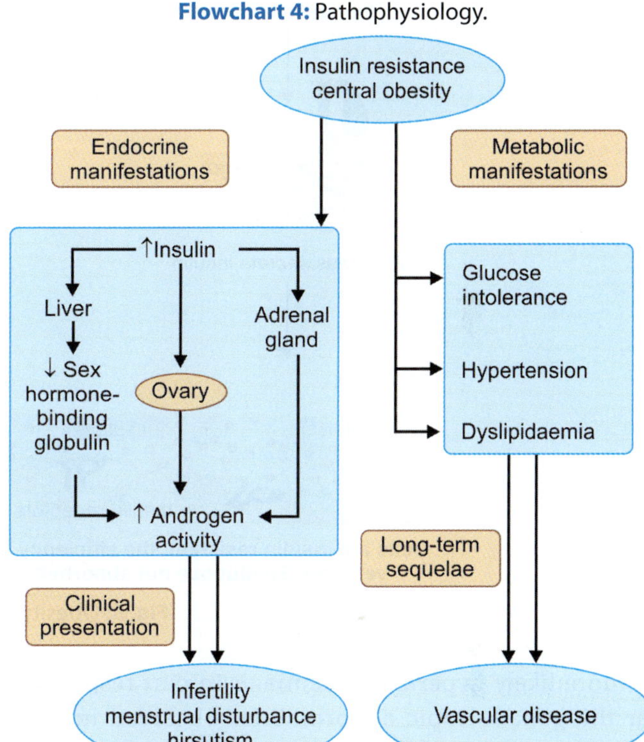

Approximately 50–70% of patients with PCOS demonstrate profound insulin resistance and secondary hyperinsulinaemia, independent of body weight. In PCOS, insulin resistance usually refers to the impaired action of insulin in stimulating glucose transport and inhibiting lipolysis in adipocytes. Insulin resistance in PCOS appears to be due to an intracellular defect of insulin signalling **(Flowcharts 3 and 4)**.

The compensatory hyperinsulinaemia, resulting from the underlying insulin resistance, augments the stimulatory action of LH on the growth and androgen secretion of ovarian thecal cells while inhibiting the hepatic production of SHBG. Treatment of patients with PCOS with insulin sensitisers may result in lower circulating levels of LH, suggesting that insulin resistance,

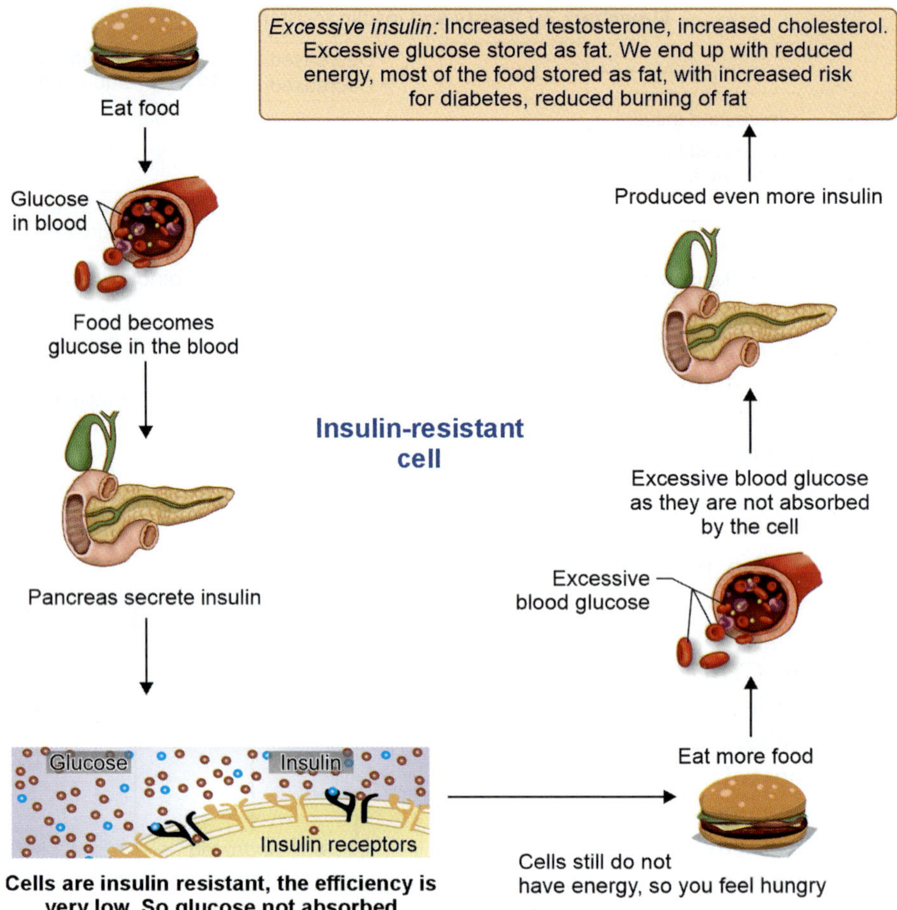

Fig. 5: Obesity and insulin resistance.

or more likely hyperinsulinaemia, is in part responsible for the gonadotropic abnormalities observed in many women with PCOS **(Figs. 5 and 6)**. Since insulin is also a mitogenic hormone, extremely elevated insulin levels may lead to hyperplasia of the basal layers of the epidermis, resulting in the development of acanthosis nigricans (a velvety, hyperpigmented change of the crease areas of the skin) and acrochordons. Overall, insulin resistance and secondary hyperinsulinaemia affect a large fraction of patients with PCOS and may cause or augment the androgen excess of these patients.

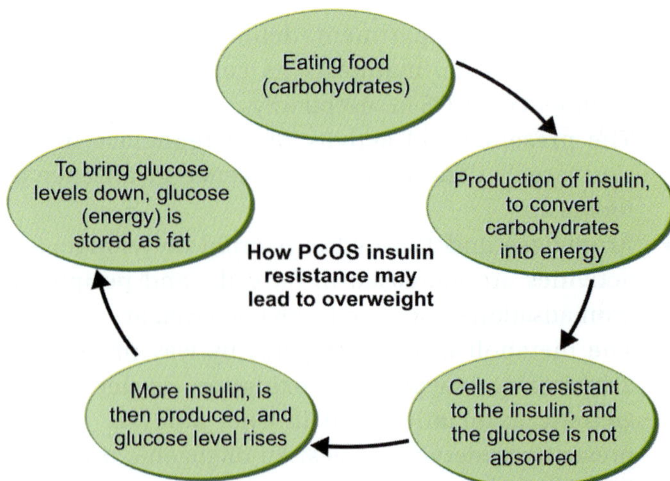

Fig. 6: Pathophysiology. (PCOS: polycystic ovary syndrome)

Insulin and the Mechanism of Anovulation in Polycystic Ovary Syndrome

The characteristic feature of anovulation **(Flowchart 5)** in PCOS is the arrest of growth of antral follicles after reaching a diameter between 5 and 8 mm. This may be caused by premature activation of LH-mediated terminal differentiation of granulosa cells, and hyperinsulinaemia makes an important contribution to this phenomenon. In the normal menstrual cycle, granulosa cells of the dominant follicle become responsive to the LH in

Flowchart 5: Anovulation.

Ovary → Granulosa cells (Decreased FSH) → Anovulation

Ovary → Theca cell stroma (Increased LH, Increased IGF-1) → Increased androgen

(FSH: follicle-stimulating hormone; IGF-1: insulin-like growth factor 1; LH: luteinising hormone)

the mid-follicle phase at a follicle diameter of 10 mm, whereas subsidiary follicles do not respond to LH. In the preovulatory phase of the cycle, LH maintains and enhances steroidogenesis but triggers terminal differentiation so that once the granulosa layer of the dominant follicle is exposed to LH, the cells undergo only two more cell divisions before growth is arrested. Theoretically, premature activation of this LH-dependent effect would result in premature arrest of growth and failure of ovulation as in PCOS. Specifically, LH-stimulated oestradiol and progesterone production in cells from follicles are as small as 4 mm in diameter. In contrast, in follicles from both ovulatory PCOS women and normal ovaries, only dominant follicles of 9.5 mm or greater responded to LH. It is believed that the remarkable amplification of LH action by insulin makes a major combination to the arrest of follicle growth. Other endemic factors, notably hypersecretion of LH and ovarian androgens, may also have a role, and an intrinsic disorder of folliculogenesis cannot be ruled out.

PATHOLOGY

Macroscopically, ovaries in women with PCOS are two to five times the normal size. A cross-section of the surface of the ovary discloses a white, thickened cortex with multiple follicles that are typically less than a centimetre in diameter. Microscopically, the superficial cortex is fibrotic and hypocellular and may contain prominent blood vessels. In addition to small atretic follicles, there is an increase in the number of follicles with luteinised theca interna. The stroma may contain luteinised stromal cells **(Figs. 7A and B)**. 'Polycystic' is a misnomer as the ovaries contain multiple follicles rather than cysts which are typically more than a centimetre in diameter.

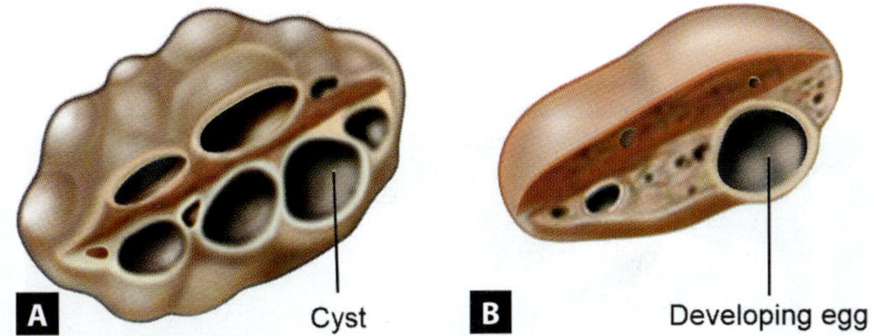

Figs. 7A and B: Pathology. (A) Polycystic ovary; (B) Normal ovary.

CLINICAL, BIOCHEMICAL AND METABOLIC FEATURES OF POLYCYSTIC OVARY SYNDROME

Menstrual dysfunction typically occurs in PCOS, ranging from oligomenorrhoea to amenorrhoea. As a rule, patients with PCOS exhibit anovulation. Even in hyperandrogenic women with regular menstrual cycles, the rate of anovulation is about 20%.

Hirsutism is the most predictive clinical sign of hyperandrogenism. Severe acne in the teenage years appears to be a common finding of PCOS. Female pattern baldness is also a feature of PCOS. All of these can be psychologically distressing features.

Obesity is found in over 50% of patients with PCOS. The body fat is usually deposited centrally (android obesity), and a higher waist-to-hip ratio indicates an increased risk of diabetes mellitus and cardiovascular disease in later life.

Insulin resistance and hyperinsulinaemia are commonly exhibited in PCOS. Insulin resistance is now recognised as a major risk factor for the development of type 2 diabetes mellitus. About one third of obese PCOS patients have impaired glucose tolerance (IGT), and 7.5–10% have type 2 diabetes mellitus.

Abnormal lipoproteins are common in PCOS and include elevated total cholesterol, triglycerides, lowdensity lipoproteins (LDLs) and low levels of high-density lipoproteins (HDLs) and apolipoprotein AI.

Other observations in women with PCOS include an increased incidence of hypertension over the years that reach a 40% incidence by perimenopause, a greater prevalence of atherosclerosis and cardiovascular disease, and an estimated sevenfold increased risk for myocardial infarction.

Women with PCOS have a significantly higher prevalence of obstructive sleep apnoea.

There is a two- to sixfold increased risk of endometrial cancer in premenopausal women with PCOS.

ULTRASONOGRAPHIC EXAMINATION

This may be a useful method for the early detection and subsequent follow-up of PCOS. Generally, ovarian size is increased. The most important ultrasonographic finding is a bilaterally increased number of microcysts measuring 0.5–0.8 cm with generally more than five microcysts in each ovary. As the number of microcysts increases and the ovarian volume enlarges, clinical and endocrine abnormalities become more obvious, and the condition becomes more severe **(Figs. 8 to 10)**.

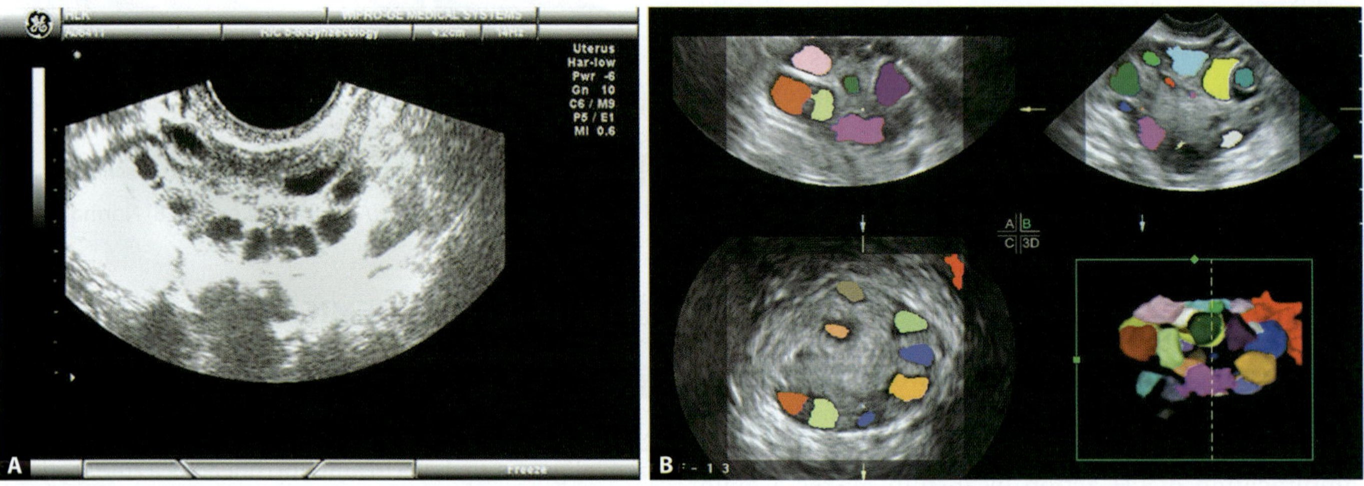

Figs. 8A and B: Ultrasonography pictures of polycystic ovary.

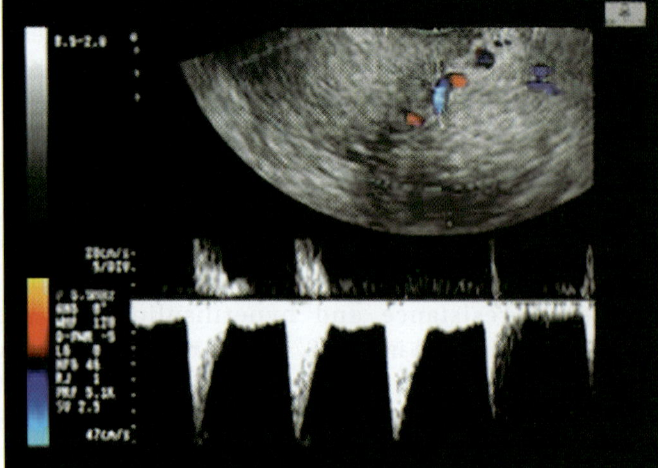

Fig. 9: Uterine artery Doppler in polycystic ovary.

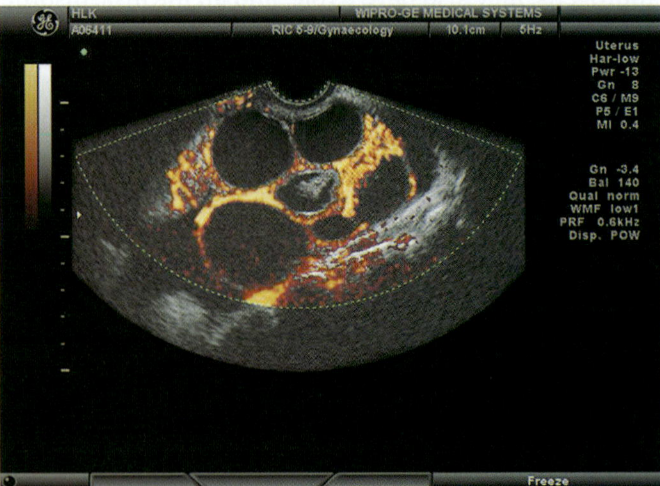

Fig. 10: Hyperstimulated polycystic ovary.

PUBERTY AND POLYCYSTIC OVARY SYNDROME

Polycystic ovary syndrome originates in puberty. Clinical observation teaches that PCOS often develops during adolescence. Excessive hair growth usually originates from before the onset of menstrual cycles. Menarche tends to be delayed. Primary amenorrhoea is diagnosed by age 15 years or >3 years post thelarche (breast development). Irregular cycles, although considered a normal phenomenon during the first gynaecological years, frequently continue into adulthood. For adolescents who have features of PCOS, but do not meet diagnostic criteria, an 'increased risk' could be considered, and reassessment is advised at or before full reproductive maturity, 8 years post menarche. Significant weight gain in adolescent years is a high-risk factor. Ultrasound and serum AMH should not be used to diagnose PCOS in adolescents.

Mechanism of Onset of Polycystic Ovary Syndrome During Puberty

Taking into account the above remarks, the following hypothesis is postulated **(Flowchart 6)**.

The onset of pulsatile growth hormone (GH) secretion during early puberty induces the release of insulin-like growth factor 1 (IGF-1) by the liver and most other tissues. GH also provokes insulin resistance, which selectively affects peripheral glucose. The resulting hyperinsulinaemia acting on IGF-1 causes ovarian hyperstimulation inducing thecal cell hyperplasia and excessive androgen production. The increased androgens cause follicular atresia and increased circulating oestrone levels because of peripheral conversion in adipose tissues.

Flowchart 6: Mechanism of onset of polycystic ovary syndrome (PCOS) during puberty.

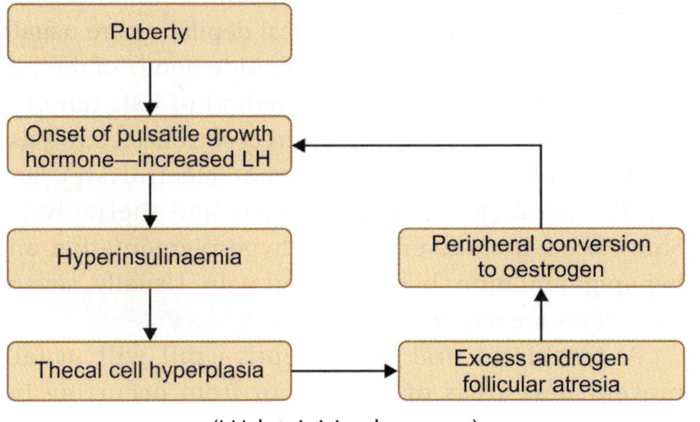

(LH: luteinising hormone)

The altered endocrine milieu provokes increased pituitary LH secretion, which aggravates the theca cell stimulation.

After puberty, the insulin and IGF-1 levels progressively decline in most patients, resulting in normalisation of the clinical and morphological picture. Only in a few cases, PCOS persists. Criteria for the metabolic syndrome in women with PCOS (three of five qualify for the syndrome). These women are more prone to metabolic syndrome X with higher levels of insulin resistance and its consequences.

Risk factor cutoff values are:

- Abdominal obesity (waist circumference >88 cm or 35 inches)
- Triglycerides >150 mg/dL
- HDL-C <50 mg/dL
- Blood pressure >130/85 mm Hg
- Fasting blood sugar of 110–126 mg/dL and 2-hour glucose from oral glucose tolerance test of 140–199 mg/dL.

MANAGEMENT

A patient with PCOS may present to a clinician at different stages of her life. During adolescence, she may present with menstrual irregularities and skin problems such as hirsutism, acne or alopecia. She may present with obesity or acanthosis nigricans. During the reproductive years, she may present with infertility. She may present in the later part of her life with problems related to long-term sequelae of PCOS, namely gynaecological cancer, diabetes or cardiovascular risk. The management of a patient with PCOS will depend on her presenting problems.

Menstrual Irregularities

Many women with PCOS will give a history of infrequent cycles and may have about three to six menstrual periods per year. As long as these are not unduly heavy or painful, no particular medical therapy may be needed **(Fig. 11)**. In obese women, weight loss should be the first line of treatment. In patients who succeed in losing >5% of their body weight, this alone may restore normal menstrual regularity. A reduction in body weight of 5–10% will cause a 30% reduction in visceral fat, which is often sufficient to restore ovulation and reduce markers of metabolic disease. Weight loss is associated with a reduction of circulating insulin and androgen levels, which can also be achieved by using insulin-sensitising drugs.

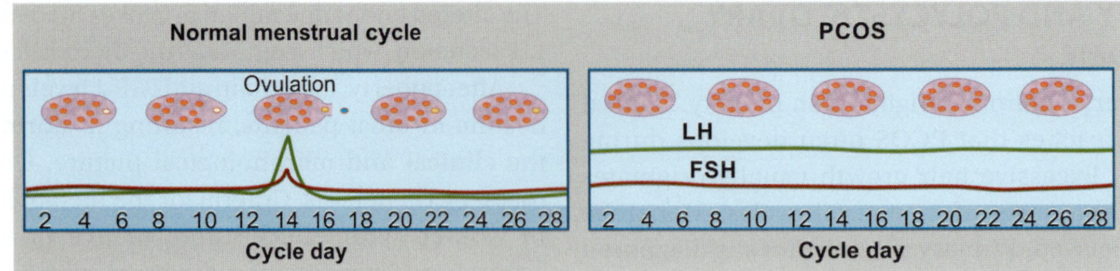

Fig. 11: A comparison between a normal menstrual cycle and a menstrual cycle of a patient with polycystic ovary syndrome (PCOS).

Often, an oral contraceptive can be a useful treatment for women with PCOS. Oral contraceptives can have the benefits of contraception, protection against endometrial cancer and improvement of skin manifestations of PCOS such as hirsutism and acne. Oral pills which contain 35 µg of ethinyloestradiol and 2 mg of cyproterone acetate (CPA) may be a good option in patients who also have hyperandrogenism (hirsutism and acne) associated with menstrual irregularity.

Skin Manifestations

Skin manifestations of PCOS include acne, hirsutism, alopecia and acanthosis nigricans.

Acne

Acne is seen in approximately one third of PCOS patients. Mild acne can be treated topically with keratolytics such as azelaic acid and retinoids or with antibacterials such as benzoyl peroxide, clindamycin 1% lotion and erythromycin 2% gel. More severe forms generally require oral antibiotics such as tetracyclines, erythromycin and trimethoprim. For severe cases, isotretinoin is prescribed and produces long-term remission in >70% of patients. However, in the reproductive age group, use of retinoids must be along with reliable contraception due to their teratogenic effects.

In PCOS, antiandrogens are most effective because acne occurs as a result of overstimulation of the pilosebaceous unit by androgens. Antiandrogens that can be used are CPA, spironolactone, flutamide and finasteride. CPA can be given as a combined oral contraceptive pill (as mentioned above). This minimal dose has proven effective in almost 100% of cases. In more severe cases, CPA in a dose of 10–100 mg/day can be given on the first 10 days of the combined oral contraceptive pill. It will take 3–5 months before any improvement can be seen. Acne will be cleared in 60% of patients in 6 months, and after 12 months, 95% should be free of acne.

Spironolactone, an aldosterone antagonist, has anti-androgen action. Flutamide, a non-steroidal antiandrogen, can be used for the treatment of hirsutism and acne. However, because of rare reports of hepatotoxicity, it is not commonly used. Finasteride acts by inhibiting 5α-reductase and can be taken orally in doses of 1–5 mg/day. It does not have much side effects. When spironolactone, finasteride and flutamide are taken, contraception is advised to avoid the potential risk of feminisation of a male foetus. It is important to inform patients that clinical response takes time and patients have to be on long-term maintenance treatment to avoid relapse. The longer the duration of treatment (at least in the ethinyl oestradiol/CPA oral contraceptive pills), the less the chance of relapse within a given period of time.

Hirsutism

A patient may present with excess hair as their main problem. Hirsutism can be treated with physical therapy such as bleaching, shaving, plucking, depilatory creams, electrolysis and laser. Bleaching of the hair with hydrogen peroxide is used to disguise pigmented facial hairs. Repeated plucking of hair is another method but may lead to permanent hair follicle matrix damage, resulting in finer, thinner hairs. Side effects include postinflammatory hyperpigmentation, folliculitis, pseudofolliculitis and, rarely, scarring **(Fig. 12)**. Chemical depilators are usually thioglycates that disrupt the disulphide bonds of the hair shaft. Electrolysis is a proven method of hair removal. Three forms exist: (1) Galvanic (direct current electrolysis), (2) thermolysis (alternate current electrolysis), and (3) the blend (galvanic electrolysis and thermolysis). Side effects include erythema, hyperpigmentation and hypopigmentation, blistering and pain. Usually, several treatments are required to improve efficacy.

A combined oral contraceptive pill will usually prevent new areas of excess hair from occurring but rarely is sufficient alone to cause regression of excess hair.

This usually necessitates the addition of an antiandrogen therapy such as CPA. Most women notice a regression of excess hair within 4–6 months, but typically treatment needs to be continued for at least 1–2 years to substantially reduce hair growth, and then maintenance therapy is required to keep the problem under control. Typically, this is a low-dose combined oral contraceptive pill. Another useful antiandrogenic treatment is spironolactone. This may be used alone or in combination with a contraceptive pill. Flutamide and finasteride are also drugs that help reduce hirsutism.

Alopecia

Some patients may present with alopecia. Treatment includes psychological support and hairstyling. Drugs such as minoxidil, CPA, spironolactone and finasteride can be used but have a limited role.

INFERTILITY

Infertility is a common presenting problem in patients with PCOS. PCOS is associated with approximately 80–90% of women who suffer from infertility due to anovulation. There are several methods for inducing ovulation and basically they are reduction of insulin concentrations, FSH stimulation or a reduction of LH concentration or a combination of these **(Fig. 13)**.

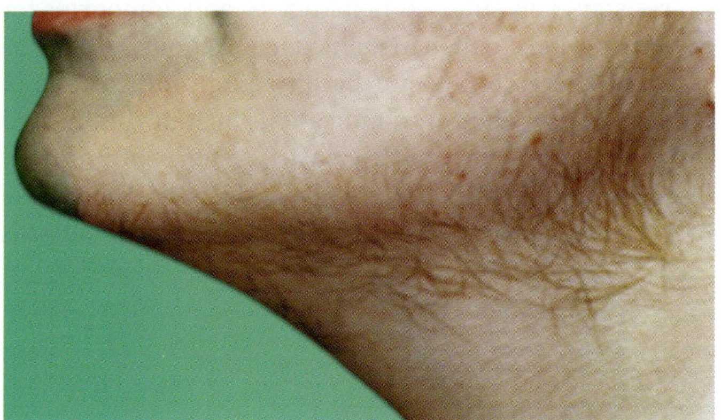

Fig. 12: Hirsutism.

WEIGHT LOSS

The first step in ovulation induction is weight loss. Obese women [body mass index (BMI) >30 kg/m^2] should be encouraged to lose weight. Even patients who are overweight (BMI >27 kg/m^2) are associated with a reduced chance of ovulation. Weight loss improves the endocrine profile and the likelihood of ovulation and a healthy pregnancy. Achieving weight reduction is, however, extremely difficult, particularly as the metabolic status of the patient with PCOS conspires against weight loss. Different strategies can be used to affect weight loss. Dieting and exercise should be encouraged.

Clomiphene Citrate

The simplest mode of ovulation induction is the use of clomiphene citrate. Patients can be started with 50 mg a day orally, for 5 days starting from day 2 to day 5 of a spontaneous or progesterone-induced bleed. Serial transvaginal ultrasound is a good method of looking at the follicles. This can be done on day 10 or 11 of her cycle and depending on the presence and size of the follicle, serial scans can be done to assist patients to determine her fertile period. Another method is the use of a urinary LH test.

There is controversy as to for how long can one be on clomiphene citrate and what is the maximum dose of clomiphene citrate that can be taken. If the patient did not ovulate with 50 mg of clomiphene citrate, then the dose can be increased to 100 mg. However, if the patient is ovulating

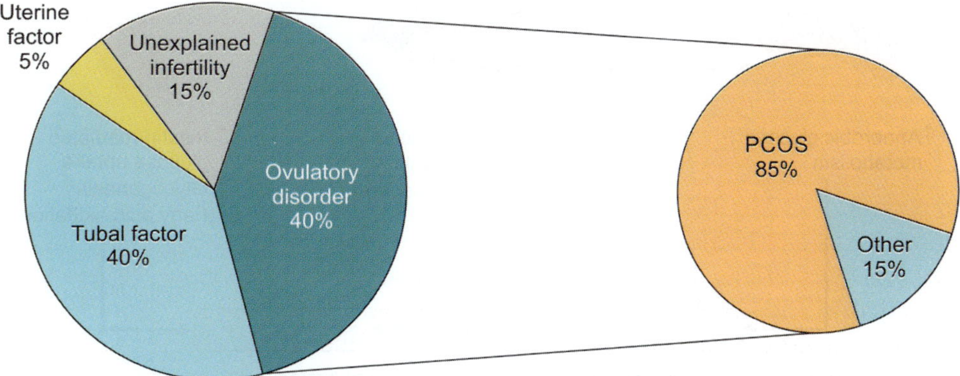

Fig. 13: Causes of female infertility. (PCOS: polycystic ovary syndrome)

with a low dose, there is no benefit in increasing the dose because a high dose has other side effects, which include thickening of the cervical mucus and antioestrogenic effect on the endometrium, and a larger dose of >150 mg/day may lead to ovarian hyperstimulation and its effects such as hyperstimulation syndrome and multiple pregnancies.

The addition of dexamethasone at the follicular phase of the cycle has given better results. Besides clomiphene citrate, the other antioestrogen that can be used is tamoxifen. Letrozole. an oral aromatase inhibitor, is another drug that may have potential in ovulation induction. Letrozole is currently considered the first-line agent by the International Evidence-Based Guidelines (2023) although in most countries, it is an off-label drug for fertility treatment.

Metformin

Metformin improves insulin sensitivity. Metformin treatment (500 mg 8 hourly) reduces hyperinsulinaemia, basal and stimulated LH levels, and free testosterone concentrations in overweight women with polycystic ovaries.

Mechanism of Action of Metformin

Metformin therapy improves insulin sensitivity shown by a reduction in fasting plasma glucose and insulin concentrations **(Fig. 14)**. It is not effective in the absence of insulin.

- Metformin decreases basal hepatic glucose output in patients, producing an important mechanism through which the drug lowers fasting plasma glucose concentration.
- It has increased glucose disposal in most studies using hyperinsulinaemic—euglycaemic and hyperglycaemic—clamp procedures, with muscle implicated as its main site of action.
- Metformin also increases the uptake and oxidation of glucose by adipose tissue as well as lipogenesis. However, the actions of metformin on peripheral tissues in vitro require high concentrations and are slow in onset.
- Metformin increases the binding of insulin to its receptors, phosphorylation and tyrosine kinase activity of insulin receptors in vivo, but this action may be due to reduced plasma glucose concentrations, since they cannot be reproduced in vitro.
- Metformin also increases the translocation of the glucose transporter (GLUT) GLUT-1 and GLUT-4 isoforms of glucose transporters in different types of cells, and it prevents the development of insulin resistance in cultured hepatocytes and adipocytes for long periods to high insulin concentrations.

First, there should not be any contraindications of metformin use. The contraindications include diminished renal function, cardiac diseases, severe pulmonary diseases, liver dysfunction, pancreatitis, concomitant use of diuretics and hypersensitivity to metformin. Patients

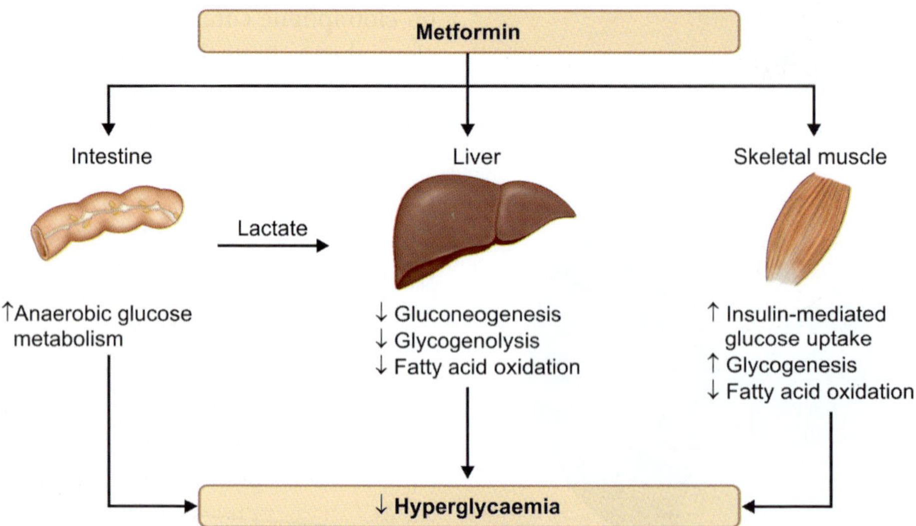

Fig. 14: Metformin: Mechanism of action.
Source: Bailey CJ, Feher MD. Therapies for Diabetes. Birmingham: Sherborne Gibbs; 2004.

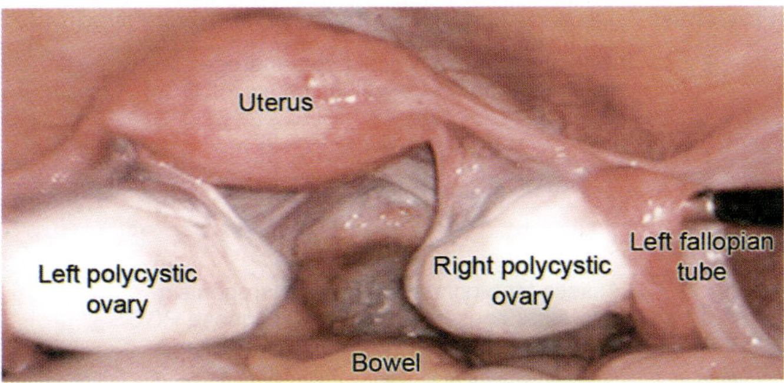

Fig. 15: Clinical image showing left polycystic ovary and right polycystic ovary.

must be informed about the adverse effects, which include gastrointestinal (GI) symptoms such as diarrhoea, nausea and vomiting, especially during the initial treatment periods. These symptoms are usually transient and resolve spontaneously. GI symptoms can be avoided if metformin is taken with meals and if the dose is increased slowly like one per day for the first week and two per day the next week and making into three per week throughout the treatment period. Probably because of the GI side effects, some patients may have weight loss. Patients may return to ovulatory cycles. Insulin-sensitising agent troglitazone appears to be of benefit to PCOS patients, but it has been withdrawn from the market because of reports of death from hepatotoxicity. The other thiazolidinedione that is being investigated is rosiglitazone. In addition to difficulty conceiving, women with PCOS are at an increased risk of miscarriage following either spontaneous or assisted conception. The intriguing question is will insulin-sensitising drugs prevent early pregnancy loss in PCOS? Some reports say that metformin therapy throughout pregnancy reduces the development of gestational diabetes in women with PCOS.

In patients who do not ovulate while on metformin, clomiphene citrate can be added to induce ovulation.

If the above attempt fails, then there are several strategies. The first is laparoscopic ovarian drilling. The other is ovulation induction with parenteral gonadotropic therapy. There is still debate as to which one should be done first.

Laparoscopic Ovarian Drilling

Laparoscopic ovarian drilling is a simple procedure whereby several punctures are made in one or both the polycystic ovaries **(Fig. 15)**. It could be second-line therapy for women with PCOS who are anovulatory and infertile, with clomiphene citrate resistance and no other infertility factors. This technique has superseded ovarian wedge resection. The controversy is how many diathermy points and at what wattage is to be used during ovarian cautery. It is now recommended that each ovary only about four per ovary for 4 seconds at 40 W. The risk of ovarian diathermy is periovarian adhesions and the possibility of ovarian failure. Abdominal lavage has helped reduce these periovarian adhesions. Besides diathermy, laser can be used to perform ovarian drilling **(Fig. 16)**.

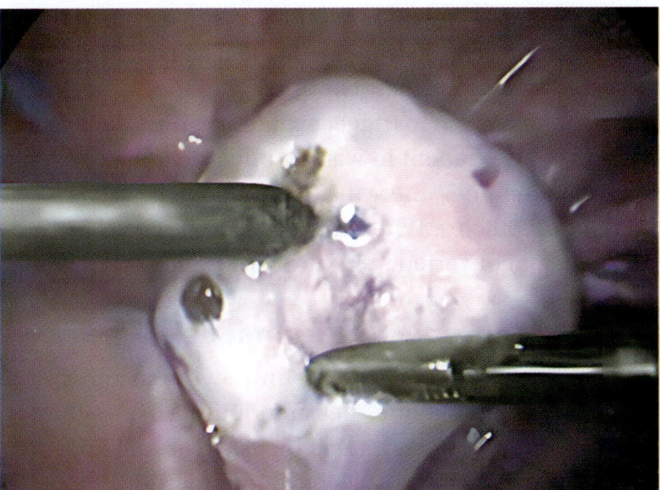

Fig. 16: Laparoscopic ovarian drilling (LEO).

Gonadotropin Therapy

Gonadotropin therapy is indicated for women with anovulatory PCOS who have been treated with antioestrogens, either if they have failed to ovulate or if they have a response to clomiphene that is likely to reduce their chance of conception (e.g. persistent hypersecretion of LH or negative postcoital tests due to the antioestrogenic effect on cervical mucus). The aim is for unifollicular development, and this can be challenging. There are many protocols available, but the more recent and probably the best protocol is the sequential step-up, step-down protocol. Patients are started with very low-dose gonadotropin (FSH), and the dose is gradually increased. When the leading follicle reaches 14 mm, the FSH threshold dose is reduced by half. This protocol appears to reduce the number of lead follicles when compared with a classic step-up protocol. The aim of this low-dose step-up protocol is to reduce the risk of both multiple pregnancies and ovarian hyperstimulation syndrome (OHSS), both of which are increased in women with PCOS compared with normal ovaries. Treatment cycles can be very long, up to 28–35 days. When the leading follicle reaches 17 mm in its largest diameter, human chorionic gonadotropin (hCG) 10,000 units is given to trigger ovulation. Some believe that there may be a benefit in waiting until the follicle reaches 20 mm. Sometimes, there may be a sudden increase in the number of follicles. When this happens, the cycle can be cancelled or converted to in vitro fertilisation (IVF).

Artificial Reproductive Techniques

In some patients, IVF or even intracytoplasmic sperm injection (ICSI) may be the only option for pregnancy. Patients with PCOS with tubal blockage or male partners with low sperm counts may have to undergo IVF or IVF-ICSI. Many protocols are available when performing IVF. The safest protocol in PCOS is a short protocol or antagonist protocol, as this is shown to reduce the risk of OHSS.

Long-term Monitoring

There have been suggestions in the literature that women with PCOS are at an increased risk of developing a number of chronic conditions and that, consequently, their health should be monitored.

Insulin resistance and resulting hyperinsulinaemia have been recognised features of PCOS for many years. It is now believed that insulin resistance is the underlying disorder of PCOS. Women with PCOS may be at an increased risk of developing non-insulin-dependent diabetes mellitus (NIDDM).

Clinicians have been concerned for some time about the possibility of an increase in cardiovascular disease in women with PCOS, due to the disturbance in insulin resistance and lipid profiles that often accompany this diagnosis. Lipid studies showed that there are poorer lipid profiles among women with PCOS compared with control women.

The association between exposure to unopposed oestrogens and an increased risk of endometrial cancer has been well established. Obesity has been shown consistently to be an important risk factor for endometrial cancer and is therefore likely to contribute to cancer risk in overweight women with PCOS. Diabetes and hypertension have been associated with an increased risk of endometrial cancer in some studies, but, overall, the findings have been inconsistent and the relationship is not well defined. So, whether PCOS per se increases the risk of endometrial cancer is inconclusive but with added obesity and diabetes, the risk is increased.

Flowchart 7: Diagnostic pathway for polycystic ovary syndrome.

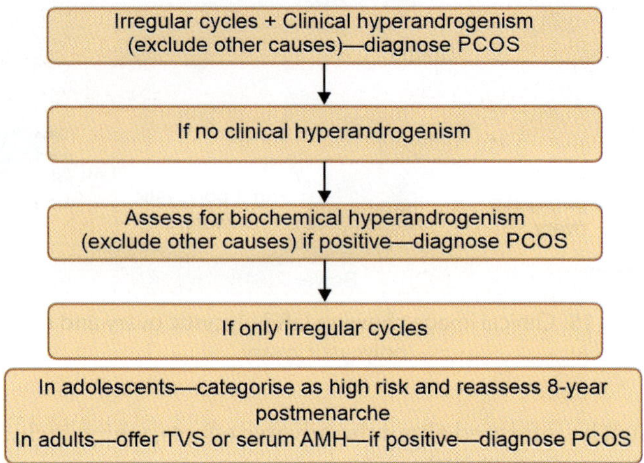

(AMH: anti-Müllerian hormone; PCOS: polycystic ovary syndrome)

There is also probably no association between PCOS and breast cancer. The risk of ovarian cancer in women with PCOS is not well studied.

SUMMARIES

Diagnosis

Refer to **Flowchart 7**.

Nonfertility Management

- *Lifestyle:* Weight loss and exercise
- Regularise periods—with combined oral contraceptive pills
- *Insulin resistance:* Metformin particularly in those with high BMI and other risk factors such as family history of type 2 diabetes
- Dermatological and pharmacological management with antiandrogens in acne, hirsutism and alopecia
- Screen for obstructive sleep apnoea and treat
- Management of psychological health, body image issues and detection and treatment of eating disorders
- Antiobesity pharmaceuticals and antiobesity surgery in BMI >40 kg/m^2 or high-risk metabolic risks in BMI >35 kg/m^2

Fertility Management

- *First line:* Lifestyle, weight loss and oral ovulation induction with letrozole/clomiphene citrate with or without metformin

- *Second line*: Gonadotropin ovulation induction and laparoscopic ovarian drilling
- *Third line*: IVF with PCOS as the only cause for subfertility. If there are other factors, they may be considered earlier.

SUGGESTED READING

1. Khomami BM, Boyle JA, Tay CT, Vanky E, Teede HJ, Joham AE, et al. Polycystic ovary syndrome and adverse pregnancy outcomes: current state of knowledge, challenges and potential implications for practice. Clin Endocrinol (Oxf). 2018;88(6):761-9.
2. Palomba S, de Wilde MA, Falbo A. Pregnancy complications in women with polycystic ovary syndrome. Hum Reprod Update. 2015;21(5):575-92.
3. Regidor PA, Schindler AE, Lesoine B, Druckman R. Management of women with PCOS using myo-inositol and folic acid. New clinical data and review of the literature. Horm Mol Biol Clin Investig. 2018;2:20170067.
4. Smyka M, Grzechocinska B, Wielgos M. The role of lifestyle changes in the treatment of polycystic ovary syndrome. Neuro Endocrinol Lett. 2018;38(8):521-7.

25

CHAPTER

Hirsutism

Deepak Goenka, Shamantaka Somayaji, Muralidhar V Pai

Chapter Outline

- Types of Hair
- Physiology of Hair Growth
- Androgens Physiology
- Aetiology
- Diagnosis of Hyperandrogenism
- Laboratory Evaluation
- Treatment

INTRODUCTION

Firstly, we will understand some basic definitions.

- *Hirsutism:* It is defined by the presence of excess terminal hair growth (dark, coarse hair) in androgen-dependent areas (e.g. upper lip, chin, midsternum, upper and lower abdomen, upper arms, upper and lower back and inner thigh/buttocks) in which women typically have little or no hair. It occurs in approximately 5–10% of women in the reproductive age group.
- *Hyperandrogenism:* Elevated serum concentrations of androgens in women are referred to as hyperandrogenism and manifest as hirsutism, acne, androgenetic alopecia and virilisation. Hirsutism is the most commonly used clinical diagnostic criterion of hyperandrogenism.
- *Virilisation:* It is defined as the presence of signs of masculinisation in women. It is rare, occurs only with severe hyperandrogenism and includes the appearance of sagittal, temporal and frontal balding, clitoromegaly and severe hirsutism. Furthermore, if androgen levels are extremely elevated for a substantial period of time, the features of virilisation may be accompanied by masculinisation of the body habitus, with atrophy of the breasts, an increase in muscle mass, a redistribution of body fat and a deepening of the voice.
- *Unwanted hair:* Excess hair that is not true hirsutism, i.e. is not dark, coarse, and in androgen-dependent areas, does not need biochemical evaluation and does not respond to the pharmacologic therapies for androgen-dependent hair.

TYPES OF HAIR

There are approximately 50 trillion hair follicles covering the body, of which 100,000–150,000 are on the scalp; the remaining follicles are on fascial and other body sites. The only areas free of hair follicles are the soles of the feet, palms of the hands and the lips.

Structurally, there are three types of hair:

1. *Lanugo:* These are soft hair, densely covering the skin of the foetus, which are shed between the first and the fourth month postpartum.
2. *Vellus hair:* These are also soft fine hair but larger than and longer than lanugo hair. Vellus hair are usually nonpigmented, generally measuring <2 mm in length, and cover the apparently hairless areas of the body. These are androgen-independent hair.

   Hypertrichosis: The excessive growth of androgen-independent hair that is vellus, prominent in nonsexual areas and most commonly familial or caused by systemic disorders (hypothyroidism, anorexia nervosa, malnutrition, porphyria and dermatomyositis) or oral medications (phenytoin, penicillamine, diazoxide, minoxidil, or cyclosporine).
3. *Terminal hair:* These are longer, pigmented and coarse in texture. These hair make up the eyebrow, eyelashes, scalp hair and pubic and axillary hair in both sexes, and much of the body and fascial hair of men. These are androgen-dependent hair.

PHYSIOLOGY OF HAIR GROWTH

The hair follicle and its sebaceous gland together make up the pilosebaceous unit. The hair follicle begins to develop within the first 2 months of gestation, and by birth, a child possesses all of the hair follicles he or she will ever have. Hair first appears as vellus hair, which is fine, short and lightly pigmented. During puberty, adrenal and ovarian androgen levels rise, converting vellus hair to terminal hair, which is coarse, long and more heavily pigmented.

Hair grow in a cyclic pattern. The three phases of the cycle are as follows:

1. *Anagen (growth):* It is an active growth phase where there is a rapid proliferation of cells in the epithelial matrix at the base of the hair follicle, elongating in length towards the dermis and the surface of the skin.
2. *Catagen (rapid involution):* Where the hair column rapidly shrinks and the hair bulb shrivels.
3. *Telogen (inactivity):* Where hair is loosely attached to the bulb. During this phase, hair are shed as new hair displaces it.

The length of each hair is determined by the relative duration of anagen and telogen and varies with different locations on the body, although each hair follicle has its own growth cycle independent of adjacent hair follicles. The growth and development of the hair follicle may be influenced by several factors. First, the pilosebaceous unit is sensitive to the effects of sex hormones, especially androgens. During puberty, androgen levels rise which can initiate growth and increase both the diameter and pigmentation of hair.

Genetic factors may also influence the pilosebaceous unit. Although males and females are born with equal numbers of hair follicles, racial and ethnic differences are noted in the concentration of hair follicles. Caucasians have a greater number of hair follicles than African-Americans, who in turn have a greater number than Asians. Different ethnic groups within each race may also exhibit differences in hair follicle concentrations.

ANDROGENS PHYSIOLOGY

Androgenic hormones stimulate terminal hair growth and cause voice and muscle changes, hair loss, clitoral enlargement and reduction in breast size. Androgens are secreted from adrenals and ovaries. Circulating androgens are as follows:

- Testosterone
- Dihydrotestosterone (DHT)
- Dehydroepiandrosterone (DHEA)
- Dehydroepiandrosterone-sulphate (DHEA-S)
- Androstenedione

TABLE 1: Source of common androgens in the body.

Androgen	*Source*
Testosterone	• 25% Adrenals • 25% Ovaries • 50% Peripheral conversion of androstenedione
Androstenedione	• 50% Ovaries • 50% Adrenals
DHEA	• 90% Adrenals • 10% Ovaries
DHEA-S	100% Adrenals
DHT	Converted from testosterone by 5α-reductase

(DHEA: dehydroepiandrosterone; DHEA-S: dehydroepiandrosterone-sulphate; DHT: dihydrotestosterone)

The ovary produces testosterone, androstenedione and DHEA. The adrenal glands produce testosterone, androstenedione, DHEA and DHEA-S. The most common androgens are testosterone and androstenedione. The most biologically active form of androgen is DHT followed by testosterone. Others are weak androgens **(Table 1)**.

- *Testosterone:* It is the most potent androgenic hormone. Source:
  - 25% is secreted by the ovaries.
  - 25% is secreted by the adrenals.
  - The remaining 50% is produced by the peripheral conversion of androstenedione.

Normal circulating concentrations of testosterone in women range from 20 to 60 ng/dL. This range is far lower than the concentrations found in men, which range from 300 to 800 ng/dL. Testosterone binds to sex hormone-binding globulin (SHBG) and albumin. Approximately 80% of testosterone is bound to SHBG, and 19% of the remaining testosterone is loosely bound to albumin, which leaves approximately 1% in the free (unbound) and active form. The free testosterone is elevated in 60–70% of hirsute women.

- *Dihydrotestosterone:* Testosterone is converted to DHT by 5 alpha-reductase, an enzyme found in many androgen-sensitive tissues such as skin. DHT is a very potent androgen and is primarily responsible for androgenic effects on hair follicles.
- *Androstenedione:* It is produced in equal amounts by the adrenal glands and the ovaries, and most of the androstenedione secreted is converted to testosterone.

Androstenedione is a less potent androgen than testosterone, but it can produce significant androgenic biological effects when present in excess amounts. The normal serum concentration of androstenedione in women ranges from 60 to 300 ng/dL.

- *Dehydroepiandrosterone and dehydroepiandrosterone-sulphate:* Most of DHEA and all of DHEA-S are produced by the adrenal glands. DHEA is metabolised quickly. As a consequence, the measurement of its serum concentration does not reflect the adrenal gland activity. DHEA-S has a much longer half-life than DHEA, and the measurement of its serum level is used to assess adrenal function. Levels of DHEA-S in women vary widely, with a normal range of 38–338 μg/dL.
- *Sex hormone-binding globulins:* Since androgenicity is determined mainly by an unbound testosterone, the circulating concentration of SHBG influences the hormonal state. Testosterone and insulin both decrease SHBG levels, whereas oestrogen and thyroid hormone increase its levels. Symptoms of hyperandrogenism may be seen in a patient with a normal total testosterone level if the level of SHBGs is decreased enough to significantly increase the free testosterone concentration.

In order of potency, DHT > testosterone > androstenedione > DHEA-S. The mechanism of excess hair growth in hirsute women involves an increased level of soft testosterone, which binds to the androgen receptor on hair follicles. This activation of 5α-reductase causes the activation of testosterone to DHT, which in turn causes proliferation and growth of the terminal hair.

AETIOLOGY

- Hyperandrogenism
- Increased sensitivity of hair follicles to normal circulating androgens
- Idiopathic
- Causes of hyperandrogenism:
  - Increased productions of androgens:
    - Ovarian hyperandrogenism
    - Adrenal hyperandrogenism
  - Increased proportion of unbound androgens due to decrease in SHBG levels:
    - Ovarian hyperandrogenism:
      - Polycystic ovary syndrome (PCOS)
      - Hyperandrogenic insulin-resistant acanthosis nigricans (HAIR-AN) syndrome
      - Ovarian stromal hyperthecosis
      - Luteomas of pregnancy
      - Tumours: Leydig cell tumours, Sertoli–Leydig cell tumours, gynandroblastomas and steroid (lipoid) cell tumours.

PCOS: This is the most common cause of hyperandrogenism. The characteristic presentation is that of a young girl with obesity, menstrual irregularity, hyperandrogenism, infertility and hirsutism. Insulin resistance and dyslipidaemia are common.

Hyperandrogenism in PCOS is the result of several abnormalities, namely:

- Increase in luteinising hormone (LH) secretion by the pituitary and increased responsiveness of the ovarian tissue to LH result in the stimulation of the ovarian stroma, theca and granulosa cells to produce more testosterone and androstenedione.
- The adrenal glands secrete more DHEA-S due to hyper-responsiveness to the circulating adrenocorticotropic hormone (ACTH).
- In addition, obesity and the associated insulin resistance lead to hyperinsulinaemia. This stimulates ovarian androgen production.
- An increase in 5α-reductase production has been demonstrated in the peripheral tissue.

Hyperandrogenic insulin-resistant acanthosis nigricans (HAIR-AN) syndrome: This condition is considered a variant of PCOS, and clinically, it is difficult to distinguish between the two. Insulin resistance and the resultant hyperinsulinaemia are more severe; hence, acanthosis nigricans is more pronounced. Hyperinsulinaemia stimulates ovarian androgen production. Features of virilisation may be present in some.

Ovarian stromal hyperthecosis: Ovarian stromal hyperthecosis refers to the presence of luteinised theca cells in the ovarian stroma, which secrete increasing amounts of testosterone.

- Ovaries are enlarged with an increase in the ovarian stroma, to about 6–7 cm, but not polycystic.
- Women with this disorder initially present with hirsutism, acne and virilisation, insulin resistance and hyperinsulinaemia. Obesity may or may not be present. The disorder is more common in postmenopausal women. In premenopausal women, it may be difficult to differentiate it from PCOS.

- The androgens are converted to oestrogens in the peripheral tissues, increasing the risk of endometrial hyperplasia and cancer, especially in postmenopausal women.

Luteoma of pregnancy: This is a benign hyperplasia of the ovary that causes virilisation in the foetus and mother. The condition regresses spontaneously after delivery.

Androgen-producing tumours of the ovary: Androgen-producing tumours of the ovary are mostly sex cord-stromal tumours (SCSTs) and are uncommon.

- Leydig cell tumours (hilus cell tumours) and stromal luteomas occur in the postmenopausal age and are benign.
- Sertoli–Leydig cell tumours are low-grade malignant tumours and are usually diagnosed at an early stage. They occur in the reproductive age.
- Steroid cell tumours are rare SCSTs, composed of cells that resemble steroid hormone-secreting cells.
- Gynandroblastomas are rare tumours containing ovarian and testicular elements.
    - *Adrenal hyperandrogenism:*
        - Congenital adrenal hyperplasia (CAH)
        - Nonclassic CAH
        - Cushing's syndrome
        - Adrenal tumours—adenomas and carcinomas

Congenital adrenal hyperplasia:

- Congenital adrenal hyperplasia is an autosomal recessive disorder that results from an enzymatic defect in the cortisol synthesis pathway.
- Deficiency of 21-hydroxylase is the most common, but 11β-hydroxylase defects and 3β-hydroxysteroid dehydrogenase deficiencies can also occur.
- Deficiency of 11β-hydroxylase is the second most common. It is associated with hypertension due to the accumulation of 11-deoxycortisol and deoxycorticosterone, which are weak mineralocorticoids.
- Deficiency of 3β-hydroxysteroid dehydrogenase is rare.
- The classic form of 21-hydroxylase deficiency is congenital and manifests as sexual ambiguity and electrolyte disturbances in the newborn.

Nonclassic congenital adrenal hyperplasia:

- The milder form of 21-hydroxylase deficiency usually referred to as nonclassic congenital adrenal hyperplasia (NCCAH) presents at or after puberty and accounts for 1.5–2% of cases of hirsutism. These patients also have menstrual irregularity, acne and obesity. Hirsutism is more marked than in PCOS, and there is associated virilisation.
- Nonclassic CAH can easily be mistaken for PCOS unless virilisation is looked for.

When 21-hydroxylase is deficient, the substrates, namely DHEA and 17α-hydroxyprogesterone, accumulate in the system. DHEA is converted to testosterone in the peripheral tissues. The lack of cortisol leads to a compensatory increase in ACTH production, and the androgen production increases further. Elevation of serum 17α-hydroxyprogesterone (early morning sample is a diagnostic of 21-hydroxylase deficiency).

Cushing's syndrome: Cushing's syndrome refers to the effects of excess of circulating glucocorticoids as a result of exogenous administration or endogenous production. The most common cause of excessive endogenous production is Cushing's disease, which is an excessive production of glucocorticoids by the adrenal gland secondary to increase in ACTH levels. This can cause hirsutism and menstrual irregularity. This is because ACTH stimulates adrenal androgen production as well. These women have other clinical features of Cushing's disease such as obesity, purple abdominal striae, nuchal fat pad, proximal weakness, bone pains, menstrual irregularity, secondary diabetes mellitus and hypertension. In these patients, hirsutism and virilisation, if present, tend to be mild, and the other clinical features of Cushing's disease dominate the clinical picture. The condition can be mistaken for PCOS, and further evaluation by dexamethasone suppression tests is required to establish the diagnosis.

Adrenal tumours: They are adenomas and carcinomas and secrete DHEA-S and androstenedione, which get converted into testosterone peripherally. Markedly elevated levels of DHEA-S usually indicate adrenal tumour. They can be visualised on computed tomography (CT) scan or magnetic resonance imaging (MRI). These tumours of the adrenal glands are rare.

- Increased proportion of unbound androgens: This is generally due to a reduction in SHBG. Oestrogens increase the SHBG level, but androgens decrease it. Hyperinsulinaemia also decreases hepatic synthesis of SHBG. Therefore, conditions that cause hyperandrogenism also reduce the SHBG levels and cause further increase in serum levels of the free testosterone.

DIAGNOSIS OF HYPERANDROGENISM

History and physical examination play an important part in the management of hirsute women. Important points in history taking are as follows:

- *Menstrual history:* Age at menarche, cycle-regularity, oligomenorrhoea/amenorrhoea and sudden changes in weight
- *Drug history:* Use of oral contraceptive preparations (OCPs), methyltestosterone, anabolic drugs, diazoxide, danazol, cyclosporine and hormone replacement therapy (HRT)
- Recent or current pregnancy
- Rapidly increasing hirsutism: Suggestive of androgen producing tumour
- History of acne/seborrhoea/temporal balding
- History of easy bruising/striae/thin skin: Symptom of Cushing's syndrome
- Family history of PCOS and hyperandrogenism.

Hyperandrogenism may be diagnosed on physical examination if biological signs of androgen excess are present. These signs include excessive sexual hair growth, acne, male pattern baldness, deepening of the voice, enlargement of the clitoris, reduction in breast size and male muscular development. A careful breast examination should be performed to look for galactorrhoea. Body mass index (BMI) should be calculated. Symptoms of thyroid disorder should be investigated. Signs of hyperinsulinaemia such as the presence of acanthosis nigricans should be sought. Any mass palpable per abdomen should be evaluated to rule out ovarian tumours.

Hirsutism and normal menstrual cycles: Women with hirsutism and normal menstrual cycles are most likely to fall into the category of PCOS or idiopathic hirsutism and are unlikely to have a more serious cause for their hirsutism. Measuring of serum total testosterone would be sufficient in these patients.

Hirsutism with oligomenorrhoea/amenorrhoea: Women with hirsutism and irregular menstrual cycles have an underlying endocrine disorder. Many, if not most, women will be diagnosed with PCOS. Measuring serum total testosterone as well as a routine evaluation for oligomenorrhoea/amenorrhoea [human chorionic gonadotrophin (hCG), prolactin, follicle-stimulating hormone (FSH) and thyroid-stimulating hormone (TSH)] and an early morning 17-hydroxyprogesterone (around 8 am) may be necessary. Although the menstrual dysfunction will almost always be due to PCOS or, in some cases, NCCAH due to 21-hydroxylase deficiency, the possibilities of pregnancy, hyperprolactinaemia, primary ovarian insufficiency and thyroid disease should not be overlooked.

The distribution and extent of hirsutism should be documented by the *modified Ferriman-Gallwey score*. This scoring system quantitates the hair growth in nine androgen-sensitive areas; each area gives scores from 0 to 4, adding up to a total score of 36.

- Upper lip
- Chin
- Chest
- Upper abdomen
- Lower abdomen
- Upper arm
- Thighs
- Upper back
- Lower back

A score of 8 or more is considered as hirsutism **(Fig. 1)**. Hirsutism is graded as mild (score 8–15), moderate (score 16–25) and severe (score >25).

It is important to ask the woman when she last removed hair before scoring and assessment of hirsutism.

LABORATORY EVALUATION

- *Serum total testosterone:* It is best assessed by liquid chromatography-tandem mass spectroscopy (LC-MS/MS), an accurate and specific method. With LC-MS/MS, the upper limit of normal for serum testosterone in women is in the range of 45–60 ng/dL (1.6–2.1 nmol/L). The immunoassays that are available in most hospital laboratories are not suitable to accurately measure testosterone in women. Women with PCOS have serum testosterone concentrations that may be in the normal range [up to the upper limit of normal, which varies between 45 and 60 ng/dL depending upon the laboratory (0.69–2.1 nmol/L)], or elevated but <150 ng/dL (5.2 nmol/L). Although the degree of hyperandrogenaemia may not correlate well with the severity of hirsutism, it does appear to correlate with metabolic risks observed in women with PCOS. Total testosterone values above 150 ng/dL (5.2 nmol/L) should prompt additional evaluation for a testosterone-secreting ovarian or adrenal tumour as well as ovarian hyperthecosis. Both disorders are seen more commonly in postmenopausal women but occur occasionally in premenopausal women.

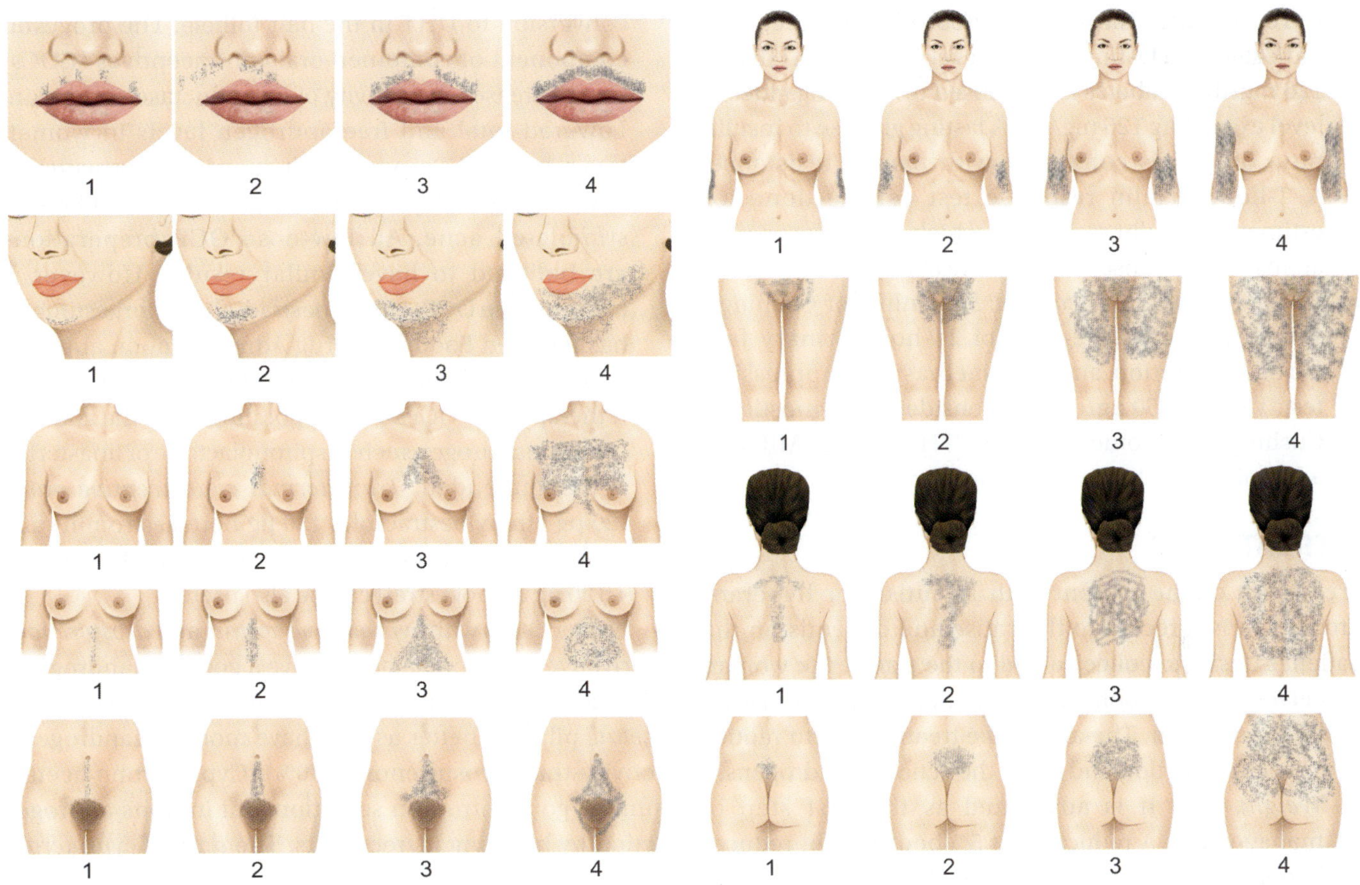

Fig. 1: Grading severity of hirsutism in patients.

- *17-hydroxyprogesterone:* Testing for NCCAH due to 21-serum hydroxylase deficiency in hyperandrogenic women by measuring an 8 am 17-hydroxyprogesterone level. This is measured in the mornings to avoid later elevated values due to a diurnal pattern of ACTH secretion. The most common form of CAH is 21-hydroxylase deficiency. For women who have some spontaneous menstrual cycles, this should be done in the early follicular phase, while for those without cycles, it can be drawn on a random day. A morning value of 17-hydroxyprogesterone >200 ng/dL in the early follicular phase strongly suggests the diagnosis, which may be confirmed by a high-dose (250 μg) corticotrophin (ACTH) 1-24 (cosyntropin) stimulation test. The response to cosyntropin is exaggerated, with most patients having values exceeding 1,500 ng/dL (43 nmol/L) 60 minutes after administration of cosyntropin.
- *Free testosterone:* Not routinely measured. However, free testosterone (0.3–6 pg/mL) measured by equilibrium dialysis is a sensitive test for detecting hyperandrogenic disorders, but it must be performed in a specialty laboratory. Free testosterone by the analogue method ('direct') is not accurate and should not be ordered. It increases from 1 to 2% in women with an ovulation and PCOS.
- *Serum DHEA-S:* Mildly elevated levels of DHEA-S are unlikely to affect management. Levels >700 ng/dL are considered markers for abnormal adrenal function.
- *Serum TSH and prolactin:* Hypothyroidism and hyperprolactinaemia cause reduced SHBG, which leads to increased free testosterone. Hyperprolactinaemia and thyroid disorders may produce hyperandrogenism directly by affecting androgen production and indirectly by creating an anovulatory state.
- *Insulin function:* Because hyperandrogenism and hyperinsulinaemia are often associated, a comprehensive workup includes the *assessment of insulin function*. Diabetes mellitus may be excluded by determining that the fasting glucose level is

<116 mg/dL. Impaired glucose tolerances are indicated by a fasting glucose level of between 116 and 126 mg/dL. Diabetes is diagnosed by a fasting glucose level exceeding 126 mg/dL. A fasting glucose to insulin ratio of <4.5 is consistent with insulin resistance. A 2-hour insulin response test can be done for estimating insulin resistance, which is diagnosed with an insulin response of 100–150 μU/mL.

- *24-hour urinary free cortisol:* Screening for Cushing's syndrome—measurement of 24-hour urinary free cortisol excretion and dexamethasone suppression test. Values >250 μg/day are considered diagnostic for Cushing's syndrome. Plasma ACTH, pituitary MRI and adrenal CT can be done in suspected cases.

TREATMENT

Treatment of the patient with hirsutism or hyperandrogenism is directed to the cause and depends on the patient's desire to conceive and to the extent, the woman perceives it as a problem. Most patients have increased levels of androgen. The aim of the treatment is to reduce androgen production and block the action of androgens.

- *Weight loss:* It is advocated as the first step of management. A reduction of 5% body weight reduces hyperinsulinaemia and androgen levels.
- *Removal of source of androgen production:* Adrenal and ovarian tumours secreting androgens should be surgically removed. Cushing's disease can be treated by adrenalectomy. ACTH-producing tumours can be removed by trans-sphenoidal surgery.

If pregnancy is not desired, then the therapy is directed towards stopping the development of new hair growth, removing existing excessive hair growth and regulating the menstrual cycle. Hirsutism is slow to respond to hormone suppression, and results may not be seen for up to 6 months. In addition, previously established hair patterns do not change with androgen suppression. *Mechanical methods of hair removal* such as shaving, waxing, depilatories and electrolysis should also be considered.

- *Oral contraceptive preparations:* Combined OCPs containing oestrogen+progesterone diminish circulating gonadotrophin levels and increase SHBG levels. Lowering of gonadotrophin levels results in decreased ovarian androgen secretion, which produces lower circulating levels of androgens. Increasing SHBG levels (due to the oestrogen component of combined OCPs) result in less free testosterone available for conversion to DHT in the hair follicle. The progestin component of combined oral contraceptives (COCs) also decreases the activity of 5α-reductase at the skin. Lowered total and free androgen levels in women treated with OCPs cause a reduction in the formation of new androgen-dependent hair growth and androgen-stimulated acne. All low-dose OCP preparations are believed to have similar results. However, a combination OCP (ethinyloestradiol and norgestimate) has received Food and Drug Administration approval to be prescribed specifically for the treatment of acne. If therapy with OCPs is disappointing, then the addition of an antiandrogen such as spironolactone or finasteride is recommended. *Transdermal contraceptive patch* (20 μg ethinyloestradiol + 150 μg norelgestromin) and *vaginal contraceptive ring* (15 μg ethinyloestradiol + 120 μg etonogestrel) can be also used.

Newer OCPs with *cyproterone acetate* and *drospirenone* (derivative of spironolactone) have a good antiandrogenic effect and are helpful in managing hirsutism. *Cyproterone acetate* pills are better as they have more antiandrogenic activity than drospirenone (30%). Cyproterone acetate inhibits gonadotrophin secretion and inhibits androgen action by blocking its receptors. The *dose of cyproterone acetate is 50–100 mg from day 5 to 14 of cycles plus 30–50 μg ethinyloestradiol per day from day 5 to 25 of cycles.* Improvement in facial hirsutism is noted after 2–3 months of use. Side effects include fatigue, weight gain, mastalgia and loss of libido.

- *Medroxyprogesterone acetate:* If combination OCPs are contraindicated or not desired, then the medroxyprogesterone acetate, given as 10 mg for 10–12 days every month or every other month, may be used to produce regular withdrawal bleeding to reduce the risk of menorrhagia or endometrial hyperplasia or both. Patients should be cautioned that, unless contraception is used, pregnancy is possible with cyclical progestin therapy.
- *Spironolactone therapy:* It is often initiated if OCP use is not an option for the treatment of hirsutism or if results from OCP therapy are not optimal. An aldosterone antagonist, having structural similarity with progestins, spironolactone, is an asteroid compound originally dispensed as an antihypertensive agent. Its activity as an antiandrogen was detected after men receiving the compound developed gynaecomastia. Spironolactone inhibits the binding of DHT to its receptor and directly

inhibits 5α-reductase. Spironolactone also decreases androgen synthesis by inhibiting 17α-hydroxylase and 17, 20-lyase. After 6 months of therapy at 100–200 mg/day, a reduction in the diameter of the terminal hair and cessation of new terminal hair growth are observed. Doses may be tapered down to a maintenance dose of 25–50 mg/day. Because of potential adverse effects on the development of the external genitalia of male foetuses, spironolactone should be used together with contraception in sexually active women. Side effects include diuresis, fatigue, dysfunctional uterine bleeding, hyperkalaemia and breast enlargement.

- *Flutamide:* It is a nonsteroidal antiandrogen that blocks the binding of androgen to its receptor. It was developed initially for the treatment of prostate disease. When administered in a dosage of 250 mg/day, decreased terminal hair diameter and cessation of new hair growth are observed. Side effects include dry skin and a rare but severe hepatotoxicity. Liver function should be monitored. During pregnancy, flutamide may have a detrimental effect on male foetal development. Therefore, concurrent therapy with OCPs or other contraception is encouraged.
- *Finasteride:* An inhibitor of type II 5α-reductase, finasteride, was developed initially as a treatment for prostate hypertrophy and cancer. By inhibiting 5α-reductase, the drug decreases the DHT activity at the hair follicle. Two types of 5α-reductase enzyme activity exist, type I and type II. Although finasteride treatment prevents new hair growth and decreases the terminal hair shaft diameter, it does not appear to completely inhibit type-I 5α-reductase, which is present in the skin. Finasteride is orally dosed at 5 mg daily. Apart from dizziness, weakness and occasional headaches, no major side effects have been associated with this drug. There is a potential risk in the male foetus during pregnancy as DHT participates in the development of male external genitalia. Adequate contraception should be used. Finasteride is also available in a lower-dose preparation, 1 mg (Propecia), and has been approved for the treatment of hair loss in men.
- *Cimetidine:* 300 mg QDS—improves hirsutism by androgen receptor-blocking agent.
- *Ketoconazole:* 400 mg/day blocks androgen synthesis by inhibiting the cytochrome P450 system.
- *Newer agents: Eflornithine hydrochloride, 13.9% cream:* Twice daily application—it is an inhibitor of ornithine decarboxylase which is a dermal papillary enzyme essential for hair growth. Best for mild facial hirsutism. Improvements occur in the first week of application. When combined with laser therapy, better and rapid responses are achieved.

LASER and pulsed light therapies: Selectively target the hair bulb. Four to six therapies are required at 6-weekly intervals. If pregnancy is desired by individuals with hyperandrogenemic chronic anovulation syndrome, then assistance with ovulation induction frequently is required.

Cosmetic treatment of hirsutism: It is useful when permanent hair have grown.

- *Glucocorticoid agents:* Individuals diagnosed with late-onset adrenal hyperplasia may be treated by administration of glucocorticoid agents to restore ovulation. This treatment also reduces circulating androgen levels. Glucocorticoid administration is therefore appropriate therapy for infertility or hirsutism in individuals with late-onset adrenal hyperplasia. In patients with 21-OH deficiency, prednisone, 5 mg before bedtime, is used to suppress endogenous ACTH. Alternatively, the same hormone therapy indicated for individuals with hyperandrogenemic chronic anovulation may be used in individuals with late-onset adrenal hyperplasia. OCPs or antiandrogens may be used successfully to treat hirsutism, alone or in combination with dexamethasone. Ovulation-inducing drugs may also be used to treat infertility.
- *Surgical:* Androgen-producing ovarian or adrenal tumours usually are treated surgically. Depending on the type of tumour, additional treatment with chemotherapy or radiation therapy may be required.

CONCLUSION

- Hirsutism is the excessive growth of terminal hair in a male distribution. Hirsutism is the result of excessive androgen production by the adrenal glands or ovaries.
- Out of all the circulating androgens, only the free fraction of testosterone is biologically active.
- Polycystic ovarian syndrome is the most common cause of hyperandrogenism and hirsutism.
- Adrenal androgen production increases in CAH and adrenal tumours.

- Serum total testosterone levels must be measured as the initial step in the diagnostic workup of hirsutism.
- The management of hirsutism is by cosmetic and physical measures and medications.

SUGGESTED READING

1. Derksen J, Nagesser SK, Meinders AE, Haak HR, van de Velde CJ. Identification of virilizing adrenal tumors in hirsute women. N Engl J Med 1994;331(15):968.
2. Ferriman D, Gallwey JD. Clinical assessment of body hair growth in women. J Clin Endocrinol Metab. 1961;21:1440.
3. Friedman CI, Schmidt GE, Kim MH, Powell J. Serum testosterone concentrations in the evaluation of androgen-producing tumors. Am J Obstet Gynecol. 1985;153(1):44.
4. Martin KA, Anderson RR, Chang RJ, Ehrmann DA, Lobo RA, Murad MH, et al. Evaluation and treatment of hirsutism in premenopausal women: an endocrine society clinical practice guideline. J Clin Endocrinol Metab. 2018;103(4):1233.
5. Meldrum DR, Abraham GE. Peripheral and ovarian venous concentrations of various steroid hormones in virilizing ovarian tumors. Obstet Gynecol. 1979;53(1):36.
6. O'Driscoll JB, Mamtora H, Higginson J, Pollock A, Kane J, Anderson DC. A prospective study of the prevalence of clear-cut endocrine disorders and polycystic ovaries in 350 patients presenting with hirsutism or androgenic alopecia. Clin Endocrinol (Oxf). 1994;41(2):231.
7. Rosenfield RL. Clinical practice. Hirsutism. N Engl J Med. 2005;353(24):2578.
8. Rosner W, Auchus RJ, Azziz R, Sluss PM, Raff H. Position statement: utility, limitations, and pitfalls in measuring testosterone: an Endocrine Society position statement. J Clin Endocrinol Metab. 2007;92(2):405.
9. Rosner W, Vesper H, Endocrine Society, American Association for Clinical Chemistry, American Association of Clinical Endocrinologists, Androgen Excess/PCOS Society, et al. Toward excellence in testosterone testing: a consensus statement. J Clin Endocrinol Metab. 2010; 95(10):4542.
10. Wild RA, Carmina E, Diamanti-Kandarakis E, Dokras A, Escobar-Morreale HF, Futterweit W, et al. Assessment of cardiovascular risk and prevention of cardiovascular disease in women with the polycystic ovary syndrome: a consensus statement by the Androgen Excess and Polycystic Ovary Syndrome (AE-PCOS) Society. J Clin Endocrinol Metab. 2010;95(5):2038.
11. Wilson RC, Nimkarn S, Dumic M, Obeid J, Azar MR, Najmabadi H, et al. Ethnic-specific distribution of mutations in 716 patients with congenital adrenal hyperplasia owing to 21-hydroxylase deficiency. Mol Genet Metab. 2007;90(4):414.

26

CHAPTER

Epithelial Abnormalities of the Genital Tract

Shyamala Guruvare, Muralidhar V Pai

Chapter Outline

Vulva
- Senile Atrophy
- Lichen Sclerosus
- Vulvar Intraepithelial Neoplasia

Vagina
- Vaginal Intraepithelial Neoplasia

Cervix
- Cervical Intraepithelial Neoplasia

Uterine Corpus
- Endometrial Hyperplasia without Atypia
- Endometrial Hyperplasia with Atypia

Fallopian Tube

INTRODUCTION

The clinical and histological appearances of the various parts of the genital tract can vary considerably, although in many instances, the pathological changes are part of a continuing process. In some cases, this process may be reversible; in others, it may be static, while in some, it may be irreversible and the possibility of malignant change increased **(Figs. 1 and 2)**.

The skin of the vulva is commonly the site of chronic and resistant changes, the pathogenesis of which is obscure. Comparable changes are seen in the male and affect the scrotum and phallus.

Epithelial abnormalities of the vulva may appear clinically as white patches or plaques (so-called leucoplakia from the Greek, 'leuco' meaning white and 'plax' meaning a flat plate), as reddened areas, or as a combination of both. The naked eye appearances give little clue **(Fig. 3)** to the underlying histological features and yet it is these which will determine the outcome. The term leucoplakia, which is commonly used to describe the clinical appearance of the vulva, should not be used as a definitive diagnosis. It is imprecise and as such may be easily misinterpreted.

To avoid this ambiguous term, Professor Jeffcoate in 1966 introduced the term dystrophy into the nomenclature of benign vulvar epithelial lesions. The term dystrophy is no longer used either. The vulvar lesions are categorised as inflammatory, cysts, non-neoplastic proliferations and neoplasms. The inflammatory lesions can be lichenoid or acanthotic. The squamous epithelial abnormalities which are characterised by epithelial growth and maturation are grouped under the general term—non-neoplastic epithelial disorders of skin and mucosa at the recommendation of the International Society for the Study of Vulvovaginal Disease (ISSVD) **(Box 1)**. The epithelial neoplasia of the vulva are classified broadly as human papillomavirus (HPV) associated lesions and HPV-independent lesions as per the 2020 World Health Organization (WHO) classification **(Table 1)**.

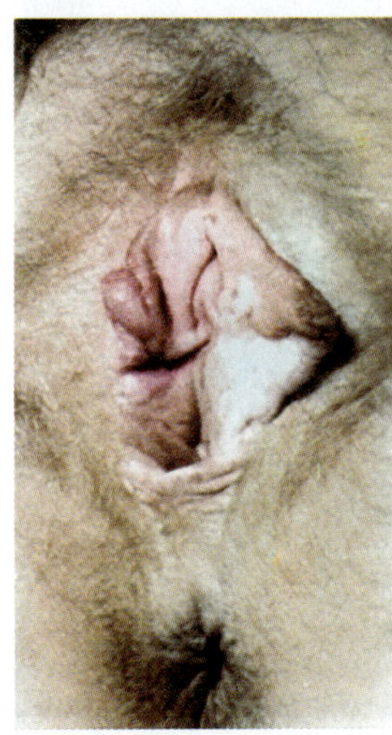

Fig. 1: A hyperkeratotic form of chronic vulvar epithelial disorder, the classical appearance of what in the past was called clinical leukoplakia. This vulva on section showed in different areas histological appearances varying from atrophic epithelium to invasive cancer **(Figs. 2A to D)**.

SENILE ATROPHY

Atrophy and shrinkage of the labia in old age, with some contracture of the introitus, is a normal physiological

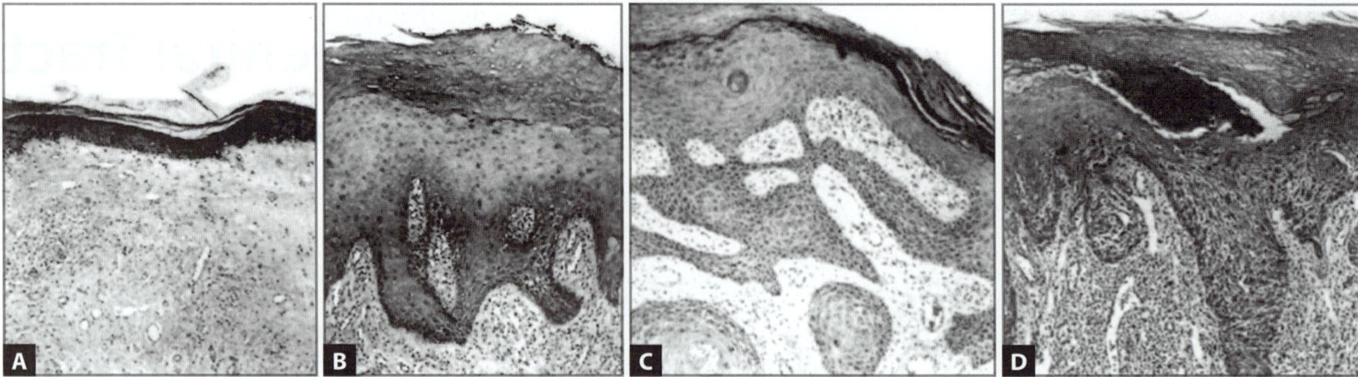

Figs. 2A to D: Varying histological appearances in different parts of the vulva shown in **Figure 1**. (A) An atrophic but hypertrophic epithelium with subepithelial degenerative changes and hyalinisation. The picture is typical of lichen sclerosus; (B) This area shows hyperkeratosis and a thicker acanthotic epithelium; (C) A higher power view showing epithelial cells exhibiting pleomorphism, lack of orientation and atypia; a picture of vulvar intraepithelial neoplasia (VIN); (D) This field shows changes indicative of invasive squamous carcinoma.

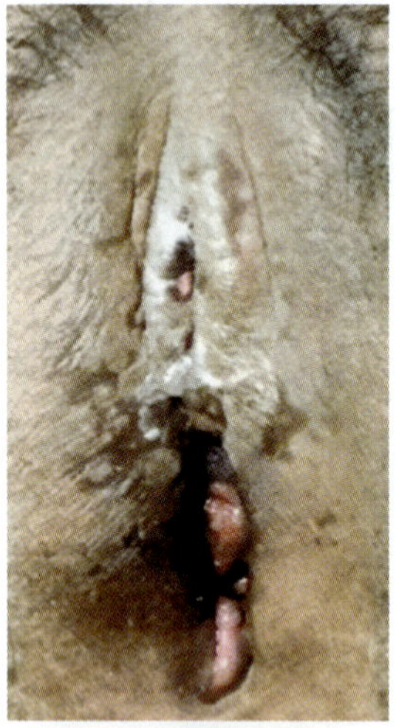

Fig. 3: A chronic vulvar epithelial disorder showing hyperkeratosis and contracture around the clitoris and the foreparts of the vulva. Elsewhere the skin is atrophic. Patchy ulceration from scratching is shown. This appearance might, in the past, have been described as atrophic leucoplakia, kraurosis or primary atrophy.

change attributable to withdrawal of the hormone influences of the ovary and adrenal. The histological features are indicative of atrophy of the epidermis and dermis. Except that, it causes dyspareunia, senile atrophy of the vulva, usually associated with a similar change in the vagina and is symptomless.

LICHEN SCLEROSUS

Lichen sclerosus is the most common white lesion of the vulva. It is most often seen in postmenopausal women. It appears as white, glistening sheets with clearly defined

BOX 1: Classification of epithelial vulvar disease (ISSVD 1989).

- Non-neoplastic epithelial disorders of the skin and mucosa:
  - Lichen sclerosus (formerly hypoplastic dystrophy)
  - Squamous cell hyperplasia (formerly hyperplastic dystrophy)
  - Other dermatoses
- Mixed non-neoplastic and neoplastic epithelial disorders
- Intraepithelial neoplasia:
  - Squamous intraepithelial neoplasia:
    - VIN I
    - VIN II
    - VIN III
  - Non-squamous intraepithelial neoplasia:
    - Paget's disease
    - Tumours of melanocytes, non-invasive
- Invasive tumours

(ISSVD: International Society for the Study of Vulvovaginal Disease; VIN: vulvar intraepithelial neoplasia)

TABLE 1: The 2020 World Health Organization tumor classification.

	Classification
HPV-associated squamous intraepithelial lesions	• Low-grade squamous intraepithelial lesion of the vulva • High-grade squamous intraepithelial lesion of the vulva
HPV-independent VIN	• Differentiated vulvar intraepithelial neoplasia • Differentiated exophytic vulvar intraepithelial lesion • Vulvar acanthosis with altered differentiation

(HPV, human papillomavirus; VIN, vulvar intraepithelial neoplasia)
Source: https://pmc.ncbi.nlm.nih.gov/articles/PMC8494521/figure/FI15454279en-1/

margins and involves the labia, the perineum and the perianal region. The labia minora are adherent to the labia majora, the clitoris is buried and the introitus shrinks. Although the epithelium is not thickened, the naked-eye picture clearly resembles that of what is often called leucoplakia; an alleged difference is that leucoplakia does not extend around the anus.

Histologically, lichen sclerosus shows not only a thin and inactive epithelium but also hyperkeratosis, loss of elastic tissue, hyalinisation of the collagen layer and subepithelial infiltration with leucocytes. Extravasated red cells are commonly seen.

Some say that lichen sclerosus can transform to intraepithelial neoplasia and this in turn to cancer; the majority, however, take the view that lichen sclerosus is never a forerunner of malignant change.

Skin which shows gross injury—with excessive keratinisation and destruction of the dermis—may have reached a stage from which recovery is impossible. This change may represent a permanent degree of damage from ischaemia. Indeed, the development of male and female genital—leucoplakia to a stage of irreversibility has been studied in cases of ariboflavinosis occurring in the tropics.

Table 1: WHO classification of squamous epithelial neoplasias of vulva.

AETIOLOGY

Familial incidence is well recognised and may involve both sexes, e.g. a father and a daughter. It has also been seen in identical and nonidentical twins.

The unusual character of the skin changes in non-neoplastic epithelial disorders is probably explained by environmental factors. The skin in other sites exposed to warmth and moisture tends to react in a similar way. The lesions produced by fungus and other infections between the toes and around the arms closely resemble those of clinical leucoplakia. The mouth and tongue have a similar environment and suffer similar diseases variously described as leucoplakia and lichen. Skin anywhere can be made—leucoplakic by exposure to warm wet poulticing. Finally, it has been shown that grafts of skin from an extragenital site, when used to cover the raw area after vulvectomy for epithelial disorders, often develop the disease. Even more important, abnormal skin transplanted from the vulva to an extragenital site can spontaneously return to normal.

The factors that initiate changes in the vulvar skin are not known for certain, but investigations and therapeutic trials indicate the following possibilities.

Chronic Mechanical Irritation

Constant scratching and rubbing produce lichenification of the skin, the appearances of which are quite different from those of any of the epithelial abnormalities. Although a scratch habit can produce local injury and even neurodermatitis, it is not the cause of an epithelial abnormality. It is the epithelial abnormalities which make a woman scratch, not the reverse, and the resulting lesions are easily distinguished.

Deficiency States

Various external genital epithelial disorders (in males and females) can accompany states of deficiency in iron, folic acid, vitamin B_{12}, riboflavin and possibly other essential factors. Thus, they are seen in cases of anaemia and pellagra. The deficiency can arise from errors in diet, as in the case of the elderly living alone. They can also result from malabsorption syndromes, achlorhydria and chronic diarrhoea.

Autoimmunisation

A weak link with autoimmunisation is established.

Metabolic Upsets

Diabetes mellitus, in addition to causing diabetic vulvitis, is sometimes associated with leucoplakic changes in the vulva.

Infection

Many women with epithelial abnormalities have evidence of fungus infection elsewhere, on the hands and feet particularly **(Fig. 4)**. Digital lesions are rarely caused by Tinea, more often by *Candida* or *Corynebacterium minutissimum*. Vulvar and vaginal candidiasis is often demonstrable by culture. Whenever the perianal skin is involved, an alimentary or local fungus infection should be presumed. Sometimes, it is the patient's husband who has athlete's foot or some other fungal lesion.

Candidiasis can cause hyperkeratotic skin abnormalities and is well shown by the fact that *Candida balanitis* in the male can result in leucoplakic or lichen-like lesions on the glans penis which persist for weeks

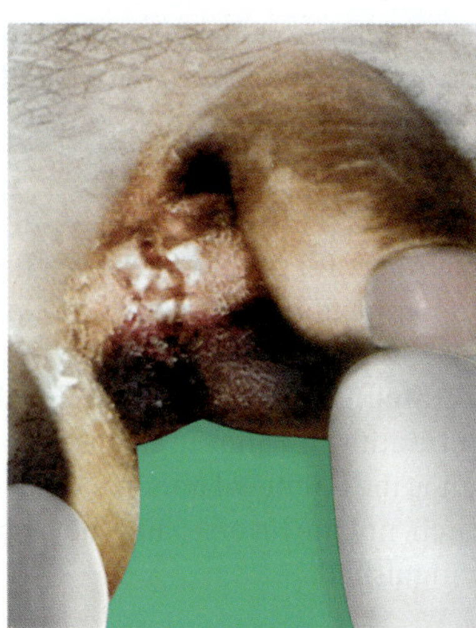

Fig. 4: A chronic interdigital infection (fungus) associated with a chronic vulvar epithelial disorder. The photograph shows the space between two toes, these being held apart by the examining fingers. The skin is hyperkeratotic, sodden, cracked and peeling, producing a lesion very similar in appearance to the one on the vulva. This sort of condition is commonly found in women suffering from vulvar and perianal epithelial changes and pruritus.

despite applications of fungicides. In the case of Tinea pedis infections, the associated vulvar epithelial disorder is more likely to represent an epidermophytide reaction than a spread of the fungus to the vulva. The spirochaete *Borrelia burgdorferi* was implicated in the causation of lichen sclerosus, but this has not been fully substantiated.

SYMPTOMS

Some epithelial abnormalities are symptomless and progress insidiously for many years without the patient's knowledge. Usually, they cause pruritus which is intense and persistent. When the skin cracks, or is broken by scratching, it becomes secondarily infected and painful. Dyspareunia can result from this or contracture of the introitus. The average age at which the patient presents for treatment is 45 years. Nevertheless, vulvar epithelial disorders, and especially lichen sclerosus, are described in childhood when they may or may not cause itching. These usually undergo spontaneous cure at puberty.

DIAGNOSIS

Non-neoplastic epithelial disorders must be distinguished from leucoderma, a condition of patchy depigmentation of otherwise normal skin. More clearly defined skin diseases such as psoriasis have also to be excluded.

The first step in the investigation of a non-neoplastic epithelial disorder is to take portions of affected skin from several sites for histological examination. This is primarily to exclude vulvar intraepithelial neoplasia (VIN), invasive cancer and epithelial activity which carry a threat of cancer in the future. It may also sometimes distinguish the vulvar lesion from a recognised skin disease such as psoriasis. Biopsy is essential in all long-standing lesions, irrespective of their appearance. It is best taken with the 4- or 6-mm Keyes punch under local anaesthesia. Knife biopsies tend to be tangential and often do not reach the deeper layers.

The second step is to attempt to determine a possible underlying cause of the abnormality; the more carefully this is done the more likely it is to be successful. Attention should be paid to the points already mentioned under aetiology while taking the history. Full physical examination should include a search for extragenital lesions, especially in the mouth and ears, and on the hands and feet. The appearance of the vulva itself is not particularly diagnostic. The skin may be white or red or both in patches; it may be thin or thick. Special investigations to be performed in all cases are repeated examination of vaginal and vulvar swabs for *Trichomonas vaginalis* and *Candida albicans*, examination of the blood, tests for achlorhydria, glucose tolerance test, tests for folate and vitamin B12 deficiencies and skin sensitivity tests.

TREATMENT

Treatment depends on the cause and on whether biopsy reveals VIN or epithelial atypia which carries a threat of cancer.

General Treatment

It is important to prevent the patient from scratching and to ensure sleep by giving sedatives, if necessary. During the day, cold cream applications or washing with 1% sodium bicarbonate can provide temporary comfort. The vulva should be kept cool and free from sweat by the wearing of loose and light cotton underclothing. Nylon and similar materials should be banned. At night, a free circulation of air to the vulva should be ensured by supporting the bedclothes with a cradle.

Medical Treatment of the Cause

Treatment is directed primarily to eliminating any aetiological factor discovered. Anaemia is corrected, folic acid or vitamin B_{12} administered if a deficiency is present, glycosuria controlled, candidiasis eradicated and proven antigens avoided. Fungus infections of the feet of either the patient or her husband are treated with fungicides.

When a possible cause is not found, as happens in at least 50% of cases, empirical treatment becomes necessary.

Empirical Measures

Corticosteroids

Clobetasol propionate 0.05% ointment is the definitive treatment of lichen sclerosus. Its safety and efficacy have been documented in a dose not exceeding 30 g over a period of 3 months. The skin immune response and reversal of squamous hyperplasia have been demonstrated in biopsies of treated patients. Monitoring is important. The response is usually sustained. A combination of steroids with antibacterial agents may be required in cases with secondary infection. Treatment may need to be continued for 6–12 months in some patients. After completion of therapy, an emollient cream may be applied regularly.

Oestrogens and Testosterone

Oestrogen therapy only helps to clear up a secondary infection of the vulva in postmenopausal women.

Testosterone propionate 2% in petrolatum was considered the standard treatment for lichen sclerosus, applied twice daily for 3–6 weeks and then once or twice a week. However, nearly 70% of patients have been found to discontinue therapy because of a lack of response as compared to only 10% with clobetasol propionate. Even when a response does occur, it is not sustained if therapy is discontinued. Overdosage can result in virilisation.

Local Analgesia

Anaesthetic ointments containing procaine or similar agents should never be used; they give little symptomatic relief and very often produce severe local reactions. The local injection of anaesthetic solutions is also best avoided; it involves a high risk of abscess formation and does not usually improve symptoms.

Division of Cutaneous Nerves: Nerve Block

Division of all the cutaneous nerves by a circular incision around the vulva gives relief; the effect usually only lasts for 3–6 months but occasionally, and perhaps because it breaks a scratch habit, it is permanent.

Multiple injections of absolute alcohol, presumably to block or damage cutaneous nerves, have been advocated but are rarely effective in the long term.

Vitamins

Large doses of vitamin A or riboflavin can be given orally or by injection. The results are unsatisfactory except when a deficiency state is proven. Atretin and etretinate have been effective orally. However, they have significant side effects.

Fungicides

Whenever a lesion is associated with evidence of an extragenital fungus infection, applications of fungicidal ointments to the vulva are worth trying and can have good results.

Other Local Applications

When the skin is hard and tends to crack, emollient applications to the vulva help. Examples are crude cod liver oil, an emulsion of equal parts of lanoline and arachis oil and a cream made up of zinc oxide (40 parts) and olive oil (60 parts). Whatever treatment is applied, every patient suffering from an epithelial disorder requires continuous supervision for an indefinite period. If the lesion persists or recurs, further biopsies at intervals are required to exclude the possibility of changes in epithelial activity, if not cancer **(Figs. 5A and B)**. One of the remarkable things revealed by late follow-up is that sometimes when a patient, after years of misery, abandons all hope of cure and all treatment, a long-standing epithelial disorder disappears spontaneously.

Vulvectomy

When a non-neoplastic epithelial disorder is localised, local excision or partial vulvectomy may be the best method of biopsy. Otherwise, vulvectomy should be reserved mainly for those cases in which atypical epithelial activity is found histologically **(Figs. 5A and B)**. In these cases, it is clearly indicated and need not be accompanied by lymphadenectomy.

Whenever vulvectomy is performed, it should be followed by treatment of any aetiological factors revealed by investigation, and by regular supervision of the patient for an indefinite period. Invasive carcinoma can supervene despite vulvectomy. If there is no threat of cancer, empirical vulvectomy should be avoided. It is mutilating and gives

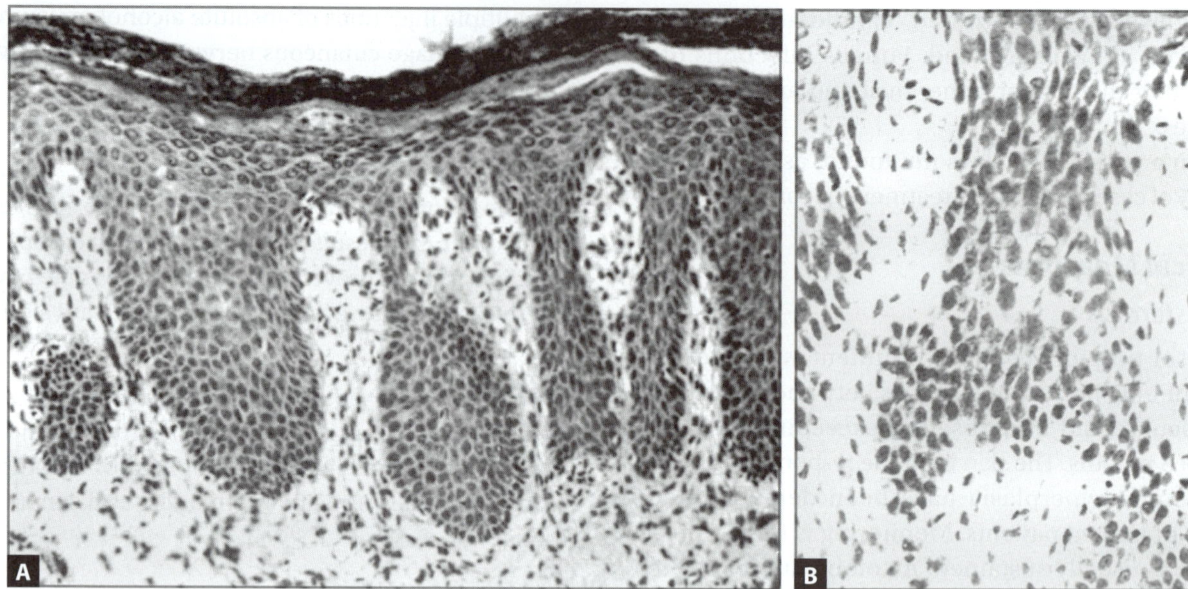

Figs. 5A and B: Moderate vulvar intraepithelial neoplasia (VIN II). (A) There is a layer of keratin on the surface and the underlying epithelium shows a disturbance of normal stratification, which is most severe in the basal two thirds of the epithelium; (B) A high-power photomicrograph shows mitotic figures as well as hyperchromatic nuclei and pleomorphism. Hence, the necessity for mandatory multiple biopsies when a vulvar epithelial disorder is present.

poor results. The disorder recurs sooner or later in 50% of cases treated by vulvectomy, and in skin which, had it been left in its normal site (well outside the labia), would not have become affected. There is no role of vulvectomy in children with lichen sclerosus.

VULVAR AND ORAL EPITHELIAL ABNORMALITIES

Traditional leucoplakia of the vulva is often regarded as being a disease different from leucoplakia of the buccal cavity and tongue. Clinical leucoplakia of the external genitalia is rarely seen in conjunction with oral leucoplakia in the same individual, male or female. Nevertheless, there are some extraordinary bonds between these two areas of the body. Both are erogenous zones; both are common sites for fungal infection; both are subject to recurrent (cyclical) ulceration and both show epithelial changes in deficiency states such as anaemia and ariboflavinosis.

VULVAR INTRAEPITHELIAL NEOPLASIA

Incidence and Aetiology

Vulvar intraepithelial neoplasia is now being discovered with increasing frequency and this may be the result of the modern practice of submitting non-neoplastic epithelial disorders to biopsy, which is the means of bringing most cases to light. The increase appears to be among young, rather than old, women. In 40% of reported cases, the patients were under 40 years of age. It is suggested that the modern involvement of the young is related to their acquiring sexually transmitted virus and other infections. In particular, the HPV is postulated as a causal agent. It is also seen more commonly in smokers.

Pathology

The diagnosis is essentially a histological one and the microscopic patterns fall into two main groups, these having been regarded as separate diseases **(Box 1)**.

Squamous intraepithelial neoplasia ISSVD 2015: Terminologies of vulvar squamous intraepithelial lesions:

- Low-grade squamous intraepithelial lesion (LSIL) of the vulva or vulvar LSIL, encompassing flat condyloma or HPV effect
- High-grade squamous intraepithelial lesion (HSIL) or vulvar high-grade squamous intraepithelial lesion (VHSIL) (which was termed 'VIN usual type' in the 2004 ISSVD terminology)
- VIN, differentiated type

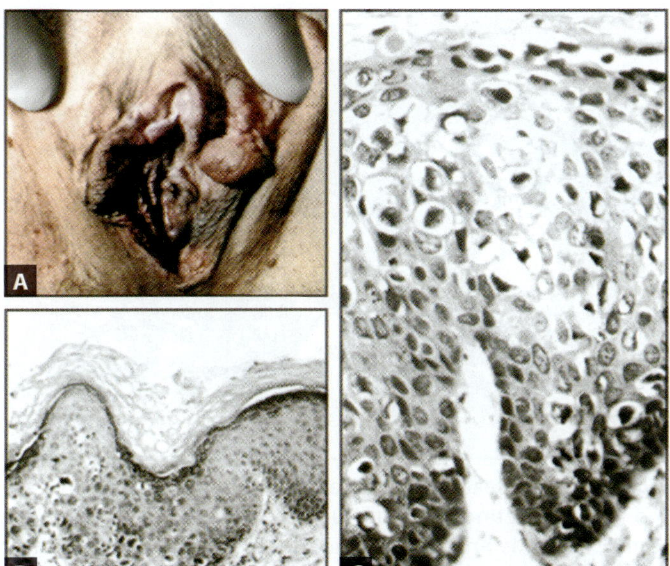

Figs. 6A to C: Vulvar intraepithelial neoplasia (VIN III) of the vulva in a woman aged 35 years who had pruritus for 5 years. Originally, she was treated for proven *Trichomonas* and *Candida* infection with improvement in symptoms; 3 years and 6 months later she returned and the vulva was then rather pale and thickened with one hyperkeratotic plaque which lies medial to the examiner's thumb and condylomatous areas in (A); (B) Photomicrograph of a biopsy specimen showing the junction of hyperkeratotic epithelium and a focus of Bowenoid VIN III. The epithelium shows a loss of stratification, and pleomorphic cells with hyperchromatic nuclei, mitotic figures and koilocytes; (C) A higher power view to emphasise these features. Subsequent simple vulvectomy revealed multiple abnormal foci scattered throughout the vulva on both sides, even in completely normal-looking skin.

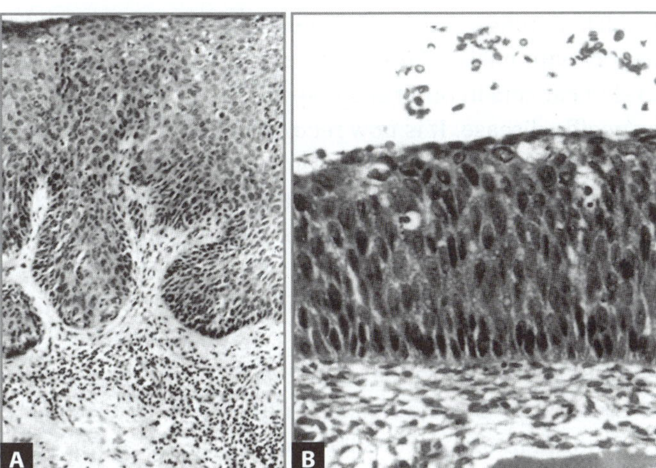

Figs. 7A and B: Vulvar and cervical intraepithelial neoplasia in the same woman who was aged 47 years. She had no complaints but had a routine cervical smear when she attended a special clinic and was also noted to have one small pale area on one labium. When the diagnosis was established, she was treated by cone excision of the cervix and simple vulvectomy. (A) VIN III: One of the many separate foci found throughout the vulva; (B) CIN III: The entire thickness of the epithelium is occupied by darkly staining, hyperchromatic cells with high nucleocytoplasmic ratios, and there is no normal stratification. These are separate lesions but they commonly coexist. Intraepithelial or invasive carcinoma of the cervix or vagina or both is found in 20–25% of cases of VIN, reflecting a field change. (CIN: cervical intraepithelial neoplasia; VIN: vulvar intraepithelial neoplasia)

2020 WHO Terminology

Human papillomavirus-associated squamous intraepithelial lesions: LSIL of the vulva; HSIL of the vulva.

Human papillomavirus-independent VIN: Differentiated vulvar intraepithelial neoplasia (dVIN); differentiated exophytic vulvar intraepithelial lesion (DEVIL); vulvar acanthosis with altered differentiation (VAAD).

The pattern here is similar to that of dysplasia or in situ squamous cell cancer in any site. Depending on whether the lesion is VIN I (mild dysplasia), VIN II (moderate dysplasia) or VIN III (severe dysplasia or carcinoma in situ), changes are seen predominantly in the lower one third, two thirds or the whole thickness of the epidermis, respectively. The cells have malignant characteristics, showing pleomorphism, large irregular and hyperchromatic nuclei and mitotic activity **(Figs. 6 and 7)**. There is a disorderly arrangement of the cells with a loss of stratification. Hyperkeratosis and parakeratosis are variable findings. The recent classification no longer uses the terminology of VIN; VIN I is called LSILs and VINs II and III come under HSILs. This ensures uniformity in the classification of squamous epithelial lesions at all the parts of the lower genital tract and anal region as well. Besides, the lesions of the highest clinical importance, i.e. the lesions likely to progress to invasive cancer are grouped as HSIL.

An essential feature is failure of the cancer cells to penetrate the basement membrane. As in the case of the same condition in the cervix, a stage of microinvasion is described but is more closely related in behaviour to an invasive carcinoma. The term Bowen's disease has often been applied to some cases of intraepithelial neoplasia when large bloated—Bowen's cells and sometimes—corps ronds appear amongst the ordinary cancer cells. The former are large cells showing perinuclear vacuolation and nuclear fragmentation; the latter have small hyperchromatic nuclei and a cytoplasm which stains deeply with eosin. These features, also sometimes found in skin cancers in other sites, were once thought to denote a specific disease. It is now recognised that the large cells represent nothing more than malignant epithelial cells which have undergone degenerative change and nuclear clumping, and there is, therefore, no need to continue using the term—Bowen's disease of the vulva. It is a pattern of VIN found in association with HPV infection, usually type 16.

Vulvar intraepithelial neoplasia occurs by itself but is sometimes a histological finding alongside invasive carcinoma in about 20–30% of cases. HSIL can progress to invasive cancer in <8 years, the incidence being significantly higher in untreated than in treated cases (87.5% vs. 3.8%).

Paget's Disease

Paget's disease of the vulva is a nonsquamous intraepithelial neoplasia associated with proliferation of atypical glandular cells of the apocrine type. In this condition, the epidermis contains large secretory cells arranged singly or in groups, often called—Paget's cells. Their nuclei are polymorphic and hyperchromatic; their cytoplasm is pale and vacuolated and contains a mucopolysaccharide (mucin) similar to that normally secreted by apocrine glands **(Fig. 8)**. This shows up with special stains such as periodic acid-Schiff (PAS). It was once believed that Paget's disease of the vulva was similar to Paget's disease of the nipple in that the special cells are migrants to the epidermis from an underlying or neighbouring adenocarcinoma. Only 30–40% of cases of Paget's disease of the vulva are associated with an adnexal carcinoma. The remainder is intraepithelial neoplasms and the behaviour and treatment of the two groups are therefore different. Paget's disease tends to recur, not necessarily because it is multifocal but because it is an in situ change and because excision is difficult as the edges are ill-defined and the cells extend beyond the apparent clinical limits. So, Paget's disease of the vulva is nothing more than a variant of vulvar intraepithelial neoplasia.

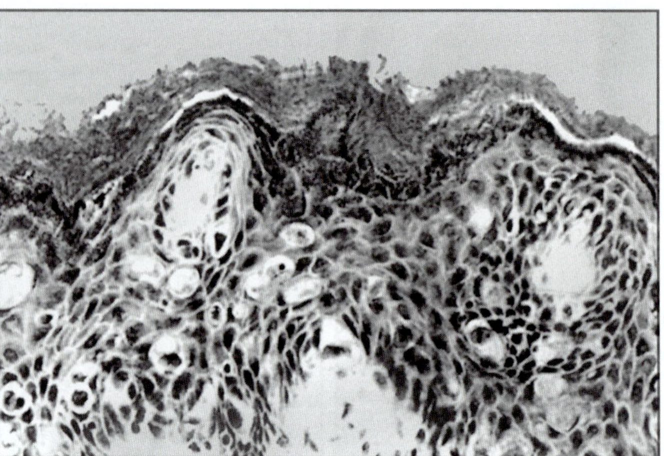

Fig. 8: Paget's disease of the vulva. The section is from an extensive red lesion affecting the introitus of a multiparous woman. The lesion, which is an epithelial adenocarcinoma, recurred after repeated excision for 10 years without ever becoming invasive. In contrast to Paget's disease of the breast, where an underlying carcinoma is the rule, in only about 30% of cases of vulvar Paget's disease is an underlying invasive neoplasm identified. Large Paget's cells with clear cytoplasm which were positive for mucin can be seen within the epidermis.

Clinical Features

Vulvar intraepithelial neoplasia occurs at any age. It is not infrequently associated with a past or present history of intraepithelial neoplasia or invasive cancer, of the vagina or cervix or both. This must reflect widespread epithelial unrest affecting the whole lower genital tract (field change). In keeping with this idea is the fact that the lesions on the vulva are often multifocal.

The patient may complain of pruritus vulvae or slight soreness; she is sometimes aware of a change in colour or consistency of the skin. VIN I is never visible macroscopically while higher grades are nearly always visible.

Characteristically, the lesion appears as a bright scarlet, slightly raised and velvety plaque with clearly defined serpiginous edges. This can be a feature of any of the histological types of the disease but is especially likely with Paget's disease. It explains why carcinoma in situ was sometimes called erythroplasia of the vulva and in practice, care is necessary to distinguish the disease from psoriasis.

Although this is the classical picture, the affected skin can look completely normal, brownish, thickened or white and hyperkeratotic **(Fig. 6)**.

Vulvar intraepithelial neoplasia can arise in any part of the vulva but is mostly found around the introitus. From there, it may spread internally to involve the urethral meatus and laterally to the skin of the groins. It is also not uncommon to find the perineal and perianal areas implicated, without much in the way of macroscopic skin change.

Diagnosis

The diagnosis can only be made by histological examination of excised tissue. Cytology for diagnostic or follow-up purposes is generally useless; the cancer cells are not desquamated and are rarely picked up in scrapings of the skin. Areas likely to be affected may be identified by their staining reaction to nuclear stains, specifically 1% toluidine blue and tetracycline fluorescence, which make areas of increased metabolic activity show up. However, the test is of limited value, being nonspecific and unreliable. Colposcopic assessment after the application of 5% acetic acid is of limited value as a screening procedure in demarcating areas before conservative surgery.

If there are multicentric lesions, a skinning vulvectomy with or without skin grafting can be done. In this procedure, the involved skin is excised leaving the subcutaneous tissue intact. A split-thickness skin graft taken from the buttocks or the inner aspect of the thigh may be substituted in its place. This procedure gives excellent cosmetic and functional results. Recurrences of VIN usually occur in the remaining areas of original vulvar skin and are seldom seen in the grafted area. Results are satisfactory in most patients, even without grafting.

The skinning vulvectomy and skin graft procedure requires bed rest for a week, with its consequent potential for morbidity. In the elderly patient, therefore, a simple vulvectomy may be preferred. This also takes into account the likelihood of multiple microscopic foci but does not guarantee against future recurrence.

Destructive therapy using electrocautery, cryotherapy and laser ablation has been tried. This treatment leaves behind a painful ulcer, which may take up to 3 months to heal. The best results are with the carbon dioxide (CO_2) laser but great expertise is required to control the depth of destruction. This depth should be <1 mm in non-hairy and 3 mm in hairy areas. General anaesthesia may be required for large lesions. Postlaser management includes keeping the vulva clean and dry (a hair drier is recommended for this purpose), local application of topical steroids and analgesia—the severest pain occurs 3–4 days postoperatively.

Before treatment, the patient should be told about the possibility of recurrence. She should also be informed about the future risk of invasive cancer and the importance of life-long follow-up. Recurrence occurs in 20–30% of cases.

Treatment

For dVIN, an excisional procedure must always be adopted. For VHSIL, both excisional procedures and ablative ones can be used. The latter can be considered for anatomy and function preservation and must be preceded by several representative biopsies to exclude malignancy. Topical imiquimod (off-label use) is also a choice.

Recent studies favour an approach of using imiquimod in vulvar Paget's disease. Surgery must take into consideration that the extension of the disease is usually wider than what is evident in the skin. A 2 cm margin is usually considered necessary. A wide local excision with 1 cm free surgical margins is recommended for melanoma in situ. Given the relatively slow rate of progression, women with a complete response to therapy and no new lesions at follow-up visits scheduled 6 months and 12 months after initial treatment should be monitored by visual inspection of the vulva annually thereafter. Follow-up should be modulated according to the risk of recurrence (type of lesion, patient age and immunological conditions and other associated lower genital tract lesions)

Immunisation with the quadrivalent or 9-valent HPV vaccine, which is effective against HPV genotypes 6, 11, 16 and 18 and 6, 11, 16, 18, 31, 33, 45, 52 and 58, respectively, has been shown to decrease the risk of VHSIL (VIN usual type) and should be recommended for girls aged 11–12 years with catch-up through age 26 years if not vaccinated in the target age. There are no screening strategies for the prevention of vulvar cancer through early detection of vulvar HSIL (VIN usual type). Detection is limited to visual assessment with confirmation by histopathology when needed.

In young patients, sometimes nothing more than regular supervision is called for. In mild cases, spontaneous cure can be an outcome, but close follow-up is essential.

Topical 5-fluorouracil has been used but is painful and ineffective. Topical gamma interferon may give better results. Radiotherapy is not indicated.

Recurrences of VIN are common, but these probably represent new lesions arising in an unstable epithelium. These may require repeated treatment over the course of many years.

Although VIN always carries a threat of invasive cancer, this rarely develops. However, microinvasive lesions should always be regarded as invasive cancer.

VAGINA

Epithelial abnormalities of the vagina are rare. Basal cell hyperplasia, hyperplasia and vaginal intraepithelial neoplasia (VAIN) of the squamous epithelium can occur in single or multiple patches, at any site.

The first is usually regarded as a reactive response to inflammation; the latter is often associated with intraepithelial neoplasia or invasive cancer of the cervix or vulva, and then represents not extensions of these conditions but independent lesions which reflect a widespread epithelial unrest affecting the whole of the lower genital tract. These epithelial abnormalities are symptomless and the affected epithelium may look normal to the naked eye. Occasionally, they cause red patches on the vaginal wall and often they can be identified by a negative Schiller's iodine test or colposcopy.

Vaginal Intraepithelial Neoplasia

Pathology and Aetiology

Vaginal intraepithelial neoplasia can have a localised or patchy distribution in the vagina, be extensions of cervical intraepithelial neoplasia (CIN) or be associated with similar but separate lesions on the cervix or vulva. HPV infection may occur by way of abrasions from coitus or tampons. In such a situation, the abrasion heals with metaplastic squamous cells which are similar to the immature epithelial cells of the transformation zone (TZ) and HPV may begin its growth here. It may, rarely, be seen many years after radiotherapy for cervical carcinoma. Its histological features are the same as those of CIN. Untreated, or inadequately treated, VAIN may progress to invasive cancer in about 3% of cases.

Clinical Features

To the naked eye, the disease may appear as discrete red areas but often the epithelium looks normal. In the latter case, the lesion is then only discovered accidentally or as the result of routine vaginal cytology or colposcopy examination, especially with associated CIN. Its site may be revealed by failure of the epithelium to stain brown with Lugol's iodine. International Federation for Cancer Prevention and Colposcopy (IFCPC) guidelines for the classification of vaginal intraepithelial lesions allow for structured documentation as well as uniform treatment for vaginal lesions.

Treatment

The treatment of VAIN varies with the circumstances. A clearly defined lesion can be excised or treated by laser vaporisation. Since the disease is often multifocal, adequate surgery may involve total vaginectomy. In the majority of cases, especially in relatively young women, this is unnecessarily radical. In these, and if the disease is symptomless, no treatment other than regular colposcopy assessment is usually indicated.

When treatment is required, the possibilities include local excision, cryotherapy, laser therapy and topical imiquimod.

Vaginal Adenosis

Adenosis of the vagina is a very unusual condition in which columnar epithelium, sometimes multilayered, replaces the squamous lining. It has a patchy distribution, the affected areas having a dull-red granulomatous appearance and failing to stain with Lugol's or Schiller's iodine. The epithelium is cervical in type and secretes mucus. The patient's complaint, if any, is leucorrhoea. Clinically, the condition can be mistaken for intractable vaginitis; histologically, it has to be distinguished from adenocarcinoma.

- Vaginal adenosis results from faulty differentiation or distribution of Müllerian duct tissue during the development of the vagina, one of the causes of this being exposure of the young foetus in utero to oestrogens. If the foetal vagina is exposed to large amounts of a nonsteroidal oestrogen, as used to happen when recurrent abortion was treated by giving the mother massive doses of diethylstilboestrol (DES), it can be permanently affected. The consequence is the finding of vaginal adenosis when the child grows to adolescence or early maturity. This is sometimes associated with minor degrees of vaginal stricture formation, just below the level of the cervix. Today, in the postdiethylstilbestrol era, vaginal adenosis usually occurs in women exposed to other hormones, drugs, trauma, inflammation, vulvovaginal involvement by Stevens-Johnson syndrome (SJS) or toxic epidermal necrolysis (TEN), laser, radiation or chemotherapy (5-fluorouracil).

The chance of this happening is calculated to be very small statistically, but it is serious, because the adenosis may be associated with, or be the forerunner of, a clear cell adenocarcinoma.

Vaginal adenosis can undergo spontaneous cure by metaplasia into squamous epithelium. Failing this, it always needs to be kept under observation and, if it causes symptoms, the appropriate treatment seems to be ablation of the lesions in the hope that squamous epithelium will grow over the raw areas. Progestogen therapy is also advised by some. For extensive and resistant lesions, excision of large areas of the vaginal wall, followed by skin grafting, is reported.

CERVIX

Ectopy

Pathology

A cervical ectopy is a condition in which the squamous covering of the vaginal aspect of the cervix is replaced by columnar epithelium, which is continuous with that lining the endocervix. It is not an area denuded of epithelium as the name implies. Small areas of ulceration sometimes seen microscopically are the results of secondary infection and local trauma or are artefacts. An ectopy has a bright-red appearance with a clearly defined edge, the colour is explained by the underlying vascular tissue showing through a thin epithelium. The columnar epithelium may be arranged in a regular pattern but is sometimes proliferated and heaped up to form villous projections—a papillary ectopy. Beneath the epithelium, the tissues often show round cell infiltration and glandular proliferation **(Fig. 9)**. Some assume that these signs are indicative of a chronic infection which precedes and causes the ectopy (see further). Any inflammatory process, however, is more likely to be secondary, the columnar epithelium having less power of resistance to infection than the normal stratified covering.

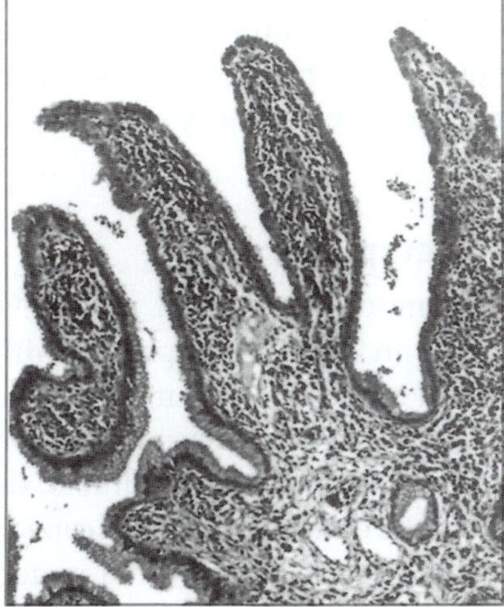

Fig. 9: Cervical ectopy. The squamocolumnar junction lies to the left. The surface of the exposed endocervical tissue is thrown into a series of villus-like structures, which may be seen colposcopically. This is normal (photomicrograph 120×).

An ectopy is not a static condition and the line of demarcation between the two types of epithelium moves to and from the external os. The junctional zone is referred to as the—TZ of the squamocolumnar junction. When it is advancing towards the os, the ectopy is said to be healing. In this process, the proliferating squamous epithelium can obstruct the ducts and produce Nabothian cysts; it may also extend down into the crypts to produce the condition of epidermidisation of the crypts. This phenomenon, however, is better explained by metaplasia of the reserve cells in the endocervix (see further).

An ectopy was formerly thought to predispose to cancer of the cervix, but this view is no longer acceptable. The junctional zone is, however, the site from which cervical smears should be taken.

Aetiology

Congenital and developmental: The stratified epithelium on the surface of the cervix and the endocervical columnar epithelium may have separate origins. Alternatively, and more likely, they represent different types of differentiation of the same parent (Müllerian) tissue. The squamocolumnar junction ordinarily coincides with the external os but may lie either within the cervical canal or outside the external os. In the latter case, the result is a congenital ectopy. This is not a pathological state and is said to be found in at least one third, some say all, female babies at birth, possibly because of exposure to maternal oestrogen in utero. The ectopy tends to disappear during childhood only to reappear at or soon after puberty in one third of teenage girls. This, again, may be an oestrogen effect.

Hormonal: In the adult, as in the foetus and adolescent, a cervical ectopy is determined by the amounts of progesterone and oestrogen in circulation, the probable operative factor being oestrogen. So, even if not present previously, an ectopy commonly and normally develops during pregnancy and then tends to undergo squamous metaplasia during the subsequent 3–6 months. The finding of an ectopy, a few weeks after delivery was formerly thought to be evidence of low-grade puerperal infection and to require treatment. It is now generally recognised that it is a physiological reaction. This concept is confirmed by the fact that the taking of oestrogen-progestogen oral contraceptives often causes an ectopy or makes one more obvious (the so-called—pill ectopy). Indeed, these preparations sometimes result in gross proliferation of the columnar epithelium of the cervix, causing it to move away from the external os. The TZ in the reproductive phase of life is a dynamic area and changes in relation to endogenous and exogenous hormone levels.

All this explains why a cervical ectopy is rarely, if ever, seen in a postmenopausal woman.

Infection: An ectopy of the cervix was once regarded as always being indicative of chronic cervicitis, and surprisingly, there are still some who, in view of the evidence, hesitate to discard this concept. It was, and still is, postulated that the initial infection, operating directly or by altering the vaginal pH and bathing the cervix in discharge, destroys the squamous epithelium around the external os leaving a denuded or potentially denuded area. At the same time, it stimulates overactivity of the endocervical epithelium which grows down and out to cover the raw area. This is pure theory and quite out of keeping with the known natural life history of cervical ectopy. Moreover, it is ruled out by the fact that whenever an area of the portio vaginalis is deliberately denuded, it is the squamous and not the columnar epithelium, which grows in to cover it. Indeed, this is the basis of treating an ectopy by destroying the columnar epithelium with a cautery, diathermy, cryotherapy or laser.

Symptoms

Nearly all ectopies are symptomless. When symptoms are present, the possibilities are as follows:

Discharge: This is essentially an increase of the normal cervical secretion (leucorrhoea) brought about by overgrowth, overactivity and exposure of cervical crypts. It becomes mucopurulent if infection gains entry through the columnar epithelium or if there is coincidental cervicitis. It may even be bloodstained for a few days premenstrually when the tissues are most congested.

Contact bleeding: The epithelial area is fragile and sometimes bleeds on coitus and during defaecation. This symptom, however, should always raise the question as to whether the ectopy is in fact a carcinoma.

Physical Signs and Diagnosis

An ectopy is easily recognised on inspection as a bright red area continuous with the endocervix and with a clearly defined outer edge. Hyperaemia resulting from acute cervicitis, on the other hand, fades gradually into the normal tissues. Surface infection which is part of vaginitis shows as multiple lesions lacking continuity with the endocervix. An ectopy is not tender unless complicated by infection. It often bleeds from multiple pinpoint areas when touched or rubbed with a swab. It feels soft, granular and velvety.

An ectopy has to be distinguished from carcinoma, tuberculosis, syphilitic and other ulcers of the cervix. Although a cervical smear may be helpful, the distinction may not be possible except by colposcopy or biopsy. A common happening, however, is confusion between ectopy and ectropion in which the lips of the cervix are curled back to expose the red endocervix. Such exposure can also be produced as an artefact, merely by opening wide a bivalve vaginal speculum.

Treatment

An ectopy which is symptomless does not ordinarily require treatment. The cauterisation of ectopies discovered on routine postnatal examination is unnecessary and harmful. When symptoms are present and infection and dysplasia are excluded or treated, an ectopy can be treated by electrocautery, cryotherapy using a special probe cooled with nitrogen or CO_2 or CO_2 laser vaporisation. The resulting raw area takes 6–8 weeks to become covered with squamous epithelium. As coitus should be avoided until healing has taken place, this may be an opportunity to temporarily stop oral contraceptive therapy.

Squamous Metaplasia

In theory, squamous epithelium may develop in the cervical canal as an error in the primary differentiation or distribution of Müllerian and urogenital sinus tissues. When found in the adult, however, it is usually the result of metaplasia. Although in tissue cultures, the columnar epithelial cells of the endocervix show a capacity to change to squamous cells, it seems likely that metaplasia stems mostly from a proliferation of the reserve cells which lie deep to the endocervical epithelium **(Figs. 10A to D)**. Initially, these become arranged as a plaque, several layers thick, beneath the surface columnar cells but the latter

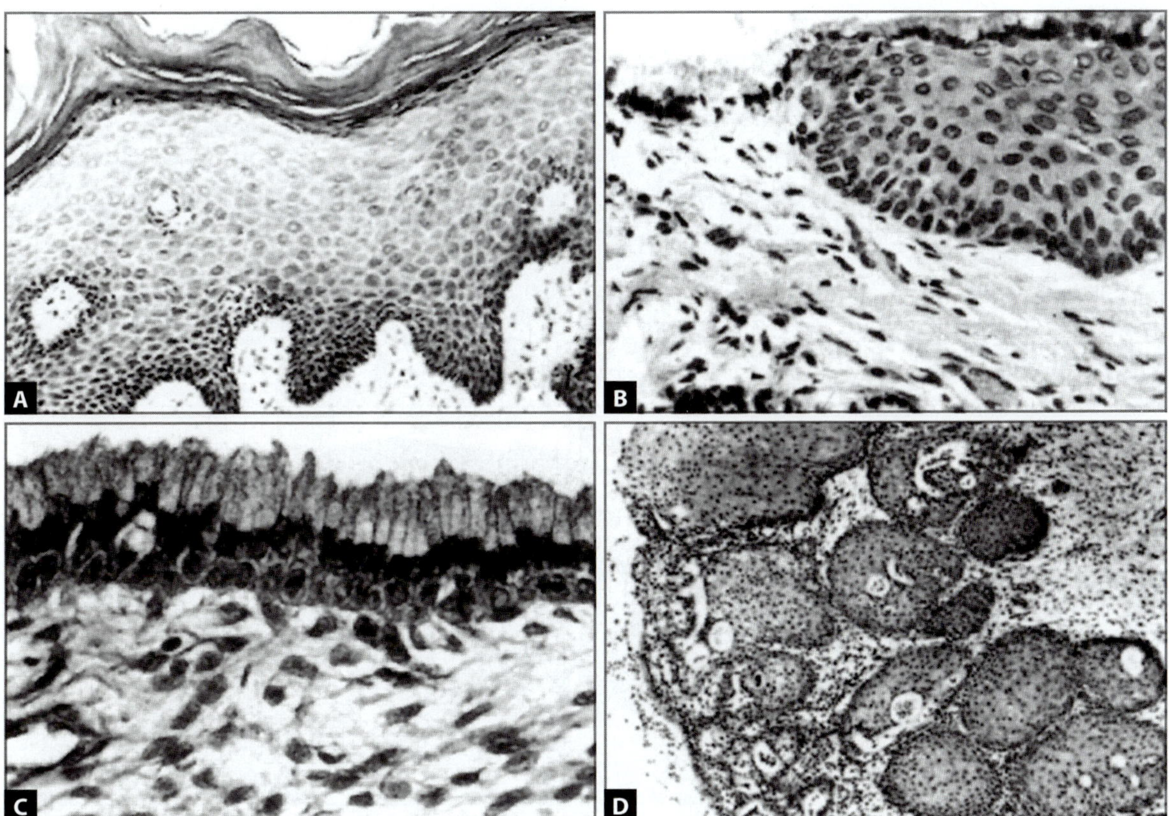

Figs. 10A to D: Benign epithelial changes in the cervix. (A) Reactive squamous cell hyperplasia. An orderly thickening of the epithelium with keratinisation; (B) Reserve cells—a single layer of orderly reserve cells lies beneath the columnar epithelium of the endocervix; (C) Metaplasia—a sheet of immature squamous epithelium, the result of reserve cell proliferation, lies under an intact columnar epithelium; (D) Complete metaplasia—mature squamous epithelium replaces all the columnar epithelium but the outlines of the crypts remain. The picture should not be mistaken for downgrowths of cancer.
Source: Reproduced with permission from Dr Claud Taylor. J Obstet Gynaecol Br Commonw and J Clin Pathol.

tend to break down in areas which then become lined by stratified squamous cells. At this stage, the metaplasia is described as incomplete. In complete metaplasia, which is the same as epidermidisation, there are no columnar cells remaining in affected areas and the squamous epithelium also grows down into the crypts whose columnar epithelium is replaced. In microscopic sections, the resulting islands of squamous cells can be mistaken for malignant downgrowths of carcinoma **(Figs. 11A to D)**. In fact, the proliferation of reserve cells is always regular and devoid of excessive mitosis, nuclear changes and other features of malignancy. So, metaplasia of any degree in the cervix is completely benign.

It is suggested, however, that during the process of metaplasia of columnar cells or of hyperplasia of reserve cells, the tissues are especially prone to virus infections and to take in foreign nucleic acids and that this may start mutations which lead to an increased risk of carcinoma of the cervix. Proliferation of the reserve cells is also postulated as a possible mechanism whereby the raw area of the cervix resulting from cauterisation of an ectopy becomes covered by squamous epithelium. The causes of metaplasia are unknown but one of the stimulating factors is probably the hormone environment of pregnancy; this would explain why it is sometimes found in newborn babies. Local irritants, infections and factors such as alterations in the pH differential at the external os are also suggested. Metaplasia is not uncommonly found in cervical polyps.

Squamous Cell Hyperplasia

This is a benign and orderly hyperplasia of the squamous cell covering the cervix. The whole epithelium can be thickened and microscopically some degree of

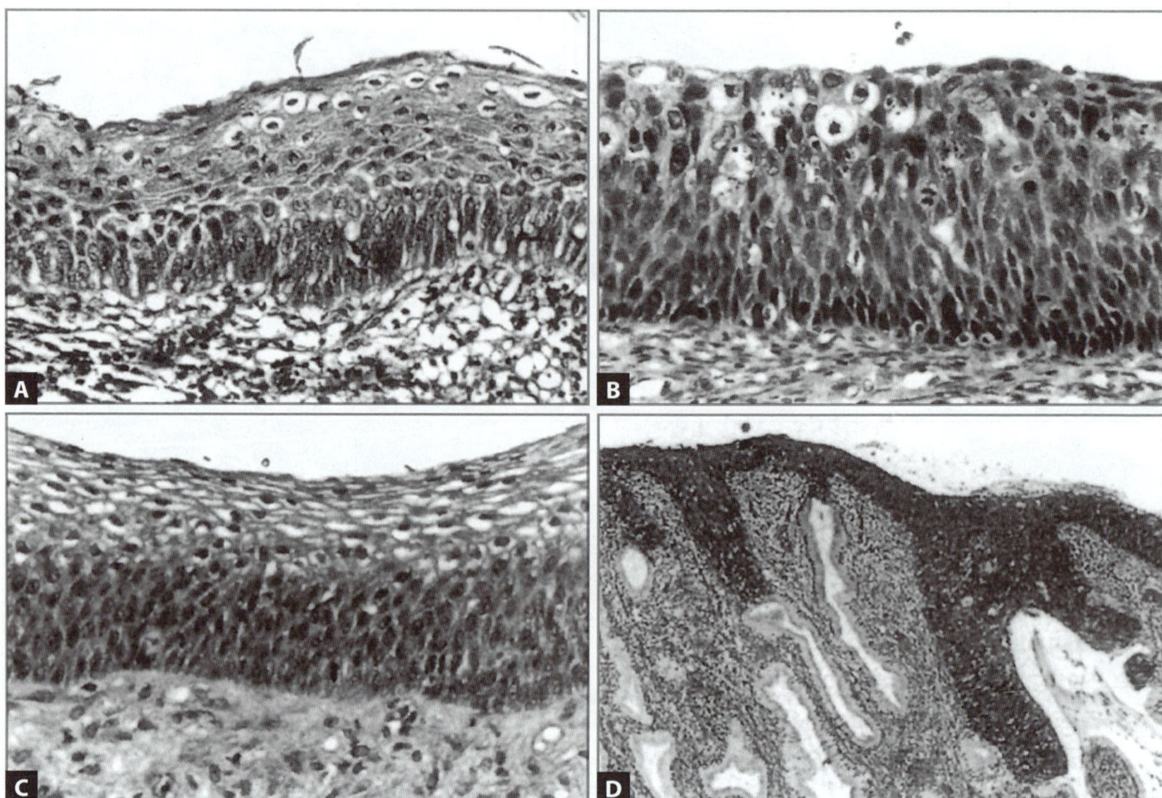

Figs. 11A to D: (A) Cervix, CIN I—the basal third of the squamous epithelium is occupied by cells with high nucleocytoplasmic ratios, lacking stratification. Cytoplasmic maturation occurs in the upper two thirds of the epithelium where there is cellular stratification but nuclear abnormalities persist throughout (photomicrograph 300×); (B) Cervix, CIN II—the cells in the lower half of the epithelium lack stratification have high nucleocytoplasmic ratios and show irregularities of nuclear chromatin distribution. Cytoplasmic maturation and stratification are seen only in the upper half of the epithelium (photomicrograph 300×); (C) Cervix, CIN III—in this example, the full thickness of the epithelium is occupied by abnormal cells with high nucleocytoplasmic ratios, abnormal dispersion of nuclear chromatin and lacking cytoplasm: Mitoses are seen in the middle and upper layers of the epithelium in contrast to their normal basal distribution (photomicrograph 300×); (D) Cervix, CIN III—the surface of the cervix is covered by darkly stained epithelium with the features of CIN III. The atypical epithelium dips down to line several of the endocervical crypts. This appearance should not be mistaken for stromal invasion (photomicrograph 75×). (CIN: cervical intraepithelial neoplasia)

hyperkeratosis, parakeratosis and lengthening of the rete ridges may be seen. The cells, however, do not show atypia. This change can result from local irritation, mechanical in the case of a prolapsed cervix and infective in the case of chronic *Trichomonas* or *Candida* vaginitis. The condition is therefore called reactive hyperplasia **(Figs. 10A to D)**.

In basal cell hyperplasia, the basal cells proliferate to form several layers instead of the usual one or two and they look rather active, tending to have larger nuclei which are hyperchromatic. There is nothing to suggest disorderly behaviour in these cells, and the middle and superficial zones of the squames show good stratification. Both reactive and basal cell hyperplasia are entirely benign and reversible states. Another benign state of reserve cell hyperplasia is described; this can involve gland crypts and can be mistaken for cancer. It is morphologically identical to early squamous metaplasia described above, but metaplasia is not an inevitable sequel.

Cervical Intraepithelial Neoplasia: Dysplasia and Carcinoma In Situ

A range of intraepithelial abnormalities of varying degrees have been described in the cervical epithelium which are characterised by perversion of squamous cell maturation and differentiation, pleomorphic and hyperchromatic nuclei and an abnormal number of chromosomes. Active mitosis may be apparent in microscopic sections.

The term CIN was introduced to emphasise the unity of those conditions formerly designated dysplasia or carcinoma in situ. CIN has been divided into three grades: (1) CIN I corresponds to mild dysplasia, (2) CIN II corresponds to moderate-to-severe dysplasia and (3) CIN III corresponds to severe dysplasia and carcinoma in situ. CIN is regarded as a single disease and begins at the squamocolumnar junction in the epithelium of the TZ. The interpretation of the histological appearances of the tissue is still subject to individual variation despite the more uniform criteria regarding CIN **(Figs. 11A to D)**. The natural history of CIN is difficult to predict because it is modified by diagnostic procedures and by treatment itself. Genuine regression to normal probably only occurs with CIN I because, in this grade, true CIN will be difficult to distinguish from inflammatory or infective changes. About one quarter of the cases of CINs I and II will progress to a more severe lesion without treatment and over a half of the untreated cases of CIN III will eventually develop invasive carcinoma. The aetiological factors involved are the same as for carcinoma of the cervix.

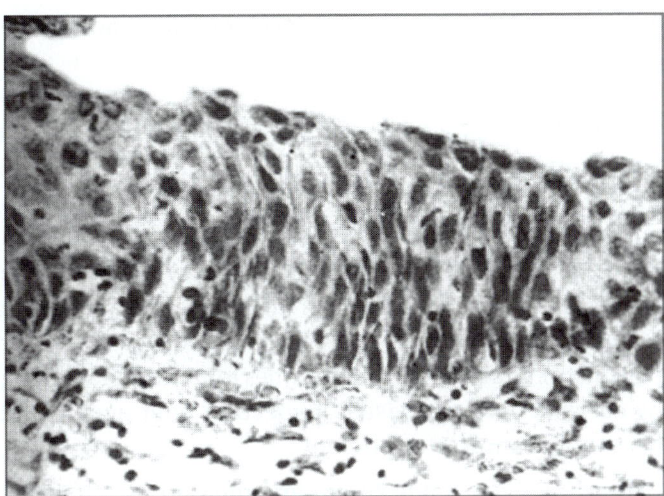

Fig. 12: Cervical intraepithelial neoplasia (CIN) to show the origin of cells seen in **Figure 13**.

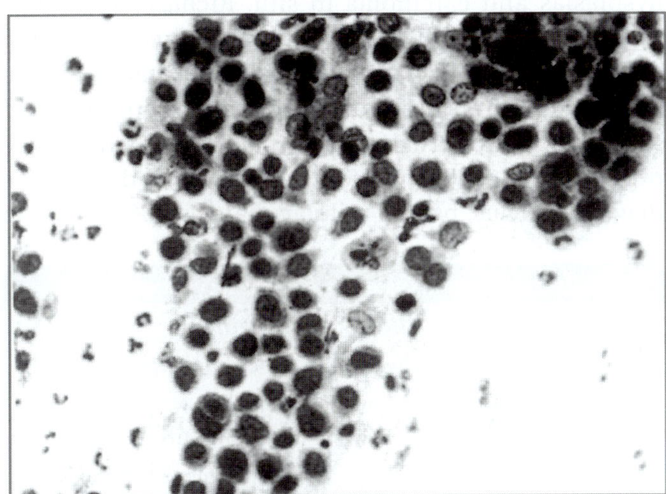

Fig. 13: Cervical smear of cells shed from CIN III shown in **Figure 12** (CIN: cervical intraepithelial neoplasia).

Pathology

Cervical intraepithelial neoplasia is graded according to the proportion of epithelium occupied by undifferentiated cells. In CIN I (mild dysplasia), only the basal third or less of the epithelium is occupied by the undifferentiated cells. A lesion is classified as CIN II (moderate dysplasia) if the cells occupy between one third and two thirds of the epithelium. If more than two thirds of the epithelial thickness is occupied by undifferentiated cells, a diagnosis of CIN III is made (severe dysplasia or carcinoma in situ). In the most severe form of CIN III, atypical cells that occupy the full thickness of the epithelium and mitotic figures, often abnormal, are seen at all levels.

The main histological criteria of CIN III are: A disorderly and disorientated arrangement of closely packed cells throughout the whole thickness of the epidermis with loss of stratification. A few cells on the surface may be flattened, but this does not imply stratification; an intact basement membrane with absence of rete ridges; variation in size and shape of cells; variation in size, shape and staining qualities of nuclei and usually but not always frequent mitoses **(Figs. 11 to 13)**. The nuclei also invariably show a high percentage of abnormal chromosome patterns. The abnormal epithelium of CIN III often extends down into the endocervical crypts.

Frequency and Significance

Among women aged >25 years, CIN III is found in 0.2–0.4%. This is a considerably higher incidence than might be expected if all such lesions progressed to invasive cancer. The discrepancy is explained by the fact that it becomes invasive in not >20–30% of cases. Some put the figure lower, some higher, but observation in either direction can easily be prejudiced.

It takes 1–17 years for an in situ lesion to become invasive, with an average of 10 years. So, the mean age at which carcinoma in situ is found is 35 years and invasive cancer at 53 years, respectively. There is another peak of invasive carcinoma between 30 and 40 years, and in these younger women, the change from an in situ to an invasive lesion appears to be much faster (weeks or months rather than years). Coexisting human immunodeficiency virus (HIV) infection, smoking and immune deficient states may accelerate the pace of the disease.

Diagnosis

Squamous metaplasia, squamous cell hyperplasia and CIN are symptomless conditions, which may show no naked-eye signs of their presence. Indeed, the affected cervix usually looks remarkably healthy. The disease is therefore discovered either incidentally during the histological examination of cervices removed for other reasons, or as a result of programmes for routine screening by cervical cytology, visual inspection after acetic acid (VIA) application or colposcopy.

Cervical cytology: **Table 2** compares the various systems of cytologic classification. Papanicolaou's initial description of five classes was replaced by the WHO system of grading dysplasias and carcinoma in situ. Richart introduced the term CIN to emphasise the continuum of changes. The Bethesda system of cytologic classification, while giving statements about specimen adequacy and general categorisation (normal, benign cellular change or epithelial cell abnormality), also gives descriptive diagnoses. Thus, benign cellular changes may be due to infection or reactive changes. Epithelial cell abnormalities of squamous cells are classified as atypical squamous cells of undetermined significance (ASCUS), LSIL, atypical squamous cells-high grade cannot be excluded (ASCs-H), HSIL and squamous cell carcinoma.

Similarly, glandular cells may be endometrial cells, cytologically benign, atypical glandular cells of undetermined significance (AGCUS) or adenocarcinoma.

Low-grade intraepithelial lesion is a term that includes flat condyloma, CIN I and LSILs. These are usually HPV-related. High-grade intraepithelial lesion is a diagnosis reserved for those cases truly considered precancerous, i.e. CIN II and III **(Flowchart 1)**. Aneuploidy is often seen in these lesions, and these are the ones clinically most relevant to be picked up during screening. Both low-grade and high-grade CINs may involve the glands, but this is of no significance clinically and should not affect the management.

Low-grade CIN mostly reverts to normal, and in some, may persist, or progress to high-grade CIN. Patients with low-grade CIN are at some risk of developing high-grade CIN, but it is not clear whether all high-grade CIN starts as low-grade CIN, or whether some may arise de novo. However, high-grade CIN is undoubtedly a true cervical cancer precursor.

The results of cervical cytology: The accuracy of cytodiagnosis depends on the quality of the smear, the way in which it was obtained as well as on the skill and experience of the cytologist. As many as 10% of smears, prepared from cervical scrapings made by untrained doctors or nurses may have to be discarded. This figure falls to 0.3% when a gynaecologist is responsible. An adequate smear is one which contains cells from the entire TZ and which, therefore, shows squamous metaplastic cells and endocervical cells. It should have adequate cell numbers, be properly fixed and not be obscured by blood or inflammatory exudate.

Using conventional techniques, most of the cells are left behind on the sampling device (and this may include most abnormal cells). The smears are often not spread evenly. Liquid-based preparations are being developed to enhance the quality of the smear by transferring the entire sample onto the slide; the sampling implement is rinsed in a liquid preservative which is transported to the laboratory where a subsample, thin-layer preparation is made (thin prep). This is expected to minimise the wastage of samples. Besides, liquid-based cytology has the advantage of the sample being available for reflex HPV testing or for repeat smears.

TABLE 2: Classification systems for cervical cytology.

WHO	*CIN*	*Bethesda*
Negative for cancer	Negative	Within normal limits
Atypical squamous cells	Negative	Infection (specify organism)
		Reactive/reparative changes
	Atypical cells HPV atypia	Atypical squamous cells of undetermined significance (ASCUS)
Mild dysplasia	CIN I	Low-grade squamous intraepithelial lesion
Moderate dysplasia	CIN II	ASC-H High-grade squamous intraepithelial lesion
Severe dysplasia Carcinoma in situ	CIN III	
		Atypical glandular cells of undetermined significance (AGCUS)
Invasive carcinoma	Invasive carcinoma	Invasive carcinoma

(ASC: atypical squamous cell; CIN: cervical intraepithelial neoplasia; HPV: human papillomavirus; WHO: World Health Organisation)

Flowchart 1: Standards of cytodiagnosis—histologically proved (CIN I–III, adenocarcinoma and invasive cancer).

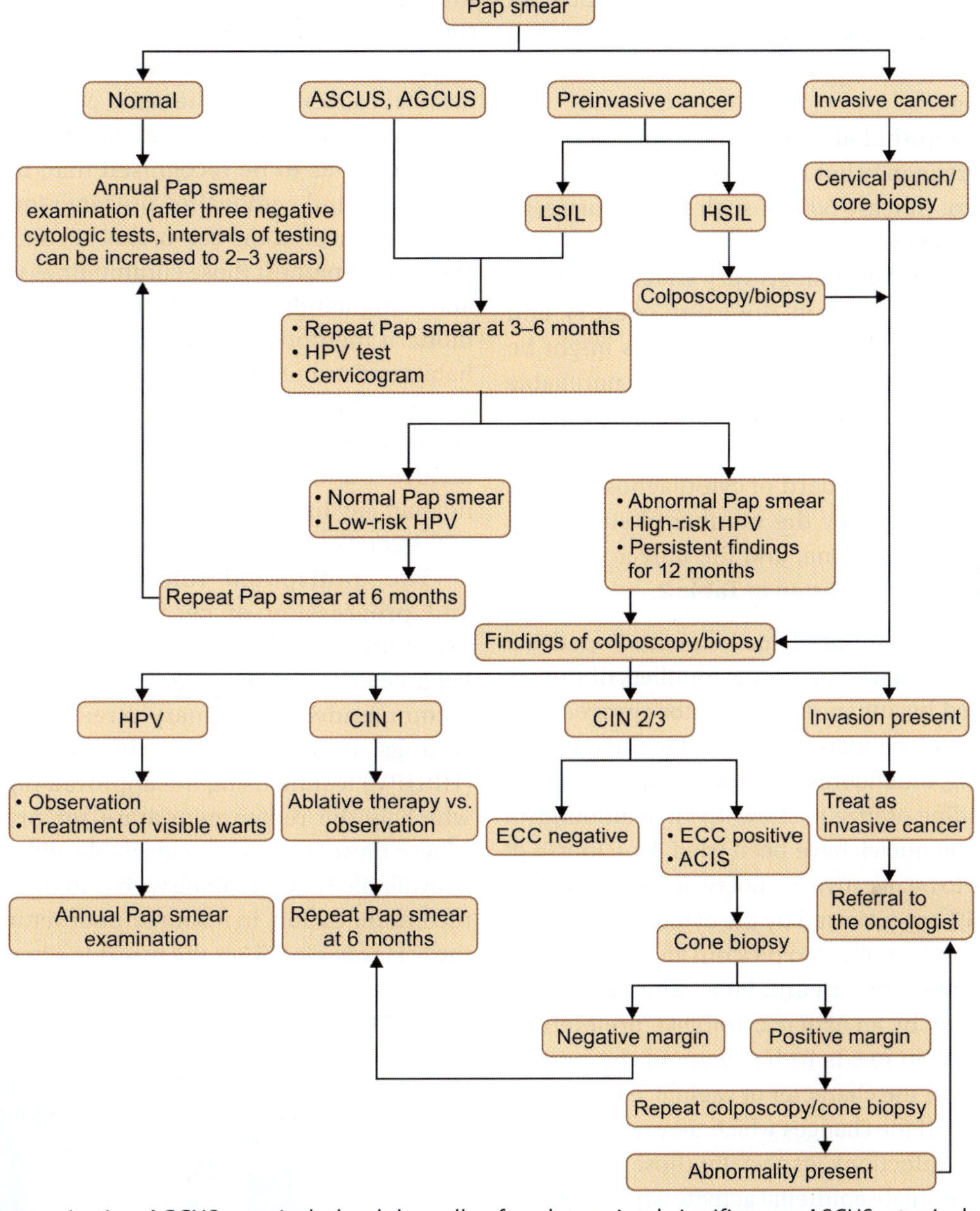

(ACIS: adenocarcinoma in situ; AGCUS: atypical glandular cells of undetermined significance; ASCUS: atypical squamous cells of undetermined significance; CIN: cervical intraepithelial neoplasia; ECC: endocervical curettage; HPV: human papillomavirus; HSIL: high-grade squamous intraepithelial lesion; LEEP: loop electrosurgical excision procedure; LSIL: low-grade squamous intraepithelial lesion)
Source: WHO Guidelines for Treatment of Cervical Intraepithelial Neoplasia 2–3 and Adenocarcinoma in situ: Cryotherapy, Large Loop Excision of the Transformation Zone, and Cold Knife Conization. Geneva: World Health Organization; 2014. Available from: https://www.ncbi.nlm.nih.gov/books/NBK206775/

These findings apply only to women who do not have clinically recognisable cancer of the cervix. In those who do, cervical smears, even when repeated, show a false-negative rate of 10%. The reason is that, with established cancer, the actively growing cells are deeply situated; those which are exfoliated from the growth are often necrotic and obscured by inflammatory cells. This high false-negative rate in cases of cancer emphasises that cervical smears should only be taken by someone who is competent to judge the health of the cervix clinically, and that cytodiagnosis is for the woman who is free from symptoms or signs of malignant disease. When such are present, it is essential to proceed to colposcopy, cervical biopsy, endocervical evaluation irrespective of the cytological findings.

Cervical intraepithelial neoplasia is occasionally present during pregnancy but disappears spontaneously in the puerperium. At least, 50% of such lesions undergo reversal after pregnancy.

The standards of cytodiagnosis vary widely from one laboratory to another, even in the same country and amongst those where consistently high levels might be expected. In many cases, the reporting is more unreliable than the histological diagnosis of CIN III. The common error is to classify too many smears as malignant or suspicious. Indeed, the standard of cytodiagnosis in any laboratory can be judged by the number of suspicious returns. There should be none, and the only acceptable diagnoses are the categories listed in **Table 2**.

Interpretation of cervical smears: It has long been hoped that the workload of dealing with very large numbers of smears might be lightened by automating laboratory procedures. Automatic electronic scanners which react to the intensity of nuclear staining, and fluorescent microscopy of smears stained with acridine orange to show up large amounts of nucleic acids in the nuclei, have been tried. One fourth of slides most likely to be negative are not reviewed manually, the remaining 75% are reviewed by the cytotechnologist.

Technicians can be trained to pick out all the obviously normal smears and this means 90%. The remaining 10% require a study by an expert cytologist, preferably a histopathologist, who needs to be aware of the normal cyclical variations in the character of vaginal, cervical and endometrial cells and the changes which they undergo with pregnancy. Local infections, especially those caused by *T. vaginalis*, also simulate epithelial activity which can be a trap for the inexperienced. The expert cytologist, however, has little difficulty in distinguishing inflammatory and hormone reactions from atypical or malignant activity.

The significance of a positive cervical smear: When cervical smears contain cells indicative of CINs II and III or malignancy, the next step is to carry out colposcopy since this will determine the site for a direct punch biopsy.

In those areas where a large section of the female population has been regularly subjected to cervical cytology for several years, the incidence of cervical invasive carcinoma has fallen. Decreases of 30% in 5–15 years have been reported from British Columbia and Ontario, for example. Yet it is not established that such a change is the result of routine cytodiagnosis, which in turn leads to the elimination of CIN III. Similar falls in the incidence of cervical cancer during the same period are reported from cities and areas where cytodiagnosis was not practiced. Indeed, it has to be recognised that, irrespective of the discovery and removal of precancerous or preinvasive lesions, cancer of the cervix was becoming less common, especially amongst those communities where educational and living standards were being raised. On the other hand, modern methods of contraception and changing sexual habits and morals are associated with a more virulent form of cervical cancer in women under 40 years of age. As a consequence, there have been only small reductions in incidence and number of deaths. Cervical cytology has also not had any impact on the prevention of adenocarcinoma of the cervix **(Annexures 1 and 2)**.

The undisputed role of HPV in the initiation and progression of cervical epithelial changes has revolutionised the screening protocols. Conventional Papanicolaou smear or liquid-based cytology is no longer recommended for primary screening in good resource settings. It is rather high-risk human papillomavirus (HRHPV) testing using the approved high-standard tests, which is the recommendation for primary screening. Where these tests are not available, either contesting, that is, available HPV kits along with cytological screening is the recommendation. In resource-poor settings where none of these is feasible, VIA is the possible screening modality.

It was the German virologist Harald zur Hausen **(Fig. 14)** who proved the link between HPVs and

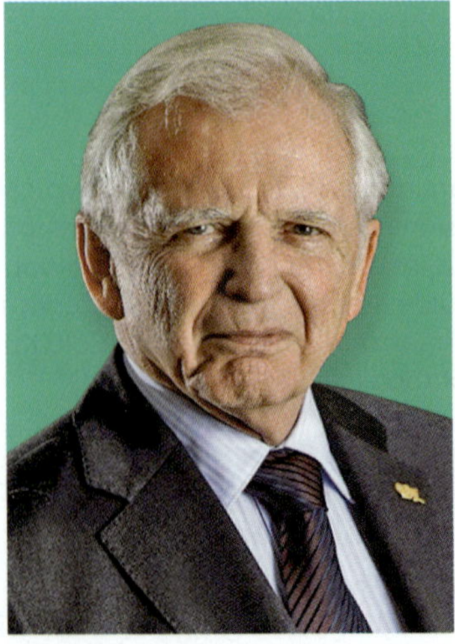

Fig. 14: German virologist Harald zur Hausen.

cervical cancer. His researches paved the way for the invention of HPV vaccine, which is presently one of the most important strategies in cervical cancer prevention. In 2008, zur Hausen was awarded the Nobel Prize in Physiology or Medicine.

Nearly all cases of cervical cancer are associated with HPV infection, with two types, (1) HPV16 and (2) HPV18, present in 70% of cases. Persistent HPV infection increases the risk for developing epithelial abnormalities and cancer. Viral early region proteins E6 and E7 play the major role in oncogenesis by suppressing P53 and Rb proteins which are responsible for apoptosis and tumour suppression, respectively. The cells are rendered immortal by this process and there will be tumorigenesis. In addition, there are various epigenetic changes and DNA methylation processes, and the participation of microRNAs in these processes.

Primary HRHPV screening with or without typing is recommended from the age of 30 years onward, once in 5–10 years (once in 3–5 years for retropositive women) till the age of 65 years, provided prior three consecutive reports were normal. It is important to choose the prequalified/approved HPV test platforms for this purpose; and where such test platforms are not available, cotesting (HPV test plus cytology) every 5 years or cytological screening or VIA every 3 years are the choices. It is observed that HPV is prevalent in cervicovaginal environment in majority of women between 20 and 30 years, and this infection usually clears off in 2 years. Persistence of HRHPV infection is associated with epithelial neoplastic changes and cancer.

In resource-constrained settings, VIA plays an important role in screening. This is a simple test involving visualising the cervix after application of freshly prepared 3–5% acetic acid. VIA is usually reinforced with visual inspection after Lugol's iodine (VILI) and/or visual inspection with magnification (VIAM). Recently, scientists have been exploring the usefulness of the latest technology such as artificial intelligence, image transfer via cloud and tele reporting.

Colposcopy and colpomicroscopy: These techniques in which the cervix is visualised through optical instruments are used to detect changes in the surface pattern and vascularity of the covering epithelium. The magnification of the colposcope is 10–20 times and that of the colpomicroscope 100–300 times. So, the latter offers microscopy in vivo. The evaluation of the TZ is of great importance as this is where the majority of cancers originate. TZ is classified as types 1, 2 and 3 depending on the complete visibility of inner squamocolumnar junction as type 1, visibility on opening the ectocervix as type 2 and nonvisibility despite opening the ectocervix as type 3. Type 3 TZ mandates further assessment of endocervix as there can be a lesion much inside. The endocervical canal can be evaluated with the help of an endocervical speculum and an endocervical curettage can be done. In assessing the grade of a lesion on colposcopy, the colposcopist looks at the surface contour, the arrangement of the surface capillaries, the distance between them and the presence of areas of leucoplakia.

The first step is to visualise the cervix under magnification. Any discharge present can be removed gently with saline. Leucoplakia must be looked for before applying acetic acid otherwise it cannot be differentiated from acetowhite epithelium (see further) **(Fig. 15)**. Leucoplakia is a white area of thickened epithelium seen on the portio by the naked eye or by means of a colposcope. As in the case of the vulva, the white colouration, while denoting a deposit of keratin, is not indicative of any particular type of epithelial behaviour underneath. Histologically, apart from patchy keratinisation, the underlying epithelium may be normal, shows features of CIN or even invasive disease and should therefore be biopsied.

Condylomatous reactions caused by HPV may appear frond-like or can lead to leucoplakia. Biopsies should be taken, especially when they arise from the TZ.

Frank invasive carcinoma can be identified before the application of acetic acid by the presence of the following: microexophytic epithelium—the surface is irregular,

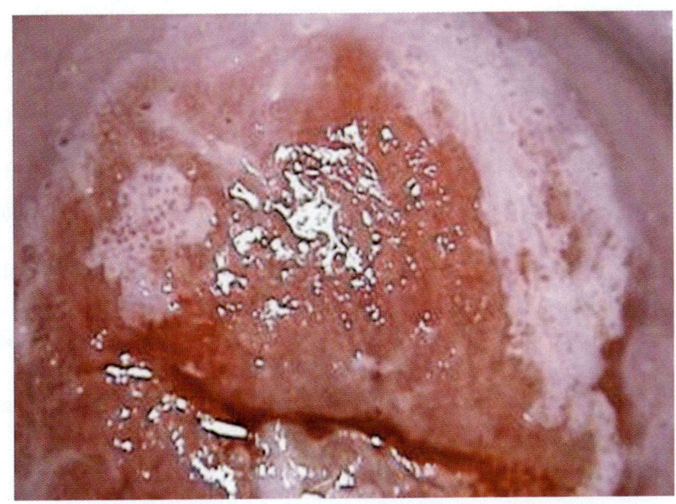

Fig. 15: Leucoplakia—a white area of thickened epithelium.

raised or ulcerated; atypical corkscrew or comma-shaped vessels of irregular calibre and branching pattern are seen. Viewing the lesion through a green filter allows a clearer demonstration of the vasculature.

The second step in the colposcopic examination is to apply 5% acetic acid gently but liberally.

In dysplastic epithelium, the nucleocytoplasmic ratio is increased and the increased nucleoproteins are precipitated by acetic acid about 30 seconds after application to make this area look opaque compared to the normal epithelium, hence the term acetowhite epithelium. Terminal capillaries may surround circular or polygonal areas of acetowhite epithelium to give the appearance of a mosaic. Punctations may be seen within the acetowhite areas. These are the terminal ends of dilated capillaries.

Biopsies may be taken from suspicious areas under colposcopic guidance. Bleeding can be controlled with the application of Monsel's or silver nitrate solution or by a pack. The application of Lugol's iodine used to be done routinely in the past—abnormal epithelium did not take up the stain as the dysfunctional dysplastic cells were devoid of glycogen. However, this is not mandatory if a thorough colposcopic examination has been done.

The reliability of colposcopy depends on whether the field was adequate (complete cervix seen) or not, and whether TZ was seen completely or not (TZ types 1/2/3).

The colposcopy findings are to be documented as per IFCPC guidelines **(Table 3)**, and the scoring can be done using Swede's score **(Table 4)**. The colposcopy diagnosis is done using the score.

TABLE 3: 2011 IFCPC Nomenclature
Accepted in Rio World Congress, July 5, 2011
Nomenclature Committee chairman: Jacob Bornstein MD

2011 IFCPC colposcopic terminology of the cervix			
General assessment		• Adequate/inadequate for the reason … (i.e.: cervix obscured by inflammation, bleeding, scar) • Squamo-columnar Junction visibility: Completely visible, partially visible, not visible • Transformation zone types 1,2,3	
Normal colposcopic findings		*Original squamous epithelium:* • Mature • Atrophic *Columnar epithelium:* • Ectopy	*Metaplastic squamous epithelium:* • Nabothian cysts • Crypt (gland) openings Deciduosis in pregnancy
Abnormal colposcopic findings	General principles	*Location of the lesion:* Inside or outside the T-zone, Location of the lesion by clock position *Size of the lesion:* Number of cervical quadrants the lesion covers, Size of the lesion in percentage of cervix	
	Grade 1 (Minor)	• Thin aceto-white epithelium • Irregular, geographic border	• Fine mosaic • Fine punctation
	Grade 2 (Major)	• Dense aceto-white epithelium • Rapid appearance of acetowhitening • Cuffed crypt (gland) openings	• Coarse mosaic • Coarse punctuation • Sharp border • Inner border sign • Ridge sign
	Non-specific	• Leukoplakia (keratosis, hyperkeratosis) • Erosion • Lugol's staining (Schiller's test): Stained/non-stained	
Suspicious for invasion		Atypical vessels *Additional signs:* Fragile vessels, irregular surface, exophytic lesion, necrosis, ulceration (necrotic), tumor/gross neoplasm	
Miscellaneous finding		• Congenital transformation zone • Condyloma • Polyp (Ectocervical/endocervical) • Inflammation	• Stenosis • Congenital anomaly • Post treatment consequence • Endometriosis

Source: Bornstein J, Bentley J, Bösze P, Girardi F, Haefner H, Menton M, et al. 2011 IFCPC colposcopic nomenclature.https://ifcpc.org/Colposcopy-guidelines-and-Terminology

TABLE 4: Swede score.

	Score		
	0	*1*	*2*
Aceto uptake	Zero or transparent	Shady, milky (not transparent not opaque)	Distinct, opaque white
Margins/surface	Diffuse	Sharp but irregular, jagged, "geographical" satellites	Sharp and even, difference in surface level incl "cuffing"
Vessels	Fine, regular	Absent	Coarse or atypical
Lesion size	<5 mm	5–15 mm or 2 quadrants	>15 mm or 3–4 quadrants or endocervically undefined
Iodine staining	Brown	Faintly or patchy yellow	Distinct yellow

Source: https://ifcpc.org/Colposcopy-guidelines-and-Terminology

Cone biopsy: By using colposcopy, it is possible to define which lesions are appropriate for laser therapy or cryotherapy or thermoablation. For those which are not totally visible, a cone biopsy is indicated, because the abnormal area extends into the cervical canal, or there is a suggestion of invasion. A cone biopsy removes not only the whole of the squamocolumnar junction but also a considerable part of the endocervix **(Figs. 16 and 17)**. The tissue so obtained is divided into 12–16 segments and each one is blocked and sectioned separately.

Following removal of the cone, the raw area is fulgurated using a ball cautery, or be covered immediately with flaps of the vaginal epithelium, paying careful attention to haemostasis. Many techniques are used, from leaving the area raw, to packing and to suturing the cervix laterally. The descending arteries on each lateral aspect of the cervix should be controlled by deeply placed sutures.

Cone biopsy can result in immediate or secondary severe haemorrhage. Delayed complications include stenosis and cervical incompetence.

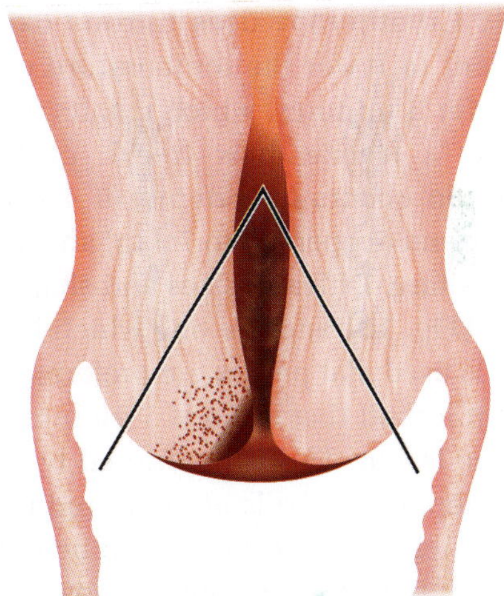

Fig. 16: A diagrammatic illustration of the common site of origin of a squamous cell carcinoma of the cervix and the tissue removed in the course of cone biopsy.

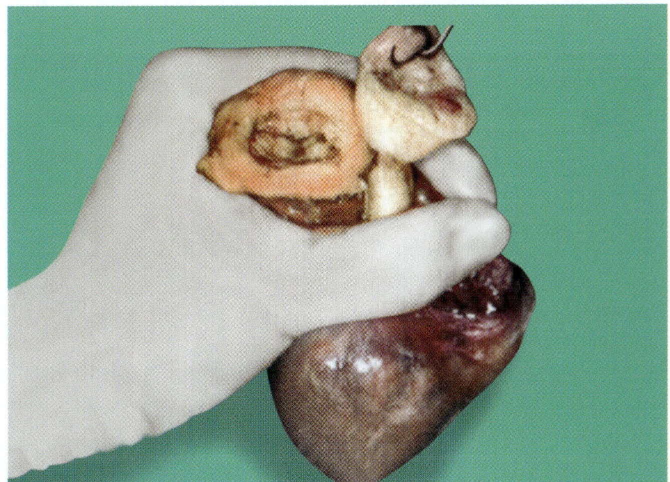

Fig. 17: Cervical cone biopsy demonstrated on a hysterectomy specimen. The single black suture, placed at 12 o'clock position before the incision is made, permits the histopathologist to orientate the specimen in the laboratory.

Treatment

Low-grade intraepithelial lesions patients can be kept under observation and monitored by Pap smear. However, 5–10% of cases may be underdiagnosed and 0.1% of these may even have invasive or an endocervical cancer.

When opting for conservative measures, it is important to ensure patient follow-up. Where this is doubtful, it is safer to treat all patients with abnormal Pap smears with a colposcopically identifiable lesion. Without an identifiable lesion, the patient is followed by Pap smear until a lesion is identified or until three negative smears are obtained.

All high-grade intraepithelial lesions require treatment. Treatment modalities vary depending on the age of the patient, nature of the epithelial lesion, desire for future fertility and facilities available.

Curative punch biopsy: In young women with low-grade lesions and a small unifocal lesion located within the TZ, punch biopsy can be curative. To enhance the accuracy, it can be done under colposcopic guidance and the base curetted well. If the disease persists on follow-up, other treatments can be undertaken.

The treatment options are either ablative procedures or excisional techniques. The criteria for ablation are as follows: TZ completely visible (type 1), lesion occupying <75% of cervix and invasive carcinoma ruled out.

Excisional techniques are loop electrosurgical excision procedure (LEEP), cold knife conization or laser conisation.

Cryotherapy: Cryotherapy uses nitrous oxide or CO_2 as a refrigerant to lower the temperature of the tissue below -22°C for 3 minutes, which results in cell death. Alternatively, a freeze-thaw-freeze cycle is used. Cryodestruction occurs to a depth of 4–5 mm. Some lesions may extend deeper (up to 7 mm) and are the cause of treatment failure. Different sizes and shapes of probes are available **(Fig. 18)** and the one which is best suited to the lesion is used; flat probes are preferred. The aim is to produce an iceball that extends 5-10 mm beyond the margins of the lesion. This is confirmed by colposcopy. Multiple overlapping iceballs are required to treat large lesions adequately. The procedure can be done without anaesthesia. Only minor cramps are experienced, but postoperatively the patient often has profuse, watery discharge, which requires the use of a sanitary napkin. Electrolyte replacement is recommended. Light spotting may occur after 2 weeks when the char separates.

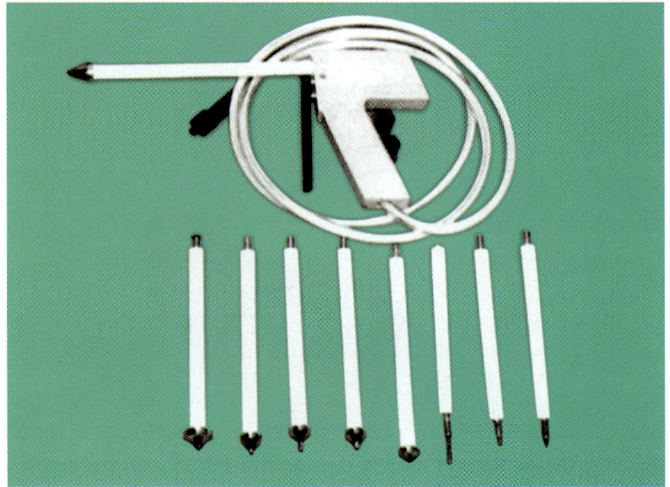

Fig. 18: Cryotherapy gun with probes of different sizes and shapes.

Fertility is not impaired subsequent to the procedure, but some patients may have cervical stenosis or cervical dystocia. In some patients, the squamocolumnar junction may recede into the endocervical canal and subsequent evaluation may be difficult. This is especially likely if a probe with an endocervical extension is used. The success rate is about 93–97%.

Carbon dioxide laser: This is a useful modality but is available at only very few centres in developing countries. It can be used both for ablation and for cutting, but in cervical lesions, it is used to ablate those lesions confined to the portio. In all destructive techniques, it is important to first rule out invasive disease by colposcopy-directed biopsy and endocervical curettage. The depth of destruction can be better controlled with laser.

Lesions extending into the endocervical canal can be subjected to laser conisation to rule out invasive disease.

Results of laser ablation are comparable with cryotherapy, but vaginal discharge is less and the TZ is maintained. Cervical stenosis rates are the same. However, it is very expensive, and special skills are required for performing the procedure.

Thermocoagulation: It is safe and more convenient in field settings. Hand-held battery-operated devices are used to treat the lesions during screen-and-treat or screen-see-and-treat protocols in community settings.

Excisional procedures: These are suitable for high-grade lesions with extensive involvement if cerix (>75%). Based on the type of TZ and need for excluding endocervical epithelial abnormality, the excisional procedure, either *LEEP* or cold knife conisation, is chosen.

Loop electrosurgical excision procedure (large loop excision of the transformation zone): LEEP, also known as large loop excision of the transformation zone (LLETZ), has become the procedure of choice for the management of CIN in many countries.

Loop electrosurgical excision procedure can be learned easily; it can be performed under colposcopic control, i.e. residual margins can be examined and residual lesions excised; it yields tissue for histopathological examination, although the surgical margins may be charred. Different sizes of loops are available for LEEP and the appropriate loop is selected **(Fig. 19)**. The use of a very large loop may result in amputation of the cervix with subsequent obstetric complications. The procedure is contraindicated in pregnancy.

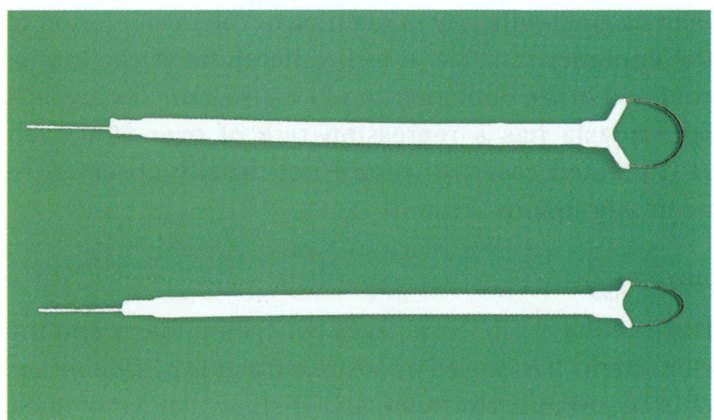

Fig. 19: Two sizes of loops for loop electrosurgical excision procedure (LEEP).

Cervical conisation: Traditional cold knife conisation is the time-honoured technique, which continues to be used in most parts of the developing world to excise lesions that extend into the endocervical canal. Indeed, the cone biopsy essential for the diagnosis of the disease is usually curative. If the lesion is not suitable for ablative therapy, this is often the appropriate treatment for younger women and for older women as well.

Before accepting that cone excision of the tissues around the external os and the endocervix, or amputation of the cervix, is adequate for the treatment of any case, an assurance from the histopathologist that the line of incision is outside the diseased area is required. Moreover, regular follow-up of the patient, with repeat cervical smears at 3-month intervals at first, is essential.

When the patient treated by cone biopsy subsequently conceives, one worry is whether the stimulus of pregnancy will light up the disease, but this does not seem to occur. If the original cone has included the internal os, cervical incompetence resulting in abortion may ensue. Another possible complication is cervical dystocia during labour consequent upon scarring. In practice, trouble rarely occurs.

Total hysterectomy: If margins are positive after coinisation, or if follow-up smear becomes positive after conservative surgery, total hysterectomy is indicated, but the ovaries need not be removed if the woman is premenopausal. There is also a place for total hysterectomy as an elective procedure when microinvasion is found on biopsy, or when the patient is over 40 years of age. Some gynaecologists advise hysterectomy in all cases. This may be justified if they are dealing with women likely to default from follow-up, but not otherwise. In fact, regular follow-up cytology is as important after total hysterectomy as it is after conservative surgery. The woman who suffers from CIN III is the one most likely to develop similar lesions in the vagina.

A cuff of vagina should be removed only if there is clear evidence of disease in the vaginal vault. Most in situ lesions found in the vagina after hysterectomy represent new and separate developments and not extensions from the cervical cancer. It is established that routine removal of a vaginal cuff does not improve the overall results.

Hysterectomy is never indicated merely on the finding of a positive cervical smear. Preliminary colposcopy and cervical biopsy are essential, because cytodiagnosis is not completely reliable and does not permit a distinction between CIN III, microinvasive and invasive cancer; treatment of the last requires more than hysterectomy.

UTERINE CORPUS

Endometrial Hyperplasia

Endometrial hyperplasia is extremely common. It occurs at all ages, even in postmenopausal women.

Pathology

The disease occurs in two main forms: (1) Hyperplasia with atypia or (2) hyperplasia without atypia. Hyperplasia with atypia is a premalignant condition, hence requires detailed evaluation of uterus by MRI/hysteroscopy to rule out coexistent endometrial cancer, possibility of this being 40%.

Since the underlying cause is a prolonged oestrogen secretion unopposed by progesterone, the myometrium simultaneously undergoes hypertrophy to cause diffuse uterine enlargement.

The combination of endometrial and myometrial hypertrophy constitutes generalised myohyperplasia **(Fig. 20)**.

Atypical hyperplasia: The nuclei are unusually large, pleomorphic, hyperchromatic with parachromatin clumping, increased nuclear-cytoplasmic ratios and prominent nucleoli **(Figs. 21A to C)**.

Usually, the risk of hyperplasia progressing to carcinoma is related to the presence and severity of cytologic atypia **(Figs. 22A to C)** and the risk is around 29%. Certain risk factors are known to affect the risk of progression: Age, obesity, endocrinopathy, ovarian disease, endogenous hormone exposure (oestrogens, tamoxifen), etc.

In 17–28% of patients with atypical hyperplasia, an unexpected carcinoma might be found on hysterectomy, the risk of such an event being greater in postmenopausal women.

It has been proposed that the term endometrial intraepithelial neoplasia (EIN) be used to describe atypical hyperplasia. However, it is generally agreed that there is great difficulty in defining a true in situ lesion of the endometrium, i.e. a well-differentiated carcinoma confined to the endometrium, because complex atypical hyperplasia has a regression rate of over 50% even in untreated cases, a feature not usually observed in neoplastic lesions.

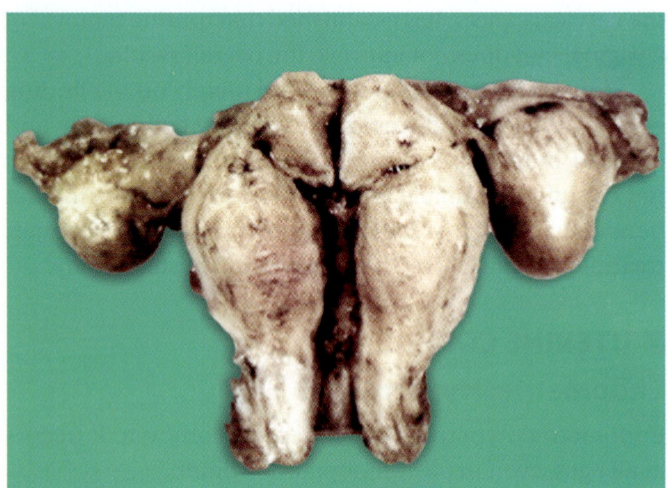

Fig. 20: Generalised myohyperplasia of the uterus in a woman aged 52 years who suffered from recurrent episodes of irregular bleeding. The myometrium and the endometrium both show hypertrophy, the cause being an unopposed oestrogen secretion by the follicular cyst in the right ovary.

Aetiology

Hyperplasia occurs at all ages between puberty and the climacteric. It is caused by oestrogen acting in the absence of progesterone. Hormone assays show that sometimes, in hyperplasia, the oestrogen level is maintained for long periods of time at a moderate level. In other cases, there are fluctuations between abnormally low and high levels. Hyperplasia results under any circumstances which determine a prolonged, increased or unopposed oestrogen production; these include follicular cysts, polycystic ovary syndrome (PCOS), granulosa and theca cell tumours of the ovary. It can readily be induced by the administration of oestrogens of any kind.

Clinical Features

Endometrial hyperplasia can exist without causing any complaint hyperplasia; however, especially if associated with fluctuating oestrogen levels, typically causes prolonged and heavy uterine bleeding with intervening

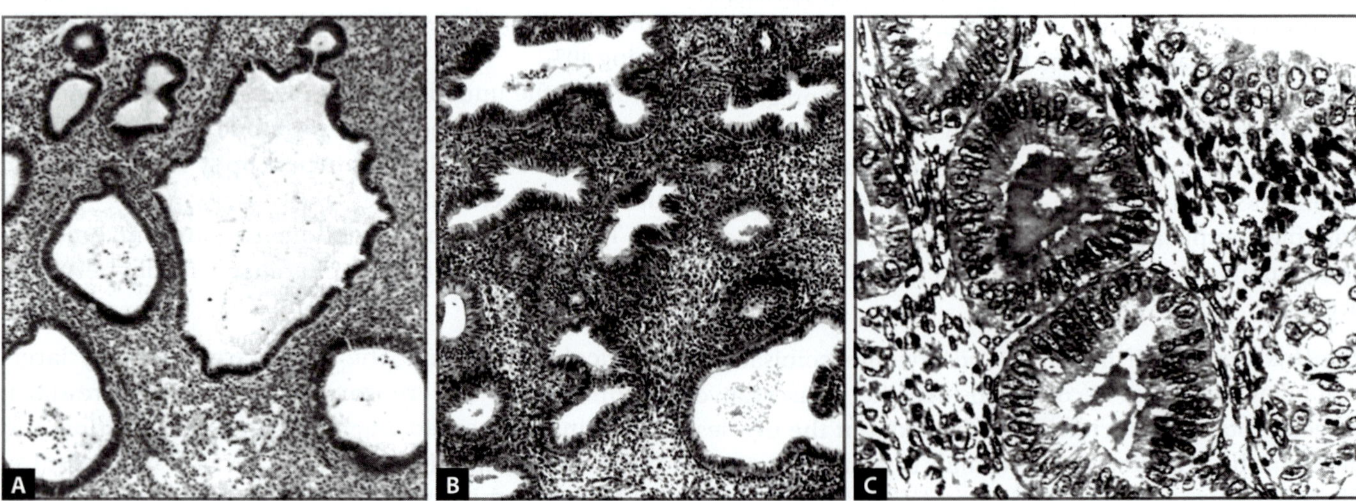

Figs. 21A to C: Endometrial hyperplasia. (A) Simple hyperplasia (cystic glandular) is characterised by enlarged nonsecretory glands, with variations in the size of glands and a compact stroma; (B) Endometrial glandular hyperplasia with architectural atypia. The glands are irregular in outline, with infoldings of their lining epithelium and out-pouchings. There is no cytological atypia in this example (photomicrograph 150×); (C) Endometrial glandular hyperplasia with cytological atypia. The glands on the left are lined by epithelium of fairly normal appearance whilst that on the right is multilayered and shows loss of nuclear polarity and abnormalities of chromatin pattern (photomicrograph 370×).

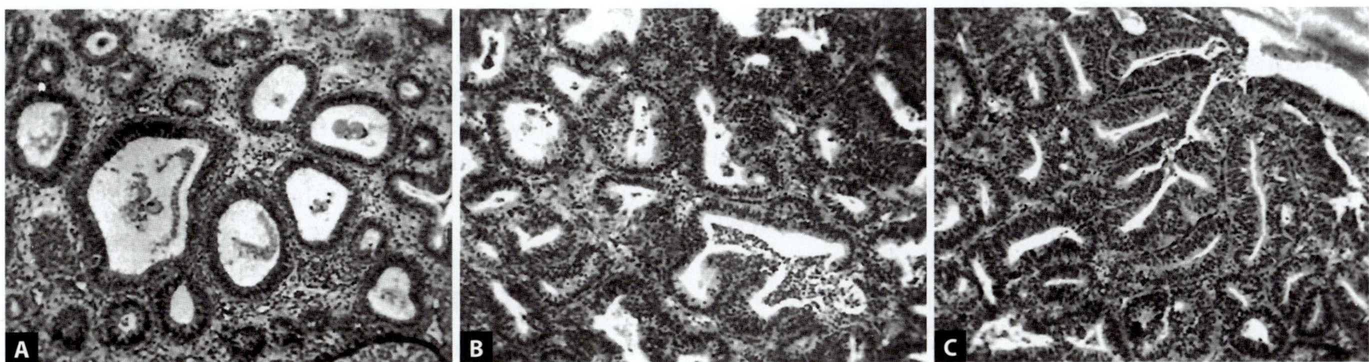

Figs. 22A to C: Aspects of atypical endometrial hyperplasia. (A) Minimal glandular architectural atypia; (B) Minor degree of glandular architectural atypia with a moderate degree of cytological atypia; (C) Severe architectural and cytological atypia.

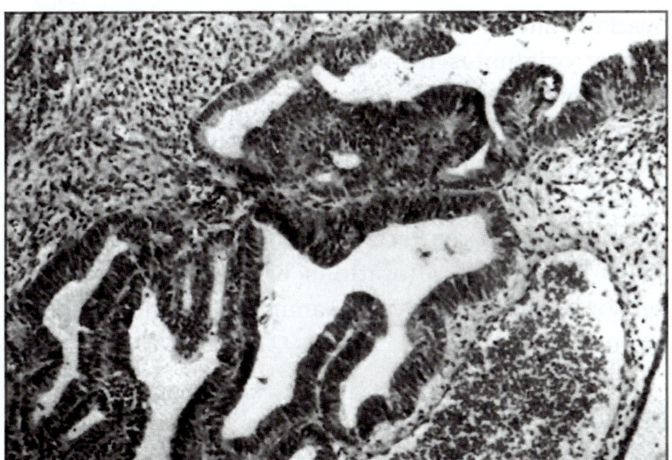

Fig. 23: Endometrium with the features of architectural atypia and moderate cytological atypia. This endometrium was obtained from a woman aged 30 years who presented with the polycystic ovary syndrome and had alternating phases of oligomenorrhoea and menorrhagia. The endometrial picture remained the same for 5 years after which time the uterus was removed because of the cancer threat. Sometimes the histological appearance regresses following progestogen therapy.

short periods of amenorrhoea. Because of an underlying faulty ovarian function, or of the endometrial abnormality itself, infertility can be a symptom of both types. It does not give rise to significant physical signs, although the uterus may be palpably symmetrically enlarged. Hysteroscopy aids the localisation of an abnormal endometrium which is seen to be hyperplastic and may have abnormal vascular patterns but the diagnosis of endometrial hyperplasia is essentially a histological one **(Fig. 23)**.

Treatment

If an abnormal oestrogen influence is the background, the cause of this has to be removed. Functional ovarian upsets resulting in endometrial hyperplasia may undergo spontaneous cure. Meanwhile, a normal endometrial picture can be induced by cyclical hormone therapy. When the fault in the hormone stimulus is corrected, hyperplasia is reversible.

Young women who desire fertility may receive ovulation induction. If pregnancy is not an immediate issue, cyclical progestogen therapy with medroxyprogesterone acetate or megestrol acetate 21 days a month for 3 months provides relief in over 80% of patients. Such patients, however, need to be kept under supervision and have a repeat endometrial aspiration after 3 months. Treatment may need to be continued for 6–9 months.

Local progesterone administration by means of a levonorgestrel intrauterine contraceptive device (IUCD) has also been successful. Combined use of gonadotrophin-releasing hormone analogues and high-dose progestogens has been found to be effective. It is important to exclude atypia or malignancy. Endometrial ablation is not recommended as the tissue cannot be subjected to histopathological evaluation.

In the presence of atypia, response to progesterone therapy is poorer and the relapse rate is high. Nearly one third of them will progress to cancer and one fourth may already have associated undiagnosed cancer. Close vigilance with transvaginal ultrasound, endometrial aspiration or hysteroscopy-guided biopsy is required in this group if conservative therapy is chosen. The persistence of atypical epithelial activity may call for hysterectomy.

In women approaching or past menopause, hysterectomy is a safer choice in those with atypical hyperplasia.

Squamous Cell Metaplasia of the Endometrium

Pathology

Squamous metaplasia of the columnar epithelium of the endometrium (ichthyosis uteri) is interesting but less common. It affects mainly the surface, but squamous cells can grow into and around the glands or develop in them. Various degrees of cellular activity are present; sometimes squamous metaplasia is associated with hyperplasia or endometrial polyps.

Aetiology

Squamous metaplasia is mostly seen in women aged >40 years, often they are postmenopausal. It is a possible response to pyometra, especially one caused by senile endometritis. In younger women, it is described in association with tuberculous endometritis, and following prolonged exposure of the endometrium to mechanical or chemical irritants. Squamous cell metaplasia can be a response to any type of IUCD. When it is present, it usually disappears spontaneously; this can happen despite continued use of the device. Squamous cell metaplasia in these circumstances is to be regarded as a protective or reparative phenomenon. Squamous metaplasia also occurs in the absence of pyometra or other irritants, especially in older women, for reasons unknown, but a vitamin A or other deficiency state is postulated. Metaplasia is associated with adenomatous hyperplasia or endometrial polyps.

This condition is, by itself, symptomless and is usually discovered because of studying endometrium removed for other reasons. It then must be distinguished microscopically from the intrauterine surface spread of cancer of the cervix and also from the accidental inclusion of cervical epithelium amongst curettings. The last is a common happening.

Treatment

Squamous metaplasia does carry a threat of cancer, but generally, there is very little risk.

Other Forms of Endometrial Metaplasia

Other tissues found in the uterus, possibly because of metaplasia induced by the same sort of factors as squamous cell metaplasia, include cartilage, bone and neuroglia. Their discovery, however, creates a need to exclude their being part of a mixed Müllerian tumour or, even more likely, the aftermath of instrumental termination of pregnancy. In this operation, foetal tissues can be left in the uterus and maintain some sort of life, resulting in discharge or abnormal bleeding dating from the abortion.

FALLOPIAN TUBE

It was of the impression that epithelial abnormality of the endosalpinx is described as an incidental histological finding of little significance. However, in the recent years, it has been observed that the deadliest type of ovarian cancer, high-grade serous epithelial carcinoma, in fact originates from the tuboperitoneal junction. Three main lesions—(1) p53 signatures, (2) serous tubal intraepithelial lesions (STILs) and (3) serous tubal intraepithelial carcinomas (STICs)—have been defined in the fallopian tubes, based on the immunohistochemistry (IHC) pattern of p53 and Ki67 markers and the architectural alterations of the cells, using the Sectioning and Extensively Examining the Fimbriated End protocol.

SUGGESTED READING

1. Bornstein J, Bentley J, Bösze P, Girardi F, Haefner H, Menton M, Perrotta M, et al. 2011 colposcopic terminology of the International Federation for Cervical Pathology and Colposcopy. Obstet Gynecol. 2012;120(1):166-72.
2. Fellegara G, Carcangiu ML, Rosai J. Benign epithelial inclusions in axillary lymph nodes: report of 18 cases and review of the literature. Am J Surg Pathol. 2011;35(8):1123-33.
3. Gibb RK, Martens MG. The impact of liquid-based cytology in decreasing the incidence of cervical cancer. Rev Obstet Gynecol. 2011;4(Suppl 1):S2-11.
4. Höhn AK, Brambs CE, Hiller GGR, May D, Schmoeckel E, Horn LC. 2020 WHO classification of female genital tumors. Geburtshilfe Frauenheilkd. 2021;81(10):1145-53.
5. La Vignera S, Condorelli RA, Russo GI, Morgia G, Calogero AE. Endocrine control of benign prostatic hyperplasia. Andrology. 2016;4(3):404-11.
6. Nicholson TM, Ricke WA. Androgens and estrogens in benign prostatic hyperplasia: past, present and future. Differentiation. 2011;82(4-5):184-99.
7. Preti M, Joura E, Vieira-Baptista P, Van Beurden M, Bevilacqua F, Bleeker MCG, et al. The European Society

of Gynaecological Oncology (ESGO), the International Society for the Study of Vulvovaginal Disease (ISSVD), the European College for the Study of Vulval Disease (ECSVD) and the European Federation for Colposcopy (EFC) consensus statements on pre-invasive vulvar lesions. J Low Genit Tract Dis. 2022;26(3):229-44.
8. The American College of Obstetricians and Gynecologists (the College) and the American Society for Colposcopy and Cervical Pathology Number 675 (Replaces Committee Opinion Number 509, 2011. Reaffirmed 2024). [online] Available from https://www.acog.org/clinical/clinical-guidance/committee-opinion/articles/2016/10/management-of-vulvar-intraepithelial-neoplasia [Last accessed May, 2025].
9. Wisztorski M, Aboulouard S, Roussel L, Duhamel M, Saudemont P, Cardon T, et al. Fallopian tube lesions as potential precursors of early ovarian cancer: a comprehensive proteomic analysis. Cell Death Dis. 2023; 14:644.
10. Wisztorski M, Aboulouard S, Roussel L, Duhamel M, Saudemont P, Cardon T, et al. Fallopian tube lesions as potential precursors of early ovarian cancer: a comprehensive proteomic analysis. Cell Death Dis. 2023; 14:644.

ANNEXURES

ANNEXURE 1: FLOWCHARTS FOR SCREEN-AND-TREAT STRATEGIES (NEGATIVE OR UNKNOWN HUMAN IMMUNODEFICIENCY VIRUS STATUS)

Screen with a Human Papillomavirus Test and Treat with Cryotherapy or Loop Electrosurgical Excision Procedure when not Eligible for Cryotherapy

When a human papillomavirus (HPV) test is positive, treatment is provided. With this strategy, visual inspection with acetic acid (VIA) is used to determine eligibility for cryotherapy.

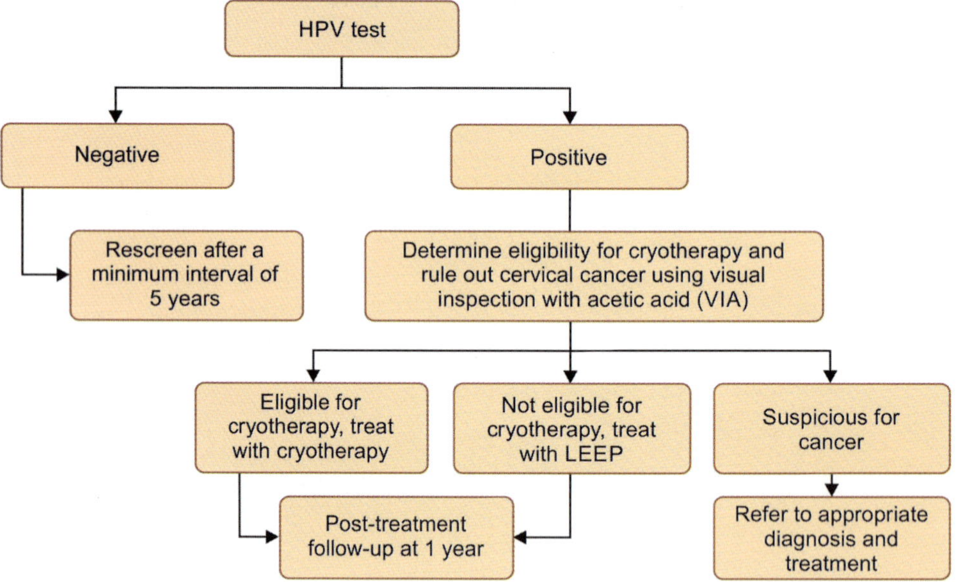

(HPV: human papillomavirus; LEEP: loop electrosurgical excision procedure)

Screen with a Human Papillomavirus Test Followed by Visual Inspection with Acetic Acid and Treat with Cryotherapy or Loop Electrosurgical Excision Procedure when not Eligible for Cryotherapy

When an HPV test is positive, then VIA is provided as a second screening test to determine whether or not treatment is offered. Treatment is only provided if both the HPV test and VIA are positive.

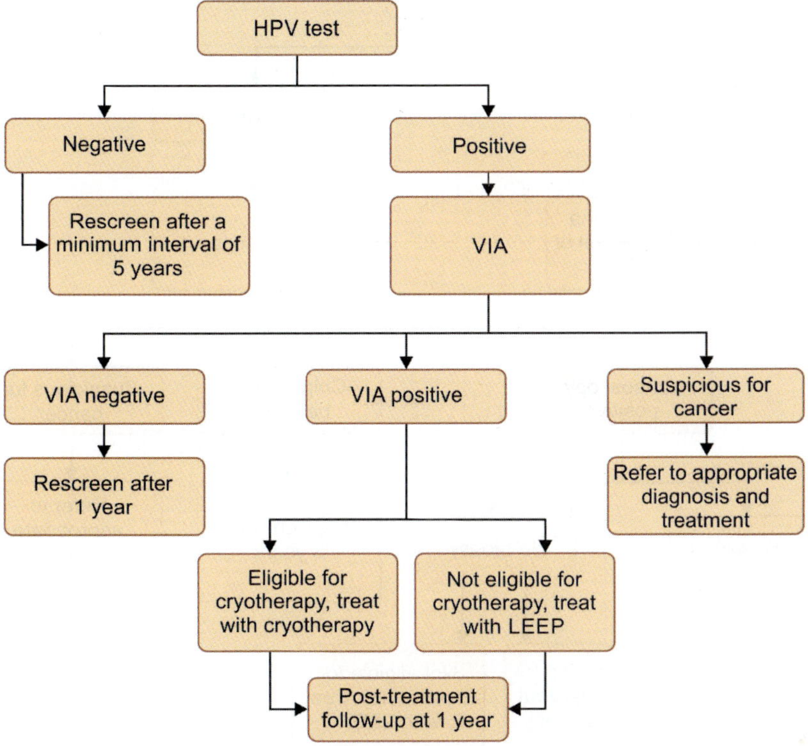

(HPV: human papillomavirus; LEEP: loop electrosurgical excision procedure; VIA: visual inspection with acetic acid)

Screen with Visual Inspection with Acetic Acid and Treat with Cryotherapy or Loop Electrosurgical Excision Procedure when not Eligible for Cryotherapy

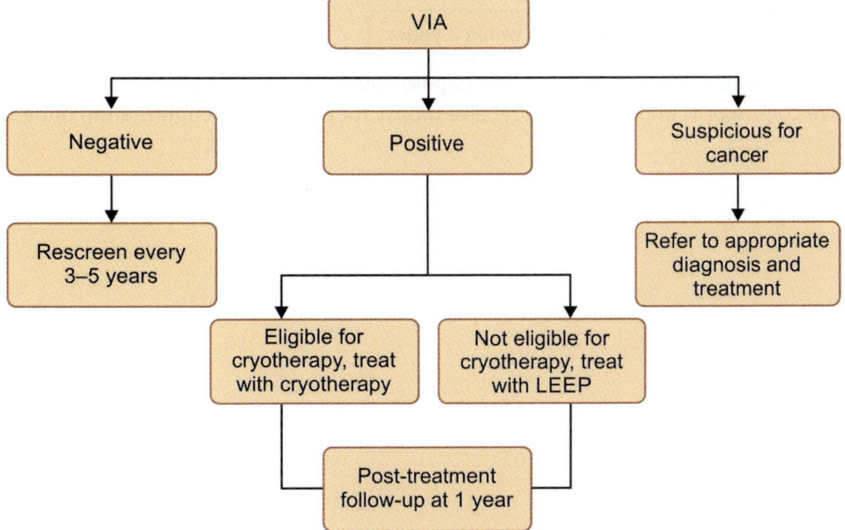

(LEEP: loop electrosurgical excision procedure; VIA: visual inspection with acetic acid)

Screen with a Human Papillomavirus Test Followed by Colposcopy (with or without Biopsy)[1] and Treat with Cryotherapy or Loop Electrosurgical Excision Procedure when not Eligible for Cryotherapy

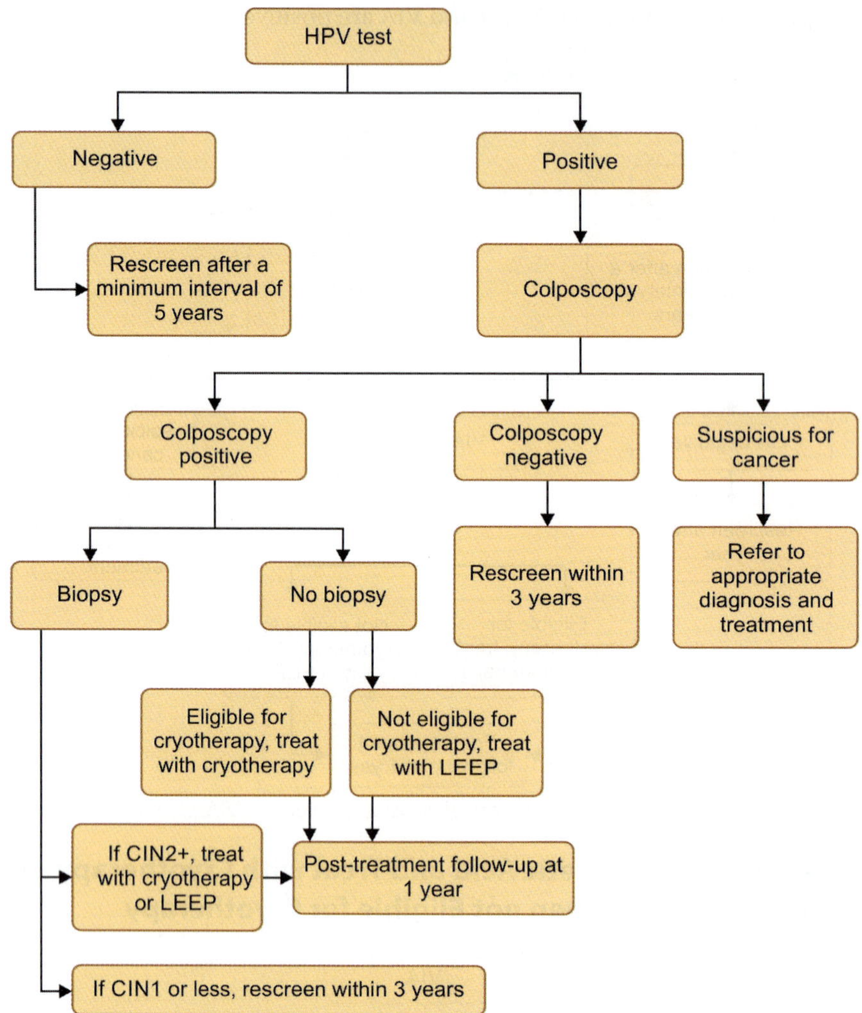

(CIN: cervical intraepithelial neoplasia; HPV: human papillomavirus; LEEP: loop electrosurgical excision procedure)

[1]Women with positive colposcopic impression can receive biopsy for histological confirmation or be treated immediately.

Screen with Cytology Followed by Colposcopy (with or without Biopsy)[1] and Treat with Cryotherapy or Loop Electrosurgical Excision Procedure when not Eligible for Cryotherapy

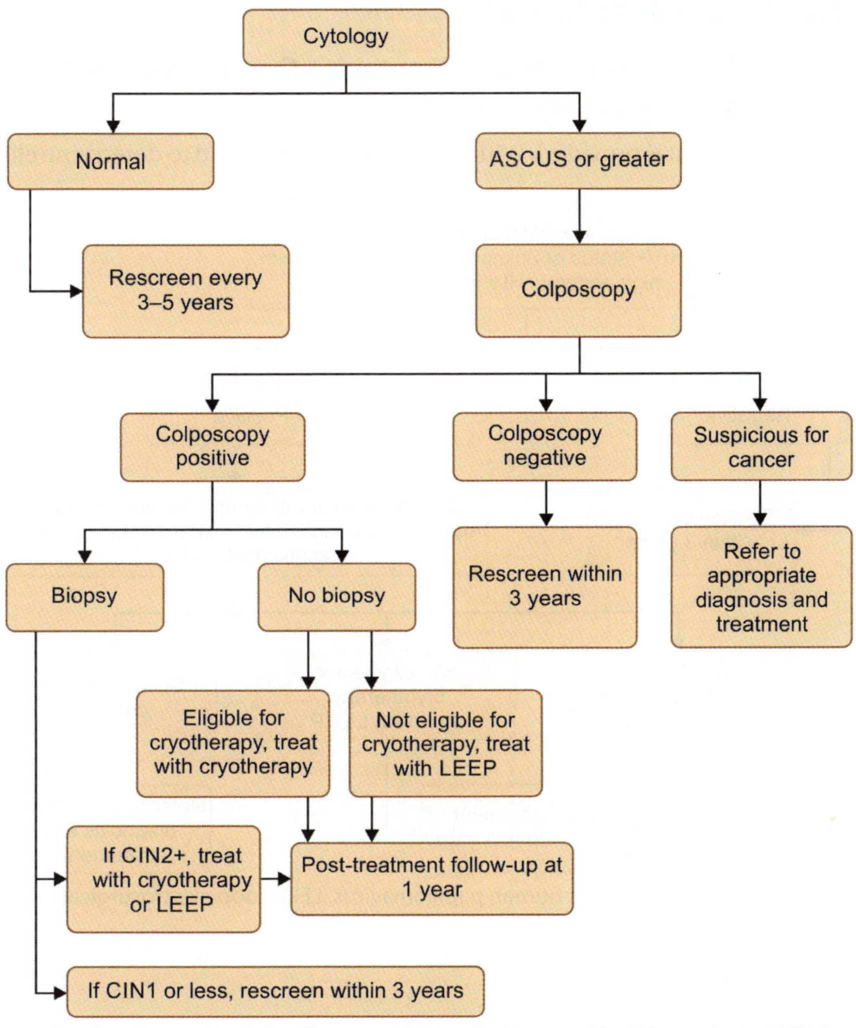

(ASCUS: atypical squamous cells of undetermined significance; CIN: cervical intraepithelial neoplasia; LEEP: loop electrosurgical excision procedure)

[1]Women with positive colposcopic impression can receive biopsy for histological confirmation or be treated immediately.

ANNEXURE 2: FLOWCHARTS FOR SCREEN-AND-TREAT STRATEGIES (HUMAN IMMUNODEFICIENCY VIRUS-POSITIVE STATUS OR UNKNOWN HUMAN IMMUNODEFICIENCY VIRUS STATUS IN AREAS WITH HIGH ENDEMIC HUMAN IMMUNODEFICIENCY VIRUS INFECTION)

Screen with a Human Papillomavirus Test and Treat with Cryotherapy or Loop Electrosurgical Excision Procedure when not Eligible for Cryotherapy

When an HPV test is positive, treatment is provided. With this strategy, VIA is used to determine eligibility for cryotherapy.

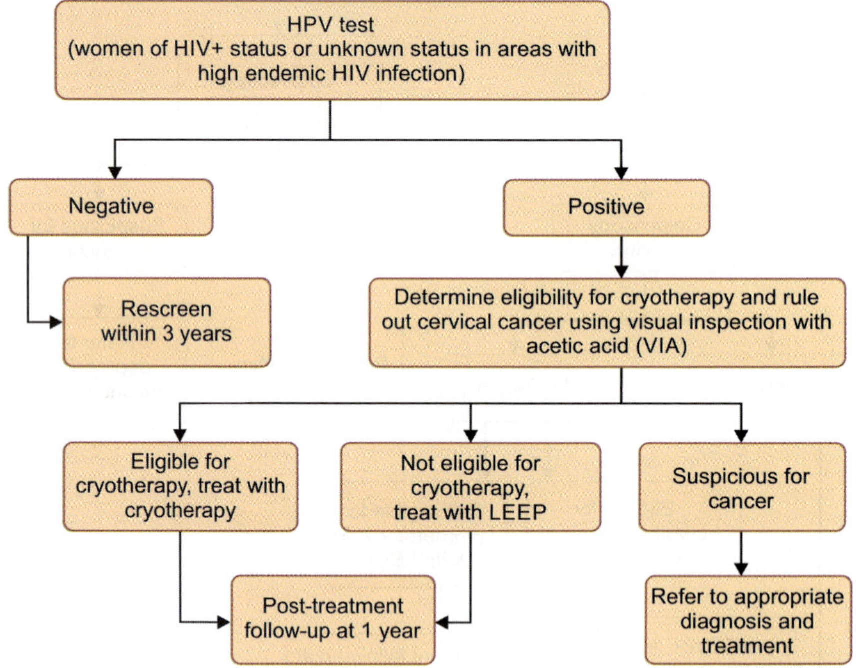

(HIV: human immunodeficiency virus; HPV: human papillomavirus; LEEP: loop electrosurgical excision procedure)

Screen with a Human Papillomavirus Test Followed by Visual Inspection with Acetic Acid and Treat with Cryotherapy or Loop Electrosurgical Excision Procedure when not Eligible for Cryotherapy

When an HPV test is positive, then VIA is provided as a second screening test to determine whether or not treatment is offered. Treatment is only provided if both the HPV test and VIA are positive.

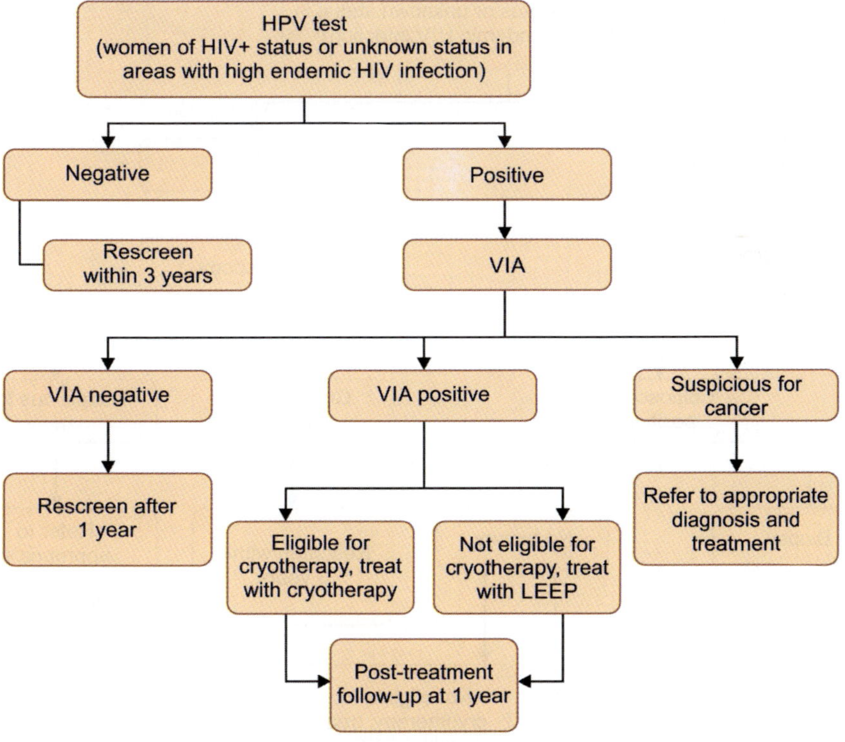

(HIV: human immunodeficiency virus; HPV: human papillomavirus; LEEP: loop electrosurgical excision procedure; VIA: visual inspection with acetic acid)

Screen with Visual Inspection with Acetic Acid and Treat with Cryotherapy or Loop Electrosurgical Excision Procedure when not Eligible for Cryotherapy

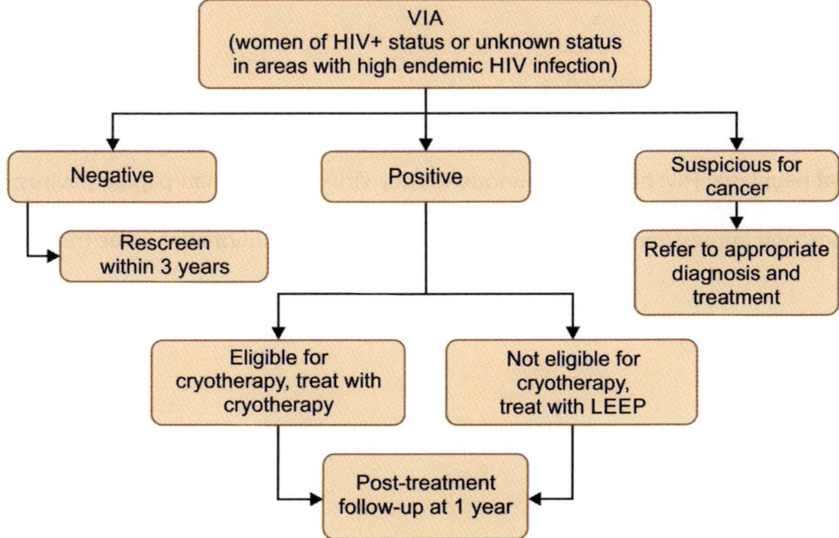

(HIV: human immunodeficiency virus; LEEP: loop electrosurgical excision procedure; VIA: visual inspection with acetic acid)

Screen with a Human Papillomavirus Test Followed by Colposcopy (with or without Biopsy)[1] and Treat with Cryotherapy or Loop Electrosurgical Excision Procedure when not Eligible for Cryotherapy

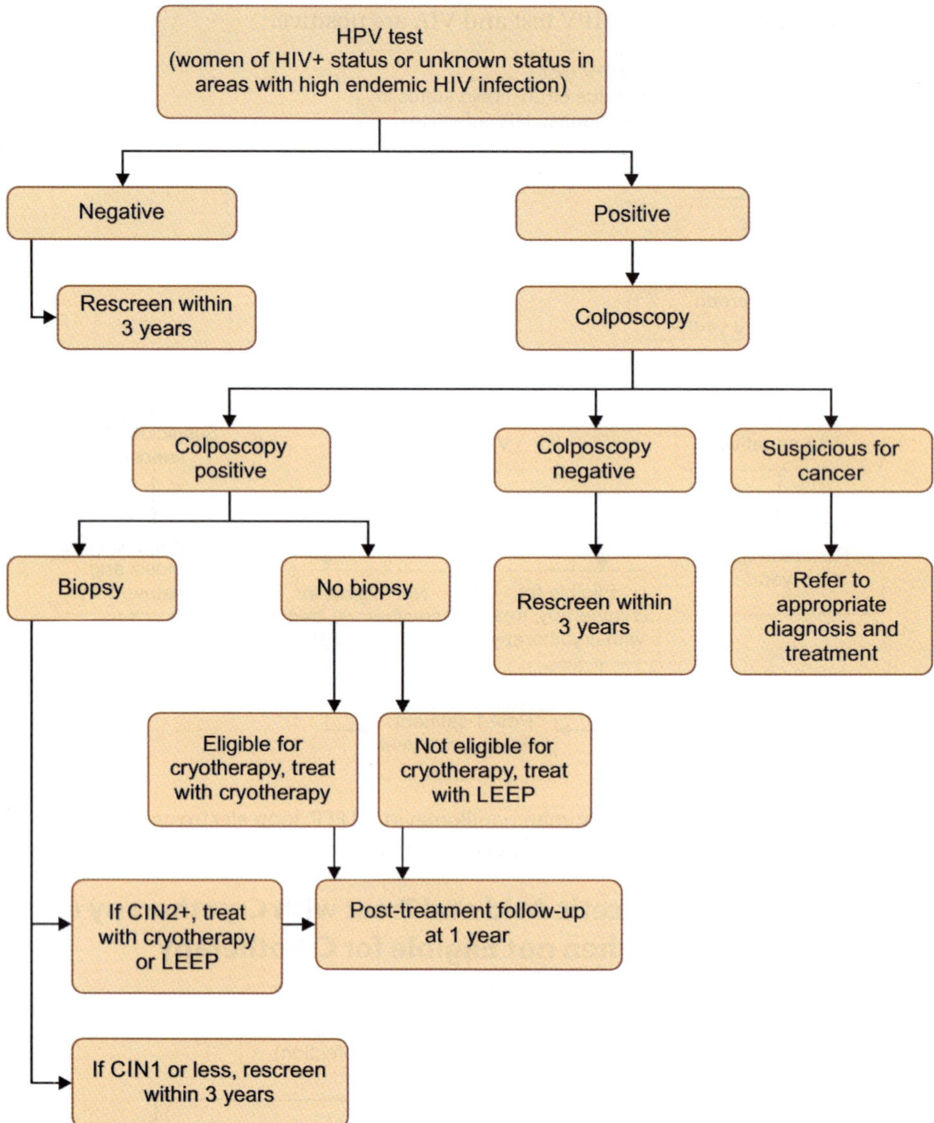

(CIN: cervical intraepithelial neoplasia; HIV: human immunodeficiency virus; HPV: human papillomavirus; LEEP: loop electrosurgical excision procedure)

[1]Women with positive colposcopic impression can receive biopsy for histological confirmation or be treated immediately.

Screen with Cytology Followed by Colposcopy (with or without Biopsy)[1] and Treat with Cryotherapy or Loop Electrosurgical Excision Procedure (when not Eligible for Cryotherapy)

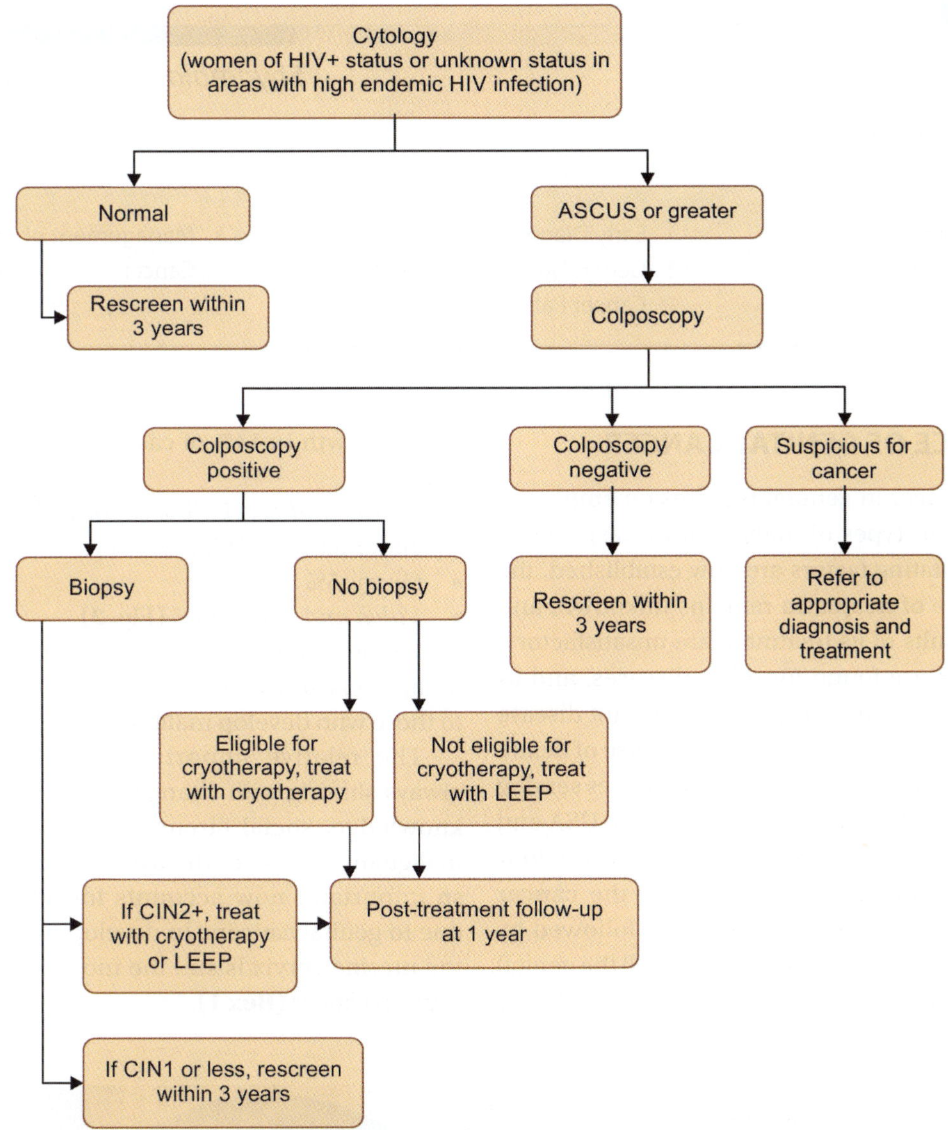

(ASCUS: atypical squamous cells of undetermined significance; CIN: cervical intraepithelial neoplasia; HIV: human immunodeficiency virus; LEEP: loop electrosurgical excision procedure)

[1]Women with positive colposcopic impression can receive biopsy for histological confirmation or be treated immediately.

27

CHAPTER

Genital Cancers

Shyamala Guruvare, Muralidhar V Pai

Chapter Outline

- Significance of Genital Cancer
- Treatment and Results
- Prevention of Pelvic Cancer
- Early Diagnosis
- General Management of the Cancer Patient
- Management of Advanced Pelvic Cancer

SIGNIFICANCE OF GENITAL CANCER

The problem of cancer in general requires no emphasis. Although for certain types of malignant disease, aetiological and precipitating factors are now established, the fundamental cause of neoplasia remains unknown, and the nature and results of its treatment are unsatisfactory. Moreover, as cures are found for other diseases, and as more individuals live to the *cancer age*, malignant disease is becoming relatively more important as a cause of death. In developed countries with good medical services serving communities such as those found in the UK, the USA and Australia, cancer now accounts for one out of every four deaths occurring amongst women and, of the cancer deaths, breast cancer is the foremost cause followed by lung cancer, both in greater proportions than all the genital cancers grouped together. The genital tract is the primary site of growth in 14% of cases. This figure is made up as follows:

- *Uterus and cervix:* 8% (approaching 1:1 in favour of endometrium) **(Fig. 1)**
- *Ovary:* 5%
- *Vulva and vagina:* 1% **(Fig. 2)**

Women who suffer from cancer of the breast are often nulliparous and well-to-do; as a group, they are opposite to those who develop malignant disease in the cervix.

The relative importance of different cancers is always shifting with changes in life expectancy, medical knowledge, social circumstances, and lifestyle. Thus, malignant disease of the ovary, formerly regarded as not so important, now accounts for 50–55% of the deaths due to genital cancers. In developing countries, cancer of the uterine cervix is still the most common, followed by ovarian cancer **(Box 1)**.

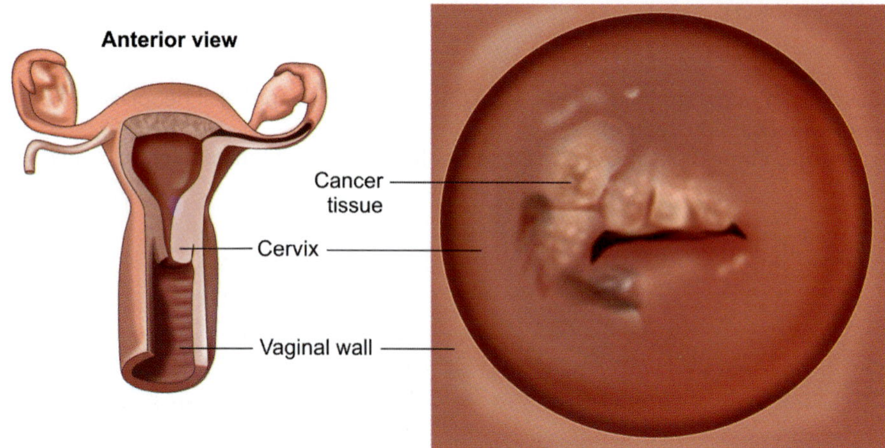

Fig. 1: Carcinoma cervix.

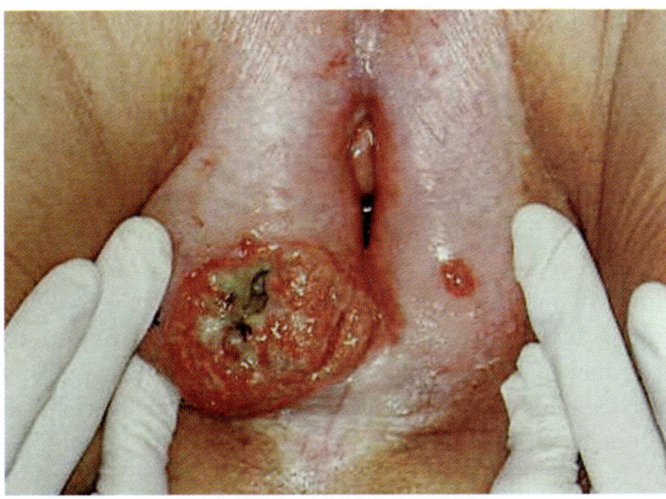

Fig. 2: Vulvar cancer.

BOX 1: Female genital cancer.

- Cervical cancer
- Uterine cancer
- Ovarian cancer
- Vulvar cancer
- Vaginal cancer
- Fallopian tube cancer
- Gestational trophoblastic neoplasia

TREATMENT AND RESULTS

The treatment of cancer falls mainly under the headings of surgery and radiotherapy, or combinations of the two-plus chemotherapy.

Both surgery and radiotherapy depend on the complete destruction or removal of the primary growth for their success at one time, radical vulvectomy with extensive groin dissection was the practice. The women used to suffer significantly due to wound complications and prolonged time taken for wound healing. Radiotherapy too had major complications crippling the quality of life. In the present-day practice, approach has shifted to less radicality, emphasis on quality of life without compromising on the disease-free survival/overall survival. To achieve this, there are various newer treatment options like sentinel lymph node detection and site-specific surgeries, laparoscopic approach and so on. Even techniques of radiotherapy have evolved to a great extent such that only tumour tissue is specifically targeted and the surrounding normal tissues are spared thus minimising the complications.

Improvements in the development of chemotherapeutic agents with fewer side effects may make drug treatment much more appropriate in the future. Immunotherapy and other targeted therapies have emerged as game changers in several cancers. Proto-oncogenes and tumour suppression genes have been recognised. It is now known that the *p53* gene is mutated in up to 50% of solid tumours. BRCA 1 mutations are associated with an 80–90% risk of breast cancer and a 50% risk of ovarian cancer. Gene therapy is an exciting possibility for the future in the prevention and treatment of cancers.

The assessment of the results of treatment in terms of the length of survival of the patient raises the vital question—when is cancer cured? The very question is a condemnation of the present outlook, encouraged by statistics, which concerns itself with the disease and not the patient. The object of treating cancer is the elimination of every cancer cell; the object of treating the patient is to ensure physical and mental well-being for as long as possible. As things are, the woman with half her viscera removed, or with a rectal stricture or with urinary incontinence, knowing that she has had cancer and living in dread of its return, is regarded as cured. One who lives, albeit for a shorter time, in blissful ignorance of her fate and with her physical functions not too much impaired, is regarded as a therapeutic failure.

The cure for cancer, which will inevitably be found sooner or later, will presumably have a genetic or immunological basis—something which will attack the special metabolism of the cancer cell wherever it may be, leaving the normal metabolism of the healthy cell unimpaired.

On the other end of the spectrum, the main hope for the individual at present lies in the prevention of malignant disease or in its earlier diagnosis and treatment.

PREVENTION OF PELVIC CANCER

As more is learned about the factors associated with malignant disease of the female genital tract, there is hope of preventing certain types. The elimination or control of what are believed to be causal agents, some viruses, for example, could have an effect. The wider extension of better living conditions and higher standards of personal hygiene, male as well as female, and the avoidance of promiscuity and coitus at an early age, probably have much to offer so far as carcinoma of the cervix is concerned.

Vulvectomy for dysplasia of the vulvar epithelium has its place, but does not always prevent squamous cell carcinoma in that site. Wholesale hysterectomy for all

Flowchart 1: Prevention of pelvic cancer.

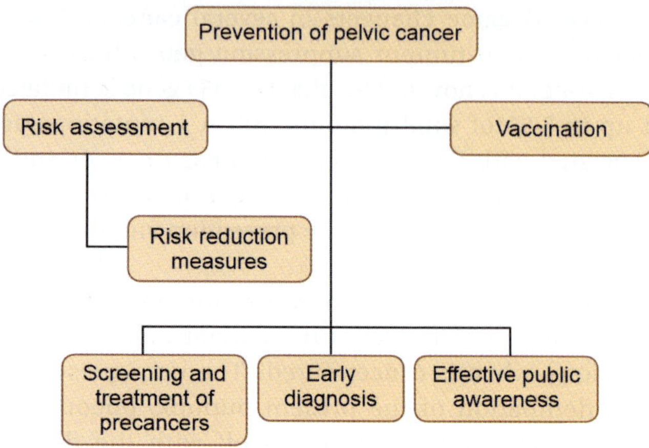

women showing cervical epithelial dysplasia, or suffering from postmenopausal bleeding or discharge, or whose family is complete, could well reduce the number of cancers of the cervix or corpus. Such an approach, however, is likely to involve operative mortality and morbidity rates; hence, risk-reducing measures are to be recommended for those who are identified to have high risk for specific malignancies. Reason and safety impose strict limits on the place of prophylactic surgery in the prevention of cancer of the vulva, uterus, tubes and ovaries.

Flowchart 1 summarises the various ways to prevent pelvic cancer.

EARLY DIAGNOSIS

It is generally accepted that an early cancer is more amenable to cure than one which has been present for some time. Therefore, it is important to pay heed to the first suspicious symptoms or signs presented by the patient, for example, irregular uterine bleeding or discharge occurring after the age of 40 years.

Although early diagnosis and treatment must offer the patient a better chance of survival, they do not always make as much difference as might be expected. Stage I, cases of cancer of the cervix can do badly, while more advanced ones sometimes respond well to treatment. This is because certain growths invade the vascular channels at a very early stage, whereas others remain localised for months and years. Some women appear to have little inherent tissue resistance. Others can come to terms with their cancer—even to the extent of inactivating malignant cells liberated into the blood or lodged in the bone marrow and elsewhere. The first type is rarely cured, no matter how early the attack; the second is nearly always cured, no matter how long treatment is deferred.

The results of therapy according to the stage of cancer of the cervix clearly show that the less the clinical extent of the disease, the better the outlook; but it is all too often assumed that the extent of a cancer represents its age. That this is not the case is shown by relating cures to duration of symptoms. It can then be shown that women who have symptoms for >6 months before being treated often show better 5-year survival rates than those with symptoms for only 3–6 months. This is because those women who delay taking advice either die before treatment is instituted, or they have a cancer which is only slowly progressive. This also explains why the clinical stage of cancer of the cervix is not necessarily proportional to the duration of symptoms.

Nevertheless, the earlier the patients report, the greater the relative number of stage I growths and the better the overall 5-year survival rate. Even this argument, however, may be deceptive. Let it be supposed that a woman with a stage I carcinoma of the cervix is treated in 1989 and dies in 1995; her survival for >5 years is then credited to early treatment. If the same woman neglects her symptoms and fails to take advice until 1994, the cancer has then progressed to stage IV; she is treated but only survives until 1995, and thus, contributes to the poor figures for stage IV growths. In this case, the day of her death is uninfluenced by early diagnosis and treatment. This is hypothetical, but the fact remains that there is as yet no evidence to show even approximately how many more women would be saved by early treatment of invasive carcinoma of the cervix. Some of those whose lesion is only discovered microscopically following screening in *well-women clinics* and who receive prompt treatment still die of the disease.

Effective Public Awareness

Women themselves are often slow to report symptoms; in developed countries, the usual interval between the onset of symptoms and the taking of medical advice in cases of cancer of the cervix is:

- <3 months: 25–50%
- 3 months to 1 year: 20–45%
- >1 year: 30%

For this reason, those who believe that early treatment will have a dramatic effect on the results often advocate propaganda to ensure that all women are aware of the early symptoms of cancer of the genital tract and breast. Unfortunately, some women are resistant to education by the mass media and are more likely to accept what they are told by friends than by doctors. Often it is the overanxious, introspective woman who takes notice of such propaganda, and she is forever producing symptoms which have no basis except fear. The woman with genuine symptoms often avoids taking advice because she does not wish to have her fears confirmed. She would rather remain in doubt because, whatever else she may have heard, she refuses to believe that cancer can be cured.

Despite the acknowledged risks of smoking, girls and young women are now amongst the heaviest smokers in the West. The lung cancer rate has more than tripled in women in the past three decades. To date, health education does not appear to have been heeded, although there has been some reduction in those who smoke during pregnancy.

That delay is not caused by ignorance, as shown by the fact that women doctors and nurses wait just as long as do the laity before reporting suspicious symptoms.

In developing countries, it is commonly observed, especially in the lower socioeconomic strata, that postmenopausal women are reluctant to report symptoms of bleeding and discharge to their families because of embarrassment, although they recognise their symptoms as being abnormal.

Screening (Table 1)

One possible method of improving the results is to discover malignant disease before it has become invasive or, if already invasive, while it is still microscopic and asymptomatic. This means the routine screening of all apparently normal women who are at risk. Arrangements for this, however, usually concentrate on the detection of cervical cancer to the exclusion of other diseases which may be equally, if not more, injurious to health.

Since, in the West, cancer of the breast kills five times as many women as does the cancer of the cervix, it can be argued that regular examination of the breasts is more important than routine tests on the cervix. Malignant conditions of the ovary, although less common, are mostly fatal unless detected in their early asymptomatic stage. Again, diseases such as chronic hypertension, diabetes and even obesity alone may be potentially far more dangerous to a woman than is cervical intraepithelial neoplasia.

These observations mean that cancer detection clinics, or clinics devoted only to cervical or uterine cytodiagnosis, are of limited value. If the best results are to be obtained, cervical smears need to be taken merely as part of a full pelvic and general examination carried out by someone who is competent to recognise pelvic and other diseases by their clinical manifestations, and to give expert medical advice.

TABLE 1: Screening tests.

Cervical cancer	*Endometrial cancer*	*Ovarian cancer*
• Pap test – Traditional Pap smear – Liquid-based cytology • HPV test	• Endometrial tissue sampling – Endometrial biopsy – Dilatation and curettage • Hysterectomy • Transvaginal USG	• Transvaginal USG • CA-125

(CA-125: cancer antigen 125; HPV: human papillomavirus; USG: ultrasonography)

From the standpoint of detecting genital cancer in its early and preinvasive stage, cytology and colposcopy have proven their worth. CA-125 has been developed as a reasonably satisfactory tumour marker for ovarian cancer, which helps in the clinical management of certain cases, but it is neither a cost-effective method for widespread screening nor is it sufficiently specific. Similarly, transvaginal ultrasound and colour flow studies are useful but not suitable for large-scale screening *(see further).*

Cytodiagnosis

Cytodiagnosis depends on the fact that surface cells are being shed continually from the epithelium lining the genital tract. They can therefore be collected and examined to see if they show cytological evidence of unusual, if not malignant, activity. Basically, cytology is not a method for diagnosing cancer; it is a means of screening apparently healthy and symptom-free women to discover those who deserve further investigation to see if they have malignant disease. Cancer can only be diagnosed with reasonable certainty by histological examination of tissue; such a diagnosis is an essential prerequisite for instituting cancer therapy.

Techniques

Vaginal cytology: The secretions lying in the upper vagina normally contain cells desquamated from the vaginal wall, the vaginal aspect of the cervix, the endocervix, the endometrium and sometimes the tubes. The examination of material in the vaginal pool, first suggested and used by Papanicolaou, may therefore be the earliest means of detecting misbehaviour in the epithelium in any of these sites but especially the cervix and the endometrium.

A specimen is collected from the posterior vaginal fornix in a pipette fitted with a rubber bulb to apply suction **(Figs. 3A and B)**. It is smeared onto a grease-free microscope slide and immediately (while still wet) fixed by spraying with 90% alcohol and is transfered to the laboratory. There it is stained usually by the Papanicolaou technique.

This method of collecting material has the advantage that it can be done blindly by anyone, even the woman herself. Since the smear contains endometrial as well as cervical cells, its examination may give a lead to cancer in either site. On the other hand, the admixture of cells means that the cytologist finds it more difficult and time-consuming to interpret. So, since it is the detection of cervical lesions which is more important, the cervical scrape method for obtaining material is preferable.

Cervical scrape: This method is the current gold standard. It involves scraping of the superficial cells from the external os and lower endocervix by means of a special wooden spatula **(Fig. 4)**. Accurate application of the spatula to the *squamocolumnar epithelial junction* throughout its whole circumference is essential; this means direct vision of a well-exposed cervix. A smear is made from the material thus obtained and handled in the same way as described above.

The Ayre's *scrape technique* is unreliable in picking up endometrial cells but is more efficient than the Papanicolaou method in collecting cervical cells. Moreover, the resulting smear can be assessed more easily and more quickly in the laboratory.

The Ayre's spatula occasionally yields an insufficient number of endocervical cells. The extended tip spatula with a longer endocervical limb has been found to have a higher rate of satisfactory smears. The Ayre's spatula can also be combined with the endocervical cytobrush to improve the yield of endocervical cells **(Fig. 4)**.

This is the technique to be employed for the routine screening of apparently well women. It can be applied during pregnancy and is not ruled out if the woman is menstruating or bleeding for other cause. If the patient cannot return later, the blood or discharge can be gently wiped away from the external os and the specimen subsequently taken gives quite reliable findings in the hands of an expert in the field.

Intracervical and intrauterine aspiration techniques: These are not for routine screening purposes but for the investigation of women suspected on clinical grounds of harbouring malignant disease within the cavity of the uterus. The collection of endometrial cells on rotating brushes and other gadgets is now supplanted by endometrial lavage under negative pressure. Indeed, it is potentially dangerous to insert into the cavity of the uterus

Figs. 3A and B: The original methods for taking cervical and vaginal material to make 'smears' for the purpose of cytology. For Papanicolaou's technique, vaginal pool specimens are collected by some form of suction pipette.

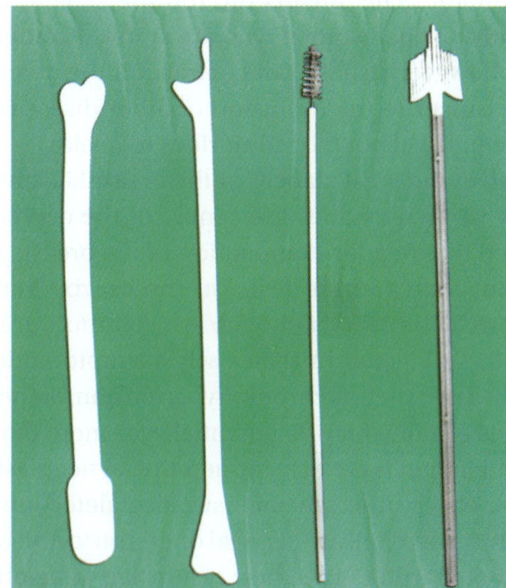

Fig. 4: Sampling devices for cervical cytology. From left to right: Ayre's wooden spatula, extended tip plastic spatula, endocervical cytobrush, Cervex-Brush®.

any instrument if there is a possibility of corporeal cancer or pyometra. Suction curettage by the Vabra aspirator is an effective method of obtaining endometrial tissue using negative pressure. The endometrial biopsy curette used for the investigation of patients with infertility, or the Karman-type cannula, can also be used. Aseptic techniques are essential, but these can be applied without anaesthesia and without the need to admit the patient to the hospital.

Suction aspiration of this type carries an accuracy rate of 90% in the diagnosis of endometrial carcinoma and can sometimes reveal a growth missed by conventional diagnostic curettage.

Screening for Cervical Epithelial Abnormalities

Ideally, cervical cytology should be carried out on all sexually active women, but this is impractical. If the first smear is reported free from abnormal cells, the test should be repeated within 1 year and preferably earlier. This is because a single negative finding, as with all laboratory procedures, carries a 10% risk of being wrong. The explanation is not only mistakes on the part of the cytologist, but also those made during the collection, labelling and handling of specimens at all stages of the test.

If a second smear is reported as being negative the chance of error is extremely small and the test need then be repeated only at 1- to 3-yearly intervals. If a woman has had prior three consecutive negative smears by the age of 65 years, there is no necessity of further cervical smears as she is not likely to develop carcinoma of the cervix.

When the cytologist reports the presence of abnormal or suspicious cells, further evaluation should be carried out. Even minor cytological variations are associated with major histological changes. Repeat smears for confirmation are therefore no longer recommended.

In practice, and no matter where facilities for cervical cytology are provided, only a proportion of women take advantage of them. These are mostly the women who are better educated, intelligent and belong to the higher socioeconomic group—the women who are least likely to develop carcinoma of the cervix. The sarne type of women attend postnatal clinics, whereas those at greater risk tend to default. A programme designed to cover all or most women should therefore include routine cervical cytology as part of antenatal and postnatal supervision. Indeed, if all women attending antenatal care, and all those seen in gynaecological, infertility, STD and family planning clinics were tested, many of those at risk would be included.

In developing countries, an extreme paucity of medical services, lack of access to these services and trained cytotechnicians and laboratories means that the majority of women will never undergo a Pap smear. At a minimum, it is recommended that all women should have at least one cervical smear by the age of 40 years. Successful programmes for the clinical downstaging of cervical cancer have been developed—midwives and other paramedical staff are trained to do a speculum examination of the cervix and identify a suspicious cervix. All women thus identified then have a Pap smear. Thus, limited resources are targeted at the high-risk population. The incidence of invasive cancer is reported to be 29/1,000 in women with an abnormal cervix but only 1.53/1,000 in those with a healthy cervix.

Visual Inspection after Acetic Acid (VIA)/ Lugol's Iodine (VILI)

The clinicians as well as trained health workers can inspect the uterine cervix after applying freshly prepared 3–5% acetic acid. The abnormal area will appear acetowhite/ iodine negative. The test is used as a screening method in low-resource settings. With the help of technology assistance, such as image capture, transfer to an expert, expert reporting on the images, this modality can be made more acceptable and reliable. The addition of artificial intelligence-based applications for image analysis and reporting is also likely to make the modality more robust.

Human Papillomavirus Testing

In the year 2018, World Health Organization (WHO) called for the elimination of cervical cancer by 2030, and for the same, strategies were proposed with guidelines. Screening at least 70% of the eligible women has been one of the strategies. For this purpose, one can adopt any of the available screening modalities depending on the resources. Women between 30 and 55 years having cervical screening at least once or twice using a high-performance screen test is expected to reduce the cancer burden significantly.

High-risk human papillomavirus (HPV) testing in the cervicovaginal secretions is the presently recommended test for cervical screening. A US Food and Drug Administration (FDA)-approved or WHO-preauthorised test platform can be used for primary screening. The sample may be collected by a clinician performing a speculum examination or by self-sampling. This test in future is expected to take the screening to homes, thereby empowering women to do their testing themselves. Client participation in this form will also boost the community awareness.

Colposcopy

Colposcopy is not a practical means for screening large numbers of asymptomatic women. It is useful for the further study of women whose cervical smears are reported as positive or doubtfully positive, and of those whose cervix is clinically suspicious despite negative cytological findings. Colposcopy is the next level test for the women diagnosed as HPV 16/18 positive. Colposcopy then indicates the need and site for cervical biopsy and possible suitability for ablative therapy. The colposcope can also be used to visualise the vulva and vagina under magnification.

Cervicography

Cervicography has been designed as a substitute for colposcopy in those areas where medical services are available but not the services of a skilled colposcopist. In such a situation, two photographs of the cervix are taken with a especially designed camera, following the procedure of colposcopy. These are then sent to a specialised centre where they are developed as 35 mm slides, projected and reported by a specialist viewer. Further management is planned accordingly. More than 90% of colposcopically diagnosed lesions can be correctly detected with cervicography. More importantly, cases of invasive cancer are accurately diagnosed. Thus, this is a viable alternative to colposcopy for patients in remote areas.

Ultrasound

Ultrasonic scans, especially by the transvaginal route, have been suggested as having a role in screening for ovarian and to evaluate the endometrium to identify endometrial hyperplasia or cancer. The principal difficulty lies in recognising those at risk, and such as breast carcinoma, a cancer will be present, so the lesion will not be diagnosed before it is already invasive. Nevertheless, it should be done annually in women with a family history of epithelial ovarian cancer or a history of prolonged therapy for the induction of ovulation. Addition of colour flow Doppler studies and serum markers like CA-125 *(see further)* improves the sensitivity. However, these techniques are expensive, not widely available and are unsuited to large-scale screening programmes.

Ultrasound has a major role to play in the diagnosis of trophoblastic disease and the differential diagnosis of pelvic and abdominal masses.

Tumour Markers

Tumour markers are useful in the management of ovarian malignancy and gestational trophoblastic tumours but have not been found useful as a screening test for the general population.

Cancer antigen 125 (CA-125) is a tumour-associated antigen expressed by about 80% of patients with epithelial ovarian cancer. It is not suitable for screening for ovarian cancer in the general population, because it is elevated in many benign conditions with ascites and in nongynaecologic malignancies where there is involvement of the pleura or peritoneum. When combined with clinical assessment and ultrasound, it may help to differentiate benign pelvic masses from malignant ones and is useful in the follow-up of malignancy and the detection of recurrence. Other tumour markers that have been used in ovarian malignancy are *human epididymis protein 4* (HE4), TAG 72 and CA 15-3. Similarly, alpha-fetoprotein (AFP), beta-human chorionic gonadotrophin (hCG) and lactate dehydrogenase (LDH) are useful markers for germ cell tumours of the ovary. β-hCG is a very sensitive marker for gestational trophoblastic tumours.

GENERAL MANAGEMENT OF THE CANCER PATIENT

Attention to General Health

No matter what the site and type of genital cancer, and whether surgery, radiotherapy or chemotherapy is contemplated, the patient's prospects are considerably improved if her nutritional state is at its best and if anaemia and cachexia are corrected and diabetes controlled before treatment.

Should the Patient be Told the Diagnosis?

It has for generations been held that, with few exceptions, it is not in the interest of the patient to tell her that she suffers from cancer, and this view was reached by doctors who were more expert in the art of medicine than is the profession of today. Within recent years, there has grown a body of opinion which takes the opposite view.

It is easy for both doctor and relatives to tell the truth and thus be spared much dissembling, trouble and even criticism when the patient is not making the progress she expects. It makes for personal comfort to shift responsibility, even at the expense of depriving the dying of all hope or of making the healthy live in fear of the recurrence which may never come. The conscience can always be quietened with a glib assertion that it is unethical or immoral not to tell the patient the truth. Are those who take this standpoint equally candid about their errors in diagnosis or mishaps during operations? Do they tell a very sick man that he is suffering from pneumonia or heart failure? Or do they describe these conditions in the softer terms of congestion and weakness?

There are some who advocate telling the diagnosis to only those women who can be cured of their cancer. These patients, by advertising the good result, can then correct the public impression that cancer is incurable. But who can foretell which patient will be cured? Other doctors argue that they reveal the diagnosis to all patients in order to ensure their readiness to attend follow-up clinics. One tactic which can be employed from this standpoint is to describe the lesion in terms of inflammation, which, if neglected, might possibly develop into a growth. This gives the excuse necessary to ensure continued observation and leaves the patient happy at the thought that she has avoided the dreaded disease. Prevarication or distortion of the truth is made all the easier by the fact that the woman herself is alert to accept any innocent explanation. This is true even for members of the medical or nursing professions. Even though they know or suspect the diagnosis, many wish to have it denied, not confirmed.

The reactions of patients vary, and undoubtedly change with a wider dispersal of medical knowledge. One follow-up enquiry amongst those who had been told of the presence of cancer showed that some were grateful to have the knowledge, some resented it, but many denied having received it. The last had deliberately closed their minds to the situation.

Unquestionably, there are some people whose mental fibre is such that they are happier when their doubts are removed, but these do not include the ones who, with outward bravado, say, "Tell me the truth, doctor, I can take it". It is impossible to recognise those women who might be happier to know the diagnosis, even with considerable experience. It is preferable to keep the whole truth from the women unless a very radical operation is required. All patients who are going to have a colostomy (temporary or permanent) or urinary diversion, for example, and their immediate relatives, must be informed why such procedures are necessary.

The matter is clearly one on which there may be an honest difference of opinion, and on which procedure must vary from patient to patient. It is essential always to explain the exact state of affairs to the nearest relative at the earliest possible moment.

MANAGEMENT OF ADVANCED PELVIC CANCER

A problem commonly facing the medical attendant is the woman with advanced pelvic cancer—often a return of growth following ineffectual surgery or radiotherapy, with complications of treatment added. Such women are in a miserable plight which may last for months and years; their management and treatment are as much a challenge to the art as to the science of medicine.

Palliative Approach

This approach is to recognise that nothing more can be done to cure the patient, and to concentrate on relieving symptoms as they arise and on making the woman's remaining life and ultimate death as comfortable as possible. Death itself is not a dreadful thing; it is the manner of it which counts. In the terminal phases, nature usually takes a hand and invokes uraemia to induce oblivion during the last few hours or days. When this or any other happening betokens the end, there should be no meddling with nature by renal dialysis, resuscitation, intensive care or other modern gadgetry.

General Care

Morale is best maintained if the patient does not realise the situation and if she is encouraged to lead as normal a life as possible for as long as possible. There is no reason for denying any reasonable wish. Once she becomes bedridden, the problems mount because constant attendance and expert nursing are required if bed sores are to be avoided. Despite this, and provided that help and conveniences are available, the woman is happier to remain at home. For anorexia and nausea, antiemetics, alcohol and small doses of prednisolone are helpful. Cachexia can be counteracted by parenteral nutrition. Abdominal distension and dyspnoea caused by fluid effusions can be relieved by *tapping*. Hospice care is an alternative for the terminal cancer patient who requires intervention and cannot be treated at home. It allows comprehensive management by a skilled team of doctors and paramedical staff aided by specialised counsellors, psychiatrists, music therapists, religious priests, etc. in an atmosphere of peacefulness and cleanliness to allow the terminal cancer patient an atmosphere of dignity and comfort.

Relief of Pain

The pain, which is nearly always present in the later stages of pelvic cancer, is of two kinds; both are sometimes present in the same case.

Visceral

This is often a diffuse type of pelvic pain, which may be described by the patient as a dull ache or *bursting*. Sometimes, it is colicky and intermittent. It arises most commonly in the bladder or rectum, but its origin can be uterine (as in the case of pyometra), intestinal (as in obstruction) or renal and ureteric (when the lower ureter is obstructed).

Somatic

This pain is localised to certain nerves or groups of nerves and is shooting or throbbing; it tends to be worse at night. It originates mainly from the sacral plexus but can have an obturator nerve distribution. It may result from infiltration of soft tissues, bones or nerves by the tumour.

Treatment for cancer pain is usually done in a stepwise fashion. The primary management involves assessment (by history, examination and investigation) of the likely cause of pain. The first step is to administer mild analgesics such as paracetamol or aspirin. Nonsteroidal anti-inflammatory drugs (NSAIDs) are particularly useful in cases of bony metastases where pain is mediated through prostaglandin release, but they are useful in other cases as well. Many cancer patients may be receiving other drugs as well, so drug interactions and side effects must be kept in mind while prescribing palliative therapy.

Next, the addition of a tranquilliser or an antidepressant decreases anxiety, potentiates the effects of analgesics, and raises the threshold to pain. Along with the care and concern of loved ones as mentioned above, music therapy and religion also play an important role here.

With advanced cancers, this therapy may not suffice to provide adequate pain relief. A wide range of opioids is available for the third step of treatment. Milder ones such as codeine or dextropropoxyphene, are used initially. Morphine is a stronger opioid. It is now available in oral as well as parenteral preparations. The oral route is the simplest. If there are problems of gastrointestinal absorption, the subcutaneous route is sometimes required. The intramuscular and intravenous routes are seldom used. The latter, especially, gives only short-lived benefit and may be hazardous.

A proportion of patients may develop addiction to morphine, but this is of little consequence. Caregivers are sometimes concerned that there may be no stronger analgesic available later when the disease (and the pain) worsens, and need adequate counselling and reassurance. Indeed, the dose of morphine does need careful initiation and titration for effective results. It is started at a dose of 5–10 mg orally every 4 hours and increased as required. The usual dose requirement is 30–60 mg 4-hourly, but some patients need doses of 100 mg. Controlled-release tablets have the advantage of twice-daily administration. Some patients develop severe constipation, which may increase their discomfort, and symptomatic relief may be needed. Oxycodone is tolerated better than morphine by some patients, but pethidine can itself cause neurotoxicity when used in high doses for prolonged periods and is not recommended.

The last step is the relief of neuropathic pain. Regular small doses of corticosteroids can relieve nerve root pains, reduce tumour oedema and produce euphoria. Antidepressants, anticonvulsants and regional anaesthesia blocks with long-acting anaesthetics are useful in these cases.

The rule is to choose a small range of drugs and to become an expert in their use, alone or in combination. It is important, too, to administer analgesics regularly, which may be <4 hourly, not just when there is another bout of pain. They should never be given *as a favour,* and there is much to be said for letting the patient help herself to them as much and as often as she wishes. For these reasons, it is best to keep to oral medication for as long as possible.

Surgical measures may sometimes be called for, e.g. drainage of a pyometra or an abscess or the relief of ureteric obstruction *(see further).*

Haemorrhage

When haemorrhage occurs from incurable malignant ulcers in the vulva, vagina and uterus, drastic remedies may not be indicated. Death from haemorrhage is one of the more comfortable escapes from misery. Radiotherapy can control recurrent haemorrhage, but cannot be used if the patient has had previous radiotherapy. In that case, painting of the ulcer with acetone or coagulating its surface with diathermy not only stops the bleeding but temporarily clears up the troublesome offensive discharge. Acetone is an old remedy, the value of which now tends to be overlooked. Another alternative sometimes used is packing, with the application of Monsel's solution. Arterial embolisation may be possible if the main bleeder is identified.

Swelling of the Leg

Oedema of the legs can be counteracted by posture and elastic bandaging. Often, however, it is the result of deep phlebothrombosis; this, sometimes followed by embolism, is not uncommon in advanced pelvic cancer. Embolism may offer a quick release for the patient and, in these circumstances, anticoagulant therapy is generally not indicated.

Urinary Tract Symptoms

Hydronephrosis leading to subsequent infection, pain and obstructive uropathy is often seen with advanced gynaecological cancers, especially of the cervix. Some of these may be candidates for nephrostomy or insertion of a stent. Surgery has a place in those patients where the expectation of life is not short. Medical means to reduce oedema and improve patency include the administration of corticosteroids.

Advanced pelvic cancer often means a urinary fistula, and for this, it may be best to transplant the ureters into the colon. The disadvantages of this operation—the risks of pyelonephritis and of electrolyte imbalance—do not matter because the treatment is merely symptomatic for a woman with only a short time to live. Before operation, it is important to exclude the presence, or the impending presence, of a rectovaginal fistula; in such cases, the ureters can be transplanted into an ileal conduit.

If these operations are contraindicated by active growth or impending death, it becomes a matter of preventing excoriation of the skin of the vulva by applying a barrier cream or grease, and of controlling the dribbling by liberal applications of cotton wool. Female urinals, in the form of bags which fit the vulva, are nearly always unsatisfactory. The leak from a high fistula can sometimes be controlled by inserting a Foley catheter into the vagina, or by packing the vagina with a sponge whose lower part fits into a soft wide-bore rubber tube.

Incontinence of Faeces

A vaginal faecal fistula is not usually as troublesome as a urinary one, provided that diarrhoea is avoided. The patient learns to empty the lower bowel regularly and to douche the vagina clear of faeces immediately afterwards. If the incontinence is distressing, and especially if it is accompanied by dyschezia, colostomy is indicated. But if the patient suffers from radiation enteritis, the frequent fluid motions can make a colostomy intolerable.

Chemotherapy

A large variety of drugs have been tried to combat malignant disease. Those which have established merit in the treatment of cancer of the female genitalia and which are in common use are mentioned below. They are given individually or in various combinations, as supplements to surgery or radiotherapy, as prophylactics against recurrence after surgery, and to control or modify advanced cancer. In the last circumstance, chemotherapy can prolong life, and sometimes give comfort.

Chemotherapeutic agents may be cell cycle-specific or nonspecific; the drugs which are cycle-specific act on cells in a particular phase of the cell cycle only and other cells are spared, e.g. actinomycin D acts on the Gl phase, adriamycin and methotrexate on the S, etoposide on the G2 and the vinca alkaloids on the M phase. Cells in the G0 phase are not affected. Cycle nonspecific drugs can kill cells in all phases of the cell cycle.

Many of the details of the usage of some of the drugs already appear in other chapters under the heading of treatment of individual malignant states. What follows aims to summarise these and to give a broad picture.

Cell Growth Cycle

To understand how chemotherapy works, one must first understand the cell growth cycle. Most of the cells in a tumour are in the resting or G0 phase. In response to certain factors, normally growth factors or steroids, cells are induced to enter the growth cycle, which is divided into two growth phases (Gl and G2), a phase of synthesis (S) and a mitotic phase (M). The Gl phase varies from cell to cell, ranging from 8 to 100 hours and in this phase, there is hectic activity resulting in the synthesis of various enzymes and proteins, which will be needed in the next phase of synthesis.

In the S phase, DNA is synthesised and thus doubled. This phase lasts about 10 hours and is followed by the G2 phase. This is a shorter phase, about 5 hours in duration, during which RNA and protein synthesis occur, which provides for the requirements of the two daughter cells. During the G2 phase, DNA replication errors are also corrected.

The last phase is the phase of mitosis, which lasts about an hour and results in the generation of two daughter cells.

Types of Drugs

All the following groups, except hormones, act by destroying actively dividing cells or preventing their propagation. They are classified on the basis of their biochemistry **(Flowchart 2)**.

Alkylating agents: These crosslink DNA strands and deprive the cell of substances essential to mitosis, respiration and glycolysis, such as nucleoproteins and enzymes. They include the nitrogen mustards, chlorambucil, cyclophosphamide, melphalan, ethyleneimines such as thiotepa, and the newer agents, ifosfamide and treosulfan. All are used for any form of pelvic malignant disease, but especially for those arising in the ovaries and also for the breast and various sarcomas. Whilst chlorambucil and cyclophosphamide can be given orally, they are best given intravenously.

Since they cause bone marrow suppression, careful monitoring of the white cells and platelets is required. Cyclophosphamide and ifosfamide cause alopecia and a severe chemical cystitis unless the uroprotector mesna (sodium 2-mercaptoethane sulphonate) is simultaneously administered.

Alkylating-like agents: Cis-dichlorodiammineplatinum (commonly known as cisplatin), carboplatin and dacarbazine (DTIC) are classified as alkylating-like agents. Their precise mode of action is uncertain, but they do have an alkylating effect, although they may have other modes of action too. They are used in the therapy of ovarian carcinoma, germ cell tumours and cervical cancer. DTIC has been used in the treatment of uterine and soft tissue sarcomas.

Cisplatin causes severe nephropathy, nausea, vomiting, dose-related peripheral neuropathy and anaemia. It also produces tinnitus and hearing loss. Carboplatin has less neurotoxicity, ototoxicity and nephrotoxicity than cisplatin but may have greater myelosuppression, especially thrombocytopaenia.

Antimetabolites: These can be divided into three groups:

1. *Folate antagonists*, such as methotrexate, which are particularly valuable in the treatment of choriocarcinoma; they act by inhibiting the enzyme dihydrofolate reductase and by depriving dividing cells of coenzymes essential to the synthesis of nucleic acids. Methotrexate is generally a very safe drug. The most common side effect is mouth ulcers. However, in patients with renal compromise or ascites, it can be very toxic.
2. *Pyrimidine antagonists*, such as 5-fluorouracil (5-FU), block thymidine synthesis and the incorporation of uracil into DNA. Myelosuppression and mucositis are the most common side effects. They are rarely employed systemically, but are sometimes applied locally in the treatment of vulvar intraepithelial neoplasia (VIN III).
3. *Purine antagonists*, which have no established role in gynaecological cancer. Antimetabolites are often used in combination when they exert a complementary effect because of their cycle-specific behaviour.

Antitumour antibiotics: Of these, actinomycin D and doxorubicin (adriamycin) are used for the treatment of malignant disease of the female genitalia, mostly trophoblastic tumours, ovarian cancer and sarcomas in the pelvis. Bleomycin has been used in cases of carcinoma of the cervix and of the vulva, as well as in testicular and bladder cancer. It has a pulmonary toxicity, and careful monitoring is required to avoid severe complications. Mitomycin C has been used to treat tumours of the breast, cervix and ovary. They form irreversible complexes with DNA and interfere with its replication.

Doxorubicin causes myelosuppression and marked alopecia. More importantly, it is very irritating if injected

Flowchart 2: Classification of chemotherapy drugs.

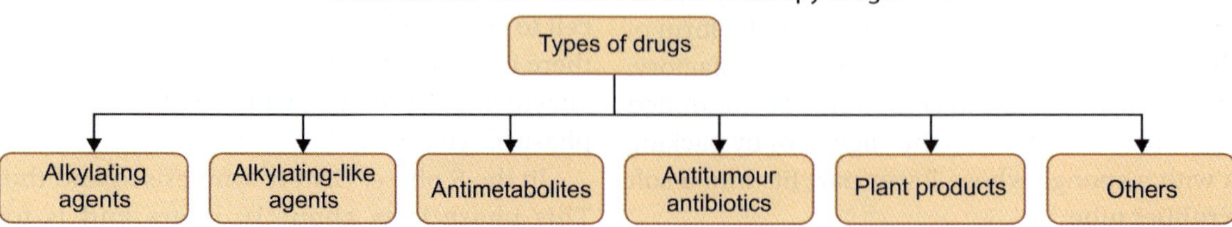

subcutaneously inadvertently, and it should be given in a rapidly running drip. The total dose is limited to 450 mg/m^2; cardiomyopathy can result from higher doses. *Epirubicin* and *mitoxantrone* are newer drugs in this group, which are less cardiotoxic. Bleomycin causes a dose-related pulmonary fibrosis, usually at doses >300 mg/m^2.

Plant products: Plant alkaloids such as vinblastine and vincristine have a specific blocking effect on mitosis and are effective against sarcomas, ovarian germ cell tumours and cervical cancer. Derived from the common periwinkle plant (Vinca rosea), the vinca alkaloids bind intracellular microtubular proteins, destroy the mitotic spindle and arrest mitosis.

Peripheral and autonomic neuropathy are the main side effects, especially with vincristine. Local irritation may be encountered at the injection site, so they should be administered into a rapidly running drip. However, they are not myelotoxic.

Paclitaxel, an extract from the bark of the Pacific Yew tree, disrupts microtubule function and has been found to be extremely useful in the treatment of ovarian carcinoma and breast cancer. It causes myelosuppression, nausea, severe alopecia and hypersensitivity reactions. When combined with platinum agents, it should be administered first, and when combined with doxorubicin, it should be administered last to promote synergistic action and decrease toxicity. Docetaxel is the first semisynthetic analogue of paclitaxel.

Epipodophyllotoxins are extracts from the mandrake plant. The active principle etoposide (VP-16) is useful in the treatment of gestational trophoblastic tumours. It does not inhibit the mitotic spindle, but acts by causing breaks in the DNA. It causes severe myelosuppression, nausea, vomiting and alopecia.

Other agents: Hexamethyl melamine is an oral drug used in protocols for ovarian and breast cancer; the mechanism of action is poorly understood.

Dangers

All chemotherapeutic agents have real dangers and need to be carefully controlled. Cytotoxic drugs attack normal as well as neoplastic tissues, especially those which are always actively replacing themselves, namely the bone marrow, the intestinal mucosa and hair follicles. Hence, anaemia and leucopoenia are inevitable effects, and nausea, vomiting, wasting, stomatitis, conjunctivitis, ulceration of the mouth, gut and anus, skin rashes and alopecia are all common. The platelet level also falls, and this can result in blood coagulation defects and haemorrhage.

Chemotherapy is controlled essentially by repeated examination of the blood. In general, maximum myelosuppression usually occurs 10–14 days after treatment has been initiated. If the white cell count falls below 3,000/mL or the platelet count falls below 100,000/mL, treatment is suspended until the counts recover. Renal function has to be checked carefully when cisplatin and its analogues are used, and respiratory function must be monitored during bleomycin treatment.

During treatment, the patient should be protected as far as possible by vitamin and iron supplements added to her diet, and by blood, red cell or platelet transfusions as and when required. Because her resistance to infection is lowered, routine antibiotic therapy may be indicated.

If given during the first trimester of pregnancy, cytotoxic and antimetabolic agents may kill or maim the foetus, especially the antimetabolites and alkylating agents. A higher abortion rate is reported. Chemotherapy in the second or third trimester is not reported to cause foetal abnormality, but it may induce in the foetus side effects experienced by the mother, e.g. leucopoenia and thrombocytopenia. Intrauterine growth restriction and prematurity have been observed, but it is unclear whether this can be attributed to the chemotherapy or to other factors associated with the disease.

Treatment Regimens

The objective of cancer chemotherapy is to provide the patient with the maximum therapeutic benefit with the minimal amount of morbidity. Since most drugs used are only relatively selective for tumour cells compared to normal cells, most of the drugs have a narrow therapeutic range. Those involved in cancer chemotherapy have therefore to choose dosages within a narrow range because of the dose-response relationship and low therapeutic index of most drugs used. Short courses in full doses are generally preferred to long-term, continuous small-dose therapy. However, determination of the most appropriate dose is a complex clinical skill, based on the anticipated response of the patient and characteristics of the drug(s) used compared with the morbidity of the treatment and the potential benefits. In a patient with advanced disease who will die, if untreated, in a short period of time, highly aggressive use of the drugs is justified if a significant potential for survival exists. If survival without treatment is expected to be prolonged, then caution is required in the use of drugs. Considerable clinical expertise is therefore necessary to make a decision regarding an individual patient's potential tolerance to chemotherapy and the proposed treatment.

All antineoplastic agents kill a constant fraction of cells, not a constant number, producing successive log falls in tumour burden with successive courses.

With the exception of gestational trophoblastic tumours, single-agent therapy rarely results in a cure.

The use of cancer chemotherapeutic agents in clinical practice now relies heavily on combinations of drugs. As a consequence, combinations of two to five drugs may be used. The revised drug regimens have increased the efficacy and enhanced the antitumour capabilities of the presently available drugs. Further advances may be expected with continuing research in basic pharmacology, biochemistry and toxicology, as well as into the intricate behaviour of the tumour cell.

The best results with chemotherapy have been seen with trophoblastic tumours and germ cell ovarian tumours. In other genital cancers, chemotherapy does not always cure a patient, so a proper balance of the advantages, potential or actual, and the disadvantages, namely the adverse effects, must be maintained by all those involved in treating patients.

Hormone Therapy

Hormone receptor assays can be done on biopsies of hormone-responsive tumours, e.g. of the endometrium and therapy is planned accordingly. Oestrogens are valueless in the treatment of genital cancer. Androgens merely have an anabolic effect. Progestogens, however, appear sometimes to arrest endometrial carcinoma and its metastases and are worth trying in the treatment of recurrent malignant disease of the uterus. The response is almost certainly related to whether the tumour contains progesterone receptors. Antioestrogens such as tamoxifen may be used for oestrogen-dependent tumours but are more commonly used in carcinoma of the breast.

Targeted therapy: In gynaecologic malignancies, potential therapeutic targeted agents include antiangiogenic agents, poly (ADP-ribose) polymerase (PARP) inhibitors, tumour-intrinsic signalling pathway inhibitors, selective oestrogen receptor downregulators and immune checkpoint inhibitors. bevacizumab, olaparib, rucaparib, niraparib, and pembrolizumab have been approved by the FDA for selected patients with recurrent, metastatic, or high-risk diseases.

Radical Surgery

Some take the view that it is wrong to accept what appears to be inevitable and that, if surgery is sufficiently radical, even the apparently hopeless case of pelvic cancer can sometimes be cured. The cure, however, is at the expense of injury to, or removal of, the ureters, bladder and rectum.

Exenteration

This operation is mainly carried out for central recurrence of cancer of the cervix after radiotherapy, but sometimes as a primary treatment for advanced pelvic cancer of all kinds. It relieves pain, discharge, incontinence (but only by changing the site of incontinence) and can sometimes cure. Exenteration is technically possible when the growth is confined to the pelvis and is not fixed to the bony walls. Unfortunately, it is often not possible to judge the extent without laparotomy, and this may mean only one exenteration operation for every three abdomens opened. The presence of oedema of the leg or of hip pain referred to the leg, is the warning against attempted exenteration. Poor renal function is also a contraindication. If pelvic nodes are involved, the 5-year survival rate is <5%, and the procedure should therefore be abandoned if any of the lymph nodes show evidence of metastatic disease.

The total operation consists of the excision of all the pelvic viscera, fascia and lymphatics, the woman being left with a separate colostomy and ileal loop bladder. In anterior exenteration, the rectum is not removed, and in posterior exenteration, the bladder and ureters are spared, and all other viscera are removed. Because it is often impossible to conserve the rectum or bladder and ureters without leaving potential lymphatic spread, a total exenteration may be preferred for cure, which should be the aim of the operation. No exenteration operation should ever be carried out as a palliative procedure, except possibly in the presence of a vesicovaginal fistula.

These major operations, especially total exenteration, carry a high risk, even in the hands of those with special experience and facilities. For the total operation, the average surgeon can expect a primary mortality rate of 3–10% and a 5-year survival rate varying from 0 to 70%, depending upon the extent of the disease, with an average of 25–35%. Successful salvage is more likely in patients who have recurrence following primary surgery than in those following primary radiotherapy and whose tumour size is <3 cm. The patients most likely to benefit are those who have central pelvic recurrence at least 1 year, but preferably longer, after initial therapy.

Providing the selection is good, then this ultraradical surgery is justifiable for a few women who have not only courage and fortitude but also some special incentive to live longer. Recurrence may be expected in up to one-third of patients. Any woman for whom exenteration is contemplated should be aware of all its implications, and the medical attendant should beware of striving too hard to keep her alive. There is a difference between life and existence.

SUGGESTED READING

1. Bergman C, Boente M. Surgery for gynecologic malignancies. Curr Opin Oncol. 1998;10(5):434-8.
2. Chai W, Gong F, Zhang W, Wen Y, Cui L. Multiple primary cancer in the female genital system: Two rare case reports and a literature review. Medicine (Baltimore). 2017;96(47):e8860.
3. Gottwald L, Akoel KM, Wójcik-Krowiranda K, Bieńkiewicz A. Malignant tumors of the female genital track in the elderly. Ginekol Pol. 2003;74(9):714-7.
4. Lawton F, Smith R. Surgery for gynecologic cancer. Curr Opin Oncol. 1994;6(5):519-23.
5. Patibandla JR, Fehniger JE, Levine DA. Small cell cancers of the female genital tract: Molecular and clinical aspects. Gynecol Oncol. 2018;17.
6. Wang Q, Peng H, Qi X, Wu M, Zhao X. Targeted therapies in gynecological cancers: a comprehensive review of clinical evidence. Signal Transduct Target Ther. 2020;5(1):137.

28

CHAPTER

Tumours of the Vulva

Rekha Upadhya, Muralidhar V Pai

Chapter Outline

- Swellings of the Vulva
- Varicose Veins
- Oedema
- Retention Cysts
- Benign Neoplasms
- Malignant Neoplasms of Vulva
- Tumours of Bartholin's Gland
- Urethral Tumours
- Tumours of the Inguinal Canal

INTRODUCTION

Vulvar tumours including both benign and malignant growths are the neoplasms of the female external genitalia, in the region of vulva. Vulvar cancer is an uncommon malignancy, however it is important to understand its early detection and effective management.

SWELLINGS OF THE VULVA

A complaint of swelling of the vulva may be caused by the following conditions:

- *Development abnormalities:*
  - Hypertrophy of the clitoris
  - Phimosis or paraphimosis with oedema of the glans clitoris
  - Unilateral or bilateral hypertrophy of the labium minus
  - Accessory nipple or breast
- *Injury*:
  - Haematoma
- *Displacements*:
  - Vaginal or uterine prolapse, inversion of the uterus vaginal, cervical and uterine tumours projecting through the introitus
- *Vascular changes*:
  - Oedema of the vulva
  - Varicose veins
  - Elephantiasis and false elephantiasis
- *Infections*:
  - Acute vulvitis, infective or chemical
  - Furuncle and carbuncle
  - Condylomata acuminata (warts)
  - Syphilitic condylomas
  - Hypertrophic tuberculosis
  - Smegma concretions
- *Retention cysts*:
  - Sebaceous cyst
  - Epidermoid cyst (inclusion dermoid)
  - Hymeneal and clitoral cysts (Wolffian remains)
- Endometriotic deposits and cysts
- *Benign neoplasms*:
  - Papilloma, fibromyoma, neuroma, neurofibroma, lipoma, angioma, lymphangioma and myoblastoma
  - Hidradenoma (sweat gland tumour)
  - Adenoma of Wolffian duct origin
- *Malignant neoplasms*:
  - Squamous cell carcinoma (SCC)
  - Melanoma
  - Sarcoma
  - Metastases, bloodborne from any site, including choriocarcinoma and lymphoma
- *Enlargement of Bartholin's gland*:
  - Bartholinitis; Bartholin abscess
  - Bartholin cyst
  - Adenoma
  - Adenocarcinoma
- *Urethral conditions*:
  - Prolapse of the urethra, acute or chronic
  - Caruncle
  - Carcinoma
  - Cyst of Skene's tubules
  - Diverticulum of the urethra
- *Conditions of the inguinal canal and round ligament*:
  - Inguinal hernia
  - Hydrocele of the canal of Nuck

- Varicocele of the round ligament
- Tumours of the round ligament, including endometriosis.

VARICOSE VEINS

Varicose veins commonly occur on the vulva during pregnancy **(Figs. 1 and 2)** but disappear afterwards. As a significant clinical entity, they are rare in the nonpregnant woman, even one who has a badly affected leg. Symptom-producing varicosities in nonpregnant women are treated by the injection of sclerosing fluids or ligation of the long saphenous vein at a high level.

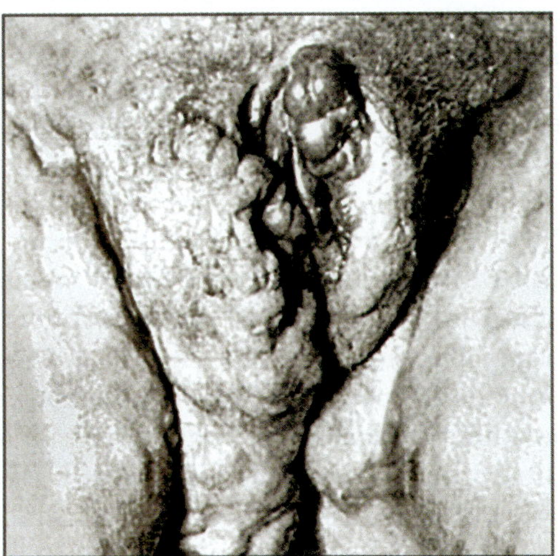

Fig. 1: Varicosities of the vulva during pregnancy.

OEDEMA

Oedema of the vulva has the same causes as bilateral oedema of the legs—heart failure, renal failure, large abdominal tumours, ascites, anaemia, malnutrition and the like. Its association with a pelvic or abdominal mass nearly always means that the tumour is malignant. Oedema of the vulva is common in pregnancy, especially as part of the syndrome of pre-eclampsia **(Fig. 3)**.

The cure of vulvar oedema depends on removing its cause. Symptomatic relief is achieved by the patient resting in a bed, the foot of which is elevated. If this fails, multiple punctures of the skin with a sharp needle can have a dramatic effect (although performed rarely, this is still very effective).

RETENTION CYSTS

Sebaceous Cysts

Sebaceous and apocrine glands are present in the labia majora and minora and in the mons; cysts arise in them if their ducts are blocked by debris or fibrosis **(Fig. 4)**. These rarely exceed a grape in size and, in the labia minora, they tend to be tiny and multiple. Secondary infection is not uncommon.

Epidermoid Cyst; Implantation Dermoid

Small cysts containing creamy yellow laminated keratinous debris material and lined by stratified epithelium are often found in the perineum and posterior vaginal wall and sometimes in other parts of the vulva. They are rarely

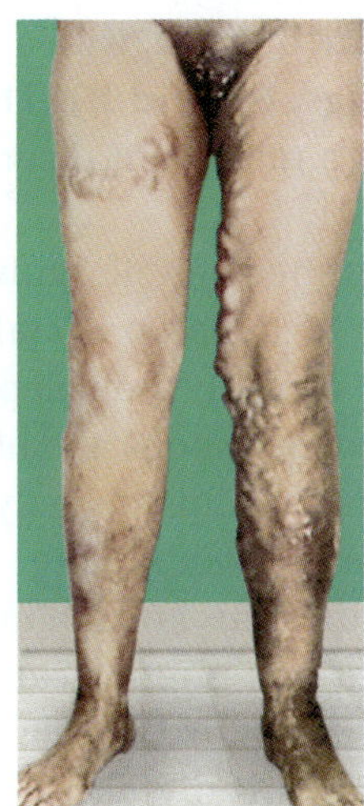

Fig. 2: A severe degree of varicose veins of the legs (and vulva) associated with pregnancy.

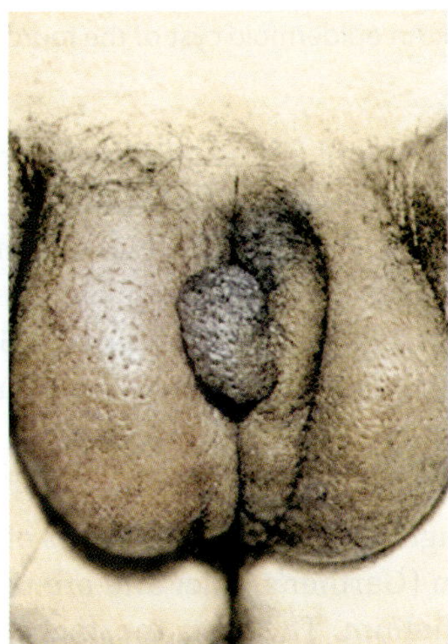

Fig. 3: Oedema of the vulva. The cause in this case was pre-eclampsia.

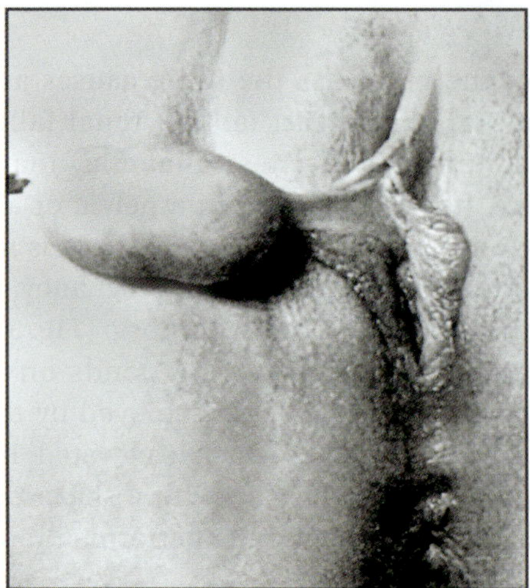

Fig. 4: A sebaceous cyst of the labium minus. Treatment is by excision or incision, depending on whether the cyst is infected.

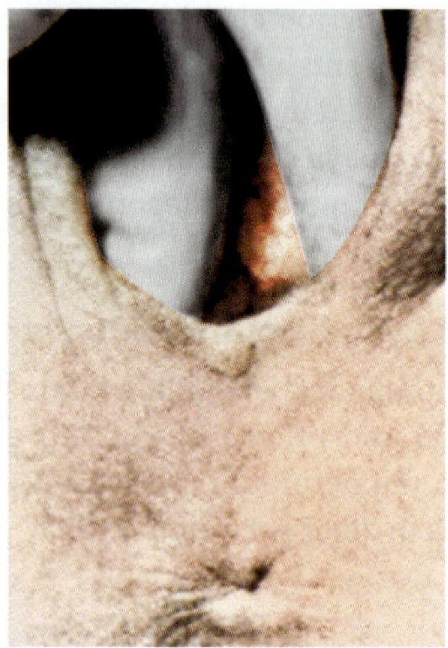

Fig. 5: An epidermoid cyst of the fourchette.

bigger than a pea and are usually symptomless. Most of these cysts arise from small portions of perineal skin which become buried at the time of obstetrical injuries. Congenital inclusions are also a possible source; when they are, the cysts are always in the midline **(Fig. 5)**. Epidermoid cysts are easily excised if they cause symptoms.

Hymeneal and Clitoral Cysts

These are thought to arise from remnants of the lower part of the Wolffian (Gartner's) duct and are usually lined by cuboidal epithelium. The cysts mostly cause trouble by becoming infected and leading to recurrent abscesses or persistent sinuses.

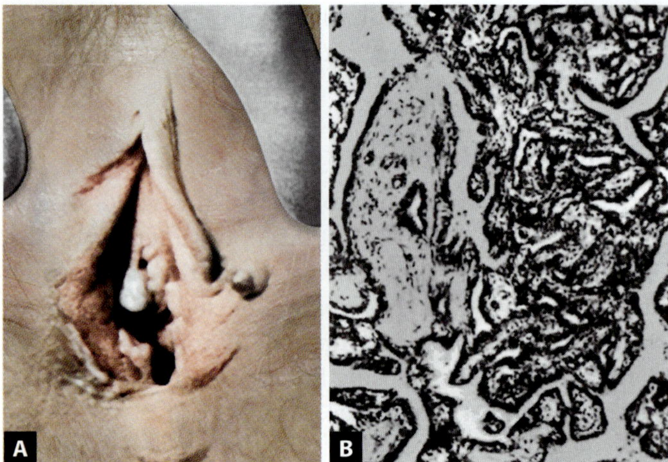

Figs. 6A and B: Hidradenoma (sweat gland tumour) of the vulva. (A) The position and size of the tumour are typical. The red-topped umbilication is a well-recognised feature but is not always present; (B) Microscopic section showing the benign adenomatous structure of the tumour.

BENIGN NEOPLASMS

Benign growths may be composed of any of the tissues which make up the vulva. The most common are the fibroma and lipoma, and these can reach large sizes. Others include the papilloma, pigmented mole, myoma, myoblastoma, haemangioma, lymphangioma, myxoma and neurofibroma. Adenomas are rare and are mostly small in size. They arise from sweat glands (hidradenoma) and Wolffian remains. Tumours of the latter are mostly found on the anterolateral aspect of the introitus, near the urethra and clitoris. The hidradenoma is usually found on the foreparts of a labium majus. Typically, it forms a raised nodule, about the size of a pea, with a red and sometimes umbilicated top **(Figs. 6A and B)**. The last features are rather suggestive of a malignant ulcer, but the tumour is quite benign.

Although sometimes sessile, vulvar tumours show a strong tendency to develop a stalk and to become polypoidal **(Figs. 7 and 8)**; their dependent parts then become congested, oedematous and ultimately ulcerated.

The patient usually complains only of the swelling, or bleeding and discharge from it. Large tumours, however, can cause difficulty in coitus and labour.

The treatment of any tumour causing symptoms, or whose nature is in doubt, is by excision. Its structure is usually determined only by subsequent microscopic examination; such an examination is important if only to exclude malignant disease.

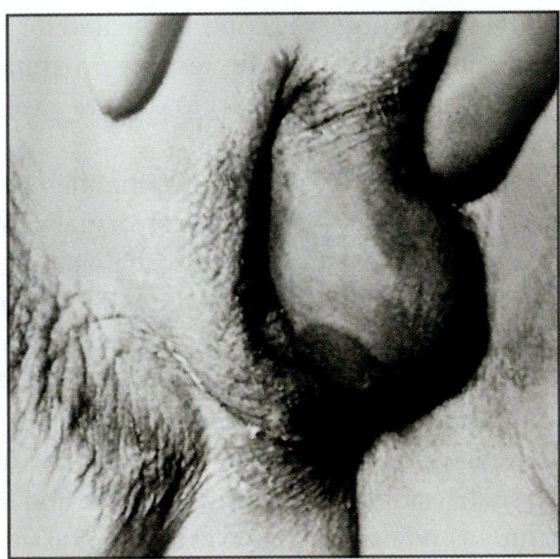

Fig. 7: A sessile leiomyoma in a woman aged 69 years. The surface ulceration at first suggested malignant disease but proved to be mechanical and ischaemic in origin.

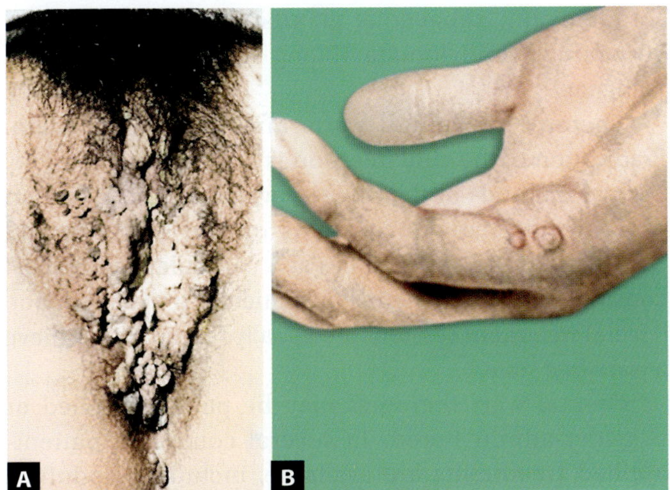

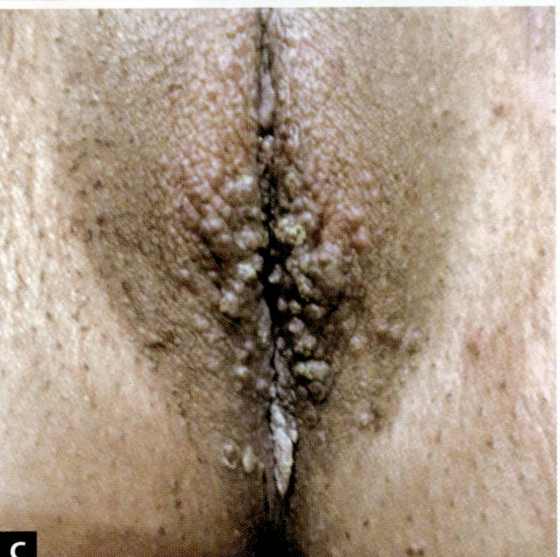

Figs. 9A to C: Multiple warts (condylomata acuminata) of the vulva. These, like warts elsewhere, are caused by a virus, but their particular character in this site is determined by warmth and moisture. (A) The vulvar lesions in a woman aged 24 years and pregnant; (B) This patient also had typical warts at the base of the fifth finger, but vulvar warts commonly occur without lesions elsewhere; (C) Vulvar regions in a woman aged 30 years and nonpregnant.

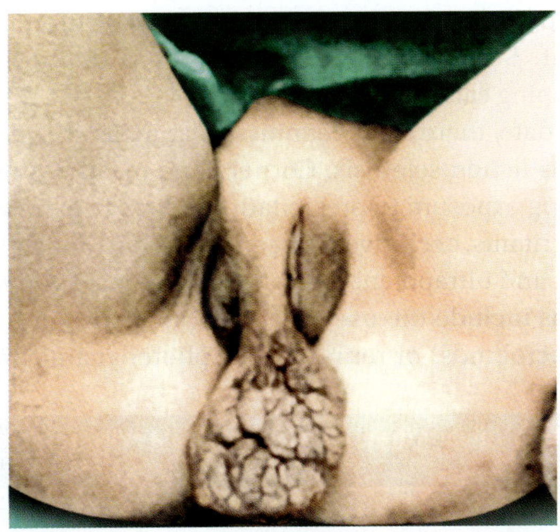

Fig. 8: A pedunculated fibroma of the vulva.

Condylomata Acuminata (Vulvar Warts)

Condylomata are papillary or verrucous lesions caused by human papillomavirus (HPV) infection. Types 6 and 11, the nononcogenic types, are usually responsible for genital warts. On the vulva, they are nearly always multiple. The virus can be transferred to this site from other parts of the body, so warts elsewhere may be associated **(Figs. 9A to C)**.

They can also be transmitted sexually and are highly contagious, affecting 75% of sexual partners. Vaginal discharge provides an environment, which causes them to flourish and during pregnancy. This environment of warmth and moisture, with little exposure to air, explains why vulvar condylomata assume a form different from that of those found on the hands. Typically, they are finely branched structures with a narrow stalk. They grow in clusters to give a cauliflower appearance, but they can be broad-based and coarse.

Condylomata acuminata are found on any part of the vulva and around the anus but most commonly on the posterior fourchette and lateral areas; they spread within the introitus and sometimes involve the upper vagina and cervix. Their differential diagnosis is from syphilitic condylomata lata, SCC, skin tags, molluscum contagiosum, sebaceous glands and lichen planus. Very rarely, condylomata of long standing can become malignant.

Therapy for genital warts aims to remove them. Eradication of the viral infection is not presently feasible. Several methods of therapy are available, and selection of a specific regimen depends on the site, size and number of warts, the facilities at a particular centre, cost considerations and whether the patient is pregnant or not. Several treatment sessions are usually required to achieve a wart-free state.

Genital wart therapies may be patient-applied or provider-administered. In several countries, patient-applied treatments are available, including podofilox solution and gel and imiquimod cream. The provider-administered methods include topical, excisional or injectable treatments. Podophyllum resin has been commonly used for multiple condylomata which, when applied to them directly, causes them to shrivel and drop off within about 7 days. Various preparations are used, but the common one is a 10–25% emulsion in spirit or tincture benzoin compound. This has to be applied accurately to each wart with a cotton-tipped applicator taking care to avoid the surrounding skin. It is important to wash it off in 1–4 hours. If the need arises, and it often does when the warts are many in number, treatment is repeated once or twice a week for up to 6 weeks. Each application is limited to 0.5 mL or an area of 10 cm^2 to decrease the potential for systemic effects, e.g. bone marrow depression.

Podophyllin is cytotoxic and can be absorbed from the vulvar skin, so its use is contraindicated in the first 3 months of pregnancy. It should also not be applied to warts within the vagina. These, like warts in any site, including the vulva, can disappear spontaneously. Condylomata—which resist podophyllin therapy and those which are coarse with thick stalks are best snipped or shaved off under local anaesthesia and their bases cauterised. Trichloroacetic acid (TCA) 80–90% solution has been used to treat small moist warts. Sodium bicarbonate can be used to remove the unreacted acid from the normal skin. Treatment is repeated weekly for up to 6 weeks. TCA can also be used to cauterise the bases of the warts after cutting. It is not as toxic as podophyllin and can safely be used in pregnancy. Tiny warts can be destroyed with the cautery, diathermy or cryotherapy. This sort of surgical approach is also appropriate for warts situated within the vagina. Laser has been used in patients who do not respond to other regimens. Thermal methods are more effective than therapy, but electrosurgery is contraindicated for patients with cardiac pacemakers or with lesions proximal to the anal verge. Injections of 5-fluorouracil are rarely used because of their side effects.

Recurrences are common with all modalities, occurring in at least one third of patients. These are usually the result of reactivation of pre-existing subclinical infection. Sexual partners need treatment if they have manifest warts and should also be counselled regarding transmission risks.

As shown in **Table 1**, the terminology and definitions for premalignant or precursor lesions of vulvar cancer have been reviewed and changed in the last few decades. Currently, such lesions arising from the vulva and the anus are all included and named as 'lower anogenital squamous intraepithelial lesions'.

Under this classification, three subtypes are distinguished for the vulva: (1) Low-grade squamous intraepithelial lesions (LSILs), (2) high-grade squamous intraepithelial lesions (HSILs) and (3) differentiated variant. Such distinction correlates with the risk of developing cancer over time.

To date, there is no definitive treatment for conditions such as lichen sclerosis. Cornerstone measures include avoiding exposure to precipitating factors (e.g. trauma by local irritants, occlusive moist environment) and the use of potent and ultrapotent topical corticosteroids. Alternative options include the use of topical calcineurin inhibitors (e.g. tacrolimus) or retinoids and photodynamic therapy

TABLE 1: Vulvar intraepithelial neoplasia (VIN) terminology changes.

ISSVD 1986	*ISSVD 2004*	*Lower Anogenital Squamous Terminology (LAST) 2012*
VIN 1	Flat condylomata or HPV effect	LSIL
VIN 2 and VIN 3	VIN, usual type: • VIN, warty type • VIN, basaloid type • VIN, mixed	HSIL
Differentiated VIN (dVIN)	VIN, differentiated type	dVIN

(HPV: human papillomavirus; HSIL: high-grade squamous intraepithelial lesion; ISSVD: International Society for the Study of Vulvovaginal Disease; LSIL: low-grade squamous intraepithelial lesion)

Source: Hoang et al.; Bornstein et al.; Sideri et al.

for selected cases and/or cases resistant to corticosteroid therapy.

Surgical treatment was previously restricted to excision of scars in women where scarring had led to functional impairment. In a recent review, Eshtiaghi et al. indicated the potential benefit of mesenchymal stem cells, including adipose-derived stem cells and autologous platelet-rich plasma, in the treatment of lichen sclerosis.

Differentiated vulvar intraepithelial neoplasia (dVIN) represents <5% of preneoplastic lesions of the vulva. However, it is characterised by a higher rate of progression to squamous vulvar carcinoma, shorter time interval to progression and higher recurrence rate than HSIL. It is rarely associated with persistent HPV infection (<2%). Excision (with 0.5–1 cm margins) constitutes the treatment of choice to allow proper evaluation and exclusion of occult invasion. Multiple treatment modalities exist for the management of HSIL, but simple excision with 5-mm margins and 4-mm depth is the most common. Excision has the advantage of excluding invasion histologically, but the lack of preservation of vulvar skin results in psychosexual morbidity, particularly in younger women. An alternative option to preserve anatomy is ablation, e.g. with carbon dioxide laser, but this lacks the assessment of occult invasion. A less destructive option is the use of imiquimod 5% to avoid scarring and sexual dysfunction, particularly in multifocal lesions. Moderate quality evidence shows that response rates with imiquimod and cidofovir, another topical treatment, are similar at 6 months compared with surgical management or laser vaporisation. There is very little evidence of the effectiveness of topical treatment for HSIL among immunocompromised women. Independent of chosen treatment and margin status, there is a risk of recurrence (up to 30–40%). Therefore, close follow-up is recommended for at least 2–3 years.

Prevention

Primary Prevention (Vaccination)

As for cervical premalignant lesions predisposing to cervical cancer, persistent HPV infection, particularly by HPV 16 subtype, has been associated with the long-term development of HSIL and SCC of the vulva. The introduction of HPV vaccination as a primary prevention strategy in cervical cancer has also been shown to reduce the prevalence of noncervical premalignant lesions among vaccinated women who were not initially infected with high-risk HPV types or types included in the vaccines, with vaccine efficacies of >90%. Long-term trend analyses by the Cancer Registry of Norway also show promising estimates of reduction in HPV-associated cases of vulvar cancer in future years among HPV-vaccinated communities.

Secondary Prevention (Screening)

There is no evidence for specific screening for vulvar cancer. Self-examination in women with lichen sclerosis, a condition related to vulvar cancer development, should be encouraged. In addition, there should be early evaluation of any patient with symptoms (e.g. chronic vulvar pruritus) or signs (e.g. pigmented lesions, irregular ulcers), who may be a candidate for skin biopsy. Finally, women who are known to have squamous intraepithelial lesion (SIL) of the cervix, vagina or anus should have inspection of the vulva as part of their follow-up colposcopy visits.

Tertiary Prevention (Management of Premalignant Lesions)

An effective strategy to reduce vulvar cancer incidence is the opportune treatment of predisposing and preneoplastic lesions associated with vulvar cancer development.

There are two main pathological pathways that lead to vulvar SCC given as follows:

1. Keratinising SCC usually occurs in older women and is often associated with lichen sclerosis and/or dVIN.
2. Warty/basaloid SCC, generally occurs in younger women, is caused by persistent infection with oncogenic strains of HPV (particularly HPV 16, 18, 31 and 33) and has SIL as its precursor lesion. Lesions are frequently multifocal and may be associated with SIL in other parts of the lower genital tract (e.g. cervix, vagina and anus). Human immunodeficiency virus (HIV) infection and cigarette smoking are also common predisposing factors.

Investigations

- Cervical cytology, and colposcopy of the cervix and vagina, if applicable, due to the association of HPV-related cancers with other SILs
- Full blood count, biochemical profile, liver profile and HIV testing
- Chest X-ray
- CT or MRI scan of the pelvis and groins may be helpful, especially for locally advanced tumours, to detect any enlarged lymph nodes in the groins or pelvis, erosion

into underlying bone or other metastases. In addition, CT or MRI could be useful in further treatment planning.

- 18F-fluorodeoxyglucose (18F-FDG) positron emission tomography with computed tomography (PET-CT) can more effectively assess and detect inguinofemoral lymph node involvement compared with CT, influencing the planning of primary surgery and inguinal lymph node dissection to determine the optimum surgical extent without sentinel lymph node dissection and use of frozen sections. Additionally, PET-CT might be used with larger tumours when metastatic disease is suspected or in the recurrence scenario, particularly when exenteration is contemplated.

MALIGNANT NEOPLASMS OF VULVA

Malignant neoplasms of vulva are rare, about 3.7/100,000 women with crude mortality rate of 1.3/100,000 women. It is ranked as 20th most common cancer.

Histology

Types of Vulvar Cancer

Histopathological types: SCCs account for most vulvar cancers (>80%), and melanomas are the next most common cancer. Rarer histological types include:

- Basal cell carcinoma
- Verrucous carcinoma
- Adenocarcinoma related to extramammary Paget's disease
- Bartholin gland carcinoma (squamous, adenocarcinoma or transitional cell carcinoma)
- Sarcoma

Histological grades:

- GX: Grade cannot be assessed
- G1: Well differentiated
- G2: Moderately differentiated
- G3: Poorly or undifferentiated

Squamous Cell Carcinoma (Invasive)

Invasive cancer of the vulva accounts for only 4% of cases of female genital cancer, and most gynaecologists probably see <50 patients during their lifetime.

Pathology

Cancer of the vulva can arise in normal skin or within lesions of lichen sclerosus, squamous hyperplasia or VIN. The lesion resembles skin cancer elsewhere, both macroscopically and microscopically. It usually appears as an ulcer with a sloughing base and raised edges, but fungating papillomatous forms and flat plaques are also seen **(Figs. 10 to 14)**. The disease affects any part of the vulva, but the most common sites are the labium majus and the clitoris. Multiple growths are not uncommon; sometimes, there are labial *kiss ulcers* whose appearance suggests that the lesion spreads from one side to the other by direct contact, a disputed explanation. A widespread epithelial *field change* in the skin of the vulva probably accounts for multiple primaries as well as a number of recurrences after treatment.

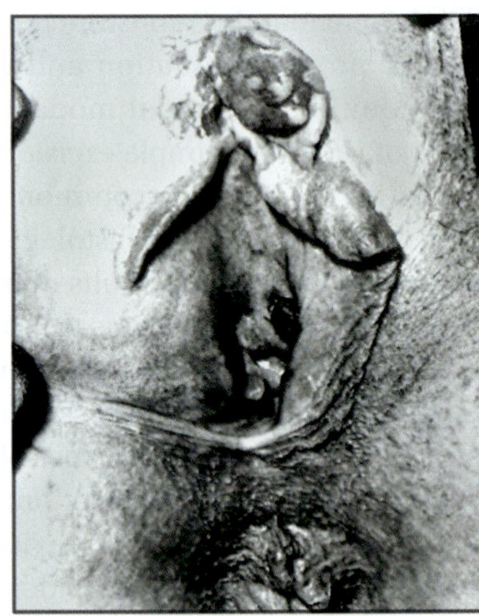

Fig. 10: Carcinoma of the clitoris. The white appearance of the surrounding skin is due to highlighting, not leucoplakia.

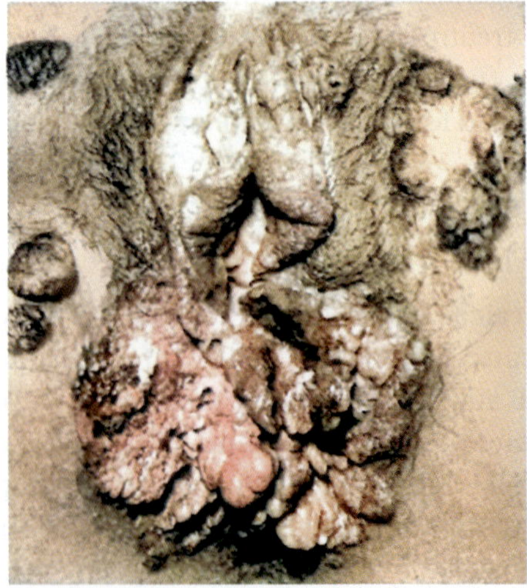

Fig. 11: Multiple carcinomatous lesions of the vulva. Invasive, like in situ, cancer tends to be multifocal.

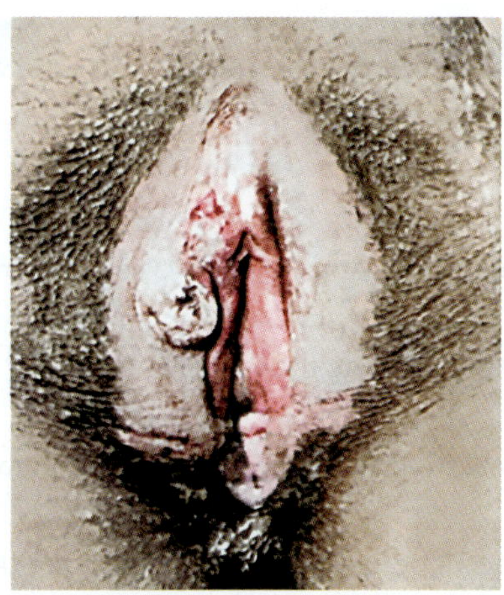

Fig. 12: An early ulcerative squamous cell carcinoma arising on skin which is affected by leucoderma, not leucoplakia. The skin is normal except for the absence of pigment.

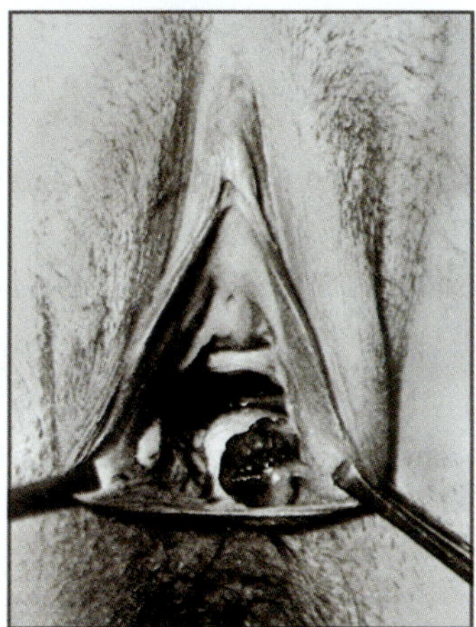

Fig. 13: A relatively early exophytic and almost pedunculated squamous cell carcinoma arising just within the introitus; this is an unusual site.

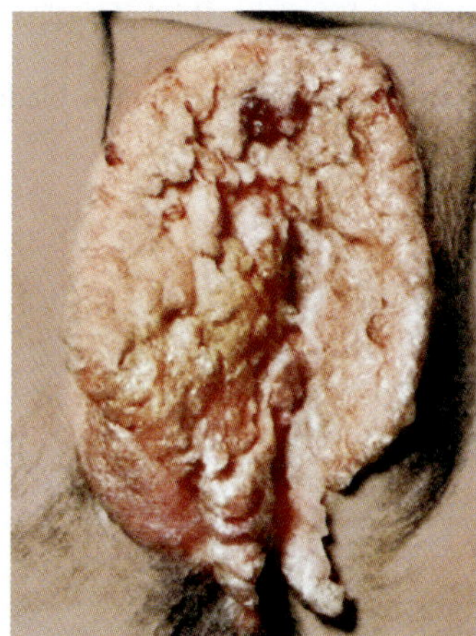

Fig. 14: An extensive proliferative cancer destroying all the tissues of the vulva. Involvement of the pubic bones prevented its complete excision.

Aetiology

Although recorded before the age of 20 years, vulvar cancer is essentially a disease of old age. It mostly arises between the ages of 50 and 80 years, with an average of 62 years. The cause of the cancer is unknown, but it is reasonable to suppose that any long-standing irritative agent—chemical, infective or mechanical, especially if combined with poor hygiene—can be an aetiological factor. Before they were adequately protected, women workers in cotton and woollen mills suffered repeated exposure to mineral oil and then proved more liable to develop cancer of the vulva.

Malignant change is also associated with chronic inflammatory diseases such as the venereal granulomas and vulvar warts of 20–30 years' standing, often with an intermediate phase of epithelial atypism. Where these conditions are common, as in the West Indies, vulvar cancer is said to be relatively more common and occur in young women. HPV is suspected to play a role in the aetiology of SCCs of the vulva.

Chronic vulvar epithelial disorders rarely lead to cancer unless they are accompanied by histological evidence of epithelial unrest and overactivity.

Spread

Extension of the growth occurs by direct spread to the vagina, urethra, groin and anus. More important is dissemination by the lymph stream to the superficial inguinal nodes on both sides. From here, the deep inguinal (femoral) and external iliac nodes become involved. Drainage to both groins occurs from midline structures, i.e. the clitoris and the perineum, but even other parts of the vulva may have some degree of contralateral spread. It has long been said that a cancer of the clitoris, even a small one, carries a bad prognosis because the rich blood and lymph networks in that site favour early dissemination directly to the deep femoral node of Cloquet, but modern observations do not confirm this.

Staging

In 1974, the International Federation of Gynaecology and Obstetrics (FIGO) approved a clinical classification for invasive SCC of vulva **(Table 2)**. This was based on analysis of tumour (T) by size and location, node (N) status by palpation, distant metastasis (M) as assessed by general and pelvic examination, evaluation of bladder or rectum or both and radiological investigation.

TABLE 2: The FIGO and TNM staging of cancer vulva.

FIGO stage	*TNM classification*[a]	*Clinical/pathologic findings*
Stage I		Tumour confined to the vulva
Stage Ia	$T_{1a}N_0M_0$	Lesions ≤2 cm in size, confined to the vulva or perineum and with stromal invasion ≤1 mm.* No nodal metastasis
Stage Ib	$T_{1b}N_0M_0$	Lesions >2 cm in size or with stromal invasion >1 mm confined to the vulva or perineum.* No nodal metastasis
Stage II	$T_2N_0M_0$	Tumour of any size with extension to adjacent perineal structures (lower one-third urethra, lower one-third vagina, anus) with negative nodes
Stage III		Tumour of any size with or without extension to adjacent perineal structures (lower one-third urethra, lower one-third vagina, anus) with positive inguinofemoral nodes
Stage IIIa	$T_{1or2}N_{1b}M_0$ $T_{1or2}N_{1a}M_0$	• With one lymph node metastasis (≥5 mm) • One to two lymph node metastasis(es) (<5 mm)
Stage IIIb	$T_{1or2}N_{2b}M_0$ $T_{1or2}N_{2a}M_0$	• With two or more lymph node metastases (≥5 mm) • Three or more lymph node metastases (<5 mm)
Stage IIIc	$T_{1or2}N_{2c}M_0$	With positive nodes with extracapsular spread
Stage IV		Tumour invades other regional (upper two-thirds urethra, two-thirds vagina) or distant structures
Stage IVa	$T_3N_{any}M_0$ $T_{any}N_3$	Tumour invades any of the following: • Upper urethral and/or vaginal mucosa, bladder mucosa, rectal mucosa or fixed to pelvic bone • Fixed or ulcerated inguinofemoral lymph nodes
Stage IVb	$T_{any}N_{any}M_1$	Any distant metastasis, including pelvic lymph nodes

*The depth of stromal invasion is measured from the epithelial–stromal junction of the adjacent most superficial dermal papilla to the deepest point of invasion.

[a]TNM classification:

- T: Primary tumour
- T_x: Primary tumour cannot be assessed
- T_0: No evidence of primary tumour
- T_{is}: Carcinoma in situ (preinvasive carcinoma)
- T_{1a}: Lesions ≤2 cm in size, confined to the vulva or perineum and with stromal invasion ≤1 mm
- T_{1b}: Lesions >2 cm in size or any size with stromal invasion >1 mm, confined to the vulva or perineum
- T_2: Tumour of any size with extension to adjacent perineal structures (lower one third of urethra, lower one third of vagina, anal involvement)
- T_3: Tumour of any size with extension to any of the following: Upper two thirds of urethra, upper two thirds of vagina, bladder mucosa, rectal mucosa or fixed to pelvic bone
- N: Regional lymph nodes (femoral and inguinal nodes)
- N_x: Regional lymph nodes cannot be assessed
- N_0: No regional lymph node metastases
- N_1: One or two regional lymph node metastases with the following features:
  - N_{1a}: One or two lymph node metastases each <5 mm
  - N_{1b}: One lymph node metastasis ≥ 5 mm
- N_2: Regional lymph node metastases with the following features:
  - N_{2a}: More than or equal to three lymph node metastases, each <5 mm in diameter
  - N_{2b}: More than or equal to two lymph node metastases ≥ 5 mm
  - N[MB2] $[MB2]_{2c}$: Lymph node metastases with extracapsular spread
- N_3: Fixed or ulcerated regional lymph node metastasis
- M: Distant metastasis
- M_0: No distant metastasis
- M_1: Distant metastasis (including pelvic lymph node metastasis)

(FIGO: International Federation of Gynaecology and Obstetrics; TNM: tumour-node-metastasis)

TABLE 3: New (2021) FIGO staging for carcinoma of the vulva.

Stage	Description
I	Tumour confined to the vulva IA tumour size ≤2 cm and stromal invasion ≤1 mm[a] IB tumour size >2 cm or stromal invasion >1 mm[a]
II	Tumour of any size with extension to lower one third of the urethra, lower one third of the vagina and lower one third of the anus with negative nodes
III	Tumour of any size with extension to upper part of adjacent perineal structures or with any number of nonfixed, nonulcerated lymph node
IIIA	Tumour of any size with disease extension to upper two thirds of the urethra, upper two thirds of the vagina, bladder mucosa, rectal mucosa or regional lymph node metastases ≤5 mm
IIIB	Regional[b] lymph node metastases >5 mm
IIIC	Regional[b] lymph node metastases with extracapsular spread
IV	Tumour of any size fixed to bone, or fixed, ulcerated lymph node metastases or distant metastases
IVA	Disease fixed to pelvic bone or fixed or ulcerated regional lymph node metastases
IVB	Distant metastases

[a]Depth of invasion is measured from the basement membrane of the deepest, adjacent, dysplastic, tumour-free rete ridge (or nearest dysplastic rete peg) to the deepest point of invasion.
[b]Regional refers to inguinal and femoral lymph nodes.
Source: Olawaiye AB, Cuello MA, Rogers LJ. Cancer of the vulva: 2021 update. Int J Gynecol Obstet. 2021;155(Suppl 1):7-18.

In 1988, the FIGO approved a surgical staging system. Vulval cancer has been staged surgicopathologically using the FIGO staging system since 1994. The staging has been revised in 2009 and 2021 revised staging with role of imaging **(Table 3)**.

Paralleling the change in the FIGO staging, the American Joint Committee on Cancer (AJCC) significantly modified the vulval cancer tumour-node-metastasis (TNM) classification with release of the 2009 edition of the AJCC Cancer Staging Manual **(Table 3)**.

- While stage Ia remains unchanged as the only group of patients with a negligible risk of lymph node metastases, former stages I and II have been combined into stage Ib.
- The new stage II segregates patients whose tumours involve the lower adjacent perineal structures from those with positive lymph nodes.
- For stages III and IV, the number and morphology of the involved nodes are taken into account, and the bilaterality of lymph nodes is discounted.

The above staging is based on clinical observations, not operative findings. Of all cases of invasive cancer coming to operation, malignant cells are found in the superficial inguinal nodes in 30–40% and deep nodes in 10–15%. Larger the area of the primary growth, more likely is lymph node involvement.

Diagnosis

Diagnosis requires a wedge biopsy specimen. If the lesion is about 1 mm in diameter, excisional biopsy is preferable. The biopsy should include sufficient underlying dermis to assess for microinvasion.

Clinical Features

The patient may suffer from pruritus or discomfort in the vulva or be aware of a small tumour. Quite often, she regards the lesion as a small septic spot or wart, which she neglects until ulceration causes some bleeding and discharge. The growth appears as an eroding ulcer with everted edges or as a dirty discharging hypertrophic mass **(Figs. 10 to 14)**. It is hard and friable, bleeds easily and may be fixed to underlying tissues. These are the typical features, but atypical lesions of all kinds are seen, and only safe rule is to subject any persistent ulcer or nodule to histological scrutiny **(Figs. 15 and 16)**.

If the inguinal lymph nodes are enlarged, it is often impossible without microscopical examination to

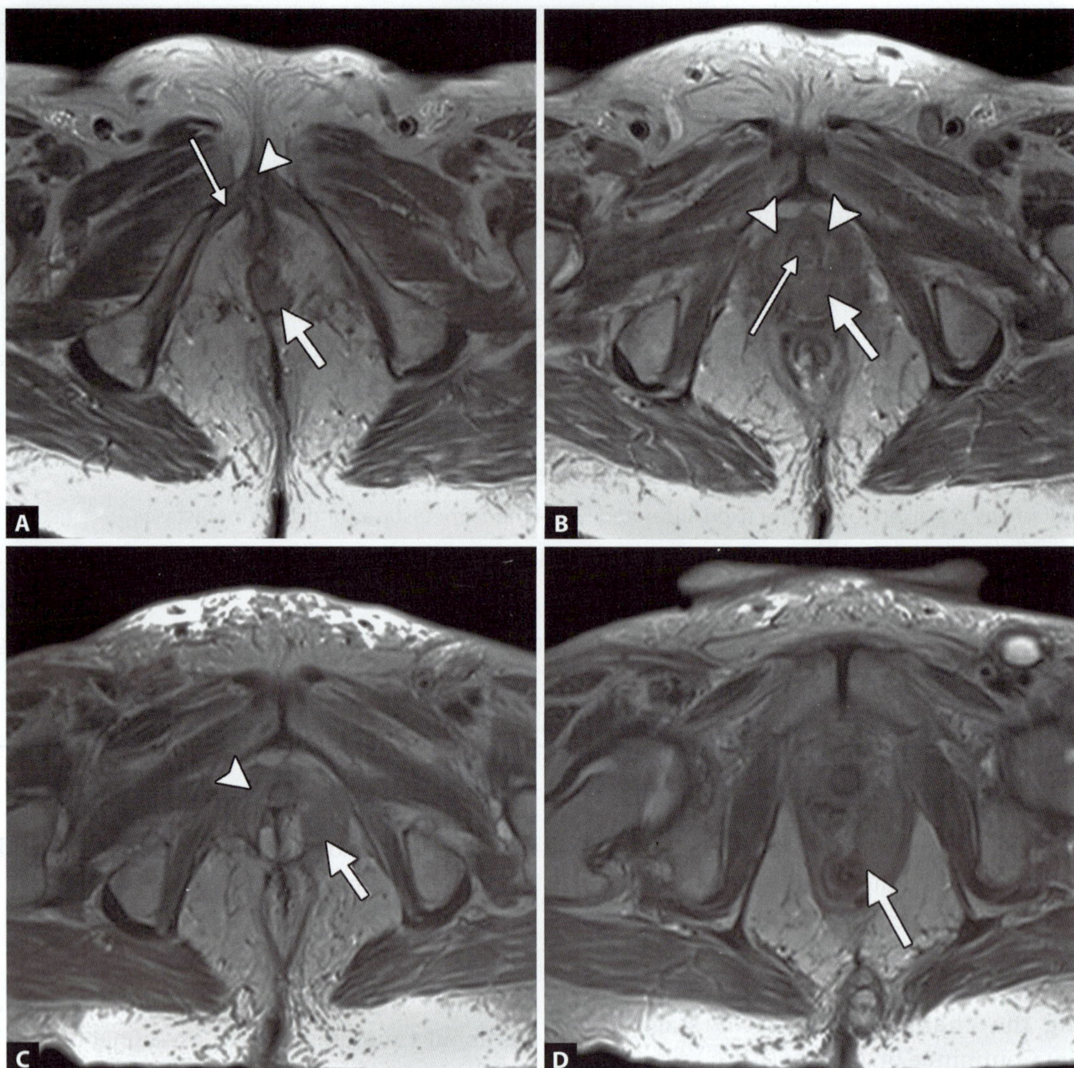

Figs. 15A to D: A 65-year-old woman with mass in labia majora. (A) Axial T2-weighted image obtained at level of perineum shows lobulated 2.6 cm mass (thick arrow) with intermediate high signal intensity in vulva, clitoral crura (thin arrow), clitoral body (arrowhead) and urethral orifice; (B) Axial T2-weighted image at the level of symphysis pubis shows vulvar mass extended into lower vagina (thick arrow) and invades left bulb of vestibule. Urethra (thin arrow) is spared. Inverted U-shaped bilateral bulbs of vestibule (arrowheads) are evident. Patient was treated with radical local excision, including local vaginectomy and left inguinofemoral lymphadenectomy. Lesion was surgically confirmed stage II; (C) Axial T2-weighted MR image obtained at the level of symphysis pubis level 5 months after surgery shows recurrent mass (arrow) with intermediate high signal intensity at left perineum. Remaining right bulb of vestibule (arrowhead) and urethra are evident. Left bulb of vestibule and lower vagina were resected and replaced by fat; (D) Axial T2-weighted MR image at high level shows recurrent mass (arrow) abutting anal sphincter. Area of high signal intensity at left femoral region is site of left inguinal lymphadenectomy with small fluid collection. Neoadjuvant chemoradiation was used for further treatment.

determine whether the enlargement is a manifestation of secondary infection or invasion by tumour cells.

Treatment

Prevention: Chronic non-neoplastic epithelial disorders and other skin diseases of the vulva precede cancer in only a small percentage of cases. Nevertheless, the investigation, regular observation and treatment of these are the chief hopes of preventing cancer at present. Those characterised by epithelial atypism may call for prophylactic vulvectomy, but this is not an absolute safeguard.

Surgical: The standard treatment for established disease has been radical excision of the vulva with block dissection of the inguinal and femoral nodes on both sides, even in

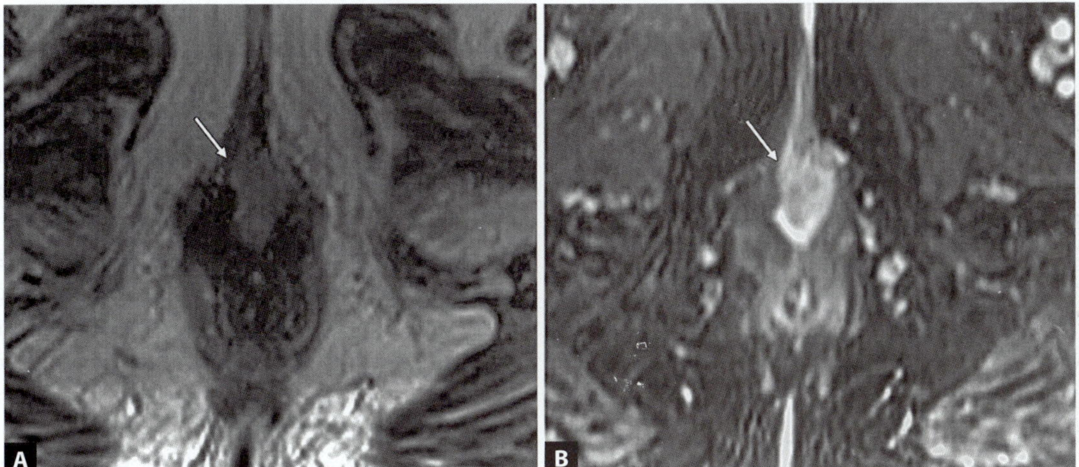

Figs. 16A and B: A 68-year-old woman with stage II vulvar carcinoma. T2-weighted (A) and contrast-enhanced T1-weighted (B) MR images show 3 cm T2 hyperintense and enhancing vulvar mass (arrows) arising from left labia minora and confined in perineum without invasion of adjacent organs. There is no evidence of nodal metastasis.

cases with unilateral lesions, because the lymphatics from one side are thought to communicate freely with the other. It is now recognised, however, that a flexible approach to the treatment of these patients may decrease the morbidity of the standard procedure while maintaining comparable survival rates.

In planning an operation, it has to be remembered that squamous carcinoma of the vulva is generally a well-differentiated growth of relatively low-grade malignancy; its owner is often an old woman, ill-fitted to withstand a radical procedure, and whose expectation of life is in any case limited. *Wide excision of the primary growth* sometimes means removing the lower part of the urethra, vagina or bowel and leaving an area uncovered by skin which can take 2–3 months to heal unless skin grafts are used. When the wound is closed under tension, there is a high breakdown rate. The most important modification of the standard *en bloc* excision has been the development of the three-incision technique in which the vulvectomy is the first and the bilateral groin incisions are the other two incisions **(Fig. 17)**. This method leaves a bridge of tissue between the incisions and spares the mons pubis. Groin wound breakdown is reduced by 50%. This method may be considered in patients with early disease with clinically negative inguinofemoral nodes.

There is an increased risk of venous thromboembolism and later of chronic oedema of the legs, following radical vulvectomy. Other problems include the possibility of urinary or faecal incontinence. The vulva may be left

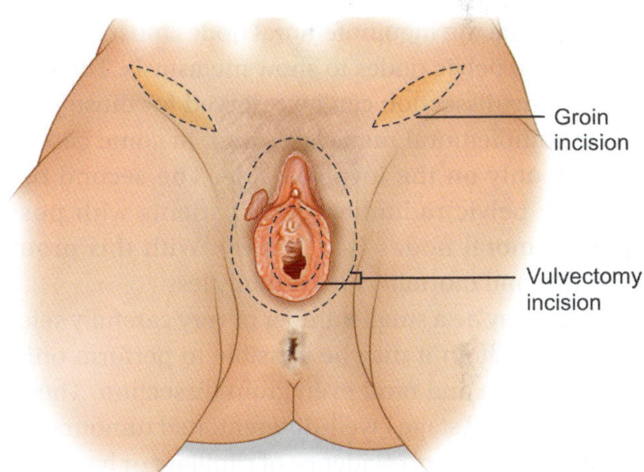

Fig. 17: Three-incision technique of vulvectomy. Modified hemivulvectomy with unilateral groin dissection has been tried in patients with an early well-lateralised tumour, with no capillary or lymphatic space involvement and with negative ipsilateral inguinal nodes. However, patients with tumours involving the perineum, clitoris, vagina and labia minora have a high risk of contralateral lymph node metastases.

gaping or stenosed with a high incidence of psychosexual problems. But young women have conceived, and delivered normally, after this operation **(Fig. 18)**.

Another important modification has been in the management of the regional nodes. Some surgeons used to advocate extending the dissection to include the external iliac and common iliac nodes in all cases, but such an extensive operation carries a high morbidity rate, and it is

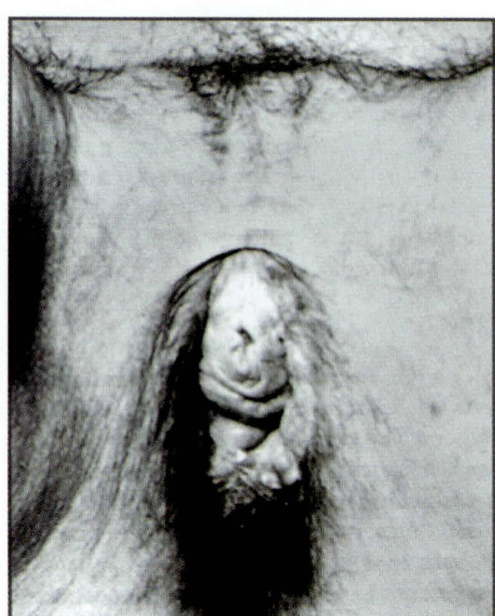

Fig. 18: The ultimate distortion resulting from radical vulvectomy for cancer, even though not all the hair-bearing skin of the pubes was removed. Photograph taken 6 years after operation during which time the patient had a normal vaginal delivery.

now clear that the inguinofemoral nodes must be involved for the deep pelvic nodes to show metastasis. Thus, pelvic lymph node dissection can be reserved for those patients with inguinofemoral metastases and, in some cases, can be done only on the involved side. The second option is to give pelvic radiotherapy to patients with positive inguinofemoral nodes (*see further*). With this protocol, morbidity and mortality are certainly less.

There may be a small number of very carefully selected patients in whom it may be possible to perform only the local resection and omit even groin dissection. These are low-risk clinical stage I well-differentiated tumours, which are unilateral with no evidence of capillary or lymph space involvement and up to 5 mm of invasion. Some have restricted this to an invasion of 1 mm. It must be noted that there are reports of 20% groin node positivity with invasion up to 5 mm, so this method of treatment should be used with caution.

In view of the type of patient involved, a primary operative mortality rate of 1–3% is likely, but the overall results of radical vulvectomy for carcinoma of the vulva are good. The 5-year survival rate is 60–65% of all cases treated and can be as high as 80–90% in cases where the nodes are not involved. When nodes are involved, the survival rate falls to 25–45%; the lower figure being obtained if the pelvic nodes are implicated. These assessments are based on a case operability rate of 90–95%.

Radiotherapy: The vulvar tissues are unusually sensitive to ionising radiations, and a cancericidal dose produces a violent and persistent reaction in the surrounding skin. For this reason, radiotherapy is not usually recommended. At present, radiotherapy is restricted to the following situations.

Preoperative radiotherapy is recommended for patients who are medically unfit for surgery; patients with advanced disease who are otherwise candidates for pelvic exenteration and young patients with small primary tumours, especially clitoral or periclitoral, who are psychologically unfit for surgical resection.

Postoperative radiotherapy is indicated for treating the groin if there are two or more positive lymph nodes, treating the pelvic lymph nodes and in patients with evidence of disease in an area ≤5 mm of the surgical margins. In all cases, therapy is aimed at preventing recurrences.

Improvements in radiotherapy techniques and the development of interstitial needles will further improve the scope of radiotherapy. Chemotherapy has been combined with radiotherapy to reduce the size of the tumour preoperatively in patients with central disease.

Treatment of recurrent cancer of the vulva: Local vulvar recurrences correlate with the number of positive groin nodes (>3) and the size of the primary tumour (>4 cm). Local lesions can be excised and covered with a myocutaneous flap, e.g. the gracilis. Radiotherapy (external beam with interstitial needles) has also been used but may have the delayed sequelae of necrosis.

Regional and distant recurrences have a poor prognosis. Surgery and radiotherapy are used for recurrences in the groin. Chemotherapy is used for distant metastases.

Diathermy coagulation: When the disease is advanced or the patient is old, quite good results can be obtained by fulgurating the growth with coagulation diathermy. This can be repeated if necessary to keep the growth and its offensive discharge in check.

Basal Cell Carcinoma

The vulva is an unusual site of this lesion (2% of vulvar malignancies), but, when it occurs, the features are similar to those of rodent ulcer of the face.

It is sometimes described as a type of intraepithelial neoplasia of the vulva. This it is not. A basal cell carcinoma is an invasive squamous cell growth which penetrates into the dermis and deeper tissues seen most commonly on the labia. But its spread is slow and limited, and it does not metastasise, so it is nearly always cured by adequate local excision.

Malignant Melanoma; Sarcoma

These are among the rare tumours of the vulva, but about 30% occur premenopausally.

Melanoma

Melanoma is the second most common malignancy of the vulva. It shows varying degrees of malignancy; some are entirely benign, and others are virulent and metastasize quickly. It presents as a patchily or diffusely pigmented slightly raised area usually located on the labia **(Fig. 19)** or clitoris and is occasionally pedunculated. If malignant, it tends to ulcerate. The diagnosis can only be made by biopsy, and, unless ulceration is present, this is indicated despite old arguments to the effect that it disseminates tumour cells.

The treatment, even for malignant melanomas, is generally by wide local excision or radical vulvectomy. Survival rates are good if the lymph nodes are negative, but all patients with positive nodes succumb to the disease.

Rare Vulvar Malignancy

Paget's Disease of the Vulva

Extramammary Paget's disease is rare and can affect the apocrine glands of the vulva. There are two types: (1) The primary form begins as an intraepithelial lesion, but (2) the secondary form is due to invasion from an underlying adenocarcinoma, which may be anorectal, urothelial or genital tract carcinoma (e.g. endocervical or endometrial). Vulvar Paget's disease occurs predominantly in postmenopausal women who present with vulvar pruritus and pain, and, on examination, an eczematoid weeping lesion is often seen. Diagnosis is usually confirmed by biopsy, which will also help to differentiate between an intraepithelial and an invasive lesion. The treatment of choice for intraepithelial Paget's disease is wide local excision. It is challenging to achieve clear margins, as histological changes often extend far beyond what is visible macroscopically; even with adequate margins, recurrence rates are high. Due to the high recurrence rate and surgical morbidity, there is a current move to perform less radical resection for intraepithelial lesions, with re-excision at a later date lesions should recur. Lesions involving the urethra or anus also present a management challenge and may require laser therapy. Another conservative treatment option is local imiquimod. A Cochrane meta-analysis that investigated treatment options concluded that there was no 'best' intervention for vulvar Paget's disease. If an underlying adenocarcinoma is present, treatment should be radical wide local excision with margins of at least 1 cm. Inguinofemoral lymphadenectomy should be performed, with adjuvant radiation for the same indications as for squamous carcinomas. Women with Paget's disease of the vulva should have long-term follow-up in a specialist vulvar clinic.

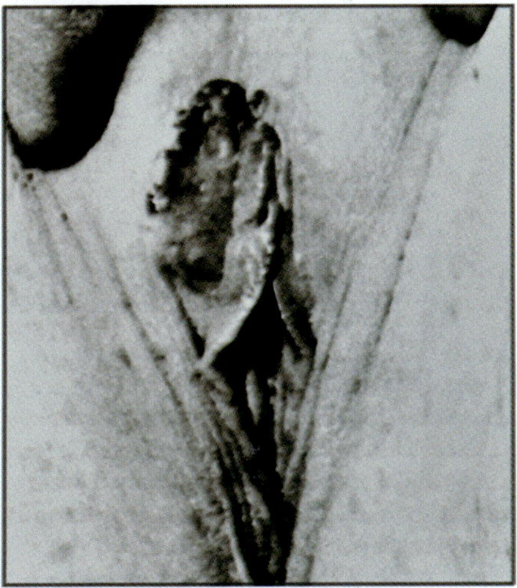

Fig. 19: Melanoma of the vulva. The tumour is linear and affecting the right labium majus. On biopsy, the melanoma was reported to be malignant. Further examination of the tissues after vulvectomy led to a conclusion that the condition was benign.

Sarcoma

Sarcomas represent 2% of vulvar malignancies. They vary in type and malignancy, as they do elsewhere. The most common are leiomyosarcomas. Other histologic types seen are rhabdomyosarcomas and epithelioid sarcomas. Rare variants include fibrosarcomas, neurofibrosarcomas, liposarcomas and malignant schwannomas. The appropriate treatment is by local excision; the lymph nodes should not be removed, as sarcoma metastasises via the bloodstream. Rhabdomyosarcomas may be managed with chemotherapy, with or without radiotherapy.

Metastatic Tumours

It is rare to see metastatic growths in the vulva, but they can arise from any site and are usually bloodborne. For example, a small tumour of the vulva may prove to be the first evidence of recurrence of carcinoma of the breast treated surgically several years previously.

The vulva may be involved by non-Hodgkin's lymphoma or leukaemia. Other rare tumours include the endodermal sinus tumour, Merkel cell carcinoma and dermatofibrosarcoma protuberans.

TUMOURS OF BARTHOLIN'S GLAND

Bartholin's Cyst

Pathology

Bartholin's cyst is the most common cyst of the vulva. There are two types: (1) A cyst of the duct and (2) a cyst of the gland. They can only be distinguished on microscopic section, the difference being in their lining epithelium (refer to **Fig. 5** of Chapter 2: Anatomy) **(Fig. 20)**. The majority of cysts represent a dilatation of the duct, the gland itself lying closely adherent to the cyst on its posterolateral aspect. The typical content is glairy colourless Bartholin's gland secretion, although it is often brownish from contamination with old blood.

Aetiology

Cyst formation requires obstruction of the main duct or the opening of an acinus. The cause of the obstruction is usually fibrosis which follows either infection or trauma. It was formerly believed that the infection was invariably gonococcal, but almost any organism can be responsible. Moreover, the original bartholinitis may be so slight as to pass unnoticed.

Complete and sudden obstruction of the duct by division or ligation, which must happen frequently during operations and confinements, does not appear to be followed by cyst formation. The type of injury which operates is more in the nature of repeated minor friction. The left gland is more often affected than the right, but both are often involved, not necessarily simultaneously.

Clinical Features

The cyst rarely exceeds the size of a hen's egg and is often so small and symptom free that it passes unnoticed by the examiner as well as the patient. If it is large, the woman becomes conscious of the swelling, and it may interfere with coitus. The tumour is painless, nontender and fluctuant, and its origin is determined by its position. Like all swellings of Bartholin's gland or duct, it distends the posterior and middle parts of the labium majus and opens up the base of the labium minus. Its projection inwards makes the vulvar cleft S-shaped **(Fig. 21)**.

Complications

Bartholin's cysts are liable to become secondarily infected; they then become acutely painful, throbbing and tender and present all the features of a Bartholin's abscess **(Fig. 22)**. When the pus has been released by simple drainage, the cyst usually reforms in a few weeks or months. Marsupialisation is the best way to avoid this.

Treatment

Excision of the cyst was the traditional treatment if symptoms were present, if the cyst was large and if there was a history of having been infected in the past. The operation is not so simple as it might appear. The technical problems are haemorrhage from the extremely vascular tissues and obliteration of the dead space. Unless these are adequately solved, haematoma formation leads to

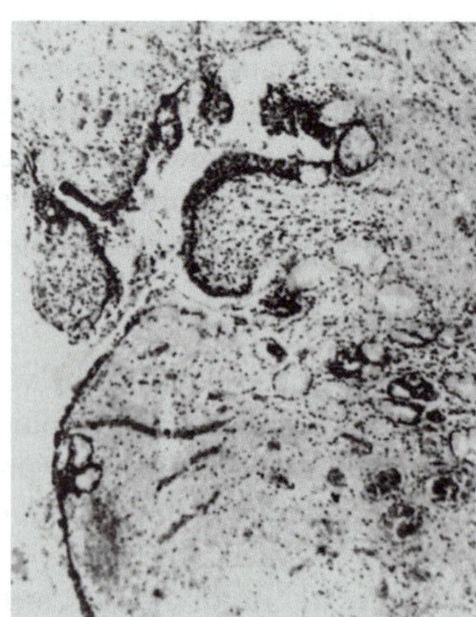

Fig. 20: Part of the wall of a cyst of Bartholin's duct lined by multilayered columnar epithelium. Acini of the gland can be seen alongside.

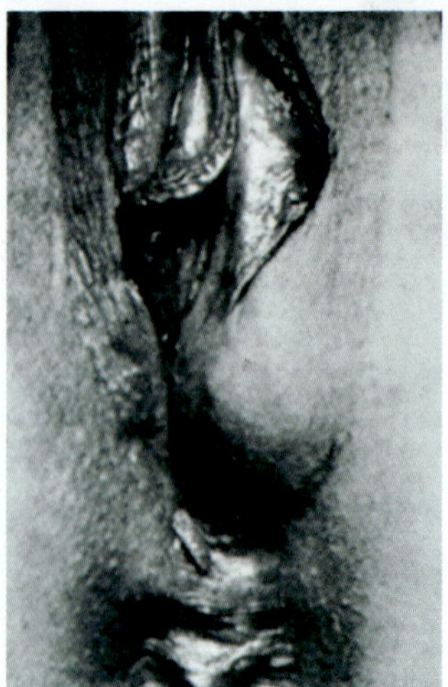

Fig. 21: A left-sided Bartholin's cyst showing the typical position with the base of the labium minus spread out over the dome of the tumour.

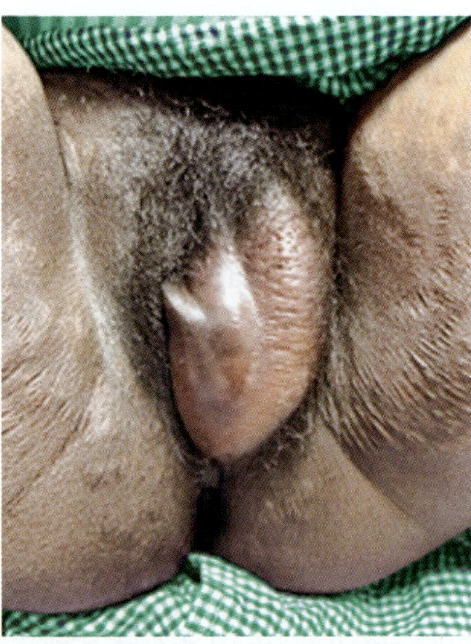

Fig. 22: Bartholin abscess in a 28-year-old woman at 32-week gestation, treated conservatively with antibiotics and $MgSO_4$ dressing. Spontaneous drainage of abscess and relief of symptoms. Patient was delivered at term without any residual lesions.

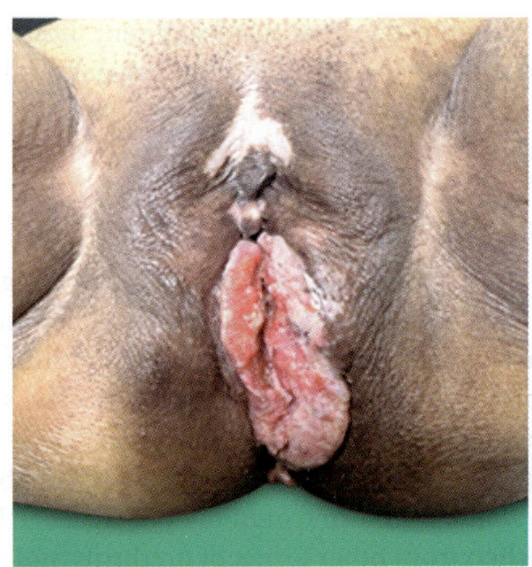

Fig. 23: A 77-year-old woman presented with foul smelling discharge and vaginal itching. On examination, 6 × 5 cm ulceroproliferative growth involving labia majora, labia minora and lower half of vagina. Anteriorly extending to 0.5 cm from urethral meatus, posteriorly up to upper third of anal opening. Urethral meatus is free. Cervix appears normal, cytology sent. Rectal mucosa and rectovaginal septum free. Biopsy taken from vulvar and vaginal growth. Histopathological diagnosis, vulval growth biopsy shows squamous cell carcinoma, HPV independent, grade 2. IHC, p16/INK4a does not exhibit a block positive staining pattern. Vaginal biopsy also suggestive of squamous cell carcinoma, HPV independent, grade 2. (HPV: human papillomavirus; IHC: immunohistochemistry)

breakdown of the wound. To avoid this, a tiny drain should be left for 24 hours. It is desirable to remove the gland as well as the cyst, and care is necessary to avoid injury to the vaginal wall. Fear of rupture of the cyst during dissection is groundless because the contents are invariably innocuous. Indeed, deliberate opening of the cyst makes dissection easier.

If the cyst is actively infected when the patient seeks advice, it is not possible to excise it. It is then treated like acute bartholinitis.

To avoid the technical difficulties described above and with the added advantage of preserving the function of the gland, simple incision into the cyst can be followed by marsupialisation of the cut edges of its wall to those of the skin. This can be done no matter whether the cyst is infected or not and gives a short convalescence with good prospects for a permanent cure. This type of operation now takes precedence over excision.

Neoplasms of Bartholin's Gland

These are exceptionally rare and are more likely to be malignant than benign. They take the form of a columnar cell adenoma or carcinoma. A malignant growth requires radical vulvectomy with block dissection of the inguinal glands on both sides **(Fig. 23)**.

URETHRAL TUMOURS

Prolapse of the Urethra

Acute

Acute urethral prolapse is seen mostly in old age and childhood, so a lack of oestrogen may be a predisposing aetiological factor. The accident is often precipitated by straining at stool, coughing or crying. The whole circumference of the lower endourethra prolapses and becomes strangulated to form a purple-coloured tumour of variable size. The complaints are pain, dysuria, frequency of sudden onset and sometimes reflex retention. After a few days, the prolapsed tissue becomes ulcerated and may bleed. The diagnosis is usually easy, although the condition may be confused with acute urethritis, caruncle, carcinoma and choriocarcinoma.

Treatment by replacing the prolapse and inserting a self-retaining catheter for several days may be curative in children, but in old women, it usually gives only temporary relief. In both, a better result can be obtained by the ligation of the extruded tissues around the catheter leaving them to slough away. The best treatment, however, is to amputate the prolapsed epithelium surgically, taking care not to allow the endourethral lining to retract and to suture this to the external meatus.

Chronic

Chronic urethral prolapse is common in old age, when atrophy causes the external meatus to gape and allows some part of the urethral lining (usually the posterior rim) to project as a small tumour. This has the same red colour as the normal urethral epithelium. The condition is asymptomatic unless the exposed tissue becomes infected, when dysuria and frequency are likely. It has to be distinguished from other forms of urethritis and caruncle and carcinoma.

No treatment is required unless symptoms are present; though rare if present, a plastic operation on the posterior aspect of the urethral meatus is an easy and satisfactory procedure.

Diverticulum of the Urethra

A diverticulum with a narrow communication to the lumen of the lower urethra can result from a congenital error, an abscess of the periurethral glands which bursts into the urethra or obstetrical and surgical injury. It forms a swelling on any aspect of the urethra, but it is most often posterior or posterolateral. A posterior diverticulum projects into the vagina and from the introitus **(Fig. 24)**. It can extend up the vaginal wall around the base of the bladder, and its size varies according to whether it fills or empties itself of urine. The opening into the urethra is often valve-like, so material cannot always be expressed. Infection is almost inevitable, and calculus formation is not uncommon.

The likely symptoms are local discomfort, dysuria, dribbling of urine and dyspareunia. The condition has to be distinguished from a cyst of Gartner's duct or Skene's tubules and from a urethrocele. The diagnosis of a urethral diverticulum is made by keeping the condition in mind: The urethral escape of pus or urine on pressure over the tumour, urethroscopy and a lateral urethrography during voiding.

Treatment is by excision of the diverticulum with closure of the small urethral defect, a procedure neither difficult nor dangerous if reasonable care is taken. It is important to carry out a histological examination of the tissue removed for; on rare occasions, carcinoma can develop in a diverticulum.

Cysts of Skene's (Paraurethral) Tubules

Cysts form when the openings of these structures are blocked by a previous infection. They present as small swellings low down on the anterior wall of the vagina rather than on the vulva **(Fig. 25)**. The cyst can become infected to cause a *paraurethral abscess*. Treatment is by excision at a time when infection is quiescent.

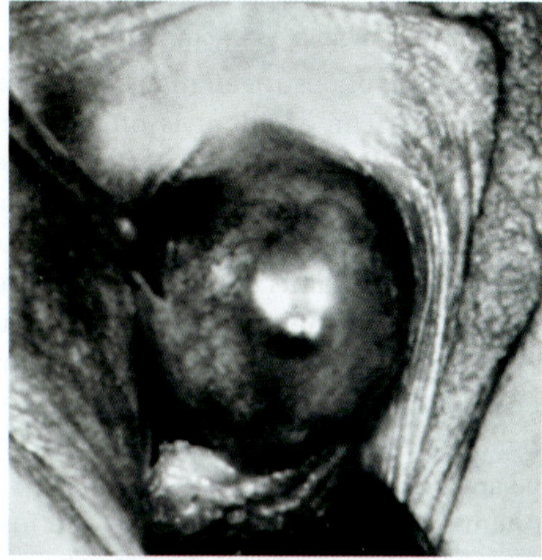

Fig. 24: A diverticulum of the urethra, the urethral meatus being indicated by a sound. The diverticulum filled and discharged intermittently. It was excised without difficulty and with a good result.

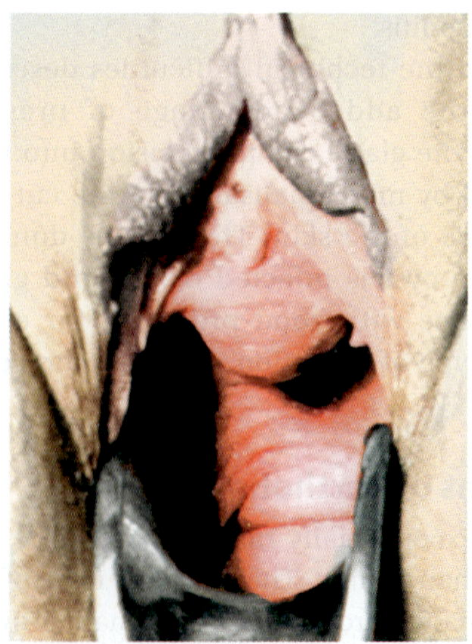

Fig. 25: A cyst of Skene's (paraurethral) tubules, producing an irreducible tumour on the lower anterior vaginal wall.

Urethral Caruncle

The nature of this lesion was much disputed in the past, but any remaining difficulty over its pathology, diagnosis and treatment is caused by confusion between two conditions—(1) A true caruncle and (2) a chronic inflammatory reaction.

True Caruncle

Pathology

A true caruncle is not so common as generally supposed. It consists of a scarlet polyp, which always has a narrow pedicle attached to the posterior margin of the urethral meatus. It varies in size from a pinhead to a pea; its colour indicates its extreme vascularity, which is also evident on section. The tumour is a papilloma of the urethra and is covered with transitional epithelium; this is arranged in folds and crypts, which can give a false impression of malignant downgrowths **(Fig. 26)**. In fact, caruncles are rarely malignant, although they show a tendency to local recurrence. Microscopic examination also reveals that most caruncles are secondarily infected, and some are well supplied with nerves.

Clinical Features

Carundles arise at any age but generally after the menopause. Most but not all are exquisitely tender, so the patient complains of pain on sitting and walking, dyspareunia and dysuria. Other possible symptoms include slight bleeding and the presence of a swelling. The diagnosis rests on the colour, site and strictly localised polypoid nature of the tumour.

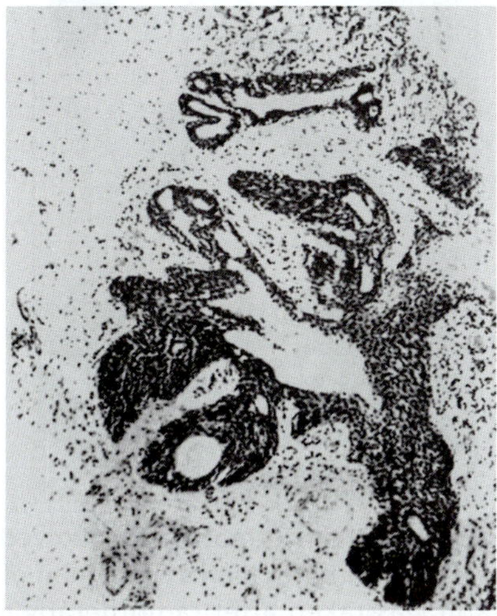

Fig. 26: A true urethral caruncle showing its essentially papillomatous structure with some secondary leucocytic infiltration of the connective tissue. The transitional epithelium is arranged in folds which, on section, give the false impression of downgrowths.

Treatment

To obtain a permanent cure, it is necessary to make a wedge excision of the area from which the caruncle arises, including the tumour itself. Moreover, the site should then be coagulated with a cautery or diathermy. Thereafter, it is preferable to cover the area with epithelium brought in from the sides.

Granulomatous Caruncle or Diffuse Caruncle

Pathology

This non-neoplastic, nonpolypoidal condition is much more common and is often mistakenly labelled and treated as a caruncle. It is a granulomatous lesion affecting the external urethral meatus, notably on its posterior lip but extending around the sides. Although the margin of the urethral opening is raised and pouting, the *tumour* is without a pedicle, is dull red rather than cherry red and not so tender as a caruncle.

On the section, it shows the usual histological features of tissue reaction to chronic infection.

A granulomatous caruncle is a relatively localised form of chronic urethritis; it may sometimes be nothing more than secondary infection of a slightly prolapsed endourethra, possibly associated with senile vaginitis. In the majority of cases, however, it is a manifestation of a chronic *Trichomonas* infestation. This possibility should be excluded in all cases by culture of material taken from the urethra and vagina.

Since the lesion is a response to infection and is not clearly demarcated, it usually recurs after excision or cauterisation, and this mostly explains why caruncles in general have an evil reputation in this respect.

Clinical Features

The symptoms produced are similar to those of caruncle, but they are not so bothersome.

Treatment

It is essential to determine the type of infection present and to treat it accordingly. Even when the presence of *Trichomonas vaginalis* organisms is not confirmed, a prolonged and intensive course of treatment with metronidazole should always be given empirically. Postmenopausal patients sometimes benefit from oestrogen therapy, applied locally or in the form of vaginal pessaries. Local applications of antiseptic preparations can also be of help. In long-standing cases, it may be necessary to excise the affected area. Cauterisation or diathermy coagulation without excision always gives unsatisfactory results.

Other Urethral Papillomas

These take the form of small skin-coloured pedunculated tags arising from just within the external urethral meatus **(Fig. 27)**. Occurring at all ages, sometimes in childhood, they are usually symptomless but can cause local discomfort. They are easily treated by excision.

Carcinoma of the Urethra

Pathology

The urethra can be involved in the direct extension of a cancer of the vulva. Primary carcinoma of the urethra is rare, and most gynaecologists see not more than five or six cases in a lifetime. Although an adenocarcinoma of the paraurethral glands is a possibility, most tumours are epidermoid and arise from the transitional epithelium. The growth nearly always develops low in the urethra, so its lymphatic dissemination is the same as that of carcinoma of the vulva.

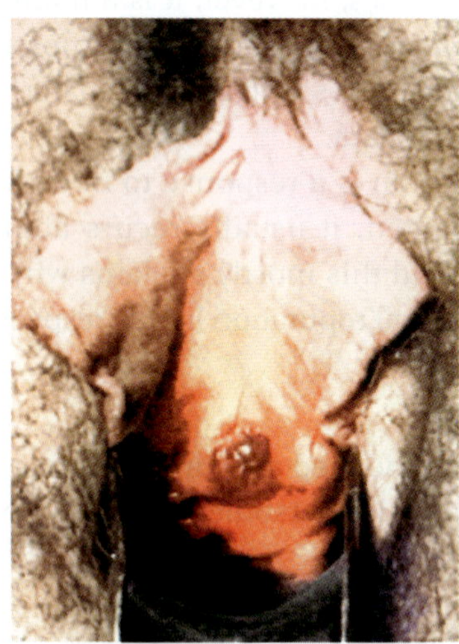

Fig. 27: A bilobed papilloma arising from the posterior margin of the urethral meatus. This might be regarded as a true caruncle, but the tumour was fleshy coloured, not red, and was symptomless.

Clinical Features

The usual complaints are dysuria, frequency and haematuria, and sometimes bleeding apart from micturition. Urinary retention is a late symptom. Unless the growth is fungating at the meatus, the only physical sign is palpable enlargement and hardening of the urethra as judged by rolling it against the symphysis pubis. The diagnosis is made certain by histological examination of urethral scrapings and biopsy.

Treatment

Each case has to be treated according to its circumstances **(Fig. 28)**, the possibilities being: Insertion of radium needles as a palisade around the urethra, with or without inguinal lymphadenectomy; excision of the urethra (and possibly the bladder) together with the anterior vaginal wall, the adjacent parts of the vulva and the inguinal nodes—this also involves transplantation of the ureters; local excision of the growth; and combinations of surgery and radiotherapy.

The majority of carcinomas in the distal half of the urethra are treated by local excision or radiotherapy. The 5-year survival rate is 30–50%.

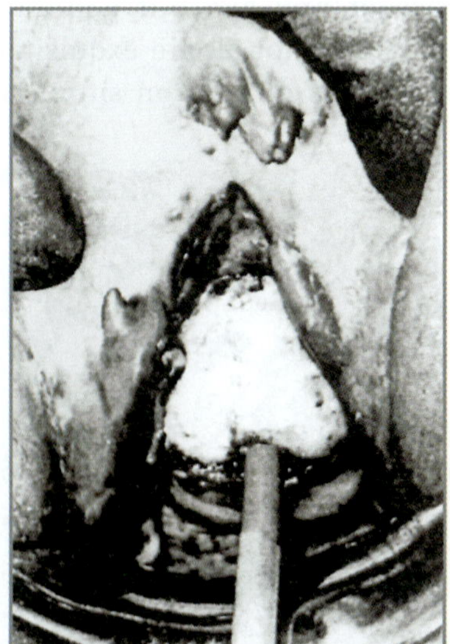

Fig. 28: Carcinoma of the urethra which involved the inferior ramus of the pubis. A catheter marks the lumen of the urethra. This photograph was taken after radiotherapy covering the whole of the urethra, and this has destroyed the foreparts of the labia minora and caused necrosis of the growth. The lesion, together with the urethra and the lower part of the bladder, was subsequently excised, the ureters being transplanted into the colon. The patient survived for another 7 years.

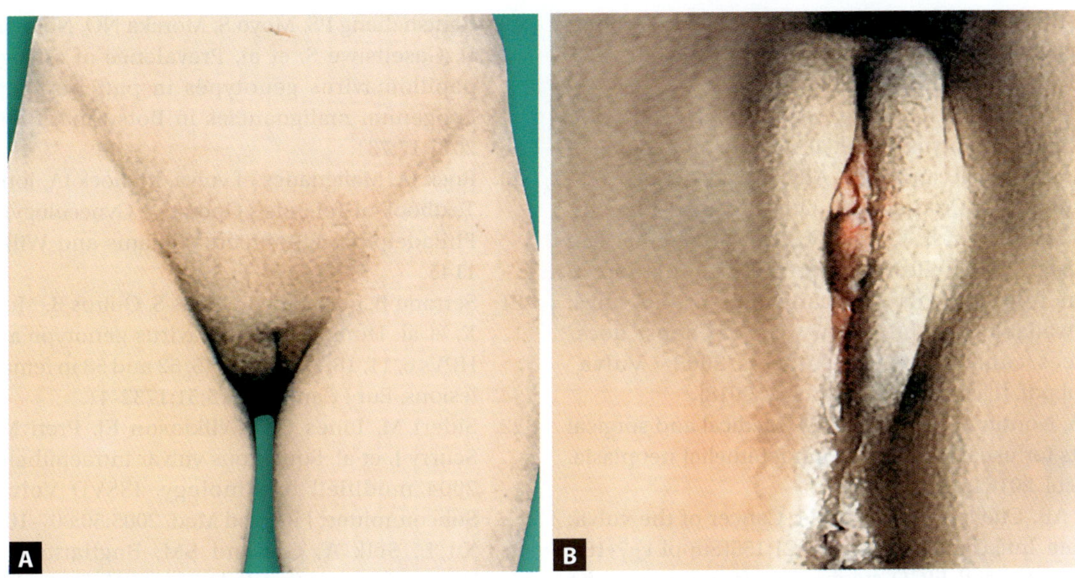

Figs. 29A and B: A right-sided inguinal hernia presenting as a tumour of the labium majus.

TUMOURS OF THE INGUINAL CANAL

An obliterated peritoneal pouch extends down the inguinal canal with the round ligament. A hydrocele of the canal of Nuck is a fluid distension of a portion of this rudimentary structure and may present as an irreducible cystic swelling in the forepart of the labium majus. It has to be distinguished from an inguinal hernia which also can extend far into the labium **(Figs. 29A and B)**. A fibroma or endometriosis of the round ligament can give rise to a hard swelling at the insertion of the ligament into the subcutaneous tissues of the mons, the endometrioma having a characteristic behaviour. A varicocele of the round ligament is mostly seen during pregnancy and simulates an inguinal hernia; active treatment for it is rarely necessary.

SUGGESTED READING

1. Allbritton JI. Vulvar neoplasms, benign and malignant. Obstet Gynecol Clin North Am. 2017;44:339-52.
2. Black D, Tornos C, Soslow RA, Awtrey CS, Barakat RR, Chi DS. The outcomes of patients with positive margins after excision for intraepithelial Paget's disease of the vulva. Gynecol Oncol. 2007;104:547-50.
3. Bornstein J, Bogliatto F, Haefner HK, Stockdale CK, Preti M, Bohl TG, et al. The 2015 International Society for the Study of Vulvovaginal Disease (ISSVD) terminology of vulvar squamous intraepithelial lesions. Obstet Gynecol. 2016;127:264-8.
4. Cancer Research UK. (2018). Vulval cancer incidence statistics. [online] Available from http://www.cancerresearchuk.org/cancer-info/cancerstats/types/vulva/incidence/. [Last accessed April, 2025].
5. Cancer Research UK. (2018). Vulval cancer mortality statistics. [online] Available from http://www.cancerresearchuk.org/cancer-info/cancerstats/types/vulva/mortality/. [Last accessed April, 2025].
6. Edey KA, Allan E, Murdoch JB, Cooper S, Bryant A. Interventions for the treatment of Paget's disease of the vulva. Cochrane Database Syst Rev. 2019;6(6):CD009245.
7. Eshtiaghi P, Sadownik LA. Fact or fiction? Adipose-derived stem cells and platelet-rich plasma for the treatment of vulvar lichen sclerosus. J Low Genit Tract Dis. 2019; 23:65-70.
8. Eva LJ, Ganesan R, Chan KK, Honest H, Luesley DM. Differentiated-type vulval intraepithelial neoplasia has a high-risk association with vulval squamous cell carcinoma. Int J Gynecol Cancer. 2009;19:741-4.
9. Fistarol SK, Itin PH. Diagnosis and treatment of lichen sclerosus: an update. Am J Clin Dermatol. 2013;14: 27-47.
10. Garland SM, Paavonen J, Jaisamrarn U, Naud P, Salmerón J, Chow SN, et al. Prior human papillomavirus-16/18 AS04-adjuvanted vaccination prevents recurrent high grade cervical intraepithelial neoplasia after definitive surgical therapy: post-hoc analysis from a randomized controlled trial. Int J Cancer. 2016;139:2812-26.
11. Hampl M, Sarajuuri H, Wentzensen N, Bender HG, Kueppers V. Effect of human papillomavirus vaccines on vulvar, vaginal, and anal intraepithelial lesions and vulvar cancer. Obstet Gynecol. 2006;108:1361-8.
12. Hoang LN, Park KJ, Soslow RA, Murali R. Squamous precursor lesions of the vulva: current classification and diagnostic challenges. Pathology. 2016;48:291-302.

13. Karam A, Dorigo O. Treatment outcomes in a large cohort of patients with invasive extramammary Paget's disease. Gynecol Oncol. 2012;125:346-51.
14. Kim KW, Shinagare AB, Krajewski KM, Howard SA, Jagannathan JP, Zukotynski K, et al. Update on imaging of vulvar squamous cell carcinoma. AJR. 2013;201:W147-57.
15. Krishnamurti UG, Crothers BA, Otis CN, Birdsong GG, Movahedi-Lankarani S, Klepeis V, College of American Pathologists. (2009). Protocol for the examination of specimens from patients with carcinoma of the vulva. [online] Available from http://www.cap.org/apps/ docs/ committees/cancer/cancer_protocols/2009/ Vulva_ 09protocol.pdf. [Last accessed February, 2018].
16. Lawrie TA, Nordin A, Chakrabarti M. Medical and surgical treatments for usual-type vulvar intraepithelial neoplasia. JAMA Oncol. 2016;2:1647-8.
17. Olawaiye AB, Cuello MA, Rogers LJ. Cancer of the vulva: 2021 update. Int J Gynecol Obstet. 2021;155(Suppl 1):7-18.
18. Pecorelli S. Revised FIGO staging for carcinoma of the vulva, cervix, and endometrium. Int J Gynaecol Obstet. 2009;105(2):103-4.
19. Rantshabeng PS, Moyo S, Moraka NO, Ndlovu A, MacLeod IJ, Gaseitsiwe S, et al. Prevalence of oncogenic human papillomavirus genotypes in patients diagnosed with anogenital malignancies in Botswana. BMC Infect Dis. 2017;17:731.
20. Rock JA. Malignancy of vulva. In: Rock JA, Jones HW (Eds). Textbook of TeLinde's Operative Gynecology, 10th edition. Philadelphia: Lippincott Williams and Wilkins; 2011. p. 1145.
21. Serrano B, de Sanjosé S, Tous S, Quiros B, Muñoz N, Bosch X, et al. Human papillomavirus genotype attribution for HPVs 6, 11, 16, 18, 31, 33, 45, 52 and 58 in female anogenital lesions. Eur J Cancer. 2015;51:1732-41.
22. Sideri M, Jones RW, Wilkinson EJ, Preti M, Heller DS, Scurry J, et al. Squamous vulvar intraepithelial neoplasia: 2004 modified terminology, ISSVD Vulvar Oncology Subcommittee. J Reprod Med. 2005;50:807-10.
23. Xu L, Selk A, Garland SM, Bogliatto F, Kyrgiou M, Weyers S, et al. Prophylactic vaccination against human papillomaviruses to prevent vulval and vaginal cancer and their precursors. Expert Rev Vaccines. 2019;18:1157-66.

29

CHAPTER

Tumours of the Vagina

Rekha Upadhya, Muralidhar V Pai

Chapter Outline

- Swellings of the Vagina
- Vaginal Cysts
- Benign Neoplasms
- Malignant Neoplasms

INTRODUCTION

Vaginal tumours including both benign and malignant, are abnormal growths in the region of vagina which may arise from different cell types. Benign tumours are more common and malignant are rare but can spread to surrounding tissues. The most common type of vaginal cancer is squamous cell carcinoma, mostly associated with HPV infection and elderly women, but also occur among younger women.

SWELLINGS OF THE VAGINA

A complaint of swelling or fullness in the vagina may be caused by the following:

- Retained fluid—haematocolpos, pyocolpos
- Prolapse of the vaginal walls or uterus
- A congenitally short vagina with a relatively low cervix
- Varicose veins, which are usually low on the anterior wall and are mostly seen during pregnancy
- Vaginitis of any kind
- Tumours of the urethra
- Enlargement of the cervix
- Any tumour that is impacted in the pelvis
- Vaginal cysts
- Benign neoplasms
- Malignant neoplasms.

This chapter is concerned with the last three groups of conditions.

VAGINAL CYSTS

Since the vaginal epithelium is normally devoid of glands, most cysts arise from included or adjacent structures. Their nature and origin are therefore determined clinically by their position.

Cysts of Vestigial Structures Types

- *Müllerian:* Tiny cysts, single or multiple, lined by tissue similar to that of the cervical epithelium and containing mucinous material, sometimes occur near the cervix. They are thought to arise from displaced cervical glands or Müllerian duct diverticula and their remnants.
- *Wolffian:* The majority of vaginal cysts arise from Gartner's duct; their origin is deduced by their position on a line running down the lateral or anterolateral wall of the vagina from the cervix to the region of the urethra and clitoris **(Fig. 1)**. The cysts are usually small and multiple but can attain the size of a foetal head; in the lateral fornix they are in close association with the ureter. Their lining is a single layer of flattened columnar or cuboidal epithelium, but can be transitional; their fluid content is free from mucin **(Fig. 1)**.

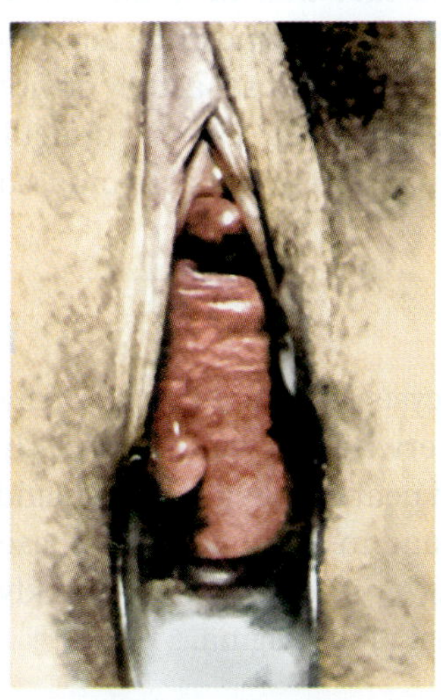

Fig. 1: A cyst in the anterolateral wall of the vagina probably arising from the remnants of the Wolffian duct, as judged from its site.

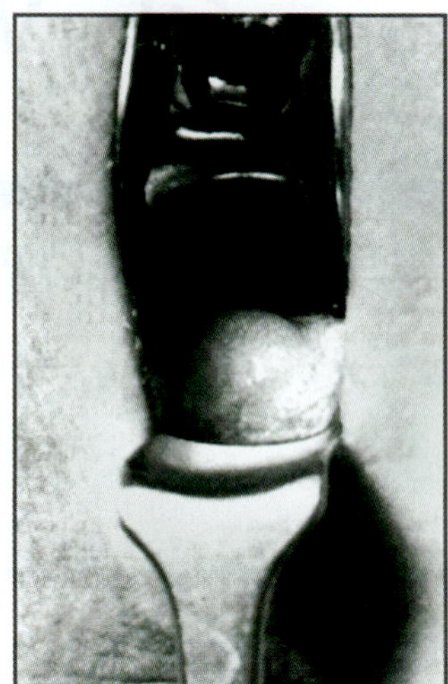

Fig. 2: A cyst in the lower part of the posterior vaginal wall or a nulliparous woman complaining of infertility. It was asymptomatic and was therefore not removed. So, its pathology remains uncertain. The midline site suggests a developmental inclusion cyst.

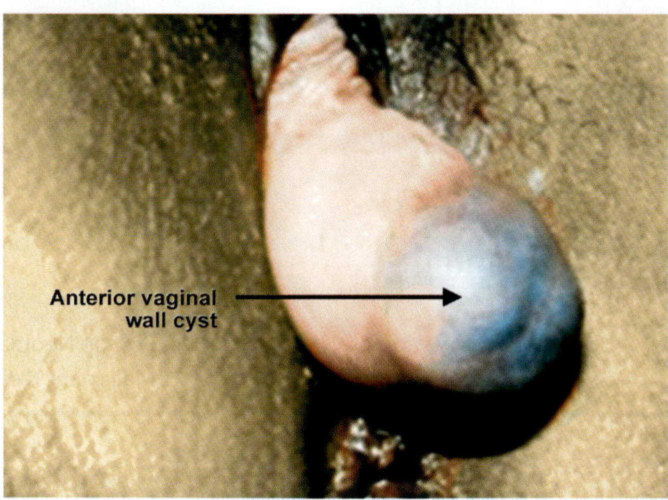

Fig. 3: This was the case of anterior vaginal wall cyst. In figure, this is seen as a bluish discolouration projection, shown by an arrow. Cervix is not seen in this picture.
Courtesy: Dr Narayan M Patel.

- *Others:* Midline cysts in the posterior vaginal wall may arise from the remains of the tongue of coelom **(Fig. 2)**.

Clinical Features

Small cysts are usually symptomless, large ones cause dyspareunia, infertility, dystocia or a sensation of fullness in the vagina. They are distinguished from a urethrocele, cystocele, urethral diverticulum and other cysts by their position; by the fact that they do not disappear with pressure or with change in posture; and by demonstrating with a sound or other means that they do not communicate with the bladder or urethra. It can be difficult to distinguish a vaginal cyst from a paravaginal lipoma, soft fibroma and myxoma.

Treatment

Asymptomatic cysts discovered incidentally do not require treatment. Otherwise, they are excised. If, however, the cyst is large and near the ureter or the bladder, it is safer to remove its top and to marsupialise its base to the vaginal wall; the lining epithelium then quickly assumes the characters of that of the vagina.

Cyst of Skene's Tubules

Discussed in Chapter 28: Tumours of the Vulva.

Diverticulum of Urethra

Discussed in Chapter 28: Tumours of the Vulva.

Epidermoid Cyst and Implantation Dermoid

These arise from accidental implants of fragments of sebum-producing skin, such as that of the perineum. They therefore usually follow obstetrical injuries or perineorrhaphy, and their only common vaginal site is the lower part of the posterior wall. These cysts cannot develop from implants of vaginal epithelium (which does not secrete sebum). They are small and rarely produce symptoms or require treatment.

Endometriotic Cysts

These can arise in scars in any position in the vagina; otherwise, they are mostly seen in the posterior fornix in association with endometriosis of the rectovaginal septum or in episiotomy scars.

Anterior Vaginal Wall Cyst

Figures 3 to 11 show the anterior vaginal wall cyst.

BENIGN NEOPLASMS

Benign neoplasms of the vagina may be sessile or pedunculated. Some are paravaginal rather than vaginal; in that they arise from tissue in the paracolpos.

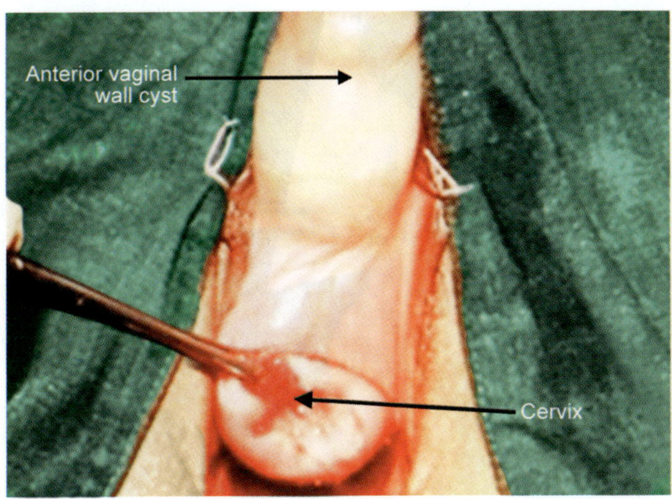

Fig. 4: On lifting up the cyst, the cervix is seen, as shown by an instrument and also by an arrow. Speculum is in position. This slide clearly shows that cyst is in anterior vaginal wall.
Courtesy: Dr Narayan M Patel.

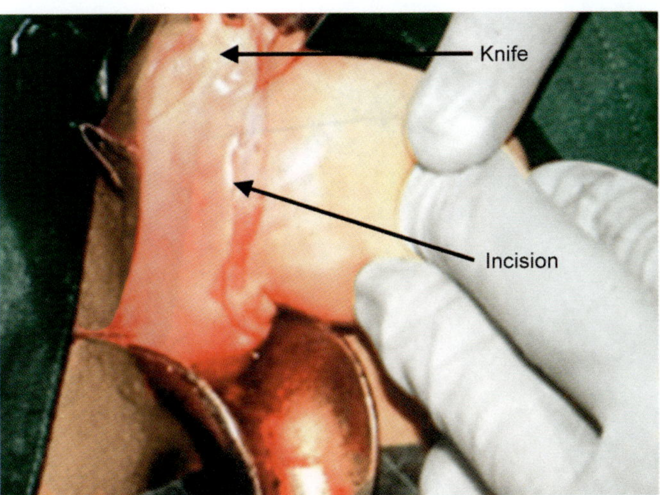

Fig. 6: An incision is put on the wall of cyst, deep enough to reach up to the vaginal wall. A similar incision was put on the other side, pulling the cyst to the right side of the patient.
Courtesy: Dr Narayan M Patel

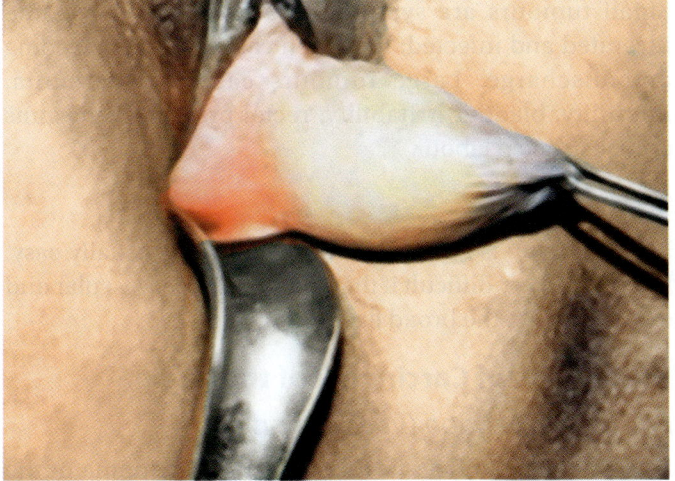

Fig. 5: The cyst is grasped by Allis forceps and pulled on left side of the patient to define its base. Speculum is in position.
Courtesy: Dr Narayan M Patel

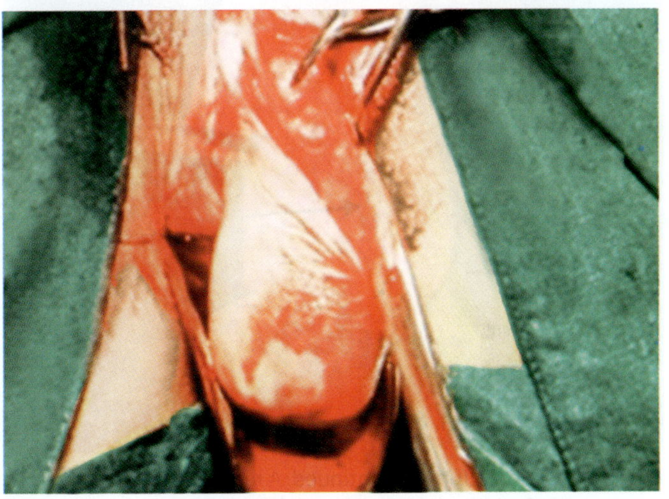

Fig. 7: The cyst is being dissected on the left side of the patient, remaining in the cleavage.
Courtesy: Dr Narayan M Patel.

Types

- *Papilloma:* True papillomas (including multiple warts) do occur (refer to Chapter 20: Infections Including Sexually Transmitted Diseases), but most tumours of this type are skin tags remaining from obstetrical injuries or operations.
- *Angioma:* An angioma is a congenital malformation of the blood vessels, usually seen under the lateral walls.
- *Adenoma:* This rare tumour arises in association with Gartner's duct and therefore has an anterolateral site. The lesions are often small and multiple. When they occur in children, they are sometimes confused with carcinoma.
- *Adenosis:* Discussed in Chapter 26: Epithelial Abnormalities of the Genital Tract.
- *Fibroma and lipoma:* These arise from the outer coats of the vagina or from the paracolpos. They can reach large dimensions and can extend into the broad ligament and into the ischiorectal fossa.
- *Myxoid soft-tissue tumours:* These are soft, fluctuant, almost cystic tumours containing myxomatous and

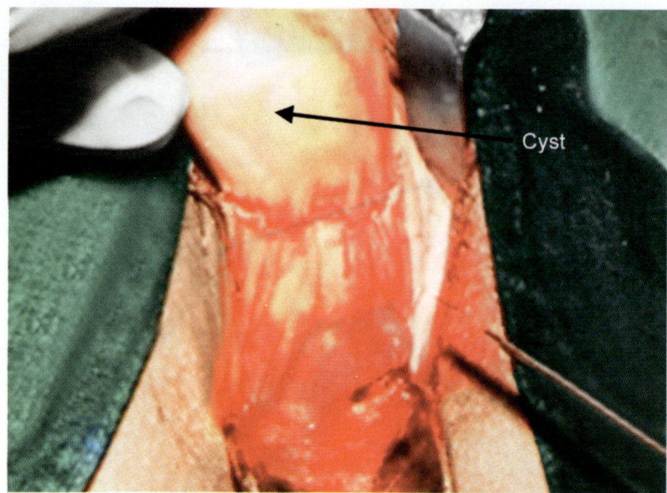

Fig. 8: The cyst is lifted up and dissected posteriorly from cervix, trying to remain in cleavage.
Courtesy: Dr Narayan M Patel.

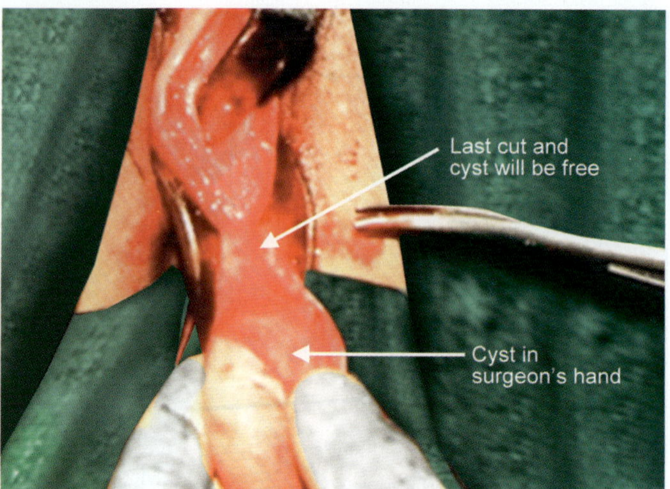

Fig. 10: Final cut is given to cyst.
Courtesy: Dr Narayan M Patel.

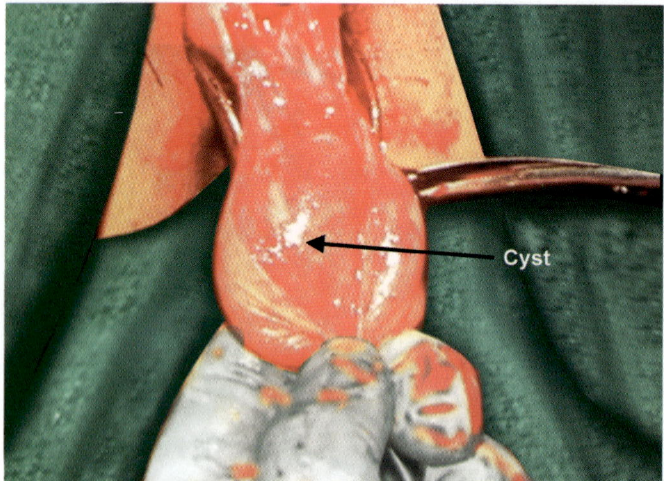

Fig. 9: Dissection is further continued. A retractor is used to stretch the tissue to find out the lower limit of the cyst.
Courtesy: Dr Narayan M Patel.

fibrous or fatty tissue elements. The common sites are the ischiorectal fossa and the subcutaneous tissue of the buttock. But they are also seen arising in, or extending to, the paracolpos **(Figs. 12A and B)**. They do not metastasise but are locally recurrent and may ultimately become frankly sarcomatous.

- *Granuloma:* Discrete and often polypoidal areas of granulation tissue are not uncommonly found in vaginal scars, especially those following colporrhaphy and total hysterectomy. They are not neoplasms, but they sometimes persist for months and years after operation and can be mistaken for malignant disease.

Clinical Features

Small tumours are symptomless unless they become ulcerated and infected; they then cause contact bleeding and discharge. Large tumours cause dyspareunia, infertility, bladder irritability, rectal pressure, tenesmus and obstructed labour.

Treatment

Local excision is generally indicated. This is usually easy, but can be very difficult if the tumour is large, vascular and extending into the broad ligament.

Prevention of Carcinoma of the Vagina

Primary Prevention (Vaccination)

Like premalignant cervical lesions and carcinoma of the cervix, persistent human papillomavirus (HPV) infection—particularly the HPV 16 subtype—has been associated with the long-term development of high-grade squamous intraepithelial lesion (HSIL) and carcinoma of the vagina. The introduction of HPV vaccination as a primary prevention strategy in cervical cancer has also been shown to reduce the prevalence of noncervical premalignant lesions among vaccinated women. Long-term trend analyses from the Norwegian Cancer Register also show promising estimates of reduction in HPV-associated cases of vaginal cancer in future years among HPV-vaccinated communities.

Secondary Prevention (Screening)

There is no evidence to indicate routine screening for vaginal cancer after hysterectomy for benign disease.

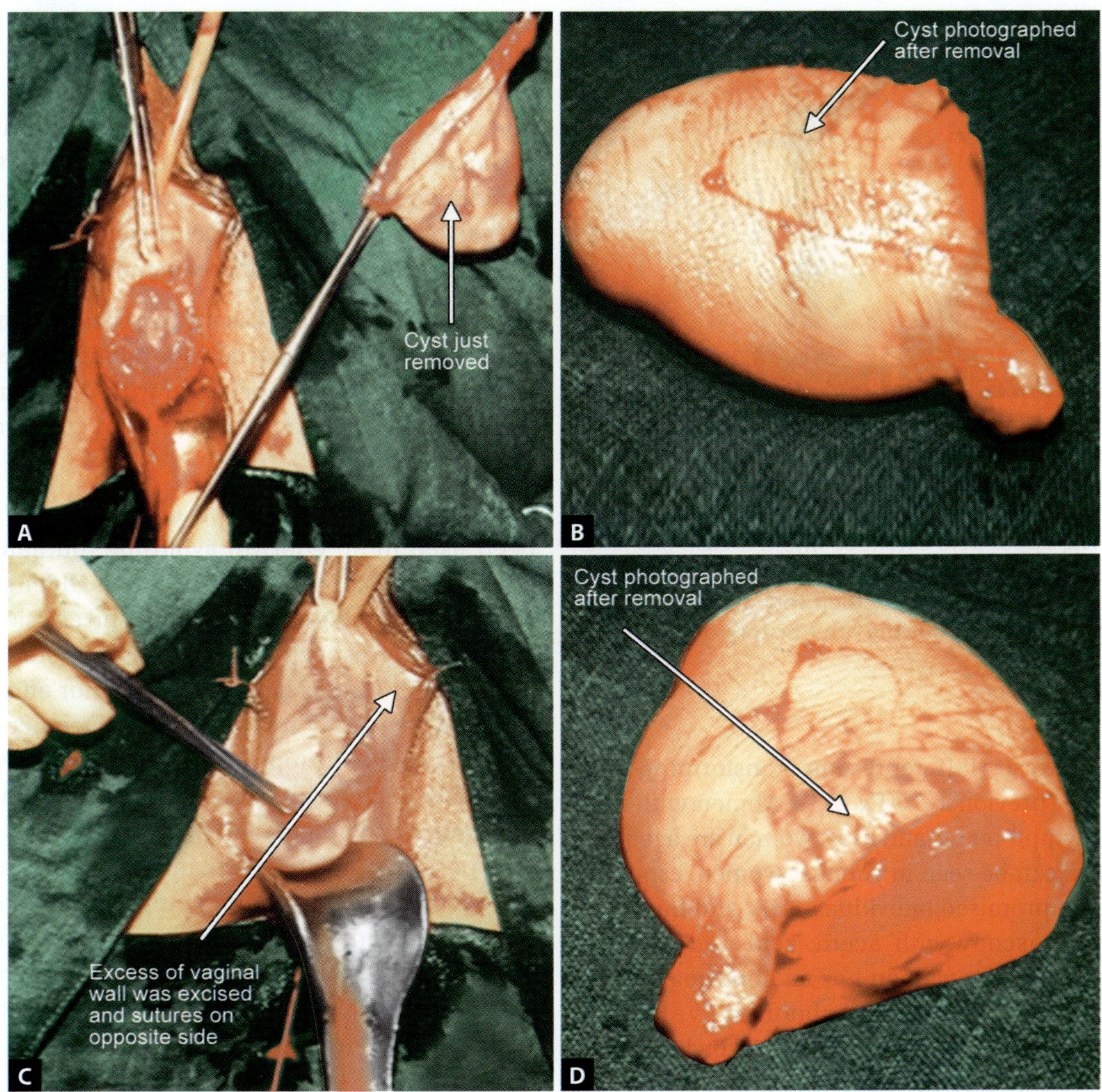

Figs. 11A to D: Cyst is removed.
Courtesy: Dr Narayan M Patel.

If a hysterectomy has been performed for persistent HSIL after repeated excisional procedures of the cervix, vault smears and colposcopy are recommended for long-term follow-up. In those cases where screening for vaginal cancer is indicated, HPV tests adequately correlate with cytological findings. Independently of that, co-testing seems to offer better accuracy in the diagnosis of recurrent disease, as observed during follow-up after treatment of premalignant cervical lesions.

Tertiary Prevention (Management of Precancerous Lesions)

As the majority of vaginal cancers are of squamous histology, a common aetiology is shared with cervical cancer. This is the persistence of high-risk/oncogenic HPV infections. Co-factors include immunosuppression and cigarette smoking. Smoking in combination with high-risk HPV increases the risk of progression to vaginal HSIL when compared with nonsmokers. The terminology for precancerous HPV-associated vaginal lesions has changed over time.

In 2014, the WHO classification replaced the three-tiered classification used previously [vaginal intraepithelial neoplasia (VAIN) 1–3] with squamous intraepithelial lesion (SIL). This is divided into two categories: Low grade (LSIL) and high grade (HSIL). LSIL (VAIN 1) may be associated with either low-risk or high-risk HPV, and it represents productive or transient infections that may

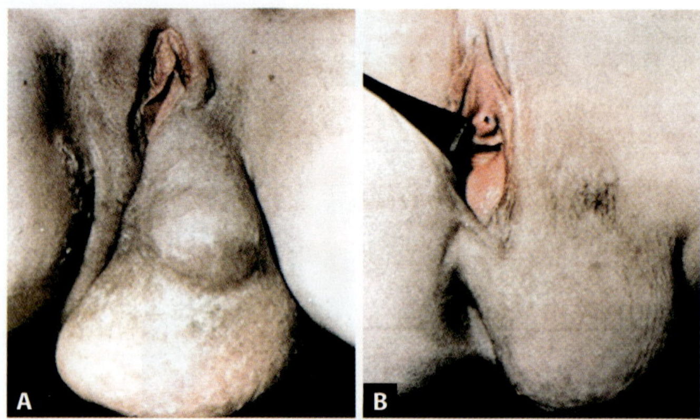

Figs. 12A and B: A paravaginal fibromyxoma in a multiparous woman aged 35 years: (A) The original tumour, when excised, proved to extend from the vulva through the ischiorectal fossa to the paracolpos; (B) A recurrence of the tumour 3 years after its removal. The upper pole extended into the base of the left broad ligament. Its extent and the fact that the myxoma was soft and poorly encapsulated made excision very difficult. A further recurrence seemed likely, but the after history of this case is unknown.
Courtesy: Mr E Parry Jones.

regress. In contrast, HSIL represents transforming high-risk infections (previously VAIN 2–3). Women with HSIL are usually asymptomatic, and most women are aged over 60 years. HSIL can be seen in younger women, especially in immunocompromised individuals (HIV and transplant patients). Colposcopy with acetic acid and/or Lugol iodine is indicated if a woman has an abnormal vaginal cytological smear and no gross abnormality. Biopsies of colposcopically abnormal areas (acetowhite areas with punctation and/or punctation and mosaicism) are essential for the diagnosis. The risk of progression of HSIL to invasive cancer has been found to range between 2% and 12%. Treatment of precancerous lesions of the vagina must be individualised. Biopsy-proven LSIL lesions can be followed up with observation only (repeat smears and colposcopy), especially if women have nononcogenic strains of HPV. The various modalities of treatment for HSIL lesions include laser ablation, surgical excision and topical treatments such as imiquimod and topical chemotherapy with 5-fluorouracil (5-FU). Choice of treatment depends on the number and location of the lesions, and the degree of suspicion for an invasive cancer, as well as the availability of various treatment options, the cost of treatment and the skill of the treating doctor.

Surgical excision: The advantages of excising HSIL of the vagina is that it provides a pathological description of the tissue removed, especially when there is a suspicion of microinvasion on colposcopic evaluation. Most HSIL lesions are in the vault or upper third of the vagina and excision is ideal in this situation. Morbidity can be associated with the proximity of structures such as the bladder and rectum, as well as associated dyspareunia as a result of vaginal shortening and stenosis. Women should be extensively counselled preoperatively.

CO_2 laser vaporisation: Laser vaporisation is an alternative option to excision, especially for multifocal lesions. Since there is no histologic specimen with this procedure, it is imperative to ensure that there is no concern regarding cancer.

Topical 5-fluorouracil: Topical application of 5-FU has been used in an effort to avoid the mutilating adverse effects of excision and laser ablation. Older studies have shown comparable efficacy to laser and excision. However, these are retrospective in nature with small numbers. More recent studies have shown inferior efficacy. A 2018 retrospective study reviewed the recurrence rate in 576 women treated with topical 5-FU, excision, or laser ablation. The statistically significant factors that contributed to recurrence and progression were the presence of high-risk HPV positivity and treatment modality. Laser and excision were found to be superior to topical management with 5-FU in reducing recurrences. It was also found that laser was more effective than excision in reducing recurrences of multifocal lesions, whereas surgical excision was preferable with unifocal HSIL.

Topical 5% imiquimod: Imiquimod (applied topically either in creams or drug-embedded tampons) is an immune response modulator that activates the innate immune response and subsequently induces proinflammatory factors such as interferons. It provides an alternative noninvasive and safe method for treating women with vaginal HSIL, especially young women with multifocal lesions or older women who wish to avoid surgical modalities. Studies on imiquimod are few, but a 2016 randomised controlled trial (RCT), as well as a systematic review and meta-analysis (including this RCT) in 2017, found that this is a safe and effective treatment with regression rates similar to laser. HPV clearance rates were >50%, which was superior to laser. In general, independent of the therapy chosen, most patients require more than one therapy for adequate control. Since the recurrence rate is high with any single therapy, close and extended follow-up is recommended in all cases. As in treated premalignant cervical lesions, both HPV testing and cytology are recommended.

Management of Invasive Cancer of the Vagina

Women usually present with bleeding or a malodorous discharge. Locally advanced disease may also result in pain, and symptoms of disseminated disease depend on the site of metastases. Diagnosis of vaginal cancer is made with directed biopsy of the lesion and a clinical assessment that ensures there is no evidence of tumour on the cervix or the vulva. Biopsy can be performed in an outpatient setting; however, sometimes examination under anaesthesia is required for diagnosis and adequate assessment, particularly in young girls and elderly women, where the exam can become painful or limited by the narrowness of the introitus. As primary vaginal cancer is rare, treatment is complex, often individualised, and much of the management is extrapolated from cervical cancer owing to its similar aetiology and anatomical location. Therefore, it is recommended that women diagnosed with primary vaginal cancer are referred to a tertiary unit whenever possible. Accordingly, outcomes are influenced by the experience of the medical team in treating this type of rare tumour.

Patterns of Spread

Direct extension: A vaginal tumour may extend to the surrounding pelvic soft tissue structures, including paravaginal tissue, parametria, urethra, bladder and rectum. Most tumours occur in the upper third of the vagina, especially the posterior wall.

Lymphatic spread: The lymphatic drainage of the vagina is complex. The upper vagina drains by lymphatics to the pelvic lymph nodes. This includes the obturator, internal iliac (hypogastric) and external iliac nodes. Spread to the para-aortic lymph nodes is rare. The lower vagina drains to the inguinal and femoral nodes (groin nodes). Cancer in the mid-vagina may follow both pelvic and groin node routes.

Haematogenous spread: Haematogenous dissemination to the lung, liver and bone is usually a late manifestation.

Histologic subtypes: The predominant histologic subtype in primary vaginal cancer is squamous carcinoma, which comprises 90% of cases. Adenocarcinoma accounts for about 8–10% of cases. Lymphomas, sarcomas and melanomas of the vagina are extremely rare. All malignancies must be confirmed histologically. Since 80% of cases are metastatic or secondary tumours, it is important to ensure that there is no other primary site by careful examination and appropriate investigations. Although biopsy can be obtained under local anaesthesia, in many instances, examination under sedation or general anaesthesia should be performed to undertake an adequate exam and obtain a biopsy. By definition, tumours in the vagina that touch or extend to the external os of the cervix should be classified as cervical cancer.

Grading

- GX: Grade cannot be assessed
- G1: Well differentiated
- G2: Moderately differentiated
- G3: Poorly or undifferentiated

MALIGNANT NEOPLASMS

Primary

The majority, i.e. 92% of primary vaginal cancers, are reported to be squamous cell carcinomas. Other tumours seen are the clear cell adenocarcinomas, malignant melanomas, embryonal rhabdomyosarcomas and endodermal sinus tumours.

Vaginal Intraepithelial Neoplasia

For patients with an abnormal Pap smear and no gross abnormality, vaginal colposcopy and use of Lugol's iodine to stain the vagina are necessary. Excision of colposcopically abnormal areas is usually necessary under anaesthesia. This is particularly true for lesions involving the vaginal vault, where occult carcinoma may be found in up to 28% of patients with VAIN.

Treatment of VAIN is individualised and depends on the extent, location and general medical condition of the patient. Numerous treatment methods, ranging from the various methods of local tissue destruction or ablation through to more extensive surgery and including total vaginectomy, as well as intracavitary radiotherapy, have been used to treat VAIN. Selection of appropriate treatment is usually based on a careful study of several factors, including the general medical condition of the patient, histology of the lesion and location and extent of disease, as well as the experience of the treating surgeon with the specific treatment methods.

The proximity of the urethra, bladder and rectum to the vaginal epithelium is an important factor to be considered, particularly when local destructive or surgical excision methods are used. Damage or injury to these structures can occur with possible fistula formation, particularly when the patient has had prior radiation therapy.

The use of topical 5-FU is a relatively simple ambulatory treatment, which does not require anaesthesia or complicated equipment. This approach may be especially valuable for patients with widespread multifocal lesions, which would require extensive surgical procedures. Side effects with this therapy during treatment are usually minimal as long as it is not used more than twice a week. Imiquimod cream 5% might represent an alternative method of management in young, HPV positive women with multifocal high-grade lesions (VAIN 2/3).

Laser vaporisation with a CO_2 laser is an effective treatment for VAIN. This technique generally requires local or general anaesthesia.

Excisional procedures, either with electrosurgical loops or a scalpel excision, have also been used to treat VAIN. Surgical excision is particularly appropriate for vault lesions. Also on occasion, total vaginectomy and split thickness skin grafting may be necessary to treat extensive lesions that involve virtually the entire length of the vaginal tube and where other conservative methods have been unsuccessful.

Squamous Cell Carcinoma

Incidence and aetiology: Primary invasive squamous cell carcinoma of the vagina is rare and is found only once for every 30–50 cases of carcinoma of the cervix, accounting for only 1–2% of genital malignancies. The growth usually begins high on the posterior vaginal wall opposite to the external os **(Figs. 13A and B)** and this, in the past, gave rise to a suggestion that it is caused by irritating discharges from the cervix. Long-standing prolapse or the prolonged wearing of a pessary could also determine neoplastic change. In the past, a history of exposure to a pessary, not necessarily a neglected one, was obtained in 25% of cases. In these, the disease sometimes had an annular distribution.

Since the vagina is thin walled, the growth quickly involves adjacent organs and the prognosis is therefore poor.

Spread: Carcinoma of the vagina spreads by direct extension to the bladder, the rectum, the cellular tissues

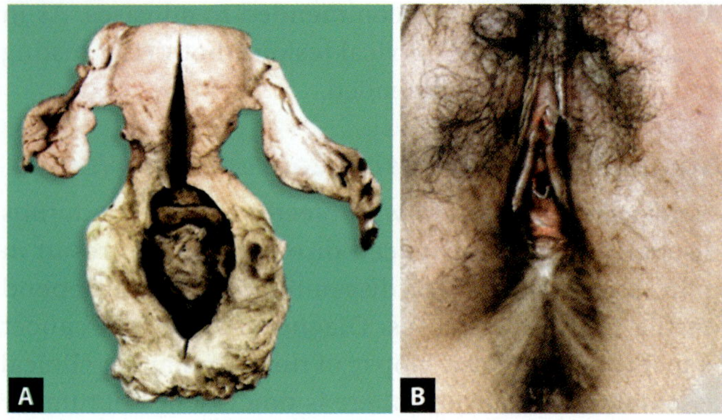

Figs. 13A and B: (A) A specimen of carcinoma of the upper posterior vaginal wall obtained by abdominoperineal excision of all the internal genital organs and the rectum (posterior exenteration); (B) The local result 6 months after the operation. The patient concerned died from metastases 18 months later.

of the uterosacral and broad ligaments, the cervix and the vulva. When the growth is in the upper vagina, the lymphatic spread is the same as in carcinoma of the cervix; if it is situated lower, the vulvar as well as the cervical lymphatic drainage fields are implicated. This explains why the higher growths justify a slightly better prognosis.

Clinical features, diagnosis and staging: The patient suffering from invasive squamous carcinoma of the vagina is usually over the age of 40 years and mostly within the range of 60–80 years. Her symptoms are irregular bleeding, contact bleeding and offensive discharge. The diagnosis is made by seeing and feeling the malignant growth. This usually takes the form of an ulcer with a hard base and raised edges, which becomes fixed to underlying structures at an early stage. Its surface is friable and bleeds easily on touching.

Carcinoma of the upper vagina has to be distinguished from vault endometriosis and granulomatosis, from malignant disease of the rectum and from a primary growth on the cervix. When the lower vagina is involved, it can be difficult to say whether the lesion is primary in the vagina or in the vulva. For the purpose of international consistency in recording, it is recommended that any growth which involves the cervix should be classified as cervical and not vaginal.

To be classified as a primary vaginal cancer, there must be no clinical evidence that the vaginal tumour is metastatic.

Diagnosis is made by a generous, full-thickness biopsy and histopathology. Colposcopy identifies coexisting VAIN, if any, and helps in planning treatment.

TABLE 1: Comparison of staging systems for vaginal cancer.

AJCC stage	***Stage grouping (TNM)***	***FIGO stage (2009)***	***Stage description***
IA	T1a N0 M0	I	The cancer is only in the vagina and is no >2.0 cm (4/5 inch) (T1a). It has not spread to nearby lymph nodes (N0) or to distant sites (M0)
IB	T1b N0 M0	I	The cancer is only in the vagina and is >2.0 cm (4/5 inch) (T1b). It has not spread to nearby lymph nodes (N0) or to distant sites (M0)
IIA	T2a N0 M0	II	The cancer has grown through the vaginal wall, but not as far as the pelvic wall and is no >2.0 cm (4/5 inch) (T2a). It has not spread to nearby lymph nodes (N0) or to distant sites (M0)
IIB	T2b N0 M0	II	The cancer has grown through the vaginal wall, but not as far as the pelvic wall and is >2.0 cm (4/5 inch) (T2b). It has not spread to nearby lymph nodes (N0) or to distant sites (M0)
III	T1 to T3 N1 M0 or	III	The cancer can be any size and might be growing into the pelvic wall, and/or growing into the lower one-third of the vagina and/or has blocked the flow of urine (hydronephrosis), which is causing kidney problems (T1 to T3). It has also spread to nearby lymph nodes in the pelvis or groin (inguinal) area (N1) but not distant sites (M0)
	T3 N0 M0	III	The cancer is growing into the pelvic wall, and/or growing into the lower one-third of the vagina and/or has blocked the flow of urine (hydronephrosis), which is causing kidney problems (T3). It has not spread to nearby lymph nodes (N0) or to distant sites (M0)
IVA	T4 any N M0	IVA	The cancer is growing into the bladder or rectum or is growing out of the pelvis (T4). It might or might not have spread to lymph nodes in the pelvis or groin (inguinal area) (any N). It has not spread to distant sites (M0)
IVB	Any T any N M1	IVB	The cancer has spread to distant organs such as the lungs or bones (M1). It can be any size and might or might not have grown into nearby structures or organs (Any T). It might or might not have spread to nearby lymph nodes (any N)

(AJCC: American Joint Committee on Cancer; FIGO: International Federation of Gynaecology and Obstetrics)

Table 1 describes the various staging systems for vaginal cancer.

Staging and Role of Imaging Techniques in Diagnosis, Staging and Treatment

Vaginal cancer is currently staged clinically, as is cervical cancer. Modern imaging techniques such as computed tomography (CT), magnetic resonance imaging (MRI) and positron emission tomography (PET) are encouraged to guide management; however, these tests should not be used to change the initial clinical staging. In this regard, the FIGO Gynaecologic Oncology Committee recommends that, wherever available, imaging should be used to better define tumour volume and extension of disease. The Committee also encourages the registering of imaging findings and their influence on therapeutic decisions as a complement to the assigned clinical FIGO stage. This will allow further analyses that could change the current staging system.

Magnetic resonance imaging: As extrapolated from cervical cancer, MRI is more sensitive in detecting tumour size, as well as paravaginal or parametrial involvement. In primary vaginal tumours, clinical assessment may be difficult and MRI may be a useful tool in individual cases owing to its superior soft tissue resolution.

PET-CT: As in cervical cancer, the use of PET-CT in primary vaginal cancer has been found to be superior compared with other imaging modalities for detecting nodal disease. It is also useful in detecting recurrent disease.

Evaluation and Treatment

The treatment of carcinoma of the vagina depends primarily on histology, tumour volume, anatomical localisation of the lesion, stage of the disease and age of the patient. Adversely, owing to anatomical localisation, both reproductive potential (young women) and sexual function (any age) can be affected. Different modalities of treatment can be offered to patients affected by this disease, including surgery, radiotherapy, chemotherapy or a combination of some or all of the above.

Surgery: The role of surgery is limited in primary vaginal cancer since the primary tumour is in close proximity to the bladder, urethra and rectum. In general, primary treatment with surgery is limited to early and small lesions confined to the vaginal mucosa (<2 cm). There are no RCTs, and most of the literature is retrospective in nature. There may be a role for surgical treatment in certain additional situations beyond early disease, as listed here.

- *Surgical management of stage I disease (early disease):*
  - Upper vaginal disease:
    - The tumour is limited to the mucosa in stage I disease.
    - If the uterus is in situ, radical hysterectomy, vaginectomy aiming for 1 cm disease-free margins, and pelvic lymphadenopathy should be offered. If the uterus has been removed, radical vaginectomy as above, with pelvic lymphadenopathy, can be performed.
  - Lower vaginal disease:
    - Radical wide local excision with 1 cm margins can be offered, in addition to bilateral groin node dissection.
- *Ovarian transposition during surgery and preradiation:* In young women with vaginal cancer requiring radiation as primary treatment, ovarian transposition can be offered prior to definitive radiation treatment in an effort to prevent the adverse effects of radiation-induced menopause. In selected cases, laparoscopic or extraperitoneal removal of bulky lymph nodes can be offered as part of staging and treatment planning.
- *Central recurrence after radiation treatment:* Pelvic exenteration is a possibility if the recurrence is central and isolated. These patients require extensive counselling regarding the risks and morbidity of surgery, as well as the impact on quality of life and body image.
- *Palliative management of recurrent or advanced disease*: In women with advanced (Stage IV disease) or recurrent disease who present with vesicovaginal or rectovaginal fistula, a palliative urinary diversion or colostomy can be offered to improve quality of life before definitive management with radiation treatment.

Radiation: In the majority of cases and especially in advanced stages, radiation constitutes the cornerstone of treatment for this disease. This is a combination of external beam radiation (EBRT) and intracavitary radiotherapy or brachytherapy (ICRT). The principal advantage of radiation is organ preservation. As in other pelvic malignancies, MRI has become an essential component for properly defining tumour volume and the spatial relationship of the tumour with neighbouring organs during treatment planning. EBRT to the pelvis includes the external iliac and obturator nodes as per standard of care. In addition, the inguinal nodes may be included if the tumour is in the distal vagina. Brachytherapy is used to deliver a boost of high-dose radiation to the residual tumour, and the use of brachytherapy is associated with longer overall survival. Image-guided or adaptive brachytherapy with CT or MRI offers the potential to give higher doses of radiation to the residual tumour and decrease radiation dose to surrounding healthy organs. The optimal or lower threshold dose is 70 Gy, which has been shown to improve outcomes. Doses higher than 70 Gy result in significant grade three and four toxicities. Intensity modulated radiation therapy (IMRT) is an advanced form of radiation that allows for higher dosages of radiation to be delivered to the cancer. Although studies in vaginal cancer are limited, this form of radiation may allow improved dosages to the cancer, with fewer adverse effects because dose to the adjacent structures is limited.

Concurrent chemotherapy with radiation: Modern management of vaginal cancer often combines concurrent chemotherapy such as cisplatin or 5-FU. This has been extrapolated from the successful outcomes of this treatment with cervical cancer. However, most studies using chemoradiation in vaginal cancer are limited owing to the small numbers of cases and lack of comparison to radiation on its own. Chemoradiation may be considered in the treatment of vaginal cancer following a 2013 retrospective review, suggesting a potential improvement in overall and disease-free survival. Although this was a small review (71 patients), it showed a significant difference between both overall survival and disease-free survival when comparing women who received radiation alone versus chemoradiation as primary treatment (3-year overall survival of 56% versus 79% and 3-year disease-free survival of 43% versus 73%). The combination of EBRT and brachytherapy to a total dose of 70–80 Gy with concomitant weekly cisplatin-based chemotherapy is the current standard of care for locally advanced vaginal cancer.

Treatment

Invasive carcinoma: Patients should all be referred to referral units, because of the limited experience with these lesions. All treatment must be individualised, and will vary depending on the stage of disease and the site of vaginal involvement.

Adenocarcinoma

A vaginal adenocarcinoma can arise in relics of the Wolffian duct and then has the histological features of a clear cell adenocarcinoma. It is extremely rare and, when it does occur, forms a tumour deep to the lateral vaginal wall—the position of the tissue of origin. The clinical features and management are as for squamous cell carcinoma.

Adenocarcinoma can also be of Müllerian duct origin, arising possibly in misplaced cervical glands, but more likely as a result of metaplasia or as a consequence of the potential for Müllerian duct tissue to differentiate in different ways.

A special form of this type of adenocarcinoma has appeared in the last three decades and, because of its histological features, is designated the clear cell adenocarcinoma. The large, clear cells contain glycogen, the nuclei have a hobnail appearance, and the malignant cells are arranged in clumps and in tubules, suggestive of renal carcinoma. The tumour is not a mesonephroma or of Wolffian duct origin, because it usually arises high on the anterior vaginal wall, and it is very superficial, often polypoidal.

This condition is found in girls <25 years of age, mostly in their early teens, and in 80% of cases, there is a history of exposure in utero to oestrogens which were administered to their mothers before the 18th week of pregnancy. The oestrogens have all been of the synthetic nonsteroidal type, mostly diethylstilboestrol. In 80% of cases there is associated vaginal adenosis and the lesions, benign or malignant, are often multiple (refer to Chapter 13: Malformations and Maldevelopments of the Genital Tract and Chapter 26: Epithelial Abnormalities of the Genital Tract). There is also usually cervical ectopy. Another common associate, indicative of interference with Müllerian duct development, is congenital transverse ridging and stricture of the upper vagina.

It is reckoned that <1 in every 1,000 girls exposed to the oestrogen influence in utero develops a clear cell adenocarcinoma of the vagina or cervix.

Clear cell adenocarcinoma of the vagina may be symptomless but, if the surface is ulcerated, the girl complains of bleeding and discharge. Vaginal cytology gives negative findings in 20% of cases.

Bearing in mind the young age of the patient and the superficial site of the growth, local excision followed by measures described for vaginal adenosis is often the best treatment. However, for multiple lesions, vaginectomy and even more radical procedures have been carried out. Most are located in the upper vagina and are treated as cervical lesions. Radiotherapy by itself gives poor results. Those for surgery alone cannot yet be assessed, although 20% of patients are known to die within 2–3 years of operation. In many cases, combinations of radiotherapy and radical surgery have been used.

Melanoma

The origin of the melanoma is disputed. Some consider that a vaginal tumour of this type is always secondary to a lesion elsewhere. Others postulate a primary development as a result of metaplasia or misplacement of mesodermal and epithelial tissues **(Fig. 14)**.

Melanoma of the vagina is rare and carries a poor prognosis (5-year survival rate 7%), depending on the depth of the epithelial invasion. Its clinical features and treatment are similar to those of squamous cell carcinoma of the vagina; however, treatment is ineffective if it is deeply invasive as it metastasises early through the bloodstream. It does not respond to chemotherapy.

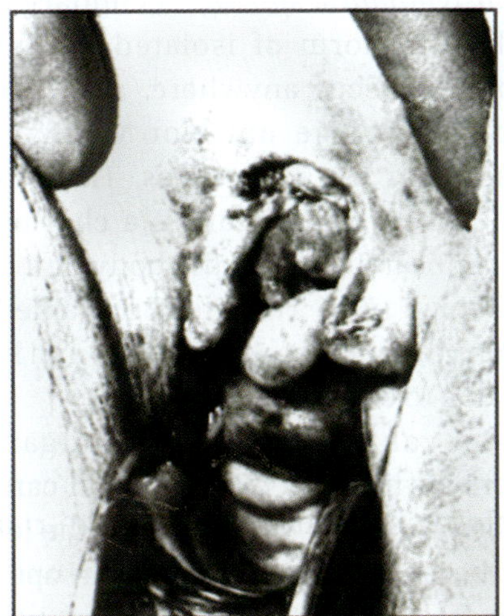

Fig. 14: Multiple melanomas of the anterior wall of the vagina in a woman aged 79 years. The lymph nodes in both groins were involved, but no evidence of an extragenital primary was found. Only palliative treatment was possible.

Sarcoma

Sarcoma botryoides is a highly malignant tumour of the rhabdomyoblasts. These neoplasms are found in infants and children and usually present with discharge, bleeding or a visible mass at the introitus.

In the past, exenterative surgery was used for these lesions, but survival was poor. More recently, conservative surgery has been used in conjunction with preoperative or postoperative chemotherapy and radiotherapy, with significantly improved survival. Most reported chemotherapeutic experience has been with vincristine, actinomycin D and cyclophosphamide (VAC).

If the lesion is small and can be resected with organ preservation, surgery should be the initial approach. For bulkier lesions, preoperative chemotherapy or radiotherapy should be given.

Extended radiotherapy fields are not recommended as they may produce significant developmental problems with the bony pelvis by destroying or interfering with growth centres in these structures.

Secondary

Malignant disease of the vagina is usually secondary to a primary growth elsewhere. The mechanisms of spread are as follows:

- *Direct extension:* This occurs from the cervix, vulva, urethra, bladder, rectum and occasionally from malignant deposits in the pouch of Douglas, which invade the posterior fornix.
- *Blood and lymphatic spread:* Secondary carcinoma often takes the form of isolated nodules which, although they occur anywhere, are nearly always disposed low in the anterior vaginal wall, i.e. suburethrally or in the fornices. This is especially noticeable when the primary is a choriocarcinoma and an adenocarcinoma of the body of the uterus or of the fallopian tube. The site is explained by direct connections through the azygos veins and lymphatics; spread is due to embolism.

Metastases can arise from any organ. Vaginal metastases are particularly likely in renal carcinoma; in such cases the primary is more often in the left than the right kidney, because the left ovarian vein opens into the left renal vein.

- *Seeding:* Carcinoma secondary to growth in the body of the uterus, occurring after hysterectomy, is occasionally caused by detached fragments of growth becoming implanted into the vaginal vault or elsewhere **(Fig. 15)**.

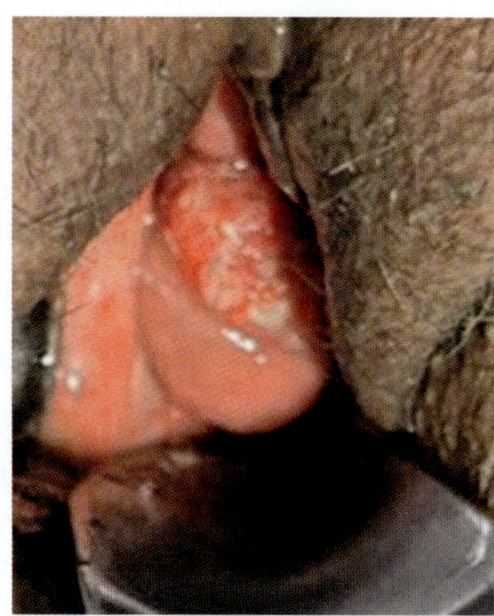

Fig. 15: Vaginal growth punch biopsy in a 77-year-old multiparous woman with postmenopausal bleeding had outside report of HSIL, invasion cannot be ruled out. Cervix appeared healthy. Repeat biopsy of the vaginal growth on the lower half of vagina for confirmation showed histopathological examination (HPE) of an invasive tumour, arranged in nests, trabeculae and islands composed of malignant squamous cells showing enlarged pleomorphic vesicular nuclei, prominent nucleoli, irregular nuclear contour, vesicular chromatin, moderate eosinophilic cytoplasm and brisk mitotic figures (19–20/10 HPF) along with few areas of dyskeratosis, surrounded by desmoplastic stroma, containing lymphocytic and few neutrophilic infiltrate and blood vessels. Immunohistochemistry (IHC) and immunofluorescence (IF) for HMB-45 were negative. Moderately differentiated squamous cell carcinoma.
Source: Department of Obstetrics and Gynecology, Kasturba Medical College, Manipal, MAHE, Karnataka.

SUGGESTED READING

1. Adams TS, Rogers LJ, Cuello MA. Cancer of the vagina: 2021 update. Int J Gynecol Obstet. 2021;155:19-27.
2. Ballon SC, Roberts JA, Lagasse LD. Topical 5-fluorouracil in the treatment of intraepithelial neoplasia of the vagina. Obstet Gynecol. 1979;54:163-6.
3. Bansal M, Austin RM, Zhao C. Correlation of histopathologic follow-up findings with vaginal human papillomavirus and low-grade squamous intraepithelial lesion Papanicolaou test results. Arch Pathol Lab Med. 2011;135:1545-9.
4. Bipat S, Glas AS, van der Velden J, Zwinderman AH, Bossuyt PM, Stoker J. Computed tomography and magnetic resonance imaging in staging of uterine cervical carcinoma: a systematic review. Gynecol Oncol. 2003;91:59-66.
5. Boonlikit S, Noinual N. Vaginal intraepithelial neoplasia: a retrospective analysis of clinical features and colpohistology. J Obstet Gynaecol Res. 2010;36:94-100.
6. Campagnutta E, Parin A, De Piero G, Giorda G, Gallo A, Scarabelli C. Treatment of vaginal intraepithelial neoplasia (VAIN) with the carbon dioxide laser. Clin Exp Obstet Gynecol. 1999;26:127-30.

7. Cardenes HR, Schilder JM, Roth LM. Vagina. In: Barakat RR, Markman M, Randall ME, (Eds). Principles and Practice of Gynecologic Oncology. Philadelphia: Lippincott Williams & Wilkins; 2009: pp. 591-622.
8. Dodge JA, Eltabbakh GH, Mount SL, Walker RP, Morgan A. Clinical features and risk of recurrence among patients with vaginal intraepithelial neoplasia. Gynecol Oncol. 2001;83:363-9.
9. Farghaly H, Bourgeois D, Houser PM, Padmanabhan V, Lage JM, Hoda RS. Routine vaginal Pap test is not useful in women status-post hysterectomy for benign disease. Diagn Cytopathol. 2006;34:640-3.
10. Gardner CS, Sunil J, Klopp AH, Devine CE, Sagebiel T, Viswanathan C, et al. Primary vaginal cancer: role of MRI in diagnosis, staging and treatment. Br J Radiol. 2015;88:20150033.
11. Garland SM, Paavonen J, Jaisamrarn U, Naud P, Salmerón J, Chow SN, et al. Prior human papillomavirus-16/18 AS04-adjuvanted vaccination prevents recurrent high grade cervical intraepithelial neoplasia after definitive surgical therapy: Post-hoc analysis from a randomized controlled trial. Int J Cancer. 2016;139:2812-26.
12. Hampl M, Sarajuuri H, Wentzensen N, Bender HG, Kueppers V. Effect of human papillomavirus vaccines on vulvar, vaginal, and anal intraepithelial lesions and vulvar cancer. Obstet Gynecol. 2006;108:1361-8.
13. Hodeib M, Cohen JG, Mehta S, Rimel BJ, Walsh CS, Li AJ, et al. Recurrence and risk of progression to lower genital tract malignancy in women with high grade VAIN. Gynecol Oncol. 2016;141:507-10.
14. Hricak H, Gatsonis C, Chi DS, Amendola MA, Brandt K, Schwartz LH, et al. Role of imaging in pretreatment evaluation of early invasive cervical cancer: results of the intergroup study American College of Radiology Imaging Network 6651-Gynecologic Oncology Group 183. J Clin Oncol. 2005;23:9329-37.
15. Hui Y, Hansen K, Murthy J, Chau D, Sung CJ, Quddus MR. Relevance of the Pap test: a report of HPV-DNA test-negative high-grade squamous intraepithelial lesions of the female lower genital tract. Acta Cytol. 2016;60:445-50.
16. Kim MK, Lee IH, Lee KH. Clinical outcomes and risk of recurrence among patients with vaginal intraepithelial neoplasia: a comprehensive analysis of 576 cases. J Gynecol Oncol. 2018;29:e6.
17. Krebs HB. Treatment of vaginal intraepithelial neoplasia with laser and topical 5-fluorouracil. Obstet Gynecol. 1989;73:657-60.
18. Lamoreaux WT, Grigsby PW, Dehdashti F, Zoberi I, Powell MA, Gibb RK, et al. FDG-PET evaluation of vaginal carcinoma. Int J Radiat Oncol Biol Phys. 2005;62:733-7.
19. Lamos C, Mihaljevic C, Aulmann S, Bruckner T, Domschke C, Wallwiener M, et al. Detection of human papillomavirusinfection in patients with vaginal intraepithelial neoplasia. PLoS One. 2016;11(2):e0167386.
20. Patibandla JR, Fehniger JE, Levine DA, Jelinic P. Small cell cancers of the female genital tract: Molecular and clinical aspects. Gynecol Oncol. 2018;149(2):420-7.
21. Perrotta M, Marchitelli CE, Velazco AF, Tauscher P, Lopez G, Perematеu MS. Use of CO2 laser vaporization for the treatment of high-grade vaginal intraepithelial neoplasia. J Low Genit Tract Dis. 2013;17:23-7.
22. Rajaram S, Maheshwari A, Srivastava A. Staging for vaginal cancer. Best Pract Res Clin Obstet Gynaecol. 2015;29: 822-32.
23. Rapi V, Dogan A, Schultheis B. Melanoma of the vagina: case report and systematic review of the literature. Anticancer Res. 2017;37(12):6911-20.
24. Reich O, Regauer S, Marth C, Schmidt D, Horn LC, Dannecker C, et al. Precancerous lesions of the cervix, vulva and vagina according to the 2014 WHO classification of tumors of the female genital tract. Geburtshilfe Frauenheilkd. 2015;75:1018-20.
25. Rome RM, England PG. Management of vaginal intraepithelial neoplasia: a series of 132 cases with long-term follow-up. Int J Gynecol Cancer. 2000;10:382-90.
26. Scott K, Trainor J, McVeigh G. Human papillomavirus (HPV)-associated lymphoepithelioma-like carcinoma of the vagina and anal canal: a rare variant of squamous cell carcinoma. Int J Gynecol Pathol. 2017;18.
27. Serrano B, de Sanjosé S, Tous S, Quiros B, Muñoz N, Bosch X, et al. Human papillomavirus genotype attribution for HPVs 6, 11, 16, 18, 31, 33, 45, 52 and 58 in female anogenital lesions. Eur J Cancer. 2015;51:1732-41.
28. Sherman JF, Mount SL, Evans MF, Skelly J, Simmons-Arnold L, Eltabbakh GH. Smoking increases the risk of high-grade intraepithelial neoplasia in women with oncogenic human papillomavirus. Gynecol Oncol. 2008;110:396-401.
29. Tainio K, Jakobsson M, Louvanto K, Kalliala I, Paavonen J, Nieminen P, et al. Randomised trial on treatment of vaginal intraepithelial neoplasia-Imiquimod, laser vaporisation and expectant management. Int J Cancer. 2016;139:2353-8.
30. Tranoulis A, Laios A, Mitsopoulos V, Lutchman-Singh K, Thomakos N. Efficacy of 5% imiquimod for the treatment of vaginal intraepithelial neoplasia-a systematic review of the literature and a meta-analysis. Eur J Obstet Gynecol Reprod Biol. 2017;218:129-36.
31. Videlefsky A, Grossl N, Denniston M, Sehgal R, Lane JM, Goodenough G. Routine vaginal cuff smear testing in post-hysterectomy patients with benign uterine conditions: when is it indicated? J Am Board Fam Pract. 2000;13:233-8.

30

CHAPTER

Tumours of the Cervix Uteri

Priya Ganeshkumar

Chapter Outline

- Benign Neoplasms of the Cervix
- Benign Tumours of the Cervix
- Carcinoma of the Cervix
- Screening for Cervical Cancer
- Other Malignant Tumours of the Cervix

BENIGN NEOPLASMS OF THE CERVIX

The causes of benign changes of the cervix are:

- Cervical mucous polyp
- Nabothian cyst
- Cervical fibroid
- Condyloma
- Tuberculosis

The causes of malignant neoplasms of the cervix are:

- Squamous cell carcinoma and adenocarcinoma
- Adenosquamous carcinoma
- Neuroendocrine tumours
- Others—melanoma and metastases

BENIGN TUMOURS OF THE CERVIX

Cysts of Embryonic Tissues

Wolffian duct cysts similar to those in the vagina are found in the sides of the cervix. Cervical cysts can also arise from diverticula of the Müllerian duct. Sometimes, they represent the rudimentary and incompletely canalised cervix of a bicornuate uterus **(Fig. 1)**.

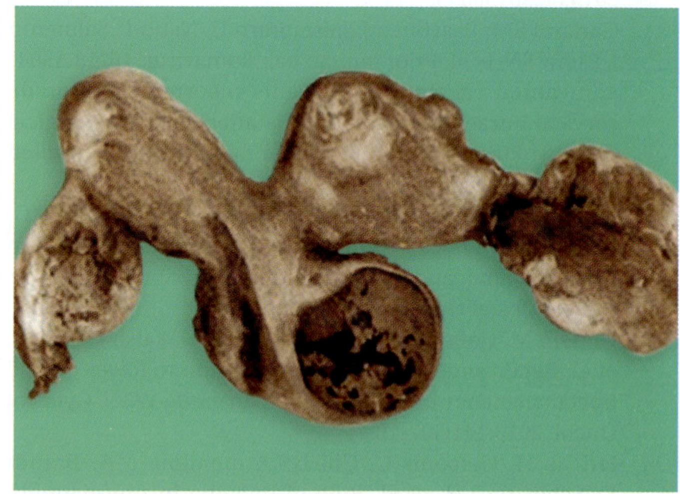

Fig. 1: A bicornuate uterus with a large blood cyst in the cervix and a haematosalpinx on the same side. There appears to be only one cervix, but the collection of blood possibly represents retention of menstrual discharge in a second, imperforate cervix.

Cervical Polyp

Cervical mucous polyps are the most common benign tumours of the cervix **(Fig. 2)**. They arise from endocervical canal and rarely become symptomatic. In case of a big polyp, women may present with pain in lower abdomen, dyspareunia, contact bleeding, etc. Treatment is polypectomy. Rarely polyps turn into malignancy and require management in the line of invasive cancer.

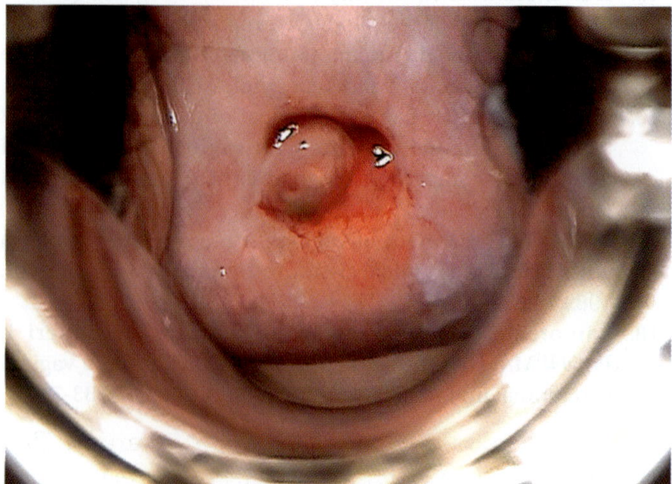

Fig. 2: Cervical mucous polyp.

Nabothian Follicles or Cysts

Nabothian cysts often develop on the surface of the cervix **(Fig. 3)**. The mucus-producing endocervical cells

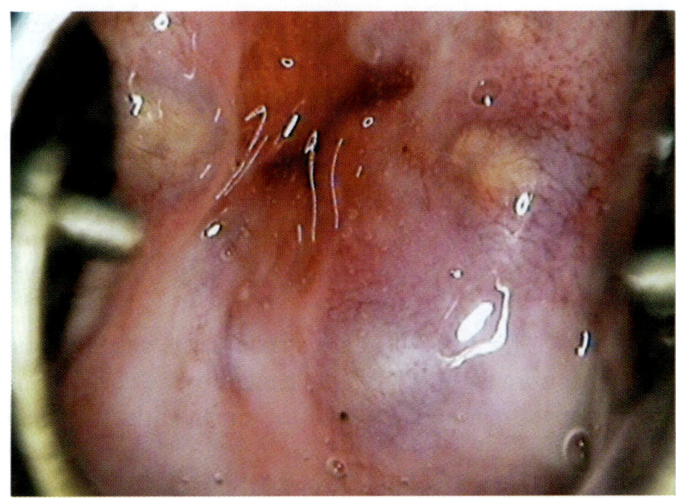

Fig. 3: Multiple nabothian cysts of the cervix.

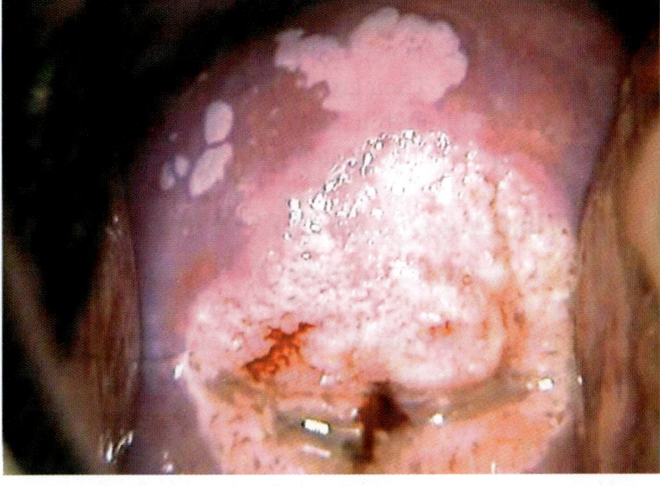

Fig. 4: Multiple condylomas of cervix.

sometimes get trapped during the squamous metaplastic changes occurring on the ectocervix which extends inside the endocervix. The cyst is lined by columnar epithelium and is usually of a few millimetres in size. Rarely due to chronic retention of mucus, the size increases and makes pelvic examination difficult. The condition is benign and almost never requires treatment. In case of large cysts, one can drain the cyst by simple cauterisation, puncture of the cyst wall or marsupialisation.

Condyloma/Papilloma

Condylomas are sometimes found on the ectocervix **(Fig. 4)**. Condylomas are strongly associated with non-oncogenic human papillomavirus (HPV) type 6 and type 11 infection and are usually asymptomatic. Size of the lesion varies widely from flat condylomas/benign papillomas to large condyloma accuminata causing obstruction in vaginal birth. In majority of cases, they rarely require treatment as the infection gets cleared on its own. Biopsy and if required removal of the condylomatous/papillomatous growth is suggested as the condylomas may be associated with low-grade squamous intra-epithelial lesions (LSILs) of cervix.

Leiomyoma

Cervix leiomyomas are smooth, benign neoplasms seen as interstitial or submucous (polypoidal) variety. They usually coexists with multiple myomas arising in the upper part of the uterus **(Fig. 5)**.

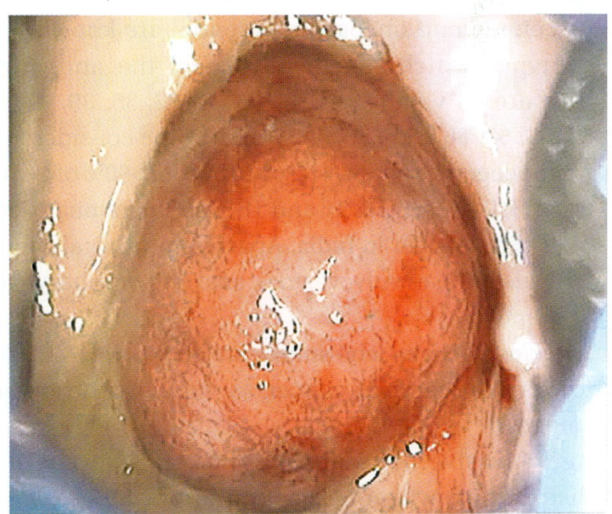

Fig. 5: Cervical leiomyoma.
Courtesy: Dr Priya Ganeshkumar.

Clinical Features

Cervix myomas are rare. Cervix myomas become symptomatic when size of the tumour increases causing lower abdominal pain; bleeding per vagina; urinary symptoms such as frequency, urgency and retention of urine and bowel disturbances.

Treatment

Treatment is usually medical or surgical with myomectomy or hysterectomy according to the age and desire of fertility.

Angioma and Allied Tumours

Haemangiomas of the cervix are seen as small superficial lesions but are rare. Their growth is said to be encouraged by pregnancy. Although usually asymptomatic, they can cause irregular bleeding, postcoital bleeding.

CARCINOMA OF THE CERVIX

Carcinoma of the cervix is the most common genital malignancy in females. It is one of the leading causes of cancer mortality in India, accounting for 17% of all cancer deaths among women aged between 30 and 69 years.

Aetiology

- *Human papillomavirus infection*: It is the most important risk factor for cervical cancer. At least 100 subtypes of HPV with distinguished variations in its genetic and oncogenic potential are known. The subtypes which specifically affect the anogenital tract are HPV subtypes 16, 18, 31, 33, 35, 39, 45, 51, 52, 56, 58, 66 and 69. HPV 6 and 11 are considered as nononcogenic subtypes responsible for >90% of genital warts. HPV serotypes 16 and 18 account for nearly 80% of cervical cancer in India. Apart from cervical cancer, HPV also causes vulvovaginal, anal and oropharyngeal cancers.
- *Smoking:* Women who smoke are about twice as likely to develop cervical cancer as women who do not smoke.
- *Age:* Invasive cervical cancer has a binomial age distribution with one peak at about 35 years and another at about 60 years, following which there is a reduced incidence.
- *Immune system deficiency:* Women with lowered immune systems have a higher risk of developing cervical cancer. A lowered immune system can be caused by immune suppression from corticosteroid medications, organ transplantation, treatments for other types of cancer or the human immunodeficiency virus (HIV), which is the virus that causes acquired immunodeficiency syndrome (AIDS). When a woman has HIV, her immune system is less able to fight off early cancer.
- *Socioeconomic factors:* Cervical cancer is more common among groups of women who are less likely to have access to screening for cervical cancer. Those populations are more likely to include Black women, Hispanic women and American Indian women. Detailed studies have revealed that low standards of hygiene (including penile hygiene), coitus or marriage at an early age, frequency of sexual intercourse and promiscuity of both partners are associated with high incidence of cervical cancer. Men in jobs which require frequent travel and those whose first wives died of cancer of the cervix constitute a group termed as *high-risk males.*
- *Coitus:* The sexually active woman is two to four times more likely to develop cancer of the cervix than the sexually inactive woman. Cancer of the cervix is almost unknown in groups of nuns, whereas cancer of the corpus occurs as frequently in these as in any other section of the population. Indeed, the practice of coitus is now established as being a prime cause of cervical malignant disease, intraepithelial or invasive. Earlier the age of first intercourse, more the partners and more promiscuous the partners, greater the risk. The incidence of positive cervical smears amongst girls and women attending special [sexually transmitted disease (STD), genitourinary medicine] clinics is two or three times higher than that for all women of similar age.

  Persistence of high-risk HPV is primarily the main cause of cervical cancer and precancerous lesions. It has been observed that HPV infection is a very common infection with at least 50% of sexually active people will become HPV positive. HPV usually regresses after 1 year, but on two consecutive smears of 6-month interval, the person is HPV positive with the same stain, then it is called persistent infection. This persistent HPV infection causes certain dysplastic changes in the squamous metaplastic cells, which are the dividing cells. HPV, being an epitheliotropic virus, requires dividing cells to survive and further progress to high copy numbers creating precancerous lesions, condylomas and sometimes cancers.
- *Multiparity:* About 95% of invasive cancers occur in multiparae; but 70–80% of mature women are parous. Any association with the bearing of children, or the bearing of many children, is not accounted for by cervical injury or infection during labour but by the sexual intercourse, which results in the pregnancies. High parity usually means frequent coitus during many years, starting at a young age, and is often associated with poor socioeconomic conditions.

- *Cervical irritation and infection:* Cervical trauma, chronic cervicitis and ectopy are no longer considered as aetiological factors in cervical intraepithelial neoplasia (CIN) or invasive cancer. It has now been established that mixed sexually transmitted infections (STIs) such as chlamydia, gonorrhoea and herpes simplex virus (type 2) along with HPV are greater risk factors for precancerous and cancer lesions. The main factor associated with the presence of coinfections is the chronic inflammation caused by these microorganisms.

  This can act as a promoter of carcinogenesis inducing the occurrence of significant cellular and molecular changes.

  The proliferation, recruitment of inflammatory cells and increased production of reactive oxygen species (ROS) during the inflammatory process can lead to damage and inhibition of DNA repair.

  These changes induced make the cervical epithelium more susceptible to mutations by activating oncogenes, inactivating tumour suppressor proteins and, thus, facilitating the action of HPV in the induction of tumour lesions.
- *Oral contraceptive pills (OCPs):* While excessive and unbalanced oestrogen stimulation favours the development of cancer of the cervix in certain lower animals, this is not established for women. Indeed, the disease occurs commonly after ovarian activity has ceased—even after surgical removal of both ovaries.

  Some research studies suggest that oral contraceptives may be associated with an increase in the risk of cervical cancer due to the association of ectopy with OCPs. Columnar epithelium which is a single-layered epithelium is highly prone to trauma and HPV infection.
- *CIN:* Most CIN spontaneously regresses. Left untreated, >90% of CIN 1 lesions and 50% of CIN 2 lesions regress within 2 years without any treatment. Progression to invasive cancer occurs in 10–12% cases of CIN 3; hence, CIN 3 is considered as true precursor of invasive cancer.
- *Diethylstilboestrol (DES) exposure:* Women whose mothers were given this drug during pregnancy to prevent miscarriage have an increased risk of developing a rare type of cancer of the cervix or vagina. DES was given for this purpose from about 1940 to 1970. Clear cell adenocarcinoma may be associated with exposure to DES.

Histological Classification

Cancer of the cervix can be broadly divided into two histological variants: (1) Cancer arising from epithelial component and (2) cancer arising from squamocolumnar junction. The nonepithelial part arises from the mesenchymal or germ cell component of the cervix **(Table 1)**.

Cancer nearly always starts at the squamocolumnar epithelial junction and in 80–90% of cases, it is of squamous cell type. In about 5–10% of cases, it is entirely columnar cell in pattern (adenocarcinoma). The predominance of squamous cell tumours in older women and the occurrence of mixed patterns is rather in keeping with the idea that most cancers arise in reserve cells.

Squamous Cell Carcinoma

Squamous cell carcinoma usually starts in the area of the squamocolumnar junction (transformation zone) as described earlier. Occasionally, however, it arises in the endocervix, sometimes deep to the lining. Even if not all squamous cell growths begin in reserve cells, those developing in the endocervix almost certainly do.

Some invasive cancers of the cervix are hypertrophic or exophytic, producing a cauliflower-like mass; others are mainly eroding and ulcerative or infiltrative **(Figs. 6 and 7)**. An early growth can simulate erosion.

About 20% of the tumours are of the well-differentiated type (often known as 'large cell keratinising tumours'). Moderately differentiated tumours (large cell nonkeratinising tumours) constitute about 60% of the total. The remaining 20% are poorly differentiated (small cell nonkeratinising tumours). However, biopsies taken from different areas of the same tumour often show different degrees of differentiation and different predominant cell types.

Two distinctive histological variants of cervical squamous cell carcinoma merit mention; some, usually of the well-differentiated type, have cells which contain abundant glycogen and, thus, appear as 'clear' cells, whilst, occasionally, poorly differentiated tumours assume a spindle-shaped cell form and so resemble a sarcoma.

World Health Organization 2020 classification of squamous cell carcinoma:

- Squamous cell carcinoma—HPV associated
- Squamous cell carcinoma—HPV independent
- Squamous cell carcinoma not otherwise specified (NOS).

TABLE 1: Histological classification of invasive cancer of the cervix.

Epithelial tumour				
Nonglandular	***Glandular***	***Other, including mixed***	***Nonepithelial tumour***	***Miscellaneous***
Squamous cell cancer	Adenocarcinoma	Adenosquamous	Carcinosarcoma	Melanoma
Verrucous carcinoma	Mucinous adenocarcinoma	Glassy cell carcinoma	Leiomyosarcoma	Lymphoma
Papillary squamous	Endometroid adenocarcinoma	Mucoepidermoid	Embryonal rhabdomyosarcoma	Primitive neuroectodermal tumour
Sarcomatoid	Villoglandular adenocarcinoma	Adenoid cystic	Nongestational choriocarcinoma	
	Adenoma malignum	Adenoid basal	Mature teratoma	
	Clear cell adenocarcinoma	Small cell carcinoma	Yolk sac tumour	
		Classical carcinoid		
		Gestational choriocarcinoma		

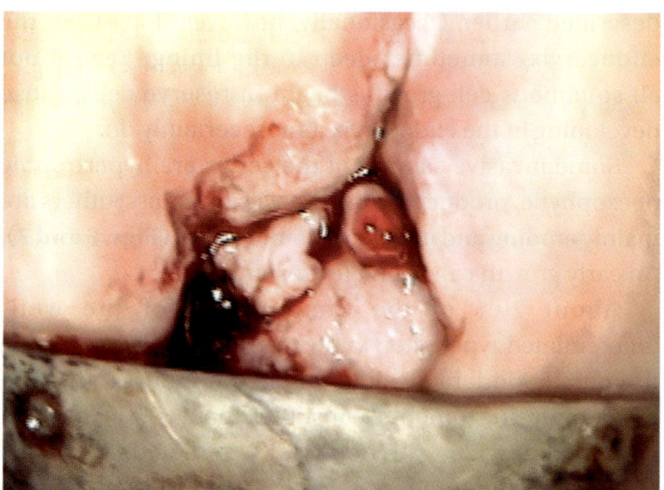

Fig. 6: An early invasive cancer of the cervix.

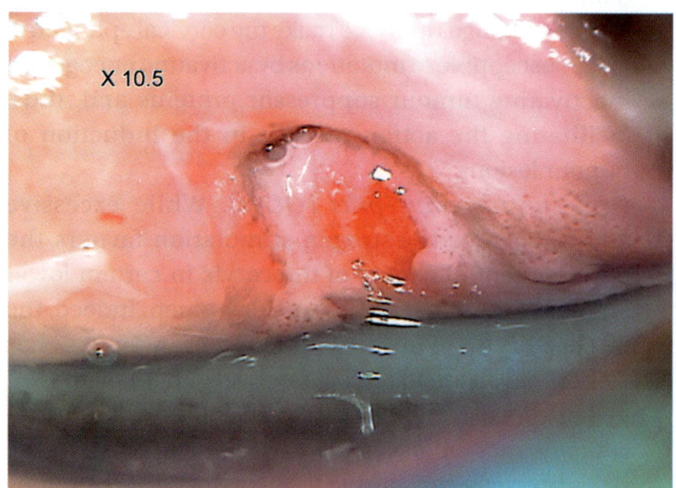

Fig. 7: Microinvasive cancer of the cervix.

Adenocarcinoma

Adenocarcinoma usually arises in the endocervix suggesting that its origin may be the columnar cells normally found there. It is usually ulcerative and infiltrative, leading to a hard, indurated, barrel-shaped cervix **(Fig. 8)**. The histological appearances vary. The cells are essentially columnar in shape; they may contain mucin and form acini. Anaplasia is common, and it is sometimes difficult to distinguish a columnar from an undifferentiated squamous cell cancer. However, if mucin stains, electron microscopy and other methods are used; the correct diagnosis can usually be made or the tumour is classed as undifferentiated.

In some cases, a cancer arising low in the corpus or the isthmus is mistaken for, or is indistinguishable from, a primary cervical lesion.

A few adenocarcinomas of the cervix arise from the Wolffian duct, and these are sometimes described as mesonephromas. Endometriotic carcinomas have the best and glassy cell carcinomas the worst prognosis among the variants of adenocarcinoma.

World Health Organisation 2020 classification of adeno-carcinoma:

- HPV-associated cervical adenocarcinoma
- HPV-independent cervical adenocarcinoma
- Gastric type

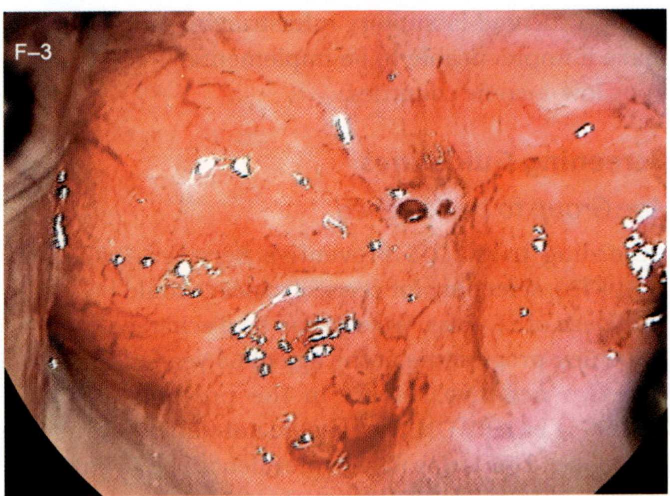

Fig. 8: Adenocarcinoma of the cervix.

- Mesonephric type
- Clear cell type
- Other adenocarcinoma

Spread

- *Direct extension*: By this mechanism, the growth spreads to the body of the uterus, the vaginal wall, the bladder and the cellular tissues of the broad and uterosacral ligaments.
  Direct invasion of the rectum is rare, because the pouch of Douglas intervenes. In the broad ligament, the growth surrounds and constricts the lower ends of the ureters, but does not invade them. Similarly, when it reaches the pelvic wall and the sacral plexus, it causes sciatic pain, but the nerves and their sheaths are never demonstrably penetrated.
- *Lymphatic permeation and embolism*: Spread by the lymphatics in the bases of the broad ligaments and in the uterosacral ligaments is an early feature, the nodes most commonly involved being the obturator, external iliac and those at the bifurcation of the common iliac vessels. Others are the internal iliac, common iliac, sacral and ultimately the para-aortic nodes.
- *Bloodstream*: This route is much less frequently used, but embolic metastases are occasionally seen in the ovary, brain, bones and lungs. The occurrence of distant metastases without simultaneous involvement of the lungs is explained by the transfer of cancer cells by the vertebral venous plexus.

Symptoms

In its very early stage, invasive carcinoma of the cervix causes no symptoms and is only discovered on per speculum examination or as a result of positive screening tests. Symptoms come with either surface ulceration or an increased size of the growth and consist only of irregular uterine bleeding or discharge or both, these being peri- or postmenopausal in half the cases. The first episode of bleeding commonly follows coitus, straining at stool or any circumstance, which exposes the cervix to trauma and may be slight. Later, the losses can be alarmingly heavy. The discharge is at first creamy or white but subsequently resembles dirty brown water; it has a particularly offensive and characteristic odour. The odour is caused by an infection of necrotic tissue with saprophytes.

Any other symptoms usually occur so late that they are to be regarded as evidence of advanced (late-stage) cancer. They include frequency of micturition, dysuria, urinary incontinence, rectal pain, deep pelvic ache, low backache, sciatica, ureteric colic, oedema of the legs, loss of weight, anorexia and malaise. Liver metastases may present as right upper quadrant pain and fullness; lung metastases as haemoptysis and a persistent cough; supraclavicular lymph node metastasis as neck swelling and pain.

A remarkable feature of carcinoma of the cervix is that most of those who suffer from it do not present early for treatment, despite propaganda and health education. This is partly explained by the fact that the irregular bleeding or discharge is dismissed as being insignificant. Even those women who report symptoms immediately do not necessarily have the consolation of knowing that their growth is amenable to treatment because the duration of symptoms is not proportional to the extent of the disease.

Physical Signs

In the early stages, the cervix may appear normal, eroded or chronically infected. Suggestive signs are hardness, irregularity and bleeding on examination.

When the disease is established, the patient's general state is usually good, but the cervix may be enlarged, misshapen, ulcerated and excavated, completely destroyed or replaced by a hypertrophic mass. The cardinal signs are hardness, visible growth, friability, fixation and bleeding on examination. Whenever cancer is suspected, vaginal examination should be gentle lest it precipitate the most violent haemorrhage. If this should happen, the vagina should be packed tight with gauze, and the woman kept lying flat with the foot of the couch raised.

The diagnosis is difficult if the growth is entirely endocervical. The external os then looks normal, but the cervix as a whole feels big, broad and barrel shaped. Fixation occurs relatively early, but bleeding on examination is not a prominent sign in such cases. In most cases, a rectal examination is more useful in determining the extent of spread within the pelvis.

SCREENING FOR CERVICAL CANCER

India alone accounts for one quarter of the worldwide burden of cervical cancers and yet lacks an organised screening programme in the country. Different screening tests such as Pap smear cytology, visual inspection with acetic acid (VIA) and HPV DNA test are available for early detection of cervical precancers and cancer. Cervical cytology is the most used method of cervical cancer screening in developed countries. Requirement of laboratory infrastructure, trained cytologists and cytotechnicians and considerable financial, technical and logistic inputs make implementation of cytology-based cervical cancer screening programme difficult, especially in low- and middle-income countries such as India. VIA is one of the alternative methods for cervical cancer screening that has been widely investigated. However, the biggest advantage of visual tests is that it can be implemented through primary healthcare workers, it does not require a laboratory infrastructure and the results are obtained immediately following testing, allowing diagnosis and treatment to be instituted during the same visit. Evidence from Indian study suggests that even a single round of VIA is capable of reduction of cervical cancer incidence by 25% and a 35% reduction in mortality over 7 years of follow-up. Indian studies of testing for HPV DNA indicate higher sensitivity and comparable specificity to visual inspection and cytology. However, the requirement of sophisticated laboratory infrastructure and high cost make it impracticable to be implementable in resource-poor, low-income countries.

Screening Guidelines

Age Group to be Screened

According to the US Preventive Services Task Force (USPFTS), screening for cervical cancer should be started at the age of 21 years. Women can be discharged from the screening programme at the age of 65 years if they have had two negative smears in the previous 10 years. Screening by HPV DNA test should not start before the age of 30 years. This is due to high prevalence of HPV infection in age < 30 years. In this group of women, cytology-based screening is recommended.

Frequency of Screening

For cytological tests, it has been seen that higher incidence of women develops cancer if the time from the previous smear is extended beyond 3 years. The World Health Organization (WHO) recommends minimum 5-year interval if HPV DNA test is used as primary screening method. In immunocompromised patients, screening interval is 3 years by HPV DNA test.

Various screening recommendations and approaches for HPV are mentioned in **Flowcharts 1 to 4, Table 2 and Figure 9**.

Management of Abnormal Pap Smear

Management of abnormal Pap smear has been discussed in **Flowchart 5**.

Management of atypical squamous cells of undetermined significance (ASC-US): Management of ASC-US has been discussed in **Flowchart 6**.

Flowchart 1: Screening recommendations according to resource settings.

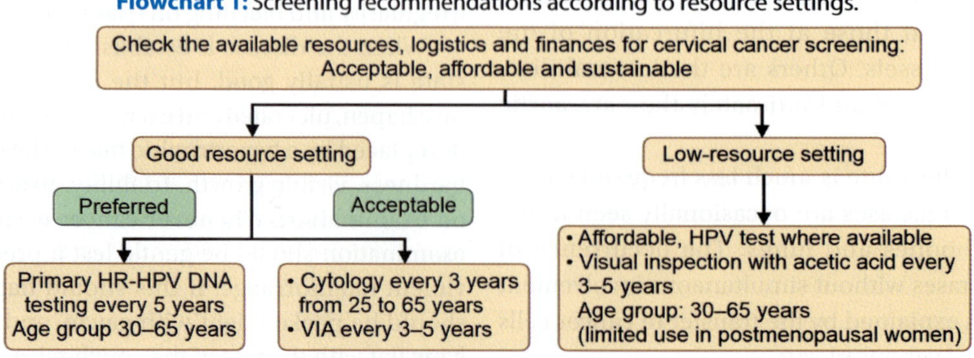

(HPV: human papillomavirus; VIA: visual inspection with acetic acid)

Flowchart 2: Screen-and-treat approach.

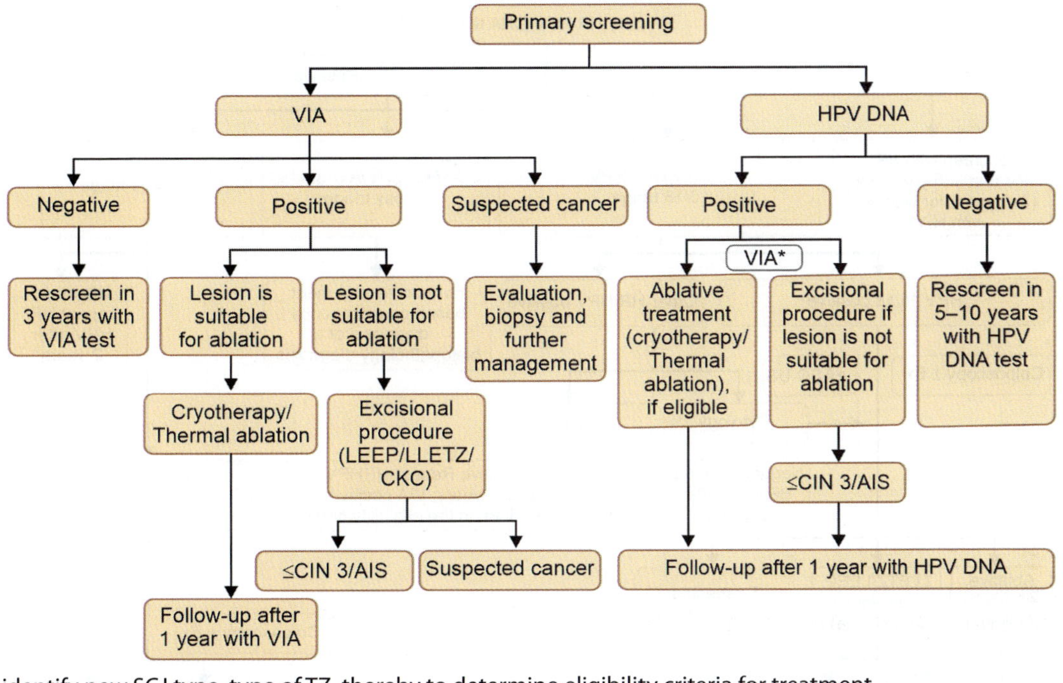

*VIA is used to identify new SCJ type, type of TZ, thereby to determine eligibility criteria for treatment.

(AIS: adenocarcinoma in situ; CIN: cervical intraepithelial neoplasia; CKC: cold knife conisation; HPV: human papillomavirus; LEEP: loop electrosurgical excision procedure; LLETZ: large loop excision of the transformation zone; VIA: visual inspection with acetic acid)

Flowchart 3: Screen-triage-and-treat approach (primary cytology screening and colposcopy triage).

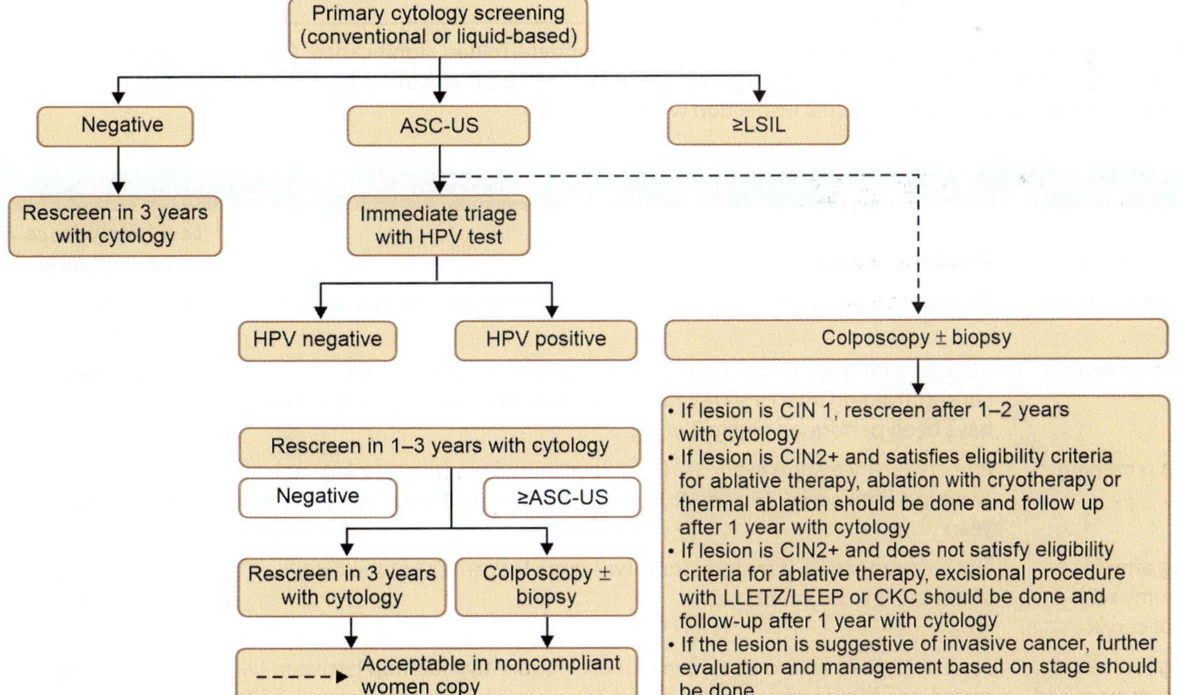

(ASC-US: atypical squamous cells of undetermined significance; CIN: cervical intraepithelial neoplasia; CKC: cold knife conisation; HPV: human papillomavirus; LEEP: loop electrosurgical excision procedure; LLETZ: large loop excision of the transformation zone; LSIL: low-grade squamous intraepithelial lesion)

Flowchart 4: Screen-triage-and-treat approach (primary HPV DNA screening and HPV 16/18 or colposcopy or VIA triage).

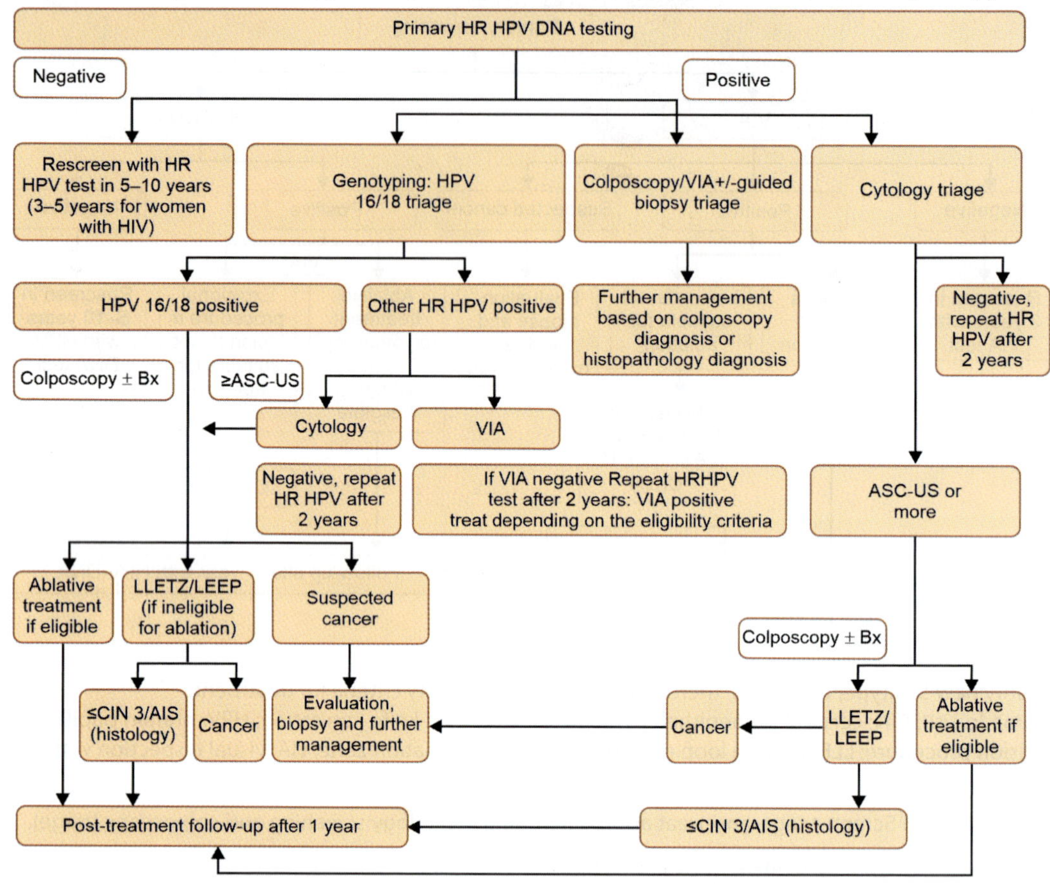

(AIS: adenocarcinoma in situ; ASC-US: atypical squamous cells of undetermined significance; CIN: cervical intraepithelial neoplasia; HIV: human immunodeficiency virus; HPV: human papillomavirus; LEEP: loop electrosurgical excision procedure; LLETZ: large loop excision of the transformation zone; VIA: visual inspection with acetic acid)

TABLE 2: FOGSI screening recommendations.

	Recommendation	*Level of evidence, grade of recommendation*
Age to start screening	25 years in a good resource setting, universal recommendation: 30 years	Level 1, strong recommendation
Age to end screening	65 years with three consecutive negative cytology results or two consecutive negative HPV test within 10 years. The most recent test should have been performed within 5 years	Level 1, strong recommendation
Tests with screening interval	Primary hrHPV testing every 5–10 years; in limited-resource settings at least twice in a lifetime, i.e. 35 and 45 years; cytology every 3 years VIA every 3–5 years	Level 1, strong recommendation
Screening after hysterectomy with removal of cervix	Not recommended. If hysterectomy was done for cancer or precancer, screening is to be continued	Level 1, strong recommendation
Screening for immunocompromised women	Start at 25 years and to be screened more frequently; duration between two screenings should not extend beyond 3 years, preferable to screen with HPV tests	Level 1, strong recommendation

(FOGSI: Federation of Obstetric and Gynaecological Societies of India; HPV: human papillomavirus; VIA: visual inspection with acetic acid)

FOGSI-ICOG

Good Clinical Practice Recommendations (GCPR)

Prevention and Management of Cervical Cancer

Convenor—Priya Ganeshkumar *Co-Convenor*—Bhagyalaxmi Nayak

Mentors—Hrishikesh D Pai, Madhuri Patel, Laxmi Shrikhande

Advisors—Sanjay Gupte, Hema Divakar

National Coordinators—CN Purandare, Rishma Dhillon Pai, Nandita Palshetkar, Jaydeep Tank

Coordinator—Surekha Tayade

Gynaecologic Oncology Committee

Fig. 9: FOGSI-ICOG Good Clinical Practice Recommendations (GCPR) prevention and management of cervical cancer. (FOGSI: Federation of Obstetric and Gynaecological Societies of India)
Source: Federation of Obstetric and Gynaecological Societies of India. (2024). FOGSI GCPR on Prevention and Management of Cervical Cancer. [online] Available from https://www.fogsi.org/fogsi-gcpr-on-prevention-and-management-of-cervical-cancer-june-2024/. [Last accessed April, 2025].

Changes in the Management of Cervical Cytology Results

In 2012, consensus guidelines for the management of abnormal cervical cancer screening tests and cancer precursors recommendations were updated, and the changes were as follows:

- Cytology reported as negative but lacking endocervical cells can be managed without early repeat
- Cervical intraepithelial neoplasia 1 (CIN 1) on endocervical curettage should be managed as CIN 1, not as a positive endocervical curettage.
- Cytology reported as unsatisfactory requires repeat even if HPV negative

Flowchart 5: Management of abnormal Pap smear.

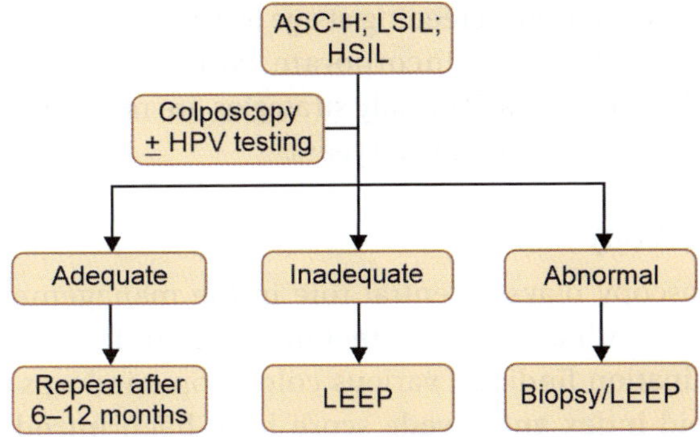

(ASC-H: atypical squamous cells-cannot exclude high-grade squamous intraepithelial lesion; HPV: human papillomavirus; HSIL: high-grade squamous intraepithelial lesion; LEEP: loop electrosurgical excision procedure; LSIL: low-grade squamous intraepithelial lesion)

Flowchart 6: Management algorithm of ASC-US cytology.

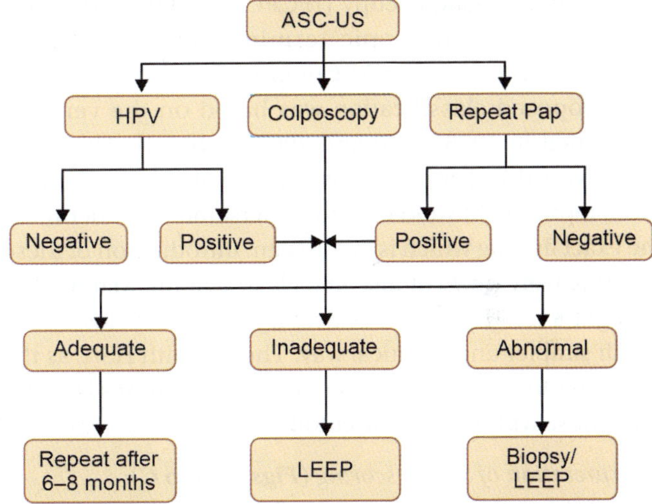

(ASC-US: atypical squamous cells of undetermined significance; HPV: human papillomavirus; LEEP: loop electrosurgical excision procedure)

- Genotyping triages HPV-positive women with HPV type 16 or 18 to earlier colposcopy only after negative cytology; colposcopy is indicated for all women with HPV and ASC-US, regardless of genotyping result.
- For ASC-US cytology, immediate colposcopy is not an option. The serial cytology option for ASC-US incorporates cytology at 12 months, not 6 and 12 months and then if negative, cytology every 3 years.
- HPV-negative and ASC-US results should be followed with cotesting at 3 years rather than 5 years.

- HPV-negative and ASC-US results are insufficient to allow exit from screening at age 65 years.
- More strategies incorporate cotesting to reduce follow-up visits. Pap-only strategies are now limited to women younger than 30 years.

Colposcopy

Colposcopy plays a central role in the management of patients with abnormal screening tests. To improve the examination findings, various colposcopic indexes such as Reid index and Swede score have been introduced to interpret colposcopic findings followed by with or without biopsy as the gold standard. For Swede scoring of colposcopy findings, the total score ranges between 0 and 10, assigning each colposcopy finding parameter a score between 0 and 2 **(Table 3)**. A score of ≥5 is reported to identify all high-grade squamous intraepithelial lesions (HSILs). In 2011, the International Federation for Cervical Pathology and Colposcopy (IFCPC) presented the new international colposcopic terminology/classification system at the 14th World Congress in Rio de Janeiro. The proposed classification was based on the versions developed in 1975, 1990 and 2002 **(Table 4)**. The main objective of this classification is to make colposcopy findings more reproducible and easy to understand and document the exact finding which is being seen. Introduction of these two relatively new colposcopic classification systems has brought a new approach in dealing with cervix lesions in much simpler and practical way. Though with HSIL as the cutoff, performance of the comprehensive indexes is better than those with LSIL as the cutoff.

Interpretation of Swede scoring ***(Figs. 10A to C)***:

- 0–1: Chronic cervicitis
- 2–4: LSIL/CIN 1
- 5–7: CIN 2 HSIL
- 8–10: CIN 3 HSIL

Complications

- *Pyometra:* The cancer obstructs the cervical canal and is also a nidus of infection; pyometra is, therefore, common.
- *Intractable haemorrhage:* Due to large tumour growth, patient may present with massive intractable haemorrhage resulting in severe anaemia. To control the bleeding, surgical management by tying the internal iliac artery or by high-dose radiation therapy (RT) in the form of haemostatic RT should be considered.
- Vesicovaginal and vesicocervical fistulas.
- *Rectovaginal fistula:* This is seen in untreated cases.
- Hydronephrosis and pyonephrosis caused by ureteric obstruction.
- *Uraemia:* This is caused by renal failure due to obstructive uropathy as well as infection. The ultimate causes of death in their order of frequency and importance used to be uraemia, cachexia associated with recurrent haemorrhage, infection and interference with nutrition, complications of treatment and remote metastases in vital organs (rare). With improved radiotherapy, uraemia is less common in developed countries as the main cause of death.
- *Intestinal obstruction:* Rare, due to widespread metastasis resulting in bowel obstruction.

Staging of Disease

Staging of cervical cancer is essentially based on the clinical stage of the disease. Staging is determined at the time of the primary diagnosis and cannot be altered, even at recurrence. Only if the rules for clinical staging are strictly observed, it is possible to compare results among clinics and by differing modes of therapy.

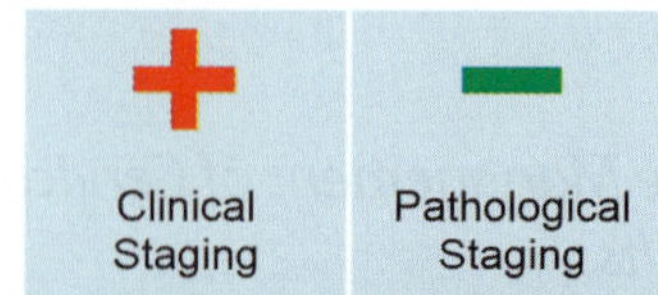

TABLE 3: Swede score for interpretation of colposcopy findings.

	Score		
	0	*1*	*2*
Uptake of acetic acid	0 or transparent	Shady, milky	Distinct, stearin like
Margins and surface	0 or diffuse	Sharp, but irregular, jagged, 'geographical' satellites	Sharp and even, difference in surface level such as 'cutting'
Vessels	Fine, regular	Absent	Coarse or atypical
Lesion size	<5 mm	5–15 mm or spanning two quadrants	>15 mm or spanning three to four quadrants or endocervically undefined
Iodine staining	Brown	Faintly or patchy yellow	Distinct yellow

TABLE 4: IFCPC 2011 colposcopy terminology classification.

General assessment		• Adequate/inadequate(reason) • *SCJ visible:* Completely visible/partially visible/not visible • *Transformation zone:* 1/2/3	
Normal colposcopic findings		*Original squamous epithelium:* • Mature • Atrophic *Columnar epithelium:* • Ectopy *Metaplastic squamous epithelium:* • Nabothian cysts • Crypt openings • Deciduosis in pregnancy	
Abnormal colposcopic findings	General principles	*Location of the lesion:* Inside or outside the T-zone • Location of the lesion • Inside/outside T-zone • Clock position *Size of the lesion:* • Number of quadrants involved by the lesion • Percentage of cervix involved by the lesion	
	Grade 1 (minor)	• Thin AW epithelium • Irregular, geographic border	• Fine mosaic • Fine punctuation
	Grade 2 (major)	• Dense AW epithelium • Rapid appearance of acetowhitening • Cuffed crypt openings	• Coarse mosaic • Coarse punctuation • Sharp border • Inner border sign • Ridge sign
	Nonspecific	• Leucoplakia • Erosion • Stained/nonstained	
Suspicious for invasion		• Atypical vessels • *Additional signs*: Fragile vessels, irregular surface, exophytic lesion, necrosis, ulceration (necrotic) and tumour/gross neoplasm	
Miscellaneous finding		• CTZ • Condyloma • Polyp/Inflammation	• Stenosis • Congenital anomaly • Post-treatment • Endometriosis

(AW: acetowhite; CTZ: chemoreceptor trigger zone; IFCPC: International Federation for Cervical Pathology and Colposcopy; SCJ: squamo-columnar junction)

- *Clinical staging:* Staging of cervical cancer is based on clinical evaluation; therefore, careful clinical examination should be performed in all cases, preferably by an experienced examiner and under anaesthesia. The clinical staging must not be changed because of subsequent findings. When there is doubt as to which stage a particular cancer should be allocated, the earlier stage is mandatory. The following examinations are permitted: palpation, inspection, colposcopy, endocervical curettage, hysteroscopy, cystoscopy, proctoscopy, intravenous urography and X-ray examination of the lungs and skeleton; suspected bladder or rectal involvement should be confirmed by biopsy and histologic evidence. Invasive cancers so identified are to be included in the reports. Findings of optional examinations, e.g. laparoscopy, ultrasound, computed tomography (CT) scan, magnetic resonance imaging (MRI) and positron emission tomography (PET)-CT scan are of value for planning therapy, but because they are not generally available and the interpretation of results is variable, the findings of

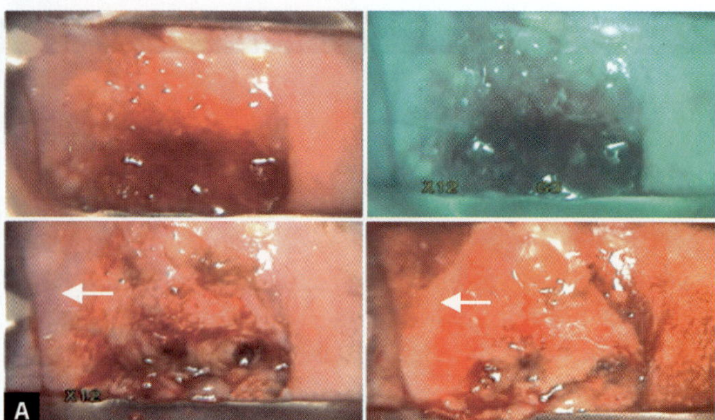

Thin acetowhite area from 6 o'clock to 10 o'clock position with lugol's positive Swede scoring 6-cin 2

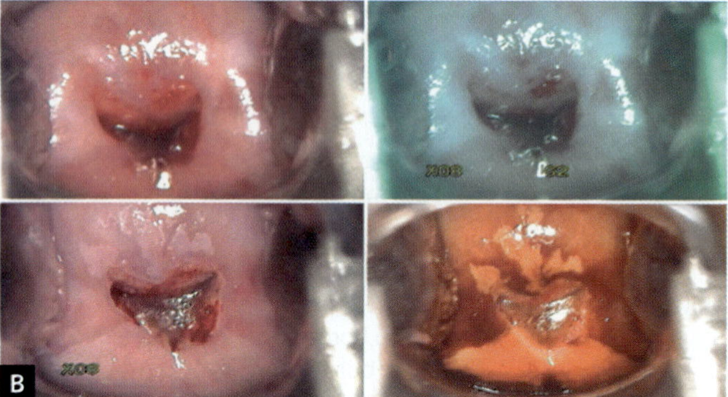

Dense acetowhite epithelium, Lugol's positive, fine punctation, covering three quadrants
Swede 2+2+0+2+1=7

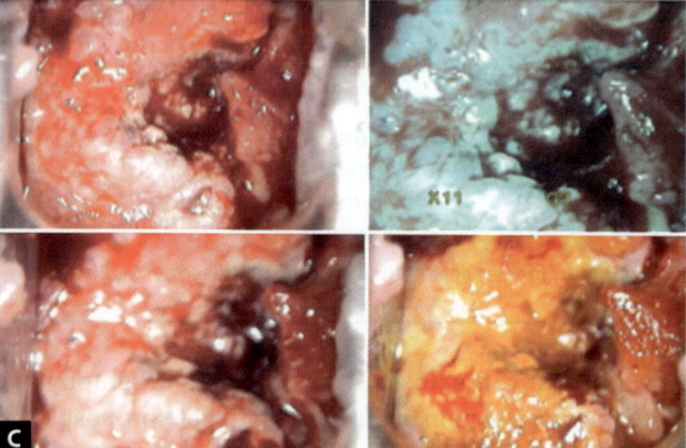

Dense opaque acetowhite area with raised margin and mustard iodine staining swede 2 + 2 + 2 + 2 + 2 = 10 HPE-Adenocarcinoma

Figs. 10A to C: Interpretation of the Swede scoring.
Courtesy: Dr Priya Ganeshkumar, India.

such studies should not be the basis for changing the clinical staging. Fine needle aspiration (FNA) of scan-detected suspicious lymph nodes may be helpful in treatment planning.

- *Pathological staging:* In cases treated by surgical procedures, the pathologist's findings in the removed tissues can be the basis for extremely accurate statements on the extent of disease. The findings should not be allowed to change the clinical staging but should be recorded in the manner described for the pathologic staging of disease. The tumour-node-metastasis (TNM) nomenclature is appropriate for this purpose. Infrequently, it happens that hysterectomy is carried out in the presence of unsuspected extensive invasive cervical carcinoma. Such cases cannot be clinically staged or included in therapeutic statistics, but it is desirable that they be reported separately.

The staging procedures are shown in **Tables 5 to 7**.

Prognosis

Irrespective of the type of treatment, the prognosis depends on the following:

- *Extent of growth at the time of treatment:* This is the single most important factor.
- *Site:* An endocervical growth is potentially more dangerous than one which grows on the vaginal surface, because it is diagnosed relatively late, and it spreads to the broad ligaments and to lymph nodes relatively early.
- *Size of the tumour:* The hypertrophic, florid, growth >4 cm in size is considered to be as a bulky disease and usually carries a bad prognosis—even if it does not appear to have spread much beyond the cervix.
- *Histology:* An adenocarcinoma offers relatively unfavourable prospects, not because it is less radiosensitive than a squamous cell growth as was once believed. Groups of cases of adenocarcinoma certainly show a much inferior salvage rate, but this is because they include cancers in young women and more cancers in an advanced stage. Since adenocarcinoma is usually endocervical in site, it is discovered and treated relatively late. If the results of treatment are properly controlled by matching cases by age of patient, stage of growth and other factors, there is no difference between those of the two cell types. The same applies to mixed adenosquamous growths in older women but not in women under 40 years of age. Among the squamous cell growths, the well differentiated are to be preferred, because they grow slowly and metastasise late. It is sometimes suggested that they are more radiosensitive, but the widely accepted view

TABLE 5: New FIGO staging 2018.

Stage	*Description*
I	The carcinoma is strictly confined to the cervix (extension to the uterine corpus should be disregarded)
IA	Invasive carcinoma that can be diagnosed only by microscopy, with maximum depth of invasion <5 mm[a]
IA1	Measured stromal invasion <3 mm in depth
IA2	Measured stromal invasion ≥3 mm and <5 mm in depth
IB	Invasive carcinoma with measured deepest invasion ≥5 mm (greater than stage IA), lesion limited to the cervix uteri[b]
IB1	Invasive carcinoma 25 mm depth of stromal invasion and <2 cm in greatest dimension
IB2	Invasive carcinoma ≥2 cm and <4 cm in greatest dimension
IB3	Invasive carcinoma ≥4 cm in greatest dimension
II	The carcinoma invades beyond the uterus, but has not extended onto the lower third of the vagina or to the pelvic wall
IIA	Involvement limited to the upper two thirds of the vagina without parametrial involvement
IIA1	Invasive carcinoma <4 cm in greatest dimension
IIA2	Invasive carcinoma ≥4 cm in greatest dimension
IIB	With parametrial involvement but not up to the pelvic wall
III	The carcinoma involves the lower third of the vagina and/or extends to the pelvic wall and/or causes hydronephrosis or nonfunctioning kidney and/or involves pelvic and/or para-aortic lymph nodes
IIIA	The carcinoma involves the lower third of the vagina, with no extension to the pelvic wall
IIIB	Extension to the pelvic wall and/or hydronephrosis or nonfunctioning kidney (unless known to be due to another cause)
IIIC	Involvement of pelvic and/or para-aortic lymph nodes, irrespective of tumour size and extent (with r and p notations)[c]
IIIC1	Pelvic lymph node metastasis only
IIIC2	Para-aortic lymph node metastasis
IV	The carcinoma has extended beyond the true pelvis or has involved (biopsy proven) the mucosa of the bladder or rectum (a bullous oedema, as such, does not permit a case to be allotted to stage IV)
IVA	Spread to adjacent pelvic organs
IVB	Spread to distant organs

[a]Imaging and pathology can be used, where available, to supplement clinical findings with respect to tumour size and extent, in all stages.
[b]The involvement of vascular/lymphatic spaces does not change the staging. The lateral extent of the lesion is no longer considered.
[c]Adding notation of r (imaging) and p (pathology) to indicate the findings that are used to allocate the case to stage IIIC. Example: If imaging indicates pelvic lymph node metastasis, the stage allocation would be stage IIIC1r, and if confirmed by pathologic findings, it would be stage IIIC1p. The type of imaging modality or pathology technique used should always be documented.
(FIGO: International Federation of Gynaecology and Obstetrics)
When in doubt, the lower staging should be assigned.

is that the anaplastic tumours have the advantage in this respect. The presence of lymphovascular space invasion (LVSI) is associated with a poorer prognosis.

- *Age:* The younger the patient, the more likely is the growth to be poorly differentiated in type and the worse the outlook.
- *Ureteric obstruction:* If, at the outset of managing a case, pyelography reveals unilateral or bilateral ureteric obstruction, the ultimate outlook is poor.

Imaging

The major role of imaging in cancer cervix is as follows:

- Evaluation of the tumour size
- Delineate parametrial involvement
- Vaginal involvement
- Differentiating cervix versus endometrial cancer
- Evaluation of pelvic wall or adjacent organ evaluation
- Lymph node evaluation
- Distant metastasis

TABLE 6: TNM and FIGO classification for cervical cancer staging.

TNM Categories	*FIGO Stages*	*Surgicopathological findings*
Tx		Primary tumour cannot be assessed
T0		No evidence of primary tumour
Tis		Carcinoma in situ (preinvasive carcinoma)
T1	I	Cervical carcinoma confined to the cervix (disregard extension to the corpus)
T1a	IA	Invasive carcinoma diagnosed only by microscopy; stromal invasion with a maximum depth of 5.0 mm measured from the base of the epithelium and a horizontal spread of 7.0 mm or less; vascular space involvement, venous or lymphatic, does not affect classification
T1a1	IA1	Measured stromal invasion ≤3.0 mm in depth and ≤7.0 mm in horizontal spread
T1a2	IA2	Measured stromal invasion >3.0 mm and ≤5.0 mm with a horizontal spread ≤7.0 mm
T1b	IB	Clinically visible lesion confined to the cervix or microscopic lesion greater than T1a/IA2
T1b1	IB1	Clinically visible lesion ≤4.0 cm in greatest dimension
T1b2	IB2	Clinically visible lesion >4.0 cm in greatest dimension
T2	II	Cervical carcinoma invades beyond uterus but not to pelvic wall or to lower third of vagina
T2a	IIA	Tumour without parametrial invasion
T2a1	IIA1	Clinically visible lesion ≤4.0 cm in greatest dimension
T2a2	IIA2	Clinically visible lesion >4.0 cm in greatest dimension
T2b	IIB	Tumour with parametrial invasion
T3	III	Tumour extends to pelvic wall and/or involves lower third of vagina and/or causes hydronephrosis or nonfunctional kidney
T3a	IIIA	Tumour involves lower third of vagina, no extension to pelvic wall
T3b	IIIB	Tumour extends to pelvic wall and/or causes hydronephrosis or nonfunctional kidney
T4	IV	Tumour invades mucosa of bladder or rectum and/or extends beyond true pelvis (bullous oedema is not sufficient to classify a tumour as T4)
T4a	IVA	Tumour invades mucosa of bladder or rectum (bullous oedema is not sufficient to classify a tumour as T4)
T4b	IVB	Tumour extends beyond true pelvis
Regional lymph nodes		
NX		Regional lymph nodes cannot be assessed
N0		No regional lymph node metastasis
N1		Regional lymph node metastasis
Distant metastasis		
M0		No distant metastasis
M1		Distant metastasis (including peritoneal spread; involvement of supraclavicular, mediastinal or para-aortic lymph nodes and lung, liver or bone)

(FIGO: International Federation of Gynaecology and Obstetrics; TNM: tumour-node-metastasis)

Computed Tomography

This can be used to demonstrate tumour spread. It can visualise enlarged lymph nodes (although it cannot differentiate enlargement due to tumour from that caused by infection) and distortion of tissue spaces or planes by tumour or surgery. It is helpful for assessing recurrence of disease after surgical treatment of carcinoma of the cervix. It provides more information about involvement outside the pelvis **(Fig. 11)**.

TABLE 7: Staging procedures.

Physical examination[a]	• Palpate lymph nodes • Examine vagina • Bimanual rectovaginal examination (under anaesthesia recommended)
Radiological studies[a]	• Intravenous pyelogram • Barium enema • Chest X-ray • Skeletal X-ray
Procedures[a]	• Biopsy • Conisation • Hysteroscopy • Colposcopy • Endocervical curettage • Cystoscopy • Proctoscopy
Optional studies[b] FIGO staging criteria recommend inclusion of these imaging techniques when possible, their use remains optional	• Computerised axial tomography • Lymphangiography • Ultrasonography • Magnetic resonance imaging—more sensitive and specific than CT scan • Positron emission tomography • Radionucleotide scanning • Laparoscopy

[a]Allowed by the International Federation of Gynaecology and Obstetrics (FIGO).
[b]Information that is not allowed by FIGO to change the clinical stage.

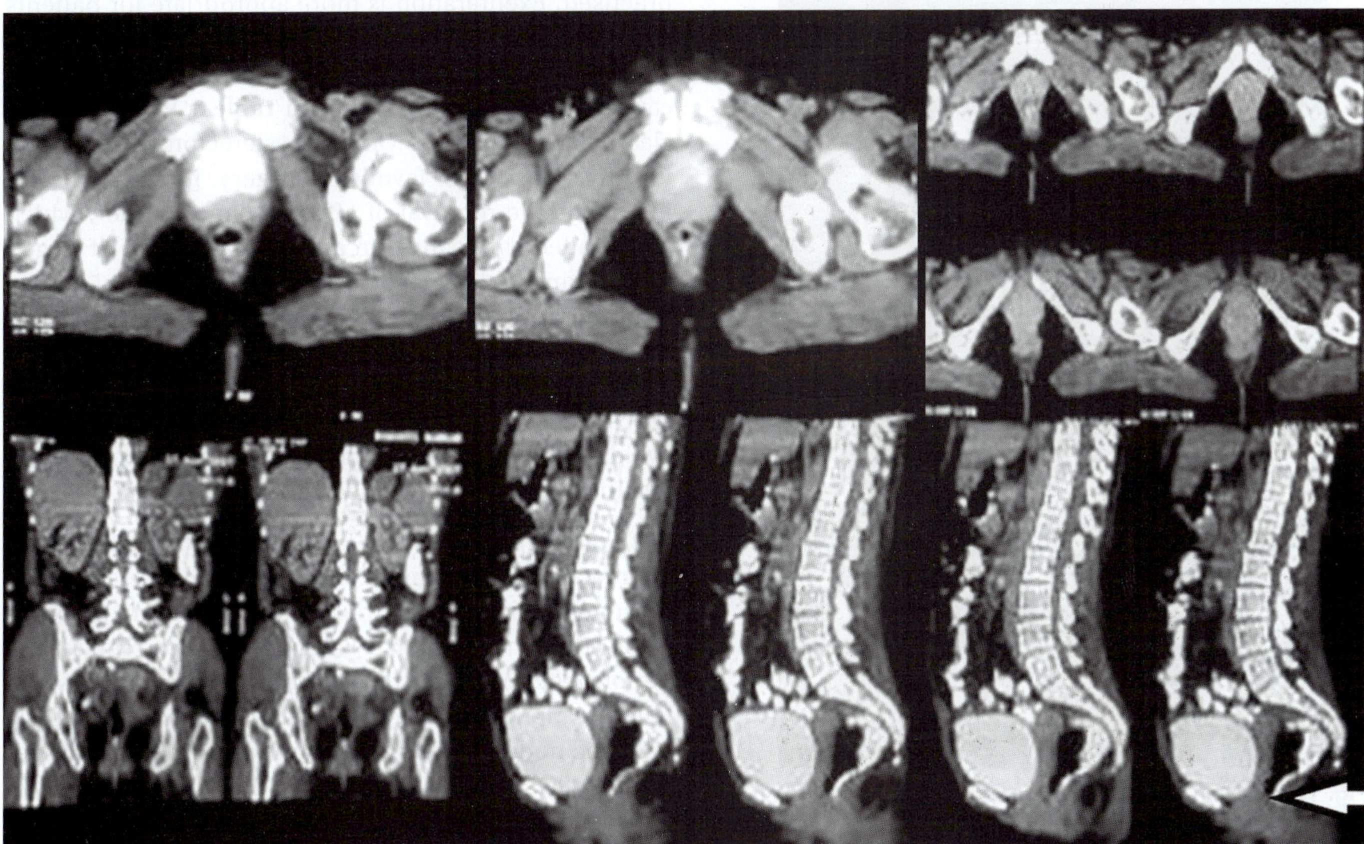

Fig. 11: Contrast-enhanced computed tomography (CECT) of the abdomen reveals cervical mass with vaginal wall involvement.

Magnetic Resonance Imaging

Magnetic resonance imaging is the best method of imaging to determine the size and extent of a tumour, especially if an endovaginal receiver is used. MRI more accurately defines tumour borders and discriminates between cervical and endometrial cancers. However, even with MRI, small metastatic deposits in the lymph nodes are likely to be missed.

Positron Emission Tomography-Computed Tomography Scan

Positron emission tomography-CT scan is a functional method, combined with CT as a morphological method. It is mainly used to determine the following features of cancer cervix **(Fig. 12)**:

- Determining relapse
- Detection of occult primary
- Detection of involved nodes and other active metastatic foci
- Differentiate between benign and malignant lesions.

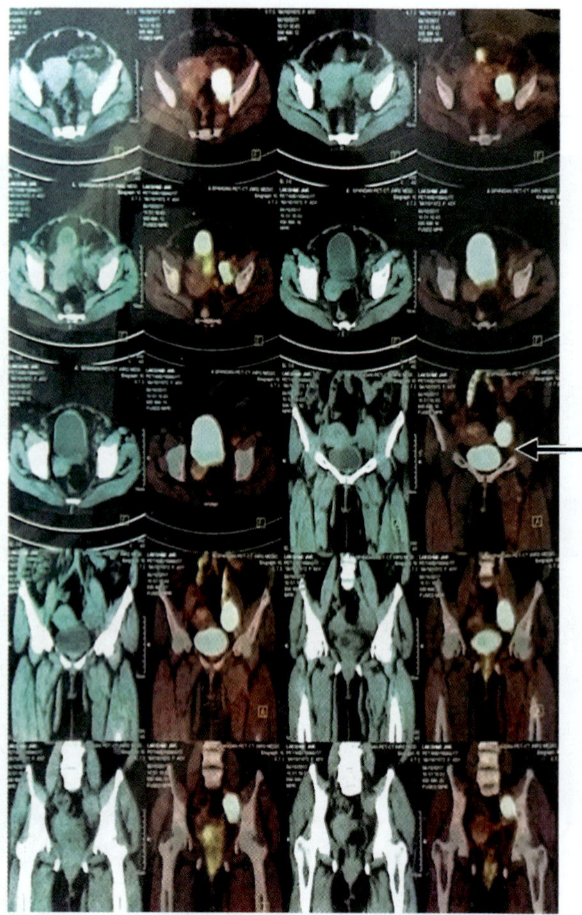

Fig. 12: Positron emission tomography-computed tomography (PET-CT) scan reveals nodal recurrence in a case of postradiated cancer of cervix.

Treatment of Invasive Cancer of the Cervix

Treatment is by radiotherapy, surgery, chemotherapy or by combinations of these. It is now highly specialised, and the best results can only be obtained by a multidisciplinary approach. Moreover, these require complicated and expensive equipment as well as trained nursing and technical staff, so centralisation of the facilities in any one area becomes more and more desirable. The tendency to follow a fixed plan of treatment for all cases has an advantage when it comes to assessing results.

Surgery

Surgery can be carried out as a primary procedure, in stages I and IIA, especially in young women to conserve ovarian function, or when carcinoma of the cervix shows a poor response to radiotherapy, or if it recurs after such treatment. For advanced and failed radiotherapy cases, ultraradical surgery such as exenteration is sometimes practised. Exenteration is more appropriate for patients with recurrent central disease occurring at least 2 years after radiotherapy. The primary surgery for cancer of cervix is summarised in **Table 8**. Piver–Rutledge classification classifies various hysterectomy procedures into five classes. In favour of surgery, it is argued that it permits the removal of affected lymph nodes, which are invaded with cancer in approximately 15% of stage I growths and which may not receive a cancericidal dose of radiotherapy. Moreover, some women are happier with the thought that the disease has been removed rather than *treated*. Nevertheless, radical surgery is one which requires special skill and experience and one which even the expert avoids when the cancer sufferer is obese, in poor general health, or has associated medical disorders.

Sentinel lymph node (SLN) biopsy: SLN biopsy is a new approach in the treatment of early-stage cancer of cervix. Mostly based on clinical trials, a successful SLN mapping is the adherence to the SLN algorithm which requires the performance of a side-specific nodal dissection in cases of failed mapping and removal of any suspicious or grossly enlarged nodes regardless of mapping. Things to consider for a successful SLN are optimal timing, best site and appropriate tracer material. More trials are required to establish the role of SLN biopsy in cancer of cervix.

TABLE 8: Surgical management of invasive cancer of cervix.

	Primary treatment (fertility sparing)	*Primary treatment (nonfertility sparing)*
Stage Ia1 (no LVSI)	Conisation with negative margins	• Conisation with negative margins • Extrafascial hysterectomy • Conisation with positive margins for cancer • Extrafascial hysterectomy/modified radical hysterectomy + Pelvic lymphadenectomy
IA1(with LVSI) and stage IA2	Conisation with negative margins + Pelvic lymphadenectomy Or Radical trachelectomy + Pelvic lymphadenectomy	Modified radical hysterectomy + Pelvic lymphadenectomy Or Pelvic radiotherapy
Ib1 and IIA1		Radical hysterectomy + Pelvic lymphadenectomy Or Pelvic RT
Ib2 and IIA2 (bulky disease)		Pelvic RT + Concurrent cisplatin-containing chemotherapy + Brachytherapy Or Radical hysterectomy + Pelvic lymphadenectomy Or Pelvic RT + Concurrent cisplatin-containing chemotherapy + Brachytherapy + Adjuvant hysterectomy
IIB, IIIA, IIIB and IVA		Pelvic RT + Concurrent cisplatin-containing chemotherapy + Brachytherapy
Stage IVB		Systemic therapy with or without individualised RT

(LVSI: lymphovascular space invasion; RT: radiation therapy)

Piver–Rutledge classification of extended hysterectomy:

- *Class I:* All cervical tissue (extrafascial)
- *Class II:* Modified radical (Wertheim's hysterectomy)
- *Class III:* Radical classical hysterectomy
- *Class IV:* Extended radical
- *Class V:* Pelvic exenteration

The ovaries are involved in <1% of patients with squamous cell carcinoma of the cervix; hence, they may be conserved in women younger than 40 years of age if they appear grossly normal. However, they should be transposed above the pelvic brim into the paracolic gutters and anchored there with a permanent suture, so that they can be spared the effect of radiotherapy should it be required subsequently. The discovery at laparotomy that the para-aortic lymph nodes are positive for cancer may prompt the operator to discontinue the operation and to opt for radiotherapy instead. Tumour extension into the bladder base which cannot be detected cystoscopically may prevent adequate mobilisation of the bladder flap, leading to the procedure being abandoned. For this reason, this part of the operation is undertaken early on opening the abdomen. Okabayashi described his technique of radical hysterectomy in 1921 **(Fig. 13)**. This technique aimed at improving the operability rate even in those patients with advanced disease, with a more radical dissection of the parametrial and paracervical tissue.

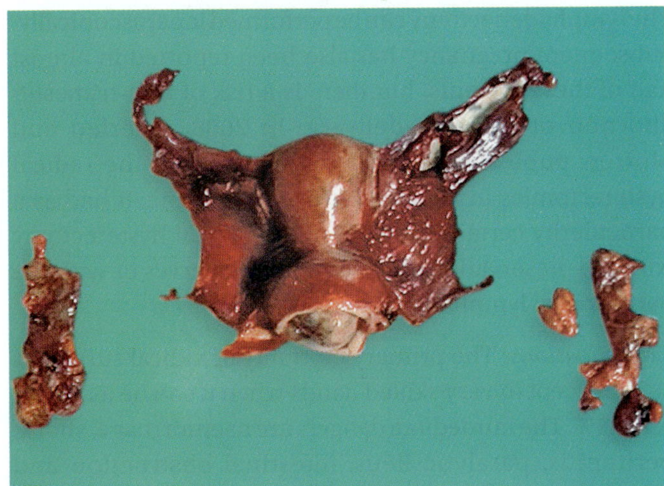

Fig. 13: Specimen of type III radical hysterectomy.

Sakamoto et al. further modified this (Tokyo method). They attempted to preserve the base of the cardinal ligaments which contain the pelvic nerve bundles and also treated the ureters differently, leaving a protective sheath. Both these technical differences resulted in a decreased incidence of bladder dysfunction, which is the main advantage of the Tokyo method. Several other modifications in the Wertheim's procedure have been reported from time to time; most of these have been attempts to decrease the rate of ureteric fistula formation. A rather less extensive operation (so far as node dissection is concerned) can be carried out by the vaginal route (Schauta or Schauta-Amreich operation), but it is only popular in a few centres. Mitra from India modified the operation and added bilateral extraperitoneal lymphadenectomy through two separate abdominal incisions to correct this deficiency. Nowadays, the Schauta procedure can be combined with laparoscopic lymphadenectomy to decrease the morbidity of the procedure. In selected young women with early stage I disease confined to the ectocervix, who desire to preserve fertility, radical trachelectomy has been described, in which the cervix is removed along with the cardinal and uterosacral ligaments and paracervical tissue, followed by suturing of the uterus to the vagina. Lymphadenectomy is either done previously at a separate sitting or the lymph nodes are assessed by frozen section to be free of disease. The lymphadenectomy can be performed laparoscopically. Subsequent pregnancy has also been reported in almost half of these patients, but there is a risk of mid-trimester abortion or preterm delivery. In 2008, Querleu and Morrow published another classification of the radical hysterectomies in Lancet Oncology magazine. It had as a particularity certain subtypes of the radical hysterectomy with the preservation of the autonomic nerves or with the paracervical lymphadenectomy.

Complications: The primary mortality of radical surgery is 1–2%, except in very skilled hands when it can be as low as 0.1–0.5%. The immediate dangers are haemorrhage, shock, peritonitis, paralytic ileus, intestinal obstruction and thromboembolism. The operation involves considerable risk of direct injury to the bladder, ureters and rectum. Ureteric fistula, previously a major complication, is now relatively uncommon as a result of improved operative technique, especially in selected centres where experienced gynaecologists do these operations regularly. Febrile morbidity is a common complication. Atony of the bladder, incomplete emptying, cystitis and pyelitis complicate 20% of operations, and there is generally a need for postoperative bladder drainage. Minor degrees of hydronephrosis and hydroureter occur in some cases, but these changes usually disappear within 1 year. Nevertheless, ureteric incompetence, with reflux of urine from the bladder, persists in some cases, and troublesome stress incontinence can be a problem. Late sequelae include stenosis of the ureter by surrounding fibrosis and lymphocyst formation. The latter, which occurs in 1–5% of cases if lymphadenectomy is routinely carried out, can be mistaken for recurrent cancer; it is a cystic dilatation of the remaining but interrupted lymph channels and can be left untreated if small, aspirated under ultrasonic control or marsupialised into the abdominal cavity if large. Secondary infection requires drainage. It is not, however, in the interests of the individual patient, and the aim should be to choose and to modify treatment to suit the circumstances of each case. It may even be necessary to change treatment if the initial response is not satisfactory. If it is concluded that radiotherapy is not effective, it can be abandoned in favour of surgery. Unfortunately, the evidence suggests that poor responders to radiotherapy do equally badly with surgery.

Assessment of the case before treatment: Preliminary pelvic examination under anaesthesia may be necessary in order to estimate the extent of the disease, the size of the uterus and vaginal fornices and to obtain material for histological study. Cystoscopy, intravenous pyelography and an estimation of the blood urea level are essential. The presence of remote metastases should be excluded as far as possible. Anaemia and malnutrition should be corrected, even at the expense of delaying treatment. A normal blood picture improves the results of radiotherapy considerably, possibly because it means better oxygenation of the malignant tissues; it is a prerequisite for safe surgery.

Radiotherapy

Radiotherapy for carcinoma of the cervix is delivered both with external beam radiotherapy (EBRT) and intracavitary brachytherapy (ICRT). EBRT treats the whole pelvis and parametria, and ICRT primarily treats the central disease, i.e. cervix, vagina and medial parametria. EBRT is delivered before ICRT in the following circumstances:

- In case of bulky cervical lesions to improve the geometry
- In exophytic easily bleeding tumours
- In tumours with necrosis and infection
- In cases with parametrial involvement

External beam radiotherapy portals for conventional radiotherapy: Portal includes:

- *Anterior–posterior fields:*
    - Superior border is taken at L4–L5 interspace in order to include the common iliac nodes.
    - Inferior border is at lower border of obturator foramen. In case of vaginal involvement, entire length down to introitus is included in the portal.
    - Lateral border is taken 2 cm lateral to the bony pelvis on either side. In cases of involvement of lower one-third vagina, inguinal nodes are covered.
- *Lateral fields:*
    - *Superior and inferior:* Same as anterior–posterior fields.
    - Anterior border of the lateral portal is taken at 1 cm anterior to the pubic symphysis in order to adequately cover the external iliac nodes.
    - Posterior border is between the S2 and S3 vertebrae (mid-sacrum); maximum care should be given to the posterior extension of the tumour, and a margin of at least 1–2 cm should be given to the tumour.

Lateral fields allow a decrease in dose to small bowel and a portion of the low rectum, but care must be taken to include all structures of interest **(Figs. 14A and B)**.

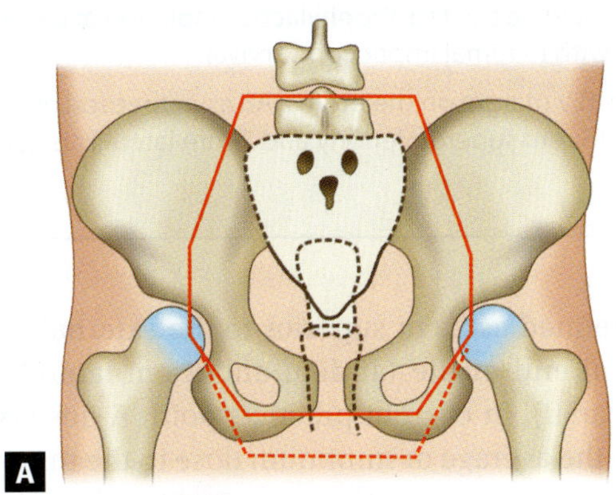

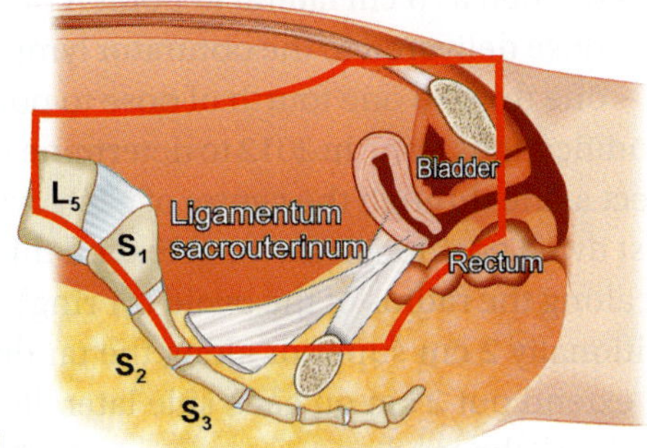

Figs. 14A and B: Anteroposterior and lateral portals of conventional four-field radiation therapy for uterine cervix and pelvic lymph nodes.

External beam radiotherapy with three-dimensional conformal image-guided radiotherapy: Three-dimensional (3D) conformal radiotherapy using CT-based planning with image guidance is highly recommended wherever the facility is available to improve the delineation of target structures and exclusion of normal tissues, including bowel, bladder and bone marrow. Target volumes for definitive RT using CT-based planning are summarised in **Table 9 and Figure 15**.

Brachytherapy: The American Brachytherapy Society (ABS) strongly recommends that:

- Definitive irradiation for cervical carcinoma must include brachytherapy as a component.
- Precise applicator placement is essential for improved local control and reduced morbidity.
- Interstitial brachytherapy should be considered for patients with disease that cannot be optimally encompassed by ICRT.
- Total treatment duration should be <8 weeks (exceeding beyond 8 weeks can reduce local control and survival by about 1% per day of prolongation).

Types of treatment and clinical techniques also vary according to the source loading by preloading (no longer used because of radiation hazards to caregivers) or after loading and dose rate as low-dose rate (LDR) < 2 Gray (Gy) per hour, medium-dose rate 2–12 Gy per hour or high-dose rate (HDR) >12 Gy per hour (practically, much higher dose rate is used). Presently, there is a move towards HDR brachytherapy from traditional LDR systems due to the following reasons:

- Eliminates radiation exposure hazard for caregivers and visitors
- Allows shorter treatment times
- Less risk of applicator movement during therapy
- Allows greater displacement of nearby normal tissues
- Possible to treat larger number of patients
- Allows use of smaller diameter sources than are used in LDR
- Physically easier to insert applicator into the cervix
- Makes treatment-dose-distribution optimisation possible.

Historically used brachytherapy systems are Stockholm system, Paris system and the Manchester system. Out of these, Manchester system designed to deliver a constant dose rate to defined points near cervix, irrespective of variation in size and shape of uterus/vagina **(Table 10)**.

Point A: Originally defined as 2 cm superior to the lateral vaginal fornix and 2 cm lateral to the cervical canal

TABLE 9: Target volumes for definitive radiation therapy using CT-based planning.

Target	*Description*
Primary cervical tumour	*Gross tumour volume primary (GTV-P)* is the primary cervical tumour with its extensions to parametria, uterosacral ligaments and vagina visible on imaging (a vaginal marker is placed at the lower extent of vaginal disease while taking CT)
	Clinical target volume (CTV) includes the GTV-P, uterine cervix, uterine corpus, parametria, vagina and ovaries. The uterine corpus, entire cervix and the vagina are contoured along with the gross disease (GTV-P) as a single structure *(CTV P1)*. If upper vagina is involved by the tumour, then upper two thirds are included in the CTV, and in case of extensive involvement, entire vagina is included. If there is minimal and no vaginal involvement, the contouring is stopped few slices above the lower border of the obturator foramen, so that when 1.5 cm internal margin [internal target volume (ITV)] is given over the uterus, the lower border does not extend beyond the lower border of obturator foramen. To delineate the parametrium *(CTV P2)*, connective tissue extending from the cervix to the pelvic wall is included, along with the visible linear structures that run laterally (e.g. vessels, nerves, fibrous structures). Posteriorly, parametrium is contoured only till the anterior part of the mesorectal fascia. In case of significant parametrial invasion (IIIB)/uterosacral ligament involvement, entire mesorectum is included
	Planning target volume (PTV): 1 cm margin is taken around the CTV P1 + P2 to account for the setup variability
Regional lymphatics	*GTV-N:* Includes grossly involved lymph nodes
	CTV-N: Includes GTV-N and relevant draining nodal groups (common iliac, external iliac, internal iliac, obturator and presacral lymph nodes. Inguinal nodes are included if lower one third of vagina is involved). All the visible nodes are given a margin of 1 cm. Pelvic blood vessels are uniformly given a margin of 7 mm
	PTV-N: 1 cm margin around CTV-N to account for setup variability
Para-aortic nodes	In para-aortic LN-positive cases, para-aortic field should be treated. Prophylactic irradiation of para-aortic nodes is not recommended as it increases toxicity with minimal impact on survival
ITV and final PTV	• The uterine motion is accounted for by giving an ITV margin on the uterus. An asymmetrical margin with ITV expansion of 15 mm anteroposteriorly, 15 mm superoinferiorly and 7 mm laterally is taken from the uterus (CTV P1) • Final PTV includes PTV and PTV-N along with the ITV

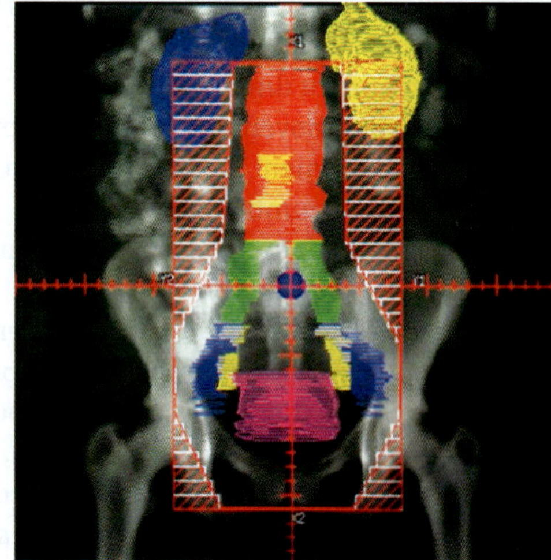

Fig. 15: Anterior digitally reconstructed radiograph of an extended pelvic and para-aortic external beam field in advanced cancer of the cervix.

(later redefined as 2 cm superior to the external cervical os/cervical end of the tandem and 2 cm lateral to the cervical canal). In current practice, point A dose is used to denote the average or minimum dose to the tumour.

Point B: It is defined as 3 cm lateral to point A (intended to quantify the dose delivered to the obturator lymph nodes). It receives ~ one third to one fourth of dose to point A.

The modifications done in 2012 to determine point A by ABS connect a line through the centre of each ovoid or the lateral most dwell position in the ring. Extend this position superiorly along the radius of the ovoid (or ring), and then move additionally 2 cm superior along the tandem. From this point, extend out 2 cm on each side laterally on a line perpendicular to the tandem.

Applicator selection: The most frequently used applicator for cervical cancer patients worldwide is tandem and

TABLE 10: Common radioactive sources for gynaecological brachytherapy.

Source	*Half-life*	*Energy (MeV)*	*Remarks*
Ra^{226}	1,620 years	2.45 (maximum)	Naturally occurring. Extensively used in the past for cervical brachytherapy with preloaded sources. No longer used
Cs^{137}	30 years	0.662	Fission product. Replaced radium as the isotope of choice for LDR brachytherapy in cervical cancer
Co^{60}	5.26 years	1.17 and 1.33	Product of neutron activation. Used for HDR brachytherapy in gynaecological cancer
Ir^{192}	74 days	0.38 (mean)	Product of neutron activation. Major isotope for HDR brachytherapy in gynaecological cancer

(HDR: high-dose rate; LDR: low-dose rate)

Source: Banerjee R, Kamrava M. Brachytherapy in the treatment of cervical cancer: a review. Int J Womens Health. 2014;6:555-64.

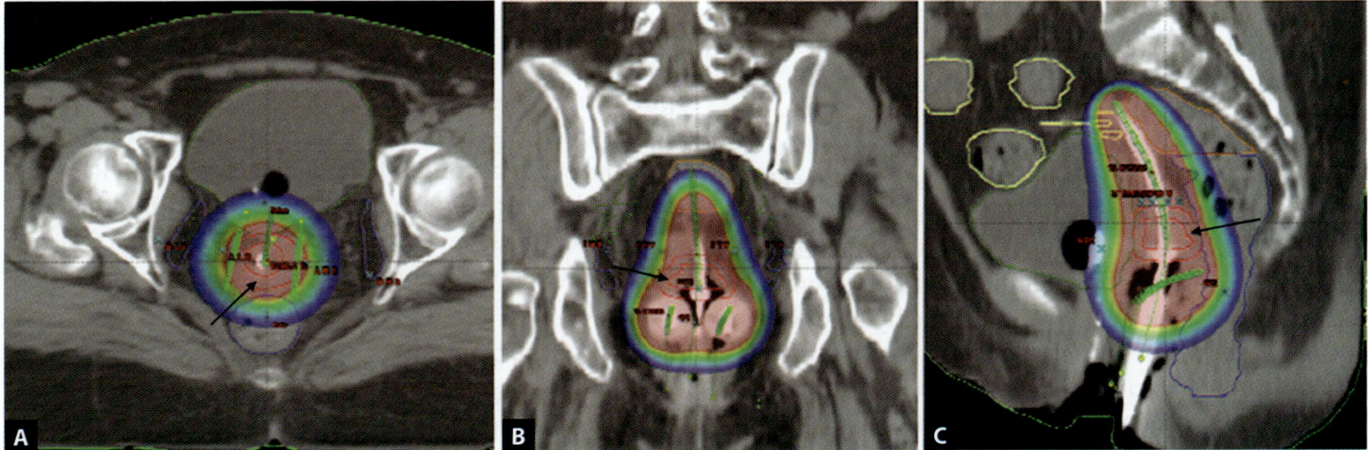

Figs. 16A to C: Classic pear-shaped dose distribution for intracavitary brachytherapy application with tandem and ovoids. (A) Axial; (B) Coronal; (C) Sagittal images.

ovoid applicator, which provides radiation dose covering the cervix, uterus, inner parametria and approximately 1–2 cm of the upper vagina.

The tandem and ring applicator has a slightly narrower dose distribution, but with HDR, the dose distribution may be optimised and mimics that obtained with tandem and ovoid applicator. For patients with large tumours with residual bulky disease after EBRT or those with vaginal extension or pelvic sidewall invasion, a combination of tandem/ring or ovoid with interstitial applicator or tandem/interstitial applicator alone may be inserted.

Dose specification: Due to the limited availability of 3D imaging worldwide and 100-year history of plane film radiography, the majority of institutions used point-based dosimeter based on the ICRU 38 nomenclature, defining point A rather than prescribing dose to a tumour volume.

Interstitial brachytherapy: It is a complex, multistep procedure with special diametric advantages and patient management requirements. In certain clinical situations, such as bulky lesions, a narrow vaginal apex, inability to enter the cervical os, extension to the lateral parametria or pelvic sidewall and lower vaginal extension, interstitial brachytherapy can achieve better dose distribution than intracavitary methods and may be the treatment of choice for some cases. In addition to interstitial needles, a tandem should be placed whenever possible to dose the cervix, uterus and parametrial tissues adequately.

Three-dimensional image-based brachytherapy treatment planning precisely defines the tumour and aids with the precision of radiation dose delivery, which may reduce the dose to the normal tissues and reduce toxicity. Over the last 10 years, there have been considerable advances in computer software along with the availability of CT- and MR-compatible applicators. These concepts have been developed recently and are detailed in the GEC-ESTRO recommendations that define target volumes using MRI **(Figs. 16A to C and Table 11)**.

TABLE 11: Definition of target volumes according using MRI.

Volume (GEC-ESTRO recommendation)	*Definition*
Gross tumour volume-brachytherapy (GTV_B)	Macroscopic tumour at the time of brachytherapy
Gross tumour volume-at diagnosis (GTVd)	Macroscopic tumour extension at diagnosis as detected by clinical examination and as visualised on MRI
High-risk clinical target volume (HRCTV)	Includes GTV_B + Whole cervix + Presumed extracervical tumour extension
Intermediate-risk clinical target volume (IRCTV)	Based on the macroscopic tumour extension at diagnosis (GTV_d)
Organs at risk (OAR)	Bladder, rectum, sigmoid and small bowel

Stagewise management with radiotherapy: The ABS recommends a total treatment duration of 8 weeks for EBRT and brachytherapy, as a 1% per day decrease in local control, and survival has been noted with extended treatment. Every attempt should be made to complete radiotherapy treatment (EBRT plus brachytherapy) in an 8-week time frame. With very large primary tumours, it may be beneficial to complete EBRT before initiation of brachytherapy to allow for maximal tumour shrinkage and optimal implant geometry. In these cases, brachytherapy treatments should be scheduled twice weekly if possible.

As a standard of practice, radiation oncologists attempt to maintain patient haemoglobin levels at generally 10 g/dL during treatment of cervical cancer. Lower haemoglobin levels adversely affect patient quality of life and may affect the ability to tolerate aggressive chemo-RT. The impact of optimal haemoglobin levels on outcome in terms of tumour control is still not certain.

Microinvasive cancer (IA1 and IA2): In patients of stage IA1 disease with no LVSI on the cone specimen, and who either refuse or are unfit for surgery, radiotherapy in the form of one or more ICRT insertions alone may be considered. Doses to point A range from 65 to 75 Gy in LDR equivalents, with a maximal vaginal surface dose of 100–120 Gy depending on the extent of microinvasive disease, size of cervix and normal tissue anatomy.

Similarly, in women with stage IA1 with LVSI or IA2 disease who have medical contraindications to surgery or refuse the surgical option, brachytherapy along with 40–45 Gy of pelvic EBRT to a cumulative total dose of 70–80 Gy to point A is delivered.

TABLE 12: Sedlis criteria regarding the requirement of adjuvant radiotherapy.

LVSI	*Stromal invasion*	*Tumour size (cm) (determined by clinical palpation)*
+	Deep one third	Any
+	Middle one third	≥2
+	Superficial one third	≥5
-	Middle or deep one third	≥4

(LVSI: lymphovascular space invasion)

The 5-year cancer-specific survival rates for IA1 and IA2 are ≥98% and ≥95%, respectively.

IB1 and IIA1: Patients with stage IB1 and IIA1 lesions can be treated with either radical surgery or pelvic EBRT plus brachytherapy to a cumulative dose up to 80 Gy to point A. The results of either modality are equivalent. The randomised trial comparing radical surgery with RT alone reported 5-year overall survival of 87% for the International Federation of Gynaecology and Obstetrics (FIGO) stages IB to IIA (tumours < 4 cm) treated with primary surgery compared with 90% for patients with definitive RT.

Indications of adjuvant radiotherapy: In node-negative, margin-negative and parametria-negative cases, Sedlis criteria are followed for decision regarding adjuvant radiotherapy **(Table 12)**.

In patients with positive surgical margin or node positive or positive parametrial disease, adjuvant concurrent chemoradiotherapy (CCRT) is recommended. Vaginal vault brachytherapy is given if vaginal margin is positive.

The National Cancer Institute (NCI) consensus conference in 1996 concluded that 'primary therapy should avoid the routine use of both radical surgery and radiotherapy'. If clinical evaluation reveals risk factors that would require pelvic RT after radical hysterectomy, RT should be considered the primary treatment choice to minimise the morbidity related to multimodality treatment.

IB2, IIA2, IIB and IIIB: Patients in these groups should be treated with radical radiotherapy (pelvic EBRT plus brachytherapy) and concurrent cisplatin-based chemotherapy with a total point A dose of 80–85 Gy.

Chemoradiation: It has been a standard of care for locally advanced disease since the NCI, United States, alert in 1999 that was based on the results of five phase III clinical trials. Collective results of these five trials along with the NCI Canada trial showed cumulative and statistically significant 36% reduction in the risk of death favouring combined cisplatin-based concurrent chemoradiation. The most commonly used regimen is weekly cisplatin 40 mg/m^2 up to five to six cycles concurrent with EBRT.

IVA: Concurrent RT/CT is an option in selected patients with good general and renal status who are not suitable for surgical exenteration. But majority of patients in this stage have poor general condition and have extensive disease and are best treated with palliative RT alone.

IVB: Stage IV B patients are treated with palliative intent. Radiotherapy can be used for palliation of distant painful bony metastases or symptomatic brain metastases. Additionally, symptoms due to extensive central disease such as pain, bleeding and tenesmus can be effectively palliated with radiotherapy.

Radiotherapy dose: External beam radiotherapy doses are in the range of 45–50.4 Gy in 1.8 Gy fractions. For brachytherapy, point A doses of 30–40 Gy (LDR equivalent) are recommended to achieve a cumulative point A dose of 80 Gy for small volume tumours or ≥85 Gy for larger tumours.

Sequelae of radiation therapy:

Acute:

- Fatigue, nausea, diarrhoea, abdominal cramping, bladder irritation and dysuria, rectal discomfort, occasionally, rectal bleeding
- Pruritus, erythema, pigmentation and dry/moist desquamation in perineum or intergluteal fold
- Radiation vaginitis/superficial ulceration of vagina/vaginal stenosis
- Acute effects occur to some degree in most patients undergoing RT and are typically magnified by concurrent chemotherapy. However, acute effects can often be managed with medications and supportive care, and they resolve soon after completion of treatment.

Late:

- Rectovaginal/vesicovaginal fistula: 1–2%
- Proctitis/cystitis (3–5% stage I–IIA, 10–15% for stage IIB–III)
- Ureteral stricture (1–3%)
- Intestinal obstruction or perforation (<5%)
- Vaginal stenosis
- Anal incontinence
- Femoral neck fractures/lumbosacral plexopathy (extremely rare).

These late complication data come from the older literature and with the advent of modern technology and image-based 3D treatment planning for both EBRT and brachytherapy, the treatment-related complications can be minimised to a great extent with both improved dose conformity to the target volume with reduction in dose to the organs at risk.

Combined Radiotherapy and Surgery

Intraoperative radiotherapy (IORT) is a specialised technique that delivers a single highly focused radiation to a tumour bed at risk or isolated unresectable residual during an open surgical procedure. The bowel is retracted out of the field, and RT is administered.

Chemotherapy

Chemotherapy has not been shown to cure cervical cancer, but it can cause significant tumour regression. Single agents used are cisplatin, bleomycin, ifosfamide and methotrexate. The best response rates have been observed with cisplatin-based combinations. Neoadjuvant chemotherapy has been used in cases with bulky tumours preoperatively and in combination with radiotherapy. However, it has not been shown to improve survival rates. Anti-vascular endothelial growth factor (VEGF) such as bevacizumab (BV) commercially available as Avastin acts against circulating VEGF and, therefore, arrests angiogenesis and disease progression. The use of BV as a second-line chemotherapy in persistent, recurrent or metastatic cervical cancer in combination with chemotherapy has been proven in various clinical trial settings.

Relapse

Management of patients who relapse after primary treatment: Treatment decisions should be based on the performance status of the patient, the site of recurrence and/or metastases, the extent of metastatic disease and the prior treatment. In regional recurrence, following are the options:

- *Radical surgery:* Pelvic exenteration may be an alternative (particularly if a fistula is present) to radical radiotherapy and concurrent chemotherapy in selected patients without pelvic sidewall involvement.
- RT is indicated in patients with locally recurrent cervical cancer following radical surgery.

- Concurrent chemotherapy with either 5-fluorouracil and/or cisplatin with radiation should be considered and may improve outcome.

In case of distant metastasis, treatment is for palliative intent only, and the patient should be encouraged to take part in clinical trials. The options are systemic chemotherapy, local ablation and localised radiotherapy according to the site of distant metastasis. The prognosis is better for patients with a disease-free interval >6 months, a recurrence 3 cm or less in diameter and no sidewall fixation. The 5-year survival for patients selected for treatment with pelvic exenteration is in the order of 30–60%, and the operative mortality should be <10%.

Post-treatment Surveillance

Whatever the method of treatment, the patient treated for invasive cancer of the cervix should thereafter be examined routinely every 3 months in the first 2 years, 6 monthly for the next 3 years, and yearly thereafter. At each visit, assessment of the situation is made by analysis of symptoms and physical signs, by cytology, renal function tests and sometimes, with large central tumours, by endocervical curettage. A chest X-ray may be done annually in patients with advanced disease. Intravenous pyelography is indicated if a pelvic mass is detected or if there are urinary symptoms. CT scan may be done at 6–12 months in surgically treated patients with a high risk of recurrence to allow for early institution of radiotherapy. It is sometimes difficult to distinguish recurrence of cancer from later radiation reaction in the parametrium on cytology. As a general rule, however, it is wise to assume that any woman who, after a period of complete freedom after treatment, has a return of symptoms, or develops symptoms referable to the pelvic organs, has a return of growth. Most recurrences occur within the first 2 years after therapy.

Premenopausal patients may require counselling for sexual dysfunction and can be given hormone replacement therapy.

Stump Carcinoma

The possible development of cancer in the cervical stump after subtotal hysterectomy is one of the reasons why this operation had virtually disappeared from gynaecological practice. Sometimes, the malignancy represents a recurrence of carcinoma of the corpus (or even of the cervix) which was present at the time of operation and passed unrecognised. Otherwise, the carcinoma (usually squamous cell) develops de novo, and is especially likely when the hysterectomy has been performed for pelvic infection. The incidence naturally varies with the standards of gynaecology in any area. Where subtotal hysterectomy is carried out exceptionally, and then only after a negative cervical smear, stump carcinoma is rare. The tumour behaves like any cancer of the cervix but carries a less favourable prognosis because the peritoneal cavity, the bladder and the rectum are all at the top of the stump. So, they become invaded early and do not allow the vital high intrauterine dose of radiotherapy. Radical surgery is more difficult and less complete in these cases because of the disturbed anatomy. The 5-year survival rate for all cases of stump carcinoma after any method of treatment was formerly only 20–30%, but the prospects have improved with modern radiotherapeutic apparatus and combinations of radiotherapy and radical surgery. 5-year survival rates of up to 60% are obtained in most advanced clinics.

Carcinoma of the Cervix Complicated by Other Pelvic Conditions

Carcinoma of the Cervix and Pregnancy

Cases of invasive cancer of the cervix discovered during pregnancy are usually stage I or stage II. The prognosis for those with advanced disease is relatively unfavourable, because the patient is relatively young, the hormonal and vascular changes in pregnancy encourage rapid growth and early dissemination and the presence of the pregnancy hinders treatment. Diagnosis is usually made by a colposcopy-directed biopsy if the Pap test is positive. However, if this is not possible, a diagnostic conisation may be necessary, and this should be done in the second trimester only if the Pap smear is strongly suggestive of invasive cancer, as the procedure carries a high risk of abortion. Treatment depends on the stage of disease, the period of gestation and the wishes of the patient. In stage IA with no LVSI, patients may be delivered vaginally at term followed by hysterectomy 6 weeks later if no further childbearing is required or a conisation if further childbearing is required.

In stage IA1 with LVSI and stage IA2, delivery is at term but by caesarean section, and modified radical hysterectomy with pelvic node dissection is carried out at the same time. The tissue planes separate easily during pregnancy so dissection is facilitated, but there may be troublesome haemorrhage from engorged veins around the vagina.

In stage IB, delivery can be delayed for a maximum of 4 weeks in the interest of improving foetal lung maturity. In tertiary care institutions, the foetus can be delivered after 32 weeks by classical caesarean section and radical hysterectomy with pelvic lymph node dissection. In stages II through IV, radiotherapy is the treatment of choice. In the first trimester, treatment is started with EBRT; the treatment of malignant tumour takes precedence over continuation of pregnancy, and spontaneous abortion may occur after the first few fractions and usually results before the delivery of 40 Gy. In the second trimester, the patient's wishes and the available facilities need to be taken into consideration before deciding the timing.

In the third trimester, treatment is by classical caesarean section after foetal maturity is attained. This is followed by external irradiation and intracavitary therapy. The treatment is usually commenced 4–21 days after delivery of the child.

The overall 5-year survival rate is slightly better for patients with carcinoma of the cervix in pregnancy, because they are usually in an early stage of the disease.

Carcinoma of the Cervix Associated with Uterine Leiomyomas and Ovarian Cysts

An ovarian cyst can be removed first, radiotherapy being given 2–4 weeks later. If large uterine leiomyomas interfere with adequate irradiation, a radical hysterectomy, or a combination of this with radiotherapy, is clearly indicated. In some cases, it may be possible to carry out radiotherapy in full, leaving the removal of the second tumour until later; the disadvantage is that the cyst or myoma may undergo necrosis.

Carcinoma of the Cervix Associated with Salpingo-oophoritis

Because of probable exacerbations with peritonitis and abscess formation, the presence of an inflammatory lesion in the adnexa, even a quiescent one, is a contraindication for radiotherapy. Radical surgery is preferable if it is technically possible. If it is not, it may be necessary to operate on the tubal disease first (bilateral salpingectomy or salpingo-oophorectomy) and to follow this by radiotherapy 4–6 weeks later.

OTHER MALIGNANT TUMOURS OF THE CERVIX

These include growths which have spread or metastasised from elsewhere, usually from the body of the uterus or from the vagina. Rare primary tumours include the melanoma. Sarcoma and mixed Müllerian tumours are considered similar tumours arising in the body of the uterus.

SUGGESTED READING

1. Brown DC, Cole D, Gatter KC, Mason DY. Carcinoma of the cervix uteri: an assessment of tumour proliferation using the monoclonal antibody Ki67. Br J Cancer. 1988;57(2): 178-81.
2. Cocuzza CE, Martinelli M, Sina F, Piana A, Sotgiu G, Dell'Anna T, et al. Human papillomavirus DNA detection in plasma and cervical samples of women with a recent history of low grade or precancerous cervical dysplasia. PLoS One. 2017;12(11):e0188592.
3. Kamphuis EI, Naber SK, Danhof NA, Habbema JDF, de Groot CJM, Mol BWJ. Effect of cervical cancer screening programs on preterm birth: a decision and cost-effectiveness analysis. Obstet Gynecol. 2017;130(6):1207-17.
4. Koc N, Arinkan SA, Ozbay NO, Selcuk S. Colloid carcinoma of the uterine cervix and its immunohistochemical analysis: a case report. J Pathol Transl Med. 2018;52(1): 56-60.
5. Radiopaedia. (2018). WHO histological classification of tumours of the uterine cervix. [online] Available from https://radiopaedia.org/articles/who-classification-of-tumours-of-the-uterine-cervix-5th-edition?lang=us. [Last accessed April, 2025].
6. World Health Organisation. (2018). WHO histological classification of tumours of the uterine cervix. [online] Available from http://screening.iarc.fr/atlasclassifwho.php. [Accessed April, 2025].

31

CHAPTER

Tumours of the Corpus Uteri

Saritha Shamsunder, Sufian Zaheer, Shivani Verma

Chapter Outline

- Enlargement of the Uterus
- Uterine Polyps
- Benign Neoplasms
- Malignant Neoplasms
- Molecular Classification
- Adjuvant Treatment
- Endometrial Stromal Tumours

ENLARGEMENT OF THE UTERUS

The causes of enlargement of the body of the uterus are as follows **(Table 1)**:

- *Pregnancy or recent pregnancy:* This is the most common and the first possible cause to be considered in the reproductive age group.
- *Retained products of conception:* Incomplete abortion and placental polyp. Delayed and incomplete involution
- *Distension by fluid:* Haematometra; pyometra; hydrometra
- *Hypertrophy (myohyperplasia):* Developmental or idiopathic; active or passive congestion; excessive oestrogen or oestrogen/progestogen stimulus; adenomyosis
- *Cysts:* These, it is believed, arise from Müllerian diverticula and are exceptionally rare.
- *Benign neoplasms:*
  - Leiomyoma
  - Rarities such as the haemangioma, glioma and fibro-osteochondroma (<100 cases reported)
- *Malignant neoplasms:*
  - Carcinoma
  - Sarcoma
  - Choriocarcinoma
  - Mixed mesodermal tumours
  - Metastatic growth from any site, including melanoma
  - Rarities such as lymphoma and diffuse large B-cell lymphoma (DLBCL) are the most common and haemangiopericytoma.

TABLE 1: Diseases associated with enlargement of the body of the uterus.

Disease	*Differentiating signs/symptoms*	*Diagnostic tests*
Adenomyosis	Congestive dysmenorrhoea	Distinguished by histopathological examination, imaging with pelvic USG and MRI
Endometrial polyp	Spasmodic dysmenorrhoea, intermenstrual spotting	Sonohysterography (SHG), MRI
Endometrial hyperplasia	Heavy and irregular bleeding per vaginum with passage of clots	Hysteroscopic guided endometrial biopsy and curettage followed by histopathology
Endometrial carcinoma	Abnormal vaginal bleeding or discharge	Endometrial sampling, dilatation and curettage
Uterine sarcoma	Rapid growth of the tumour	Serial MRI
Pregnancy	Symptoms of pregnancy and missed menstrual period	Pelvic USG, blood or urine beta-hCG

(hCG: human chorionic gonadotrophin; MRI: magnetic resonance imaging; USG: ultrasonography)

UTERINE POLYPS

Many tumours of the uterus present as polyps within its cavity; the common causes are:

- *Benign:*
  - Adenoma (mucous)
  - Leiomyoma (fibroid)
  - Placental (or foetal)
- *Malignant:*
  - Carcinoma
  - Sarcoma; mixed Müllerian tumours
  - Choriocarcinoma

BENIGN NEOPLASMS

Adenoma

Pathology

A true adenoma occurs with or without associated endometrial hyperplasia and is invariably polypoidal (mucous polyp) **(Fig. 1)**. Polyps can be single or multiple; they rarely exceed a grape in size. On histopathology, it shows endometrial glands and stroma, and these may or may not show reaction to ovarian hormones by exhibiting the menstrual phases. The cause of single mucous polyps is unknown. Single endometrial polyps are common, especially in the postmenopausal uterus, when they are mostly asymptomatic; they are often surprise findings on opening the excised organ.

Multiple polyps have a strong tendency to recur as they are generally a manifestation of endometrial hyperplasia with a persisting background of hypoestrogenism.

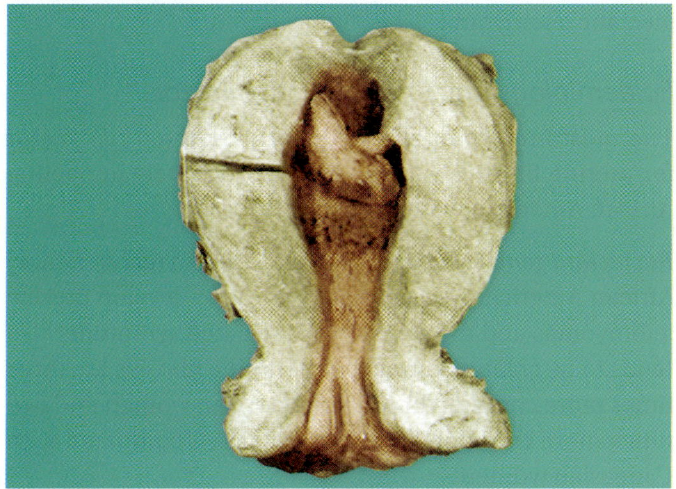

Fig. 1: An endometrial polyp.

Clinical Features

Symptoms are more likely when the tip of the polyp becomes necrotic and ulcerated; these include menorrhagia, intermenstrual (or postmenopausal) discharge, bleeding after coitus and, occasionally, dysmenorrhoea. The presence of a polyp may be suspected from the history and by finding the cervix patulous with the polyp at the os.

Transvaginal ultrasound reveals a thickened endometrial shadow **(Fig. 2A)**. The endometrial polyp may be outlined at saline infusion sonography **(Fig. 2B)** or hysterography. The diagnosis is made for certain by hysteroscopy or if the polyp is removed by curettage.

Treatment

Curettage can be done, but this is not always satisfactory, because one or more polyps may elude the polyp forceps. Hysteroscopy-guided polypectomy is the gold standard; rarely, hysterectomy may be required if there is associated endometrial pathology.

Leiomyoma (Myoma and Fibromyoma)

Pathology

Leiomyoma is the most common of all pelvic tumours, present in 20% of women in the reproductive age group, and increasing with age. It is composed essentially of muscle tissue although there is a variable amount of fibrous connective tissue as well, especially in the older and larger tumours **(Fig. 3)**. It is also termed *myoma* or *fibromyoma* and is popularly called a fibroid. Various types of fibroids are shown in the **Figures 4 to 7** and are classified by their location **(Flowchart 1)**.

Each individual uterine leiomyoma is monoclonal. It arises from a somatic mutation in a progenitor myocyte. Multiple chromosomal abnormalities are detected in approximately 50% of leiomyomas by cytogenetic analysis; the most common being translocation between the long arms of chromosomes 12–14, followed by deletion on the long arm of chromosome Y.

Leiomyomas are frequently multiple and as many as 200 may be found in one uterus **(Fig. 8)**. More often, the number is between 5 and 30. The tumours tend to be spherical in shape, although their surface can be lobulated **(Figs. 8 and 9)**. They are surrounded by a pseudo capsule **(Fig. 5)**, which consists of compressed normal uterine wall. Except when modified by degeneration, they are hard

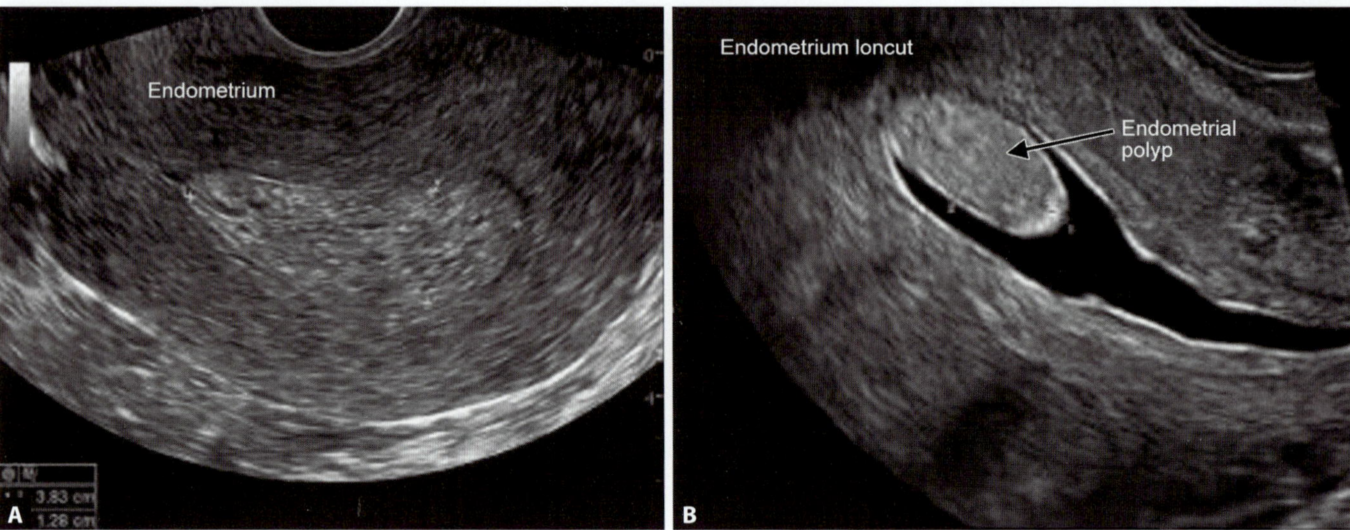

Figs. 2A and B: (A) Transvaginal sonogram shows an appearance of a thickened endometrium; (B) Saline infusion sonography. A polyp is seen projecting into the endometrial cavity. This was confirmed and resected at hysteroscopy.

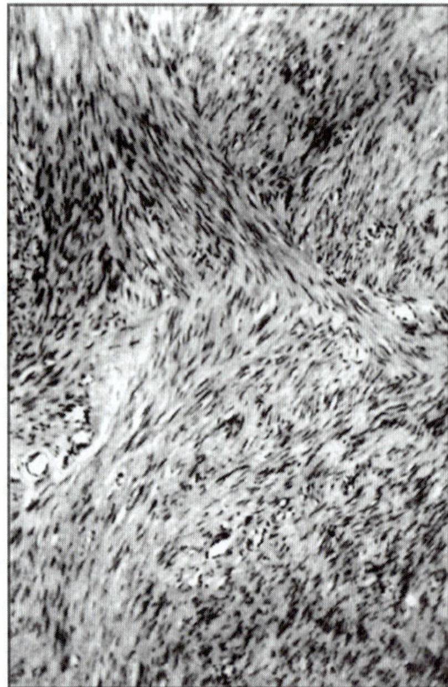

Fig. 3: Microphotograph of a leiomyoma of the uterus showing the interlacing bonds of smooth muscle and fibrous tissue.

in consistency and their cut surface presents a white and whorled appearance. They can grow to a large size, filling the whole abdomen. With the availability of ultrasound, they are detected earlier; however, mammoth tumours are rarely found **(Figs. 10 and 11)**.

Leiomyomas are slow to grow, and the rate of growth varies from patient-to-patient and from time-to-time in the same patient. There may be waves of growth interspersed with phases of quiescence, and a degenerative change can cause a rapid and gross enlargement of any tumour **(Fig. 12)**. An arrest or slowing of activity is most likely after the menopause, but at least 10% of leiomyomas continue to grow after this time.

The tumours themselves are relatively avascular, the main blood vessels being distributed in their capsules. Occasionally, a tumour has numerous blood or lymph vessels, with large cavernous spaces throughout its substance; it is then called a telangiectatic or a lymphangiectatic leiomyoma.

Epidemiology and Risk/Protective Factors

The most important and frequently reported risk factor for uterine fibroids is race, disproportionately impacting African American women **(Table 2)**.

Racial and genetic factors: Women of certain races, notably African American, are especially prone to develop uterine leiomyomas and the severity of associated symptoms also tends to be greater among them. Uterine fibroids are three times more common in African American women and two times more common in Hispanic women compared with Caucasian women.

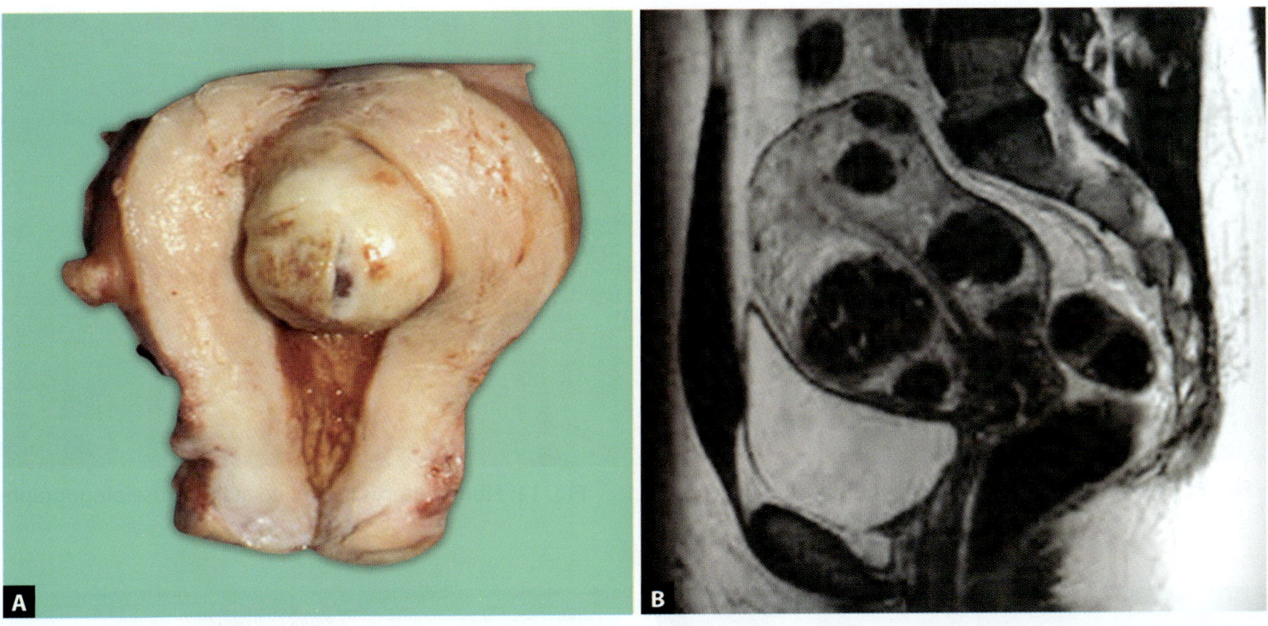

Figs. 4A and B: Fibroids.

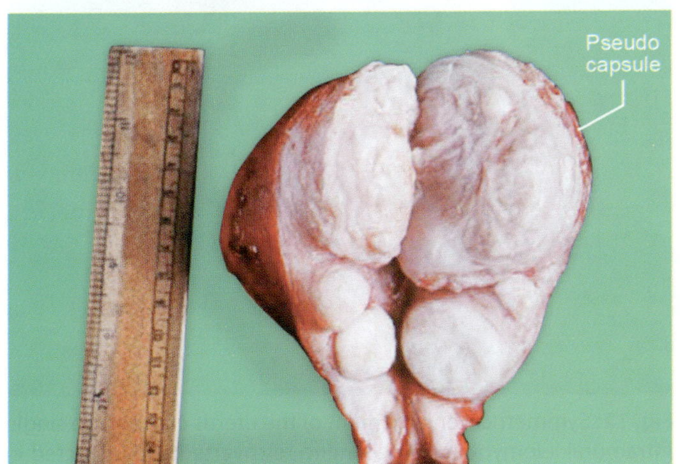

Fig. 5: Fibroid.

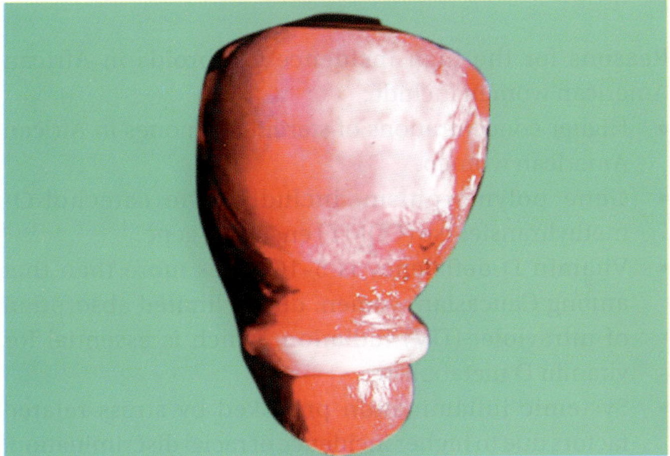

Fig. 6: Fibroid polyp.

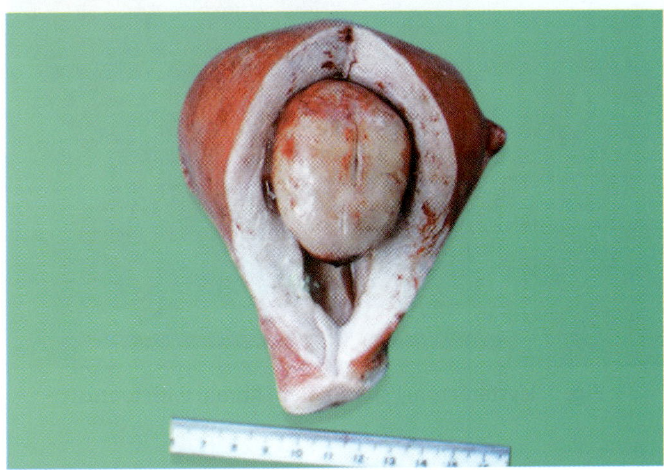

Fig. 7: Fibroids intracavitary.

Flowchart 1: Uterine fibroids.

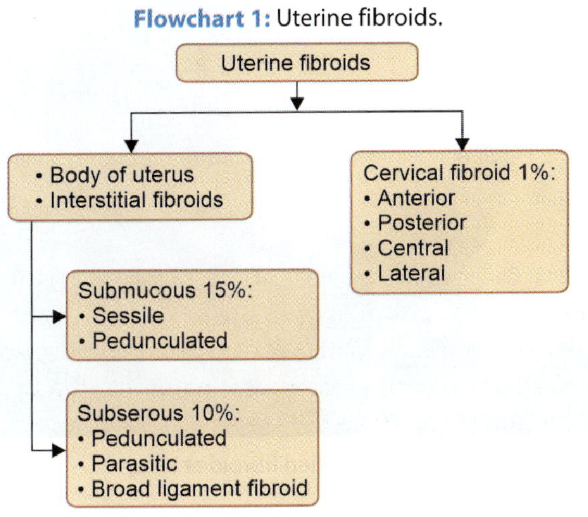

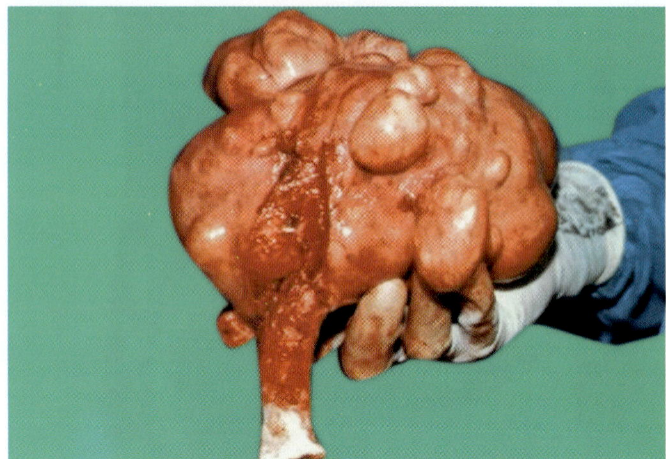

Fig. 8: Hysterectomy specimen with multiple fibroids.

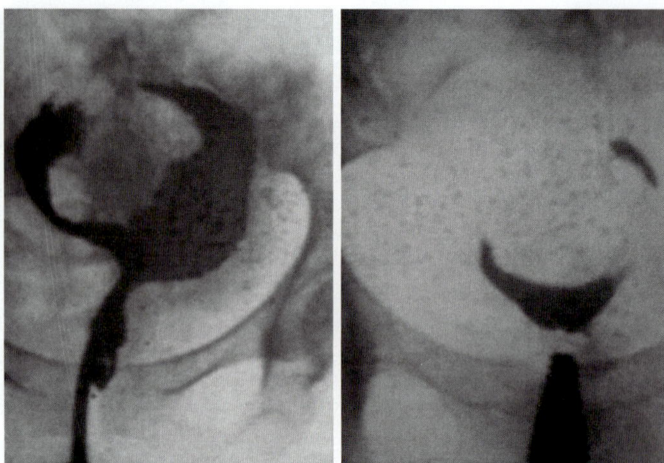

Fig. 11: Fibroid uterus identified at hysterosalpingography.

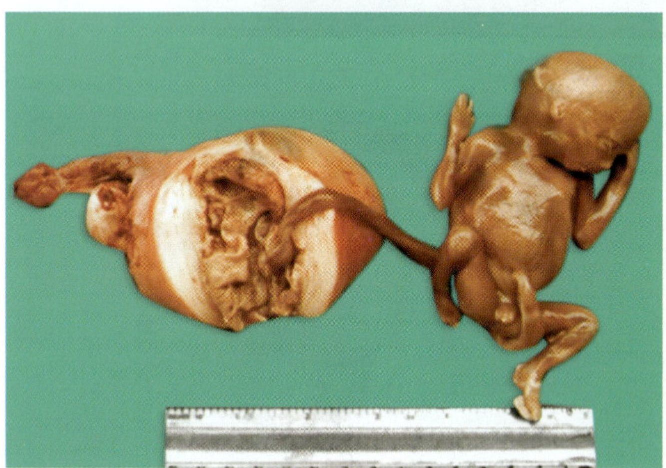

Fig. 9: Hysterectomy specimen of fibroid with foetus.

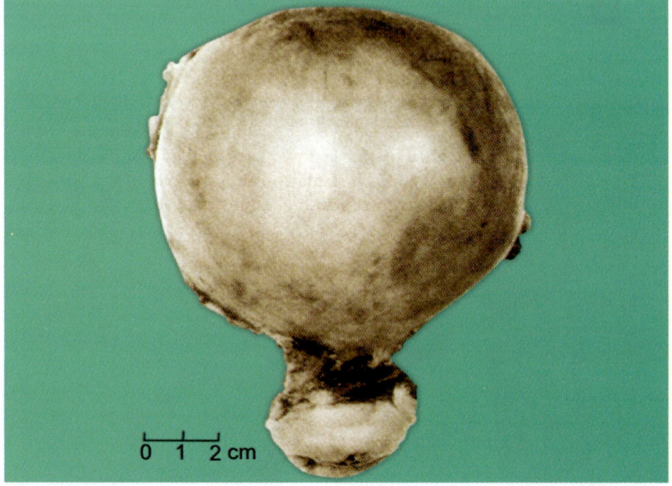

Fig. 12: Symmetrical enlargement of the uterus caused by a single intramural leiomyoma. By becoming retroverted and impacted in the pelvis, this uterus caused acute retention of urine in a woman aged 44 years.

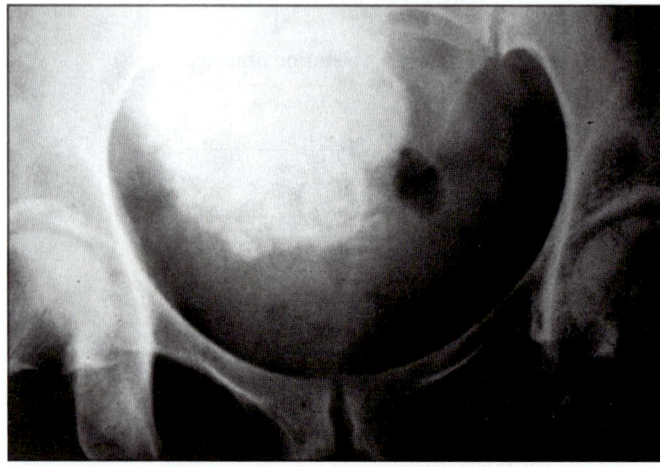

Fig. 10: Calcified fibroid at X-ray.

Reasons for the high incidence of fibroids in African American women include:

- Higher concentrations of steroid hormones in African American women.
- Gene polymorphism, including the catechol-O-methyltransferase (COMT) encoding gene.
- Vitamin D deficiency is 5–10 times more than that among Caucasian women, due to limited absorption of ultraviolet (UV) radiation, which is essential for vitamin D metabolism.
- Systemic inflammation provoked by stress-related factors due to higher incidence of racial discrimination.

TABLE 2: Risk factors and protective factors.

Risk factors	***Protective factors***
Race (African American > Caucasian)	Combined oral contraception
Older age	Injectable medroxyprogesterone acetate in the depot form
Premenopausal state	Smoking in women of low mass
Nulliparity	Multiparity
Family history of uterine fibroids	Diet rich in citrus fruits
Hypertension	Green vegetables, fruit and fish
Food additives such as butylated hydroxytoluene (BHT), Bisphenol A	
Frequent consumption of soybean milk	
Obesity	
Vitamin D deficiency	
Excessive vitamin E levels	
Altered reproductive tract biome	
Exposure to endocrine disrupting chemicals (organophosphate esters and plasticisers)	

Age: Uterine leiomyomas are rare before the age of 20 years but are to be found, if only as single tiny tumours, in approximately 20% of women over 20 years of age and in 40% of women over the age of 40 years. They most commonly cause symptoms between the ages of 35 and 45 years but probably exist in microscopic form before the age of 30 years. Sporadic cases have been reported in adolescents, and they were recognised to have a translocation between chromosomes 12 and 14, which is a confirmed risk factor for uterine fibroids. The use of hormonal replacement therapy in menopausal women with asymptomatic fibroids may cause them to regrow and induce the first clinical symptoms of uterine fibroids.

Obesity: Metabolic functions of adipose tissues play a significant role in obese women for uterine fibroids development. Adrenal androgens are mostly metabolised by aromatase in adipose tissues to oestrogens. There is an associated decline in the production of the sex hormone-binding globulin (SHBG), which binds circulating hormones and disrupts the hormonal activity.

An increase in the body mass index (BMI) by one-unit, abdominal visceral fat, higher waist-to-hip ratios and body fat percentage exceeding 30% increase the risk for uterine fibroids.

Obese women with type 2 diabetes are more likely to develop uterine fibroids due to elevated concentrations of insulin-like growth factor (IGF-1) and associated insulin resistance. Uterine fibroids occur frequently in obese postmenopausal women and those who have undergone hormonal replacement therapy.

Parity: Leiomyomas are more common in nulliparous or relatively infertile women, but it is not known whether infertility causes leiomyomas or vice versa, or whether both conditions have a common cause. Steroid hormone exposure during pregnancy and remodelling of the uterine tissues after each pregnancy may be attributable to a decrease in uterine fibroid formation.

Hypertension: Women suffering from hypertension are five times more likely to develop uterine fibroids and earlier diagnosis of hypertension is a significant factor. Development of fibroids is attributed to the chronic destruction of the myometrium due to increased blood flow and cytokines secreted by injured myometrial cells. Increased diastolic blood pressure is associated with a higher risk of uterine fibroids, despite the use of antihypertensive drugs.

Caffeine and alcohol: An association has been reported between alcohol and caffeine intake and an increased risk of developing uterine fibroids in a study concerning the health of women of African origin.

Uterine Fibroids Driver Mutations

The application of advanced genomic technologies in the past decade, including sequencing methodologies, has led to the identification of recurrent and mutually exclusive genetic alterations (so-called *drivers*) responsible for the formation of uterine fibroids. Among these, somatic mutations in the *Xq13* gene encoding the ribonucleic acid (RNA) polymerase II (Pol II) mediator subunit MED12 are the most prevalent, occurring in 45–90% of cases of uterine fibroids depending upon patient ethnicity. A smaller fraction of uterine fibroids has been attributed to genetic alterations leading to overexpression of *HMGA2*, disruption of the *COL4A5-COL4A6* locus and biallelic loss of *FH* encoding the tricarboxylic acid (TCA) cycle enzyme fumarate hydratase. Recurrent deletions and rearrangements involving chromosomes 6p21, 7q22, 22q and 1p have also been observed. These mutations generally co-occur with other genetic alterations, suggesting that they represent secondary driver events restricted to a subpopulation of tumour cells.

Sites

Leiomyomas are described as being subserous, interstitial or submucous, according to their relationship to the peritoneal coat and to the endometrium **(Fig. 13)**. Their site is determined by the position of their origin and by the direction in which they grow; an interstitial leiomyoma can, by development, become submucous or subperitoneal. Subserous and submucous leiomyomas often become pedunculated.

Most leiomyomas are situated in the body of the uterus but in 1–2% of cases they are confined to the cervix, usually to its supravaginal portion. A cervical leiomyoma is commonly single and is either interstitial or subserous **(Fig. 14)**. Rarely, does it become submucous and polypoidal. The subserous tumour usually grows out into the broad ligament. Cervical leiomyoma presents special clinical features because, being extraperitoneal, it remains fixed in the pelvis and displaces the bladder and ureters; its removal is hence difficult.

Extrauterine leiomyomas may develop in the broad ligament or at other sites where smooth muscle exists **(Fig. 15A)**. A myoma developing in the cervical stump after subtotal hysterectomy is rare but possible and can create a surgical problem **(Fig. 15B)**.

In 2011, The International Federation of Gynaecology and Obstetrics (FIGO) published a classification system for categorising the location of uterine fibroids, which

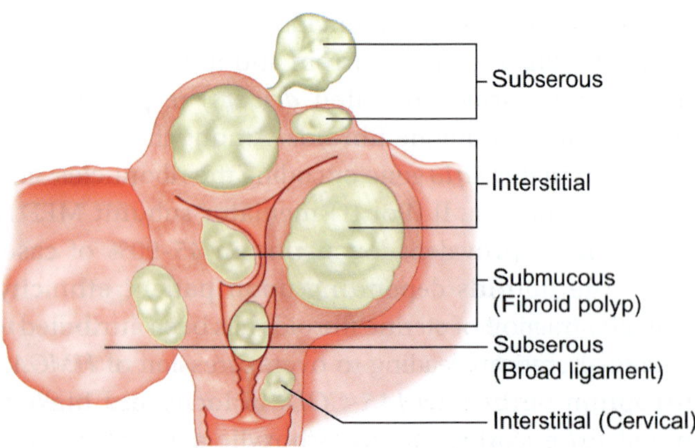

Fig. 13: The sites of uterine leiomyomas.

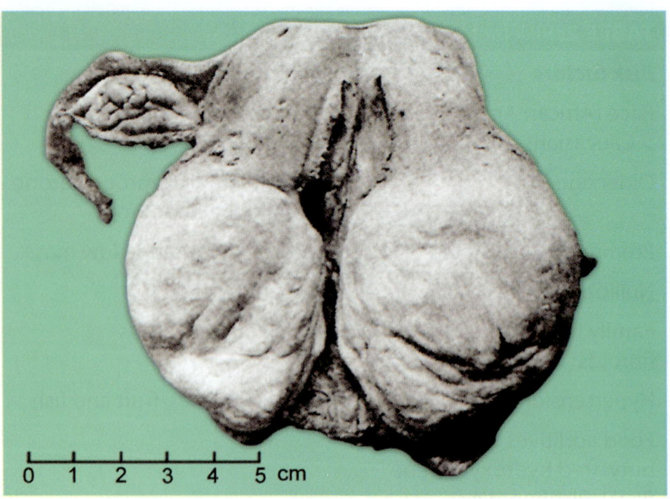

Fig. 14: An interstitial cervical leiomyoma.

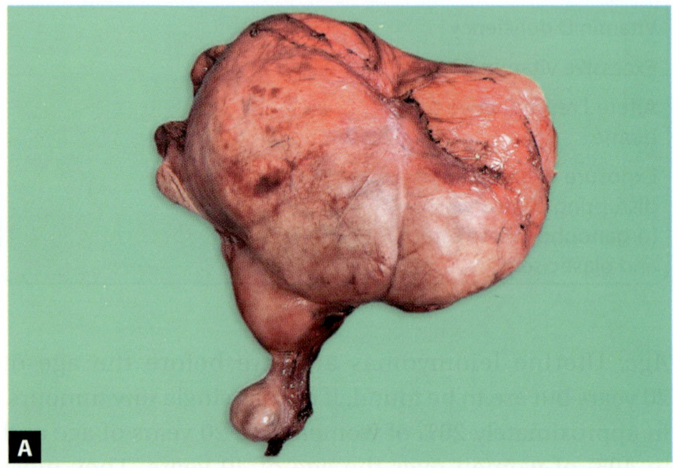

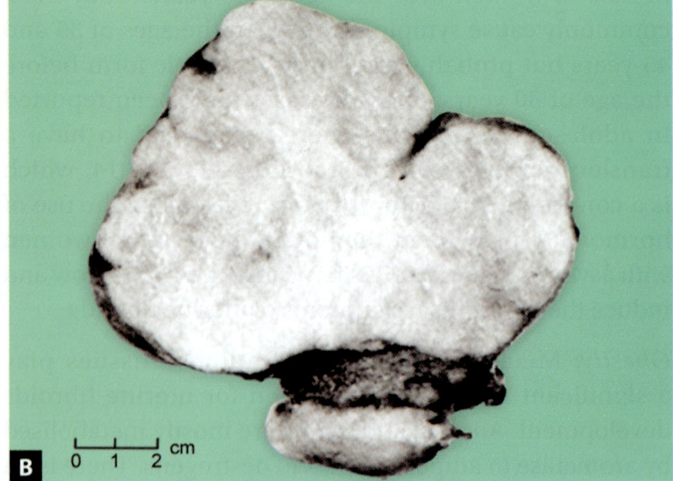

Figs. 15A and B: (A) Broad ligament leiomyoma arising from the lateral wall of the uterus; (B) A myoma growing from the cervical stump after previous subtotal hysterectomy.

TABLE 3: FIGO classification of fibroids.

Localisation	***Type***	***Description***
Submucosal	0	Pedunculated intracavitary fibroid (i.e. submucosal fibroid without intramural extension)
	1	Submucosal fibroid with intramural extension <50%
	2	Submucosal fibroid with intramural extension >50%
Intramural	3	Intramural fibroid in contact with the endometrium but not extending into the uterine cavity or serous surface
	4	Intramural fibroid without contact with the endometrium and without extension into the uterine cavity or serous surface
Subserosal	5	Subserosal fibroid with intramural extension >50% and <50% subserosal
	6	Subserosal fibroid with intramural extension <50% and >50% subserosa
	7	Subserosal pedunculated fibroid
Other	8	Other types of fibroids (e.g. cervical, broad ligament and parasitic fibroids)
Hybrid type	2–5	Hybrid classification used when a fibroid extends from the endometrial cavity to the serosa, composed of two numbers, separated by a hyphen, the first characterising the relationship between the fibroid and the endometrium and the second characterising its relationship with the serosa

(FIGO: International Federation of Gynaecology and Obstetrics)

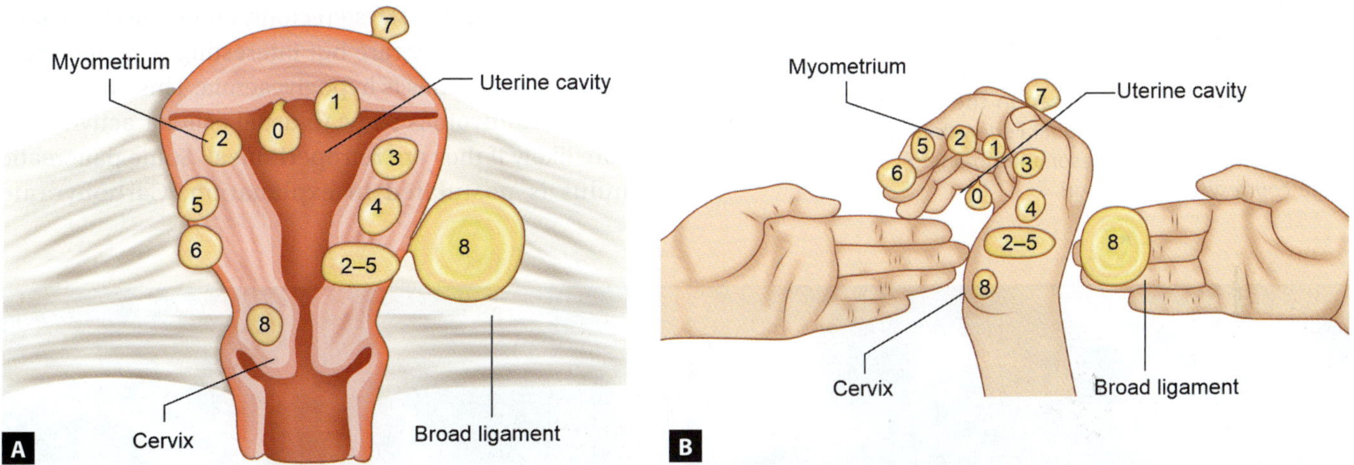

Figs. 16A and B: The 'Hand as Foot' teaching method in fibroids demonstrating FIGO classification of fibroids. (FIGO: International Federation of Gynaecology and Obstetrics)

includes a total of nine types of fibroids—types 0 through 8 (as presented in **Table 3 and Figs. 16A and B**).

The FIGO classification system was revised in 2018 and suggests that an estimate of the total uterine volume should be provided in the ultrasound report, and report should include the estimated total number of fibroids. In addition, the report should include the estimated volumes of up to four fibroids and their locations, described as anterior, posterior, right, left or fundus. The relationship between the endometrium and fibroids should be recorded in accordance with the FIGO classification system **(Figs. 17 to 20)**.

Symptoms

The majority of small leiomyomas and some large ones are symptomless.

The nearer the leiomyoma to the endometrial cavity, the more likely it is to cause symptoms, especially menstrual symptoms **(Box 1)**.

A leiomyoma does not cause pain unless it is complicated by: Extrusion from the uterus as a polyp—in this case, the pain is caused by uterine colic, which *aborts* the myoma; torsion of its pedicle or of the uterus; degeneration; sarcomatous change; or adhesions to other organs. One of the latter is being extruded through the cervix.

Pain that accompanies uterine leiomyomas is often caused by an associated lesion, especially endometriosis.

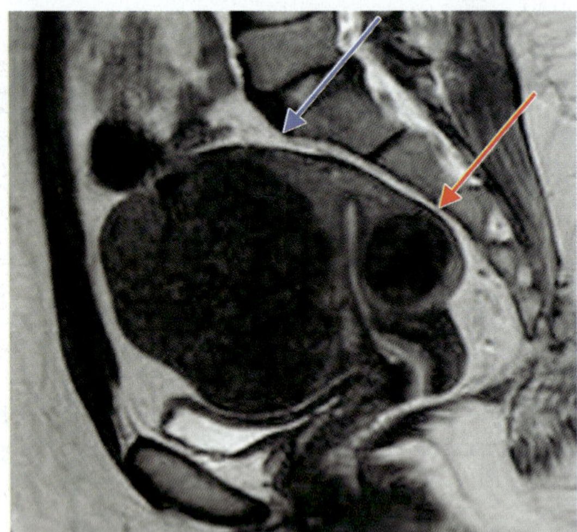

Fig. 17: A 44-year-old lady with complaint of abdominal discomfort, on MRI sagittal plane T2-weighted images, showing a large subserosal fibroid with >50% intramural component (FIGO type 5), arising from anterior myometrium (blue arrow). Another small intramural fibroid is seen in the posterior myometrium (red arrow). (FIGO: International Federation of Gynaecology and Obstetrics; MRI: magnetic resonance imaging)
Image courtesy: Dr Neha Bagri.

General Effects

Manifestations of anaemia, such as palpitation, lassitude and even loss of weight, are common and can constitute the presenting symptoms; they result from menorrhagia.

A rare finding is polycythaemia, which disappears when the leiomyoma is removed. In such cases, the myoma is usually, if not always, large and situated in the broad ligament. The site may be important because polycythaemia is also known to complicate other types of broad ligament tumours, which can be explained as:

- The tumour is itself erythropoietic—islands of extramedullary erythropoiesis have been documented in leiomyomas; a high level of erythropoietin activity has been reported within uterine leiomyomas.
- Arteriovenous shunts have also been found in these tumours and these may also play a role; the tumour presses on the ureter and affects the erythropoietic function of the kidney.

Polycythaemia increases the risk of thromboembolism, with or without surgery. Hysterectomy cures polycythaemia.

Another extremely rare but interesting systemic effect of uterine leiomyomas is hypoglycaemia. This only occurs when the leiomyomas show unusual cellular activity and is more likely if they are retroperitoneal. Some pancreatic stimulus is postulated in explanation. Carbohydrate

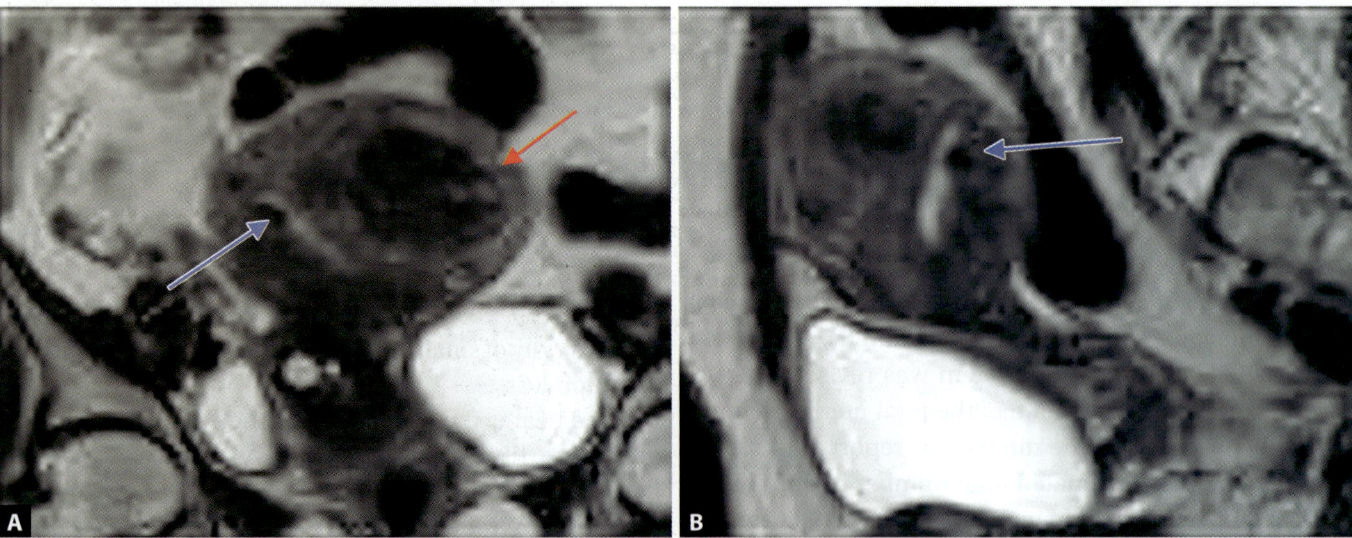

Figs. 18A and B: A 43-year-old lady with complaints of irregular menstrual bleeding. On MRI pelvis, (A) coronal T2 and (B) sagittal T2 images showing a small submucosal fibroid >50% intramural (blue arrow). The red arrow in A showing a large intramural fibroid. (MRI: magnetic resonance imaging)
Image courtesy: Dr Neha Bagri.

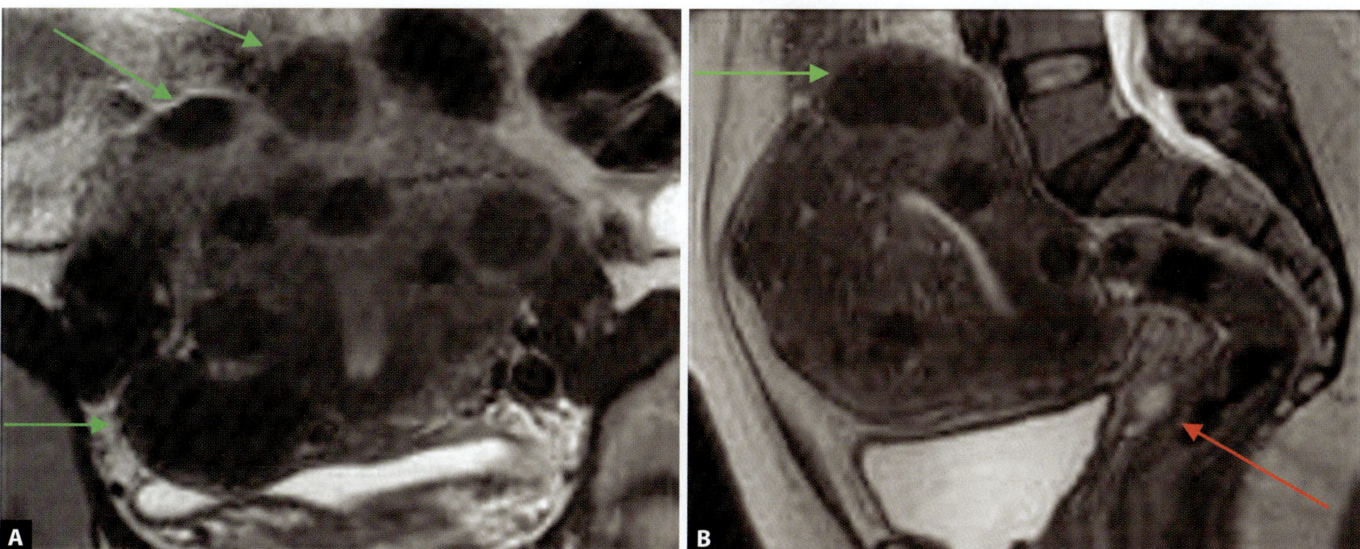

Figs. 19A and B: A 39-year-old lady with complaint of lower back pain and AUB. On MRI pelvis, (A) coronal T2 and (B) sagittal T2 images showing multiple subserosal fibroids with >50% intramural component (FIGO type 5, green arrows). The red arrow in B showing a Gartner's duct cyst: An incidental finding. (AUB: abnormal uterine bleeding; FIGO: International Federation of Gynaecology and Obstetrics; MRI: magnetic resonance imaging)
Image courtesy: Dr Neha Bagri.

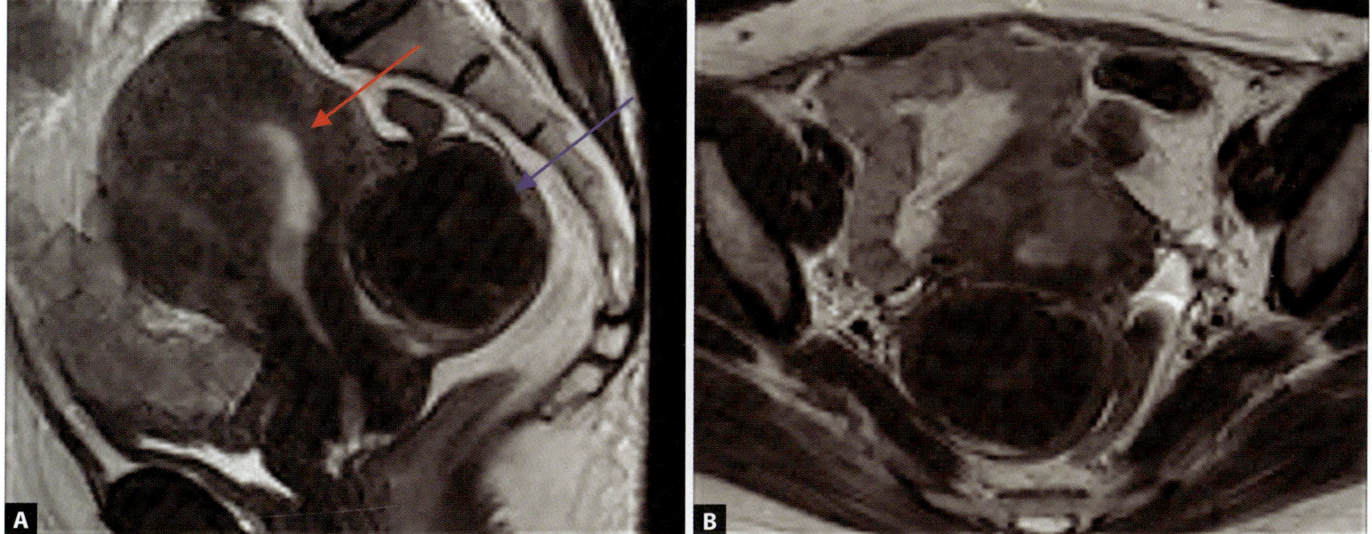

Figs. 20A and B: A 36-year-old lady with complaint of lower back pain. On MRI pelvis, (A) sagittal T2 and (B) axial T2 images showing a large subserosal fibroid with <50% intramural component (FIGO type 6) seen arising from the posterior myometrium. (A) The blue arrow showing fibroid, and the red arrow showing endometrium. (FIGO: International Federation of Gynaecology and Obstetrics; MRI: magnetic resonance imaging)
Image courtesy: Dr Neha Bagri.

BOX 1: Spectrum of clinical symptoms of fibroid.

- *Incidental finding:* Asymptomatic
- *Gynaecological:* Abnormal uterine bleeding (AUB)
- *Reproductive problems:* Infertility
- *Obstetric problems:* EPL, RPL, PTL, PPROM, IUGR, pain, red degeneration, malpresentation, dysfunctional labour, LSCS and PPH
- *Pressure symptoms:* Urinary tract obstruction, bowel symptoms
- *Generalised symptoms:* Anaemia, poor health
- *Rare symptoms:* Ascites, polycythaemia, benign metastasising uterine fibroids with renal cell carcinoma
- *Malignant change:* Sarcomatous change

(EPL: early pregnancy loss; IUGR: intrauterine growth retardation; LSCS: lower segment caesarean section; PPH: postpartum haemorrhage; PPROM: preterm premature rupture of membranes; PTL: preterm labour; RPL: recurrent pregnancy loss)

metabolism returns to normal after removal of the tumour. Hypokalaemia has also been reported.

Menstrual Disturbances

The characteristic symptom of leiomyomas is *abnormal uterine bleeding (AUB)*, which is usually heavy, with increased blood loss at normally spaced intervals, gradual in onset and progressive. The duration of the period may be normal or prolonged; the loss being heaviest on the second and the third day of the cycle. Amenorrhoea in a woman with leiomyoma may be due to pregnancy or postmenopause.

The factors causing heavy menstrual bleeding are an increase in size of the endometrial cavity and of the bleeding surface; increased vascularity of the uterus; associated endometrial hyperplasia; hypoestrogenism; compression of veins by the tumour(s) with consequent dilatation and engorgement of venous plexuses in the endometrium and myometrium; and interference with uterine contractions which are alleged to control the blood flow through the uterine wall (theoretical).

Spasmodic dysmenorrhoea is possible when a submucous tumour stimulates expulsive uterine contractions, but it is not common. Dysmenorrhoea of an unusual character, severe but one-sided, can be caused by a single but quite small leiomyoma, which happens to be sited at the uterotubal junction, from which uterine contraction waves arise. Congestive dysmenorrhoea may occur because of the associated pelvic congestion.

Continuous and irregular bleeding and discharge in association with leiomyomas is seen when there is surface ulceration of a submucous leiomyoma, polypoidal leiomyoma, sarcomatous change in a leiomyoma (rare), coincidental endometrial carcinoma or endometrial polyp.

Every woman suffering from leiomyomas who has continuous or irregular bleeding should have an endometrial aspiration before her treatment is planned.

Pressure Symptoms

Presence of tumour: A leiomyoma has to attain the size of a 14-week pregnancy or more before a woman is conscious of swelling of the abdomen or of the presence of a hard tumour. Smaller ones can cause a sensation of weight in the pelvis.

Alimentary tract: Large leiomyomas filling up the abdomen can cause dyspepsia; constipation from pressure on the rectum can occur rarely due to rectal compression.

Bladder: An anterior wall leiomyoma commonly causes bladder irritability with diurnal frequency. A cervical leiomyoma or a corporeal one that becomes impacted in the pouch of Douglas can cause retention of urine. The onset of retention is acute and usually occurs immediately before menstruation when the uterus is further enlarged by congestion, or during early pregnancy.

Veins and lymphatics: Oedema and varicosities of the legs are sometimes seen with large leiomyomas going into the broad ligament and compressing the veins and lymphatics.

Nerves: Pain from pressure on the nerves of the sacral plexus or on the obturator nerve is extremely rare, even when leiomyomas are impacted in the pelvis. Any pelvic tumour causing such pain is generally malignant.

Symptoms Related to Pregnancy

Infertility: Fibroids can impair fertility through several possible mechanisms:

- Alteration of the local anatomy (anatomic distortion of the uterine cavity), which can impair implantation
- Functional changes, such as increased uterine contractility and impairment of the endometrial and myometrial blood supply
- Changes to the local hormone milieu and paracrine molecular changes induced by fibroids, which could impair gamete transport and/or reduce blastocyst implantation

Those who believe that leiomyomas lower fertility point out that 40% of women with the opportunity to conceive after myomectomy. Those who take the opposite view point out that 30–50% of all women attending an infertility clinic subsequently conceive, no matter what treatment is given. There is obviously a vicious circle; deferment of pregnancy encourages leiomyomas, and the leiomyomas then discourage pregnancy. However, leiomyomas have been reported as a sole cause in <3% cases of infertility.

Many women with leiomyomas succeed in becoming pregnant. Often the tumours are only discovered during routine antenatal examination. The pregnancy usually proceeds without serious complications, especially if the leiomyomas are not submucous. Even very large subserous tumours do not usually disturb pregnancy.

Abortion and premature labour: These complications occur when the leiomyoma interferes with enlargement of the uterus, initiates abnormal uterine contractions, prevents efficient placentation or causes impaction of the uterus in the pelvis. Inflammatory pathways, associated or not with other reproductive disorders, may impair pregnancy outcomes. Fibroids are significantly associated with preterm delivery (<37 weeks), primary caesarean section, breech presentation and lower birthweight infants.

Malposition and malpresentation of the foetus: These can result if the leiomyoma distorts the shape of the uterus or prevents engagement of the head.

Obstructed labour: As pregnancy advances, most leiomyomas lift into the abdomen and do not complicate delivery. Labour can be obstructed, however, by cervical and broad ligament tumours, which are fixed in the pelvis, and by pedunculated subserous leiomyomas, which become trapped in the pouch of Douglas.

Abnormal uterine action: Inertia due to leiomyomas is only a theoretical possibility, not supported by experience. These tumors can lead to adherent/retained placenta which may implant on a submucosal leiomyoma. They can also delay the involution of the uterus.

Effect of Pregnancy on Leiomyomas

Increased growth of tumour: Leiomyomas enlarge due to congestion and oedema and usually return to their original size afterwards. Similar changes are sometimes seen during pseudopregnancy induced by oestrogen-progestogen preparations.

Degeneration: Red degeneration is rather special to pregnancy, but other types are more common. Degeneration of any kind is said to occur because the enlarging uterus puts tension on the capsule of the tumour and thus reduces its blood supply.

Physical Signs

Physical signs depend on the size and site of the leiomyoma. The uterus may be uniformly enlarged, or irregularly enlarged due to multiple leiomyomas. Subserous leiomyomas may be pedunculated and felt as a freely mobile firm mass, and mistaken for an adnexal mass. A broad ligament leiomyoma is felt as a firm mass adjacent to the uterine body. A cervical leiomyoma stretches the lower segment of the uterus and pushes the uterine fundus upwards.

Differential Diagnosis

Leiomyomas have to be distinguished from all other causes of enlargement of the uterus; adenomyosis causes a uniform enlargement, and leiomyomas may cause a uniform enlargement if single intramural, and irregular enlargement if multiple.

One horn of a bicornuate uterus can be mistaken for a leiomyoma.

The means of distinguishing between a uterine and an ovarian, or other pelvic and abdominal tumours are described in **Chapter 35**.

Occasionally, leiomyomas are first diagnosed by the finding of calcification in the tumour during radiological examination of the trunk for another purpose (womb-stone) **(Fig. 21)**.

Management

No treatment: Small symptomless leiomyomas discovered accidentally do not require treatment, although the patient should be kept under observation. It is only justifiable to operate on a symptomless tumour when it is larger than a 12–14-week pregnancy, if it is growing rapidly, if it is subserous and pedunculated and prone to torsion of its pedicle, if it is likely to complicate a future pregnancy, or if there is doubt about its nature. If the complaint is infertility alone, single or multiple tiny subserous leiomyomas are best left undisturbed; but intramural or submucous tumours, even of moderate size, deserve removal if no other cause is found **(Flowchart 2)**.

General treatment: If there is anaemia due to AUB, it is important to correct it before any surgical intervention.

Medical Therapy for Fibroids

Goals of medical therapy:

- Treat symptoms
- Prevent occurrence in women genetically disposed to develop myomas
- Postpone or avoid surgery
- Prevent recurrence after surgery in women at high risk (young age and family history)

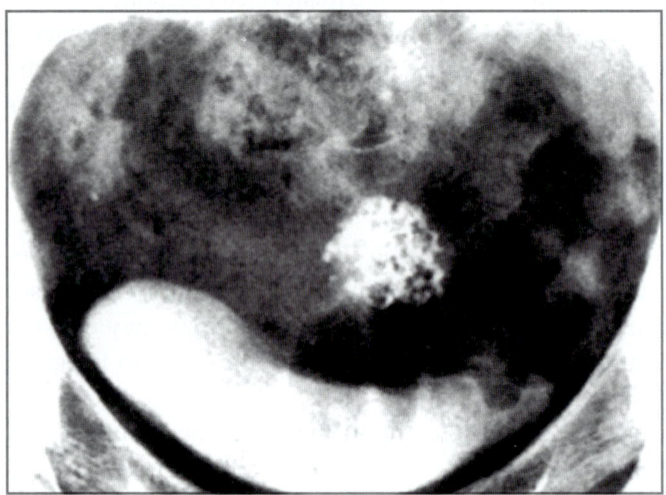

Fig. 21: Diffuse calcification in a small uterine leiomyoma, its position being orientated by instilling radio-opaque fluid into the bladder.
Image courtesy: Mr CH Walsh.

Gonadotrophin-releasing Hormone Agonists

Gonadotrophin-releasing hormone (GnRH) agonists have a direct action on the pituitary, thereby inducing a state of hypoestrogenism and amenorrhoea, and have been shown to decrease the volume of the uterus and the leiomyoma by 40–60%. Thus, they are used before myomectomy and have also been used to make vaginal hysterectomy, hysteroscopic resection or laparoscopic destruction more feasible. However, they can alter the tissue planes and make dissection difficult. The administration of a single dose of leuprolide acetate depot 3.75 mg to anaemic women improves the haemoglobin level and also reduces intraoperative blood loss, thereby decreasing the incidence of blood transfusion. GnRH agonists are also used where there are medical contraindications to surgery, or where surgery is to be delayed for any reason.

In a woman approaching the age of the menopause, active treatment of symptom-producing leiomyomas is often delayed in the hope that cessation of ovarian function would lead to control of the menorrhagia and eventually to atrophy of the tumours. GnRH agonists are useful in selected patients in this group. They cannot be used for long periods of time because of their side effects, which include hot flushes and bone loss. There is modest evidence that add-back therapy (tibolone, raloxifene, oestriol and ipriflavone) can help reduce bone loss and that medroxyprogesterone acetate (MPA) and tibolone

Flowchart 2: Management of fibroids.

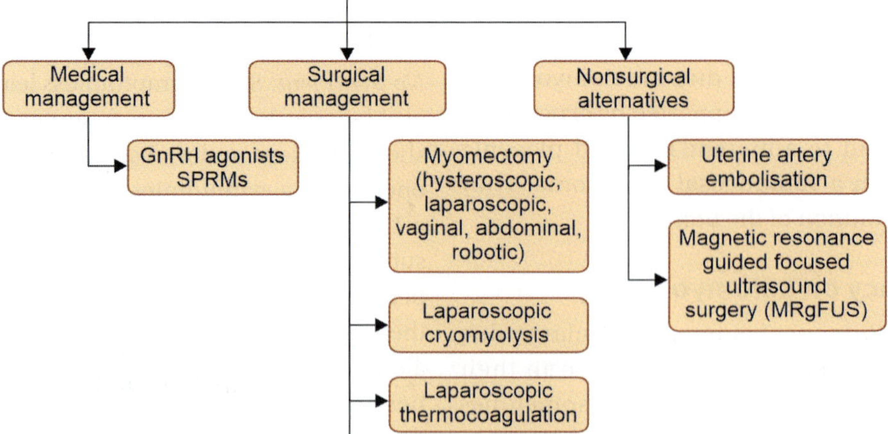

(GnRH: gonadotrophin-releasing hormone; SPRMs: selective progesterone receptor modulators)

Flowchart 3: Medical treatment of leiomyomas.

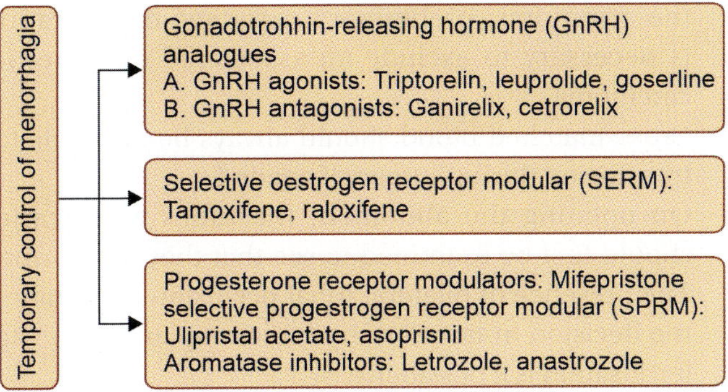

may moderate vasomotor symptoms **(Flowchart 3)**. Leiomyomas will recur in 50% of women thus treated.

Selective Progesterone Receptor Modulators

Selective progesterone receptor modulators (SPRMs) have a direct effect on fibroids and reduce their size by inhibition of cell proliferation and induction of apoptosis. They also inhibit ovulation by maintaining mid-follicular phase levels of oestradiol. The direct effect of SPRMs on endometrium stops uterine bleeding and is associated with benign and reversible changes in endometrial tissue 'progesterone receptor modulator associated endometrial changes (PAEC).'

Four members of the SPRM family which have been evaluated for use in fibroids include mifepristone, asoprisnil, ulipristal acetate (UPA) and telapristone acetate. All have shown to decrease leiomyoma size by up to 30% and reduce uterine bleeding in a dose-dependent manner.

Ulipristal acetate is given as 5 mg dose per day for 3 months, initiated during the first 7 days of cycles and can be repeated after a gap of 1 month. UPA is contraindicated in women with underlying liver disorders. Before initiation of each treatment course, a liver function test is performed, and UPA is not initiated in women with baseline alanine transaminase (ALT) or aspartate aminotransferase (AST) more than two times the upper limit of normal (ULN). During the first two treatment courses, liver function tests are performed every month and every 2–4 weeks after completion of treatment.

Progesterone receptor modulator (mifepristone) can be used for 3 months at a dosage of 10 or 25 mg.

Progesterone: Progesterone (Norethisterone acetate) can be used to control the bleeding while building up the haemoglobin before surgery. Alternatively, an oestrogen–progestogen preparation is also used for contraception purposes, and while awaiting surgery **(Flowchart 4)**.

Flowchart 4: Progesterone receptor modulators (PRMs).

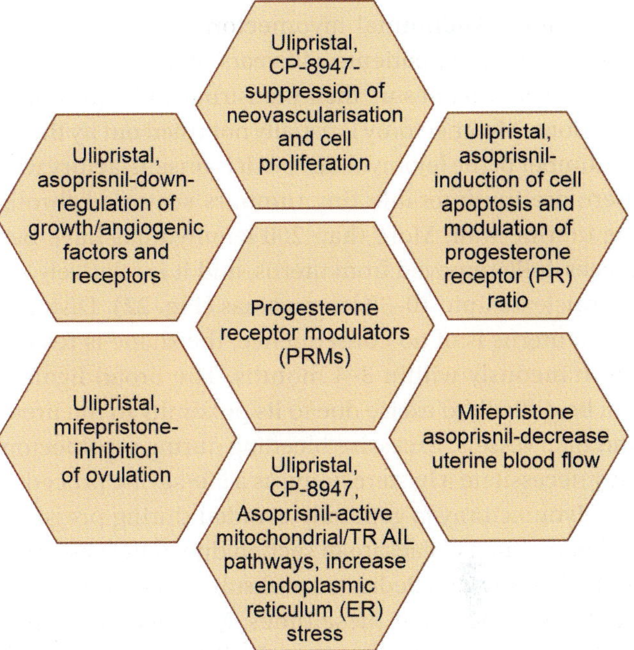

Curettage or Endometrial Aspiration

It is performed as a diagnostic procedure to exclude an associated endometrial carcinoma before myomectomy or hysterectomy. It is especially indicated when uterine bleeding is irregular or continuous. However, it has no therapeutic effect on menorrhagia caused by leiomyomas.

Polypectomy and Vaginal Myomectomy

Tumours presenting at or through the vaginal cervix are removed vaginally, taking care to exclude associated uterine inversion. Pedunculated or submucous intra-uterine tumours can be removed hysteroscopically.

Myomectomy is indicated in infertile women if:

- The myoma is causing significant distortion of the uterine wall or endometrial cavity.
- There is obstruction or distortion of the fallopian tube by a myoma.
- Symptomatic leiomyomas when the woman wants to retain the uterus

Myomectomy can be done by open, laparoscopic or hysteroscopic technique.

Abdominal Myomectomy

Indications: Abdominal myomectomy is the operation of choice in most patients <40 years of age, and in some older ones who treasure their menstrual and reproductive functions. Myomectomy is usually not ruled out by the size or number of the leiomyomas, but it is unsatisfactory when there are innumerable tiny tumours scattered through the uterine wall. More than 200 leiomyomas have been successfully removed from uterus, and it is relatively easy to enucleate upto 10–30 leiomyomas **(Fig. 22)**. Distortion of the uterus is of no consequence: the shape is restored spontaneously within 3–4 months. The broad ligament can be difficult to excise due to its proximity to the ureters and iliac vessels. Excessive bleeding during myomectomy may necessitate a hysterectomy as a life-saving procedure.

Myomectomy is generally avoided during pregnancy and at the time of caesarean section due to the vascularity of the leiomyoma. Pedunculated subserous tumours can safely be removed at these times. Myomectomy can be performed 3 months later, at which time the myoma is smaller and its bed less vascular.

Technique: Every myomectomy is different, but should be planned according to the following principles:

- The patient must be warned previously that myomectomy may prove so difficult and dangerous that it may have to be abandoned in favour of hysterectomy. This is rarely necessary with experienced operators.
- If infertility is the problem, the operation should be preceded by semen analysis on the partner. A finding of azoospermia may contraindicate myomectomy.
- If continuous or irregular bleeding and discharge are the symptoms, preliminary curettage or aspiration is necessary to exclude an associated endometrial carcinoma.
- Cross-matched blood should always be available for transfusion during surgery if needed.
- On opening the abdomen, the tubes and ovaries should first be examined to see that they are normal. The presence of bilateral tubal occlusion may change the decision in favour of hysterectomy unless in vitro fertilisation is a possibility.
- Dilute vasopressin can be infiltrated around the leiomyoma to decrease the blood loss.
- Bleeding from the uterine wall should be controlled by Bonney's myomectomy clamp **(Fig. 23)**, or a rubber tube tourniquet, placed around the lower part of the uterus. Provided the metal blades are covered with pieces of rubber tubing, the clamp is both safe and useful. It usually offers a bloodless operating field and is always a means of lifting and fixing the uterus. However, the tourniquet and clamp should be released intermittently to facilitate perfusion and prevent necrosis. Deliberate and meticulous surgery is thus facilitated. Neither the clamp nor the tourniquet can be used if a cervical leiomyoma is present, or not until it has been shelled out. The ovarian vessels can be controlled temporarily by sponge holders, but this is not usually necessary.
- Incisions in the uterus should be as few as possible. Each should be so planned that as many leiomyomas as possible can be reached through it by burrowing in the uterine wall.

Fig. 22: A group of leiomyomas obtained by myomectomy from a woman aged 39 years who complained of infertility.

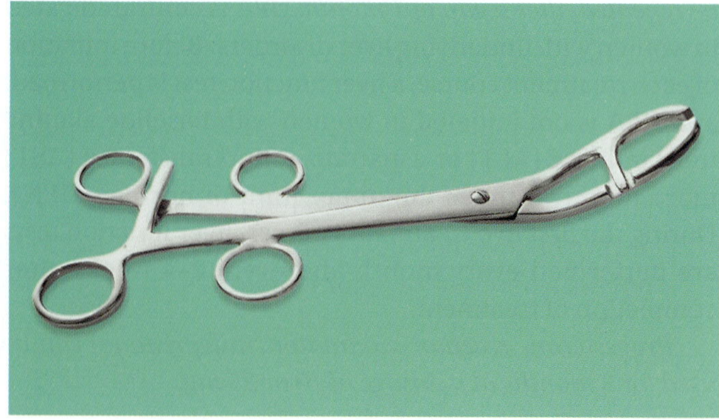

Fig. 23: Bonney's myomectomy clamp.

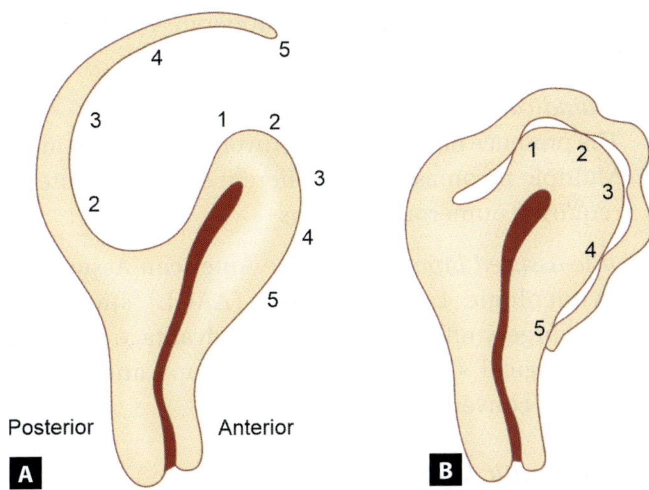

Figs. 24A and B: The Bonney's hood technique. A fundal posterior incision is made to enucleate the myomas. After reapproximating the uterine muscle, the excess serosa is draped over the fundus and fixed to the anterior surface of the uterus with fine suture. This creates a functional anterior uterine incision out of a posterior incision.

- Incisions in the anterior and posterior walls should be midline and vertical, in the least vascular area. Incisions on the peritoneal aspect of the posterior wall, however, involve risks of postoperative intestinal adhesions and should be avoided as far as possible. Interstitial leiomyomas in the posterior wall can usually be approached via the anterior wall and uterine cavity.
- An interstitial tumour high on the posterior wall is sometimes best enucleated through a transverse fundal incision. The edge of the capsule is then brought forwards and stitched low on the anterior wall to form a *Bonney's hood* **(Figs. 24A and B)**.
- In planning incisions, enucleating tumours and suturing cavities, it is important to avoid injury to, or occlusion of, the intramural portions of the tubes.
- The uterine cavity need not be opened if transvaginal sonohysterography and/or hysteroscopy have not shown the presence of any intrauterine polyps. If these facilities are not available, the cavity should nearly always be opened and a search made for intrauterine polyps—mucous or leiomyomatous. The omission of this step is only justified when the patient is not complaining of menorrhagia and the leiomyoma is obviously single and subserous.
- All tumour cavities should be carefully obliterated to avoid dead space and haematoma formation.
- Although some say it has the danger of producing ischaemic necrosis, the author finds it best to close large cavities with mattress sutures.
- Meticulous attention to haemostasias is important at all stages.
- The uterine serosal layer should be closed with a fine suture, preferably using a modified baseball suture technique, which will leave a minimal amount of suture material on the surface and thereby lead to minimal adhesion formation.
- Plication of round ligaments helps in preventing retroversion of the uterus and adhesion formation postsurgery.
- *Results:* Myomectomy is said to be more dangerous than hysterectomy but this is not true for present-day surgery. The immediate mortality should not be higher than 0.2%. Low-grade postoperative pyrexia is the rule and should not be treated by antibiotics. It is indicative of slight extravasation of blood into the uterine wall or peritoneal cavity and settles spontaneously in 7–14 days. Late sequelae, especially if the incisions are multiple and badly closed, are omental and intestinal adhesions to the uterus.

A disadvantage of myomectomy is that menorrhagia persists after operation in 1–5% of cases. This is either because the myomas were not responsible for the original complaint, or because an intrauterine polyp or leiomyoma was overlooked at operation. The recurrence rate of leiomyomas after myomectomy is 5–10%. The reappearance of tumours within 5 years probably means that tiny seedlings were not recognised and removed during the original operation. Most recurrences occur after myomectomy in young women, those <35 years of age.

About 20–25% of women subjected to myomectomy ultimately come to hysterectomy after completion of their family.

Pregnancy after myomectomy: Of all women subjected to myomectomy, 25–30% subsequently become pregnant. It usually takes 3–6 months for the uterine scar to undergo healing.

Effects on pregnancy:

- *No effect:* This is the rule.
- *Rupture of the scar:* The scar of myomectomy hardly ever ruptures, either in pregnancy or labour, no matter how long the incision may have been and irrespective of its encroachment on the cavity.

- *Treatment:* Delivery should be in a fully equipped hospital. Vaginal delivery should be the aim but, since the patient is likely to be advancing in years with a previous history of infertility, caesarean section is indicated if the uterine cavity is breached. The risk of uterine rupture in subsequent pregnancy after myomectomy is reported to be 0.7–1%.

Laparoscopic Myomectomy

In both conditions, laparoscopic myomectomy followed by uterine repair is comparable or superior to the uterine closure of abdominal myomectomy.

The advantages over abdominal myomectomy are less severe postoperative morbidity, faster recovery and no significant difference between reproductive outcomes after laparoscopic or abdominal myomectomy.

Limitations to laparoscopic myomectomy: If myomas are large and multiple, operative time and blood loss may be more. If myoma is embedded deeply in the myometrium, proper repair of the uterine wall is difficult or even impossible.

Retrieval of the resected myoma may also pose problems. Large myomas have to be morcellated in an endobag and retrieved through the posterior vaginal fornix or through the abdominal wall through separate incisions.

Open/uncontained morcellation of the uterus and myomas has been scrutinised because of the possible spread of an unsuspected leiomyosarcoma while using a power morcellator during a hysterectomy or myomectomy. In February 2020, the Food and Drug Administration (FDA) released an updated Safety Communication recommending that laparoscopic power morcellation for myomectomy or hysterectomy be performed only with a tissue containment system that is legally marketed in the United States for use during laparoscopic power morcellation and is compatible with only specifically designated laparoscopic power morcellators. Additionally, the FDA's February 2020 guidance stated that laparoscopic power morcellators for the removal of uterine tissue containing suspected leiomyomas should not be used in patients who are postmenopausal or older than 50 years, or 'candidates for removal of tissue (*en bloc*) through the vagina or via a mini-laparotomy incision.'

An important disadvantage of myomectomy is the risk of postoperative pelvic adhesions, which adversely affect fertility. It causes pain and increases the risk of ectopic pregnancy and intestinal obstruction. Studies have demonstrated that the risk of postoperative adhesions is more with laparoscopic myomectomy.

Contraindications to laparoscopic myomectomy:

- The presence of an intramural myoma >10–12 cm in size
- Multiple myomas (≥4) in different sites of the uterus, requiring numerous incisions

Robotic-assisted laparoscopy: The American Association of Gynecologic Laparoscopists (AAGL) states that robotic surgery offers no significant advantage in benign gynaecological surgery over laparoscopy and is more costly than conventional surgery.

Hysteroscopic Myomectomy

Advances in instruments and techniques have promoted hysteroscopic myomectomy to the rank of a standard minimally invasive surgical procedure for submucous myomas. Small fibroids (<2 cm) can be routinely removed in an outpatient setting according to the technique described by Bettocchi.

Techniques of hysteroscopic myomectomy:

- The first involves cutting the base of pedunculated fibroids with either the resectoscopic loop or laser fibre. The base of the pedicle is cut, and the fibroid is extracted by forceps or may be left in place.
- The second alternative is a complete excision of fibroids by a one-step procedure. The most commonly used approach is the slicing technique. Repeated and progressive passage of the cutting loop allows the surgeon to cut the myoma into small chips.
- Hysteroscopic resection is effective and safe and should be considered the technique of choice for type 1 myomas. The development of intrauterine morcellators has facilitated the implementation of hysteroscopic myomectomy. If the myoma is large (>3 cm in diameter), there is an increased risk of operative complications (perforation, bleeding and fluid intravasation) and damage to the surrounding myometrium due to the use of electrosurgery.
- The third alternative is myomectomy by a two-step procedure (for large type 1–3 myomas). After resection or ablation of the protruded portion of the myoma during first-step hysteroscopy, the residual intramural component rapidly migrates to the uterine cavity, with a parallel increase in myometrial thickness, allowing complete and safe myoma excision during second-step hysteroscopy.

Complications of hysteroscopic myomectomy:

- Risk of fluid (glycine) absorption while using monopolar energy. This risk is avoided by the use of bipolar or laser energy with saline solution.
- Hysteroscopic myomectomy is effective for control of bleeding, but failures are reported and are often related to the growth of fibroids in other sites, the association of fibroids with adenomyosis and the incomplete treatment of large intramural (partially submucous) myomas.

Laparoscopic Cryomyolysis and Thermocoagulation

Both techniques have the same goal: Reduction or suppression of the primary blood supply and induction of myoma shrinkage by causing scleral hyaline degeneration (by very low or very high temperatures). For cryomyolysis, a cryoprobe is inserted into the myoma and cooled to a temperature of <90°C.

For laparoscopic thermocoagulation, either a monopolar or bipolar probe is inserted into the myoma before delivering the electrical current. Laser fibres (YAG) have also been used.

The limitation of all of these techniques is the lack of histological evaluation of the fibroids.

Uterine Artery Embolisation

Uterine artery embolisation (UAE) using polyvinyl alcohol or gel foam pellets, being a minimally invasive therapy, is gaining popularity. It can obviate the need for surgical procedures in patients suffering from symptomatic leiomyomas.

UAE is indicated for patients with symptomatic myoma who are not fit or desirous of surgical therapy.

There is limited experience of pregnancy following this therapy, but it is possible that patients have reduced fertility as a consequence of injury to the uterus or ovaries, placental insufficiency resulting from inadequate blood flow through the uterus, or uterine rupture during pregnancy from UAE-induced myoma necrosis.

It also appears to increase the risk of preterm delivery, malpresentations, spontaneous abortions and postpartum haemorrhage compared with laparoscopic myomectomy. This procedure is contraindicated in pregnancy, acute pelvic infection, severe contrast medium allergy, arteriovenous malformations, desire for future pregnancy, adenomyosis or pedunculated myoma and undiagnosed pelvic mass.

The success rate of this procedure is 96–98%. About 80–90% of embolised patients had improvement in menorrhagia bulk-related symptoms. Myoma showed an average volume reduction of 60–65%.

Laparoscopic Occlusion of the Uterine Arteries

Laparoscopic occlusion of the uterine arteries appears to have no specific advantage over vaginal occlusion, as it requires a laparoscopic approach. When compared to the UAE, the outcomes were found to be inferior in terms of myoma size reduction and devascularisation.

High-frequency Magnetic Resonance-guided Focused Ultrasound Surgery

Magnetic resonance-guided focused ultrasound surgery (MRgFUS) is thermal ablation using magnetic resonance imaging (MRI) to visualise the myoma and define the target. Ultrasonic energy is directed to a point inside the fibroid and coagulation tissue necrosis is induced in the myoma. Damage to surrounding tissue is minimal, but the impact on critical neighbouring structures cannot be excluded.

The principal limitations to the use of MRgFUS are that:

- Only a fraction of patients with fibroids meet the inclusion criteria.
- Future fertility may be compromised.
- The financial burden may be too heavy.

Vaginal Occlusion of the Uterine Arteries

Occlusion of the uterine arteries with a clamp-like device that remains in place for 6 hours leads to myoma ischaemia by interfering with the blood supply to the uterus. However, this technique is not recommended for women wishing to conceive in the future.

In a study by Vilos et al., dominant fibroid volume decreased by 24%, and heavy bleeding symptoms decreased by 51%. Research with larger populations is needed to prove the efficacy of the technique.

Hysterectomy

This is the best treatment for uterine leiomyomas in women over the age of 40 years and in those who are not anxious for more children. The cervix as well as the corpus should be removed in most cases but the ovaries, if normal, should be conserved in premenopausal women. The operation can be carried out vaginally when the myomas are small but this route is not to be advocated when the uterus is larger than that of a 12-week pregnancy even though its bulk can be reduced.

Laparoscopic hysterectomy has become the ideal surgical approach to replace laparotomy. A uterine volume of ≥13–14 weeks represents a relative contraindication to laparoscopic approach.

Complications of Leiomyomas

Torsion: Torsion of the pedicle of a subserous pedunculated leiomyoma interrupts first the venous and then the arterial supply, leading first to extravasation of blood and then to gangrene. The accident usually causes acute symptoms calling for an emergency operation.

In certain cases of torsion in which the diagnosis is overlooked, or when the twist is intermittent, the tumour degenerates; its roughened surface then forms adhesions to the omentum and other structures. It obtains an additional blood supply through these and occasionally this becomes the only blood supply, the original connection with the uterus being severed. Hence, a *parasitic leiomyoma* is formed, which can be found anywhere in the abdomen but most often attached to the omentum.

Haemorrhage: The rupture of a large vein on the surface of a leiomyoma is an uncommon accident, resulting in the clinical picture of intraperitoneal haemorrhage and requiring urgent treatment. Haemorrhage into the substance of a tumour is unusual except in association with torsion of the pedicle.

Ascites; pseudo-Meigs' syndrome: Very mobile tumours, usually pedunculated subserous ones, can cause ascites, presumably by mechanical irritation of the peritoneum. Rarely, the ascites is accompanied by a right-sided hydrothorax to produce a pseudo-Meigs' syndrome.

Infection: A submucous leiomyoma nearly always becomes ulcerated and infected at its lower pole. Infection of myomas in other sites is generally preceded by necrosis. It only occurs following abortion or labour, when the tumour is adherent to the bowel, or when it becomes involved in appendicitis, diverticulitis and the like.

Malignant Change

Sarcomatous change is found in only 0.2% of tumours coming to operation but is a risk which cannot be discounted. The malignant process usually begins towards the centre of the tumour and the diagnosis is only made by histological examination of a removed myoma **(Fig. 25)**. Sarcomas with a malignant behaviour have 10 or more mitoses per high-power field (HPF).

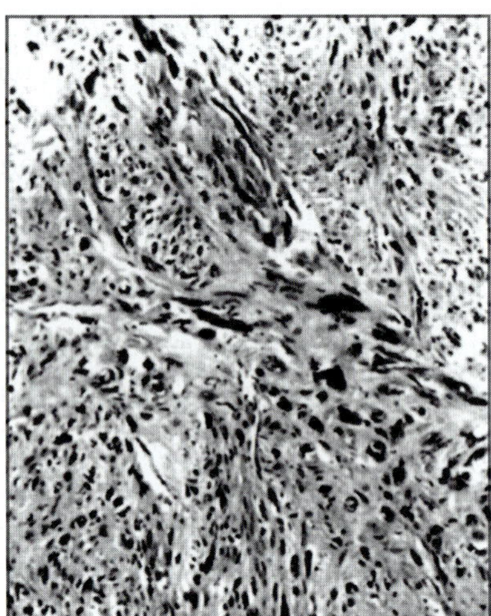

Fig. 25: Bizarre changes in a leiomyoma which may be confused histologically with sarcoma by the inexperienced histopathologist.

Atypical Smooth Muscle Tumours (STUMP)

Uterine smooth muscle tumours that show some worrisome histologic features (i.e. necrosis, nuclear atypia or mitoses), but do not meet all diagnostic criteria for leiomyosarcoma, fall into the category of atypical smooth muscle tumours [smooth muscle tumours of uncertain malignant potential (STUMP)]. They have 5–9 mitoses/10 HPF that do not demonstrate nuclear atypia or giant cells; or 2–4 mitoses/10 HPF with nuclear atypia or giant cells. Most tumours classified as STUMP have been associated with favourable prognosis and, many cases, only follow-up of the patients is recommended.

Progression to sarcoma: The development of sarcoma may be suspected clinically when a leiomyoma, usually in a postmenopausal woman, becomes painful and tender and grows rapidly, producing systemic upset and pyrexia. The overall 5-year survival rate for patients with sarcoma is only 20–30%.

Degeneration

All leiomyomas that attain or exceed the size of an orange, and many that are smaller, show some form of degenerative change. The immediate cause of degeneration is an interference with the capsular circulation and, while the process is active, the tumour becomes painful, tender, softened and enlarged.

Atrophy: Alleged postmenopausal atrophy is insignificant and unimportant.

Oedema: Oedema may be only microscopic but is sometimes obvious to the naked eye. The fluid collects between tumour cells to form pools and *cysts*.

Hyaline degeneration: This, the most common degeneration, first affects fibrous tissue cells, which are replaced by a homogeneous substance, which stains pink with eosin **(Fig. 26)**. The muscle fibres and bundles then become isolated and die, so that large areas of the tumour become structureless. Ultimately, the hyaline material liquefies, leaving ragged cavities filled with colourless or bloodstained fluid **(Fig. 26)**.

Cystic degeneration: This is the end result of either oedema or hyaline degeneration **(Fig. 27)**.

Myxomatous degeneration: This is rare.

Fatty degeneration; calcification: Sometimes, and usually in association with partial necrosis, a leiomyoma contains fat. A later stage in this process is the deposition of calcium, first in the form of calcium soaps. The calcium may be diffused throughout the tumour, a change, which ultimately produces a *womb stone* **(Fig. 28)**, or it may have a peripheral *eggshell* distribution. The former happens when the persistence of some circulation permits multifocal deposits in the centre of the leiomyoma and the latter happens when it is completely avascular and necrotic.

A calcified subserous leiomyoma can become detached from the uterus and be found wrapped in omentum or elsewhere in the abdominal cavity **(Fig. 28)**.

Red degeneration; necrobiosis: This is mostly seen during pregnancy and the puerperium but can occur at other times. It manifests itself typically about mid-pregnancy

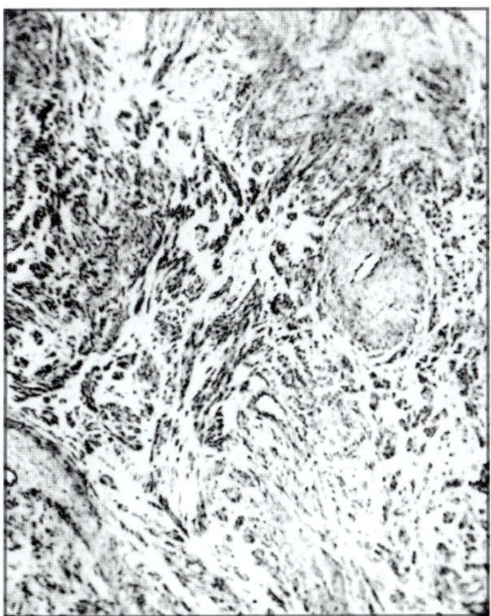

Fig. 26: Early hyaline degeneration in a leiomyoma. It is the fibrous tissue elements, which undergo hyaline change, leaving islands of muscle tissue. Their isolation means that they ultimately die.

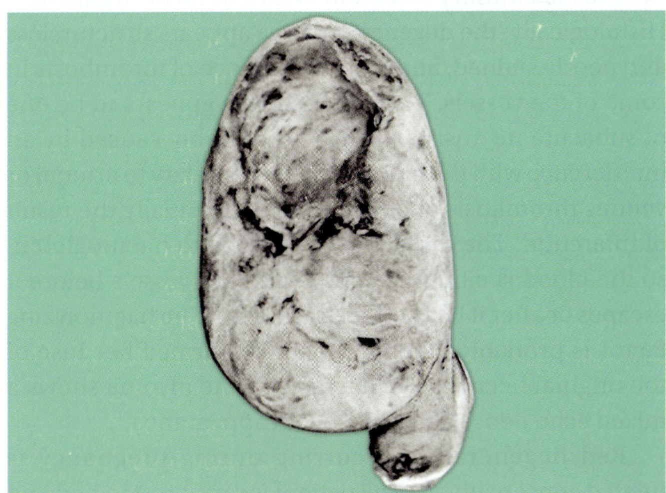

Fig. 27: A uterus containing a single subserous leiomyoma which, on section, shows one large and several small ragged cavities, which are the result of hyaline degeneration followed by liquefaction of the necrotic tissues.

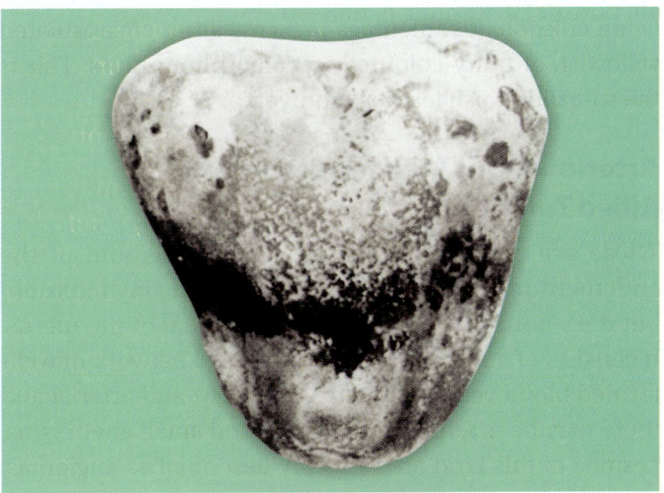

Fig. 28: A *womb stone*, which consists of a smooth calcified body found at autopsy in the tissues adjacent to but separate from the uterus. The structure almost certainly represents a calcified and parasitic leiomyoma.

when the leiomyoma suddenly becomes acutely painful, enlarged and tender. The patient may vomit and become generally ill with malaise and slight pyrexia. The condition can be mistaken for torsion of the pedicle of a leiomyoma or ovarian cyst, *abruptio placentae*, acute pyelitis or any abdominal catastrophe.

The changes in the tumour are striking. It is soft and homogeneous or necrotic, especially in its centre, and is diffusely stained red or salmon pink. A fishy smell, described in the past, is rare and probably denotes secondary infection with coliform organisms. Histologically, the degenerated area appears structureless and poorly stained, and there is evidence of thrombosis in some of the vessels. The initial change appears to be one of subacute necrosis, which is presumably caused by an interference with the blood supply, secondary to arterial or venous thrombosis and the lesion is essentially the result of infarction. The discolouration is due to haemoglobin, so the blood is either haemolyzed in the vessels before it escapes or after it has been extravasated. The haemolyzing factor is probably a lipoid substance formed because of the original necrosis. On ultrasound, the myoma shows a mixed echo dense and echo lucent appearance.

Red degeneration occurring during pregnancy is treated conservatively. The patient is put at rest in bed and given analgesics to relieve the pain. The acute symptoms subside gradually during the course of 3–10 days and the pregnancy then usually proceeds uneventfully.

When a leiomyoma which has suffered red degeneration or partial necrosis is removed several months after the acute episode, it sometimes presents as an encapsulated yellowish or putty-coloured soft amorphous mass. This is the so-called wash leather leiomyoma.

Arteriovenous Malformations and Allied Tumours

These are rare; beginning as a haemangioma of the endometrium, usually spread to involve the myometrium but does not cause significant enlargement of the uterus. It consists of a complicated but localised network of well-formed blood vessels—venous, capillary, and arterial and there may be arteriovenous shunts and small aneurysms. Lesions of this kind are variously described as angiomas, cricoid aneurysms and hamartomas.

The main, if not the only, symptom is excessive uterine bleeding, which can be alarmingly heavy and does not respond to any of the usual remedies. Ultrasound scan and Doppler reveal the abnormal blood vessels. If the diagnosis is suspected on analysis of the symptoms, it may be confirmed by angiography, and it can then be successfully treated by embolisation.

Other Rare Benign Tumours

These include tumours consisting of gliomatous, cartilaginous or osseous tissue. They can be the outcome of endometrial metaplasia but most often they represent pieces of foetal tissue left in the uterus after instrumental termination of pregnancy. Such tissue cannot only remain alive but also can proliferate and become polypoidal to cause bleeding and discharge from the uterus. Since the lesions are superficial, curettage alone is often curative.

MALIGNANT NEOPLASMS

Carcinoma of the Endometrium

Incidence

Endometrial carcinoma occurs in women in the sixth and seventh decades of life. 75% of cases occur in women over 50 years. The risk of endometrial cancer is increased three times in women who are moderately overweight and 10 times more in grossly overweight. The incidence of endometrial carcinoma is about 2–3%. Risk factors for endometrial cancer are shown in **Table 4**.

Aetiology

Endometrial cancer appears to have two distinct pathogenetic types. The first and more common variety

TABLE 4: Risk factors for endometrial cancer.

Characteristic	*Relative risk*
Nulliparity	2–3
Late menopause	2.4
Obesity	
21–50 lb. overweight	3
>50 lb. overweight	10
Diabetes mellitus	2.8
Unopposed oestrogen therapy	4–8
Tamoxifen therapy	2–3
Atypical endometrial hyperplasia	829
HNPCC syndrome	20

(HNPCC: hereditary nonpolyposis colorectal cancer)

is seen in younger, perimenopausal women, is oestrogen dependent, starts in a background of endometrial hyperplasia and is better differentiated with a more favourable prognosis. Most of the risk factors identified for endometrial cancer are related to prolonged, unopposed oestrogen stimulation of the endometrium and are related to this type. The second type is seen in older, postmenopausal, thin women with no source of oestrogen stimulation of the endometrium, is associated with endometrial atrophy, is less differentiated and has a poorer prognosis. This type is seen more often in African and Asian women.

Some of the risk factors are discussed here.

Age

Carcinoma of the body of the uterus occurs at a later age than carcinoma of the cervix, the peak incidence being in women aged 60 years. Nevertheless, it arises before the menopause in 25% of cases, sometimes in the comparatively young.

Parity

Unlike carcinoma of the cervix, it is often seen in nulliparous women and in virgins. From 25% to 50 of cases occur among nulliparae, the relative risk being two to three times, and many of the others among women who have had few pregnancies. The low fertility association probably explains why leiomyomas and carcinoma of the body of the uterus sometimes occur together **(Fig. 29)**.

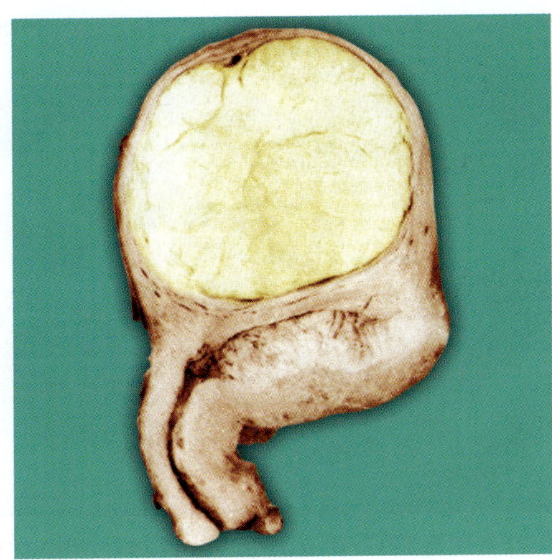

Fig. 29: A carcinoma of the endometrium filling the uterine cavity with its common associate—a leiomyoma.

Race

Unlike malignant disease of the cervix, endometrial carcinoma is more common in Jews than in women of other races.

Diabetes Mellitus and Metabolic Errors

There is a significant association between diabetes and endometrial cancer. 50% of patients suffering from endometrial carcinoma can be shown to have abnormal glucose tolerance curves, and 10–30% are frankly diabetic, the relative risk being 1.3–3 times. A disturbed glucose metabolism can often be demonstrated in menopausal and postmenopausal women known to have endometrial hyperplasia **(Figs. 30A and B)**. It is the obese diabetic woman who is most vulnerable; indeed, obesity alone is a predisposing factor. Women who are 10–20 kg overweight have a 3-fold risk, which increases to 10-fold if they are >25 kg overweight, because of the increased peripheral conversion of androstenedione to oestrone by aromatisation in fat. The combination of diabetes, obesity and hypertension, in association with endometrial carcinoma, is sometimes called the corpus cancer syndrome. A causal relationship between hypertension and hypothyroidism has not been confirmed.

Oestrogens: Endometrial Intraepithelial Neoplasia

Hyperplasia of the endometrium is often found in association with carcinoma, and all histological stages between simple hyperplasia and anaplastic carcinoma can be demonstrated.

According to the 2014 World Health Organization (WHO) classification, there are two types of endometrial intraepithelial neoplasia [atypical hyperplasia **(Fig. 31)** and endometrial hyperplasia without atypia **(Fig. 32)**]. Hyperplasia without atypia are benign changes, which regress again after the endocrine milieu has normalised. However, in 1–3% cases, progression to invasive disease may occur if the endocrine disorder (persistent oestrogen exposure or progesterone deficiency) persists over the long term.

Approximately 40% of cases of atypical hyperplasia with cellular atypia, particularly if of severe degree, progress to invasive carcinoma, the increase in risk being 8–29 fold.

A woman who suffers from menopausal bleeding is said to have a three times increased chance of developing adenocarcinoma of the corpus uteri subsequently.

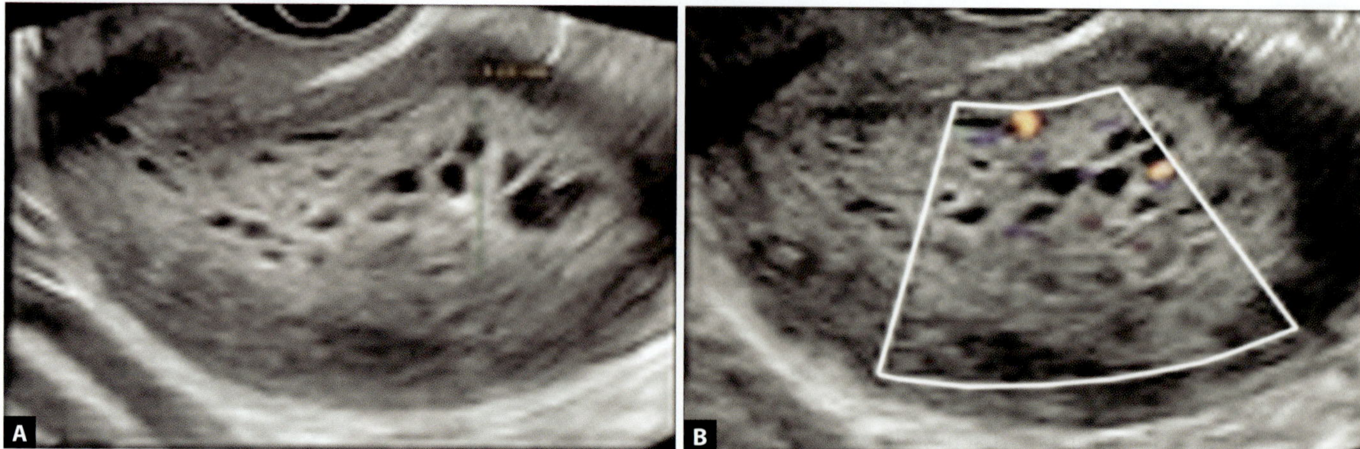

Figs. 30A and B: A TVUS of a 55-year-old lady with postmenopausal bleeding showing heterogenous thickened endometrium (endometrial thickness—31.1 mm) with irregular cystic areas, irregular endomyometrial junction and minimal vascularity. Histopathological examination of endometrial biopsy is suggestive of endometrial hyperplasia without atypia. (TVUS: transvaginal ultrasound)
Image courtesy: Dr Neha Bagri.

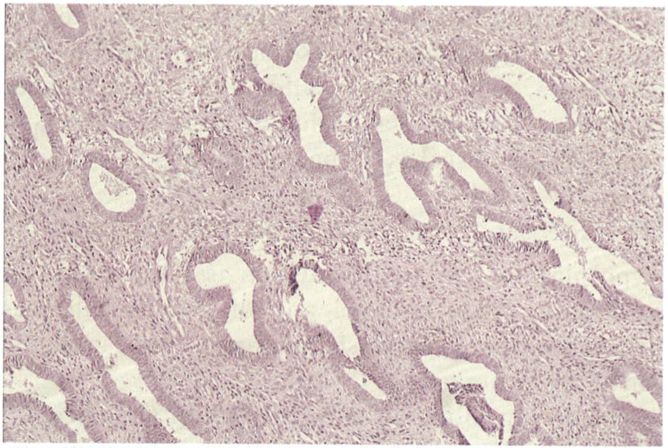

Fig. 31: *Endometrial hyperplasia without atypia* on haematoxylin and eosin stain showing overgrowth of the endometrial glands relative to the stroma, but without cytological abnormalities in the glandular cells. The glands are significantly *increased in number* and appear crowded, leading to a higher gland-to-stroma ratio compared to a normal endometrium.
Image courtesy: Dr Sufian Zaheer.

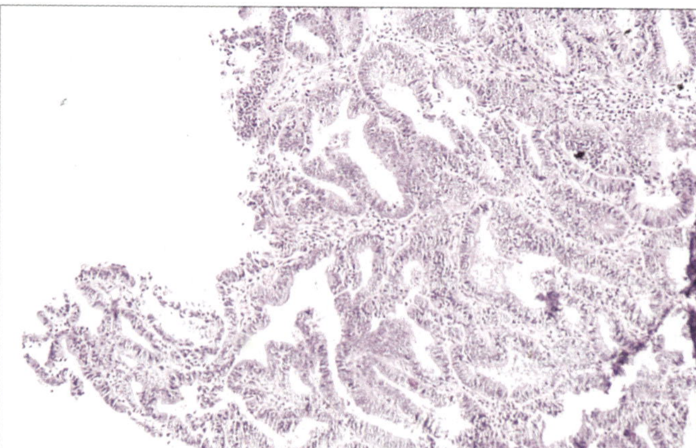

Fig. 32: *Endometrial hyperplasia with atypia [endometrial intraepithelial neoplasia (EIN)]* on haematoxylin and eosin stain showing increased gland-to-stroma ratio, with glands appearing crowded and complex. Glands exhibit irregular shapes and sizes, with back-to-back arrangements in focal areas. Cells lining the glands show nuclear enlargement with hyperchromasia (dark-staining nuclei). Nuclear pleomorphism, with variation in size and shape, is evident.
Image courtesy: Dr Sufian Zaheer.

The incidence of endometrial carcinoma increases in any group of women given oestrogen alone as hormone replacement therapy (RR 4–8). It is for this reason that all hormone replacement therapy includes a progestogen in women with an intact uterus.

Tamoxifen

The use of the anti-oestrogen tamoxifen as long-term adjunctive therapy in patients of breast cancer has been associated with a large number of cases of endometrial hyperplasia and a two- to threefold increased risk of endometrial cancer. However, these cancers are usually well differentiated.

Invasive Carcinoma of the Endometrium

Histology

Histopathological findings are central to the 2023 FIGO staging of endometrial carcinoma.

The following different histological types of endometrial carcinoma have been recognised:

- Endometrioid carcinoma (EEC), of low grade (grades 1 and 2) or high grade (grade 3)
- Serous carcinoma (SC)
- Clear cell carcinoma (CCC)
- Mixed carcinoma (MC)
- Undifferentiated carcinoma (UC)
- Carcinosarcoma (CS)
- Other unusual types, such as mesonephric-like
- Gastrointestinal mucinous type carcinomas

Nonaggressive histological types are composed of low-grade (grades 1 and 2) EECs, while aggressive histological types are composed of high-grade EECs (grade 3), SC, CCC, MC, UC, CS and mesonephric-like and gastrointestinal type mucinous carcinomas. The different histological types have different molecular features, microscopic appearance, precursor lesions and natural history.

Pathology

The vast majority of endometrial neoplasms are adenocarcinomas **(Box 2)**.

Adenocarcinoma

Macroscopically, endometrial cancer can be predominantly polypoidal into the cavity or invasive. Sometimes, it is found only in a polyp. It may occupy a small area and be completely removed during curettage, so that subsequent hysterectomy produces a uterus in which no cancer can be found. Multiple foci of origin in a growth are not uncommon.

The growth bleeds and becomes infected, and the senile myometrium cannot easily expel the resulting discharges, especially when the cervix is stenosed or obstructed by debris. Pyometra and haematometra are therefore common complications **(Figs. 33 and 34)**.

Histologically, most adenocarcinomas are well-differentiated columnar-celled cancers, which preserve

BOX 2: Classification of endometrial carcinoma.

- *Endometrioid adenocarcinoma*:
  - Well-differentiated
  - Villoglandular/papillary
  - Secretory
  - With squamous differentiation
- Mucinous adenocarcinoma
- Papillary serous carcinoma
- Clear cell carcinoma
- Squamous carcinoma
- Poorly differentiated carcinoma

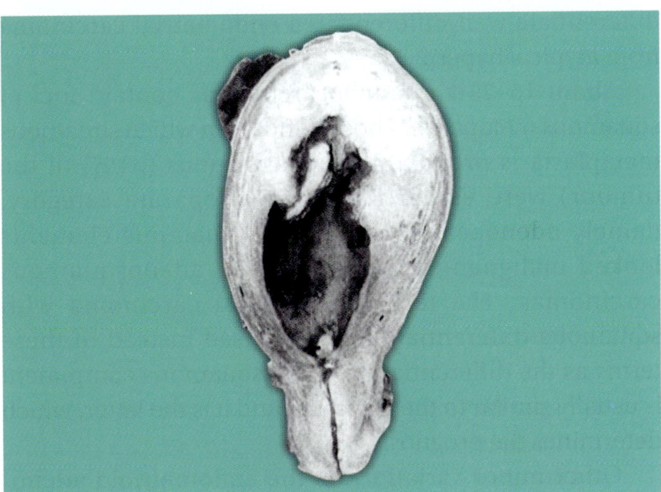

Fig. 33: An ulcerative carcinoma of the body of the uterus with deep invasion of the myometrium. The cavity of the uterus below the growth is distended, because it is the seat of a pyohaematometra.

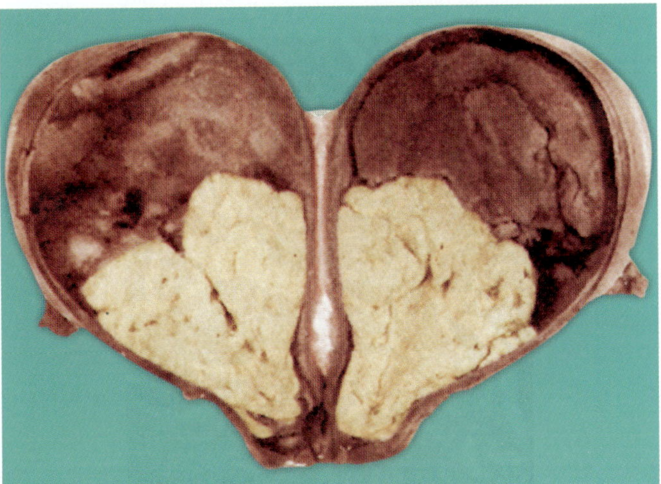

Fig. 34: An adenocarcinoma arising in the region of the isthmus of the uterus and blocking the cervix to cause a haematometra above the growth.

their glandular pattern but invade both stroma and myometrium **(Fig. 35)**. Areas of necrosis, haemorrhage and leucocytic infiltration are common. A minority of endometrial adenocarcinomas are less well differentiated and tend to show areas of solid growth, less gland formation, and more cytologic atypia, while a few are completely anaplastic.

Back-to-back arrangement of glands without intervening stroma, desmoplastic stroma, extensive papillary pattern and squamous epithelial differentiation are criteria that indicate the presence of invasion and are used to diagnose carcinoma. However, it may be difficult to differentiate well-differentiated endometrial carcinoma from atypical hyperplasia.

About 15–25% of adenocarcinomas contain foci of squamous metaplasia. Those tumours in which squamous metaplasia is prominent or conspicuous (>10% of the tumour) were earlier placed in a separate category, namely adenoacanthoma. If the squamous elements looked malignant, they were called adenosquamous carcinomas. The term endometrial carcinoma with squamous differentiation is now used instead of these terms as the differentiation of the squamous component is usually similar to the glandular and it is the latter, which determines the prognosis.

Other minor variations of the endometrioid adenocarcinomas are those with the villoglandular or papillary configuration (2%) and the secretory carcinoma (about 1%). The villoglandular carcinoma needs to be differentiated from the papillary serous carcinoma, which has a poorer prognosis, and the secretory from the clear cell carcinoma.

All the above are types of endometrioid adenocarcinomas that account for 80% of endometrial malignancy. Other endometrial carcinomas are the mucinous, papillary serous, clear cell, squamous, undifferentiated and mixed carcinomas.

Mucinous adenocarcinomas comprise about 5% of endometrial carcinomas. Over half the tumour has cells with intracytoplasmic mucin. The tumour has a good prognosis and needs to be distinguished from endocervical adenocarcinoma. A primary endometrial tumour can be diagnosed by the following: Merging with areas of normal endometrium, presence of endometrioid carcinoma, squamous metaplasia or foamy endometrial stromal cells; positive perinuclear immunohistochemical staining with vimentin.

Papillary serous carcinomas comprise 3–4% of endometrial carcinomas. They have branching papillae with a thin fibrovascular core and columnar cells with nuclear atypia **(Fig. 36)**. They have a very poor prognosis and are usually seen in elderly hypoestrogenic women. They account for up to half the deaths from endometrial carcinoma. They resemble serous carcinoma of the ovary and fallopian tube morphologically. Behaviourally, they are often associated with lymph vascular space and

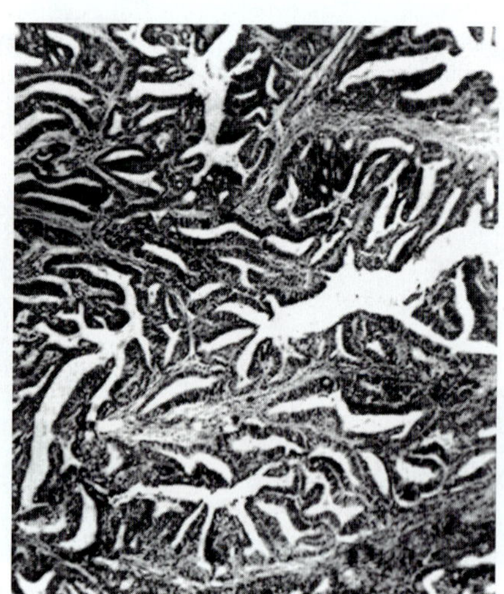

Fig. 35: A well-differentiated adenocarcinoma of the endometrium.

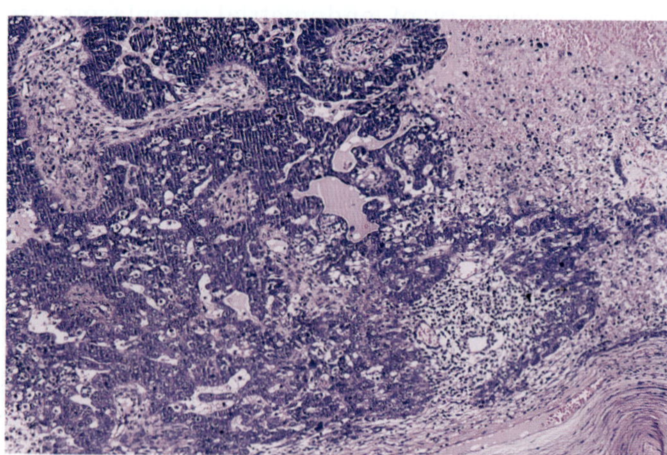

Fig. 36: *High-grade serous carcinoma endometrium* on haematoxylin and eosin stain showing papilla with fibrovascular core, solid nests and glandular formations. Individual tumour cells depict marked nuclear atypia, coarse chromatin and prominent nucleoli. Nuclei are disproportionately large compared to scant cytoplasm. *Image courtesy:* Dr Sufian Zaheer.

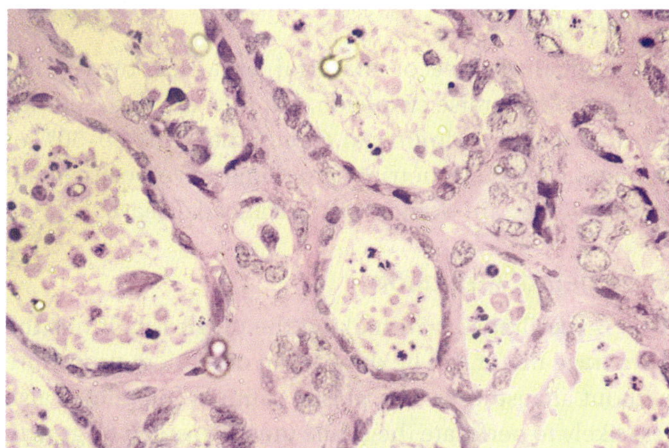

Fig. 37: *Clear cell carcinoma endometrium* on haematoxylin and eosin stain showing cells arranged in a glandular arrangement with a high nucleocytoplasmic ratio. Cells have pale eosinophilic to clear cytoplasm.
Image courtesy: Dr Sufian Zaheer.

deep myometrial invasion, and, like ovarian carcinoma, spread intra-abdominally. The presence of lymph node metastases, positive peritoneal cytology and intraperitoneal tumour does not correlate with the degree of myometrial invasion.

Less than 5% of endometrial carcinomas are of the clear cell type. It usually has a mixed histological pattern including tubules, papillae, solid sheets and glands **(Fig. 37)**. This tumour also occurs in older women and has a poorer prognosis than the papillary serous carcinoma.

Squamous Carcinoma

This is rare and has to be distinguished from cervical cancer: There should be a connection with the cervical epithelium in the latter case. It has a very poor prognosis.

Spread

Direct Invasion

The tumour usually grows slowly, especially when it is well differentiated and when it occurs in old age. It gradually infiltrates the myometrium but may take several years to reach the peritoneal coat. This indolence is sometimes attributed to a barrier of polysaccharides in the uterine wall.

Ultimately, the tumour protrudes on the outer surface of the uterus and invades the broad ligament and adjacent organs. Downwards spread to the endocervix can occur.

Lymphatic

Permeation of lymphatics probably accounts in part for some of the local spread, to the tubes and ovaries for example, and possibly to the upper vagina.

Involvement of the lymph nodes occurs relatively late, although not so late as was formerly believed. The nodes affected are the para-aortic group via the ovarian lymphatics, and the internal, external and common iliac groups via the uterine lymphatics. Occasionally, the route follows the round ligaments to the superficial inguinal nodes. Pelvic wall lymph node involvement is reported in 10–15% of cases coming to operation. It varies from nil, when the cancer is limited to the endometrium, to up to 40% if it invades the myometrium to within 1–2 mm of its peritoneal coat. The chance of finding cancer cells in the nodes also increases with the degree of anaplasia shown by the tumour. Thus, for tumours infiltrating the inner third of the myometrium the risk of pelvic node metastasis is substantial for grade 3; for tumours infiltrating the middle third of the myometrium the risk is substantial for grades 2 and 3; and for tumours infiltrating the outer third of the myometrium the risk is substantial for all grades of tumour.

Bloodstream

Embolism accounts for remote secondaries and for certain deposits in the pelvis, notably those which occur low on the anterior vaginal wall.

Seeding

Tubal washings in cases of carcinoma of the uterus frequently show the presence of malignant cells, and retrograde spill was once favoured as the mechanism of metastases in the ovaries and tubes. Lymphatic permeation is a more popular theory, if only because ovarian deposits are deep seated and not on the surface. Peritoneal washings from the pouch of Douglas may reveal malignant cells on cytological examination.

Cancer cells also spill from the undisturbed uterus into the vagina and can be picked up on vaginal cytology. It was once believed that cellular spill accounts for the development of vaginal metastases. Those in the lower vagina, however, undoubtedly represent vascular embolism.

Metastases

Vaginal metastases develop in 10–15% of cases. Those in the lower vagina are almost invariably suburethral in site and can arise before or after hysterectomy; those in the upper vagina only occur after this operation. The appearance of postoperative metastases in either site may be delayed for 3–4 years, but, in 50% of cases, it is within 1-year.

Ovarian secondaries, nearly always bilateral, are found in 3–5% of cases coming to surgery. Some may not be *secondaries,* however, and the same is true for rare cancers of the tube associated with endometrial cancer.

Extra pelvic metastases in the lungs, brain and elsewhere are rare and usually late manifestations.

Clinical Features

The only symptom of endometrial cancer, as a rule, is irregular bleeding and discharge occurring in a perimenopausal or postmenopausal woman. About 10% of cases of postmenopausal bleeding have endometrial cancer, but over 90% of cases of endometrial cancer present with abnormal bleeding. In approximately 1% of cases, the discharge is free from blood (hydrorrhoea); otherwise, it is brown, watery and offensive. The bleeding is not usually heavy, as it is in carcinoma of the cervix. Occasionally, the patient passes a piece of polypoid growth *per vaginum.*

Pain of an extraordinary character (Simpson's pain) is noted by 15% of patients. Referred to the hypogastrium or to both iliac fossae, it is not severe and tends to appear at the same time each day, lasting only 1–2 hours. It is probably caused by expulsive uterine contractions. Less than 5% of patients are asymptomatic, or detected by Pap smear, at ultrasound, computed tomography (CT) scan or hysterectomy for some other problem.

General physical examination is directed towards looking for obesity, hypertension, breast lesions and peripheral lymphadenopathy (supraclavicular, axillary and inguinal). Per speculum examination may reveal a polypoidal mass in case of an endocervical extension.

On bimanual examination, the uterus is usually small but may be enlarged with a big growth or haematopyometra. Palpation of the perineum, vagina, adnexa and of the parametrium by rectovaginal examination is important to assess the spread of the disease.

Diagnosis

Endometrial carcinoma has to be distinguished from endometrial hyperplasia, carcinoma of the cervix and all other causes of irregular bleeding and discharge. Every woman presenting with suggestive symptoms requires further investigation to establish the diagnosis.

Cytodiagnosis

Cytological studies of material obtained by vaginal aspiration may raise suspicion, but they are not methods for diagnosing endometrial carcinoma. Only 30–50% of patients with endometrial carcinoma have positive Pap tests, and they are women with advanced disease.

Endometrial Aspiration

This is the first step in making the diagnosis. It has the advantage that it can be done as an outpatient procedure without anaesthesia. The plastic cannula (pipelle) is also less likely to perforate the senile uterus invaded by growth than is the metallic curette. The diagnostic accuracy is 92–98% when compared with subsequent dilatation and curettage (D&C) or hysterectomy. Endometrial aspiration is combined with endocervical curettage to rule out cervical pathology.

Hysteroscopy and Dilation and Curettage

Hysteroscopy and D&C are not recommended routinely. D&C is advised in patients with cervical stenosis, if the specimen obtained is inadequate, especially if the clinical suspicion of malignancy is high, or if bleeding recurs after a negative report on endometrial aspiration. In the last-mentioned situation, if small growths are missed with the curette or where polyps are present, hysteroscopy aids by allowing direct visualisation and a guided biopsy.

The curettings are subjected to histological examination but to the expert, their naked-eye characteristics can be diagnostic. Malignancy is suggested if the curettings are profuse and friable, if they appear as cheesy lumps rather than strips, and if they are dark in colour. Failure of the uterine wall to *grate* in response to the curette is also suspicious.

Transvaginal Ultrasound and Saline Infusion Sonography

Transvaginal ultrasound is more accurate in delineating endometrial lesions and in evaluating myometrial invasion than is the transabdominal route. The finding of an endometrium >4 mm in thickness, a polypoid mass or a collection of fluid within the uterus is helpful in differentiating those patients who need further endometrial evaluation from those whose bleeding is likely to be caused by atrophy **(Figs. 38A and B)**. The instillation of fluid into the endometrial cavity (sonohysterography

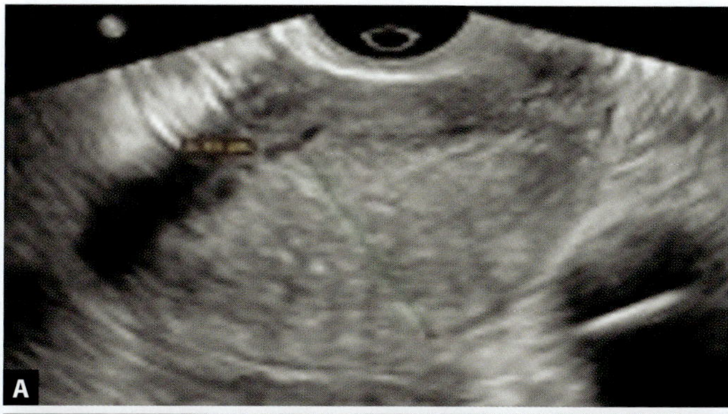

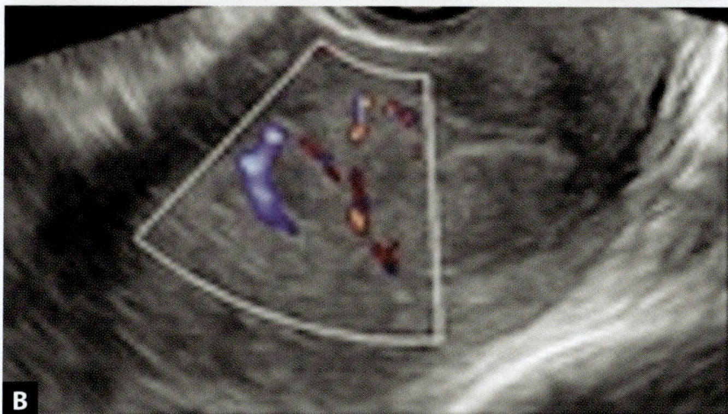

Figs. 38A and B: A TVUS image of a 55-year-old lady with postmenopausal bleeding, showing heterogenous thickened endometrium (Endometrial thickness: 35.3 mm) with moderate vascularity and indistinct endomyometrial interface. Minimal intracavitary fluid is also seen. Histopathological examination of endometrial biopsy is suggestive of endometroid cancer, squamous differentiation FIGO Stage II. (FIGO: International Federation of Gynaecology and Obstetrics; TVUS: transvaginal ultrasound)
Image courtesy: Dr Neha Bagri.

or saline infusion sonography) helps in the diagnosis of endometrial polyps.

There are concerns that the instillation of fluid during hysteroscopy and sonohysterography may aid the dissemination of malignant cells into the peritoneal cavity and lead to positive peritoneal cytology. However, it is not included in the staging but is of prognostic value. These procedures are best avoided when there is a high index of suspicion for malignancy, unless absolutely necessary for diagnosis.

Computed Tomography Scan and Magnetic Resonance Imaging

Computed tomography scan of the abdomen and pelvis is not routinely recommended. It can be used for staging of the disease in those women who are not suitable for surgery. MRI has the best sensitivity for assessing myometrial invasion. Thus, both ultrasonography and MRI can be used to plan the surgical procedure.

Serum Cancer Antigen-125

Serum cancer antigen-125 (CA-125) levels are usually normal in stages I and II. With extrauterine spread and peritoneal involvement, higher levels are found.

Staging of Endometrial Cancer

Endometrial cancer is surgically staged and pathologically examined. The latest FIGO staging system for endometrial cancer in 2023 defines the pathology and molecular findings related to endometrial carcinoma, which is inclusive of new treatments, results of clinical trials and prognostic and survival data **(Table 5)**.

Micrometastases are considered to be metastatic involvement [pN1 (mi)]. According to TNM8, macrometastases are >2 mm in size, micrometastases are >0.2–2 mm and/or >200 cells and isolated tumour cells are ≤0.2 mm and ≤200 cells.

For EECs, grade is based on the proportion of solid areas:
- Low grade = Grade 1 (≤5%) and grade 2 (6–50%)
- High grade = Grade 3 (>50%).

Nuclear atypia excessive for the grade raises the grade of a grade 1 or 2 tumour by one.

The presence of unusual nuclear atypia in an architecturally low-grade tumour should prompt the evaluation of p53 and consideration of serous carcinoma.

Adenocarcinomas with squamous differentiation are graded according to the microscopic features of the glandular component.

Lymphovascular Space Invasion

Lymphovascular space invasion (LVSI) should be assessed at the invasive front of the tumour. Focal LVSI is defined by the presence of a single focus around the tumour, substantial LVSI as multifocal or diffuse arrangement of LVSI or the presence of tumour cells in five or more lymph vascular spaces.

Myometrial Invasion

Myometrial invasion has been recognised as an essential prognostic risk factor. It is recommended that the assessment of the percentage of myometrium involved should be expressed as the percentage of the overall

TABLE 5: 2023 FIGO staging of cancer of endometrium.

Stage	*Description*
Stage I	*Confined to the uterine corpus and ovary*
IA	Disease limited to the endometrium OR nonaggressive histological type, i.e. low-grade endometroid, with invasion of less than half of the myometrium with no or focal lymphovascular space invasion (LVSI) OR good prognosis disease
IA1	Nonaggressive histological type limited to an endometrial polyp OR confined to the endometrium
IA2	Nonaggressive histological types involving less than half of the myometrium with no or focal LVSI
IA3	Low-grade endometrioid carcinomas limited to the uterus and ovary
IB	Nonaggressive histological types with invasion of half or more of the myometrium, and with no or focal LVSI
IC	Aggressive histological types are limited to a polyp or confined to the endometrium
Stage II	*Invasion of cervical stroma without extrauterine extension OR with substantial LVSI OR aggressive histological types with myometrial invasion*
IIA	Invasion of the cervical stroma of nonaggressive histological types
IIB	Substantial LVSI of nonaggressive histological types
IIC	Aggressive histological types with any myometrial involvement
Stage III	*Local and/or regional spread of the tumour of any histological subtype*
IIIA	Invasion of uterine serosa, adnexa or both by direct extension or metastasis
IIIA1	Spread to ovary or fallopian tube (except when meeting stage IA3 criteria)
IIIA2	Involvement of the uterine subserosa or spread through the uterine serosa
IIIB IIIB1 IIIB2	Metastasis or direct spread to the vagina and/or to the parametria or pelvic peritoneum Metastasis or direct spread to the vagina and/or the parametria Metastasis to the pelvic peritoneum
IIIC	Metastasis to the pelvic or para-aortic lymph nodes or both Metastasis to the pelvic lymph nodes
IIIC1	IIIC1i micrometastasis IIIC1ii macrometastasis
IIIC2	Metastasis to para-aortic lymph nodes up to the renal vessels, with or without metastasis to the pelvic lymph nodes IIIC2i micrometastasis IIIC2ii macrometastasis
Stage IV	*Spread to the bladder mucosa and/or intestinal mucosa and/or distant metastasis*
IVA	Invasion of the bladder mucosa and/or the intestinal/bowel mucosa
IVB	Abdominal peritoneal metastasis beyond the pelvis
IVC	Distant metastasis, including metastasis to any extra- or intra-abdominal lymph nodes above the renal vessels, lungs, liver, brain or bone

(EEC: endometrioid carcinoma; FIGO: International Federation of Gynaecology and Obstetrics)

myometrial thickness infiltrated by carcinoma using three categories: None; <50%; or ≥50%.

MOLECULAR CLASSIFICATION

Molecular features can be used to estimate the risk of recurrence and hence survival. Genetic testing of the endometrial tissue by next-generation sequencing is needed to identify the mutation.

The most impactful molecular classification is that proposed by The Cancer Genome Atlas (TCGA), which classifies endometrial carcinomas into four categories:

1. *POLE/ultra-mutated,* with somatic inactivating hotspot mutations in the *POLE* exonuclease domain and a very high mutational burden (ultra-mutated). Irrespective of grade, *POLE*-mutated tumours have an excellent prognosis

2. *Microsatellite instability (MSI)-high/hypermutated,* characterised by EECs or undifferentiated carcinomas with mismatch repair protein deficiency (MMRd)/ MSI, have an intermediate prognosis.
3. *Somatic copy-number alteration high/serous like (SCNA-high),* with a low mutation rate, nearly universal (95%) *TP53* mutations, and a highly unfavourable prognosis. Most of these tumours are serous carcinomas, but up to 25% are endometrioid (mostly high grade) and carcinosarcomas.
4. *Somatic copy-number alteration low (SCNA-low),* which includes EECs and CCCs with low copy—number alterations and low mutational burden.

Molecular classification is encouraged in all endometrial carcinomas, especially high-grade tumours **(Table 6)**. High-grade EEC (grade 3) is a prognostically, clinically and molecularly heterogeneous disease, and the tumour type that benefits most from applying molecular classification. POLE mutation analysis may be omitted in low-risk and intermediate-risk endometrial carcinoma with low-grade histology.

Immunohistochemistry: The morphologic features of the genetic mutations can be detected by special immunohistochemistry stains on the endometrial cancer tissue. The diagnostic algorithm that is currently used, widely available and cost-effective is based on three immunohistochemical markers and a molecular test [p53, mismatch repair markers MutS homologue 6 (MSH-6) and post-meiotic segregation increased 2 (PMS-2) and a mutation analysis of the exonuclease domain of polymerase-ε (POLE)] **(Figs. 39 and 40)**. The use of immunohistochemistry (IHC) markers helps to identify the prognostic categories equivalent to those obtainable with the molecular classification proposed by the TGCA. Prospective clinical trials have all consistently confirmed the prognostic relevance of the diagnostic algorithm in high-grade endometrial cancers.

Other IHC markers, such as L1 cell adhesion molecule (L1CAM) overexpression **(Fig. 41)** and the loss of oestrogen receptors (ERs) and/or progesterone receptors (PRs) are associated with poor prognosis and a high risk

TABLE 6: FIGO endometrial cancer stage with molecular classification.

Stage designation	Molecular findings in patients with early endometrial cancer (stages I and II after surgical staging)
Stage IAmPOLEmut	*POLEmut* endometrial carcinoma, confined to the uterine corpus or with cervical extension, regardless of the degree of LVSI or histological type
Stage IICmp53abn	p53abn endometrial carcinoma confined to the uterine corpus with any myometrial invasion, with or without cervical invasion, and regardless of the degree of LVSI or histological type

(FIGO: International Federation of Gynaecology and Obstetrics; LVSI: lymphovascular space invasion)

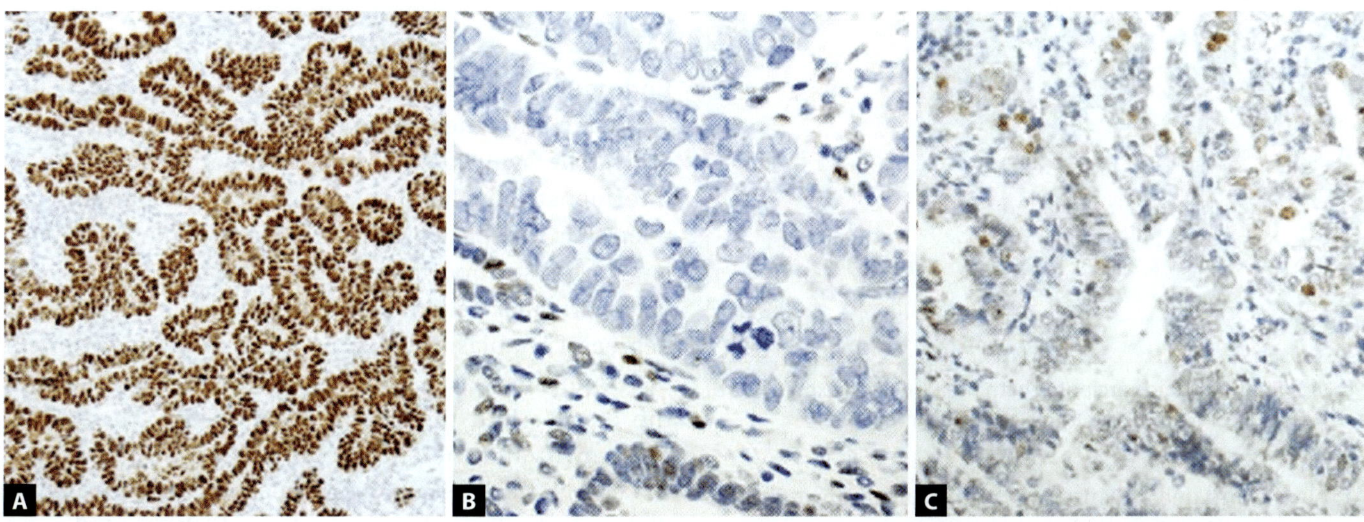

Figs. 39A to C: Mutation-type p53 immunoexpression in endometrial serous carcinoma is defined as: (A) Either diffuse strong nuclear staining in >80% of tumour cells or (B) complete absence of any staining in tumour cells; (C) p53 staining in grade 1 endometrioid carcinoma is weak and patchy (wild-type immunoreactivity).

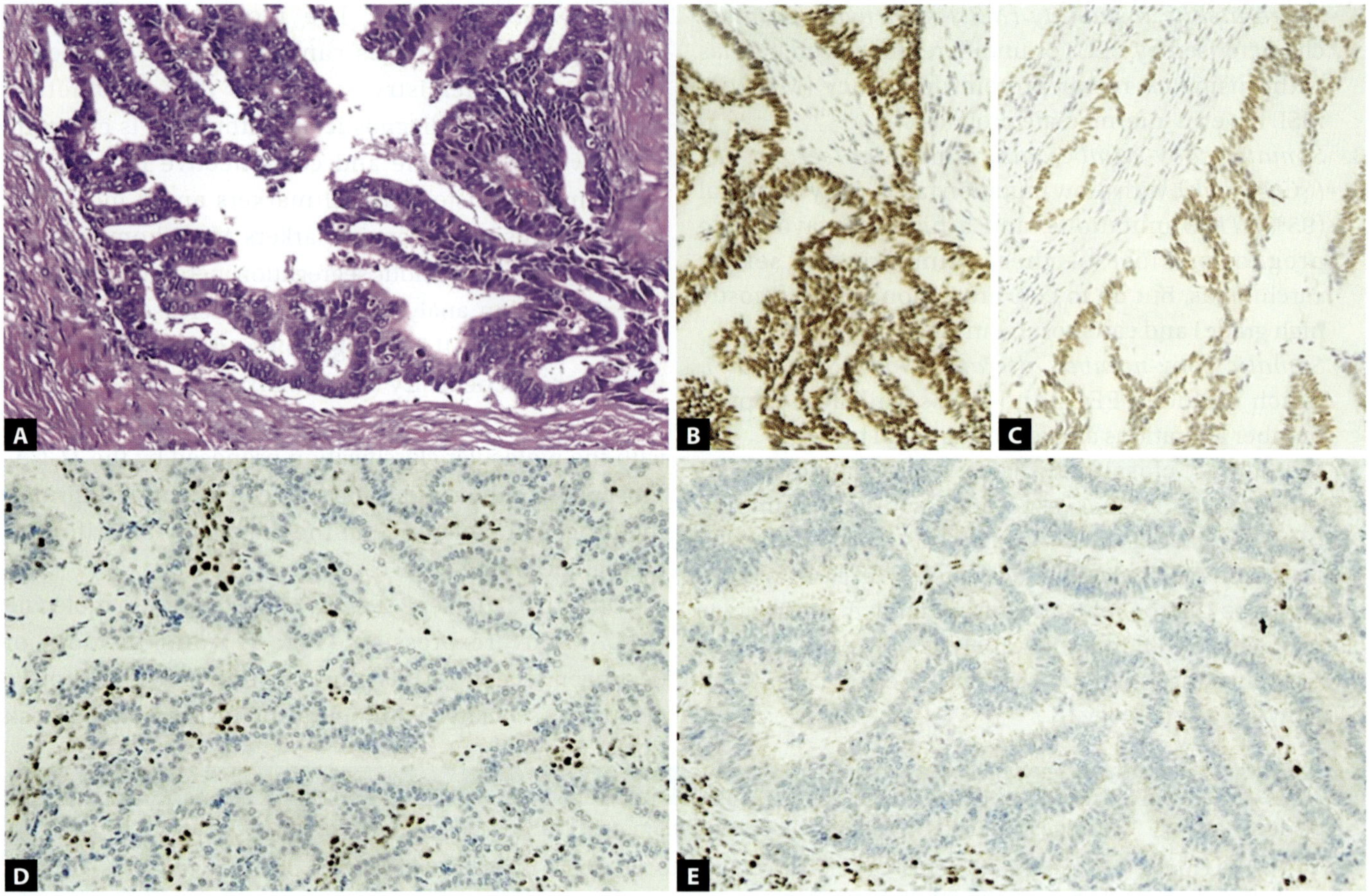

Figs. 40A to E: *MMR deficient endometrial Ca:* (A) Haematoxylin and eosin-stained section illustrating an endometrioid carcinoma of moderate grade (G2). By immunohistochemistry, neoplastic cells showed positive staining for MSH6 (B) and MSH2 (C) and negative staining for MLH1 (D) and PMS-2 (E). (MMR: mismatch repair; MLH1: MutL homologue 1; MSH6: mutS homologue 6; PMS-2: post-meiotic segregation increased 2)

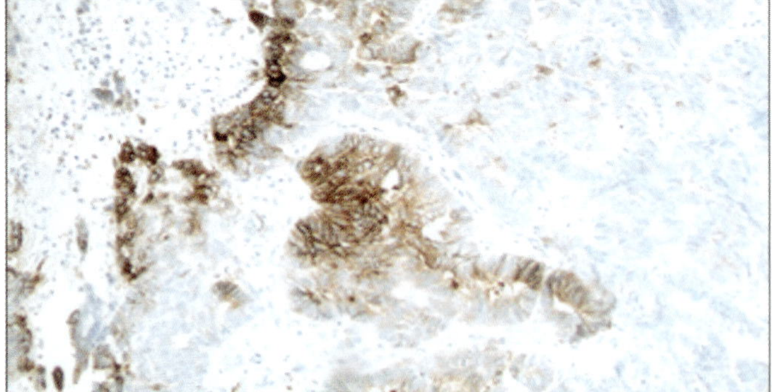

Fig. 41: Endometrioid carcinoma with membranous expression of L1CAM. (L1CAM: L1 cell adhesion molecule)

of relapse and death. Mutations of the tumour protein p53 are associated with L1CAM expression, but not universally.

Table 7 outlines the classification of disease risk by Gynecologic Oncology Group.

Prognosis

Endometrial carcinoma offers better prospects for cure than any other malignant growth in any site in the body. The symptoms of postmenopausal bleeding or intermenstrual bleeding also mean that patients are referred to the specialist earlier, usually within 3 months.

The most important factors governing the outlook for a particular patient are: The stage of the disease; the degree of anaplasia shown by the growth; involvement of lymph nodes, which is determined by the stage of the disease and the degree of anaplasia; the size of the growth and the encroachment of the tumour into the cervix; the presence of associated diseases such as diabetes, obesity and hypertension, which may influence treatment; and the availability of the best therapeutic facilities.

TABLE 7: Classification of disease risk by Gynecologic Oncology Group (GOG).

Disease risk	*Criteria*
Low-risk disease	MMRd or NSMP positive stage 1A tumours without any or only focal lymph vascular invasion or *POLE*mut stage 2 disease or less
Intermediate-risk disease	Any evidence of myometrial invasion, MMRd or NSMP positive stage 2 disease or less, or grade 2 or 3 disease
High-intermediate risk	PORTEC classifies individuals with two of the following factors within this category: 1. Age 60 or older and grade 3 disease 2. Myometrial invasion ≥50% GOG divides individuals by age and risk factors consisting of grades 2 and 3 with MMRd or NSMP subtyping, lymph vascular space invasion and invasion to the outer one third of the myometrium into the following subgroups: • Age 70 and older with at least 1 risk factor • Age 50 and older with ≥2 risk factors • Younger than 50 with all 3 risk factors
High-risk disease	Stage 3 disease or clear cell and serous carcinoma tumours of any stage; invasive, high-grade stage 1 endometrioid carcinoma is also placed in this group by some experts also

(MMRd: DNA mismatch repair protein deficiency; NSMP: no specific molecular profile; *POLEmut*: polymerase epsilon exonuclease domain mutated; PORTEC: postoperative radiation therapy in endometrial cancer)

Treatment

Pretreatment evaluation of the patient includes complete blood counts, serum chemistry, renal and liver function tests, urinalysis, blood type, chest X-ray, electrocardiogram and CA-125 levels. Ultrasound or MRI can assess myometrial invasion accurately. Unlike cervical cancer, cystoscopy, proctosigmoidoscopy, intravenous pyelography and CT scanning of the abdomen and pelvis are not indicated unless suggested by the clinical features or laboratory tests. Management of patients with endometrial carcinoma is shown in **Flowcharts 5A and B**.

Surgery

Surgical Management of Apparent Stage I/II Endometrial Carcinomas

Minimally invasive surgery is the preferred surgical approach, including patients with high-risk endometrial carcinoma. Standard surgery is total hysterectomy with bilateral salpingo-oophorectomy without vaginal cuff resection. The procedure includes peritoneal cytology, thorough exploration of the abdomen and pelvis and biopsy of extrauterine lesions followed by hysterectomy and bilateral salpingo-oophorectomy. Tumours with metastases outside the uterus and cervix (excluding lymph node metastases) are relative contraindications for minimally invasive surgery. Any intraperitoneal tumour spillage, including tumour rupture or morcellation (including in a bag), should be avoided. Staging infracolic omentectomy should be performed in clinical stage I serous endometrial carcinoma, carcinosarcoma and undifferentiated carcinoma and can be omitted in clear cell and endometrioid carcinoma in stage I disease. The cut section is examined for tumour size, depth of myometrial invasion and extension to the cervix.

Sentinel lymph node biopsy can be considered for staging purposes in patients with low-risk/intermediate-risk disease. It can be omitted in cases without myometrial invasion. Surgical lymph node staging should be performed in patients with high-intermediate-risk/high-risk disease. When a systematic lymphadenectomy is performed, pelvic and para-aortic infrarenal lymph node dissection is suggested. If pelvic lymph node involvement is found intraoperatively, further systematic pelvic lymph node dissection should be omitted. However, debulking of enlarged lymph nodes and para-aortic staging can be considered.

The specimen is sent for histopathological examination and, if possible, for measurement of steroid hormone receptors and flow cytometry.

Total hysterectomy with bilateral salpingo-oophorectomy and lymph node staging is the surgical standard of care in patients with stage II endometrial carcinoma, and more extensive procedures, such as radical hysterectomy, should only be performed if required to achieve free surgical margins.

Flowcharts 5A and B: Surgical management algorithm.

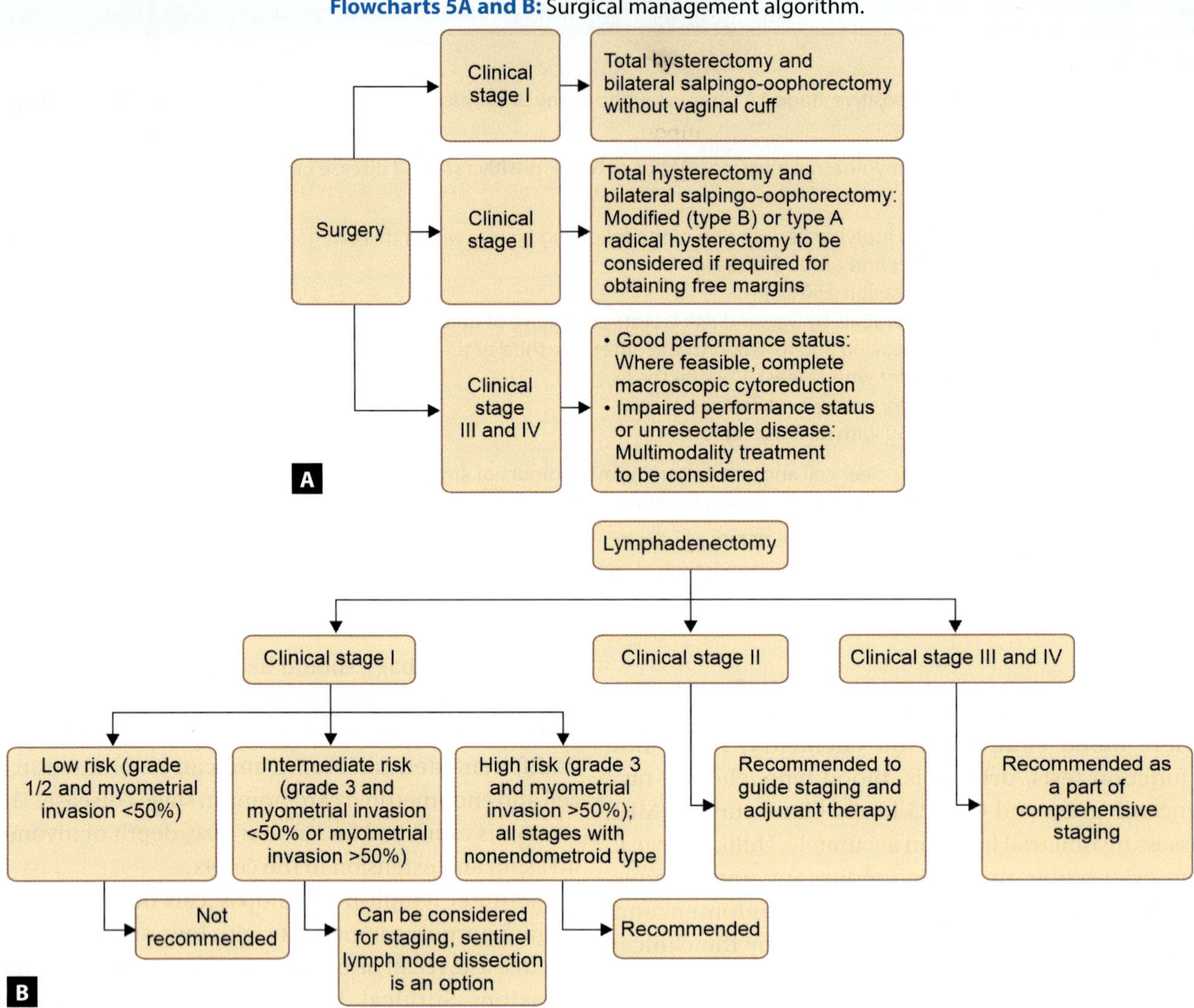

Surgery/Radiotherapy for Clinically Overt Stage III and IV Disease

In stage III and IV endometrial carcinoma (including carcinosarcoma), surgical tumour debulking, including enlarged lymph nodes, should be considered when complete macroscopic resection is feasible with an acceptable morbidity and quality of life profile. Primary systemic therapy should be used if upfront surgery is not feasible or acceptable. In cases of a good response to systemic therapy, delayed surgery can be considered. Systematic lymphadenectomy is not recommended, and only enlarged lymph nodes should be resected.

For unresectable tumours, a multidisciplinary approach should be taken and definitive radiotherapy with external beam radiation therapy (EBRT) and intrauterine brachytherapy, or neoadjuvant chemotherapy prior to surgical resection or definitive radiotherapy, depending on response, should be considered. Image-guided brachytherapy is recommended to boost intrauterine, parametrial or vaginal disease. Chemotherapy should be considered after definitive radiotherapy **(Flowcharts 5A and B)**.

ADJUVANT TREATMENT

- For patients with low-risk endometrial carcinoma, no adjuvant treatment is recommended.
- In intermediate-risk endometrial carcinoma, adjuvant brachytherapy can be recommended to decrease the vaginal recurrence rate. Omission of adjuvant brachytherapy can be considered, especially for patients

aged <60 years. For p53abn carcinomas restricted to a polyp or without myometrial invasion, adjuvant therapy is generally not recommended.

- In high-intermediate risk endometrial carcinoma (pN0 after lymph node staging), i.e. stage IA endometrioid carcinomas with substantial LVSI, stage IB low-grade endometrioid with substantial LVSI, stage IB high-grade endometrioid carcinomas regardless of LVSI and stage II endometrioid carcinomas, adjuvant brachytherapy/EBRT can be recommended to decrease the vaginal recurrence.
- In high-risk endometrial carcinomas (stages III and IVA without residual disease or stage I–IVA p53abn or non-endometrioid carcinomas without residual disease with myometrial invasion), EBRT with concurrent and adjuvant chemotherapy or alternatively sequential chemotherapy and radiotherapy is recommended.

Radiotherapy

Radiotherapy should preferably commence within 6–8 weeks of surgery or be scheduled in relation to chemotherapy. It is used in 5–15% of patients who are unfit for operative treatment or when the growth is too advanced for surgery.

Intensity-modulated radiation therapy (IMRT)/volumetric modulated arc therapy (VMAT) techniques are recommended, because the more conformal dose distribution increases normal tissue-sparing compared with a four-field conventional or 3D-conformal plan. The clinical target volume (CTV) includes the pelvic nodes (external iliac, internal iliac, obturator, distal common iliac), parametria and upper vagina. The upper common iliac and subaortic, presacral lymph nodes are included when there is cervical stromal involvement and/or pelvic lymph node involvement. The CTV should be individualised when there is a positive resection margin, pelvic peritoneal disease or vaginal involvement. Treatment with a comfortably full bladder reduces the volume of irradiated small bowel and bladder.

The prescription dose is commonly 45–50.4 Gy in 25–28 fractions over 5–6 weeks.

An integrated or sequential EBRT boost is given to residual lymph node disease, sites of extracapsular nodal spread and positive lateral resection margins with a total dose of 55–60 Gy for microscopic residual disease, or up to 66 Gy for macroscopic/bulky disease. Concurrent and adjuvant chemotherapy may be considered for stage III disease, serous histology and/or recurrent disease. The results of radiotherapy alone are generally inferior to those obtained with other methods, and most centres can obtain no >45–60% (65% for stage I) apparent 5-year cure rates. It has to be accepted that the patients are preselected as being advanced cases or poor surgical risks.

Chemotherapy and Hormone Therapy

Disseminated metastatic disease found either at the initial operation or as a recurrence requires systemic therapy. The efficiency of progestogen therapy in producing objective responses has been reported in approximately 30% of patients with metastatic endometrial carcinoma.

Hormone therapy is the preferred front-line systemic therapy for patients with low-grade carcinomas without rapidly progressive disease.

Progestogens (MPA 200–300 mg and megestrol acetate 160 mg) are recommended. Alternative options for hormonal therapies include aromatase inhibitors, tamoxifen and fulvestrant.

The standard chemotherapy treatment is carboplatin area under the curve (AUC) 5–6+ paclitaxel 175 mg/m^2 every 21 days for six cycles. Partial response rates of 38–76% are reported, with a median survival of <12 months. In patients with a long platinum-free interval, reintroduction of platinum can be considered.

Anti-PD1-based immune therapy with pembrolizumab could be considered for second-line therapy of MSI/MMRd carcinomas.

Follow-Up for Endometrial Cancer

For low-risk endometrial cancer, the proposed surveillance is at least every 6 months, with physical and gynaecological examination for the first 2 years and then yearly until 5 years. For the high-risk groups, physical and gynaecological examinations are recommended every 3 months for the first 3 years, and then every 6 months until 5 years.

A CT scan or positron emission tomography-computed tomography (PET-CT) could be considered in the high-risk group, particularly if node extension was present. Nearly 80% of recurrences can be detected by clinical methods. Regular exercise, healthy diet and weight management should be promoted with all endometrial cancer survivors.

The 5-year survival rate is >95% for patients with stage 1 endometrial cancer, and >80% of patients are diagnosed early in the disease process. Endometrial cancer has a good prognosis overall, though some molecular subtypes have better survival rates than others. Patients with endometrial cancer of the *POLE* molecular subtypes have a 5-year relapse-free survival rate of 98%, while the rate of those with p53abn subtypes, which is associated with the highest risk for metastasis, is 46.6%. For those in stages IIB and IIIA, survival rates vary between 55 and 77%, depending on the grade. It decreases to 42–59% in stage IIIC and 18–35% in stage IV.

Uterine Sarcoma

Uterine sarcomas are a heterogeneous group of malignancies that arise from mesenchymal tissue within the uterus. They account for approximately 1% of all female genital tract malignancies and 3–7% of all uterine cancers. Their rarity and histopathological diversity have contributed to the lack of consensus on risk factors for poor outcome and optimal treatment. Various preoperative diagnostic tests for the evaluation of suspicious uterine tumours have been developed and each test has varying degrees and ranges of accuracy—endometrial biopsy, 58–64%; pelvic ultrasonography, 11–56%; pelvic MRI, 35.3–80%; lactate dehydrogenase (LDH); and sensitivity, 0.47. The use of these tests in combination with patient demographics, such as age and menopausal status, has been proposed for use independently or as part of an algorithm to determine a 'preoperative risk score' for uterine tumours.

Prolonged exposure to tamoxifen is associated with a three times risk of sarcoma development. Radiation-induced sarcomas occurring long after treatment for other cancers have been reported.

Carcinosarcoma has been reclassified, largely based on its spreading pattern, as a dedifferentiated or metaplastic form of endometrial carcinoma and is now staged under endometrial carcinoma **(Flowchart 6)**.

The new FIGO staging system developed in 2009 for uterine sarcomas has two divisions, one for leiomyosarcoma and endometrial stromal sarcoma (ESS), and one for adenosarcoma.

Leiomyosarcomas

Leiomyosarcoma has become the most common subtype of uterine sarcoma, even though it accounts for only 1–2% of uterine malignancies. Approximately 1 in every 800 smooth muscle tumours of the uterus is leiomyosarcoma. It occurs in women over 40 years of age. Up to 4% of patients may have received pelvic radiotherapy previously.

Flowchart 6: Classification of uterine sarcomas (WHO 2014).

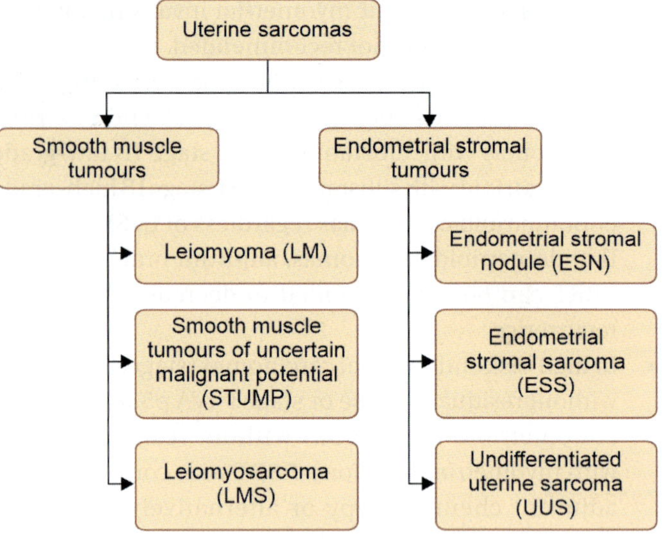

(WHO: World Health Organization)

Women usually present with abnormal vaginal bleeding, a palpable pelvic mass and pelvic pain. Signs and symptoms resemble those of leiomyoma and preoperative distinction between the two tumours may be difficult. Malignancy should be suspected by the presence of tumour growth in postmenopausal women who are not using hormonal replacement therapy, although it is rare for a leiomyosarcoma to present as a rapidly growing tumour **(Figs. 42 and 43)**.

Two-thirds of leiomyosarcomas are intramural, poorly circumscribed and cannot be shelled from the surrounding myometrium. The cut surface is bulging, soft, fleshy, focally necrotic and haemorrhagic and lacks the whorled appearance.

On histology, the most clinically malignant smooth muscle tumours of the uterus exhibit the constellation of hypercellularity, severe nuclear atypia and high mitotic rate generally exceeding 15 mitotic figures per 10 high power fields (MF/10 HPF).

Supportive clinicopathologic features such as peri- or postmenopausal age, extrauterine extension, large size (over 10 cm), infiltrating border, necrosis and atypical mitotic figures are frequently present.

Epithelioid and myxoid leiomyosarcomas are two rare variants that may be difficult to recognise microscopically, due to mild nuclear atypia and low mitotic rate (<3 MF/10 HPF). In the absence of severe cytologic atypia and high mitotic activity, both tumours are diagnosed as sarcomas based on their infiltrative borders.

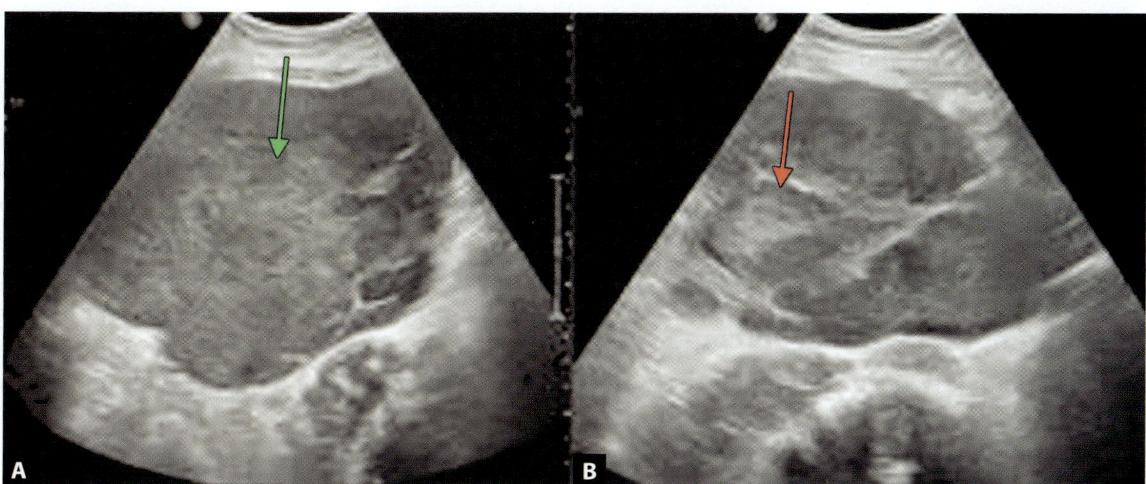

Figs. 42A and B: Ultrasound pelvis showing a large heterogeneous uterine mass diffusely infiltrating the myometrium (green arrow) and extension in the endometrial cavity (red arrow). Histopathological examination of the uterine mass is suggestive of leiomyosarcoma.
Image courtesy: Dr Neha Bagri.

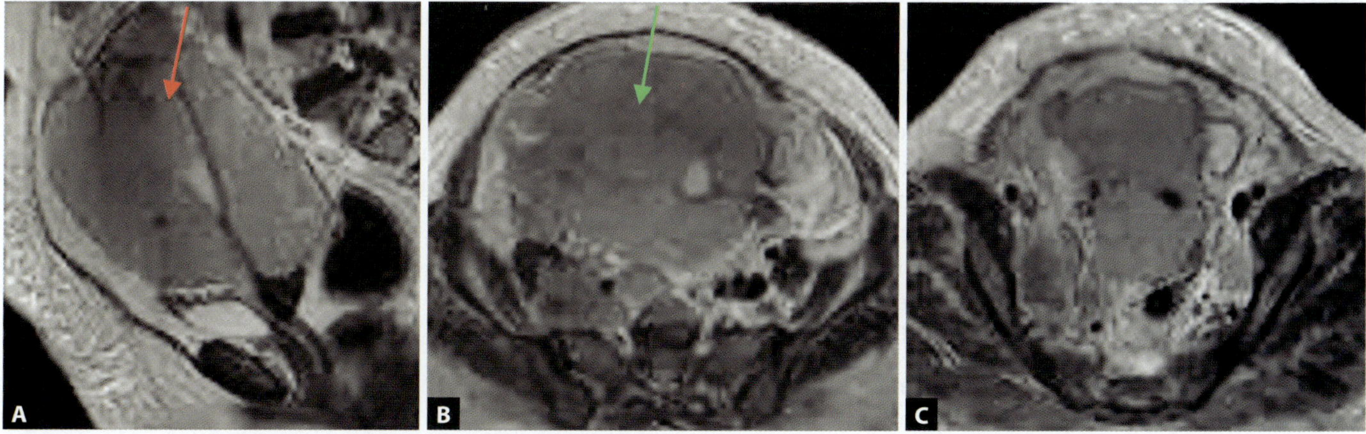

Figs. 43A to C: (A) MRI pelvis (T2 sagittal and axial) showing a large heterogeneous uterine mass diffusely infiltrating the myometrium (green arrow) and (B) extension in the endometrial cavity (red arrow); (C) Histopathological examination of the uterine mass is suggestive of leiomyosarcoma. (MRI: magnetic resonance imaging)
Image courtesy: Dr Neha Bagri.

Treatment of Leiomyosarcomas

Treatment includes total abdominal hysterectomy and debulking of the tumour if present outside the uterus. Removal of the ovaries and lymph node dissection remains controversial as metastases to these organs occur in only a small percentage of cases and are frequently associated with intra-abdominal disease.

In completely resected organ-confined disease (stages I and II), the influence of adjuvant systemic therapy or radiotherapy on survival is uncertain. Docetaxel/gemcitabine, doxorubicin and ifosfamide are all reasonable options for advanced or recurrent disease.

Targeted therapies such as trabectedin and olaratumab have been investigated as treatment in advanced-stage or metastatic leiomyosarcoma.

Prognosis of leiomyosarcomas: Leiomyosarcomas are associated with poor prognosis even when confined to the uterus at the time of diagnosis, with a recurrence rate ranging from 53 to 71%.

The first recurrence occurs in the lungs in 40% of patients and in the pelvis in only 13%. Overall, 5-year survival rate ranges from 15 to 25% with a median survival of only 10 months. All patients with tumour spread outside the pelvis died within 5 years.

ENDOMETRIAL STROMAL TUMOURS

Endometrial stromal tumours account for <1% of all uterine tumours and represent the second most common category of mesenchymal uterine tumours.

Low-grade Endometrial Stromal Sarcoma

Low-grade ESSs frequently occur in women between 40 and 55 years of age and >50% of patients are premenopausal. Around 25% of women are asymptomatic, and common presentation is usually with AUB, pelvic pain and dysmenorrhoea.

Extrauterine pelvic extension, most commonly involving the ovary, is found in up to one third of patients at the time of presentation. This nonencapsulated tumour extends into the broad ligament and shows a peculiar tendency to permeate veins and lymphatics. When the uterus is removed, these extensions can be pulled out from the broad ligament as worm-like threads.

Microscopically, ESSs consist of well-differentiated endometrial stromal cells exhibiting mild nuclear atypia and characteristically invade the lymph vascular spaces of the myometrium. On IHC, the tumour cells are strongly immunoreactive for CD10, usually positive for smooth-muscle actin and less frequently for desmin (30%), but they are negative for h-caldesmon and HDAC8.

Treatment: Surgical treatment in the form of hysterectomy and bilateral salpingo-oophorectomy can be considered. Lymph node dissection does not seem to have a role in the treatment of these tumours. Patients may also receive adjuvant radiation or hormonal treatment with progestational agents or aromatase inhibitors. Post-treatment hormone (oestrogen) replacement therapy is discouraged.

Although distant metastases are uncommon, the local recurrence rate is between 40 and 80% and 5–25% of the women die of the disease. Late recurrences may occur up to 25 years after the original diagnosis. Recurrences usually occur when the tumour has reached or breached the serosa. 5-year survival for patients with stage I and II tumours is 90% compared with 50% for stages III and IV.

High-grade Stromal Sarcoma

These rare tumours have features that are intermediate between low-grade ESSs and undifferentiated sarcomas. Patients range in age from 28 to 67 years (mean 50 years). Tumours may appear as intracavitary polypoid or mural masses. The cut surface is fleshy with extensive areas of necrosis and haemorrhage. Microscopically, they consist mainly of high-grade round cells that are sometimes associated with a low-grade spindle cell component that is most commonly fibromyxoid **(Fig. 44)**. Mitotic activity is typically >10 per 10 HPF. Necrosis is usually present. On IHC, high-grade ESSs are CD10, ER and PR negative but show strong diffuse cyclin D1 immunoreactivity (>70% nuclei). They are also typically c-kit positive but DOG1 negative.

Compared with low-grade ESSs, patients with high-grade ESSs have earlier and more frequent recurrences (often <1 year) and are more likely to die of the disease. Advanced or recurrent tumours should be treated aggressively with a combination of radiation and chemotherapy.

The 5-year survival rate is approximately 25%.

Spread

Apart from local invasion, sarcoma of the uterus spreads by the bloodstream, the common site for metastases being the lungs.

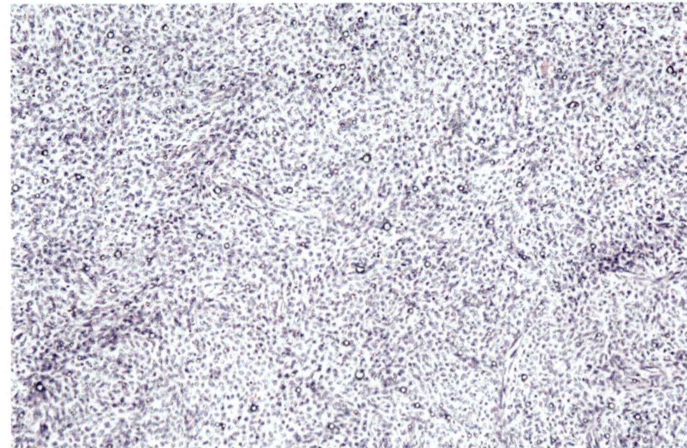

Fig. 44: *Endometrial stromal sarcoma (ESS)* on haematoxylin and eosin stain showing cells resembling proliferative-phase endometrial stroma with a uniform, small, spindle-shaped appearance. There is minimal nuclear pleomorphism with relatively bland nuclei. Nuclei are oval to round in shape with evenly dispersed chromatin and small, indistinct nucleoli. The cytoplasm is scant and lightly eosinophilic.
Image courtesy: Dr Sufian Zaheer.

Follow-Up of Sarcomas

Follow-up is determined by the risk of recurrence. Metastasis of sarcomas to the lungs is common, and efforts must be made to rule these out.

Low-grade sarcoma patients may be followed for local relapse every 4–6 months for the first 3–5 years, then yearly.

High-grade tumours can be followed up every 3–4 months for the first 2–3 years, twice a year for the next 2–3 years, and then annually.

Mixed Müllerian Tumours

This group of tumours is considered here, because it is uncertain whether they originate primarily in the endometrium or myometrium. Rarely, these tumours can also develop in the cervix and ovary. They are identical regardless of their origin.

The tumours arise from Müllerian mesenchymal cells, which differentiate into stromal and epithelial elements. If both components are benign, the tumour is known as a Müllerian adenofibroma, but if both components are malignant, the tumour is called a malignant mixed Müllerian tumour (or mixed mesenchymal sarcoma, mixed mesodermal sarcoma, among other names). If the epithelial element of a mixed tumour is benign and the stromal element malignant, it is called a Müllerian adenosarcoma; the alternative combination is rare.

The epithelial component of a mixed Müllerian tumour is usually of a type found in the uterus, but whilst the stromal component can differentiate into smooth muscle or endometrial stroma—like cells, it can differentiate into other tissues such as cartilage, striated muscle or bone **(Fig. 45)**. The heterogeneous structure of these tumours reflects the capacity of the mesoderm of the Müllerian ducts to differentiate in many directions, a potential retained by adult tissues.

Clinical Features

Despite their complexity, malignant mixed Müllerian tumours occur principally in older women, the median age of incidence being 62 years. The presenting symptom is usually vaginal bleeding but pelvic pain and vaginal discharge are also common symptoms and fragments of necrotic tumour may be passed per vaginum.

On examination, the uterus is invariably enlarged by a bulky, soft, fleshy, polypoidal tumour mass, which tends to fill the uterine cavity and sometimes passes through the cervical canal to present in the vagina. The tumour contains foci of haemorrhage and necrosis.

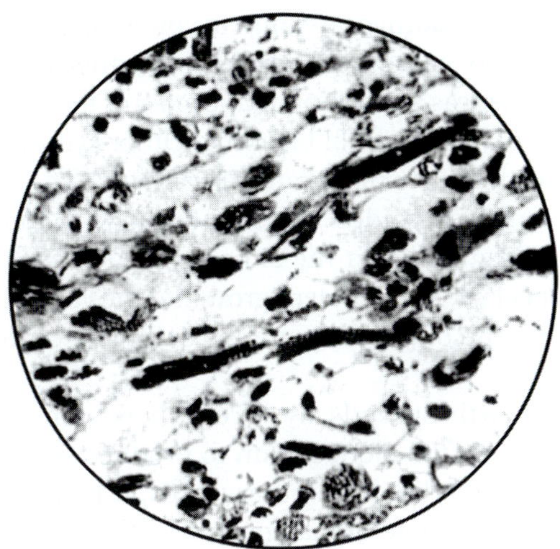

Fig. 45: A malignant mixed Müllerian (mesodermal) tumour with heterologous elements. A variety of malignant cells including conspicuous strap—like muscle cells with cross striations: these are rhabdomyosarcomatous elements.

The pattern of spread is similar to that for endometrial adenocarcinoma, but the rate of progression is faster, and for mixed Müllerian tumours, it is highly aggressive. It is common for the tumour to have spread outside the uterus before the diagnosis is made and to involve the pelvic peritoneum and lymph nodes. Death is almost certain and rapid if the tumour has spread outside the uterus.

Treatment protocol is as for the high-grade ESS, i.e. total abdominal hysterectomy and bilateral salpingo-oophorectomy followed by radiotherapy and chemotherapy, but response to chemotherapy is very poor.

The Müllerian adenosarcoma is a much less malignant neoplasm and, although often developing in the same age group, tends to occur in younger women. The adenosarcoma is of relatively low-grade malignancy and, while pelvic or vaginal recurrences occur in about half the patients after hysterectomy, distant metastases are uncommon. Those patients with local recurrence often survive for prolonged periods.

Occasionally, a mixed Müllerian tumour is limited to a uterine polyp, and there is no invasion of the myometrium. In these cases, there may be a favourable outcome.

Overall, the 5-year survival rate is 20–30%.

Rhabdomyosarcomas

These occur in two locations in the female genital tract. Some are confined to the uterine myometrium and others arise in the cervix and vagina.

Vaginal rhabdomyosarcomas in young girls are usually referred to as sarcoma botryoides (grape-like). They usually present as an asymptomatic mass or the presenting symptom may be vaginal bleeding. Other symptoms are usually secondary to metastatic disease.

Sarcoma botryoides is an embryonal rhabdomyosarcoma originating in the subepithelial tissues of the vagina or cervix. As the polyps grow into the vaginal cavity, they retain the original squamous epithelial covering of the vagina.

The growth spreads by direct extension to other organs, and via the bloodstream to produce secondaries, especially in the lungs; in other words, it behaves like a sarcoma. The degree of malignancy varies but is usually high. The typical sarcoma botryoides seen in children is often fatal, irrespective of treatment.

Other Rare Uterine Tumours

Melanoma

Melanoma of the uterus is always a secondary growth, even though it is sometimes difficult to locate the primary. It is a pathological curiosity.

Haemangiopericytoma

Both benign and malignant forms of this tumour of the uterine wall are described. It arises from pericytes and consists of masses of blood vessels, each surrounded by one or more layers of round, oval or spindle cells.

Depending on its site, on encroachment of the uterine cavity, and on its benign or malignant nature, the condition causes symptoms similar to those of adenomyosis or endometrial carcinoma. The uterus is often palpably enlarged, so the clinical diagnosis is usually leiomyoma or adenomyosis.

The true nature of the lesion is only revealed by histological examination of the specimen resulting from hysterectomy.

Leukaemic and Lymphadenomatous Growths; Lymphomas

These, formerly extremely rare, are occurring with increasing frequency. This is because the modern chemotherapy of leukaemias and of Hodgkin's disease is so efficient as to prolong life and ensure remissions without always producing a cure. There is, therefore, much more opportunity for masses of leucoblastic or lymphomatous tissues to develop in the pelvic organs.

The most common sites are the ovaries and tubes, which become involved in large fixed tumours. The uterus, too, can be a site; the growths infiltrate its wall and extend into the broad ligaments and other tissues to produce physical signs similar to those of advanced carcinoma of the cervix. The development of ascites is often the lead to the lymphomatous tissue in the adnexa. Symptoms similar to those of cancer of the cervix or corpus draw attention to uterine involvement. Knowledge that the patient is suffering, or has suffered, from leukaemia or lymphoma strongly suggests the diagnosis, and this can be confirmed by biopsy of any growth which is accessible. The only treatment is as for the primary disease.

SUGGESTED READING

1. Al-Hendy A, Salama SA. Catechol-O-methyltransferase polymorphism is associated with increased uterine leiomyoma risk in different ethnic groups. J Soc Gynecol Investig. 2006;13(2):136-44.
2. Berek JS, Matias-Guiu X, Creutzberg C, Fotopoulou C, Gaffney D, Kehoe S, et al. FIGO staging of endometrial cancer: 2023. Int J Gynecol Obstet. 2023;162:383-94.
3. Bettocchi S, Ceci O, Nappi L, Di Venere R, Masciopinto V, Pansini V, et al. Operative office hysteroscopy without anesthesia: analysis of 4863 cases performed with mechanical instruments. J Am Assoc Gynecol Laparosc. 2004;11:59-61.
4. Boynton-Jarrett R, Rich-Edwards J, Malspeis S, Missmer SA, Wright R. A prospective study of hypertension and risk of uterine leiomyomata. Am J Epidemiol. 2005;161(7):628-38.
5. Brooks RA, Fleming GF, Lastra RR, Lee NK, Moroney JW, Son CH, et al. Current recommendations, and recent progress in endometrial cancer. CA Cancer J Clin. 2019;69(4):258-79.
6. Concin N, Matias-Guiu X, Vergote I, Cibula D, Mirza MR, Marnitz S, et al. ESGO/ESTRO/ESP guidelines for the management of patients with endometrial carcinoma. Int J Gynecol Cancer. 2021;31:12-39.
7. Eltoukhi HM, Modi MN, Weston M, Armstrong AY, Stewart EA. The health disparities of uterine fibroid tumors for African American women: a public health issue. Am J Obstet Gynecol. 2014;210(3):194-9.
8. Emons G, Beckmann MW, Schmidt D, Mallmann P. Uterus commission of the Gynecological Oncology Working Group (AGO). New WHO classification of endometrial hyperplasias. Geburtshilfe Frauenheilkd. 2015;75:135-6.
9. Exacoustos C, Zupi E, Marconi D, Romanini ME, Szabolcs B, Piredda A, et al. Ultrasound-assisted laparoscopic cryomyolysis: two- and three-dimensional findings before, during and after treatment. Ultrasound Obstet Gynecol. 2005;25:393-400.
10. Fischer K, McDannold NJ, Tempany CM, Jolesz FA, Fennessy FM. Potential of minimally invasive procedures

in the treatment of uterine fibroids: a focus on magnetic resonance-guided focused ultrasound therapy. Int J Womens Health. 2015;7:901-12.

11. Kapp DS, Shin JY, Chan JK. Prognostic factors and survival in 1396 patients with uterine leiomyosarcomas: emphasis on impact of lymphadenectomy and oophorectomy. Cancer. 2008;112:820-30.
12. Koppikar S, Oaknin A, Govind Babu K, Lorusso D, Gupta S, Wu LY, et al. Pan-Asian adapted ESMO Clinical Practice Guidelines for the diagnosis, treatment and follow-up of patients with endometrial cancer. ESMO Open. 2023;8(1):100774.
13. Lee M, Chung YJ, Kim HK, Hwang H, Park JY, Shin I, et al. Estimated prevalence and incidence of uterine leiomyoma, and its treatment trend in South Korean women for 12 years: a national population-based study. J Women's Health. 2021;30(7):1038-46.
14. Leon-Castillo A, De Boer SM, Powell ME, Mileshkin LR, Mackay HJ, Leary A, et al. Molecular classification of the PORTEC-3 trial for high-risk endometrial cancer: impact on prognosis and benefit from adjuvant therapy. J Clin Oncol. 2020;38:3388-97.
15. Makker V, MacKay H, Ray-Coquard I, Levine DA, Westin SN, Aoki D, et al. Endometrial cancer. Nat Rev Dis Primers. 2021;7(1):88.
16. Markowski DN, Bartnitzke S, Löning T, Drieschner N, Helmke BM, Bullerdiek J. MED12 mutations in uterine fibroids–their relationship to cytogenetic subgroups. Int J Cancer. 2012;131(7):1528-36.
17. McGuire MM, Yatsenko A, Hoffner L, Jones M, Surti U, Rajkovic A. Whole exome sequencing in a random sample of North American women with leiomyomas identifies MED12 mutations in majority of uterine leiomyomas. PLoS One. 2012;7(3):e33251.
18. Moroni RM, Martins WP, Ferriani RA, Vieira CS, Nastri CO, Candido Dos Reis FJ, et al. Add-back therapy with GnRH analogues for uterine fibroids. Cochrane Database Syst Rev. 2015;3:CD010854.
19. Munro MG, Critchley HOD, Broder MS, Fraser IS; FIGO Working Group on Menstrual Disorders. FIGO classification system (PALM-COEIN) for causes of abnormal uterine bleeding in nongravid women of reproductive age. Int J Gynaecol Obstet. 2011;113:3-13.
20. Piulats JM, Guerra E, Gil-Martín M, Roman-Canal B, Gatius S, Sanz-Pamplona R, et al. Molecular approaches for classifying endometrial carcinoma. Gynecol Oncol. 2017;145:200-7.
21. Qiwei Y, Michal C, Maria VB, Mohamed A, Hoda E, Thomas GB, et al. Comprehensive review of uterine fibroids: developmental origin, pathogenesis, and treatment. Endocrine Rev. 2021;43(4):678-719.
22. Shen Y, Xu Q, Xu J, Ren ML, Cai YL. Environmental exposure and risk of uterine leiomyoma: an epidemiologic survey. Eur Rev Med Pharmacol Sci. 2013;17(23):3249-56.
23. Tristan M, Orozco LJ, Steed A, Ramírez-Morera A, Stone P. Mifepristone for uterine fibroids. Cochrane Database Syst Rev. 2012;8:CD007687.
24. van der Putten LJ, Visser NC, van de Vijver K, Santacana M, Bronsert P, Bulten J, et al. L1CAM expression in endometrial carcinomas: an ENITEC collaboration study. Br J Cancer. 2016;115:716-24.
25. Van Gool IC, Stelloo E, Nout RA, Nijman HW, Edmondson RJ, Church DN, et al. Prognostic significance of L1CAM expression and its association with mutant p53 expression in high-risk endometrial cancer. Mod Pathol. 2016;29:174-81.
26. Vilos GA, Allaire C, Laberge PY, Leyland N. The management of uterine leiomyomas. J Obstet Gynaecol Can. 2015;37:157-81.
27. Yang Y, He Y, Zeng Q, Li S. Association of body size and body fat distribution with uterine fibroids among Chinese women. J Womens Health (Larchmt). 2014;23(7):619-26.

32

CHAPTER

Adenomyosis

Anjali Mundkur, Muralidhar V Pai

Chapter Outline

- Associated Pathology
- Aetiology
- Diagnosis
- Differential Diagnosis
- Management
- Complications

INTRODUCTION

Adenomyosis is a condition in which there is a growth of endometrial cells inside the uterine myometrium (usually >2.5 mm beneath the basal endometrium). It is associated with myometrial hypertrophy and may be either diffuse or focal (adenomyoma). Microscopically, there are ectopic, non-neoplastic endometrial glands and stroma, surrounded by hypertrophic and hyperplastic myometrium.

The majority of cases of adenomyosis is diagnosed following histological examination of hysterectomy specimens showing a prevalence varying between 5% and 70%. The prevalence in the general population, however, remains unclear. The majority of cases is reported among women in the age group of 40–50 years, and there is a positive association with parity. Multiparas between the ages of 30 and 50 years are most commonly affected with this disease. No association has been observed with age at menarche, menopausal status, or age at hysterectomy or its indication.

ASSOCIATED PATHOLOGY

Nearly 80% of women with adenomyomas may also have other lesions, the most common being leiomyomas. Other lesions that may frequently occur in these cases include endometrial polyps, endometrial hyperplasia (with or without atypia), adenocarcinoma and pelvic endometriosis. Presence of adenomyosis, however, has no adverse effect on cancer survival.

AETIOLOGY

Abnormal in growth and invagination of the basal endometrium into the subendometrial myometrium at the endometrial–myometrial interface are likely to result in development of adenomyosis. In case of adenomyosis, the margins are poorly defined because the endometrial glands and stroma are in direct contact with the myometrium. Hence, these lesions cannot be enucleated. Though the exact cause of adenomyosis remains unknown, various factors, such as hormonal, genetic and immunological, are likely to play a role in the pathogenesis of adenomyosis. Some likely causes are as follows:

- *Uterine trauma:* Various causes of uterine trauma that may break the barrier between the endometrium and myometrium include surgical procedures such as caesarean section, tubal ligation and pregnancy termination. Pregnancy is another factor that can break this barrier.
- *Oestrogen dominance:* Conditions associated with the localised production of excessive oestrogens may predispose the woman to develop adenomyosis.
- *Abnormal level of various cytokines:* Increased levels of interleukin 18 (IL-18) receptor messenger RNA (mRNA) and the ratio of IL-18 binding protein to IL-18, and dysregulation of leukaemia inhibitory factor.
- *Misplaced pluripotent Müllerian remnants:* This is supported by various studies that describe proliferative and biological properties of ectopic and eutopic endometrium with distinct characteristics. The response to hormones, secretory changes and cyclic properties are not similar to eutopic endometrium.
- *Invagination of myometrial basalis:* This proceeds along the myometrial lymphatic system leading to adenomyosis.
- *Origin from the bone marrow derived stem cells:* This theory suggests that bone marrow-derived stem cells contribute to the regeneration of the endometrium.

- *Tissue injury induced by uterine hyperperistalsis/ dysperistalsis (TIAR) causes adenomyosis.*
- *Epigenetic theory: Alterations:* Increased expression of deoxyribonucleic acid methyltransferases enzyme was found in ectopic endometrium from patients with adenomyosis compared with controls.

DIAGNOSIS

The diagnosis of adenomyosis can only be confirmed by a pathologist.

Clinical Presentation

Nearly 35% of women with adenomyosis uteri are asymptomatic. Commonly occurring symptoms include menorrhagia (unresponsive to hormonal therapy or uterine curettage) and progressively increasing dysmenorrhoea. Menorrhagia can occur in nearly 40–50% of cases, dysmenorrhoea in 10–30% of cases and metrorrhagia in 10–12% of cases. Menorrhagia may be due to dysfunctional contractility of the myometrium, endometrial hyperplasia and anovulation. Other symptoms may include pelvic pain, backache, dyspareunia, dyschezia and subfertility. Older women tend to be more symptomatic in comparison to younger women.

Pelvic Examination

- Uterus may become diffuse and enlarged in cases of diffuse adenomyosis. Uterus may be enlarged to about 12–14 weeks in size and may be tender to touch, soft and boggy.
- Adenomyosis is associated with uterine fibroids in about 6–20% of cases.

Investigations

Presently, there is a lack of a reliable, noninvasive diagnostic test for diagnosing adenomyosis. No serum markers for the diagnosis of adenomyosis are currently available. Some investigations, which are commonly performed, include the following:

- *Ultrasound examination*: Transvaginal sonography (TVS) is better than transabdominal sonography (TAS) in demonstrating the subtle features suggestive of adenomyosis uteri. Some features suggestive of adenomyosis on TVS are listed in **Box 1**. Presently, there is no consensus regarding whether one or some of these criteria should be used for making the diagnosis of adenomyosis. Most authorities presently use three or more of these criteria for making the diagnosis of adenomyosis. A recent meta-analysis has indicated that ultrasound features such as presence of myometrial cysts, linear myometrial striations, poor delineation of the endomyometrial junction and a heterogeneous myometrium are associated with an increased probability of the presence of disease **(Fig. 1)**.

BOX 1: Criteria used to diagnose adenomyosis using transvaginal sonography (TVS).

- Globular uterine enlargement in the absence of leiomyomas
- Asymmetric enlargement of the anterior or posterior myometrial wall
- Heterogeneous, poorly circumscribed anechoic areas within the myometrium
- Hyperechoic islands or nodules, finger-like projections or linear striations, indistinct endometrial stripe
- Anechoic lacunae or cystic spaces of varying sizes, which may be blood-filled
- Focal or diffuse thickening of the junctional zone
- Low-signal intensity uterine mass with an ill-defined border
- Junctional zone thickness: 12 mm
- Indistinct endometrial–myometrial border
- Localised high signal foci within an area of low signal intensity
- Myometrial linear striations
- Parallel shadowing
- Bright foci in endometrium of similar intensity to the myometrium (T1-weighted)
- Ratio of maximal junctional zone thickness to myometrium thickness: 40%
- Subendometrial halo thickening

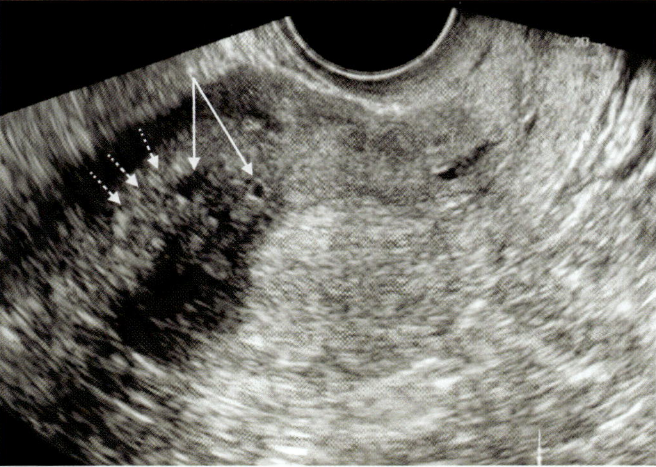

Fig. 1: Ultrasound showing mottled texture of the myometrium and presence of hypoechoic areas within the hyperechoic area (as depicted by broken arrows) in the fundal region, which is suggestive of adenomyosis.

- *Morphological uterus sonographic assessment (MUSA) statement* is a consensus statement on terms, definitions and measurements that may be used to describe and report the sonographic features of the myometrium using grey-scale sonography, colour/ power Doppler and three-dimensional ultrasound imaging. MUSA adenomyosis ultrasound features: Asymmetrical thickening, fan-shaped shadowing, cyst, hyperechoic island, echogenic subendometrial lines and buds, translesion vascularity, irregular junctional zone and interrupted junctional zone.
- In the normal woman, the myometrium has three distinct sonographic layers, of which the middle layer is the most echogenic and the inner layer is hypoechoic relative to the middle and outer layers. This hypoechogenicity is responsible for producing the subendometrial or myometrial halo. The presence of adenomyosis uteri can cause alterations in the sonographic appearance of these zones. Studies regarding the accuracy of TVS for the detection of adenomyosis have reported the rates of sensitivity varying between 53% and 89% and specificity varying between 50% and 99%. Three-dimensional ultrasonography is likely to offer higher accuracy in determining uterine volume and pathology.
- *Magnetic resonance imaging:* This is superior to ultrasound for the diagnosis of adenomyosis. There has been growing evidence to support the use of magnetic resonance imaging (MRI) in the diagnosis of adenomyosis uteri. MRI may be considered when findings on TVS appear to be inconclusive. However, its high cost and limited availability may impede its routine use. The presence of heterotopic endometrial glands and stroma in the myometrium appears as bright foci within the myometrium on T2-weighted MR images **(Fig. 2)**. Adjacent smooth muscle hyperplasia may present as areas of reduced signal intensity on MRI. On MRI examination, there is considerable variation in the thickness of the junctional zone, ranging from 2 to 8 mm. The appearance of diffuse or focal widening of the junctional zone on MRI is suggestive of adenomyosis uteri. Several studies that have compared the accuracy of TVS and MRI have found both these techniques to have comparable sensitivities and specificities. Nevertheless, MRI is less observer-dependent. MRI has proved to be superior to TVS in the presence of associated leiomyomas or additional pathologies. MRI is more useful in distinguishing adenomyosis from fibroids in an enlarged uterus.

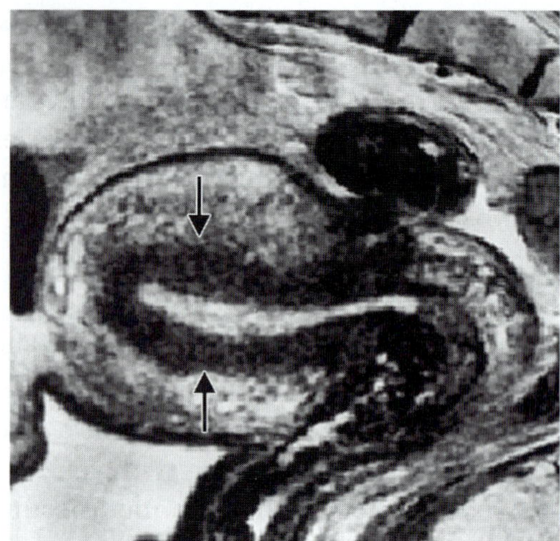

Fig. 2: Sagittal T2-weighted MR image showing diffuse, even thickening of the junctional zone (as depicted by arrows) that is consistent with the diagnosis of diffuse adenomyosis.

- *CA-125:* The level of CA-125 in the peripheral blood may be raised.
- *Histopathological examination:* The final diagnosis is established by histopathological examination of the hysterectomy specimen.

DIFFERENTIAL DIAGNOSIS

Leiomyomas: Adenomyosis is most commonly confused with leiomyomas. TVS is an effective, noninvasive and relatively inexpensive procedure for establishing the diagnosis of adenomyoma preoperatively.

MANAGEMENT

Different surgical and medical modalities of treatment have been used for the management of cases of adenomyosis uteri. Management is often directed at the treatment of symptoms. Presently, there is limited evidence regarding the use of medical, nonhormonal therapy for the treatment of cases of adenomyosis. These treatment strategies are likely to result in a variable and unpredictable degree of symptomatic relief, which is usually limited to the duration of treatment.

Medical Therapy

Medical treatment for cases of adenomyosis comprises nonsteroidal anti-inflammatory drugs (NSAIDs), hormone therapy, danazol, gonadotrophin-releasing hormone (GnRH) agonists and Mirena® intrauterine contraceptive device (IUCD). Medical nonhormonal therapy, including mefenamic and tranexamic acid, may be effective for the symptomatic relief of menorrhagia in patients with uterine adenomyosis. Symptomatic relief is also obtained using hormonal treatment, including progestogens, the combined oral contraceptive pills (OCPs) and GnRH analogues.

Combined oral contraceptive pills: Use of low-dose, continuous combined oral contraceptives with withdrawal bleeding after every 4–6 months may be effective in relieving menorrhagia and dysmenorrhoea associated with adenomyosis. However, there is no specific study related to this therapy in cases with adenomyosis.

Gonadotrophin-releasing hormone analogues: Use of GnRH analogues is also likely to be useful for the treatment of adenomyosis uteri by reducing uterine volume and providing symptomatic relief. However, these benefits are rapidly reversed following the cessation of treatment. Moreover, they are also likely to cause skeletal and general side effects. There could be a role for long-term use of GnRH therapy in association with add-back therapy as described with uterine fibroids and endometriosis.

Danazol: The use of danazol has largely become outdated due to its androgenic side effects. Danazol-loaded intrauterine device has been used as a noninvasive method for the treatment of infertile women with adenomyosis uteri. This method is likely to result in pregnancy following the discontinuation of treatment. Moreover, it is associated with preservation of both menstrual and ovulatory functions and a significant decrease in dysmenorrhoea.

Levonorgestrel intrauterine system: Levonorgestrel intrauterine system (LNG-IUS) has been tried as the treatment option for moderate or severe dysmenorrhoea and/or menorrhagia associated with adenomyosis. There is some evidence that the presence of deep lesions of adenomyosis is associated with the failure of endometrial ablation. In these situations, LNG-IUS has also been successfully used for the treatment of adenomyosis-associated menorrhagia, especially when inserted immediately after endometrial ablation. In these situations, LNG-IUS has also been successfully used for the treatment of adenomyosis-associated menorrhagia, especially when inserted immediately after endometrial ablation.

Dienogest, a novel 19-nortestosterone derivative, is a synthetic oral progestin, highly selective for progesterone receptors. Effective in reducing the pain of adenomyosis, well tolerated and drawback of irregular bleeding is the common reason for discontinuation of treatment.

Surgical Management

Hysterectomy

Total hysterectomy with or without bilateral salpingo-oophorectomy is the treatment of choice in elderly patients who are past their childbearing age or those who have completed their childbearing. The decision to perform a hysterectomy is usually based on the presence of other pathologies such as leiomyomas or failure of medical or conservative management in cases of menorrhagia. Conservative surgery may be performed in the younger patients.

Conservative Surgery

Uterine Artery Embolisation: Uterine artery embolisation (UAE) is presently developing as an effective and safe method for the treatment of adenomyosis. UAE, by causing a reduction of the uterine blood flow by blocking the uterine artery, has been shown to reduce the symptoms associated with adenomyosis uteri and to improve the quality of life. However, the recurrence rate of adenomyosis following the procedure has not yet been evaluated. UAE can be considered as a recognised and effective treatment option for women with adenomyosis having concurrent fibroids. However, there is limited evidence regarding the efficacy of UAE in cases where the predominant lesion is adenomyosis, and all patients undergoing UAE should be counselled regarding the chances of treatment failure, recurrence rates and the requirement for hysterectomy in the future. The chances of a subsequent successful pregnancy following the procedure are unclear.

Endomyometrial Ablation: Endometrial ablation or resection can be considered as an option for women with superficial adenomyosis, presenting with the complaints of menorrhagia. However, the option of endometrial ablation cannot be used in women desiring future pregnancy. Moreover, this procedure is likely to be associated with an increased failure rate in patients with heavy menstrual bleeding in case of deep adenomyosis.

Magnetic Resonance-guided Focused Ultrasound: Magnetic resonance-guided focused ultrasound (MRgFUS) has also been tried as a noninvasive option for the treatment of adenomyosis. However, further studies are required in the future for assessment of the overall safety and long-term effectiveness of MRgFUS for the treatment of adenomyosis.

Adenomyomectomy: Laparoscopy or open conservative surgical techniques of removal of adenomyoma have been proposed. However, no randomised controlled trials (RCTs) are available to know the recurrence, efficacy and reproductive outcomes.

COMPLICATIONS

- Adenomyosis can be associated with considerable morbidity due to the presence of debilitating symptoms such as menorrhagia, dysmenorrhoea, chronic pelvic pain, etc.
- Reduced fertility
- Coexistence of pelvic abnormalities such as uterine fibroids, endometrial hyperplasia and endometrial adenocarcinoma.

SUGGESTED READING

1. Ascher SM, Arnold LL, Patt RH, Schruefer JJ, Bagley AS, Semelka RC, et al. Adenomyosis: prospective comparison of MR imaging and transvaginal sonography. Radiology. 1994;190(3):803-6.
2. Atri M, Reinhold C, Mehio AR, Chapman WB, Bret PM. Adenomyosis: US features with histologic correlation in an in-vitro study. Radiology. 2000;215(3):783-90.
3. Azziz R. Adenomyosis: current perspectives. Obstet Gynecol Clin North Am. 1989;16(1):221-35.
4. Bazot M, Cortez A, Darai E, Rouger J, Chopier J, Antoine JM, et al. Ultrasonography compared with magnetic resonance imaging for the diagnosis of adenomyosis: correlation with histopathology. Hum Reprod. 2001;16(11): 2427-33.
5. Bergholt T, Eriksen L, Berendt N, Jacobsen M, Hertz JB. Prevalence and risk factors of adenomyosis at hysterectomy. Hum Reprod. 2001;16(11):2418-21.
6. Brosens JJ, de Souza NM, Barker FG, Paraschos T, Winston RM. Endovaginal ultrasonography in the diagnosis of adenomyosis uteri: identifying the predictive characteristics. Br J Obstet Gynaecol. 1995;102(6):471-4.
7. Dartmouth K. A systematic review with meta-analysis: the common sonographic characteristics of adenomyosis. Ultrasound. 2014;22(3):148-57.
8. Dueholm M. Transvaginal ultrasound for diagnosis of adenomyosis: a review. Best Pract Res Clin Obstet Gynaecol. 2006;20(4):569-82.
9. Fedele L, Bianchi S, Dorta M, Zanotti F, Brioschi D, Carinelli S. Transvaginal ultrasonography in the differential diagnosis of adenomyoma versus leiomyoma. Am J Obstet Gynecol. 1992;167(3):603-6.
10. Fedele L, Bianchi S, Raffaelli R, Portuese A, Dorta M. Treatment of adenomyosis- associated menorrhagia with a levonorgestrel-releasing intrauterine device. Fertil Steril. 1997;68(3):426-9.
11. Grow DR, Filer RB. Treatment of adenomyosis with long-term GnRH analogues: a case report. Obstet Gynecol. 1991;78(3 Pt 2):538-9.
12. Hall JB, Young RH, Nelson JH. The prognostic significance of adenomyosis in endometrial carcinoma. Gynecol Oncol. 1984;17(1):32-40.
13. Hauth EA, Jaeger HJ, Libera H, Lange S, Forsting M. MR imaging of the uterus and cervix in healthy women: determination of normal values. Eur Radiol. 2007; 17(3):734-42.
14. Hirai M, Shibata K, Sagai H, Sekiya S, Goldberg BB. Transvaginal pulsed and color Doppler sonography for the evaluation of adenomyosis. J Ultrasound Med. 1995;14(7):529-32.
15. Igarashi M, Abe Y, Fukuda M, Ando A, Miyasaka M, Yoshida M, et al. Novel conservative medical therapy for uterine adenomyosis with a danazol-loaded intrauterine device. Fertil Steril. 2000;74(2):412-3.
16. Kim MD, Kim S, Kim NK, Lee MH, Ahn EH, Kim HJ, et al. Long-term results of uterine artery embolization for symptomatic adenomyosis. AJR Am J Roentgenol. 2007;188(1):176-81.
17. Lee JK, Gersell DJ, Balfe DM, Worthington JL, Picus D, Gapp G. The uterus: in vitro MR-anatomic correlation of normal and abnormal specimens. Radiology. 1985;157(1):175-9.
18. Lohle PN, De Vries J, Klazen CA, Boekkooi PF, Vervest HA, Smeets AJ, et al. Uterine artery embolization for symptomatic adenomyosis with or without uterine leiomyomas with the use of calibrated tris-acryl gelatin microspheres: midterm clinical and MR imaging follow-up. J Vasc Interv Radiol. 2007;18(7):835-41.
19. Maheshwari A, Gurunath S, Fatima F, Bhattacharya S. Adenomyosis and subfertility: a systematic review of prevalence, diagnosis, treatment and fertility outcomes. Hum Reprod Update. 2012;18(4):374-92.
20. Maia H, Maltez A, Coelho G, Athayde C, Coutinho EM. Insertion of mirena after endometrial resection in patients with adenomyosis. J Am Assoc Gynecol Laparosc. 2003;10(4):512-6.
21. McCausland AM, McCausland VM. Depth of endometrial penetration in adenomyosis helps determine outcome of rollerball ablation. Am J Obstet Gynecol. 1996;174(6): 1786-94.
22. Mehasseb MK, Habiba MA. Adenomyosis uteri: an update. Obstet Gynaecol. 2009;11(1):41-7.
23. Moghissi KS. Treatment of endometriosis with estrogen-progestin combination and progestogens alone. Clin Obstet Gynecol. 1988;31(4):823-8.

24. Neriishi K, Hirata T, Fukuda S, Izumi G, Nakazawa A, Yamamoto N, et al. Long-term dienogest administration in patients with symptomatic adenomyosis. J Obstet Gynaec Research. 2018;44(8):1439-44.
25. Pados G, Gordts S, Sorrentino F, Nisolle M, Nappi L, Daniilidis A. Adenomyosis and infertility: a literature review. Medicina (Kaunas). 2023;59(9):1551.
26. Parazzini F, Vercellini P, Panazza S, Chatenoud L, Oldani S, Crosignani PG. Risk factors for adenomyosis. Hum Reprod. 1997;12(6):1275-9.
27. Rabinovici J, Inbar Y, Eylon SC, Schiff E, Hananel A, Freundlich D. Pregnancy and live birth after focused ultrasound surgery for symptomatic focal adenomyosis: a case report. Hum Reprod. 2006;21(5):1255-9.
28. Rabinovici J, Stewart EA. New interventional techniques for adenomyosis. Best Pract Res Clin Obstet Gynaecol. 2006;20(4): 617-36.
29. Reinhold C, Atri M, Mehio A, Zakarian R, Aldis AE, Bret PM. Diffuse uterine adenomyosis: morphologic criteria and diagnostic accuracy of endovaginal sonography. Radiology. 1995;197(3):609-14.
30. Reinhold C, McCarthy S, Bret PM, Mehio A, Atri M, Zakarian R, et al. Diffuse adenomyosis: comparison of endovaginal US and MR imaging with histopathologic correlation. Radiology. 1996;199(1):151-8.
31. Rusda M, Hayati R. Morphological uterus sonographic assessment criteria for adenomyosis diagnostic: a case report. Open Access Maced J Med Sci. 2022;10(T7):20-2.
32. Sheng J, Zhang WY, Zhang JP, Lu D. The LNG-IUS study on adenomyosis: a 3-year follow-up study on the efficacy and side effects of the use of levonorgestrel intrauterine system for the treatment of dysmenorrhea associated with adenomyosis. Contraception. 2009;79(3):189-93.
33. Siskin GP, Tublin ME, Stainken BF, Dowling K, Dolen EG. Uterine artery embolization for the treatment of adenomyosis: clinical response and evaluation with MR imaging. AJR Am J Roentgenol. 2001;177(2):297-302.
34. Tamaoka Y, Orikasa H, Sakakura K, et al. Direct effect of danazol on endometrial hyperplasia in adenomyotic women: treatment with danazol containing intrauterine device. Hum Cell. 2000;13(3): 127-33.
35. Uduwela AS, Perera MA, Aiqing L, Fraser IS. Endometrial-myometrial interface: relationship to adenomyosis and changes in pregnancy. Obstet Gynecol Surv. 2000;55(6):390-400.
36. Vavilis D, Agorastos T, Tzafetas J, Loufopoulos A, Vakiani M, Constantinidis T, et al. Adenomyosis at hysterectomy: prevalence and relationship to operative findings and reproductive and menstrual factors. Clin Exp Obstet Gynecol. 1997;24(1):36-8.

33

CHAPTER

Tumours of the Fallopian Tubes

Sanjay Kumar KR, Muralidhar V Pai

Chapter Outline

- Benign Neoplasms
- Primary Malignant Neoplasms
- Secondary Malignant Neoplasms
- Prevention of Fallopian Tube Cancer
- Recurrent Disease
- Coping with Disease

INTRODUCTION

Fallopian tubes are an important part of the female reproductive system. Tumours of fallopian tubes are as such a rare entity. Diagnosis is most of the time incidental.

BENIGN NEOPLASMS

Benign tubal tumours are exceptionally rare. They are:

- Fibroma
- Leiomyoma
- Haemangioma
- Adenomatoid tumour
- Mucosal polyps

These are asymptomatic and small in size. Diagnosis is incidental during operation and sometimes on histopathological examination of the tubes removed after surgery.

Polyps are within the intramural portion of tubes revealed by salpingography, salpingoscopy, falloposcopy or at micro-surgery. These intraluminal polyps can cause infertility.

PRIMARY MALIGNANT NEOPLASMS

These are more frequent at mean age of 55–60 years. These are most common tumours of fallopian tubes. Fallopian tube cancers account for 0.3–4% of all cancers and 1–2% of female genital tract cancer. Cancer of fallopian tube is abnormal growth of fallopian tubes.

Primary malignant tumours are:

- *Sarcomas:* This tumour arises from smooth muscles in fallopian tubes.
- *Transitional cell carcinoma:* It arises from stretchy cells found in the tubal lining.
- *Papillary serous adenocarcinoma:* It grows from the lining of fallopian tubal cells.
- *Choriocarcinoma:* This tumour can arise after tubal pregnancy.
- Clear cell carcinoma
- Endometrioid carcinoma
- Germ cell tumours
- Lymphoma

Predisposing Factors

- *Family history:* Having two or more close relatives suffering from ovarian and breast cancer. Mother or sister with ovarian or fallopian tube cancer
- *Genetic mutation: BRCA 1* and *BRCA 2* gene mutations can contribute to 10–20% of cases.
- *Chronic infection of genital tract:* Leads to chronic inflammation and malignant changes.
- *Inherited conditions:* Lynch syndrome, Peutz-Jeghers syndrome.
- Nulliparity, early menarche, late menopause and obesity.

Signs and Symptoms

Symptoms are almost similar to ovarian malignancy. Symptoms might include:

- Irregular vaginal bleeding
- *Hydrops tubae profluens:* Watery and blood-stained excessive vaginal discharge is in 50% of the cases. It is intermittent discharge from a large hydrosalpinx.
- *Spasmodic pelvic pain—due to tubal distension and forced peristalsis, relieved by vaginal discharge.*
- Infertility

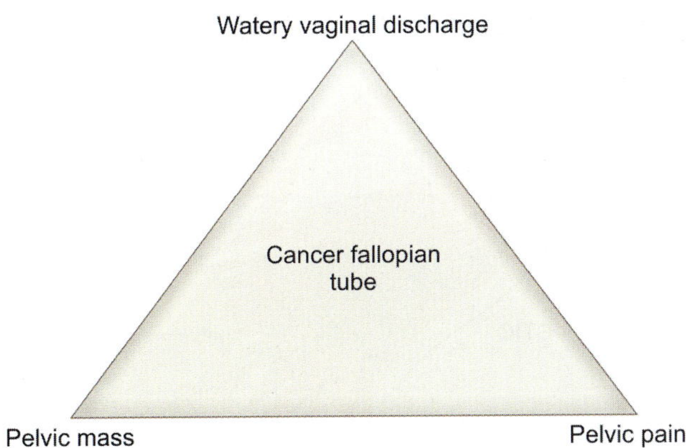

Fig. 1: Classical triad of symptoms (Latzko's triad).

- Heaviness in the lower abdomen
- Pelvic mass
- Nonspecific symptoms

The classical triad of symptoms is watery vaginal discharge with hydrops tubae profluens, pelvic pain and pelvic mass **(Fig. 1)**. It occurs in 15% of cases. Otherwise, most of the features are nonspecific. Clinician should think the possibility of occult tubal cancer in a perimenopausal or postmenopausal women presenting with unexplained vaginal discharge pain and mass with vague complaints. There may also be ascites.

Diagnosis

- Adnexal mass on pelvic examination.
- Ultrasound is the most common modality for diagnosis. A pelvic mass in adnexal region separates from ovary. It may be of in determined nature.
- Incidental findings of malignant cells in cases of endometrial or cervical involvement on Pap smear.
- Raised cancer antigen 125 (CA 125) levels, though not diagnostic, but are raised in some cases.
- A CT scan or an MRI of pelvis is done to confirm the nature of the mass seen on ultrasonography. Imaging diagnosis of primary fallopian tube cancer is important, because it can help plan adequate initial surgery and avoid second-look laparotomy. Imaging findings of primary fallopian tube carcinoma are usually nonspecific, and a tubo-ovarian abscess or ovarian tumour may appear the same, but a sausage or C-shaped mass suggests tubal nature **(Figs. 2 and 3)**.
- At the time of surgery, an incidental finding.
- On examination of ascetic fluid, malignant cells can be found.

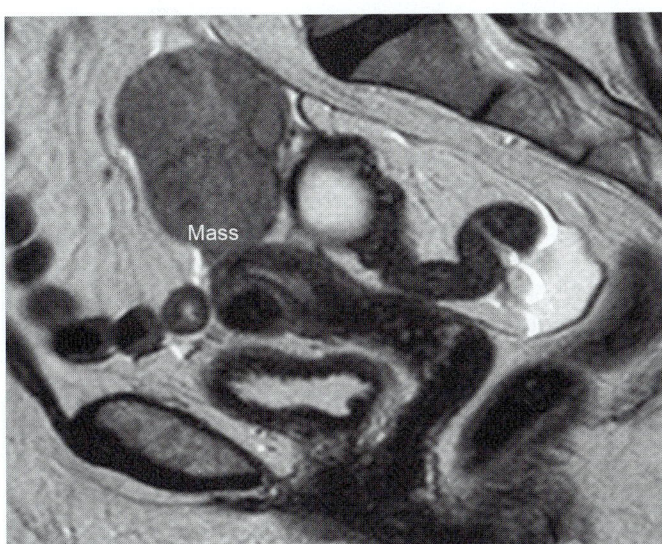

Fig. 2: T2-weighted image of solid tubal mass, suggestive of malignancy.

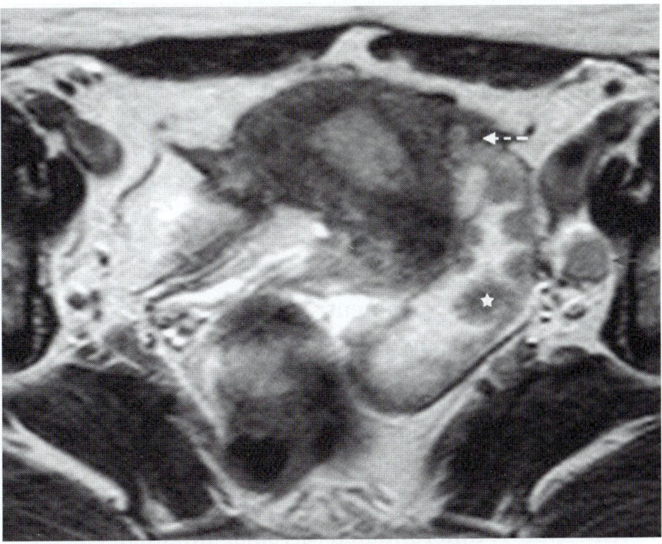

Fig. 3: MRI scan showing C-shaped tubal mass as highlighted by broken arrow and asterisk.

- Positron emission tomography (PET) scan can finally tell the malignant nature by showing a hot spot in the mass, helpful in judging the extension of disease and recurrence.

Misdiagnosis or Lesions Mimicking Tubal Malignancy

- Tiny peritoneal cysts and pseudo-peritoneal cysts on the tubal surface can be misdiagnosed as fallopian tube tumours.

TABLE 1: Stages of malignant diseases.

Stage 0	Carcinoma in situ
Stage I	Growth is limited to the fallopian tubes
Stage II	Growth involving one or both fallopian tubes with extension to the pelvis
Stage III	Tumour involving one or both fallopian tubes with spread outside the pelvis
Stage IV	Growth involving one or more fallopian tubes with distant metastases

TABLE 2: Pathologic criteria for primary fallopian tube malignancy.

1.	The tumour arises from the endosalpinx
2.	The histologic pattern reproduces the epithelium of the tubal mucosa
3.	There is a transition from benign to malignant epithelium
4.	The ovary and endometrium are either normal or with a tumour smaller than the tumour in the tube

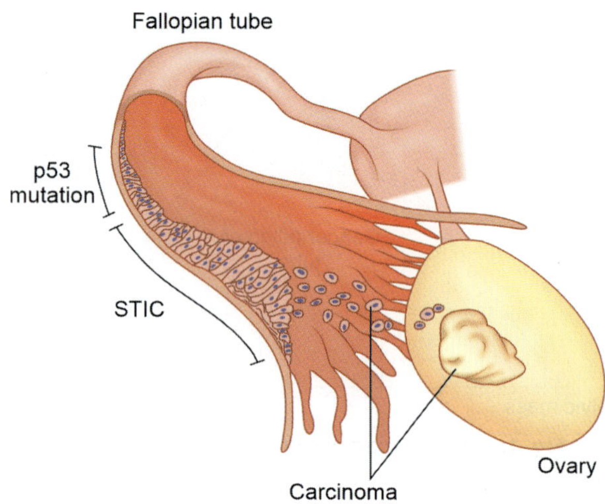

Fig. 4: The first step is the evolution of a single cell p53 mutant epithelial layer that then develops into serous tubular intraepithelial carcinoma (STIC) lesion. STIC lesion either invades locally into the tubal stroma (fallopian carcinoma) or exfoliates into surface of ovary or peritoneum (ovarian or primary peritoneal carcinoma).

- Tuberculosis of fallopian tube with hyperplastic tubal epithelium may be misdiagnosed as tubal carcinoma.

Staging

As in other malignant diseases, staging is done depending upon the **Tables 1 and 2**:

- Histological features
- Lymph node involvement
- Presence or absence of metastasis

Histological grades:

- GX—grade cannot be assessed
- G1—well differentiated (papillary)
- G2—moderately differentiated (papillary-alveolar)
- G3—poorly differentiated (alveolar-medullary).

Lymph nodes (N):

- NX—regional lymph nodes cannot be assessed
- N0—no regional lymph node metastasis
- N1—regional lymph node metastasis.

Distant metastasis (M):

- MX—distant metastasis cannot be assessed
- M0—no distant metastasis
- M1—distant metastasis.

Pathophysiology

The tumour is usually a papillary adenocarcinoma situated in the middle or outer third of the tube **(Fig. 4)**. It is bilateral in 5–10% of cases. When it is bilateral, growth is usually found in the uterus as well and may be the primary.

The origin of the fallopian tube carcinoma is explained in **Figure 4**.

The tube walls are so thin that they are rapidly invaded, and the growth encroaches on the peritoneal cavity either directly or by sprouting through the abdominal ostium. The latter, however, is often closed, so a hydrosalpinx is present. The disease also spreads by lymphatics to the para-aortic and pelvic lymph nodes by seeding. Sub-urethral vaginal metastases, which are not uncommon, represent venous embolism either directly from the tube or via the uterus.

The prognosis, therefore, is poor and by the time the diagnosis is made, the situation is often hopeless. Indeed, almost the only cases cured are those in which the cancer is found accidentally at operation while it is still in an asymptomatic stage.

Spread Pattern

Fallopian tubes are thin-walled structures that lead to the fast and easy spread of cancer.

- Tubal cancer usually spreads by trans-coelomic route, i.e. spread across a body cavity. From tube, there is exfoliation of cells that implant throughout the peritoneal cavity. In 80% of the patient's metastases are found in peritoneal cavity **(Fig. 5)**.

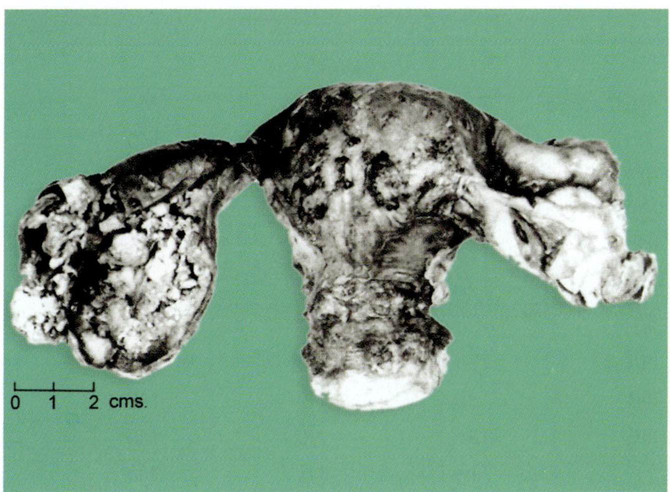

Fig. 5: A specimen showing bilateral adenocarcinomas of the fallopian tubes. The left tube is cut open to show the coarse papillomatous nature of the growth.

- Fallopian tubes being richly permeated with lymphatics, there is easy spread to the pelvic lymph nodes and para-aortic lymph nodes. Nodal involvement is seen in 35% of the patients.

Screening Test for Fallopian Tube Cancer

Currently nitric oxide screening test for the detection of tubal cancer is available; however, regular health check-ups and not ignoring the untoward symptoms are crucial.

Treatment

Treatment is based upon the following factors:

- Stage of the disease
- Age
- Medical history
- Need for reproductive function
- Current health status of the patient
- Personal preference.

The main goal is to eradicate cancer, if possible, save the reproductive function where it is required, and that too with minimal side effects. A gynaecological oncologist is the ideal person for treating such patients.

Treatment options are as follows:

- Surgery
- Radiation therapy
- Chemotherapy.
- Novel targeted therapies

Surgery

In early stages of the disease, salpingo-oophorectomy, unilateral or bilateral, is done with peritoneal biopsies. Salpingo-oophorectomy is the removal of ovary with fallopian tube.

In advanced stages of the disease, multiple surgical procedures such as total hysterectomy, bilateral salpingo-oophorectomy, omentectomy, appendicectomy, peritoneal washings and biopsy and lymphadenectomy are needed. In patients with very advanced stage of disease where above said surgery is not possible, cytoreductive surgery, that is, debulking of the tumour, is done, which will reduce the tumour load. Adjuvant therapy is given in advanced stages.

Retrospective analysis has suggested that advanced stages at presentation and the presence of residual tumour at the end of treatment with chemotherapy are associated with poorer prognosis. Therefore, carefully done surgical staging at presentation is paramount in the treatment of early fallopian cancer. The para-aortic nodes above the inferior mesenteric artery are the most frequently involved retroperitoneal nodes. For advanced disease, there should also be optimal removal of the primary tumour and involved adjacent organs. The following must be performed through a midline incision:

- Careful evaluation of the entire abdominopelvic cavity to delineate the extent of disease
- Total abdominal hysterectomy and bilateral salpingo-oophorectomy
- Sampling of the pelvic and para-aortic lymph nodes
- Infra-colic omentectomy
- Washing of the peritoneal cavity
- Biopsies of any suspicious areas, including the abdominal and pelvic peritoneum.

Histopathology of fallopian tube cancer: Carcinomas of the fallopian tubes are microscopically similar to ovarian carcinomas. In order to establish the tumour as tubal in origin, there should be limited tumour in the ovary and no similar type of carcinoma in the uterus **(Tables 3 and 4)**.

Microscopically, serous carcinoma dominates. Less common subtypes are endometrioid, mucinous, clear cell, transitional cell and undifferentiated carcinomas. The mixed epithelial and mesenchymal tumours, such as carcinosarcoma, is sometimes seen as primary tubal cancers **(Figs. 6 and 7)**.

Serous tubal intraepithelial carcinoma is characterised by replacement of the tubal epithelium by malignant

TABLE 3: Carcinoma of the fallopian tube—staging.

FIGO	*Definition*	*TNM*
	The primary tumour cannot be assessed	TX
0	No evidence of primary tumour	T0
	Carcinoma in situ (preinvasive carcinoma)	Tis
I	Tumour confined to the fallopian tube (s)	T1
IA	Tumour limited to one tube, without penetrating the serosal surface; no ascites	T1a
IB	Tumour limited to both tubes, without penetrating the serosal surface; no ascites	T1b
IC	Tumour limited to one or both tubes, with extension onto/through the tubal serosa; or with positive malignant cells in the ascites or positive peritoneal washings	T1c
II	Tumour involves one or both fallopian tubes with pelvic extension	T2
IIA	Extension and/or metastasis to the uterus and/or ovaries	T2a
IIB	Extension to other pelvic organs	T2b
IIC	IIB/C with positive malignant cells in the ascites or positive peritoneal washings	T2c
III	Tumour involves one or both fallopian tubes with peritoneal implants outside the pelvis and/or positive regional lymph nodes	T3 and/ or N1
IIIA	Microscopic peritoneal metastasis outside the pelvis	T3a
IIIB	Macroscopic peritoneal metastasis outside the pelvis, 2 cm or less in greatest dimension	T3b
IIIC	Peritoneal metastasis >2 cm in greatest dimension and/or positive regional lymph nodes	T3c and/ or N1
IV	Distant metastasis beyond the peritoneal cavity	M1

(FIGO: International Federation of Gynaecology and Obstetrics; TNM: tumour, node and metastasis)

TABLE 4: Carcinoma of the fallopian tube—stage grouping.

	UICC		
FIGO stage	*T*	*N*	*M*
IA	T1a	N0	M0
IB	T1b	N0	M0
IC	T1c	N0	M0
IIA	T2a	N0	M0
IIB	T2b	N0	M0
IIC	T2c	N0	M0
IIIA	T3a	N0	M0
IIIB	T3b	N0	M0
IIIC	T3c	N0	M0
	Any T	N1	M0
IV	Any T	Any N	M1

(FIGO: International Federation of Gynaecology and Obstetrics; TNM: tumour, node and metastasis; UICC: Union for International Cancer Control)

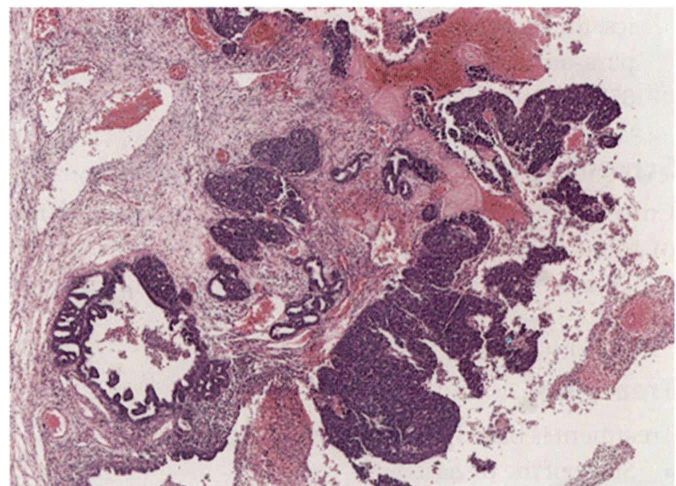

Fig. 6: Stained slide of serous papillary tubal carcinoma.

glandular epithelial cells with pleomorphic nuclei, florid epithelial proliferation. Excessive epithelial proliferation sometimes occurs even in salpingitis and should not be mistaken for carcinoma in situ. At times, histology of the fallopian tube is normal, but immunostaining reveals mitotic activity.

Chemotherapy

These drugs are used to kill cancer cells left after surgery that is why chemotherapy is advisable prophylactically thereafter. Drugs can be given IV or IP, that is intraperitoneal, as per the recommended regimes.

Combined chemotherapy regimens are used for ovarian carcinoma.

The success of the paclitaxel and carboplatin combination in ovarian cancer has led to greater usage of

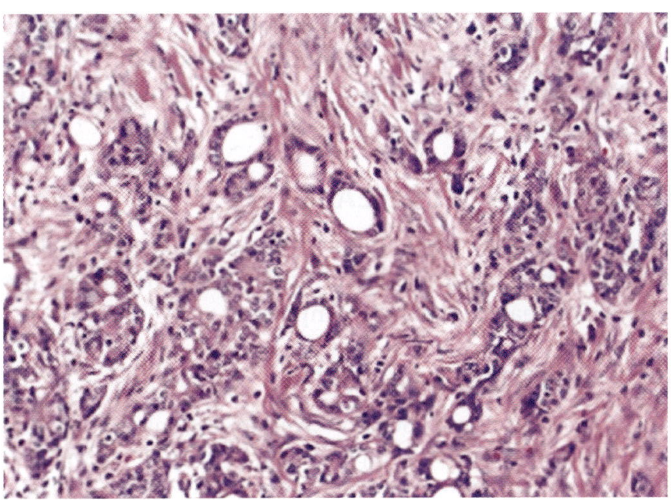

Fig. 7: Primary adenocarcinoma of the ampullary region of the tube in high magnification. An incidental finding in hysterectomy specimen.

this combination in fallopian cancer. Other drugs used are docetaxel, cisplatin and gemcitabine.

Radiation Therapy

It refers to the use of high-energy X-rays to kill the malignant cells. It is not a primary treatment. It can be used prior to surgery to shrink the tumour mass or in cases where chemotherapy is contraindicated. It has low efficacy and more side effects.

Novel Treatment Options

- *Vascular endothelial growth factor (VEGF) antibody:* Bevacizumab. FDA-approved for adjuvant therapy, as monotherapy in maintenance therapy and recurrent cancer.
- *PARP inhibitors:* PARP is a protein (enzyme) found in our cells. It stands for poly-ADP ribose polymerase. It helps damaged cells to repair themselves. As a cancer treatment, PARP inhibitors stop the PARP from doing this repair work in cancer cells and the cell dies. They are more efficacious in patients with BRCA gene mutation where repair is already faulty. Olaparib, rucaparib, niraparib are few PARP inhibitors.
- *Hyperthermic intraperitoneal chemotherapy (HIPEC):* Single intraoperative administration of warmed chemotherapy during cytoreductive surgery, causing direct cell damage.
- *Immunotherapy:* Few cases may be helped by such therapy.

Flowchart 1: Follow-up of primary malignant neoplasms.

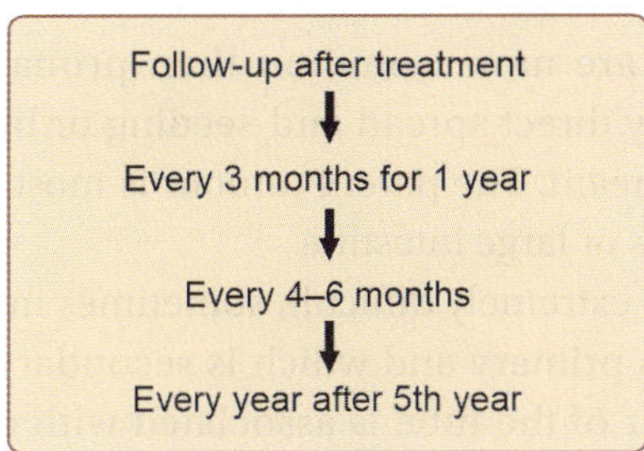

Survival after Treatment

The 5-year survival rate is approximately 40% of all cases. The very early ones (Stage I) discovered accidentally will have a survival rate of about 65%. Stage 2 patients have a 5-year survival of 50–60%, but it is only 10–20% in stage 3 and stage 4 disease.

Follow-up (Flowchart 1)

The objectives of follow-up are as follows:

- Determination of the patient's immediate response to the treatment employed
- Early recognition and prompt management of any treatment-related complications, including any psychological sequelae
- Early detection of persistent or recurrent disease
- Collection of data regarding the efficacy of treatment
- For patients with early disease, screening for breast cancer and for patients treated with conservative surgery, cervical cancer screening should be done in follow-up.

In general, during the first year following treatment, patients should be seen every 3 months with a gradual increase in intervals to every 4–6 months and annually after the fifth year.

At each follow-up visit: The patient should have her history retaken and a complete physical examination (including breast, pelvic and rectal examination) should be performed to exclude any clinical signs of recurrence. The serum CA 125 titre may also be checked at regular intervals, especially if it was raised at primary diagnosis, although the literature in this area is unclear as to the impact of such a practice on survival. But if it was positive earlier, it can definitely suggest recurrence. Radiological tests such as ultrasonography of the pelvis, CT scans or MRI scans should only be performed when the clinical findings or the tumour markers suggest possible recurrence.

SECONDARY MALIGNANT NEOPLASMS

Metastases are more common than primary growths; they arise by direct spread and seeding or by the lymph and bloodstream. The parent tumour is most often in the ovary, uterus or large intestine.

It can be extremely difficult, sometimes impossible, to say which is primary and which is secondary, especially when cancer of the tube is associated with endometrial carcinoma, with certain ovarian tumours or with the rare primary peritoneal carcinomatosis. Cancer cells pass along the tubes and the lymphatic channels, in either direction.

PREVENTION OF FALLOPIAN TUBE CANCER

The disease is not preventable. Incidence can be lowered to some extent by the use of *birth control pills* (30–50% reduction after 3–5 years of use) or *by childbirth or breastfeeding*. If there is a family history of tubal malignancy and gene *BCRA1* is positive or genes related to Lynch syndrome present, more closer monitoring is recommended. Patients with *BRCA1/BRCA2* mutation should consider removal of the tube and ovaries as a prophylactic measure *[Risk reduction salpingo-oophorectomy (RR-BSO)]. Opportunistic salpingectomy during hysterectomy or pelvic surgery, or for sterilisation, could also be considered in genetically prone patients.*

RECURRENT DISEASE

- The role of secondary cytoreductive surgery is there, especially if 6 months have passed and the patient's general condition is stable to withstand another surgery.
- Drugs such as bevacizumab, which is anti-angiogenic, may be beneficial for maintenance therapy.
- Combination chemotherapy regimens are helpful in controlling the recurrent disease.

COPING WITH DISEASE

It requires proper psychological counselling and healthy family support. Knowledge of the disease and awareness about the treatment are also important.

SUGGESTED READING

1. American Cancer Society. Ovarian, Fallopian Tube, and Peritoneal Cancer: Symptoms and Signs. [online] Available from https://www.cancer.net/cancer- types/ovarian-fallopian-tube-and-peritoneal-cancer/symptoms-and-signs [Last accessed April, 2025].
2. Cancer Research UK. Fallopian tube cancer. [online] Available from http://www.cancerresearchuk.org/about-cancer/ovarian-cancer/types/fallopian-tube [Last accessed April, 2025].
3. Choi SM, Choi MY, Kang WD, Choi HS, Kim SM. Serous borderline tumor of the fallopian tube. Obstet Gynecol Sci. 2014;57(4):334-7.
4. National Cancer Institute. Ovarian, Fallopian tube, and primary peritoneal cancers screening (PDQ®)–Health professional version. [online] Available from https://www.cancer.gov. [Last accessed April, 2025].
5. OncoLink. All About Fallopian Tube Cancer. [online] Available from https://www.oncolink.org/cancers/gynecologic/information-about-gynecologic-cancers/fallopian-tube-cancer/all-about-fallopian-tube-cancer [Last accessed April, 2025].
6. Pectasides D, Pectasides E, Economopoulos T. Fallopian tube carcinoma: a review. The Oncologist. 2006;11:902-12.
7. Stasenko M, Fillipova O, Tew WP. Fallopian tube carcinoma. J Oncol Pract. 2019;15(7):375-82.

34 CHAPTER

Tumours of the Pelvic Ligaments

Sanjay Kumar KR, Muralidhar V Pai

Chapter Outline

- Cysts of the Broad Ligament and Associated Structures
- Neoplasms of the Pelvic Ligaments and Connective Tissues
- Neoplasms of the Peritoneum

CYSTS OF THE BROAD LIGAMENT AND ASSOCIATED STRUCTURES

Pathology

Some broad ligament cysts are really ovarian cysts which, during growth, open up the leaves of the mesovarium and then bulge more and more into the broad ligament to become retroperitoneal tumours.

Primary cysts of the broad ligament arise by distension of one or other part of the rudimentary Wolffian system, or by neoplasia in these structures.

Epoophoron and Paroophoron

- These are common and typical broad ligament cysts that arise from one of these structures, usually the epoophoron (paraovarium).
- The epoophoron is the remnant of the mesonephric tubules found next to the ovary and tube.
- Paroophoron consists of a few rudimentary tubules lying in the broad ligament between the epoophoron and the uterus.
- Paraovarian cysts form 10% of all adnexal masses.
- It is sited near the attachment of the mesovarium and, as it grows, separates the ovary from the fallopian tube, stretching the tube and the fimbriae over its upper pole **(Figs. 1 and 2)**.
- Such cysts are variously termed *paraovarian or fimbrial,* although they certainly do not arise from the fimbria. Although usually smaller than ovarian cysts, they can attain a very large size, filling the whole abdominal cavity. In such a case, the lesion probably represents benign neoplasia rather than distension. Indeed, some paraovarian cysts develop intracystic papillae, and this has led to a suggestion that they can arise from misplaced ovarian tissue.

The paraovarian cyst is nearly always unilocular and thin-walled; it contains a watery colourless fluid in which cholesterol crystals can be found. Most paraovarian cysts are asymptomatic and are discovered accidentally; sometimes they cause symptoms enlargement or torsion.

The lining epithelium is usually a single layer of flat or cuboidal cells, some of which may be ciliated. Indeed, the histological appearance is similar to that of a serous cystadenoma of the ovary, and for this reason, it has been suggested that the cyst arises from Walthard cells. The wall of a paraovarian cyst frequently contains smooth muscle, and this helps to distinguish it from an ovarian cyst on microscopy.

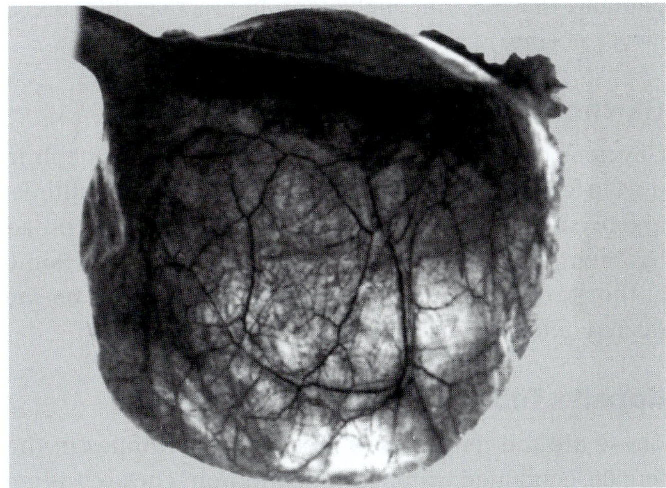

Fig. 1: A paraovarian (sometimes called fimbrial) cyst with the tube stretched over its upper pole. The presence of vessels crossing each other in the capsule tells the surgeon that the tumour may be extraperitoneal. The vessels belong to the peritoneum and to the true capsule of the cyst, so the cyst is easily shelled out of its peritoneal coat.

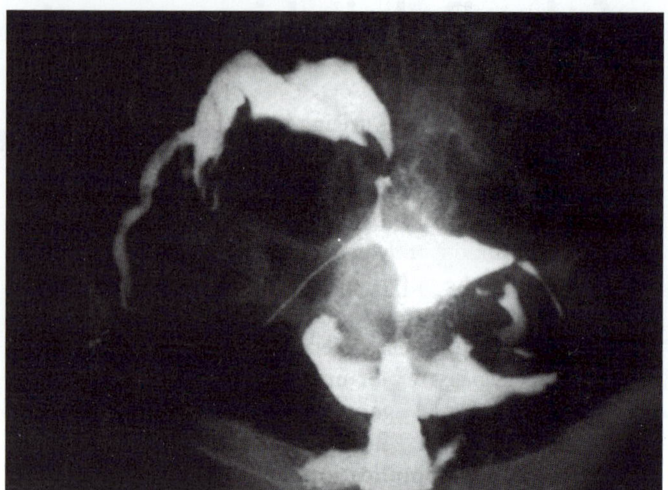

Fig. 2: Salpingography in the case of paraovarian cyst. The right tube is stretched out over and around the tumour.

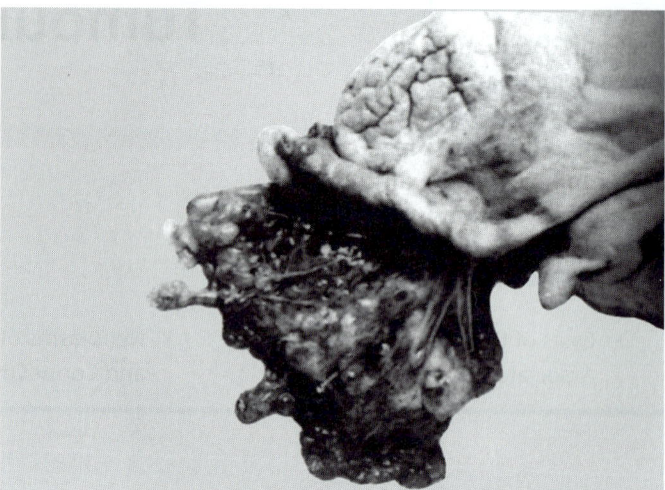

Fig. 3: A multicystic structure growing from the anterior leaf of the outer part of the broad ligament and immediately below the tube. It is probably arising from Kobelt's tubules.

At operation, the cyst is found to have two coverings, the peritoneum of the broad ligament being closely applied to the cyst wall proper. The sight of blood vessels crossing each other tells the surgeon immediately that he or she is dealing with an extraperitoneal tumour **(Fig. 1)**. Its extraperitoneal site raises important anatomical considerations. The lower pole of the cyst may remain in the pelvis and displace the uterus to one side. If it does, it also comes into close relation with the ureter, which is pushed outwards.

In theory, a paraovarian cyst, especially one with papillae, may become malignant. In practice, this rarely, if ever, occurs.

Gärtner's Duct

Gärtner's duct is a vestigial remnant of the mesonephric duct in females. These cysts are small, sometimes multiple, and occur at any point on the line of the duct. In the broad ligament, they are of little practical importance. Some authorities consider the hydatid of Morgagni to be the dilated outer end of the duct.

Kobelt's Tubules

These are the remnants of mesonephric tubules in the female, contained within the epoophoron. These cysts are also small and merely of academic interest. They lie on the posterior aspect of the outer part of the broad ligament. Very rarely, a moderate-sized bunch of innumerable tiny cysts is found in this area and probably represents a benign neoplastic change **(Fig. 3)**.

Complications

Broad ligament cysts are the same as ovarian cysts. Pregnancy complicating a paraovarian cyst is considered.

Clinical Features

Broad ligament cysts tend to arise at a rather younger age than do ovarian cysts, but otherwise the symptoms and signs are similar. It may therefore be impossible to distinguish between the two types, but *a broad ligament origin should be suspected whenever a cyst is fixed in the pelvis and especially when it displaces the uterus laterally.* The close proximity of the tumour to the uterus sometimes suggests that it is uterine in origin. Confusion can arise over a soft leiomyoma, uterine or broad ligament in site, and over a pelvic kidney.

Treatment

Operative treatment is indicated in nearly all cases and consists of shelling out the cyst from its extraperitoneal bed. If the lower pole is deep in the pelvis, the ureter is at risk during this process. Routine removal of any paratubular or paraovarian cyst discovered at laparoscopy is advocated as the cyst may interfere with sonography during ovulation induction. Laparoscopic treatment is often feasible.

NEOPLASMS OF THE PELVIC LIGAMENTS AND CONNECTIVE TISSUES

Extensions of growths arising in the bladder, uterus, cervix, vagina, ovary and bowel are extremely common, and have

TABLE 1: Clues to rule out non-broad ligament origin of tumour.

Exclude	***Sign to disprove***	***What to look for***	***Examples***
Ovarian origin	*'Phantom organ' sign*	Recognise ovarian tissue independently from the tumour, as an undetectable ovary suggests that as the origin of the tumour	
	'Beak' sign	The interface of the ovary and the mass should have dull edges, instead of a 'beak' shape, suggesting that the tumour compresses but does not arise from the ovary	
	'Embedded organ' sign	The ovary should be compressed and deformed into a crescent shape by the tumour, in contrast to an ovarian tumour, which embeds the ovary	
	'Ovarian vascular pedicle' sign	There should be no asymmetries of the gonadal veins, pointing to an ovarian tumour	
Uterine origin	*'Claw' sign*	There should be no uterine tissue, particularly with a 'claw-like' shape, embedding the tumour	
	'Bridging vessel' sign	There should be no bridging vessels in the interface between the uterus and the lesion, indicating a uterine origin	
Tubal origin	The tumour must not have a tubular shape, folded configuration or the presence of incomplete septum, suggesting a fallopian tubes origin		

already been covered. Leaving these aside, and also broad ligament cysts, some of which are undoubtedly neoplastic (*see above*), primary tumours of the pelvic ligaments include the leiomyoma, fibroma, teratoma and various sarcomas. Only the first of these deserves description.

Primary Broad Ligament Tumours

To be considered a tumour from the broad ligament, it must occur on or in the broad ligament, but be completely separated from, and in no way connected, with either the uterus or the ovary, as proposed by Gardner et al. Imaging clues to diagnose primary broad ligament tumour, excluding ovarian, uterine or tubal origin, are mentioned below in **Table 1**.

Leiomyomas are not uncommon in the round, ovarian and broad ligaments. They are often found in association with similar uterine tumours, and their pathology and complications are the same.

Broad ligament leiomyomas are of two types:

1. False broad ligament leiomyoma—a uterine tumour (usually cervical) which grows into the broad ligament but preserves a uterine attachment **(Fig. 4)**.
2. True (Primary) broad ligament leiomyoma arising from the subperitoneal connective tissue of the ligament.

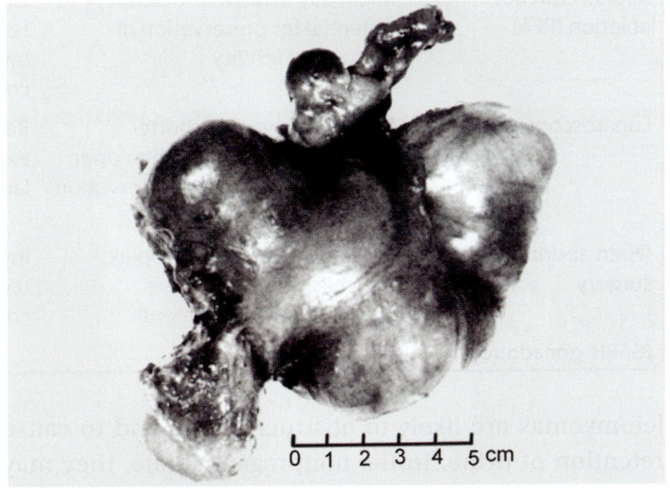

Fig. 4: A broad ligament leiomyoma growing from the right wall of the uterus, elevating the tube and ovary and displacing the cervix to the left.

It is the anatomy of these tumours, which makes them important clinically. They are extraperitoneal and therefore remain fixed in the pelvis, displacing the uterus to one side. The true broad ligament tumour may lie lateral to the ureter, but the false broad ligament tumour is always medial to it. This is important in estimating the course of the ureter during surgery. In pregnancy, broad ligament

TABLE 2: Various treatment options for broad ligament leiomyoma.

Treatment options	***Advantages***	***Disadvantages***	***Effectiveness***
Observations	Noninvasive, avoids potential risks and complications associated with treatment interventions	May not alleviate symptoms or prevent the growth of myoma	Does not directly treat the myoma
Medical therapy	Nonsurgical approach may reduce symptoms and shrink myomas	Temporary effects. Potential side effects (e.g. menopausal symptoms with GnRH agonists), myoma regrowth	Variable effectiveness; may provide temporary relief
Myomectomy	Preserves the uterus and fertility if desired	Surgical procedure with associated risks and potential complications, longer recovery time	High success rate in symptom relief and myoma removal
Hysterectomy	Definitive treatment eliminates the risk of myoma recurrence	Loss of fertility, an irreversible procedure, longer recovery time	Highly effective in eliminating symptoms and preventing recurrence
Uterine artery embolisation (UAE)	Nonsurgical approach, preserves the uterus, shorter recovery time	Potential complications (e.g. pain, infection), risk of postembolisation syndrome, myoma regrowth	Effective in symptom relief and myoma size reduction in many cases
MRI-guided focused ultrasound (MRgFUS)	Noninvasive, no incisions or radiation exposure, preserves the uterus	Limited availability. Potential for incomplete myoma removal, high cost	Effective in symptom relief and myoma size reduction in many cases
Radiofrequency ablation (RFA)	Minimally invasive procedure, potential for preservation of uterus and fertility	Limited availability, long-term effectiveness still under investigation, potential complications	Promising results in small, accessible myomas
Laparoscopic surgery	Minimally invasive, shorter recovery time compared to open surgery, potential for preservation of the uterus	Requires specialised surgical expertise. May not be suitable for large or complex myomas	Effective in symptom relief and myoma removal in appropriate cases
Open abdominal surgery	Suitable for large or complex myomas, comprehensive evaluation and treatment	Invasive procedure with longer recovery time, potential for complications	Highly effective in symptom relief and myoma removal

(GnRH: gonadotrophin-releasing hormone)

leiomyomas are likely to obstruct labour and to cause retention of urine. In the nonpregnant state, they may cause hydronephrosis. The symptoms they cause are those resulting from pressure on adjacent organs, or the patient may notice a lower abdominal tumour. Their removal can be difficult and hazardous chiefly because of the risk to the ureter.

Parasitic or wandering fibroid: It is a subserosal fibroid, which has undergone torsion, and the blood supply is established from the adjacent organ after detachment from the original site. They pose diagnostic problems due to unusual locations. As per the International Federation of Gynaecology and Obstetrics (FIGO) classification system, parasitic fibroids have been categorized as type eight with no myometrial involvement and uterine attachment.

Various treatment options for broad ligament leiomyoma are listed in **Table 2**.

NEOPLASMS OF THE PERITONEUM

The peritoneum is commonly involved in the advanced stages of malignancies of abdominal and pelvic organs. Primary tumours are rarely seen.

Peritoneal Carcinomas

Primary peritoneal carcinoma simulates ovarian cancer in its clinical features, and is seen especially in women who have previously undergone hysterectomy and bilateral salpingo-oophorectomy.

At laparotomy, extensive disease is seen in the upper abdomen, particularly in the omentum. Microscopic or small macroscopic cancer deposits are seen on the surface of the ovaries, but more extensive involvement of the uterosacral ligaments, pelvic peritoneum or omentum is seen.

Histologically, peritoneal serous carcinomas resemble moderately to poorly differentiated serous ovarian carcinoma. Primary peritoneal endometrioid carcinoma is less common.

Treatment is by chemotherapy and/or radiotherapy with intraperitoneal radioisotopes and external beam therapy.

Mesotheliomas

Peritoneal malignant mesotheliomas are uncommon tumours. They may be fibrosarcomatous, papillary-alveolar, carcinomatous or mixed. They can also develop after hysterectomy and bilateral salpingo-oophorectomy for benign disease. Grossly, they appear as multiple masses intraperitoneally. The differential diagnosis is from ovarian tumour implants and primary peritoneal Müllerian neoplasms.

SUGGESTED READING

1. Barek JS. Benign diseases of the female reproductive tract. Novack's Gynaecology, 15th edition. New Delhi: Lippincott Williams and Wilkins, Wolters Kluwer (India); 2007. p. 470.
2. Fasih N, Prasad Shanbhogue AK, Macdonald DB, Fraser-Hill MA, Papadatos D, Kielar AZ, et al. Leiomyomas beyond the uterus: unusual locations, rare manifestations. Radiographics. 2008;28:1931-48.
3. Nikolaos K, Craig S, Peter V. Pregnancy-related pelvic girdle pain: an update. BMC Med. 2011;9:15.
4. Oliveira JD, Cun ha TM, Tereso A. Tumors of the broad ligament: what and when to suspect such rare location. Radiol Bras. 2020;53(5):349-55.
5. Saremi AT, Nateghi MR, Abbasi B, Karimi Mansoorabad E. Broad ligament myoma: a review on epidemiology, clinical presentation, diagnosis, and treatment. Sarem J Reprod Med. 2023;7(4):222-8.
6. Yousefi Z, Sharifhi N, Hasanzadeh M, Mottaghi M, Bolandy S. Peripheral primitive neuroectodermal tumor of the pelvis. Iran J Med Sci. 2014;39(1):71-4.

35

CHAPTER

Tumours of the Ovary

Pralhad Kushtagi

Chapter Outline

- Clinical Diagnosis of Ovarian Tumours
- Complications of Ovarian Tumours
- Features Suggestive of Malignancy in Ovarian Tumour
- Pathology of Ovarian Tumours
- Non-neoplastic Ovarian 'Tumours'
- Neoplastic Ovarian Tumours
- Staging
- Nonepithelial Ovarian Tumours
- Germ Cell Tumours
- Treatment of Malignant Germ Cell Tumours

INTRODUCTION

The word tumour comes from the Latin word *tumeo*, meaning 'to swell'. According to Merriam-Webster, a tumour is a new growth of tissue that is abnormal, benign or malignant, possesses no physiological function and arises from uncontrolled usually rapid cellular proliferation. It can also refer to swollen or distended part. Ovary is a peculiar organ in human body. It is a gonad and has elements of all three dermal layers, originates elsewhere and situated anatomically somewhere else, possesses cells that secrete hormones periodically orchestrated by hypothalamus-pituitary and controlling other organs and even another life. Ovarian tumour can be a 'tumour' and symptomatic without being enlarged, and a palpable pelvic mass could be present without it being symptomatic. These may occur at any age from childhood to senescence. Depending upon patient's age, physiological and pathological manifestations, the implications and management strategies will have to vary. Most of the ovarian tumours are cystic and remain asymptomatic. Symptoms arise because of the enlarged size compressing adjacent structures, infiltrates or it elaborates hormones.

CLINICAL DIAGNOSIS OF OVARIAN TUMOURS

The ability to achieve early diagnosis remains an unsolved problem. There are different types of neoplasms that occur in different age groups. Whenever an ovarian tumour/mass/cyst is found, in order to provide optimal care, clinician needs to have a high index of suspicion regarding it being malignant and to rule out the possibility. Cystic enlargement of one or other of the normal ovarian structures is common in reproductive age group and is more often physiological. The senile ovary is usually free of cysts. Whenever the tumour is non-cystic or reported as containing noncystic elements, malignancy needs to be excluded. Borderline tumours occur most commonly in the perimenopausal age group.

The clinical problems that any gynaecological cases present with are mass, pain, bleeding, discharge and fertility issues–all or any. For ovarian tumours, the leading finding is the mass and sometimes pain. The mass may not be obvious at early phase of disease. Pelvic ultrasound may find the mass, bimanual palpation may detect or swelling could be obvious on abdominal examination. The associated ascites and/or pressure effects to lymph and venous tracts in some stages of the disease will add to it. Ovarian mass *per se* may not be associated with pain. Rapid increase in size due to bleeding into it, torsion of the pedicle, pressure on other organs or infiltration at later stages of malignancy can be the causes of abdominal or pelvic pain. Ovarian tumours when found in reproductive age group do not affect ovarian function and cause menstrual disturbances, unless the particular type of tumour is hormone producing or the enlargement is related to hormonal effect. As for the fertility issue, there are reports of occurrence of ovarian tumours linked to subfertility. Ovarian tumours require to be distinguished from all the conditions that present with abdominal or pelvic mass.

Even a distended urinary bladder can be a source of confusion. The plethora of conditions such as pregnancy, pseudocyesis and phantom tumours, ectopic pregnancy, uterine leiomyoma, broad ligament tumours, endometriosis, pyosalpinx or hydrosalpinx, pelvic abscess, an appendix abscess, retroperitoneal tumours, tumours of the colon and rectum, a mesenteric cyst, a large hydronephrosis, pelvic kidney, an enlarged liver or spleen, hydatid (echinococcal) cysts, diverticulitis, obesity and ascites need to be kept in mind.

It is always a good practice to rule out pregnancy and to ensure empty urinary bladder before abdomen and pelvic examination. During abdominal examination, paying attention to percussion may provide pertinent clinical information. Auscultation can be helpful. A peritoneal rub distinguishes an ovarian cyst from ascites. A soufflé means that the tumour is more likely to be uterine than ovarian. The foetal heart sounds are a proof of pregnancy. At pelvic examination, determining whether the swelling is attached to (or part of) the uterus, moves with the cervix will provide clue to the primary affected organ. A good guide is the presence or absence of a sharp cleft between the uterus and the lower pole of the tumour **(Figs. 1A and B)**. The pulsating uterine vessels felt through vaginal fornix reduce the possibility of the mass being ovarian.

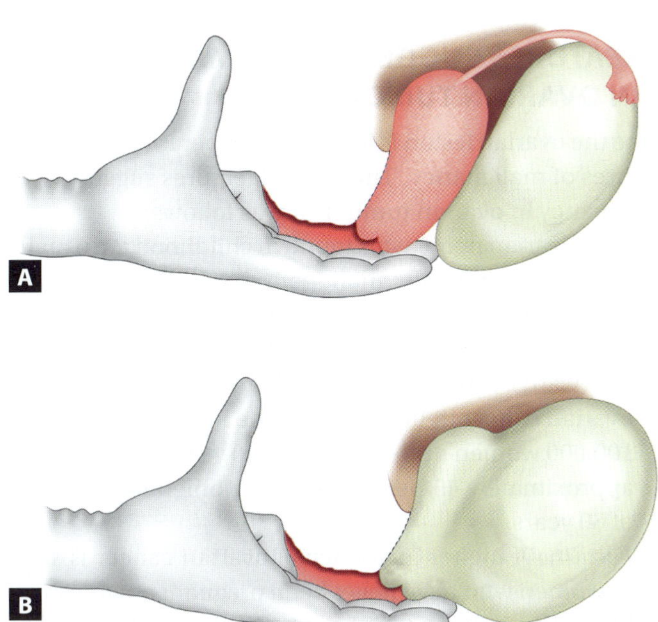

Figs. 1A and B: Diagrammatic demonstration to show (A) presence of cleft or wedge between extrauterine mass and uterus and (B) absence of such a notch in uterine mass at pelvic vaginal examination.

Sometimes, the diagnosis of ovarian mass is discovered after an ultrasound or radiological studies carried out for other reasons. For example, X-ray of the abdomen, intravenous (IV) urography or barium studies may reveal the evidence of foetal skeleton, calcification in a leiomyoma or teeth in a mature cystic teratoma (dermoid cyst) **(Figs. 2A and B)**.

COMPLICATIONS OF OVARIAN TUMOURS

The complications of ovarian mass are as follows:

- *Torsion of the pedicle:* Axial rotation is more likely to involve smaller mobile tumours with longer pedicles, e.g. dermoid cysts **(Fig. 3)**. The restricted movements with tumours of larger size may not aid torsion. The clinical features, causes and treatment of axial rotation are described in Chapter 19: Torsion of Pelvic Organs.

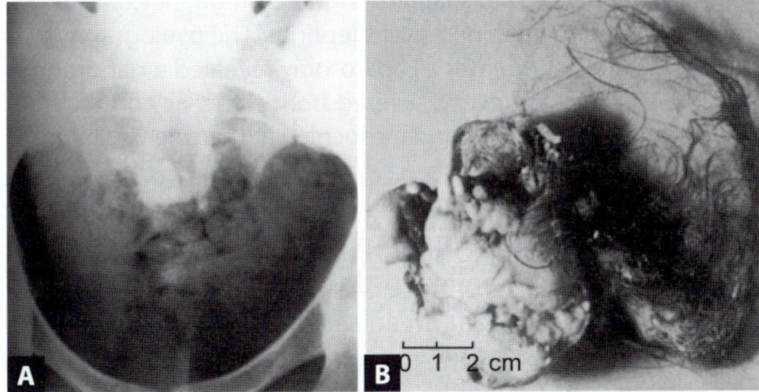

Figs. 2A and B: The mature cystic teratoma (dermoid cyst) picked up by radiography. (A) An area of calcification recognisable as tooth in the pelvis; (B) The well-formed tooth, as shown in Figure A, in the specimen after removal. From the nodal point in the cyst, tuft of hair is also seen.

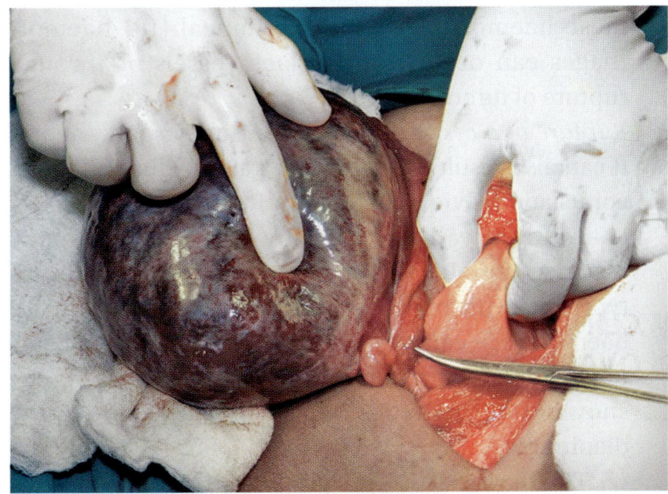

Fig. 3: Axial torsion of the pedicle of ovarian cyst.

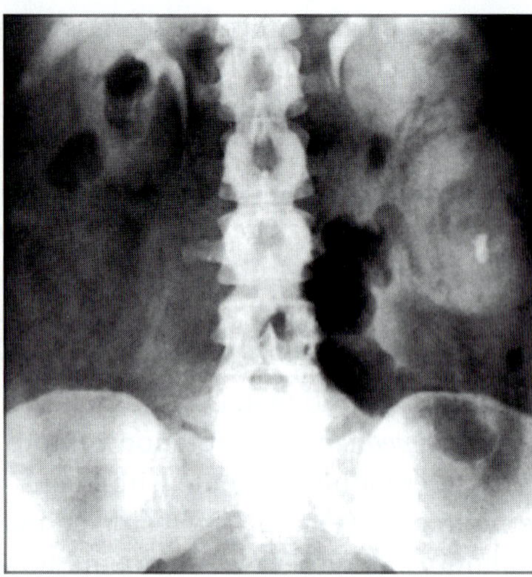

Fig. 4: A parasitic mature cystic teratoma (dermoid cyst) visible on the radiograph as a round soft-tissue shadow containing a tooth, high in the abdomen on the left. The patient in this case suffered from repeated attacks of pain during late pregnancy, and these were attributed to left-sided pyelonephritis. The pyelography was carried out after her delivery. Laparotomy revealed a gangrenous dermoid cyst and left ovary, severed from all pelvic connections, and adherent to the colon and mesocolon at the splenic flexure.

Intermittent and incomplete torsion can lead to degenerative changes in the cyst wall making them adherent to adjacent organs and omentum. New blood supply through adhesions may sustain the tumour even after it is severed making it parasitic **(Fig. 4)**.

- *Haemorrhage into or from a cyst:* Small haemorrhages into the cavity of a cyst are common. They do not cause pain and tenderness in the tumour at the time of their occurrence. The bleeding is self-limiting. The discolouration in tumour or fluid is the result of these haemorrhages. Intraperitoneal (IP) haemorrhages can occur from surface vessels or through rupture of tumour.
- *Rupture of a cystic tumour:* It is usually spontaneous. It can also result from external trauma, during labour, coitus and pelvic examination. Rupture is more likely in the cyst wall damaged by previous ischaemic degeneration. It is also seen in cysts of papilliferous type and with malignant tumours. Rupture with IP haemorrhage can present with acute abdomen. Signs of peritoneal irritation can be present including the shoulder-tip pain resulting from fluid under the diaphragm.

  The diagnosis is difficult unless the patient had a record of earlier cyst. Noticeable reduction in size and presence of free fluid in the peritoneal cavity will lead to the diagnosis.

  The leakage of the sebaceous contents of a dermoid cyst can result in oleic or chemical peritonitis. The initial picture is of acute abdomen often accompanied by pyrexia. The subsequent effect is to produce dense adhesions, whereas the rupture of a mucinous cystadenoma leads to the condition called pseudomyxoma peritonei.
- *Degeneration:* Fibromas are subject to the same types of degeneration as are uterine fibroids, except the red degeneration. Most large solid tumours show evidence of central necrosis and haemorrhage.
- *Infection:* Necrosis following torsion of the pedicle is a common forerunner to infection of an ovarian tumour. The banished practice of cyst aspiration, abdominal or vaginal, can result in infection. Adherent infiltrated bowel loops with ischaemia or compromised wall can infect the tumour.
- *Intestinal obstruction:* This rarely occurs with benign tumours. It is very likely with malignant ovarian tumours due to involvement in spread and adhesions with loops of small intestine. It is the common mode of death from ovarian cancer.
- *Malignancy:* Benign ovarian tumours can turn malignant.

FEATURES SUGGESTIVE OF MALIGNANCY IN OVARIAN TUMOUR

Once the ovarian lesion is found, it is imperative to look for features of malignancy. The clinical features suggestive of malignancy in ovarian tumours are as follows:

- *Age:* Ovarian neoplasms found in childhood are usually malignant or locally malignant. Excluding them, the risk of malignancy is roughly proportional to age and ranges from 20% before the menopause to 50–60% afterwards. A woman has a 1-in-70 risks of developing ovarian cancer in her lifetime. The incidence is 1.4 per 100,000 women under the age of 40 years, increasing to approximately 45 per 100,000 for women over the age of 60 years.
- *Fertility:* A higher incidence of ovarian cancer is seen in women who have never been pregnant or who are of low parity. Women who have had either breast or colon cancer or have a family history of these cancers also are at higher risk of developing ovarian cancer. Protective factors include multiparity, contraceptive use, a history of breastfeeding and anovulatory disorders.

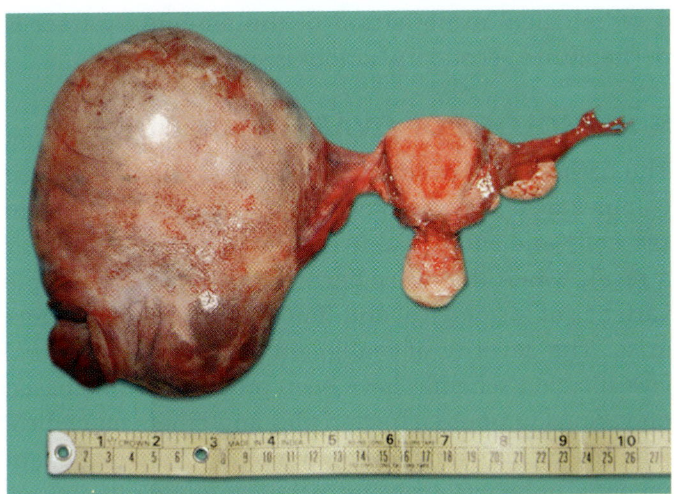

Fig. 5: Ovarian tumour with variegated consistence—cystic and solid areas.

- *Pain and tenderness:* A dull aching pain (as distinct from a sudden acute pain caused by torsion or rupture) and tenderness over one or other aspects of the tumour is very suggestive of malignant change. This is often the first and most reliable evidence. Sacral nerve root pains strongly indicate very advanced malignancy.
- *Tumour characteristics:*
  - *Rapidity of growth:* A rapidly growing tumour is suggestive of malignancy.
  - *Consistence:* Solid, nodular and irregularly-shaped growths are more likely to be malignant than smooth cystic ones **(Fig. 5)**.
  - *Bilaterality:* 75% of malignant tumours are bilateral compared with 15% of benign ones.
  - *Fixity:* This is an ominous sign but can also be caused by impaction of the tumour and by an associated lesion such as endometriosis.
  - *Ascites:* The presence of free fluid in the abdominal cavity usually means peritoneal metastases or at least that the tumour has perforated the ovarian capsule. It is more significant if the fluid is bloodstained. In benign tumours such as fibroma or cystadenomas of the papilliferous type, clear exudate is often found.
  - *Oedema feet and/or vulva, varicosities:* Obstruction of the venous or lymph return practically never occurs with a benign tumour.

Ultrasound scanning will help in delineating the site and size of the mass. Several ultrasonographic criteria have been used to devise scoring systems and algorithms for differentiating benign from malignant tumours. In general, benign lesions are likely to be unilateral, unilocular, thin walled with no papillae or solid areas. Septae, if present, are also thin. In contrast, malignant lesions are often multilocular with thick walls, thick septae and a mixed echogenicity because of the presence of solid areas.

Doppler flow studies help to increase the specificity of diagnosis. In malignant tumours, the resistance to flow is usually low (<0.4), and there is a high peak velocity.

Computed tomography (CT) and magnetic resonance imaging (MRI) can be used to evaluate the tumour and extent of spread but are more useful in monitoring the progress of disease.

- *Tumour markers:* Various tumour markers have been developed, which may help in differentiating benign from malignant lesions. More importantly, if serum levels are elevated preoperatively, they are useful in follow-up and for the detection of recurrence **(Table 1)**.

For epithelial ovarian tumours, the most important of these biomarkers is serum cancer antigen 125 (CA-125), a surface glycoprotein. Elevated values of >35 U/mL are found in over 80% of patients with nonmucinous epithelial ovarian cancers but in only 1% of the general population. CA-125 can also be elevated in inflammatory conditions involving the peritoneum, e.g. tuberculosis and endometriosis, though to a lesser level. Other markers can be used in combination with CA-125 to improve the predictive value, e.g. CA 15-3 is elevated in breast cancers but not in ovarian cancers; CA 19-9 is elevated in mucinous ovarian malignancy and in gastrointestinal cancers. Carcinoembryonic antigen (CEA) levels higher than 5 mg/L are seen in 88% of mucinous cancers but in only 29% of epithelial cancers. Macrophage colony-stimulating factor (M-CSF) and monoclonal antibody ovarian XI (OV XI) have been found to be indicative of a positive second-look laparotomy even if CA-125 is normal. Human epididymis protein 4 (HE4) is considered to have potential as better biomarker than CA-125 in discriminating malignant from benign masses. Utilising risk stratification, a panel of biomarkers, including HE4, may ultimately be useful for detecting ovarian cancer. For stromal tumours, oestrogen, androgens and inhibin have been used as tumour markers. In germ cell tumours, the value of tumour markers has been proved for a long time. Alpha-fetoprotein (AFP), human chorionic gonadotropin (hCG), lactate dehydrogenase (LDH) and even CA-125 are used. AFP can be elevated in all except dysgerminoma

TABLE 1: Tumour markers.

Tumour	*Tumour markers*
• *Epithelial ovarian tumours:* – Serous tumours – Mucinous tumours	• CA-125, CEA, CA19-9, and HE4: – CA-125 – CEA and CA19-9
• *Malignant germ cell tumours:* – Endodermal sinus (yolk sac) tumours, embryonal carcinomas, polyembryomas and immature teratomas – Choriocarcinomas, embryonal carcinomas, polyembryomas and, in low levels, in some dysgerminomas – Dysgerminoma	• AFP, beta-hCG and LDH: – AFP – Beta-hCG – LDH, placental alkaline phosphatase
• *Sex cord-stromal tumours:* – Granulosa cell tumour – Leydig cell tumour – Fibroma – Thecoma – Sertoli cell tumour – Leydig cell tumour	• Inhibin, oestradiol, testosterone and AFP: – Oestradiol, inhibin, calretinin, CD56 and FOXL2 – Testosterone and AFP – Calretinin – Oestrogen – AFP – Alpha-inhibin, vimentin and cytokeratin
Mesenchymal tumours	CA-125, vimentin and laminin
Carcinosarcoma	CA-125

(AFP: alpha-fetoprotein; CA-125: cancer antigen 125; CEA: carcinoembryonic antigen; FOXL2: Forkhead box protein L2; hCG: human chorionic gonadotrophin; HE4: human epididymis protein 4; LDH: lactate dehydrogenase)

and choriocarcinoma and hCG in all except embryonal sinus tumour and immature teratomas. The list of tumour markers and in immunohistochemistry is endless. Other tumour markers such as lipid-associated sialic acid (LSA), NB/70K and TAG-72, and many others need to find their place in clinical practice.

- *Laparoscopy:* If the nature of the tumour is in doubt, laparoscopy will aid the diagnosis. It provides an opportunity to carry out required treatment in the same sitting for benign and non-neoplastic lesions.

Once an ovarian neoplasm is diagnosed, the next step is to determine whether it is primary or metastatic. A full clinical examination is, therefore, essential, and a radiological examination of the alimentary tract is desirable, if a secondary tumour is suspected.

PATHOLOGY OF OVARIAN TUMOURS

The pathology of ovarian neoplasms is one of the most complex areas of gynaecology. Ovaries consist of totipotent sex cells and multipotent mesenchymal cells, and as a result, when the ovary becomes neoplastic, multiple varieties of histological and functional types of tumours arise. The severity of malignancy also varies. Several classification schemes have been proposed, some based on various tumour characteristics and others on clinical features such as functioning tumours or the malignant potential or behaviour. None of them is found satisfactory. For the purposes of uniformity and comparison of clinical experience, the one proposed by the World Health Organization (WHO) is recommended for the ovarian tumour classification **(Table 2)**. It takes into account the histological cell of origin, severity of malignancy (benign, borderline or malignant) and histological grade with some varieties.

In the present chapter, only the commonly described tumours are discussed, and it does not include all the conditions listed in **Table 2**. Conditions listed as 'tumour-like lesions' by the WHO are not malignant, and these are first dealt under 'non-neoplastic tumours of the ovary' in this chapter. These non-neoplastic 'tumours' are either hormone effect related, pregnancy related or infection related **(Box 1)**.

NON-NEOPLASTIC OVARIAN 'TUMOURS'

Clinical Features

Symptoms

- *Menstrual disturbance:* There may not be any changes with menstruation pattern with most of the non-neoplastic ovarian cysts, except when they are due to the associated hormonal effect or when they are related to inflammatory process. The aberrant menstrual patterns that can be found are:
    - *Frequent cycles or frequent cycles with increased flow:* These are mostly seen when multiple small cysts are associated with conditions causing ovarian hyperaemia as in infection-related conditions. Ovulation continues despite the cysts.
    - *Delayed menstruation followed by irregular bleeding:* Corpus luteum cysts and conditions

TABLE 2: WHO classification of ovarian tumours.

Epithelial tumours:

Type of tumour	***Benign***	***Borderline***	***Malignant***
Serous	Cystadenoma, adenofibroma and surface papilloma	Serous borderline/ atypical proliferative, micropapillary/ noninvasive low-grade serous	Low-grade, high-grade carcinoma
Mucinous	Cystadenoma, adenofibroma	Mucinous borderline, atypical proliferative	Carcinoma
Endometroid	Cystadenoma, adenofibroma	Endometroid borderline, atypical proliferative	Carcinoma
Clear cell (mesonephroid)	Cystadenoma, adenofibroma	Clear cell borderline/ atypical proliferative	Carcinoma
Brenner	Benign	Brenner borderline/ atypical proliferative	?
Seromucinous	Cystadenoma, adenofibroma	Seromucinous borderline/atypical proliferative	Carcinoma
Undifferentiated	–	–	Carcinoma

Mesenchymal tumours:
- Low-grade endometroid stromal sarcoma
- High-grade endometroid stromal sarcoma

Mixed epithelial and mesenchymal tumours:
- Adenosarcoma
- Carcinosarcoma

Sex cord-stromal tumours:

Pure stromal tumours	***Pure sex cord tumours***	***Mixed sex cord-stromal tumours***
Fibroma, cellular fibroma, thecoma, luteinised thecoma with sclerosing peritonitis, fibrosarcoma, sclerosing stromal, signet-ring stromal, microcystic stromal, Leydig cell and steroid cell (benign and malignant)	Granulosa cell (adult and juvenile), Sertoli cell and sex cord tumour with annular tubules	Sertoli–Leydig cell—well differentiated, moderately differentiated (with and without heterologous elements), poorly differentiated (with and without heterologous elements) and retiform (with and without heterologous elements) Sex cord-stromal tumours NOS

Germ cell tumours:
- Dysgerminoma
- Yolk sac tumour
- Embryonal carcinoma
- Choriocarcinoma
- Mature teratoma
- Immature teratoma
- Mixed germ cell tumour

Contd...

Contd...

Monodermal teratoma and somatic-type tumours arising from dermoid cyst:
- Struma ovarii—benign and malignant
- Carcinoid—strumal and mucinous
- Neuroectodermal-type tumours
- Sebaceous tumours—adenoma, carcinoma
- Other rare monodermal teratomas
- Carcinomas—squamous cell, others

Germ cell-sex cord-stromal tumours:
- Gonadoblastoma, including malignant
- Mixed germ cell-sex cord-stromal tumour, unclassified

Miscellaneous tumours: Tumours of rete ovarii—adenoma, adenocarcinoma; Wolffian tumour; small cell carcinoma—hypercalcaemic, pulmonary; Wilms' tumour; paraganglioma; solid pseudopapillary neoplasm; mesothelial tumours—adenomatoid, mesothelioma and soft-tissue tumours—myxoma, others

Tumour-like lesions: Follicle cyst, corpus luteum cyst, luteinised follicle cyst, hyperreactio luteinalis, pregnancy luteoma, stromal hyperplasia, fibromatosis, oedema, Leydig cell hyperplasia and others

Lymphoid and myeloid tumours—lymphoma, plasmacytomas and myeloid neoplasms

Secondary tumours

(NOS: not otherwise specified; WHO: World Health Organisation)

Source: Adapted from International Agency for Research on Cancer (IARC) and World Health Organisation. Female Genital Tumours. WHO Classification of Tumours, 5th edition. Switzerland: WHO; 2020.

BOX 1: Non-neoplastic tumours.

- *Hormone related:* Follicular and luteal cysts, corpus luteum cysts, theca lutein cysts, polycystic ovaries and endometriotic (chocolate) cyst
- *Pregnancy related:* Luteoma, ovarian ectopic pregnancy
- *Infection related:* Oophoritis, salpingo-oophoritis

producing oestrogen or progesterone continuously (e.g. endometrioma) will be associated with this presentation.

- *Infrequent cycles with/without scanty flow or amenorrhoea* are found in women with 'cystic ovaries' that are androgenic as in polycystic ovary syndrome (PCOS).

- *Subfertility:* When cystic change is associated with suppression of ovulation as in PCOS, infertility of long or short duration is present.
- *Pain:* An ovarian cyst does not cause pain unless haemorrhage occurs or it is involved in pelvic adhesions. Inflammatory lesions may be associated with pelvic pain, with cyclic exaggeration. Increase in size of ovaries *per se* is not associated with pain since the tunica albuginea is ill formed and nonresistant. An ovarian cyst buried in peritoneal adhesions and the resistance offered to distension can cause pelvic pain. Rupture of haemorrhagic corpus luteal cyst can cause peritoneal irritation and pain. Torsion of ovary when it occurs will present with acute abdomen.

Signs

Small ovarian tumours lying in the pelvis are palpable on bimanual (vaginal) or rectal examination. They usually lie behind the uterus and possibly, but not always, a little to one side. If one is found in the uterovesical pouch, it is probably either a dermoid cyst or its pedicle has undergone torsion.

When an ovarian tumour emerges from the pelvis, it comes to lie behind the abdominal wall displacing the intestines above and to the side and the uterus below and behind its lower pole. On abdominal examination, therefore, an ovarian tumour is always dull to percussion, with areas of resonance in the flanks.

Cysts are often so tense that they give the impression of being solid, especially if they are multilocular. Presence of thin-walled cyst and flaccid due to watery content could exhibit fluid thrill. Patch of resonance at percussion will help to differentiate encysted fluid from ascites. It is difficult to determine the side of affected ovary for tumour based on physical examination. Even if the tumour is in the pelvic cavity and is lying well to one side, it may still arise from the opposite ovary. A tumour reaching the abdominal cavity tends to lie in the midline **(Figs. 6A to D)**.

Presence of ascites can mask tumour palpability. Removal of some of the peritoneal fluid will facilitate interpretation of bimanual examination finding by making ovarian mass palpable. When paracentesis is carried out,

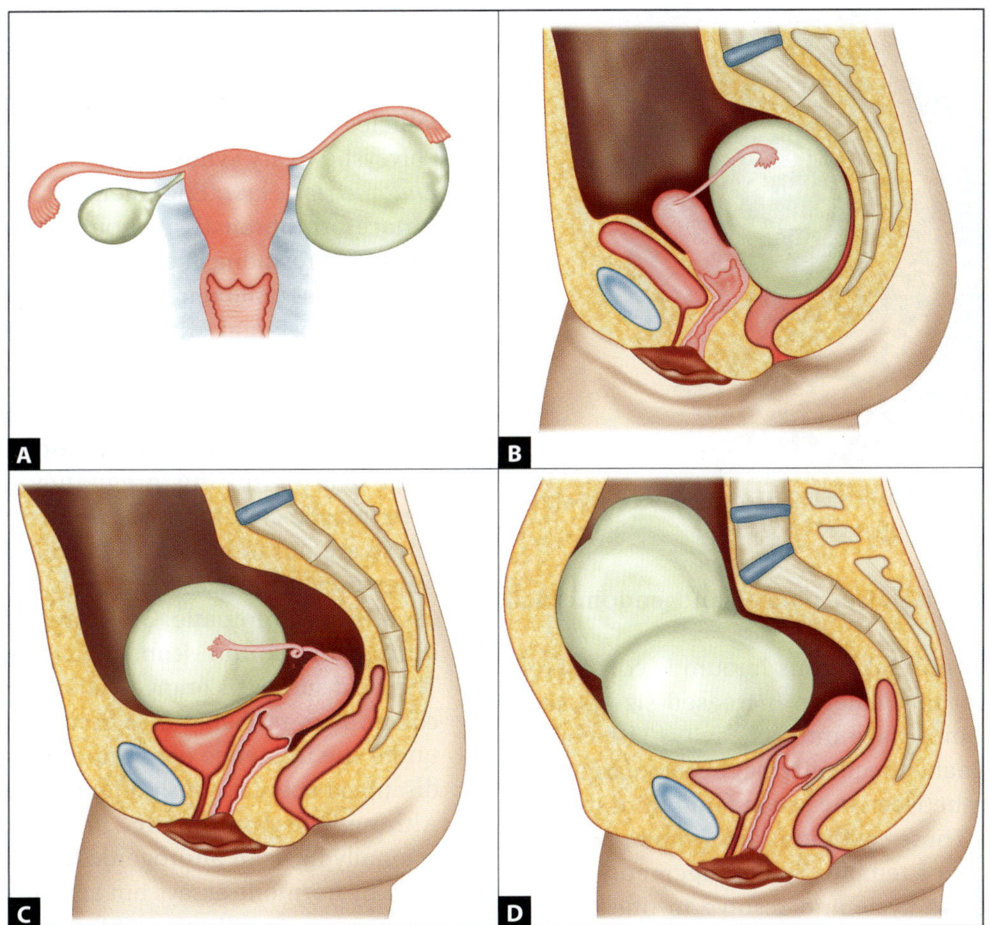

Figs. 6A to D: The common positions of ovarian tumours in relation to the uterus. (A) A small tumour lies to the side; (B) A medium-sized tumour lies behind; (C) A small- or medium-sized tumour which lies in front is likely to have its pedicle twisted; (D) A large tumour lies above and in front of the uterus, immediately behind the abdominal wall.

microscopic examination of the centrifuged fluid is an important pointer to rule out malignancy.

Hormone related: Cystic changes in ovarian follicles are common and are more often under the influence of hormones. They do not usually grow beyond 2 cm, and such ovarian findings are referred to as 'cystic ovary' in clinical practice. It is better to avoid the use of this term. The Graafian follicle itself or any of its products such as the corpus luteum, corpus albicans and corpus fibrosum may remain cystic for some time prior to their ultimate replacement by fibrous tissue. The cysts are usually small and multiple and may be lined by granulosa cells, granulosa lutein cells, theca lutein cells, connective tissue or hyaline tissue. They are normally found in small numbers at all ages before the menopause; they have no pathological significance and are symptomless. The majority of these 'cystic ovaries' are symptomless and are incidental discoveries. When associated with symptoms, they are due to either hormonal effect or secondary to inflammatory hyperaemia.

- *Follicular cysts:* Follicular cysts possibly represent enlargements due to unruptured Graafian follicles. The ovum degenerates and disappears, but the granulosa and theca cell lining persist and remain functional for a variable time **(Fig. 7)**. As more follicular fluid is produced, the follicle increases in size, and its lining epithelium may ultimately become flattened or disappear. These cysts can be single or multiple. In the latter case, they commonly affect both ovaries equally. They are always small and, even when they occur singly, usually have a diameter of up to 3–5 cm and rarely >10 cm. They can persist for several menstrual cycles. These are more likely to resolve in 16 weeks' time. They may occasionally produce oestrogen

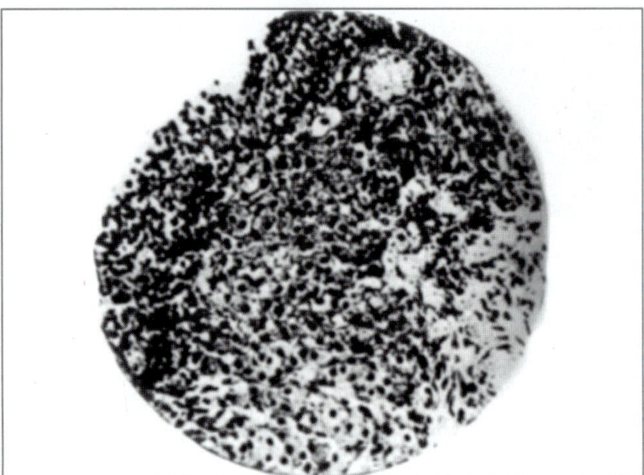

Fig. 7: The wall of a follicular cyst lined by granulosa cells with theca lutein cells outside.

causing menstrual disturbances and endometrial hyperplasia.

- *Luteal cysts:* A normal corpus luteum is considered cystic if >3 cm in diameter. Increased size is seen following haemorrhage into its cavity. The corpus luteum of pregnancy frequently may become larger, and it degenerates between the second and third months of pregnancy. These conditions are symptomless, are manifestations of temporary derangements in the pituitary–ovarian cycle and resolve in due course. Sometimes, the corpus luteum of menstruation not only becomes cystic; the lining of granulosa lutein and paralutein cells continues to produce progesterone and oestradiol for a longer time than normal.

They occasionally cause short periods of amenorrhoea (rather a delayed period) followed by prolonged uterine bleeding to produce a clinical picture simulating early pregnancy, abortion or even ectopic pregnancy. Rupture of haemorrhagic corpus luteal cyst is one of the causes of haemoperitoneum. The endometrium in this condition will be in secretory phase.

- *Theca lutein cysts:* They are usually bilateral, multicystic and can be as large as 25 cm in diameter. Excessive luteinisation is the result of the high output of gonadotrophins. They are associated with molar pregnancy, choriocarcinoma, multiple pregnancies and in ovarian hyperstimulation syndrome (OHSS) seen following ovulation induction with clomiphene citrate or gonadotrophins. No treatment is required for these cysts. Treatment of the cause will resolve abnormal luteal tissue. In case of OHSS fluid and electrolyte status needs attention.
- *Polycystic ovaries:* The PCOS, a condition of ovarian hyperandrogenism, more often will have moderately enlarged ovaries. It is due to peripherally aligned follicles like 'string of pearls' (refer to Chapter 24: Polycystic Ovary Syndrome).
- *Endometriotic cyst:* Endometriotic foci on the ovarian surface form fibrous tissue around the accumulated fluid and blood resulting in cyst formation. These cysts vary from several millimetres to 10 cm in size (Chapter 23: Endometriosis and Chronic Pelvic Pain).

Pregnancy related:

- *Luteoma of pregnancy:* Luteomas are multiple foci of solid luteal tissue found sometimes in one or both ovaries during pregnancy. They represent hyperplastic conditions rather than true neoplasms. These are not to be confused with corpus luteum of pregnancy. The sizes vary from 8 to 20 cm and are usually asymptomatic. They are incidental findings during ultrasound scan or at caesarean delivery. Their cut surface is orange-yellow to greyish-yellow in colour. They probably arise from theca or stromal cells under the influence of chorionic gonadotrophin and disappear spontaneously after pregnancy.

Although asymptomatic, luteomas of pregnancy occasionally have an androgenic function, as evidenced not only by hormone assays but also by the occurrence of minor degrees of virilisation of the mother or her female child.

- *Ovarian pregnancy:* The clinical findings of ovarian pregnancy are similar to tubal ectopic pregnancy or ruptured corpus luteum. The condition is rare, and the factors leading to occurrence of ovarian pregnancy are not clear. The diagnosis is often made by the pathologists using Spiegelberg criteria that specify that the fallopian tubes, including fimbria, must be intact and separate from ovary, the gestational sac must occupy the normal position of ovary, ovary must be attached to uterus through the utero-ovarian ligament and there must be ovarian tissue attached to the pregnancy in the specimen (placental tissue has to be mixed with ovarian cortex). These are surgical criteria, and all cannot be established by ultrasonography (Chapter 9: Ectopic Pregnancy and Pregnancy of Unknown Location).

Infection related:

- *Oophoritis:* Oophoritis is seen as a part of residual ovarian syndrome. It is usually a perio-ophoritis due to cyclical expansion of the conserved ovary after hysterectomy, encased in adhesions making a thickened ovarian capsule. Whenever there is ovarian infection, it is usually with the salpingitis, a combined salpingo-oophoritis. It is said that only oophoritis could be seen with mumps infection, and the condition disappears with resolution of the viral infection. Ovarian abscesses can occur as part of tubo-ovarian abscess or after gynaecological surgery and are less accessible to antimicrobial treatment. Calor (pyrexia), dolor (pelvic pain), rubor as ovarian/pelvic hyperaemia (menstrual aberration) and tumour (adnexal mass due to inflammatory enlargement) of inflammatory process are the presenting symptoms.

- *Salpingo-oophoritis:* Adnexal mass is usually due to inflammation of fallopian tubes and ovaries resulting from bacterial infection in pelvic inflammatory disease. Ovary is involved in inflammatory process of fallopian tube because of anatomic juxtaposition and shared blood supply. The pelvic inflammatory disease is dealt elsewhere in detail (Chapter 20: Infections Including Sexually Transmitted Diseases).

Management of Non-neoplastic Tumours

If ovarian cysts are infection-related, appropriate antimicrobial treatment will be sufficient. If there is an abscess, more often a tubo-ovarian abscess when not responding to antimicrobials, tense or ruptured would require surgical intervention—drainage and lavage or even adnexectomy.

In the absence of gross pelvic disease, the treatment of ovarian cysts is self-curative. If left alone, the cysts become inactive and disappear. If there is a worrisome menstrual disturbance, appropriate ovarian steroidal hormones-combined oestrogen and progesterone pills or luteal phase support with progesterone will be acceptable.

Polycystic ovaries do not require any treatment. In the management of subfertility, ovarian drilling may be offered.

NEOPLASTIC OVARIAN TUMOURS

Ovarian neoplasm continues to have the highest mortality of all gynaecological cancers. They are the least able to be diagnosed in early stages. About 70–80% of primary ovarian tumours are of epithelial origin, 10% of stromal origin and 5% of germ cell origin, while the remainder fall into the other groups.

Epithelial Ovarian Tumours

Epithelial ovarian tumours arise from surface epithelium of the ovary. Ovary develops from the coelomic epithelium (mesothelium) of the embryonic gonad. Coelomic epithelium is continuous with the epithelium that penetrates the underlying mesenchyme to form Müllerian duct and mesonephric duct. This proximity is reflected in the various directions of Müllerian differentiation pursued by the surface epithelium such as fallopian tube, endometrium, endocervical epithelium, clear cells of the kidney and transitional epithelium of bladder when the surface epithelium turns neoplastic in the postnatal ovary. The result is the manifestation of different histological types of epithelial ovarian tumours. Serous tumours appear similar to the epithelium of the fallopian tube, mucinous tumours to the endocervical mucosa, endometrial tumours to the endometrium, similarity of clear cell tumours to renal cell cancers and cells in Brenner tumours suggestive of the transitional epithelium of the bladder or urothelium. Many present a mixed histological appearance to include several of the epithelial tumour types. Although common epithelial tumours may arise directly from surface epithelium and grow exophytically, more commonly, they appear to originate from its inclusion glands accounting for the cystic or endophytic nature of most of these tumours. Epithelial ovarian tumours could be benign, malignant or one in between as borderline. It is not always a disease of continuum.

Borderline epithelial ovarian tumours are tumours of low malignant potential (LMP) and are seen in younger premenopausal women between the ages of 30 and 50 years. Borderline tumours remain confined to the ovary for a longer time, but they also metastasise. Metastases may be noninvasive or invasive. Sometimes, metastases occur as a late event, and patients may die from borderline tumours some 10–30 years after the primary surgery.

Serous and mucinous cystadenocarcinoma are the most common types of invasive epithelial ovarian cancers. Mixed tumours are more common. They comprise 60% of all primary tumours of the ovary, and 9% of those that are malignant. The ratio of serous to mucinous cystadenocarcinoma varies between 4:1 and 10:1 in different parts of the world. They may also contain tissue of the endometrioid variety, although endometrioid carcinomas can be distinguished separately (2% of ovarian tumours). Malignant Brenner tumours are extremely rare. Clear cell ovarian tumours or mesonephric tumours are highly malignant tumours, and two histological patterns are recognised—(1) The solid clear cell pattern and (2) the hobnail pattern. The borderline and benign varieties of clear cell tumours are uncommon. Clear cell carcinomas and endometrioid carcinomas have often been described to have association with endometriosis.

Benign Epithelial Tumours

Benign Serous Tumours

Serous tumours account for 20% of benign ovarian neoplasms and are the second most common in this category, the most common being the benign cystic teratoma.

These may be cystic, papillary or adenofibromatous, and each type may occur singly or in combination. The serous cystadenoma occurs as a thin-walled, often translucent cyst, which is usually unilocular. It may have a few daughter cysts in the wall. The cyst may vary in size from 20 to 30 cm in diameter and is often unilateral. The papillary serous cystadenoma can occur in combination with a cyst and the papillae on the inner wall or on the outer surface (exophytic). The exophytic tumours are often associated with ascites, and there may be implantation of fragments of tumour on the peritoneal surfaces, thus giving a false impression of malignancy at surgery. 5–10% have borderline malignant potential. The serous adenofibroma occurs as a lobulated, hard knobby solid mass that occurs alone but is more often associated with a serous cyst when it forms a fibrous thickening or nodule in the cyst wall. The serous adenofibroma is essentially a fibrous neoplasm.

Histologically, serous cystadenomas are lined by a single layer of flattened or cuboidal cells, but in places, the cells may be more columnar and resemble those lining the fallopian tubes. The tubal nature of the epithelium is particularly evident over the papillae. Stroma of some of these tumours shows psammoma bodies, but they are not a specific diagnostic feature and are not indicative of malignancy. These are areas of fine calcific granulation dispersed throughout the tumour, detectable on X-ray.

Mucinous Cystadenoma

These are also common and account for up to 20% of all ovarian tumours. In approximately 10% of cases, the tumour is bilateral. They may attain a very large size and may be multilocular **(Fig. 8)**. The growing point of the cyst is marked by a mass of small locules, and some of the large locules may result from a breakdown of partitions. Intracystic papillae, if present, are small and few, and the inner walls are generally smooth. The outer wall varies in thickness and is white, grey or silvery-blue in colour. Adhesions to adjacent tissues are not present unless there have been degenerative changes in the wall.

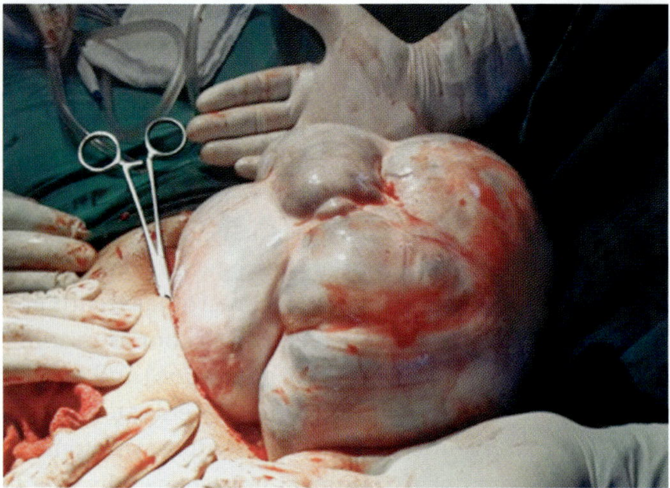

Fig. 8: Mucinous cystadenoma.

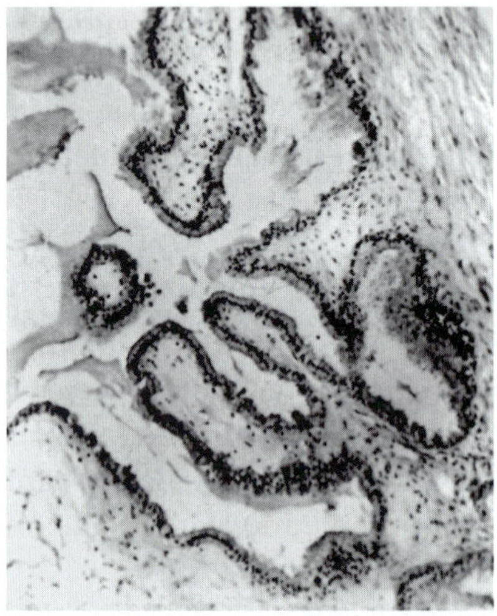

Fig. 9: Photomicrograph of a mucinous cystadenoma showing the single-layered lining of secretory cells.

The cysts are lined by tall columnar cells, and these secrete a mucus material—a glycoprotein with a high content of neutral polysaccharides. The appearance of the epithelium is remarkably like that of the glands of the cervix or of the intestine **(Figs. 9 and 10)**. The fluid content is thick in consistency and glary and is colourless, yellow, green or brown depending on the presence of blood pigments derived from previous intracystic haemorrhages.

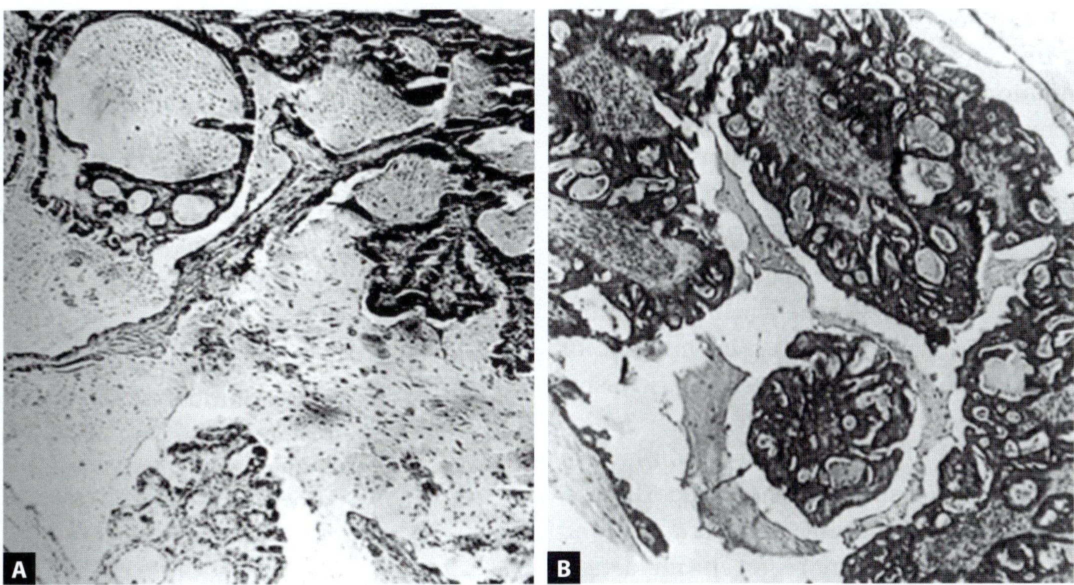

Figs. 10A and B: (A) Photomicrograph of mucinous ovarian tumour that had gross appearances typical of cystadenoma and histological features of borderline malignancy. She had bilateral salpingo-ovariectomy with hysterectomy; (B) Photomicrograph of metastasis excised from the umbilicus, 2 years after the removal of the ovaries.

A unique complication of rupture of an active cyst is pseudomyxoma peritonei, a condition in which the epithelial cells of the tumour invade the omentum and spread as a film over the visceral and parietal peritoneum. These sites secrete semisolid mucin into the abdominal cavity, resulting in distension, pain and vomiting. Possibly, due to induction of mucinous metaplasia of the peritoneum, the abdomen refills. Pseudomyxoma peritonei could occur as a complication of a mucocele or adenocarcinoma of appendix or colon. Appendicular diseases and a cystadenoma of the ovary sometimes coexist in these cases.

Brenner Tumour

It is nearly always benign. The growth is found as part of a fibroma or in the wall of a mucinous cystadenoma. It may occur bilaterally. Brenner tumours range in size from being microscopic to as big as 30 cm in diameter and are asymptomatic.

Grossly, the tumour is solid, slight lobulated cut surface, with grey white or yellow colour. Microscopy shows a characteristic pattern of circumscribed epithelial cell nests having coffee-bean appearance in fibromatous stroma. The epithelium consists of columns of squamous or transitional cells with a central core lined by columnar cells. Occasionally, calcium deposits are seen in stroma. The squamous cell elements could have origin from epithelium of the urinary tract, derived from the rete tubules. The columnar cells resemble those of the endocervix. The histogenesis of the Brenner tumour remains in doubt since none of the theories explains all the characteristic features of the tumour. Some tumours may exhibit endocrine activity, oestrogenic activity resulting in endometrial hyperplasia and uterine bleeding, and few others may have androgenic activity. The biological or mechanical stimulation-induced theca cell reaction in the tissues alongside its surface is the probable reason for the hormonal activity.

Treatment of benign epithelial tumours usually is resection of the tumour, and this may involve a cystectomy or salpingo-ovariectomy with or without a hysterectomy, depending on patient's age and reproductive desires.

Benign *endometrioid* and *clear cell tumours* are rare.

Borderline Epithelial Tumours

Borderline epithelial tumours are of LMP and show only atypical proliferation of cells. Hence, they are referred to as tumours of LMP or atypical proliferating tumours. They are seen in younger women, 10 years younger than their malignant counterparts, remain confined to the ovary for long periods and have a good prognosis. Women with low parity, who had ovulation inductions and those who failed to lactate, have increased risk of developing borderline tumours. Smokers are also prone.

The diagnosis is histological, and criteria for the diagnosis of borderline tumours are epithelial proliferation with papillary formation and pseudostratification, nuclear atypia and increased mitotic activity and absence of true stromal invasion.

The serous and mucinous tumours largely form this histological group. Endometrioid, mesonephroid and Brenner tumours of borderline malignancy are rare.

Serous borderline tumours present with or without micropapillary features, and they can be invasive or noninvasive. Serous borderline tumours with invasive implants have 5-year survival rates of 60%.

Mucinous borderline tumours tend to be confined to ovary and have good prognosis. In advanced stage disease, there is association with pseudomyxoma peritonei, and survival drops to 50%. They may represent metastatic disease from gastrointestinal tract.

Endometrioid borderline tumours are sometimes recognised, either as adenofibromas in which there is a prominent fibromatous component and the endometrial-like epithelial component. It shows some degree of irregular proliferation or areas of atypical proliferation in foci of endometriosis.

Mesonephroid borderline tumours are invariably adenofibromas.

Brenner borderline tumour is also known as a proliferating Brenner tumour. These are large tumours that are wholly or partly cystic and, in the majority of cases, behave in a benign fashion, though occasional instances of metastasis are reported.

Overall, about 15–25% of borderline tumours behave in a malignant fashion, invading locally and even metastasising. Histological grading of the degree of severity of the epithelial proliferation and atypia prove to have some prognostic benefits.

Management is individualised dependent on age, parity and desire to conserve fertility. Surgery is the cornerstone in management, and ovarian cystectomy, ovariotomy and salpingo-ovariectomy with or without hysterectomy are the surgical options. In a mucinous tumour, simultaneous appendicectomy is suggested. No adjuvant chemotherapy or radiotherapy is required. However, follow-up is mandatory as recurrence of up to 30% is reported. Chances of progression to invasive malignancy is <1%. It is said that patient of borderline tumour may die with the disease but not because of the disease.

Malignant Epithelial Tumours

Epithelial ovarian carcinomas account for 80–90% of all ovarian malignancies. The various malignant forms of the epithelial tumours of the ovary are grouped and studied together. They are all adenocarcinomas. They tend to occur in women aged 45–60 years and are commonly asymptomatic until they have reached a considerable size.

Risk Factors

Race, environmental factors, diet, hormonal, genetic and hereditary factors and number of pregnancies have been associated with the development of ovarian cancer.

White women have the highest incidence of ovarian cancer. Women from America, Europe or any industrialised Western country have higher incidence than in women of Asian countries. Increasing incidence among Asians is reported.

Incidence of ovarian cancer increases with increasing age possibly due to extended time available to accumulate random genetic alterations in the ovary. Incidence increases up to mid-70s.

Nulliparity, early menarche and late menopause associated with long periods of repetitive ovulation are the risk factors. Risks decrease with each live birth. Protective effect of pregnancy may be due to prolonged anovulation and possibly inducing shedding of premalignant ovarian cells. Early menopause and the use of oral contraceptives have been associated with lowering the risk.

Tubal ligation and hysterectomy are associated with risk reduction attributed to blocking of ascent of carcinogen through vagina.

Family history of ovarian cancer in first-degree relative, non-polyposis colorectal cancer has increased risk of inheriting ovarian carcinoma. Breast–ovarian cancer syndrome is linked to inherited mutation of *BRCA1* and *2* genes.

Screening

There is no effective screening programme for ovarian cancer. Studies using routine CA-125 estimation in serum, pelvic examination and ultrasound of pelvis have not been helpful in low-risk population. For women with familial ovarian cancer syndrome who wish to maintain their reproductive capacity, transvaginal ultrasonography, analysis of levels of CA-125 in serum, in combination with periodic pelvic examinations may be considered.

Current recommendations for the management of women at high risk for ovarian cancer are as follows:

- Women who appear to be at high risk for ovarian or breast cancer should undergo genetic counselling and, if with substantial risk, genetic testing for *BRCA1* and *BRCA2*.
- Women who wish to preserve their reproductive capacity can undergo frequent screening by transvaginal ultrasonography every 6–12 months, although the efficacy of this approach is not clearly established.

Diagnosis

In early stages, epithelial ovarian cancer does not produce symptoms or signs that would alert the clinician to the diagnosis. Therefore, the detailed medical history to ascertain possible risk status and high index of suspicion is required for all women after their age of 40 years. To help preoperative determination of likelihood of adnexal mass being malignant, various scoring systems to calculate the risk of malignancy are in vogue. Some use menopausal status, sonomorphological score and CA-125 levels with different weightages given to these variables for calculation. Risk of malignancy algorithm that uses levels of HE4 with CA-125 and menopausal status is claimed to have 94% accuracy in identifying epithelial ovarian cancers. The imaging group has come out with stepwise categorisation of adnexal masses to interpret ultrasound images using the International Ovarian Tumor Analysis (IOTA) system. It follows a simple strategy of first identifying it as ovarian, then recognising the pattern and thereafter arriving at risk status, to help plan the further course of action.

An abdominal swelling may be noticed by the patient or discovered during routine medical examination. Dyspepsia of some kind is the only symptom of ovarian tumours. The patients admit to having early satiety rather than loss of appetite on enquiry. The usual complaints are of increasing abdominal girth, lower abdominal pain or discomfort and the presence of a pelvic mass. A dull aching pain in the abdomen localised to the tumour is often reported. There is no plausible explanation for this localised pain, since it occurs even before the growth erodes the surface and irritates peritoneum. A large tumour with bowel infiltration or associated ascites presents with indigestion and vomiting. Urinary symptoms due to pressure on the bladder are quite frequent, while disturbances of the menstrual cycle or postmenopausal bleeding are unusual. Nevertheless, 30% of postmenopausal women suffering from ovarian tumours report having had some, albeit slight, uterine bleeding. It is due either to the effect of the tumour on the surrounding ovarian stroma or by associated changes in the vascularity of the pelvic organs.

Features suggestive of malignancy and investigations required for workup are outlined earlier. In peri- and postmenopausal women, an adnexal mass must be presumed to be malignant unless proven otherwise. For preoperative assessment in addition to a complete blood count, renal and liver function tests, it is necessary to obtain serum levels of CA-125 and CEA. The chest X-ray may reveal pleural effusion or may suggest lung parenchymal disease that would alter the extent of tumour resection. Pelvic and abdominal ultrasounds are useful and necessary. Other radiological investigations, CT or MRI scans, are not mandatory. Intestinal evaluation with radiological upper gastrointestinal series is indicated, if clinical features suggest or stools show occult blood.

Elevated serum CEA is a marker associated with gastrointestinal primary cancers but can also occur in patients with mucinous ovarian malignancies. A ratio of serum CA-125 to CEA of >25 has been proposed for differentiating ovarian cancer from colorectal cancer and for corroborating ovarian cancer diagnosis in patients under consideration for neoadjuvant therapy. For patients with mucinous ovarian cancer, CEA may be useful for monitoring of recurrent disease. CA19-9 is another marker that is elevated more often in mucinous tumours compared with other ovarian cancer types. It may be useful for monitoring for recurrence, especially in patients with mucinous ovarian cancers, and in those with high CA19-9 levels prior to treatment.

Pathology of Malignant Epithelial Ovarian Tumours

Malignant Serous Tumours

Up to one fourth of serous tumours are malignant. They account for 75% of epithelial cancers. Serous adenocarcinomas are usually fairly large, and in over half of the cases, both ovaries are involved. About a quarter of these carcinomas are primarily cystic, and about two thirds are semi-solid, with only a small proportion being solid. The tumour may be adherent to the bowel, the pelvic organs or pelvic wall, and the peritoneum may be studded with widespread deposits, especially if papillae are present on the outer surface of the tumour. On section, areas of haemorrhage and necrosis are frequently seen, and the fluid in a cystic portion of the tumour is often bloodstained.

Histologically, the tumours show a wide variety of patterns. Papillary, adenopapillary or diffuse patterns are the principal types noted in well-differentiated tumours. Most tumours have a mixed pattern of differentiation, and it can be difficult to diagnose the precise type of tumour.

Malignant Mucinous Tumours

These are mostly large, unilateral and multilocular masses and are heterogeneous. They contain areas of cystadenoma and atypical proliferative tumour admixed with areas of carcinoma. Cystic and solid areas are evenly distributed throughout ovary without discrete nodularity.

Stromal invasion could be infiltrative or expansile. Glands are usually of intestinal type. The one with endocervical type of glands will usually have other components such as serous, endometrioid and squamous. Most mucinous tumours are well differentiated.

Endometrioid Tumours

Endometrioid adenocarcinomas account for 2% of epithelial cancers. The primary neoplasms of the ovary histologically closely resemble tumours of the uterine endometrium. They may develop either from pre-existing ovarian endometriosis or from the surface epithelium of the ovary via a process of Müllerian metaplasia along endometrial lines. The proportion of cases that arise from each of these sources is uncertain.

They are generally large and measure between 10 and 25 cm in diameter. The outer surface is usually smooth, but there may occasionally have papillary outgrowths. On section, the tumours may be solid, partially cystic or wholly cystic, and the latter usually showing abundant papillary ingrowths. The cystic areas can contain clear, mucoid or haemorrhagic fluid.

Histologically, these tumours have cuboidal or columnar epithelial cells arranged in a glandular or acinar pattern; a proportion of these neoplasms have a papillary form. Most of the tumours are well differentiated, have clear or vacuolated cytoplasm, and squamous metaplasia is common.

Clear Cell (Mesonephroid) Tumours

Histologically, the mesonephroid tumours have to be distinguished from the endodermal sinus tumour, the endometrioid carcinoma, papillary serous cystadenocarcinoma and the lipoid cell tumour. These are usually unilateral. Size varies from subcentimetre to 30 cm in diameter. They have variable appearance on cut surface. Surface involvement is seen in about 10% of cases.

Microscopically, mesonephroid tumours show low cuboidal, polyhedral, hobnail or flattened cells arranged in different patterns such as papillary, tubulocystic and solid. Admixture of papillary and tubulocystic patterns is more common.

Metastases of Malignant Ovarian Tumours

The direct, transcoelomic and lymphatic spread are the main ways of ovarian cancer metastasis. IP metastasis occurs by direct spread to adjacent organs in pelvis and transcoelomically to omentum, peritoneum and intestines. Secondary deposits are usually seen on the omentum and on the visceral and parietal peritoneum (including the under surface of the diaphragm) which becomes studded with small nodules. A common site for these is the pouch of Douglas, and they are often palpable on rectal examination.

The lymph nodes most likely to be involved are the aortic groups and the iliacs. The supraclavicular nodes are sometimes enlarged and should always be examined. Inguinal nodes get infiltrated via round ligament when tumour has spread to uterus and tubes.

Secondary nodules are occasionally seen in the umbilicus, the cancer cells reaching through the lymphatics of the obliterated hypogastric arteries and of the urachus **(Figs. 10A and B)**. Vaginal metastases are rare and usually denote blood-borne emboli. The finding of a hydrothorax does not necessarily mean pulmonary deposits, even when the ovarian tumour is malignant.

Sarcomas and teratomas spread by the bloodstream to the lungs. The liver is relatively immune to metastasis.

STAGING

The prognosis of ovarian cancers is affected by the extent of spread of the disease (stage) at the time of diagnosis and the volume of residual disease after primary surgery. The histological subtype and grade also influence the outcome. In this light, the initial surgical exploration of abdomen and pelvis assumes importance. This exploration, the surgical staging, helps not only to document the extent of disease but also to decide on the need for adjuvant therapy. Despite disease being confined to ovaries on gross examination, it is possible to have occult dissemination. Therefore, the surgical staging process includes the histological component to make it comprehensive. The techniques or the steps to be followed for surgical staging are described very well in most of the textbooks **(Table 3)**.

The staging of ovarian cancers according to the International Federation of Gynaecology and Obstetrics (FIGO) with equivalent tumour, node and metastasis (TNM) classifications is provided for reference **(Table 4)**.

Treatment

Comprehensive surgical staging is the initial approach in the care of ovarian cancers. It may serve as the complete treatment in some early ovarian cancers. For cases with advanced disease, it not only establishes the diagnosis but also allows planning the appropriate adjuvant care. Primary treatment of malignant ovarian tumours consists of comprehensive surgical staging (including bilateral salpingo-ovariectomy, total hysterectomy and

TABLE 3: Evaluation steps during surgical staging of ovarian cancer.

Preoperative preparation	• Mechanical bowel preparation with/without antimicrobial bowel preparation • Systemic prophylactic antimicrobials • Arrange for frozen section evaluation, especially if operating on young patient where disease appears confined to one ovary and fertility preservation is planned
Abdominal incision	• Midline or paramedian preferred • Low transverse, if made inadvertently, divide/detach rectus muscles from pubic symphysis; can extend the incision cephalad on right side
Exploration	Inspection and palpation of: • Ovaries and pelvis—document whether: – Capsule is intact, ruptured already, or rupture occurred during manipulation – Excrescences present over the surface or not present • Intra-abdominal surfaces and viscera—proceed in a clockwise direction: Caecum, paracolic gutter, right kidney, liver, gall bladder, under surface of diaphragm, entrance to lesser sac, left side of falciform ligament, spleen, left kidney, entire length of small intestine from ligament of Treitz to cecum, including peritoneal surfaces of intestinal mesentery and large intestine (ascending, transverse and descending colon)
Sampling	• Tumour confined to ovaries and pelvis; if no macroscopic evidence of tumour beyond pelvis: – Sample all sites in upper abdomen – Retrieve ascitic fluid, if present; obtain peritoneal washings when there is no or sufficient ascitic fluid after instilling 50–100 mL of normal saline at different sites—pelvic cul-de-sac, each paracolic gutter, under each half of diaphragm* – Multiple random peritoneal biopsies from the above sites of pelvic cul-de-sac, paracolic gutters, under surfaces of the diaphragm,† peritoneum over bladder and rectum and small intestinal mesentery – Biopsy from adhesions and irregularities – Exploration of retroperitoneal spaces, resection of enlarged lymph nodes, if nodes are not enlarged obtain representative nodal tissue from para-aortic area and iliac area (along external, internal and common iliac vessels) • Young patient, disease confined to one ovary, fertility preservation is planned—send for frozen section evaluation and obtain results, in addition to above to obtain biopsy from contralateral ovary • In advanced disease with abdominal involvement and ascites—collection of peritoneal washings, peritoneal biopsies are not required
Surgery considered	• Bilateral salpingo-ovariectomy, total hysterectomy, omentectomy (at least infracolic), maximum tumour resection. Resection of suspicious and/or enlarged nodes, identified on preoperative imaging or during surgical exploration, if possible (resection of clinically negative nodes is not required) • In fertility preservation—removal of affected ovary with fallopian tube, infracolic omentectomy (contralateral ovary, fallopian tube and uterus are preserved)

*Collection can be facilitated by the use of rubber catheters attached to a bulb syringe; alternatively, surface smear with a spatula/brush can be obtained such as in Pap smear.

†Laparoscope-facilitated biopsy.

Source: Adapted from: P Kushtagi. Malignant Ovarian Tumours. In: Obstetrics and Gynaecology for Postgraduates. Volume (2) 3rd edition; Eds. S Arulkumaran, S Gopalan, P Kumar. Universities Press (India) Pvt Ltd., 2010; Ch. 22, pp. 354-70.

TABLE 4: Staging of carcinoma of ovary—FIGO and equivalent TNM staging.

Staging is based on findings at clinical examination and surgical exploration. The final histological findings (cytological, when required) after surgery are to be considered in staging.

Stage	*Extent of disease*	*TNM*
I	Growth limited to ovaries:	T1
	• Growth limited to one ovary, no malignant cells in ascites or peritoneal washings (on cytology), no tumour on external surface, capsule intact	T1a-N0-M0
	• Growth limited to both ovaries, no malignant cells in ascites or peritoneal washings (on cytology), no tumour on external surface, capsule intact	T1b-N0-M0
	• Tumour of 1A or 1B, with any of the following:	
	– Surgical spill	T1c1-N0-M0
	– Capsule ruptured before surgery or tumour on surface	T1c2-N0-M0
	– Malignant cells in ascites or peritoneal washings	T1c3-N0-M0
II	Growth involving one or both ovaries with pelvic extension, no malignant cells in ascites or peritoneal washings:	T2
	• Extension and/or implants on uterus/fallopian tube/ovaries	T2a-N0-M0
	• Extension to other pelvic intraperitoneal tissues	T2b-N0-M0
III	Growth involving one or both ovaries with cytological or histological confirmed spread to outside pelvis and/or lymph node metastases:	T1-3-N1-M0
	• Positive (cyto- or histological) retroperitoneal nodes only:	
	– Lymph nodes ≤10 mm in the greatest dimension	T1/T2-N1a-M0
	– Lymph nodes >10 mm in the greatest dimension	T1/T2-N1b-M0
	• Microscopic extrapelvic (above pelvic brim) peritoneal involvement with or without retroperitoneal lymph nodes metastasis	T3a2-N0/N1-M0
	• Macroscopic peritoneal metastasis beyond pelvis >2 cm in the greatest dimension, with or without retroperitoneal lymph node metastasis	T3b-N0/N1-M0
	• Macroscopic peritoneal metastasis ≤2 cm in the greatest dimension, with or without retroperitoneal lymph node metastasis, including extension of tumour to capsule of liver and spleen without parenchymal involvement	T3c-N0/N1-M0
IV	Distant metastasis excluding peritoneal metastases:	T any-N any-M1
	• Pleural effusion with positive cytology	Ta-Na-M1a
	• Parenchymal metastases and metastases to extra-abdominal organ, including inguinal lymph nodes and lymph nodes outside abdominal cavity	Ta-Na-M1b

(FIGO: International Federation of Gynaecology and Obstetrics; TNM: tumour, node and metastasis)
Source: Prat J. FIGO Committee on Gynecologic Oncology. Staging classification for cancer of the ovary, fallopian tube, and peritoneum. Int J Gynaecol Obstet. 2014;124(1):1-5.

omentectomy), debulking (cytoreductive) surgery and in most cases appropriate chemotherapy.

Stage I: Low Grade, Low Risk

- *Stage IA, fertility desired:* Comprehensive surgical staging and *unilateral* salpingo-ovariectomy. Women require regular periodic follow-up with pelvic examination and determination of serum CA-125 levels. Completion of surgery and removal of uterus with the other tube and ovary are suggested after completion of desired childbearing.
- *Stage IB, fertility desired:* Comprehensive surgical staging and *bilateral* salpingo-ovariectomy. Women require regular periodic follow-up with pelvic examination and determination of serum CA-125 levels. Removal of uterus is suggested after completion of desired childbearing.

Other Cases

The remaining stage I cases and women with stage II disease will be amenable to the planned primary cytoreductive surgery at the time of surgical staging. The higher stages of III and above may not always be operable with optimal removal of the disease. Hence, in them, the operability upfront will be the variable to consider before undertaking surgical approach.

- *Stage I high grade/high risk and stage II:* Comprehensive surgical staging and bilateral salpingo-ovariectomy followed by adjuvant chemotherapy.
- *Advanced stages (III and IV):*
  - *Surgical candidate, optimal tumour reduction likely, fertility not desired:* Bilateral salpingo-ovariectomy and total hysterectomy, omentectomy, para-aortic and pelvic lymph node sampling/ lymphadenectomy with optimal cytoreduction followed by adjuvant chemotherapy.
  - *Poor surgical candidate, low likelihood of optimal tumour reduction:* Neoadjuvant chemotherapy and dependent on:
    - *Response with tumour regression, improved operability*: Interval debulking surgery with completion bilateral salpingo-ovariectomy and total hysterectomy
    - *Stable disease, no change in operability status*: Continue chemotherapy to complete six courses and reassess
    - *Progressive disease*: Cytotoxic combination chemotherapy or single agent targeted therapy

The combinations of primary chemotherapy vary dependent upon type of tumour and the stage. However, paclitaxel and carboplatin remain the common components across the candidates receiving primary chemotherapy.

Surgery

Primary Cytoreductive or Debulking Surgery

In patients with advanced-stage epithelial ovarian cancer, the objective at initial exploratory laparotomy will be to perform cytoreductive surgery to remove all visible macroscopic diseases. In addition to salpingo-ovariectomy with total hysterectomy and omentectomy, the maximum surgical efforts might involve intestinal resection, peritonectomy, diaphragmatic resection, retroperitoneal nodes resection and splenectomy done without increasing the morbidity. Among all the surgical procedures performed in a cytoreductive surgery, only the extensive peritoneum surgery is predictive of survival. The surgical morbidity, however, is high (25–30%) with this approach, but the survival rate in a successful surgery makes the morbidity tolerable.

The optimal cytoreduction is the surgical strategy that aims to reduce the disease to microscopic levels. For practical purposes, the debulking is considered optimal when residual tumour nodules are <1 cm in maximum diameter. Procedures that may be considered for optimal surgical cytoreduction (in all stages) include bowel resection and/or appendectomy, stripping of the diaphragm or other peritoneal surfaces, splenectomy, partial cystectomy and/or ureteroneocystostomy, partial hepatectomy, partial gastrectomy, cholecystectomy and/ or distal pancreatectomy.

The removal of bulky tumour masses may reduce the volume of ascites present. Often, ascites will completely disappear after removal of the primary tumour and omental cake. It often alleviates the nausea and early satiety that many patients experience. Removal of intestinal metastases may restore adequate intestinal function, leading to an improvement in the overall nutritional status of the patient and facilitate patient's ability to tolerate subsequent chemotherapy. Tumour-involved areas are poorly vascularised. They contain higher proportion of cells in non-multiplying resting phase. Thus, cytoreduction will help to improve availability and effectiveness of chemotherapeutic agents at target areas improving vascularity and removing tumour areas with nonmultiplying phase.

The resectability of the metastatic tumour is usually determined by the location of the disease. Optimal cytoreduction is difficult to achieve in the presence of extensive disease on the diaphragm, in the parenchyma of the liver, along the base of the small-bowel mesentery, in the lesser omentum or in the porta hepatis.

The ability of cytoreductive surgery to influence survival is limited by the extent of metastases before cytoreduction presumably because of the presence of phenotypically resistant clones of cells in large metastatic masses. A patient whose metastatic tumour is large (i.e. >10 cm before cytoreductive surgery) has a shorter survival than those with smaller areas of disease. Extensive carcinomatosis, the presence of ascites and poor tumour grade irrespective of the size may also shorten the survival.

When attempting pelvic tumour resection, it is worth remembering that epithelial ovarian cancers tend not to infiltrate peritoneum of pelvic wall deeply or invade the lumina of bladder or colon. Adopting approach of entering retroperitoneum laterally along the surface of psoas makes surgery easier and helps to avoid injuring iliac vessels and ureter. The technique of reverse or retrograde hysterectomy will help to approach through the site of weak adhesions, opening the vagina and proceeding in reverse direction. This technique is helpful in such cases having obliterated pouch of Douglas with the primary tumour.

For omentectomy in advanced epithelial ovarian cancers, one prefers to severe attachment of infracolic omentum to the transverse colon. It is done by lifting the omental cake cephalad to incise peritoneum along serosa of transverse colon and separating omentum from the greater curvature of stomach while ligating both gastroepiploic and short gastric arteries.

Secondary Cytoreduction

The term secondary cytoreduction is used interchangeably with interval debulking. It is applied to the tumour reductive surgery done on cases (1) with recurrence after optimal cytoreduction and chemotherapy, (2) women in whom optimal primary surgery was not performed and received chemotherapy, (3) after induction chemotherapy in between courses of chemotherapy and (4) partial responders on first-line chemotherapy. In patients with residual lesions of >10 mm after primary cytoreductive surgery, secondary debulking significantly increases the progression-free and overall survival.

Procedures that may involve during interval debulking in candidates of neoadjuvant chemotherapy are visualisation of all peritoneal surfaces, selective excision biopsy of suspicious (for harbouring metastasis) peritoneal surface or adhesions, bilateral salpingo-ovariectomy, hysterectomy, omentectomy and resection of suspicious and/or enlarged lymph nodes. In patients with recurrence and partial responders, removal of lymph nodes noted to have potential metastasis at the time of primary cytoreductive surgery should be carried out. For optimal cytoreduction, it may be necessary for bowel resection and/or appendectomy, stripping of diaphragm or other peritoneal surfaces, splenectomy, partial cystectomy and/or ureteroneocystostomy, partial hepatectomy, partial gastrectomy, cholecystectomy and/or partial distal pancreatectomy.

Second-look Exploration

Second-look exploration is an attempt for documenting response to therapy in those patients with ovarian cancer who are clinically (sonography included) free of disease at that time. A negative second-look is one that documents no pathological (both cytological and histological) evidence of persistent disease. It must be remembered that the report of negative second-look is no guarantee against recurrence later. The reported recurrence rates after negative second-look range from 12 to 36% over 1–2 years. The main intention of second look appears to be to decide discontinuation of therapy. It would be wise and logical to consolidate the gain of no evidence of disease after primary therapy with some kind of consolidation therapy. If no such subsequent therapy is planned, a case can be made for omission of second-look exploration. Associated surgical morbidity also precludes recommendation for second-look surgery.

Chemotherapy

Chemotherapy prolongs remission and survival. Type of chemotherapy, dosage and drug combinations and length of treatment vary depending on type of tumour, stage of disease, operability and patient tolerability.

Combination chemotherapy is chosen to reduce the dose of individual drugs, increase effectiveness by acting at different cell cycle phases, improve drug tolerance and lower toxicity. It has the advantage of having drugs with different modes of action. The combination, in addition, has the advantage of decreasing development of drug resistance. The chosen drug combinations are administered at interval of 2–3 weeks. This interval provides time for cells with collateral damage to recover. Large variety of regimens and approaches are tested and are in use. Most of these regimens are intravenous (IV) and some with oral therapy. IP chemotherapy is also used. Systemic chemotherapy is discussed in detail in Chapter 36: Chemotherapy in Gynaecological Malignancies.

Adjuvant Chemotherapy

Adjuvant chemotherapy is the systemic chemotherapy advised after primary surgery to reduce risk of recurrence and/or eliminate any remaining cancer cells. Various chemotherapeutic agents and their combinations are active in the management of ovarian cancer. Platinum-based therapy has been the mainstay of treatment over the years. With the advent of effective molecules, improved universal availability and simplification of administration, the combination with taxanes has become the combination of choice. Most of the drugs chosen with combination are administered IV. An episode of administration of chosen combination chemotherapy more often intravenously is called 'a cycle'. At an interval of 3 weeks, six cycles are given. The limit of six cycles appears to have been decided empirically. Different combinations have been in use at different times at different treatment centres with the sole intention to attain disease-free status and long survival benefit with respect to the determining variables of availability, affordability and tolerability of drugs. The widely used situations are:

- *Stage I serous high grade, endometroid grades 2 or 3 and clear cell types:* Combination chemotherapy with carboplatin and paclitaxel (CP) is recommended.
- *Stage II–IV:* Choice of IV versus IP platinum and taxane chemotherapy with the addition of bevacizumab should be individualised.

Neoadjuvant Chemotherapy

Initiation of upfront chemotherapy for three to four cycles, performing cytoreduction (interval debulking) surgery, and completing the remaining cycles of chemotherapy is termed as neoadjuvant chemotherapy. Pathological confirmation of diagnosis by biopsy is necessary prior to offering patients, the neoadjuvant chemotherapy. It is considered in patients with advanced ovarian cancer in whom optimal cytoreduction is less likely at staging attempt and/or in those who could be a high perioperative risk. Neoadjuvant chemotherapy reduces tumour bulk, ascites and pleural effusion, if any, and facilitates maximal cytoreduction. It also decreases the blood loss during cytoreductive surgery. It is associated with lower perioperative morbidity, may be because they require less radical procedures. However, dense adhesions between the uterus and adjacent organs are often encountered. Women with stage IV disease and tumour extensiveness higher than 45 mm have shown a better survival rate. In women with stage III disease and metastatic lesions, <45 mm is likely to survive better and longer with primary cytoreductive surgery.

Intraperitoneal Chemotherapy

The supposed advantage of adjuvant IP chemotherapy is local administration to the surgical bed, higher reach because of large surface area of peritoneal cavity and instillation of higher dosage with lesser systemic effects. Several randomised controlled trials have opined that IP administration of carboplatin or cisplatin with paclitaxel in the primary therapy of optimally resected stage III ovarian cancer is an acceptable alternative. It is best suited to patients with good performance status. An important limitation appears to be very limited tissue penetration of few millimetre. Extensive adhesions, gross contamination of bowel contents from a left-sided bowel resection and significant obesity may limit successful IP access and distribution of drug. In patients who received IP chemotherapy, the survival benefit was significant.

Hyperthermic Intraperitoneal Chemotherapy

Hyperthermic IP chemotherapy is one-off dose instillation into peritoneal cavity of chemotherapeutic agent(s) after cytoreductive surgery in hyperthermic conditions. Effective cytoreductive surgery remains of primary importance, and hyperthermic IP chemotherapy is only an adjuvant therapy. Heating is thought to enhance the penetration of chemotherapy agent at peritoneal surface, increases sensitivity of cancer cells by impairing DNA repair and induces activation of systemic immune response. It is offered to patients who are candidates of neoadjuvant chemotherapy during their interval cytoreductive surgery. The advantages of this timing are that it allows for shorter gap between chemotherapy treatments as interval surgery interrupts chemotherapy cycles, could be effective against remaining chemotherapy-resistant cancer cells and that there will be lower volume of disease immediately following surgery. Despite encouraging published results from the trials, its use remains contentious.

Radiotherapy

Role of radiotherapy is very much limited in the management of ovarian tumours, and the reader is directed to Chapter 37: Radiotherapy in Gynaecological Malignancies for the detailed account on this modality. Radiotherapy finds its application as palliative treatment for metastatic bone or brain lesions for localised recurrence to alleviate the pain. It is one of the options in treating recurrent germ cell tumours, especially dysgerminomas.

Follow-up Care Plan after Completion of Treatment

Objective of the follow-up is to determine patient's immediate response to the treatment, early recognition and prompt management of treatment-related complications and detection of recurrence. The patients are usually advised follow-up every 2–4 months for 2 years, every 6 months for next 3 years and yearly thereafter. It should involve clinical examination and investigation profile of complete blood counts, kidney and liver biochemistry and CA-125 estimation. Imaging studies can be carried out, if clinically indicated.

There is no evidence to show that intensive clinical monitoring in asymptomatic women has any positive impact on overall survival or quality of life.

NONEPITHELIAL OVARIAN TUMOURS

Nonepithelial malignant ovarian tumours account for about 10% of ovarian tumours. They include malignancies from sex cord, stromal, germ cell origin, sarcomas and metastatic tumours. Their management approach is different from that of epithelial ovarian tumours.

Sex Cord-Stromal Tumours

They are grouped as pure stromal (e.g. fibroma, thecoma, Leydig cell and tumours arising from different stromal elements), pure sex cord (granulosa cell and Sertoli cell tumours) and mixed sex cord-stromal, including gynandroblastoma. These could be benign (thecoma and fibroma) or malignant (granulosa cell tumour, Sertoli–Leydig cell tumour and steroid cell malignant). Granulosa cell tumours form the majority of the sex cord-stromal tumours and are the more likely one to be malignant. The sex cord tumours are of low-grade malignancy.

These are functional tumours with acyclical oestrogen and/or androgen production. The demonstration of clinical hormonal activity by an ovarian tumour does not necessarily indicate that the tumour is of sex cord or stromal origin, because many metastatic tumours interact with the ovarian tissue to result in a significant hormonal production. Nor does the hormonal activity reflect the likely clinical outcome, but it may be useful as a tumour marker. Fibroma is the only inert tumour from the group. Levels of oestrogen, progesterone, testosterone and AFP should be obtained when sex cord-stromal tumours are suspected. The other substances showing sensitiveness as tumour marker and immunohistochemistry markers are calretinin, inhibin, CD56 (in cases that are inhibin and calretinin negative), Forkhead box protein L2 (*FOXL2*), epithelial membrane antigen (EMA) (as a discriminator for epithelial tumours), melanin A, cytokeratin, Müllerian-inhibiting substance and relaxin-like factor.

In these patients, preoperative evaluation of the uterus by hysteroscopy and endometrial aspiration is recommended to rule out a coexisting endometrial adenocarcinoma. Principles of staging and surgical treatment of malignant sex cord-stromal tumours are similar to epithelial tumours.

In this chapter, common sex cord-stromal tumours of some particular types are described. Benign and malignant varieties are considered together.

Fibroma

Fibroma affects all ages, being more common in women of 40–60 years. It is unilateral and multinodular. From being, an incidental finding at histopathology because of nonpalpable size, ones as big as 15–20 cm, can also be found. Cut surface has whorled appearance. Spindle-shaped cells in storiform pattern with hyalinisation and intracellular oedema are found on microscopy.

There are two described associations: (1) Pelvic mass with hydrothorax and ascites, known as Meigs syndrome and (2) with a hereditary basal cell nevus syndrome, characterised by early-appearing basal cell carcinomas, keratocysts of the jaw, calcification of the dura and mesenteric cysts.

Fibromas are inert tumours and are inhibin negative. Calretinin is a sensitive marker for fibromas. Treatment involves surgical removal with or without hysterectomy. In the young and fertility desirous women, ovarian cystectomy (enucleation) or ipsilateral salpingo-ovariectomy is sufficient. In patients with Meigs syndrome, the hydrothorax and ascites usually resolve after resection of the pelvic tumour.

Meigs Syndrome

It was first described by Demons and Tait. The exudative ascites could be the result of peritoneal reaction to mobile hard mass of the tumour. The hydrothorax is mostly right-sided probably due to ascitic fluid tracking through a defect in the diaphragm.

Thecoma

Thecomas usually occur in the postmenopausal women. They are oestrogen-producing tumours and present with abnormal or postmenopausal uterine bleeding. They could be of insignificant size and nonpalpable. They are solid unilateral tumours and can even be of 15 cm in diameter with smooth outer surface. The cut section reveals lobulated appearance with yellow hue and often a cystic change. Microscopically, tumour is laden with round or oval cells with lipid-containing cytoplasm. Luteinised thecoma is found in younger women.

Elevated oestrogen levels hint at the diagnosis. The acyclic oestrogen production may lead to endometrial adenocarcinoma and needs to be ruled out by endometrial biopsy before treating the patient.

Treatment is resection of the tumour with salpingo-ovariectomy or ovarian cystectomy for women desiring fertility and bilateral salpingo-ovariectomy with total hysterectomy in others.

Sertoli Cell Tumour

These are rare tumours and are mostly benign; possess estrogenic activity, when functional. Androgenic and progestogenic effects can also occur. Present as circumscribed unilateral pelvic mass. Cut surface shows closely packed hollow or solid tubules lined by Sertoli cells with significant cytoplasmic lipid. Association with Peutz–Jeghers syndrome (non-cancerous hamartomatous polyps in gastrointestinal tract with hyperpigmented macules on lips and mouth) is reported.

Malignant Sertoli cell tumours are rare. Nearly two thirds of Sertoli cell tumours are oestrogenic and rest are androgenic; present with excessive prolonged or irregular uterine bleeding and some associated with virilisation features. AFP is a useful tumour marker. Conservative surgery should be a sufficient care. The poorly differentiated ones have aggressive behaviour and rapidly turn fatal.

Leydig Cell Tumour

These tumours could arise from hilus or ovarian stroma and present with oestrogenic and androgenic manifestations. Although most of these tumours are benign, cases with malignant tumours are also found.

They are functioning ovarian tumours occurring in postmenopausal women. They may present with hirsutism, virilisation and postmenopausal bleeding because of oestrogenic activity. Endometrial hyperplasia and carcinoma need exclusion. They are unilateral and small solid tumours of size <5 cm. The cut surface is lobulated and yellow, orange or red-brown coloured. Microscopic features are steroidal cells filled with bright or eosinophilic cytoplasm having protein inclusions as Reinke crystals. Mitotic index is usually low. The positive immunohistochemical staining of alpha-inhibin and vimentin helps to establish the diagnosis. Positive reactions are also observed with cytokeratin, actin and EMA.

They are usually detected early in stage I and have positive prognosis. Hysterectomy with adnexal removal and comprehensive staging constitutes primary treatment. In advanced cases, the adjuvant combination chemotherapy with either bleomycin/etoposide/cisplatin, vinblastine/doxorubicin/cisplatin or paclitaxel/cisplatin can be recommended. If the tumour relapses, recurrent surgery, radiotherapy and/or hormone therapy are used.

Granulosa Cell Tumour

Granulosa cell tumours are found commonly after the menopause and before puberty. These are feminising tumours. They metabolise oestrogens as in the normal ovary. The production of oestrogen by these tumours is from surrounding stromal tissue. The resultant negative feedback on hypothalamic-pituitary system is manifest in low gonadotrophins. The unopposed acyclic secretion of oestrogen is responsible for uterine hyperplasia, uterine bleeding **(Fig. 11)**, an active vulvar and vaginal epithelium, enlargement of the breasts and even increased libido. Depending on the age of occurrence, precociousness in child, abnormal uterine bleeding in young adult and rejuvenation of the elderly would be the outcome. Carcinoma of the body of the uterus is sometimes seen in association with these tumours.

Histologically, the granulosa cell tumour consists of cuboid cells with deeply staining nuclei, arranged diffusely, in columns, cords or rounded masses, separated by hyaline tissue. Depending on the particular cell arrangement, the histological patterns are termed as folliculoid, cylindromatous and the like **(Fig. 12)**. Development of cysts and small collections of fluid within the rosettes of cells formed under the influence of secretory activity give

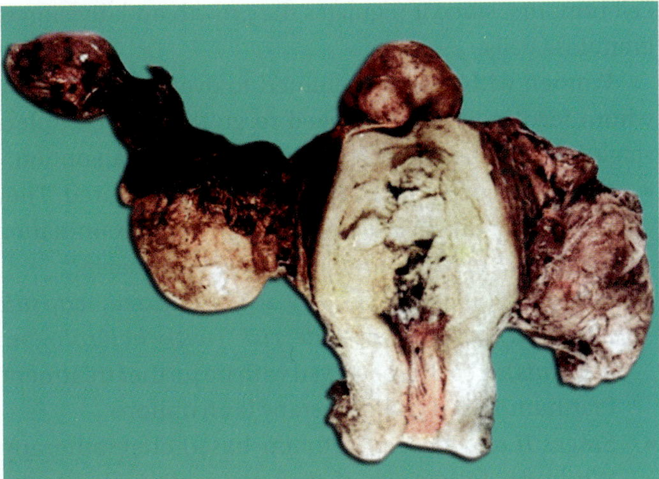

Fig. 11: Granulosa cell tumour showing myohyperplasia of the uterus and endometrial polyposis on cut section. The patient was 39 years of age and complained of intractable menorrhagia. She remained well for 11 years after primary surgery. She developed a recurrence of the granulosa cell tumour on the floor of the pelvis.

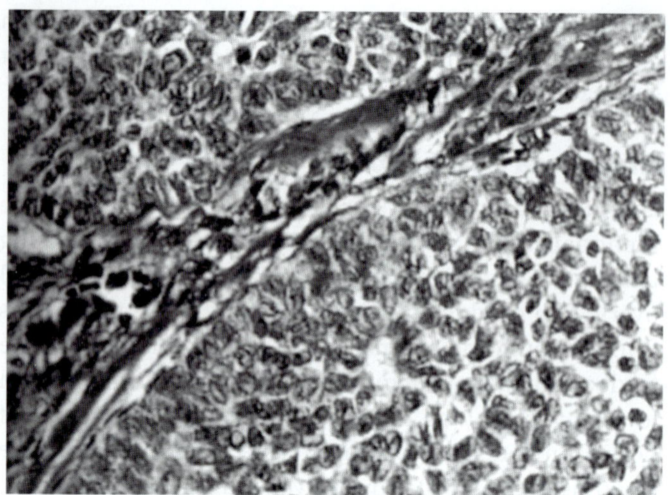

Fig. 12: Photomicrograph (370×) of granulosa cell tumour showing insular pattern and rosette-like Call–Exner bodies.

rise to the appearance of *Call–Exner bodies.* Liquefaction of clumps of tumour cells could also be responsible for some cysts.

Granulosa cell tumours can produce inhibin, and inhibin expression level in tumour tissue and serum can be considered as diagnostic markers. Serum levels of inhibin A and B, particularly inhibin B, will be of help in long-term follow-up because of correlation with extent of disease, decreasing during treatment and then increasing again prior to relapse. *FOXL2,* a gene encoding protein, is another sensitive and specific marker for adult granulosa cell tumours, since it regulates the growth and division of granulosa cells.

Women with disease confined to ovary, and those in whom fertility is desired, need to go through complete staging and in them fertility-sparing surgery is an option.

- *Stage I, low risk*: No further treatment is required. They need to be on surveillance with physical examination every 6–12 months, tumour marker and imaging.
- *Stage I, high risk (poorly differentiated, capsule ruptured) or intermediate risk (with heterologous elements):* It can be observed with no further treatment. Platinum-based chemotherapy is an option.
- *Stages II and above:* Platinum-based chemotherapy. While on follow-up, if there is a clinical relapse, secondary cytoreduction is to be considered. If there are isolated pelvic recurrences, pelvic irradiation may help to palliate.

Juvenile Granulosa Cell Tumour

Juvenile granulosa cell tumour is manifest in first decade of life. Juvenile tumour is associated with pseudoprecocious puberty, haemangiomatosis with enchondromatoses (Maffucci syndrome) or without enchondromatoses (Ollier syndrome). Their morphological features are similar to adult tumour. The differences from adult tumour are: (1) Hyperchromatic tumour cells are without grooves, (2) luteinisation of both granulosa and theca cells, (3) immature follicles and (4) absence of Call–Exner bodies.

Sertoli–Leydig Cell Tumours

Sertoli–Leydig cell tumours contain a mixture of Sertoli and Leydig cells and were previously known as androblastoma or arrhenoblastoma. It is thought that the Sertoli cells are responsible for differentiation in stromal cells to function like Leydig cells.

These occur at any age, being common in age group of women younger than 35 years. Endocrinological disturbances dominate the clinical picture. Well-differentiated Sertoli–Leydig cell tumours are common. About 90% of them are androgenic and produce clinical virilisation, and few tumours could be oestrogenic. The gross appearance of these tumours is not characteristic. They are often well circumscribed and may appear to be encapsulated. The outer surface is usually smooth or bosselated and on section, the tumour may be solid, partially cystic or wholly cystic. Histologically, there is a very wide spectrum of differentiation. Well-differentiated tumours are composed of tubular structures lined by Sertoli-like cells and Leydig cells in variable numbers between the tubules. Less well-differentiated tumours have a distinguishable epithelial component set in a mesenchymal stroma. The epithelial component consists of Sertoli-type cells arranged in solid tubules, true tubules, trabeculae or solid cords. The abundant mesenchymal element contains spindle cells and collagen in varying proportions. Mature Leydig cells will be seen in stroma as sheets or clusters or sometimes occur singly. Poorly differentiated tumours consist largely of sheets of closely packed spindle-shaped cells in which occasional irregular cord-like structures or imperfectly formed tubules may be recognised, and small groups or clusters of Leydig cells are seen.

The well-differentiated tumours behave in a benign fashion. Despite pursuing benign course, other tumours recur or metastasise within 12 months and are fatal in 2 years of the initial diagnosis.

Some Sertoli–Leydig cell tumours contain heterologous elements such as gastrointestinal epithelium, striated muscle, fat, bone or cartilage. Presence of these elements could be due to mesenchymal metaplasia. These subtypes being of teratomatous origin cannot be ruled out. The clinical and endocrinological behaviour of these neoplasms is not different than others in the group.

Mixed type of tumours with both granulosa cells and Sertoli–Leydig cell types were earlier referred to as gynandroblastoma. These are rare, benign and may be purely androgenic or solely oestrogenic. A few, however, do appear to secrete both oestrogens and androgens.

Sex Cord Mesenchymal Tumour with Annular Tubules

Sex cord tumour with annular tubules is a rare tumour. They occur in young age and are considered separately because of having intermediate phenotypical expression of pluripotent sex cord cell of the gonads. These tumours are separate entities than Sertoli cell tumours. There are two types of tumours depending on association with Peutz–Jeghers syndrome. The ones associated are multifocal, bilateral, very small and calcified. Those not associated with the syndrome are normally unilateral, unifocal and larger in size.

They like other tumours in the group present with hyperestrinism, amenorrhoea and postmenopausal bleeding. They could be solid, cystic or mixture of solid and cystic. They appear as yellow or brown tumours of any size. Microscopically, they are typically characterised by circumscribed columnar epithelial nests composed of ring-shaped tubules, which are encircled by acidophilic hyalinised basement membrane-like material and some with calcification.

Mostly, these tumours run a benign course. Those with malignant characteristics show stromal and vascular space invasion by individual tumour cells and tumour cell clusters and with or without capsular infiltration. Malignant tumours seem to spread mainly via the lymphatics and commonly involve the pelvic, para-aortic and supraclavicular lymph nodes.

Recurrence and metastases tend to occur several months to years after removal of the primary tumour. A recurrence rate of almost 50% is reported and may have repeated recurrence.

Steroid Cell Tumours, not Otherwise Specified

These previously referred to as lipid or lipoidal cell tumours and are formed of large oval or polygonal cells resembling steroid-secreting cells such as lutein, Leydig and adrenal cortex. These are solid, well-circumscribed tumours of <10 cm. They may look yellowish orange in colour. These are rarely malignant and about 10% of them tend to recur or metastasise. Surgical management is like that for epithelial ovarian tumours.

GERM CELL TUMOURS

Germ cell tumours are derived from the primordial germ cells of the ovary and represent the neoplastic transformation of them at various stages of differentiation. They include many types of tumours from teratomas to dysgerminomas. These tumours can be grouped as those with embryonic differentiation (e.g. teratomas), extraembryonic differentiation (viz. choriocarcinoma, yolk sac tumour and embryonal cell carcinoma) and those without any differentiation (e.g. dysgerminoma). They constitute the most common gynaecological malignancy in young women and account for about 15% of all ovarian tumours at all ages, and nearly 90% of them occurring before puberty.

Most of the germ cell tumours are unilateral, except the malignant dysgerminoma.

The germ cell tumours grow rapidly and present with pelvic pain due to capsular distention following haemorrhage or necrosis. The onset of symptoms can be acute. There can be a palpable adnexal mass. Since many patients are premenarchal, abdominopelvic ultrasound and examination under anaesthesia would be required.

Levels of AFP and beta-hCG may help with intraoperative diagnosis to determine whether fertility-sparing surgery is an option. High serum AFP levels and poor decline in serum AFP levels after treatment appear to be associated with worse outcomes in patients with germ cell tumours. High serum beta-hCG is also associated with poorer prognosis. High levels of serum LDH are found with more extensive disease and poor outcomes in some others. AFP and hCG are commonly used to monitor for recurrence in patients with germ cell tumours.

Germ Cell Tumours with Embryonic Differentiation

Teratomas

Teratomas are tumours consisting of tissues representative of all three primary embryological layers. They may develop from the ovum itself by varied differentiation of a totipotent cell. Teratomas are considered as mature and immature as the prognosis of any individual tumour arising from its components is determined by the degree of maturity of the constituent tissues and not by criteria of malignancy. Increasing degrees of tissue immaturity are associated with a progressive tendency towards malignant behaviour. The term 'malignant' is reserved for those cases in which malignant change has occurred in mature tissues.

Mature Cystic Teratoma

Mature cystic teratoma is commonly referred as a dermoid cyst. It occurs at an early age and can be found complicating pregnancy. These could be bilateral and may be multiple in one ovary. Often, they coexist with mucinous cystadenomas.

A dermoid cyst is mostly unilocular, has greyish-yellow thick capsule and smooth surface **(Fig. 13)**. They are filled with thick sebaceous material **(Fig. 14)**. Chemical changes in the sebaceous material and fragmentation of the hairs sometimes result in the formation of balls and pellets of fat and hair **(Fig. 15)**. The lining epithelium is stratified squamous and contains the cutaneous elements such as sebaceous glands, hair follicles and sometimes teeth **(Fig. 16)**. Tissues of the central nervous system, even the choroid plexus, are often present. Cartilage and gastrointestinal epithelium are not uncommon. These tissues are mainly distributed around the nodal point in one part of the cyst wall. The epithelium of its other constituents such as transitional or columnar can be found and sometimes is replaced by granulation tissue with foreign body giant cells.

Malignant change can occur in mature tissues of mature cystic teratoma. For example, there can be sarcomas arising from mesodermal contents, neuromas and gliomas from nerve tissue elements. The wall of a dermoid cyst can develop a squamous cell carcinoma and

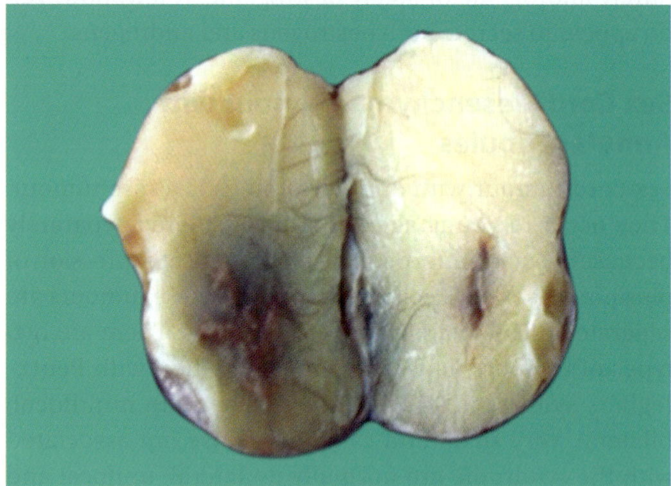

Fig. 14: Dermoid cyst cut open showing cheesy pultaceous material and hair.
Source: Dr Nikhil Kumar, Department of Pathology, IQ City Medical College (IQCMC), Durgapur, West Bengal.

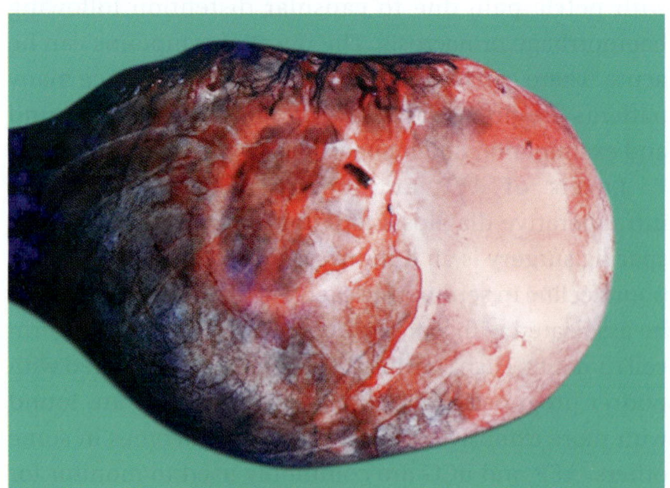

Fig. 13: Dermoid cyst of ovary.

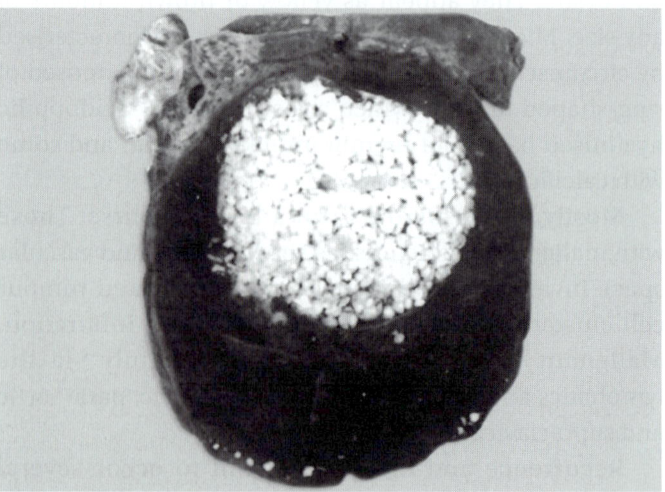

Fig. 15: Cut section of dermoid cyst showing sebaceous balls and pellets. It was a case with torsion of its pedicle.

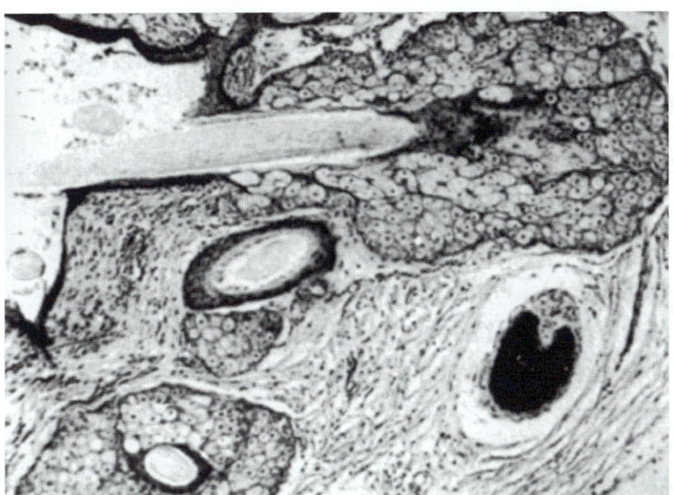

Fig. 16: The wall of a mature cystic teratoma (dermoid cyst) showing stratified squamous cell epithelial lining and hair follicles.

possibly a melanoma. The struma ovarii can become the seat of a thyroid cancer.

Immature Teratoma

The immature teratoma is usually solid and consists of a haphazard mass of rapidly dividing cells of all types without the formation of tissues. Presence of immature neuroepithelium correlates with survival and, therefore, is the basis for grading these tumours. Immature teratomas may be associated with gliomatosis peritonei, a result of induced metaplasia of pluripotent Müllerian stem cells in peritoneum. It is a highly malignant neoplasm and is seen mostly in childhood and adolescence. It spreads by the bloodstream to the lungs. There has been some success with chemotherapy.

These tumours are typically confined to the affected ovary, and, hence, routine resection biopsy of contralateral ovary is not required even when fertility sparing is not opted.

Germ Cell Tumours with Extraembryonic Differentiation

Choriocarcinoma

Choriocarcinoma is the malignancy arising from ovarian germ cells with extraembryonic differentiation into trophoblast and is a nongestational choriocarcinoma. The tumour can be of variable size and nodular. The cut section shows a variegated appearance with extensive areas of necrosis and haemorrhage. The histological features show both malignant cytotrophoblast and syncytiotrophoblast. The tumour produces hCG. The prognosis is very poor, with rapid pelvic invasion, intra-abdominal spread and extensive lymphatic and haematogenous dissemination. The nongestational choriocarcinoma responds relatively poorly to the chemotherapeutic regimen. Most of these choriocarcinomas are combined with other malignant germ cell elements resulting in a mixed tumour, a probable reason for poor response to chemotherapy.

Yolk Sac Tumour

Yolk sac tumour are also referred to as endodermal sinus tumour and represent germ cell differentiation into extraembryonic mesoblast and yolk sac endoderm. They synthesise only AFP. Endocrine disturbance is not a feature of the pure yolk sac tumour and commonly presents with nonspecific symptoms. These unilateral tumours form large, encapsulated, smooth or nodular masses of rubbery consistency. The cut surface is yellowish-grey with conspicuous areas of haemorrhage and necrosis together with small gelatinous cysts. The histological appearance is complex. The characteristic feature is the endodermal sinus or the Schiller–Duval body, a cystic space with a layer of flattened or irregular epithelium with glomerulus-like tufts having central vascular core projecting into them.

These tumours are malignant. The progress of the tumour and the development of recurrences can be monitored by serial estimations of serum AFP levels.

Embryonal Carcinoma

Embryonal carcinomas may secrete oestrogen, and the young child may have precocious puberty or if later in age with abnormal uterine bleeding. The tumours are large with about 60–70% being unilateral. These are solid soft tumours with grey-white cut surface. Areas of haemorrhage and necrosis may be present. Microscopy shows sheets of undifferentiated cells with vesicular nuclei. Syncytiotrophoblastic giant cells are frequent. These tumours synthesise both hCG and AFP.

Germ Cell Tumours without Any Differentiation

Dysgerminoma

Dysgerminoma is the most common type of the germ cell tumour. The dysgerminoma of the ovary is identical with the seminoma of the testis.

Placental alkaline phosphatase and LDH are elevated in dysgerminomas. Karyotyping of girls with malignant dysgerminomas has shown that the patients could be:

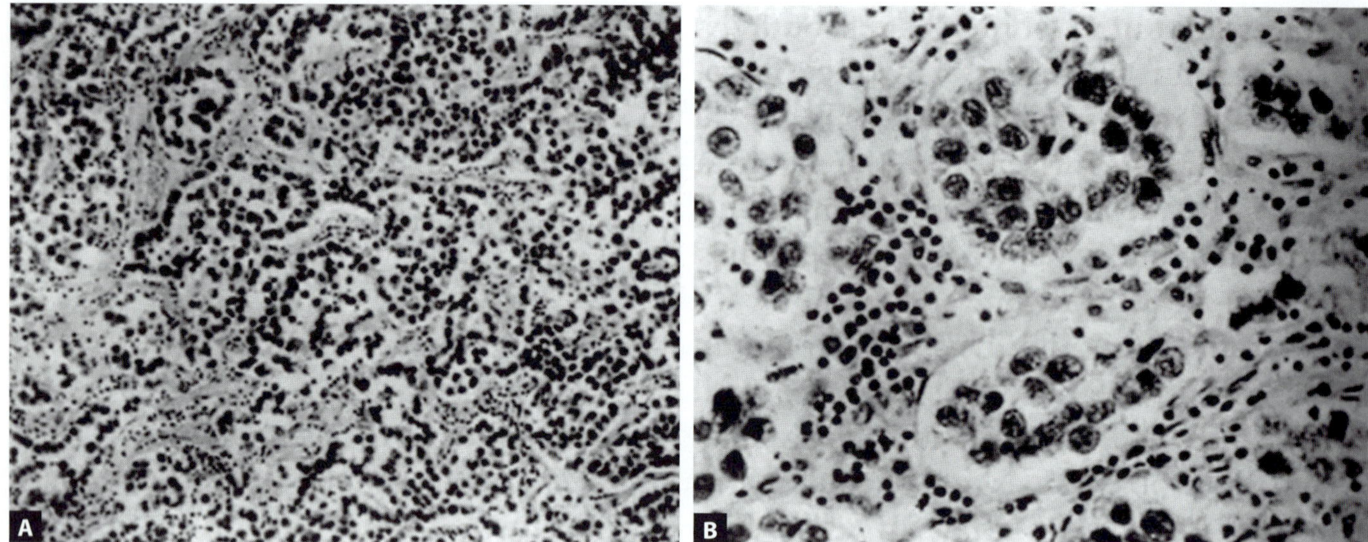

Figs. 17A and B: Photomicrographs of a dysgerminoma. (A) A low-power view showing the general appearance; (B) A higher-power view showing clusters of germ cells separated by characteristic bands of connective tissue infiltrated with lymphocytes.

(1) Pure gonadal dysgenesis with bilateral streak gonads with 46, XY, (2) mixed gonadal dysgenesis with unilateral streak gonad and contralateral testis or (3) androgen insensitivity syndrome with 46, XY testicular feminisation and, therefore, karyotyping is a necessary step in the workup of a patient.

In pure dysgerminomas, palpable or detected pelvic mass in a girl is the only presenting feature. The size of dysgerminomas varies from 5 to 15 cm in diameter. Some tumours are not pure dysgerminomas. They can be the seat of a primary choriocarcinoma that secretes hCG. Other admixtures are theca, Leydig and Sertoli cells. If these are present, the tumour could exhibit mildly oestrogenic or androgenic effects. Otherwise, the pure dysgerminoma is without any endocrine activity. Macroscopically, the tumour is solid except for any degenerative cystic change. It has the consistency of a soft fibroma, and its cut surface has a homogeneous appearance. They are bilateral in one third of the cases.

Microscopically, sections show large cells arranged in bundles or alveoli, separated by network of connective tissue infiltrated with lymphocytes **(Figs. 17A and B)**. Cells may be multinucleated. The appearances mimic those of the gonad at a very early stage of its development, and the large tumour cells resemble primitive ova.

Most dysgerminomas are malignant. The treatment is primarily surgical. If there is desire for fertility, contralateral ovary with fallopian tube and uterus can be left behind even in the presence of metastasis, since these tumours are chemosensitive. It is imperative to remove both the gonads, if karyotyping has revealed Y-element. It will be appropriate to perform hysterectomy with bilateral adnexectomy, if fertility is not to be preserved. Recurrences are known to occur. These tumours are highly radiosensitive.

Mixed Germ Cell Tumours

Mixed germ cell tumours contain two or more elements of the germ cell tumours. A significant proportion of germ cell tumours show a mixed pattern, with combinations such as dysgerminoma with endodermal sinus tumour, choriocarcinoma or immature teratoma and immature teratoma with endodermal sinus tumour. Polyembryoma is a part of mixed germ cell neoplasm characterised by embryoid bodies that resemble presomite embryos. Even syncytiotrophoblast cells are noted. AFP, hCG and sometimes human placental lactogen (HPL) are detected. Size of the primary tumour and relative size of the most malignant components are the determinants of prognosis. Primary tumour size of <10 cm and the component malignant element less than one third are associated with very good prognosis.

Monodermal Teratoma and Somatic-type Tumours Arising from Dermoid Cyst

The structures in a cystic teratoma are predominantly ectodermal. This is not always the case in more solid growths, which can contain single specialised tissue type.

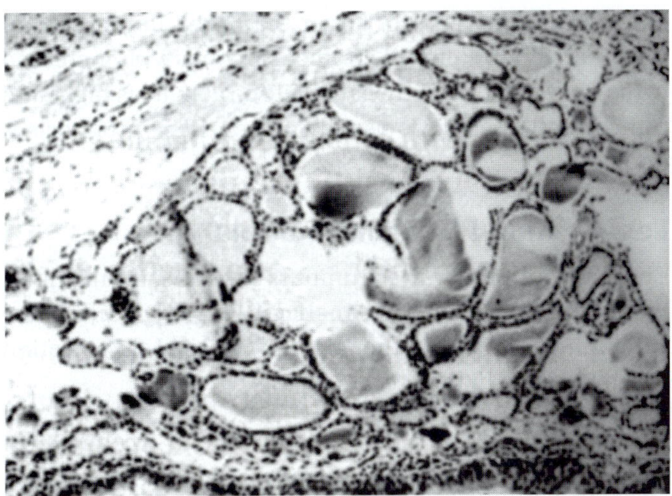

Fig. 18: Struma ovarii showing typical structure of the thyroid gland.

Struma ovarii: This is the mature cystic teratoma consisting tumour of thyroid tissue. Cut surface shows gelatinous red to green colloid. Microscopy is similar to thyroid tissue. The thyroid tissue may be functional and cause hyperthyroidism **(Fig. 18)**. The thyroid gland enlargement is occasionally seen. Malignant changes of follicular histology can occur. The treatment is similar to thyroid carcinoma.

Strumal carcinoids: These are the tumours arising from argentaffin cells of gastrointestinal or bronchial tissue present in mature cystic teratoma. These are hormonally active secreting serotonin, bradykinin and other peptides. Derivative of intestinal elements in the wall of a dermoid cyst can present as the carcinoid tumour causing the carcinoid syndrome. Strumal carcinoids are 5 cm or bigger in diameter. Frequent attacks of flushing, cyanosis and abdominal cramps in a patient with adnexal mass should alert the diagnosis. The serotonin from the tumour fails to be metabolised since ovary does not drain through liver, and the symptoms are exaggerated despite absence of metastasis.

Other examples are the tumours arising in dermoid such as lipoma, myoma, chondroma and osteoma.

Germ Cell-sex Cord-stromal Tumours

These include gonadoblastomas and mixed germ cell-sex cord-stromal tumours.

Gonadoblastoma

These arise in dysgenetic gonads of patients with Y chromosome and are rarely associated with androgen and oestrogen secretions. These are benign tumours with no metastatic potential. They could be precursors to germ cell cancers - dysgerminomas, teratomas, embryonal carcinomas or endodermal sinus tumour. Patients report with primary amenorrhoea, virilisation or developmental abnormalities of genitalia.

They are found in right gonad more often than in left and is bilateral in one third of the cases. Their size varies from being microscopic to 8–10 cm in diameter. Microscopic examination shows nests of mixture of germ cells and immature sex cord-stromal cells with hyaline bodies and calcification. The consistence varies from being soft, fleshy to firm and hard. In patients with Turner in whom there is no evidence of spread, uterus may be preserved for adopting artificial reproductive technologies when fertility is desired.

Mixed Germ Cell-Sex Cord-Stromal Tumours

Various combinations of germ cell and sex cord-stromal elements can be found in a tumour. These are mentioned with some of the individual entities in the previous paragraphs.

TREATMENT OF MALIGNANT GERM CELL TUMOURS

Most of the malignant ovarian tumours occur in young women. At the initial surgery, irrespective of the stage, if fertility is desired, fertility-preserving procedure and comprehensive staging are offered. If fertility is not a concern, patient should undergo complete staging surgery. For women who have had prior incompletely staged surgery, needs to be restaged.

No adjuvant chemotherapy is required for stage I dysgerminoma and stage I, grade I immature teratoma, whereas all other situations would require adjuvant chemotherapy. The regimen preferred is bleomycin/etoposide/cisplatin for three to four cycles at 3-weekly interval. Patients with risk require the additional cycle of adjuvant chemotherapy. If there is recurrence, high-dose chemotherapy with paclitaxel/ifosfamide/cisplatin is chosen.

Mesenchymal Tumours

Pure mesenchymal tumours of the ovary are a subset of rare ovarian tumours that are composed of mesenchymal tissue without an epithelial, germ cell or sex cord-stromal element. These tumours have an uncertain histogenesis, and the notion of a 'pure' ovarian mesenchymal tumour is disputed. These may be associated with endometriosis.

Low-grade Endometrioid Stromal Sarcoma

Most patients present with abdominal distension and/or pain, back pain, palpable mass or elevated serum CA-125 level. Tumours can be unilateral or bilateral. Tumour extension beyond the ovary at the time of exploratory laparotomy is a frequent finding. These tumours are solid, solid and cystic or, rarely, predominantly cystic. The cysts are usually filled with haemorrhagic fluid. The cut surfaces are tan or yellow-white and have a soft consistency.

Low-grade endometrioid stromal sarcoma is typically composed of sheets of small, closely packed cells resembling the stromal cells of the proliferative endometrium, with scanty cytoplasm, round to oval nuclei and small blood vessels resembling the spiral arterioles of late secretory endometrium. Secondary changes, including storiform fibrosis, a 'starburst' pattern of hyaline plaques, foamy cell change, sex cord-like differentiation and myxoid change, may occur. Focally, a few benign-appearing endometrioid glands may be present that resemble endometriotic lesion.

These tumours display a characteristic vascular pattern and lack expression of alpha-inhibin and calretinin. Approximately one third of the cases are accompanied by a similar tumour in the uterus, and most likely the ovarian involvement is metastatic.

Hysterectomy with bilateral salpingo-ovariectomy is the primary treatment of choice. Delayed recurrences may occur. Radiation, chemotherapy and progestin treatment have been used for the treatment of recurrent disease. Patients with widespread disease respond favourably to progestin treatment.

High-grade Endometroid Stromal Sarcoma

These are mesenchymal tumours with some evidence of endometrial stromal differentiation but showing high-grade cytologic atypia with brisk mitotic activity. In the high-grade regions, a resemblance to proliferative endometrial stromal cells seen in low-grade areas is lost. These tumours demonstrate only the modest endometrial stromal differentiation without marked nuclear pleomorphism.

The tumour cells are larger than the tumour cells of low-grade endometrioid stromal sarcoma with increased cytoplasm and nucleomegaly. Mitotic activity is high, and tumour cell necrosis is usually present. The prognosis is poor.

Less Common Ovarian Tumours

The less common ovarian tumours such as seromucinous, mixed epithelial and mesenchymal tumours and other carcinomas grouped in the WHO histological classification are not briefed in the present chapter.

Carcinosarcoma

Ovarian carcinosarcoma, previously known as mixed malignant Müllerian tumour, is an uncommon, highly aggressive cancer of the female genital tract. These are biphasic, comprising malignant epithelial (carcinomatous) and malignant mesenchymal (sarcomatous) populations. Since molecular studies have revealed a clonal relationship between these two malignant cell populations, they are grouped as a single entity.

Carcinomatous elements may be of any ovarian high-grade carcinoma type (high-grade serous, endometrioid, clear cell and mucinous). The sarcomatous compartment may be classified as homologous demonstrating either nonspecific appearance or differentiation native to the female genital tract or heterologous showing differentiation physiologically foreign to the adnexa. The most common heterologous sarcomatous elements are chondroid (chondrosarcoma) and rhabdoid differentiation (rhabdomyosarcoma), with other heterologous elements noted only in rare cases (angiosarcoma, osteosarcoma and liposarcomas).

The average age of onset is between 60 and 70 years. At the time of diagnosis, they are in advanced stages of III and IV. About half the patients will have ascites, pelvic and para-aortic lymph node metastasis. CA-125 will be elevated to above 75 U/mL. The treatment of newly diagnosed and relapsed ovarian carcinosarcoma follows the model of epithelial ovarian cancer. The prognosis is poor.

Metastatic (Secondary) Ovarian Tumours

The ovary is a common site for metastases because of its vascular and lymphatic connections. Approximately 5% of all malignant growths found in the ovary during life are secondary to a primary lesion elsewhere. Autopsy examination of cancer subjects reveals an even higher incidence. For example, 20–25% of women dying from cancer of the breast have secondaries in the ovaries, and 80% are bilateral.

Secondary deposits in the ovary can arise in women suffering from leukaemias or lymphoma. These are common with Hodgkin's disease and Burkitt's lymphoma. With other lymphomas, ovarian involvement is much rare and with leukaemias, it is extremely infrequent.

Although carcinoid tumours account for <2% of ovarian metastatic tumours, it is important to remove the ovaries in peri- and postmenopausal women during surgery for intestinal carcinoid.

The most common sites for the primary carcinoma are the stomach, colon, breast, uterus, fallopian tube and the opposite ovary. The breast is the most frequent. In the case of a primary ovarian tumour, there is some dispute as to whether the contralateral tumour is metastatic or it is another primary focus. Ovarian metastases can be found several years after apparent cure of breast carcinoma. Sometimes the primary growth in the alimentary tract could escape recognition, while ovarian mass is the presentation.

Although the ovary can be involved by direct extension of growth from adjacent organs, cancer cells ordinarily travel to it by way of blood vessels or lymphatics as emboli or by permeation. Transcoelomic and retrograde spread is also possible. From the body of the uterus, cancer cells may travel along the lumina of the tubes to spill on the ovaries, but a lymph or bloodstream spread is the more likely mechanism.

Metastatic cancers are nearly always bilateral **(Fig. 19)**. They are often larger than the primary lesion. Their surface is usually smooth, lobulated and free from adhesions. They are essentially solid with a waxy consistency **(Fig. 20)** and may contain degenerative cystic spaces. Microscopically, they show islands of malignant cells and morphologically similar to those in the primary growth and scattered throughout the ovary as multiple foci.

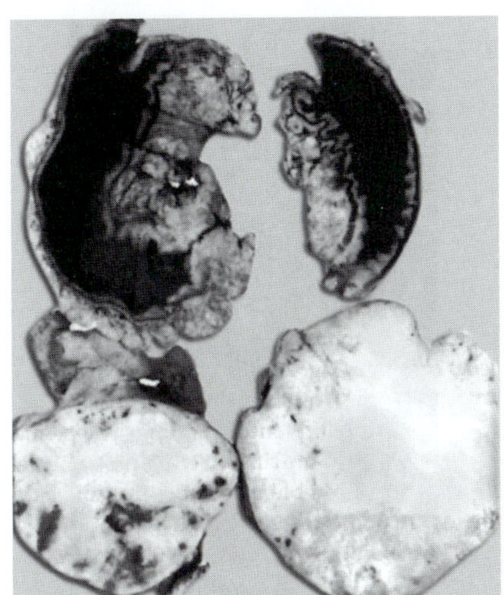

Fig. 19: Carcinoma of the colon with metastases in both ovaries.

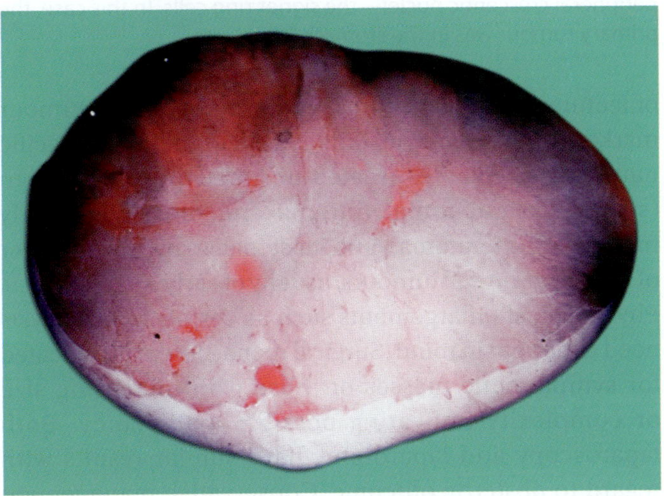

Fig. 20: Secondary ovarian tumour (Krukenberg tumour) with waxy consistence, smooth and no surface adhesions.

Krukenberg Tumour

Krukenberg tumour accounts for 30–40% of metastatic cancers. The histological features are characteristic. It consists of clumps and cords of epithelial cells in a proliferating stroma. The epithelial cells secrete mucin that mostly remains within their cytoplasm to give them a bloated appearance and an eccentric nucleus, signet ring cells **(Fig. 21)**. The mucin sometimes escapes into the stroma. The primary growth is always in mucin-secreting tissue, usually the stomach or colon but sometimes the gallbladder or breast. In some cases, a primary tumour is not found. Rarely, it may be in the cervix or bladder.

Treatment is directed to the primary tumour. It is better to remove the ovarian masses to reduce the tumour burden.

Ovarian Tumours and Pregnancy

Ovarian tumours in pregnancy pose a diagnostic and management challenge. While most masses are benign and resolve spontaneously, there are others that persist and indicate the need for surgical management. Ultrasound not only detects asymptomatic masses but also helps to guide their management based on presence or absence

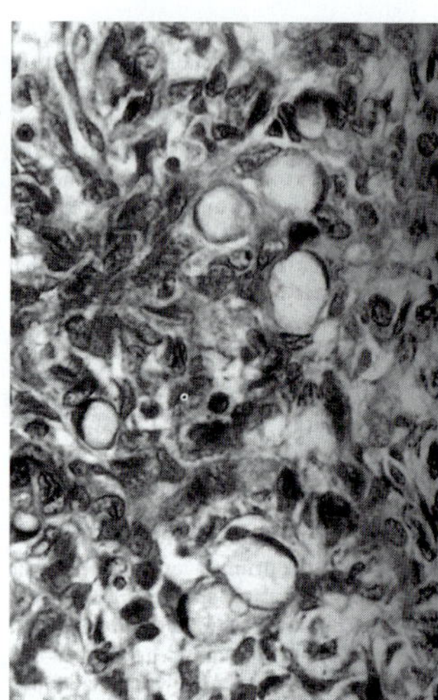

Fig. 21: Photomicrograph (750×) of ovarian Krukenberg tumour showing several large cells with clear, vacuolated cytoplasm and peripheral crescentic nuclei—the signet ring cells. In this case, the primary tumour was in the stomach.

of features suspicious of malignancy. The role of tumour markers in pregnancy is limited due to their nonspecific nature. Most masses treated in pregnancy are benign (serous cystadenoma, fibroma and most commonly mature cystic teratoma), and most malignancies are either of LMP or germ cell tumours, usually of early-stage disease. Physiological enlargements such as corpus luteum cysts need to be kept in mind. Surgical management is indicated for symptomatic masses or those with increasing size or complexity indicating possible malignancy. Both laparoscopy and laparotomy have similar results with regard to obstetric outcome. Conservative management is preferred in the remainder. MRI may help in better characterisation of doubtful masses. The advent of ultrasound and its use in obstetric care for assessing foetal viability in early pregnancy and later for assessing foetal growth or checking for anomalies has resulted in increased detection of ovarian masses.

The corpus luteum cyst disappears by the 12–16th weeks of pregnancy. Tumour detection does not interfere with either pregnancy or labour. Common complications with the tumour are torsion, impaction and rupture of the ovarian tumour.

Masses persisting after the first trimester or found during the second trimester require removal: (1) To prevent torsion or rupture during pregnancy, (2) to prevent possible obstruction during labour and (3) to exclude malignancy. However, the risk of ovarian malignancy is rare in pregnancy.

Torsion of the pedicle of the tumour occur around 12–14 weeks of pregnancy and in the puerperium. After 12 weeks of pregnancy, uterus rises into abdomen and takes ovary along. This provides more space for ovary, and the bowel movements and jerks can propel ovarian pedicle to undergo axial torsion. After 16–20 weeks of pregnancy, further growth of uterus will restrict space for movement of the ovary. Immediate postpartum, the sudden reduction in size of uterus, enacts similar situation as in early second trimester.

Impaction of the tumour in the pelvis posterior to uterus may result in retention of urine during pregnancy and may cause obstruction of labour. Presence of large tumour may result in malpresentation of the foetus.

Rupture of the cyst can occur at any time during pregnancy or labour. The tumour may be malignant or may become malignant during pregnancy.

The conditions most likely to be confused with an ovarian tumour during pregnancy are paraovarian cyst, uterine leiomyomas, the nonpregnant horn of a bicornuate uterus, pelvic kidney, retroperitoneal tumour, ectopic pregnancy and a retroverted gravid uterus.

If the patient is examined in the Trendelenburg position, all these conditions remain in the pelvis, whereas an ovarian tumour tends to ride out and feels separate from the uterus in most of the cases.

Size of tumour, suspicion of malignancy, duration of pregnancy, period of pregnancy when diagnosed and presence of complications determine the planning of intervention.

- *Tumour size <10 cm in diameter and not solid:* If the cyst appears benign on ultrasound, it is generally treated conservatively. If the cyst persists past puerperium, surgery may be considered.
- *Tumour found in the first trimester of pregnancy:* If the tumour is persisting or found, intervene around 14–16 weeks of pregnancy. By this time, the placenta would have taken over its function. Corpus luteum cysts will more often disappear by second trimester. Ovarian cystectomy or ovariectomy can be considered.
- *Tumour found in third trimester of pregnancy:* An ovarian tumour can be removed easily and safely until the 28–30 weeks of pregnancy. Thereafter, manipulation to remove the tumour might become difficult and may precipitate preterm labour. Such patients are managed conservatively until delivery, and tumour is removed during the postpartum period. If found obstructing labour or at caesarean delivery, tumour is removed after extraction of the baby.

- *Axial torsion of the tumour* or rupture of the cyst with haemorrhage should receive immediate attention irrespective of the duration of pregnancy.
- *Tumour with evidence of malignancy:* Diagnosed in first and second trimesters of pregnancy are operated with or without termination of pregnancy. Women diagnosed in their third trimester of pregnancy can be offered option for delaying the treatment of ovarian tumour until 34 weeks of pregnancy and delivery.

SUGGESTED READING

1. Gibbs RS, Karlan BY, Haney AF, Nygaard IE. Danforth's Obstetrics and Gynecology, 10th edition. Philadelphia: Lippincott Williams & Wilkins; 2008.
2. Berek JS, Berek DL. Berek & Novak's Gynecology, 16th edition. Philadelphia: Lippincott Williams & Wilkins; 2019.
3. Coppleson M. Gynecologic Oncology: Fundamental Principles & Clinical Practice, 1st edition. Edinburgh: Churchill Livingstone; 1981.

36

CHAPTER

Chemotherapy in Gynaecological Malignancies

Sourjya Banerjee, Pratik Kumar Chatterjee

Chapter Outline

- Chemotherapy and the Cell Cycle
- Therapeutic Agents used in the Treatment of Gynaecological Cancer
- Chemotherapy Toxicity
- Systemic Therapy in Gynaecological Malignancies
- Assessment of Response to Chemotherapy

INTRODUCTION

In gynaecological malignancies, systemic therapy, when employed, is primarily administered in the adjuvant setting to eradicate micrometastatic disease; concurrently when indicated along with external beam radiotherapy (EBRT); in the neoadjuvant setting in advanced epithelial ovarian cancer (EOC) if upfront surgery is predicted to result in sub-optimal debulking; or with palliative intent in the event of unresectable recurrence or metastatic disease. The only gynaecological malignancy with high cure rates with chemotherapy is choriocarcinoma, wherein complete disease eradication is frequently achieved even in the metastatic setting. To a lesser extent, germ cell tumours, particularly dysgerminoma, are also significantly chemosensitive.

CHEMOTHERAPY AND THE CELL CYCLE

In most solid tumours, the doubling time of cancer cells is significantly longer than the corresponding normal cells. Actively proliferating cells are most vulnerable to cytotoxic chemotherapy, whereas the growth fraction in most solid malignancies, including the gynaecological ones, is only about 20%.

The effects of cancer chemotherapy on tumour cell populations demonstrate first-order kinetics, i.e. chemotherapy follows an exponential (log-kill) model. Chemotherapy may be said to have a specific exponential, or log-kill, potential. For example, a log kill of two reduces a theoretical human tumour burden of 10^9 cells to 10^7 cells. Although this represents a reduction of 99%, at least 10 million (10^7) viable cells remain. A log kill of three achieves a reduction of 99.9%, but 1 million (10^6) cells remain. Theoretically, therefore, such fractional reductions by antineoplastic agents can never reduce a tumour cell population to zero. This fact prevents the complete eradication of malignant diseases by systemic therapy alone.

Cisplatin, carboplatin and the alkylating agents are lethal throughout the cell cycle but are particularly active in G2 and at the G1/S boundary. Antimetabolites such as 5-fluorouracil (FU) and methotrexate are most active against cells in the S phase. Etoposide, vinca alkaloids and taxanes are most effective against cells in the G2/M phases of the cell cycle.

Therapy must also take into account the length of time a therapeutic concentration of the drug is maintained. The maximal effectiveness of some oncolytic drugs depends mainly on peak tissue concentration, whereas that of others depends on the duration of exposure.

A therapeutic concentration of phase-specific drugs is best maintained by prolonged exposure, e.g. antimetabolites such as methotrexate and 5-FU. In contrast, the cell cycle phase-nonspecific drugs are best administered as an intravenous bolus of the highest tolerable dose, and the dose is repeated when normal target tissues have recovered. Since tumours are composed of numerous cell clones that vary in their sensitivity to drugs, the use of multiple agents should lessen the chance of the development of resistance and repopulation of the tumour by a resistant cell clone. Drugs with different dose-limiting toxicities and different modes of action may increase the fractional cell kill without a parallel rise in damage to normal tissues. Indeed, combination chemotherapy has proved superior to single-agent therapy in most gynaecological cancers.

THERAPEUTIC AGENTS USED IN THE TREATMENT OF GYNAECOLOGICAL CANCER

Alkylating Agents

Deoxyribonucleic acid (DNA) replication is inhibited by this group of drugs by the drug-forming covalent bonds with DNA bases. Some are bifunctional and react with two strands of DNA to produce cross-linkage. Cyclophosphamide and ifosfamide have activity against gestational trophoblastic neoplasm (GTN) and certain subtypes of ovarian malignancy. However, both these drugs produce a metabolite called acrolein, which can lead to haemorrhagic cystitis.

Platinum Agents

These drugs are probably the most important chemotherapeutic agents in the treatment of gynaecological cancer at present. Platinum compounds form DNA cross-links by an action similar to the bifunctional alkylating agents. Cisplatin is the most active agent in this class and is used in the treatment of cervical cancer in conjunction with radiotherapy. Its major adverse effects include nephrotoxicity, ototoxicity, dyselectrolytemia and severe vomiting. Carboplatin has a milder adverse effect profile in terms of the above and is therefore better tolerated; it, however, results in greater bone marrow suppression than cisplatin. Oxaliplatin is used in mucinous carcinoma of the ovary in conjunction with an oral prodrug of 5-FU known as capecitabine.

Antimetabolites

Methotrexate is an antifolate, and its major biochemical action is to block the enzyme dihydrofolate reductase. The toxicity of methotrexate can be inhibited by the timely administration of leucovorin, also known as folinic acid. Methotrexate is very useful in gestational trophoblastic tumours. 5-FU acts against the enzyme thymidylate synthetase and can be incorporated into ribonucleic acid (RNA) and DNA, directly leading to inhibition of nucleic acid production. Its prodrug, capecitabine, is used along with oxaliplatin in mucinous carcinoma of the ovary.

Antitumour Antibiotics

The most important members of this drug class in gynaecological malignancies are anthracyclines, doxorubicin (and its pegylated liposomal form), dactinomycin and bleomycin. Anthracyclines inhibit DNA synthesis through a complex series of actions. Doxorubicin is used in the treatment of uterine sarcomas and is also effective against ovarian cancer. Dactinomycin is used in GTN. Bleomycin can produce strand breaks in both the DNA of the nucleus and the mitochondria and is most commonly used in the treatment of germ-cell tumours.

Taxanes

Taxanes act against microtubules to induce a sustained block in mitosis. Two of the most common drugs in this class are paclitaxel and docetaxel. The former causes significant peripheral neuropathy; the latter exhibits myelotoxicity. This class, especially paclitaxel, is used in all gynaecological malignancies under various settings such as neoadjuvant, adjuvant or palliative.

Antiangiogenics

Angiogenesis is a significant hallmark of cancer and is a major driving force in EOC. Bevacizumab, a humanised monoclonal antibody against the vascular endothelial growth factor, has shown significant improvement in progression-free survival when used along with carboplatin-paclitaxel and subsequently as a monotherapy maintenance or in conjunction with poly [adenosine diphosphate (ADP)-ribose] polymerase (PARP) inhibitors in certain subtypes of epithelial ovarian malignancy.

PARP Inhibitors

Olaparib and niraparib interfere in the base excision repair process of single-stranded DNA and subsequently in the repair of double-stranded DNA, especially in the setting of BRCA mutations, which are a driving force behind several types of epithelial ovarian malignancies.

Immunotherapy

The immune pathway most commonly targeted in gynaecological malignancies is the interaction between Programmed Death 1 (PD-1) receptors present on T lymphocytes and Programmed Death Ligand-1 (PDL-1), a transmembrane protein expressed by various tumour cells. In simple terms, when PDL-1 binds to the PD-1 receptor, it prevents the immune-mediated destruction of cancer cells. Averting this interaction by monoclonal antibodies against PD-1 (e.g. pembrolizumab) therefore unleashes the immune system against the malignant cells and brings about their demise. Less commonly, anti-PDL-1 antibodies such as avelumab are effective in certain circumstances.

CHEMOTHERAPY TOXICITY

Bone Marrow Suppression

Many chemotherapeutic agents affect the rapidly dividing cells in the bone marrow, leading to temporary bone marrow suppression. The lowest white cell and platelet counts (Nadir values) are usually seen 10 days after treatment. Cisplatin is considerably less myelosuppressive than carboplatin. The vinca alkaloids and bleomycin are particularly nonmyelosuppressive.

Nausea and Vomiting

Cisplatin, doxorubicin and ifosfamide are amongst the most emetogenic drugs used in gynaecological malignancies.

Alopecia

Temporary hair loss is a side effect of cyclophosphamide, doxorubicin, etoposide and taxanes. Carboplatin and cisplatin chemotherapy are not usually associated with hair loss.

Renal Toxicity

Both methotrexate and cisplatin can cause severe damage to the renal tubules. Renal damage can be largely prevented during cisplatin administration by adequate pre- and postchemotherapy hydration with saline. A small number of patients treated with cisplatin develop hypomagnesemia. Carboplatin is considerably less nephrotoxic compared to cisplatin.

Cardiotoxicity

Doxorubicin can cause cardiomyopathy, leading to conduction problems in the heart and congestive cardiac failure. This is not usually seen until the cumulative dose of doxorubicin approaches 450–550 mg/m^2. The doxorubicin analogue, epirubicin, is less cardiotoxic.

Second Malignancies

Etoposide predisposes patients to acute myeloid leukaemia; PARP inhibitors result in myelodysplastic syndrome in 1–2% of patients.

Immunotherapy-associated Toxicities

This includes immune-mediated endocrinopathies, pneumonitis, pericarditis, hepatitis, nephritis and potentially fatal immune-mediated colitis.

SYSTEMIC THERAPY IN GYNAECOLOGICAL MALIGNANCIES

Endometrial Cancers

Endometrial Carcinoma

In those patients in whom adjuvant EBRT is indicated, even in the early stage [e.g. stage IB grade 2 if the age is ≥60 years and/or if lymphovascular space invasion (LVSI) is present; stage IB, grade 3, and all grades of stage II disease], concurrent cisplatin at a dose of 50 mg/m^2 body surface area should be administered once weekly in the first and fourth week of EBRT. This should be followed by four cycles of adjuvant chemotherapy with a combination of carboplatin, area under the curve (AUC) 5 and paclitaxel, 175 mg/m^2, at three weekly intervals as per the evidence observed from the PORTEC-3 trial.

In stage IA grade 3 disease, while EBRT is indicated (albeit with a lower level of evidence) if the age is ≥70 years or LVSI is present, concurrent and adjuvant chemotherapy may be omitted in the elderly age group.

In stages III and IV, systemic therapy takes precedence over radiotherapy.

Six cycles of carboplatin-paclitaxel form the backbone of systemic therapy for all histological subtypes of endometrial carcinoma when indicated. The addition of pembrolizumab to this combination significantly improves progression-free survival in this subset, irrespective of deficient or proficient mismatch repair status. However, pembrolizumab is not approved in carcinosarcoma, which is the high-risk variant of adenocarcinoma that represents a stable disruption of epithelial-to-mesenchymal transition. Dostarlimab (a monoclonal antibody against PD-1) or durvalumab (a monoclonal antibody against PDL-1) can also be used along with carboplatin-paclitaxel. Dostarlimab is used in stage IIIC1, carcinosarcoma, clear cell or mixed histology. Durvalumab is currently approved only in the deficient mismatch repair subset of patients. Her-2-positive serous carcinoma or carcinosarcoma is eligible for trastuzumab along with carboplatin-paclitaxel. All these drugs can be used as maintenance after 6–8 cycles of the carboplatin-paclitaxel combination.

In recurrent or metastatic settings, bevacizumab can be added to the carboplatin-paclitaxel backbone. Lenvatinib (a small molecule multikinase inhibitor with significant activity against vascular endothelial growth factor) can be added to pembrolizumab in proficient mismatch repair tumours. Her2 2+ or 3+ tumours that progress on trastuzumab may benefit from Fam-trastuzumab deruxtecan nxki. Ifosfamide combined with paclitaxel shows benefit in terms of progression-free survival in carcinosarcoma.

Low-grade endometrioid histologies with a low tumour burden significantly benefit from hormonal therapy. Megestrol acetate alternating with tamoxifen is the preferred regimen. Oestrogen receptor (ER)-positive tumours may benefit from letrozole combined with cyclin-dependent kinase 4 and 6 inhibitors such as ribociclib or abemaciclib.

Uterine Sarcoma

Gynaecologic mesenchymal malignancies warrant molecular profiling for accurate classification. In metastatic settings, neurotrophic tyrosine receptor kinase (NTRK) gene, microsatellite instability (MSI) and tumour mutation burden (TMB) should be assessed as a bare minimum.

Low-grade endometrial stromal sarcoma (ESS) or adenosarcoma without sarcomatous overgrowth benefit from anti-oestrogenic hormonal therapy in stages II, III, IVA and IVB. Aromatase inhibitors are preferred in this setting. Radiation has lower evidence of benefit in this subset of patients. In adenosarcoma with sarcomatous overgrowth, systemic therapy is recommended for patients with residual measurable disease or those who present in stage IVB.

In high-grade ESS, undifferentiated uterine sarcoma (UUS) and leiomyosarcoma, additional postoperative systemic therapy should be considered from stage II to IVA and also in stage IVB, the latter being palliative in intent. Observation is a valid option for stages II and III if an R0 resection has been achieved.

The optimal regimen remains a matter of investigation; however, a combination of doxorubicin with trabectedin followed by maintenance trabectedin is the preferred first-line regimen in metastatic leiomyosarcoma, demonstrating an overall survival benefit at the cost of significant toxicity. Another option is a combination of adjuvant gemcitabine with docetaxel. Other choices include doxorubicin, either alone or in combination with ifosfamide or dacarbazine.

Neurotrophic tyrosine receptor kinase fusion-positive tumours benefit from Larotrectinib and Entrectinib. Anaplastic lymphoma kinase (ALK) translocated tumours benefit from crizotinib and ceritinib. Tumour mutation burden-high (TMB-H) tumours benefit from pembrolizumab, and BRCA-altered leiomyosarcomas benefit from PARP inhibitors such as Olaparib.

In the second-line setting, sequential single agents not used in the first line are better tolerated. Trabectedin is preferred in prior anthracycline-exposed patients if not administered earlier. Other agents include liposomal doxorubicin, epirubicin and pazopanib.

Gestational Trophoblastic Neoplasia

These include benign pathologies (hydatidiform mole and partial mole), low-grade malignancy (invasive mole), intermediate-grade lesions [placental site trophoblastic tumour (PSTT) and epithelioid trophoblastic tumour (ETT)] and high-grade choriocarcinoma.

In patients with complete or partial hydatidiform mole, after suction dilation and curettage, human chorionic gonadotrophin (hCG) levels are assessed every 1–2 weeks while the patient is kept on oral contraceptives. If the levels are normal for three consecutive assays, the frequency of assessment can be increased to once in 3 months. However, if the levels plateau for four consecutive values over 3 weeks (i.e. fall by <10%) or rise for three values over 2 weeks, a pelvic Doppler should be performed to confirm the absence of pregnancy and characterise the tumour. A contrast-enhanced computed tomography (CT) scan of the thorax, abdomen and pelvis should also be performed to arrive at the International Federation of Gynaecology and Obstetrics (FIGO) stage and prognostic score as shown in **Tables 1 and 2**.

In the absence of extrauterine disease, repeat dilation and curettage may suffice if the prognostic score is ≤4.

TABLE 1: FIGO staging system for gestational trophoblastic neoplasia.

Stage	*Criteria*
I	Tumour confined to uterus
II	Tumour extends to other genital structures (ovary, tube, vagina and broad ligaments) by metastasis or direct extension
III	Lung metastasis
IV	All other distant metastases

(FIGO: International Federation of Gynaecology and Obstetrics)

TABLE 2: Prognostic scoring index for gestational trophoblastic neoplasia.

Prognostic factor	*Risk score*			
	0	*1*	*2*	*4*
Age (years)	<40	≥40	–	–
Antecedent pregnancy	Hydatidiform mole	Abortion	Term pregnancy	–
Interval from index pregnancy (months)	<4	4–6	7–12	>12
Pretreatment hCG (IU/L)	$<10^3$	10^3 to $<10^4$	10^4 to 10^5	$\geq 10^5$
Largest tumour size, including uterus (cm)	<3	3–5	>5	–
Site of metastases	Lung	Spleen, kidney	Gastrointestinal tract	Brain, liver
Number of metastases identified	0	1–4	5–8	>8
Previous failed chemotherapy	–	–	Single drug	Two or more drugs

Note: The total score for a patient is obtained by adding the individual scores for each prognostic factor.
(hCG: human chorionic gonadotrophin)

These patients may alternatively be treated with single-agent antineoplastics as for low-risk GTN (<7 prognostic score) with extrauterine disease as below.

- Methotrexate 1 mg/kg intramuscular injections on days 1, 3, 5 and 7

  Alternating with

- Leucovorin 15 mg orally on days 2, 4, 6 and 8 (30 hours after each administration of methotrexate)

The cycle is repeated once every 14 days.

The other alternative is a fixed dose of dactinomycin 0.5 mg intravenous (IV) daily for 5 days, repeating every 14 days. This is used for patients with effusions, as methotrexate tends to accumulate in the third space, leading to an increase in its plasma half-life and resultant toxicity. During this treatment, hCG assays must be checked at the beginning of each cycle. If the hCG normalises, the regimen should be continued for three more cycles past the point of normalisation. Thereafter, hCG should be tested every month for 12 months. During this, the patient should also be kept on oral contraceptives.

If, after an initial good response, the hCG falls by <10% for three cycles, but the value remains <1,000 IU/mL, the patient should undergo hysterectomy with salpingectomy, and the single agent should be replaced with the one that was not used earlier. The patient should be followed up as before with hCG assays. If at this point the hCG changes by <10% for two cycles or rises by >10% after one cycle, the patient should be evaluated for metastasis and switched to etoposide, methotrexate, actinomycin D, cyclophosphamide and vincristine (EMA-CO). The switch to EMA-CO should also be done in case of poor response to initial therapy, i.e. hCG rises by >10% for two cycles of initial treatment for low-risk disease or rapidly rises to ≥1,000 IU/mL after an initial good response. In the event of histopathologically proven choriocarcinoma or high-risk GTN with a prognostic score ≥7 or stage IV at presentation, treatment proceeds directly with EMA-CO, with hCG monitoring prior to each cycle. The chemo regimen is as shown below.

- Etoposide 100 mg/m^2/day IV on day 1 and 2
- Dactinomycin 0.5 mg IV push on day 1 and 2
- Methotrexate 300 mg/m^2 IV over 12 hours on day 1 after adequate alkalinisation of urine
- Leucovorin 15 mg orally × 4 days once every 12 hours, beginning 24 hours after the start of methotrexate infusion.

Day 8:
- Cyclophosphamide 600 mg/m^2 IV
- Vincristine 0.8 mg/m^2 IV over 10 minutes (maximum dose not to exceed 2 mg)

The regimen is repeated once every 2 weeks till hCG is normalised and then for an additional 6–8 weeks. Thereafter, the patient is followed up with monthly hCG levels for 12 months.

In case of initial good response followed by an hCG plateau, or poor response to treatment, or relapse after remission (the criteria for these events being the same as those mentioned in low-risk GTN), the regimen is changed to etoposide, methotrexate, actinomycin-D, etoposide

and cisplatin (EMA-EP), which is similar to EMA-CO with the following differences:
Etoposide and dactinomycin are administered on day 1 alone.

Day 8 chemo consists of etoposide 100 mg/m^2 and cisplatin 75 mg/m^2.

For those who present with upfront brain metastasis, the methotrexate in EMA-CO is increased to 1,000 mg/m^2 over 24 hours instead of 12 hours. Leucovorin, 15 mg orally, is also given for 12 doses, with a frequency of once every 6 hours. This is initiated 32 hours after the start of methotrexate infusion. Alternatively, stereotactic radiation or whole-brain radiation may be used.

All patients treated with EMA-CO or EMA-EP should be considered for prophylactic granulocyte colony-stimulating factor to prevent potentially fatal neutropenia.

For patients who present with a prognostic score >12, treatment is started with a regimen of etoposide 100 mg/m^2 and cisplatin 20 mg/m^2 on day 1 and day 2, once every week for 1–3 courses prior to switching to EMA-CO. This is to reduce the likelihood of a very rapid tumour shrinkage, which may be associated with catastrophic tumour bleed.

For intermediate trophoblastic tumour (i.e. PSTT and ETT): In the non-metastatic setting, the patient can be kept on follow-up with hCG assays after surgery if the interval from index pregnancy is <2 years, the tumour showed superficial invasion without necrosis, and it had a mitotic count of ≤5/10 high-power fields (HPFs). All other non-metastatic patients and all metastatic cases should be treated with EMA-CO; platinum-based regimens are preferred for the metastatic setting.

Epithelial Ovarian Cancer, Fallopian Tube Cancer and Primary Peritoneal Carcinoma

These malignancies are grouped together because of common origin, common natural history and treatment. Further discussion shall proceed under the heading of EOC. Surgical staging with optimal cytoreduction remains the goal and bedrock of treatment. Surgical principles are outside the scope of this chapter.

Early Stage (Stage I and II) Epithelial Ovarian Cancer

For completely staged stage IA or 1B grade 1 disease, adjuvant systemic therapy can be omitted. Adjuvant chemotherapy is recommended in stage 1A and 1B grade 2 disease, but the level of evidence is low.

All patients with grade 3-early stage EOC, carcinosarcoma, clear cell histology and all completely staged patients with stage 1C and stage II disease should receive adjuvant chemotherapy.

A combination of carboplatin, AUC 5 to 6 and paclitaxel 175 mg/m^2 is administered once every 3 weeks for a total of six cycles for stage I patients in whom adjuvant chemotherapy is indicated. For patients who are intolerant to taxanes, pegylated liposomal doxorubicin can be used as a substitution. Those with mucinous carcinoma can alternatively receive a combination of capecitabine and oxaliplatin. Those with low-grade serous or endometrioid histology requiring adjuvant systemic therapy may derive benefit from the addition of letrozole to the carboplatin-paclitaxel backbone.

All stage II EOC may derive a benefit in their progression-free survival by the addition of bevacizumab to the chemotherapy backbone and continuing bevacizumab for an additional 12 cycles thereafter. BRCA-mutated patients benefit from the addition of PARP inhibitor olaparib to bevacizumab. Olaparib can be continued for a total of 2 years in the absence of disease progression. Another PARP inhibitor, niraparib, is approved as maintenance for up to 3 years irrespective of BRCA mutation if the patient has responded to platinum-based chemotherapy.

All incompletely staged patients, such as those who underwent surgery for ovarian torsion and other presumed benign conditions and were then diagnosed to have EOC by histopathology, should undergo complete surgical staging. However, this may be omitted in grade 3 or clear cell tumours, where all patients are required to receive adjuvant chemotherapy irrespective of the restaging procedure outcome.

If the restaging procedure is not possible for any reason, ALL incompletely staged patients should receive adjuvant chemotherapy. The same principles as mentioned above hold good. The dose of carboplatin may be increased to an AUC of 7.5 if the three weekly regimen is chosen.

Stage III and IV Epithelial Ovarian Cancer

Optimal cytoreduction remains the goal of therapy, followed by adjuvant systemic therapy. However, for those in whom optimal cytoreduction, i.e. achieving a residual disease of <1 cm, is anticipated to be unachievable, neoadjuvant chemotherapy (NACT) is administered.

Such situations include metastatic deposits or nodes at the porta hepatis, presence of hepatic parenchymal or lung metastasis at presentation, and those who have massive ascites or extensive malignant deposits over the bowels or the peritoneal surfaces and mesentery (Stage III C1 and III C2).

Principles of adjuvant therapy are the same as for early-stage EOC; however, a dose-dense regimen with carboplatin AUC 5 to 6 on day 1 and paclitaxel 80 mg/m^2 on day 1, day 8 and day 15 once every 3 weeks, repeated for a total of six cycles, may provide greater benefit in those who underwent upfront surgery but have a residual disease >1 cm. This regimen is significantly more toxic than the conventional three-weekly regimen and therefore, in medically frail patients, a modified regimen may be given in the form of weekly carboplatin AUC 2 and paclitaxel 60 mg/m^2 for a total of 18 weeks. The results of this combination are a similar progression-free survival and an equal probability of survival at 24 months compared to the standard three-weekly regimen.

Combined intraperitoneal and intravenous regimen is an option in optimally debulked patients, but its role in the era of bevacizumab and PARP inhibitors is unclear. For all suboptimally debulked patients, IV chemotherapy alone is preferred over a combination of intravenous and intraperitoneal regimens.

For those in whom NACT is indicated, the standard regimen is three cycles of carboplatin, AUC 5 to 6, combined with paclitaxel 175 mg/m^2 at three weekly intervals. Bevacizumab can be added to this regimen in those who present with pleural effusion or ascites. Post-NACT, heated intraperitoneal chemotherapy (HIPEC) is suggested at the time of surgery when optimal debulking is achieved. Commonly, 100 mg/m^2 of cisplatin at 40°C over 90 minutes is used.

Management of recurrent disease depends on the platinum-free interval (PFI), i.e. the duration between completion of platinum-based therapy and detection of relapse. If relapse is only identified based on rising cancer antigen 125 (CA-125) without gross disease on imaging, such patients can be kept on oral tamoxifen 20 mg twice daily till the time of progression. If the PFI is >6 months, combined modality therapy is used where carboplatin is used along with paclitaxel as before or with gemcitabine or pegylated liposomal doxorubicin for six cycles with or without Bevacizumab. Bevacizumab, if used, should be continued beyond the chemotherapy cycles as maintenance therapy till further progression or unacceptable toxicity. In platinum-resistant disease, where PFI is <6 months, or platinum-refractory disease, which progresses while on a platinum-based chemotherapy regimen, sequential single-agent drugs such as pegylated liposomal doxorubicin, gemcitabine, and topotecan are used, but the progression-free interval between agents continues to decrease sequentially, and the overall prognosis is dismal.

Malignant Germ Cell Tumours and Malignant Sex-cord Stromal Tumours

Following surgery, patients with stage I dysgerminoma or stage I grade 1 immature teratoma may be kept on regular follow-up with imaging and serum tumour marker assays. Patients with all other stages and grades of these two pathologies and all stages of embryonal tumour, endodermal sinus tumour and non-gestational choriocarcinoma should receive four cycles of bleomycin, etoposide and platinum (BEP) as the standard regimen after pulmonary function has been found to be adequate. This is especially important for patients with poor-risk disease, such as those with logarithmic elevation of beta hCG, and those with liver and brain metastasis. While three cycles may be administered to patients with lower risk or stage I disease who require chemotherapy, the level of evidence for this approach is low. The chemotherapy regimen is as follows:

- Bleomycin 30 units IV on days 1, 8 and 15
- Etoposide 100 mg/m^2 IV daily on days 1–5
- Cisplatin 20 mg/m^2 IV daily on days 1–5

The cycle is repeated every 3 weeks, chemotherapy should not be delayed, nor the doses modified in the event of neutropenia.

Recurrent disease can be potentially cured by high-dose chemotherapy followed by stem cell rescue. A combination of paclitaxel, ifosfamide and cisplatin may alternatively be used.

Among patients with malignant sex-cord stromal tumours, those with low-risk stage I disease may be kept on follow-up after surgery. All others should receive a combination of paclitaxel and carboplatin at the same dosage as used in EOC. A combination of cisplatin and etoposide is used in the recurrent setting. Other alternatives are hormonal agents such as tamoxifen and letrozole. Leuprolide or Goserelin may be beneficial in granulosa cell tumour.

Cervix, Vulva and Vagina

All patients who receive definitive or adjuvant radiotherapy in these diseases should also receive cisplatin concurrently at a dose of 40 mg/m^2 once a week during the course of external beam radiation; chemotherapy should never be administered concurrently with brachytherapy. However, this may be omitted in cervical carcinoma of stage 1A. Locally advanced cervical carcinoma patients may derive additional benefit by administering pembrolizumab in addition to the above-mentioned regimen.

The combination of carboplatin and paclitaxel forms a backbone in recurrent and metastatic settings. Erlotinib and gemcitabine are useful as second-line agents. In these settings, pembrolizumab is beneficial in TMB-H, PDL-1-positive and deficient DNA mismatch repair (dMMR) tumours.

ASSESSMENT OF RESPONSE TO CHEMOTHERAPY

In order to cure any patient with chemotherapy, there needs to be a complete response to treatment. This is seen as disappearance of all measurable or evaluable disease, signs, symptoms and biochemical changes related to the tumour for at least 4 weeks. Partial response is taken when there is a reduction of >50% of the original mass in 4 weeks. Typical response rates for elective chemotherapy regimens such as full-dose carboplatin or carboplatin and paclitaxel in ovarian cancer are 60–70%. The smallest detectable tumour measuring 1 cm^3 contains about 1,000,000,000 (10^9) cancer cells. Not all of these cells are viable and it is the clonogenic cell component that must be sterilised. If there was initially 10^{11} cells, 10^6 cells will remain. A million cancer cells may be clinically undetectable but, in time, this tumour will regrow. In some cases, however, all of the clonogenic cells are sterilised, resulting in a clinical cure.

ACKNOWLEDGMENT

I would like to express my sincere gratitude to Dr Pratik Kumar Chatterjee, Associate Professor of Physiology, Kasturba Medical College, Mangalore, Manipal Academy of Higher Eduction, Manipal, India. For his invaluable assistance in preparing the manuscript for Chapter 36. His expert contributions and support were instrumental in the development of this chapter.

SUGGESTED READING

1. da Costa AA, Baiocchi G, Guimarães AP. Progression-free survival in the ICON8 trial. Lancet. 2020;396(10253):756-7.
2. Eskander RN, Sill MW, Beffa L, Moore RG, Hope JM, Musa FB, et al. Pembrolizumab plus chemotherapy in advanced endometrial cancer. N Engl J Med. 2023;388(23):2159-70.
3. Feldman DR, Lorch A, Kramar A, Albany C, Einhorn LH, Giannatempo P, et al. Brain metastases in patients with germ cell tumors: prognostic factors and treatment options—an analysis from the Global Germ Cell Cancer Group. J Clin Oncol. 2016;34(4):345-51.
4. González-Martín A, Pothuri B, Vergote I, DePont Christensen R, Graybill W, Mirza MR, et al. Niraparib in patients with newly diagnosed advanced ovarian cancer. N Engl J Med. 2019;381(25):2391-402.
5. Hensley ML, Ishill N, Soslow R, Larkin J, Abu-Rustum N, Sabbatini P, et al. Adjuvant gemcitabine plus docetaxel for completely resected stages I–IV high grade uterine leiomyosarcoma: results of a prospective study. Gynecol Oncol. 2009;112(3):563-7.
6. Joly F, Ray-Coquard I, Fabbro M, Donoghoe M, Boman K, Sugimoto A, et al. Decreased hypersensitivity reactions with carboplatin-pegylated liposomal doxorubicin compared to carboplatin-paclitaxel combination: analysis from the GCIG CALYPSO relapsing ovarian cancer trial. Gynecol Oncol. 2011;122(2):226-32.
7. Lorusso D, Xiang Y, Hasegawa K, Scambia G, Leiva M, Ramos-Elias P, et al. Pembrolizumab or placebo with chemoradiotherapy followed by pembrolizumab or placebo for newly diagnosed, high-risk, locally advanced cervical cancer (ENGOT-cx11/GOG-3047/KEYNOTE-A18): overall survival results from a randomised, double-blind, placebo-controlled, phase 3 trial. The Lancet. 2024;404(10460):1321-32.
8. Mahul B Amin. AJCC Cancer Staging. 8th Edition. Chicago: Springer; 2017.
9. Neugut AI, Bates SE. Highlights of ASCO 2023. Oncologist. 2023;28(9):739-42.
10. Oza AM, Cook AD, Pfisterer J, Embleton A, Ledermann JA, Pujade-Lauraine E, et al. Standard chemotherapy with or without bevacizumab for women with newly diagnosed ovarian cancer (ICON7): overall survival results of a phase 3 randomised trial. Lancet Oncol. 2015;16(8):928-36.

11. Ozols RF, Bundy BN, Greer BE, Fowler JM, Clarke-Pearson D, Burger RA, et al. Phase III trial of carboplatin and paclitaxel compared with cisplatin and paclitaxel in patients with optimally resected stage III ovarian cancer: a Gynecologic Oncology Group study. J Clin Oncol. 2003;21(17):3194-200.
12. Pignata S, Scambia G, Katsaros D, Gallo C, Pujade-Lauraine E, De Placido S, et al. Carboplatin plus paclitaxel once a week versus every 3 weeks in patients with advanced ovarian cancer (MITO-7): a randomised, multicentre, open-label, phase 3 trial. Lancet Oncol. 2014;15(4): 396-405.
13. Ray-Coquard IL, Pautier P, Pignata S, Pérol D, González-Martín A, Sevelda P, et al. Phase III PAOLA-1/ENGOT-ov25 trial: Olaparib plus bevacizumab (bev) as maintenance therapy in patients (pts) with newly diagnosed, advanced ovarian cancer (OC) treated with platinum-based chemotherapy (PCh) plus bev. Ann Oncol. 2019;30: v894-5.
14. Somarelli JA, Shetler S, Jolly MK, Wang X, Bartholf Dewitt S, Hish AJ, et al. Mesenchymal-epithelial transition in sarcomas is controlled by the combinatorial expression of microRNA 200s and GRHL2. Mol Cell Biol. 2016;36(19):2503-13.

37

CHAPTER

Radiotherapy in Gynaecological Malignancies

Sourjya Banerjee, Pratik Kumar Chatterjee

Chapter Outline

- Biological Basis of Radiotherapy Treatment
- Radiation Dosage
- Therapeutic Ratio
- Radiotherapy Machines
- Brachytherapy
- Radiotherapy in Carcinoma of the Cervix
- Radiotherapy in Endometrial Cancer
- Radiotherapy in Vulvar Cancer
- Brachytherapy in Carcinoma of the Cervix
- Chemoradiation in Locally Advanced Carcinoma of the Cervix
- Radiotherapy in Vaginal Cancer

INTRODUCTION

Radiotherapy is the art of using ionising radiation to destroy malignant tumours whilst minimising damage to normal tissues.

BIOLOGICAL BASIS OF RADIOTHERAPY TREATMENT

In medical practice, the reasons why tumours are destroyed and normal tissues recover following radiotherapy are complex and poorly understood. The mechanism of action of radiation is that radiation kills cells by the production of secondary charged particles and free radicals, which interact with the nucleic acids. A number of double-stranded DNA breaks produced in the nucleus is related to cellular lethality. The sensitivity of tissues to radiotherapy seems to depend on their ability to repair radiation damage, repopulate and reoxygenate. The capacity to repair double- and single-strand DNA breaks varies between normal tissue and different tumours. The ability to repopulate is important, as cells can divide rapidly to replace cells killed by radiation. Normal tissues such as the buccal mucosa in the mouth and bone marrow have a considerable number of cells in the G0 resting phase of the cell cycle that can be rapidly stimulated to divide to replace dead cells. Unfortunately, well-differentiated and moderately differentiated squamous carcinomas have a marked ability to repopulate, and this may account for radiation failure in the treatment of some of these tumours. As tumours grow, new blood vessels develop to feed the neoplasm. By and large, the new blood vessels are primitive in nature, and the blood supply is inadequate to supply the growing tumour. Necrotic areas develop within such tumours. These areas contain hypoxic cells, which are a source of radio resistance. However, following a course of radiation treatment, cells that were initially hypoxic can reoxygenate and become more radiosensitive.

RADIATION DOSAGE

It is necessary to understand the radiation absorption and the dosage. The interaction of radiation with tissues is measured as the absorbed dose, which is the quantity of energy absorbed per unit mass. In the SI system of units, this is measured as joules per kilogram. 1 J/kg is 1 Gray (Gy). 1 Gy equals 100 rad, the unit used previously. The side effects caused by radiation limit the radiation dose given in an attempt to cure a tumour is the risk of normal tissue damage. This damage is seen initially as acute radiation effects in rapidly proliferating cells such as skin epithelium, mucosal lining of the upper digestive tract or the surface lining of the small bowel. This may manifest itself as moist desquamation of the skin, mucositis or diarrhoea. This damage normally heals. What is more worrying is the risk of late damage, which appears 9 months to 5 years after treatment, owing to the effects on slowly proliferating tissue, particularly vascular endothelium. This leads to necrosis, fistulae or stricture. The serious complication rate for patients treated for carcinoma of the cervix by radical radiotherapy is about 5%.

THERAPEUTIC RATIO

The therapeutic ratio has been defined as the relationship between the desired and undesired effects of therapy. One method to reduce the risk of normal tissue injury and increase the therapeutic ratio is to fractionate treatment. The total radiation dose is divided into 20–30 separate treatments and delivered over 4–6 weeks, 5 days a week. Another method of increasing the therapeutic ratio is the use of continuous low-dose-rate radiation. Such treatments are usually referred to as brachytherapy.

RADIOTHERAPY MACHINES

The most important and useful machine of the modern radiotherapy departments is the linear accelerator, which is used to produce X-rays with energies of 4–20 million electron volts (MeV). Such X-rays have major clinical advantages over low-energy X-rays generated by older kilovoltage machines. Megavoltage X-rays are relatively 'skin sparing'. It is fairly easy to treat deep-seated tumours with a homogeneous radiation beam, and the radiation dose to bone is no higher than surrounding tissues. Older kilovoltage apparatus generates X-rays of 100,000 to 300,000 electron volts (KeV). These machines look similar to diagnostic X-ray units and produce X-rays, which are only two or three times more energetic than those used to take diagnostic radiographs. The maximum energy of kilovoltage X-rays is deposited on the skin surface, and moist desquamation of the skin is often dose limiting. The dose received by the bone is higher than soft tissues. It is difficult to treat deep-seated tumours as these X-rays are rapidly attenuated; therefore, at present, kilovoltage machines are relegated to low-dose palliative treatments or the treatment of superficial tumours. An alternative to a linear accelerator is a cobalt machine, which produces a gamma ray with similar physical characteristics to a 4 MV X-ray beam. Cobalt machines are much simpler than linear accelerators, but the source requires replacement about every 3 years.

BRACHYTHERAPY

The radiocurability of gynaecological malignancies hinges upon the high radiation tolerance of the organs involved. The uterus and cervix can tolerate >200 Grays, while the upper vagina can tolerate 140 Grays. The distal vagina can tolerate up to 100 Grays.

Brachytherapy involves placing a radiation source in contact with or very close to the tumour. In the past, the sources used to be low-dose rate (LDR), providing anywhere between 0.4 and 2.0 Grays/h. However, in the present era, high-dose-rate (HDR) brachytherapy has gained precedence. The reasons are as follows: LDR requires the patient to be immobile for a very long period of time, often for >24 hours. On the other hand, HDR provides the same biological effect within a matter of minutes. Also, the applicators used for HDR brachytherapy are much smaller and therefore contribute to increased patient comfort and compliance.

Present-day HDR sources include iridium-192, a source, which requires to be replaced once every 3–4 months. It is for this reason that an HDR cobalt source has become more popular; The long half-life of Cobalt-60 allows the same source to be used for 5 years or even more.

RADIOTHERAPY IN CARCINOMA OF THE CERVIX

While cervical carcinoma up to stage IB1 can be treated with definitive surgery, radiation alone can be curative in these early stages. Surgical techniques are outside the scope of this chapter. Therefore, to summarise the role of radiation; 'very early cervical cancer, such as medically inoperable stage IA1 or IA2, can be treated with brachytherapy alone to an EQD2 dose of 75–80 Grays. EQD2 is a concept that expresses any numerical dose in equivalent terms if it had been delivered in fractions of 2 Grays each. Adjuvant radiation therapy in patients who undergo hysterectomy for cervical carcinoma is determined by the Sedlis criteria, as depicted in **Table 1**.'

'For patients with carcinoma serving stage IB2 to stage IVA, definitive external beam radiation to a dose of 45–50 Grays is prescribed. Subsequently, positive nodes, if any, are boosted by an additional 10 Grays,

TABLE 1: Sedlis criteria for external pelvic radiation after radical hysterectomy in node-negative, margin-negative, parametria-negative cases.

Lymphovascular space invasion	*Stromal invasion*	*Tumour size (cm)*
+	Deep one-third	Any
+	Middle one-third	≥2
+	Superficial one-third	≥5
–	Middle/deep one-third	≥4

using the intensity-modulated radiation therapy (IMRT) technique. The primary tumour itself is boosted by brachytherapy, according to the following rules, patients with a complete response to external beam radiotherapy, along with concurrent chemotherapy or those who have residual disease of <4 centimetres, should receive a dose of >80 Grays EQD2 to point A (*described later in the chapter*). However, for those with a residual disease of >4 centimetres at the time of brachytherapy, the dose needs to be escalated to EQD2 of 85 to 90 Grays at point A.'

Treatment Volumes for External Beam Radiotherapy

The radiation treatment volume for external beam radiation therapy (EBRT) should include the gross disease, if present, along with the parametria, uterosacral ligaments and a sufficient vaginal margin of at least 3 centimetres from the gross disease. In addition, it should include the presacral nodes and other nodal regions at risk. In cases where surgical or radiologic imaging indicates negative nodes, the radiation field must cover the entire external iliac, internal iliac, obturator and presacral nodal basins. For patients identified as having a higher risk of lymph node involvement, such as those with larger tumours or suspected or confirmed nodes limited to the lower true pelvis, the radiation volume should be expanded to include the common iliac nodes as well. Elective para-aortic nodal basin irradiation should be considered for patients with even a single metastatic node in the common iliac station or three or more nodes in the pelvic basins. In instances where there is confirmed involvement of the common iliac and/or para-aortic nodes, it is advisable to implement extended-field pelvic and para-aortic radiotherapy, reaching up to the renal vessels or further, depending on the distribution of the involved nodes. Furthermore, for patients with involvement of the lower third of the vagina, coverage of the bilateral groins is also necessary.

RADIOTHERAPY IN ENDOMETRIAL CANCER

Radiation in endometrial carcinoma is primarily used in the postoperative adjuvant setting either in the form of vaginal brachytherapy (VBT) alone or in combination with EBRT. Only if the patient is deemed medically inoperable, radiation is used as the primary modality of locoregional treatment.

Flowchart 1: Treatment schema for endometrioid carcinoma endometrium stage I and II.

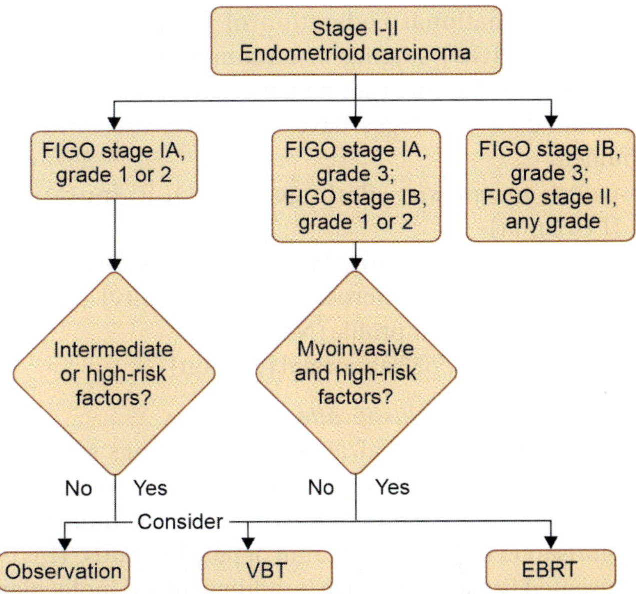

- Intermediate-risk factor = Age ≥ 60 years and focal lymphovascular space involvement (LVSI)
- High-risk factor = Substantial LVSI, especially in the absence of surgical nodal staging
- Focal LVSI = A single focus of LVSI around the tumour
- Substantial LVSI = Diffuse or multifocal LVSI around the tumour

(EBRT: external beam radiation therapy; FIGO: International Federation of Gynaecology and Obstetrics; Myoinvasive: myometrial invasion; VBT: vaginal brachytherapy)

Details of surgical techniques are beyond the scope of this chapter.

Treatment schema for endometrioid carcinoma of the endometrium, stage I and II, is depicted in **Flowchart 1**.

High-risk histologies refer to the following:

- Serous carcinoma
- Clear cell carcinoma
- Carcinosarcoma
- Dedifferentiated carcinoma
- Undifferentiated carcinoma
- Mixed histology carcinoma (One of the components includes a high-risk histology).

As a general principle, randomised controlled trials are not feasible for these histologies owing to their rarity. As a general rule, for stage IA, IB and II, postoperative vaginal brachytherapy is indicated for all such patients; in case of positive peritoneal washings, EBRT along with systemic therapy is added to the VBT.

In stages III and IVA of all histologies, systemic therapy takes precedence over radiation as adjuvant management.

The International Federation of Gynaecology and Obstetrics (FIGO) staging of endometrial cancer was updated in 2023 by incorporating molecular classification; the individual substages have also been substantially modified:

- *Good prognosis:* Pathogenic POLE mutation (POLEmut)
- *Intermediate prognosis:* Mismatch repair deficiency, i.e. MMRd/MSI (microsatellite instability) and no specific molecular profile (NSMP)
- *Poor prognosis:* p53 abnormal (p53abn)

When the molecular classification is known:
Histological and surgical/anatomical findings serve as the foundation for FIGO stages I and II. The FIGO stage is altered in the early stages of the disease if the molecular categorisation indicates POLEmut or p53abn status. This is represented in the FIGO stage by adding 'm' for molecular categorisation and a subscript to indicate POLEmut or p53abn status. Although early FIGO stages are unaffected by MMRd or NSMP status, these molecular classifications ought to be noted for data gathering purposes. It should be noted as stage ImMMRd or stage ImNSMP and stage IImMMRd or stage IImNSMP when molecular categorisation indicates MMRd or NSMP.

Anatomical and surgical findings provide the basis of FIGO stages III and IV. Although molecular categorisation does not change the stage category, if it is known, it should be noted. For data collection purposes, it should be noted as stage IIIm or stage IVm with the relevant subscript when the molecular categorisation is available. For instance, p53abn should be noted as stage IIImp53abn or stage IVmp53abn when molecular classification indicates it.

In view of these changes in the staging system, the American Society for Radiation Oncology (ASTRO) recommends the following:

Chemotherapy and radiation therapy are advised for patients with FIGO stage I-IIIC2 TP53 mutant uterine cancer. Since dMMR patients did not benefit from systemic therapy in the relevant PORTEC-3 trial, radiation without chemotherapy is advised for patients with IB-IIIC2 dMMR endometrial malignancy. Radiation therapy without chemotherapy is advised for patients with stage IB-IIIC2 POLE mutant endometrial cancer. However, at present, the amount of supporting evidence is regarded as minimal, and it is crucial to remember that all recommendations are conditional.

Treatment Volumes

The postoperative bed (with consideration to intestinal movement, bladder and rectal filling)/intact uterus in a medically inoperable patient and the lower common iliacs, external iliacs, internal iliacs, obturators, parametria, upper vagina/paravaginal tissue and presacral lymph nodes (in patients with cervical involvement) should all be included in the volume receiving pelvic EBRT. In addition, extended-field radiation therapy (required in stage III disease) also encompasses the entire common iliac chain and the para-aortic lymph node region. Depending on the clinical circumstances, the upper boundary of the extended field should be at least 1–2 cm above the renal arteries. This volume is treated to 45–50.4 Grays at 1.8–2 Grays per fraction. Grossly metastatic nodes, if any, are boosted up to 60 Grays by IMRT to respect the radiation tolerance limits of adjacent bowel loops.

The postoperative vaginal vault being the most common site of recurrence, this region is boosted by brachytherapy using vaginal cylinders: the greatest diameter that fits comfortably should be used.

The upper two-thirds of the vagina are treated by brachytherapy; in cases of extensive lymphovascular space invasion (LVSI) or positive margins, a greater length needs to be treated.

If postoperative VBT is used alone, 7 Grays (HDR) × 3 fractions is prescribed 5 mm from the vaginal surface.

If VBT is used to boost the EBRT, doses of 4–6 Grays (HDR) in 2–3 fractions are prescribed to the vaginal mucosa.

RADIOTHERAPY IN VULVAR CANCER

During staging, the vulvar tumour is surgically excised with a clinical gross margin of at least 1 cm. For a unifocal tumour <4 cm in diameter, at least 2 cm from the vulvar midline with a clinically negative inguinofemoral basin, unilateral sentinel lymph node biopsy (SLNB) or inguinofemoral dissection is appropriate. Tumours within 2 cm of the midline warrant bilateral inguinofemoral SLNB/dissection. Groin dissection can be omitted for patients with stage IA disease with clinically negative groins.

It must be noted that the inguinofemoral nodes are considered the sole regional basin for vulvar tumours; pelvic nodes, if involved, must be considered as distant metastases.

As such, lymph nodal status is the single most important determinant for survival.

Radiotherapy volumes include the primary disease or postoperative bed with a margin along with bilateral inguinofemoral basins, internal and external iliac stations.

Treatment Doses

- Gross primary vulva disease = 60–70 Gray
- Primary surgical bed (postoperative, negative margins) = 45–50 Gray
- Primary surgical bed (postoperative close or positive margins) = 54–60 Gray
- Clinically and/or radiographically uninvolved inguinofemoral lymph nodes (LNs) = 45–50 Gray
- Inguinofemoral LNs (positive, no extracapsular extension or gross residual disease) = 50–55 Gray
- Inguinofemoral LNs (with extracapsular extension) = 54–64 Gray
- LNs (gross residual or unresectable disease) = 60–70 Gray.

BRACHYTHERAPY IN CARCINOMA OF THE CERVIX

Initially, three systems for intracavitary brachytherapy were developed: the Paris, the Stockholm and the Manchester systems. The systems differed in the type of applicator used, the strength of the source and the time of administration. Today, most systems are derivations of the Manchester technique. Point A is 'Classically' defined as being 2 cm above the mucous membrane of the lateral vaginal fornix and 2 cm lateral to the centre of the uterine canal, which corresponds to the paracervical triangle, in the medial edge of the broad ligament, where the uterine vessels crossed the ureters. Point B, defined as 5 cm from the midline at the same level as point A, was intended to quantify the dose delivered to the obturator nodes **(Fig. 1)**.

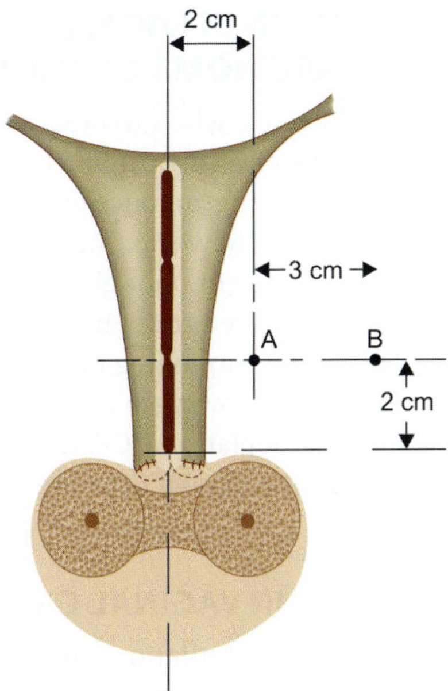

Fig. 1: Manchester system: definition of points 'A' and 'B'.

Presently, point A dose is used to approximate the average or minimum dose to the tumour. A later definition 'revised' point A as being 2 cm above the distal end of the lowest source in the cervical canal and 2 cm lateral to the tandem. Point A represents the location where the uterine artery crosses the ureter and is the dose-limiting point within the paracervical triangle. The brachytherapy dose in the 'Point A' based system must be so adjusted that radiation-induced necrosis does not occur at this point while delivering a curative dose to the high-risk clinical target volume. In the current era, brachytherapy is delivered under image guidance such that the high-risk clinical target volume consists of the entire cervix and presumed extra cervical extensions into the parametrium and vagina as determined by prebrachytherapy MRI and clinical examination. While delivering curative doses, the rectal dosage must be limited to <75 Grays–2 cc of the rectal volume at an equivalent dose of 2 Grays per fraction. Similarly, bladder dose must be constrained to <90 Grays–2 cc at an equivalent dose of 2 Grays per fraction. This caveat is mentioned because, while HDR brachytherapy (the current standard of care) uses anywhere between 4 and 9 Grays per fraction over 2–5 fractions, the biological effect of each such treatment is much greater than what the numerical value suggests. In practice, the os is radiographically demarcated by the tandem collar, whereas the lateral fornix is indicated by the colpostat surface. Various applicators have been designed based on the Manchester system with minor modifications. For example, Williamson-Fletcher, Howard, Delclos suit, etc.

Ideally, the tandem should be in the midline, as equidistant as possible from the lateral pelvic wall, crossing the mid long axis of the ovoids, and the vaginal colpostats should be symmetrically positioned against the cervix in relation to the tandem. However, this holds good only if residual disease after external beam radiotherapy is limited to the cervical os, the medial halves of bilateral parametria or the fornices. If the extent of residual disease is greater than this, brachytherapy is delivered through interstitial needles inserted into the cervix, parametria and vagina through the perineal skin using a Syed-Neblett template or Martinez universal perineal interstitial template (MUPIT).

CHEMORADIATION IN LOCALLY ADVANCED CARCINOMA OF THE CERVIX

All patients above stage IA, when treated with definitive radiotherapy, should receive concurrent chemotherapy in the form of cisplatin at 40 mg/m^2 once every week during the course of EBRT. This, however, may sometimes not be possible in the presence of poor glomerular filtration rate secondary to hydroureteronephrosis in stage IIIB or enlarged lymph nodes impinging upon the ureters in stage III C1 or IIIC2 disease, owing to the inherent nephrotoxicity of cisplatin. Carboplatin AUC-2 as per the Calvert formula is an option but is known to be less effective than cisplatin.

RADIOTHERAPY IN VAGINAL CANCER

The primary treatment is radiation instead of surgery because it allows for better preservation of the organ. This is generally combined with concurrent weekly cisplatin.

Treatment volumes: This includes the primary disease with a margin of 1–2 cm along with the entire vagina, paravaginal tissue, cervix and bilateral parametria together with common iliac, internal and external iliac, presacral and obturator nodes. Inguinal nodes are included if the lower third of the vagina is involved. Presacral and mesorectal basins are included if the posterior wall of vagina or rectovaginal septum are involved. Para-aortic basin is treated only if gross nodes are present in the common iliac and/or para-aortic stations.

Treatment doses: The above volume is treated up to 50 Grays at 2 Grays per fraction. 'Gross nodes, if any, are boosted to 60–70 Grays using IMRT. Care needs to be taken in accounting for the internal target motion, which can be as much as 2 cm in the region of the upper vagina; the lower vagina is immobile.

The primary disease is further boosted by brachytherapy up to 80 Grays (EQD2) for upper vaginal disease and 70 Grays (EQD2) for lower vaginal disease, to respect radiation tolerance limits of local tissue. Brachytherapy is usually delivered by intravaginal cylinders for tumours <5 mm thick. Thickness above 5 mm warrants the employment of hollow interstitial needles through which the radiation source is passed and kept at specific locations for a specified duration as determined by highly sophisticated software in order to deliver the required dose.

ACKNOWLEDGMENT

I would like to express my sincere gratitude to Dr Pratik Kumar Chatterjee, Associate Professor of Physiology, Kasturba Medical College, Mangalore, Manipal Academy of Higher Eduction, Manipal, India. For his invaluable assistance in preparing the manuscript for Chapter 37. His expert contributions and support were instrumental in the development of this chapter.

SUGGESTED READING

1. Berek JS, Matias-Guiu X, Creutzberg C, Fotopoulou C, Gaffney D, Kehoe S, et al. FIGO staging of endometrial cancer: 2023. Int J Gynecol Obstet. 2023;162(2):383-94.
2. Brower JV, Bregar AJ, Klopp AH. Path to precision: refining radiation therapy guidelines for early stage endometrial cancer through incorporation of primary tumor size, lower uterine segment invasion, and molecular markers. Pract Radiat Oncol. 2024;14(2):154-60.
3. Harkenrider MM, Abu-Rustum N, Albuquerque K, Bradfield L, Bradley K, Dolinar E, et al. Radiation therapy for endometrial cancer: an ASTRO clinical practice guideline. Pract Radiat Oncol. 2022:S1879-8500.
4. Pötter R, Tanderup K, Kirisits C, de Leeuw A, Kirchheiner K, Nout R, et al. The EMBRACE II study: the outcome and prospect of two decades of evolution within the GEC-ESTRO GYN working group and the EMBRACE studies. Clinical and translational radiation oncology. 2018;9:48-60.
5. Sedlis A, Bundy BN, Rotman MZ, Lentz SS, Muderspach LI, Zaino RJ. A randomized trial of pelvic radiation therapy versus no further therapy in selected patients with stage IB carcinoma of the cervix after radical hysterectomy and pelvic lymphadenectomy: a gynecologic oncology study group. Gynecol Oncol. 1999;73:177-83.

38

CHAPTER

Immunotherapy in Obstetrics and Gynaecology

Pralhad Kushtagi

Chapter Outline

- Immune system—Some Basics
- Immunotherapy in Gynaecologic Cancers
- Immunotherapy in Reproductive Medicine
- Immunotherapy in other situations
- Immunotherapy in Pregnancy

INTRODUCTION

William Coley wrote a preface to immunotherapy with his inadvertent discovery that postoperative infections with pyogenic *Streptococcus* could induce tumour regression in sarcoma patients. It was back in 1893. Initially, immunotherapy was applied to the field of oncology. Since virtually all diseases have some form of direct or indirect relation with the immune system, the scope of immunotherapy has extended beyond to treat a wide array of diseases related to immune molecules, immune cells and the immune system itself.

Immunotherapy is a biological therapy defined as the prevention and/or treatment of diseases by inducing, enhancing or suppressing immune response. It includes a variety of treatments that work in different ways—some intended to boost immune system defences and others helping to train the immune system to recognise and attack.

IMMUNE SYSTEM—SOME BASICS

The immune system in humans is a complex system capable of discriminating self from non-self and mounting appropriate allogeneic immune responses to protect themselves from that is non-self. Immune response defence is made up of a nonspecific innate response that humans are born with and do not require antigenic recognition and a specific humoral response that involves B- and T-cells that are capable of mounting responses to a particular threat with immense specificity.

Innate Immune Response

Some of the known innate immune cells are macrophages, dendritic cells (DCs) and neutrophils. These constitute the first line of defence, and they recognise, engulf and destroy the non-self or the insurgent. They exhibit their function through receptors. Since these sensors sense the signals from damage-associated molecular pattern molecules (DAMP), they are called as pattern recognition receptors (PRRs). DAMPs are phospholipids, carbohydrates, proteins and nucleic acids released by dying cells in necrotic or apoptotic processes. DCs are a heterogeneous population of immune cells that populate almost all the tissues of our body. They are very mobile and readily migrate from peripheral tissues to draining lymph nodes. These cells have both phagocytic and specialised antigen-presenting functions. Once stimulated by DAMPs, DCs undergo a complex process of maturation/activation, which allows them to present in an immunogenic manner the antigens captured in the periphery and initiate immune responses. DCs are thus multifunctional cells and link the innate immune response to adaptive immune response.

Adaptive Immune Response

The adaptive immune process is a gradual response involving a specific reaction to an antigen, and it follows the activation of innate immune cells in the presence of a danger signal. Innate cells start the process by producing inflammatory cytokines and other signal molecules that recruit granulocytes and antigen-presenting cells (APCs) such as DCs to the site of injury. The classical response involves the APCs, mainly DCs, travelling to draining lymph nodes and displaying the antigen to naïve T lymphocytes. Several cytokines, such as interleukin (IL)-2, 4, 6 and 10, as well as various cell surface molecules, including CD40, CD19 and CD21, are necessary for the interaction between T-cells and APCs. Finally, the production of high-affinity antigen-specific B cells and the generation of memory cells accompany the antigen-stimulated proliferation of B cells. These events result in return to tissue homeostasis.

Both of these systems interact with each other to protect effectively and efficiently. Immunosurveillance describes the processes and is used to indicate the host immune response to foreign antigens, which will result in their destruction. Logically, any failure in immunosurveillance would lead to the diseases. Immunosurveillance involves immunoediting, immune checkpoint pathways, immunomodelling, adaptive immune resistance and immunosuppression. Immunomodelling acts in three phases of elimination, equilibrium and escape.

The host immune system has evolved as a powerful tool that if better harnessed could significantly enhance the efficacy of chemotherapeutics and improve outcomes. Recent developments in immunology and biotechnology have led to an increasing number of clinically available cellular and immune therapies that require administration of biologics and cells of different origins. For inducing protection against diseases, the active immunotherapy with use of vaccines and the passive immunotherapy in the form of serum from recovering patients, the use of antitoxins and pooled immunoglobulin therapy is well established in medical practise. Molecular technology has added the development and the use of defined monoclonal antibodies against factors involved in the pathogenesis of diseases.

The present chapter attempts to review the applicability and present status of immunotherapy in the field of obstetrics and gynaecology.

IMMUNOTHERAPY IN GYNAECOLOGIC CANCERS

Immuno-oncology has assumed a status of branch of medicine since the role of immune system in controlling tumourigenesis and tumour progression is established. It is understood that when a T-cell encounters a tumour antigen, this results in activation, clonal proliferation/expansion and a cytolytic response. Creating an immunosuppressive microenvironment is the basis of the application of immunology in cancer treatment. The innate and adaptive immune systems interact to mediate the anticancer immune surveillance and immune editing. The application of knowledge about immunomodulation in cancer therapy is shown in **Figure 1**.

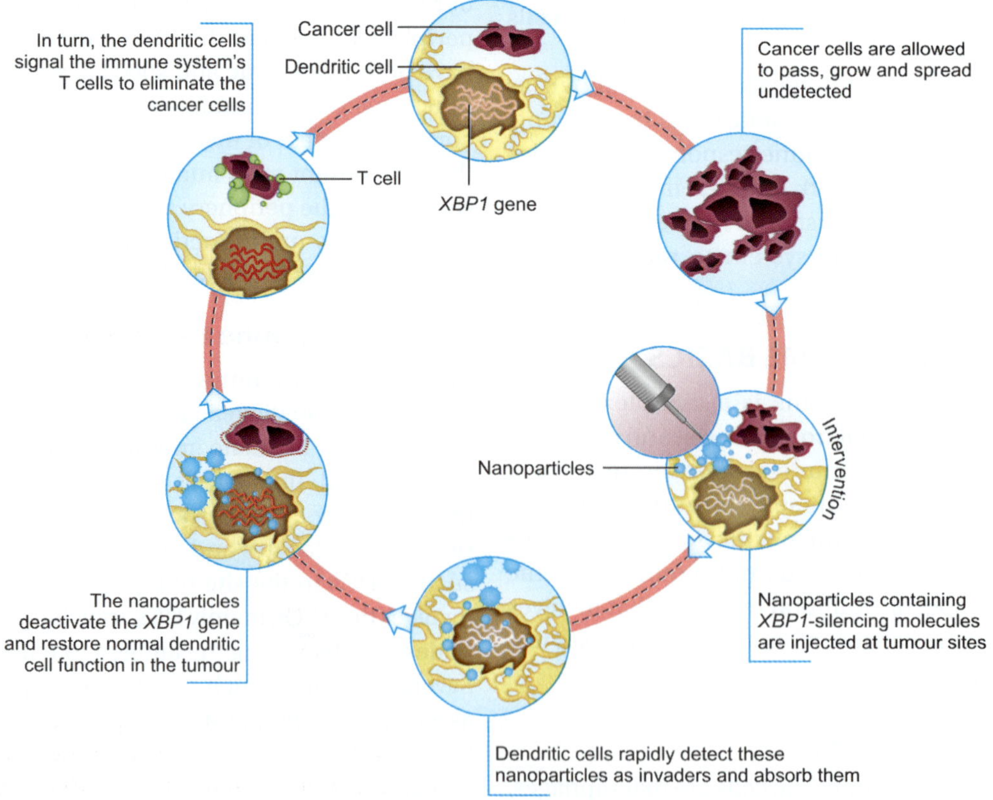

Fig. 1: Harnessing the immune system to fight cancer.

Each tumour is identified by the host immune system because of unique tumour antigens presented on it, and they are called tumour-associated antigens (TAAs) and can be grouped as self or non-self-antigens. Self-antigens form a group of antigens that are generated from native molecules and maintain their original amino acid sequences. This group includes repressed or silent antigens such as carcinoembryonic antigen (CEA), alpha-foetoprotein (AFP) and overtly expressed antigens such as human epidermal growth factor receptor 2 (HER2)/NEU. Non-self-antigens include products of genetic mutation and oncogenic and other pathogenic viruses or other microorganisms. Genetic mutations such as point mutation or translocation may lead to the development of altered novel peptides such as oncogene RAS and tumour suppression gene *p53*. Oncogenic viruses may be deoxyribonucleic acid (DNA) or ribonucleic acid (RNA) viruses that integrate their genome into human cells resulting in the expression of foreign proteins that form potential TAAs. For example, human papillomaviruses (HPVs), Epstein–Barr virus and hepatitis B and C viruses.

Successful immunotherapy for gynaecologic cancers will require multimodal approaches that target different aspects of the antitumour immune response, including tumour antigen recognition, T-cell activation and blockade of immune inhibitory mechanisms. Active immunotherapy uses the immune system to recognise and target specific cancer antigens, e.g. vaccines, which stimulate the patient's immune response, or chimeric antigen receptor T-cell (CAR-T) therapy; collected from the patient and genetically engineered immune cells with the ability to recognise antigens or target therapy; and a specific antibody designed to eliminate the specific target. Passive immunotherapy enhances the activity of a patient's immune system response, e.g. checkpoint inhibitors or cytokines. Immunomodulatory therapy that blocks the suppressive signals of checkpoint proteins (checkpoint blockade), or selectively targets immunosuppressive cells in the tumour microenvironment (such as Tregs), allows for activation and proliferation of tumour-specific T-cells that will be able to identify and eliminate cancer cells. Strategies for the development of oncoimmunotherapy can be outlined as presented in **Figure 2**.

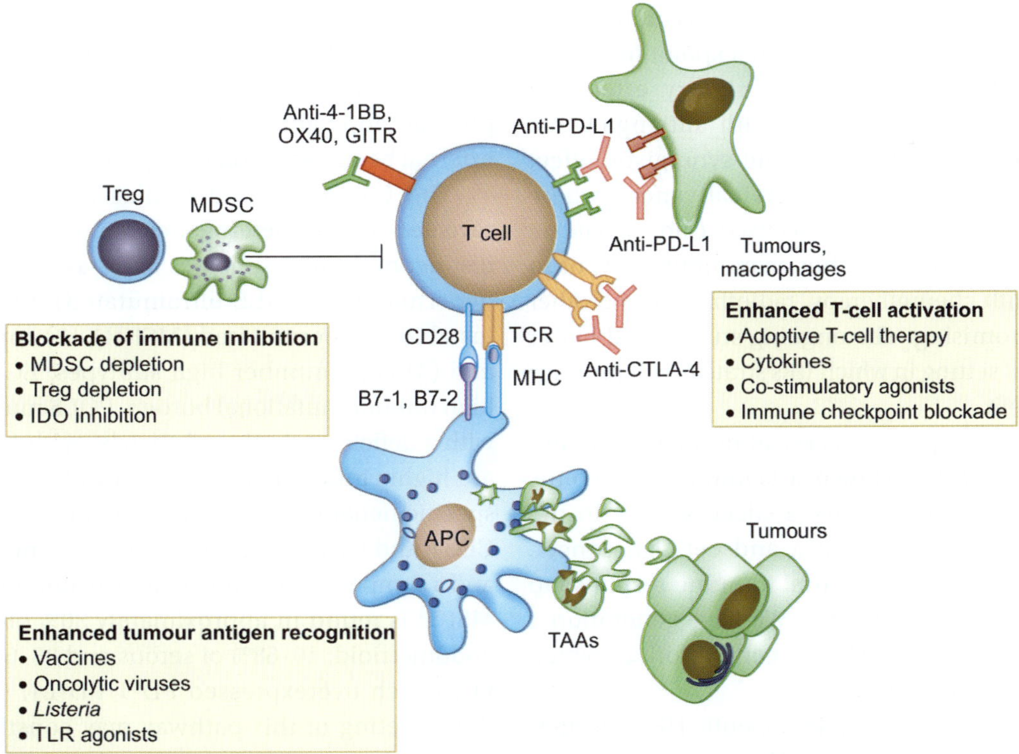

Fig. 2: Opportunities for immunotherapy in gynaecologic malignancies. (APC: antigen-presenting cell; CTLA-4: cytotoxic T-lymphocyte-associated antigen 4; GITR: glucocorticoid-induced tumour necrosis factor receptor-related protein; IDO: indoleamine 2,3-dioxygenase; MDSC: myeloid-derived suppressor cell; MHC: major histocompatibility complex; TAAs: tumour-associated antigens; TCR: T-cell receptor; TLR: toll-like receptor; Treg: regulatory T-cell)

Immunotherapy in Cervical Cancer

Treatment approaches and outcomes for cervical cancer patients are highly dependent on disease stage at diagnosis. Treatment options for early-stage cancer include radical hysterectomy or radical trachelectomy with pelvic lymphadenectomy and for invasive cervical cancers concurrent chemotherapy and radiation therapy are the mainstay of management. For distant metastatic cervical cancer, the treatment focuses on systemic therapies. With the low cure rates for advanced disease and side effects of current therapies, new therapeutic options for cervical cancer patients are needed. Immunotherapy as an anticancer strategy that aims to modify and recruit the host immune system to more effectively and specifically target cancer cells is hoped to offer improved cervical cancer treatment and survival.

Persistent HPV infection is the recognised cause of almost all cervical cancers. HPV escapes the immune system in different ways. Reports of elevated rates of PD-1/PD-L1 expression in up to 80% of cervical tumours support a decisive role in immunotherapy to restore the immune response against cervical cancer. PD-1 inhibitors, pembrolizumab and nivolumab, alone or in combination, are under trial. These are immune checkpoint inhibitors (ICIs). Knowing the immunomodulatory effects of bevacizumab, ICIs are combined with antiangiogenic drugs in order to capture a possible synergistic effect of the association in advanced cervical cancer, where antiangiogenic drugs are already licensed. Clinical data on the use of immunotherapy either as monotherapy, or in combination with chemotherapy, radiotherapy and other ICIs, appear promising. The ongoing studies will better address the best setting in which this strategy will produce the higher benefit.

For persistent atypia and cervical dysplasia, the use of interferon alpha has shown a favourable outcome. Prophylactic HPV vaccines are a success story in the prevention of cervical dysplasia and cervical cancer. It is based on inducing a humoral immune response to generate neutralising antibodies. We have generation 1 (bivalent and quadrivalent) and generation 2 (which covers nine strains) vaccines.

There are efforts to develop therapeutic HPV vaccines targeting E6 and E7 oncoproteins. The most promising of these appears to be the ADXS11-001, axalimogene filolisbac: A live attenuated *Listeria monocytogenes* (*Lm*) vaccine containing E7 oncoprotein from HPV-16; ADXS11-001 is under evaluation in different trials. Although there are many clinical trials and preclinical investigations regarding the use of immunotherapy for the control of cervical cancer, so far only pembrolizumab is approved for clinical use for advanced cervical cancer. Immunotherapeutic approaches targeting different aspects of the immune environment, as depicted in **Figures 3A to D** when materialised, can improve the control of cervical cancer.

Immunotherapy in Endometrial Cancer

Endometrial cancer (EC) patients are diagnosed at early-stage disease with a 5-year overall survival of 80%, and advanced-stage patients present a dismal prognosis with a 5-year survival of about 15%. Traditionally, EC is categorised into two types based on Bokhman's concept. Type I is the most common, accounting for 60–70% of cases and includes endometrioid cancer with grades of 1 and 2 differentiation and the strong expression of hormonal receptors. Type II includes high-grade endometrioid cancer and other histological types such as serous or clear cell carcinoma. These cancers are typically negative for hormone receptors and carry a worse prognosis. Currently, for locally advanced cancer, surgery is the main therapeutic option, and the assessment is surgicopathological. If postoperative adverse factors are present, adjuvant treatment is recommended, such as external beam radiation therapy and brachytherapy.

The Cancer Genome Atlas (TCGA) research has revealed disease heterogeneity and identified four main distinct molecular subtypes of EC as the (1) endometrial hypermutated (POLE ultramutated), (2) microsatellite instability hypermutated (MSI-H), (3) copy number low and (4) copy number high subtypes. EC subtypes with high tumour mutational burden, POLE mutant and MSI-H with a deficiency in the mismatch repair (dMMR) system, are highly immunogenic. They exhibit elevated tumour-specific neoantigens, resulting in an enlarged number of CD3+ and CD8+ tumour-infiltrating lymphocytes (TILs) and a compensatory upregulation of immune checkpoints. MSI-H is found in approximately 30% of EC; 40–80% of endometrioid, 10–68% of serous and 23–69% of clear cell EC, which overexpressed PD-1/PD-L1, suggesting that the targeting of this pathway may constitute a hopeful strategy to increase antitumour immune response, and ongoing studies are focussed on enhancing clinical responses through immunotherapy techniques. Efforts are required to increase the role of active and/or passive

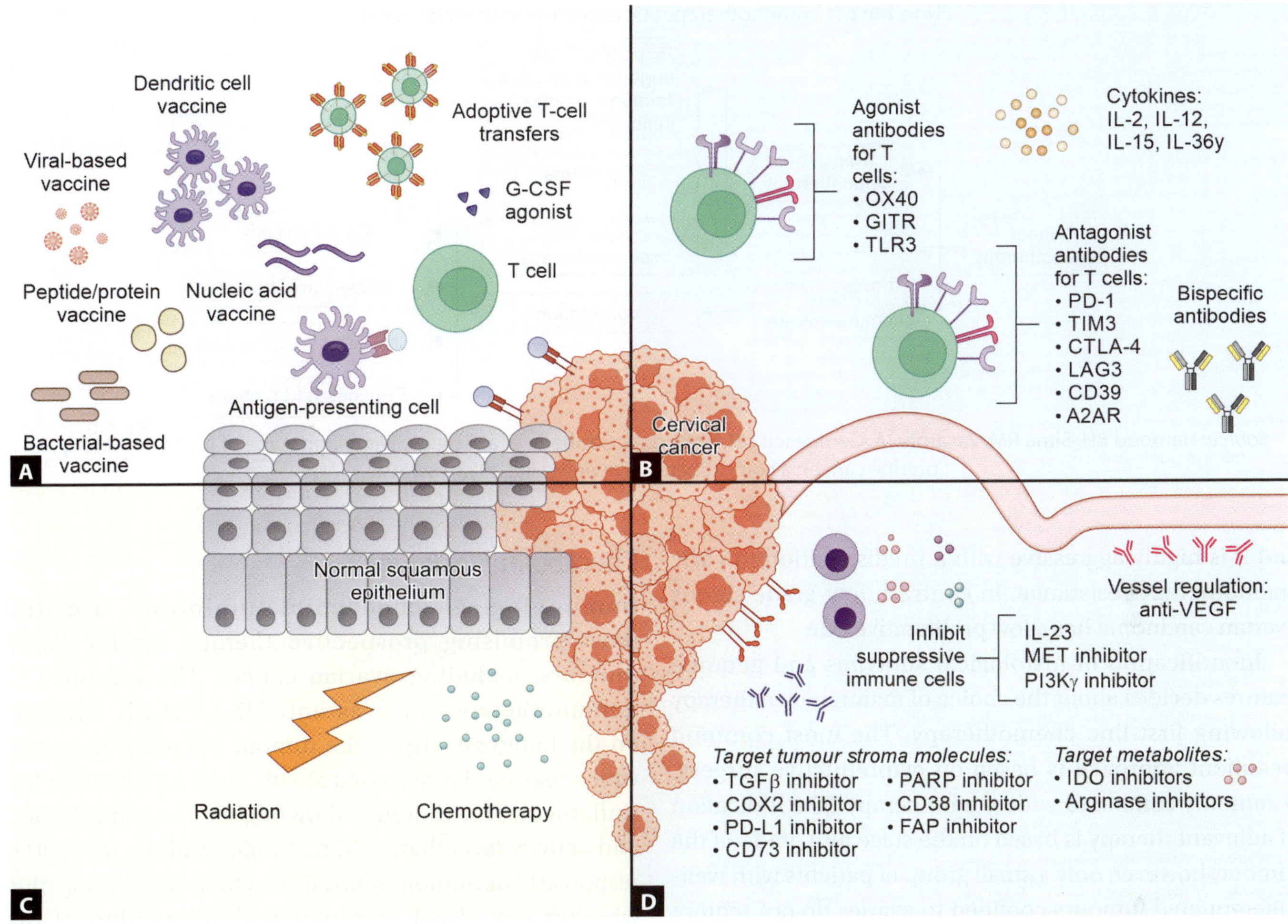

Figs. 3A to D: Schematic overview of cancer immunotherapies to target cervical cancer. (A) Strategies to generate and enhance cervical cancer-specific T-cells; (B) Strategies to augment effector immune cells in the TME; (C) Conventional cervical cancer therapies; (D) Strategies to target immunosuppressive factors in the TME. (A2AR: adenosine 2A receptor; COX-2: cyclo-oxygenase-2; CTLA-4: cytotoxic T-lymphocyte-associated protein 4; FAP: fibroblast activation protein; G-CSF: granulocyte colony-stimulating factor; GITR: glucocorticoid-induced tumour necrosis factor receptor-related protein; IDO: indoleamine 2,3-dioxygenase; IL-2: interleukin-2; LAG3: lymphocyte activation gene 3; MET: mesenchymal–epithelial transition; PARP: poly(ADP-ribose) polymerase; PD-1: programmed cell death protein 1; PD-L1: programmed cell death ligand 1; PI3K: phosphoinositide 3-kinase; TGF-β,: transforming growth factor-β; TIM3: T-cell immunoglobulin and mucin domain-containing 3; TLR3: toll-like receptor 3; VEGF: vascular endothelial growth factor)
Source: Ferrall L, Lin KY, Roden RBS, Hung CF, Wu TC. Cervical cancer immunotherapy: facts and hopes. Cancer Res. 2021;27(18):4953-73.

immunotherapy in treating the patients with metastatic or recurring disease **(Flowchart 1)**. Preclinical and phase I trials (with pembrolizumab and dostarlimab) evaluating the effectiveness of immunotherapy in such patients have shown positive immunologic responses. Clinical responses have been limited. This has led to concerns about proving therapeutic efficacy in a group of extensively pretreated patients with advanced illness and short follow-up. The key challenges in determining the effectiveness of immunotherapy for EC are identifying the subgroup of patients most likely to respond to immunotherapy, identifying biomarkers that can predict treatment success and finding therapeutic combinations that can improve medication performance while reducing toxicity.

Immunotherapy in Ovarian Cancer

Ovarian cancer is often diagnosed in its advanced stages, due to the lack of initial symptom specificity and screening methods. The vast majority of ovarian neoplasms develop from epithelial tissues, and there are various histology subtypes. High-grade serous ovarian carcinoma (HGSOC) is the most common epithelial subtype (around 75%),

Flowchart 1: Immunotherapeutic approach to uterine cancer.

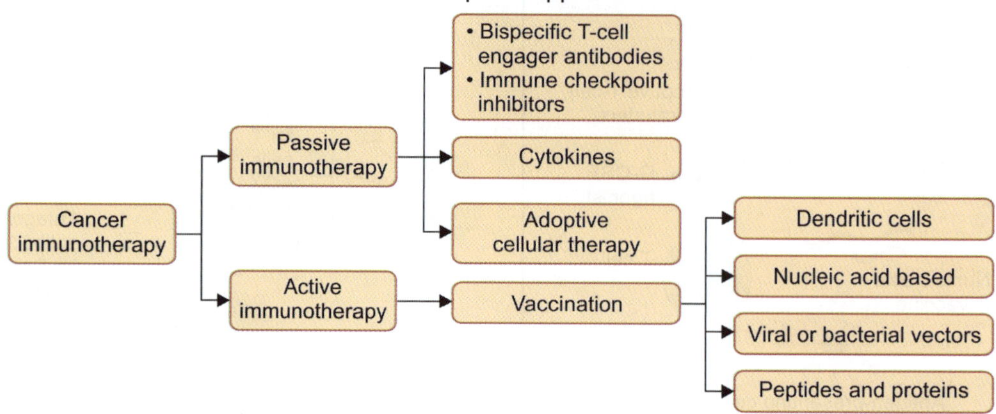

Source: Hamoud BH, Sima RM, Vacaroiu IA, Georgescu MT, Bobirca A, Gaube A, et al. The evolving landscape of immunotherapy in uterine cancer: a comprehensive review. Life. 2023;13:1502.

and it is highly aggressive with a predisposition to early chemotherapy resistance. In contrast, low-grade serous ovarian carcinoma has a low proliferative rate.

Identification of histological subtypes and genome features decides about the choice of maintenance therapy following first-line chemotherapy. The most common treatment approach is based on cytoreductive surgery, commonly combined with chemotherapy. The indication of adjuvant therapy is based on the stage and grade of the tumour; however, only a small group of patients with well-differentiated tumours confined to ovaries do not require systemic treatment. First-line chemotherapy is often a combination of platinum (carboplatin or cisplatin) and taxane (paclitaxel) compounds. The neoadjuvant therapy is applied when the optimal cytoreduction surgery is not possible.

Following systemic chemotherapy, there are options for maintenance treatment. Antiangiogenic agent, bevacizumab, which affects vascular endothelial growth factor (VEGF), is clinically used in combination with chemotherapy in adjuvant and recurrence treatment. Inhibitors of the poly(ADP-ribose) polymerase (PARP) enzyme, such as olaparib or niraparib, are effective in patients with homologous recombination deficit, especially in a group with BRCA mutations. There are studies confirming a significant progression-free survival benefit of bevacizumab and olaparib combination in the group of patients with homologous recombination deficit. The innovative strategy of immunotherapy could overtake systemic chemotherapy in ovarian cancer **(Fig. 4)**.

Checkpoint Blockade

Immunological checkpoint inhibitors are the most promising prospective therapy for incurable tumours, including ovarian cancer. The response to immunotherapy, such as anti-PD-1/PD-L1, depends on the heterogeneity of the tumour microenvironment, which may be characterised as cold (non-inflamed) or hot (inflamed). Hot tumours show higher T-cell infiltration and activity level than cold tumours, resulting in a better response to immunotherapy. Researchers are investigating whether combined therapies and stimulation of the tumour's immune system can enhance the response to immunotherapy. Monotherapy with nivolumab presented a low tumour response in ovarian cancer. Pembrolizumab administered as a single agent was found effective only in a small fraction of patients with recurrent ovarian cancer. The overall response rate varies depending on the number of previous platinum regimens.

Combination Therapies

Combining immunotherapies that exploit different mechanisms may have a complementary effect.

- Combination therapy with anti-CTLA-4 (ipilimumab) and anti-PD-1 (nivolumab) delivered promising results, demonstrating greater efficacy compared to monotherapy with a higher rate of response and greater prolongation of progression-free survival.
- Therapies with a primary nonimmune mechanism of action may make tumours susceptible to immunotherapy. Triggering of antitumour immune

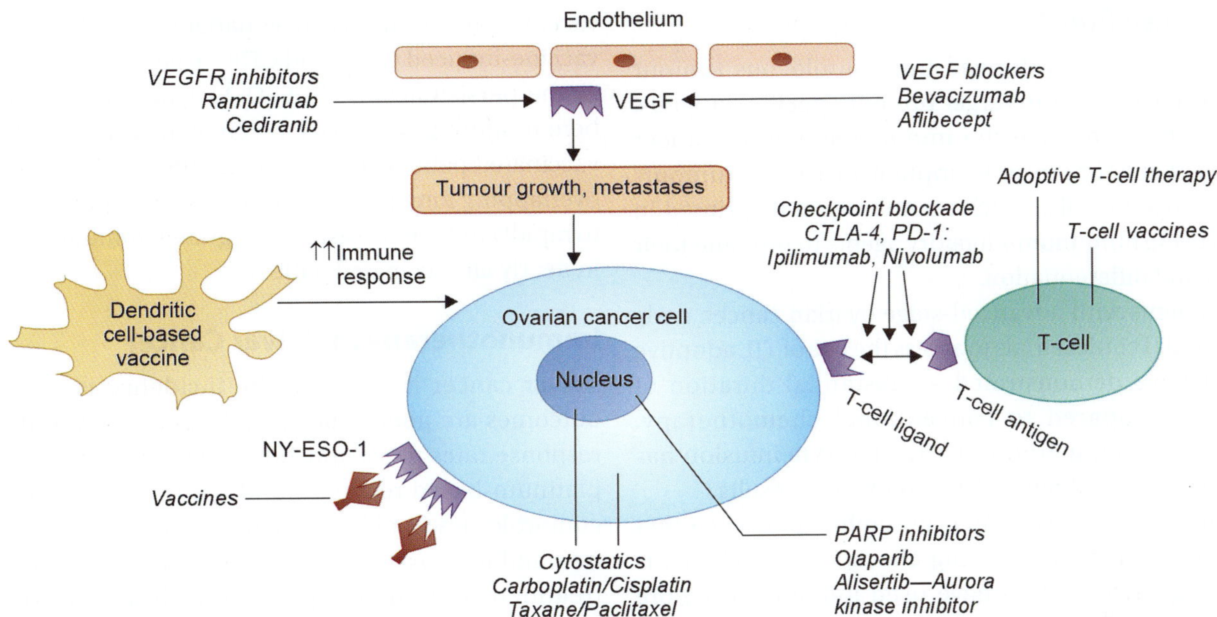

Fig. 4: Current immunotherapy approaches to ovarian cancer treatment. (CTLA-4: cytotoxic T-lymphocyte-associated protein 4; NY-ESO-1: New York oesophageal squamous cell carcinoma-1; PD-1: programmed cell death protein 1; VEGFR: vascular endothelial growth factor receptor)
Source: Siminiak N, Czepczyński R, Zaborowski MP, Iżycki D. Immunotherapy in ovarian cancer. Arch Immunol Ther Exp (Warsz). 2022;70:19.

response leading to DNA damage in BRCA1-deficient ovarian cancer cells can be enhanced by combining PARP inhibitors (such as niraparib) with pembrolizumab, the anti-PD-1 antibody in the treatment of recurrent platinum-resistant ovarian cancer.

- VEGF plays an important role in angiogenesis and dissemination in ovarian cancer. VEGF also inhibits DCs and TILs. The combination of VEGF inhibitor—bevacizumab with pembrolizumab—has been shown to be safe and effective in ovarian cancer in a phase 2 clinical study.
- Pembrolizumab in combination with pegylated liposomal doxorubicin is being evaluated in platinum-resistant ovarian cancer.

Assessing response to immunotherapy:

- *Expression of PD-L1:* The expression of PD-L1 is used as the most predictive marker to predict responsiveness to and efficacy of immunotherapy. It is measured as the percentage of tumour cells that express PD-L1 or a number of PD-L1-positive tumour cells, lymphocytes, and macrophages divided by the total number of viable tumour cells. Higher PD-L1 expression (combined positive score >10) is considered as predictive of a better response to pembrolizumab therapy in ovarian cancer. Nevertheless, the cutoff value, which may be used in ovarian cancer, is still under investigation.
- *Status of microsatellite instability:* In advanced or recurrent EC, the susceptibility to anti-PD-1 therapy is determined based on hallmarks of microsatellite instability. It leads to the increase of DNA replication errors that result in the generation of new aberrant cell surface proteins. Those neoantigens are well recognised and rejected by the host immune response. At some point, however, cancer cells suppress this effect via PD-L1 signalling. For this reason, anti-PD-1 molecules, such as dostarlimab or pembrolizumab, are effective in restoring antitumour response. The status of microsatellite instability is determined based on the immunohistochemical staining for proteins involved in mismatch repair (MLH1, PMS2, MSH2, and MSH6). This assay serves as a biomarker to identify responders to the anti-PD-1 immunotherapy. In contrast to EC, however, microsatellite instability is rare in ovarian cancer.
- *Biomarkers in peripheral blood:* The activity of cytotoxic cells was determined by measuring the expression of granzyme B in peripheral blood mononuclear cells. This assay revealed that many patients with ovarian cancer have suppressed cytotoxic responses. The effect was even more pronounced in higher-stage diseases.

Adoptive Cell Transfer

Lymphocytes, either derived from autologous tumour tissue or engineered to target tumour-specific antigens, can be infused to help the immune system of cancer patients. Leukapheresis is applied to isolate tumour-reactive effector cells, which are subsequently primed in culture using immunomodulatory agents to promote their survival and differentiation.

In patients with advanced-stage ovarian cancer, early phase I and II clinical trials to assess the use of TIL adoptive transfer have demonstrated a substantial duration of response compared to conventional chemotherapy. Furthermore, intraperitoneal T-lymphocyte infusion has also been evaluated but with less promising results.

Adoptive cell transfer (ACT) in combination with other therapeutic options, including checkpoint blockade, is also being tried. Studies have used ipilimumab before surgery to activate T-cells immune response and infusion of nivolumab after tumour resection.

Chimeric Antigen Receptor T-cell Therapies

Chimeric antigen receptor T-cells are genetically engineered, patient-derived, white blood cells, which are programmed to identify tumour cell surface antigens and activate a specific immune response. The most common target antigens in ovarian cancer CAR-T include MUC16, mesothelin, HER2 and folate receptor-alpha (FR-α). Despite the great potential of CAR T-cell therapy and its success in haematology, there are no satisfactory effects in solid tumours and ovarian cancer.

Therapeutic Cancer Vaccines

Peptide vaccines and DC therapies can activate the patient's anticancer immunity system to inhibit tumour growth and/or recurrence using modulated immune responses. Vaccines, including mutated p53 peptides, New York oesophageal squamous cell carcinoma-1 (NY-ESO-1) and mesothelin, have been investigated in ovarian cancer. Genetic abnormalities of the p53 protein are observed in most advanced ovarian cancer patients, but the p53 vaccines have not provided enough improvement in subsequent chemosensitivity or progression-free survival. The cancer testis/cancer germline antigen, named NY-ESO-1, has shown to be present in epithelial ovarian cancer and can be a potential vaccine target. Expression of NY-ESO-1 in epithelial ovarian cancer is associated with phenotypically aggressive disease. The results of NY-ESO-1 vaccination in ovarian cancer patients have demonstrated vaccine-induced CD4+ and CD8+ T-cell responses, as well as the persistence of NY-ESO-1+ lymphocytes. Survival benefit among NY-ESO-1 vaccinated compared to non-vaccinated patients is suggested. The NY-ESO-1 synthetic overlapping long peptide vaccine is shown to be safe and to rapidly induce consistent integrated immune responses in nearly all vaccinated patients.

Immunotherapy in Vulvar Cancer

Vulvar cancer is rare, but the incidence is rising, and outcomes are poor in advanced disease. Given the poor response rates to second-line chemotherapy after initial platinum-based regimens and the presence of frequent comorbidities in older patients, there is a clear need for new and less toxic therapeutic options. There are limited treatment options for patients with advanced vulvar cancer. However, several ICIs that have shown clinical benefit in certain patients are a promising therapeutic option. Pembrolizumab therapy may elicit a tumour response and potentially contribute to prolonged survival in patients with advanced, recurrent or metastatic vulvar cancer, especially when administered as second- or later-line treatment. The therapeutic efficacy of pembrolizumab may be more pronounced particularly when administered in combination with a second ICI or with chemotherapy, offering a valuable treatment modality for individuals with limited alternative therapeutic options. The role of ICIs in vulvar cancer is mainly extrapolated from trials in cutaneous squamous cell and cervical cancers.

Immunotherapy in Gestational Trophoblastic Neoplasia

Patients with low-risk gestational trophoblastic neoplasia (GTN) are likely to respond to methotrexate or actinomycin D, and, in cases of chemoresistance, the sequential use of these agents leads to high cure rates. Complete remissions with the use of pembrolizumab in polydrug treated are noted. With avelumab in low-risk GTN, human chorionic gonadotrophin (hCG) normalisation was seen in half of the patients treated. Anti-PD-1 has shown to be more effective than anti-PD-L1.

Endoglin is a co-receptor of transforming growth factor-beta (TGF-β) family and is essential for vascular remodelling. Durable remission in a refractory choriocarcinoma treated with antiendoglin monoclonal antibody and bevacizumab is reported. Increased

PD-1 expression on cytotoxic T-cells is observed with antiendoglin treatment. Combination of antiendoglin with anti-PD-L1 may throw up better results. Other pathways of PTEN and PI3K-Akt are the potential targets for study. Immunotherapy can, at the most, be considered as a third line for low-risk GTN. In high-risk patients, who require an intensive polydrug regimen, to reduce toxicity, there is a need to evaluate it as a frontline option.

It is still early days with oncoimmunotherapy and sufficient response rates are not obtained. Dysregulation of the immune system caused by this approach might result in immune-related adverse effects. Hence, when introducing immunotherapy, it is necessary to establish a suitable treatment regimen and a possible combined therapy, as well as manage the potential side effects.

IMMUNOTHERAPY IN REPRODUCTIVE MEDICINE

Immunology tries to find answers to many of the common problems that are faced in reproductive medicine, including issues with implantation, infertility, miscarriage and later pregnancy. The paradox of the foetus not being rejected by the maternal immune system where the uterus accepted a semiallogeneic graft even though the immune system had not been exposed previously to the paternal antigens found in the embryo is recognised. The role of natural killer (NK) cells, decidual macrophages, DCs, regulatory T-cells, major histocompatibility complex molecules and an array of cytokines and other immune regulators is thought of. It is known that immune mechanisms may play a role in male factor infertility.

Immunotherapy for Recurrent Pregnancy Loss

Several immunologic treatments are advocated based on evidence that pretransplant blood transfusions decreased rejection of organ allografts. The most popular attempts at maternal immunomodulation have employed transfusion of paternal leucocytes prior to conception or passive immunisation with intravenous immunoglobulin (IVIG) during pregnancy. Other interventions include third-party donor white cells or trophoblast membrane transfusions, intralipid (20% intravenous fat emulsion) and the use of growth factors such as granulocyte colony-stimulating factor (G-CSF) (filgrastim) to enhance placental and foetal growth and increase subsequent live births. The rationale for using IVIG to treat women with recurrent pregnancy loss (RPL) is based on reports that it downregulates systemic NK cells and abrogates NK cell activity at the implantation site. Immunisation with paternal white cells or third-party donor white cells is postulated to prevent miscarriage in a similar manner as pretransplant blood transfusions to improve kidney graft survival. Neither immunisation with paternal leukocytes nor treatment with IVIG are found to improve the live birth rate in women with unexplained RPL. It may be due to the fact that, presently, it is not known as to how many recurrent early pregnancy losses are the result of an embryonic or chromosomally abnormal conceptuses, anatomic or structural abnormalities and how many are embryonic or foetal deaths. It is likely that some unexplained early losses are due to yet undefined subchromosomal genetic abnormalities impairing early development of the conceptus.

Immunotherapy in Assisted Reproductive Technology

Adjuvant immunotherapy treatments in in-vitro fertilisation (IVF) aim to improve the outcome of assisted reproductive technology (ART) in both the general ART population as well as subgroups such as patients with recurrent miscarriage or implantation failure. Successful outcomes in ART cycles depend on the developmental competence of the transferred embryo(s) and endometrial receptivity. Multiple factors influence endometrial receptivity, including the hormonal preparation of the endometrium, contractility of the myometrium and the interaction between the embryo and endometrium, the latter inherently involving immunological mechanisms. In an effort to improve outcomes in ART cycles in general and in patients with recurrent implantation failure and/or pregnancy loss, adjuvant immunotherapies are introduced into IVF treatment cycles with the hope that they may correct an immunological imbalance resulting in improved and sustained implantation of the developing embryo, ultimately leading to improved live birth outcome.

Granulocyte Colony-stimulating Factor and Granulocyte/Macrophage Colony-stimulating Factor F

Discovery of granulocyte/macrophage colony-stimulating factor (GM-CSF) and G-CSF production and receptors in reproductive tissues raised hope that these cytokines supplementation of embryo cultures could improve IVF outcomes. There is no sufficient evidence to recommend for or against local G-CSF to improve endometrial thickness in women with a thin endometrium or clinical pregnancy rates with IVF.

Intravenous Fat Emulsions

Intravenous fat emulsions used for parenteral nutrition have been shown to inhibit proinflammatory mediators. In an early murine model, the rate of spontaneous abortion was significantly reduced with the administration of intravenous fat emulsions, possibly by reducing the activity of NK cells within the endometrium. There is insufficient evidence to recommend intravenous fat emulsions for infertile women pursuing IVF, as a routine.

Intravenous Immunoglobulin

Anti-inflammatory and immunomodulating properties of IVIG have been considered as a potential treatment for failed IVF and RPL given the hypothesised role of inflammatory bias in these conditions. There is insufficient evidence to recommend IVIG administration as part of IVF to improve IVF outcomes.

Adalimumab

Considerable success in the treatment of autoimmune diseases with disease-modifying agents such as adalimumab [tumour necrosis factor alpha (TNF-α) blocking antibody] raises hope that patients with abnormally high TNF secretion may benefit from treatment in conjunction with IVF. However, there is insufficient evidence to recommend to improve IVF outcome.

Peripheral Mononuclear Cells

Successful embryo implantation requires a receptive endometrium with an optimal level of local inflammation. Aberrant cell signalling leading to immune dysfunction has been implicated in implantation failure, especially in cases of repeated failed IVF-embryo transfer (ET). One possible mechanism may involve poor lymphocyte recruitment within the endometrium. Intrauterine infusion of peripheral blood mononuclear cells (PBMCs) has been investigated as a possible therapy for patients with recurrent implantation failure, based on the rationale that maternal immune cells are necessary to achieve immune tolerance to embryonic implantation and placentation. It is suggested that treatment with PBMCs may improve live birth rate in women with more than four failed transfers and those with endometrial thickness between 7 and 8 mm. However, the evidence is insufficient to recommend intrauterine infusion prior to ET to improve IVF outcome.

Seminal Plasma

Instillation of seminal plasma into the uterus and/or cervix at the time of ovum pickup for IVF in order to improve endometrial receptivity and/or immune tolerance, could as a strategy, improve pregnancy rates in fresh ET cycles. Available randomised controlled trials (RCTs) investigating the use of seminal plasma insemination have shown an insignificant increase in pregnancy rates compared to either placebo or no intervention.

Spermatozoa, Antibody-free Preparation

Antibody-free preparation of spermatozoa was a technique followed to reduce the potential impact of antisperm antibodies on fertilisation rates in couples with antisperm antibody-positive male partners, prior to the development of intracytoplasmic sperm injection (ICSI). Study with chymotrypsin–galactose treatment of sperm in patients with over 50% antisperm antibodies immunoglobulin G (IgG), immunoglobulin A (IgA) or both found improvement in fertilisation rate and apparent increase in pregnancy rate compared to the inseminations with sperm incubated in culture medium. Other researchers did not reproduce these results. With ICSI in the armamentarium, the procedure is obsolete.

Tacrolimus

The establishment of a healthy pregnancy requires maternal immune tolerance to the invading trophoblast to ensure successful implantation and adequate placentation and foetal growth. Th1 and Th2 mediate immune rejection and tolerance, with recurrent implantation failure being associated with a high peripheral blood Th1/Th2 ratio. A Th1 immune response is associated with allograft, as well as embryo rejection. Tacrolimus, an immunosuppressive drug that inhibits antigen-induced lymphocytic proliferation, cytotoxic T-cell formation, IL-2 receptor expression and the production of IL-2 and interferon gamma, was thought to be useful in treating patients with recurrent implantation failure. The treated cohorts did show significantly higher clinical pregnancy and live birth rates in a nonrandomised trial for IVF outcome.

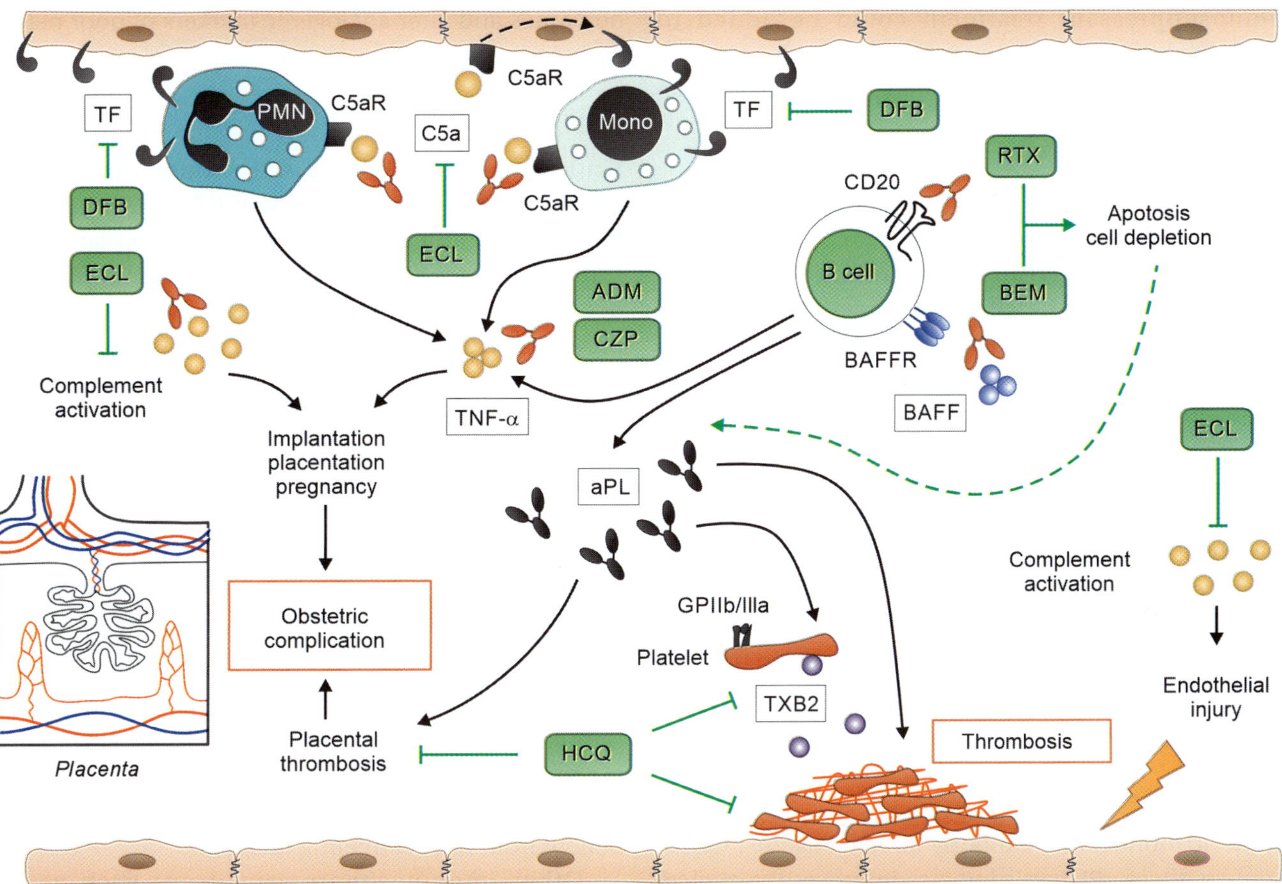

Fig. 5: Pathogenetic pathways in antiphospholipid syndrome (APS) and possible molecular targets of the immunological therapy. (ADM: adalimumab; BEM: belimumab; CZP: certolizumab; ECL: eculizumab; DFB: defibrotide; GPIIb/IIa: glycoprotein IIb/IIIa; HCQ: hydroxychloroquine; RTX: rituximab; TF: tissue factor; TXB2: thromboxane B2)
Source: Mormile I, Granata F, Punziano A, de Paulis A, Rossi FW. Immunosuppressive treatment in antiphospholipid syndrome: is it worth it? Biomedicines. 2021;9:132.

Immunotherapy in Antiphospholipid Syndrome

The antiphospholipid syndrome (APS) is characterised by the development of venous and/or arterial thrombosis and pregnancy morbidity in patients with persistent antiphospholipid antibodies (aPL). Early pregnancy losses (<10 weeks) seem to be more frequent than late foetal losses (>10 weeks). Obstetric manifestations described in APS are pre-eclampsia, eclampsia and abruptio placentae. Treatment strategies for the management of APS can be differentiated into primary thromboprophylaxis in patients with persistent aPL with no prior thrombotic events (TEs) and secondary thromboprophylaxis in patients with previous TEs.

It has been demonstrated in vitro that aPL are involved in activating endothelial cells, platelets and syncytiotrophoblast cells. The main candidate receptors for beta-2GPI on cell membranes are toll-like receptors (TLRs), apolipoprotein E receptor 2 and several cellular receptors. By investigating the role of immune cells in pathogenetic mechanisms of APS, the potential therapeutic windows have opened up. These include antiinflammatory, immunomodulatory interventions **(Fig. 5)**.

Immunotherapy is generally not recommended in APS unless required to manage the underlying autoimmune condition or treat the catastrophic variant. The suppression of the aPL titre through immunotherapy or plasmapheresis is only temporary, and it is not the main aim of the management since the role of the aPL level reduction on APS clinical manifestations is not entirely understood. Reproductive health is a critical issue whose importance is addressed by several recent publications.

Immunosuppressant treatment could be added to conventional therapy in pregnant women with recurrent foetal losses despite treatment with heparin and low-dose aspirin.

Hydroxychloroquine

Hydroxychloroquine (HCQ) is an antimalarial with immunomodulating, anti-inflammatory and antithrombotic effects. Its inflammatory action is due to the inhibition of cytosolic phospholipase A and the reduction of cytokines IL-6 and TNF-α. Therapeutic interest of HCQ for the management of APS obstetric complications is based on the premise that anti-beta2GP1 antibodies decrease trophoblastic differentiation via TLR4. Studies have shown the benefit of HCQ addition in patients with refractory obstetrical APS as demonstrated by a decrease in pregnancy losses and an increase in live births. As of now, although HCQ is not routinely recommended in patients with primary APS, it can be considered in patients with refractory APS symptoms achieving a poor outcome despite conventional therapy.

Rituximab

A chimeric monoclonal antibody directed against CD20, not only reduces aPL levels but also improves the clinical manifestation of APS. A well-documented use of rituximab in APS is the management of noncriteria manifestations. Rituximab may be an effective alternative treatment in catastrophic APS or APS patients with haematologic and/or microthrombotic manifestations when there is poor disease control with conventional therapies. Due to insufficient documentation concerning foetal safety, rituximab requires discontinuation before a planned pregnancy.

Tumour Necrosis Factor-alpha Blockers

Tumour necrosis factor-alpha is a pivotal mediator of inflammation. TNF-α antagonists can be effective in treating inflammatory disorders in which TNF-α plays a central pathogenic role. TNF-α is associated with inflammatory mechanisms related to implantation, placentation and pregnancy evolution, and it is involved in aPL-related placental injury and miscarriages. Studies have tried to evaluate the addition of certolizumab to usual treatments (a heparin agent and low-dose aspirin) in pregnant women with APS to determine whether TNF-α blockers can reduce the rate of adverse pregnancy outcomes and alter angiogenic markers of poor placental vascularisation.

Eculizumab

Eculizumab is a humanised monoclonal antibody against complement component C5, which inhibits the formation of C5a and C5b, limiting further complement activation. Evidences regarding the possible effectiveness of eculizumab on thrombotic APS are scarce. Eculizumab may be safe in pregnancy since it is not present in breast milk, and the levels observed in umbilical cord blood samples are not sufficient to affect the concentrations of complement in newborns. However, the use of eculizumab for managing obstetric complications in APS is limited to a single case report. Olendalizumab (ALXN1007) another molecule of humanised monoclonal antibody has potential for use in the treatment of primary APS since it targets the complement inflammatory pathway.

Belimumab

Belimumab is a human immunoglobulin G1-lambda monoclonal antibody that inhibits B-cell-activating factor (BAFF). A subset of patients with APS, refractory cases may benefit from BAFF-targeting therapies.

Other immunosuppressant drugs such as corticosteroids, IVIGs, azathioprine, cyclophosphamide, sirolimus and defibrotide have been previously used to treat APS patients. Lifelong anticoagulation remains the cornerstone of therapy for thrombotic APS. Immunosuppressant drugs may be a therapeutic choice in patients with refractory APS symptoms experiencing recurrent TEs despite standard therapy. Innovative therapeutic approaches targeting inflammatory and intracellular signalling pathways involved in aPL-mediated pathogenic effects have also been shown to be effective in managing non-criteria manifestations of APS and catastrophic APS, as well as refractory obstetrical complications.

Immunotherapy in Endometriosis

Endometriosis is a common disease of the female reproductive system, a benign disease with erosive growth characteristics leading to severe pelvic pain and female subfertility. Unfortunately, several aspects of the pathogenesis of endometriosis are still unclear, and the clinical therapeutic methods are unsatisfactory. The recurrence rate of endometriosis is high. Accumulating evidence suggests that the onset and development of endometriosis are closely related to the abnormal function of the female autoimmune system, especially the function of some immune cells such as the aggregation of neutrophils, abnormal differentiation of macrophages, decreased cytotoxicity of NK cells and abnormal function of T- and B-cell lines. Therefore, immunotherapy is probably a novel therapeutic strategy for endometriosis besides surgery and hormone therapy **(Flowchart 2)**.

An increasing number of studies have suggested that the medical methods targeting these immunologic factors inhibit the development of endometriosis across different aspects. Some of the interventions such as immune cell inhibitors or stabilisers (PD-1 inhibitors, loratadine), immune cytokine modulators (anti-TNF agents, IL-12 and IL-37, anti-TGF preparations, nuclear factor kappa B-targeted inhibitors), other immunomodulators such as interferon (recombinant INF-2beta), complement

Flowchart 2: Immunotherapeutic methods for endometriosis.

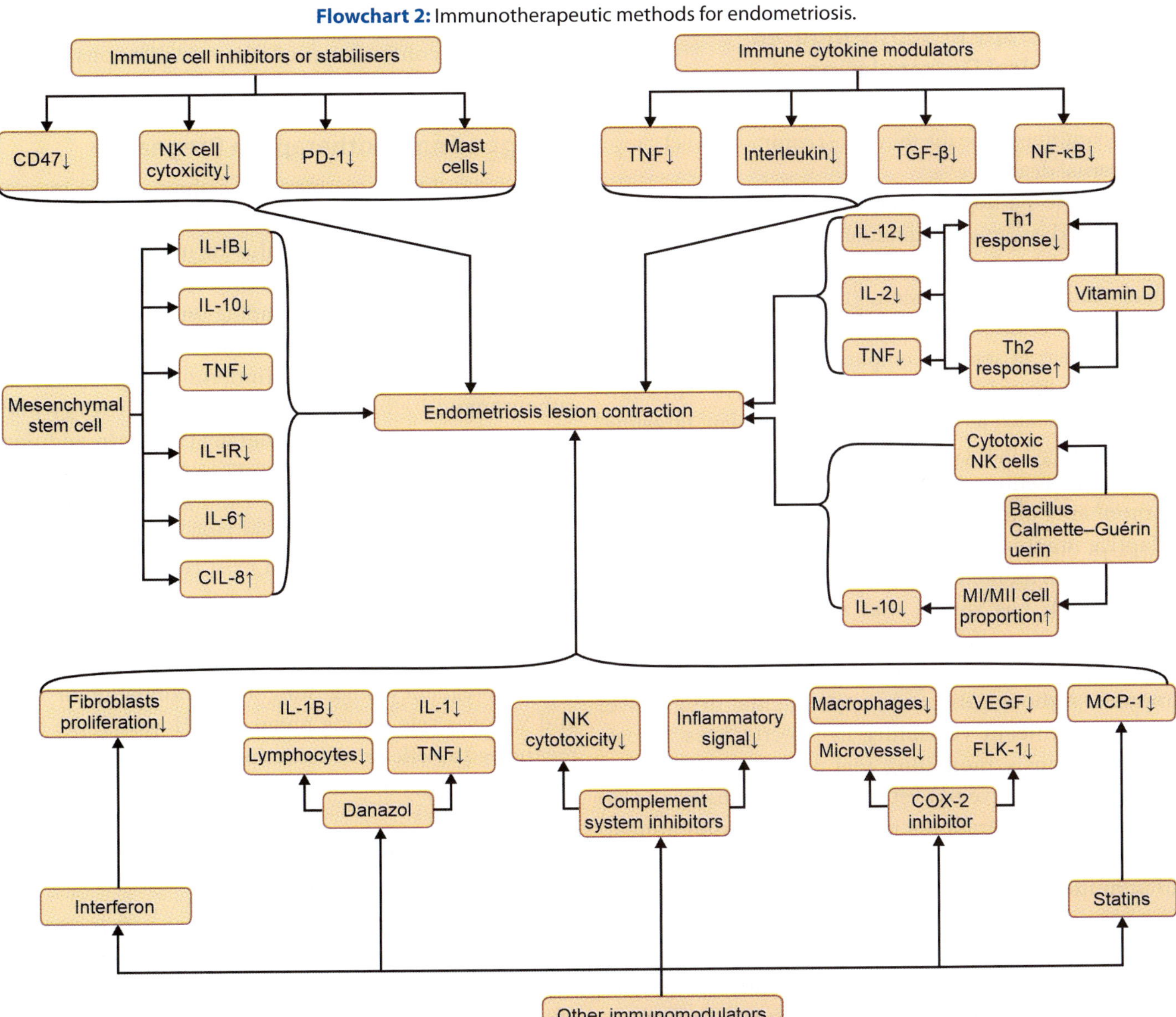

(COX-2: cyclo-oxygenase-2; IL-10: interleukin-10; NK: natural killer; PD-1: programmed cell death protein 1; TNF: tumour necrosis factor; VEGF: vascular endothelial growth factor)

Source: Li W, Lin A, Qi L, Lv X, Yan S, Xue J, et al. Immunotherapy: a promising novel endometriosis therapy. Front Immunol. 2023;14:1128301.

system inhibitors, cyclo-oxygenase-2 (COX-2) inhibitors (naproxen, diclofenac, celebrex, glycyrrhizin and puerarin), statins (atorvastatin), mesenchymal stem cells, vitamin D and Bacillus Calmette–Guérin inoculations who in some way or the other might play a role in tackling this enigmatic disease. However, information on the clinical application of immunotherapy in endometriosis is very limited, and detailed mechanisms require further investigation.

IMMUNOTHERAPY IN OTHER SITUATIONS

Immunotherapy in Sepsis-induced immunological Dysregulation

Despite advances in various sectors of living, maternal sepsis continues to be the third most common direct cause of maternal death.

The core pathophysiological mechanism of sepsis involves a dysregulated immune response characterised by acute-phase hyperinflammation followed by late-phase immune suppression, triggered by pathogens. This suggests the feasibility of immunotherapy in the management of sepsis. Compared to bundle therapies, immunotherapy can modulate disease through mechanisms such as cytokine level adjustment, targeting immune checkpoints/blocking programmed cell death and supplementing immunoglobulins. This adjusts the components and functions of the patient's innate and adaptive immune systems, thereby facilitating the rapid restoration of immune homeostasis.

Research has shown that immunotherapy offers some protective effects against the severity of disease, organ dysfunction and mortality in sepsis models in animals. Although the same experimental drugs have shown significant variability in effectiveness across different sepsis modelling techniques, some drugs found effective have not yet successfully transitioned to clinical trials. Overall, the positive results from animal studies provide preliminary indications for the potential of immunotherapy in clinical trials targeting cytokines, complements, immune checkpoints and mesenchymal stem cells **(Fig. 6)**.

Although recent research into the use of immunotherapy for treating sepsis has made preliminary progress, issues such as the therapy's stability, long-term efficacy and potential side effects remain to be validated.

IMMUNOTHERAPY IN PREGNANCY

Allergic diseases such as asthma and allergic rhinitis constitute a significant burden of disease among women of childbearing age and those who are pregnant. Autoimmune conditions also occur more often among women of childbearing age. Immunomodulating drugs are being used with increasing frequency for a variety of diseases because of their demonstrated efficacy. The other group of women are organ transplant acceptors on immunosuppressant drugs contemplating or reporting with pregnancy. Decision needs to be taken regarding initiation or continuation of these medications during pregnancy.

Allergen Immunotherapy in Pregnancy

The conventional treatment of asthma in pregnancy consists of salbutamol and inhaled corticosteroids (budesonide in particular) plus or minus long-acting beta-2 agonists, as well as theophylline and leukotriene antagonists as adjuncts, depending on severity. Another widely used modality for the treatment of asthma and allergic rhinitis is allergen immunotherapy (AIT) as subcutaneous allergen immunotherapy (SCIT) and sublingual allergen immunotherapy (SLIT). In addition to asthma and allergic rhinitis, AIT in the form of venom immunotherapy (VIT) is also commonly used for the treatment of *Hymenoptera* allergy. Despite the widespread use of AIT, however, few data exist regarding its safety in pregnancy. Existing evidence shows no significant difference in the incidence of prematurity, hypertension (HTN)/proteinuria or congenital malformations in current pregnancy, suggesting that continuation of SCIT and VIT was safe during pregnancy. However, the data regarding the effects of initiation of allergen treatment during pregnancy are scarce, and hence, it is discouraged.

Immune Modulating Therapies in Pregnancy and Lactation

Immunomodulating drugs are being used with increasing frequency for a variety of autoimmune diseases because of their demonstrated efficacy. These conditions occur more often among women of childbearing age. Optimisation of disease management in the women and the pregnancy outcomes, demands decision making about initiation

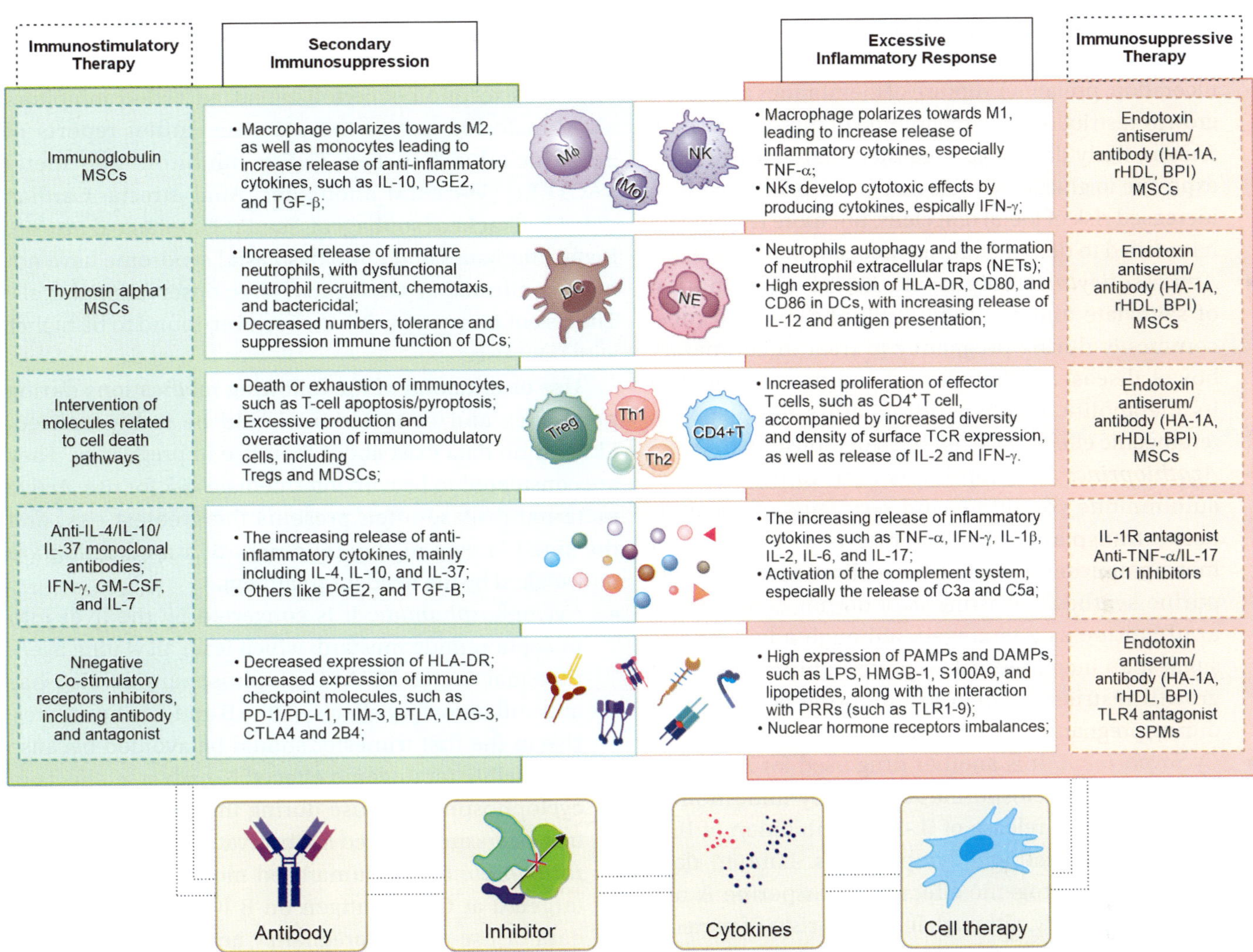

Fig. 6: Immunotherapy for sepsis: The central portion of the illustration presents alterations in immune cells and components within the host under different immune states (with excessive inflammatory responses on the right and secondary immune suppression on the left), alongside corresponding immunotherapeutic strategies. The lower section of the illustration summarizes the four primary types of immunomodulatory agents, including antibodies, inhibitors, cytokines and cellular therapies. (BPI: bactericidal/permeability-increasing protein; CTLA-4: cytotoxic T-lymphocyte-associated protein 4; GM-CSF: granulocyte-macrophage colony-stimulating factor; HA-1A: human monoclonal antiendotoxin antibody; rHDL: reconstituted high-density lipoprotein; SPMs: specialised proresolving mediators)
Source: Wu Y, Wang L, Li Y, Cao Y, Wang M, Deng Z, et al. Immunotherapy in the context of sepsis-induced immunological dysregulation. Front Immunol. 2024;15:1391395.

or continuation of these medications for them during pregnancy, without placing the foetus at undue risk.

Many commonly prescribed drugs can be used safely during pregnancy without risk of teratogenicity or pregnancy complications, whereas a few are strictly contraindicated. For immunomodulators considered appropriate to use during pregnancy, the common clinical practice of stopping their use at approximately 32 weeks of gestation because of theoretical concerns regarding the immune system of the foetus is not supported by currently available data.

- *Glucocorticoids*: Oral corticosteroids, such as prednisone, prednisolone or methylprednisolone, are recommended during pregnancy because of their conversion to relatively inactive forms by the abundance of 11β-hydroxysteroid dehydrogenase found in the human placenta. Long-term glucocorticoid treatment during pregnancy may increase the risk of HTN, pre-eclampsia, weight gain, hyperglycaemia, immunosuppression, gastrointestinal ulceration, prelabour rupture of membranes and foetal growth restriction. The magnitude of these risks is not known. Early data have suggested that first-trimester exposure to glucocorticoids may be associated with an increased risk of foetal oral clefts, but more recent data have failed to demonstrate an association.

- *Aminosalicylate*: Sulphasalazine, a combination of salicylate and a sulpha antibiotic, is used most commonly during pregnancy to treat inflammatory bowel disease. Although both sulphasalazine and its metabolite, sulphapyridine, cross the placenta, teratogenic effects have not been demonstrated.
- *Azathioprine:* Azathioprine is used to treat several autoimmune conditions and recipients of organ or tissue transplants. Azathioprine is a derivative of mercaptopurine. It blocks DNA replication and inhibits purine synthesis. Existing data do not demonstrate azathioprine as a teratogen, although a few reports suggest an increased risk of preterm birth and foetal growth restriction when azathioprine is continued during pregnancy.
- *Cyclosporine A:* It is another drug used for immunosuppression. Cyclosporine A works by inhibition of production and release of IL-2 and inhibition of IL-2 activation of resting T lymphocytes. Limited data suggest no teratogenic effect of cyclosporine A use during pregnancy, although increased risks of preterm birth and foetal growth restriction have been reported. Ophthalmic cyclosporine A does not produce detectable amounts of drug in the serum and is not expected to confer any foetal risk.
- *HCQ:* It is an antimalarial drug with anti-inflammatory effects and often is used for maintenance therapy for autoimmune conditions. Although its mechanism of action is unclear, multiple studies have demonstrated no evidence of teratogenicity. HCQ may be more effective than glucocorticoids in disease flare prevention during pregnancy and should be continued in patients using this therapy.

Immunomodulating medications, various preparations of TNF-α inhibitors, are being used in clinical practice because of their highly effective disease-modifying effects as maintenance medications for autoimmune disease. The data regarding safety of these medications are emerging, but currently available data would suggest that they can be considered as of low-risk category to continue or initiate in pregnancy. The drugs currently used are infliximab, etanercept, adalimumab, certolizumab and golimumab. With the exception of certolizumab, all TNF-α inhibitors are transferred across the placenta. Initial reports of an association between TNF-α inhibitors and foetal VACTERL (Vertebral anomalies, Anal atresia, Cardiac defects, Tracheoesophageal fistula, Esophageal atresia, Renal anomalies and Limb dysplasia) syndrome have not been confirmed in subsequent large observational trials. The risk of preterm birth was, however, found to be higher with their use.

Use or initiation of the following medications during pregnancy and/or lactation should be individualised. Little or no data exist about their use in pregnancy. They are considered to be with intermediate risk for use. Active maternal disease often presents the greatest risk, and the small known or theoretic risks of a medication are outweighed by the need for treatment.

- *Cyclophosphamide:* It is converted by the liver into phosphoramide mustard, which is an alkylating agent that inactivates DNA. Cyclophosphamide also has anti-inflammatory effects on the B and T lymphocytes. Use in the first trimester should be avoided because of possible teratogenic effects. No adverse effects of cyclophosphamide use during the second and third trimesters are reported in observational studies.
- *Rituximab:* It is a humanised monoclonal antibody targeted at CD20 antigen on B lymphocytes. Safety data of use during pregnancy and 6 months before pregnancy are limited. Safety of rituximab during lactation is not studied.
- *Belimumab:* It is an inhibitor of B-lymphocyte survival as well as B-cell conversion to immunoglobulin-secreting cells. A single case report of use during pregnancy describes good disease control of systemic lupus erythematosus but mild Ebstein's anomaly in the infant.

The following are the high-risk medications and are typically not continued or initiated in pregnancy:

- *Methotrexate:* It is commonly used to provide long-term maintenance immunosuppression in patients with autoimmune conditions. Its use during pregnancy is contraindicated because of abortogenic and teratogenic effects. It is suggested that women delay pregnancy for 1–3 months after discontinuation of methotrexate because of persistence of drug for up to 4 months in the liver.

- *Mycophenolate:* It is frequently used as maintenance therapy in patients with lupus nephritis. It works by inhibition of purine biosynthesis. It is abortogenic and teratogenic and is associated with cleft lip and palate, micrognathia, microtia and auditory canal abnormalities. It is better to delay pregnancy for at least 6 weeks after discontinuing mycophenolate.
- *Leflunomide:* It works by inhibition of dihydroorotate dehydrogenase, an enzyme necessary for pyrimidine biosynthesis. It is routinely used to treat inflammatory arthritis and lupus-related skin manifestations. Use is contraindicated during pregnancy because of its teratogenic effects of facial malformations. The metabolite of leflunomide, teriflunomide, remains detectable as long as 2 years after drug discontinuation.

Breastfeeding and Infant Considerations

The amount of medication transmitted into breast milk and the potential effect on the neonate are important considerations when the use of immunomodulating drugs is being considered for women who are lactating. In general, immunomodulating drugs that are not contraindicated in pregnancy are compatible with breastfeeding. Data describing the amount of immunomodulators that are detectable in breast milk are limited. It is unlikely that these medications are present at any significant level in breast milk, if they are detectable. However, the concern exists that the immune system of infants born to women who received immunomodulating therapies during pregnancy or while breastfeeding might be negatively affected.

It is critical that counselling should occur in the prepregnancy and interpregnancy periods to review the individual risks and benefits as they relate to disease management and pregnancy-associated risks with high-risk medication. There may be selected circumstances when continued treatment is the safest option.

Immunotherapy is rapidly evolving as the therapeutic entity against a variety of disease conditions, including cancers. Advancement in the field is highly dependent on a better understanding of the immune system and the advent of newer agents. However, like any other therapeutic modality, it has its own set of adverse effects and toxicities. Therapeutic enhancement of immune response itself may lead to autoimmune disorders. Cardiotoxicity with use of ICIs and CAR T-cell therapy, dermatological toxicities, thyroid disorders, paraneoplastic neurological syndromes and even emergence of ovarian cancer call for patient and physician education when initiating therapy. Immunotherapy is still in its infancy, with a better understanding of the working of immune system and as specific therapies are standardised, the ratio of benefits to risks may increase significantly.

SUGGESTED READING

1. Naing A, Hajjar J (Eds). Immunotherapy, 4th edition. Cham: Springer; 2021. p. 447.
2. Rich RR, Fleisher TA, Schroeder HW, Weyand CM, Corry DB, Jennifer M, et al. (Eds). Clinical Immunology: Principles and Practice, 6th edition. Amsterdam: Elsevier; 2022. p. 1344.

39 CHAPTER

Amenorrhoea, Hypomenorrhoea, and Oligomenorrhoea

Pratik Tambe, Muralidhar V Pai

Chapter Outline

- Amenorrhoea
- Aetiology
- Treatment
- Hypomenorrhoea
- Oligomenorrhoea

INTRODUCTION

Menstrual irregularities are some of the commonest complaints that women present with. Irregular periods, delayed periods and scanty bleeding may appear innocuous but may obfuscate and conceal a deeper endocrinological, genetic or extensive infectious pathology which need thorough investigation. In this chapter, we tackle the common and rarer causes of amenorrhoea, hypomenorrhoea and oligomenorrhoea which are encountered in day to day clinical practice.

AMENORRHOEA

Amenorrhoea means *without menstruation*. Primary amenorrhoea is the absence of menstruation by 16 years of age in the presence of normal secondary sexual characteristics or by 14 years of age if secondary sexual characteristics have not developed. Secondary amenorrhoea is the absence of menstruation for three normal cycles or for 6 months. Any woman who complains of amenorrhoea may be suffering from either of the following:

- *False amenorrhoea:* In this condition, menstruation is taking place but the patient is unaware of it because the outflow is obstructed at the level of the cervix, vagina or vulva. This is hidden menstruation or *cryptomenorrhoea* and has already been considered in Chapters 13 and 15.
- *True amenorrhoea:* This condition is the subject of this chapter. It is one in which the menstrual function is suppressed, and the explanation may be physiological or pathological.

AETIOLOGY

Physiological Amenorrhoea

Before Puberty

Amenorrhoea is normal during childhood and is explained mainly by a low output of gonadotropin-releasing factor(s). Menstruation is usually established by the age of 16 years but may not appear until the age of 18 years (and sometimes later) without there being an abnormality (constitutional amenorrhoea).

Adolescence

Initial menstrual cycles are often anovulatory and therefore irregular. Periods of amenorrhoea lasting 2–12 months during the first 1–2 years after the menarche are so common that they should be regarded as normal. They occur in 20% of girls without subsequent ill effect on their fertility.

Pregnancy

Pregnancy is the most common cause of secondary amenorrhoea, and suppression of menstruation is the leading symptom of early pregnancy. The amenorrhoea is caused by a continuous production of large quantities of oestrogen and progesterone by the chorion. Therefore, it is important to rule out pregnancy as a cause of secondary amenorrhoea before proceeding to further investigations **(Flowchart 1)**.

Lactation

Menstruation is suppressed for varying periods after abortion and labour, but especially by lactation when

Flowchart 1: Pregnancy test in a case of secondary amenorrhoea.

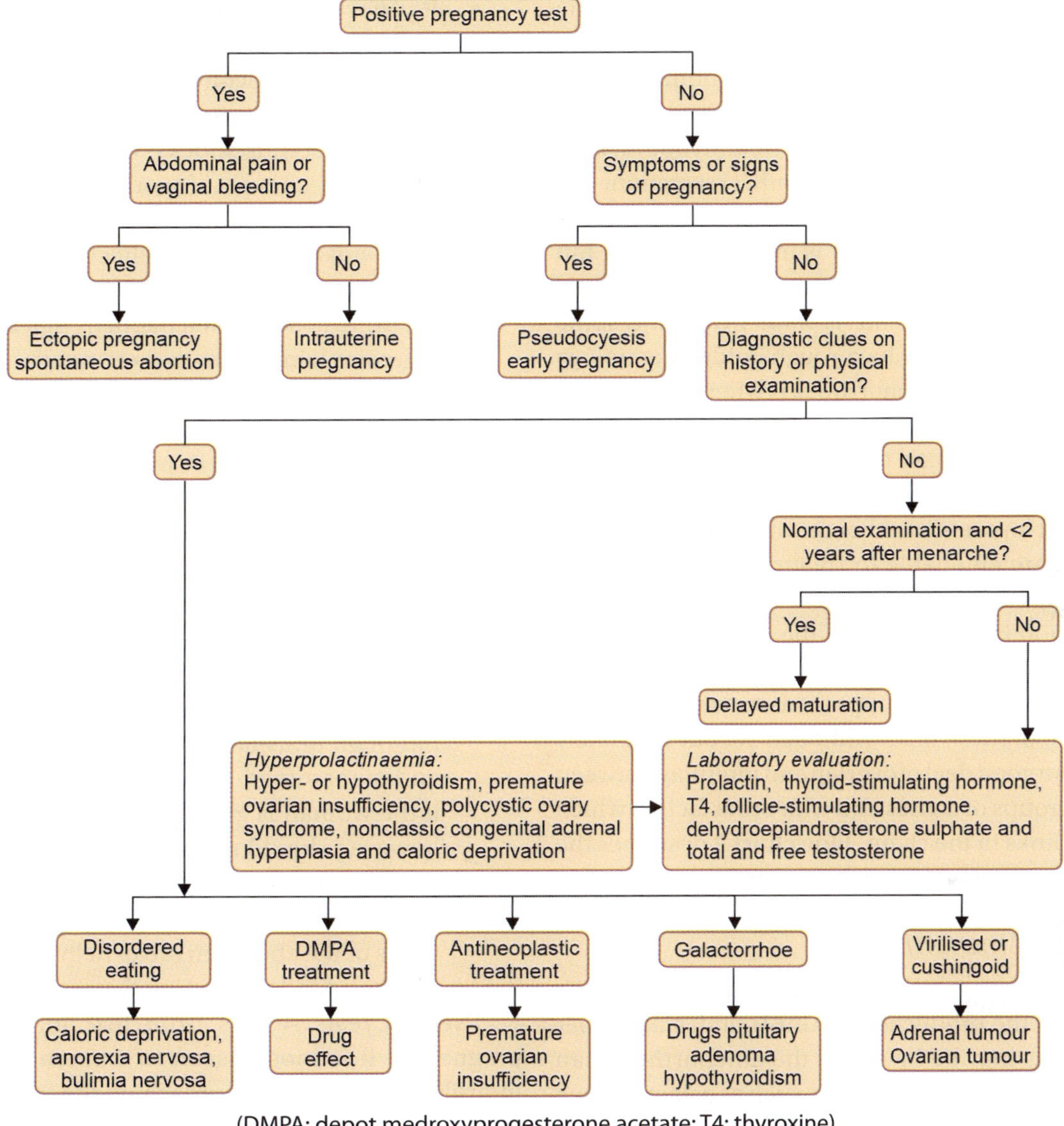

(DMPA: depot medroxyprogesterone acetate; T4: thyroxine)

the hypothalamic-pituitary system concentrates on the production of prolactin rather than gonadotropins.

Menopause

The menopause comes about because the ovaries cease to react to the gonadotropic stimulus when all their Graafian follicles have disappeared. It occurs usually between the ages of 45 and 55 years and can occasionally occur naturally before the age of 40 years, viz. in case of premature ovarian insufficiency. Periods of physiological amenorrhoea lasting 3–6 months often precede the menopause itself.

Pathological Amenorrhoea

Three types are given as follows:

1. Amenorrhoea without secondary sexual characteristics
2. Amenorrhoea with secondary sexual characteristics and anatomic abnormalities
3. Amenorrhoea with secondary sexual characteristics and nonanatomic causes.

In order to detect the cause of amenorrhoea, it is useful to determine whether secondary sexual characteristics are present. The absence of secondary sexual characteristics indicates that a woman has never been exposed to oestrogen stimulation. If the secondary sexual characteristics are present, i.e. when the findings of the physical examination are normal, anatomic abnormalities may still be considered. If the secondary sexual characteristics are present with nonanatomic causes, it could be connected to ovarian failure, pituitary and hypothalamic lesions, and abnormal hypothalamic gonadotrophin-releasing hormone (GnRH) secretion.

Amenorrhoea is a symptom, not a disease, and has a variety of causes. A complete list is impossible here, but groups of causes can usefully be recognised. The division of amenorrhoea into *primary* and *secondary* types has some clinical value in that it may be a rough guide to aetiology and prognosis. Primary amenorrhoea is when a female has never had menses. Secondary amenorrhoea, for example, is more likely than primary to be the result of pregnancy or acquired disease; it is less likely to be caused by a gross error in the development of either the uterus or ovaries and is therefore more amenable to treatment. Nevertheless, the possible causes of both types are essentially the same.

Menstruation is dependent on the proper functioning of a chain made up of hypothalamus → pituitary → ovary → uterus; amenorrhoea presupposes a weakening or break in one or more of these links. Although set out separately below, there is a good deal of overlap and interplay between the different groups of causes and with other factors which influence the links in the chain. **Flowchart 2** describes the approach to a patient with primary amenorrhoea.

Hypothalamic Amenorrhoea

Disturbances of the hypothalamus cause amenorrhoea by interfering with the production of GnRH and, since other releasing factors may be involved, the amenorrhoea can be accompanied by other symptoms such as galactorrhoea and errors in physical growth. The hypothalamus has centres controlling appetite and metabolism, so overeating, undereating, obesity or wasting, and faults in fluid balance can be associated with suppression of menstruation. The consequence is that amenorrhoea is a feature of syndromes such as *pituitary infantilism*, Chiari–Frommel and Forbes syndromes (*see* Chapter 11) and dystrophia adiposogenitalis (*Frohlich's syndrome*). In the last, genital hypoplasia is combined with obesity and sleepiness.

Upsets in hypothalamic function can be caused by the following:

- *Disease or injury in the region of the midbrain:* These include encephalitis, meningitis, tumours and fractures of the base of the skull.
- *Cerebral cortex influences:*
    - *Psychoses*: Amenorrhoea is a common feature of depressive mental disorders and is also seen following electroconvulsive therapy.
    - *Emotional upsets and stresses*: Examples of these include nervous shocks, the death of a friend or relative, a change of work or abode, separation from close acquaintances, travel abroad, a love affair and marriage. The effect of nervous tensions is seen not only in causing amenorrhoea but also in curing it. So, it often happens that a woman with this complaint begins to menstruate spontaneously on the day she has planned to take medical advice.
    - *Pseudocyesis*: In this rare condition, a woman imagines that she is pregnant and accordingly suppresses her menstrual function and develops other symptoms and signs of pregnancy such as nausea and vomiting, breast changes, increase in weight and swelling of the abdomen. She may even allege that she can feel foetal movements and, ultimately, that she is in labour. The enlargement of the abdomen is *not* the result of gaseous distension but of an unusual use of the muscles of the trunk and an assumed lordosis; it therefore disappears if the woman is given a general anaesthetic. This, however, should not be necessary to demonstrate that the tumour is a phantom; resonance on percussion is conclusive evidence. Ultrasonic views of the abdomen are of help in confirming the diagnosis and convincing the patient.

  Pseudocyesis results from fear of, or desire for, pregnancy. It is mostly seen in women suffering from infertility and in those approaching the menopause, who either see their last chance of conception disappearing or suddenly realise what an embarrassment another pregnancy at that age would be.

  The syndrome is not always complete, and amenorrhoea can occur without other clinical manifestations. Moreover, in most cases, menstruation is not entirely suppressed, and the patient will, under pressure, admit to scanty cyclical losses.
    - Anorexia nervosa
    - Polycystic ovary syndrome (PCOS)
- *Drugs:* These include the phenothiazine derivatives, reserpine and ganglion-blocking agents, all of which affect the hypothalamus by reducing the prolactin-inhibiting factor (PIF) levels, thereby resulting in an elevated prolactin level. Amenorrhoea is also seen

Flowchart 2: Approach to a patient with primary amenorrhoea.

- Primary amenorrhoea
  - Normal secondary sexual characteristics
    - Pelvic USG
      - Uterus absent
        - Karyotype
          - 46,XX → Müllerian agenesis
          - 46,XY → Androgen insensitivity syndrome
      - Uterus present
        - Outflow tract obstruction
        - Normal anatomy
          - FSH/LH/prolactin estimation
            - Normal → Hypothalamic
            - Elevated LH/FSH → PCOS
            - FSH ↑ LH ↑ → Resistant ovary
            - Prolactin ↑ → Hyperprolactinaemia
  - Poor/absent secondary sexual characteristics
    - Height
      - Normal
        - FSH/LH
          - Low → Hypogonadotropic hypogonadism
          - High
            - Karyotype
              - 46,XX → Primary ovarian/failure resistant ovary gonadal agenesis
              - 46,XY → Androgen insensitivity testicular feminization syndrome
      - Short
        - FSH/LH
          - Low → Hypothalamic–pituitary dysfunction and intracranial lesions
          - High
            - Karyotype
              - 45,XO 45,XO/46,XX → Gonadal dysgenesis

(FSH: follicle-stimulating hormone; LH: luteinising hormone; PCOS: polycystic ovary syndrome; USG: ultrasonography)

with drug addiction of various types and with certain chemotherapeutic agents, especially alkylating agents.

The most important of the drugs which cause amenorrhoea, sometimes with galactorrhoea, are the *oestrogen–progestogen oral contraceptives*, which can produce what is called the *oversuppressive syndrome or postpill amenorrhoea*. The occurrence is not related to the length of time during which the woman has taken the pill; it seems that some women have a hypothalamic–pituitary system which is unusually sensitive to the inhibition which these hormones provide. Although many women experience a brief delay in the onset of menstruation after they stop the pill, only a small proportion develop secondary amenorrhoea of 6 months' duration. Approximately 80% of women resume a normal menstrual pattern within 3 months of stopping the pill and 95–98% are ovulating regularly within 1 year. The degree of risk involved in developing postpill amenorrhoea of at least 6 months' duration is estimated at <1%. In some women, it is recognised that the amenorrhoea which follows stopping taking the pill is merely a stage in the progression of a previous oligomenorrhoea.

Although the amenorrhoea associated with the taking of oral contraceptives is assumed to be due to the suppression of hypothalamic–pituitary function, an organic change must be excluded for certain **(Figs. 1A and B)**. Certainly, care is necessary in excluding other causes. It has been shown that whenever a diagnosis of postpill amenorrhoea (of 6 months or longer) is made, there is a 10% chance of missing premature ovarian failure, a 20% chance of missing hyperprolactinaemia and a 30% chance of missing weight-related amenorrhoea.

While amenorrhoea persists, the levels of follicle-stimulating hormone (FSH), luteinising hormone (LH) and oestrogens in body fluids are low and the ovaries are inactive.

Spontaneous cure is the outcome in 25% of cases, and this can happen even after 1 year; it is recorded as late as after 6 years. Otherwise, ovulation and menstruation can be induced artificially and pregnancy can result. Thereafter, menstruation sometimes returns but not always.

Pituitary Amenorrhoea

True pituitary amenorrhoea is not common and when it occurs, it can be accompanied by other evidence of disturbed pituitary function. An *isolated pituitary gonadotropin deficiency syndrome* is described, but its one symptom of amenorrhoea can be cured by administering GnRH, so it now appears that the trouble is in the hypothalamus.

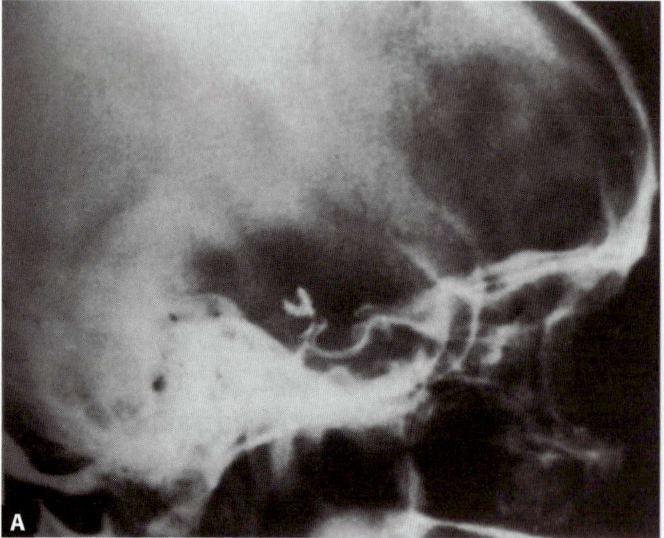

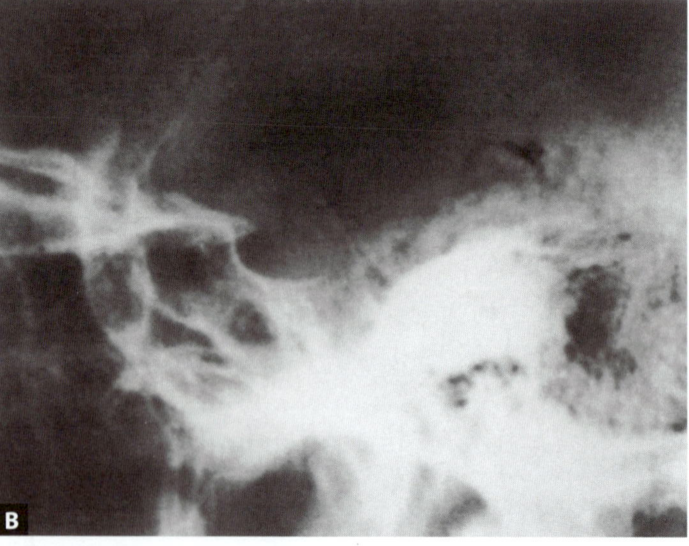

Figs. 1A and B: Diseases of the midbrain and pituitary causing amenorrhoea without other symptoms. (A) A craniopharyngioma causing primary amenorrhoea in a woman aged 25 years. The lesion is indicated by the area of calcification just above and behind the posterior clinoid process, the patient facing to the right; (B) A probable pituitary tumour indicated by enlargement of the pituitary fossa and destruction of the posterior clinoid processes, the patient facing to the left. In this case, a parous woman complained of secondary amenorrhoea following the taking of an oestrogen–progestogen contraceptive pill for 3 years. Until this radiograph was taken, it was assumed that the amenorrhoea was the result of continued inhibition of the hypothalamus following the therapy.

Upsets in the function of the anterior pituitary can be caused by the following:

- *Tumours in or near the pituitary gland:* It is now recognised that pituitary adenomas are more common than originally thought because of the sophisticated methods available to diagnose them.

  The clinical effects depend on tumour size, rate of growth and hormonal secretion, but endocrinological symptoms such as amenorrhoea appear long before the neurological symptoms **(Figs. 1A and 2A and 2B)**. In about three quarters of these adenomas, there is an excess production of prolactin, but growth hormone may be produced in excess leading to acromegaly. In general, tumours outside the pituitary fossa will produce neurological symptoms before endocrine abnormalities. Progressive lesions (tumours, granulomas or infections) will impair both pituitary and hypothalamic function in time. One condition which has to be excluded when looking for a pituitary microadenoma is an empty sella turcica in which the amenorrhoea is due to hypopituitary function.
- *Disease of the anterior pituitary*: Any destructive disease can reduce or eliminate the gonadotropic and other functions of the gland to produce a clinical picture similar to that of *Sheehan's syndrome*. This syndrome, however, is characteristically caused by ischaemic necrosis of most of the anterior pituitary which results from spasm in its arterioles occurring at the time of severe haemorrhage or shock (usually postpartum) complicating childbirth.

  This peculiar reaction to shock is hardly ever seen except in the parturient woman and in explanation it is suggested that normally during labour, the blood supply to the pituitary gland is modified to the advantage of the posterior lobe and disadvantage of the anterior lobe. When spasm occurs, therefore the posterior lobe is protected and the anterior lobe is vulnerable. The risk of this ischaemic injury occurring in women suffering postpartum haemorrhage and shock depends on the speed and efficiency with which blood loss is controlled and replaced. Nevertheless, even where maternity services are highly developed, it is reckoned that 4% of women who lose >800 mL of blood in the third or fourth stages of labour suffer some degree of damage to the anterior pituitary. The figures rise to 8% for moderate and 50% for severe postpartum haemorrhage and shock.

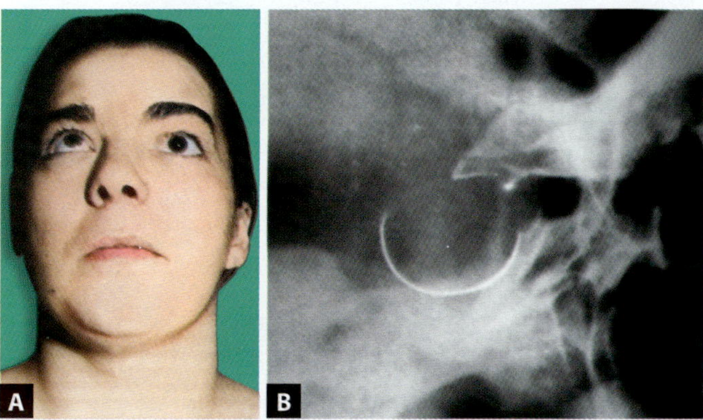

Figs. 2A and B: A pituitary tumour causing amenorrhoea for 9 months in a primipara aged 24 years. She had been given oestrogens which produced cyclical uterine bleeding and had also been treated by an ophthalmologist for defective vision. (A) Examination revealed fixation of the left eye and swelling of the lower lid; (B) Radiological examination of the skull showed a grossly enlarged sella turcica with so much erosion of the bones that the outline of the fossa is shown here in white ink. The patient is facing to the right.

In the fully developed syndrome (Simmond's) which is only seen when 95% of the anterior pituitary is destroyed, all functions—lactogenic, gonadotropic, thyrotropic, corticotropic and somatotropic—are impaired. Lactation does not occur after the causal delivery, and later there develop amenorrhoea, loss of libido and evidence of hypothyroidism, although the blood cholesterol level usually remains normal. The woman becomes sensitive to cold and is apathetic; hence in cold climates, she sits by the fire and develops severe *erythema ab igne*. Insulin tolerance is reduced and spontaneous hypoglycaemia is common.

Acute crises can develop and coma may be caused by hypoglycaemia, hypothermia and hypothyroidism; death under anaesthesia is used to be common.

Signs of adrenal cortical failure include absence of axillary sweating, loss of axillary and pubic hair, and decrease in skin pigmentation. The last mainly accounts for the striking pallor of these women, but they also have a moderate degree of anaemia which is caused by lack of the pituitary erythropoietic factor. There is no significant decrease in weight.

The plasma levels of FSH, LH, thyroid-stimulating hormone (TSH), adrenocorticotropic hormone (ACTH), oestrogens, and urinary 17-keto- and ketogenic steroids are considerably reduced and may be negligible. All the genital organs show extreme atrophy; the uterus becomes smaller than it does in the normal postmenopausal state.

Although dormant, the ovaries retain their ova until the natural age of the menopause, when they disappear. Meanwhile, however, they respond readily to gonadotropin therapy to result in ovulation, menstruation and conception. If the woman has another pregnancy as a result of such treatment, it seems sometimes to lead to an improvement of pituitary function afterwards.

Less extensive destruction of the anterior pituitary can lead to an incomplete, or delayed, onset of Sheehan's syndrome. In such a case, lactation may not fail, and menstruation may continue regularly or intermittently for several years after the causal childbirth. Weakness and apathy are often the only complaints, but the clinical features and hormone levels are directly related to the amount of remaining functional pituitary tissue.

Ovarian Amenorrhoea

In this group, the hormonal disturbance causing amenorrhoea appears to arise primarily in the ovary.

- *Underproduction of oestrogen and progesterone (hypergonadotropic amenorrhoea):* An obvious example of this mechanism is the amenorrhoea which follows surgical removal of both ovaries or exposure of the follicular apparatus to radiation or sometimes after chemotherapy, especially with alkylating agents. The natural menopause itself is another illustration of primary ovarian failure, and there are cases of ovaries which are resistant to gonadotropic stimuli (resistant ovary syndrome). In these patients, follicles are present deep within the ovary and can be demonstrated either by ultrasound or by a full-thickness biopsy at laparotomy. Premature ovarian failure is associated with other autoimmune diseases.

  The ovary, although present, may never develop a capacity to respond to the gonadotropin stimulus or, having very few ova, may do so for only a few years or intermittently. This usually betokens an abnormal sex chromosome pattern such as 47, XXX, 46, XX/45, XO or deletion of fragments and isochromosomes. More commonly, however, unreactive gonads are *streak* or even testes in an apparent woman (see Chapter 14). Thirty percent of all women presenting with *primary* amenorrhoea have demonstrable chromosome anomalies; if those who have another obvious cause for their symptom are excluded, the figure is 40–45%. Rarely, patients with galactosaemia may have fewer oogonia because of the effect of galactose on germ cell migration; they may also have defective carbohydrate moieties which render the FSH and LH inactive.
- *Continuous production of oestrogen and progesterone:* Menstruation depends on the cyclical withdrawal of steroid hormones so when these are produced continuously rather than intermittently, amenorrhoea can result. There may, therefore, be an amenorrhoeic phase in cases of follicular cysts, persisting luteal cysts, and granulosa and theca cell tumours. Amenorrhoea in the woman who has previously had a trophoblastic tumour means persisting or renewed trophoblastic activity with luteinisation of the ovaries.
- *Overproduction of androgens:* Androgens inhibit endometrial and follicular activity, so masculinising tumours of the ovary cause amenorrhoea, usually of the secondary variety. This is accompanied by other signs of virilism.
- *PCOS:* The oestrogen, progesterone and androgen normally produced by the ovary are chemically interchangeable, androgens being intermediate products in the biosynthesis of oestradiol. Ovarian metabolic errors may therefore explain certain anomalies in hormone production which are associated with amenorrhoea.

The best example is the PCOS. In this, the patient typically complains of amenorrhoea or oligomenorrhoea, is infertile and has slightly enlarged and polycystic ovaries which have a smooth pearly coloured and thickened capsule. There is a failure to ovulate, the follicles becoming cystic and showing, on section, hyperplasia of the theca interna **(Figs. 3 and 4)**. The syndrome is seen in the second and third decades of life and, in about 50% of cases,

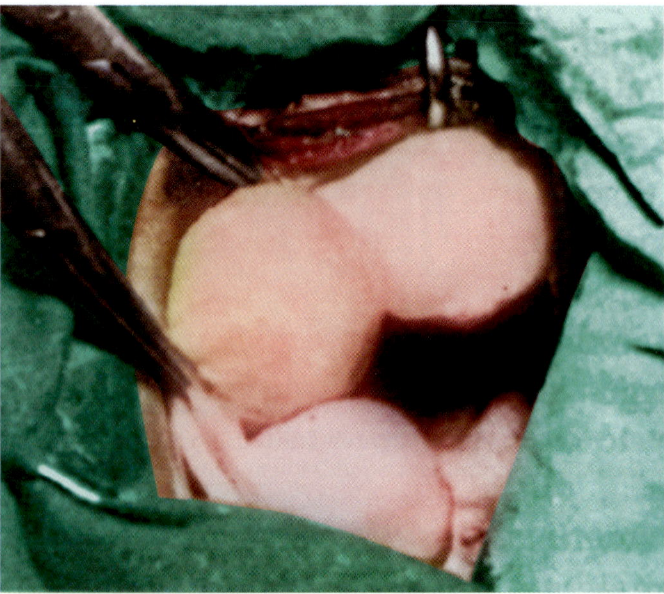

Fig. 3: The large, pale, thin-coated ovaries, typical of the polycystic ovary syndrome lying on either side of the fundus of the uterus at the time of laparotomy.

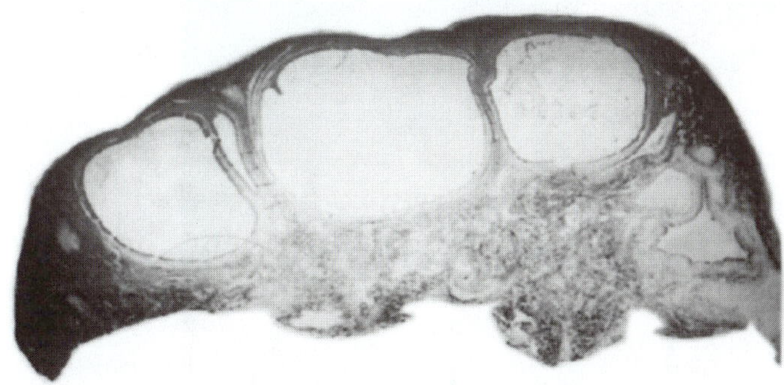

Fig. 4: A slice of the ovarian cortex of a polycystic ovary.
Source: Reproduced with permission from Dr KV Bailey, J Obstet Gynaecol Br Emp.

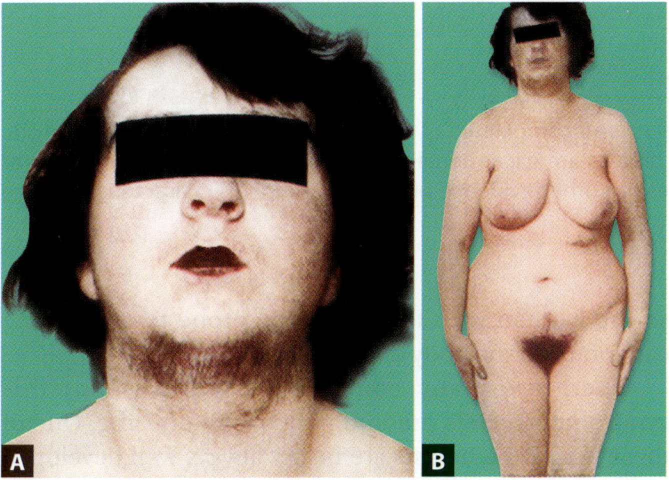

Figs. 5A and B: The polycystic ovary syndrome. This girl, aged 18 years, complained of secondary amenorrhoea and facial hirsutism. She was also overweight, with good breast development. Menstruation returned after wedge resection of polycystic ovaries which is no longer practiced in modern medicine.

includes obesity, hirsutism and acne. Hyperinsulinaemia is associated. The lipoprotein pattern is similar to that in males. These patients are at an increased risk of endometrial and breast cancer, cardiovascular disease and diabetes mellitus as a long-term consequence of androgen excess associated with PCOS. Advances in ultrasound have improved the diagnosis of PCOS **(Figs. 5A and B)** which is found to be prevalent in up to 20% of normal women but in up to 60% of women with hirsutism, acne and menstrual disturbances. However, ultrasonography is not mandatory for the diagnosis of PCOS—clinical and biochemical evidence of androgen excess may be sufficient for the same.

It is supposed that hyperthecosis is related to an overproduction of androgens which reduces granulosa cell proliferation and maturation, as well as stimulating fibrosis of the surrounding stroma and capsule. In fact, there are no specific histological features which characterise the ovary in PCOS. Follicular as well as theca lutein cysts may be present; moreover, ripening follicles and occasionally an active corpus luteum can be found **(Figs. 6A to C)**. This means that ovulation may occur intermittently, despite the thick capsule.

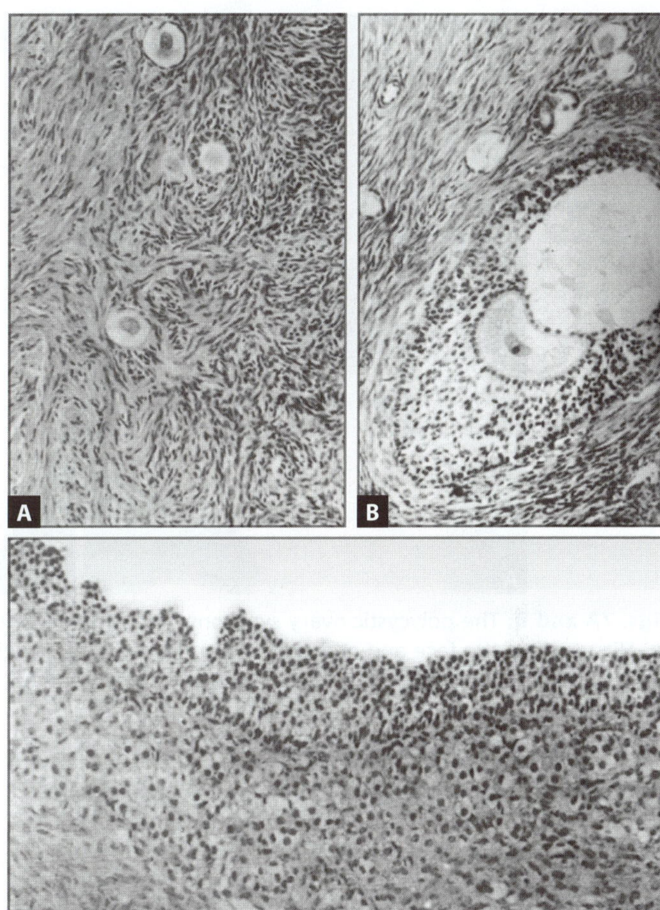

Figs. 6A to C: The variable microscopic appearances of the ovary in the polycystic ovary syndrome. The three sections illustrated were obtained from the same ovary of a woman whose oligomenorrhoea and infertility appeared to be cured by wedge resection of polycystic ovaries. (A) Normal primordial and primary follicles in masses of theca tissue; (B) A ripening Graafian follicle; (C) The wall of one of the cysts lined by granulosa cells with theca outside; the latter shows evidence of luteinisation.
Source: By permission of the Editor, Am J Obstet Gynecol.

Irrespective of the microscopic appearances, however, it is clearly established that there is no defect in the hypothalamic-pituitary-ovarian axis. Normal function is, however, masked by inhibition of ovarian follicular

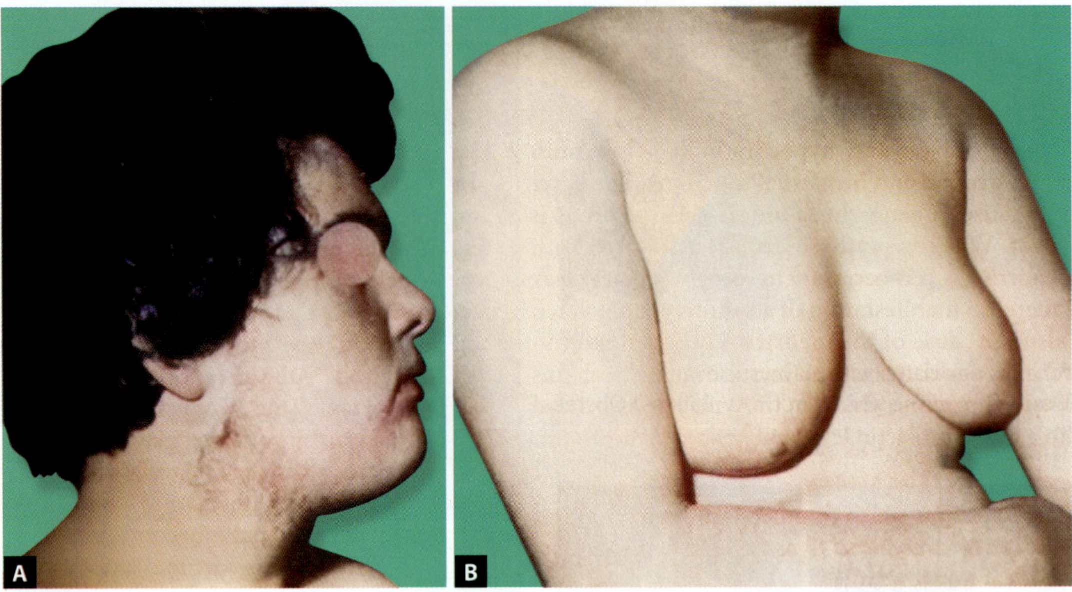

Figs. 7A and B: The polycystic ovary syndrome in a girl aged 12 years who complained of secondary amenorrhoea and hirsutism. (A) Hirsutism of the face and neck; (B) The arms are hairy, but the breasts are exceptionally well developed with a suggestion of Montgomery's tubercles on the areola. Good bust development, despite other evidence of defeminisation, is characteristic of the syndrome (see text).
Source: By permission of the Editor, Am J Obstet Gynecol.

development and inappropriate feedback to the pituitary. The high oestrogen production is largely due to the conversion of androgens to oestrogen in the ovary and peripherally. This causes an increase in LH and a decrease in FSH, the LH level being multiple times the FSH level on day 2 of the cycle. A vicious circle is established, for the increase in LH induces thecal hyperplasia and increased androgen synthesis in the ovary.

High levels of androgen result in an increase in the peripheral production of oestrogen and a reduction in the sex hormone-binding globulin. This leads to an increased level of free androgens to produce hirsutism and to be converted to oestrogens. There is also anovulation as a result of the effect of the androgens on follicular maturation. The degree of hyperandrogenism is proportional to the degree of hyperinsulinaemia. Another consequence of the raised oestrogen levels is the target organ effect on adipose tissue formation and endometrial hyperplasia.

As might be expected from the above, the vagina and the uterus do not show signs of atrophy, despite the amenorrhoea. Vaginal cytology and endometrial histology can show evidence of high or low oestrogen production. The endometrium is sometimes unstimulated, occasionally secretory and sometimes hyperplastic. In the latter circumstance, atypical hyperplasia can be found, so the woman with PCOS may be prone to developing carcinoma of the body of the uterus.

There are many conflicting features about this syndrome which is predominantly defeminising. One of these is that the breasts are nearly always well developed and, quite often, they show areolar and other changes which mimic those seen in pregnancy **(Figs. 5 and 7A and B)**. These, associated as they generally are with episodes of amenorrhoea, often give rise to a clinical suspicion that the woman has conceived.

Although we have a greater knowledge and understanding of the hormonal effects, the cause of the PCOS remains unknown. It is accepted as a clinical entity, but the starting point in the circle of endocrine disturbances is debatable. It is suggested that there may be a disturbance of adrenocortical function in the prepubertal and postpubertal phases of life initially, followed by a shift to ovarian dominance which is associated with a noncyclical pattern of ovarian function. The end result would be the increased androgen production in the ovary and the increased peripheral (nonovarian) production of oestrogen. Another suggestion has been that there is a familial or genetic role in some cases.

The clinical picture and possible causes of the syndrome are so variable that there is good reason to doubt its being a clinical entity or, at least, to conclude that many differing syndromes are at present being included under one heading. Any process capable of producing a cyclical oestrogen production will produce clinical and endocrine features resembling the PCOS. Two out of three criteria are required for the diagnosis of PCOS: Evidence of hyperandrogenism, clinical (hirsutism, acne, male pattern balding) or biochemical (elevated serum androgen level); polycystic ovaries on ultrasound and the exclusion of other diseases. Examples of these include Cushing syndrome, androgen-producing tumours of the adrenal or ovary and congenital adrenal hyperplasia.

The objectives of therapy are to reduce endometrial hyperplasia, to control hirsutism and to induce ovulation (if fertility is required).

If an amenorrhoeic patient does not wish to become pregnant and is not bothered by hirsutism, the long-term problem of endometrial hyperplasia remains, for which a progestogen (e.g. medroxyprogesterone acetate 10 mg/day) for 10–14 days every 6–8 weeks will produce withdrawal bleeding as well as reduce endometrial hyperplasia. In some patients, progestogen may need to be administered for 20 days in each cycle.

Hirsutism can be improved by suppression of ovarian function or by increased binding of circulating androgen. Both are achieved by giving a combined oestrogen-progestogen contraceptive pill, preferably one of the newer progestogens, e.g. those containing drospirenone.

Medical and surgical methods of induction of ovulation in the infertile patient have been discussed in Chapter 5.

It is again emphasised that these ovaries are very easily overstimulated. Metformin administered to those patients who have hyperinsulinaemia improves the outcome.

Amenorrhea Due to the Defects of the Outflow Tract

Müllerian Agenesis (Mayer–Rokitansky–Küster–Hauser Syndrome)

This may be the probable diagnosis in an individual with primary amenorrhoea and no apparent vagina **(Figs. 8A and B)**. There is usually an absence or hypoplasia of the internal vagina and absence of fallopian tubes and uterus. The syndrome occurs due to a defect in fusion of the Müllerian ducts resulting in absence of proximal one-third of vagina with or without the uterus. Since the ovaries are not Müllerian structures, they are normal. The cause of this syndrome is unknown and is probably related to the mutations in the gene for anti-Müllerian hormones or the gene for anti-Müllerian hormone receptor. Other anomalies, including the renal tract anomalies such as ectopic kidney, renal agenesis, horseshoe kidney and abnormal collecting ducts, are frequently present. Extirpation of the Müllerian remnants, if any present, is not required unless they are causing some problems such as fibroid growth, haematometra and endometriosis.

Treatment of the condition usually involves progressive dilatation using Frank's dilators. Initially, the dilatation is begun in the posterior direction and then after 2 weeks, it is changed to upward direction in the line of vaginal axis. This must be performed daily for 20 minutes to the point of modest discomfort. By utilising increasingly larger sized dilators, a functional vagina can be created within a period of several months. Operative treatment is used in the patients in whom Frank's method is unacceptable or fails. It is important for the gynaecologist to provide adequate reassurance and support in these cases. Adequate

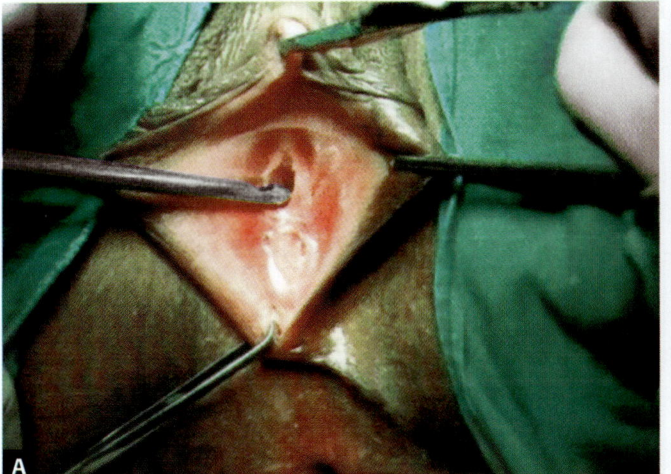

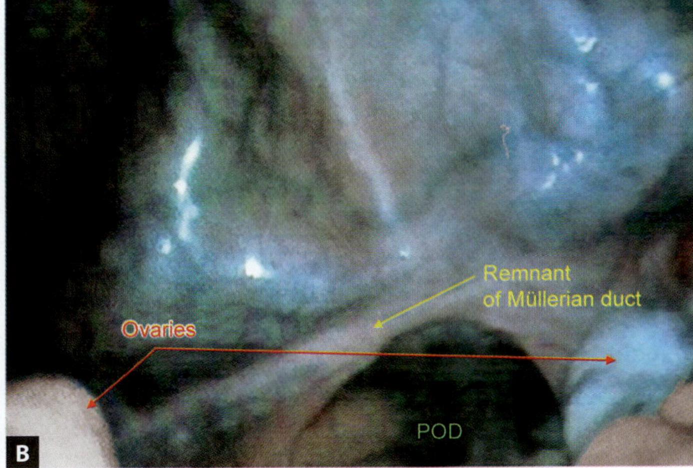

Figs. 8A and B: Mayer–Rokitansky–Küster–Hauser (MRKH) syndrome. (A) Vaginal agenesis; (B) Laparoscopic view of Müllerian agenesis.

counselling helps in avoiding problems with altered body image, which are likely to develop in these cases.

Creating an artificial vagina through the use of either Frank's dilators or surgical procedure (McIndoe vaginoplasty) at the time the patient plans to get married helps in ensuring that she and her partner would be able to obtain adequate sexual enjoyment following their marriage. Having regular sexual intercourse helps in maintaining the patency of a newly created artificial vaginal orifice. Though the patient remains infertile, she can lead an almost normal life. Genetic offspring can be achieved by collecting oocytes from a genetic mother, fertilising them with sperms obtained from a genetic father and their placement in a surrogate carrier.

Androgen Insensitivity Syndrome

Androgen insensitivity syndrome is another condition, which is commonly associated with a blind vaginal canal and absent uterus **(Figs. 9A to D)**. This was formerly known as testicular feminisation syndrome. The patients with this syndrome are male pseudohermaphrodites. This implies that the patient is genetically a male, i.e. has a male karyotype (46, XY). Since the karyotype is male, the patient has male gonads or testes. Pseudohermaphrodite implies that the genitalia are opposite of the gonads. The individual is phenotypically a female with absent or scant pubic and axillary hair. In these cases, the receptors are insensitive to androgens, due to which there is failure of normal masculinisation of the external genitalia in individuals who are genetically male. As a result, the patient is phenotypically a female. The pubic hair and axillary hair fail to develop, as testosterone is unable to exert its action. The testes may remain undescended. Affected individuals have normal testes with normal production of testosterone and normal conversion to dihydrotestosterone (DHT), unlike 5-alpha reductase deficiency, which is characterised by reduced levels of DHT. The transmission of this disease is via X-linked recessive inheritance. The gene responsible for androgen intracellular receptor is defective. A karyotype analysis is

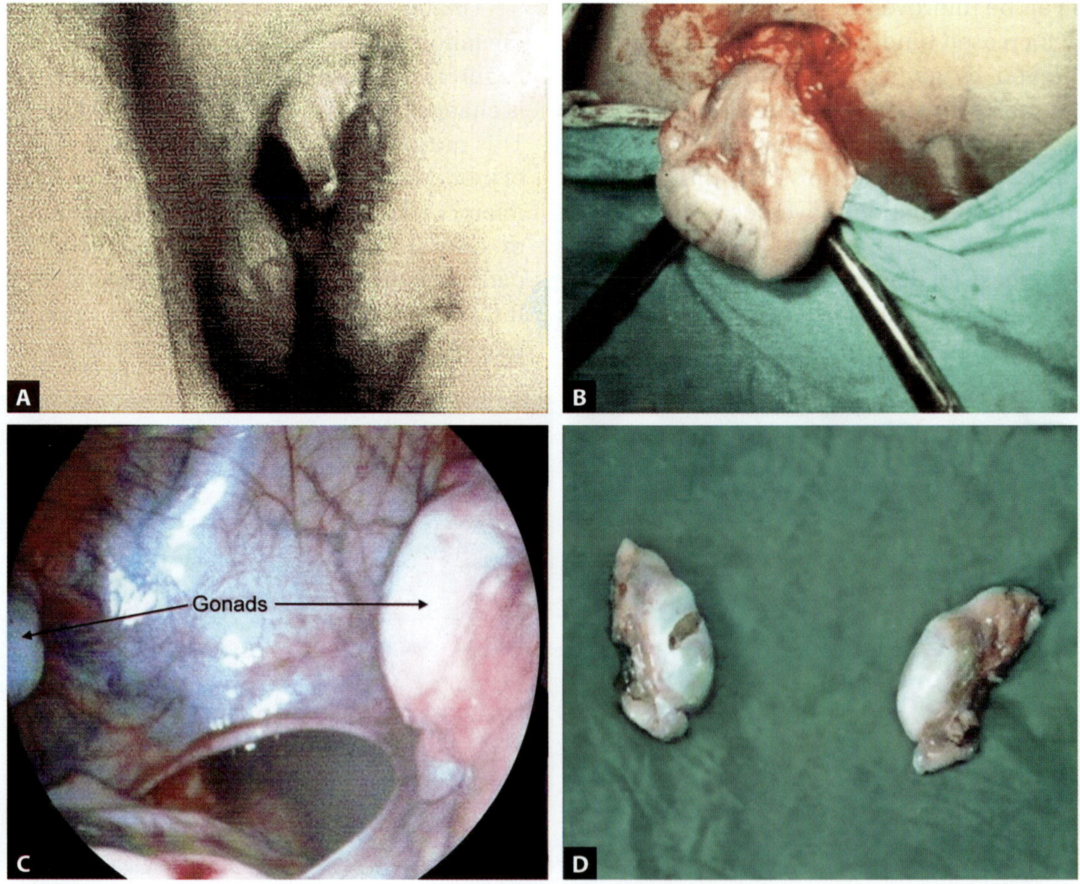

Figs. 9A to D: Androgen insensitivity syndrome. (A) Clitoromegaly with partial labial fusion; (B) Gonads being removed; (C) Laparoscopic view of intra-abdominal gonads and absent uterus; and (D) Removed gonads (testes).

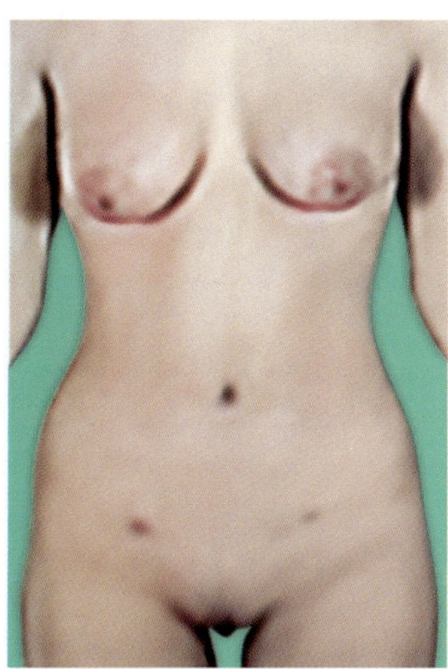

Fig. 10: Androgen insensitivity.

required to reach the proper diagnosis in these cases. The female child may present with inguinal hernia because the testes are frequently partially descended.

While the growth and development are normal, there may be a eunuchoidal tendency (long arms, big hands and big feet). The breasts are large as testosterone gets converted into oestrogens, which stimulate their growth **(Fig. 10)**. However, the breasts are abnormal as the glandular tissue is not abundant, nipples are small and the areolae are pale. Female internal genitalia (uterus and fallopian tubes) are either rudimentary or absent. In such a patient, the testes may be intra-abdominal or present in the form of hernia. However, even if present, the testes are immature and do not show any spermatogenesis. Due to high incidence of malignancy in the gonads with Y chromosomes, they must be removed at the age of 16–18 years once full development has been attained after puberty. The plasma levels of testosterone are within normal to high male range. As a result of failure of action of testosterone, the critical steps in sexual differentiation, which require testosterone, fail to take place.

Uterine Amenorrhoea

Amenorrhoea is not difficult to understand if the uterus is congenitally absent or has been removed at operation, if it is grossly underdeveloped or it has been damaged by radiotherapy. It can even result from heavy curettage in the presence of postabortal infection—*Asherman syndrome.* Sometimes, the endometrium is completely destroyed by infection and inflammation, as in the case of tuberculous endometritis.

Flowchart 3: Types of endocrine disorders.

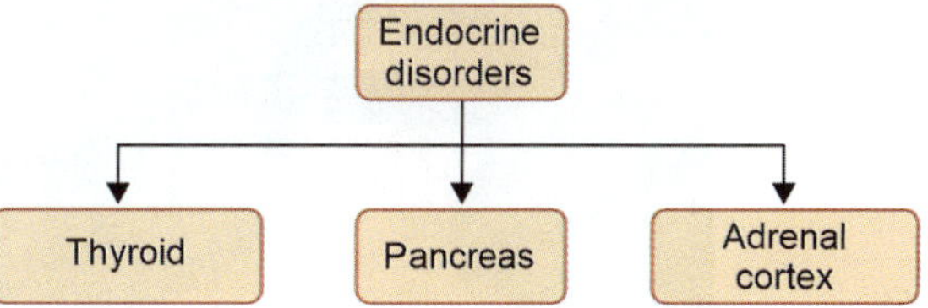

Other Aetiological Factors

Every case of amenorrhoea, physiological or pathological, is explained by one or other of the above mechanisms, but they can be brought into play by many factors other than those mentioned.

Endocrine Disorders

Endocrine disorders are of three types **(Flowchart 3)**:

1. Thyroid
2. Pancreas
3. Adrenal cortex

Thyroid

Hypothyroidism and hyperthyroidism can both depress ovarian and menstrual functions. The latter never causes amenorrhoea unless exophthalmos is present. When hyperthyroidism is associated with amenorrhoea, it is necessary to recognise that it may be merely a manifestation of a pituitary fault which is also the cause of the menstrual upset. Hypothyroidism is associated with an increase in thyrotropin-releasing hormone which, in turn, may be associated with a raised prolactin level and hence amenorrhoea.

Pancreas

Diabetes mellitus which commences in childhood and adolescence causes, or is associated with, amenorrhoea if not controlled.

Adrenal Cortex

Congenital adrenal hyperplasia or tumour formation results in amenorrhoea (*see* **Fig. 28** *in Chapter 14*; **Figs. 11A and B)**. In these conditions, it is accompanied by other evidence of virilism.

The administration of corticoids to women with normal ovarian and menstrual cycles sometimes causes amenorrhoea. Amenorrhoea and failure to ovulate are, on the other hand, sometimes seen in Addison's disease

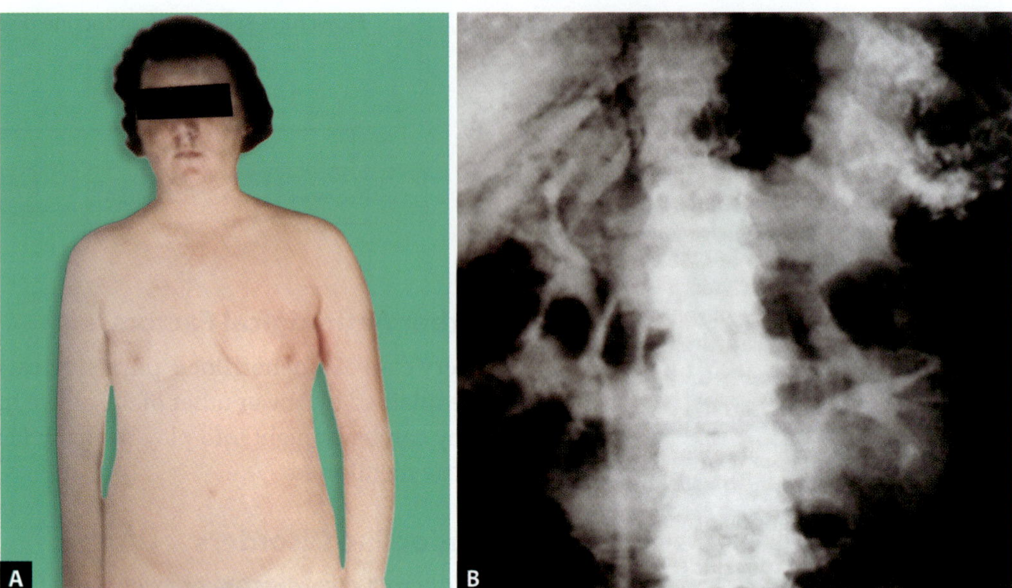

Figs. 11A and B: Amenorrhoea as part of Cushing syndrome caused by an adrenal cortical tumour. This girl, aged 22 years, complained of secondary amenorrhoea and increasing weight. She had slight hypertension in addition to obesity with striae on the hips and flanks. The radiograph shows a calcified tumour of the left adrenal displacing the kidney downwards. The tumour proved to be malignant and the patient died from metastases 6 months after its removal.

(total adrenal failure) and can then be cured by giving corticosteroids.

General Constitutional Upset and Disease

Any Acute Illness

Such conditions can cause a short period of amenorrhoea.

Chronic Diseases

These cause more lasting suppression of menstruation. It is particularly seen in tuberculosis, lymphoma and Crohn's disease. However, anaemia never causes amenorrhoea.

Nutrition

- *Malabsorption syndrome:* Gross and prolonged dietetic deficiencies during childhood are alleged to cause amenorrhoea, which can be permanent, in later life. Such a happening after the deficiency has been corrected must be rare, but it has been called *alimentary castration.*

  Malabsorption syndromes such as steatorrhoea can cause amenorrhoea which is associated with demonstrably reduced activity of the anterior pituitary.
- *Starvation:* Starvation in the adult, such as occurs during wars and famines, can also be followed by suppression of menstruation. Although proteins are essential to the production of gonadotropins, no special article of food is usually concerned; it is a general deficiency that seems to operate.

  There is good reason to doubt, however, whether it is lack of food or the stress of the situation that is more important. Thus, women in concentration camps during wartime often quickly develop amenorrhoea. Yet, later, when they are really suffering from the effects of starvation, menstruation may return. This is because they have become emotionally conditioned to their adverse circumstances. Starvation amenorrhoea may, therefore, derive from the cerebral cortex rather than from the faulty nutrition; no doubt, both are concerned.
- *Anorexia nervosa:* This is a syndrome resulting from a girl or woman deliberately starving herself. It is mostly seen in teenagers and women in their twenties but can occur much later **(Fig. 12)**. In minor degrees, when the only features are amenorrhoea accompanied by moderate loss of weight, it is much more common than is generally realised.

  The classical picture is one of secondary amenorrhoea in an extremely emaciated patient whose weight is between 25 and 45 kg, the weight loss being about 25% of the body weight or 15% below the normal for her age and height. The patient is of lively disposition, insisting that she is well and is reluctant

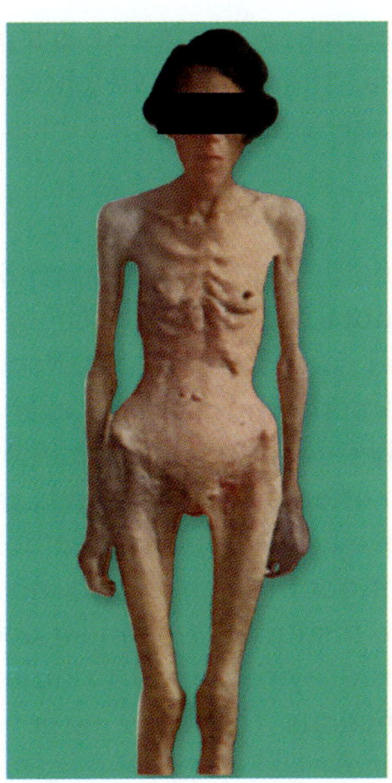

Fig. 12: Anorexia nervosa in a woman aged 41 years whose only complaint was amenorrhoea for 5 years. She weighed 30 kg. Treatment of various kinds during several years proved ineffective and the cachexia ultimately resulted in a spontaneous fracture of the neck of one femur and, later, in a similar accident on the other side.

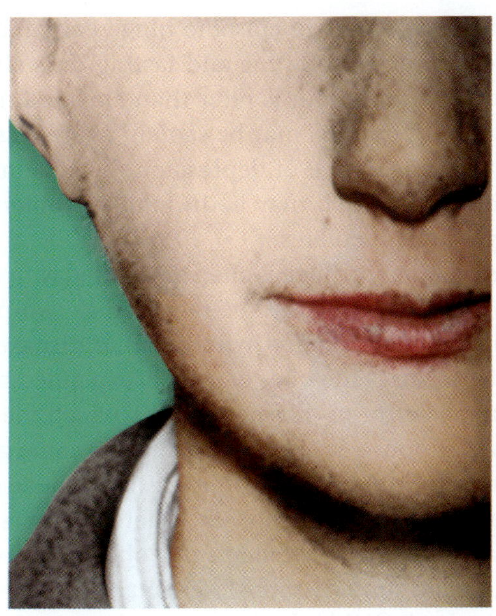

Fig. 13: This photograph shows the growth of fine downy hair on the cheek of a woman suffering from anorexia nervosa. This is a characteristic finding, and the downy hair appears also on the trunk and limbs. The patient was aged 22 years and unmarried. Her only complaint was secondary amenorrhoea for 2 years, but she admitted to considerable loss of weight. The background of the trouble was a desire to escape responsibility for the care of her parents.

to take medical advice. She says she is eating normally and often deceives observers by hiding food or making herself regurgitate. Sometimes, she attempts meals but finds it impossible to continue because of flatulence and distension. Constipation is the rule.

Although alert, affected girls and women have bradycardia, hypotension and cold blue extremities. An interesting and diagnostic sign is a growth of fine downy hair on the face, trunk and limbs **(Fig. 13)**; it is said that this represents a lower animal reflex to cold and a sluggish metabolism. The whole of the genital tract is generally atrophic. The ovaries lie dormant but can be stimulated to ovulate with gonadotropins. Diabetes insipidus may develop.

Although free thyroxine (T4) levels and adrenal functions may remain unaffected, the levels of gonadotropins and oestradiol are very low. An observation of great significance is that the administration of GnRH brings about the secretion of gonadotropins. The hypothalamus must therefore be at the root of the trouble. Some might argue that it is a hypothalamic disturbance which causes the loss of appetite, but most clinical observations indicate that the refusal to eat is deliberate or the result of an emotional upset.

It has been suggested that sufferers from anorexia nervosa have a frank psychosis such as schizophrenia. A few may develop these ultimately, but the disease usually starts as a bad habit consequent to unnecessary and *crash* dieting in adolescence or represents a *self-destructive flight* from problems and responsibilities. It can also represent a subconscious desire to attract attention.

In all cases, it is the underlying psychological factor which is the cause of the hypothalamic upset. Unless this is eliminated, the amenorrhoea persists, even though the patient resumes eating and recovers her weight. However, weight gain indicates emotional recovery, and menstruation usually resumes when a critical weight for the individual patient is achieved.

Anorexia nervosa is very resistant to treatment and is a serious condition. It is said to have an ultimate mortality rate of 7–10%. Death often comes suddenly from myocardial failure which is the result of either muscle atrophy, paralysis associated with hypokalaemia or occult (and therefore untreated) but severe infection.

- *Bulimia nervosa:* Amenorrhoea can be caused by overeating as well as undereating. Bulimia nervosa is marked by secretive, episodic binge eating followed by self-induced vomiting and fasting. It is also seen in young women but is rarer than anorexia nervosa. Episodes of bulimia may be seen in anorectics. There is a high incidence of depression in bulaemics, the aetiology of which may lie in family problems. The body weight fluctuates.

- *Obesity:* Amenorrhoea is often associated with obesity. This combination might be regarded as two-pronged evidence of a primary hypothalamic disease, but it rarely is. Nor is the obesity usually explained by some metabolic error or 'hormone upset' which the patient likes to suppose. While recognising that some girls and women (and men) *run to fat* easily because of their inherent type of metabolism, whereas others always remain thin; the fact remains that obesity is always the result of an unnecessarily large intake of food for that particular individual. Moreover, whatever its cause, it can always be corrected by a low-calorie intake and if it is, the associated amenorrhoea disappears spontaneously.

It is of interest to study fat children and adults in public places such as airports and railway stations. They are always eating—sweets, sandwiches, ice cream or something—no matter whether they are sitting, standing or walking. Yet, if asked in the consulting room, they always deny that they eat more than others.

Children can acquire the habit of overeating by following the practice of parents and other members of the family. Some mothers cannot resist giving their children the best of everything, doing so with the best of intentions.

Environment

Changes of climate, occupation and living conditions frequently cause amenorrhoea in susceptible women, operating through the psyche and the hypothalamus. Work involving institutional life, long hours of study and worry over examinations is particularly prone to having this effect. About 25–50% of student nurses and resident college students develop short periods of amenorrhoea at some time during their training. Air hostesses on international routes commonly have a similar problem until they become acclimatised to rapidly changing environments.

Exercise-related Amenorrhoea

Exercise-related amenorrhoea is being noted more frequently, especially in long-distance runners. Detailed studies reveal low gonadotropins and low oestrogens, but impaired LH secretion is suggested as a primary factor in the amenorrhoea. Altered diet, weight loss and stress are also factors in many amenorrhoeic athletes.

Investigation

It is never justifiable to treat amenorrhoea without first making an attempt to determine its cause and to assess its significance, and care is required in deciding when, and to what extent, amenorrhoea should even be investigated. This is especially true for primary amenorrhoea in young girls who are so often suffering merely from a late onset of what will prove to be an otherwise normal menarche. If there is doubt about such a case, no harm comes of waiting. Delay in instituting treatment does not prejudice the ultimate result with regard to either menstrual or reproductive functions. The following general rules can be applied in practice.

If menstruation has not commenced by the age of 16 years, an examination should be carried out to exclude systemic disease and stigmas of gross endocrine dysfunction and also to make sure the case is not one of cryptomenorrhoea. If any of these is found, a detailed investigation is indicated at once. If the physical and sexual developments appear normal, nothing further need to be done except to advise the girl on diet, exercise, work, leisure and health in general. If, however, menstruation has not commenced by the age of 18 years, further investigation should be arranged.

The avoidance of *unnecessary* investigation and overenthusiastic treatment is equally important in older patients. When amenorrhoea is of short duration and appears to be associated with a temporary physical or mental upset or with a change of environment, it is usually wise to await a spontaneous cure. On the other hand, when there is no reasonable explanation for the cessation of menstruation, the fullest possible investigation should be instituted before any conclusion is reached.

Clinical Examination

This is the most valuable of all investigations. A clear guide to the cause of amenorrhoea can often be deduced from a careful family and personal history of the patient and from the presence or absence of associated symptoms. The age of the patient and the previous menstrual habit are important. Was the onset of amenorrhoea dramatic or preceded by oligomenorrhoea? Has there been an increase or decrease in weight or any change in the voice? Is the woman pregnant? Has she been taking oral contraceptives?

Is there any evidence of galactorrhoea? Amenorrhoea due to primary ovarian failure, especially if it comes after a phase of normal ovarian activity, is accompanied by an outpouring of excessive amounts of gonadotropin by a pituitary released from oestrogen inhibition; this results in climacteric symptoms. Hypothalamic, pituitary and uterine amenorrhoea, on the other hand, are not associated with menopausal flushes. These *never* occur, e.g. in Sheehan's syndrome or anorexia nervosa. The answer to a simple question on this matter is of great value in elucidating the cause.

The stature and build of the patient should be noted. The development of the breasts and other secondary sex characters is assessed. If this is normal for the age, primary amenorrhoea is almost certainly due to the absence or gross underdevelopment of the uterus or to cryptomenorrhoea. The vulva and vagina reflect accurately the functional capacity of the ovaries. The presence of the uterus may be indicated by vaginal or rectal examination.

Special Investigations

Whenever the clinical features and simple tests do not reveal a clear cause for the amenorrhoea, and sometimes when they apparently do, special investigations are indicated. These include the following, and the choice rests on the circumstances of each case.

Tests for Pregnancy

These are advisable whenever the amenorrhoea is secondary and of short duration.

Radiology

Radiological examination of the pituitary gland is recommended in all cases. A coned-down view of the sella was done in cases of galactorrhoea. More detailed studies are required if this is abnormal or the prolactin level is significantly raised. Small pituitary adenomas are best detected by computed tomography (CT) scan or magnetic resonance imaging (MRI) **(Fig. 14)**.

Ophthalmology

Examination of the retina and visual fields should be done if a pituitary tumour is suspected.

Urinalysis

A check for glycosuria should be carried out and, if possible, a glucose tolerance test.

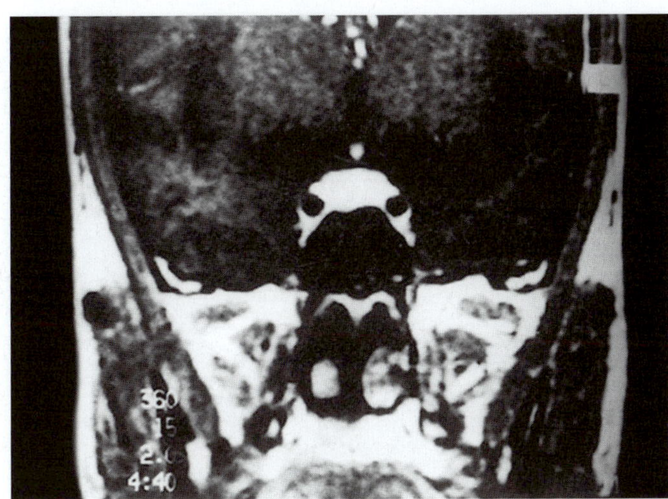

Fig. 14: T1-weighted coronal MR image after gadolinium enhancement showing a right-sided hypointense lesion in the anterior lobe of the pituitary gland, suggesting pituitary microadenoma.

Hormone Assays

These assays aim to cover pituitary, thyroid, adrenal and gonadal functions. If facilities are available, the plasma levels of FSH, LH and prolactin should be determined and thyroid function tests [TSH, free triiodothyronine (T3), T4 levels] carried out; other tests may be indicated on clinical grounds or following initial test results.

If the level of gonadotropins is raised, it strongly suggests a primary ovarian fault; if it is lowered, the trouble lies in the hypothalamic-pituitary system. Evidence of adrenal, cortical or thyroid dysfunction may call for supplementary tests involving suppression or stimulation of the particular gland. These show whether the upset is primary or secondary and also help to exclude tumour formation. Serum FSH levels are required to determine whether the patient has hypergonadotropic, hypogonadotropic or eugonadotropic amenorrhoea. A circulating FSH level of >40 mIU/mL indicated on at least two blood samples is indicative of hypergonadotropic amenorrhoea. Hypergonadotropism signifies that the cause of amenorrhoea is at the level of the ovary.

In patients under 30 years of age with hypergonadotropic amenorrhoea, a karyotype is required to rule out the presence of a Y cell line.

It is important to identify Y chromosomal material so it may be removed to prevent malignant degeneration.

There is much debate regarding the extent of an autoimmune workup required for a patient with ovarian failure.

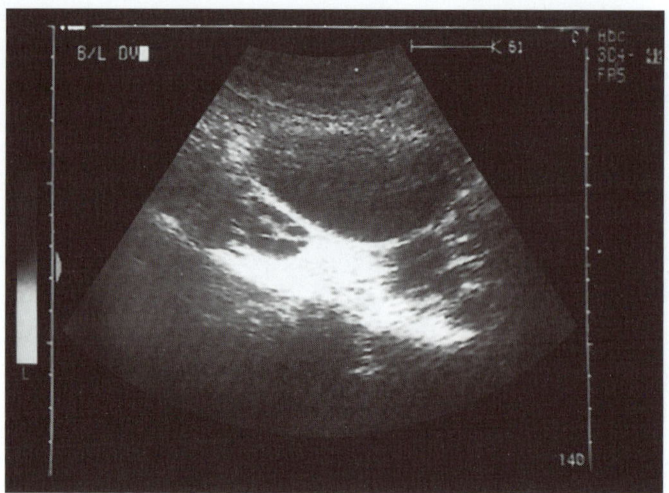

Fig. 15: Polycystic ovary seen on ultrasound.

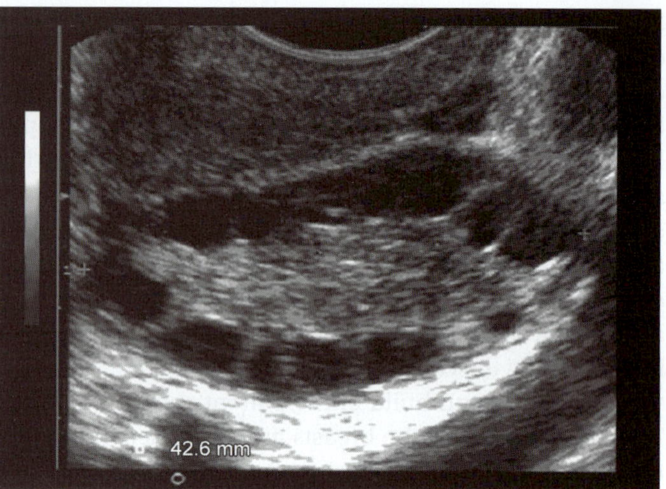

Fig. 16: Polycystic ovary syndrome.

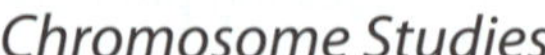

Chromosome Studies

The sex chromatin pattern is determined by the examination of buccal smears and the sex chromosome makeup by culturing leucocytes or skin (*see* Chapter 14). These investigations are essential, if the amenorrhoea is primary but rarely when it is secondary and the patient has no other physical stigmata.

Ultrasound

Ultrasound is used to document the presence of the uterus and ovaries and to study their morphology. This is useful in cases of primary amenorrhoea to rule out congenital anomalies, to see the thickness of the endometrial echo which reflects the oestradiol level and to evaluate the size of the ovaries, the number and arrangement of the follicles and the appearance of the stroma. In a case of polycystic ovaries, the follicles are arranged around the periphery with stromal hyperplasia **(Figs. 15 and 16)**.

In hypoestrogenic states, e.g. anorexia nervosa, the endometrial thickness is <4 mm; the converse obtains with prolonged unopposed oestrogen stimulation and endometrial hyperplasia. The widespread availability of ultrasound, aided by the development of MRI, laparoscopy and hormone assay, has almost done away with the need for examination under anaesthesia in cases of amenorrhoea.

Laparoscopy

Laparoscopy is done to exclude the presence of streak gonads, testes and small ovarian tumours and to recognise polycystic ovaries. Abnormal gonads can be removed at the same sitting. Polycystic ovaries can be 'drilled' if medical treatment has been unsuccessful.

Therapeutic Tests

When investigations leave doubt as to which link of the hypothalamus → pituitary → ovary → uterus chain is primarily at fault, therapeutic tests are of great value. The first of these is to assess uterine sensitivity to ovarian hormones. After excluding pregnancy, hyperprolactinaemia and hypothyroidism, a progestogen challenge test is administered: 10 mg medroxyprogesterone acetate daily for 5 days or 200 mg parenteral progesterone. The former is generally preferred. If the patient has a withdrawal bleeding, it indicates the presence of a functional outflow tract and also the presence of sufficient circulating endogenous oestrogen which has 'primed' the endometrium, and the diagnosis is anovulation.

If, on the other hand, the patient does not have withdrawal bleeding in response to the progestogen challenge, a combination of oestrogen and progestogen is given, either sequentially using conjugated oestrogens for 20 days with medroxyprogesterone acetate in the last 10 days or a combined oral contraceptive pill is administered daily for 21 days. If there is still no bleeding, the course is repeated. A negative response indicates a defect in the outflow tract, i.e. uterine amenorrhoea. If, however, bleeding occurs, it points to a defect in the production of both oestrogen and progesterone.

Serum FSH and LH levels are measured. If these are raised, the cause is ovarian failure, whereas if they are low or normal, the cause is hypothalamic.

TREATMENT

Treatment of the Cause

The treatment of amenorrhoea is largely dependent on its cause. If this is due to some general disease such as diabetes, that alone requires treatment. Pelvic tuberculosis calls for antituberculous drugs. An adrenal cortical adenoma or an androblastoma of the ovary can be removed and menstruation, even if it has been suspended for many years, quickly and spontaneously returns. Equally good results sometimes follow the treatment of psychological disturbances and systemic disease, but this is by no means the rule. Young women persuaded to discontinue a strict reducing diet may have to wait a long time before their menses return. Environmental amenorrhoea can be very persistent. In all such instances, however, it is more than likely that the underlying psychological or other cause is not corrected to the extent suggested by other features of the case.

Anorexia nervosa is particularly difficult to treat successfully, the prognosis depending to some extent on the duration of the syndrome. Hospitalisation, often for as long as 2–3 months, and sometimes including isolation, is essential. In the hospital, the approaches vary. One of the most common approaches is *behaviour modification*. This involves withdrawal of privileges and a stepwise reinstatement of these in reward for weight gain. The patient is encouraged to consume a minimum of 2,600 kcal/day. Some physicians advocate forced feeding supplemented by psychiatric measures; others aim to eliminate the patient's inhibition by giving large doses of tranquilisers such as chlorpromazine over long periods. Gentle and considerate counselling and an explanation of the problem to the patient are, however, often sufficient to stimulate patient response. Even though the patient responds well to institutional care, she requires regular supervision and psychiatric support thereafter. Despite this, however, relapse is common, and readmission to hospital becomes necessary in one third of the cases. If amenorrhoea persists when nutrition has been improved, ovulation for conception can be induced with gonadotropin therapy and sometimes with clomiphene. Pregnancy is well tolerated and may help in the cure.

General Treatment

This includes the correction of errors in diet, working conditions, home environment and the use of leisure. When amenorrhoea is associated with obesity, reduction of weight can be achieved by strict adherence to a low-calorie diet. An intake of not >1,500 kcal a day will cause a loss of 15–20 kg in 3 months; if it does not, then the patient has departed from instructions. Lest she becomes discouraged, she should be warned that loss of weight is often not apparent until after the first 2 or 3 weeks of treatment.

It is remarkable that weight reduction alone is not infrequently followed by cure of amenorrhoea and oligomenorrhoea, and this is true even when the woman presents features of a recognised syndrome such as PCOS. Associated with weight reduction and loss of adipose tissue is altered oestrogen metabolism as is a change in the function of the adrenal cortex.

In a large number of cases in which the amenorrhoea is not the result of organic disease; for example, when it reflects a temporary derangement of the neuroendocrine system caused by environmental or other factors, it cures itself spontaneously. Such an outcome should always be awaited before resorting to hormone or other special treatment.

Meanwhile, it is important to give the patient a rational explanation of the state of affairs and to reassure the harmlessness of amenorrhoea from the standpoint of general health. Ancient myths die slowly, and it is still common for women to fear that what they regard as a failure to excrete noxious materials will lead to ill-health. The basis of these fears is the long-known association between amenorrhoea and ill-health; unfortunately, the laity reverse the cause-and-effect relationship.

Hormone Therapy

Thyroid

Although only a few patients with amenorrhoea will be diagnosed to have hypothyroidism, the replacement of T4 in these women produces a dramatic relief in symptoms.

Corticosteroids

Corticosteroids, in the form of prednisone, prednisolone or dexamethasone, cure amenorrhoea which is a feature of congenital adrenal hyperplasia. But they are rarely of value when given empirically. The rare dramatic successes attending such *blind* therapy are explained by the amenorrhoea being the result of latent undiagnosed adrenal failure (Addison's disease) or polycystic ovaries.

Oestrogen and Progestogen

Cyclical treatment with oestrogens and progestogens can be given for up to three cycles as a diagnostic measure to test uterine reactivity. In most cases, especially when amenorrhoea is primary, menstruation ceases as soon as treatment is withheld.

One has to remember that the use of oral contraceptive preparations is *relatively contraindicated* in patients with amenorrhoea or oligomenorrhoea because it temporarily masks the symptom and is then followed by *postpill amenorrhoea*.

It is sometimes advised that oestrogen therapy should not be commenced until it is reasonably certain, by radiological study of the bony epiphyses that no more physical growth is to be expected. In fact, oestrogens probably play little part in closing epiphyses; they can even cause a spurt in physical growth, such as is normally seen at puberty.

If the effect of cyclical oestrogen–progestogen therapy proves to be only temporary so far as uterine bleeding is concerned, and the amenorrhoea appears to be constitutional, it should not be continued indefinitely merely to produce what the patient regards as menstruation.

When primary amenorrhoea is associated with infantilism and poorly formed secondary sex characteristics, as in cases of streak gonads and intersex, a reason for giving oestrogens (along with progestogens) over long periods is to promote facial maturity, breast development and the growth of body hair. Oestrogen will also develop the vagina to permit satisfactory coitus. This hormone does not always succeed in these objectives, especially so far as body hair is concerned. In these patients and in cases of premature ovarian failure, long-term oestrogen and progestogen therapy is recommended to avoid the problems of osteoporosis.

Clomiphene

Clomiphene is only effective when the hypothalamic–pituitary system is capable of function. The likelihood of response to clomiphene is determined by the basal oestrogen level. Its main indication is infertility (with amenorrhoea) associated with PCOS, postpill amenorrhoea and the Chiari–Frommel syndrome. Some women with postpill amenorrhoea who have no other cause for their amenorrhoea ovulate following a single course of clomiphene, hence the descriptive term clomiphene-responsive amenorrhoea. This is preferable to the term hypothalamic amenorrhoea for there is no evidence of a hypothalamic disorder although hypothalamic function is suppressed.

In recent years, letrozole, an aromatase inhibitor, has replaced clomiphene as first-line therapy for ovulation induction in women with diagnosed PCOS as it promotes monofollicular development and is not detrimental to endometrial thickness as is the case with clomiphene with its antioestrogenic properties.

Gonadotropins

Gonadotropins are indicated only when the overriding complaint is infertility, when anovulation is caused by a proven failure in pituitary function, as shown by a persistent low output of gonadotropins, and when the gonads contain responsive ova. The effect of this treatment is limited to the period of its application, the details of which are given in Chapter 5.

Clomiphene and Gonadotropins

See Chapter 5.

Gonadotrophin-releasing Hormone Agonists

Induction of ovulation by GnRH agonists has an important place in the treatment of infertility and amenorrhoea whose basic cause lies in the hypothalamus and cerebral cortex.

Agents Influencing the Hypothalamus

Amenorrhoea with a hypothalamic basis, such as that associated with the taking of oral contraceptives and hyperprolactinaemia, sometimes responds well to L-dopamine. More often used in these circumstances is bromocriptine, which can have a dramatic effect restoring ovulation as well as menstruation while suppressing lactation. This ergot alkaloid is effective even in cases of pituitary tumour (for actions and dosage). In recent years, cabergoline administered once weekly is adequate as opposed to multiple daily doses of bromocriptine.

Surgical Treatment

See Chapter 5.

Results

It is difficult to assess the overall results of treating amenorrhoea because its causes are so many and varied, some amenable to appropriate treatment, some not. If replacement therapy of one kind or another results in isolated episodes of ovulation and menstruation or even in pregnancy, without restoring the cycle, is this to be regarded as a cure?

Moreover, many *cures* of amenorrhoea of uncertain origin are spontaneous and independent of treatment. Thus, although *primary* amenorrhoea in women aged over 20 years is rarely treated successfully, no matter what method is employed, in those who are younger the results are better because in many the menses would have started spontaneously had they been given time.

Similarly, in *secondary* amenorrhoea, the prognosis depends to some extent on its duration; this usually means that the longer the amenorrhoea, the less likely is a spontaneous cure. In the majority of cases, investigation will reveal a cause and appropriate therapy can be instituted. Among cases for which no organic cause is found, the results for psychotherapy, oestrogens, progestogens, T4 and corticosteroids, indeed, for no treatment at all, are identical—a 60% cure rate for secondary amenorrhoea of 1–2-year duration.

Pessimism is generally unwarranted, and it is extraordinary how often menstruation returns sooner or later or even begins when least expected.

Let this section conclude with a case which illustrates a common situation.

A medical student presented with amenorrhoea of 1-year duration. The uterus was rather small, but the physical signs were otherwise unremarkable; her early life had been unhappy; she had been dieting unnecessarily and was studying hard. A therapeutic test with cyclical oestrogens failed twice but produced a feeble response on the third occasion. The girl was told that general factors were responsible and was seen annually. Menstruation returned unexpectedly on the first day of her written final examination papers.

She had infrequent periods in the following years but despite this, she ovulated spontaneously, for she subsequently had three children without difficulty. This was despite a gloomy outlook given by gynaecologists in other cities she worked in and emphasis on the necessity of drugs to induce ovulation.

The diagnostic workup is summarised in **Box 1 and Table 1**.

Assessment of the serum FSH level should be performed, as the initial laboratory test unless the history and physical examination suggest otherwise. The FSH level differentiates hypergonadotropic and hypogonadotropic forms of hypogonadism **(Fig. 17)**. If the FSH level is elevated, a karyotype is obtained. An elevated FSH level in combination with a 45,XO karyotype confirms the diagnosis of Turner syndrome **(Fig. 18)**. Partial deletion of the X chromosome, mosaicism, pure gonadal dysgenesis and mixed gonadal dysgenesis are diagnosed by obtaining a karyotype.

Because of the association of coarctation of the aorta and thyroid dysfunction, patients with Turner syndrome should undergo echocardiography and thyroid function studies.

If the karyotype is normal and the FSH is elevated, it is important to consider the diagnosis of 17α-hydroxylase deficiency because it may be a life-threatening disease, if untreated. This diagnosis should be considered when testing indicates elevated serum progesterone levels (>3 ng/mL), a low 17α-hydroxyprogesterone level (<0.2 ng/mL) and an elevated serum deoxycorticosterone (DOS) level. The diagnosis is confirmed with an ACTH stimulation test. After ACTH bolus administration, affected individuals have markedly increased levels of serum progesterone compared with baseline levels and no change in serum 17α-hydroxyprogesterone levels.

If the screening FSH level is low, the diagnosis of hypogonadotropic hypogonadism is established.

If the history suggests the presence of a central nervous system lesion or galactorrhoea, imaging of the head using CT or MRI is helpful in the diagnosis. Suprasellar or intrasellar calcification in an abnormal sella is found in approximately 70% of patients with craniopharyngioma.

BOX 1: History of diagnostic workup.

- *Chemotherapy or radiation:* Brain, pituitary and ovary dysfunction
- Family history of delayed menarche
- Galactorrhoea—pituitary adenoma
- Hirsutism and acne
- Illicit or prescription drug use—consider the effect on prolactin
- Menarche and menstrual history
- Rule pregnancy
- Significant headaches or vision changes
- Temperature intolerance, palpitations, diarrhoea, constipation, tremor, depression and skin changes
- *Vasomotor symptoms:* Primary ovarian insufficiency and natural menopause
- Weight loss, excessive exercise, poor nutrition, psychosocial stress and diets—hypothalamic amenorrhoea

TABLE 1: Abnormal thyroid examination and characteristics of thyroid disorder.

Abnormal thyroid examination	***Thyroid disorder***
Anthropomorphic measurements and growth charts	Turner syndrome and constitutional delay of puberty
	High: PCOS
Body mass index	
	Low: Functional hypothalamic amenorrhoea
Dysmorphic features (webbed neck, short stature, low hairline)	Turner syndrome
Male pattern baldness, increased facial hair and acne	Hyperandrogenism, PCOS, ovarian or adrenal tumour, CAH and Cushing syndrome
Pelvic examination	
Absence or abnormalities of cervix or uterus	Rare congenital causes
Clitoromegaly	Androgen-secreting tumour and CAH
Presence of transverse vaginal septum or imperforate hymen	Outflow tract obstruction
Reddened or thin vaginal mucosa	Decreased endogenous oestrogen
Striae, buffalo hump, central obesity and hypertension	Cushing syndrome
Tanner staging abnormal	Turner syndrome, constitutional delay of puberty and rare causes
Complete blood count and metabolic panel abnormalities	Chronic disease

(CAH: congenital adrenal hyperplasia; PCOS: polycystic ovary syndrome)

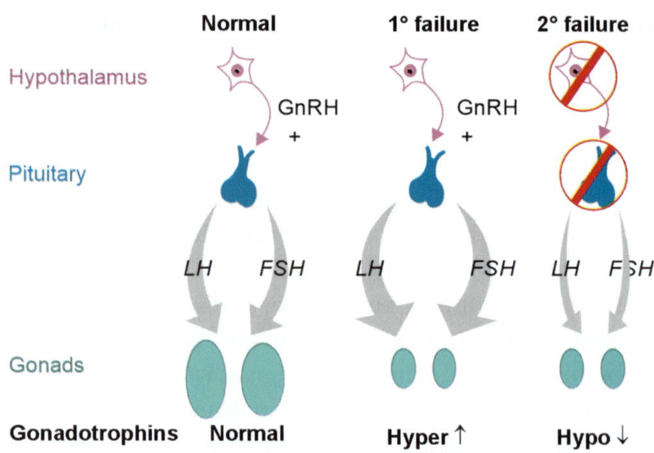

Fig. 17: Hormonal levels in hypergonadotropic and hypogonadotropic hypogonadism. (FSH: follicle-stimulating hormone; GnRH: gonadotrophin-releasing hormone; LH: luteinising hormone)

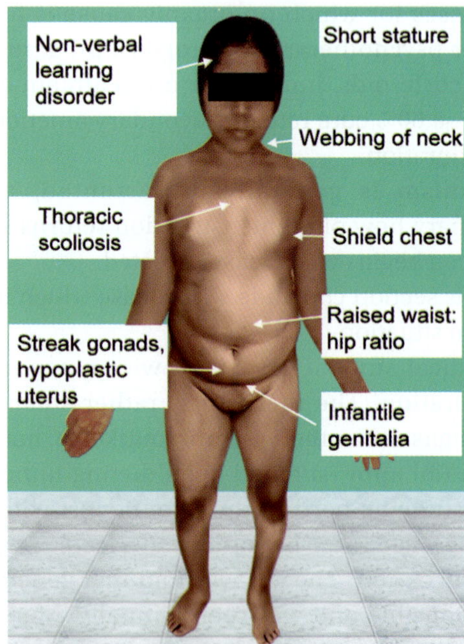

Fig. 18: Hypergonadotropic hypogonadism: Turner syndrome. A 25-year-old girl studying in 6th standard.

Physiologic delay is a diagnosis of exclusion that is difficult to distinguish from insufficient GnRH secretion. The diagnosis can be supported by a history suggesting physiologic delay, a radiograph showing delayed bone age and the absence of a central nervous system lesion on CT or MRI scanning. Gonadotropin-deficient patients can usually be distinguished from patients with physiologic delay by their response to GnRH stimulation. Patients with physiologic delay have a normal LH response to GnRH stimulation for their bone age, in contrast to gonadotropin-deficient patients, in whom the LH and FSH responses are low. **Flowcharts 4 and 5** describe the various diagnostic modalities and the management options in cases of amenorrhoea.

HYPOMENORRHOEA

Definition

Uterine bleeding may be slight in amount, short in duration or both, but the menstrual function varies so widely

Flowchart 4: Various diagnostic modalities and the management options in cases of amenorrhoea.

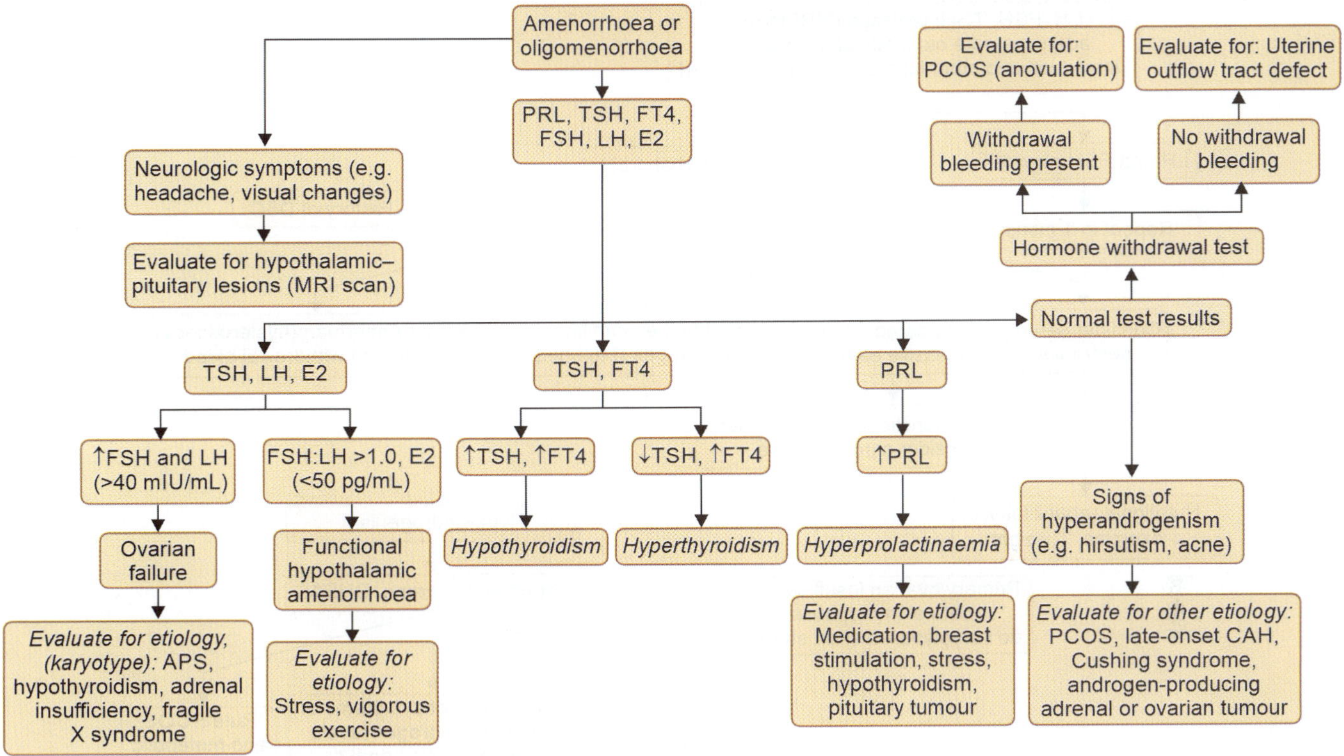

(CAH: congenital adrenal hyperplasia; E2: oestradiol; FSH: follicle-stimulating hormone; FT4: free thyroxine; LH: luteinising hormone; PCOS: polycystic ovary syndrome; PRL: prolactin; TSH: thyroid-stimulating hormone)

within normal limits that the definition of an abnormally scanty loss is a matter of opinion. Bleeding which lasts 2 days or less is unusual, if not pathological, and is termed *hypomenorrhoea* **(Fig. 19)**.

Causes

Constitutional

In most cases, scanty menstruation characterises the whole menstrual life of a woman and is to be regarded as a constitutional trait of no significance. Even when it precedes or follows a phase of full menstrual loss, it rarely has a pathological basis. Bleeding which lasts only a few hours is not incompatible with full fertility, the ovarian and endometrial cycles usually being normal.

Constitutional scanty menstruation is perhaps best explained by assuming the presence of an unusual arrangement, or relative insensitivity, of the endometrial vascular apparatus.

Uterine

Scanty loss sometimes means that the bleeding surface is smaller than normal and is occasionally seen when the endometrial cavity has been reduced too much during myomectomy or other plastic operation on the uterus, by intrauterine adhesions or by chronic endometritis, e.g. tubercular. The finding of endometrial tuberculosis almost always means that the tubes are infected, although not necessarily closed. The endometrium is involved in approximately 50–60% of women with genital tuberculosis. On hysteroscopy, synechiae are present in 25% of patients of whom 40% may have a positive endometrial biopsy. Therefore, a hysteroscopic examination should be performed routinely, before admitting patients with genital tuberculosis into an in vitro fertilisation (IVF) program. The preliminary evaluation reduces the failure rate and increases the cancellation rate. A history of tubercular endometritis represents a special indication for a preliminary hysteroscopy before IVF.

The preferred treatment for synechiae is lysis of adhesions at hysteroscopy, followed by immediate insertion of an intrauterine device for a short duration to prevent further adhesions. Use of oestrogens or a combination of oestrogen and progestogen for rapid endometrial growth is recommended for three to six cycles depending on the extent of the adhesions/severity of Asherman syndrome.

Flowchart 5: Management of elevated LH, FSH, TSH and prolactin levels.

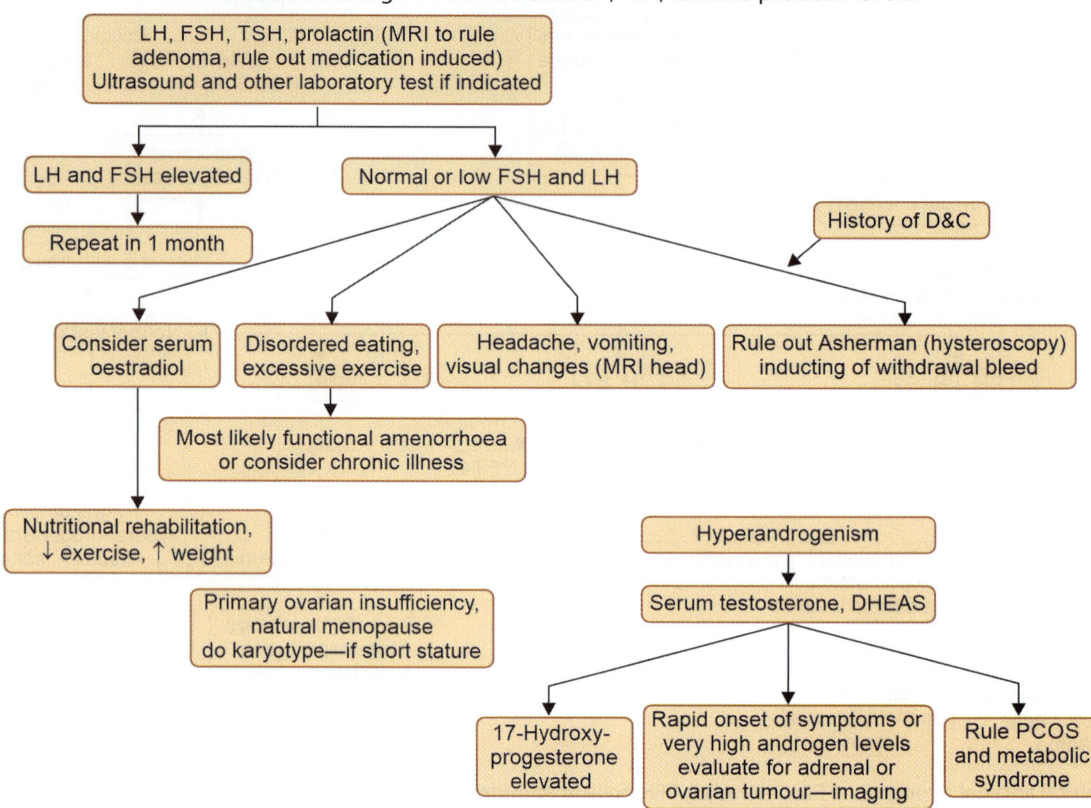

(DHEAS: dehydroepiandrosterone sulphate; FSH: follicle-stimulating hormone; LH: luteinising hormone; PCOS: polycystic ovary syndrome; TSH: thyroid-stimulating hormone)

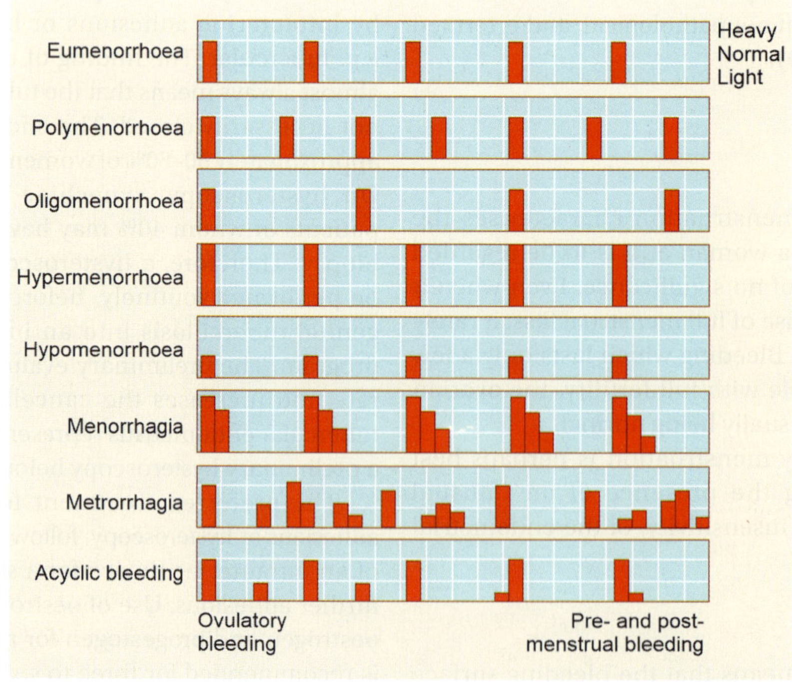

Fig. 19: Menstruation: Abnormalities as shown in Kaltenbach chart.

The success of treatment regarding term deliveries and rate of abortions depends on the severity of adhesions. The antitubercular treatment consists of initial multidrug medical therapy for a period of 9 months to 1 year.

Hormonal

Disturbances of the endocrine system do not ordinarily lead to scanty menstruation without altering the cycle at the same time (*see* oligomenorrhoea). Scanty menstruation is, however, occasionally seen as a forerunner to amenorrhoea and then has the same causes. It can also occur with long-term use of low-dose oral contraceptives as a result of progressive endometrial atrophy.

Nervous and Emotional

Psychological factors may fail to suppress a stable ovarian and uterine cycle completely and sometimes succeed only in reducing the amount of flow. The best example is pseudocyesis which is frequently characterised by scanty periods rather than amenorrhoea.

Treatment

Unless a significant causal abnormality is found, no treatment other than reassurance is necessary. So far as health and fertility are concerned, it usually does not matter whether menses last half an hour, half a day or half a week.

OLIGOMENORRHOEA

Definition

Oligomenorrhoea can only be defined arbitrarily as one in which the cycle lasts longer than 35 days. Menstruation may be both infrequent and irregular or may be regularly infrequent. In either case, the error is in the ovary and its controlling factors rather than in the uterus; for this reason, the symptom tends to have more significance than hypomenorrhoea. *Infrequent menstruation and amenorrhoea are essentially similar symptoms with identical causes*—the difference is only one of degree. Indeed, when menstruation only occurs at intervals of 3 or more months, it is a matter of opinion as to whether the condition is described as one or the other.

Causes (Fig. 20)

Constitutional and Physiological

In the majority of cases, infrequent menstruation represents a peculiarity of the individual and is not out of keeping with health and good fertility. It can be familial. The bleeding can be ovular in type, which means that the ovarian cycle is drawn out or temporarily arrested at some phase. As a rule, the luteal phase tends to be fairly constant at 14 days; it is the follicular phase which is either lengthened or slow to commence.

Infrequent menstruation sometimes follows the menarche and precedes the menopause; it then marks a gradual waxing and waning of the endocrine cycle and is physiological. Adolescent oligomenorrhoea tends to cure itself within a few years but may persist until the first pregnancy, after which it is often replaced by a more normal cycle.

Hormonal

If there is any abnormality, it is essentially one in which the ovary is underactive, and this is reflected in the

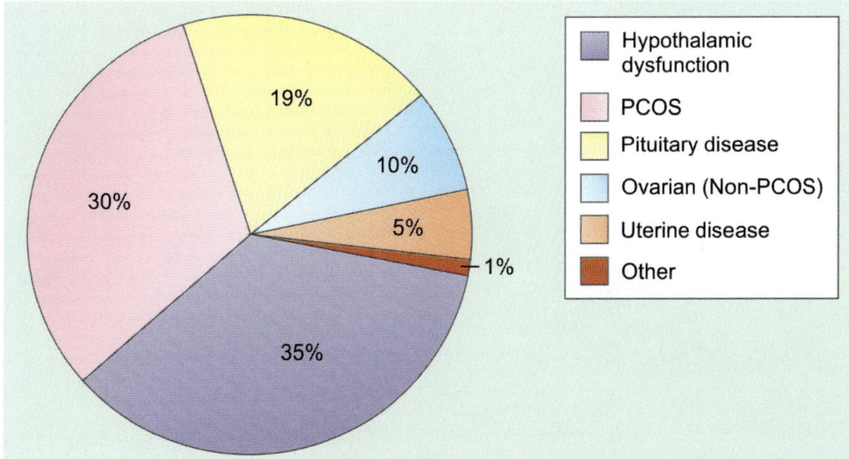

Fig. 20: Causes of oligomenorrhoea/secondary amenorrhoea (excluding pregnancy). (PCOS: polycystic ovary syndrome)

secondary sex organs. Hypoplasia of the uterus and vagina, and a history of a late menarche, is, therefore, to be expected. The ovarian disturbance is often secondary to hypothalamic, pituitary, thyroid or adrenal dysfunction, so the patient may have other stigmas of endocrine upset such as obesity, squat figure, hirsutism and low fertility. Obesity and oligomenorrhoea are close companions so are oligomenorrhoea and hirsutism, but the basis may still be genetic and familial. Otherwise, these combinations may be a part of the PCOS.

Chromosomal

An underlying sex chromosome abnormality, such as an XXX arrangement, is occasionally found.

Treatment

The investigation and treatment of oligomenorrhoea are the same as those for amenorrhoea, but the prognosis is better because gross abnormalities of the ovary and uterus are less likely to be present. There is no need for any treatment except reassurance in the majority of cases, i.e. those in which the condition appears to be constitutional and is unassociated with impaired fertility. Overtreatment should also be avoided, particularly in young girls in whom a spontaneous cure can be expected.

If, in addition, infertility is a problem, treatment may be required to induce or increase the frequency of ovulation. Counselling regarding the time of intercourse is difficult with erratic or infrequent menstrual cycles.

SUGGESTED READING

1. Insulite Health PCOS. (2018). Is Unpredictable Menstruation Complicating your Life, Impacting your Daily Activities, and Making it Difficult for you to Plan Ahead? [online] Available from https://pcos.com/menstrual-irregularities-or-oligomenorrhea-and-pcos/. [Last accessed April, 2025].
2. Long WN. Abnormal vaginal bleeding. In: Walker HK, Hall WD, Hurst JW (Eds). Clinical Methods: The History, Physical, and Laboratory Examinations, 3rd edition. Boston: Butterworths; 1990.
3. Seltzer VL, Benjamin F, Deutsch S. Perimenopausal bleeding patterns and pathologic findings. J Am Med Womens Assoc (1972). 1990;45(4):132-4.

40

CHAPTER

Abnormal and Excessive Uterine Bleeding

Jayaraman Nambiar M, Muralidhar V Pai

Chapter Outline

- Terminology in Abnormal Uterine Bleeding
- PALM-COEIN Classification of Abnormal Uterine Bleeding
- Causes of Abnormal Uterine Bleeding—PALM-COEIN
- Wamsteker Classification
- STEPW Classification of Myoma
- Approach to a Patient with Abnormal Uterine Bleeding
- Special Clinical Types of Bleeding

INTRODUCTION

Abnormal uterine bleeding (AUB) affects 3–35% of women and is an important cause of morbidity. It is a major part of the gynaecological workload in clinical practice.

TERMINOLOGY IN ABNORMAL UTERINE BLEEDING

The previous definition of abnormal and excessive uterine bleeding is no longer in use. Terms such as menorrhagia are no longer used. Instead, abnormal bleeding patterns are described objectively based on frequency, duration, regularity, etc. The terminology is described in **Table 1**.

For all patients with AUB, the pattern of bleeding is described as per **Table 1**. For regularity of bleeding, the interval is different for different age groups. Between 18 and 25 years of age ≤9 days, 26 and 41 years of age ≤7 days and between 42 and 45 years ≤9 days are considered as normal.

TABLE 1: Terminology of abnormal uterine bleeding.

Parameter	*Normal*	*Abnormal*
• Absent • Infrequent (>38 days) • Normal (≥24 to ≤38 days) • Frequent (<24 days)		
Duration	• Normal (≤8 days) • Prolonged (>8 days)	
• Regularity • Irregular	• Normal (interval between longest and shortest cycle: ≤7–9 days), 18–25 years ≤9 days, 26–41 years ≤7 days, 42–45 years ≥9 days • Shortest to longest cycle interval: ≥8–10 days	
Flow volume (as described by the patient)	• Light • Normal • Heavy	
Intermenstrual bleeding	None	• Early cycle • Mid cycle • Late cycle
Unscheduled bleeding on oestrogen ± progesterone (pills, rings, patches or injections)	• Not applicable • None	Present

PALM-COEIN CLASSIFICATION OF ABNORMAL UTERINE BLEEDING

Abnormal uterine bleeding is more often diagnosed with symptoms and examination now since the causes of bleeding are found to be overlapping. The International Federation of Gynaecology and Obstetrics (FIGO) in 2011 developed the classification PALM-COEIN for causes of AUB in the nonreproductive age group. It was modified in 2018 **(Fig. 1)**. In the PALM-COEIN classification system, causes that can be identified by imaging and histopathology are classified under the PALM category. Causes that cannot be identified by imaging are classified under the COEIN category, which is due to nonstructural causes.

The term dysfunctional uterine bleeding (dub) is obsolete now and no longer in use. DUB is due to ovulatory and endometrial causes.

Many causes of bleeding are strongly suggested by history alone. Note the amount of menstrual flow, the length of the menstrual cycle and menstrual period, the length and number of episodes of intermenstrual bleeding and any episodes of contact bleeding. Note also the last menstrual period, age at menarche and menopause, and any changes in general health. The patient must keep a record of bleeding patterns to determine whether bleeding is abnormal or only a variation of normal. However, most women have an occasional menstrual cycle that is not in their usual pattern. Depending on the patient's age and the pattern of bleeding, observation may be all that is necessary.

Abnormal bleeding is divided into acute, chronic and intermenstrual AUB. These three can be presented as separate entities or acute or chronic episodes.

1. *Acute* is an episode of heavy bleeding in sufficient quantity to require immediate intervention.
2. *Chronic* is where the abnormal bleeding pattern is present for >6 months at least.
3. *Intermenstrual* has replaced the initial terminology of *menometrorrhagia or metrorrhagia.*

CAUSES OF ABNORMAL UTERINE BLEEDING—PALM-COEIN

P—Polyps

Polyps are included in this classification irrespective of their number, size, and location. Polypoidal-looking endometrium is excluded from this category. Polyps cause menorrhagia in about 8–10% of the population. The exact aetiology is unknown; polyps are thought to be focal areas of stromal and glandular overgrowth. Diagnosis is usually made by transvaginal sonography, sonohysterography or hysteroscopy.

Treatment modality depends on the age of the patient, symptoms and desire to retain fertility. Treatment is mainly done by using hysteroscopy with scissors or bipolar electrode or Collins knife. When fertility is concerned, it is wise to use scissors rather than an electrical modality to avoid thermal endometrial damage. Cornual polyps are more of a concern than any other site. The size of polyps <1.5 cm usually does not affect fertility outcome **(Fig. 2)**.

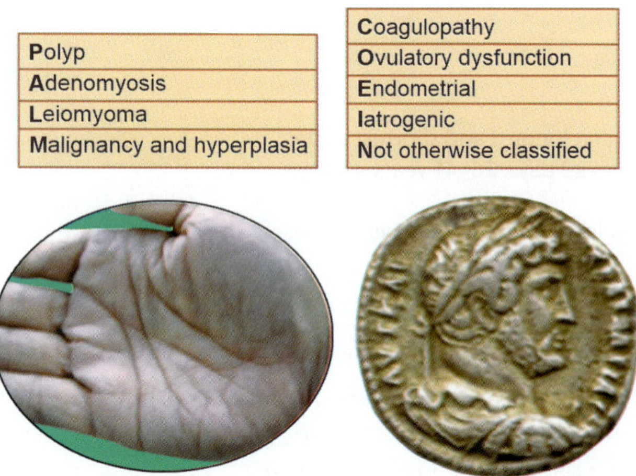

Fig. 1: Classification of PALM-COEIN for causes of AUB in the nonreproductive age group.

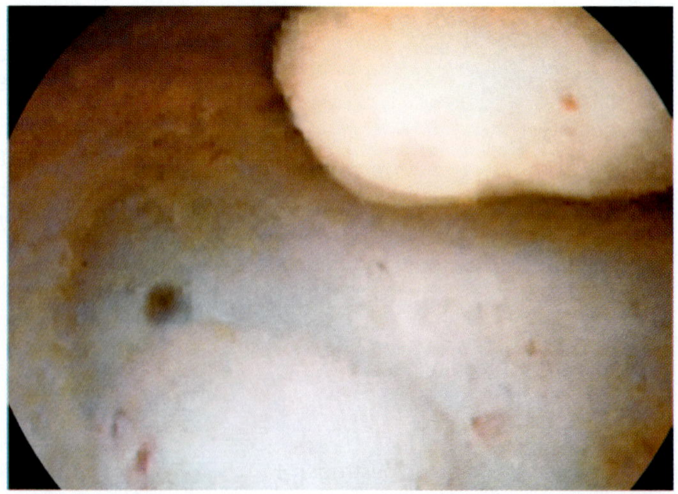

Fig. 2: Multiple polyps with left-sided (LT) ostia.

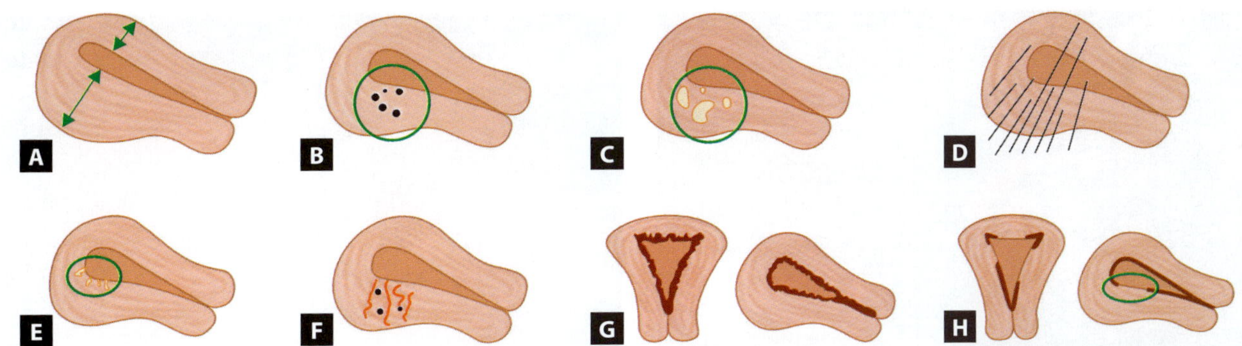

Figs. 3A to H: MUSA criteria. (A) Asymmetric thickening; (B) Myometrial islands; (C) Hyperechoic islands; (D) Fan-shaped shadows; (E) Echogenic subendometrial lines; (F) Vascularity; (G) Irregular junctional zone; (H) Interrupted junctional zone.

A—Adenomyosis

There is no direct correlation between adenomyosis and AUB, but about 5–20% may find a correlation between the two. Adenomyosis may be locally called adenomyoma or may be diffuse. The only confirmation is by doing histopathology.

Adenomyosis can reliably be diagnosed by ultrasound criteria. Transvaginal sonography is as sensitive as MRI for the diagnosis. Morphological uterine sonographic assessment (MUSA) criteria have suggested eight criteria to diagnose adenomyosis. These include asymmetrical myometrial thickening, myometrial cysts, hyperechoic islands, fan-shaped shadowing, echogenic subendometrial lines, translesional vascularity, irregular junctional zone and interrupted junctional zone **(Figs. 3A to H)**. Using transvaginal sonography, a diagnosis of adenomyosis can be reliably made with MUSA criteria. Adenomyosis can be diffuse or focal.

Figure 4 shows an ultrasound picture of diffuse adenomyosis.

- Treatment of adenomyosis includes medical and surgical treatment. The medical line of treatment includes the use of oral contraceptive (OC) pills or progesterone or non-steroidal anti-inflammatory drugs (NSAIDs). Levonorgestrel-releasing intrauterine system (LNG-IUS) is also an option for patients with adenomyosis. Aromatase inhibitors such as letrozole have also been used in the treatment. For patients who want to preserve fertility, uterus sparing resection of adenomyoma can be done. The definitive treatment of adenomyosis is hysterectomy.

L—Leiomyoma

- Incidence of fibroids causing AUB is about 10–15%.
- AUB in cases of fibroids is due to:

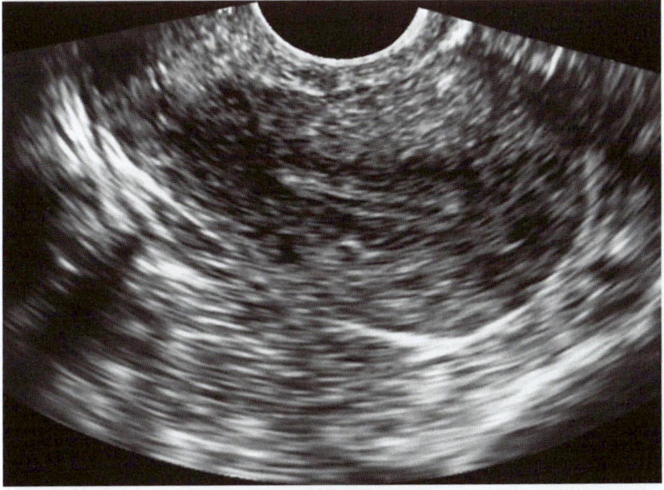

Fig. 4: Diffuse adenomyosis.

  - Fibroid polyps coming out of the cervical canal, causing intermenstrual bleeding
  - In the case of submucous fibroids, due to an increase in surface area as well as intrinsic oestradiol production, these fibroids can cause heavy bleeding.
  - Increased uterine cavity as well as uterine contractility
  - Imbalance between prostaglandin production

Diagnosis

- Clinical history and menstrual history
- Ultrasonography-transvaginal scan (USG-TVS) with use of Doppler, 3D and 4D **(Figs. 5 and 6)**.
- Sometimes, sonohysterography and hysteroscopy may be needed to diagnose small submucous myoma **(Fig. 7)**.

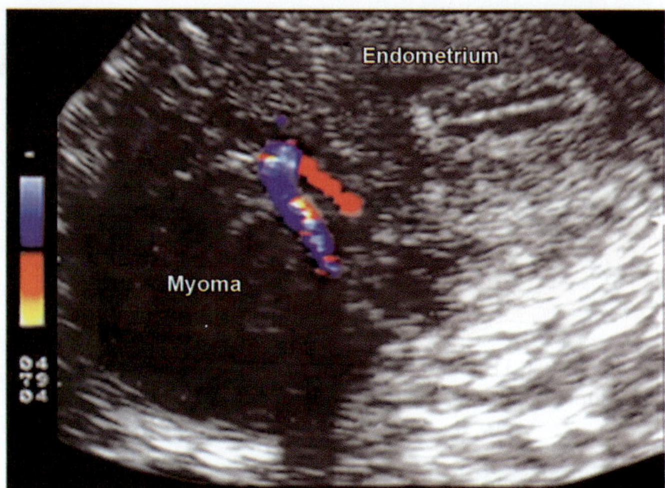

Fig. 5: Colour Doppler showing the presence of subserosal fibroid with peripheral vascularisation.

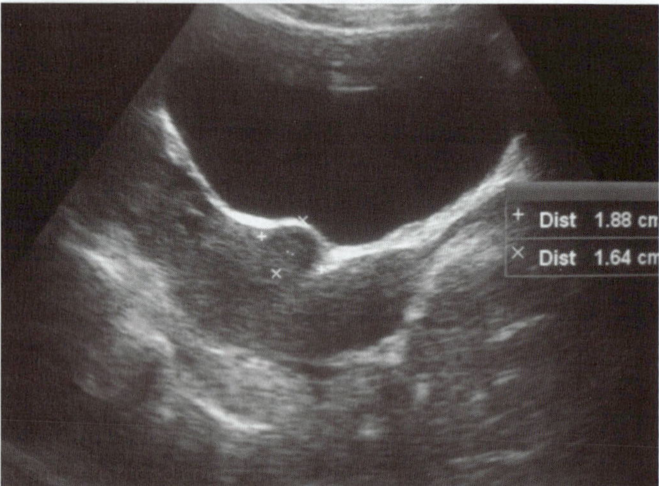

Fig. 6: Intramural myoma.

- MRI may also sometimes be needed to determine the exact location of the fibroid or sometimes to differentiate it from adenomyosis.

WAMSTEKER CLASSIFICATION (FIG. 8)

Wamsteker classification describes myomas in relation to endometrium into different types. Types 0, 1, 2 and 3 lie near endometrium and are most likely to give rise to AUB. Types 0 and 7 are defined as myomas where the stalk is <10% of the diameter of myoma. If the stalk is >10%, it is classified as type 1 or 6 depending on their location. Hysteroscopy sometimes may be needed to differentiate between a type 2 and type 3 myoma.

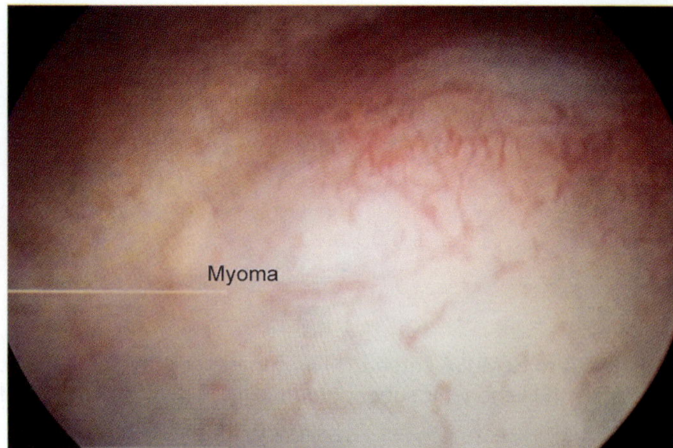

Fig. 7: Submucous myoma.

STEPW CLASSIFICATION OF MYOMA

This classification aims at predicting successful hysteroscopic myomectomy. STEPW (size, topography, extension of the base, penetration, and lateral wall position) classification is used to predict the feasibility of hysteroscopic myomectomy. In groups 1 and 2, hysteroscopic myomectomy may be tried. In group 3, hysteroscopic myomectomy will be difficult. Before attempting hysteroscopic myomectomy, a STEPW score should be done, and surgery is approached with respect to the score **(Table 2)**.

- Treatment depends upon the size of myoma, location and number as well as the age of the patient and desire to preserve fertility.
- Medical management
- Nonhormonal treatment:
  - *Prostaglandin synthetase inhibitors:* There is evidence that prostaglandin E compounds are increased in menorrhagia although the mechanism is unclear.
  - Mefenamic acid, 250–500 mg three times daily, is effective in reducing menstrual loss by 20–50% in 75% of patients, although it has little effect on cycle length. There are few side effects and, as administration is restricted to the time of the blood loss, it is often preferred to oestrogen-progestogen preparations by the patients. It may well be the first choice for those over the age of 35 years. Diclofenac, ibuprofen and naproxen are also useful.
  - *Antifibrinolytic agents:* For menorrhagia (and for bleeding caused by an intrauterine contraceptive device), symptomatic treatment can be given

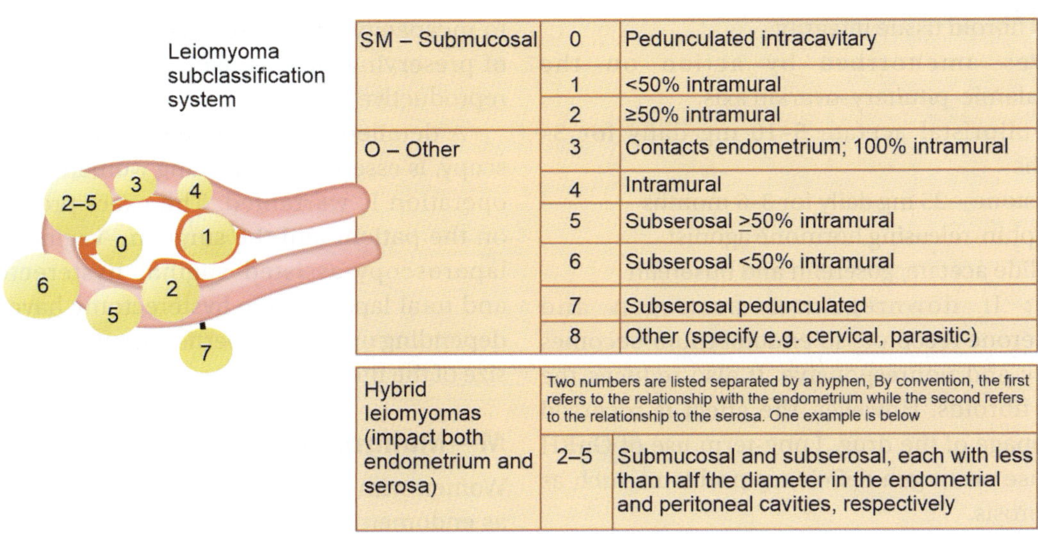

Fig. 8: Subclassification of leiomyoma.

TABLE 2: STEPW classification of myoma.

Points	*Size*	*Topography*	*Extension of the base*	*Penetration*	*Lateral wall*
0	<2 cm	Low	<1/3	0	1
1	2–5 cm	Middle	1/3–2/3	<50%	
2	>5 cm	Upper	>2/3	>50%	
Score	***Group***	***Complexity and therapeutic options***			
Score 0–4	Group I	Low complexity hysteroscopy myomectomy			
Score 5–6	Group II	High complexity hysteroscopy myomectomy, two-step hysteroscopy myomectomy, GnRH agonist			
Score 7–9	Group III	An alternative to hysteroscopy myomectomy to be considered			

(GnRH: gonadotrophin-releasing hormone; LMs: leiomyomas)

with antifibrinolytic agents administered orally for 3–6 days during each period. These include e-aminocaproic acid (EACA) 3 g, 4–6 times daily, or tranexamic acid, 1 g, 2–4 times daily. Tranexamic acid is a synthetic derivative of the amino acid lysine in the chemical structure of trans-4 (amino methyl) cyclohexane carboxylic acid.

- Tranexamic acid competitively *inhibits activation of plasminogen, thereby reducing plasmin*. It blocks lysine-binding sites of plasminogen molecule, which is required for binding to fibrin reversibly. Tranexamic acid acts by inhibiting tissue plasminogen activator, a fibrinolysis enzyme, which has raised levels. It prevents fibrinolysis or lysis of blood clot or thrombus, therefore used in controlling blood loss. It is also an anti-inflammatory agent given in a dose of 3–6 g. It can reduce menstrual loss by about 50% during therapy. This may be tried when oestrogens and progestogens are contraindicated or unsatisfactory, although a history of thromboembolism is a contraindication for their use.

- *Hormonal treatment:*
  - Combined oral contraceptive (COC)
  - Progestogen-only contraceptive pill (POP)
- *Selective progesterone receptor modulators (SPRM) such as ulipristal and mifepristone:*
  - *Action:* It is a selective progesterone receptor modulator; it blocks progesterone receptors and hence decreases growth of fibroids as well as size up to 60–70% and achieves amenorrhea in 90–95% within 3–7 days.
  - Inhibits proliferation of leiomyoma cells
  - Induces apoptosis
  - Downregulates vascular endothelial growth factor (VEGF) and suppresses neovascularisation

- Impairs fibroid tissue integrity
- Achieves amenorrhea by action on the hypothalamic–pituitary–ovarian axis.
- Dose—ulipristal acetate 5–10 mg daily for 3–6 months
- Mifepristone—25 mg daily for 3–6 months

- Gonadotrophin-releasing hormone agonist
  - Leuprolide acetate, goserelin and buserelin
  - *Action:* It downregulates oestrogen and progesterone receptors so endometrium becomes atrophic and nonresponsive. It also reduces the size of fibroids. However, the effect is reversed on stoppage of the drug. Long-term use of GnRH can cause oestrogen deficiency problems such as osteoporosis.
  - *LNG-IUS*
  - May be used in cases where there is no distortion of uterine cavity and uterine size is not large
  - Fertility-preserving surgical treatment
  - *Myomectomy:* Hysteroscopic myomectomy can be done by using a monopolar hook or bipolar electrode. If the majority of myoma is intramural, double setting myomectomy is advised.
  - Laparoscopic myomectomy can be done in cases of intramural as well as subserous fibroids. There is no contraindication nowadays regarding the size and number of fibroids to be removed laparoscopically.
  - Magnetic resonance-guided focused ultrasound surgery improves clinical symptoms in 70–80%. It is performed as an OPD procedure without anaesthesia. Depending on the size, location and fibroid compressing on other side of tissue structure, low to high energy sonication is delivered to the actual target spot. Each sonication duration varies from 20 to 30 seconds, followed by a cooling period. It decreases size by causing thermal necrosis.

Hysterectomy

When the patient is over 40 years of age, and when the haemorrhage fails to respond to simpler measures, hysterectomy is indicated. It is the treatment of choice in all cases of persistent or recurrent bleeding. Hysterectomy can usually be carried out easily by the vaginal route and this involves little risk.

In younger women, this is to be avoided whenever possible. Even in these, there comes a time when hysterectomy with conservation of the ovaries is preferable to incapacity prolonged indefinitely merely for the sake of preserving what is likely to be a very unsatisfactory reproductive function.

A detailed preoperative workup, including hysteroscopy, is essential in all young women to be sure that this operation is warranted. The exact procedure depends on the patient and the surgeon—vaginal, abdominal or laparoscopy-assisted vaginal hysterectomy (LAVH), and total laparoscopic hysterectomy have all been used depending upon the expertise of surgeon and location and size of the uterus.

M—Malignancy

Women with premalignant or malignant conditions, such as endometrial carcinoma and hyperplasia, are classified in this group. Endometrial sampling is needed in women with a family history of malignancy or based on other risk factors such as obesity. Endometrial sampling is always to be done in women over 45 years of age. If transvaginal sonography shows increased endometrial thickness, endometrial sampling is indicated. If AUB is persistent and not responding to treatment, it is always better to do an endometrial sampling to rule out malignancy.

C—Coagulopathy

Any blood disorder characterised by coagulation defects or by excessive capillary fragility can cause endometrial haemorrhage. Such bleeding may be one of the *first* manifestations of thrombocytopenic purpura, aplastic anaemia, leukaemias, von Willebrand's disease, and Christmas disease, for example, and can be so severe as to threaten life. Anticoagulants, which increase the blood flow, are also classified as iatrogenic rather than coagulopathy in the 2018 modification of the AUB classification. Approximately 13% of AUB can occur from coagulation abnormalities, the most common of them being von Willebrand's disease. All women must be screened for coagulopathy based on history, and if the screening history is positive, then investigations are done to rule out coagulopathy as a cause of bleeding.

Increased fibrinolytic activity of the endometrium is a postulated but unproven cause of menorrhagia. Some observers claim to have demonstrated an increase in fibrin degradation products in the uterine and systemic veins in certain cases; others deny this finding. If the level is raised, it is more likely to be the result than the cause of menorrhagia; that is, the endometrium is being called upon to deal with more clots than normal.

Treatment depends on the cause, in consultation with a haematologist.

O—Ovulatory Dysfunction

Predictable regular menstruation suggests ovulation whereas if cycles are irregular, it means anovulation. Midluteal measurement of progesterone may be done to confirm ovulation. Histopathological finding of secretory endometrium also confirms ovulation. Ovulatory causes of AUB are usually seen in adolescence and at extreme of reproductive age.

Treatment

Treatment of ovulatory disorders includes treatment of any underlying cause such as hyperprolactinemia, if present. Combined oral contraceptive pills may be used to regularise ovulation. Cycle progesterone can be given to prevent endometrial hyperplasia. LNG-IUS is an option. Weight loss can improve ovulatory function in women with PCOS.

I—Iatrogenic

This category includes side effects of hormonal drugs or the use of medicated uterine devices. Previously, in 2011 classification use of anticoagulants was considered as coagulopathy, but now, in the 2018 modifications, anticoagulants are reclassified under iatrogenic causes.

E—Endometrial Causes

In women with regular cycles and AUB when all other causes are ruled out, the cause of bleeding is probably endometrial. Imbalances in prostaglandins and endometrial inflammation can all lead to AUB.

Hysteroscopic-guided targeted endometrial biopsy is the gold standard for both diagnosis and treatment of endometrial lesions. The addition of hysteroscopy has greatly improved diagnostic accuracy in the evaluation of focal intrauterine lesions. It allows for visual inspection of the endometrial cavity and gives the physician the opportunity to perform directed biopsies. Endometrial polyps or submucosal leiomyomas can easily be identified by hysteroscopy and removed in the same sitting. As with many high-technology approaches, however, hysteroscopy requires appropriate training and equipment to ensure patient safety. If hysteroscopy is unavailable, dilation and curettage remains an accepted method for evaluation of the endometrium in a low-resource setting.

N—Not Otherwise Specified

This category has been renamed as "not otherwise specified" in the 2018 classification. AV malformations and bleeding from the uterine niche fall under this category.

APPROACH TO A PATIENT WITH ABNORMAL UTERINE BLEEDING

A patient with AUB may have more than one cause of AUB, and all factors must be assessed in a woman with AUB.

General Assessment

Pregnancy-related causes always need to be ruled out, preferably by scan and a pregnancy test. Women should be tested for anaemia. Thorough clinical assessment should be done to rule out local pathology in vagina, vulva, etc. Abdominal, speculum and pelvic examination should be done.

Determination of Ovulatory Status

Regular predictable cycles usually suggest ovulation. Midluteal progesterone levels may be done to confirm ovulation. Endometrial biopsy if done for any reason and shows secretory endometrium again suggests ovulation.

Screening for Coagulation Abnormality

Structured screening by history has a high sensitivity to detect coagulopathy. If any of the following criteria is positive, women must be tested for coagulation abnormality **(Box 1)**.

BOX 1: Screening for bleeding disorders.

Initial screening for an underlying disorder of haemostasis in patients with excessive menstrual bleeding should be by a structured history

A positive screening result comprises any of the following:

- Heavy menstrual bleeding since menarche
  - One of the following:
    - Postpartum haemorrhage
    - Surgical-related bleeding
    - Bleeding associated with dental work
- Two or more of the following symptoms:
  - Bruising 1–2 times per month
  - Epistaxis 1–2 times per month
  - Frequent gum bleeding
  - Family history of bleeding symptoms

If women are positive for coagulopathy by screening in history, they should be evaluated for abnormalities with the help of a haematologist. Screening by history has a high sensitivity to diagnose coagulation disorders.

Evaluation of Endometrium

Endometrial evaluation is needed if the woman is >45 years, obese or in the presence of a family history of malignancy. Women who have failed to respond to therapy or have irregular bleeding should also undergo an endometrial evaluation of endometrium. If transvaginal sonography shows increased endometrial thickness, such women should have endometrial sampling to rule out malignancy.

Evaluation of Endometrial Cavity

Initially, a transvaginal sonography is done. If it is normal, nothing is needed. If findings are abnormal, sometimes sonohysterography or hysteroscopy may be needed to rule out a polyp or submucosal myoma.

Myometrial Assessment

Sonography is used primarily to diagnose a myoma. To know the exact location and type of myoma, sometimes MRI, hysteroscopy or sonohysterography may be needed. Adenomyosis, as described before, can be diagnosed by MUSA criteria. MRI is also useful in differentiating myoma from adenomyosis.

Management of Acute Bleeding

Sometimes women can present with acute bleeding, which may need immediate control. Acute bleeding can be arrested with conjugated equine oestrogen 25 mg given intravenously every 4 hours. Combined pills can be given one tablet three times a day for 7 days to control bleeding. Progesterone, such as norethisterone, can be given 5 mg three times a day to control bleeding. Dilatation and curettage can control bleeding in an acute setting of bleeding. Sometimes, unresponsive bleeding, uterine artery embolisation or even hysterectomy may have to be done.

SPECIAL CLINICAL TYPES OF BLEEDING

Ovulation Bleeding

Ovulation bleeding is not strictly abnormal; it is a common, if not regular, cyclical phenomenon in all women. However, both patient and attendant may fail to distinguish it from menstruation and thus mistake what is an essentially normal cycle for polymenorrhoea.

Clinical Features

Some individuals appear more susceptible to overt ovulation bleeding than others, but even in these, its occurrence is inconsistent. It may be present in some for months and not in others, and can disappear for years. The bleeding usually lasts only a few hours and rarely for longer than 2 or 3 days. It is small in amount, often consisting of nothing more than "spotting" or of a red tinge in the mucoid ovulatory discharge from the cervix. It is said that all women experience this phenomenon and that most are not aware of it because the loss is literally microscopic. Ovulation bleeding may or may not be accompanied by ovulation pain. Its diagnosis rests on the time and character of the loss.

Causes

The bleeding usually occurs from the endometrium and is probably the result of a temporary oestrogen deprivation during the changeover from the follicular to the luteal phase in the ovary. Normally, there is a fall in the blood oestrogen level at this time. Ovulation bleeding is said to be more likely when the pelvic organs are congested. Another view is that the blood-stained discharge originates from the ovary at the time of ovulation and is picked up by the tubes to be passed through the uterus.

Treatment

Ovulation bleeding is a physiological phenomenon which does not ordinarily require any treatment other than explanation.

Prepubertal Bleeding

Prepubertal bleeding is arbitrarily defined as bleeding before the age of 10 years (some say 8 or 9 years).

Precocious Puberty

The bleeding may be menstrual and due to precocious puberty; it is then accompanied by other evidence of sexual maturation.

Nonmenstrual Bleeding

Vaginal bleeding in childhood without concomitant development of secondary sex characters always calls for careful investigation because it is probably not menstrual in type. The causes include foreign bodies in the vagina, vaginitis and neoplasms of the vagina, cervix and uterus.

Genital Crisis in the Newborn

Slight uterine bleeding, sometimes amounting to no more than a single blood-stained smear on a napkin, occurs in 10% of female babies 2 or 3 days after birth. This is an oestrogen withdrawal phenomenon, the foetal uterus having been stimulated before birth by placental oestrogen. No treatment is necessary; the discharge ceases in a few hours or days.

Pubertal Bleeding

Pubertal bleeding is arbitrarily defined as excessive bleeding occurring between the menarche and the age of 20 years. The first one or two periods are commonly profuse, prolonged and irregular in time of onset, but such disturbance generally cures itself quickly, and medical advice is usually not sought. Sometimes, however, the bleeding is so heavy as to produce anaemia and even to threaten life (near-fatal menarche). There may be several such episodes during the 2 or 3 years before a regular cycle is established, and any can call for blood transfusion. Extreme, alarming and persistent forms of pubertal bleeding are mostly seen in spoiled, often only children with overanxious parents. Sometimes, a normal loss may be claimed to be excessive. Pubertal bleeding is usually anovulatory in type.

Perimenopausal Bleeding

Perimenopausal bleeding is the excessive bleeding which commonly occurs at the age when menopause might be expected.

The menopause is never normally heralded by increasing menstrual loss, and the only safe rule is to regard any bleeding which is heavier in amount, longer in duration, or acyclical, occurring in a woman over 40 years of age, as requiring immediate and careful investigation. Essentially, this means pelvic examination, cervical and endometrial cytology, cervical biopsy and curettage, with the possibility of malignant disease ever in mind. In fact, cancer of the uterus is found in less than 5% of women complaining of premenopausal bleeding.

Often, shortening of the menstrual cycle because of a shortened follicular phase is the first change of menopause. In some cases, the bleeding proves to be dysfunctional and anovulatory in type, but often no endometrial abnormality is found. For a full list of possible causes, see postmenopausal bleeding (*see below*).

One basis for excessive and prolonged bleeding around the time of the menopause is the injudicious use of oestrogens. These are prescribed for real or imagined climacteric symptoms, arthritis, emotional instability, pruritus vulvae and the like; they operate no matter whether they are given by injection, orally or in the form of ointments and gels. Moreover, an admixture of an androgen does not always prevent it from stimulating the endometrium. In a susceptible woman, one tube of an oestrogen ointment applied to the vulva may be enough to cause uterine bleeding. Careful inquiry about the use of any remedies, bearing in mind that proprietary preparations containing oestrogen can be obtained by the public without a medical prescription, is essential in all cases.

When AUB occurs in middle-aged women taking oestrogens, how should the case be managed? Ideally, endometrial aspiration should always be carried out to exclude malignant disease. Nevertheless, this is not always practicable and the compromise solution is to exclude a gross abnormality by vaginal examination, cytology and ultrasound and to discontinue the oestrogen. All bleeding should then clear within 1 month; if it does not, or if it recurs after that time, hysteroscopy and endometrial sampling are essential.

Postmenopausal Bleeding

Bleeding from the genital tract occurring after menopause is much more sinister than premenopausal bleeding. In defining postmenopausal bleeding, the question arises as to when menopause can be regarded as established. An arbitrary time limit of 1 year's amenorrhoea is generally set, but some prefer to reduce the period to 6 months. Even without amenorrhoea or irregularity, menstruation continuing after the age of 55 years should be investigated.

Causes

Postmenopausal bleeding is more likely to be caused by pathologic disease than is bleeding in younger women, and it must always be investigated. Nongynaecologic causes must be excluded; these are also more likely to be caused by pathologic disease in older women, and the patient may be unable to determine the site of bleeding. The source of bleeding should not be assumed to be nongynaecologic unless there is good evidence or proper evaluation has excluded gynaecologic causes.

Neither normal (functional) bleeding nor dysfunctional bleeding should occur after menopause. Although pathologic disorders are more likely, other causes may also occur. Atrophic or proliferative endometrium is not unusual. Secretory patterns should not occur unless the patient has resumed ovulation or has received progesterone therapy.

After nongynaecologic causes of bleeding are excluded, gynaecologic causes must be considered.

The most common cause of bleeding occurring after menopause is the *indiscriminate use of oestrogens* for hormone replacement therapy (HRT). If this is excluded, 10% of all patients and 30–50% of those in whom the bleeding is continuous or occurs more than once, are accounted for malignant disease of the cervix or of the body of the uterus.

The possible causes of postmenopausal bleeding are listed *below*, and, except for the senile states, they apply equally to premenopausal bleeding:

- Oestrogen therapy
- Atrophic vaginitis
- Fibroid polyps
- Benign and malignant neoplasms of the vulva, vagina, cervix, corpus and fallopian tubes
- Ovarian tumours—oestrogen-producing tumours—any tumour of a large size affecting the vascularity of the uterus, "misfit tumours".
- *Infections:*
  - *Vaginitis: Trichomonas, Candida, Chlamydia* and senile
  - *Endometritis:* Tuberculous, senile pyometra and hematometra
- *Dysfunctional uterine bleeding:*
  - Anovulatory
  - Ovulatory
- *Injuries:*
  - Direct trauma
  - Decubital ulceration
  - Foreign bodies such as supporting pessaries
  - Postradiation ulceration
- Diseases of the blood and the capillaries
- *Bleeding from the urethra, bladder and rectum (mistaken for vaginal bleeding):*
  - Urethral caruncle
  - Papilloma and carcinoma of the bladder
  - Haemorrhoids and fissure in anovulatory
  - Carcinoma of the rectum
- No cause found (? vascular or psychogenic basis).

In approximately 10% of cases, the bleeding proves to be either "dysfunctional" or caused by a reawakening of ovarian function. Thus, anovulatory bleeding and endometrial hyperplasia without bleeding can occur 1 and 2 years after menopause. In these cases, continued production of steroid hormones by the hilus or stromal cells is postulated. An ovarian source is suggested by the fact that oophorectomy lowers the hormone levels. Indeed, the production of oestrogens by ovarian stromal cells for as long as 25 years after the menopause is reported. Nevertheless, whenever the endometrium is found to be hyperplastic, and the vulva and vagina look under the influence of oestrogens, two questions arise: (1) Is the hormone exogenous? (2) Is there a small granulosa or theca cell tumour in the ovary? Occasionally, postmenopausal bleeding is ovulatory and is then presumably the result of the belated ripening of a stray ovum—a phenomenon which has been called "flash in the pan" menstruation. This is usually seen soon after menopause.

Postmenopausal hyperplasia carries a stronger threat of cancer than does premenopausal hyperplasia. It is also an indication for testing blood sugar.

In patients who have had only one episode of slight postmenopausal bleeding, it is common (12–50% of cases) not to find any abnormality. In these, as well as in women with dysfunctional bleeding, a sudden emotional shock or other upset may be in the background. The bleeding must result from a break in endometrial blood vessels, and it appears more likely in hypertensive women.

Of patients with negative findings who have bled only once before curettage, 70–80% do not bleed again afterwards.

Investigation and Treatment

Postmenopausal bleeding or discharge calls for immediate investigation, even though there is only a single episode. Even when there is a history of oestrogen therapy, transvaginal ultrasonography, endometrial aspiration and possibly hysteroscopy and colposcopy-guided cervical biopsy are necessary. Endometrial cancer is rare when the endometrial thickness is <4 mm. This is true even if vaginal and cervical smears and endometrial aspirates are negative for cancer cells; it is true even when an adequate cause for bleeding such as a cervical polyp or senile vaginitis is found. The presence of such lesions does not exclude the presence of carcinoma of the uterus; indeed, a cervical polyp stands in the same relation to carcinoma of the body of the uterus as do haemorrhoids to carcinoma of the rectum.

If standard tests do not show the lesion, there is a case for doing a CT scan or an MRI of the pelvis to exclude a genital lesion.

When a cause is found, treatment is directed to it. When no cause is found in the genital tract and the bleeding occurs, abnormal and excessive uterine bleeding, repeatedly, its origin from another site has to be excluded. This means a full study of the urinary system and lower bowel, including cystoscopy and sigmoidoscopy. The recurrence or persistence of bleeding per vaginum after all investigations have given negative findings always calls for laparotomy with a view to hysterectomy. This may be the only means of detecting an early carcinoma of the uterus, the tube or the ovary.

SUGGESTED READING

1. Bakour SH, Timmermans A, Mol BW, Khan KS. Management of women with postmenopausal bleeding: evidence-based review. Obstet Gynaecol. 2012;14:243-9.
2. Eden J, O'Neill S. The management of perimenopausal abnormal uterine bleeding. Obstet Gynaecol Reprod Med. 2019;29(12):359-63.
3. Khafaga A, Goldstein SR. Abnormal uterine bleeding. Obstetrics and Gynecology Clinics. 2019;46(4):595-605.
4. Munro MG, Critchley HO, Broder MS, Fraser IS. FIGO classification system (PALM-COEIN) for causes of abnormal uterine bleeding in nongravid women of reproductive age. Int J Gynaecol Obstet. 2011;113(1):3-13.
5. Munro MG, Critchley HOD, Fraser IS. The two FIGO systems for normal and abnormal uterine bleeding symptoms and classification of causes of abnormal uterine bleeding in the reproductive years: 2018 revisions. Int J Gynaecol Obstet. 2018;143(3):393-408.

41

CHAPTER

Dysmenorrhoea

Brihathi Pranavi Dasari, Muralidhar V Pai

Chapter Outline

- Primary Dysmenorrhoea
- Secondary Dysmenorrhoea
- Membranous Dysmenorrhoea
- Other Conditions Simulating Dysmenorrhoea

INTRODUCTION

Dysmenorrhoea means painful menstruation, restricting the patient's daily activity. Dysmenorrhoea is of two types:

1. Primary, idiopathic or true dysmenorrhoea
2. Secondary dysmenorrhoea

Every patient complaining of dysmenorrhoea must be asked:

- When do you feel the pain?
- Does it ever occur apart from menstruation?
- What is its relation to the first day of the period?
- On which days is it most intense?
- How long does it last?
- Where is the pain situated?

Primary dysmenorrhoea is essentially a first-day pain *(spasmodic dysmenorrhoea)*, while secondary dysmenorrhoea may continue throughout the flow or may be worse premenstrually and is relieved during the flow *(congestive)*. A pain which is equally severe before, throughout and after menstruation is likely to have its origin in the psyche; no pelvic lesion can cause such a pain.

PRIMARY DYSMENORRHOEA

Primary dysmenorrhoea refers to the presence of spasmodic and painful cramps in the lower abdomen that begin shortly before or at the onset of menses but with no visible pelvic pathology. *It is a common condition which may be seen in 50% of post-pubertal women aged 18–25 years.*

Aetiology

Behavioural and Psychological Factors

Just before and during menstruation, most women are less efficient physically and more unstable emotionally; these factors alone lower the pain threshold. *A dysmenorrhoeic mother usually has a dysmenorrhoeic daughter.* It is often very difficult to separate the respective contributions of physiological and psychological factors, and they make dysmenorrhoea worse even if they do not cause it. A complete psychosocial history may suggest other causes for abdominal pain, such as depression, substance abuse, or stress secondary to abuse or other trauma.

Muscular Incoordination and Uterine Hyperactivity

Spasmodic dysmenorrhoea could be due to incoordinate muscle action of the uterus as a whole. It could be explained by sympathetic overactivity leading to hypertonus of the circular fibres of the isthmus and the internal os. This would also explain the other manifestations of autonomic upset, such as bowel and bladder tenesmus, which accompany dysmenorrhoea.

Hormone Imbalance

Spasmodic dysmenorrhoea has some connection with the progesterone stimulus to the uterus. It only occurs in ovular cycles, and it is suggested, but not proved, that the occurrence of anovular menstruation explains the absence of dysmenorrhoea during the few years following menarche and the occasional painless period even at a later age due to immaturity of the hypothalamo-pituitary axis. Another observation is that progesterone induces high tone in the isthmus and upper cervix. An exaggeration of this could therefore be the basis of the incoordinate action of the uterus.

Prostaglandins

Prostaglandin E2 and prostaglandin F2 alpha in menstrual fluid and endometrial tissue are elevated in patients with primary dysmenorrhoea and correlate with the severity of pain resulting from endometrial sloughing at the beginning of menses. They play a major role in inducing uterine contractions, which are nonrhythmic or incoordinate, occur at a high frequency (more than four or five per 10 minutes), often begin from an elevated basal tone (>10 mm Hg), and result in high intrauterine pressures (frequently >150–180 mm Hg, sometimes exceeding 400 mm Hg). When uterine pressure exceeds arterial pressure, uterine ischemia develops, and anaerobic metabolites accumulate, which stimulate type C pain neurons, resulting in dysmenorrhoea. Activation of stretch receptors and central sensitisation of pain likely play a role in pain perception.

Prostaglandin synthetase inhibitors relieve the symptoms in about 80% of patients with dysmenorrhoea, which supports the view that excessive prostaglandin activity is a major factor in its aetiology.

Other Factors

Vasopressin, leukotrienes and endothelins also increase myometrial contractility, but their role in dysmenorrhoea is unclear.

Clinical Features

In primary dysmenorrhoea, the pain sensation arises in the uterus and is related to muscle contractions. It is experienced a few hours before and after the onset of menstruation and rarely lasts in a severe form for longer than the first 2 days. It is colicky in type, associated with backache, causing a patient to *double up*. The pain is felt in the hypogastrium and is referred to the inner and front aspects of the thighs; *It never extends below the level of the knee and is never experienced in the back of the leg.* The cutaneous areas of pain reference are innervated by the iliohypogastric and ilioinguinal nerves (T12, L1 and L2).

During a severe attack, the patient may experience nausea, sweating and vomiting. There may be diarrhoea and rectal and bladder tenesmus due to an imbalance in the autonomic nervous system.

Despite its high prevalence and impact on daily activities, it is often inadequately treated, as many women consider it an embarrassment and a taboo and also perceive the pain as an inevitable response to menstruation that should be tolerated.

In at least 50% of cases, the pain does not arise until 6–12 months after the menarche. A description of intense pain dating from the menarche should raise doubts about its reality. Primary dysmenorrhoea reaches a maximum between the ages of 18 and 24 years, and thereafter diminishes. Moreover, it is nearly always cured by pregnancy. It is postulated that nerve endings in the muscle and cervix are destroyed by pregnancy and this may explain how primary dysmenorrhoea is often cured after the birth of a baby.

Treatment

A sympathetic approach to the patient, including consideration of psychological and behavioural elements, will help in a positive outcome. **Flowchart 1**—up-to-date treatment of dysmenorrhoea in adult females—shows an approach to the management of a case of dysmenorrhoea.

The goal of treatment is to provide adequate relief of pain that permits them to perform their usual activities, improves their quality of life, and decreases their academic or work-related absenteeism.

Prevention

Unfavourable environmental factors, malnutrition and general ill health should be corrected. Regular physical activity is to be encouraged both between and during menstruation.

Drugs

Prostaglandin synthetase inhibitors: The nonsteroidal anti-inflammatory drugs (NSAIDs), are active inhibitors of prostaglandin synthetase **(Table 1)**. The drugs are required for 1–3 days from the onset of menses. Continuous therapy during the period, every 6–8 hours, prevents the reformation of prostaglandin byproducts and is very effective for pain relief. If given for 3–6 cycles, it gives better results. The fenamates (mefenamic acid and flufenamic acid) are the most effective and are virtually free from side effects, which act by inhibiting both prostaglandin synthetase and block the action of prostaglandins that are already formed. Their use is contraindicated in women with gastrointestinal ulcers, bronchial asthma and hypersensitivity to aspirin. Side effects include nausea, vomiting, diarrhoea, abdominal pain, constipation, heartburn and dizziness. Less commonly, patients may have bronchospasm, melena, hearing disturbances, drowsiness, skin rash haematologic and renal function abnormalities.

Flowchart 1: Management of dysmenorrhoea.

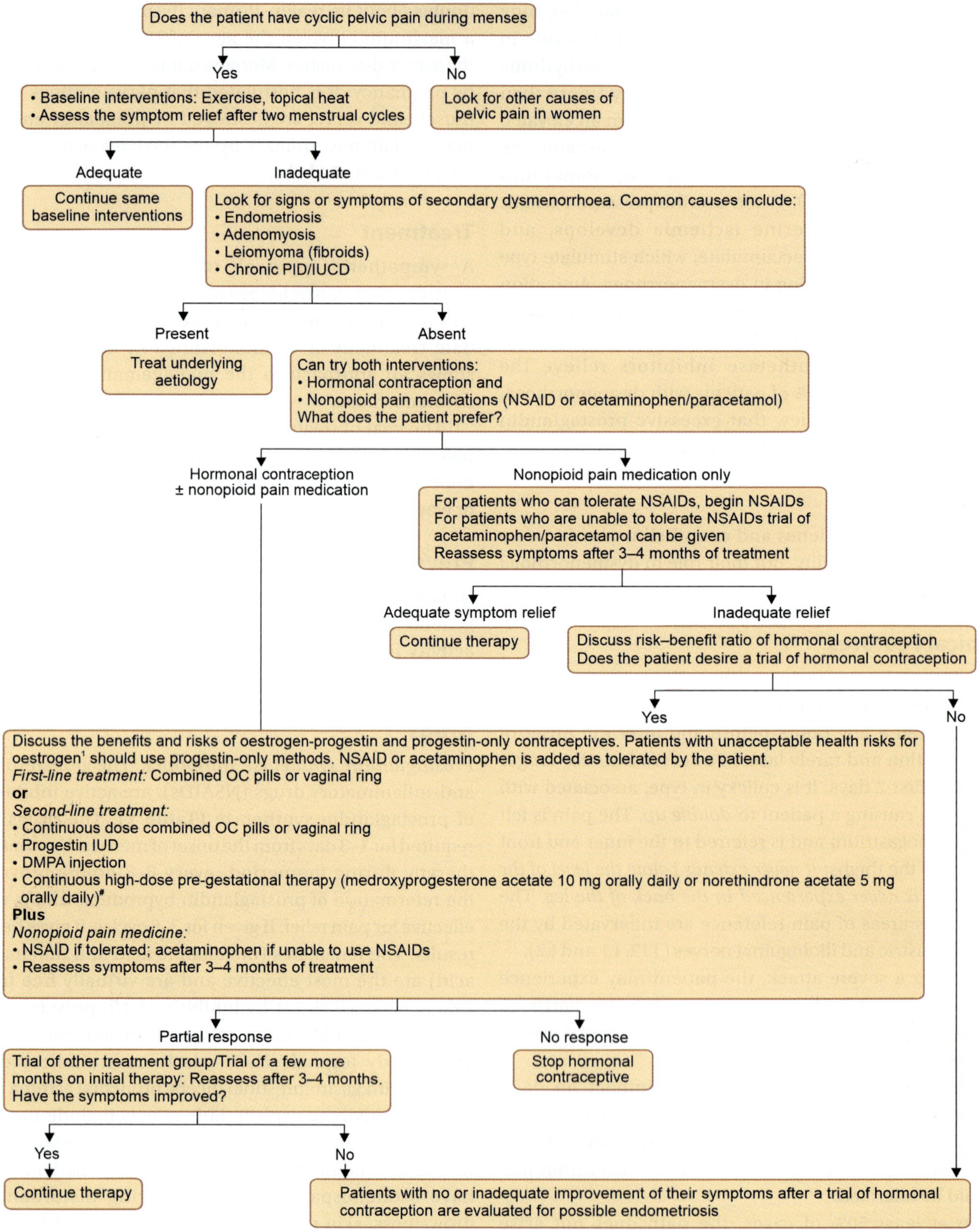

Does the patient have cyclic pelvic pain during menses

Yes

- Baseline interventions: Exercise, topical heat
- Assess the symptom relief after two menstrual cycles

No

Look for other causes of pelvic pain in women

Adequate

Continue same baseline interventions

Inadequate

Look for signs or symptoms of secondary dysmenorrhoea. Common causes include:
- Endometriosis
- Adenomyosis
- Leiomyoma (fibroids)
- Chronic PID/IUCD

Present

Treat underlying aetiology

Absent

Can try both interventions:
- Hormonal contraception and
- Nonopioid pain medications (NSAID or acetaminophen/paracetamol)

What does the patient prefer?

Hormonal contraception ± nonopioid pain medication

Nonopioid pain medication only

For patients who can tolerate NSAIDs, begin NSAIDs
For patients who are unable to tolerate NSAIDs trial of acetaminophen/paracetamol can be given
Reassess symptoms after 3–4 months of treatment

Adequate symptom relief

Continue therapy

Inadequate relief

Discuss risk–benefit ratio of hormonal contraception
Does the patient desire a trial of hormonal contraception

Yes

Discuss the benefits and risks of oestrogen-progestin and progestin-only contraceptives. Patients with unacceptable health risks for oestrogen[1] should use progestin-only methods. NSAID or acetaminophen is added as tolerated by the patient.
First-line treatment: Combined OC pills or vaginal ring
or
Second-line treatment:
- Continuous dose combined OC pills or vaginal ring
- Progestin IUD
- DMPA injection
- Continuous high-dose pre-gestational therapy (medroxyprogesterone acetate 10 mg orally daily or norethindrone acetate 5 mg orally daily)[#]

Plus
Nonopioid pain medicine:
- NSAID if tolerated; acetaminophen if unable to use NSAIDs
- Reassess symptoms after 3–4 months of treatment

Partial response

Trial of other treatment group/Trial of a few more months on initial therapy: Reassess after 3–4 months. Have the symptoms improved?

Yes

Continue therapy

No

No response

Stop hormonal contraceptive

No

Patients with no or inadequate improvement of their symptoms after a trial of hormonal contraception are evaluated for possible endometriosis

Contd...

Contd...

#Oral medroxyprogesterone acetate and norethindrone acetate are not labelled for contraception. Thus, patients desiring contraception should be counselled to use an additional contraceptive method.

[1]Patients with unacceptable health risks for oestrogen:

- Age ≥35 years and smoking ≥15 cigarettes/day
- Multiple risk factors for arterial cardiovascular disease (such as older age, smoking and hypertension)
- Hypertension (systolic ≥160 mm Hg or diastolic ≥100 mm Hg)
- Venous thromboembolism
- Known ischaemic heart disease
- History of stroke
- Complicated valvular heart disease (pulmonary hypertension, risk for atrial fibrillation and history of sub-acute bacterial endocarditis)
- Current breast cancer
- Severe (decompensated) cirrhosis
- Hepatocellular adenoma or malignant hepatoma
- Migraine with aura
- Diabetes mellitus of >20 years duration or with nephropathy, retinopathy or neuropathy

(DMPA: depot medroxyprogesterone acetate; IUD: intrauterine device; NSAID: nonsteroidal anti-inflammatory drug)

TABLE 1: Commonly used nonsteroidal anti-inflammatory drugs.

Drug	*Dosage*
Mefenamic acid	250–500 mg 2–4 times daily
Flufenamic acid	100–200 mg 8 hourly
Ibuprofen	400 mg 8 hourly
Naproxen sodium	250 mg 8 hourly
Ketoprofen	50 mg 8 hourly
Piroxicam	20 mg once/twice daily
Indomethacin	25 mg 3–4 times daily

Newer NSAIDs are selective COX-2 inhibitors that relieve pain with similar efficacy, have fewer gastrointestinal side effects, but heart attack, stroke have been reported by their use.

Transdermal use of *nitric acid donor, glyceryl trinitrate,* results in uterine relaxation and is used currently as a new therapeutic alternative. Headache has been reported with its use.

Pethidine, morphine and the newer powerful analgesics should *never* be prescribed.

Hormone therapy: Anovulatory cycles are always painless; so, suppression of ovulation gives certain relief from primary dysmenorrhoea. This is best achieved by means of one of the *oestrogen-progestogen oral contraceptive (cyclical/extended cycle) preparations.* Prolonged suppression of the endometrium reduces the prostaglandin content and makes the endometrium relatively atrophic with low-prostaglandin menstruation, free of pain.

Oral contraceptive pills: They have been shown to be equally effective as NSAIDs. It is suggested that any combination oral oestrogen-progestin contraceptive pill is likely to reduce dysmenorrhoea by causing endometrial regression, atrophy, decidualisation and prevention of ovulation.

Vaginal rings and transdermal patches: As transdermal and vaginal oestrogen-progestin contraceptives are newer than oral contraceptives, few trials have evaluated their efficacy for treatment of primary dysmenorrhoea. The endometrial effects of oestrogen-progestin contraceptives are similar regardless of the method of delivery; therefore, the route of administration should not significantly affect efficacy.

Hormone therapy (combined oestrogen-progestogen pill) is the treatment of choice for the woman who desires contraception and for older teenagers who have achieved their full stature when prostaglandin inhibitors fail or are contraindicated.

Calcium-channel blockers: Patients with intractable dysmenorrhoea with no demonstrable pelvic pathology often respond well to nifedipine.

Surgical Treatment

Surgery for primary dysmenorrhoea is considered only when medical treatment has failed, and when a significant psychological or pathological basis is excluded. It is rarely indicated, and hardly ever before the age of 18 years.

Laparoscopy: A diagnostic laparoscopy should be considered to rule out any pelvic lesions causing secondary dysmenorrhoea for a patient with failed medical therapy over 4–6 cycles. If present, these can be treated simultaneously.

Transcutaneous electric nerve stimulation (TENS) has also been used for dysmenorrhoea, but the results are not good.

Presacral neurectomy ***(Fig. 1):*** Obsolete

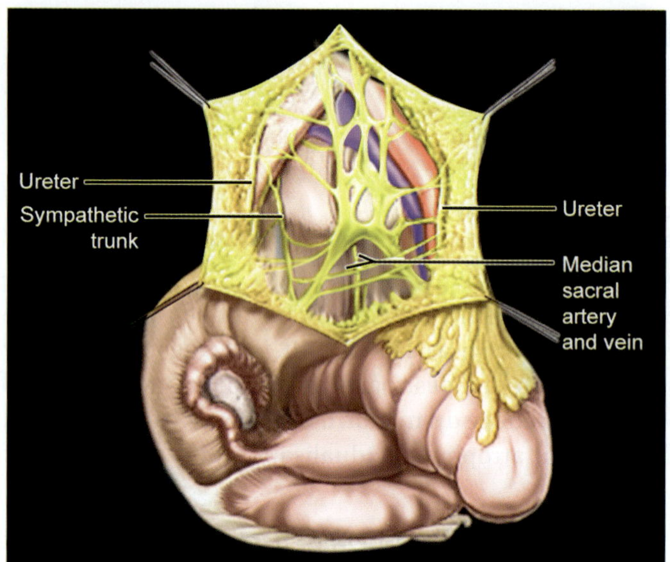

Fig. 1: The presacral nerves exposed as in the operation of presacral neurectomy. The peritoneum over the bifurcation of the aorta and the promontory of the sacrum has been incised vertically to show not only the sympathetic nerves, but also the other retroperitoneal structures in close relation to them.

Flowchart 2 enumerates which cases are to be selected for surgical therapy.

Currently, *laparoscopic ultrasound nerve ablation (LUNA)* is done in patients with intractable dysmenorrhoea along with laparoscopic surgery for endometriosis, but long-term results are still awaited.

Results

A good medical management is effective in 80–95% of cases.

Complementary and Alternative Treatment

Drugs: Thiamine 100 mg daily, vitamin E 2,500 IU taken once daily, and omega-3 polyunsaturated fatty acids intake, but evidence is limited.

Medicinal herbs, acupuncture, acupressure and yoga can also reduce dysmenorrhoea, but there is limited evidence.

SECONDARY DYSMENORRHOEA

Secondary dysmenorrhea is a pain which is associated with uterine or pelvic pathology.

Aetiology

Pelvic lesions at various sites can result in secondary dysmenorrhoea. The common causes are endometriosis, acute and chronic pelvic inflammatory disease, adenomyosis, leiomyoma, polyp, intrauterine

Flowchart 2: Management of a case of dysmenorrhoea after failed first-line therapy.

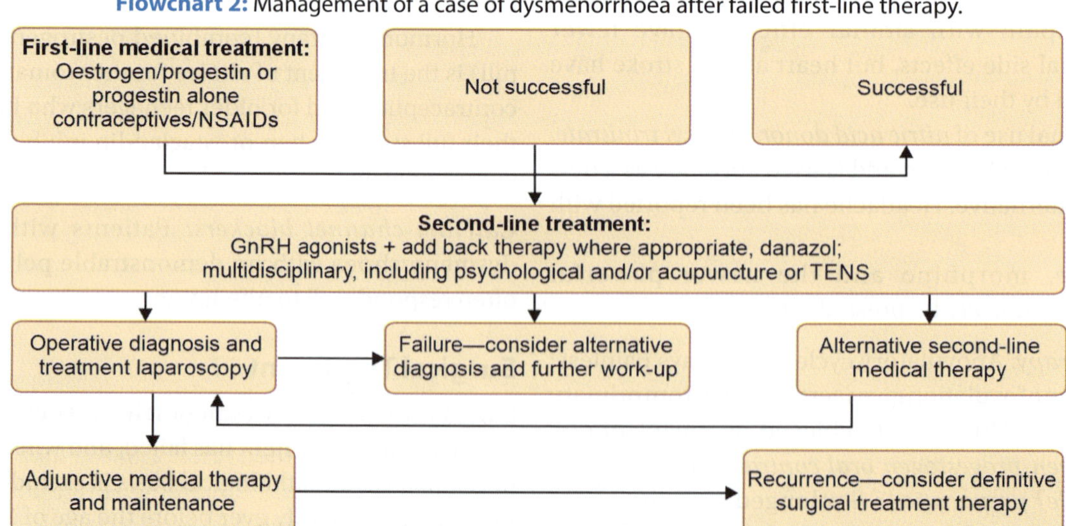

(GnRH: gonadotrophin-releasing hormone; NSAIDs: nonsteroidal anti-inflammatory drugs; TENS: transcutaneous electrical nerve stimulation)

contraceptive device (IUCD) and congenital malformations of the uterus.

One-sided spasmodic dysmenorrhoea in a young patient should always raise the possibility of a uterine malformation. Cervical stenosis, imperforate hymen or transverse vaginal septum cause cyclical pain once a haematometra develops.

Secondary dysmenorrhoea arising after the age of 30 years always suggests the possibility of endometriosis. It is experienced as an increasing ache for 2 or 3 days premenstrually but reaches its peak *during or at the end of the period.* Unlike spasmodic dysmenorrhoea, the pain persists for several days and only ceases completely after the period is over.

The *Allen–Masters syndrome* and pelvic congestion involve the peritoneum and cause secondary dysmenorrhoea.

Accessory and cavitated uterine mass (ACUM) is a condition defined by the presence of a noncommunicating uterine mass close to the insertion of the round ligament and is diagnosed by the presence of a central cavity in the uterus, lined by functional endometrium, and surrounded by a ring of smooth muscle on ultrasound **(Fig. 2)**.

Case report: Two young women presented with medically refractory dysmenorrhoea. They were initially diagnosed with subserosal fibroid and rudimentary uterine horn **(Fig. 3)**, respectively. After failure of all forms of medical treatment for dysmenorrhoea, they underwent laparoscopy. Intraoperatively, they were diagnosed with accessory and cavitated uterine masses (ACUMs) and successfully underwent complete laparoscopic excision of ACUM and remained symptom-free after that.

It is a congenital anomaly that may present at any age, may be misdiagnosed, and is unresponsive to medical therapy. It requires a high degree of suspicion, proper evaluation with preoperative imaging, and first-line surgical management for prompt relief.

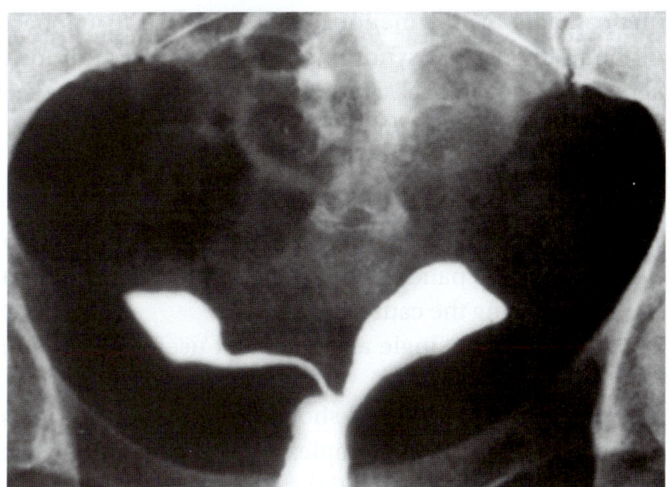

Fig. 2: Blood casts from the uterus in a case of spasmodic dysmenorrhoea associated with the passage of clots.

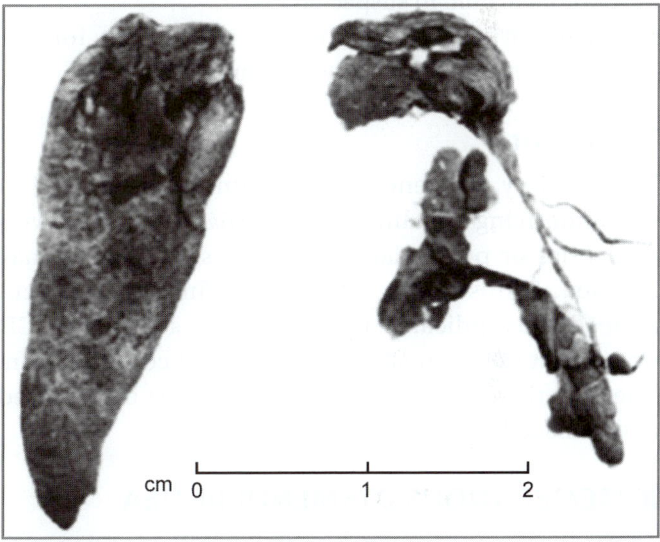

Fig. 3: Hysterogram showing unequal development of the two horns of a bicornuate uterus. In such a case, spasmodic dysmenorrhoea, if present, might be unilateral. But the pain would most likely arise from the better-developed horn. A rudimentary horn only causes dysmenorrhoea when it fails to communicate with the cervix and becomes the seat of a haematometra.

Clinical Features

Secondary dysmenorrhoea usually develops after a phase of painless cycles and is seen at an older age. However, endometriosis can rarely occur at or shortly after menarche. History and physical examination aid in elucidating most of the etiological factors. The pain may be spasmodic or congestive. Congestive dysmenorrhoea (Taylor syndrome) is a diffuse dull ache in the pelvis, often accompanied by backache, and is thought to be the result of increasing tension in the pelvic tissues associated with inflammation exacerbated by premenstrual engorgement. The pain is therefore maximum in the premenstrual phase (2–3 days prior) and is slowly relieved as congestion is reduced with the onset of menstruation. It is frequently associated with menorrhagia or polymenorrhoea, and often forms part of the premenstrual syndrome. Orthopaedic conditions affecting the lower back can cause premenstrual backache and should be ruled out.

Investigations

- *Secondary dysmenorrhoea:* Diagnosis is based on the history of the patient. Important investigations to help in identifying the cause are:
- Laparoscopy—single and the most useful diagnostic procedure
- Pelvic ultrasound—will show ovarian endometriosis and demonstrate the complexity of the ovaries in pelvic inflammatory disease (PID)
- Hysterosalpingogram—useful in identifying intrauterine adhesions
- Microbiological cultures—from endocervix or peritoneal fluid in suspected PID
- Magnetic resonance imaging is the best for the diagnosis of congenital uterine anomalies.

Treatment

In secondary dysmenorrhoea, treatment is directed to the underlying condition. Supportive measures with analgesics or prostaglandin synthetase inhibitors may be used. If this is not sufficient, definitive treatment is needed as indicated in the relevant sections. IUCD users must select an alternate method of contraception. The underlying cause of menorrhagia must be explored and managed.

MEMBRANOUS DYSMENORRHOEA

This is a very rare condition with a familial incidence in which the endometrium, instead of being fragmented, strips off in large pieces or even as a whole cast of the uterus; the passage of these is preceded and accompanied by severe colic. Its pathogenesis is obscure. The traditional explanation is that an overmature corpus luteum induces an excessive decidual reaction to make the surface endometrium so compact that it will not easily disintegrate. In certain cases, the fault may lie in the sensitivity of the endometrium rather than in its hormone stimulus.

It is refractory to all treatment, including curettage. Suppression of ovulation by means of an oestrogen-progestogen preparation, administered cyclically for 1–2 years, is said to be effective in some cases.

OTHER CONDITIONS SIMULATING DYSMENORRHOEA

Menstrual Pain of Ovarian Origin

Corpus Luteum Haematoma

It is a rare condition where there is haemorrhage into and from the corpus luteum. It may be spontaneous or by direct injury, such as that sustained during coitus or physical exercise. The patient experiences an acute onset of sharp lower abdominal pain followed by a feeling of faintness. Severe collapse can occur if there is much intraperitoneal bleeding, simulating a ruptured ectopic pregnancy. Other similar features are a palpable small but tender swelling of one adnexa, generalised tenderness and distension of the lower abdomen. The pain is also usually followed by uterine bleeding, which in this condition is the premature arrival of a menstrual period due to the failure of corpus luteum function. Even at laparotomy, the haematoma may be diagnosed as an ovarian pregnancy, the true nature of the lesion only being recognised on histological examination. Rupture of an endometriotic cyst and torsion of a small ovarian tumour can also be confused preoperatively.

The clue to the diagnosis is that the symptoms begin during the second half of a previously regular cycle. It may be added, however, that the corpus luteum of early pregnancy can also bleed into its substance or into the peritoneal cavity. In that case, it may be impossible, before operation, to distinguish the syndrome from ectopic pregnancy clinically. Ultrasound and serum human chorionic gonadotrophin (hCG) titres may help with the diagnosis.

If the diagnosis of corpus luteum haematoma is made, and it is clear that the haematoma is small and self-limiting, no treatment other than analgesics and continuous observation is necessary.

Ovulation Pain

Clinical Features

Mid-cycle pain *(mittelschmerz)* is present from time to time during the menstrual life of almost 50% of women, although it may go unnoticed. The discomfort appears between day 10 and 15, is experienced in the hypogastrium or in the iliac fossa, and is occasionally referred to the rectum. It varies in severity but rarely lasts longer than 12–24 hours.

Cause

Ovulation pain is said to be caused by contractions of the tube or uterus; increased tension in the Graafian follicle or the ovary; irritation of the peritoneum by the discharge of fluid and blood from the follicle; and muscle cramps in the caecum or pelvic colon. Its occurrence during the menstrual cycle is variable. Sometimes precedes ovulation and subsides before ovulation.

Treatment

Ovulation pain is rarely severe enough to merit more than reassurance and explanation.

Orthopaedic Conditions Simulating Dysmenorrhoea

Disc lesions and arthritic changes in the spine are possible findings, but in nearly all cases of premenstrual and menstrual backache, the patient is suffering only from a chronic muscular or ligamentary strain.

Pain in the knees with each menstrual period is an interesting but less well-known syndrome. It begins premenstrually only lasts a few days, and is the result of fluid retention associated with high levels of steroid hormones. This causes swelling of the infrapatellar pads of fat, which then becomes nipped in the joints.

SUGGESTED READING

1. Dawood MY. Primary dysmenorrhea: advances in pathogenesis and management. Obstet Gynecol. 2006;108(2):428-41.
2. Gupta N, Corrado S, Goldstein M. Hormonal contraception for the adolescent. Pediatr Rev. 2008;29(11):386-96.
3. Habibi N, Huang MS, Gan WY, Zulida R, Safavi SM. Prevalence of primary dysmenorrhea and factors associated with its intensity among undergraduate students: a cross-sectional study. Pain Manag Nurs. 2015;16(6):855-61.
4. Harada T. Dysmenorrhea and Endometriosis in Young Women. Yonago Acta Med. 2013;56(4):81-4.
5. Iacovides S, Avidon I, Baker FC. What we know about primary dysmenorrhea today: a critical review. Hum Reprod Update. 2015;21(6):762-78.
6. Juang CM, Yen MS, Twu NF, Horng HC, Yu HC, Chen CY. Impact of pregnancy on primary dysmenorrhea. Int J Gynaecol Obstet. 2006;92(3):221-7.
7. Michelle P. Diagnosis and management of dysmenorrhoea. BMJ. 2006;332(7550):1134-8.
8. Morrow C, Naumburg EH. Dysmenorrhea. Prim Care. 2009;36(1):19-32.
9. Panwar A, Davis A, Lata K, Sharma S, Kriplani A. Laparoscopic management of accessory cavitated uterine mass: a report of two cases and review of literature. J Gynec Surg. 2020;36(5):285-8.
10. Petraglia F, Parke S, Serrani M, Mellinger U, Römer T. Estradiol valerate plus dienogest versus ethinylestradiol plus levonorgestrel for the treatment of primary dysmenorrhea. Int J Gynaecol Obstet. 2014;125(3):270-4.
11. Wong CL, Farquhar C, Roberts H, Proctor M. Oral contraceptive pill for primary dysmenorrhoea. Cochrane Database Syst Rev. 2009;2009(4):CD002120.

42

CHAPTER

Premenstrual Syndrome and Other Menstrual Phenomena

Kaushik Naik V, Muralidhar V Pai

Chapter Outline

- Clinical Features
- Natural History
- Laboratory Findings
- Aetiology
- Differential Diagnosis
- Treatment
- Menstrual Migraine
- Premenstrual Mastalgia
- Recurrent (Cyclical) Buccal and Vulvar Ulceration
- Pelvic Allergy
- Vicarious Menstruation
- Cyclical Haemothorax and Pneumothorax
- Menstrual Epilepsy

INTRODUCTION

The premenstrual syndrome (PMS) is characterised by the presence of both physical and behavioural symptoms that occur repetitively in the second half of the menstrual cycle and interfere with some aspects of woman's life. Premenstrual dysphoric disorder (PMDD) is a severe form of PMS in which symptoms of anger, irritability and internal tension are prominent.

CLINICAL FEATURES

Most well-adjusted women experience minor psychological and somatic changes for a few days preceding menstruation. This menstrual molimina gives way to a sensation of relief and well-being once menstruation is established. In some women, these manifestations become exaggerated to constitute a PMS. This is extremely common at all ages, but especially in women aged 30–45 years, the reported prevalence ranges from 5 to 95%. It is wrongly attributed to an approaching menopause. The age incidence of PMS is said to be due to the fact that stresses are most severe in the third and fourth decades. The problem is a feature of modern conditions of life in Western civilised communities. It used to be rarely encountered in, or complained of, by women in Eastern countries, but changing lifestyles this pattern is changing. It is certainly the cause of much individual misery and family disharmony, absenteeism and even criminal acts such as murder and suicide.

NATURAL HISTORY

Premenstrual syndrome symptoms begin any time after menarche but usually by one's early 20s and typically continue throughout reproductive life. Some women experience more severe symptoms in their late reproductive years. Women with premenstrual disorders appear to be at higher risk for developing mood disorders during menopausal transition. PMS resolves completely after menopause and transiently during pregnancy or during any disruption of ovulatory cycles.

The symptoms can be any of those discussed above, accentuated to a pathological degree and present for as long as 7–10 days premenstrually. In some instances, the symptoms are so severe that the woman fails to cope with her ordinary day-to-day life. If the onset of a period is delayed, the symptoms become even more intense. The main complaints are headache, depression, insomnia, emotional outburst, intestinal distension, colonic spasm and congestive dysmenorrhea.

The patient herself is conscious of nervous tension and has a bloated feeling, often accompanied by an actual increase in girth and weight. In certain cases, there is an obvious swelling of legs caused by oedema **(Table 1)**.

Not all the various discomforts are present in each case; sometimes, one is so prominent as to overshadow the others and to justify it being regarded as a special clinical entity such as menstrual migraine, menstrual oedema and premenstrual mastalgia.

The affected individual is often full of restless energy, cleaning the house when it is already spotless, fussing and nagging the children and worrying when there is no need. The husband cannot understand the periodic outbursts and moods; the resulting quarrels make the situation worse. It is the imaginative women 'living on her nerves' who are likely to suffer.

TABLE 1: Diagnostic criteria for premenstrual dysphoric disorder.

Timing of symptoms	In the majority of menstrual cycles, at least five symptoms must be present in the final week before the onset of menses, start to improve within a few days after the onset of menses, and become minimal or absent in the week post menses
Symptoms	• One or more of the following symptoms must be present: (1) Marked affective lability (e.g. mood swings, feeling suddenly sad or tearful, increased sensitivity to rejection); (2) Marked irritability or anger or increased interpersonal conflicts; (3) Markedly depressed mood, feelings of hopelessness or self-deprecating thoughts and (4) Marked anxiety, tension and/or feelings of being keyed up or on edge. • One (or more) of the following symptoms must additionally be present to reach a total of 5 symptoms when combined with symptoms from above: 1. Decreased interest in usual activities 2. Subjective difficulty in concentration 3. Lethargy, easy fatigability or marked lack of energy 4. Marked change in appetite; overeating or specific food cravings 5. Hypersomnia or insomnia 6. A sense of being overwhelmed or out of control 7. Physical symptoms such as breast tenderness or swelling, joint or muscle pain and a sensation of 'bloating' or weight gain
Severity	The symptoms are associated with clinically significant distress or interference with work, school, usual social activities or relationships with others
Other psychiatric disorders	The disturbance is not merely an exacerbation of the symptoms of another disorder, such as major depressive disorder, panic disorder, persistent depressive disorder (dysthymia) or a personality disorder (although it may co-occur with any of these disorders)
Confirmation of the disorder	• The above criteria must be confirmed by prospective daily ratings during at least two symptomatic cycles (although a provisional diagnosis may be made prior to this confirmation) exclude other medical conditions • The symptoms are not attributable to the physiological effects of a substance (e.g. drug abuse, medication, other treatment) or another medical condition (e.g. hyperthyroidism)

Examination is usually not helpful. Various questionnaires have been developed in an attempt to quantify the problem. These are designed to measure the severity of symptoms, underlying psychological dysfunction and the degree of disruption of normal functioning. Commonly used methods include visual analogue scales and psychiatric questionnaires, e.g. the General Health Questionnaire and Moos Menstrual Distress Questionnaire.

LABORATORY FINDINGS

There are no specific biochemical abnormalities associated with the disorder. Daily serum concentrations of gonadotrophins and sex steroids are no different in women with PMS than the women without PMS. A serum thyroid-stimulating hormone (TSH) may be done to rule out hyper-/hypothyroidism, as both can cause mood symptoms.

AETIOLOGY

At the present time, despite intensive study, the aetiology remains unknown, and there are many theories but no real explanation. There are undoubtedly physiological and psychological factors or components, which act to varying extents in different individuals.

The underlay of over anxiety and emotional instability present in some cases makes it necessary with regard to the condition as a psychosomatic disorder.

The aetiology of PMS is uncertain. Since PMS symptoms occur simultaneously with the hormonal fluctuations of the menstrual cycle, hormonal disproportions such as oestrogen surplus and progesterone deficiency have been proposed. Symptoms are also associated with serotonin to link as a key aetiological factor.

Oestrogen comprises three major hormones: (1) Oestrone, (2) oestradiol and (3) oestriol; oestradiol is the most potent. Oestrogen levels that fluctuate during the luteal phase are what is responsible for women's mood changes. Clinical trials have shown that serotonin precursors significantly increase between days 7–11 and 17–19 of the menstrual cycle. This indicates that PMS is closely associated with mood disorders through oestrogen–serotonin regulation.

Neurotransmitters play a role. The luteal phase levels of beta-endorphins have been shown to be low in women with PMS and can lead to anxiety, food craving and physical discomfort. Low serotonin levels have also been demonstrated in red blood cells and platelets. Treatment with fluoxetine, a selective serotonin reuptake inhibitor (SSRI), is effective in improving symptoms. Vitamin B6 is a cofactor in the synthesis of serotonin and dopamine from tryptophan, but its deficiency has not been clearly proven.

Aetiology and Pathophysiology

The exact cause of PMS remains elusive; however, several theories have been proposed given as follows:

- *Hormonal fluctuations:* Sensitivity to normal hormonal changes during the menstrual cycle may play a role in PMS development.
- *Neurotransmitter abnormalities:* Alterations in neurotransmitter systems, particularly serotonin, have been implicated in PMS, suggesting a link between mood regulation and symptom manifestation.
- *Biopsychosocial factors:* A comprehensive review highlights the interplay of biological, psychological and social factors in the aetiology of PMS, emphasising the need for a multifaceted approach to understanding and managing the syndrome.

Although more than one mechanism may be concerned in the production of symptoms, an increase in extracellular fluid throughout the body is one, which is often blamed. This explains why some affected women gain 1.8–2.3 kg weight just before a period. The oedema is said to be associated with sodium retention and this in turn with high levels of both oestrogen and progesterone in circulation during the second half of the menstrual cycle. Oophorectomy, either surgically or medically [by administration of gonadotrophin-releasing hormone (GnRH) analogues], eliminates the symptoms of PMS, whereas several postmenopausal women who take hormone replacement therapy (HRT) develop them, especially during the progesterone phase of cycle. Another view is that it is a relative deficiency of progesterone, which is the causal factor, but it is more likely that the swings in hormone level cause it. The subjective sensation of bloatedness may be due to gut distension.

However, most women who suffer from PMS do not put on weight. Controlled observations show that the incidence and intensity of symptoms are not related to weight gain. The tendency, therefore, is to credit the syndrome to a hypothalamic–pituitary disturbance. Such a basis would explain the cases in which fluid retention is a feature, as well as those in which it is not. It would also account for certain symptoms, which have been attributed to neurovascular instability and hypoglycaemia.

Defective essential fatty acid or prostaglandin metabolism is postulated to result in an exaggerated response to normal ovarian hormone levels through a change in the receptor status at the cellular level.

Other theories to explain PMS include excess prolactin secretion and an increased production of aldosterone. There are no really good control-based studies due to the wide variations in the syndrome.

DIFFERENTIAL DIAGNOSIS

Psychiatric problems, familial disharmony and hyperthyroidism may lead to irritability and behavioural change. A premenstrual pelvic pain may be caused by pelvic inflammatory disease or endometriosis. Underlying breast lesions should be ruled out in cyclical mastalgia.

Lethargy may be due to hypothyroidism or anaemia, which must be looked for and treated.

TREATMENT (TABLE 2)

General Symptoms

The treatment goals for patients with premenstrual disorders are to relieve symptoms and improve functional impairment. The most important line of treatment is the correction of environmental causal factors. A sympathetic inquiry into personal problems and worries, and a reasonable explanation of the situation to both the patient and her husband, may do better than any specific medical remedies. Since woman is overdriving herself, nervously if

TABLE 2: Treatment options for premenstrual syndrome with varying efficacies.

Treatments with demonstrated efficacy	*Treatments with probable efficacy*	*Ineffective treatments*
SSRIs	Cyclical OCPs not containing drospirenone	Progesterones
Drospirenone containing cyclical OCP	Alprazolam	Vitamin supplements
Continuous OCPs (any progestin)	Exercise	Dietary restrictions
GnRH agonists		

(GnRH: gonadotrophin-releasing hormone; OCPs: oral contraceptive pills; SSRIs: selective serotonin reuptake inhibitors)

not physically, reorganisation of her life or her outlook on her life is often necessary. A mid-day nap for 2 hours every day is particularly helpful.

A number of lifestyle measures (exercise and relaxation techniques) and medications (SSRIs) are effective for women with PMS or PMDD. These therapies have largely supplanted earlier approaches that had little or no scientific evidence to support their efficacy.

Cognitive-behavioural therapy (CBT) is an approach that emphasises the correction of unsettled disruptive thoughts, behaviours, and emotions. CBT helps in the recognition of these behaviours and helps develop coping strategies to improve daily functioning.

Mild Symptoms

For women with mild premenstrual symptoms that do not cause distress or socioeconomic dysfunction, lifestyle measures such as regular exercise and stress reduction techniques are helpful.

A number of vitamins and dietary supplements, including vitamin B6, vitamin E, calcium, and magnesium, have been studied as therapeutic agents for PMS. These have not been found to be more effective than placebo.

Moderate-to-severe Symptoms

These are best treated with pharmacological intervention.

The two main treatment approaches are given as follows:

1. Targeting the serotonin system by increasing central serotonergic transmission [SSRIs and serotonin-norepinephrine reuptake inhibitors (SNRIs)]
2. Suppressing the hypothalamic-pituitary-ovarian axis to abolish cyclic changes in gonadal steroids [oral contraceptives (OCs) and GnRH agonists]

Elimination of Fluid

In those cases in which a temporary increase in weight is a feature, the prevention of the accumulation of fluid in the tissues is the best form of symptomatic treatment. For this, the intake of fluid should be limited for 7–10 days premenstrually, and at the same time, diet should contain as little sodium as reasonably possible. When fluid retention is considerable, a therapeutic trial of spironolactone may be tried for 10–14 days prior to the expected period. As there is no conclusive evidence that diuretics are effective in the relief of premenstrual tension, patient must be cautioned against addiction and indiscriminate use.

Serotonin Reuptake Inhibitors

Selective serotonin reuptake inhibitors have been found to be effective with good long-term results. Commonly used drugs are fluoxetine in a dose of 20 mg daily and sertraline in a dose of 50–150 mg daily. SSRIs are effective for premenstrual symptoms whether taken continuous or luteal phase only. Response is seen in 2–3 months.

Second-line therapies: A number of other drugs may be used when SSRIs are only partially effective, ineffective or difficult to tolerate.

Oral contraceptives: The simplest method of inducing anovulation is the use of OC pills; an OC containing progestin drospirenone and the use of 4-day rather than 7-day pill-free interval is found to be more effective.

Gonadotrophin-releasing hormone agonists: In women with severe symptoms who have not responded to or cannot tolerate SSRIs or OCs, GnRH agonists are used. This medical oophorectomy has significant side effects. Combining it with oestrogen-progesterone add-back may not only decrease the side effects but also the efficacy of treatment of PMS.

Other Drugs

Bromocriptine has been tried, but it best relieves cyclical breast symptoms. While some of the other symptoms are relieved or made tolerable, the overall benefit is not significantly greater than that obtained by the combination of placebo therapy and a caring physician.

When there is emotional instability and anxiety, mild tranquilisers are beneficial. Most proprietary remedies contain mixtures of vitamins and micronutrients, while others contain tranquilisers, antihistamine stimulants and progestogens as well.

The fruit extract *Vitex agnus-castus* (VAC) is the only herbal medicine that is proven to control PMS-associated mood swings and irritability.

Surgery

In some extreme cases, relief may not be obtained with any medication. Total abdominal hysterectomy with bilateral salpingo-oophorectomy has been recommended for those women, followed by HRT with the unopposed oestrogen. However, since this is an extreme step, a test with GnRH analogue should be done to confirm that the procedure will indeed be effective. Adequate counselling is essential.

MENSTRUAL MIGRAINE

Menstrual migraine is a specific subtype of migraine that occurs in relation to the menstrual cycle, predominantly affecting women during their reproductive years. These migraines are often more severe, longer lasting and less responsive to treatment compared to nonmenstrual migraines. Understanding the pathophysiology, clinical presentation, diagnostic criteria and management strategies is crucial for effective patient care.

Clinical Features

The patient ordinarily susceptible to migraine is most liable to attacks before and at the time of menstruation, but the term menstrual migraine is usually restricted to those cases in which attacks occur only at the time of menses. The condition is often familial. The headaches are localised to one area and are severe enough to be incapacitating; they are often accompanied by nausea and vomiting but are not usually preceded by visual, sensory and speech disturbances as in the case of classical migraine.

Menstrual migraines typically occur without aura and are closely linked to the menstrual cycle. They can be classified into two categories given as follows:

1. *Pure menstrual migraine:* Migraine attacks occur exclusively within a 5-day window, starting 2 days before menstruation and continuing through the first 3 days of bleeding, with no attacks at other times of the cycle.
2. *Menstrually-related migraine:* While attacks predominantly occur during the same 5-day perimenstrual window, additional migraines may happen at other times throughout the menstrual cycle.

These migraines are often more intense, last longer and are more resistant to treatment compared to nonmenstrual migraines.

Pregnancy usually brings temporary relief after the first trimester, but migraine can be very troublesome during lactation. The menopause does not necessarily cure them, and headaches may continue as a part of a climacteric syndrome.

Aetiology

The aetiology of menstrual migraine is multifactorial and similar to migraine in general. An attack is more likely if the individual is overtired, overworked or overwrought; excessive smoking is a contributory factor in some cases.

The cause of headache can be attributed to an allergic reaction to gonadotrophin, swelling of the pituitary gland, cerebral congestion and oedema, increased intracranial pressure, a local release of serotonin, cerebral ischaemia and psychological factors.

The exact mechanisms underlying menstrual migraines are not entirely understood; however, hormonal fluctuations, particularly involving oestrogen, play a significant role. Oestrogen influences various neurotransmitters, including serotonin and dopamine, which are integral to pain modulation and vascular regulation. The precipitous decline in oestrogen levels just before menstruation is believed to trigger migraine attacks in susceptible individuals. This hormonal drop may lead to increased release of calcitonin gene-related peptide (CGRP), a neuropeptide associated with vasodilation and neurogenic inflammation, both key components in migraine pathogenesis.

Additionally, oestrogen receptors are present on trigeminal nerve fibres, suggesting that fluctuations in oestrogen levels can directly sensitise these nerves, contributing to migraine development. It is possible that changes in the hormonal milieu produce the setting for vascular headaches. A fall in oestrogen levels may lead to cerebral vascular spasm.

Diagnosis

Accurate diagnosis requires a detailed headache diary maintained over at least three menstrual cycles, documenting the timing, duration and characteristics of headaches in relation to menstrual periods. The International Classification of Headache Disorders (ICHD) provides specific criteria for diagnosing menstrual migraines, emphasising the temporal association with menstruation and the absence of aura **(Box 1)**.

Treatment

General

Attention to general health and change in lifestyle are important. Regular exercise, adequate sleep, stress management and dietary considerations may help mitigate migraine frequency and severity. Visual defects, sinusitis and dental diseases must be excluded.

Hormone Therapy

Since menstrual headaches occur in response to cyclic variations in circulating levels of oestrogen

BOX 1: Diagnostic criteria according to the International Classification of Headache Disorders.

Pure menstrual migraine:
- Attacks in a menstruating woman fulfilling the criteria for migraine without aura
- Attacks occur 2 days before and last till the third day of menstruation:
  - Occur in at least two out of three menstrual cycles
  - Do *not* occur at other times of the cycle

Menstrually related migraine:
- Attacks in a menstruating woman fulfilling the criteria for migraine without aura
- Attacks occur 2 days before and last till the third day of menstruation
  - Occur in at least two out of three menstrual cycles
  - *Can* also occur at other times of the cycle

and progesterone, daily administration of exogenous hormones, i.e. combined OC pill or medroxyprogesterone acetate, is effective in preventing migraine headaches in many women. Tamoxifen and danazol have also been reported to be effective. The true severe migraine headaches with aura should not be treated with hormones and are, in fact, an indication for discontinuing OCs.

Symptomatic

An attack may be prevented by giving drugs such as phenobarbitone, belladonna and chlorpromazine, singly or in combination on the day before or at the onset of a period.

If, despite these and other measures described above, an attack of migraine occurs, earlier that treatment is given, better the result. With the patient at rest in a darkened room, the drugs of first choice to relieve pain are aspirin, paracetamol or nonsteroidal anti-inflammatory drugs (NSAIDs). The occurrence of vomiting, however, limits their usefulness.

A specific remedy is ergotamine tartrate (a serotonin agonist) with or without caffeine, which can be given orally.

A 2-mg dose is followed by 1 mg every 30 minutes, if required, up to a maximum of 4–6 mg. The weekly dose should not exceed 10 mg.

Antiemetics such as metoclopramide by mouth, or if vomiting is likely, by intramuscular (IM) injection, relieve the nausea associated with migraine attacks. Phenothiazine and antihistamine antiemetics may also be used. Sumatriptan, a serotonin receptor agonist, is used in oral doses of 25–100 mg per attack. Preloaded syringes carrying 6 mg of drug are available in some countries for self-administration subcutaneously. A safe and equally effective drug is clonidine hydrochloride, one tablet of 0.025 mg by mouth two or three times daily. It is, however, more often used to prevent attacks.

Artificial Menopause

The patient sometimes demands the induction of menopause, which she believes will lead to permanent relief. This treatment should be avoided because, to be effective, ovarian function has to be destroyed, and, in the type of woman under consideration, the end result may be climacteric headaches and other symptoms, which can be even more troublesome.

PREMENSTRUAL MASTALGIA

Premenstrual mastalgia, also known as cyclical mastalgia, refers to recurrent breast pain associated with the menstrual cycle, predominantly affecting women of reproductive age. This condition is characterised by bilateral, diffuse breast pain that typically intensifies during the luteal phase and subsides with the onset of menstruation. While often considered a component of PMS, emerging research suggests that premenstrual mastalgia may represent a distinct clinical entity.

Clinical Features

Approximately 80% of women experience slight fullness, tingling and tenderness of the breast during the week preceding menstruation. When this is exaggerated, it becomes part of PMS and is termed premenstrual mastalgia. Approximately 8–10% of premenopausal women experience moderate-to-severe perimenstrual breast pain monthly. The breasts may feel tense, knotty and tender, and there is some relationship to fibroadenosis. Indeed, women who suffer from the latter often relate their discomfort to the premenstrual phase.

Premenstrual mastalgia is probably restricted to ovular cycles and can be used as evidence of ovulation. As in all breast conditions and because of unequal development and activity, it is uncommon for the pain to be unilateral or worse on one side than the other.

Aetiology

The precise aetiology of premenstrual mastalgia remains incompletely understood. Hormonal fluctuations, particularly involving oestrogen and progesterone, are believed to play a pivotal role. Additionally, latent hyperprolactinaemia, resulting from insufficient dopaminergic inhibition of prolactin secretion, has been implicated in the pathogenesis of cyclical mastalgia. Lifestyle factors such as smoking, caffeine consumption and perceived stress have also been associated with an increased risk of mastalgia, suggesting a multifactorial aetiology.

Treatment

- The patient should be reassured, especially about the absence of cancer.
- The breasts should be well supported, and the patient discouraged from handling them to see if tenderness or nodules are present.
- *Lifestyle modifications*: Given the associations between mastalgia and factors such as smoking, caffeine intake and stress, lifestyle modifications addressing these elements may contribute to symptom relief. However, further research is necessary to establish the efficacy of such interventions.
- Premenstrual restriction of fluid and salt, as PMS is worthy of trial.
- Bromocriptine and progestogens such as dydrogesterone for 7–10 days premenstrually are sometimes of value.
- Other drugs used for the treatment of PMS are sometimes helpful.
- *Vitex agnus-castus (chasteberry):* A systematic review and meta-analysis encompassing 25 studies demonstrated that VAC effectively alleviated breast pain intensity in women aged 18–45 years with cyclical mastalgia. The typical dosage ranged from 20 to 40 mg/day over a treatment duration of 3 months. VAC was also found to lower elevated serum prolactin levels, with a moderate effect size favouring VAC over placebo. The treatment was generally safe, with only mild and reversible adverse events reported.

RECURRENT (CYCLICAL) BUCCAL AND VULVAR ULCERATION

Clinical Features

Recurrent buccal ulceration (aphthous ulcers) is sometimes cyclical and related to menstruation, the ulcers developing during the middle of the cycle or during the premenstrual phase, healing during and after menstruation. In the typical case, occurring in a woman during active reproductive life, the ulcers disappear during pregnancy and lactation but return afterwards. There may be simultaneous ulceration of the vulva, lower vagina and anus; genital ulceration can occur without oral lesions.

Aphthous ulcers of mouth are common; on the vulva, they are not uncommon. They may first appear in adolescence but rarely become really troublesome until early adult life.

In the majority of cases of alleged cyclical ulceration, the lesions have no relationship to menstruation and are not cyclical. They appear intermittently, last for a few days or weeks, and then slowly heal. The dissociation of this syndrome from menstruation is emphasised by the fact that it is seen in men as well as in women, though less commonly. The lesions in mouth and on genitalia usually take the form of extremely painful small shallow ulcers, which have a central yellow slough surrounded by a scarlet rim. These occur singly or in crops and are roughly circular with a diameter of up to 1 cm in size. They represent the breakdown of an initial papule and, in appearance, are similar to herpetic ulcers.

In the mouth, the two forms of disease are sometimes termed 'minor' and 'major' aphthous ulcers. The lesions develop on the insides of lips and cheeks, on the tongue, the floor of the buccal cavity and the fauces.

Recurrent oral and genital ulceration can be accompanied or followed by recurrent iridocyclitis to form Behçet's syndrome. The interval before the appearance of iridocyclitis may be as long as 10 years. Rare additional manifestations of this syndrome are other skin lesions such as pyoderma, thrombophlebitis, joint pains, hepatomegaly, splenomegaly and degenerative changes in the central nervous system. The last, which appear late, are serious; they are mostly found in the mid-brain, cerebellum and brainstem. Erythema nodosum is also a recognised association. Most of the manifestations of this syndrome appear to have vasculitis as a basis.

Aetiology

The cause of this extraordinary trying condition is unknown, but there are several theories postulated and certain aetiological factors established.

Genetic Factors

The operation of these is suggested by the fact that the disease can have a familial incidence. Genes encoding tumour necrosis factor have been implicated.

Allergy

A personal or family history of asthma, hay fever and other allergic states are often seen. Among the possible antigens are foodstuffs.

An immunological disorder is also favoured by the finding of histiocytes, plasma cells and eosinophils in the tissue adjacent to the ulcer and by generally good response to treatment with corticosteroids and immunosuppressives.

Virus Infection

The herpetic appearance of one form of ulceration raises this possibility, but a specific virus has never been demonstrated.

Hormonal Influences

Some connection with sex hormones is suggested by the occasional relationship between ulceration and menstruation and by its disappearance during pregnancy. It has been postulated that various hormones can act as antigens, but the evidence for this is lacking.

Psychological Factors

These are the most important of all the known associations. Whatever other agents may be involved, a background of nervous stress, unhappiness, sexual misadventures and marital unhappiness is a frequent finding. An attack of ulceration is often precipitated by an emotional crisis, and this can be clearly established in at least one third of cases. For such reasons, the oral lesions were once (100 years ago) called 'neurotic ulcers of mouth'.

The part played by the psyche and nervous stress could well explain the cyclical occurrence of ulceration premenstrually, when tension is at height, and the disappearance of ulceration during pregnancy when most women are placid and content.

Treatment

This is generally unsatisfactory only because it is empirical. Measures, which have been and are used, include the following:

- Attention to general health, mental as much as physical. This, together with correction of background factors and the giving of sympathetic psychological supports, is more important than anything else in preventing relapses.
- Tranquilisers given regularly at night
- Dental and oral hygiene
- *Local antiseptics and astringents:* These include hydrogen peroxide mouthwashes and lotions and application of 1% silver nitrate, salicylate gels or tincture benzoin compound to the ulcers wherever they may be. They sometimes relieve local discomfort.
- *Hormones:* All the sex hormones have been tried and, if any are of value, it is oestrogens. This cornifies the buccal mucosa and corrects neutropaenia. When given cyclically, preferably with the progestogens, they sometimes appear to help.
- *Corticosteroids:* Given systemically, these are of little value in preventing or curing the ulcers, but, when applied locally as early as possible in an outbreak, they constitute the best available means of reducing tissue reaction, relieving pain and encouraging healing of lesions. It is said that after several courses of treatment, relapse is less common, but this is certainly not always true.
- For genital ulcers, regular applications of hydrocortisone ointment is best; for buccal ulcers, pellets of hydrocortisone hemisuccinate sodium are held against them until the pellets dissolve. Tablets of 0.4 mg betamethasone are also given for sublingual absorption, but these depress adrenal function.
- *Colchicine and azathioprine:* These have been used singly or in combination with corticosteroids.
- Newer therapeutic approaches include the use of cyclosporine, interferon, acyclovir, cyclophosphamide pulse therapy and thalidomide. Thalidomide has now been recognised as a potent anti-inflammatory drug, but its teratogenicity necessitates the use of effective contraception, when used in child-bearing age group.
- Antihistamine preparations, given orally or parenterally, rarely help.
- *Antibiotics:* These are generally useless except when applied locally to clear up secondarily infected ulcers.

PELVIC ALLERGY

Allergic reactions described in relation to menstruation are herpetic eruptions on lips, skin rashes, menstrual coryza, cyclical conjunctivitis and menstrual asthma. Some asthmatic subjects are especially liable to attacks premenstrually, and these may not always be precipitated by nervous tension at the time. Oestrogens induce an attack in some subjects at any time; in others, they are curative. Cyclical conjunctivitis (menstrual red eye) may be related to menstrual coryza, in that swelling of nasal mucosa in response to oestrogens could be cause of both.

The treatment of cyclically occurring allergic states is generally unsatisfactory. Some treat them as they would the PMS; others use tranquilisers, antihistamines and corticosteroids.

VICARIOUS MENSTRUATION

Clinical Features

This is a rare condition in which extragenital bleeding occurs at regular intervals corresponding to the menstrual period. If the bleeding replaces normal menstruation, it is substitutional; this is reported to have occurred sometimes after hysterectomy with conservation of the ovaries. Usually, extragenital bleeding accompanies a uterine flow and is supplementary. Vicarious menstruation occurs most often at the extremes of menstrual life and in individuals with nervous and vascular instability. It ceases with menopause.

The most common form of vicarious bleeding is epistaxis, and this is a feature of at least 30% of cases. Other sites affected are the alimentary tract, lungs, breasts, gums, lips, kidney, rectum, retina and conjunctiva. Older writers described 'bloody sweat' and 'bloody tears'.

Cause

In many cases, the bleeding is not exactly cyclical, and a local lesion is ultimately found to account for it. Indeed, with the increasing facilities for investigation, the diagnosis of vicarious menstruation is made much less frequently than in past. Nevertheless, the phenomenon occurs and is the result of a vascular or cellular response of certain tissues to ovarian hormones. The epithelium over the inferior turbinate bones is readily influenced by oestrogen, hence the frequency of epistaxis. Extragenital endometriosis should always be considered as a possible basis. Cyclical haemoptysis, for example, can be manifestation of pulmonary endometriosis.

Treatment

A primary blood disorder and an organic lesion in the affected organ must be excluded as far as possible. When this has been done, no special treatment is necessary unless the bleeding is heavy and uncontrollable. Accessible bleeding points, as in the nose, can be cauterised. Empirical remedies of unproven merit include calcium and vitamins C and K.

In very exceptional cases, for example, when retinal haemorrhages threaten sight, suppression of ovarian function may have to be considered.

CYCLICAL HAEMOTHORAX AND PNEUMOTHORAX

Cyclical Haemothorax

A rarity of great interest is the sudden development of haemothorax during menstruation, with resolution between each period. This causes chest pain, faintness, respiratory embarrassment, pyrexia and constitutional upset—clinical features which gradually subside when the period is over. Although cyclical haemothorax can be suspected as being a form of vicarious menstruation, it is probably always a manifestation of endometriosis. Moreover, the haemothorax is invariably right sided and is associated with pelvic endometriosis. It, therefore, seems likely that the blood does not arise from ectopic endometrium in the pleura but tracks from the abdominal cavity. Removal of pelvic endometriosis is followed by the cure of haemothorax. The right sidedness probably has the same anatomical basis as same as seen in Meigs syndrome.

Cyclical haemothorax can be controlled temporarily by suppressing menstruation with large doses of progestogen or danazol. Its cure rests on the treatment of associated pelvic endometriosis. In this, a radical approach of bilateral oophorectomy, rather than hormone therapy alone, is often required.

Cyclical Pneumothorax

An even rarer and more mysterious condition is the sudden development of pneumothorax with collapse of lung with each period. This resolves in the intermenstrual interval. The patient complains of acute chest pain followed by dyspnoea at onset of each menstrual period, and discomfort only subsides during the ensuing 14 days. It is predominantly associated with thoracic endometriosis, where ectopic endometrial tissue is present within the thoracic cavity.

The explanation of this phenomenon is uncertain. Professor Jeffcoate reported one case in which the pneumothorax was right sided and occurred in every menstrual cycle during 13 months of observation. The patient was treated by thoracotomy (repeated) to obliterate the space between two layers of pleura. She remained well and free from symptoms 10 years later.

In this case, rupture of emphysematous bullae was certainly not responsible for the recurrent pneumothorax (a theory which has been put forwards). It is probably significant that in most of the recorded cases, as in Professor Jeffcoate's, the pneumothorax was right sided. This raises the possibility of air tracking from peritoneal cavity through a defect in the diaphragm, having gained access to the former via the genital tract at the onset of menstruation.

Unfortunately, in Professor Jeffcoate's case, radiographs never showed any evidence of pneumoperitoneum.

MENSTRUAL EPILEPSY

Clinical Features

Less is heard of this condition now than in the past—when hysteroepilepsy was recognised as a special form of epilepsy in which the uterus (or at least the activity of the pelvic organs) was said to be the cause. It mostly affected girls and young women, and the fits were said to occur only during menstrual periods. It was even treated by hysterectomy and oophorectomy in the first quarter of this century.

It is now clear that classical idiopathic epilepsy often makes its first appearance at puberty, and its manifestations are much more likely at the time of menstruation and also at the mid-cycle coinciding with oestrogen peak. Oestrogen has been shown to increase seizure activity in animals, whereas progesterone decreases it. The correlation with menstruation may also be because phases of stress reveal an underlying predisposition. In nearly all cases of 'menstrual epilepsy', it will be found on careful inquiry that fits occur occasionally apart from menstruation. In very few cases where attacks occur only at the time of menstruation, there is probably confusion between hysteria and petit mal.

Treatment

The treatment is that of epilepsy, although the premenstrual restriction of salt and fluid intake may make an attack during menstruation less likely.

Progesterone has a sedative effect on the central nervous system. Depot medroxyprogesterone acetate 150 mg administered every 1–2 months IM decreases the frequency of seizures by up to 50%. High doses are needed because antiepileptic drugs cause induction of hepatic enzymes and enhance metabolic clearance. Therefore, oral medroxyprogesterone acetate is not effective.

43

CHAPTER

Hormone Therapy in Gynaecology

Vidyashree G Poojari, Muralidhar V Pai

Chapter Outline

- Oestrogens
- Antioestrogens
- Progestogens
- Antiprogestogens
- Androgens
- Antiandrogens
- Types of Gonadotrophins
- Antigonadotrophins
- Hypothalamic Hormones

OESTROGENS

An oestrogen is any substance having properties similar to oestradiol, the follicular hormone of the ovary.

Natural Oestrogens

Oestradiol, oestrone and oestriol are C18 steroids synthesised in the ovary, adrenal cortex and placenta of women (refer to Chapter 3: Ovarian Functions and Chapter 7: Conception). They have in common an unsaturated A ring and a hydroxyl group at position 3 and are subject to considerable interconversion at their sites of production and in the liver. The liver is all important to the metabolism and inactivation of these oestrogens.

Before excretion, oestradiol (the most potent of the three) is mostly converted to oestrone and oestriol, and these are found in the urine and faeces in the form of biologically inactive conjugates with glucuronide and sulphate groups. Many other metabolites identified in the urine are unimportant.

Oestriol is too feebly oestrogenic to be of significant therapeutic value. Medicinally, both oestradiol and oestrone are used, mainly in the form of benzoate, propionate, sulphate and other esters. Esterification makes them more efficient in that their absorption and action are more prolonged.

Synthetic Oestrogens

These fall into two groups: (1) Semisynthetic derivatives of oestradiol, such as ethinyl oestradiol and mestranol and (2) nonsteroidal wholly synthetic preparations, such as diethylstilboestrol **(Fig. 1)**.

Both groups of synthetic oestrogens are metabolised slowly and this makes them valuable therapeutically. Moreover, they are as effective when administered orally as by any other route.

Potency

Comparison of potencies is not easy or accurate because biological activity varies according to esterification, route of administration, spacing of doses and the vehicle used for the hormone.

In practice, ethinyl oestradiol is mainly used, because it is highly potent by the oral route and cheap. When a weak oestrogenic effect is required, as for the relief of menopausal symptoms, preparations of oestrone sulphate, including conjugated equine oestrogens, can be given orally. Oestriol creams have been used vaginally.

All oestrogens act on all target organs. Differences in response are essentially due to the difference in their relative potency.

Actions

The actions of all oestrogens are similar in principle and are described in Chapter 3: Ovarian Functions.

Therapeutic Applications

General Principles

The effect of oestrogens is not seen immediately. Even if they are given intravenously, no change is manifest in <12 hours, and a full effect requires continuous treatment for 4–5 days.

- The action of oestrogens is short-lived and begins to pass off within 24–48 hours of withdrawal.

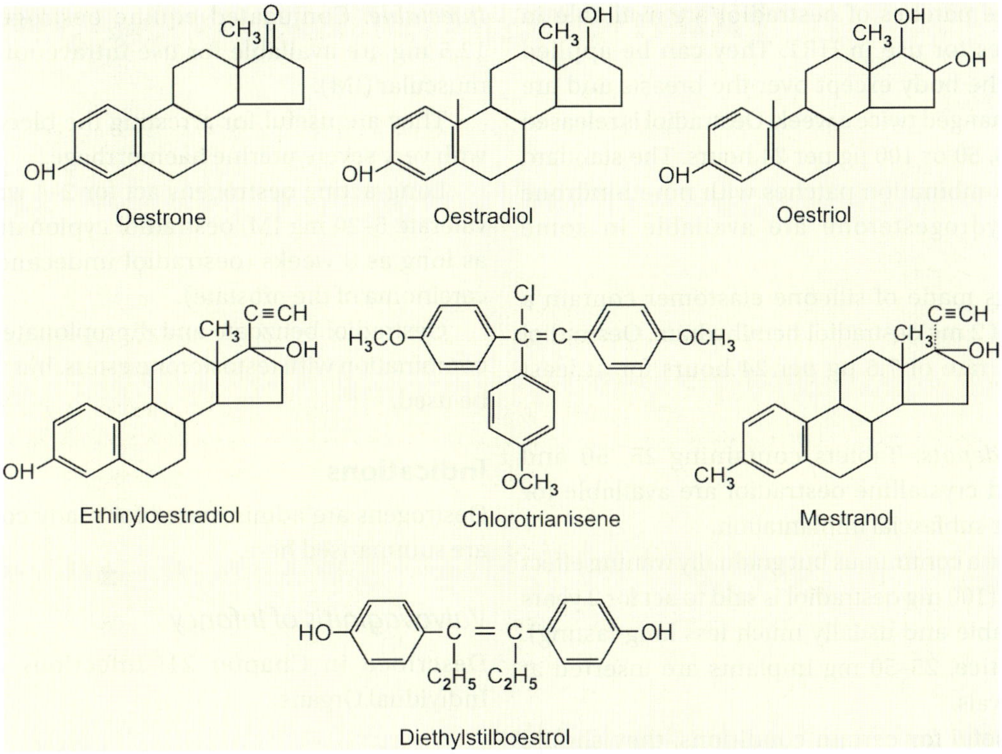

Fig. 1: Chemical structures of certain oestrogens.

- Oestrogens can be administered by mouth, by regularly spaced injections or by establishing a reservoir in the body.
- The smallest possible dose should be used to achieve its objective. It is generally best to give oestrogens intermittently, 3 weeks on and 1 week off, thus simulating the natural production by the ovary and allowing the hypothalamus and pituitary periodic relief from their inhibitory effect.
- Oestrogens are valueless if the target organs are unreceptive.
- To avoid potential carcinogenic effects, all long-term therapy should be associated with the cyclical administration of a progestogen if the uterus is intact.

Methods of Administration Oral

Ethinyl oestradiol tablets are available in strengths of 20, 50, 500 µg, 1 and 2 mg. Oral formulations are available in combination with norethindrone, levonorgestrel, norgestrel, desogestrel, gestodene and norgestimate for contraception. The strength of ethinyl oestradiol in these preparations varies from 20 to 50 µg. Ethinyl oestradiol is also available in combination with cyproterone acetate. Oestradiol valerate is available alone and in combination with levonorgestrel for hormone replacement therapy (HRT).

This route should be used if possible and is nearly always the best when synthetic preparations are given. Natural oestrogens are destroyed by gastric juices or inactivated by the liver on absorption from the stomach, so they are only one fifth as active by mouth as by injection.

Percutaneous

Oestrogens are absorbed through the skin and can be given in the form of ointments to the vagina, vulva and other areas with the idea of concentrating their action locally and limiting their general effects. Proprietary preparations contain 3–5% oestrogen and must be thoroughly rubbed in. Vaginal pessaries containing 25 mg oestradiol are also available and are used mainly for vaginitis. Some contain lactic acid in addition to one of the oestrogens. It is extremely doubtful; however, whether administering an oestrogen percutaneously or intravaginally localises its action. In fact, oestradiol gels (0.06%) are available for transdermal application for HRT. Each measure contains 1.25 g of the gel and 750 mg of oestradiol. Two measures are recommended as starting dose.

Self-adhesive patches of oestradiol are available in several countries for use in HRT. They can be applied on any part of the body except over the breasts and are required to be changed twice a week. Oestradiol is released at the rate of 25, 50 or 100 µg per 24 hours. The standard dose is 50 µg. Combination patches with norethindrone acetate and dydrogesterone are available in some countries.

Vaginal rings made of silicone elastomer contain a drug reservoir of 2 mg oestradiol hemihydrate. Oestradiol is released at a rate of 7.5 µg per 24 hours for at least 90 days.

Implants and depots: Tablets containing 25, 50 and 100 mg of fused crystalline oestradiol are available for subcutaneous or subfascial implantation.

They produce a continuous but gradually waning effect for long periods (100 mg oestradiol is said to act for 2 years but is very variable and usually much less long lasting). In clinical practice, 25–50 mg implants are inserted at 6-monthly intervals.

Although useful for certain conditions, they should never be used in women who have not had a hysterectomy carried out. Their effect on the uterus cannot be foreseen and, if severe bleeding results, it is usually impossible to find and remove the tablet. Cases are recorded where hysterectomy has had to be carried out for this complication.

Injectable: Conjugated equine oestrogens in doses of 12.5 mg are available for use intravenous (IV) or intramuscular (IM).

They are useful for arresting the bleeding in patients with very severe uterine haemorrhage.

Long-acting oestrogens act for 2–4 weeks (oestradiol valerate 5–20 mg IM, oestradiol cypionate 1–5 mg) or for as long as 8 weeks (oestradiol undecanoate 100 mg for carcinoma of the prostate).

Oestradiol benzoate and dipropionate are available in combination with testosterone esters, but these should not be used.

Indications

Oestrogens are administered for many conditions, which are summarised here.

Vulvovaginitis of Infancy

Described in Chapter 21: Infections as They Affect Individual Organs.

Secondary Sex Characters

Oestrogens help in the development of female sex characteristics in girls with gonadal dysgenesis, but certain features, such as axillary and pubic hair, require androgenic hormones, usually of adrenal origin, in addition **(Figs. 2A to C)**. They are of little value in counteracting the effects of

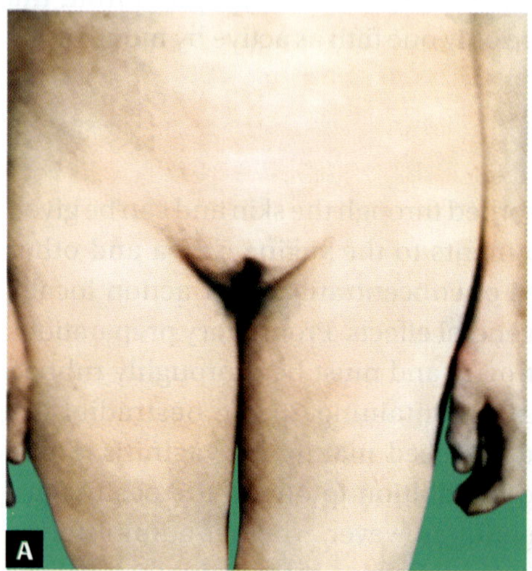

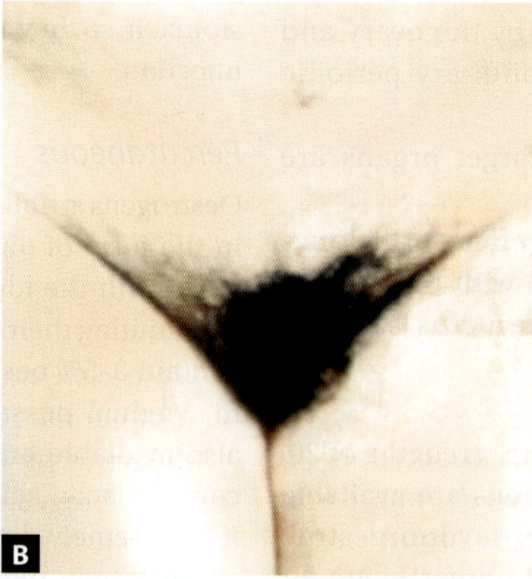

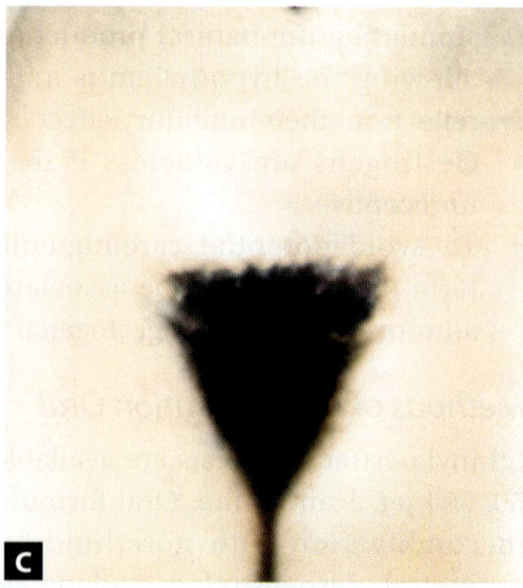

Figs. 2A to C: These photographs illustrate that the growth of pubic hair is controlled by the adrenals rather than by the ovaries and by androgens rather than by oestrogens. (A) A case of Sheehan's syndrome treated for several months with oestrogens without effect on the baldness of the pubes; (B) A similar case treated with methyltestosterone alone showing the resulting good growth of pubic hair. This, moreover, has a 'female' distribution despite the administration of an androgen; (C) The pubic hair remains luxuriant in a 44-year-old woman from whom both ovaries had been removed 5 years previously and who had not had any replacement therapy.

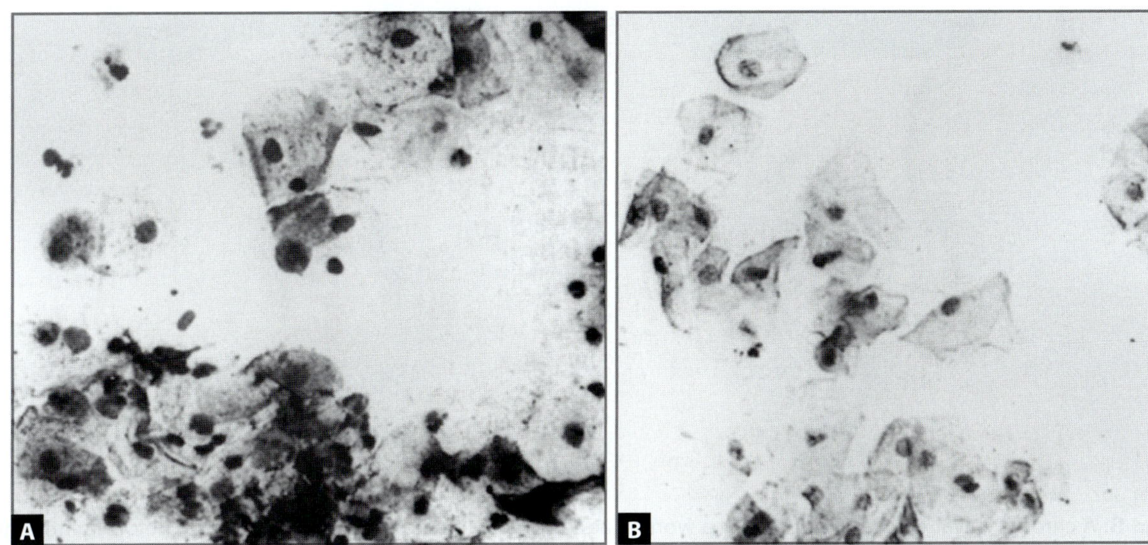

Figs. 3A and B: Senile vaginitis treated with oestrogen. (A) A vaginal smear from a 56-year-old woman suffering from vaginitis; it contains prekeratinised squamous pus cells and debris; (B) A smear obtained from the same patient 6 days later after she had taken a total of 50 mg stilboesterol; all evidence of infection has gone, and healthy cornified squamous now predominate.
Source: BMJ.

androgens in women and do not lessen the growth of facial and body hair.

To Decrease Excessive Growth

Predicted excessive tall stature (>183 cm) in girls growing excessively at the age of 11–13 years with no organic pathology may be limited by administering 0.3 mg ethinyl oestradiol daily with norethindrone 10 mg daily for 5–7 days every 4 weeks. Treatment may require to be continued for 1–3 years. The 50 µg dose does not cause epiphyseal closure.

Menopausal Symptoms and Changes

Oestrogens relieve true climacteric symptoms, i.e. those believed to be caused by an increased output of gonadotrophins or oestrogen deficiency. Short-term treatment is useful in the treatment of atrophic symptoms of the genitourinary tract **(Figs. 3A and B)** and vasomotor symptoms. On a long-term basis, they are of value for the prevention of osteoporosis, apart from benefits on skin, body fat distribution, lipid profile and a possible benefit against coronary artery disease and Alzheimer's disease. If the uterus is present and in certain special situations even after hysterectomy, they must be combined with a progestogen to prevent harmful effects.

To Improve Healing

Oestrogens are sometimes given 4–6 weeks before and after vaginal operations in the elderly to promote healing of senile tissues.

Vulvar Epithelial Disorders

Pruritus vulvae associated with these or other skin conditions is not benefited by oestrogen therapy of any kind. But, in old women, scratch lesions with secondary infection are encouraged to heal **(Figs. 4A and B)**. In a lesion showing epithelial overactivity, oestrogens might, in theory at least, determine malignant change.

Disorders of Ovulation and Menstruation

- *Amenorrhoea:* Refer to Chapter 39: Amenorrhoea, Hypomenorrhoea, and Oligomenorrhoea
- *Dysfunctional uterine bleeding:* Oestrogens are used as endometrial haemostatics to arrest an episode of heavy or prolonged bleeding but are then combined with progestogen therapy from day 15 to buildup a secretory endometrium.
- *Dysmenorrhoea:* Oestrogens only relieve dysmenorrhoea when they are given in such a way as to suppress ovulation.
- *Ovulation pain and bleeding:* Refer to Chapter 41: Dysmenorrhoea

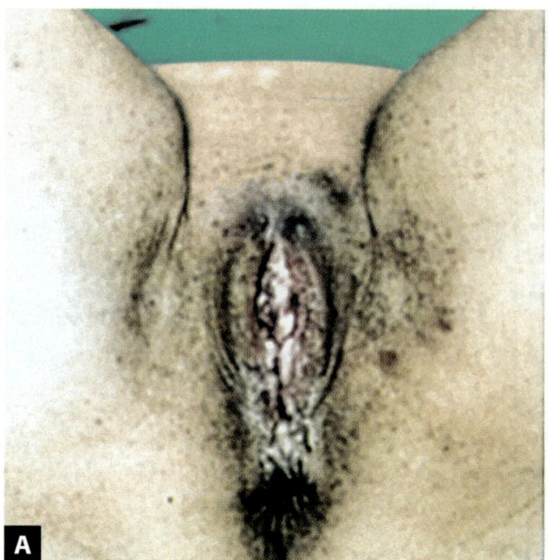

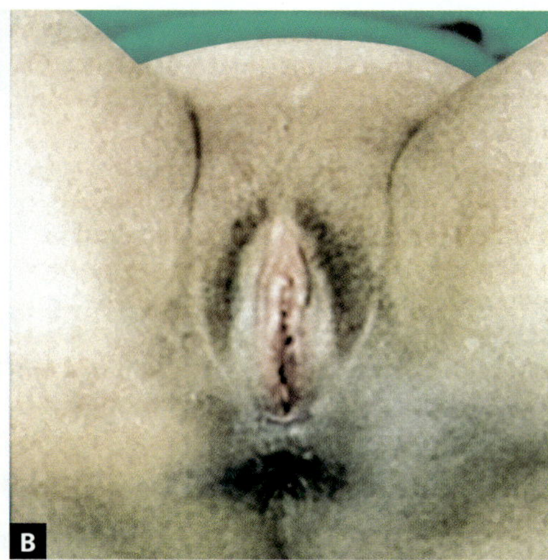

Figs. 4A and B: A chronic vulvar epithelial disorder in a woman aged 72 years treated with oestrogens. (A) Before treatment; (B) After 2 months treatment. Although the secondary infection has been eradicated, the oestrogen has had no good effect on the hyperkeratotic abnormality itself.
Source: BMJ.

- *Postponement or advancement of a menstrual period:* Refer to Chapter 5: Clinical Aspects of Menstruation and Ovulation.

Coitus and Conception

- *Frigidity:* Oestrogens only help in those cases where the condition is clearly caused by hypo-oestrogenism.
- *Contraception:* Their antiovulatory property gives oestrogens a dominant place in oral contraception. But they must be combined with a progestogen, so that unwanted side effects are counteracted.
- *In pregnancy:* There is presently no role for oestrogens in pregnancy. As a clinical test for pregnancy, with or without progestogens, they are unreliable and harmful to the foetus. They are valueless for the induction of abortion and labour, even when the foetus is dead in utero; prostaglandins give better results.

Breast Conditions

- *Inhibition of lactation; relief of breast engorgement:* This is contraindicated because of the risk of thromboembolism.
- *Development of the breast and nipples:* Oestrogens, given systemically, are useful provided that the breast tissues are sensitive to them. This is true for women and intersexes. The effect tends to be temporary so far as the gland elements are concerned, but, because of deposition of fat, the bust measurement does not reduce much when administration is discontinued.

Conditions in the Male

The main indication is carcinoma of the prostate and its metastases. Oestrogens act mainly by depressing testicular function—by 'temporary hormone castration'.

Adverse Effects

Toxicity

Many nonpregnant women cannot tolerate oestrogens and, except when very small doses are given, 20% react by nausea, vomiting, weight gain, headache, dizziness and malaise. These side effects usually subside within a few weeks or months if treatment is continued. They are less likely to occur with natural than with powerful synthetic oestrogens; their incidence being mostly determined by the biological activity of the preparation given.

Metabolic

Oestrogens tend to cause sodium and fluid retention, and this can be accompanied by oedema, an increase in weight and slight hypertension at the beginning of treatment. They raise the plasma levels of thyroxine-binding protein, corticosteroid-binding protein, sex hormone-binding globulin, renin substrate and sometimes that of cholesterol. In certain women at least, they cause hyperlipidaemia.

Glucose tolerance is reduced, possibly more by mestranol than by ethinyl oestradiol.

As revealed by the most sensitive liver function tests, oestrogens alter the blood flow and function of the liver, but this is usually of little consequence. Susceptible women can, however, develop cholestatic jaundice. Impaired liver function always contraindicates oestrogen therapy.

Inhibition of the Hypothalamus, Pituitary, Ovaries and Testes

This results from continuous oestrogen administration. Stilboesterol, 1 mg daily, is enough to have this effect; 5 mg daily results in the disappearance of all demonstrable gonadotrophins in both men and women. The comparable doses of ethinyl oestradiol are 30–50 and 200 µg.

Amenorrhoea *persisting* after suspension of treatment is a rare sequel to the inhibition.

Genital Tract

Oestrogens, unless counteracted by progestogens given simultaneously, cause endometrial hyperplasia at any age, even after the menopause and in childhood **(Figs. 5A and B)**. This can result in irregular and heavy threshold or withdrawal haemorrhage. Uterine leiomyomas may increase in size. Cervical ectropion may develop or fail to resolve, and there may be an increased tendency to vaginal candidiasis.

Thromboembolism

Oestrogens increase the coagulation factors V, VIII, X and fibrinogen in the blood. However, the risk of superficial and deep venous thrombosis, pulmonary embolism and cerebral arterial thrombosis occurring is statistically very small, especially in younger women without other predisposing factors. However, women with decreased levels of protein C, protein S, antithrombin C and smokers are at a higher risk. It is rare for natural oestrogens to cause thromboembolism.

Breasts

The breasts respond by enlargement and may become painful and tender; this may be undesirable in children, old women and men. Areas of chronic mastitis react by forming cysts; an adenoma may increase in size.

Skin

Pigmentation of the breast areolae and production of a linea nigra on the abdominal wall are common sequels to oestrogen therapy **(Figs. 6A and B)**. Chloasma is also not uncommon. The pigmentation fades in time but can take years to disappear completely. Haemorrhagic skin eruptions, erythema multiforme and erythema nodosum have been reported. Some women may have a loss of scalp hair; rarely, hirsutism may develop.

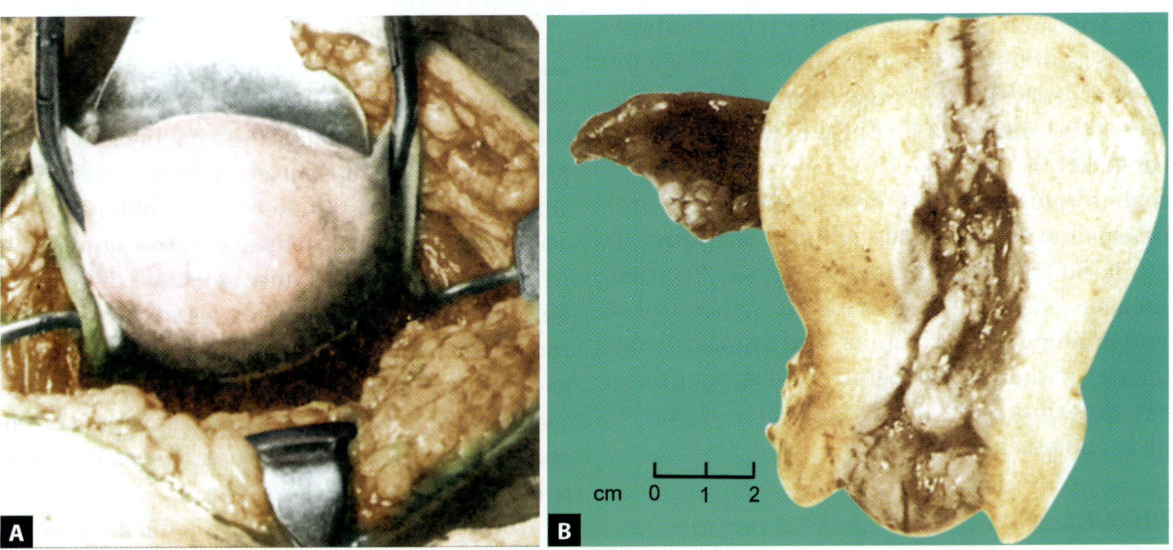

Figs. 5A and B: The effect of prolonged oestrogen therapy on the human uterus. (A) The uterus at laparotomy on a woman aged 56 years who had taken oestrogens for 3 years. It is symmetrically enlarged to the size of a 10-week pregnant uterus; (B) After removal, the same uterus shows not only diffuse thickening of the myometrium but also endometrial cancer.

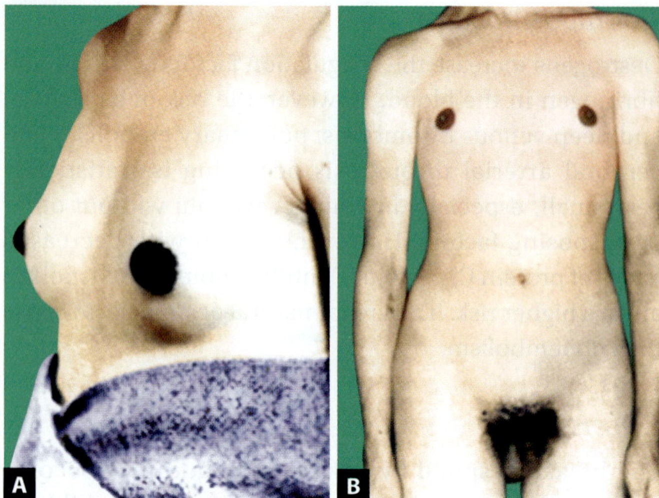

Figs. 6A and B: Pigmentation of the areolae and enlargement of the breasts caused by oestrogens. (A) The effect of 3 months' treatment with oestrogen in the case of a girl aged 20 years suffering from primary amenorrhoea and absence of breast development (cause not investigated); (B) A man aged 18 years who was given an oestrogen as the treatment of acne vulgaris. The breast areolae are almost black, although there is not much gynaecomastia.

Libido

Libido in men is decreased, but can be awakened or increased in young girls and old women, by oestrogen therapy.

Cancer

Oestrogens are such powerful epithelial stimulants that there is reason to fear that they may encourage the development of cancer in their target organs—the breasts, uterus, vagina and vulva. Local applications have caused skin cancer in certain animals.

Oestrogens also favour the development of cancer of the breast in strains of mice which are ordinarily resistant to it. So far as the human being is concerned, any carcinogenic effect is related to unopposed oestrogen therapy and endometrial carcinoma, and the knowledge that exposure of the *foetal* vagina to oestrogens can sometimes determine the occurrence of a clear cell carcinoma in adolescence.

Miscellaneous

With high doses of oestrogens, there may be changes in the corneal curvature leading to intolerance of contact lenses. Chloasma and cholestatic jaundice are rare adverse effects. Sickle cell crisis, exacerbation of symptoms of porphyria and chorea have been reported.

Contraindications

Oestrogen therapy is contraindicated in pregnancy, undiagnosed abnormal vaginal bleeding, in the presence of oestrogen-dependent cancers, e.g. those of the breast, endometrium and melanoma, and in severe systemic lupus erythematosus. Previous endometrial hyperplasia, endometriosis, active liver disease, gallstones, leiomyomas, deep vein thrombosis, severe diabetes mellitus, hypertension, migraine and otosclerosis are relative contraindications.

ANTIOESTROGENS

A number of compounds appear to have a limited ability to inhibit the action of certain oestrogens, but the concept of an antioestrogen is not simple. Antagonists may be short acting, long acting or physiological and may be pure or may have mixed agonistic–antagonistic actions.

Androgens can be considered antioestrogenic, but only because they act differently on the same target organs; this antagonism is physiological.

Some oestrogens have antioestrogenic properties; thus, diethylstilboestrol can prevent the effects which other oestrogens have on the rodent vagina. Oestriol competes with oestradiol for nuclear receptors in short-acting antagonism; therefore, short-term responses are obtained but not long term.

The two antioestrogens which have so far attracted most attention are clomiphene and tamoxifen which are mixed oestrogen agonists–antagonists of the long-acting variety. Clomiphene, a member of the triphenylethylene series, is a derivative of chlorotrianisene which is itself an oestrogen. Tamoxifen is also a member of the triphenylethylene series. The endometrium is sensitive to the agonistic response, whereas the breast is more sensitive to the antagonistic behaviour due to the differences in the type of oestrogen receptor at the two sites. The antagonistic response is essentially mediated through the depletion of hormone receptors consequent to nuclear receptor binding. Both clomiphene and tamoxifen are powerful stimulants of ovulation in selected cases.

Tamoxifen, 20 mg per day, is the adjuvant treatment of choice for breast cancer and has been shown to prolong disease-free survival. Best results are achieved in oestrogen receptor-positive tumours, but it is also effective in oestrogen receptor-negative tumours through cellular mechanisms in breast cells, fibroblasts and stromal cells. In any case, the oestrogen receptor status of breast tumours is known to change over a period of time. Currently, tamoxifen use is limited to a period of 5 years. Long-term use has been shown to be associated with endometrial agonist adverse effects, i.e. endometrial hyperplasia, endometrial polyps, endometrial cancer flare-up of endometriosis. It has a positive action on bone in postmenopausal women, though less than oestrogen or bisphosphonates, but causes bone loss in premenopausal women. Other adverse effects include hot flashes, vaginal changes, irregular menstruation and thromboembolism. Other triphenylethylene derivatives being studied for use in breast cancer include droloxifene, idoxifene and toremifene.

Raloxifene is a benzothiophene derivative which is also a mixed oestrogen agonist–antagonist with selective oestrogen receptor modulator (SERM) properties. It has minimal uterotopic properties; in the breast, it has a beneficial or neutral profile; it has beneficial effects on bones and lipids. In the bone, it inhibits interleukin-6-stimulated differentiation of osteoclasts and, thus, prevents osteoporosis. It is a promising agent for HRT. T-588 is an agent from this group which may be useful in the prevention of Alzheimer's disease. The benzopyran centchroman is also a SERM. Originally developed in India as a non-steroidal oral contraceptive, it was initially proposed as a once-a-week pill, but this was associated with unacceptable failure rates. The dose was, therefore, revised to twice weekly for the first 3 months, followed by weekly doses. It has also been tried for postcoital contraception. It inhibits osteoclast activity.

Phytoestrogens are plant-derived chemicals with oestrogenic and antioestrogenic activities. They inhibit the enzymatic conversion of endogenous oestrone to oestradiol and also possess intrinsic oestrogen activity. The isoflavones have the greatest potency along with genistein and daidzein; these are found in soy-based diets. Ginseng has also been found to have oestrogenic, antioestrogenic and androgenic properties.

Pure antioestrogens are being developed which are derivatives of oestradiol with long hydrophobic side chains. These have been termed ICI164, 384 and ICI182, 780. They inhibit breast cancer cells and cause uterine involution. They may be useful in women with tamoxifen-resistant tumours. The whole field of antioestrogens is being actively explored.

PROGESTOGENS

Types and Sources

A progestogen is a substance which produces progestational changes in an oestrogen-primed endometrium. Not all the synthetic progesterone substitutes are strongly active in this respect, and few simulate progesterone in all its effects. For example, their thermogenic, androgenic, oestrogenic and other biological properties, such as the maintenance of pregnancy in animals and support of the endometrium in women, vary widely from one to another.

Natural Progestogens

The natural product is progesterone. This is a steroid derived from cholesterol via 17α-hydroxyprogesterone and secreted by the corpus luteum, placenta and the adrenal cortex. In the last site, progesterone is an intermediate product in the formation of cortisol. In both the adrenal cortex and the ovary, progesterone can be converted to androgens and oestrogens (refer to Chapter 3: Ovarian Functions and Chapter 7: Conception).

Progesterone is rapidly metabolised by the liver, and approximately 20% is excreted in the urine as sodium pregnanediol glucuronide. The fate of the remainder is uncertain.

Synthetic Progestogens

For therapeutic purposes, progesterone is generally prepared synthetically. The synthetic progesterone substitutes which are best known and are in common usage are as follows:

- *Progesterone derivatives* such as 17α-hydroxyprogesterone caproate, medroxyprogesterone acetate, megestrol acetate and chlormadinone acetate
- *Stereoisomers of progesterone* such as dydrogesterone
- *Testosterone derivatives* such as ethisterone and dimethisterone.
- *19-norsteroids* (nortestosterone derivatives) such as norethisterone, norethisterone acetate, norethynodrel, allyloestrenol, ethynodiol diacetate and the 'newer' progestogens—desogestrel, gestodene and norgestimate—which are 'lipid-friendly'. Norgestrel is often included in this group but, although closely related, is not strictly a steroid. It is the strongest of known progestogens, except cyproterone, but this is mainly used as an antiandrogen (see further).

Of the above, dydrogesterone and norethisterone, at least, are nonthermogenic; the testosterone and 19-nortestosterone derivatives are slightly androgenic. However, little is known about the metabolism of these progestogens. In some cases, it may resemble that of testosterone, but dydrogesterone, allyloestrenol, norethisterone (acetate) and norethynodrel are in part metabolised to ethinyl oestradiol in the body to have mildly oestrogenic effects. The status of ethynodiol acetate is uncertain. None is excreted as pregnanediol.

Actions

The actions of progesterone are described in Chapter 3: Ovarian Functions. Those of the oral progestogens are basically similar but, as already noted, vary in detail and emphasis. This, as well as different methods of administration and assessment, makes it impossible to compare relative potencies.

Therapeutic Applications

General Principles

- Progestogens, such as oestrogens, take several days to produce their maximum tissue effects, although certain responses, such as a rise in temperature, occur within a few hours of their administration.
- The action of progestogens is short-lived and begins to subside within 24–48 hours of suspending treatment.
- Divided and regularly spaced doses, or continuous absorption from a depot, are necessary for efficient use. This is especially true of progesterone itself which, in the blood, has a half-life of only a few minutes.
- Progestogens are ineffective unless the target organ is previously or simultaneously primed with oestrogen.

Methods of Administration

Progesterone itself is ineffective by mouth except in the newer micronised preparation, which is available as 100/200/300/400 mg tablets to be used orally or vaginally. It may be administered by deep IM injections containing 25–50 mg/mL. Suppositories, each containing 25 mg progesterone, are available for inserting into the vagina or rectum. In some countries, progesterone is available in a gel which adheres to the vaginal mucosa. Progesterone containing intrauterine contraceptive device (IUCD) as well as in subdermal implants (Norplant) and intravaginal rings are also available.

All the progesterone substitutes except 17α-hydroxyprogesterone caproate are usually given orally. The details of dosage are given in the appropriate chapters.

Indications

Disorders of Menstruation and Ovulation

- *Amenorrhoea:* Progestogens may be given alone for secondary amenorrhoea but are usually combined with oestrogen. In primary amenorrhoea, priming with oestrogen is essential.
- *Dysfunctional uterine bleeding:* Although used for all types of dysfunctional bleeding, progestogens are chiefly indicated for anovulatory bleeding and correction of endometrial hyperplasia.
- *Spasmodic dysmenorrhoea:* Progestogens relieve true dysmenorrhoea when they are combined with oestrogen and given in such a way as to inhibit ovulation. Progestogens alone also decrease the production of prostaglandin F2α and vasopressin and relieve primary dysmenorrhoea.
- *Premenstrual syndrome (PMS):* Progestogens are widely used for this and allied conditions, but their value is debated.
- *Postponement or advancement of a menstrual period:* Refer to Chapter 5: Clinical Aspects of Menstruation and Ovulation.

Conception and Pregnancy

- *Contraception:* Mainly because they make cervical mucus hostile to spermatozoa and the endometrium unreceptive to a fertilised ovum, progestogens, with or without oestrogens, are valuable contraceptives. They can also inhibit ovulation.
- *Infertility:* Progesterone is used in cases of luteal phase defect in the secretory phase of the cycle. The empirical use of progesterone in the postovulatory phase to assist the implantation of a hypothetical early pregnancy is without proven merit. However, they have been used successfully in assisted reproduction techniques to establish a secretory endometrium.
- *Threatened and recurrent abortion:* Here again, progestogens are used, sometimes empirically, sometimes when a low level of progesterone suggests deficiency. Their value remains unproven by controlled observations when used empirically. However, in cases of proven deficiency, progesterone therapy improves

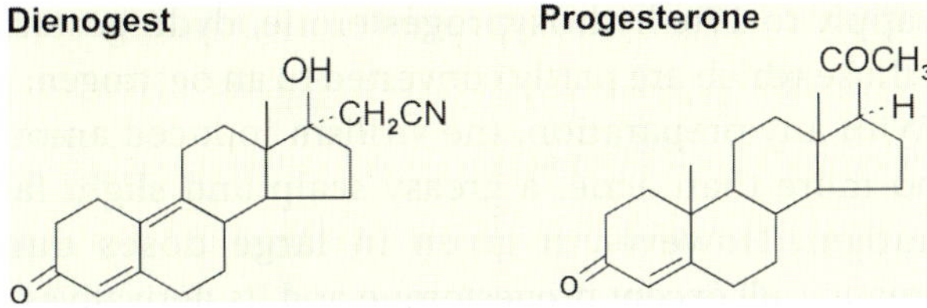

Fig. 7: Structural formula of the progestin and dienogest.

pregnancy outcomes. However, the possibility of producing virilising effects in the foetus has thrown this treatment into disrepute. There are also reports that female foetuses exposed to progestogens in utero may exhibit a 'tomboyish' behaviour.

Endometriosis

For this condition, progestogens, alone or in conjunction with oestrogens, are given continuously in large doses to produce a state of pseudopregnancy. Treatment is continuous for 6–12 months.

Dienogest: Dienogest is an oral progestin that has been investigated systematically for the treatment of endometriosis in dose-ranging, placebo-controlled, active comparator-controlled and long-term trials performed in Europe and Japan **(Fig. 7)**. Based on this trial evidence, dienogest has received approval as a monotherapy for the treatment of endometriosis in many countries.

Pharmacologically, dienogest combines the advantages of the 19-norprogestin and the progesterone derivative classes. Dienogest binds to the progesterone receptor with high specificity and produces a potent progestogenic effect related to the high circulating levels of the unbound molecule. Binding affinities of dienogest for oestrogen, glucocorticoid and mineralocorticoid receptors are negligible. Unlike other agents in the 19-norprogestin class, dienogest lacks androgenic effects; rather, dienogest has beneficial antiandrogenic properties typical of the progesterone derivatives, which are associated with minimal changes in lipid and carbohydrate levels.

Dienogest is almost completely absorbed and has a high bioavailability after oral administration, similar to other 19-norprogestins. Its relatively short half-life of 10 hours means there is no risk of accumulation after repeated dosing. The majority of orally administered dienogest is excreted within 24 hours, mainly in urine.

Dienogest reduces endometriotic lesions through a number of biological mechanisms. Dienogest is associated with relatively moderate inhibition of gonadotrophin secretion. When given continuously, dienogest induces a hypoestrogenic, hypergestagenic local endocrine environment, causing a decidualisation of endometrial tissue followed by atrophy of the endometriotic lesions. Animal studies indicate that dienogest may also reduce plasma oestradiol levels directly, through inducing apoptosis of granulosa cells in the ovary.

Dienogest and fertility considerations: The majority of women suffering from endometriosis are of reproductive age and so may require contraception. Based on the available data, dienogest provides complete ovulation inhibition at a daily dose of 2 mg. However, dienogest monotherapy was not developed as a contraceptive, and women taking dienogest as a treatment for endometriosis are advised to use nonhormonal methods of contraception.

Women with endometriosis may desire pregnancy once sufficient pain relief is achieved. Recent pharmacodynamic data in volunteers indicate that ovarian activity resumes rapidly (range 1–43 days) after cessation of dienogest. These observations support studies that describe a prompt return to fertility (e.g. mean about 30 days) and include cases of successful pregnancy in women with endometriosis following the cessation of dienogest treatment 2 mg daily for durations up to 1 year.

Hormone Replacement Therapy

In postmenopausal women with an intact uterus, the administration of oestrogen for climacteric symptoms or long-term benefit must be accompanied by the administration of progestogens to prevent the development of endometrial hyperplasia and cancer. In some cases, the administration of progestogens is recommended even in hysterectomised women. The addition of 19-norsteroids to oestrogen may also potentiate its effect in correcting osteoporosis.

Pelvic Cancer

Probably because they lead to glandular exhaustion, progestogens in large doses have an arresting effect on endometrial carcinoma and its metastases and are valuable adjuncts to surgery for this condition, especially for recurrent disease.

They are also used with less certain action for adenocarcinoma of the vagina, tube and ovary and for other types of malignant disease of the uterine corpus. They do not appear to influence squamous cell carcinoma of the cervix and lower genital tract.

Breast Conditions

Progestogens are sometimes recommended for fibrocystic disease and premenstrual mastalgia when other measures have failed.

Adverse Effects

Toxicity

Progesterone itself rarely has any immediate side effects except to cause a slight rise in body temperature. The synthetic oral progestogens, being more potent in some respects and longer acting, can produce systemic upsets such as nausea, vomiting, headache, depression, lassitude and pyrexia. The nausea is likened by the patient to that of pregnancy. Oral micronised progesterone causes somnolence and other central nervous system effects.

Jaundice is described as a complication of giving nortestosterone and testosterone derivatives, but it is very rare. These and other 19-norsteroids can, such as oestrogens, modify hepatic handling of normal metabolic products and may reflect a competitive effect for a common excretory pathway.

Uterus

Progestogens, especially when combined with a small dose of oestrogen, cause generalised enlargement of the uterus by myometrial hyperplasia and hypertrophy. They can also result in a rapid increase in the size of leiomyomas, possibly due to degenerative changes.

Menstrual Disturbance

Progestogen-only pills do not regulate the cycle as efficiently as combined pills. They cause irregular bleeding, and they may result in scanty menstruation and amenorrhoea.

Breasts

These respond by enlargement, increased vascularity, pain and tenderness.

Libido and Coitus

Progestogens tend to decrease libido, inspissate cervical mucus and make the vagina drier.

Virilism

Progesterone itself is very mildly androgenic, but many of the synthetic preparations are more so. This probably does not apply to 17α-hydroxyprogesterone, dydrogesterone and those which are partly converted to an oestrogen.

With any preparation, the virilism induced amounts to no more than acne, a greasy scalp and slight facial hirsutism. However, if given in large doses during pregnancy, all except progesterone and its derivatives can masculinise the external genitalia of the female foetus.

Hypertension

The hypertension which occasionally follows administration of the combined pill is mainly an oestrogen effect, but there are reports suggesting that levonorgestrel can raise the blood pressure.

Thromboembolism

When this complicates the taking of antiovulatory oral contraceptives, it is mostly attributable to oestrogen. But progestogens cannot be completely exonerated.

Metabolism

Most progestogens are mildly anabolic. When they cause an increase in weight, it is probably by way of increasing the appetite, which is comparable to a pregnancy reaction. Indeed, progestogens induce a state of pseudopregnancy.

ANTIPROGESTOGENS

Mifepristone (RU 486) and onapristone (ZK 98299) are antiprogestins. RU 486 is a 19-nortestosterone derivative with a dimethyl side chain at C11, which gives it its antiprogestogen action. It has a very strong binding affinity for the progesterone receptor. It has some agonistic effect, but the main effect is antagonistic, and it has proved to be an efficient and convenient abortifacient used in combination with prostaglandins in the first trimester. It is also used in emergency contraception. Its role in contraception, induction of labour, etc. is still to be fully elucidated. RU 486 binds to the glucocorticoid receptor and may be useful in the treatment of Cushing syndrome.

Antiprogestogens in combination with an antioestrogen may be of benefit in progesterone receptor-positive breast cancer. Progesterone receptors have been found in the meninges, and mifepristone has been used in the management of unresectable meningiomas.

Org 31710 and Org 31806 are newer antiprogestogens under trial. The most potent is Org 33628 with potent abortifacient, antitumour and ovulation suppressant effects.

ANDROGENS

Types and Sources

An androgen is a substance having the capacity to produce masculinity. There are many of these, some occurring naturally and some produced artificially. All tend to be anabolics as well as sex determinants, and there is a tendency to group them according to the dominant action.

Natural Androgens

Several of these are produced in the female as well as in the male. They vary in their androgenic potential, and from this standpoint, testosterone is one of major importance. In the blood, it is bound to a specific protein and in its target tissues, its effect is probably mediated by an even more active substance—dihydrotestosterone, the conversion taking place in the target organ.

Testosterone is metabolised in the liver extremely rapidly, being degraded mainly to aetiocholanolone and androsterone; these are excreted in the urine in the form of their glucuronide and sulphate esters.

In the male, testosterone is secreted mainly by the interstitial cells of the testis under the influence of luteinising hormone (LH), but a little is formed in the zona reticularis of the adrenal cortex. Other weak androgens such as androstenedione and dehydroepiandrosterone are also produced in both these sites, and these as well as testosterone being synthesised from progesterone.

In the female, identical androgens are produced in the adrenal cortex and, in amounts relatively very small compared with the testis, by the ovary.

The only naturally occurring androgen employed therapeutically is testosterone. It is administered IM. For sustained response, it is administered in the form of a subfascial tablet implant, manufactured synthetically.

Synthetic Androgens

Synthetic preparations with a mainly androgenic action are almost all derivatives of testosterone. They include its propionate and oenanthate esters for parenteral use, and methyltestosterone, fluoxymesterone and mesterolone (derived from dihydrotestosterone) for oral and sublingual administration.

Preparations which are only weakly androgenic and anabolic include the synthetic progestogens.

Those which are mainly anabolic include methylandrostenediol, oxymetholone, methylandrostanolone and norethandrolone. Although these are alleged to be free from masculinising actions in women, their use is sometimes followed by hirsutism and voice changes.

Little is known about the metabolism of any of the synthetic androgens and androgenic anabolics.

Biological Actions

Metabolic Effects in Both Sexes

Androgens conserve nitrogen and assist in the buildup of proteins. They also favour potassium, phosphorus and sulphur retention, and for these reasons, they are important to the development of muscle and the growth of bone. They, therefore, bring about an increase in weight, promote muscular strength and energy, and give a sensation of well-being. Androgens accelerate epiphyseal closure and ultimately limit stature; they also cause retention of sodium, chloride and fluid.

Actions in the Male

The effects of androgens in the male are comparable to those of oestrogens in the female. They are responsible for the development and maintenance of secondary sex organs such as the penis, prostate, vasa, seminal vesicles and characters such as hair on the face, limbs and trunk, baldness, masculine figure, deep voice and axillary sweating. Like oestrogens in the female, they are not too important for sex drive.

Testosterone may play a direct role in spermatogenesis, but testosterone in physiological amounts does not inhibit the gonadotrophic activity of the pituitary; otherwise, men would be sterile or only cyclically fertile. Any depressant effect on the hypothalamic-pituitary system and the testes requires massive and continuous dosage. Androgens can cause prostatic hypertrophy and, surprisingly, occasionally result in gynaecomastia in youths. The latter effect probably arises when the hormone administered is metabolised into an oestrogen.

Actions in the Female

Sex organs:

- *Atrophy of the tubes, vagina, vulva and breasts:* Androgens directly depress the activity of all the tissues of the female genital tract and induce atrophy and secretory quiescence of the lining epithelia. The breasts shrink, cervical secretion dries up and menstruation ceases. In the embryo, androgens interfere with the development of the external genitalia, encourage persistence of the Wolffian ducts and their derivatives, and thus cause a state of intersex in the female.

- *Suppression of uterine and tubal contractions:* These decrease both in frequency and in amplitude.
- *Ovaries:* The ovarian cycle is arrested, and ovulation and menstruation cease. This is a direct effect rather than one exerted through the hypothalamic-pituitary system. As in the male, only massive doses can possibly inhibit that system.

Secondary Sex Characters

Androgens are *normally* responsible for certain female sex characters—notably the axillary and pubic hair, axillary sweating and the activity of apocrine glands.

Therapeutic Applications

Methods of Administration

- *IM injection:* This is the route by which the esters of testosterone are administered. Their vehicle is oily, so they create depots which are effective for 7–10 days. The usual dose of the chosen preparation is of the order of 5–25 mg once weekly.
- *Orally (sublingually):* Methyltestosterone, fluoxymesterone and anabolic androgens are available in 5 and 10 mg pellets; these have a maximum effect if they are allowed to dissolve in the mouth. If they are swallowed, their action is restricted by the detoxicating action of the liver.

Mesterolone is dispensed in 25 mg tablets. For oral substitution therapy in the male, the dose is 75–100 mg daily for a few months followed by a maintenance dose of 50 mg daily.

Implants

Pellets of 100 mg testosterone are available for subcutaneous or subfascial implant but have largely been abandoned. They were employed for the purpose of substitution therapy in the male and are never to be used in the female.

Indications

In the Female

Presently, there is very little place for androgen therapy in the female. Androgens have now largely been replaced by synthetic progestogens.

Dysfunctional uterine bleeding: Androgens can control excessive uterine bleeding by decreasing the blood supply to the uterus, by causing it and its endometrium to atrophy and by depressing ovarian function. But progestogens, with or without oestrogens, are better and safer uterine haemostatics.

Premenstrual mastalgia and fibroadenosis: Small doses of androgens given premenstrually may suppress breast activity and limit discomfort, but they are rarely indicated.

Vulvar epithelial disorders: The symptoms of pruritus vulvae which occur in some cases of benign vulvar epithelial change are sometimes completely relieved by local applications of methyltestosterone solution or testosterone propionate in arachis oil. It is difficult to explain how and why this gives symptomatic relief but it does.

Uterine leiomyomas: The menorrhagia of leiomyomas can sometimes be controlled temporarily by androgens if, for some reason, the operation has to be postponed, but, again, progestogens are to be preferred for such a purpose. Androgens do not cause leiomyomas to atrophy.

Endometriosis: Androgens suppress the activity of ectopic endometrium and control the pain and bleeding associated with endometriosis. In order to produce some improvement in symptoms, the dose does not necessarily have to be large enough to suppress ovulation and menstruation. The effect is temporary, and the endometriosis usually becomes active again when treatment is suspended.

Sexual unresponsiveness: Small doses of methyltestosterone appear sometimes to increase heterosexual libido in women and are alleged to intensify orgasm. The action of androgen in this respect is not understood, but it is suggested that it promotes a feeling of well-being, increases susceptibility to psychic stimuli and makes the genitalia more sensitive. Tibolone produces this effect through its androgenic metabolites.

Metabolic errors: The less virilising androgens can be used for their anabolic effects in circumstances such as the following:

- Emaciation associated with anorexia nervosa and chronic illnesses of any kind
- To speed recovery after surgery and accidents
- Delayed physical growth in children and adolescents in constitutional delayed puberty

- States of adrenal failure
- Acute and chronic renal failure.

They are often employed, unethically, by women (and men) athletes who engage in lifting and throwing events, to increase their muscular strength.

In the Male

When the endocrine function of the testes is definitely subnormal, androgen can be used to develop secondary male characters and to relieve frigidity. Impotence in the male *with normal testes*, however, never responds to androgen therapy unless the effect is psychological. Androgens may be of help in the treatment of gynaecomastia.

The anabolic androgens can be indicated for their metabolic effects in the circumstances listed for the female above.

Adverse Effects in the Female

Toxicity

Cholestatic jaundice occasionally complicates the use of androgens with an alkyl group substituted at position 17, e.g. methyltestosterone and is an indication for discontinuing treatment immediately. The jaundice is dose related and reversible.

Fluid Retention

Oedema, swelling of the joints and other manifestations of electrolyte upset are sometimes seen during treatment.

Epiphyseal Closure

Testosterone and its derivatives not only encourage physical growth in the young, but they limit it by promoting epiphyseal closure. How far this applies to the synthetic, mainly anabolic androgens, is uncertain.

Virilism

Large doses of androgens nearly always induce virilism; small doses can do so in susceptible women. Tolerance to androgens generally increases after the age of 40 years but, before that time, varies enormously from one individual to another.

The common virilising effects of androgen therapy are deepening of the voice, acne, growth of hair on the face, increased muscular development with a decrease in subcutaneous fat, atrophy of the breasts, loss of frontal hair and enlargement of the clitoris. The last two, and deepening of the voice, are usually permanent, but the others are reversible and disappear or become less obvious when treatment is suspended.

These adverse effects are clearly undesirable and make the following guiding rules necessary:

- Never prescribe androgens for a woman without first informing the patient of the possible adverse effects
- Do not use androgens in women especially under the age of 40 years unless there is a very strong indication.

ANTIANDROGENS

Cyproterone acetate is a very powerful antiandrogen, and it seems that its antiandrogenic effects are reversible. In doses of 50 mg twice daily, it is used in the treatment of severe hypersexuality and sexual deviation in the male, as it inhibits spermatogenesis and produces reversible infertility. Consideration must be given to the risks and benefits, as hepatic tumours have been produced in animals using large doses.

Cyproterone, 2 mg, with ethinyl oestradiol, 50 μg, has been used for the treatment of severe acne refractory to other therapy. Some women with mild-to-moderate idiopathic hirsutism and polycystic ovary syndrome (PCOS) may benefit, as hair growth is also androgen dependent. Cyproterone with ethinyl oestradiol is also an effective contraceptive measure for these women or women with androgen-dependent skin conditions.

Spironolactone similarly binds to the androgen receptor and exerts mixed agonism–antagonism, but in hyperandrogenic states, only the antagonistic effect is seen.

Flutamide, a nonsteroidal pure antiandrogen, has been developed. Finasteride, a 5α-reductase inhibitor, is under clinical evaluation.

TYPES OF GONADOTROPHINS

Pituitary Gonadotrophins

The gonadotrophins secreted by the pituitary glands under the influence of the hypothalamus are described in Chapter 3: Ovarian Functions. Pituitary gonadotrophins were initially extracted from lyophilised human glands removed at autopsy, the products being termed human placental gonadotrophin (hPG), but 10 glands are required to obtain enough material to induce one ovulatory cycle in a woman. Moreover, these preparations carry the risk of contamination with the Creutzfeldt–Jakob virus.

Pituitary gonadotrophins presently available for use [human menopausal gonadotrophin (hMG)] are extracted from the urine of postmenopausal women. Preparations from this source contain both follicle-stimulating hormone (FSH) and LH. Their potencies may vary from one batch to another but usually contain 75 IU of each.

Preparations of pure FSH isolated from urine are also available (urofollitropin or uFSH) which are especially useful in the induction of ovulation in those women who have elevated levels of endogenous LH, as seen in cases of PCOS.

Chorionic Gonadotrophins

Chorionic gonadotrophins are similar but not identical to LH in chemical structure and action. They are complex glycoproteins found in the placenta, blood and urine of women throughout pregnancy. Their overall action is a luteinising one. Commercial preparations are made from the urine of pregnant women or placentas.

Recombinant Gonadotrophins

Recombinant technology has been used to clone genes for both the alpha and beta subunits of human FSH and to transfect these into Chinese hamster ovary (CHO) cells. A CHO clone has been isolated that is capable of secreting intact glycosylated FSH (follitropin), which is further purified by immunochromatography to yield an amino acid combination and sequence identical to natural FSH.

Recombinant LH and human chorionic gonadotrophin (hCG) have also been developed. The recombinant gonadotrophins have the advantage of higher purity and specific activity, batch-to-batch consistency and complete absence of contamination by other gonadotrophins. Their pharmacokinetics are very similar to the natural gonadotrophins.

Therapeutic Applications

All gonadotrophins are standardised in international units, by comparison of their biological activities with that of standard reference preparations. They are unstable in solution and are quickly destroyed by warmth and ultraviolet light.

Methods of Administration

Gonadotrophins are inactive by mouth and can only be employed parenterally. The injection is made intramuscularly. Being protein preparations, gonadotrophins can produce local and general anaphylactic reactions. For this reason, subcutaneous and IV injections should be avoided, and a preliminary small test dose is desirable. The administration of gonadotrophins always calls for careful monitoring.

Indications

In the Female

The only indication for gonadotrophin therapy with FSH and LH in the female is to induce ovulation when the complaint is infertility. Amenorrhoea alone does not justify the treatment. Moreover, the only cases in which gonadotrophins can possibly be effective are those in which the ovaries contain ova, and when failure in ovulation is the result of absent or disturbed gonadotrophic function of the pituitary.

Thus, gonadotrophins are used for the induction of ovulation and superovulation in women unresponsive to clomiphene and tamoxifen, in in vitro fertilisation (IVF) and other techniques of assisted reproduction and in hypogonadotrophic women who may have normal follicular growth but impaired oestrogen synthesis. They may be used alone or in combination with gonadotrophin-releasing hormone (GnRH) agonists.

When the dominant follicle has formed, hCG is used to mimic the LH surge to release the ovum. It is used in women with documented evidence of poor luteal function to provide luteal support in the second half of the cycle and through the first trimester of pregnancy.

In the Male

Oligozoospermia: Except when failure in spermatogenesis by potentially normal testes is caused by established pituitary failure, the value of gonadotrophins for this condition is doubtful.

Cryptorchidism: Boys aged 5–14 years in whom neither testis has descended can be given hCG. However, 80% of supposed undescended testes are merely retractile, and many authorities take the view that in those cases in which the treatment encourages descent, it is unnecessary because spontaneous cure would have occurred in time. Moreover, in most cases where spontaneous cure will not take place, there is some local anatomical error which will always require surgery.

Nevertheless, hormone therapy may lengthen the spermatic cord and enable the testes to descend before they become too large for the canals. It is worth trying as a preliminary measure or as an adjunct to surgery. Although there is much dispute, some authorities claim that, after excluding retractile testes, a cure is obtained without surgery in 33% of cases.

Gonadotrophin therapy in boys can cause troublesome, albeit temporary, precocious development and frequent erection of the phallus.

Adverse Effects

- Local reactions at the site of injection
- General anaphylactic protein reactions
- Production of antihormone antibodies
- Multiple ovulation with multiple pregnancy
- Ovarian hyperstimulation syndrome resulting in pain, cystic change, enlargement, haemorrhage into the ovary and peritoneal cavity, peritoneal and pleural effusions. Death and arterial thrombosis with loss of limb are recorded as rarities.

Contraindications

The use of gonadotrophins is contraindicated in the presence of tumours of the ovary, breast, uterus, pituitary and hypothalamus; in pregnancy (except the therapeutic administration of hCG for luteal phase defects), lactation or with undiagnosed vaginal bleeding, if there is hypersensitivity to the gonadotrophins or excipients in the formulation, if there is primary ovarian failure, if there are ovarian cysts or if the sexual organs are malformed such that pregnancy cannot occur.

ANTIGONADOTROPHINS

A variety of agents can be regarded as acting as antigonadotrophins. These include oestrogens, which depress the gonadotrophic function of the hypothalamic–pituitary system. Certain progestogens and androgens may, in large doses, have a similar effect and so lower the levels of gonadotrophins in circulation.

Danazol is a synthetic steroid derivative of ethisterone which is devoid of progestogenic and oestrogenic properties, except that it lowers the levels of FSH and LH in circulation—presumably by inhibiting the production of these hormones. The antigonadotrophic action of danazol is so strong that it can suppress ovulation and menstruation; the drug is, therefore, of value in the treatment of endometriosis. It is administered by mouth, the dose being 200–800 mg daily, depending on the indications. It has also been used for the treatment of menorrhagia, mammary dysplasia and gynaecomastia. It is mildly androgenic and anabolic and can also produce systemic side effects similar to those caused by progestogens and androgens.

Gestrinone is a 19-nortestosterone derivative which also decreases FSH and LH secretion but requires only twice-weekly administration. Indications and side effects are similar to danazol.

The isolation and synthesis of GnRH and analogues of GnRH, agonistic and antagonistic, resulted in another group of antigonadotrophin agents.

Gonadotrophin-releasing Hormone Antagonists

Gonadotrophin-releasing hormone antagonists act immediately to suppress gonadotrophin secretion. The antagonists are difficult to prepare and expensive. Many of them have severe adverse effects because they cause the degranulation of mast cells. The histamine-releasing activities of Nal-Arg, Nal-Glu and SB-75 are high. Ganirelix and A7599/8 also have relatively high histamine-releasing activity. Azaline B and antide have low histamine-releasing activities; antide forms a gel with normal saline.

Antagonists have largely been superseded by GnRH agonists in clinical practice. However, their potential role in contraception, e.g. in combination with testosterone for long-acting male contraception, is being investigated. Nal-Glu administered for 3 weeks inhibits spermatogenesis.

Elagolix marks a significant advancement as the first orally administered Food and Drug Administration (FDA)-approved treatment for endometriosis-associated pain in over a decade. Unlike GnRH agonists, which work by completely suppressing the hypothalamic–pituitary–ovarian axis to induce a hypoestrogenic state, elagolix, as a GnRH antagonist, offers a different approach. Instead of full suppression, it partially suppresses oestradiol, thereby reducing the intensity of hypoestrogenic side effects such as hot flashes, vaginal dryness, reduced bone mineral density and lipid profile changes while still maintaining its therapeutic efficacy.

What sets elagolix apart is its mechanistic difference from GnRH agonists, which often necessitate the administration of add-back hormonal therapy to counteract the hypoestrogenic effects. In contrast, elagolix's registration trials were conducted without the need for add-back hormonal therapy, showcasing its ability to manage endometriosis-associated pain effectively while minimising the burden of hypoestrogenic side effects. This nuanced approach provides patients with a treatment option that offers both efficacy and improved tolerability.

In clinical trials, elagolix has demonstrated remarkable efficacy in reducing pelvic pain associated with endometriosis, including symptoms such as dysmenorrhoea (painful menstruation), nonmenstrual pelvic pain (NMPP), and dyspareunia (pain during intercourse). Additionally, it has been shown to improve the overall quality of life for women suffering from endometriosis-associated pain. Furthermore, the need for rescue analgesics (pain-relieving medications taken as needed) was decreased among patients receiving elagolix.

Importantly, these positive outcomes were sustained over a period of 12 months of treatment, indicating the long-term effectiveness of elagolix in managing endometriosis-related symptoms. This consistency in efficacy over time underscores the reliability and durability of elagolix as a treatment option for women experiencing the debilitating effects of endometriosis-associated pain.

Gonadotrophin-releasing Hormone Agonists

Various GnRH agonists and superagonists are now available, which include buserelin, leuprorelin, nafarelin, goserelin, triptorelin, histrelin and deslorelin. They are produced by a modification of the amino acid residues at positions 6 and 10, which makes them resistant to the action of pituitary amylamidases and increases their receptor binding affinity.

Actions

Gonadotrophin-releasing hormone agonists bind to the GnRH receptor in the pituitary and provide competitive inhibition of endogenous GnRH. Initially, a supraphysiological release of FSH and LH from the pituitary occurs (flare). Repeated administration produces the paradoxical effect of decreasing the synthesis and release of both FSH and LH and therefore of the gonadal steroid hormones, along with a loss of receptors, resulting in downregulation and a state of hypogonadism. The FSH and LH levels are thus increased on days 2–3 of administration and are down to castration levels by the second to third week.

Therapeutic Applications

General Principles

Gonadotrophin-releasing hormone agonists have a short half-life of 2–6 hours.

They are not active orally and have to be administered intramuscularly, subcutaneously or intranasally.

Administration of GnRH agonists can be on a daily basis, but depot preparations are administered on a monthly basis; the interval depends on the indication. Intranasal administration is done 2–5 times per day.

Depending on the phase of the cycle in which treatment is started and the duration for which it is continued, various protocols can be used, e.g. ultra-long, long, short and ultra-short.

Methods of Administration

Orally, GnRH agonists are not effective. They are administered by subcutaneous or IM injections, as a nasal spray, sustained-release implants or injections of biodegradable microspheres. The routes of administration, dosages and relative potencies of different agents are shown in **Table 1**.

Indications

In the Female

Gonadotrophin-releasing hormone agonists cause a 'medical oophorectomy,' which has revolutionised the treatment of many conditions.

- *Precocious puberty:* In true idiopathic GnRH-dependent precocious puberty, GnRH agonists are the drugs of choice, producing amenorrhoea, a rapid and substantial regression of pubertal characteristics and a reduction in growth velocity, with increase in the final bone height if treatment is started early.
- *Endometriosis and adenomyosis:* GnRH agonists suppress the disease effectively and produce significant symptomatic relief, reduce the size of deposits and, in infertile women, have a pregnancy rate comparable with danazol but with lesser side effects. Adenomyosis has also been successfully treated with GnRH agonists.
- *Leiomyomas:* Uterine size decreases by 30–64% after 3 months of treatment with GnRH agonists, the decrease being both in the size of the leiomyomas and the uterus itself. Symptomatic relief is also obtained. GnRH agonists are used preoperatively to facilitate myomectomy, especially hysteroscopic, by bringing

TABLE 1: Route of administration, dosage, potency and chief indications of GnRH agonists.

GnRH agonist	*Route of administration*	*Dosage*	*Relative potency**	*Chief indication*
Buserelin (Suprefact)	Intranasal subcutaneous	900–1,200 μg/day 200 μg/day	100 100	Endometriosis, ART and Ca prostate
Leuprorelin (Lupron, Lucrin)	Subcutaneous Intramuscular	0.1–1.0 mg/day 3.75 mg/month	10–100 200	Endometriosis, infertility, Ca prostate and hirsutism
Nafarelin (Synarel, Nasarel)	Intranasal	400–800 μg/day	200	Endometriosis, infertility and precocious puberty
Goserelin (Zoladex)	Subcutaneous	3.6 mg/month	230	Endometriosis, pre-TCRE, Ca breast and myoma
Triptorelin (Decapeptyl)	Intramuscular	2–4 mg/month 0.1 mg/day	100	Endometriosis, Ca prostate, infertility and precocious puberty
Histrelin (Supprelin)	Subcutaneous	10 μg/kg/day	100	Central precocious puberty

*Potency of GnRH = 1
(ART: assisted reproductive technology; Ca: carcinoma; GnRH: gonadotrophin-releasing hormone; TCRE: transcervical resection of the endometrium)

about a decrease in size, endometrial atrophy, decreased vascularity and intraoperative blood loss. When hysterectomy is planned, the decrease in size may make vaginal hysterectomy feasible. Unoperated leiomyomas regain their size 3–4 months after stopping treatment. Very large submucus myomas can undergo degeneration and necrosis 5–10 weeks after starting therapy which may be symptomatic and cause significant vaginal bleeding. Regression of leiomyomatosis peritonealis disseminate can also be achieved with GnRH agonist treatment.

- *Dysfunctional uterine bleeding:* GnRH agonists are used in this condition when short-term relief is required as in a patient with renal failure awaiting transplantation, post-transplantation or with blood dyscrasias.
- *Infertility:* The role of GnRH agonists in endometriosis and leiomyomas has been discussed above. GnRH agonists have revolutionised protocols for the induction of ovulation. The use of GnRH in assisted reproductive techniques for downregulation of the hypothalamic–pituitary axis is one of the important reasons for the improved outcomes following IVF and other procedures. In the induction of ovulation, administration of 0.1 mg leuprorelin or triptorelin stimulates the LH surge, unlike hCG which mimics it.
- *PMS:* GnRH agonists are effective in treatment, but long-term treatment is not possible because of side effects. Introducing add-back therapy decreases the effect on PMS symptoms as well.
- *Hirsutism:* GnRH agonist treatment improves hirsutism because ovarian androgen production is LH dependent but requires a greater dose. Results are improved when an oral contraceptive is added, and it is more effective in severe hirsutism. Again, long-term therapy is difficult.
- *Carcinoma of the breast:* The addition of GnRH agonists to tamoxifen as adjunctive therapy in breast cancer is found to improve the outcome and is now becoming the routine practice at some centres.
- *Irritable bowel syndrome:* The use of GnRH agonists for this indication is under trial.

In the Male

- *Cryptorchidism:* Short-term intranasal nafarelin is successful where cryptorchidism is not due to anatomical blockage. It stimulates the release of gonadotrophins, thereby stimulating secretion of gonadal steroids, which mediate the descent of the testes—30% respond in 4 weeks.
- *Carcinoma of the prostate:* GnRH agonists are as effective as orchidectomy in patients with carcinoma of the prostate. However, if there are neurological symptoms or life-threatening metastatic disease, antiandrogens should be started first. GnRH agonists are combined with antiandrogens (flutamide or nilutamide) to counter the effect of testosterone of adrenal origin.

- *Benign prostatic hypertrophy:* Daily administration of leuprorelin or nafarelin decreases obstructive urinary symptoms in 1 month; although in some cases, it may take up to 6 months. Regrowth occurs within 6 months after stopping therapy.

Adverse Effects

In about 10% of patients, a local allergic reaction may be seen at the injection site. Rarely, anaphylaxis may occur.

Gonadotrophin-releasing hormone agonist use is associated with menopausal symptoms. Within 3–4 weeks of starting treatment, hot flashes, vaginal dryness, headache, joint and muscle stiffness and depression occur. One third of women experience irregular vaginal bleeding.

Osteoporosis occurs in a large proportion of patients who receive therapy for longer than 6 months, and contrary to previous belief may not be totally reversed after stopping treatment. Add-back treatment with combination oestrogen–progestogen or with tibolone as in standard HRT regimens decreases these side effects without affecting the success of therapy. This allows prolongation of therapy beyond 6 months.

The diagnosis of a leiomyosarcoma can be delayed; if the myoma is either not shrinking or is growing, it should be operated immediately.

Pregnancy can occur during therapy if there is escape from suppression, but no adverse effects on the foetus have been reported.

HYPOTHALAMIC HORMONES

It has long been known that what were once regarded as posterior pituitary hormones, notably oxytocin and vasopressin, are in fact secreted by the hypothalamus and travel from there to the pituitary gland, by way of the axons of neurons. These are mainly concerned with stimulating the contractions of certain smooth muscles and with water balance and are not considered in this chapter.

The hypothalamus is now known to control chemically the secretion of the hormones of the anterior pituitary. It governs the functions of the pituitary by actively secreting specific and independent hormones. Several of these qualify for inclusion as sex hormones in so far that, via the pituitary, they are intimately concerned with the activity of the gonads, breasts and other glands.

Types and Sources

The secretion of hypothalamic-releasing hormones is controlled either by direct feedback mechanisms or by influences from environmental factors which act via the higher cortical centres. Feedback control is usually negative or inhibitory, thus depressing both the production of the hypothalamic-releasing hormone and secretion of trophic hormone from the anterior pituitary. A positive feedback mechanism is less common but is involved in the secretion of LH. Feedback is indirect if it operates mainly upon the pituitary gland via the hypothalamus and direct if the effect is at the adenohypophysis itself. When pituitary hormones themselves inhibit secretion of releasing hormones, a short or internal negative feedback mechanism exists.

The hypothalamic regulatory-releasing hormones are thyrotrophin-releasing hormone (TRH), GnRH, growth hormone-releasing hormone (GHRH) and corticotrophin-releasing hormone (CRH). Various substances, including TRH and vasoactive intestinal peptide (VIP), are thought to act as prolactin-releasing hormone. The release-inhibiting hormones are prolactin-inhibiting factor (PIF), which is probably dopamine, growth hormone release-inhibiting hormone (GHRIH) and possibly a melanocyte-stimulating hormone (MSH) release-inhibiting hormone (MSHRIH).

Some of the hormone-releasing hormones have been synthesised and found to be low-molecular-weight peptides.

Actions

Within the central nervous system, control of the hypothalamic-releasing factors is mediated by the local synthesis of neurotransmitters—dopamine, serotonin and noradrenaline. Apart from controlling hypothalamic neurohormone secretion, these neurotransmitters are also concerned with the regulation of sexual function, behaviour and mood. The response to the neurotransmitters may be modified by drugs. Dopamine is now considered to be a PIF. Bromocriptine is a dopamine agonist, and its effect is typically seen in suppression of prolactin secretion. Also, it augments GH secretion in the normal individual but suppresses it in acromegaly. Similarly, methyldopa suppresses prolactin production and augments GH production. Beta-blocking agents augment GH responses to stress, whilst alpha-blocking agents have a reverse effect; although in anorexia nervosa, hormonal responses show quicker recovery under the effect of alpha blockade.

The actions of the hypothalamic hormones are not entirely specific to their respective pituitary hormones. For example, thyroid-stimulating hormone-releasing hormone (TSHRH) not only releases thyroid-stimulating hormone (TSH); it causes a significant rise in the output of prolactin. In men, but not in women, it also stimulates the release of LH. There are many interactions in this complex system which are still not understood, but it is known that GHRIH inhibits the LH response to TSHRH. It should not be forgotten that the hypothalamus also controls other important activities such as appetite, thirst and control of body temperature, through nervous mechanisms alone.

Diagnostic Applications

Thyrotropin-releasing Hormone

Thyrotrophin-releasing hormone is a useful diagnostic agent in difficult cases of hyperthyroidism; when injected into normal individuals, it leads to a rapid rise in thyrotropin; in patients with thyrotoxicosis, it does not rise because of the feedback mechanism of excess circulatory thyroid hormone. Many patients with hypopituitarism show a reduced or delayed rise in TSH, and a normal TSH response to TRH rules out hyperthyroidism. With the introduction of extremely sensitive assays from TSH, this test is now seldom required.

Gonadotrophin-releasing Hormone

When injected intravenously into normal individuals, GnRH leads to a rapid rise in plasma LH and FSH concentrations. This is useful in evaluating cases of precocious puberty. Cases of true precocious puberty respond to GnRH with a rise in LH levels within 2 hours following injection. Similarly, gonadotrophin deficiency can also be evaluated. The administration of GnRH should elicit a normal LH response in hypogonadotrophic patients with hypothalamic lesions and a weak or nonexistent response in pituitary disease.

Synthetic GnRH (Fertiral, Gonadorelin) is available as a 500 µg/mL ampoule. Pulsatile subcutaneous administration can induce both follicular maturation and ovulation in amenorrhoeic women with hypogonadotrophic hypogonadism. However, its administration is both difficult and expensive, and it is not used in routine clinical practice. Relefact® is available as a 100-µg ampoule for the assessment of pituitary function.

The therapeutic applications of the GnRH analogues have been discussed above.

Corticotrophin-releasing Hormone

The normal rise in plasma cortisol concentration which follows the administration of CRH does not occur in adrenocortical insufficiency. In cases of congenital adrenal hyperplasia with normal 17-OH progesterone (17-OHP) levels, the administration of CRH will produce a rise in the 17-OHP level.

SUGGESTED READING

1. Bishop P. Hormone therapy in gynaecology. Can Med Assoc J. 1947;57(4):353-7.
2. Carr B, Giudice L, Dmowski WP, O'Brien C, Jiang P, Burke J, et al. Elagolix, an oral GnRH antagonist for endometriosis-associated pain: a randomized controlled study. J Endometr Pelvic Pain Disord. 2013;5:105-15.
3. Donnez J, Taylor RN, Taylor HS. Partial suppression of estradiol: a new strategy in endometriosis management? Fertil Steril. 2017;107:568-70.
4. Karim SM. Clinical applications of prostaglandins in obstetrics and gynaecology. Ann Acad Med Singapore. 1982;11(4):493-502.
5. Leyland N, Estes SJ, Lessey BA, Advincula AP, Taylor HS. A clinician's guide to the treatment of endometriosis with elagolix. J Womens Health (Larchmt). 2021;30(4):569-78.
6. Manuilova IA. Use of different prostaglandin analogues for terminating pregnancy at different terms. Acta Med Hung. 1986;43(2):133-8.
7. Naheed B, Kuiper JH, Uthman OA. Non-contraceptive oestrogen-containing preparations for controlling symptoms of premenstrual syndrome. Cochrane Database Syst Rev. 2017;3:CD010503.
8. Practice Committee of the American Society for Reproductive Medicine. Treatment of pelvic pain associated with endometriosis: a committee opinion. Fertil Steril. 2014;101:927-35.
9. Schindler AE. Dienogest in long-term treatment of endometriosis. Int J Womens Health. 2011;3:175-84.
10. Surrey E, Taylor HS, Giudice L, Lessey BA, Abrao MS, Archer DF, et al. Long-term outcomes of elagolix in women with endometriosis: results from two extension studies. Obstet Gynecol. 2018;132:147-60.

44

CHAPTER

Vaginal Discharge

Sujatha BS, Muralidhar V Pai

Chapter Outline

- General Considerations
- Causes of Physiological Discharge
- Prognosis
- Risk Factors
- Diagnosis
- Management
- Therapy
- Prevention

GENERAL CONSIDERATIONS

The female genital tract has a complex microbial flora that varies with the site, patient age and hormonal background. The quality and quantity of cervical and vagina secretions also vary with many factors, including age, phase of the menstrual cycle and use of the oral contraceptive device. A normal physiological discharge is a white or clear, nonoffensive discharge that varies with the menstrual cycle. Prior to ovulation, oestrogen levels increase, altering cervical mucus from nonfertile (thick and sticky) to fertile (clearer, wetter, stretchy and slippery). After ovulation, oestrogen levels fall, and progesterone levels increase; cervical mucus becomes thick, sticky and hostile to sperm. Normal vaginal flora (lactobacilli) colonises the vaginal epithelium and changes according to circulating oestrogen levels. When oestrogen is present, the vaginal epithelium contains glycogen which favours colonisation. Lactobacilli and other acid-tolerant bacteria metabolise glycogen to lactic acid. This results in a pH between 3.5 and 4.7. The tough stratified squamous epithelial lining of the vagina, the presence of lactobacilli (Döderlein's bacilli) and the acidic pH play an important role in the defence mechanism against infection.

Each woman has her own sense of normality and what is acceptable or excessive for her. But women who have pathological vaginal discharge are mostly due to vaginal infection and/or irritation characterised by discharge, itching or odour and are rarely associated with dysuria and/or dyspareunia. With the availability of over-the-counter products such as dry wash or V-wash, women seek these products before an evaluation by a clinician. Despite the fact that nothing more than regular washing is necessary for hygienic purposes, women's magazines and those that advertise in them now advocate deodorant powders to be sprayed on the vulva and within the vagina in order to promote sexual attractiveness! They have the opposite effect if they destroy natural odour, and moreover, they are as harmful as they are unnecessary. Apart from inculcating a wrong mental outlook amongst girls and women, they are extremely likely to promote gross and painful local reactions, even ulceration of the vulva and vagina.

CAUSES OF PHYSIOLOGICAL DISCHARGE

The slight discharge normally seen at the vulva and in the vagina is a mixture of the following, all of which vary in amount and character with ovarian function.

- Vulvar secretions from Bartholin's, sebaceous, sweat and apocrine glands
- Vaginal discharge
- Cervical secretion
- Uterine secretion
- Fallopian tube secretion

This may also contain a contribution from peritoneal fluid.

The composition and amount of vaginal discharge changes as an individual goes through the various stages of sexual and reproductive development as described in **Table 1**.

Leucorrhoea

The term leucorrhoea should be restricted to those conditions when the normal vaginal secretions are increased in amount with no excess in leucocyte count (nonpurulent). An increase in normal vaginal secretions

TABLE 1: Various stages of sexual and reproductive development.

Stage	*Hormone responsible*	*Colour and consistency*	*pH*
Neonatal	Exposure to placental hormones	White, clear mucus	5.7
Paediatric	Lower oestrogen levels	White, clear, thinner mucus	6–8
Puberty	Higher oestrogen levels	White and thick mucus	3.5–4.7
Menstrual (proliferative)	Rising oestrogen levels/oestrogen surge	White, thick, sticky and minimal	3.5–4.7
Menstrual (ovulatory)	Oestrogens from the corpus luteum	White, clear, copious and elastic	3.5–4.7
Menstrual (secretory)	Increased progesterone levels	White, opaque and minimal	
Pregnancy	Increased oestrogen and progesterone	White or slightly grey, and musty smell	3.5–4.7
Menopause	Drop in oestrogen levels	Very minimal discharge, clear and thin	6.0–7.5

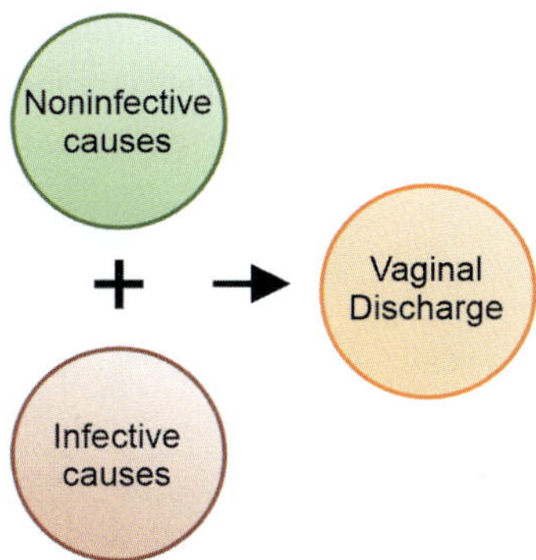

Fig. 1: Noninfective and infective causes of vaginal discharge.

is physiological at puberty, during pregnancy, at ovulation and in some women, during the premenstrual phase of the menstrual cycle.

Noninfective Causes of Vaginal Discharge (Fig. 1)

A noninfective vaginal discharge may occur secondary to:

- *Foreign body:* Intrauterine contraceptive device (IUCD), forgotten tampons, forgotten ring pessary in a postmenopausal woman
- Chemical irritation, as in excessive douching
- *Urinary or faeculent discharges:* Urine from a vesicovaginal fistula, faeces from a rectovaginal fistula
- *Serosanguinous discharge:* From carcinoma in the vagina, cervix, endometrium or rarely, the fallopian tubes
- Neoplasms such as fibroids or cervical polyp
- Endometritis
- Chronic cervicitis
- Atrophic vaginitis
- Desquamative inflammatory vaginitis
- Vulval dermatitis
- Erosive lichen planus

Infective Causes

- *Nonsexually transmitted infections:*
    - Bacterial vaginosis
    - Vulvovaginal candidiasis (VVC)
- *Sexually transmitted infections:*
    - *Chlamydia trachomatis*
    - *Neisseria gonorrhoeae*
    - *Trichomonas vaginitis*

Bacterial Vaginosis

Bacterial vaginosis (BV) is a form of vaginal dysbiosis characterised by the replacement of normal hydrogen peroxide and lactic acid-producing Lactobacillus species with elevated levels of facultative anaerobic organisms, such as *Gardnerella vaginalis, Mycoplasma hominis* and *Prevotella* species. A distinctive aspect of BV is the formation of a polymicrobial biofilm on the vaginal epithelial cells. It is the most prevalent cause of abnormal vaginal discharge in women of childbearing age, responsible for 40–50% of vaginitis cases. Approximately 70% of women with BV are asymptomatic, but 12–18% may develop symptoms over time.

Those who do experience symptoms often report a thin, grey-white, homogenous vaginal discharge **(Fig. 2A)** with a strong 'fishy' odour, which can become more pronounced after sexual intercourse and during menstruation. The presence of dysuria, itching, vulvovaginal burning or signs of inflammation (such as redness and swelling) indicates the possibility of mixed vaginitis rather than BV alone.

Bacterial vaginosis is associated with sexually active women having multiple partners, a new sex partner, douching, lack of condom use and lack of vaginal lactobacilli; women who have never been sexually active are rarely affected.

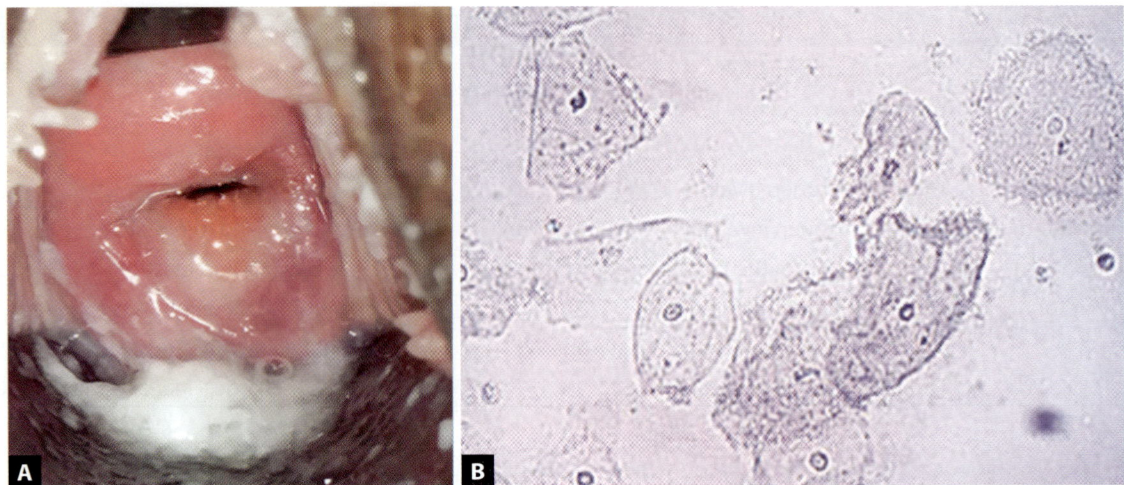

Figs. 2A and B: (A) Bacterial vaginosis; (B) Clue cells and ground-glass appearance—*Gardnerella vaginalis.*

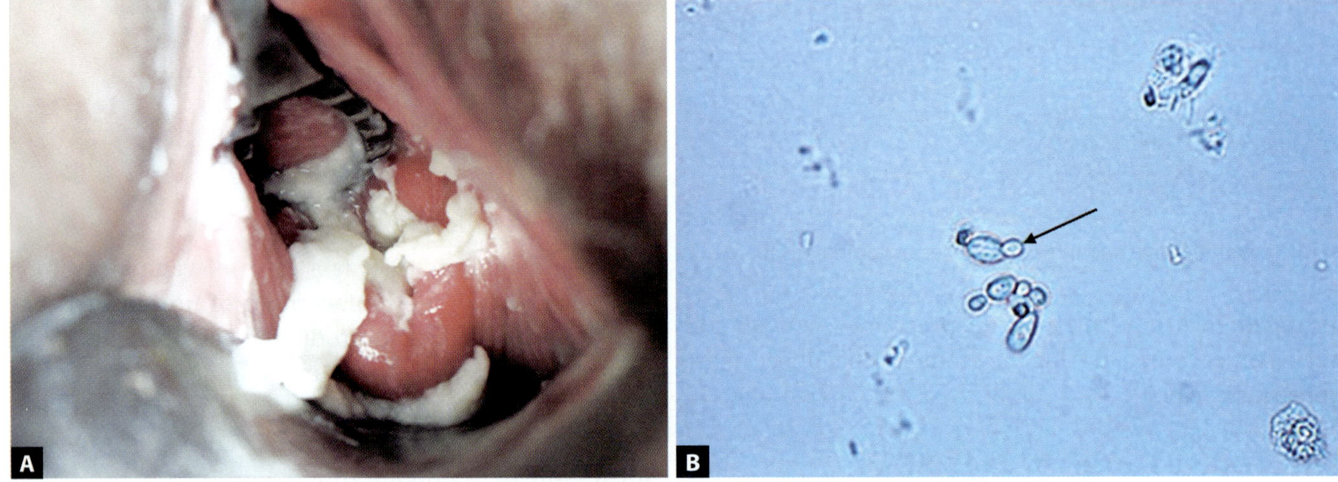

Figs. 3A and B: (A) Vaginal candidiasis; (B) *Candida albicans.*

Microscopic examination of a saline wet mount specimen **(Fig. 2B)** has a pH >4.5. It shows clumps of bacteria, total loss of normal lactobacilli and peculiar 'clue cells.' These epithelial cells with numerous coccoid bacteria attached to their surface, with misty borders and cytoplasm, resemble 'ground glass.' These bacteria are not part of the normal vaginal flora. Thus, the mere presence of these organisms is not diagnostic of BV.

Vulvovaginal Candidiasis

Vulvovaginal candidiasis is frequently caused by airborne fungi *Candida albicans* but can occasionally be caused by other *Candida* species, such as *Candida glabrata* or *Candida tropicalis*. Predisposing factors are mainly women who are pregnant, diabetic, obese, immunosuppressed, on oral contraceptives or corticosteroids or have had broad-spectrum antibiotic therapy. Patients present with pruritus, vaginal soreness, dyspareunia, external dysuria and abnormal vaginal discharge. None of these symptoms is specific for VVC. The vulval and vaginal areas are often bright red in colour, sometimes excoriated. A thick, adherent 'curdy white' or 'cottage cheese' discharge **(Fig. 3A)** is generally found. This discharge is odourless. Vagina pH is often between 4.2 and 5. Diagnosis is made by visualisation of vaginal discharge demonstrating budding yeasts, hyphae or pseudo-hyphae, blastospores, on saline **(Fig. 3B),** or 10% KOH microscopy, or a positive culture report.

The condition is classified as:

- *Uncomplicated:* When it presents as infrequent episodes, has mild to moderate symptoms or findings, suspected *Candida albicans* infection and in a nonpregnant woman without medical complications.
- *Complicated:* When episodes are recurrent (≥4 per year), symptoms and findings are severe, suspected or proven non-albicans *Candida* infection and women have predisposing factors such as diabetes, severe medical illness, immunosuppression, other vulvovaginal conditions and pregnancy.

Trichomonas vaginitis

Trichomonas vaginalis is the most prevalent nonviral sexually transmitted infection caused by a flagellate protozoan that subsists only in the vagina, Skene ducts and male or female urethra. The infection is transmitted by sexual contact. It can also occur via fomites, and the organism has been known to survive in swimming pools and hot tubs. Trichomoniasis is associated with pelvic inflammatory disease (PID), endometritis, infertility, ectopic pregnancy and preterm birth, and it often coexists with other sexually transmitted diseases and BV. Women with this infection can acquire human immunodeficiency virus (HIV) easily. Patients present with a frothy vaginal discharge that might be diffuse, foul-smelling or yellow-green with or without vulvar irritation, dysuria, dyspareunia and occasional lower abdominal pain. 10% of women will have signs such as oedema or erythema of the vulva, petechiae or strawberry patches on cervix **(Fig. 4A)**, in the upper vagina or on the cervix. Wet smear will show large numbers of mature epithelial cells, white blood cells and the flagellated parasites **(Fig. 4B)**. The coexistence of *T. vaginalis* and BV is frequently observed, with reported coinfection rates ranging from 20 to 80%. The US Centers for Disease Control and Prevention (CDC) recommends screening for *T. vaginalis* in all HIV-infected women at their initial visit and annually thereafter.

Neisseria gonorrhoeae

This sexually transmitted infection is caused by gram-negative diplococci *N. gonorrhoeae* **(Fig. 5)**. Patients with *N. gonorrhoeae* infection usually present with vaginal discharge from endocervicitis that is usually described as thin, purulent and mildly odorous. This is usually associated with PID and urethritis presenting as lower abdominal pain, intermenstrual bleeding and dysuria. Examination of these patients will reveal a mucopurulent, thin discharge with tender cervical movements and may also show an adnexal mass. Culture in New York Agar medium is the most common diagnostic test for gonorrhoea, followed by the deoxyribonucleic acid (DNA) probe and then the polymerase chain reaction (PCR) assay and ligand chain reaction (LCR). Coexisting chlamydia is present in 50% patients.

Chlamydia trachomatis

Chlamydial infection of the lower genital tract occurs in the endocervix. It can cause an odourless, mucoid vaginal discharge, typically with no external pruritus, although many women have minimal or no symptoms. An ascending infection can result in PID. Examination reveals cervicitis

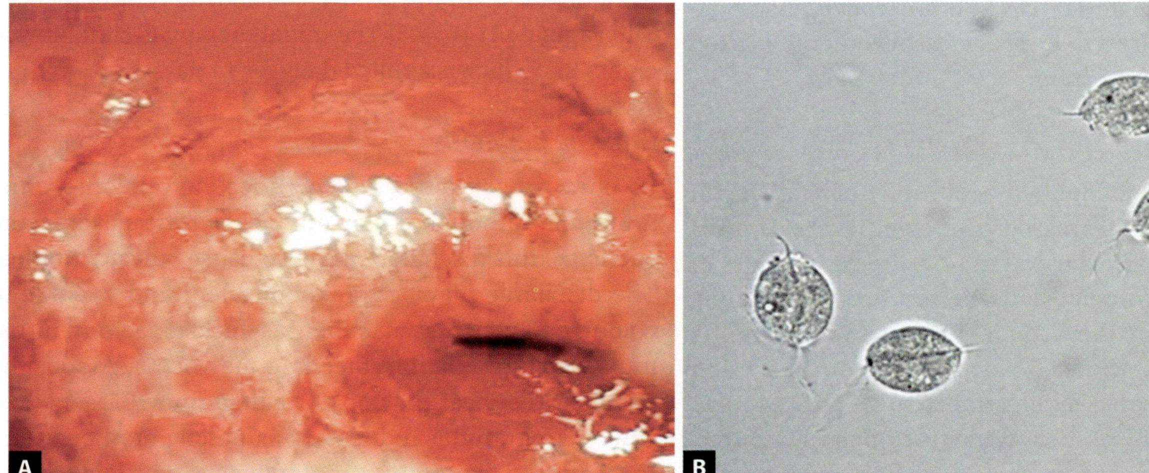

Figs. 4A and B: (A) Strawberry patches on cervix; (B) Flagellated parasites, *Trichomonas vaginalis*.

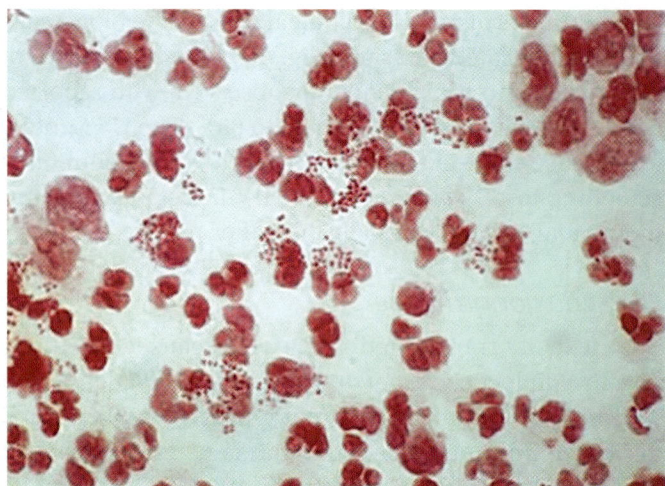

Fig. 5: Gram-negative diplococci.

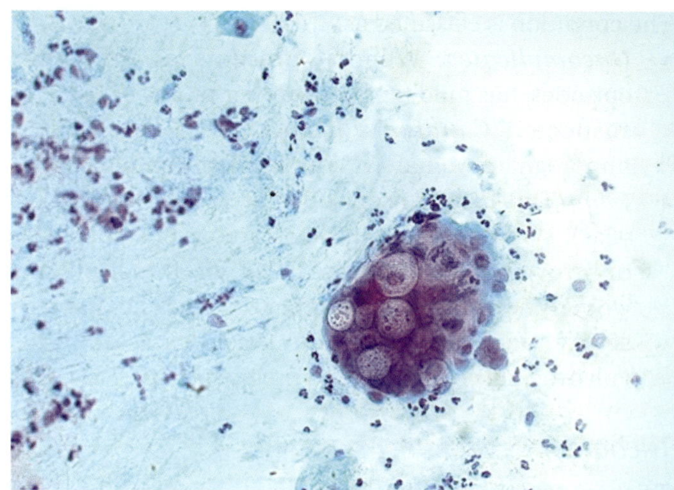

Fig. 6: *Chlamydia trachomatis.*

with a yellow or cloudy mucoid discharge from the os. The cervix tends to bleed easily on touch. Some women may develop urethritis with a urethral discharge seen on pressing over the urethra at the time of pelvic examination. Clinical microscopy and the amine test (significant odour release on addition of potassium hydroxide to vaginal secretions) can be used to help differentiate chlamydial infection from other lower genital tract infections such as urinary tract infection, BV and trichomoniasis. We must remember that chlamydial infection in the lower genital tract does not cause vaginitis. If at all vaginal findings are present, they usually indicate a different diagnosis or a coinfection. Chlamydiae are spherical or ovoid, obligate intracellular bacteria that are ubiquitous **(Fig. 6)**. Intracellular parasitism of *Chlamydia* differentiates it from other bacteria. Nucleic acid amplification tests (NAATs) find the genetic material (DNA) of *Chlamydia* bacteria. Cell culture and direct fluorescent test are other tests used in the diagnosis of infection.

Atrophic Vaginitis

Atrophic vaginitis is defined as atrophy of the vaginal epithelium due to decreased oestrogen levels. The pH of the vagina usually is elevated (4.7 or greater). Loss of elasticity in the connective tissue results in shortening and narrowing of the vagina. Women with atrophic vaginitis present with a scanty, thin, odourless and clear vaginal discharge, dryness and dyspareunia. Atrophic vaginitis is usually associated with urinary symptoms such as increased frequency of urination, burning and incontinence.

Desquamative Inflammatory Vaginitis

This is generally seen in perimenopausal and postmenopausal women and is characterised by yellowish or mucoid copious discharge, not purulent, along with exfoliation of epithelial cells with vulvovaginal burning and erythema. Desquamative inflammatory vaginitis is classified as a diagnosis of exclusion. Since there is no definitive test for this condition, it is essential to rule out other possible causes of vaginal inflammation and elevated pH, including atrophic vaginitis, erosive disorders, bacterial vaginosis and trichomoniasis. A comprehensive evaluation is crucial to accurately diagnose and address the underlying causes of symptoms such as vaginal discharge and pain.

Some cases show relatively less lactobacilli and overgrowth of Gram-positive cocci, usually streptococci. The vaginal pH is >4.5. The initial therapy is clindamycin cream 2%, which is applied daily for 14 days.

Chronic Cervicitis

In chronic cervicitis, leucorrhoea may be the chief symptom. Although it may not be as profuse as in acute cervicitis, this discharge may also cause vulvar irritation. The discharge may be frankly purulent and variable in colour, or it may present simply as thick, tenacious, turbid mucus. Intermenstrual bleeding may occur. Associated eversion (cervical erosion) or ectopy may present as a velvety to granular redness or as patchy erythema due to scattered squamous metaplasia (epithelialisation or epidermisation). Nabothian cysts in the area of the so-called transformation zone often occur. The Schiller test may show poorly staining or nonstaining areas. There is often some tenderness and thickening in the region of the uterosacral ligaments on pelvic examination, and motion of the cervix may be painful. Lower abdominal pain, lumbosacral backache, dysmenorrhoea or dyspareunia may occur occasionally, related to an associated parametritis. Colposcopy and a Pap smear are needed to rule out progressive lesions and treated later by cryosurgery.

Cervical polyps are small, pedunculated, often sessile neoplasms of the cervix. Most originate from the endocervix; a few arise from the portio vaginalis. They are composed of a vascular connective tissue stroma and covered by columnar, squamocolumnar or squamous epithelium. Asymptomatic polyps are often discovered on routine pelvic examination. Most are benign, but all should be removed and submitted for pathologic examination, because malignant change may occur. Moreover, some cervical cancers present as a polypoid mass. Polyps arise as a result of focal hyperplasia of the endocervix. It is not known whether this is due to chronic inflammation, an abnormal local responsiveness to hormonal stimulation, or a localised vascular congestion of cervical blood vessels. Endocervical polyps are usually red, flame-shaped, fragile growths and may vary in size from a few millimetres in length and diameter to larger tumours of 2–3 cm in diameter and several centimetres long. These polyps are usually attached to the endocervical mucosa near the external os by a narrow pedicle, but occasionally the base is broad. On microscopic examination, the stroma of a polyp is composed of fibrous connective tissue containing numerous small vessels in the centre. Most polyps can be removed in the physician's office. This is done with little bleeding by grasping the pedicle with a haemostat or long-grasping instrument and twisting it until the growth is avulsed. Large polyps and those with sessile attachments may require excision in an operating room setting. This will allow for anaesthesia to be administered for further visualisation, and treatment using the hysteroscope and control of any haemorrhage. If the cervix is soft, patulous or definitely dilated, and the polyp is large, hysteroscopy should be performed, especially if the pedicle is not readily visible. Exploration of the cervical and uterine cavities with the hysteroscope allows for further identification of other polyps. All tissues must be sent to a pathologist to be examined for possible underlying malignant or premalignant conditions.

PROGNOSIS

Simple removal of cervical polyps is usually curative. Any growth which is exposed to the lumen of the genital tract can cause a continuous discharge which is *at first white or creamy and nonoffensive*. Soon, however, the growth becomes ulcerated and infected as the necrotic tissue is exposed to the large number of organisms present in the vagina. The discharge then becomes purulent, offensive and blood-stained. Often, the odour is so marked that it can be appreciated as soon as the woman enters the room. Such symptoms are characteristic of a malignant neoplasm, but they may also be caused by benign lesions such as a cervical polyp or a sloughing submucous leiomyoma.

RISK FACTORS

Table 2 depicts various risk factors involved in different infections.

DIAGNOSIS

Women presenting with abnormal vulval or vaginal symptoms should be tested. If this is not possible, then examination and testing should be performed when:

- Finding of *T. vaginalis* on cervical cytology
- Diagnosis of *T. vaginalis* in a sexual partner
- Failure of vaginal discharge to respond to empirical treatment
- Severe or recurrent symptoms

All patients undergo physical examination to assess the vaginal discharge, evaluate for related findings (e.g. vulvar excoriations or oedema, erythema and cervicitis), and exclude other causes of the patient's symptoms.

Table 3 summarises a few diagnostic criteria for various infections. The definitive diagnosis of each infection is based on laboratory tests. A sample of the discharge is removed from the vaginal wall with a swab. Direct microscopy can be done immediately at the clinic if available.

Criteria for Diagnosis of Bacterial Vaginosis

- *Amsel's criteria* (the presence of three of the four criteria is required):
  1. Homogeneous grey-white discharge that smoothly coats the vaginal walls.
  2. pH of vaginal fluid >4.5

TABLE 2: Risk factors involved in different infections.

Type of vaginitis	*Risk factors*
Bacterial vaginosis	Low socioeconomic status, vaginal douching, smoking, use of an intrauterine contraceptive device, new/multiple sex partners, unprotected sexual intercourse, homosexual relationships and frequent use of higher doses of spermicide nonoxynol-9
Trichomoniasis	Low socioeconomic status, multiple sex partners, lifetime frequency of sexual activity, other sexually transmitted infections, lack of barrier contraceptive use, illicit drug use and smoking
Vulvovaginal candidiasis	Vaginal or systemic antibiotic use, diet high in refined sugars and uncontrolled diabetes mellitus
Atrophic vaginitis	Menopause, other conditions associated with oestrogen deficiency, oophorectomy, radiation therapy, chemotherapy, immunologic disorders, premature ovarian failure, endocrine disorders and anti-oestrogen medication
Irritant contact dermatitis	Soaps, tampons, contraceptive devices, sex toys, pessary, topical products, douching, fastidious cleansing, medications and clothing
Allergic contact dermatitis	Sperm, douching, latex condoms or diaphragms, tampons, topical products, medications, clothing and atopic history

TABLE 3: Diagnostic criteria for various infections.

Causative agent	*Amount of discharge*	*Appearance of discharge*	*pH*	*Amine odour on whiff test*	*Microscopic appearance*
Bacterial vaginosis: *Gardnerella vaginalis*	Increased	• Thin grey to green adherent to vaginal wall • Musty and fishy odour	>4.5	Present	• Total loss of lactobacilli • Clue cells have ground-glass cytoplasm and coccoid bacteria
Vulvovaginal candidiasis: *Candida albicans*	Sometimes increased	• Curdy white or cottage cheese • Thick and white	Normal	Absent	Presence of blastopheres, pseudohyphae and buds
Trichomoniasis: *Trichomonas vaginalis*	Increased	Grey green frothy	>4.5	Possibly present	• Mature epithelial cells • White blood cells • Flagellated parasites
Gonorrhoea *Neisseria gonorrhoeae*	Increased	White to yellow mucopurulent thin	>4.5	Absent	• Gram-negative diplococci • >10 WBCs per HPF
Chlamydia trachomatis	Increased	Yellow, cloudy mucoid	>4.5	Present	Spherical or ovoid obligate intracellular bacteria

(HPF: high-power field; WBCs: white blood cells)

3. Presence of a fishy odour when 10% potassium hydroxide (KOH) is added to a sample of vaginal discharge (positive whiff-amine test)
4. Clue cells present on saline wet mount microscopy (comprising at least 20% of epithelial cells)

- *Gram staining with Nugent score:* This is a gold standard test. It estimates the relative proportions of bacterial morphotypes on a Gram-stained vaginal smear to give a score between 0 and 10. A score of <4 is normal, 4–6 is intermediate and >6 is BV.
- *Hay–Ison criteria:* The test is based on findings on a Gram-stained smear and is better than the Nugent score.
  - *Grade 0:* Not related to BV, epithelial cells only, no lactobacilli, indicates recent antibiotics
  - *Grade 1 (Normal):* Lactobacillus morphotypes pre-dominate
  - *Grade 2 (Intermediate):* Mixed flora with some lactobacilli present, but Gardnerella or Mobiluncus morphotypes are also present

    - *Grade 3 (BV):* Predominantly Gardnerella and/or Mobiluncus morphotypes, clue cells. Few or absent lactobacilli.
    - *Grade 4:* Not related to BV, Gram-positive cocci only, no lactobacilli.
- *Newer laboratory test:*
    - *NAATs:* These are laboratory-based tests that exponentially multiply specific nucleic acid sequences through PCRs to identify vaginal pathogens, which include those specific to the diagnosis of bacterial vaginosis, vaginal candidiasis (VC) and trichomoniasis. Vaginal swabs can be collected either by a clinician or by the patient. Some of the tests are FDA-approved (BD Max vaginal panel, Aptima BV), while others are laboratory-developed tests (NuSwab VG, SureSwab BV and OneSwab BV panel) that require internal validation prior to use; all have high sensitivity and specificity (i.e. >90%). BV cannot be diagnosed by NAATs that are not specific to BV organisms. In addition to diagnosing BV, NAATs can identify VC and trichomonas vaginitis, as well as cervicitis caused by gonorrhoea and chlamydia.
    - *Point-of-care tests:* These tests can be performed in the office during the physical examination and are meant to be used alongside physical assessments, vaginal pH measurements and the whiff-amine test. Their usage has declined with the advent of NAATs.
    - *OSOM BVBlue:* The OSOM BVBlue system is a chromogenic diagnostic test that detects elevated sialidase enzyme activity in vaginal fluid samples.
    - *Affirm VP III:* The Affirm VP III test is an automated DNA probe assay designed to detect *G. vaginalis* when present in high concentrations.

Criteria for Diagnosis of Vaginal Candidiasis

- Signs include vulvar oedema, fissures, excoriations and thick curdy vaginal discharge.
- Absence of smell (in "whiff test" on speculum and in amine odour test on slide) is supportive, since candidiasis and BV/*T. vaginalis* do not usually coexist, but not diagnostic.
- Budding yeasts or pseudohyphae on wet preparation (with 10% KOH) and or/gram staining of vaginal discharge.
- Culture is not required for the routine diagnosis of VVC, because vaginal pH and microscopy are reliable tests. Also, yeast are normal colonisers of the vagina (i.e. a culture that confirms yeast may not reflect actual infection). Culture test is done in recurrent or refractory cases of VC.
- To perform a culture, a vaginal sample is collected from the lateral wall using a cotton-tipped swab and inoculated onto Sabouraud agar, Nickerson medium or Microstix-*Candida* medium, all of which yield similar results. Quantification of in vitro colony counts is not necessary for *Candida* cultures. While species identification is not required for initial diagnostic testing, since most isolates are *C. albicans*, it becomes important for managing refractory and recurrent cases.
- Repeated cultures of the same species of non-albicans *Candida*, typically *C. glabrata*, may suggest decreased sensitivity to antifungal treatments.

Criteria for Diagnosis of *Trichomonas vaginalis*

- Direct observation of the organism by a wet smear (normal saline) from the posterior vaginal fornix or endocervical swabs (sensitivity 40–70% cases) is the preferred diagnostic test. Microscopy for *T. vaginalis* should be performed as soon as possible after the sample is taken, as motility diminishes with time. The sensitivity decreases over time, with up to a 20% decrease reported 1 hour after collection.
- Culture, such as the inPouch system (BioMed Diagnostics), was considered most sensitive test will diagnose up to 95% cases.
- NAATs have been developed, and sensitivities and specificities approaching nearly 100% have been reported. Aptima *T. vaginalis* assay (Hologic) is FDA-cleared for detection in symptomatic or asymptomatic women.

Trichomonads are sometimes reported on cervical cytology; however, a meta-analysis has shown that while cytology has good specificity, the weighted mean sensitivity is only 58%. If the population prevalence of *T. vaginalis* is high, it is appropriate to treat in these circumstances; however, where a woman is unlikely to have trichomoniasis (prevalence ≤1%), it is prudent to confirm the diagnosis, preferably by the culture of vaginal secretions or NAATs if available.

MANAGEMENT

A detailed history, including sexual history, is essential to identify the necessary investigations and treatment options. Women who are in reproductive age group who are sexually active should undergo per speculum examination and if needed Pap smear or colposcopy to rule out local vaginal or cervical lesions such as polyp or a fibroid or cervical malignancy as treatment would be targeted.

Removal of a cervical polyp up to 2 cm long by 1 cm wide is a simple, painless procedure requiring little skill and is not associated with significant bleeding and can be easily done in the primary care setting. Cervical erosion, if it becomes troublesome to the patient, can be treated by discontinuing oral contraceptives, cryotherapy treatment or by using ablation treatment under local anaesthetic.

The World Health Organization (WHO) guidelines suggest two proposed approaches—*syndromic* and *empirical* for management of vaginal infections.

The WHO recommends that patients who present for primary care with symptoms that suggest sexually transmitted infections. Women assessed as being at risk of sexually transmitted infection, or who request testing, should be offered appropriate tests for *Chlamydia*, gonorrhoea, syphilis and HIV. Effective interviewing and counselling skills characterised by respect, compassion and a nonjudgemental attitude towards all patients are essential to obtaining a thorough sexual history and delivering effective prevention messages.

A high vaginal swab (HVS) is of limited diagnostic value in the management of vaginal discharge except in cases of inconclusive assessment, recurrent symptoms, treatment failure, or in pregnancy, postpartum, postabortion or postinstrumentation.

Information and Suggestions

Information, explanation and advice for the patient have been described here.

- For *T. vaginalis:* As *T. vaginalis* is a sexually transmitted organism, screening for coexistent infections should be undertaken. Sexual abstinence should be advised until treatment of all partners is completed.
- *For BV:* It should be explained that the cause is unclear and that although there is an association with sexual activity, it is not a sexually transmitted infection.

THERAPY

Table 4 depicts indications for treatment in the following three common conditions: (1) BV, (2) TV and (3) VC.

Recommended Regimens for Trichomoniasis

The nitroimidazoles comprise the only class of drugs useful for treating trichomoniasis, and most strains are highly susceptible. Due to the high rates of infection of the urethra and paraurethral glands in women, systemic chemotherapy should be given to effect a cure, and the use of metronidazole gel is not recommended. Meta-analysis and multicentric studies demonstrate that multidose metronidazole (500 mg orally twice daily for 7 days) reduces the proportion of women retesting positive at a 1-month test of cure visit by half, compared with women who received the 2-g single dose. The single dose has the advantage of improved compliance and being cheaper; however, there is some evidence to suggest that the failure rate is higher, especially if partners are not treated concurrently. There is a spontaneous cure rate in the order of 20–25%. Desensitisation was used for patients with true metronidazole allergy.

The recommended treatment for trichomoniasis in women is metronidazole 500 mg taken twice daily for 7 days. An alternative regimen is a single oral dose of tinidazole 2 g. Tinidazole is generally more expensive but achieves higher concentrations in serum and the

TABLE 4: Treatment for bacterial vaginosis (BV), *Trichomonas vaginalis* (TV) and vaginal candidiasis (VC).

BV	*TV*	*VC*
• Positive direct microscopy with/without symptoms in pregnant women (those with a history of prior idiopathic preterm birth or second-trimester loss) • Women undergoing some surgical procedures • *Optional*: Positive direct microscopy in women without symptoms • Treatment of BV is recommended for people with symptoms	• Positive test for TV regardless of symptoms • Epidemiological treatment of sexual partners	• Symptomatic women found to have *Candida* on either microscopy or culture • Asymptomatic women do not require treatment • Asymptomatic male partners do not require treatment

genitourinary tract, has a longer half-life compared to metronidazole and is associated with fewer side effects.

Healthcare providers should recommend that individuals with *T. vaginalis* infections abstain from sexual activity until both they and their partners have completed treatment and any symptoms have resolved. Additionally, testing for other sexually transmitted infections, including HIV, syphilis, gonorrhoea and chlamydia, should be conducted for those with *T. vaginalis*.

Due to the high rate of reinfection among women treated for trichomoniasis, retesting for *T. vaginalis* is advised for all sexually active women about 3 months after initial treatment, regardless of whether they think their partners have been treated. It is crucial to treat all sexual partners simultaneously to prevent reinfections.

Recurrent trichomoniasis: A recurrent infection may occur due to treatment failure (such as antimicrobial-resistant *T. vaginalis* or host-related issues), lack of adherence to the treatment plan or reinfection from an untreated partner. In cases of recurrent infection, it is important to investigate the source of the repeat infection, as most cases are likely due to reinfection. If the patient has been re-exposed to an untreated partner, a repeat course of the same treatment is recommended. For individuals with persistent infections not linked to re-exposure, clinicians should request a kit from the CDC for drug-resistance testing. Based on the results, appropriate treatment can be offered after consulting with infectious disease specialists.

Recommended Regimens for Bacterial Vaginosis

Treatment is recommended for women with symptoms. The established benefits of therapy in nonpregnant women are to relieve vaginal symptoms and signs of infection. Other potential benefits to treatment include a reduction in the risk of acquiring *C. trachomatis*, *N. gonorrhoeae*, *T. vaginalis*, HIV and herpes simplex type 2.

Recommended regimens: Metronidazole 500 mg orally twice a day for 7 days, or metronidazole gel 0.75%, one full applicator (5 g) intravaginally, once a day for 5 days, or clindamycin cream 2%, one full applicator (5 g) intravaginally at bedtime for 7 days. Abstinence from alcohol use should continue for 24 hours after completion of metronidazole or 72 hours after completion of tinidazole.

Alternative regimens for BV only intravaginal metronidazole gel (0.75%) once daily for 5 days, intravaginal clindamycin cream (2%) once daily for 7 days, or clindamycin 300 mg orally twice daily for 7 days. For BV, clindamycin and metronidazole have equal efficacy, comparing oral and vaginal formulations, both after 1 week. Most women will be cured after 5 days' treatment with metronidazole or clindamycin. Evidence suggests clindamycin is associated with fewer adverse effects than metronidazole.

Several randomised studies addressed the efficacy of vaginal clindamycin versus oral metronidazole. Eradication rates at 1 month after vaginal clindamycin cream were 66–83% versus 68–87% for metronidazole.

Vaginal versus oral clindamycin also showed similar efficacy but somewhat fewer side-effects. Clindamycin cream, as well as metronidazole gel, diminishes the strength of condoms. Barrier contraception is not considered safe during the treatment with vaginal products as these have mineral oils as their base which reduces efficacy of condoms.

Recommended Regimens for Vaginal Candidiasis

Short-course topical formulations (i.e. single dose and regimens of 1–3 days) effectively treat uncomplicated VVC. *Clotrimazole 1% cream* 5 g intravaginally daily for 7–14 days, or *Clotrimazole 2% cream 5 g* intravaginally daily for 3 days. Treatment with azoles relieves symptoms and negative cultures among 80–90% of patients after treatment is completed. Oral azoles, such as single-dose fluconazole 150 mg treatment, are as effective as longer courses.

Other oral alternative therapies that can be used, other than fluconazole 150 mg as a single dose, are itraconazole 200 mg twice daily for 1 day. Topical treatment of the vulva, though, is of no proven added benefit to intravaginal treatment, but patients get relief from emollients used. Where itching is a significant symptom, steroid-containing topical preparations may provide more rapid symptomatic relief. No substantial evidence exists to support using probiotics or homoeopathic medications for treating VVC.

Treatment of Recurrent Candidiasis

It is defined as three or more episodes of symptomatic VVC in <1 year. For women with recurrent VVC, it is important to obtain a vaginal culture or PCR to confirm the clinical diagnosis and detect non-albicans *Candida*. Since *Candida glabrata* does not form pseudohyphae or hyphae, it can be challenging to identify using microscopy.

Most cases of recurrent VVC caused by *C. albicans* respond effectively to short courses of oral or topical azole therapy. However, to ensure both clinical and mycological control, a longer initial treatment is recommended—such as 7–14 days of topical therapy or an oral regimen of fluconazole (100 mg, 150 mg or 200 mg) every third day for a total of three doses (on days 1, 4 and 7). This approach aims to achieve mycological remission before starting a maintenance antifungal treatment. The suggested maintenance regimen is a weekly dose of oral fluconazole (100 mg, 150 mg or 200 mg) for 6 months. Given the increasing resistance of *C. albicans* to azoles, susceptibility testing should be performed, if available, for symptomatic patients who remain culture positive despite maintenance therapy. These patients should be managed in consultation with a specialist.

During Pregnancy

Multiple studies and meta-analyses have not demonstrated a consistent association between metronidazole use during pregnancy and teratogenic or mutagenic effects in infants. Metronidazole can be used in all stages of pregnancy and during breastfeeding; however, high-dose regimens are best avoided in these circumstances. In lactating women who are administered metronidazole, withholding breastfeeding during treatment and for 12–24 hours after the last dose will reduce the exposure of metronidazole to the infant. Safety of tinidazole has not yet been well-evaluated. VVC occurs frequently during pregnancy. Only topical azole therapies, applied for 7 days, are recommended for use among pregnant women. Epidemiologic studies indicate a single 150-mg dose of fluconazole might be associated with spontaneous abortion and congenital anomalies; therefore, it should not be used.

Treatment for Partner

- *Bacterial vaginosis:* It should be explained that the cause is unclear and that although there is an association with sexual activity, it is not a sexually transmitted infection. Routine screening and treatment of partners is not indicated.
- *Trichomonas vaginalis:* Trichomoniasis is a sexually transmitted organism; hence, screening for coexistent infections should be undertaken. Sexual abstinence should be advised until treatment of all partners is completed. Current sexual partners should be screened for sexually transmitted infections and treated for *T. vaginalis* regardless of the results of their tests. In a male contact if found to have non-gonococcal urethritis (NGU) on screening, it is reasonable to treat for *T. vaginalis* initially and then repeat the urethral smear before diagnosing nonspecific urethritis (NSU). Patients should be instructed to avoid sex until they and their sex partners are cured.
- *Vaginal candidiasis:* Current recommendation suggests no need of screening or treatment of partner for candidiasis.

PREVENTION

- *Follow-up of cases of vaginal discharge:* Women who become asymptomatic after treatment need not come back for follow-up.
- *Prevention and counselling: T. vaginalis*: Patients should be advised that using condoms consistently will reduce the risk of acquiring trichomonal infection.

SUGGESTED READING

1. Akinbiyi AA, Watson R, Feyi-Waboso P. Prevalence of *Candida albicans* and bacterial vaginosis in asymptomatic pregnant women in South Yorkshire, United Kingdom. Outcome of a prospective study. Arch Gynecol Obstet. 2008;278:463-6.
2. Beckmann RB (Ed). Obstetrics and Gynecology, 7th edition. Baltimore, MD: Lippincott Williams & Wilkins; 2014. pp. 260.
3. Bradshaw CS, Morton AN, Garland SM, Horvath LB, Kuzevska I, Fairley CK. Evaluation of a point-of-care test, BVBlue, and clinical and laboratory criteria for diagnosis of bacterial vaginosis. J Clin Microbiol. 2005;43:1304.
4. Broache M, Cammarata CL, Stonebraker E, Eckert K, Van Der Pol B, Taylor SN. Performance of a vaginal panel assay compared with the clinical diagnosis of vaginitis. Obstet Gynecol. 2021;138:853-9.
5. Bérard A, Sheehy O, Zhao JP, Abrahamowicz M. Associations between low- and high-dose oral fluconazole and pregnancy outcomes: 3 nested case-control studies. CMAJ. 2019;191:E179-87.
6. Centers for Disease Control and Prevention. Sexually Transmitted Diseases Treatment Guidelines 2021. Bacterial Vaginosis. [online] Available from https://www.cdc.gov/std/treatment-guidelines/bv.htm [Last accessed April, 2025].

7. Centers for Disease Control and Prevention. Sexually Transmitted Diseases Treatment Guidelines 2021. Diseases Characterized by Vulvovaginal Itching, Burning, Irritation, Odor or Discharge. [online] Available from https://www.cdc.gov/std/treatment-guidelines/vaginal-discharge.htm [Last accessed April 2025].
8. Fang X, Zhou Y, Yang Y Diao Y, Li H. Prevalence and risk factors of trichomoniasis, bacterial vaginosis, and candidiasis for married women of child-bearing age in rural Shandong. Jpn J Infect Dis. 2007;60:257-61.
9. Farage MA, Miller KW, Ledger WJ. Determining the cause of vulvovaginal symptoms. Obstet Gynecol Surv. 2008;63(7):445-64.
10. Miller KE. Diagnosis and treatment of Chlamydia trachomatis infection. Am Fam Physician. 2006;73(8):1411-6.
11. Oliveira FA, Pfleger V, Lang K, Heukelbach J, Miralles I, Fraga F, et al. Sexually transmitted infections, bacterial vaginosis, and candidiasis in women of reproductive age in rural Northeast Brazil: a population-based study. Mem Inst Oswaldo Cruz. 2007;102:751-6.
12. Sherrard J, Donders G, White D, Jensen JS, et al. European (IUSTI/WHO) guideline on the management of vaginal discharge, 2011. Int J STD AIDS. 2011;22(8):421-9.
13. Sobel JD, Subramanian C, Foxman B, Fairfax M, Gygax SE. Mixed vaginitis-more than coinfection and with therapeutic implications. Curr Infect Dis Rep. 2013;15:104-8.

45

CHAPTER

Pruritus Vulvae and Vulvodynia

Sujatha BS, Muralidhar V Pai

Chapter Outline

- Definition and Incidence
- Pathophysiology
- Natural Defence Mechanisms
- Aetiological Classification of Pruritus Vulvae
- Causes of Pruritus According to Age Groups
- Evaluation of Patient with Pruritus
- Investigations
- General Measures for Women with Pruritus
- Differential Diagnosis of Pruritus
- Treatment
- Results
- Vulvodynia
- Management

DEFINITION AND INCIDENCE

Pruritus vulvae is a Latin word meaning itching of the female external genitalia. It is a common symptom and not a pathological diagnosis experienced by not <10% of women attending gynaecological clinics, although it is not always their primary complaint. Pruritus in the vulva is caused by various factors, but most often there is an identifiable cause. This condition can often cause a lot of distress to the affected woman and deserves conscientious study.

Complaints of pruritus should be distinguished from women having irritation or burning of vulva, and it is, therefore, always necessary to make certain of the sensation by asking if it arouses a desire to scratch. It is equally important to determine accurately the site of the pruritus, especially if it is vaginal, vulvar or anal. It can lead to scratching and rubbing, which can break the skin and lead to soreness, bleeding and skin infections. It is also necessary to know if other areas of the body are affected because the vulvar lesion may be merely one part of a widespread dermatological problem.

PATHOPHYSIOLOGY

The sensation of pruritus is carried by somatic pain fibres to the dorsal horn of the spinal cord to the cerebral cortex via the spinothalamic tract. Pruritus generates a spinal reflex response, the scratch, which is as innate as a deep tendon reflex. It is often exacerbated by skin inflammation, dry or hot ambient conditions, skin vasodilatation and psychological stressors; and is usually more troublesome at night.

The chemical substances found in the body which are known to induce a sensation of itching include potassium, histamine, 5-hydroxytryptamine and plasma kinins. The mechanism for pruritus might vary depending on the underlying pathology such as histamine release in atopic dermatitis or nerve paraesthesia in herpes simplex.

NATURAL DEFENCE MECHANISMS

The vagina has an acidic pH (around 4–4.5) where only Doderlein's bacilli can survive. The presence of these bacilli is associated with the production of lactic acid, which makes the vagina naturally self-sterilising. This hostile acidic pH may be raised at certain times, such as during menstruation (cervical and endometrial discharge is alkaline), after abortion or labour (lochia is alkaline) or with excessive cervical discharge. As the pH rises and becomes alkaline, nonresident pathogens are able to grow. Apart from the acidic medium, the vagina has a tough stratified squamous epithelium that presents a smooth surface against pathogens; there are no crypts, unlike the endocervix where organisms can multiply. The proximity of the urethral opening to the vaginal orifice and also to the anal orifice predisposes the potentially pathogenic micro-organisms (PPMs) to invade the urogenital tract and cause infections **(Fig. 1)**.

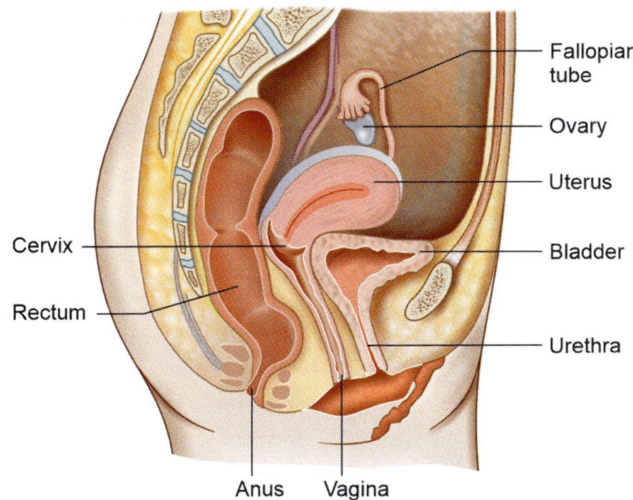

Fig. 1: Normal female urogenital anatomy.

AETIOLOGICAL CLASSIFICATION OF PRURITUS VULVAE

- *Dermatological:* The International Society for the Study of Vulvar Disease (ISSVD 2006 classification) along with hidradenitis suppurativa
- *Infections and infestations:* Candidiasis—vulvovaginal, trichomoniasis, bacterial vaginosis, herpes simplex, pubic lice (Pthirus pubis), scabies (*Sarcoptes scabiei hominis*) and threadworm (*Enterobius vermicularis*)
- *Neoplastic conditions:*
  - *Squamous:* Vulvar intraepithelial neoplasia (VIN) usual type (warty, basaloid and mixed), VIN differentiated type
  - *Nonsquamous:* Paget's disease, tumours of melanocytes
- *Hormonal:* Atrophic vaginitis, breastfeeding
- Urinary or faecal incontinence
- *Systemic causes:* Secondary to renal (chronic renal failure), haematologic (iron deficiency, polycythaemia rubra vera, hypereosinophilic syndrome, essential thrombocythaemia and myelodysplastic syndrome), hepatic (cholestasis), endocrine (hyperthyroidism, hypothyroidism, diabetes mellitus, hyperparathyroidism and hypoparathyroidism), malignancies (Hodgkin's disease, leukaemia and carcinoid syndrome) and immunosuppression leading to vulvovaginal candidiasis

Common differential diagnosis of vulvar pruritus **(Table 1)**.

- Psychosexual disorders
- *Others*: Regrowth of pubic hair after shaving

CAUSES OF PRURITUS ACCORDING TO AGE GROUPS

Prepubertal Girls: Poor Hygiene, Streptococcal Infection, *Escherichia Coli* Infection, Pinworms, Scabies, and Allergic Contact Dermatitis

- *Young women in reproductive age*: Vaginitis, allergic contact dermatitis, hidradenitis suppurativa, lichen simplex chronicus
- *Postmenopausal women:* Atrophic vaginitis, lichen sclerosus, vulvar cancer, and Paget's disease

EVALUATION OF PATIENT WITH PRURITUS

History and Examination

Detailed gynaecological history including the duration of pruritus, its severity, impact on quality of life and any past or present treatment will aid in arriving at a diagnosis. Treatment history regarding any medications and response to therapy is important as it will influence future treatment plans. History of any other atopic conditions, personal or family history of autoimmune conditions, urinary or faecal incontinence and smoking are significant.

The clinician must look into the impact of symptoms on social, psychological and sexual life. A full examination of the anogenital region and other skin and mucosal sites should also be carried out.

INVESTIGATIONS

The more careful the investigation, the more likely is the cause of the pruritus to be found and the treatment to be successful. It includes thyroid function test, blood sugars and swabs for sexually transmitted diseases. If dermatitis is suspected skin patch testing should be done. Vulval biopsy is indicated for women who do not respond to first-line therapy or if suspicion of VIN or chronic epithelial changes are there.

GENERAL MEASURES FOR WOMEN WITH PRURITUS

Women with vulval symptoms should be advised regarding general measures, which may help ameliorate their symptoms. They should use soap substitutes and a small amount of emollient to help avoid dry skin. Avoid using

TABLE 1: Common clinical presentation in pruritus vulvae and possible clinical diagnosis.

	Candidiasis	*Lichen sclerosus*	*Lichen planus*	*VIN (vulvar intraepithelial neoplasia)*	*Eczema*	*Psoriasis*
Frequency (prevalence)	10–20%	0.1–3%	0.1–0.8%	Exact prevalence unknown, incidence approximately 3/100,000 women in Germany	0.5–10%	2%
Morphological features	Red and white plaques, erosions and ulcers	• *Early form:* Erythema, erosions • *Late form:* White, firm plaques, bleeding into skin, scarring, atrophy, fissures and exaggerated skin markings	• *Early form:* Characteristic whitish reticulate (Wickham) striae • *Late form/erosive form:* Erosive erythema, scarring and extragenital involvement (e.g. oral)	Skin-coloured papules and nodules, white and red plaques, acetowhite lesions (after application of 5% acetic acid), erosions (especially with differentiated VIN)	Poorly marginated erythematous lesions on the labia majora labia minora, oedema (acute) and lichenification (chronic)	Well-demarcated, slightly scaly, erythematous red plaques, accompanying fissures and rhagades
Signs and symptoms	Pruritus, erythema and increased vaginal discharge (white, curd-like and no odour)	Pruritus, burning and dyspareunia	• *Early form:* Pruritus, burning and pain • *Late form:* Dyspareunia, burning and vaginal stenosis	Pruritus, burning, soreness and often asymptomatic	Pruritus, soreness	Pruritus
Diagnosis	• *pH value:* Normal (<4.0) • *Lactobacilli:* Yes • *Leukocytes:* Increased • *Clue cells:* None • *Microscopy:* Pseudo-mycelium and blastospores	History, clinical examination, typical figure-of-8 pattern surrounding the vulva and anus; histological confirmation by biopsy, if required	History, clinical examination, characteristic Wickham striae, vaginal involvement and histological confirmation by biopsy	Vulvoscopy, histological confirmation by biopsy	History, clinical examination; if necessary, patch test	Typical involvement of labia majora, characteristic noninvolvement of labia minora
Management	• *Acute:* Antifungal agent (e.g. oral fluconazole or topical clotrimazole preparations) • *Chronic:* Following the initial treatment, fluconazole 150 mg orally 1 x/week for at least 6 months after loading dose	• Initially ultrapotent glucocorticoids (GCs) (topical) • Life-long GC maintenance dose in reduced dose, lipid replenishment • *Second-line therapy:* Calcineurin inhibitors (off-label)	• Initially ultrapotent glucocorticoids (GCs) (topical) • Life-long GC maintenance dose in reduced dose, lipid replenishment • *Second-line therapy:* Calcineurin inhibitors (off-label)	• Laser vaporisation (standard with usual-type VIN) • Surgical excision rather with differentiated VIN (warning: occult carcinoma) • Imiquimod 5%, topical for usual-type VIN (off-label)	• Avoidance of trigger factors • Glucocorticoids (topical)	• Avoidance of mechanical stress and trigger factors • Topical treatment as for extragenital psoriasis (typically GC/ calcineurin inhibitors)

Source: Woelber L, Prieske K, Mendling W, Schmalfeldt B, Tietz HJ, Jaeger A. Vulvar pruritus—causes, diagnosis and therapeutic approach. Dtsch Arztebl Int. 2020;116(8):126-33.

sponges or flannels and gently dab and dry vulval area with a soft towel or hair dryer. They should wear loose-fitting silk or cotton underwear and sleep without underwear. Avoid fabric conditioners, biological washing powder, soaps, shower gel, scrubs, bubble bath, deodorants, baby wipes and douches.

DIFFERENTIAL DIAGNOSIS OF PRURITUS

Pruritus Associated with Vaginal Discharge

Vaginal Discharge

Infection is the most common cause of vaginal discharge. Vaginal discharge can result from vaginitis, cervicitis or both. Cervicitis can be present without symptoms. Vaginal discharge can be due to sexually transmitted infections (STIs) such as *Chlamydia* and gonococci or more commonly due to non-STIs such as *Candida*, *Trichomonas* or bacterial vaginosis (reproductive tract infections--RTIs) **(Flowchart 1)**.

Vaginal Candidiasis

Vaginal candidiasis, moniliasis, is an RTI and not an STI. It is caused by Gram-positive fungus *Candida albicans* that flourishes in the acidic vagina. Normal vaginal flora is dominated by lactobacilli. Candidiasis occurs when the normal environment in the vagina changes. This can occur after administration of broad-spectrum antibiotics, oral contraceptives or other steroids. A woman can develop a candidial infection if she is immunocompromised, such as diabetes, human immunodeficiency virus infection.

Classically, *Candida* causes intense vulval and vaginal pruritus with profuse curdy discharge. Some women may complain of superficial dyspareunia. On examination, there may be inflammation of the vulva, especially the

Flowchart 1: Vaginal discharge.

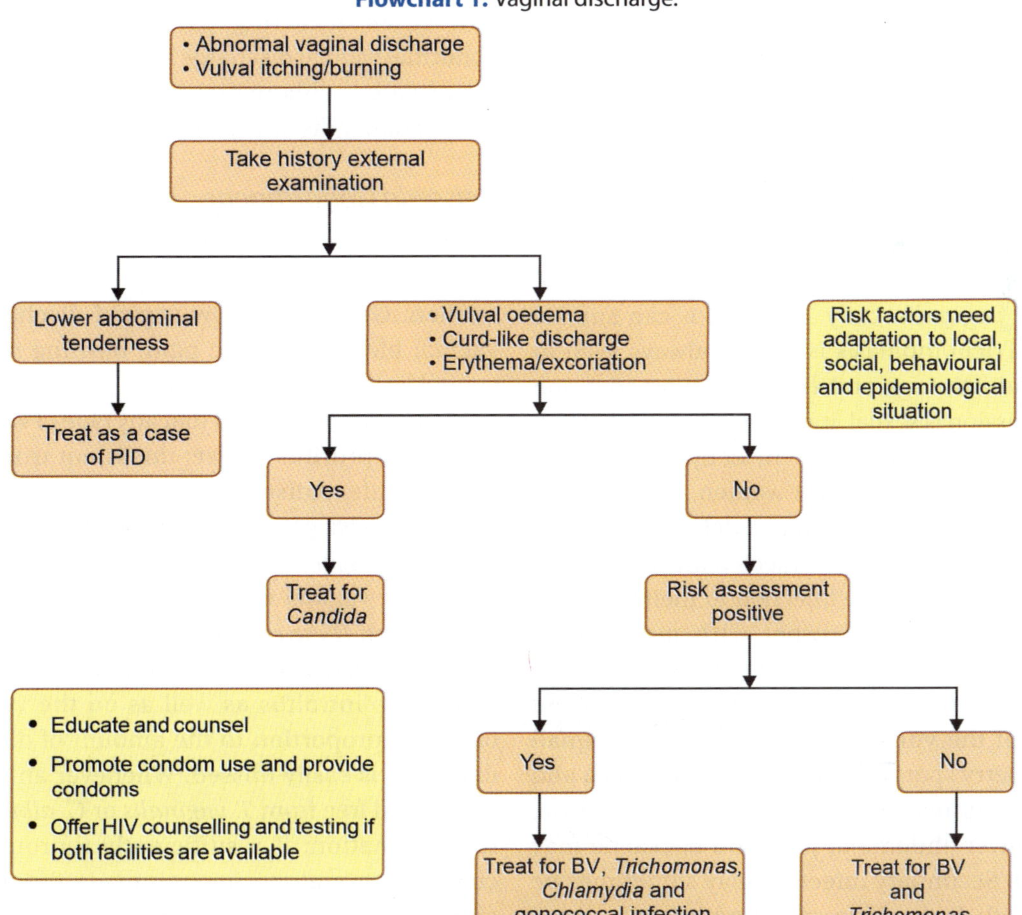

(BV: bacterial vaginosis; HIV: human immunodeficiency virus; PID: pelvic inflammatory disease)

labia minora and introitus, with excoriation. The discharge is thick, white and has the appearance of 'cottage cheese'. The discharge often adheres to the vagina in the form of white patches or plaques, and when removed, multiple petechial haemorrhagic areas are left behind. Vulvar candidiasis may produce erythema and oedema as well as satellite lesions. Other than extreme discomfort from skin irritation in severe infections, there are no complications from vaginal yeast infections. A wet saline mount with 10% KOH is diagnostic of *Candida*. Treatment is usually with topical azole (clotrimazole or miconazole) or oral triazole (fluconazole 150 mg stat dose can be given or itraconazole 200 mg twice daily for a day). Recurrent candidiasis (at least four episodes per year) can be distressing for the women and challenging for the physician. Treatment should include an induction period of 1–2 weeks, with at least 1 week of treatment either with an oral agent or with a topical antifungal lasting for 1–2 weeks. This should be followed by a maintenance treatment lasting for a period of 6 months with either oral fluconazole 100 mg weekly or topical clotrimazole 500 mg weekly.

Trichomonas Infection

In clinical practice, trichomoniasis is the most common and important vaginal infection in women. *Trichomonas* infection is an STI caused by the flagellate protozoan, *Trichomonas vaginalis*. Trichomonas is an actively motile anaerobe; three types are known, namely *T. buccalis*, *T. hominis* and *T. vaginalis*. Only *T. vaginalis* can survive in the vagina. Trichomoniasis is almost always seen in women in reproductive age, and though the most common mode of transmission is sexual, it may be acquired through improper hygiene. It may occur in conjunction with gonococcal infection. In pregnant women, trichomonas infection can cause preterm labour and delivery.

Up to 50% of women who are infected are asymptomatic, but they can still pass the infection to their partners. Patients characteristically present with malodorous vaginal discharge and pruritus. The discharge is profuse, thin, creamy or slightly green and frothy. Pruritus and inflammation of the vulva are present. Multiple small punctate strawberry spots may be seen on the vagina and portio vaginalis. Associated symptoms such as dysuria, dyspareunia, lower abdominal pain and backache may also be present. Secondary infection may sometimes be seen, usually with *Escherichia coli* or pathogenic cocci. A fresh wet film preparation showing actively motile flagellates of *T. vaginalis* or cytological smear is diagnostic.

Bacterial Vaginosis

Bacterial vaginosis is an RTI but not an STI, although it is more common among sexually active women. Bacterial vaginosis produces a disturbance of the normal vaginal flora. The normally predominant lactobacilli are reduced and replaced by a number of organisms including *Gardnerella*, *Urea plasma*, *Bacteroides* and other anaerobes. Classically bacterial vaginosis presents with white or grey fishy-smelling vaginal discharge. Bacterial vaginosis can lead to serious complications after invasive procedures such as curettage or endometrial biopsy. In pregnant women, bacterial vaginosis can cause premature rupture of membranes, preterm labour and delivery, chorioamnionitis and delivery of a low-birthweight baby.

Besides these vaginal infections, leucorrhoea can occur because of cervicitis caused by *Chlamydia* and gonococci.

Chlamydia Trachomatis

It is the most common of all bacterial STIs, with >3 million new cases occurring each year. Symptoms include abnormal vaginal discharge and burning during urination. If untreated, chlamydial infection may lead to pelvic inflammatory disease, ectopic pregnancy and infertility.

Neisseria Gonorrhoeae

Another cause of cervicitis is infection with *Neisseria gonorrhoeae*, which is a major STI in both men and women. Green or yellow vaginal discharge, abnormal vaginal bleeding, pelvic pain, burning micturition and genital lesions may be present.

It is commonly stated that any type of vaginal discharge can cause pruritus vulvae; this is not true. Purulent and mucopurulent discharges cause pain and tenderness when the vulva gets chafed, but they never induce *itching*. *The only discharges* associated with pruritus are those caused by vaginal infestation with either *T. vaginalis* or *C. albicans*; *these account for at least 80% of all cases of pruritus vulvae*. In these, the itch tends to be situated within the introitus as well as on the vulva; it may be out of all proportion to the amount of discharge, so the diagnosis is easily missed. Whenever an itchy discharge is reported free from *T. vaginalis* or *C. albicans*, it requires re-examination; if a sufficiently thorough search and culture of several specimens is made, these organisms will always be found. When there is little discharge to collect, specimens should be obtained on a swab previously moistened with Feinberg–Whittington medium. This technique is also the best for taking specimens from the urethra and from the vulvar skin, in which sites *Candida* and *Trichomonas* organisms can sometimes be found, even when they are not demonstrable in the vagina.

Sexually transmitted infections are infections that are primarily passed from person to person by sexual contact, and STIs are part of a broader group of infections known as RTIs that include all infections of the reproductive tract, including those not caused by sexual contact. The common vaginal and cervical infections that cause leucorrhoea can be classified as STIs and RTIs.

Sexually transmitted infections are a major public health problem in both developed and developing countries, but prevalence rate is higher in developing countries, where STI treatment is less accessible. The World Health Organization (WHO) has advocated the syndromic approach for the management of STIs as many healthcare providers lack time or equipment to diagnose them. This approach which bases diagnosis on a group of symptoms and signs and treats all diseases that could cause the syndrome makes diagnosis more accurate without extensive laboratory tests and allows treatment with a single approach.

Infection with an STI might lead to symptoms in the reproductive organs themselves, in the skin around the genitals or anus, or the throat or mouth. Some STIs may lead to systemic symptoms and complications, while others may be asymptomatic.

Pruritus without Vaginal Discharge

The remaining 15–20% of cases of pruritus vulvae come under this heading and are difficult clinical problems. In this group, some of the causes are clearly defined and beyond dispute but some remain hypothetical or unknown.

Generalised Pruritus

Occasionally, pruritus vulvae are only part of generalised pruritus, such as is seen in lymphoma, jaundice, uraemia and other toxic states. This possibility is merely one to be kept in mind, as is that of a drug-induced condition. These emphasise the need to ascertain the exact site or sites of the discomfort in every case.

Noninfectious Inflammatory Dermatoses

Lichen sclerosus: Lichen sclerosus is a chronic, progressive inflammation of the connective tissue of the skin and located in the anogenital area. Lichen sclerosus is a rare disease; however, it is the most common noninfectious cause of vaginal pruritus. Girls before the onset of puberty as well as adult women, especially in their postmenopausal phase, are affected. Changes in hormonal status, such as puberty and pregnancy, are suspected to influence the course of the disease, and stress and trauma can worsen the symptoms. Clinically, pruritus is the predominant symptom, which can become unbearable during the night and lead to scratch marks, excoriations and thus to secondary lichenification. However, the pruritus may also be less pronounced or completely absent, e.g. in cases where lichen sclerosus is only beginning or in only small, affected skin areas. There is the presence of white plaques and papules associated with areas of bruising usually found on the interlabial sulci, labia minora, clitoral hood, clitoris, perineal body and perineum. Scarring and narrowing of the introitus are present leading to coital problems. Even when lichen sclerosis is suspected, a vulval biopsy must be done to confirm <5% risk of developing squamous cell carcinoma.

The recommended therapy is steroids, either topical or as depot injections in the acute stages of the disease. Here, it is important to note that especially after a long-term course of the disease, the atrophic skin is so sore that ointment preparations will cause burning of the skin. Pure Vaseline with clobetasol has proven successful. It might be reasonable to start with a higher dose, e.g. 0.5% for 14 days, and to continue treatment with 0.05% for another month. Due to the dreaded atrophy of the skin by corticosteroids, long-term treatment should be avoided. Also, tacrolimus (as an ointment)—a calcineurin inhibitor—has proven successful in numerous studies.

Lichen planus: It is a chronic mucocutaneous disease seen between the third and sixth decades. Usually presents with pruritus and painful skin lesions. Various regions of the skin may be affected and appear as red, livid and flattened papules that cause severe itching (Wickham's striae). When affecting the mucosa (mucosal lichen planus), the oral cavity and genitals may be affected. Clinically, fernlike and white striae occur. In severe cases, superficial or even deep erythematous lesions of the mucosa may develop, which are very painful. Biopsy is usually necessary as squamous cell carcinoma can develop in 3% of cases. Treatment of lichen planus is the same as for lichen sclerosus, i.e. local corticosteroids or tacrolimus (as an ointment preparation). If the lesions reach within the vagina, there is a danger of adhesions and synechia, which can even cause occlusion of the vagina. Here, surgical expansion as well as intravaginal corticoid foam preparations are indicated.

Apocrine miliaria (Fox–Fordyce disease), comparable to prickly heat, is another cause of pruritus vulvae. It presents as multiple, small, discrete, skin-coloured or red papules, which are considered to be the result of obstruction of the ducts, or changes in function of the apocrine glands. This disease also occurs in the axilla and on the areola of the breast. Attacks can be precipitated by emotional upsets including sexual excitement.

Squamous cell carcinoma of the vulva causes itching in its early stage. *Carcinoma* in situ and *Paget's disease* of the vulva can cause pruritus of long standing.

Animal and Fungal Parasitic Infections

Scabies, also known as acarodermatitis, is an infectious skin disease in humans. Clinically, depending on the severity of the infection, pruritus is the main complaint. The mites are especially active at night below the warm blanket. Apart from other skin areas, the vulva can become affected due to sexual transmission. The diagnosis is confirmed by the inspection of the skin, where 1 cm long burrows are visible. With a magnifying glass or with light microscopy, the burrows, papules and vesicles can be detected. It is treated with zinc ointments and, in case of pruritus, topical corticosteroids.

Ichthyol ointments and 3% salicylic acid can soften the keratinisation process. Available topical scabicides are crotamiton, permethrin, benzyl benzoate and lindane.

Clothes and bed linen should be washed at >60°C.

Pediculosis causes pruritus pubis rather than pruritus vulvae. Candidiasis of the vulva is a not uncommon cause and is demonstrated as described above. There may be simultaneous infections of the nail beds on the hands and feet (refer to Chapter 21: Infections as they Affect Individual Organs for details).

Diseases of the Anus and Rectum

Faecal incontinence, fissure-in-ano and haemorrhoids, even if they cause pruritus ani, can be dismissed as causes of pruritus vulvae. Threadworms (*Enterobius*) only rarely migrate forward enough to cause vulvar itching.

Pruritus ani in the adult appears mostly to be caused by a fungus, usually *Candida*, or to be directly or indirectly associated with a fungal infection of the hands and feet. This sort of basis should be suspected whenever pruritus ani and pruritus vulvae occur together. In perianal candidiasis, the focus of infection is often in the bowel.

Conditions of the Urinary Tract

Bacilluria, pyuria, highly acid urine, incontinence of urine and haematuria never cause pruritus vulvae, although they may cause chafing and soreness.

The only urinary condition associated with pruritus vulvae is *glycosuria,* and this operates no matter whether it is a manifestation of diabetes or a lowered renal threshold. The characteristic features of the lesion are its distribution according to the area of contamination with carbohydrates, and its colour, which resembles that of raw beef. In long-standing cases, a hyperkeratotic epithelial disorder can develop.

In making the diagnosis of diabetes, examination of the urine should not be relied upon; this may be sugar-free if the patient has not eaten for several hours at the time of examination. The only safe rule is to carry out a glucose tolerance test in every case in which the explanation of pruritus vulvae is not clear. Another reason for this is that *hyperglycaemia without glycosuria* can cause pruritus.

In the early days of oestrogen therapy, a postmenopausal woman was referred to Professor Jeffcoate on account of pruritus vulvae. No obvious cause was found, and then, a much-acclaimed new treatment was applied. The secondary infection of the vulva cleared and the itching improved but was not cured. The patient then had a small uterine bleed which was credited to the hormone therapy. On her return from abroad, 1.5 years later, she reported that on medical advice, she had continued the oestrogens intermittently with temporary benefit and had one or more episodes of uterine bleeding. The situation appeared unchanged and Professor Jeffcoate prescribed further courses of oestrogen. Three years from the time of her first visit, this patient reported paraesthesia of the hands and feet. The urine was still sugar-free, as it had been when tested on six previous occasions. However, the fasting blood sugar was 350 mg/dL and the cause of the pruritus was at last clear. Just about the time that mystery was solved, a nodule of carcinoma was found in the vaginal wall—a metastasis from carcinoma of the body of the uterus which had probably been present for 3 years and whose symptoms had been dismissed as being due to oestrogen therapy.

Allergy and Drug Sensitivity

Skin sensitivity to various chemical constituents of toilet preparations such as soaps, bath salts, deodorants and antiseptics containing phenols or cresols, occasionally explains pruritus. Contact dermatitis from all sorts of cosmetics, even varnish on the patient's nails, is also a possibility.

The modern fashion of girls and women wearing close-fitting undergarments made of man-made fibres is a common cause of pruritus vulvae. The abrasions which such clothing sometimes causes are not, however, responsible for the itch. This is the result of skin sensitivity to nylon or similar material or, more often, to the soaps and detergents used in washing the articles, these not being thoroughly rinsed afterwards. Women not prepared to abandon fashion have therefore only to wear cotton pants beneath the tights, or to be careful to wash them only with bland soaps and to rinse meticulously, to have their symptoms relieved.

Sometimes, antiseptic preparations used in the treatment of vaginitis are the cause of pruritus or lead to its continuance after the original causal infection is under control. Preparations containing benzocaine or other local anaesthetics are especially liable to produce skin reactions and should never be applied to the vulva or vagina **(Fig. 2)**. A relationship between pruritus and coitus can often be traced to an idiosyncrasy to chemical or rubber constituents of contraceptives. Urticarial conditions of the vulva may be associated with a general skin reaction, and occasionally they form the predominant manifestation of sensitivity to medicaments of various types.

The more cases one sees of pruritus vulvae, the more important one is inclined to attach to allergy as a cause. Clinically, acute contact dermatitis is characterised by a red rash, swelling, papules, blisters or wheals. The clinical picture is polymorphic, although not all symptoms have to be present. Often, pruritus, burning and soreness are present. Chronic eczema is characterised by lichenification, desquamation and sometimes rhagades and is monomorphic.

Diagnosis is confirmed by history taking, clinical examination and a patch test.

Deficiency States

The part played by various deficiency states in causing pruritus vulvae is now generally recognised. Attention tends to be focused on avitaminosis A and B2 but other agents operate and among these may be mentioned iron, folic acid and vitamin B12. Pruritus vulvae are therefore not uncommonly a manifestation of hypochromic or macrocytic anaemia, and their investigation sometimes leads to their diagnosis. In such cases, it responds quite dramatically to the treatment appropriate to the particular type of anaemia. The vulvar lesions found in deficiency states vary from slight reddening, or pallor and oedema, to a vulvar hyperkeratotic epithelial disorder (refer to Chapter 27: Genital Cancers and **Fig. 3**). As might be expected, they are often associated with glossitis, cheilosis and angular stomatitis **(Fig. 4)**.

In developed countries, deficiency states rarely arise as a result of gross dietetic errors but these should be looked

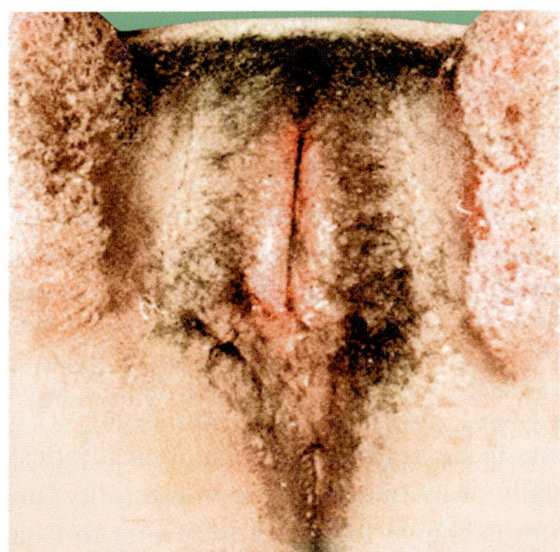

Fig. 2: Exfoliative dermatitis of the vulva occurring as an acute reaction to the application of a local anaesthetic ointment for pruritus vulvae. The ointment was prescribed empirically for itching which proved to be caused by candidal vaginitis and not only caused this skin change but made the pruritus worse.

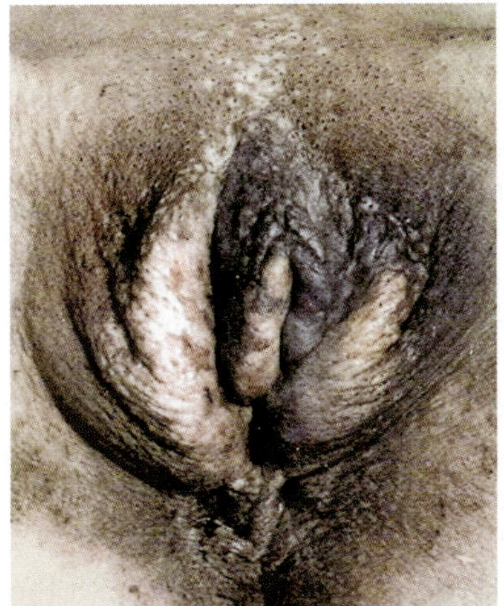

Fig. 3: A hyperkeratotic vulvar epithelial disorder, which would formerly have been labelled leucoplakia. The patient in this case, who complained of pruritus, also had histamine-fast achlorhydria but was not cured by the administration of hydrochloric acid. Once the skin changes reach this stage, they may be irreversible.

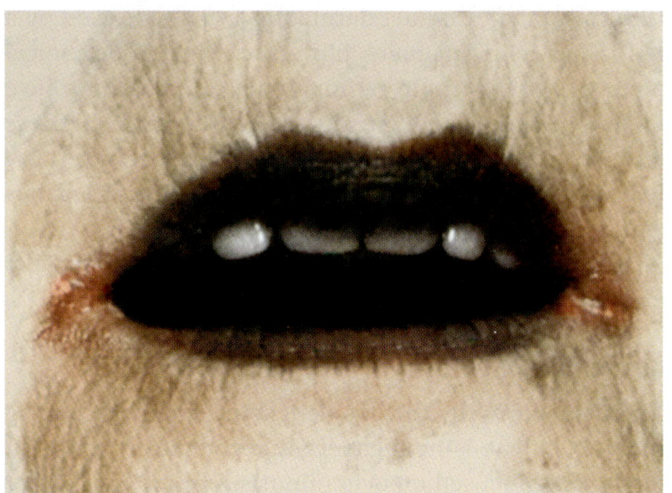

Fig. 4: Angular stomatitis associated with pruritus vulvae and indicative of a deficiency state.

for, especially in elderly women living alone who do not have trouble to prepare proper meals. More often, they are due to some disturbance of the alimentary tract, which interferes with biosynthesis or with absorption. They occur, e.g. in *chronic diarrhoea, malabsorption syndromes* and also as part of the *postgastrectomy syndrome.*

An important factor in this respect is *achlorhydria*, and a test for gastric acidity is advisable in the investigation of intractable pruritus vulvae. If hypochromic anaemia is present, iron is given in addition.

Psychological Factors

A close relationship between the mind and the skin and the part played by psychological upsets in causing skin disease are recognised by all. Moreover, many mental disturbances have a sexual basis. So, it is not surprising that the skin of the vulva can become the site for manifestations of psychoneuroses. Even when there is a local stimulus to cause pruritus, the state of the central nervous system remains important so far as the interpretation of the sensation is concerned. Under conditions of nervous fatigue, rough clothing or other surface irritants will cause itching when they would not otherwise do so. Tiredness explains in part why pruritus vulvae are always worse at night-time. It then interferes with sleep and leads to further nervous exhaustion, so that a vicious circle is created.

Again, a scratch habit is easily developed and may be started by some fleeting minor lesion which, although it heals quickly, leaves the habit behind. In such a case, the pruritus is often limited to one area of one labium, the skin of which becomes thickened and hard as a result of scratching to give rise to the lesions called neurodermatitis.

Chronic Vascular Changes

In line with the aforementioned concept, it is relevant to point out that nearly all lesions that cause itching in any part of the body have a vascular change as a basis; urticaria, nettle stings, insect bites and varicose veins are good examples. Is the same true of vulvar states associated with pruritus? Examination of the known causal factors suggests that it may well be so.

TREATMENT

When a specific and clear cause is found and treatment is directed to it, the pruritus is invariably cured or controlled. Parasitic and fungal infections can be eliminated; glycosuria can be controlled, and deficiency states can be corrected. Antigens can be avoided.

When an underlying cause cannot be discovered or is doubtful, treatment has to be tentative or empirical and the results are less than satisfactory. Otherwise, the lines of possible treatment are described in detail in Chapter 26: Epithelial Abnormalities of the Genital Tract. In summary, the best of these are antihistamines (systemically, not locally), various fungicides (even when a fungal infection is not proven), and hydrocortisone or other corticosteroid preparations locally. A combination of fungicide and corticosteroids in ointment form can be particularly helpful.

When the pruritus is perianal as well as vulvar, a course of treatment with oral fungicides, as well as local applications, is indicated. The patient should also be instructed to *wash* the affected area after each act of defaecation, for an indefinite period in the future and even when apparently cured, if she is in the habit of using toilet paper.

All remedies have to be applied regularly and pertinaciously for months if not years. Empirical treatments to be avoided are local anaesthetics applied superficially or by injection and vulvectomy (unless the epithelium is shown to be unruly) (refer to Chapter 26: Epithelial Abnormalities of the Genital Tract and **Fig. 5**). Local applications of yoghurt or proprietary preparations containing lactobacilli have not been established to be beneficial.

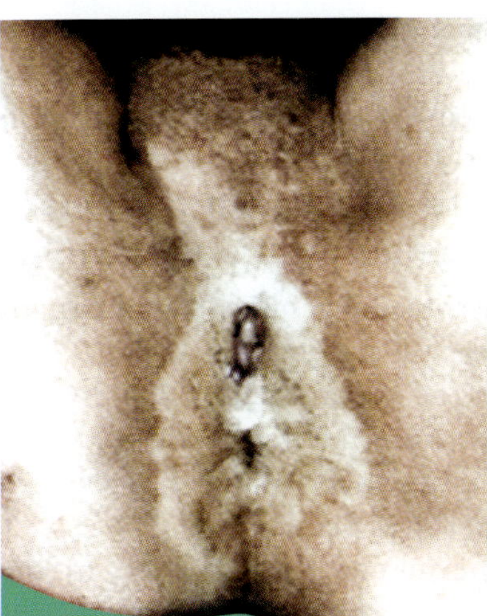

Fig. 5: The common, if not usual, end result of empirical vulvectomy for 'leucoplakia'. In this case, a woman aged 72 years has had vulvectomy carried out several years previously but her pruritus quickly recurred and became even more troublesome. There is a recurrence of a hyperkeratotic lesion and skin depigmentation, around the introitus and the anus. Investigation showed infestation with *Candida* organisms, but these might represent a secondary infection.

BOX 1: 2015 Consensus terminology and classification of persistent vulvar pain and vulvodynia.

- *Vulvar pain caused by a specific disorder*:
  - Infectious (e.g. recurrent candidiasis, herpes)
  - Inflammatory (e.g. lichen sclerosus, lichen planus and immunobullous disorders)
  - Neoplastic (e.g. Paget's disease, squamous cell carcinoma)
  - Neurologic (e.g. postherpetic neuralgia, nerve compression, or injury, neuroma)
  - Trauma (e.g. female genital cutting, obstetrical)
  - Iatrogenic (e.g. postoperative, chemotherapy and radiation)
  - Hormonal deficiencies [e.g. genitourinary syndrome of menopause (vulvovaginal atrophy), lactational amenorrhea]
- *Vulvodynia*: Vulvar pain of at least 3 months duration, without clear identifiable cause, which may have potential associated factors. The following are the descriptors:
  - Localised (e.g. vestibulodynia and ciltorodynia) or generalised or mixed (localised and generalised)
  - Provoked (e.g. insertional, contact) or spontaneous or mixed (provoked and spontaneous)
  - Onset (primary or secondary)
  - Temporal pattern (intermittent, persistent, constant, immediate and delayed)

RESULTS

The difficult and intractable case of pruritus vulvae leaves such an impression that it is easy to become pessimistic and overlook the cures. It should be emphasised that, provided a proper investigation to find aetiological factors is carried out, a cure or considerable relief can be achieved by one means or another in 90% of all cases.

VULVODYNIA

Localised vulvar pain syndrome, also known as vulvodynia, vestibulodynia, vulvar vestibulitis or focal vulvitis, is a condition characterised by persistent pain in the vulvar vestibule in the absence of relevant visible findings or a specific, clinically identifiable, neurological disorder. The pain is consistently localised to this area and has been present for at least 3 months. Various sensations such as burning, rawness, stinging or aching are described. These may or may not be associated with surface changes. In order to establish a diagnosis of vulvodynia, a thorough history and examination must exclude vulval dermatoses. The average age of occurrence of vulvodynia is approximately 30 years, although a high prevalence is observed in all decades of life until age 70 years. Based on current evidence, the prognosis for many women with vulvodynia is hopeful if an early diagnosis can be made and correct, individualised treatment given **(Box 1)**.

Aetiology

Vulvodynia is considered as a dysfunctional sensory processing in the central nervous system, involving both central and peripheral pain generators **(Flowchart 2)**. The aetiology is similar to that observed in other painful conditions (fibromyalgia, interstitial cystitis/painful bladder, irritable bowel and temporomandibular dysfunction). In 2015, representatives from various organisations developed consensus terminology for persistent vulvar pain, categorising it into two groups: Vulvar pain caused by a specific disorder and vulvodynia, which refers to persistent vulvar pain without a known cause. This classification helps in understanding and addressing diverse types of vulvar pain effectively.

Certain triggering factors have been identified for vulvodynia such as candidiasis, or any acute painful vulval, urinary or anal condition (e.g. infection and surgical procedure) may precede the occurrence of vulvodynia, especially if these physical events occur in the context of emotional stress.

Flowchart 2: Aetiology of vulvodynia.

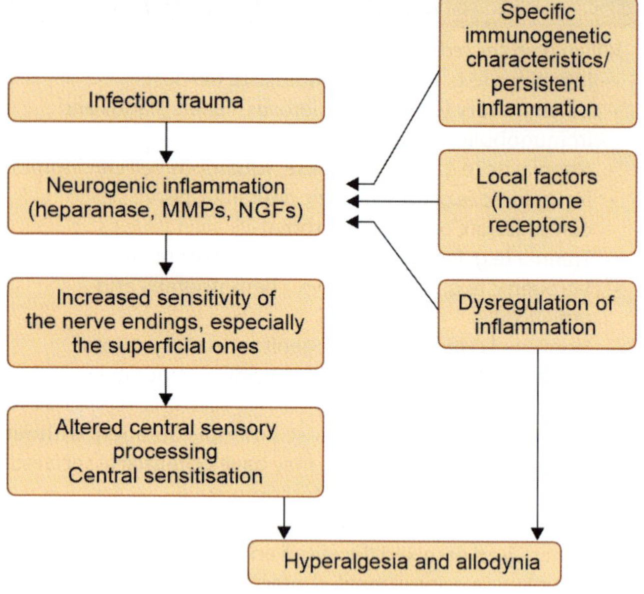

(MMPs: matrix metalloproteinases; NGFs: nerve growth factors)

Localised Provoked Vulvodynia

Localised provoked vulvodynia, also known as vestibulodynia, was formerly known as vulvar vestibulitis syndrome. Aetiology of localised provoked vulvodynia is likely to be multifactorial. A recurrent history of vulvovaginal candidiasis is the most commonly reported feature.

Unprovoked Vulvodynia

Unprovoked vulvodynia is also known as dysesthetic vulvodynia; the aetiology of unprovoked vulvodynia remains unknown and the condition is best managed as a chronic pain syndrome.

Symptoms

Burning sensation is reported by most patients but many also report tingling, stinging or rawness, which occasionally may be accompanied by itching. This discomfort can be generalised to the whole vulva and also spreads to thighs or perianal area, and in some patients, it can be localised involving one or several sites. Women experiencing moderate to severe daily chronic pain, particularly postmenopausal individuals, may report constant burning or aching pain that affects the entire vulva and can radiate to the thighs, buttocks and abdomen. This type of pain, known as generalised unprovoked vulvodynia, is characterised by its persistent nature without any apparent triggers. The pain can significantly impact daily activities such as clothing, walking, sitting for extended periods and sleeping. The most common site of involvement is the posterior aspect of vestibule termed as *vestibulodynia*.

Key Symptoms Suggesting Alternative Diagnoses for Vulvar Discomfort/Pain

Certain symptoms may indicate an alternative diagnosis for vulvar discomfort or pain, including:

- A history of vulvar itching leading to scratching (suggestive of dermatitis)
- Abnormal vaginal bleeding or discharge (potentially indicating lichen planus)
- Pain experienced while sitting or during bowel movements, which may suggest a neurological issue such as pudendal neuralgia
- A personal history of atopy or other skin conditions, pointing to a dermatologic origin for the discomfort.

It is also essential to review the patient's vulvar hygiene practices to identify any behaviours, irritants or allergens that may be contributing to the symptoms. Additionally, a history of chronic pelvic pain, dysmenorrhea or deep dyspareunia could suggest that superficial dyspareunia is secondary to an underlying primary condition, such as endometriosis.

Occasionally, the discomfort can be very severe and impact the daily life and sexual activity of the woman with consequences on her relationships.

If there are sexual problems, patients should have an adequate sexual history taken asking specifically about the presence of vaginismus, adequate lubrication during intercourse, anorgasmia and partner problems **(Box 2)**.

Signs

Inspection of the vulva reveals no relevant physical findings. This means that the vulva has a normal appearance or that, if a lesion is found, this lesion cannot explain the discomfort. In provoked vestibulodynia, tenderness is elicited by the gentle application of a cotton wool tip on the vestibule. Neurological examination is usually normal **(Box 3)**.

Diagnostic Criteria for Localised Vulvar Pain Syndrome

The criteria for diagnosing localised vulvar pain syndrome include:

- Pain localised to the vulvar vestibule, potentially involving the clitoris
- Absence of any identifiable underlying cause

BOX 2: Checklist for pain history in women with vulvodynia.

- *Onset:* Spontaneous or provoked. Presence of triggering events such as coitus, tampon insertion, cycling, long periods of sitting at work, gynaecological examination or insertion of gynaecological instruments and infection episodes such as recurrent candidiasis
- *Description of pain:* Burning, sharp stinging nature of pain. Is any associated pruritus, generalised or localised? What improves the pain, intensity of pain and impact of pain on patients' quality of life?
- *Associated symptoms:* Any skin lesions (mass, ulcer and colour change on the vulva) that are suggestive of vulval dermatosis or vulval intraepithelial neoplasia, symptoms of overlapping pain syndromes such as interstitial cystitis, low back pain, irritable bowel syndrome or fibromyalgia
- *Past medical conditions:* Herpes simplex or herpes zoster, pelvic or vulvovaginal surgeries, hip or spine surgeries and pudendal nerve injury
- *Comorbid conditions:* Irritable bowel syndrome, fibromyalgia, chronic low back pain, interstitial cystitis or anxiety, depression or stress
- *Treatment history:* Duration of therapy, dosage, side effects, compliance and reason for discontinuation, if any
- *Psychosexual history:* Dyspareunia—mild (dyspareunia present most of the time, does not prevent sexual intercourse), moderate (dyspareunia always present, intercourse possible at times), severe (dyspareunia prohibits intercourse), past and current sexual experiences, history of vaginismus and any history of sexual abuse

BOX 3: Checklist for physical evaluation and investigations in vulvodynia.

- Vulval inspection for abnormal redness, fissures, erosion, ulceration and hypopigmentation
- Cotton swab test for determining the area of tenderness and to assess the severity of pain
- Sensory neurological examination for hyperaesthesia, allodynia and stroking for bulbocavernosus reflex and anal wink to rule out peripheral neuropathy
- Vaginal examination with minimal application of pressure and narrow speculum
- Internal palpation of pelvic floor muscle for vaginismus or tenderness
- Microscopic evaluation of wet smears, vaginal pH, fungal cultures and Gram-stain to exclude vaginitis
- Testing for varicella-zoster virus and herpes simplex in the presence of ulcers or vesicular eruptions

Dermatopathologists analysed vulval biopsy in the presence of signs of vulval dermatoses, neoplasia and refractory vulvodynia.

- Symptoms persisting for at least 3 months
- Pain triggered by pressure-point testing

The onset of symptoms can be categorised as primary (occurring with initial vestibular contact) or secondary (developing after a period of normal function). The pain may present in various patterns, including intermittent, persistent (nonrelapsing) or constant (continuous), and can manifest immediately or with a delay following vestibular contact. The most common form is pain triggered by genital contact in women who are otherwise asymptomatic. Other variations include spontaneous pain or a mix of provoked and spontaneous symptoms.

MANAGEMENT

Vulvodynia is a chronic condition that necessitates ongoing management. It is crucial to set realistic expectations during the treatment process. Women should be aware that improvement can take time and that there is no one-size-fits-all solution. Finding the right therapy often involves trial and error, requiring both patience and perseverance. Collaborating closely with healthcare providers to explore various treatment options and create a personalised plan tailored to individual needs is essential. While progress may be gradual, with dedication and support, managing vulvodynia is achievable. The following steps should be taken:

- *Multidisciplinary approach:* A multidisciplinary approach to patient care comprising of a gynaecologist, dermatologist, physiotherapist, sexual therapist or counsellor, and a gynaecologic surgeon in cases of vulvodynia is recommended by the British Society for the Study of Vulval Disease (BSSVD).
- *Pain management:* One of the main aims of management in these cases is to reduce vulval or vestibular tenderness. Patients may be referred to a pain clinic in cases of treatment-resistant unprovoked vulvodynia.
- *Psychosexual counselling:* Referral to psychosexual clinic may be required if the patient needs psychosexual counselling.
- *General measures:* The patient must be reassured and adequately counselled regarding the condition. Written information in the form of leaflets should be preferably provided to the patient. The patient should be counselled to maintain strict vulval hygiene.

Localised Provoked Vulvodynia

- *Vulvar hygiene*: Maintaining proper vulvar hygiene is essential for reducing irritation and discomfort. Women should avoid using soap, fragrances or other products on the affected area, as these can potentially cause topical dermatitis. Instead, cleaning the vulvar area with lukewarm water and gentle, unscented products can help prevent further irritation and enhance overall comfort.

- *Topical agents*: Topical local anaesthetics, e.g. 5% lidocaine ointment or 2% lidocaine gel, should be cautiously used, because they can cause irritation. This gel should be applied 15–20 minutes prior to penetrative sex, and it must be washed off just before sex. In the absence of the availability of good quality evidence regarding the efficacy of a particular treatment modality for vulvodynia, lidocaine gel, along with the use of vaginal dilators, acts as the first-line treatment modality in cases of vulvodynia. Local oestrogen replacement for perimenopausal and postmenopausal women with vulvodynia is a key initial step in managing vulvar discomfort in this demographic. Research indicates that local oestrogen therapy can alleviate the adverse effects of vulvovaginal atrophy on the sexual health of postmenopausal women. Additionally, combining oestrogen with local lidocaine has been shown to effectively treat severe, unprovoked vestibulodynia in postmenopausal patients. It is essential to avoid products containing alcohol, parabens, fragrances and other irritants, as well as those that are hyperosmolar or contain warming agents. These substances can irritate the mucosa and worsen painful symptoms. Instead, choosing gentle, hypoallergenic products that are free from these potential irritants can help maintain vulvar health and comfort. Daily application of a hypoallergenic moisturiser or barrier cream to the vulva is recommended to hydrate and protect the skin. Other topical agents that are commonly used include steroid and antifungal creams. However, their use is associated with variable results.
- *Physical therapies*: This includes therapies such as pelvic floor muscle biofeedback, vaginal transcutaneous electrical nerve stimulation (TENS) and vaginal trainers.
- *Psychological counselling*: This can involve the use of cognitive behaviour therapy. Counselling sessions by a clinical psychologist can help the patient cope with pain.
- *Pain modifiers*: Benefit of drugs such as tricyclic antidepressants, gabapentin and pregabalin in cases of vulvodynia presently remains unclear. Their use may be beneficial in some women.
- *Pelvic floor physical therapy*: Pelvic floor physical therapy is widely recommended by multiple medical associations as a primary treatment for vulvodynia, supported by evidence from numerous studies. Women with vulvodynia and sexual pain often present with myofascial trigger points and increased muscle tension in areas such as the pelvis, abdomen, back and pelvic floor muscles. This therapy incorporates various techniques, including pelvic and core mobilisation, connective tissue and neural mobilisation, myofascial trigger point release, biofeedback and electrical stimulation. These methods aim to address the underlying issues contributing to vulvodynia symptoms and can be highly effective in managing the condition.
- Biofeedback therapy utilising surface electromyographic signals from the pelvic floor is likely to benefit women with vestibulodynia by addressing the dysfunction in their pelvic floor muscles.
- *Surgery*: Surgery (modified vestibulectomy) is often considered as a treatment option for women with localised, provoked vulvodynia (formerly known as vulvar vestibulitis) who have not experienced improvement with other treatment modalities. The decision to undergo surgery is typically made on a case-by-case basis, taking into account the individual's specific symptoms, medical history and response to treatment. This surgery involves the excision of a horseshoe-shaped area of vestibule and inner fold of labia followed by the dissection of the posterior vaginal wall **(Fig. 6)**. Women who respond to the application of lidocaine gel prior to sexual activity are likely to have a more successful outcome with this surgery. Postoperative psychosexual counselling is likely to improve the outcomes of this surgery further.

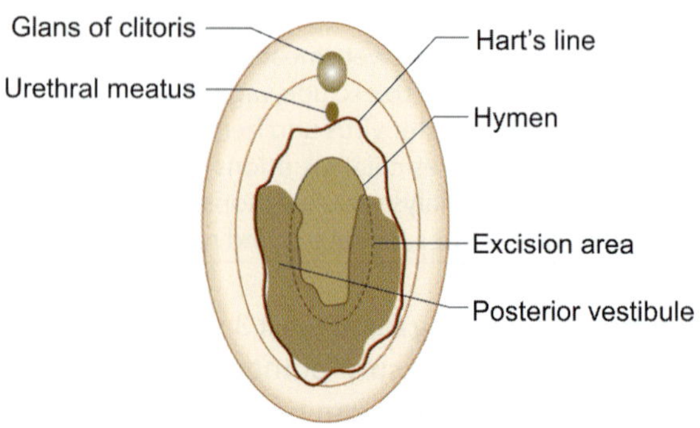

Fig. 6: Modified posterior vestibulectomy.

Unprovoked Vulvodynia

- *Topical agents*: Various topical agents such as emollient soap substitute and topical local anaesthetic agents have been tried in cases of unprovoked vulvodynia without much evidence of benefit.
- *Pain modifiers*: Tricyclic antidepressants have proved to be useful in the management of chronic pain related to unprovoked vulvodynia. Amitriptyline is frequently considered as the first-line treatment. Dosage should be increased by small increments starting at 10 mg up to 100 mg daily, based on the patient's response. However, the beneficial effect of amitriptyline has not been demonstrated by a recent randomised study. If the patient appears to be unresponsive to amitriptyline or is unable to tolerate its side effects, gabapentin or pregabalin may be used.
- Cognitive behavioural therapy and psychotherapy
- Acupuncture
- *Surgery*: Surgery is usually contraindicated in the cases of unprovoked vulvodynia.

Follow-up

Patients with vulvodynia must be followed up based on their clinical requirements. Long-term follow-up and psychological support may be required in the future.

SUGGESTED READING

1. Akopians AL, Rapkin AJ. Vulvodynia: The role of inflammation in the etiology of localized provoked pain of the vulvar vestibule (vestibulodynia). Semin Reprod Med. 2015;33:239.
2. Bornstein J, Goldstein AT, Stockdale CK, Bergeron S, Pukall C, Zolnoun D, et al. 2015 ISSVD, ISSWSH and IPPS Consensus terminology and classification of persistent vulvar pain and vulvodynia. Obstet Gynecol. 2016;127:745.
3. Edwards SK, Bates CM, Lewis F, Sethi G, Grover D. 2014 UK national guideline on the management of vulval conditions. Int J STD AIDS. 2015;26(9):611-24.
4. Nagandla K, Sivalingam N. Vulvodynia: Integrating current knowledge into clinical practice. Obstet Gynaecol. 2014;16:259-67.
5. Nardelli A, Degreef H, Goossens A. Contact allergic reactions of the vulva: a 14-year review. Dermatitis. 2004; 15(3):131-6.
6. Royal College of Obstetricians and Gynaecologists. (2011). The management of vulval skin disorders. Green-top guideline No. 58. [online] Available from https://www.rcog.org.uk/en/guidelines-research-services/guidelines/gtg58/. [Last accessed March, 2018].
7. Sadownik LA. Etiology, diagnosis, and clinical management of vulvodynia. Int J Womens Health. 2014;6:437-49.
8. Smith YR, Haefner HK. Vulvar lichen sclerosus: pathophysiology and treatment. Am J Clin Dermatol. 2004; 5(2):105-25.

46

CHAPTER

Problems of Sex and Marriage

Niraj Jadav, Poonam Mishra

Chapter Outline

- Physical Sex—Coitus
- Consummation of Marriage
- Annulment of Marriage
- Unconsummated Marriages
- Coital Difficulties in the Male
- Homosexuality
- Marriage and Sexual Problems in Females: Understanding, Challenges and Solutions
- Female Sexual Interest/Arousal Disorder
- Female Orgasmic Disorder
- Genito-Pelvic Pain/Penetration Disorder
- Vaginismus

INTRODUCTION

Sex is one of the three basic human instincts and is, therefore, strongly developed in the normal individual. Its influence on behaviour is controlled to a large extent by environment and especially by the laws, customs and outlook of a particular community which determine celibacy, promiscuity, marriage, monogamy, polygamy, polyandry and the like—the rules of society governing sexual conduct change from time to time.

In human beings, sex is an emotional as well as a physical experience and is evident to some extent in early childhood—baby girls, e.g., soon show an interest in appearance dresses and in boys. Later, childhood is generally an asexual phase, although homosexual and heterosexual love play is not uncommon at this age. Adolescence normally reveals a homosexual urge such as the violent affection that one girl has for another girl or woman and the hero worship exhibited by a boy for an older boy or man. This is quickly replaced by heterosexual impulses which become deeper and more serious as maturity is reached and which usually culminate in marriage, home building and childbearing.

The ages at which these events occur are changing, being determined by a tendency of earlier maturation and by a desire to conform to group behaviour. In Western communities, at least, girls aged 12–13 years now often have strongly developed heterosexual interests. By the age of 15 years, and if only as a status symbol, many are 'going steady' with a particular boyfriend. While a large percentage is married by the age of 20 years, there is also an increasing number of premarital and de facto relationships.

In India, the legal age of marriage is 18 years. In rural communities, the majority of women have had arranged marriages and possibly borne children by this age, but in the urban upper classes, with the benefit of education, marriage is often postponed till the age of 23–25 years or until the woman is professionally established.

There are some who regard companionship as the basis of marriage. The majority, however, accept marriage as essentially a sexual partnership with reproduction and a stable family life as its main objectives. It is, however, a partnership in which sexual acts are a demonstration of lasting affection rather than the satisfaction of a passing lust. The important feature of marriage is its permanence and this in itself gives a sexual satisfaction which is not usually obtained from a fleeting affair. Moreover, good sexual adjustment between the partner sensors permanence, because it is strong enough to override the tiffs and quarrels which are inevitable between even the closest companions. Unfortunately, sexual disorders and maladjustments are common and are the cause of much marital disharmony and divorce. On the other hand, it must be recognised that these difficulties are sometimes the result rather than the cause of incompatibility. The successful medical handling of disorders about sex cannot be taught by precept; it is largely dependent on the experience of life and comes with age and personal observation. The family doctor is usually the best one for dealing with sexual and marital problems, but some patients find it easier to tell these troubles to someone less well known to them. Whoever it is should generally interview both husband and wife but should see them separately as well.

PHYSICAL SEX—COITUS

Coitus (Sexual Intercourse)

Coitus (Latin coitio, meaning 'a coming together') is, for many of us, a vehicle for the expression of emotion and intimacy. Strictly speaking, coitus (or sexual intercourse) is the penetration of the vagina by the penis, which can be called vaginal coitus. However, the term coitus is also used for other forms of sexual contact, including oral coitus (oral-genital contact), femoral coitus (when the penis is inserted between the thighs), mammary coitus (when the penis is inserted between the breasts) and anal coitus (insertion of the penis into the rectum). There are many common slang phrases for coitus, such as 'making love', 'going to bed' and other more descriptive phrases. Legally, fornication is the voluntary coitus between an adult man and woman who are unmarried. Adultery is voluntary coitus between two people, at least one of whom is married to someone else. Sodomy means different things in different states; it usually refers to anal or oral coitus but also can mean 'acts against nature' such as coitus with an animal. Finally, masturbation, which is not a form of coitus, is the act of deriving sexual pleasure from self-stimulation of the genitals.

In anal coitus, the penis penetrates the anus and is moved within the rectum. This method of coitus is common in male homosexuals and in some heterosexual couples. A heterosexual couple should use a condom and never switch from anal to vaginal coitus before washing the penis, as the rectum contains microorganisms that could infect the female reproductive tract (refer to Chapter 17: Pelvic Organ Prolapse). The walls of the rectum are not as well lubricated as those of the vagina, and the anal sphincter is constricted. Therefore, lubrication of the anus and penis with saliva or a sterile lubricant is common.

Oral coitus is contact of the mouth with the genital organs. When the mouth of the partner touches the genitals of a female, it is called cunnilingus (Latin cunnus, meaning 'vulva'; lingere, meaning 'to lick'). Cunnilingus is practiced in several cultures. One danger of this form of oral coitus is the possibility of air being blown into the vagina, as air bubbles could enter the bloodstream and could be dangerous. Therefore, air should not be blown into the vagina.

Fellatio (Latin fellare, meaning 'to suck') is the oral manipulation of the penis or scrotum by a sexual partner. Some worry about the adverse effects of swallowing the semen, as it can contain microorganisms such as human immunodeficiency virus (HIV). Obviously, a woman cannot get pregnant from this form of coitus.

CONSUMMATION OF MARRIAGE

A marriage is not consummated until sexual intercourse has taken place. If the partners are virginal, the 'first night' generally proves a great disappointment. After the excitement and tension of the wedding day and after much hard work in preparing for it, both are emotionally, if not physically, exhausted. Add to this embarrassment, nervousness and inexperience and a common result is premature ejaculation (PE) or impotence on the part of the male. If this does not occur, the entrance to the vagina proves narrow earthen expected, or the hymen is tough, or nervousness causes vaginismus, so penetration rarely takes place on the first attempt. The experience provides more pain than pleasure. If the bridegroom realises these problems and avoids pressing his attentions on the first night, as some books advise, the bride is offended that he can resist her attractions; if he suffers impotence, she concludes that he does not love her and he finds his self-confidence shattered.

The normal couple surmounts these difficulties quickly, especially if they are prepared for them. Within a few days, they find that partial coitus is possible, although 3 or 4 weeks may elapse before intercourse is complete and satisfactory. Indeed, it may be 1 or 2 years before the wife regularly experiences a full orgasm.

After the first attempt at coitus, the hymenal edges and the introitus are usually bruised and sore; this is an indication to wait a few days before renewing the attempts. So, it is the development of honeymoon cystitis which, contrary to some statements, is rarely a manifestation of infection of the female urinary tract with gonococci or *Trichomonas vaginalis* organisms. The frequency and dysuria which characterise this syndrome are nearly always the consequence of traumatic urethritis, this being caused by injury to the vestibule and external urethral meatus during attempts to make the penis enter the vagina. The symptoms subside of their own accord within a few days, but a bacterial urethritis and/or cystitis can occur.

Frequency of Coitus

The young healthy couple practice coitus once every 24 hours during the early weeks of marriage, but, within 1 or 2 years, the frequency falls to the standard normal of two to three times a week. After many years and with advancing age and increasing responsibilities, coitus may be practiced only once a week. Thereafter, it varies with individuals and with circumstances but many couples aged 60–70 years practice coitus occasionally if not regularly. In all these matters, the partners should follow their natural inclinations.

Ordinarily, sexual desire in the female shows no special relationship to the menstrual cycle.

ANNULMENT OF MARRIAGE

If a marriage has not been consummated, it can be annulled by legal procedure.

Firstly, an annulment can be granted in the case where a marriage was never *consummated,* i.e., if the two people were unable to engage in sexual intercourse. This could be due to 'impotency' of either partner.

Secondly, a marriage could be voidable if either party had been suffering from certain *mental conditions* at the time of marriage. However, only *severe illnesses* can be considered as grounds for annulment. The person must suffer from a condition that makes them incapable of understanding marriage and marital responsibilities.

Further, if in the course of the marriage the person eventually recovers, the illness may no longer be considered as grounds for annulment. To add on, if disease is discovered later in the marriage, an annulment may be granted only if it is proven that it existed at the time of the marriage.

Thirdly, a marriage is voidable if either party was *not of marriageable age* at the time of the union (18 years for females and 21 years for males). However, a marriage annulment may not be granted if the two people continue living together and eventually reach a marriageable age.

Next, a marriage is voidable if any of the persons involved was *forced* into it or if any kind of *fraud* was involved.

Finally, a marriage can be declared void if a person was *pregnant* with a child of someone other than the spouse in question *at the time of the marriage.* However, a petition cannot be filed if the marriage is consummated after the discovery of *an existing pregnancy.*

While the description above uses the Hindu Marriage Act as a reference, annulment of Parsi, Christian and Muslim marriages follows a similar guide.

UNCONSUMMATED MARRIAGES

- Unconsummated marriage means that couple never have sexual relationship. But studies have shown that sometimes not only the intercourse cannot be consummated at the first try, but it could also be delayed for years and even would never happen; this is called an unconsummated marriage.
- Different physical, mental, social and cultural factors are effective in occurrence of this disorder, so it should be considered multidimensionally.

Aetiology

Ninety percent of the cases of unconsummated marriage in a sexual medicine clinic are because of a male partner's problem or are believed to be because of a male partner.

Most often, the female factors do not come into light. Even with the above female factors, men are being blamed for the unconsummation of marriage as the society expects the man to complete the act of consummation.

Male factors: (1) Myths and misconceptions about the size of the organ, nocturnal emissions, complex about masturbation, degree of erections, false belief about the preciousness of semen, concentration of semen, ejaculatory timings, etc.; (2) reinforced by comments of friends, relatives, media and online websites; (3) premarital sexual experience, failures because of anxiety and the comments from the experienced women during such instance; (4) lack of knowledge and ignorance, poor orientation because of lack of friends or low IQ; (5) disliking of partner or feeling inferior in front of the partner with regard to physique, wealth, education, job, stature or power; (6) forced marriage; (7) faulty position (mostly leg-stretched position); (8) PE (before insertion); (9) failure of first attempt to insert and darkness; (10) venereophobia or HIV phobia; (11) genital vitiligo; (12) halitosis, body odour and unhygienic and (13) poor self-esteem.

Female factors: (1) Disliking, appearance; (2) forced marriages or affairs with somebody else; (3) body odour and halitosis, personal uncleanliness; (4) ignorance about sex, lack of knowledge, poor information and aversion towards sex; (5) child sex abuse; (6) uncongenial family situations such as joint family, lack of privacy and gross difference between mother's house and in-law's house in facilities and habits; (7) personal conflicts between the couple; (8) faulty position causing pain during coitus; (9) vaginismus; (10) rigid hymen, atresia of vagina (rare); (11) aversion towards sex, genitals; (12) genital vitiligo and poor self-esteem and (13) poor orientation because of a lack of friends or low IQ.

Sexual Dysfunction

In the current edition of the Diagnostic and Statistical Manual of Mental Disorders, Fifth edition (DSM-5), sexual dysfunction is defined as 'a clinically significant disturbance in a person's ability to respond sexually or to experience sexual pleasure'.

The word 'significant' here means that the problem must be present for at least a few months and 'be causing the individual a degree of distress'.

Classification

The classification of sexual dysfunctions was simplified. There are now only three female dysfunctions and four male dysfunctions, as opposed to five and six, respectively, in the DSM-IV.

Female hypoactive desire dysfunction and female arousal dysfunction were merged into a single syndrome called sexual interest/arousal disorder. Similarly, the formerly separate dyspareunia and vaginismus are now called genito-pelvic pain/penetration disorder (GPPPD). Female orgasmic disorder (FOD) remains in place.

As for males, male hypoactive sexual desire disorder now has a separate entry. Male orgasmic disorder was changed to delayed ejaculation, the 'male' adjective was dropped from erectile disorder, and PE remains unchanged. Male dyspareunia or male sexual pain does not appear in the sexual dysfunctions in the DSM-5 **(Table 1)**.

COITAL DIFFICULTIES IN THE MALE

Erectile Dysfunction

Definition

The DSM-5 classifies erectile disorder as belonging to a group of sexual dysfunction disorders typically characterised by a clinically significant inability to respond sexually or to experience sexual pleasure **(Flowchart 1)**.

Criteria

In almost all or all (75–100%) sexual activity, the experience of at least one of the following three symptoms: (1) Marked difficulty in obtaining an erection during sexual activity, (2) marked difficulty in maintaining an erection until the completion of sexual activity or (3) marked decrease in erectile rigidity.

The symptoms above have persisted for approximately 6 months.

The symptoms above cause significant distress to the individual.

The dysfunction cannot be better explained by nonsexual mental disorder, a medical condition, the effects of a drug or medication or severe relationship distress or other significant stressors.

TABLE 1: Changes in diagnostic categories for female sexual dysfunctions between the DSM-IV (2000) and DSM-5 (2013).

DSM-IV diagnoses (2000)	***Changes in DSM-5 (2013)***
Female hypoactive desire disorder	Female sexual interest/arousal disorder (FSIAD)
Female arousal disorder	
Female orgasmic disorder	Same
Dyspareunia	Genito-pelvic pain/penetration disorder
Vaginismus	
Sexual aversion disorder	Deleted
Sexual dysfunction due to a general medical condition	
Substance/medication-induced sexual dysfunction	Unchanged
Sexual dysfunction NOS	Replaced by other specified sexual dysfunction and unspecified sexual dysfunction

(DSM-5: Diagnostic and Statistical Manual of Mental Disorders, Fifth edition; NOS: not otherwise specified)

Flowchart 1: Minimal diagnostic evaluation in ED.

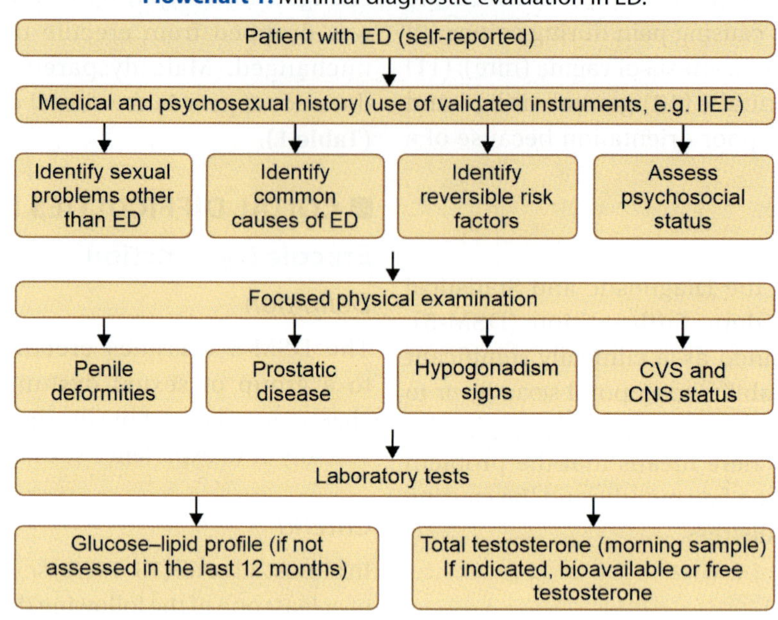

(CVS: cardiovascular system; CNS: central nervous system; ED: erectile dysfunction; IIEF: International Index of Erectile Function)

Classification

Erectile dysfunction can be classified into three subtypes **(Table 2)**:

1. Organic (iatrogenic, neurogenic, vasculogenic and hormonal)
2. Psychogenic
3. Mixed erectile dysfunction

Specialised Tests

- *Nocturnal penile tumescence and rigidity test:* Done on at least two nights.

  A functional erectile mechanism is indicated by an erectile event of at least 60% rigidity recorded on the tip of the penis that lasts for >10 minutes.
- *Intracavernous injection test:* A positive test is a rigid erectile response that appears within 10 minutes after the intracavernous injection and lasts for 30 minutes.

  Overall, the test is inconclusive as a diagnostic procedure and a duplex Doppler study of the penis should be requested.
- *Duplex ultrasound of the penis:* A peak systolic blood flow velocity >30 cm/s, an end-diastolic velocity of <3 cm/s and a resistance index >0.8 are generally considered normal. Further vascular investigation is unnecessary when a Duplex examination is normal.

Treatment for Erectile Dysfunction

Figure 1 given below.

Premature Ejaculation

- The new *DSM-5* adopted PE definition criteria similar to those adopted by the ISSM. Therefore, according to the DSM-5, the following are the criteria for a diagnosis of PE:
  A. A persistent or recurrent pattern of ejaculation occurring during partnered sexual activity within approximately 1 minute following vaginal penetration and before the individual wishes it.
  B. The symptom in criterion A must have been present for at least 6 months and must be experienced on almost all or all (approximately 75–100%) occasions of sexual activity (in identified situational contexts, or, if generalised, in all contexts).
  C. The symptom in criterion A causes clinically significant distress in the individual.
  D. The sexual dysfunction is not better explained by a nonsexual mental disorder or as a consequence of severe relationship distress or other significant stressors and is not attributable to the effects of a substance/medication or another medical condition.

TABLE 2: Psychogenic and organic erectile dysfunction.

Parameters	*Psychogenic*	*Organic*
Onset of disorder	Situational with defined onset (onset associated with a specific emotional event)	Insidious
Precipitating event	Psychogenic condition	Debilitating disease, vascular insufficiency or CNS abnormality, penile trauma or interfering drugs
Erectile function before intromission	May be present	Usually absent except in patients with pelvic steal phenomenon
Erectile function after intromission	Variable with different partners	Usually absent
Erectile response to other sexual stimuli	Usually present	Usually absent
Nocturnal or morning erections	Initially present and full, lost in long-standing dysfunction	Absent or reduced in frequency and intensity
Course of disorder	Episodic or transient loss of erection	Persistent and progressive erectile dysfunction
Associated ejaculatory disorder	Premature ejaculation and intermittent loss of ejaculation	Retrograde or absent ejaculation
Nocturnal penile tumescence • Total time • Circumferential change • Penile–brachial index (PBI) bulbocavernosus reflex latency	 • >90–180 min/night • 0.2 cm • >0.70 • <35 seconds	 • <60 min/night • 2 cm • <0.60 • >40 seconds

(CNS: central nervous system)

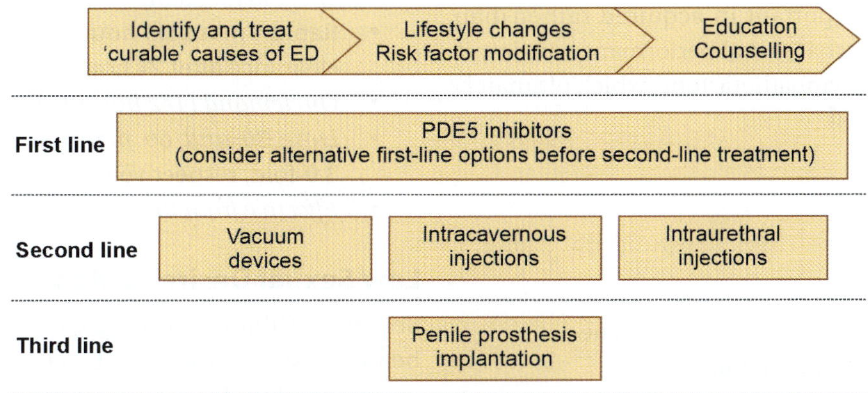

Fig. 1: Recommended treatment for ED. (ED: erectile dysfunction; PDE5: phosphodiesterase type 5)
Source: Wespes E, Eardley I, Giuliano F, Hatzichristou D, Hatzimouratidis K, Moncada I, et al. Guidelines on Male Sexual Dysfunction: erectile dysfunction and premature ejaculation. [online] Available from https://citeseerx.ist.psu.edu/document?repid=rep1&type=pdf&doi=1941c79cd09cbf456c1521510934142062f30cd0. [Last accessed May, 2025].

- Men with *lifelong PE* and an intravaginal ejaculation latency time (IELT) <1 minute, which supported the hypothesis of a genetic determination of lifelong PE.
- This ultimately led to the discussion about lifelong PE as a more neurobiologically than psychologically determined condition.

Acquired Premature Ejaculation

- *Endocrine (hormonal) factors:* Hyperthyroidism is a typical hormonal risk factor for PE.
- *Lower* prolactin and *thyroid-stimulating hormone* (TSH) levels were linked to PE, whereas lower testosterone and higher prolactin levels were linked to delayed ejaculation.

Erectile Dysfunction

Many men who are aware that rigidity starts to weaken during sexual intercourse try to speed up ejaculation before rigidity and erection are lost and coitus is terminated early.

Penile Anomalies

A short frenulum was found in 43%. After a frenulotomy under local anaesthesia, the stopwatch-measured IELT increased from 1.65 at baseline to 4.11 minutes.

Prostate Diseases

Several studies linked chronic prostatitis or chronic pelvic pain syndrome to increased PE prevalence rates.

Cognitive/Affective Factors

PE patients were preoccupied with thoughts about controlling their ejaculation, the anticipation of failure, thoughts about maintaining their erection and about the partner's satisfaction.

Anxiety

Anxiety has been associated mostly with the maintenance rather than the aetiology of PE, and it has been suggested that anxiety is more important in acquired rather than lifelong PE. It is evident that sexual performance anxiety is related to an increased sympathetic tone, which ultimately causes ED and PE as well.

Treatment

- *Behavioural:*
  - Start–stop
  - Squeeze
  - Cognitive arousal continuum technique
  - Physiological relaxation training
  - *Sensual awareness training:* Entrancement arousal
  - Pubococcygeal muscle control technique
  - Sensate focus
- *Pharmacologic:*
  - Daily use
  - On demand
  - On-demand combination drugs
  - On-demand local anaesthetics
  - There are six major pharmacological treatments for PE:
    1. Daily use of *selective serotonin reuptake inhibitors (SSRIs)* (citalopram, fluoxetine, paroxetine and sertraline)
    2. On-demand use of *dapoxetine*
    3. On-demand use of *clomipramine* [tricyclic antidepressant (TCA)]
    4. On-demand use of *topical local anaesthetics*
    5. On-demand use of *tramadol*
    6. On-demand use of *phosphodiesterase type 5 (PDE5) inhibitors* combined with above mentioned

With the exception of dapoxetine, all these treatments are off-label.

- *Long-acting antidepressants:*
  - *TCA:* Clomipramine 12.5–50 mg
  - *SSRIs:* Paroxetine (8.8-fold delay in IELT) >Sertraline >Fluoxetine >Citalopram
- *Desensitising agents:*
  - *Local anaesthetic gel:* Oldest pharmacological treatment of PE
  - Reduce the sensitivity of the glans penis, thereby delaying ejaculatory latency, but without adversely affecting the sensation of ejaculation.
  - Lidocaine–prilocaine cream: *20–30 minutes before intercourse*
- *Dapoxetine hydrochloride:*
  - *Short-acting SSRI*
  - Rapid Tmax (1.3 hours) and a short half-life (95% clearance after 24 hours)
  - *On demand (1–2 hours before coitus)*
  - *Dose 30 and 60 mg* increases IELT by 2.5- and 3.0-fold, respectively.
  - *Effective from the first dose*

Low Sexual Desire in Men

Sex drive (libido) varies greatly among men and may be decreased temporarily by conditions such as fatigue or anxiety. Libido also tends to gradually decrease as a man ages. Persistently, low libido may cause distress to a couple.

Occasionally, low libido can be a lifelong problem that results from traumatic childhood sexual experiences or learned suppression of sexual thoughts. Most often, however, low libido develops after years of normal sexual desire. Psychological factors, such as depression, anxiety, and relationship problems, are often the cause. Chronic kidney disease can decrease libido. Some drugs (such as those used to treat depression, anxiety or advanced prostate cancer) can decrease blood levels of testosterone and also lower libido.

When libido is decreased, men have fewer sexual thoughts and fantasies and less interest in sex, and they engage in sexual activity less frequently. Even sexual stimulation, by sights, words or touch, may fail to provoke interest. Men with low libido often retain the capacity for sexual function and may sometimes continue to engage in sexual activity to satisfy their partner.

Definition

According to DSM-5, a persistently or recurrently deficient (or absent) sexual/erotic thoughts or fantasies and desires for sexual activity.

No/reduced initiation of sexual activity and typically unreceptive to a partner's attempts to initiate.

A. The symptoms have persisted for a minimum duration of approximately 6 months.
B. The symptoms in criterion A cause clinically significant distress in the individual.
C. The sexual dysfunction is not better explained by a nonsexual mental disorder or as a consequence of severe relationship distress (e.g., partner violence) or other significant stressors and is not attributable to the effects of a substance/medication or another medical condition.

Diagnostic Assessment

- *History:* Masturbation, sexual fantasies, frequency of sex, initiation of love making, erection and ejaculation timings
- *Psychosocial history:* Stresses, lifestyle, relationship satisfaction and partner's sexual function
- *Genital examination*
- *Hormonal assessment:* Prolactin, total testosterone, free testosterone, sex hormone-binding globulin (SHBG), dehydroepiandrosterone (DHEA) and cortisol
- *Treatment:*
    - *Hormonal*: Testosterone replacement therapy, other hormonal treatments
    - Psychosexual

HOMOSEXUALITY

All individuals, male and female, have a potential for homosexual as well as heterosexual feelings and behaviour. Adolescent homosexual drive usually disappears with maturity or is readily resisted. Nevertheless, adult homosexuality is common in varying degrees and always has been throughout the history of the human race. Indeed, in some communities, it is accepted without disapproval. In others, the habit is regarded as antisocial, and its practice is subject to legal controls. But law, opinion and discussion generally centre on male homosexuality; female homosexuality is less discussed, possibly because any adverse effect on society is minimal.

Although usually regarded as an acquired mental illness, homosexuality may be a genetic trait. It is sometimes classified as a type of psychological intersex, but the sex chromosomes and hormone levels of affected individuals are always normal, and female homosexuals ovulate and menstruate regularly. Some combine homosexual with heterosexual activity; others do not. One could alternatively view sexual behaviour as a continuum, with pure homosexuality as a polarised extreme and pure heterosexuality as the norm, and with various degrees of bisexuality in between.

Female homosexuality in an emotional form is common but in a physical form, with a recognised sexual purpose (lesbianism), is less prevalent. Nevertheless, approximately 25% of women are said to have had experience of it in some format sometime during life, but in only 3% does it become a persistent and regular practice.

Female homosexual activity involves passionate kissing, general body contact, mutual masturbation and genital contact. Intravaginal stimulation is exceptional, and the orgasm induced is usually clitoral. One partner may be consistently active or passive; sometimes, roles are exchanged. Lesbian is misgenerally harmless except for nervous reactions centred around feelings of guilt and degradation. It can, however, arouse intense jealousy if one partner marries, and it can lead to refractory heterosexual frigidity.

The practice exists mostly among unmarried girls, spinsters and widows and is exceptional in married women. It is rife where girls are segregated in prisons and other corrective institutions. It is inherent in some girls but only acquired by others who come under the influence of a ringleader. The management of innocent puberty associations is, therefore, important lest they become permanent and pernicious.

An established lesbian who wants to remain such cannot be cured. The situation should, therefore, be accepted sympathetically, and management directed to ensure that her outlook and behaviour do not cause her to feel guilty or ashamed.

MARRIAGE AND SEXUAL PROBLEMS IN FEMALES: UNDERSTANDING, CHALLENGES AND SOLUTIONS

Introduction

Sexual intimacy is a cornerstone of marital relationships, fostering emotional connection, mutual pleasure and bonding between partners. However, sexual problems can pose significant challenges within marriages, affecting not only the individuals involved but also the overall health and stability of the relationship.

Understanding Sexual Problems in Females

Sexual problems in females encompass a range of difficulties that can affect desire, arousal, orgasm and satisfaction. These problems may be biological, psychological or relational and can arise from various factors such as hormonal imbalances, medical conditions, stress, anxiety, past traumas and relationship dynamics.

Prevalence of Female Sexual Dysfunction

General Population Studies

- The prevalence of female sexual dysfunction (FSD) varies widely across studies due to differences in definitions, methodology, cultural factors and populations studied.
- According to a meta-analysis published in the Journal of Sexual Medicine, the overall prevalence of any FSD in the general population ranges from 25 to 63%.

Classification

The DSM-5 provides criteria for diagnosing various mental health disorders, including those related to sexual functioning.

The FSDs classified by the DSM-5 are given as follows:

- Female sexual interest/arousal disorder (FSIAD)
- Female orgasmic disorder
- Genito-pelvic pain/penetration disorder
- Substance/medication-induced sexual dysfunction

These classifications are based on the DSM-5 criteria and are intended for diagnostic purposes. It is essential to remember that experiencing occasional sexual difficulties does not necessarily indicate a disorder. Only persistent, for >6 months, and distressing symptoms warrant clinical attention and potential.

FEMALE SEXUAL INTEREST/ AROUSAL DISORDER

Introduction

Female sexual interest/arousal disorder is a complex and multifaceted condition characterised by persistent difficulties with sexual interest, arousal or both, resulting in significant distress or interpersonal difficulties. It is crucial to understand the nuances of FSIAD to provide effective support and intervention for affected individuals. In this section, we will delve into the definition, diagnostic criteria, aetiology, impact and treatment options for FSIAD, drawing upon relevant literature and research in the field.

Definition and Diagnostic Criteria

Female sexual interest/arousal disorder, as defined in the DSM-5, encompasses a range of symptoms related to diminished or absent sexual interest or arousal in women. These symptoms must persist for a significant duration and cause distress or impairment in interpersonal relationships or other areas of functioning. Key features of FSIAD include:

- *Reduced sexual interest*: Women with FSIAD may experience a notable decrease in spontaneous or responsive sexual desire, leading to a lack of interest in sexual activities.
- *Diminished arousal*: FSIAD can also manifest as difficulty in becoming sexually aroused or maintaining arousal during sexual encounters, despite adequate stimulation.
- *Distress or impairment*: The symptoms of FSIAD must cause significant distress or impairment in social, occupational or other important areas of functioning to meet the diagnostic criteria.

Aetiology and Contributing Factors

The aetiology of FSIAD is multifactorial and may involve a combination of biological, psychological and interpersonal factors. Some common contributing factors to FSIAD include:

- *Hormonal imbalances:* Fluctuations in hormonal levels, such as those occurring during menopause or the postpartum period, can impact sexual desire and arousal in women.
- *Psychological factors:* Stress, anxiety, depression, body image issues and past traumatic experiences can all affect sexual interest and arousal.

- *Relationship dynamics:* Conflict, communication problems and dissatisfaction within intimate relationships can contribute to FSIAD.
- *Medical conditions:* Certain medical conditions, such as diabetes, cardiovascular disease and hormonal disorders, may interfere with sexual functioning and contribute to FSIAD.
- *Medications and substance use:* Some medications, such as antidepressants and antihypertensives, as well as substance use, can have adverse effects on sexual desire and arousal.

Treatment Options

Addressing FSIAD often requires a comprehensive and individualised approach, incorporating various treatment modalities:

- *Psychotherapy:* Cognitive behavioural therapy (CBT), mindfulness-based therapies and sex therapy can help individuals address underlying psychological factors contributing to FSIAD and develop coping strategies to enhance sexual arousal and desire.
- *Medical interventions:* Hormone therapy, such as *oestrogen replacement* therapy or *testosterone supplementation*, may be beneficial for women with FSIAD related to hormonal imbalances
  - *Phosphodiesterase type 5 inhibitors*:
    - *Overview:* Medications such as tadalafil (Cialis) and vardenafil (Levitra) are PDE5 inhibitors, similar to sildenafil (Viagra).
    - *Usage:* These drugs are primarily used to treat erectile dysfunction in men but have also been studied for their potential benefit in women with sexual dysfunction. They work by increasing blood flow to the genitals, potentially improving sexual response.
  - *Buspirone (Buspar)*:
    - *Overview:* Buspirone is an antianxiety medication that affects neurotransmitters in the brain. It has been studied for its potential to improve sexual function in women with sexual dysfunction.
    - *Usage:* It is believed to work by reducing anxiety and potentially increasing dopamine levels in the brain, which can improve sexual response.
  - *Dehydroepiandrosterone*:
    - *Overview:* DHEA is a hormone produced by the adrenal glands. It is a precursor to testosterone and oestrogen. Some studies suggest that DHEA supplementation might improve sexual function in women.
    - *Usage:* DHEA supplements are available over the counter. However, it is essential to use them under the guidance of a healthcare provider, as hormone levels need to be carefully monitored.
  - *Bupropion (Wellbutrin)*:
    - *Overview:* Bupropion is an antidepressant that is sometimes used off-label to treat female sexual disorders.
    - *Usage:* It works by affecting dopamine and norepinephrine levels in the brain, potentially enhancing sexual pleasure and function. However, like all medications, it can have side effects and should be used under the guidance of a healthcare provider.

Bremelanotide, also known as PT-141, is a medication that has been studied for the treatment of female sexual arousal and interest disorder (FSAID). It works as a melanocortin receptor agonist, affecting pathways in the brain involved in sexual response and arousal. Here is a detailed look at the treatment of FSAID with bremelanotide.

How bremelanotide works?

- *Melanocortin receptor agonist:* Bremelanotide activates melanocortin receptors in the brain, particularly in areas related to sexual function.
- *Increased dopamine release:* It increases dopamine release, which is associated with pleasure and motivation, potentially enhancing sexual desire.
- *Effects on neurotransmitters:* Bremelanotide also affects other neurotransmitters involved in sexual response, such as serotonin and norepinephrine.

Treatment protocol:

- *Assessment:*
  - Before starting bremelanotide treatment, a thorough assessment is conducted by a healthcare provider, often a gynaecologist or sexual health specialist.
  - The assessment includes a discussion of medical history, sexual history and any underlying conditions contributing to FSAID.
- *Prescription:*
  - Bremelanotide is a prescription medication and should only be used under the guidance of a healthcare provider.

- The provider will determine the appropriate dosage and treatment plan based on individual needs.
- *Administration:*
  - Bremelanotide is typically administered as a subcutaneous injection, often self-administered by the individual.
  - The injection is usually given in the abdomen or thigh, about 45 minutes before anticipated sexual activity.
- *Dosage:*
  - The recommended starting dose of bremelanotide is usually 1.75 mg.
  - The dosage may be adjusted based on individual response and tolerability, up to a maximum of 2.25 mg.
- *Frequency:*
  - Bremelanotide is not intended for daily use. It is used on an as-needed basis, with a maximum frequency of no more than one dose in 24 hours.
  - Individuals are advised not to use more than eight doses per month.
- *Timing:*
  - The timing of bremelanotide administration is important, as it takes about 45 minutes to reach peak effectiveness.
  - Individuals should plan sexual activity accordingly after administering the injection.

Benefits of bremelanotide for FSAID:

- *Increased sexual desire:* Bremelanotide aims to increase sexual desire and motivation, helping individuals with FSAID feel more interested in sexual activity.
- *Improved arousal:* By enhancing blood flow to the genital area and affecting neurotransmitters, bremelanotide can improve physical arousal and sensitivity.
- *Enhanced sexual satisfaction:* For individuals with FSAID, bremelanotide may lead to greater sexual satisfaction and pleasure during intimate encounters.

Considerations and side effects:

- *Side effects:* Common side effects of bremelanotide may include nausea, flushing, headache and fatigue.
- *Contraindications:* Bremelanotide is not recommended for use in individuals with uncontrolled high blood pressure or a history of heart disease.
- *Interactions:* It is important to discuss any other medications or supplements with a healthcare provider, as bremelanotide may interact with certain medications.
- *Patient education:* Individuals should receive thorough education on how to administer the injections, potential side effects and when to seek medical attention.

Follow-up and monitoring:

- *Response evaluation:* After starting bremelanotide, individuals and their healthcare providers should evaluate the response to treatment.
- *Adjustments:* Dosage adjustments or changes in treatment frequency may be made based on individual response and side effects.
- *Ongoing care:* Regular follow-up appointments are important to monitor the effectiveness of treatment and address any concerns.

Flibanserin, marketed under the brand name Addyi, is a medication approved by the US Food and Drug Administration (FDA) for the treatment of acquired, generalised hypoactive sexual desire disorder (HSDD) in premenopausal women. HSDD is characterised by a persistent lack of sexual desire that causes distress or interpersonal difficulties.

How flibanserin works?

Flibanserin is a multifunctional serotonin agonist and antagonist (MSAA). Unlike medications that affect blood flow (like Viagra) or hormone levels, flibanserin works on neurotransmitters in the brain, particularly serotonin and dopamine. The exact mechanism of how it works to improve sexual desire is not entirely understood, but it is believed to rebalance the levels of these neurotransmitters in a way that enhances sexual response.

Dosage and administration:

- Flibanserin is taken orally once daily at bedtime to minimise potential side effects such as dizziness and sleepiness.
- The recommended dose is 100 mg once daily.
- It can be taken with or without food.

Effectiveness:

- Studies have shown that women taking flibanserin reported modest but statistically significant improvements in sexual desire, sexual satisfaction and the number of satisfying sexual events compared to those taking a placebo.
- It is important to note that the response to flibanserin can vary among individuals, and not everyone will experience the same level of benefit.

Safety and side effects:

- *Common side effects:* The most common side effects of flibanserin include dizziness, sleepiness, nausea, fatigue, insomnia and dry mouth.
- *Alcohol interaction:* Flibanserin has a significant interaction with alcohol. Combining alcohol with flibanserin can cause severe hypotension (low blood pressure) and fainting. For this reason, it is crucial to avoid alcohol when taking flibanserin.
- *Central nervous system (CNS) effects:* Due to its effects on the CNS, flibanserin may impair our ability to drive or operate machinery. Patients are advised to avoid activities requiring full alertness until they know how flibanserin affects them.

Contraindications of flibanserin:

- Flibanserin is contraindicated in:
  - Those with a history of hypersensitivity reactions to flibanserin
  - Individuals with liver impairment
  - Those taking moderate or strong CYP3A4 inhibitors (medications that can increase flibanser in levels in the blood)

Consultation and monitoring:

- Before prescribing flibanserin, healthcare providers should evaluate patients for possible underlying causes of low sexual desire, such as relationship issues, psychological factors or other medical conditions.
- It is essential for patients to have a thorough discussion with their healthcare provider about the benefits, risks and proper use of flibanserin.
- Regular follow-ups may be necessary to assess response and monitor for side effects.

Food and Drug Administration approval and availability:

- Flibanserin was approved by the FDA in 2015 after initially being rejected twice due to concerns about its effectiveness and side effects.
- It is available by prescription only and should be obtained through a healthcare provider.
- *Lifestyle modifications*: Stress reduction techniques, regular exercise, adequate sleep and healthy lifestyle habits can promote overall well-being and sexual health.
- *Relationship counselling*: Couples therapy can help partners improve communication, resolve conflicts and enhance intimacy, thereby addressing relational factors contributing to FSIAD.

FEMALE ORGASMIC DISORDER

Introduction

Female orgasmic disorder is a condition characterised by persistent difficulty or inability to achieve orgasm despite adequate sexual stimulation. It can significantly impact a woman's sexual satisfaction, self-esteem and interpersonal relationships.

Definition and Diagnostic Criteria

Female orgasmic disorder, as defined in the DSM-5, involves recurrent or persistent difficulty or absence of orgasm following sufficient sexual stimulation. Key features of FOD include:

- *Delayed or absent orgasm:* Women with FOD may experience a delay in achieving orgasm or may be unable to reach orgasm altogether, despite engaging in sexual activity that is adequate in duration and intensity.
- *Reduced intensity of orgasmic sensations:* Even when orgasm is achieved, women with FOD may report diminished intensity or satisfaction with orgasmic sensations compared to what they desire or expect.
- *Significant distress or interpersonal difficulty:* The symptoms of FOD must cause clinically significant distress or impairment in social, occupational or other important areas of functioning to meet the diagnostic criteria.

Aetiology and Contributing Factors

The aetiology of FOD is complex and may involve a combination of biological, psychological and interpersonal factors. Some common contributing factors to FOD include:

- *Psychological factors:* Anxiety, depression, performance anxiety, past traumatic experiences and negative beliefs about sex or orgasm can all impact a woman's ability to achieve orgasm.
- *Relationship dynamics:* Conflict, communication problems and relational issues within intimate relationships can contribute to FOD.
- *Physical and medical factors:* Certain medical conditions, such as diabetes, cardiovascular disease, hormonal imbalances and neurological disorders, can interfere with sexual arousal and orgasm.
- *Medications:* Some medications, such as antidepressants, antipsychotics and certain blood

pressure medications, may have adverse effects on sexual arousal and orgasm.

Evaluation of Female Orgasmic Disorder

- *Self-report assessment tool:* Brief Index of Sexual Functioning for Women (BISF-W), Sexual Desire Inventory (SDI), Sexual Functioning Questionnaire (SFQ), Female Sexual Function Index (FSFI), etc., can aid to identify sexual problems in females.
- *Detailed sexual history from both partners:* The following questions should be asked during the taking of sexual history:
  - Initiation—who initiates? Is this her preference?
  - Frequency of coitus—how does she feel about the frequency?
  - Is the type and amount of genital stimulation adequate for her?
  - Is lubrication adequate and satisfactory for her before intercourse?
  - Length of time of intercourse—is it too long? Does it become painful?
  - Ability to achieve orgasm—Difficult? Easy? Distressed by no orgasm?
  - Does she experience any pain? If so, when? Before, during or after intercourse
  - Distractions?
- *Physical examination of both partners:*
  - *General*:
    - Overall appearance
    - Blood pressure
    - Secondary sexual characters
  - *Systemic*:
    - Cardiovascular system
    - Respiratory system
    - Abdomen
    - Central nervous system
  - *Genital examination (female)*:
    - *Breasts*: One has to check for:
      - Lumps
      - Retraction of nipples (breast cancer)
      - Axillary lymph nodes
    - *Vulva*: One has to check for:
      - *Labia*:
        - Skin lesions and ulcers
        - Enlargement of Bartholin glands
      - *Perineum*:
        - Tears/scars
        - *Introitus*:
          - Clitoral lesions
          - Urethral meatus
          - Vaginal mucosa
          - Vaginal spasm
          - Vaginal prolapse
- *Laboratory investigations:*
  - Complete blood count (CBC)
  - Thyroid and prolactin
  - Blood sugars
  - Testosterone level
  - Oestrogen level
- *Special investigations:*
  - Buccal smear
  - Nerve conduction studies
  - Other tests depending on provisional diagnosis
- Psychiatric evaluation—where necessary

Treatment of Female Orgasmic Disorder

Addressing FOD often requires a multifaceted and individualised approach, incorporating various treatment modalities:

- *Consultation:* It is crucial for women experiencing FOD to consult with a healthcare professional, preferably one who specialises in sexual medicine or gynaecology.
- *Individualised treatment:* Treatment should be tailored to the individual, taking into account any underlying medical conditions, psychological factors and overall health (giving special attention to the diet, exercise, substance abuse and sleep).
- *Sexuality education:* Providing the knowledge on anatomy and physiology of genital organs can help the couple, especially the female to reach the orgasm.
- *PLISSIT model:* A patient-centric approach consisting of:
  - *P*ermission
  - *L*imited information
  - *S*pecific *S*uggestions
  - *I*ntensive *T*reatment, can be of quite help
- *Psychological interventions:* They play the main role in the treatment of FOD.
  - *CBT*: CBT is a specialised form of psychotherapy that targets the psychological factors contributing to difficulties in achieving orgasm in women. This therapy approach aims to identify and modify negative thoughts, beliefs and behaviours related to sexuality and intimacy that may be hindering a woman's ability to reach orgasm.

- *Directed masturbation (DM)*:
    - DM training is a largely behavioural technique, usually conducted for 4–16 weekly therapy sessions.
    - It involves graded exposure to genital stimulation, which may include role-playing orgasm response, the use of sexual fantasy and/or vibrators to facilitate heightened arousal and orgasm.
    - It has shown well-established efficacy when administered in a variety of modalities: Group, individual, couples therapy and bibliotherapy.
    - The success rates for DM training (administered individually or in groups, with or without the involvement of the partner) in women with primary anorgasmia are generally high: 60–90% of the women become orgasmic with masturbation, and 33–85% will become orgasmic with partnered sexual activity.

Clitoral devices: Clitoral devices can be a part of the treatment plan for anorgasmia. These devices are designed to provide direct or indirect stimulation to the clitoris, which is a key organ for female sexual pleasure. Some different kinds of clitoral devices used for the treatment of FOD are given as follows:

- *Clitoral vibrators:*
    - Vibrators are perhaps the most well-known and widely used clitoral stimulation devices.
    - These devices produce vibrations that can stimulate the clitoris directly or indirectly through the labia and surrounding areas.
    - *Types*:
        - Bullet vibrators: Small, discreet vibrators often used for targeted clitoral stimulation.
        - Wand vibrators: Larger, more powerful vibrators that can be used for both external and internal stimulation.
        - Clitoral suction vibrators: These use pulsating air or suction to create a sucking sensation around the clitoris, mimicking oral sex.
- *Clitoral pulsators:* Pulsators are devices that create a 'tapping' or 'pulsing' sensation rather than traditional vibrations. They often have a more rhythmic and pulsating motion, which some users find more gentle and effective for clitoral stimulation.
- *Clitoral suction devices:* These devices use suction technology to create a sucking sensation around the clitoris. By gently drawing the clitoris into the device, they can increase blood flow and sensitivity, potentially leading to orgasm. Clitoral suction devices can mimic the sensation of oral sex, which many find highly pleasurable.
- *Clitoral-stimulating gels or creams:* While not devices in the traditional sense, these topical products are designed to enhance sensitivity and arousal in the clitoral area. Applied directly to the clitoris, and they can increase blood flow and sensation. Some individuals find that using a stimulating gel or cream in conjunction with manual- or device-based stimulation can enhance pleasure and make achieving orgasm easier.
- *Wearable clitoral stimulators:* These are devices that can be worn during sexual activity, providing hands-free clitoral stimulation. They are often small and discreet, fitting over or against the clitoris and surrounding area.
    - *Types*:
        - *Panty vibrators:* Designed to be worn inside underwear, these vibrators are controlled remotely for added convenience.
        - *Clitoral jewellery:* Some jewellery pieces are designed with small vibrators or stimulators built-in, providing a discreet and fashionable option.
- *Pelvic floor training devices:* While not directly stimulating the clitoris, these devices can improve overall sexual function and may indirectly help with achieving orgasm. They usually involve exercises to strengthen the pelvic floor muscles, which can enhance arousal and orgasm.
    - *Types*:
        - *Kegel balls:* Weighted balls inserted into the vagina to improve pelvic floor muscle strength.
        - *Electrostimulation devices:* These use mild electrical currents to stimulate the pelvic floor muscles, improving muscle tone.
- *Manual clitoral stimulators:* Simple devices designed for manual clitoral stimulation can be textured, shaped or ribbed for different sensations. Some individuals find that these devices offer more control and can be used in conjunction with other forms of stimulation.
- *Clitoral massagers:* These are typically ergonomically designed devices specifically for clitoral stimulation. They may have different settings for intensity and patterns of vibration or pulsation. Clitoral massagers

are often designed to be easy to hold and manoeuvre for precise stimulation.

- *Sensate focus exercises*: Engaging in sensate focus exercises, which involve gradually increasing levels of touch and intimacy with a partner, can help women enhance their awareness of sexual sensations and overcome performance anxiety.

Principles of the technique:

- Non-goal-oriented physical intimacy
- Takes the pressure off 'performance' and achieving orgasm
- Focus on the sensation of touching your partner
- Exploring sensual touching beyond the genitals

Discovering whether aspects of intimacy bring up any feelings of discomfort.

- *Systematic desensitisation*: Systematic desensitisation is a behavioural therapy technique used to treat FOD by reducing anxiety or aversion associated with sexual activity. It is based on the principle of classical conditioning, where an individual learns to associate a relaxed state with a previously anxiety-inducing situation, in this case, sexual activity.

- *Pharmacotherapy:*
  - *Hormonal treatments:*
    - *Testosterone therapy:* Testosterone is a hormone associated with libido and sexual arousal in both men and women. In some cases, low levels of testosterone may contribute to FOD. Testosterone therapy, often in the form of patches, gels or injections, can be prescribed to increase sexual desire and arousal. It is essential to note that the use of testosterone therapy in women requires careful monitoring due to potential side effects.
    - *Oestrogen therapy:* Oestrogen plays a crucial role in female sexual function, including arousal and genital tissue health. However, the direct role of oestrogen in treating FOD is less clear-cut compared to its role in other aspects of sexual health, such as vaginal dryness or pain during intercourse. Thus, oestrogen has got more important role in menopause-related FOD.
    - *Tibolone:* Tibolone is a synthetic steroid with oestrogenic, progestogenic and androgenic properties. It is primarily used in hormone replacement therapy for postmenopausal women to relieve menopausal symptoms and prevent bone loss. While tibolone's oestrogenic and androgenic effects suggest it could potentially improve vaginal health and libido, its specific role in treating FOD is not as well established as other therapies.
  - *Nonhormonal treatments:* No FDA-approved medications are available for the treatment of FOD, yet few trials with some have shown appreciable results.
    - *PDE5 inhibitors:* They have shown positive results in some populations of women.
    - *Bupropion:* A noradrenaline and dopamine reuptake inhibitor, in a dose of 150–400 mg/day, has shown positive effects on enhancing sexual arousal, orgasm and sexual satisfaction.
    - *Dietary supplements:* Combination of L-arginine, ginseng, ginkgo, damiana, multivitamins and minerals have shown benefit in orgasmic dysfunction in females.

GENITO-PELVIC PAIN/ PENETRATION DISORDER

Introduction

Genito-pelvic pain/penetration disorder is a complex and distressing condition characterised by recurrent or persistent difficulties with vaginal penetration during sexual intercourse or other vaginal penetration attempts. It encompasses various forms of pelvic pain and discomfort that can interfere with sexual intimacy and satisfaction.

Definition and Diagnostic Criteria

Genito-pelvic pain/penetration disorder, as defined in the DSM-5, involves recurrent or persistent difficulties with vaginal penetration during sexual activity, accompanied by one or more of the following symptoms:

- *Vaginal muscle tightening (vaginismus):* Involuntary contraction of the pelvic floor muscles, leading to pain or difficulty with vaginal penetration.
- *Fear or anxiety about pain during penetration:* Anticipation of pain or discomfort associated with vaginal penetration, leading to avoidance of sexual activity or attempts to prevent penetration.
- *Avoidance of vaginal penetration:* Deliberate avoidance of vaginal penetration or attempts to minimise or eliminate penetration altogether.

The symptoms of GPPPD must cause clinically significant distress or impairment in social, occupational or other important areas of functioning to meet the diagnostic criteria.

Aetiology and Contributing Factors

The aetiology of GPPPD is multifactorial and may involve a combination of biological, psychological and interpersonal factors. Some common contributing factors to GPPPD include:

- *Pelvic floor dysfunction:* Dysregulation or dysfunction of the pelvic floor muscles, leading to involuntary muscle contractions and pain during vaginal penetration.
- *Trauma or past sexual abuse:* Previous traumatic experiences, including sexual abuse or assault, can contribute to fear, anxiety and pain associated with vaginal penetration.
- *Anxiety and fear of pain:* Anticipation of pain or discomfort during penetration can trigger anxiety and fear responses, leading to muscle tension and avoidance behaviours.
- *Negative sexual scripts:* Cultural beliefs, societal norms and negative sexual scripts may contribute to feelings of shame, guilt or inadequacy related to sexual activity and penetration.

Treatment Options

Addressing GPPPD often requires a multidisciplinary and individualised approach, incorporating various treatment modalities:

- *Pelvic floor physical therapy:* Pelvic floor physical therapy, including relaxation exercises, manual therapy, biofeedback and vaginal dilator therapy, can help women alleviate pelvic floor muscle tension and improve vaginal flexibility and comfort.
- *CBT:* CBT can help individuals identify and challenge negative thoughts, beliefs and behaviours related to GPPPD; develop coping strategies for managing anxiety and fear and enhance sexual self-esteem and confidence.
- *Sex therapy:* Sex therapy can provide education, guidance and support for couples affected by GPPPD, helping them improve communication, intimacy and sexual satisfaction.
- *Medical interventions:* Medications, such as muscle relaxants or topical anaesthetics, may be prescribed to alleviate pain and discomfort associated with GPPPD. In some cases, surgical interventions may be considered for severe or refractory cases of GPPPD.

VAGINISMUS

Vaginismus is a type of female sexual dysfunction characterised by the involuntary tightening or spasm of the muscles around the vagina, making penetration difficult, painful or impossible. The muscles in the pelvic floor contract involuntarily, often in response to the anticipation of pain, fear or anxiety related to penetration. This can occur during attempts at intercourse, gynaecological examinations or even when trying to insert a tampon.

Prevalence

The prevalence of vaginismus varies across studies and populations, making it somewhat challenging to determine an exact prevalence rate. However, research suggests that vaginismus is relatively common and can affect women of all ages, and its prevalence ranges between 5% and 17% of women in the general population.

Causes of Vaginismus

Vaginismus is a complex condition with various potential causes, which can be physical, psychological or a combination of both.

Psychological Causes

- *Anxiety and fear:*
    - One of the primary psychological factors associated with vaginismus is anxiety and fear related to penetration.
    - Fear of pain during intercourse can lead to anticipatory anxiety, triggering the pelvic floor muscles to involuntarily contract.
- *Past trauma or sexual abuse:*
    - Women who have experienced sexual trauma or abuse in the past may develop vaginismus as a protective response.
    - Traumatic experiences can lead to a fear response, causing the body to react with muscle tension during attempts at penetration.
- *Negative sexual experiences:*
    - Previous painful sexual experiences, such as rough intercourse, can create a conditioned response of muscle tightening to prevent further pain.
- *Cultural and religious beliefs:*
    - Upbringing in cultures or religions with strict attitudes towards sex, virginity or sexual shame can contribute to the development of vaginismus.
    - Messages that sex is dirty or sinful can lead to anxiety and fear around sexual activity.

Physical Causes

- *Vaginal infections or irritation:*
  - Infections such as yeast infections or urinary tract infections can cause vaginal discomfort and pain, leading to muscle spasms.
  - Irritation from soaps, douches or certain products can also contribute.
- *Vaginal trauma or injury:*
  - Childbirth trauma, especially if there were tears or an episiotomy, can lead to scar tissue and pain during penetration.
  - Surgical procedures in the pelvic area, such as hysterectomy, can also contribute.
- *Hormonal changes:*
  - Fluctuations in hormone levels, such as those experienced during menopause, can lead to vaginal dryness and discomfort, triggering vaginismus.
- *Medical conditions:*
  - Conditions such as endometriosis, pelvic inflammatory disease (PID) or interstitial cystitis can cause pelvic pain and contribute to vaginismus.
- *Pelvic floor disorders:*
  - Conditions affecting the pelvic floor muscles, such as hypertonic pelvic floor dysfunction, can cause involuntary muscle spasms.
- *Genital anomalies:*
  - Rarely, structural abnormalities of the genitals can contribute to pain and muscle spasms during attempted penetration.

Lack of Sexual Education or Knowledge

- *Misconceptions about sex:*
  - Limited sexual education or misinformation about the anatomy and physiology of sex can lead to anxiety and fear of penetration.
- *Inadequate preparation:*
  - Insufficient arousal or foreplay can result in attempts at penetration before the body is ready, leading to pain and muscle tension.

Relationship Factors

- *Conflict or stress in the relationship:*
  - Relationship issues, such as unresolved conflicts, communication problems or lack of emotional intimacy, can contribute to vaginismus.
- *Partner issues:*
  - A partner's approach to sex, lack of understanding or patience or past negative experiences can impact a woman's ability to relax during intercourse.

Cognitive and Behavioural Factors

- *Conditioned response:*
  - If a woman has experienced pain during intercourse in the past, a conditioned response may develop, where the body anticipates pain and responds with muscle tension.
- *Avoidance behaviour:*
  - Over time, avoidance of sexual activity due to fear of pain can reinforce the muscle tightening response, creating a cycle of vaginismus.

Psychosocial and Cultural Factors

- *Cultural stigma:*
  - Societal or cultural stigma around women's sexuality and the expectation of pain during first intercourse (e.g., 'virginity myth') can contribute.
- *Religious beliefs:*
  - Religious teachings that frame sex as sinful or shameful can create guilt and anxiety around sexual activity.

Lamont and Pacik's Classification of Vaginismus

Dr Lamont and Dr Pacik have proposed a classification system for vaginismus based on their research and clinical experience. This classification system provides a framework for understanding the different types and presentations of vaginismus.

Primary Vaginismus

Definition: Primary vaginismus occurs when a woman has never been able to have penetrative intercourse due to involuntary muscle contractions and tightness around the vaginal opening.

Characteristics: The woman may have never been able to insert a tampon, undergo gynaecological examinations or engage in penetrative intercourse.

Symptoms typically present during the first attempt at vaginal penetration, often causing pain and making further attempts difficult or impossible.

Secondary Vaginismus

Definition: Secondary vaginismus occurs when a woman who has previously been able to have penetrative intercourse develops the condition later on.

Characteristics: The woman may have had successful penetrative intercourse in the past but begins experiencing pain and muscle spasms during attempts at penetration.

Secondary vaginismus can be triggered by factors such as trauma, childbirth, surgery, infections or psychological factors.

Situational Vaginismus

Definition: Situational vaginismus refers to a type of vaginismus where the involuntary muscle contractions and pain occur only in specific situations or contexts.

Characteristics: Symptoms may only occur during attempts at penetrative intercourse but not during other activities such as tampon insertion or gynaecological examinations.

The condition is often triggered by the anticipation of pain or fear related to certain sexual activities or partners.

Global Vaginismus

Definition: Global vaginismus is characterised by the involuntary muscle contractions and pain that occur across all situations involving vaginal penetration.

Characteristics: Women with global vaginismus experience pain and muscle spasms during attempts at intercourse, tampon insertion and gynaecological examinations.

The condition affects various aspects of the woman's life and can lead to significant distress and avoidance of sexual activities.

Spasmodic Vaginismus

Definition: Spasmodic vaginismus refers to a type of vaginismus characterised by sudden and intense muscle spasms of the pelvic floor muscles.

Characteristics: The muscle spasms can be unpredictable and occur without warning, making penetration extremely painful or impossible.

Women with spasmodic vaginismus may experience episodes of severe pain during intercourse, often leading to avoidance of sexual activity.

Idiopathic Vaginismus

Definition: Idiopathic vaginismus is a term used when the cause of vaginismus is unknown or cannot be identified.

Characteristics: Despite a thorough evaluation, including physical, psychological and medical assessments, no specific cause can be pinpointed.

Idiopathic vaginismus may present with symptoms similar to other types, such as pain, muscle spasms and avoidance of penetration.

Lamont and Pacik's Grading System

- In addition to the classification, Lamont and Pacik proposed a grading system to describe the severity of vaginismus:
  - *Grade 1 (mild):* Intercourse is possible with varying degrees of discomfort. The patient may report mild pain or tightness.
  - *Grade 2 (moderate):* Intercourse is difficult and painful, with significant muscle tightness. The patient may have difficulty with tampon insertion.
  - *Grade 3 (severe):* Intercourse is impossible, and even attempts at penetration are met with severe pain and strong muscle contractions.
  - *Grade 4 (complete):* The most severe form, where any attempt at penetration is met with an immediate, intense muscle spasm that prevents entry.

    Dr Peter Pacik, a specialist in the treatment of vaginismus, introduced a grading system that includes grade 5 vaginismus, which represents the most severe form of the condition.
  - *Grade 5 vaginismus*:
    - Definition: Grade 5 vaginismus represents an extreme and complete form of the condition where any attempt at vaginal penetration is met with an immediate and intense muscle spasm that prevents entry.

Muscles Involved in Vaginismus

Vaginismus primarily involves the pelvic floor muscles, which consist of both superficial and deep muscles.

Superficial Muscles

- *Bulbocavernosus muscle*: Located in the superficial layer of the pelvic floor, this muscle surrounds the bulb of the vestibule (the erectile tissue at the entrance to the vagina).

- *Ischiocavernosus muscle*: Also in the superficial layer, this muscle is involved in erectile function and helps compress the crus of the clitoris.
- *Superficial transverse perineal muscle*: This muscle spans the perineum (the area between the vagina and anus) and assists in supporting the pelvic organs.

Deep Muscles

- *Pubococcygeus (PC) muscle*: This is one of the primary muscles involved in vaginismus. It is a deep muscle that runs from the pubic bone to the coccyx, forming a sling-like structure supporting the pelvic organs. It plays a key role in urinary control, childbirth and sexual function.
- *Iliococcygeus muscle*: Another deep muscle, the iliococcygeus muscle attaches to the pubic bone and runs back to the coccyx, helping to form the floor of the pelvic cavity.
- *Puborectalis muscle*: This muscle loops around the rectum and is involved in maintaining faecal continence. It also contributes to the involuntary contraction of the anal sphincters.

In cases of vaginismus, the primary issue is involuntary and often painful contraction of these pelvic floor muscles, especially the PC muscle. This involuntary spasm makes penetration difficult or impossible, leading to pain and discomfort during sexual activity or attempts at penetration.

Treatment of Vaginismus

Aim of Treatment

The primary goal of treating vaginismus is to help individuals overcome the involuntary muscle spasms in the pelvic floor muscles that make penetration painful or impossible. Treatment aims to address both the physical and psychological aspects of the condition, helping individuals to achieve pain-free intercourse and improve overall sexual function.

Pelvic floor physical therapy: Pelvic floor physical therapy focuses on relaxing and retraining the pelvic floor muscles, especially the PC muscle, which is often the primary culprit in vaginismus.

- *Pelvic floor relaxation exercises:* These exercises involve learning how to consciously relax the pelvic floor muscles. Techniques such as diaphragmatic breathing and progressive muscle relaxation can be helpful.
- *Biofeedback:* This technique provides visual or auditory feedback to help individuals understand and control muscle contractions. Sensors are used to monitor muscle activity, allowing patients to see when they are tensing and learn to relax the muscles.
- *Dilator therapy:*
    - *Understanding dilators:*
        - Dilators are cylindrical objects made of smooth medical-grade plastic or silicone.
        - They come in various sizes, starting from very small (similar to the size of a pinkie finger) to larger sizes.
        - The goal is to gradually progress from smaller to larger sizes to help the vagina get accustomed to penetration without pain.
    - *How dilator therapy works:*
        - *Step-by-step approach*:
            - *Assessment*: A healthcare provider will usually start by assessing the patient's condition to determine the appropriate size of dilator to begin with.
            - *Education*: Patients are educated about their condition and how dilators can help.
            - *Preparation*: It is important to create a relaxed, private space for the therapy.
            - *Relaxation techniques*: Techniques such as deep breathing, visualisation or pelvic floor relaxation exercises may be recommended.
            - *Lubrication*: Using a water-based lubricant, apply a generous amount to the dilator and around the opening of the vagina.
        - *Using the dilator*:
            - *Insertion*: Gently insert the dilator into the vaginal opening.
            - *Hold and relax*: Once inserted, hold the dilator in place and focus on relaxing the pelvic floor muscles.
            - *Time*: The duration of each session varies but typically starts with a few minutes and gradually increases over time.
            - *Gradual progression*: As comfort increases, progress to the next size of dilator.
            - *Frequency*: Therapy sessions may be recommended several times per week.
- *Key points:*
    - The therapy should never be painful. Discomfort and pressure are normal, but pain means it is time to stop and perhaps try a smaller size or more relaxation techniques.
    - Patience is crucial. Progression may take weeks to months, depending on the individual.

Psychological counselling and education: Addressing the psychological factors that contribute to vaginismus is crucial for successful treatment. Counselling can help individuals understand their condition, manage anxiety and improve communication with their partners.

- *CBT:* CBT helps individuals identify and change negative thought patterns and behaviours related to sex and penetration. It can also address underlying anxiety or trauma that may be contributing to vaginismus.
- *Sexual education and sensate focus:* Learning about sexual anatomy, arousal and response can be empowering. Sensate focus exercises involve nongenital touching and exploration with a partner to build intimacy and reduce performance pressure.

Relaxation techniques: Learning relaxation techniques can help individuals manage anxiety and tension, which can exacerbate vaginismus symptoms.

- *Breathing exercises:* Deep breathing exercises can promote relaxation and reduce muscle tension. Techniques such as diaphragmatic breathing can be practiced regularly.
- *Mindfulness and meditation:* Mindfulness practices can help individuals become more aware of their bodies and sensations without judgement. Meditation can promote relaxation and reduce stress.

Couple's therapy: Involving a partner in the treatment process can improve communication, reduce pressure and enhance intimacy.

- *Communication skills:* Couple's therapy can help partners communicate openly about their feelings, needs and desires. Learning effective communication techniques can reduce misunderstandings and increase empathy.
- *Partner involvement in treatment:* Partners can assist with dilator therapy or sensate focus exercises, helping to create a supportive and understanding environment.

Medications: In some cases, medications may be prescribed to help manage pain, anxiety or other underlying conditions that contribute to vaginismus.

- *Topical anaesthetics:* These can be applied to the vaginal opening to reduce pain during attempted penetration.
- *Antidepressants or antianxiety medications:* These medications may be prescribed to manage anxiety or depression symptoms that contribute to vaginismus.

Gradual progression: Progress in treating vaginismus is typically gradual, and it is important to proceed at a pace that is comfortable for the individual.

- *Step-by-step approach:* Treatment often involves starting with less threatening activities, such as relaxation exercises or non-penetrative intimacy, before progressing to vaginal penetration.
- *Patience and persistence:* Overcoming vaginismus may take time, and setbacks are normal. Patience, persistence and a supportive treatment team are essential for success.

Follow-up and support: Continued support and follow-up care are crucial for long-term success and maintenance of progress.

- *Regular check-ins:* Periodic visits with healthcare providers or therapists can monitor progress and make adjustments to the treatment plan as needed.
- *Support groups:* Joining support groups or online communities can provide a sense of connection, understanding and encouragement from others going through similar experiences.

Botulinum Toxin A (Botox) Therapy for Vaginismus

Botox therapy, also known as botulinum toxin type A therapy, is a treatment option for vaginismus that involves injecting Botox directly into the pelvic floor muscles. This treatment is considered when other conservative methods such as pelvic floor physical therapy, counselling and medications have not provided sufficient relief. A detailed description of Botox therapy for vaginismus is given as follows:

- *Aim of Botox therapy:* The primary goal of Botox therapy for vaginismus is to temporarily relax the pelvic floor muscles, particularly the PC muscle, which may be involuntarily contracting and causing pain or difficulty with penetration. By temporarily paralysing these muscles, Botox can allow for easier vaginal entry and reduce pain during intercourse.
- *Procedure:*
    - *Preparation*: Before the procedure, a thorough assessment is conducted by a healthcare provider, usually a gynaecologist or urogynaecologist.

      The individual is informed about the procedure, its potential benefits, risks and what to expect during and after treatment.
    - *Injection site mapping*: The healthcare provider will identify the specific pelvic floor muscles involved in the vaginismus.

Mapping the injection sites is crucial to ensure precise placement of the Botox injections.

- *Anaesthesia*: Local anaesthesia may be used to numb the vaginal area and reduce discomfort during the procedure.
- *Injection process*: Using a thin needle, Botox is injected directly into the identified pelvic floor muscles.

  Multiple injections may be administered to cover the entire area of muscle involvement.

  The injection process is typically quick and done in an outpatient setting.
- *Monitoring*: After the injections, the individual may be monitored for a short period to watch for any immediate reactions.

How Botox works:

- *Muscle relaxation:* Botox works by blocking the release of acetylcholine, a neurotransmitter responsible for muscle contractions. This leads to temporary muscle paralysis or relaxation.
- *Targeting specific muscles:* Botox specifically targets the overactive pelvic floor muscles involved in vaginismus. By relaxing these muscles, it can reduce the involuntary spasms and tension that make penetration painful or difficult.
- *Post-treatment:*
  - *Recovery*: After the procedure, individuals can usually return home the same day.

    Some may experience mild discomfort, spotting or temporary numbness in the vaginal area.
  - *Avoiding intercourse*: It is typically recommended to avoid sexual intercourse for a period of time after the injections, usually a few days to a week.

    This allows the Botox to take effect and the muscles to relax fully.
  - *Effect duration*: The effects of Botox are temporary and usually last for several months, typically around 3–6 months.

    Over time, as the Botox wears off, the muscles gradually regain their normal function.
  - *Follow-up*: Follow-up appointments with the healthcare provider are scheduled to monitor progress.

Additional treatments may be recommended based on individual response and symptoms.

- *Potential benefits:*
  - *Pain reduction*: Botox injections can significantly reduce pain and discomfort associated with vaginismus, allowing for easier penetration.
  - *Improved sexual function*: With relaxed pelvic floor muscles, individuals may experience improved sexual function and the ability to engage in pleasurable intercourse.
  - *Increased treatment success*: Botox therapy can sometimes break the cycle of pain and tension, making it easier for individuals to engage in pelvic floor physical therapy and other treatments.
- Risks and considerations:
  - *Temporary side effects*: These may include temporary vaginal dryness, mild bleeding, bruising at the injection site or discomfort.
  - *Urinary retention*: In some cases, Botox can temporarily affect bladder function, leading to urinary retention. This is usually temporary and resolves as the Botox wears off.
  - *Rare complications*: While rare, there is a risk of more serious complications such as infection or allergic reactions to the Botox.

SUGGESTED READING

1. American Association for Marriage and Family Therapy. (2020). Sexual problems. [online] Available from https://www.aamft.org/Consumer_Updates/Sexual_Problems.aspx. [Last accessed April, 2025].
2. American College of Obstetricians and Gynecologists (ACOG). Committee Opinion No. 754: the utility of and indications for routine pelvic examination. Obstet Gynecol. 2020;135(5):e216-20.
3. American Diabetes Association (ADA). Standards of Medical Care in Diabetes—2022. Diabetes Care. 2022;45(Suppl 1):S1-255.
4. American Psychiatric Association. Diagnostic and Statistical Manual of Mental Disorders, 5th edition. Arlington, VA: American Psychiatric Publishing; 2013.
5. American Psychological Association. (2021). Female sexual dysfunction. [online] Available from https://www.apa.org/topics/female-sexual-dysfunction. [Last accessed April, 2025].
6. American Sexual Health Association (ASHA). (n.d.). Sexual history taking. [online] Available from https://www.ashasexualhealth.org/sexual-history-taking/. [Last accessed April, 2025].
7. Andreeva IS. Sociophilosophical problems of sex, marriage, and the family. Sov Stud Philos. 1980;19(2):44-67.
8. Basson R. Female sexual response: the role of drugs in the management of sexual dysfunction. Obstet Gynecol Clin N Am. 2005;32(1):107-24.
9. Basson R. Human sexual response. Handbook of clinical neurology. 2015;130:11-8.
10. Basson R. Women's sexual dysfunction: revised and expanded definitions. CMAJ. 2002;167(8):867-74.
11. Beck AT, Steer RA, Brown GK. Manual for the Beck Depression Inventory-II. Psychological Corporation; 1996.

12. Bergeron S, Binik YM, Khalifé S, Pagidas K, Glazer HI, Meana M, et al. A randomized comparison of group cognitive-behavioural therapy, surface electromyographic biofeedback, and vestibulectomy in the treatment of dyspareunia resulting from vulvar vestibulitis. Pain. 2001;91(3):297-306.
13. Blevins CA, Weathers FW, Davis MT, Witte TK, Domino JL. The Posttraumatic Stress Disorder Checklist for DSM-5 (PCL-5): development and initial psychometric evaluation. J Trauma Stress. 2015;28(6):489-98.
14. Brotto LA, Basson R. Group mindfulness-based therapy significantly improves sexual desire in women. Behav Res Ther. 2014;57:43-54.
15. Chen S, Suzuki K, MacMahon H. Development and evaluation of a computer-aided diagnostic scheme for lung nodule detection in chest radiographs by means of two-stage nodule enhancement with support vector classification. Medical physics. 2011;38(4):1844-58.
16. Clayton AH, Kingsberg SA. Female sexual dysfunction: new concepts and treatments. Curr Psych Rep. 2010;12(6):437-43.
17. Clayton AH, McGarvey EL, Clavet GJ. The Changes in Sexual Functioning Questionnaire (CSFQ): development, reliability, and validity. Psychopharmacol Bull. 1997;33(4):731-45.
18. Derogatis LR, Melisaratos N. The DSFI: a multidimensional measure of sexual functioning. J Sex Marital Ther. 1979;5(4):244-81.
19. Derogatis LR, Rosen R, Leiblum S, Burnett A, Heiman J. The Female Sexual Distress Scale (FSDS): initial validation of a standardized scale for assessment of sexually related personal distress in women. J Sex Marital Ther. 2002;28(4):317-30.
20. Garber JR, Cobin RH, Gharib H, Hennessey JV, Klein I, Mechanick JI, et al. Clinical practice guidelines for hypothyroidism in adults: cosponsored by the American Association of Clinical Endocrinologists and the American Thyroid Association. Thyroid. 2012;22(12):1200-35.
21. Goldstein AT, Pukall CF, Brown C, Bergeron S, Stein A, Kellogg-Spadt S, et al. Vulvodynia: assessment and treatment. J Sex Med. 2016;13(4):572-90.
22. Jimbo M. (2024). Decreased Libido in Men. [online] Available from https://www.msdmanuals.com/home/men-s-health-issues/sexual-function-and-dysfunction-in-men/decreased-libido-in-men. [Last accessed April, 2025].
23. Jone RE, Lopez KH. Human Reproductive Biology, 4th edition. London: Academic Press; 2014.
24. Kingsberg SA. The impact of aging on sexual function in women and their partners. Arch Sex Behav. 2015;44(3):685-97.
25. Marriage Annulment Laws In India And Everything You Should Know About What To Do (womensweb.in)
26. McCabe MP, Sharlip ID. Psychological factors and sexual dysfunctions: comorbidity and interrelationship. In: Leiblum SS, Rosen RC (Eds). Principles and Practice of Sex Therapy, 5th edition. New York: Guilford Press; 2012. pp. 25-56.
27. McCarthy BW, McCarthy KB. Rekindling Desire: A Step-by-Step Program to Help Low-Sex and No-Sex Marriages. UK: Routledge; 2019.
28. McGahuey CA, Gelenberg AJ, Laukes CA, Moreno FA, Delgado PL, McKnight KM, et al. The Arizona Sexual Experience Scale (ASEX): reliability and validity. J Sex Marital Ther. 2000;26(1):25-40.
29. Meller J, Stone GL. Marital problems in general practice. S Afr Med J. 1973;47(39):1812-4.
30. Murugan S. Unconsummation of marriage. J Psychosexual Health. 2021;3(3):283-5.
31. Myerscough PR, Blum A. Sex problems in practice: referring patients to a gynaecologist or psychiatrist and to a marriage guidance counsellor. Br Med J (Clin Res Ed). 1981;282(6276):1589-90.
32. Parish SJ, Clayton AH. Female sexual arousal disorder: therapeutic options for management. J Women Health. 2007;16(9):1246-56.
33. Porst H, McMahon CG, Althof SE, Sharlip I, Bull S, Aquilina JW, Tesfaye F, Rivas DA. Baseline characteristics and treatment outcomes for men with acquired or lifelong premature ejaculation with mild or no erectile dysfunction: integrated analyses of two phase 3 dapoxetine trials. The journal of sexual medicine. 2010;7(6):2231-42.
34. Reed BD, Harlow SD, Sen A, Legocki LJ. Prevalence and demographic characteristics of vulvodynia in a population-based sample. Am J Obstet Gynecol. 2012;206(2):170.e1-e9.
35. Rosen R, Brown C, Heiman J, Leiblum S, Meston C, Shabsigh R, et al. The Female Sexual Function Index (FSFI): a multidimensional self-report instrument for the assessment of female sexual function. J Sex Marital Ther. 2000;26(2):191-208.
36. Royal College of Obstetricians and Gynaecologists (RCOG). The Management of Dyspareunia: a report of the Royal College of Obstetricians and Gynaecologists. BJOG. 2012;119(12):1550-5.
37. Sankaranantham M. HIV-Is a cure possible?. Indian journal of sexually transmitted diseases and AIDS. 2019;40(1): 1-5.
38. Spitzer RL, Kroenke K, Williams JB, Löwe B. A brief measure for assessing generalized anxiety disorder: the GAD-7. Arch Inter Med. 2006;166(10):1092-7.
39. Starling BP, Martin AC. Improving marital relationships: strategies for the family physician. J Am Board Fam Pract. 1992;5(5):511-6.
40. Tiefer L. Sex is not a Natural Act & Other Essays, 2nd edition. Colorado: Westview Press; 2001.
41. Van Cauwenberge JR. Concerning some important sexual problems. Rev Med Liege. 1999;54(5):477-80.
42. Vermeulen A. Androgen replacement therapy in the aging male—a critical evaluation. J Clin Endocrinol Metab. 2002;87(4):1467-72.
43. Wiegel M, Meston C, Rosen R. The Female Sexual Function Index (FSFI): cross-validation and development of clinical cutoff scores. J Sex Marital Ther. 2005;31(1):1-20.
44. Workowski KA, Bolan GA. Sexually transmitted diseases treatment guidelines, 2015. MMWR Recomm Rep. 2015;64(RR-03):1-137.
45. World Health Organization (WHO). Module 4: Taking a sexual history. In Medical and Service Delivery Guidelines for Sexual and Reproductive Health. Geneva: World Health Organization; 2018. pp. 79-98.

47

CHAPTER

Male and Female Infertility Overview

Mahesh C Koregal, Muralidhar V Pai, Soumya Mahesh Koregal

Chapter Outline

- Infertility
- Frequency
- Concept of Fertility
- Causes of Infertility
- Investigation of Infertility
- Treatment

INFERTILITY

Infertility is defined as the inability of a couple to achieve conception after 1 year of unprotected coitus. Sterility is an absolute state of inability to conceive. *Secondary infertility and sterility* are the same states developing after an initial phase of fertility. All these conditions can affect either the male or female partner of a marriage. Fecundability is the probability of achieving pregnancy within a single menstrual cycle, and fecundity is the probability of achieving a live birth within a single cycle. The fecundability of a normal couple has been estimated at 20–25%. On the basis of this estimate, about 90% of couples should conceive after 12 months of unprotected intercourse.

The desire of women for children is usually stronger than self-interest in beauty and figure, and may be stronger than the claims of a career. In men, it is usually less intense. Childlessness may be a tragedy to a married woman, and can be a cause of marital upset as well as of personal unhappiness and ill health. Having children cements a marriage, and when a breakdown of the partnership is threatened—as it is at some stage in many if not most marriages—the future welfare of their offspring may deter man and wife from separating.

Childlessness may result from recurrent abortion and stillbirth, but the most common cause is a failure to conceive; it is the latter problem which forms the subject of this chapter.

FREQUENCY

About 10–15% of marriages prove to be childless. The incidence of infertility does not appear to be increasing, but more couples are seeking advice because of increased publicity. Couples do not hesitate, as they did in former times, to reveal their problem.

Since the beginning of time, human infertility has been a source of personal misery, and even of national crises. It was once, and still is in some communities, regarded as a disgrace, as a mark of Divine displeasure, as grounds for divorce and even for compulsory suicide (on the part of the woman only!). The Egyptians, Greeks and earlier civilisations all had empirical treatments—love potions, amulets, prayers, sacrifices, and the like. Although the female partner was generally blamed, the Greeks at least were aware of male infertility.

CONCEPT OF FERTILITY

Fertility is a relative rather than an absolute state, and comparatively few individuals are fully sterile or fully fertile. The majority fall somewhere between these two extremes, and the fertility of a marriage is the sum of the fertilities of the two partners. Low fertility in one can, to some extent, be balanced by high fertility in the other, whereas low fertility in both partners may result in infertility. This explains why some couples fail to reproduce yet when they separate and each takes a new mate, they both proceed to have children. Incompatibility in the sense in which it was formerly envisaged has not been demonstrated so far, although the parts played by various combinations of blood group and possible immunological reactions of the woman to a particular semen have been, and are being, studied intensively.

Fertility also varies from time to time in the same individual. In males, these are not obvious except during childhood and, less absolutely, in old age, but in females, physiological infertility is seen:

- Before puberty
- After puberty and before maturation. Although menstruation may be occurring regularly, fertility is

usually low until the age of 16–17 years. The explanation of this is unknown, although it is sometimes assumed that it is because a higher percentage of menstrual cycles are anovulatory in the earlier years.

- During pregnancy, when ovulation is suppressed
- During lactation
- Before the menopause. After the age of 34 years, fertility falls; there is a gradual decline in conception rates with age. Conception rates also depend on many factors, including in many countries, the tendency for smaller families.
- After the menopause.

CAUSES OF INFERTILITY

There are still some cases of unexplained infertility, despite the increased sophistication of tests now available. The proportion of cases of unexplained infertility seen in any clinic depends on the facilities available, varying from 6% to 60%, but is usually seen in about 10–20%. There are some factors which have still not been identified. In many cases, however, several adverse factors are operative, and if these are distributed between the partners, it may be impossible, even if it were desirable, to apportion the 'blame'. The diversity and multiplicity of possible aetiological factors emphasise the need for meticulous investigation to reveal them.

In any series of infertile marriages, the main aetiological factor is found in the female in about 40% of cases; about 35% of the husbands concerned have some degree of infertility. In 10–20% of cases, a combination of factors operates, and the rest have unexplained infertility **(Flowcharts 1 and 2)**.

Flowchart 1: Assessment of a couple with infertility.

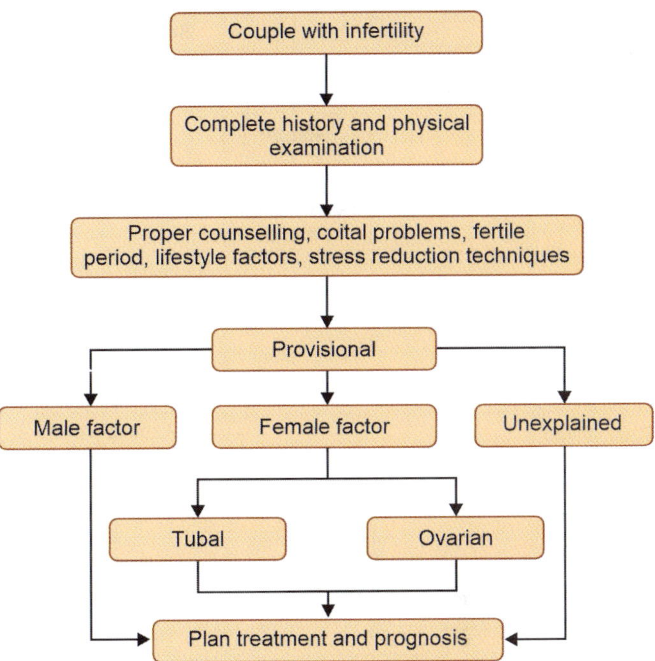

Male

Failure to Produce Spermatozoa in Sufficient Numbers and with the Capacity to Fertilise

In most cases of azoospermia and oligospermia, the underlying cause is not clear, although it is now accepted that motility and abnormal forms are at least as important as the number of spermatozoa. Established and postulated causes include the following:

- Incomplete development of the testes. The frequency of sex chromosomal aberrations among men with aplastic testes and azoospermia is probably high.
- Late descent, or nondescent, of the testes, which may or may not be the result of the former cause. In either case, the spermatogenetic function of the testis depends on its extra-abdominal site, probably because of the ill-effect of heat on the seminiferous tubules. The tissue temperature of the scrotal testis is 2°C lower than that of the rest of the body.
- Previous orchitis due to mumps or other severe infectious fevers (including influenza), or chlamydial infection occurring after the age of 14 years. Orchitis complicates 25–50% of cases of adult mumps.
- Damage to the testes resulting from operation, accident or exposure to X-rays. The injury may be to its blood supply rather than to the gonad itself.
- Exposure of the testes to heat impairs spermatogenesis, at least temporarily; frequent hot baths or the wearing of nonporous nylon underwear and suspensory garments may have this effect. Varicocele is not uncommonly found in infertile men; if its association is causal, it may be because it raises the scrotal temperature or leads to anoxia of the testicular tissues. Workers in foundries or welders may similarly be exposed to high temperatures.
- Diseases of the testes, such as tumours, tuberculosis and syphilis.
- Depression of testicular activity by disease of other endocrine glands (especially the hypothalamic-pituitary system, e.g. hypogonadism as in the Laurence–Moon–Biedl or Frohlich syndrome, thyrotoxicosis and diabetes

Flowchart 2: Assessment of male factor.

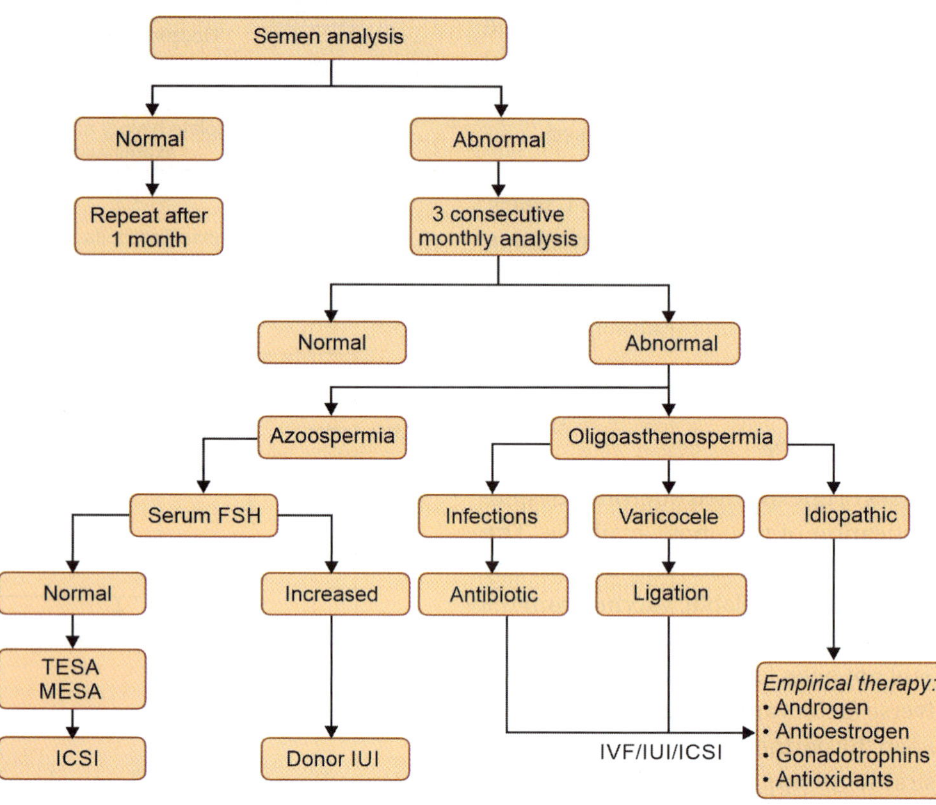

(FSH: follicle-stimulating hormone; ICSI: intracytoplasmic sperm injection; IUI: intrauterine insemination; IVF: in vitro fertilisation; MESA: microepididymal sperm aspiration; TESA: testicular sperm aspiration)

mellitus), by general ill health and by drugs and poisons. Steroids in high doses, antiandrogens, e.g. cyproterone, spironolactone, cimetidine and cannabis, depress the hypothalamo-pituitary-testicular axis. Methotrexate, colchicine, nitrofurantoin, sulfasalazine, cocaine, and alcohol act directly on the testis. Nifedipine, allopurinol and nicotine impair the fertilising capacity of the sperm, while sperm motility is impaired by lignocaine, procaine, propranolol, quinine, chlorpromazine, minocycline and tetracycline.

- *Age:* Male fertility tends to diminish after the age of 40 years, although spermatogenesis usually continues to some extent until old age. Octogenarian fathers are by no means rare.
- *Sperm agglutinins and antibodies:* In some infertile men, or following operations for reversal of vasectomy, sperm agglutinins are demonstrable in circulation, which may damage seminiferous tubules as well as cause spermatozoa to agglutinate after ejaculation. Other local and circulatory antibodies to testes, as well as to spermatozoa, are described in the male.

Bilateral Obstruction of the Epididymis, the Vas or the Ejaculatory Ducts

These may be caused by the following:

- Accident or operation, especially herniorrhaphy
- Infections, of which gonorrhoea and tuberculosis are the most important; the lesion is usually an epididymitis
- Congenital absence or gross hypoplasia of the vas
- Congenital or developmental obstruction of the epididymis, which is usually associated with congenital cystic disease of the lungs to form a definite syndrome.

Failure to Deposit Spermatozoa in the Vagina

- Impotence (including the type in which erection and penetration take place but there is no emission)
- Premature ejaculation
- Abnormalities of the penis such as hypospadias and phimosis
- Retrograde ejaculation into the bladder. This happens after prostatectomy and certain nerve resection operations. It can also occur in apparently normal men.

TABLE 1: Semen analysis as per WHO 2021 guidelines.

Semen volume (mL)	***1.4 mL***
Total sperm number (10^6 per ejaculate)	≥39 million
Total sperm concentration (10^6/mL)	≥16 million
Total motility (%)	≥42 million
Progressive motility (%)	≥30%
Non-progressive motility (%)	1%
Immotile sperm (%)	20%
Vitality (%)	≥54%
Normal forms (%)	≥4%

- Drugs which affect ejaculation include α-blockers, ganglion blockers, the tricyclic antidepressants, monoamine oxidase inhibitors, phenothiazines, β-blockers, and thiazides.

Abnormal Semen Quality (Table 1)

- An unusually high or small volume of ejaculation
- Other physicochemical anomalies, which may or may not be significant, are low fructose or high prostaglandin content, and undue viscosity.
- *Oligozoospermia:* <16 million sperm/mL
- *Asthenozoospermia:* <30% sperm with forward progression
- *Teratozoospermia:* <4% morphologically normal forms.
- *Asthenoterato-oligozoospermia:* Combinations of the above.
- *Azoospermia:* Absence of sperm in the seminal fluid; aspermia is the absence of ejaculate.

Female

Ovarian Factors

In women menstruating regularly, this is a cause operating in about 15% of cases of infertility. Regular anovulation in menstruating women can be a feature of hypothalamic anovulation, hyperprolactinaemia (due to drugs, pituitary adenoma or primary hypothyroidism), polycystic ovaries **(Fig. 1)**, subclinical adrenal failure and diabetes mellitus, luteinised unruptured follicles and luteal phase deficiency. However, it is not clear whether the last two can cause infertility.

Generally, failure to ovulate is associated with amenorrhoea or oligomenorrhoea and has the same causes. These include sex chromosome anomalies. Premature ovarian failure due to premature menopause or resistant ovary syndrome is also seen. Anovulation is also a feature of luteal phase deficiency and the luteinised unruptured follicle.

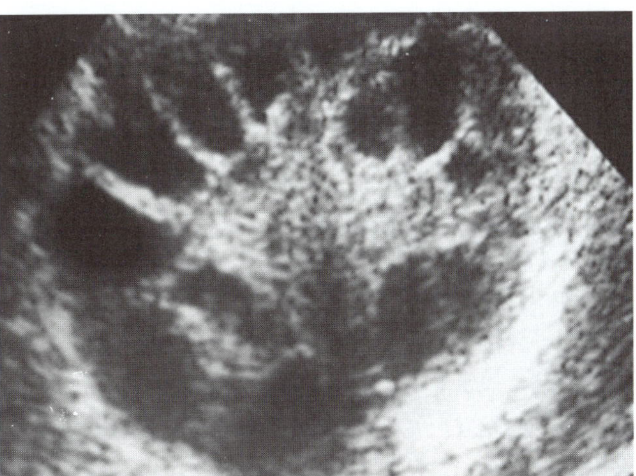

Fig. 1: Polycystic ovary on a transvaginal scan.

Luteal phase defect can be short or long, but is more often the latter. There is decreased hormone production by the corpus luteum as well as decreased levels of follicle-stimulating hormone (FSH) and luteinising hormone (LH). Some women have hyperprolactinaemia and hypothyroidism; others have unexplained infertility with normal cycles; or are habitual aborters **(Flowchart 3)**.

Peritoneal Factors

Pelvic adhesions may operate by preventing the tube from performing its 'octopus' function at the time of ovulation or by creating a mechanical barrier between the ovary and the tubal ostium. They result from pelvic peritonitis of any kind, but especially that seen in association with appendicitis, and postabortal or puerperal infections. Endometriosis is seen in at least 15% of women investigated for infertility, if all grades are considered.

Tubal Factors

Peritoneal and tubal factors may account for up to 35% of all cases of infertility. Partial or complete bilateral tubal obstruction results from previous salpingitis. Most commonly, this is postabortal, puerperal, gonococcal, chlamydial or tuberculous in nature.

Uterine Factors

- *Uterine absence, atrophy, or hypoplasia of a degree sufficient to bar the ascent of spermatozoa causes amenorrhoea as well as infertility.*
- *Tuberculous endometritis*

Flowchart 3: Assessment of ovulation.

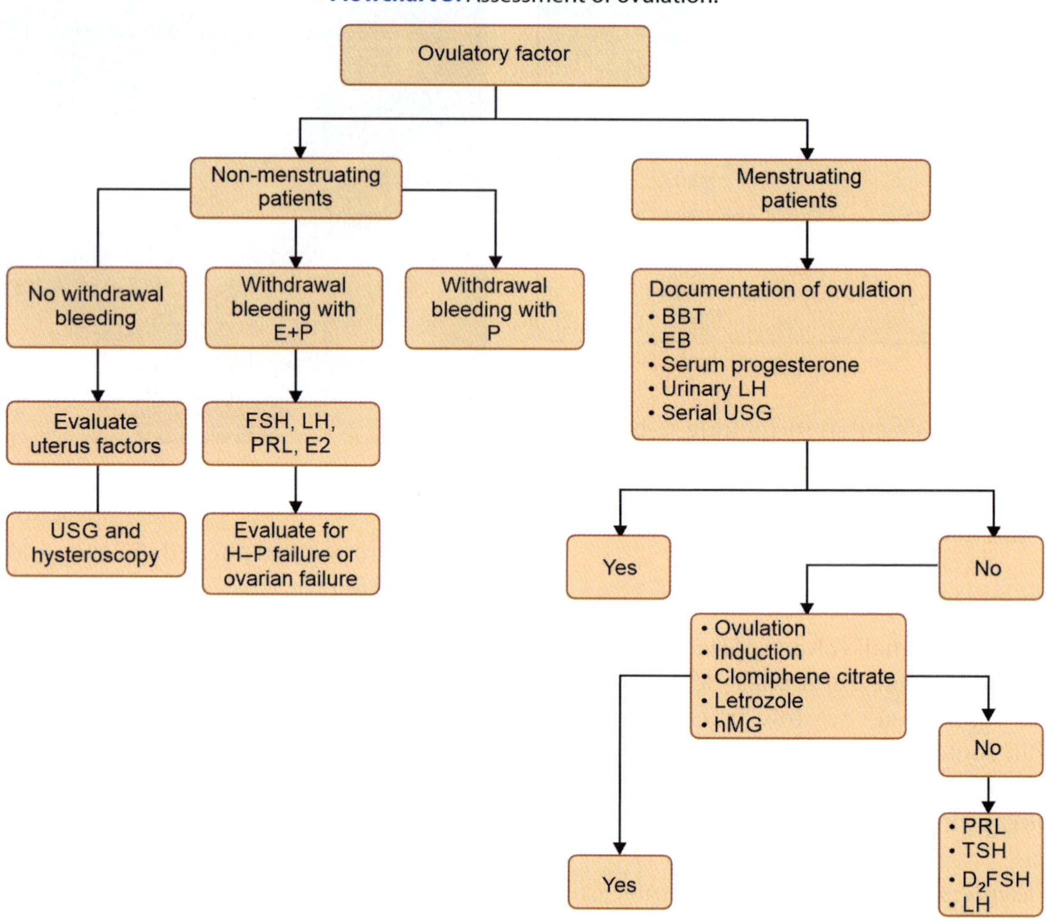

(BBT: basal body temperature; D_2FSH: day 2 follicle-stimulating hormone; E2: Oestradiol; EB: endometrial biopsy; FSH: follicle-stimulating hormone; hMG: human menopausal gonadotrophin; LH: luteinising hormone; PRL: prolactin; TSH: thyroid-stimulating hormone)

- *Intrauterine adhesions (Asherman's syndrome) due to previous overzealous curettage or previous surgery on the uterus*
- *Submucous polyp*
- *Uterine leiomyomas:* The mechanisms that apply here are discussed in Chapter 30: Tumours of the Cervix Uteri.

Cervical Factors

- Impenetrable cervical mucus or poorly penetrable mucus due to the presence of local sperm antibodies or due to low pH of the mucus at midcycle is a definite entity, the aetiology of which at present remains obscure.
- Loss of mucus due to amputation of the cervix, cone biopsies or over-enthusiastic cervical diathermy.
- Faulty direction of the cervix, such as is found in retroversion or severe prolapse.
- *Cervical stenosis:* Some of the women have a tight internal os, which may be found during procedures and needs dilatation.

Vaginal Factors

- *Purulent discharge:* This is a doubtful cause of infertility, because spermatozoa can thrive in pus under in vitro conditions. Moreover, clinical observations go to show that many women with chronic cervicitis and *Trichomonas vaginitis* conceive repeatedly without difficulty; some contract gonorrhoea and pregnancy simultaneously!
- Vaginal tumours, septa and membranes preventing the spermatozoa reaching the cervix.

Coital Errors

Apareunia and Dyspareunia

Of those women seeking advice on account of infertility, 1–2% are found not to have consummated their marriage. Many of these do not realise the fact, nor do their husbands.

Frequency and Timing of Coitus

Coitus has to take place every 48 hours during the fertile period to offer the optimum chance of conception. Too frequent coitus rarely, if ever, accounts for infertility.

Infrequency of coitus and attempts to limit it to the day of ovulation are much more important causes for failure to conceive.

Lubricants

When coitus is difficult due to a dry vagina many couples resort to using lubricants of one type or another without realising that these have a contraceptive action. Proprietary jellies are often acidic and therefore spermicidal, while greases such as soft paraffin and lanolin bring spermatozoa to a standstill.

Other Factors

Among the many factors popularly believed or alleged to lower fertility, the following deserve mention.

Orgasm

It is unnecessary for the woman to experience orgasm in order to conceive; if it were otherwise pregnancy would never result from rape.

Effluvium Seminis

Immediately after coitus most of the semen escapes from the vagina and patients often think this is the reason for infertility. *Effluvium seminis* is normal and is never a cause for infertility; there is always enough semen left behind for fertilisation. Only the spermatozoa which enter the cervical mucus are capable of fertilising an ovum, so the loss of the remainder is irrelevant. Spermatozoa only account for about 10% of the seminal fluid volume.

Anxiety and Apprehension

It is commonly believed that a nervous temperament, particularly extreme anxiety to conceive, lowers fertility. It is therefore often stated that when a couple adopt a baby, they are likely to have one of their own soon afterwards; this, however, has not been confirmed by statistics.

Familial Disposition; Genetic and Constitutional Factors

Some families appear to have a high, and others a low, conception rate but the explanation is generally not clear. The infertility which goes with obesity, heavy build, and masculine traits is merely one other manifestation of an underlying constitutional abnormality; weight (although it can affect the hypothalamic-pituitary-ovarian axis) and shape are not the direct causes of childlessness. Athletic prowess and pursuits are now recognised to lower fertility by virtue of anovulation and amenorrhoea.

Occupation and Environment

Fertility *appears* to be higher among rural than among urban dwellers, and amongst those who live by manual labour than amongst those whose work depends mostly on mental activity. Many factors may be responsible for this, including differences in the ages at which marriage takes place and in the practice of contraception in the various social classes. Statistics suggest that fertility does *not* vary *directly* with social class. However, various conditions do have a predilection for certain classes, for example, endometriosis in higher socioeconomic classes and pelvic inflammatory disease in lower socioeconomic classes; these relationships are reflected in statistics. There is also a trend in professional couples to defer pregnancy until careers are established. Attempts to conceive during the years of natural decline in fertility and a possible increase in gynaecological pathology (e.g. endometriosis) may distort the statistical analysis in future.

Diet

The diet should not be so deficient or unbalanced as to interfere with ovarian function, as in cases of anorexia nervosa. There is increasing evidence of the role of micronutrients in fertility. Deficiencies of zinc and folate are implicated in decreased spermatogenesis, possibly through defective DNA and RNA synthesis. Deficiency of dietary antioxidant micronutrients, e.g. β-carotene, lycopene, retinol, and α-tocopherol, may decrease genital tract secretions in men, leading to infertility, especially through immunological mechanisms.

Contraception

Hormonal contraceptives may sometimes result in a delay in the return of ovulation or in persistent anovulation, while intrauterine devices can cause salpingitis and tubal damage.

Postponement of childbearing by any means does, however, mean that time is passing, so even when contraception is discontinued, the age factor may be operating.

INVESTIGATION OF INFERTILITY

When should Infertility be Investigated?

A highly fertile couple practising coitus regularly takes an average of 6–7 months to achieve a pregnancy, and four out of five women conceive within 1 year of commencing regular coitus without contraception. Failure to conceive during 12–18 months despite adequate opportunity is, therefore, always acceptable as justifying full investigation. A strong case can be made for investigating infertility of only 1 year's duration—especially, if the woman is aged over 30 years or the man is aged over 40 years. A clinical examination of both partners, and possibly semen analysis, is indicated as soon as any couple becomes worried **(Flowchart 4)**.

An important preliminary to the investigation of infertility is to make certain that the woman is not suffering from a disability which might contraindicate pregnancy or make it undesirable. These conditions are present in 1% of women patients seeking advice, and it is poor practice to encourage a pregnancy which has to be terminated.

Clinical Assessment of Both Partners

History

The man and wife ideally should be questioned separately and then together, partly to have their evidence corroborated but mainly because either may have something to reveal confidentially. The special points on which information is required are as follows:

- Ages, occupations and previous marriages
- Duration of marriage and the period of time during which contraception has been practised
- Are the partners separated for significant periods of time?
- Previous illnesses and operations. Has the woman had appendicitis, peritonitis, tuberculosis in any site, or any operation on or near the genital tract? Has the man had orchitis, renal disease, bronchiectasis or any operation on or near the genital tract? Has either suffered from gonorrhoea or *Chlamydia* infection or symptoms suggesting them? Severe head injury, meningitis and encephalitis can affect the function of the hypothalamic-pituitary axis.

Flowchart 4: Diagnostic and treatment algorithm: Infertility.

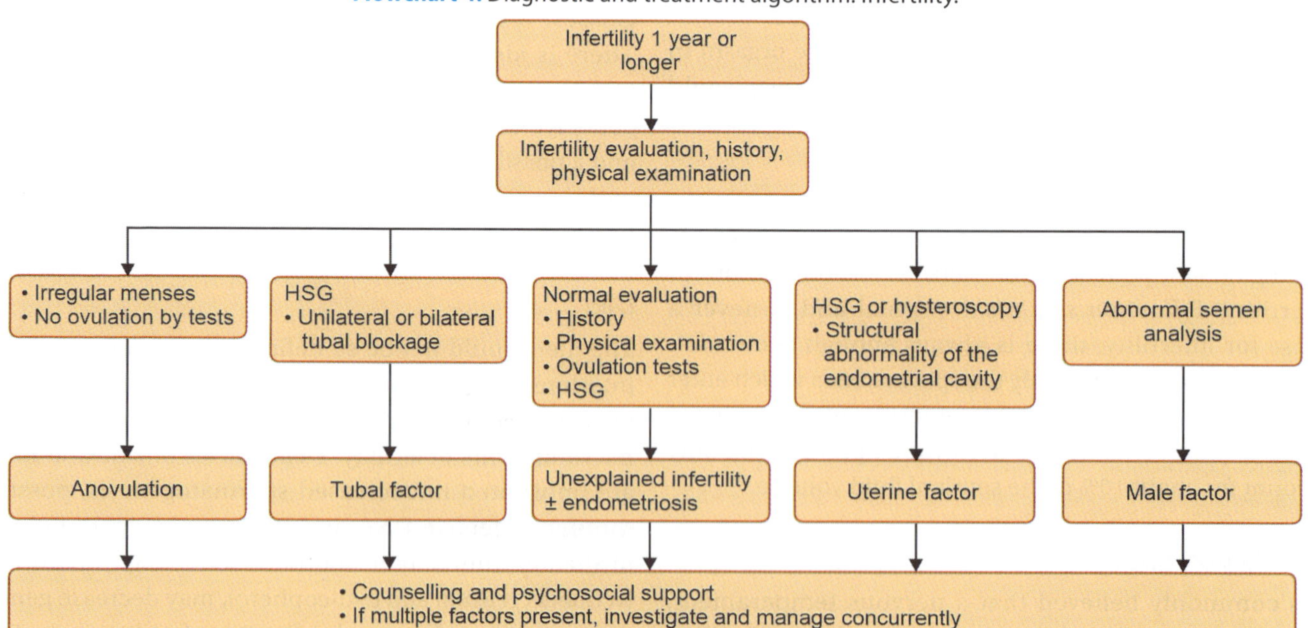

(HSG: hysterosalpingography)

- The family medical history of each, looking especially for tuberculosis on the woman's side.
- Has the woman ever been pregnant by her husband or by another man?
- Has the husband been responsible for a pregnancy in another woman?
- Is coitus normal and painless? How frequently is it practised and at what time in the cycle? Some couples have the wrong idea about the fertile period. More specific questions may be asked about their relationship and details regarding coitus, including erection, ejaculation, and penetration.
- Details of menstrual function, including factors which favour an ovulatory cycle.
- Does the woman have any other symptoms referred to the genital tract?
- Drugs, e.g. mefenamic acid taken for mittelschmerz pain, may interfere with ovulation. Drugs used for treating hypertension (e.g. guanethidine) may cause impotence, and salazopyrine (for ulcerative colitis), cytotoxic drugs, immunosuppressives and nitrofurantoin reduce the sperm count.
- Alcohol intake may reduce the potency and frequency of coitus.

Examination

This should cover all systems with particular attention to the reproductive systems where abnormalities of the penis; cryptorchidism; the size and consistency of the testes and epididymis; the presence of the vasa; a varicocele and any prostatic abnormality in the man; assessment of the vagina; the size, position and mobility of the uterus; and any enlargement or fixation of the adnexa in the woman should be looked for.

In all women with infertility, special attention must be paid to the body habitus, weight, thyroid, breast and note made of the presence of galactorrhoea, acne or hirsutism.

Assessment of Male Fertility

Clinical

Paternity is probably the best proof of male fertility, yet it can be misleading. The wide variation in results of semen analysis in fertile and infertile men at different times makes reassessment essential if a couple requests advice regarding their ability to conceive. Responsibility for two or more pregnancies, however, usually means good fertility, provided the effects of advancing years and of intercurrent disease can be excluded. There are, however, very few cases of infertile partnerships in which investigation of the male partner is not essential. Careful inquiry into past illnesses and examination of the genitalia usually reveal some abnormal finding in approximately 20–30% of infertile men. In others, it is disclosed only by semen analysis. Physical examination of the male is mandatory if semen analysis is abnormal.

Semen Analysis

The demonstration of spermatozoa in material removed from the vagina or cervix after coitus is *inadequate* for the purpose of assessing male fertility. Whatever be the findings on a postcoital test, full semen analysis is also essential.

For this purpose, semen collected in a condom during coitus is unsatisfactory because the rubber and its preservative powder are spermicidal. The specimen is best collected after 3 days of abstinence by masturbating directly into a dry and clean wide-mouthed glass container. It is kept as close as possible to body temperature (by carrying it in a hip pocket), and its examination is carried out as soon as possible after it has liquefied (this takes half an hour), preferably within 1 hour, as motility declines progressively with time. Collection under home conditions is generally preferred by the 'patient', but for optimal results, it is best carried out near the laboratory. Semen analysis should be carried out on *at least two different occasions if the first test suggests impaired fertility.*

Of all the characteristics of semen which can be studied, the essential ones are volume of fluid; number, motility, and morphology of spermatozoa **(Flowchart 5)**.

There is no such thing as a 'normal' semen because of the wide fluctuations present in anyone individual, but according to the WHO criteria, the volume should be 2–6 mL; liquefaction should be complete in 30 minutes; the sperm count should be 20 million/mL or more; 60% should have forward progressive motility or 25% or more should show rapid progression within 60 minutes of ejaculation and 70% or more must be morphologically normal. Fewer than 1 million white blood cells/mL should be present.

Computer-assisted semen analysis (CASA) was introduced to remove inconsistencies in sperm counts with

Flowchart 5: Algorithm for evaluation of semen analysis abnormalities.

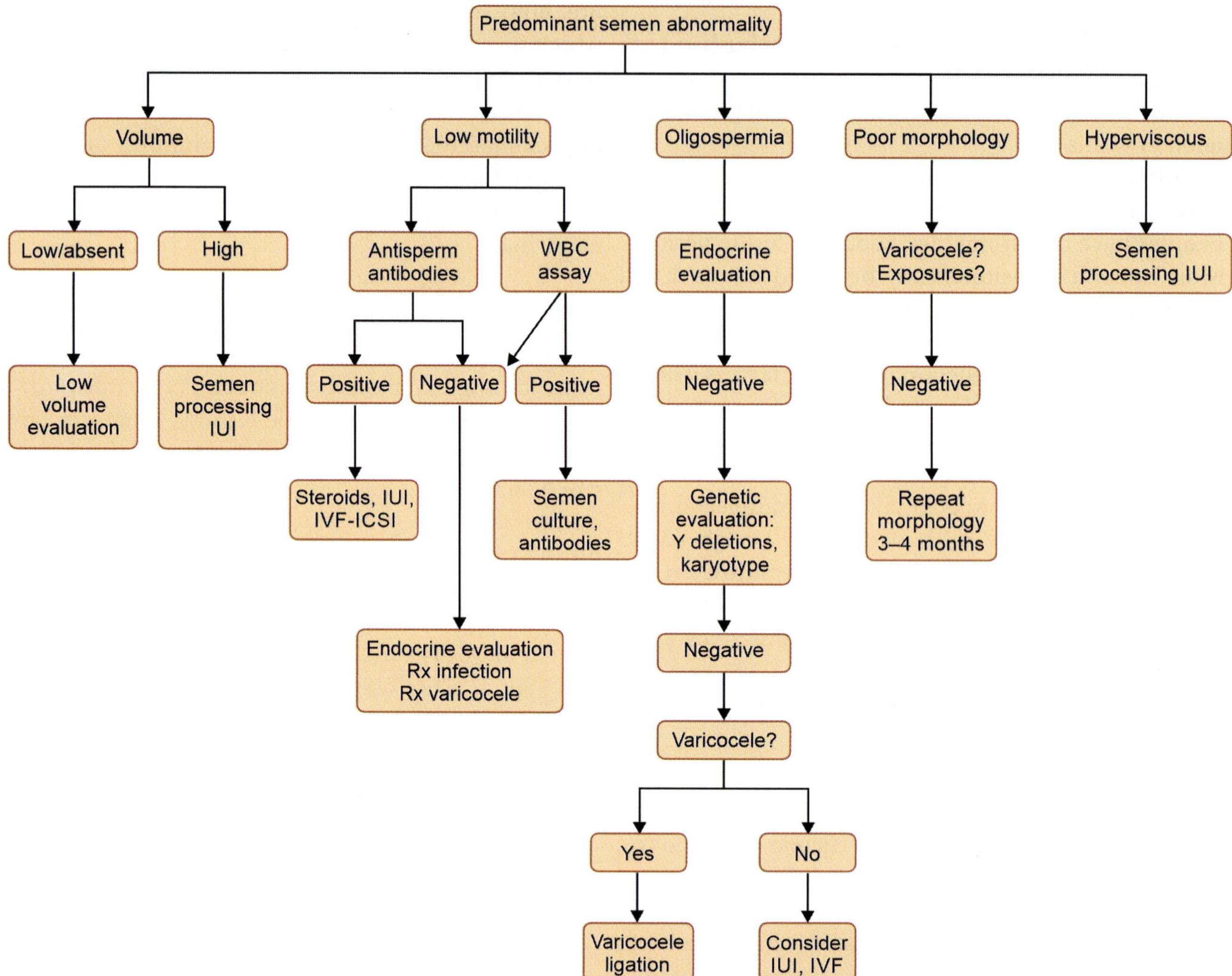

(ICSI: intracytoplasmic sperm injection; IUI: intrauterine insemination; IVF: in vitro fertilisation; WBC: white blood cell)

traditional methods. However, errors still occur, especially with low counts, when other cells can be miscounted as sperm. The CASA systems can also provide information on sperm velocity, which is suggestive.

Immature forms of spermatozoa are ranked as morphologically abnormal. Any one specimen is assessed by considering these features *in relation to each other*. For example, a low percentage of morphological abnormalities may compensate for a poor sperm count, while a small volume detracts from a high sperm density. A very high volume with resulting dilution can be a disadvantage.

Caution is necessary in interpreting the significance of the motility of spermatozoa, because this varies so much with the conditions of collection and storage of the specimen. When the number and morphology of spermatozoa are good, the finding of poor motility should be taken seriously, for it may be due to antisperm antibodies. True absence of motility *(necrospermia)* in a fresh and *otherwise* normal specimen is an extremely rare finding. Usually, 70–80% of spermatozoa are motile when the specimen is collected.

The presence of pus cells indicates an inflammatory lesion, usually in the prostate, but is not necessarily significant so far as fertility is concerned. Semen culture should be done. Urethral swabs are required for chlamydial culture. Most men with pyospermia prove fertile without treatment; nevertheless, pyospermia in an infertile man is best treated.

Fructose is secreted by the seminal vesicles and is essential to the metabolism of spermatozoa as it provides energy for their movements. At the time of ejaculation, semen contains 200–300 mg/dL fructose, but this falls to 100 mg/dL in 4–8 hours. When azoospermia is the result of an obstructive lesion, the absence of both fructose and spermatozoa indicates that the block is at or below the level of the ejaculatory ducts. Infection of the seminal vesicles also decreases the ejaculate volume, resulting in low fructose levels. Prostate infection can lead to obstructive oligozoospermia or azoospermia and a lowered zinc concentration.

When semen is not emitted and retrograde ejaculation is suspected, the urine collected immediately after orgasm should be examined for spermatozoa.

Low male fertility, as found on semen analysis, should be explained to the couple concerned, because it is impossible to interpret the results except in very general terms. An analysis from the infertility clinic in Liverpool showed that 33% of women complaining of primary infertility of not <2 years' duration, and whose husbands' sperm counts were <10 million/mL in average volume, subsequently conceived, without the male being treated or taking into consideration any female infertility factors which may also be present. However, the success rate as judged by conception in such cases is usually only about 10%.

Trial wash: It is now found that all semen samples should have sperm wash done to evaluate the motile sperm counts, and this is called a trial wash.

- Performed during semen analysis
- Evaluation of semen for various assisted conception procedures
- Helps to select suitable sperm wash methods and helps to plan treatment.

A number of motile spermatozoa inseminated (NMSI) and morphology on the success of intrauterine insemination (IUI) has been studied. When the NMSI was >5 million postwash with a normal morphology of >30%, the pregnancy rate per cycle was 18.42%, whereas if the NMSI was <5 million postwash and the morphology of <30%, the pregnancy rate per cycle was 5.43%. Hence, postwash samples with >5 million sperm count/mL of the total NMSI led to better pregnancy rates. However, in those who yield less NMSI, if a few cycles of IUI fail should be considered for assisted reproductive techniques (ART).

Sperm Function Tests

The lack of correlation between the various aspects of the semen analysis and fertility outcomes led to the development of tests for sperm function. However, these are also of limited utility because each of them tests only one aspect of sperm function. With the development of intracytoplasmic sperm injection (ICSI) (see further) their importance in clinical practice is doubtful.

Sperm function tests vary in their ability to detect defects in the complex processes leading to fertilisation, and are of limited use from a practical point of view (The ESHRE Capri Workshop 1996). Unless there is azoospermia, the predictive value of subnormal semen variables is limited. No functional test has yet been established that can unequivocally predict the fertilising capacity of spermatozoa.

Sperm Penetration Assay

Healthy sperm penetrate most, especially processed hamster ova from which the zona has been removed, and produce a significant degree of polyspermy per egg. The unhealthy sperm penetrate a lower number of ova and produce less polyspermy. A minimum of 10–30% of ova are normally penetrated. The results of the test vary from time to time in the same individual and do not correlate with eventual fertility. However, this helps in the early identification of patients who may be better suited for ICSI or donor insemination, especially in cases of unexplained infertility.

In Vitro Sperm Penetration Tests

If the postcoital test (see further) is poor, an alternative test is to place a drop of sperm on a glass slide alongside commercially available bovine mucus and to microscopically study its invasion by the spermatozoa (sperm penetration test). A modification of this type of test is to use an in vitro cross-over sperm-cervical mucus contact test (SCMCT), that is, to use mid-cycle mucus and semen of the couple under question and compare it with donor sperm and donor mucus (Kremer test). However, these are of little practical value as couples with poor postcoital tests or unexplained infertility will be treated with IUI.

Other Tests

The CASA systems can provide information on the number of spermatozoa in a hyperactivated motility state, which is suggestive of *capacitation* and on the *hypo-osmotic swelling* test, which assesses the tail membrane function. Nonmotile sperm with a positive hypo-osmotic test are reported to do better with ICSI than nonmotile and negative hypo-osmotic test sperm.

The *hemizona* assay tests the ability of the sperm to pass through the zona of the human egg. This test is no longer done following the development of ICSI.

Sperm Antibodies

Semen is known to be highly antigenic, and sperm antibodies are a known cause of infertility. Agglutination is the sticking together of sperm in variable patterns, e.g. head-to-head, tail-to-tail, mixed agglutination. It is caused by antisperm antibodies, which are usually immunoglobulin A (IgA) or IgG. Further tests, such as the immunobead or mixed antiglobulin reaction (MAR) test, can be done for the detection of these antibodies in semen. The immunobead test can also be used to detect antibodies in serum or cervical mucus. With this test, <20% of sperm should be covered with adherent particles or beads.

These tests are indicated when the semen analysis shows oligozoospermia or azoospermia, spontaneous sperm agglutination or low motility, an abnormal postcoital test, in the presence of infection, if there is failure of conception after vasectomy and in cases of unexplained infertility.

Hormonal Assessment

Up to 10% of subfertile males have endocrine abnormalities. Routine testing for endocrine dysfunction is not indicated, but should be carried out in those men found to have oligospermia or azoospermia. FSH, LH, prolactin and testosterone levels are helpful in this assessment.

A raised FSH level reflects failure of spermatogenesis. Low levels of FSH and LH are diagnostic of hypogonadotrophic hypogonadism. Normal FSH levels with normal testes but azoospermia suggest obstruction. Raised LH levels with low testosterone levels indicate Leydig cell dysfunction. A low testosterone level warrants replacement therapy.

Prolactin levels are not done routinely. Rarely, in cases of impotence or decreased libido, hyperprolactinaemia is seen without evidence of hypogonadism.

Thyroid dysfunction is so rarely a factor in men that it is not necessary to assess thyroid-stimulating hormone (TSH) levels unless clinical features indicate it.

Testicular Biopsy

Testicular biopsy is generally not recommended as the disruption of the blood-testis barrier can lead to the development of autoimmunity against spermatozoa. It is indicated in cases of azoospermia with normal FSH and inconclusive seminal markers to distinguish between a failure in spermatogenesis and an obstruction to the outflow of spermatozoa. It also reveals whether the tubules are basically normal but unstimulated or whether they are incapable of functioning. Examination of the material obtained requires a histologist with special experience.

Varicocele Assessment and Significance

A varicocele is a collection of dilated veins in the spermatic cord and is a common physical anomaly. Varicoceles are found in 11.7% of men with normal semen and 25.4% of men with abnormal semen (WHO 1992). The mechanism by which varicoceles might impair fertility and spermatogenesis is not clear. Varicoceles may be associated with decreased ipsilateral testicular volume, elevated scrotal temperature and pain, as well as impaired semen quality (WHO 1992). A review of several randomised controlled trials showed that varicocele repair did not improve pregnancy rates. Some studies on varicocele are contrary. It was found that following varicocele surgery, a rise in sperm count was seen in 31% when it was <5 million/mL prior to surgery. Hence, if there are gross varicoceles in an individual who has fluctuating levels of sperm count and motility, varicocele surgery may be worth a try. If there is an improvement in the count and motility following varicocele surgery, then the couple may benefit by IUI in some cases rather than having the only option in vitro fertilisation (IVF) or ICSI.

Other Tests

Vasography is used in cases of proximal vas deferens obstruction before microsurgical repair. Transrectal ultrasonography is combined with seminal vesiculography to demonstrate ejaculatory duct obstruction. Chromosomal analysis is indicated in men with eunuchoid features and oligozoospermia, who may have the 47, XXY complement of Klinefelter syndrome (seen in 2% of men with oligozoospermia). A high prevalence of Y chromosome submicroscopic deletions is also reported in oligozoospermic men.

Assessment of Female Infertility

Importance of Body Mass Index and Obesity

Effect of fat on hormones:

- Effects not only on gonadotrophin secretion but also 17-β-oestradiol metabolism
- It metabolises to weaker oestrogen-oestriol
- There is also conversion of androstenedione to oestrone in peripheral adipose tissue.

Body mass index (BMI):

- Obesity >30 kg/m^2
- Average = 25 kg/m^2
- Requires treatment >28 kg/m^2.

Significance of Basal Hormonal Evaluation

An elevated basal day-3 FSH is correlated with diminished ovarian reserve in women aged over 35 years and is associated with poor pregnancy rates after treatment of ovulation induction.

Basal levels <10 mIU/mL are considered normal for a normal ovarian reserve. It has been reported that pregnancy rates decline significantly as day-3 FSH rises above 15 mIU/mL. Very few pregnancies were reported when FSH exceeded 25 mIU/mL. Basal LH values of >10 IU/L are not a good value as this high LH will deteriorate the quality of oocytes.

Estimation of the Time and Frequency of Ovulation

After the basic work-up has been done, it may be wise, even in regularly menstruating women, to look for presumptive evidence of ovulation or luteinisation. The methods for assessment are described in Chapter 5: Clinical Aspects of Menstruation and Ovulation, but the one which has been overemphasised in recent years is the daily temperature record. This method has the advantage of indicating the approximate time of ovulation, and therefore the time when coitus is most likely to be fruitful. Its disadvantages are that it is a daily reminder of childlessness; it tends to make couples time their acts of intercourse with a mathematical precision and changes married love into a coldly calculated duty. When temperature recording is considered necessary, it should never be continued for longer than 3–4 months, by which time it should be possible to assess the ovulation habit. Ovulation pain (Mittelschmerz) is also an indication of ovulation.

Ultrasonography

Baseline *transvaginal ultrasound scan:* This is done to identify uterine abnormalities such as endometrial polyps, submucosal fibroids or congenital defects. The findings of a thin endometrium (<4 mm) and quiescent ovaries on the baseline scan reflect the hypo-oestrogenic state of the early follicular phase, which provide the optimal conditions with which to commence treatment. Conversely, a thick endometrium represents endogenous hormonal stimulation above normal basal levels and indicates that the patient should not initiate the cycle.

Unilocular, clear cysts may represent functional cysts or unruptured luteinised cysts. Complex ovarian cysts detected at baseline usually reflect old haemorrhagic corpus lutea and are commonly seen if the patient has been treated with gonadotrophins in the previous cycle. Nevertheless, the differential diagnoses, including endometrioma **(Fig. 2)**, benign ovarian tumour, or malignancy, must be considered. The management of ovarian cysts present at baseline is controversial. More importantly, these ovarian cysts tend to resolve spontaneously within 1–2 months. Low-dose oral contraceptive has a lower efficacy than older, high-dose oral contraceptives in preventing the formation of new cysts. Since oral contraceptives do not affect the speed of resolution of old cysts, they are not necessary in this scenario. Evidence of ovarian endometriomas can be made out.

Ultrasound is commonly used to track follicle development and is better observed with transvaginal than with abdominal ultrasound. The follicle size at ovulation is

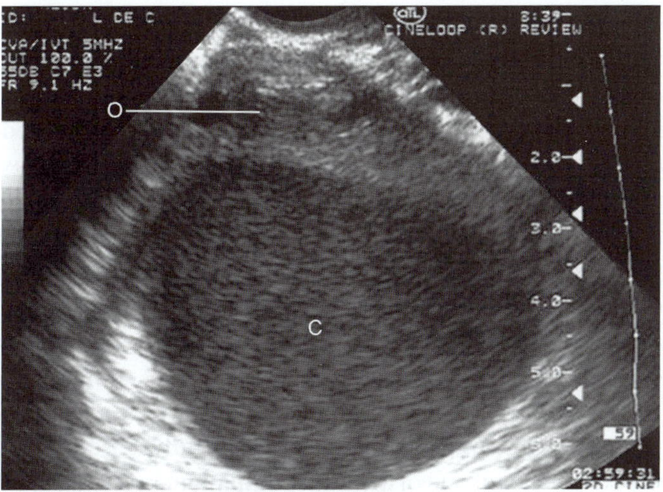

Fig. 2: Chocolate cyst.

very variable, but usually the dominant follicle is 17 mm in diameter. Follicles are larger in stimulated cycles, being 18–20 mm in diameter and larger with clomiphene than with human menopausal gonadotrophin (hMG).

The endometrium increases in thickness from a thin broken line in the early follicular phase to double its size; in the periovulatory period, it appears sonographically as a triple layer in the long axis of the uterus and is usually about 10–12 mm in diameter. The luteal endometrium loses both the hyperechogenicity and the triple-layered appearance.

The diagnosis of luteinised unruptured follicle is made on ultrasound when the follicle does not rupture, although serum progesterone rises to postovulatory levels.

Hormone Assays

Serum progesterone level measured during the mid-luteal phase is the most reliable method of confirming ovulation, the minimum level being 6.5 ng/mL and preferably over 10 ng/mL. A single low progesterone level is insufficient to judge the adequacy of the luteal phase.

Detection of the preovulatory LH surge has also been used to predict ovulation. Urinary LH kits and salivary progesterone have been used as discussed in Chapter 5: Clinical Aspects of Menstruation and Ovulation. However, hormone tests are expensive and not universally available.

Other hormones which may need to be assessed are free T3, T4 and TSH, serum FSH and LH in the immediate postmenstrual phase, and serum prolactin.

Endometrial Biopsy

There is no consensus of opinion about the diagnosis or effective treatment of luteal phase defect, and its role as a cause of infertility has been questioned. The benefit of treatment for luteal phase defect on pregnancy rates has not been established. Women should not be offered an endometrial biopsy to evaluate the luteal phase as part of the investigation of fertility problems because there is no evidence that medical treatment of luteal phase defect improves pregnancy rates. However, in a developing country where tuberculosis is suspected, and a thin endometrium is seen, there is a role for endometrial curettage in selected cases.

Endometrial aspiration or biopsy taken in the premenstrual phase can be histologically dated. This procedure is still one of the initial outpatient investigations in developing countries where genital tuberculosis is a significant problem. Alternatively, it can be carried out in conjunction with laparoscopy under general anaesthesia. If the endometrium in the second half of the menstrual cycle is found to be in a secretory phase, it can be presumed that, during that cycle at least, the woman ovulated. A diagnosis of luteal phase defect can be made if the endometrium is 2–3 days out of phase from the day of cycle on repeated biopsy, but this is not always accurate. Curetted material is also sent for bacteriological evaluation for acid-fast bacilli. Polymerase chain reaction (PCR) for *Mycobacterium tuberculosis* can be done in selected cases depending on the clinical profile.

Tubal Patency Tests

These are best carried out between the 7th and 10th day of the cycle. At that time, there is practically no risk of disturbing a fertilised ovum. The risk of embolism and of retrograde dissemination of infection and endometriosis makes it imperative not to carry out the tests while any uterine bleeding is taking place and for 2 days afterwards.

Hysterosalpingography (HSG) ***(Figs. 3 to 5):*** HSG entails injecting a nonirritant radio-opaque material through the cervix into the uterus and tubes without general anaesthesia in a radiological department.

With the cannula in place and the patient lying in the lithotomy position, the radio-opaque material is injected slowly from a syringe, the amount required varying from 2 to 20 mL. The flow through the uterus and tubes is observed by screening, with films being exposed at suitable intervals. This relatively simple procedure requires skill and experience to obtain the most instructive radiographs. In not <15% of cases in which salpingography shows apparent bilateral tubal obstruction, subsequent events and findings prove the tubes to be normal. False-positive radiographs are rare but can result if the tubes are unusually long with dilated closed extremities. Administration of atropine or nonsteroidal anti-inflammatory drugs (NSAIDs) before the procedure decreases false-positive results caused by corneal spasm.

It must be kept in mind that screening of the patient and the taking of no more than two radiographs involves some radiation exposure to the ovaries. To reduce this risk to a minimum, an image intensifier should be connected to a closed-circuit television screen.

The media presently used for injection are usually water-soluble, e.g. diatrizoate (Hypaque 60) or iothalamate (Conray 60). These are the least dangerous, but they are

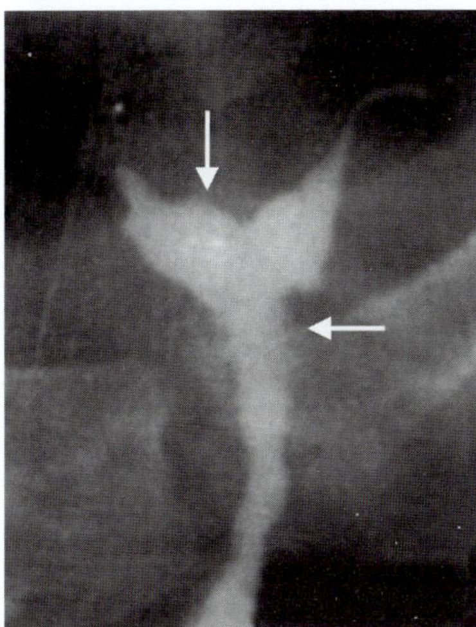

Fig. 3: Hysterosalpingography cornual block.

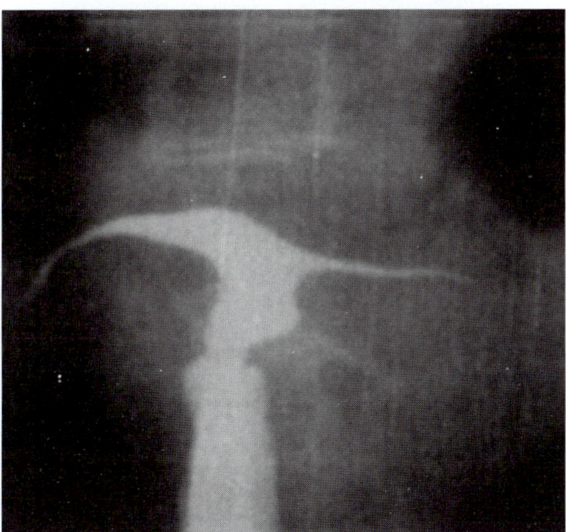

Fig. 4: Hysterosalpingography mid-tubal block.

quickly absorbed and are of less value in diagnosing peritubal adhesions than the older oily preparations, e.g. ethiodol. After screening, a film is taken; this and a repeat film 20–30 minutes later reveal all the necessary information (with oily preparations, delayed films were also taken). Sometimes the medium is seen to loculate in the pelvis; this is a valuable pointer to a diagnosis of peritubal adhesions, which interfere with the tubo-ovarian pathway **(Figs. 6 to 9)**.

Hysterosalpingography not only indicates the state of each tube and reveals the site of any obstruction **(Fig. 9C)**, but it also provides information about the uterine cavity. There may be some therapeutic benefit in the first few cycles following the procedure, but this is seen more often with oil-based dyes, which can displace the debris.

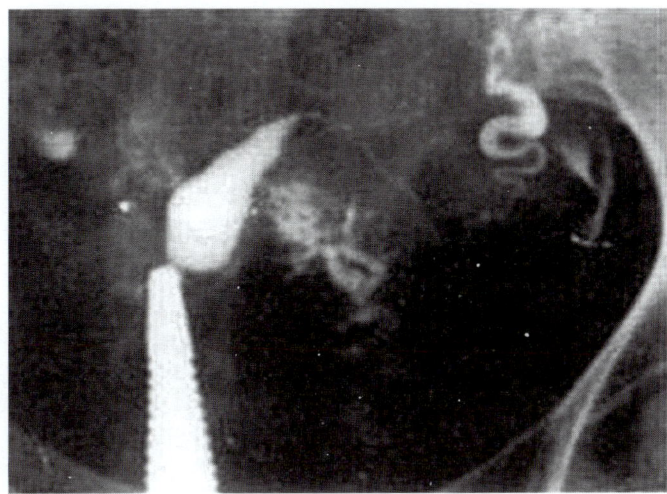

Fig. 5: Hysterosalpingography unicornuate uterus with the patent tube.

Hysterocontrast sonography (HyCoSy): In HyCoSy, a combination of air and saline or contrast medium (Echovist-200) is introduced into the uterus transcervically. The flow of the medium seen in some unanaesthetised women is more through the uterus and tubes, and its spill into the pelvis with water-soluble media than with oily or non-ionic media is monitored by ultrasound. This procedure may have certain complications, such as immediate pain, vomiting and may have hypotension and shock due to manipulation with instruments, leading to vasovagal problems.

Embolism, intravasation: The frequency of gas embolism is unknown, because it is usually subclinical and passes unrecognised. It presumably equals that of intravasation of radio-opaque material, which occurs in 1–2% of women subjected to HSG **(Figs. 10A to E)**. In this respect, oily preparations are more dangerous than aqueous ones because they cause embolism. While screening, entry of the medium into the veins can be visualised during injection and an embolism recognised at once; the injection can then be discontinued.

The occurrence of intravasation should always raise the possibility of endometrial tuberculosis and if the tubes are also obstructed, it is almost diagnostic of this disease.

Intravasation is sometimes into lymphatics and not blood vessels **(Fig. 10E)**. The resulting picture is typical and if radiographs are taken 24 hours later, collection of the medium in the pelvic lymph nodes is often demonstrable. This accident is of interest but not serious. The same is true when, at the time of laparoscopy, dye

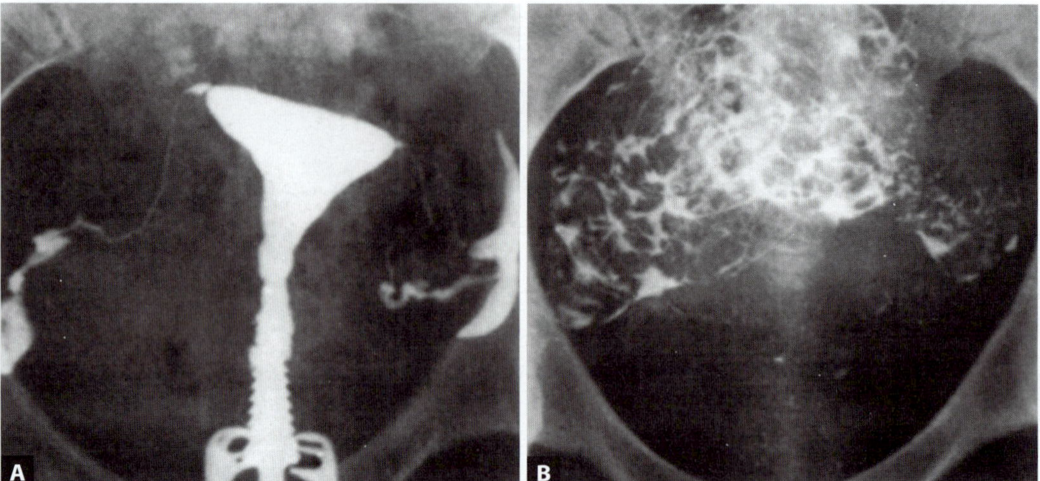

Figs. 6A and B: Hysterosalpingography showing normal tubal patency. An oily radio-opaque dye was used. (A) The initial injection shows a normal uterus except for a poor isthmic constriction. Each outer tubal junction shows a ring of muscle spasm, which is a common and insignificant finding. Both tubes are patent, and the medium is escaping into the peritoneal cavity; (B) A straight radiograph taken 24 hours later shows that the medium is freely disseminated in the pelvis.

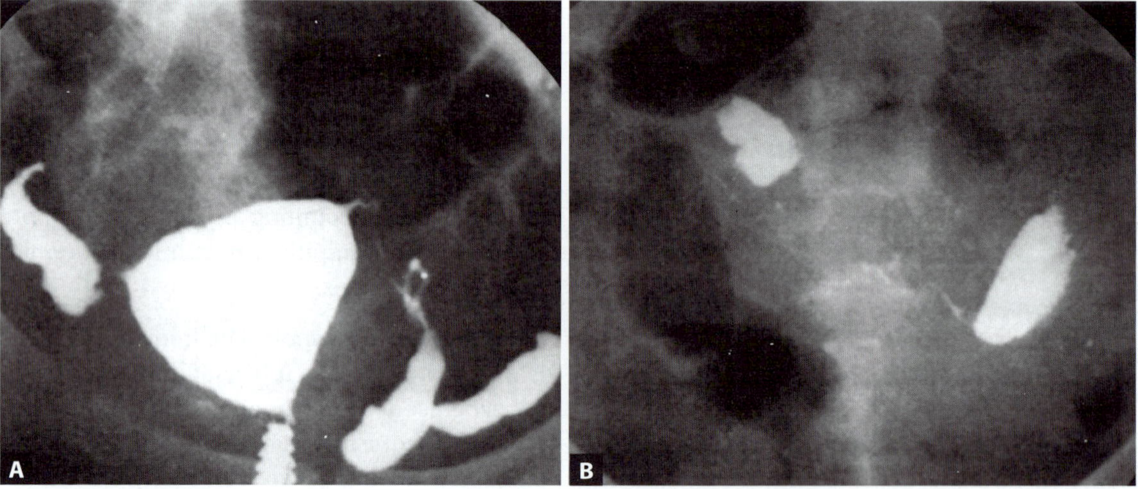

Figs. 7A and B: Hysterosalpingography showing both tubes obstructed at their outer ends and a uterine cavity which is slightly enlarged and irregular in shape as a result of small leiomyomas. The patient in this case complained of infertility and gave a history of contact with tuberculosis in adolescence. Tubal patency tests were therefore avoided until the endometrium was proved bacteriologically negative for this disease. Ultimately, however, tubercle bacilli were cultured from the tubes. (A) Radiograph at the time of injection shows dilated and closed outer ends of the tubes; (B) The medium is retained in the tubes 24 hours later.

injected through the cervix enters the circulation to produce a blue uterus and subsequently blue urine.

Peritoneal reaction and infection: Pelvic peritonitis and salpingitis follow HSG in 0.5–1.0% of cases. The infection is not usually introduced at the time of the injection but represents an exacerbation of a previously dormant salpingitis. Prophylactic antibiotics should be administered if tubal disease is discovered.

Generalised sensitivity reaction: Reactions can occur to chemicals, such as iodine, which may be in the medium. The new nonionic materials are safer in this respect but are more expensive.

Abortion: Unless care is taken, and especially when the patient has an irregular menstrual cycle, it is easy to carry out a tubal patency test in the presence of an early pregnancy. This is the reason that the 10-day rule

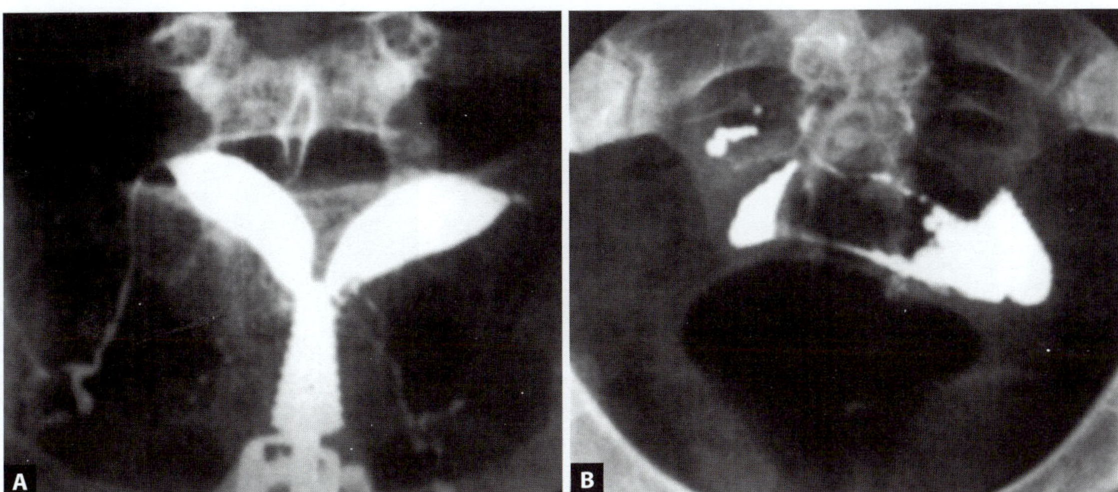

Figs. 8A and B: Hysterosalpingography in the case of a woman aged 28 years who complained of infertility following the birth of her first child 4 years previously. The labour was complicated by adherence of the placenta, which had to be removed manually. (A) This radiograph shows the uterus to be bicornuate (hence the trouble with the third stage of labour), and the right tube closed at its outer end, which is the site of a small hydrosalpinx. The left tube is doubtfully patent; (B) This radiograph, taken 24 hours later, shows the small hydrosalpinx on the right with loculation in the pelvis of medium which passed through the left tube. This means peritubal adhesions dating from puerperal infection.

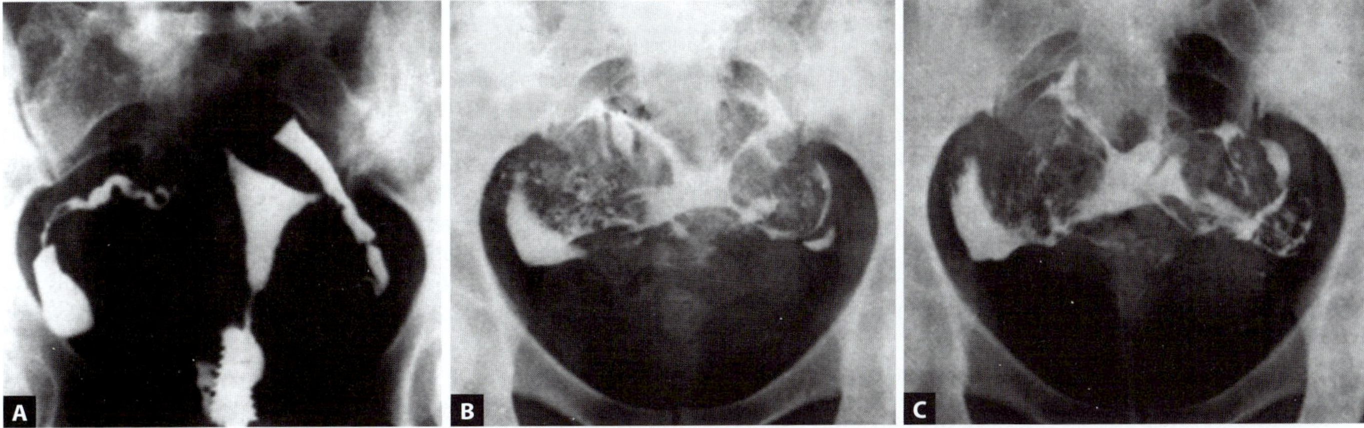

Figs. 9A to C: The diagnosis of intrapelvic adhesions by hysterosalpingography. (A) An apparently normal hysterosalpingogram showing both tubes patent; (B) A film exposed 24 hours later shows some spread, but an unusual distribution of the medium in the pelvis; (C) A radiograph taken 8 days later shows an almost identical distribution of the medium, strongly suggesting that its dissemination is impeded by adhesions.

(no X-rays after day 10 of the cycle) should be rigidly applied in infertility investigations.

Contraindications to Tubal Patency Tests

In view of the above considerations, tubal patency tests are to be avoided during and immediately before menstruation, after curettage, when there is a history of recently active salpingitis, if there is any reason to suspect the presence of active tuberculosis of the genital tract, and when there is evidence of infection of the lower genital tract, such as a purulent discharge.

Hysteroscopy and Laparoscopy

In many centres, hysteroscopy and laparoscopy are now used as the principal methods of assessment of the pelvic organs and of tubal patency. Instillation of a dye, e.g. methylene blue, through a balloon catheter or cannula in the cervix (chromopertubation) permits direct

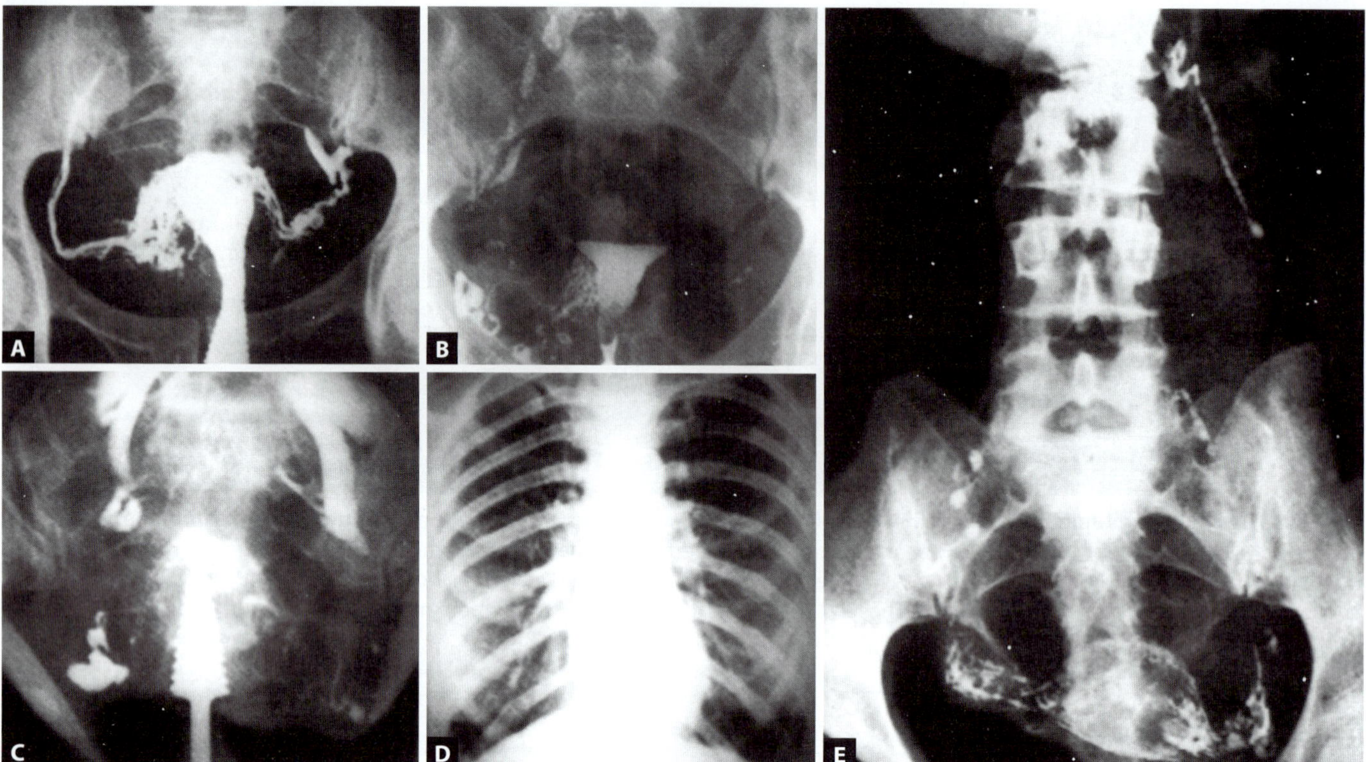

Figs. 10A to E: Some examples of intravasation of the medium during hysterosalpingography, which happens in at least 1% of cases despite all precautions. It rarely has serious consequences if screening is employed, because this allows the injection to be stopped immediately. In any case, safety is provided by the fact that no more than one ampoule of the radio-opaque fluid (20 mL) is injected. Intravasation with gas during insufflation is potentially more dangerous, because the volume is often not controlled or restricted. (A) The medium enters the wall of the fundus of the uterus and drains into the ovarian veins; (B) Medium entering the pampiniform plexus and draining via the internal and common iliac veins. Its oily nature is illustrated by its forming globules in the blood; (C) Medium diffused through the vessels of the cervix and draining into the internal iliac veins; (D) The same case as Figure 10C showing evidence of oil emboli in the lungs several hours later; the patient remained asymptomatic; (E) Lymphatic intravasation. This radiograph was taken 24 hours after salpingography and shows the medium diffused through the lymphatics of the uterine wall and broad ligament; it is also in the main trunks leading to the para-aortic nodes. The medium is slow to clear from lymphatics but clears from veins within seconds or minutes.

visualisation of its path through the tube and the exact site of block, if any. The fimbriae can be visualised directly, and the spill of the dye from each side confirmed. As the procedure is done under anaesthesia, corneal spasm as a cause of false tubal blockage is excluded. Intrauterine lesions and peritoneal and pelvic factors are better demonstrated by the simultaneous use of hysteroscopy and laparoscopy; in many cases, operative correction can be carried out at the same time.

The expense and limited availability of these techniques do not permit their universal use for initial evaluation.

Hysteroscopy should, however, be considered *mandatory* if the following are suspected on HSG or on transvaginal sonography: An intrauterine lesion, e.g. leiomyoma or endometrial polyp; a congenital uterine anomaly; intrauterine adhesions because of past history of uterine curettage, complicated forceps delivery, severe pelvic inflammatory disease, puerperal sepsis or recurrent miscarriage; and, in women undergoing IVF, failure of implantation of embryos after three cycles.

Similarly, *laparoscopy is warranted where* history or physical examination suggests the presence of pelvic disease, endometriosis, in cases of unexplained infertility or where HSG suggests tubal block or peritubal adhesions. However, neither hysteroscopy nor laparoscopy can provide information about internal tubal architecture, and HSG is indicated if, for example, salpingitis isthmica nodosa is suspected.

Salpingoscopy can evaluate internal tubal anatomy, but it is not widely available as a clinical service.

The falloposcope can be introduced through the laparoscope as well as transcervically.

On laparoscopy, an infertility factor will be found in 30–50% of women previously regarded as having normal genitalia. The unexpected findings are commonly peritubal or periovarian adhesions and endometriosis. Laparoscopy should be delayed unless symptoms indicate pelvic pathology, as many couples conceive with preliminary reassurance and simple investigations within 6 months of being seen for advice and investigation. Premature diagnosis of minimal endometriosis, for example, may hinder fertility prospects rather than aid them, by resulting in 6–9 months' 'contraceptive' hormone treatment being given.

At the time of laparoscopy, the patency of the tubes is confirmed by injecting dye through the cervix and watching its passage along the tubes and through the abdominal ostia **(Fig. 11)**.

The dye used in laparoscopy may produce a chemical peritonitis, but this is transient and settles as the dye disperses. Therapeutic procedures such as division of adhesions, salpingostomy, ovarian cystectomy or fulguration of endometrial deposits, can be undertaken at the same time. This may necessitate the use of additional puncture sites or ports. Detailed documentation of all the laparoscopic findings and the procedure executed is important for proper management subsequently. Video recordings can also be made and provided to the patients.

Postcoital Test

The postcoital test is a simple clinical test of the sperm-cervical mucus interaction.

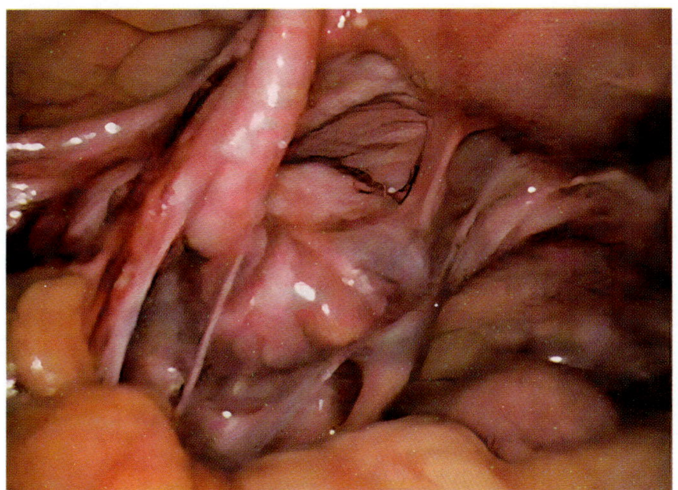

Fig. 11: Blocked tubes.

Mucus is removed from the *cervix* with a nasal polyp forceps, a pipette or a tuberculin syringe and examined at various times after coitus *(Sim's test, Hühner's test)*, to see if the mucus is invaded by spermatozoa and whether they retain their activity. The test must be carried out at the time of ovulation because at other times the cervical mucus is normally unreceptive. Preovulatory cervical mucus is normally thin, clear, abundant, and stretchable (spinnbarkeit >8–10 cm) with good tertiary ferning and low cellularity.

There is no agreement as to the criteria for a satisfactory result. Examinations are advised within 2–8 hours of coitus; the number of spermatozoa and the extent of their motility, which should be found in the mucus at those times, are matters of opinion. Some authorities say that normally, 2–8 hours after coitus, 15 spermatozoa are found in each high-power field and that these show progressive, not rotatory, activity. However, the results of the postcoital test correlate poorly with the pregnancy rates. Any purposeful forward progression should be regarded as a positive test, whereas the finding of no sperm, all dead sperm, less than three motile sperm per high-power field and sperm shaking without progression should suggest the presence of an immunological factor (or the use of vaginal lubricants). These patients can be evaluated by sperm function tests (*see* further).

The value of postcoital testing of cervical mucus for the presence of motile sperm is controversial and is a subject of continuing debate. The routine use of postcoital testing of cervical mucus in the investigation of fertility problems is not recommended, because it has no predictive value on pregnancy rate.

Screening for Chlamydia Trachomatis

Chlamydia trachomatis is present in 11% of the sexually active population aged 19 years or less. It is a major cause of pelvic inflammatory disease, leading to chronic abdominal pain, ectopic pregnancy and tubal factor infertility. Asymptomatic chlamydial infection may go unrecognised and untreated. Both doxycycline and azithromycin are effective prophylaxis and treatment for *chlamydia*. There is evidence that screening for and treating cervical chlamydial infection can reduce the incidence of pelvic inflammatory disease in women at increased risk of *Chlamydia* infection. Prophylactic antibiotics should be considered before uterine instrumentation if screening has not been carried out. Tubal disease includes tubal obstruction and pelvic adhesions due to infection, endometriosis and previous surgery. Endometriosis accounts for about 5% of female infertility. The diagnosis and severity of endometriosis are established by laparoscopy. However, disease severity has not been shown to predict the chance of pregnancy. It has been found that women with positive *Chlamydia* have more distal tubal problems, and hence it may be worthwhile considering a diagnostic laparoscopy for those women who have positive *Chlamydia* testing so that delay in the management is not present. Elevated titres of chlamydial antibodies in women are significantly associated with tubal disease.

Unexplained Infertility

Unexplained infertility is idiopathic in the sense that its cause remains unknown even after an infertility workup, usually including semen analysis in the man and assessment of ovulation and fallopian tubes in the woman. Up to 25% of infertile couples have unexplained infertility. The treatment algorithm for cases of unexplained female infertility is described in **Flowchart 6**.

TREATMENT

The objective of treatment is to eliminate as far as possible any infertility factors found in either husband or wife. Systemic diseases and other obvious diseases in the genital tracts are treated. The benefits of treatment for minimal endometriosis must be justifiable. In fact, anovulation is the only condition for which one can give a good prognosis statistically. In many other instances, an explanation of the findings and a defined period of waiting are often more appropriate. Both partners should be considered together because incurable infertility in one can sometimes be cancelled out by raising the fertility of the other.

In about 10–20% of couples, basic investigations are normal, and this is the group labelled as unexplained infertility. 60–70% of this group are found to conceive within 3 years without any further treatment.

Both Partners

Reassurance

Reassurance may be all that is necessary when couples complain of infertility too soon. They appreciate a simple account of the physiology of conception and an explanation of the fact that the mathematical chances of conception are not as high as they imagined. In all cases, *optimism should be the keynote*, tempered with realism, even when the investigations suggest that the prospects for pregnancy are poor.

Flowchart 6: Treatment algorithm for unexplained female infertility.

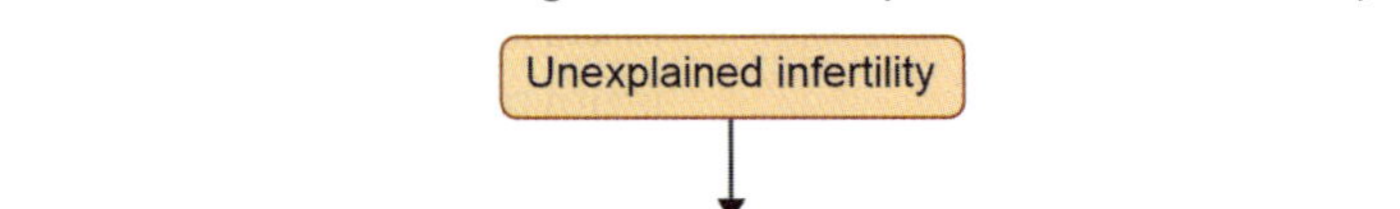

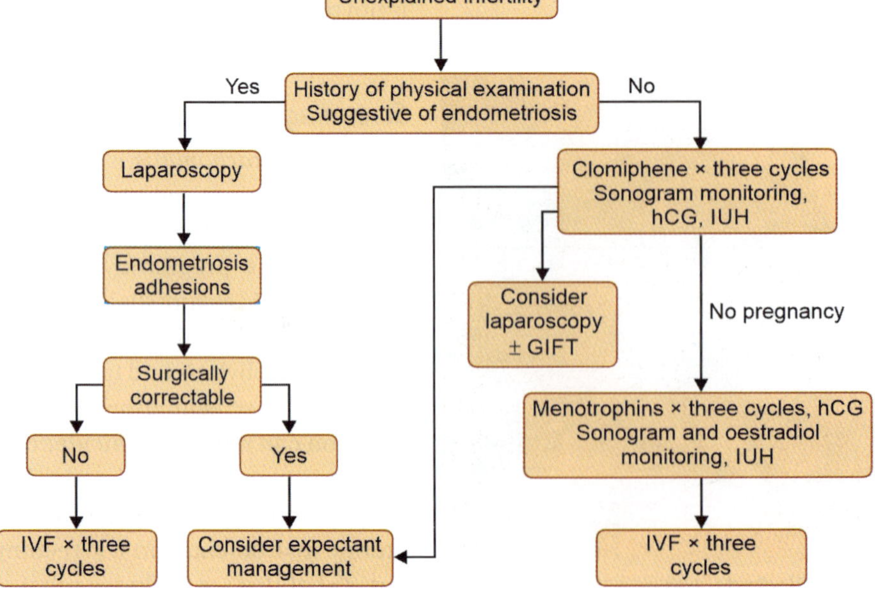

(GIFT: gamete intrafallopian transfer; hCG: human chorionic gonadotrophin; IUH: intrauterine insemination with washed husband's sperm; IVF: in vitro fertilisation

Correction of Coital Difficulties

Some couples require instruction on the difficulties of coitus, on its timing and spacing. They should not be advised to try to time coitus to coincide with ovulation and to conserve their energies at other times. They should follow their natural inclinations, but keep in mind that conception is most likely between the 10th and 18th day of a 28-day cycle, at which time coitus should be practised at 48-hour intervals.

Change in coital position can be tried in case of mechanical difficulty. Immediately after coitus, the wife should rest quietly for 10 minutes to ensure that some semen remains in contact with the cervix, though it is doubtful whether this is further encouraged by elevating the buttocks on a pillow.

Correction of General Ill Health

Under this heading are attention to matters such as overwork, anxiety, obesity and intemperance in smoking and drinking. Along carefree holiday may sometimes be the answer.

Husband

Impotence and Premature Ejaculation

Refer to Chapter 46.

Defective Spermatogenesis

The treatment of faulty spermatogenesis is not very satisfactory, and the outlook is poor. Attention to general health, obesity and mode of existence offers the best hope. Suspensory bandages and warm, tight underclothing should be avoided, and cold baths encouraged. Any infection in the prostate or other part of the urinary tract should be eradicated. Alcohol and smoking are restricted **(Flowchart 7)**. There is no consensus of opinion regarding the treatment of varicocele, although this is often done in the absence of other obvious causes of infertility. If treated surgically, care should be taken not to injure the arterial

Flowchart 7: Initial management of an infertile male.

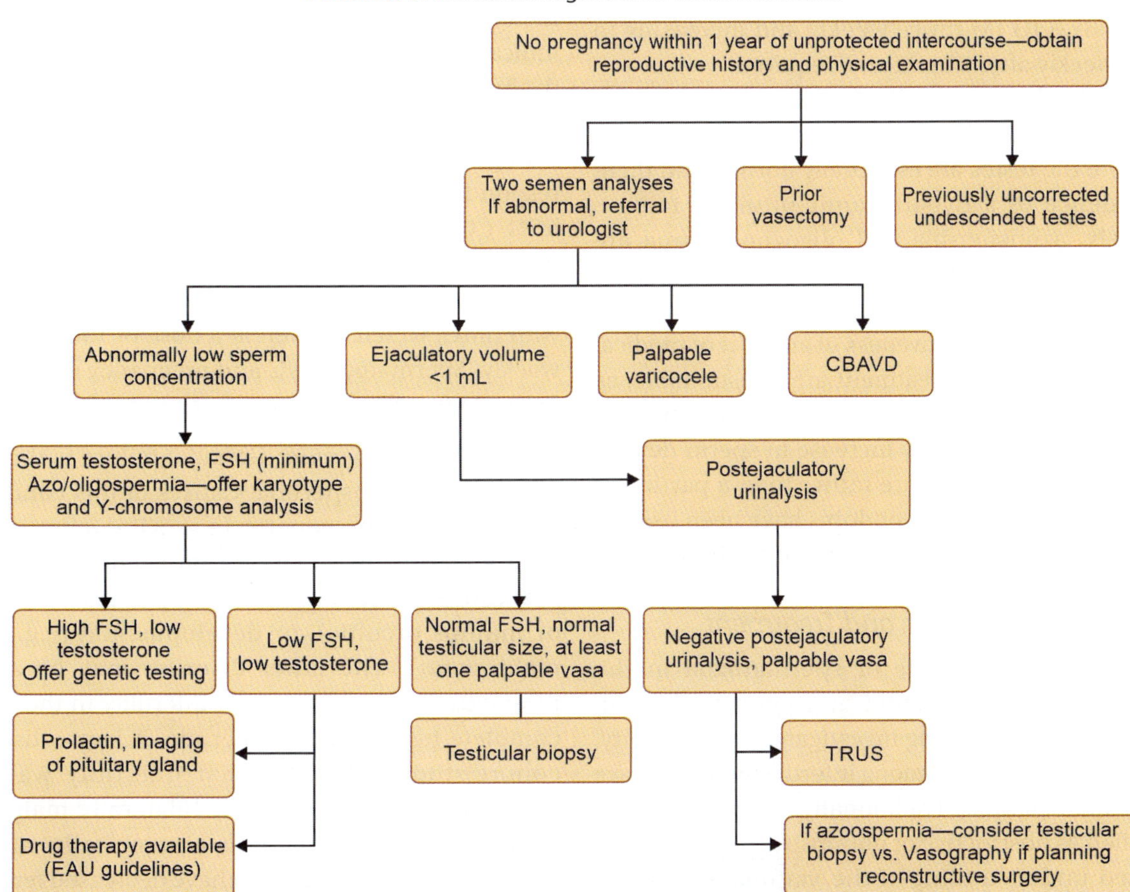

(Azo: azoospermia; CBAVD: congenital bilateral absence of the vas deferens; EAU: European Association of Urology; FSH: follicle-stimulating hormone; TRUS: transrectal ultrasound)

supply to the testes because this makes matters worse; the best technique is to ligate the spermatic vein in the inguinal canal, and this can give apparently good results. Laparoscopic surgery and embolisation techniques have also been used. Sperm density is said to continue to rise for 2 years in 80% of cases after surgery for varicocele, and pregnancy rates of 30% (uncontrolled figures) are reported. Empirical measures designed to improve spermatogenesis include the administration of vitamins E and C, which are free radical scavengers, and the administration of doxycycline or erythromycin for subclinical chlamydial infection.

Clomiphene, in a dose of 25 mg daily for 3 months, has been tried in cases of oligozoospermia but without convincing results. The most rational treatment for defective spermatogenesis in proven hypogonadotrophic hypogonadism is with gonadotrophins. FSH treatment is specific to the seminiferous tubules. Human chorionic gonadotrophin (hCG) 2,000 IU intramuscularly (IM) once or twice weekly is useful in patients with acquired or partial gonadotrophin deficiency. If there is no sperm in the ejaculate after 6–12 months of therapy, hMG is added, starting with 37.5 IU IM thrice weekly and increasing to 75 IU thrice weekly after 6 months, if required.

Treatment with gonadotrophins or gonadotrophin-releasing hormone (GnRH) can stimulate spermatogenesis in cases where the testes are essentially normal and there is clear evidence of a hypothalamic-pituitary failure. Unfortunately, azoospermia and oligozoospermia are usually manifestations of poor testicular function, and the tubules are refractory to gonadotrophins.

Most claims on the effectiveness of any sort of medical (and sometimes surgical) treatment are questionable, as the quality of semen varies spontaneously from time to time in the same man. So, any increase in sperm density is often to be credited to nature rather than a particular remedy. Glucocorticoids and condoms have been used in men with antisperm antibodies, but are of doubtful value.

Azoospermia: Classification and Treatment

Azoospermia is the absence of spermatozoa in the ejaculate. Azoospermia is found on semen analysis in about 5% of all couples being investigated for infertility, and its incidence is 10–20% among infertile men who have abnormal semen analysis. Traditionally, azoospermia has been classified as obstructive or nonobstructive. However, an increased understanding of the various aetiologies of azoospermia and treatment advances using surgical sperm retrieval and ART have prompted a reclassification. The classification system, advocated by Sharif et al., may better reflect the aetiology, prognosis, and treatment of azoospermia. It separates azoospermic patients into those with pretesticular, testicular, and post-testicular causes.

Pretesticular azoospermia: Pretesticular azoospermia represents those conditions in which the hypothalamic-pituitary axis fails to stimulate spermatogenesis within the testis. Congenital, acquired, and idiopathic aetiologies of hypogonadotrophic hypogonadism are included in this category. A full endocrine history, including information on puberty and growth and a review of endocrine systems, should guide the physician in the evaluation of the hypogonadotrophic hypogonadal patient. Laboratory investigations of particular benefit in this population include measurement of serum LH, FSH, testosterone, and prolactin levels and imaging of the pituitary gland. Low levels of gonadotrophins (LH and FSH) and low serum levels of testosterone are characteristic.

Hormonal treatment of hypogonadotrophic hypogonadism has been conclusively demonstrated to be efficacious. In fact, pulsatile GnRH therapy is both conceptually indicated and effective in infertile men with hypothalamic dysfunction, including those patients with Kallmann syndrome. Infertile males with hypogonadotrophic hypogonadism secondary to panhypopituitarism also may respond to GnRH therapy. An alternative treatment uses hCG, 1,000–2,500 IU twice a week, with the dose titrated to maintain serum testosterone and oestradiol levels within the normal range. Treatment with hCG is then combined with hMG, which is given at a dose of 150 IU three times weekly. Spermatogenesis and pregnancy can be achieved in up to 80–88% of patients after 1 year of therapy.

Testicular azoospermia: Gonadal failure is the hallmark of testicular azoospermia. Causes of this condition may be congenital or genetic (e.g. Klinefelter syndrome, microdeletion of the Y chromosome), acquired (e.g. radiation therapy, chemotherapy, testicular torsion, or mumps orchitis), or developmental (e.g. testicular maldescent). The latter disorder may be associated most closely with male factor infertility in the absence of complete testicular azoospermia. A large observational cohort study suggested that infertility was, in fact, associated with congenitally bilaterally maldescended testes, but that men with congenitally unilaterally maldescended testes did not have decreased fertility when compared with controls.

Men with hypergonadotrophic hypogonadism (elevated levels of LH and FSH with low serum levels of testosterone) generally have primary gonadal failure. A karyotype should be obtained in such cases to detect chromosomal abnormalities such as Klinefelter syndrome (47, XXY). Acquired causes of primary gonadal failure are usually evident from history, but they should be confirmed by assessment of the serum hormonal profile and biopsy. If the diagnosis of gonadal failure is confirmed on biopsy, endocrine therapy is contraindicated.

It is becoming increasingly evident that some cases of male factor infertility that have previously been categorised as idiopathic are actually the result of genetic defects on the Y chromosome. The two most commonly implicated candidate gene families are the RNA-binding motif (RBM) and the 'deleted in azoospermia' (DAZ) families, but microdeletions at various loci on the Y chromosome have been described. For example, microdeletions in Yq11.23 have been found in 10–20% of men with idiopathic azoospermia or severe oligospermia. Interestingly, 2% of fertile men also have microdeletions in the Y chromosome. These microdeletions can be transmitted to the male offspring, who may then also suffer from infertility. Therefore, screening for genetic causes is indicated in non-acquired cases of testicular azoospermia so that proper genetic counselling can be provided before treatment. Treatment is focused on the surgical retrieval of spermatozoa with subsequent fertilisation of the oocyte by ICSI. These approaches have made fertility possible for some men with testicular azoospermia.

Post-testicular azoospermia: In post-testicular azoospermia, the hypothalamic-pituitary axis and spermatogenesis are normal. No sperm appear in the ejaculate secondary to congenital absence or obstruction of the vas deferens or ejaculatory ducts, acquired obstruction of these ducts, or ductal dysfunctions, including retrograde ejaculation. Although low seminal pH or low seminal fructose may signal the congenital absence or obstruction of the vas deferens, the diagnosis is confirmed by vasography. In some cases, testicular biopsy may be indicated to differentiate between primary testicular damage and outflow obstruction. Congenital bilateral absence of the vas deferens (CABVD) is found in 1–2% of infertile men and 95% of men with cystic fibrosis. Common mutations of the cystic fibrosis transmembrane conductance regulator (CFTR) gene, which encodes a cyclic adenosine monophosphate (cAMP)-regulated chloride channel, can be found in some infertile men with CABVD, despite the absence of clinical symptoms of cystic fibrosis. Therefore, screening for mutations in the *CFTR* gene is indicated if men with CABVD plan to undergo sperm retrieval and ICSI in order to conceive using their own sperm. One cost-effective screening method addressing this problem involves screening the female partner for the three most common mutations in the *CFTR* gene. If negative, the couple has a risk of less than 1 in 1,500 for conceiving a child with cystic fibrosis, regardless of the paternal genotype.

Azoospermia caused by obstruction of the epididymis or vas: The outlook in these cases is not completely hopeless, and operations, e.g. vasovasostomy and transurethral resection of ejaculatory ducts (TUREDs), if carried out by an experienced surgeon using microsurgical technique, are occasionally successful. TURED is an outpatient procedure for ejaculatory duct obstruction. Intrauterine insemination of spermatozoa obtained by aspiration of the testis always fails because their maturation is incomplete until after they have left the gonad. ICSI may offer some hope to these patients (see further) (**Flowchart 8**).

Prevention of Male Infertility

In this respect two matters deserve mention: The efficient and early treatment of cryptorchidism; and the treatment of orchitis complicating mumps and other virus infections. If tension in the testis is reduced by incision of its capsule *early* in the course of orchitis, the ischaemia which causes tubular necrosis may be prevented. Treatment with massive doses of hydrocortisone is less likely to be effective. Vaccination against mumps in childhood may protect against postpubertal mumps orchitis.

Wife

Medical Treatment (Flowchart 9)

Hormone therapy: The only clear indication for hormone therapy is a proven failure of ovulation. In practice, this generally means infertility, which is associated with amenorrhoea or oligomenorrhoea. Even in such cases, ovulation can never be induced unless the ovaries contain ova capable of being stimulated. In such cases, the appropriate treatment is with clomiphene or similar preparations, bromocriptine, human gonadotrophins or GnRH (**Flowchart 10**). The details of these treatments are described in Chapter 5: Clinical Aspects of Menstruation and Ovulation.

Flowchart 8: Algorithm for evaluation of azoospermia or no sperm in the ejaculate.

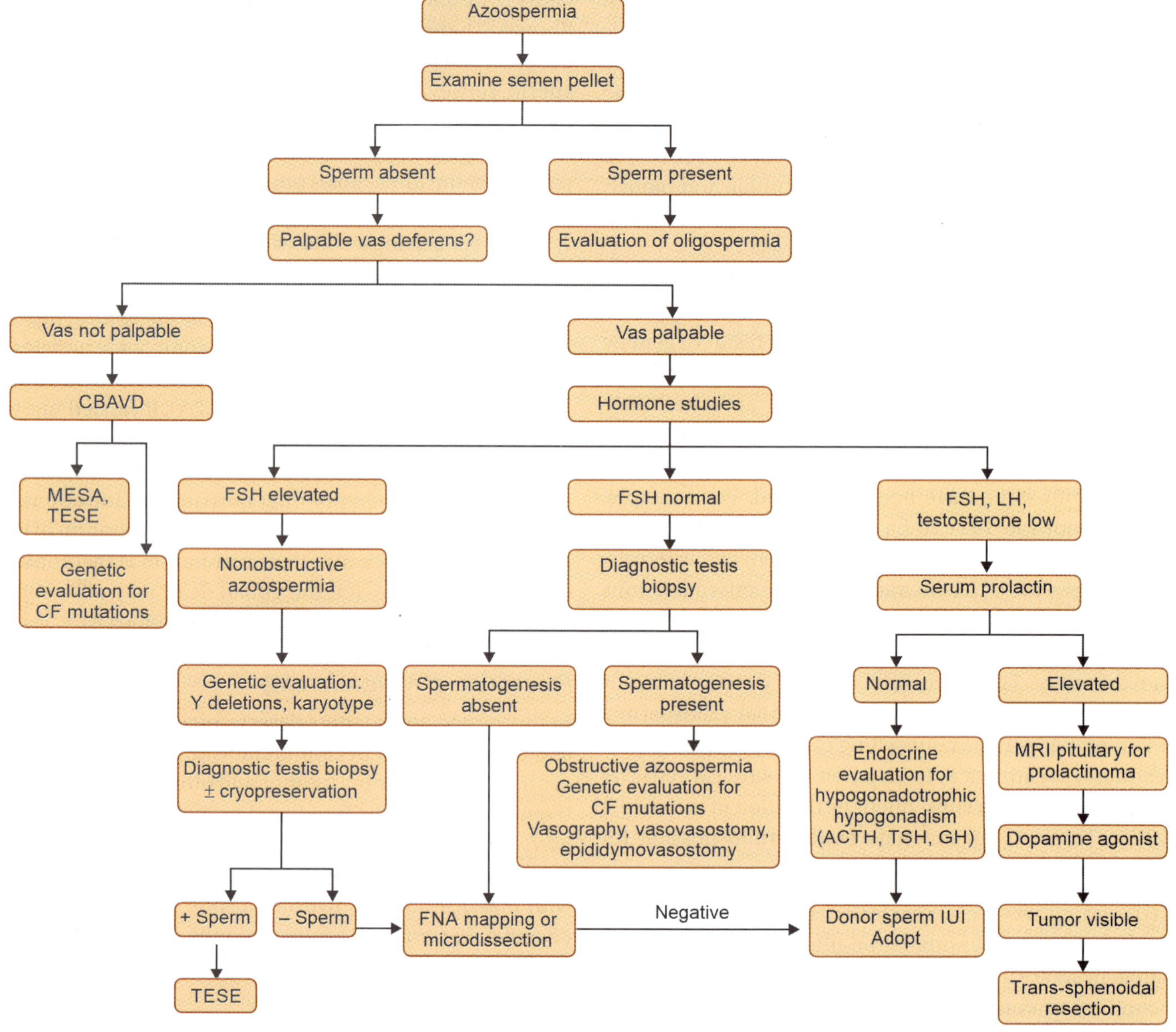

(ACTH: adrenocorticotrophic hormone; CBAVD: congenital bilateral absence of the vas deferens; CF: cystic fibrosis; FNA: fine-needle aspiration; FSH: follicle-stimulating hormone; GH: growth hormone; IUI: intrauterine insemination; LH: luteinising hormone; MESA: microepididymal sperm aspiration; MRI: magnetic resonance imaging; TESE: testicular sperm extraction; TSH: thyroid-stimulating hormone).

Source: Adapted from Nudell DM, Turek PJ. Male fertility and infertility. Clinical Manual of Urology, 3rd edition. New York: McGraw-Hill Co; 2001.

Gonadotrophin therapy requires detailed investigation to establish that the treatment is indicated, followed by strict ultrasound and laboratory control if complications, including multiple pregnancy, are to be avoided. All treatments to induce ovulation should usually be limited to six to nine proven ovulations, since the majority of successful conceptions occur within this time.

In general, women under the age of 25 years who fail to conceive within six cycles and women over the age of 25 years who do not do so in 12 cycles should be offered assisted reproduction (usually IVF).

Flowchart 9: Diagnostic and treatment algorithm: Anovulation.

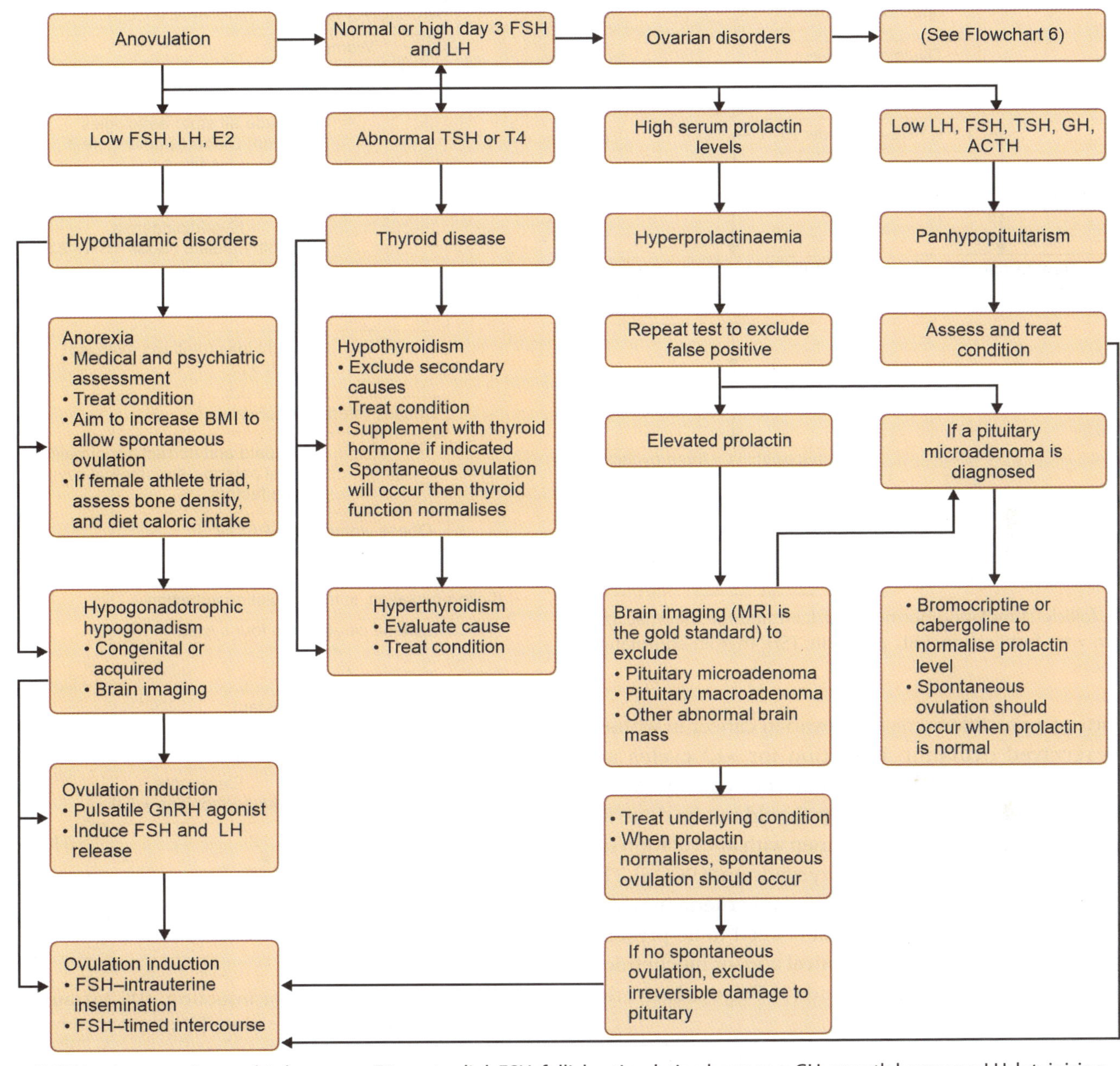

(ACTH: adrenocorticotrophic hormone; E2: oestradiol; FSH: follicle-stimulating hormone; GH: growth hormone; LH: luteinising hormone; TSH: thyroid-stimulating hormone)

The empirical administration of clomiphene to women in whom there is no reason to suppose a failure in ovulation is justified only in cases of unexplained infertility. Some of these patients may have mild alterations in hormone levels commensurate with decreased ovarian reserve. Superovulation achieved by the use of gonadotrophins and GnRH analogues coupled with IUI of washed sperm has been shown to achieve a cumulative pregnancy rate of 40% in six cycles and is a cheaper alternative to IVF. However, there are reports of a possible increase in the incidence of ovarian cancer in women who received ovulation induction for >12 cycles; the relative risk is reportedly higher in cases of unexplained infertility than of anovulation. Patients should be made aware of these reports, and, for this reason also, ovulation induction should be restricted usually to six cycles. However, the

Flowchart 10: Treatment algorithm for an infertile female with oligo-anovulation.

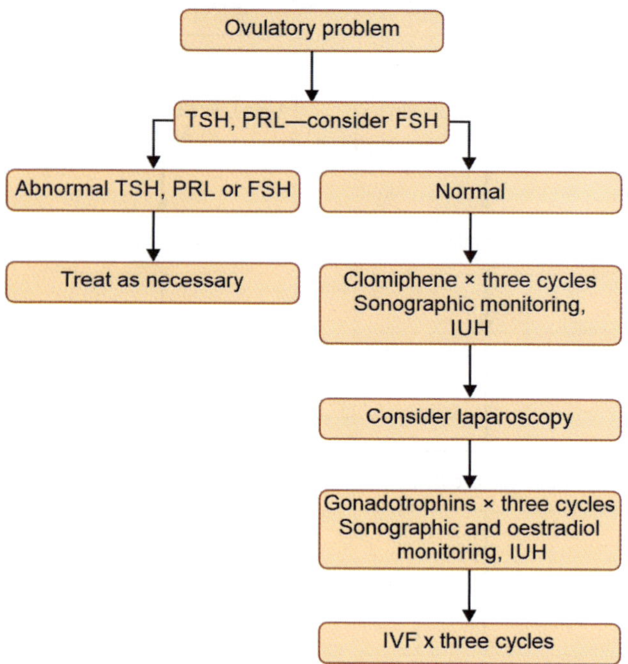

(FSH: follicle-stimulating hormone; IUH: intrauterine haematoma; IVF: in vitro fertilisation; PRL: prolactin; TSH: thyroid-stimulating hormone)

reports of a possible increase in ovarian cancer in women who received ovulation induction for >12 cycles are controversial but need to be taken into consideration. Hence, the induction of ovulation should not be done for long periods. A large group of women with anovulation fall into the category of polycystic ovary syndrome (PCOS). The syndrome is diagnosed based Rotterdam criteria in which two out of three following disorders need to be present: (1) Oligo- or anovulation, (2) Clinical and/or biochemical signs of hyperandrogenaemia and (3) Polycystic ovaries on ultrasound.

Lifestyles modifications and weight reduction play an important role in the improvement of insulin sensitivity and decreasing androgen excess, the two major derangements seen in PCOS women **(Flowchart 11)**.

The empirical use of sex hormones is useless. Oestrogens in the first half of the cycle do not overcome *supposed* uterine hypoplasia, nor do they make cervical mucus more receptive; premenstrual progestogens cannot prevent an early abortion or improve an unreceptive endometrium or poor corpus luteum function. None of these conditions is a proven cause of infertility and there is no scientific evidence to show that such remedies do

Flowchart 11: Algorithm for the treatment of infertile women with polycystic ovary syndrome (PCOS).

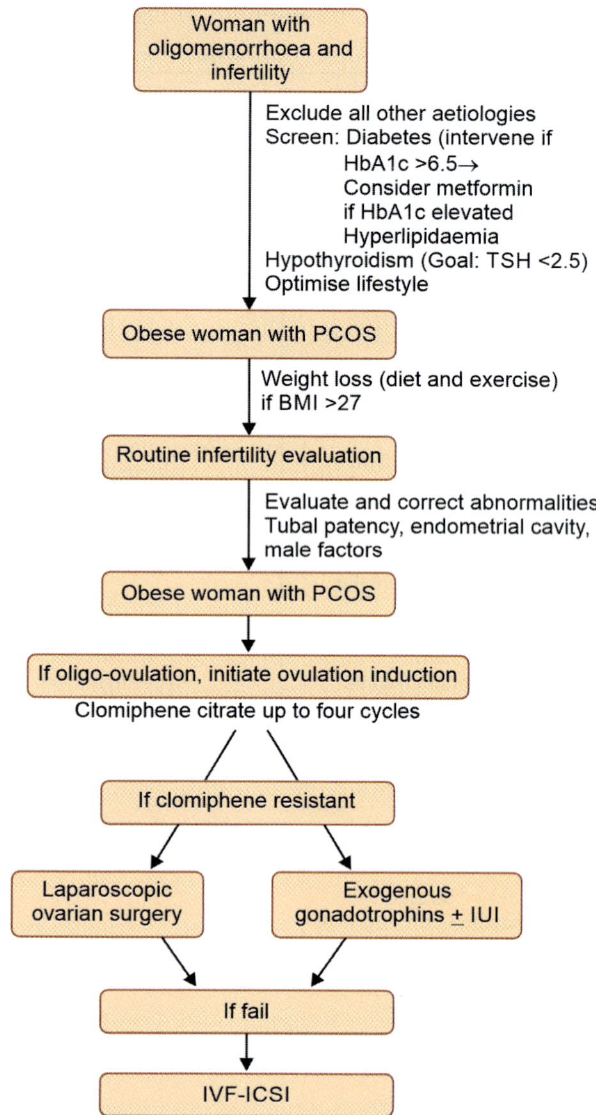

(ICSI: intracytoplasmic sperm injection; IUI: intrauterine insemination; IVF: in vitro fertilisation; TSH: thyroid-stimulating hormone)

any more than give the patient hope. Patients receiving clomiphene who have poor luteal function may benefit from hCG support started in the second half of the cycle and continued through the first trimester.

The administration of an oestrogen-progestogen antiovulatory preparation for a few months, in the hope that the subsequent rebound activity of the hypophysis and the ovaries will favour conception, is also to be deprecated. It is not only unscientific and clearly proven to be followed by no more pregnancies than can be expected by chance,

Flowchart 12: Diagnostic and treatment algorithm: Ovarian disorder.

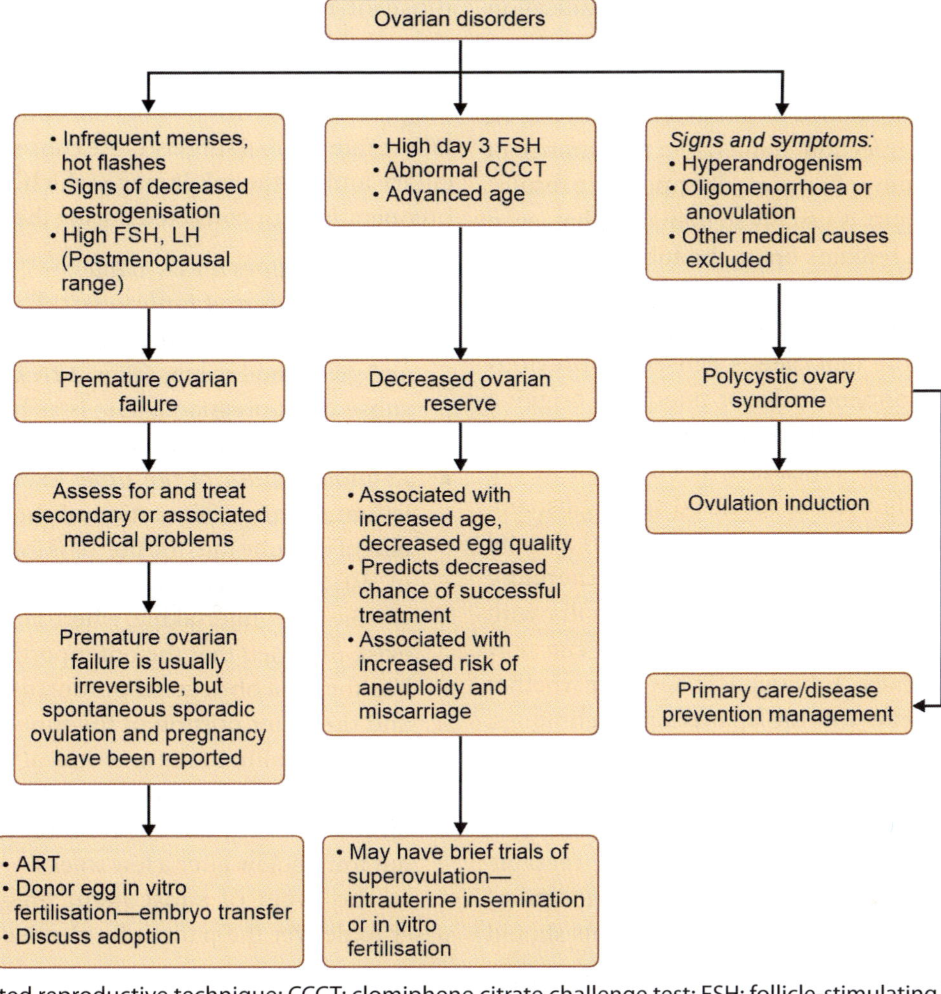

(ART: assisted reproductive technique; CCCT: clomiphene citrate challenge test; FSH: follicle-stimulating hormone; LH: luteinising hormone)

but it also often delays the search for the real cause of infertility and may permanently depress hypothalamic-pituitary function.

Bromocriptine:
Refer to Chapter 5: Clinical Aspects of Menstruation and Ovulation.

Flowchart 12 indicates various ovarian disorders and their diagnostic and treatment algorithm.

Operative Treatment

Dilatation of the cervix, tubal insufflation, HSG and laparoscopy: These procedures, although primarily diagnostic, are often said to have a definite, if small, therapeutic value. Some women conceive within a few months of having them carried out. Caution is necessary in assessing the results, for in the absence of abnormalities, conception would be expected to occur anyway, and the successes almost certainly reflect an ongoing cumulative pregnancy rate. In all cases, the use of invasive tests, which have the risk of introducing infection, apart from any risk associated with general anaesthesia, should be balanced against the need for establishing a diagnosis. As conception may occur without the need for detailed investigation, a waiting time for laparoscopy and chromotubation of 6–9 months from the time of the couple's first visit is usually reasonable if the couple is young and newly married.

Reconstruction operations on the tubes: When both fallopian tubes are found closed, the prognosis is poor but not hopeless; it depends on the site and extent of the obstruction, and on the lesion causing it. Disorganisation of the lumen for a long distance and multiple obstructions offer little hope. Treatment is not based on the causative agent, which is often unknown or not determined, but on the end result of the infection, namely the appearance of the tubes. Salpingostomy often gives disappointing results, because the endosalpinx is usually so damaged that, even if the artificial stoma remains open, the tube is devoid of cilial and peristaltic function.

The cases most suitable for reconstruction operations are those in which the blockage is caused by previous pelvic peritonitis of appendicular or puerperal origin; a mild gonococcal or chlamydial infection with only a tiny hydrosalpinx; peritubal adhesions; obstruction at the isthmus by endosalpingiosis or localised salpingitis; and surgical injury (including sterilisation operations). Careful choice of cases, analysis and evaluation are therefore essential to obtain even moderately good results with microsurgery. Many of the surgical procedures can now be done laparoscopically. Although it is not clear whether pregnancy rates are better with the laparoscopic techniques, they do reduce hospital stay and recovery time, resulting in fewer postoperative adhesions with better healing.

Surgery should generally be restricted to women aged <37 years in whom there is no other apparent treatable cause for infertility (i.e. no absolute bar to conception) and whose husbands are highly fertile. All patients should be aware of the success rates in general and especially those of the surgeon performing the operation; the risks of the surgical procedure itself; and the increased chance of subsequent ectopic pregnancy, which occurs in approximately 10–15% of conceptions. The substantial failure rate of tubal surgery is the consequence of intratubal ciliary and epithelial damage which cannot be assessed preoperatively or corrected during the operation.

Possible procedures are as follows:

- *Salpingolysis and fimbriolysis:* This involves only the separation of peritubal and periovarian adhesions, and gives good results **(Figs. 12A and B)**. The reported subsequent pregnancy rate is as high as 30–40%. This procedure can also be done laparoscopically.
- *Reimplantation of the tube:* Excision of a damaged isthmus with implantation of the remaining healthy part of the tube into the uterus is followed by pregnancy in 10–20% of cases. This operation is still well worthwhile undertaking, where facilities for IVF do not exist, provided that the outer portions of the tubes are healthy. The obstructed portion of the tube is excised, and the outer portion of the tube is implanted at the cornu to maintain the anatomical uterotubal junction. The use of splints, once routine, is now considered optional. If they are inserted, they are usually pulled out from below after a few weeks.

In the event of subsequent pregnancy, it may be wiser to deliver the patient by elective caesarean section

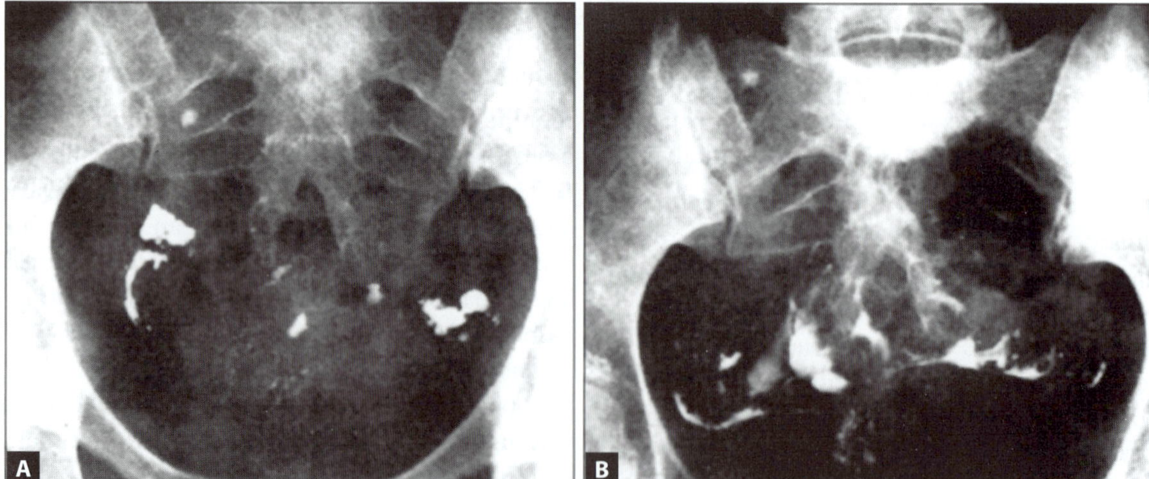

Figs. 12A and B: Salpingolysis for pelvic adhesions causing infertility by interfering with the tubo-ovarian pathway; their cause was a pelvic abscess secondary to acute appendicitis. (A) A radiograph taken 24 hours after salpingography showing loculation of the medium as evidence of peritubal adhesions; (B) A similar radiograph obtained in the same case 3 months after separation of adhesions and salpingolysis. The medium now spreads more freely, although there is still some loculation.

because of possible weakness of the uterine wall at the implantation sites. I have, however, delivered several such patients vaginally without mishap.

Hysteroscopic transcervical cannulation of the tubes has been used in cases of proximal tubal obstruction. This method has been successful in cases where there is no significant pathology but if there is endosalpingiosis or infection, this method cannot be curative. It involves the introduction of a 3-French Teflon catheter through the ostia aided by a 5.5-French outer cannula and a stainless-steel guidewire. Pregnancy rates vary from 54% to 60%, being lower if there are associated adhesions. This technique has also been used to develop the technique of falloposcopy, for transcervical placement of gamete and embryos (see further) and for intratubal insemination.

- *End-to-end anastomosis:* Without microsurgery facilities, this is usually carried out over a threaded nylon splint into the uterus, and is usually the best means of dealing with tubes whose middle portions have been obstructed or removed by a previous sterilisation procedure. The splint is often removed at the end of the operation. In such cases, the remaining portions of the tube are healthy, so a success rate as high as 50% is possible. Using microsurgical techniques, a splint is not essential, even during the operation, and success rates of up to 70–80% have been reported for sterilisation reversal operations.
- Results depend on the site of anastomosis and the residual length of the ampullary end. Isthmic-isthmic anastomosis when there is no tubal or muscular disparity gives the best results. Isthmic-ampullary anastomosis involves the approximation of lumina with different diameters. The common practice is to split the isthmic end longitudinally to increase the lumen artificially. It is usually preferable to exclude the mucosa while placing sutures, as these can cause an inflammatory endosalpingitis. However, the muscularis in the region of the ampulla is thin and it is often necessary to penetrate the lumen to get an adequate bite. Ampullary-ampullary anastomosis is rarely required. A residual ampullary length of <4 cm has been shown to be associated with poor chances of pregnancy and such patients will do better with IVF.
- *Salpingostomy:* The creation of a new stoma in the outer end of a completely closed tube is not difficult but, for reasons mentioned previously, is not often followed by pregnancy. Success rates as high as 25–50% are reported. Various techniques are employed; in all these, gentle handling of the tissues, accurate suturing and haemostasis, preferably using microsurgical techniques, are important. For large hydrosalpinges, it is sometimes best to open the tube longitudinally for a considerable length, hoping that the stoma will remain open in some part *(gutter salpingostomy)*.

For smaller hydrosalpinges and for closure only of the ampulla, the stoma is best created at the outer end of the tube and the edges rolled back to form a cuff salpingostomy or modified fimbria. Even so, in the absence of fimbria the new ostium often closes and a hydrosalpinx reforms.

The figures quoted above are those obtained by experts in these particular procedures, who also claim an overall pregnancy rate of 50% for all types of reconstruction operations. However, the average gynaecologist cannot achieve more than the occasional success. The only exception to this is where end-to-end anastomosis operations are carried out on normal fallopian tubes following sterilisation operations. In these cases, especially where the Pomeroy technique, Falope rings or Hulka clips are used for sterilisation, success rates of 70–80% are obtainable. There also appears to be a lower ectopic pregnancy rate.

All reported results need to be accepted with reserve. Sometimes the successful operations have been unilateral, the other tube being patent; sometimes salpingolysis is recorded as salpingostomy. Many tubal implants have been undertaken on completely normal tubes, spasm having been mistaken for organic obstruction during tubal patency tests.

Despite all the inherent surgical risks and complications that may occur if conception occurs, these operations are cheerfully accepted by the woman whose main concern is to have a baby. In all cases, the patient should be aware of the probable success rate as judged by pregnancies achieved before the operation. Laparoscopic surgical and microsurgical techniques now offer a better outcome but the limiting effects are a damaged endosalpinx and distorted tubo-ovarian relationships due to adhesions which may occur, or recur, postoperatively.

Correction of Uterine Position and Malformations

Retroversion and retroflexion can usually be neglected as causes of infertility until all other possibilities have been excluded; when this is so, however, the correction of the displacement is worthwhile. This is usually done by means

BOX 1: Laparoscopic ovarian diathermy indication.

- Clomiphene resistant
- Lean PCOS
- ↑ LH (>12 mIU/mL)
- <35 years
- Women from remote areas who cannot come for intensive follicular monitoring
- Cannot afford gonadotrophin therapy
- At the time of laparoscopic assessment of pelvis
- History of previous OHSS

(LH: luteinising hormone; OHSS: ovarian hyperstimulation syndrome; PCOS: polycystic ovary syndrome)

of a Hodge pessary but occasionally it may be appropriate to correct the position by ventrosuspension during surgery for pelvic adhesions or endometriosis.

The management of congenital malformations of the uterus is discussed in Chapter 13: Malformations and Maldevelopments of the Genital Tract.

Laparoscopic Ovarian Diathermy

Laparoscopic ovarian diathermy or drilling (LOD) using unipolar cautery or laser is a useful alternative to gonadotrophins in those patients who fail to respond to clomiphene; those who persistently hypersecrete LH; those who live in remote places and cannot be intensively monitored for gonadotrophin therapy; those who cannot afford or tolerate gonadotrophin therapy; those who need laparoscopic assessment of the pelvis **(Box 1)**.

This procedure has replaced wedge resection of the ovaries and increases the chances of unifollicular ovulation. Although the results are as good as those with gonadotrophins, there is a risk of postoperative pelvic adhesion formation in approximately one-fifth of patients. It has been suggested that the number of punctures be minimised, varying from 4 to 20 per ovary. Peritoneal lavage at the end of the procedure has also been correlated with a decreased incidence of adhesion formation. There is a risk of premature ovarian failure if over-cauterisation is done. Increased risk of ovarian cancer, if any, is not yet known. The effects are usually temporary.

Prevention of Female Infertility

Consideration of the causes of female infertility reveals that some of them are preventable, particularly infections causing tubal occlusion. The elimination of gonorrhoea and chlamydial infection, and of injuries and infections sustained at the time of abortion and labour, could have a significant effect on the problem.

SUGGESTED READING

1. Agarwal A, Mulgund A, Hamada A. A unique view on male infertility around the globe. Reprod Biol Endocrinol. 2015;13:37.
2. Helen K, Natalie A, Andrew T. A review of patient-reported outcome measures to assess female infertility-related quality of life. Health Qual Life Outcomes. 2017;15:86.
3. Mahshid B, Masoumeh S, Seyed A. Sexual behavior of infertile women: a qualitative study. Iran J Reprod Med. 2015;13(10):645-56.

48

CHAPTER

Assisted Reproductive Technology

Mahesh C Koregol, Soumya Mahesh Koregol, Muralidhar V Pai

Chapter Outline

- In Vitro Fertilisation and Embryo Transfer
- Controlled Ovarian Hyperstimulation
- Oocyte Retrieval
- Insemination
- Embryo Transfer
- Outcome
- Cryopreservation
- Oocyte Donation
- Embryo Donation
- Surrogacy
- Intrauterine Insemination
- Donor Insemination
- Other Assisted Reproductive Technology Methods
- Results of Treating Infertility
- Dangers of Investigating and Treating Infertility
- Complications of Assisted Reproductive Technology
- Adoption

INTRODUCTION

Assisted reproductive technology (ART) is not new. Even in mythology, there is a reference to surrogacy and artificial insemination. Certainly, artificial insemination has been practised for the last century. Assisted reproduction techniques have been established in animal husbandry. Many of the concepts have been derived from nature itself, e.g. cryopreservation which is practised by certain insects who use sugars and sugar-alcohols as cryoprotectants to withstand subzero winter temperatures; this led to the use of glycerol in animal husbandry. However, the birth of Louise Brown in 1978 in Oldham was the first real major step forward. In the words of Mr Patrick Steptoe, it was 'the end of the beginning, not the beginning of the end'.

IN VITRO FERTILISATION AND EMBRYO TRANSFER

Following success in the veterinary world, this was developed as an alternative treatment for women with severely damaged or occluded fallopian tubes. It is now used for other indications, including long-standing unexplained infertility, treated endometriosis, male factor infertility, cervical hostility and, rarely, after therapy for female cancer. Even though there are an increasing number of centres throughout the world with over half a million babies born by in vitro fertilisation (IVF), it remains a very limited service as it is expensive, very specialised and requires good laboratory facilities and a team of skilled workers.

The technique has been immensely refined and new developments are continually taking place. Superovulation is stimulated by the use of clomiphene and/or gonadotrophins so that several ova can be harvested. Gonadotrophin-releasing hormone agonists (GnRHas) are increasingly used for downregulation of the hypothalamic–pituitary–ovarian axis and have been instrumental in increasing the number of oocytes retrieved, improving endometrial receptivity and clinical pregnancy rates with a reduction in cycle cancellation rates.

CONTROLLED OVARIAN HYPERSTIMULATION

A number of controlled ovarian hyperstimulation protocols have been described, but essentially, they fall into three categories: (1) Depending on whether the patient is a normal responder, (2) a poor responder or (3) a hyper-responder (**Box 1**). For normal responders, the

BOX 1: Controlled ovarian stimulation protocols.

- Long agonist downregulation with gonadotrophin stimulation
- Antagonist downregulation with gonadotrophin stimulation
- Minimal stimulation protocol with gonadotrophin with or without clomiphene citrate combined with antagonist

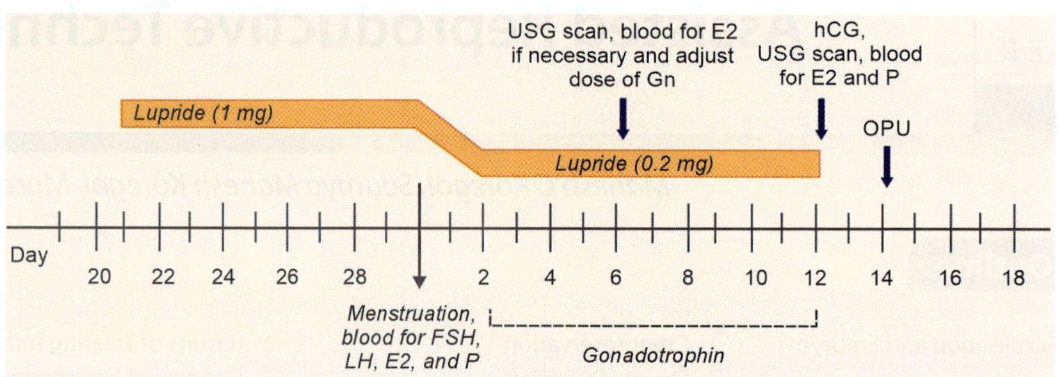

Fig. 1: Long protocol-controlled ovarian stimulation. (E2: oestradiol; FSH: follicle-stimulating hormone; Gn: gonadotrophin; hCG: human chorionic gonadotrophin; LH: luteinising hormone; OPU: ovum pick-up; P: progesterone; USG: ultrasonography)

standard *long protocol* is used. GnRHas are administered in the midluteal phase of the previous cycle, as follicle recruitment normally starts at this time in response to the falling levels of follicle-stimulating hormone (FSH), oestrogen and inhibin. Leuprolide 0.1 mg daily subcutaneously or nafarelin 200 µg BD intranasally is the usual choice. The administration is continued throughout the follicular phase till human chorionic gonadotrophin (hCG) is administered. Gonadotrophins are started after the menses. Monitoring is done by serial ultrasound and hormonal profile, i.e. serum FSH, luteinising hormone (LH), oestradiol and progesterone **(Fig. 1)**.

For poor responders, a microdose *flare protocol* can be used. Leuprolide 20 pg subcutaneously BD is started from day 2 or 3 of the cycle. Gonadotrophin administration begins on day 6. Assisted zona hatching may improve the pregnancy rates in this group.

Hyper-responders are usually patients with the polycystic ovary syndrome (PCOS). Here, a *coasting protocol* can be used. Administration of GnRHa is started from the third week of the previous cycle. Low-dose gonadotrophins (75 IU/day) are started after the menses. If the serum oestradiol is >3,000 pg/mL, gonadotrophin is discontinued regardless of follicle size, and GnRHa is continued. When the level of serum oestradiol falls to <3,000 pg/mL, hCG is administered **(Figs. 2 and 3) (Box 2)**.

OOCYTE RETRIEVAL

Oocyte retrieval, previously done at laparoscopy and percutaneously, is now almost exclusively done transvaginally under ultrasonic guidance from a transvaginal transducer. This is the easiest, most accurate and patient-friendly method. Rarely, if there is no vaginal probe available, the ovary is inaccessible vaginally, or if there is vaginal infection, a perurethral oocyte pick-up is done under the guidance of a transabdominal ultrasound probe. To prevent the ovary from slipping away, sharp and single-use disposable needles are used, and suprapubic pressure is applied with the hand or with a special abdominal pressure cuff.

It is generally preferable to make a single puncture in the vagina and the ovary. Keeping the needle in the ovary, several follicles are aspirated one after the other by careful planning and manipulation. A warmed flushing medium, either Earle's with heparin or warmed normal saline, is used. If the oocyte is not recovered, the follicle is flushed with the solution and aspirated. This procedure is repeated till the oocyte is recovered. Manipulation with the needle tip may help to dislodge the oocyte. After all oocytes have been recovered, flushing fluid and blood collected in the pouch of Douglas are aspirated.

INSEMINATION

The oocytes are inseminated in vitro by fresh or cryopreserved sperm. The technique of semen preparation is described later in this chapter. Insemination with <50,000 sperm/egg decreases the fertilisation rate, whereas the risk of polyspermy is increased with more than 500,000 sperm/egg. The sperms and oocytes are incubated under controlled conditions. After 16–18 hours, they are examined for the presence of two pronuclei which confirms fertilisation. The zygotes are returned to the incubator to allow cleavage to the two- to four-cell stage when they are ready for transfer to the uterus **(Flowchart 1)**.

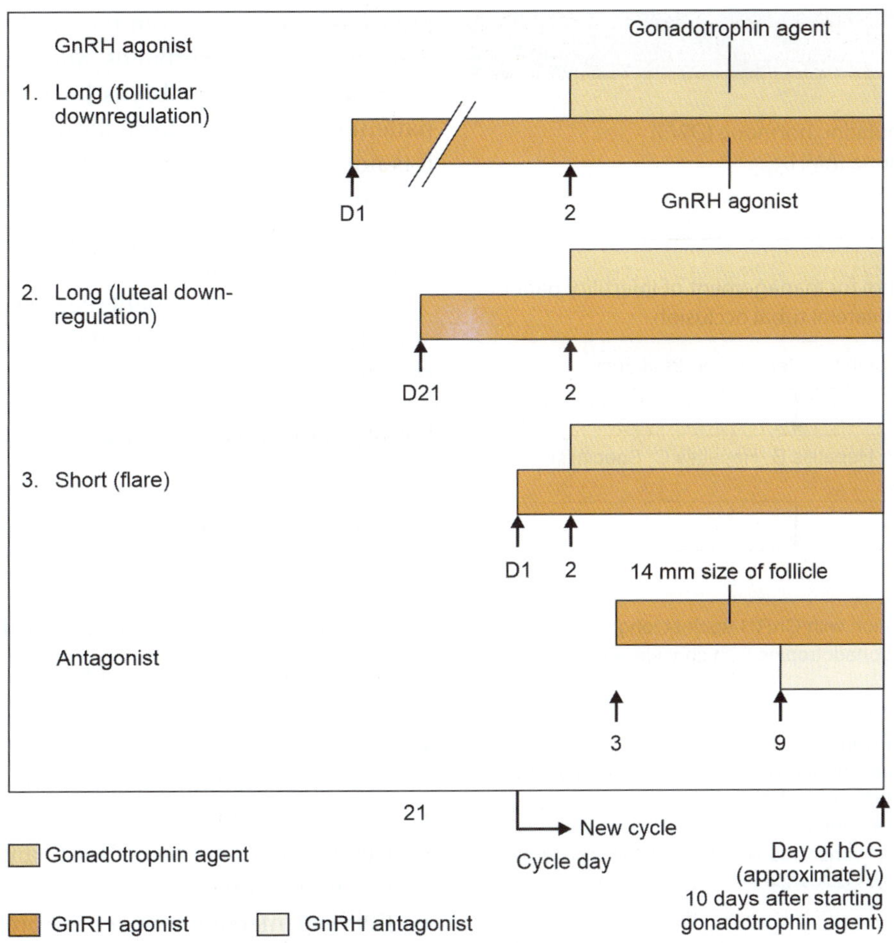

Fig. 2: In vitro fertilisation protocols using gonadotrophin-releasing hormone agonist with gonadotrophins in controlled ovarian hyperstimulation. (GnRH: gonadotrophin-releasing hormone; hCG: human chorionic gonadotrophin)

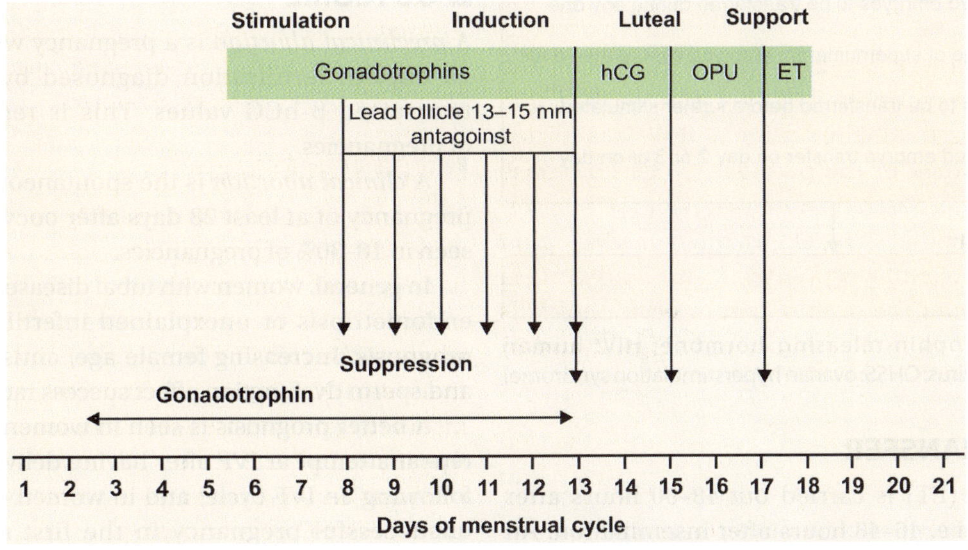

Fig. 3: Gonadotrophin-releasing hormone antagonist downregulation protocol. (ET: embryo transfer; hCG: human chorionic gonadotrophin; OPU: ovum pick-up)

BOX 2: Predictive factors for assessment of correct stimulation protocol.

- Age
- Baseline follicle-stimulating hormone (D2/3)
- Anti-Müllerian hormone (AMH)
- Basal antral follicle count
- Body mass index

Flowchart 1: Algorithm for management of infertility patient with bilateral tubal occlusion.

Procedure for in vitro fertilisation treatment

↓

1. *Offer screening:* HIV, Hepatitis B, Hepatitis C; Specialist referral if possible

↓

2. *Ovulation induction:*
   - × Natural cycle
   - ✓ Pituitary downregulation with GnRH agoinst long protocol
   - ✓ GnRH agoinst with gonadotropins with consideration to minimizing cost
   - × GnRH antagonist
   - × Growth hormone adjuvant
   - ✓ Monitor follicular development with ultrasound: Clinics should have protocols for management of OHSS
   - ✓ Oocyte maturation with human chorionic gonadotrophins
   - ✓ *Oocyte retrieval:* Offer conscious sedation (Follow Academy of Medical Royal Colleges guidance)
   - × Follicle flushing
   - × Assisted hatching

↓

3. *Embryo transfer:*
   - ✓ No more than two embryos to be transferred during any one cycle
   - ✓ Offer cryostorage of supernumerary embryos if more than two embryos
   - ✓ Frozen embryos to be transferred before further stimulated cycles
   - ✓ Ultrasound-guided embryo transfer on day 2 or 3 or on day 5 or 6

↓

4. *Luteal support:*
   - ✓ Progestrone

(GnRH: gonadotrophin-releasing hormone; HIV: human immunodeficiency virus; OHSS: ovarian hyperstimulation syndrome)

EMBRYO TRANSFER

Embryo transfer (ET) is carried out 48–50 hours after oocyte recovery, i.e. 46–48 hours after insemination. An ET catheter is used, which is flushed with Earle's medium. Two or three embryos suspended in 15–25 μL of fluid are transferred 1 cm from the fundus or lower, i.e. about 5–6 cm from the external os, and the catheter is checked to ensure that the embryos have been transferred. The patient is made to lie down for half an hour. Occasionally, it is not possible to negotiate the cervical canal. This may require the use of rigid inserters, Allis forceps, etc., and rarely the patient may require to have the ET done under general anaesthesia.

Post-transfer, the patient receives progesterone vaginal suppositories 50 mg twice daily, or intramuscular (IM) progesterone 12.5 mg daily.

Factors Affecting Embryo Transfer

- *Cervical mucus:* It may plug catheter tip leading to the retention of embryos
- *Failed negotiation of cervical canal:* Acute flexion or version
- Irritation of uterus and initiation of uterine contractions

To improve the success rate of ET:

- Dummy transfer—mock transfer
- Ultrasonography-guided transfer
- Avoiding initiation of contractions
- Using a soft malleable catheter to avoid trauma
- Cervix should not be held with any instrument to avoid irritation of uterus
- Cervical infection reduces the pregnancy rate
- Loading of embryos into catheter should be done carefully with a small volume of 30–40 μL

OUTCOME

A *preclinical abortion* is a pregnancy which ends within 28 days of fertilisation diagnosed by a minimum of two raised β-hCG values. This is reported in 9–16% of pregnancies.

A *clinical abortion* is the spontaneous termination of pregnancy of at least 28 days after oocyte pick-up and is seen in 18–30% of pregnancies.

In general, women with tubal disease, mild and treated endometriosis or unexplained infertility have a better prognosis. Increasing female age, antisperm antibodies and sperm dysfunction affect success rates adversely.

A better prognosis is seen in women who return for a repeat attempt at IVF after having delivered a live infant following an IVF cycle; and in women who have had an unsuccessful pregnancy in the first cycle, whether a miscarriage, an ectopic or a biochemical pregnancy, as compared to a woman who did not conceive at all in the first cycle. The overall clinical pregnancy rate is about 26% per retrieval. The live-birth rate varies from 9% to 26% per cycle, the overall rate is 21%. Of these, 66–72% are singleton, 22–24% twins, 26% triplets and less than 1% are higher order multiple pregnancies.

Pregnancy rates with 1, 2, 3 and 4 embryos transferred are 9.6%, 15.9%, 24.2% and 30.6% per cycle, respectively, but the multiple pregnancy rate is also correspondingly increased.

The cumulative conception rate (CCR) up to 35 years of age compares favourably with rates in the normally cohabiting fertile population. After six cycles of IVF, CCR reported from the best centres varies from 56% to 72%, whereas in the normal population, it is about 55%.

Vanishing foetuses are seen in 18% of cases, ectopic pregnancy is reported in 4–6%. Patients undergoing IVF-ET are at risk of ectopic pregnancy because of the following reasons:

- *Pre-existing tubal damage:* It was the practice earlier to occlude the tubes completely at laparoscopy to prevent subsequent ectopic pregnancy but now, with ultrasound-guided oocyte retrieval, laparoscopy is no longer mandatory. Moreover, bowel adhesions to the tube after diathermy impair oocyte recovery and the procedure does not prevent interstitial pregnancy.
- Multiple ET
- *Technique of transfer:* Increased volume of transfer fluid, use of excessive force in the transfer, placing the ET catheter beyond the mid cavity or into the tube itself
- Retrograde migration of embryos to the tubes

Bilateral tubal pregnancy is the rarest form of binovular twins. More commonly, the twin sacs are seen in the same tube or there may be simultaneous intrauterine and extrauterine gestation. In women undergoing IVF, the presence of an intrauterine gestation sac on transvaginal ultrasound (TVS) does not rule out an extrauterine pregnancy, which may be located in the cervix or the ovary.

Maternal complications include: (1) Ovarian hyperstimulation, oocyte retrieval and ET. The first category is the ovarian hyperstimulation syndrome (OHSS) (refer to Chapter 5: Clinical Aspects of Menstruation and Ovulation), which is seen in 1% of women undergoing superovulation, and ovarian cyst formation, which is seen during downregulation with GnRHa or as a result of previous gonadotrophin therapy. It usually settles with the continued administration of GnRHa. There have been a few reports of a positive association of ovulation induction with epithelial ovarian tumours, both borderline and malignant.

The second category is mainly the risks of intravenous sedation, regional anaesthesia and pelvic infection. The third category is the risk of needle damage to adjacent organs—bowel, bladder, uterus and vascular structures and pelvic infection.

Obstetric complications seen with IVF-ET are mainly multiple births, low birth weight and ectopic pregnancy. Selective foetal reduction is recommended if there are more than four foetuses. In some countries, the law prohibits the transfer of more than three embryos.

Delivery by caesarean section is common. Low birth-weight babies comprise 32% of births, mainly because of multiple pregnancy. Major congenital abnormalities occur in 2–3% of the children which is the same as in the general population. The use of cryopreserved gametes or embryos does not increase the risk of congenital abnormalities and developmental milestones are similar in all groups.

CRYOPRESERVATION

Cryopreservation of semen has been in use for over a century. Multiple follicle stimulation techniques provide oocytes or embryos in excess of the number required for fresh transfer. Embryo cryopreservation is now an accepted method for these as 60–80% of embryos survive freezing. Pregnancy rates are improved by up to 10%. No adverse effects have been seen in babies born by this technique. The procedure involves cooling of embryos in the pronucleate or early cleavage state to very low temperatures in the presence of cryoprotectants, e.g. 12-propanediol, glycerol or dimethyl sulphoxide (DMSO) with sucrose which minimises damage to the embryos. They are then stored in liquid nitrogen till required. Over half the embryos survive the thawing process. Oocyte preservation has not been successful.

OOCYTE DONATION (FIG. 4)

Oocyte donation has also emerged as a treatment modality in cases of premature ovarian failure or resistant ovary syndrome, surgical castration, following chemotherapy or radiotherapy, ovarian dysgenesis, in women with hereditary genetic disease and with abnormal oocytes during IVF treatments.

Oocytes may be obtained from volunteers or known donors, spare oocytes from IVF programmes, from sterilisation patients prepared prior to operation or,

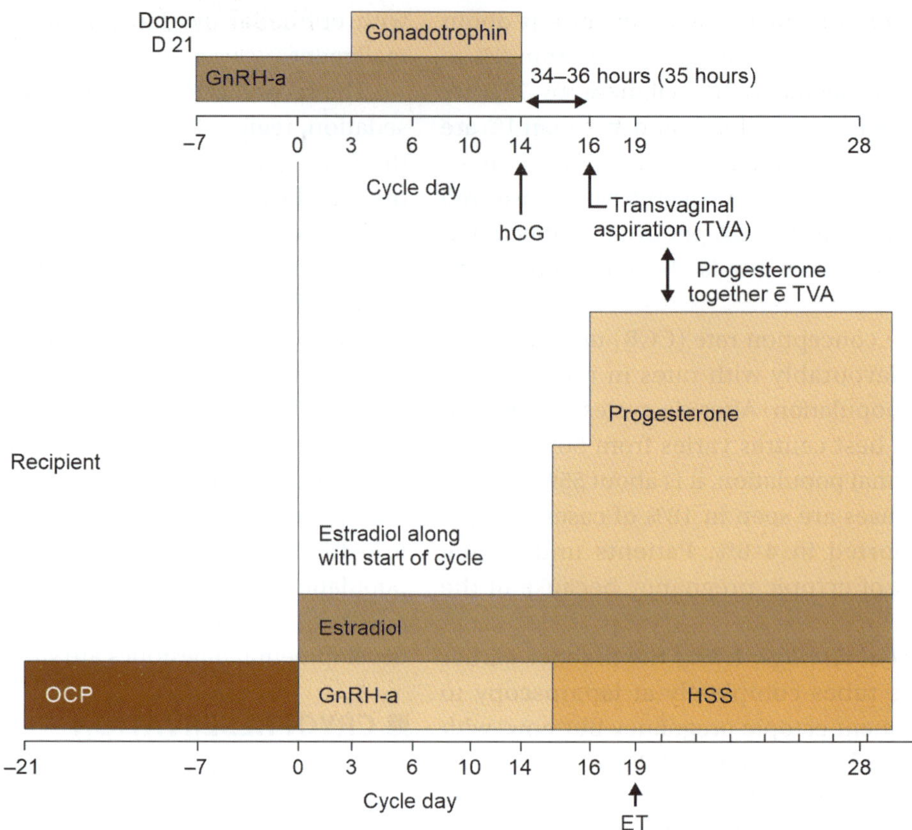

Fig. 4: Regimens of ovarian stimulation and hormone replacement used to synchronise the development of ovarian follicles in the oocyte donor and the endometrial cycle in the recipient. (ET: embryo transfer; GnRH: gonadotrophin-releasing hormone; hCG: human chorionic gonadotrophin; HSS: hyperstimulation syndrome; OCP: oral contraceptive pill)

BOX 3: Indication for oocyte donation.

- Premature ovarian failure
- Ovarian agenesis
- Surgical removal of bilateral ovaries
- Radiotherapy or chemotherapy for ovarian cancer
- Postmenopausal patient
- Risk of inheritable genetic disease in children
- Failed in vitro fertilisation due to poor oocyte quality
- Inaccessible ovaries

BOX 4: Evaluation of oocyte recipient.

- Complete medical and reproductive history
- Blood group, RH, VDRL, HIV, HbsAg, HBC and blood sugar
- Pelvic sonography to assess endometrium
- Hysteroscopy

(HBC: hepatitis B core; HbsAg: hepatitis B surface antigen; HIV: human immunodeficiency virus; RH: rhesus; VDRL: venereal disease research laboratory)

in some countries, professional donors. In the future, cadaver donation or oocyte recovery from foetuses may be possible.

Pregnancy rates are higher in cycles using donated eggs (47% per cycle). However, there is also a higher risk of first trimester bleeding, preeclampsia and intrauterine growth restriction **(Boxes 3 and 4)**.

EMBRYO DONATION

Embryo donation may be indicated in some menopausal or perimenopausal women with a subfertile partner, in cases of recurrent IVF failure or couples with genetic disease or chromosomal abnormality.

SURROGACY

Surrogacy is an option for women without a uterus but with one or both ovaries functioning, as in cases with congenital absence of the uterus or those who have undergone hysterectomy for severe haemorrhage or ruptured uterus. Some patients with recurrent miscarriages or those with medical conditions which may make pregnancy life-threatening even though long-term health prospects are otherwise good, may also prefer to opt for surrogacy.

The host mother should be normal, healthy, not >38 years of age, with at least one child. Her husband or partner should be fully aware of the implications. Investigations of the host mother are kept to a minimum. Because of the risk of human immunodeficiency virus (HIV) infection, it is recommended that frozen sperm be used after waiting to cross the stipulated window period of 6 months. The procedure is relatively simple, cheap, with fewer complications than IVF and permits better bonding with the child; although it is not genetically related. However, very few such cases are possible.

As was expected, the success of IVF has posed many ethical, social and legal problems which are being debated extensively in those countries where these procedures are carried out. Some of these issues were posed by Professor Jeffcoate in the fourth edition, well before the success of Edwards and Steptoe. The answers to some of these issues are known, but many are still not fully resolved, particularly those related to the freezing and storage of donor ova or embryos, the use of stored embryos and the disposal of those embryos not directly required in the management of infertility. At present, developments in this field are ahead of legal decisions. Public opinion is also changing; what was not acceptable a decade ago is now regarded as a normal event. It seems probable that fairly strict legislation will ultimately apply to certain infertility procedures and their performance in recognised institutions or centres.

INTRAUTERINE INSEMINATION (BOXES 5 TO 7 AND TABLE 1)

This involves the collection of semen by an emission occurring other than during coitus (usually by masturbation) and its transfer into the uterus. Intrauterine insemination (IUI) is indicated when any of the following is present: Ejaculatory failure which may be anatomical, e.g. hypospadias; secondary to spinal cord injury or other neurological problems; retrograde ejaculation as may occur in multiple sclerosis; impotence; male subfertility with oligospermia or hypospermia, asthenozoospermia or teratozoospermia [though some of these patients may require intracytoplasmic sperm injection (ICSI)] (see further); immunological factors such as antisperm antibodies in the male or female; cervical mucus hostility or poor cervical mucus; disease or deformity of the cervix making it difficult for sperm to enter and in combination with superovulation in cases of unexplained infertility, mild-to-moderate endometriosis or ovarian dysfunction. In recent times, the processed semen of an HIV-positive partner has been used to inseminate an HIV-negative woman. Efficient techniques of cryopreservation of semen now make it possible for the husband's semen to be stored prior to treatment of cancer by surgery or radiotherapy, or orchidectomy for testicular cancer, and used for IUI after

BOX 5: Indication of intrauterine insemination.

- Unexplained infertility
- Cervical factor
- Mild male factor
- Ejaculatory failure
- Immunological causes
- Mild-to-moderate endometriosis

BOX 6: Prerequisite for intrauterine insemination.

- Age <40 years
- At least one patent fallopian tube
- Occurrence of spontaneous or induced ovulation
- Postwash sperm count >5 million motile sperm

BOX 7: Steps of intrauterine insemination.

- Patient selection and workup
- Ovarian stimulation
- Semen wash
- Insemination
- Luteal support

TABLE 1: Patient workup.

Wife	*Husband*
CBC, ESR, VDRL, HIV, HbsAg and HCV	CBC, VDRL, blood sugar, HIV, HbsAg and HCV
D2/3-FSH, LH, E2, prolactin, TSH and hormonal	Semen analysis
Rule out tuberculosis	*Optional*: Semen culture, Kruger sperm morphology, sperm antibodies, FSH, testosterone, prolactin and scrotal Doppler
Hysterosalpingography or diagnostic laparoscopy, hysteroscopy, dilation and curettage	
Ovulation study: Serial vaginal ultrasound for follicular study (others: BBT, serum progesterone D21 and endometrial biopsy)	

(BBT: basal body temperature; CBC: complete blood count; E2: oestradiol; ESR: erythrocyte sedimentation rate; FSH: follicle-stimulating hormone; HbsAg: hepatitis B surface antigen; HCV: hepatitis C virus; HIV: human immunodeficiency virus; LH: luteinising hormone; TSH: thyroid-stimulating hormone; USG: ultrasonography; VDRL: venereal disease research laboratory)

cure of the disease. It can be done in natural or stimulated cycles but better results are obtained with the latter. Standard protocols of clomiphene, clomiphene/FSH or gonadotrophin alone may be used. With the development of up to four mature follicles, there are better chances of implantation. hCG is administered when the leading follicle is 18 mm in size. If monitoring by ultrasound and hormonal profile is available, better pregnancy rates are obtained.

Semen Preparation

Semen consists of seminal fluid with sperm and other cellular debris from the urogenital tract. Prostaglandins, enzymes and protease inhibitors present in the seminal fluid are detrimental to the fertilisation process in the fallopian tube or in vitro, as they provoke strong uterine contractions and impair sperm capacitation. The object of sperm preparation is to separate the sperm from the seminal fluid and provide a concentrated number of motile, capacitated sperm resuspended in a small volume of protein-supplemented medium **(Boxes 8 and 9)**.

The *swim-up technique* is commonly used and is suitable for samples with normal sperm count and motility. The semen is divided into 0.5 mL aliquots per centrifuge tube and diluted 2:1 with protein-supplemented medium to decrease viscosity and improve pellet formation. The tubes are centrifuged for 10 minutes at a speed not >400 g to avoid damage to the sperm. The supernatant is removed and the pellets are overlaid with 0.5 mL of medium. They are incubated at 37°C for 1 hour. Motile sperms swim-up into the supernatant which is collected from all the tubes and centrifuged at 300 g for 5 minutes **(Box 10)**. The final pellet is resuspended in 0.5 mL of medium.

BOX 8: Essential requirements for semen preparation.

- Motile sperm count
- Volume
- Viscosity
- Presence of leucocytes, cells and debris
- Whether it is for IUI, IVF or ICSI

(ICSI: intracytoplasmic sperm injection; IUI: intrauterine insemination; IVF: in vitro fertilisation)

BOX 9: Different methods for semen preparation.

- Direct swim-up (used for semen with normal parameters)
- Pellet and swim-up method
- Density gradient

Techniques using a *density gradient* are better for samples with a low sperm count and/or motility as they also significantly decrease bacterial contamination. Each millilitre of semen is placed on a column of silica particles or bovine albumin in centrifuge tubes and centrifuged for 20 minutes at 400 g. The sperm pellets are washed off the gradient matrix with media, combined and resuspended in 0.5 mL medium **(Box 11)**.

Sperm wash is used for severely low sperm counts and motility. In these cases, the technique described above cannot provide adequate sperms. The undiluted semen is divided into 1 mL aliquots, centrifuged at 300 g for 5 minutes, the supernatant removed and the pellet resuspended in 0.5 mL of fresh medium.

Insemination is carried out with a sterilised syringe and IUI cannula. Ordinary plastic cannulae may be toxic to spermatozoa. The washed sperm reconstituted in 0.5 mL of medium are gently injected into the uterus to avoid endometrial trauma, which can cause cramping and bleeding resulting in poorer sperm survival. Pregnancy may occur at any sperm count but most occur when the count is 50,000 to 1 million/egg. Undiluted semen is never used because of the risk of transfer of infection. The technique has the advantage of being relatively simple, cheap, effective and noninvasive. It can also be performed

BOX 10: Swim-up method for semen preparation.

- Take two test tubes, label them and put 1 mL of semen sample in each
- Add 2 mL of flushing medium in each tube and mix
- Centrifuge for 10 minutes at 1,500 rpm
- Aspirate supernatant
- Layer pellet with 1 mL flushing or culture media
- After 30–40 minutes, remove 0.5 mL of supernatant from each tube and use it for intrauterine insemination, in vitro fertilisation and intracytoplasmic sperm injection

BOX 11: Density gradient for semen preparation.

- Take two conical tubes, label them and put 1 mL of 90% sperm gradient
- Layer 1 mL of 40% sperm gradient over it
- Layer 1–2 mL of sperm on top of the two layers
- Centrifuge at 1,500 rpm for 20 minutes
- Pipette out supernatant and transfer the pellet to a new tube with 5 mL of flushing medium
- Centrifuge at 1,500 rpm for 10 minutes
- Pipette out supernatant
- Pellet is resuspended in 0.8 mL of culture media, and sample is used for intrauterine insemination, in vitro fertilisation and intracytoplasmic sperm injection

in non-IVF units. However, IVF units have the advantage that if hyperstimulation occurs, they may convert to IVF and freeze surplus embryos.

When IUI is used for retrograde ejaculation, it is attended by many practical difficulties. It necessitates alkalinising the male urine, collecting a specimen after coitus, centrifuging it for spermatozoa and then using these for insemination after washing. Though successes have been reported, ICSI can be tried if the technique fails.

The overall success rate is about 18–20% per cycle. Referral for IVF is recommended in case of failure to achieve a pregnancy in four to six cycles.

Intrauterine insemination as treatment of male factor infertility: Studies of the efficacy of IUI in the treatment of male factor infertility have been generally difficult to assess because of variations in inclusion criteria. Further, sperm function tests are neither consistently used in these studies nor is their use standardised. Considering these limitations, the benefits of IUI in male factor infertility have been accepted, because IUI appears to result in higher pregnancy rates than natural intercourse or intracervical insemination [odds ratio 2.20; 95% confidence interval (CI), 1.43–3.39]. However, the IUI pregnancy rates are generally lower in couples with male factor infertility than in couples with unexplained infertility (4.8% vs. 11.6%).

Some couples with male factor infertility fail treatment with artificial insemination, and some have initial semen parameters that make insemination a suboptimal approach. In these couples, use of ART, especially with ICSI, may be a superior treatment option. The efficacy of ICSI in ART allows almost all cases of male factor infertility to be highly treatable. ICSI only requires that viable sperm be present. Therefore, ICSI should be considered if the total motile sperm count is $<0.5 \times 10^6$, because the IUI success rates are extremely low with such sperm counts. Finally, ICSI should be recommended after a maximum of three to four IUI cycles have failed in a couple with male factor infertility.

DONOR INSEMINATION

When the woman is normal but the man is infertile, when there are familial diseases or there is severe rhesus incompatibility (to produce a rhesus-negative foetus) for the woman who has lost a series of babies as a result of isoimmunisation despite advances in perinatal medicine including intrauterine transfusions, and whose husband is homozygous (rhesus positive), the instillation of *donated* semen of good quality will nearly always result in pregnancy, if the procedure is repeated sufficiently often.

BOX 12: Donor insemination.

Donor insemination for couple with:
- Azoospermia
- Generic/infectious disease in male partner
- Severe rhesus isoimmunisation
- Severe semen defects

With the advent of microsurgical epididymal sperm aspiration (MESA), percutaneous epididymal sperm aspiration (PESA) and testicular sperm extraction (TESE) for ICSI (see further) in male infertility, with the availability of preimplantation genetic diagnosis (see further) in conditions such as haemophilia and cystic fibrosis (which allows the transfer of normal embryos only) and with the decreasing incidence of rhesus isoimmunisation in developed countries, the demand for donor insemination (DI) is decreasing except in developing countries, as the costs of these alternative procedures are much higher **(Box 12)**.

It is essential that adequate counselling of the couple concerned is done so that it can be ascertained that this method is acceptable and that they are likely to be suitable parents. The criteria are similar to those used for adoption but the upper age limit for the wife is usually 37 years. The couple should understand all the implications of DI and the risks of the pregnancy itself. Because of anonymity of the donor, genetic abnormalities cannot be looked for.

There is debate about the number of successful pregnancies, which should be allowed per donor. Although at one time 20 seemed acceptable, the increasing use of DI suggests that 5 or 10 would be more appropriate. An exception could be considered when a second child by DI is requested by a couple.

The risk of transmission of acquired immunodeficiency syndrome (AIDS) by DI suggests that fresh semen would rarely be used. Tests for freedom from infection must be repeated after 6 months before stored specimens can be used.

The general practice is to inseminate the woman for up to six or nine confirmed ovulatory cycles. The majority of successful inseminations occur within three ovular cycles, and the success rate is certainly less in women with infertility problems which required treatment.

Overall, in a large clinic, there should be a success rate of 60%.

OTHER ASSISTED REPRODUCTIVE TECHNOLOGY METHODS

Several ART methods have been developed over the years. Some of these include gamete intrafallopian transfer (GIFT), direct intraperitoneal insemination (DIPI), fallopian tube sperm perfusion (FSP) or intrafallopian insemination (IFI), peritoneal oocyte sperm transfer (POST), zygote intrafallopian transfer (ZIFT), pronuclear stage tubal transfer (PROST), tubal embryo stage transfer (TEST), tubal embryo transfer (TET), embryo intrafallopian transfer (EIFT), surgical embryo transfer (SET), transmyometrial (TM)-ET, direct oocyte transfer (DOT) and intravaginal culture (IVC). Some have been discarded in favour of IUI, IVF or ICSI (see further).

Many of the terms are self-explanatory. DIPI and IUI give similar results; the latter is a simpler technique unless there is severe cervical stenosis. FSP has been replaced by IUI or IVF. POST is a good rescue procedure for IUI or FSP if hyperstimulation develops requiring cancellation of the cycle. ZIFT, PROST, TEST, TET and EIFT have been replaced by IVF since these procedures need general anaesthesia and laparoscopy. SET or TM-ET has a place in cases of severe cervical stenosis.

Certain steps and costs of laboratory procedures can be reduced in IVC by incubating the tubes containing the gametes in the vagina, but this is not acceptable to many women. With the development of transport IVF and portable incubators, this is not required. In transport IVF, the complete clinical phase, i.e. initial oocyte recovery as well as subsequent follow-up after ET, is done at a facility near the patient's home. The oocyte is transported by the husband to the central IVF unit which takes care of the laboratory phase and ET. Thus, the wife has to come to the central IVF unit only for ET.

Higher pregnancy rates have been reported with GIFT, ZIFT and TET compared to uterine ET. However, this may be attributed to other variations in patient profile and technique, and these methods are seldom used.

Intracytoplasmic Sperm Injection (Flowchart 2)

This technique has been used in cases of aspermia, azoospermia and functional disorders of sperm. Partial zona dissection (PZD) and subzonal insemination (SUZI) have been used to improve sperm penetration but with limited success. ICSI uses special equipment with *holding* and *injection* pipettes under an inverted microscope to

Flowchart 2: Indication of intracystoplasmic sperm injection.

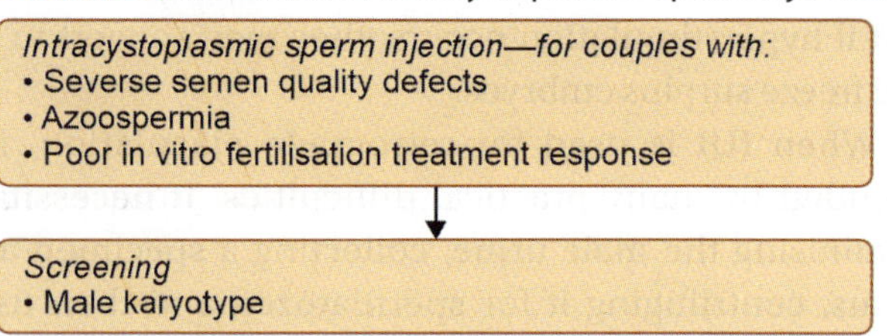

stabilise the oocyte and inject the sperm. The technique is useful in cases of oligozoospermia, where conventional IVF has failed, or in azoospermia and aspermia. In this situation, a variety of methods have been used to obtain the sperm. These include the following: rete testis aspiration (RETA), PESA, TESA, spermatocele aspiration (SPAS), MESA and TESE.

Fresh or cryopreserved sperm can be used for further ICSI cycles. The commonly used procedures are MESA, PESA and TESA. PESA usually yields enough sperms for cryopreservation. Using a mixture of methods, a 90–94% success in sperm retrieval is reported—fertilisation rates of 55% per oocyte, regardless of sperm recovery method or diagnostic category, and pregnancy rates of 21–39% per ET have been reported. Obstetric outcome is similar to that with other ARTs.

The recognised indications for treatment by ICSI include:

- Severe deficits in semen quality
- Obstructive azoospermia
- Nonobstructive azoospermia

In addition, treatment by ICSI should be considered for couples in whom a previous IVF treatment cycle has resulted in failed or very poor fertilisation.

Surgical sperm recovery for ICSI: Amongst the many surgical methods for sperm recovery, the most widely described are MESA, PESA, TESE and percutaneous testicular sperm fine-needle aspiration (TESA, also called fine-needle aspiration, or FNA). The choice of surgical sperm recovery method depends on the underlying diagnosis, whether the goal of the procedure is diagnostic or therapeutic, and whether isolated sperm will be used immediately or will be cryopreserved.

Testicular sperm extraction may be used to recover sperm in cases of post-testicular azoospermia (in which spermatogenesis is expected to be normal), with a successful sperm recovery in 96% of patients. TESA is usually well tolerated by patients. It is typically performed with a 21-gauge needle with no anaesthesia or with a 19-gauge needle or biopsy gun using local anaesthesia. Fertilisation and implantation rates have been reported to be similar in a retrospective analysis comparing TESA with open biopsy using TESA. Alternatively, if the nature of the obstruction needs to be investigated by a full scrotal exploration, or if attempted surgical correction of the obstruction will be performed at the time of sperm recovery, MESA may be the preferred procedure. MESA is performed with general or regional anaesthesia using a microsurgical approach. One advantage of MESA is that a very large number of spermatozoa is usually retrieved, so cryopreservation and avoidance of repeat surgery may be possible. Fresh and frozen-thawed epididymal or testicular spermatozoa appear to have comparable fertilisation and ongoing pregnancy rates when used for ICSI.

Sperm retrieval using PESA is another option for the treatment of post-testicular azoospermia. PESA is performed using a 19-gauge needle with local or regional anaesthesia. A sperm recovery rate of >80% has been reported with 55% fertilisation and 33% ongoing pregnancy rates after ICSI. Although this procedure appears less invasive than some of its alternatives, it is performed blindly. Bleeding and epididymal injury are possible, and postsurgical fibrosis may result. In contrast, men with testicular azoospermia or gonadal failure require TESE, and possibly multiple biopsies, to retrieve sperm. However, the sperm recovery rate with TESE is only about 50%, and clinical outcomes for ICSI after TESE amongst patients with testicular azoospermia are variable.

Lower fertilisation rates but comparable ongoing pregnancy rates have been reported for ICSI using testicular spermatozoa recovered from testicular azoospermia, compared with epididymal spermatozoa, post-testicular azoospermia. Sperm at all stages have been used to establish successful pregnancies using ICSI. However, the fertilisation and pregnancy rates associated with maturation-arrested spermatid are very low, and couples should be properly counselled regarding their prognosis and alternative options. Finally, cryopreservation of testicular tissues and spermatozoa for use in subsequent ICSI treatment cycles has been reported.

Laser-assisted Hatching

- Indium-gallium-arsenic phosphorus laser is used.
- 1.48-μm wavelength

Indications

- Thick zona pellucida
- Elderly patient
- Elevated basal FSH
- Failed implantation cycles
- Poor responders
- Unexplained infertility
- Few embryos
- IVF cycles

Laser can also be used in ICSI where it prevents excessive cell deformation during injection. Zona thinning is advantageous with no loss of blastomeres. Generally, assisted hatching is done on day 3 at six- to eight-cell stage. A laser-mounted micromanipulation is used. Multiple small holes are drilled.

Preimplantation Genetic Diagnosis

Prenatal diagnosis of genetic disorders has been further refined by the development of preimplantation genetic diagnosis. A single cell is biopsied from the embryo at the eight-cell stage and enzymes, chromosomes or specific mutations are evaluated by polymerase chain reaction (PCR) and fluorescent in situ hybridisation (FISH). If the cell shows no abnormality, the embryo is transferred to the mother. However, if any abnormality is identified, the embryo is discarded. Thus, termination of pregnancy is avoided. Healthy babies have resulted from the use of such biopsied embryos.

RESULTS OF TREATING INFERTILITY

No matter what treatment is applied or what advice is given to the infertile couple, conception will follow in a certain number of cases; this is inevitable by the laws of chance which govern conception. It is all too easy to claim a coincidence as a dramatic cure, and this is the reason why so many treatments have their advocates. Scepticism in these matters is not popular but is justified by the findings in a carefully documented series of cases. Of those women who consult a gynaecologist on account of primary infertility existing for 2 years or more, 50% have at least one pregnancy within the next 6 years. In not less than half of the cases, the occurrence of pregnancy can be shown to be unrelated to treatment. Indeed, 3–4% of patients conceive before there is time to arrange for any investigation or treatment.

The occurrence of a pregnancy after treatment does not necessarily mean that the fertility of the marriage is raised. At least half the couples who produce one pregnancy after a phase of infertility find it impossible to repeat the performance.

When pregnancy occurs in an infertile woman, it may carry special risks. The chance of tubal implantation in those with tubal disease is five times greater than normal and that of abortion is doubled. The overall chance of obstetric complications is increased by one third to a half. When, therefore, a pregnancy comes to a woman who has waited long, its management demands rigorous attention, for the loss of the child would be even more tragic than usual.

DANGERS OF INVESTIGATING AND TREATING INFERTILITY

With proper safeguards, minor operative and other procedures involved in the investigation of infertility carry little risk to life, although the danger of an exacerbation of salpingo-oophoritis and the hazards of laparoscopy cannot be disregarded. The real menace of investigating and treating infertility is that they may concentrate the patient's attention on the problem, convert a complaint into an obsession, exacerbate the already profound unhappiness, and even lead to the estrangement of the partners in marriage.

It is for these reasons that medical care should never be unduly protracted or complicated. Clinical examination, semen analysis, tubal patency tests and biochemical assessment of ovulatory status, *if properly performed and interpreted*, will either be followed by pregnancy or reveal the causes of infertility in the majority of cases. In others, laparoscopy provides the answer. Treatment should be as rational as possible and should be abandoned if not successful within a reasonable period. There is an increasing tendency for women to be referred for a third or fourth opinion regarding infertility. There is always an optimum time to call a halt, but this depends on the particular couple, who are at liberty to desist at any stage but should also have access to more specialised units for another opinion.

If the couple has had a detailed and full assessment from a specialised unit then an honest and frank appraisal of their chances of conception and pregnancy should be given. A degree of optimism is healthy, but if any abnormality is found, the couple should be kept informed and the possibility of treating or overcoming the problem explained, including the reason for limiting the period of treatment if ineffective. *Either partner* will suffer loss of esteem if infertile and each could be expected to make adjustments in accepting the infertility of the other. In practice, an absolute situation rarely exists but in a few cases where it does, e.g. azoospermia, the couple is entitled to the truth. This is important to their decision regarding further treatment by DI. The fact that the woman has completely obstructed tubes no longer means there is no chance to conceive, for IVF-ET is a possibility, although it may not be available for that particular patient. The developments in the field of infertility over the last two decades have been dramatic, and it is possible that in the next decade, we will be able to explain and perhaps overcome some of the unexplained cases of infertility which now exist.

COMPLICATIONS OF ASSISTED REPRODUCTIVE TECHNOLOGY

Twins and Higher order Multiple Gestation

Multiple gestation, especially higher order multiple gestation, is a serious complication of infertility treatment and has tremendous medical, psychological, social and financial implications. In recent years, it has been reported that only 20% of higher order multiple gestations are the result of spontaneous conceptions. The remaining 80% are attributable to reproductive interventions. Of these multiple gestations, half are attributable to ART and half to the use of ovulation drugs in non-ART cycles.

Ovarian Hyperstimulation Syndrome

Ovarian hyperstimulation syndrome is a medical complication that is both completely iatrogenic and unique to the treatment of infertility. Although the pathophysiology of OHSS is not well understood, the signs and symptoms of this disease can be attributed to local and systemic increases in capillary permeability. These changes, in turn, result in the depletion of intravascular volume at the expense of third-space fluid accumulation.

Ovarian hyperstimulation syndrome has a varied spectrum of clinical presentation. An attempt to better understand this heterogeneity led to the development of a staging system for OHSS that would reflect symptom severity. This classification categorises patients into mild, moderate and severe diseases. In mild OHSS, patients often complain of mild abdominal distension and soreness, nausea and vomiting. Ovarian enlargement can be 5–12 cm. Moderate disease is marked by the presence of abdominal ascites on ultrasound examination. Severe disease is diagnosed when there are clinical signs of tense ascites,

TABLE 2: Differences between early and late ovarian hyperstimulation syndrome.

Early ovarian hyperstimulation syndrome	*Late ovarian hyperstimulation syndrome*
Within 9 days of oocyte retrieval	After 9 days
Higher serum oestradiol	Lower serum oestradiol
Increased follicle number	Less follicle number
Increased follicular response	Multiple gestations
By exogenous human chorionic gonadotrophin	By endogenous human chorionic gonadotrophin of pregnancy

hydrothorax, shortness of breath, haemoconcentration, hypercoagulability or any complications of OHSS such as renal failure, thromboembolism or acute respiratory distress syndrome (ARDS) **(Table 2)**.

Golaris Classification of Ovarian Hyperstimulation Syndrome

- *Mild:*
  - Grade I:
- Abdominal distension pain
  - Grade II:
    - Grade I + nausea, vomiting and diarrhoea
    - Ovary enlarge (<5 cm)
    - Weight gain (<3 kg)
- *Moderate:*
  - Grade III:
    - Mild + ultrasound evidence of ascites + hyponatraemia, hypokalaemia and hypoproteinaemia
    - Ovary ≤10 cm in size
    - Weight gain 10 lbs
    - Decreased urine output
- *Severe:*
  - Grade IV:
    - Moderate + clinical ascites/hydrothorax, ARDS, ovary (>12 cm)
    - Weight gain (>5 kg)
  - Grade V:
    - Grade IV + hypovolaemia, hyponatraemia, and hyperkalaemia
    - Increased blood viscosity, hypercoagulability
    - Decreased renal perfusion, oliguria, hypertension, hypoproteinaemia, thrombosis, coagulation failure and electrolyte imbalance
    - Leucocytes >15,000/mm^3
    - Liver and kidney failure. Severe OHSS mandates hospitalisation.

Principles of Management

- *Monitor:* Fluid intake/urine output, haematocrit, electrolytes, albumin/globulin (AG)/liver function and coagulation profile
- *Replace:* Crystalloids, fresh frozen plasma (FFP) and human serum albumin
- *Aspirate:* Ascitic tapping is therapeutic
- *Operate:* Only if hematoperitoneum or torsion or life-threatening OHSS
- *Conservative in mild to moderate:*
  - Bed rest
  - Intravenous fluids
  - Anti-inflammatory, antiemetics

ADOPTION

The adoption of a child is a matter on which individual outlooks differ. Some couples cannot tolerate the idea, others find it attractive. Only the latter make suitable foster parents. I have never encountered a couple who has regretted their decision to adopt a baby, but it is possible that the venture may not always bring the happiness expected. Adoption as a solution to an infertility problem, therefore, deserves a cautious approach by those concerned. As in the case of DI, adoption should be presented as a possible option to consider. If not, the sad situation arises of the couple coming to terms with the concept of adoption only to find they are not acceptable due to their age or some other reason. They should be aware of the long waiting lists and limited availability of children, and in particular, babies for adoption.

If the husband and wife decide in favour of adoption, they should do so by the legal machinery operating in their area. No doctor should take responsibility for the arrangements.

Age and Decreased Ovarian Reserve

An association between the age of the woman and reduced fertility has been well documented, with the decline in fecundability beginning in the early 30s but accelerating during the late 30s and early 40s. Chronologic age is the strongest determinant of reproductive success in spontaneous and ART cycles, because it is a predictor of ovarian reserve.

The fecundability of women undergoing DI whose husbands are azoospermic provides insight into the effects of age on the fertility of the female alone. A French group that studied women enrolled in artificial insemination programs found that fertility rates begin to drop after 30 years of age. The pregnancy rate after 1 year of inseminations was 74% in women aged 30 years and younger, 62% in women aged 30–35 years, and 54% in women older than 35 years of age.

The physiology of declining fertility in older women is better understood in the light of data from oocyte donation programs. When embryos produced from oocytes retrieved from younger women are transferred to older women, the pregnancy rates amongst the older women approximate those of the younger women, and variations in pregnancy rates are directly dependent on the age of the donors, not that of the recipients. Several observations strongly support that it is the age of the oocyte, rather than the age of the endometrium, that accounts for the age-related decline in female fertility.

This oocyte-related decline in fertility is also known as decreased ovarian reserve. Absolute evidence of decreased ovarian reserve often can be ascertained only after ART treatment shows decreased ovarian responsiveness to controlled ovarian hyperstimulation. In ART, decreased ovarian reserve is reflected by an increased requirement for gonadotropins (FSH ± LH), small numbers of ovarian follicles and oocytes, and low serum oestradiol levels during exogenous stimulation of folliculogenesis. These clinical outcomes probably reflect a decreased number of ovarian antral follicles as well as poor quality of granulosa cells and oocytes. Although age is the best predictor of ovarian reserve as reflected by ovarian responsiveness to controlled ovarian hyperstimulation, there is a subset of women who demonstrate an ovarian reserve that is prematurely diminished based on their chronologic age. Similarly, there are women who respond well to controlled ovarian hyperstimulation and achieve pregnancies despite their advanced age. Therefore, tremendous efforts have been expended to identify an ovarian reserve test that can be used to counsel patients and guide their management.

Ovarian reserve screening tests that have been proposed include serum day 3 FSH, clomiphene citrate challenge test (CCCT), serum inhibin B, and TVS to assess antral follicle number or ovarian size. Measurement of day 3 FSH is based on evidence that a small increase in basal serum FSH levels correlates with the decreased fecundability seen amongst women in their late 30s. Counting of antral follicles is a good method and if a woman has less than four antral follicles, they usually are poor responders.

Recently, serum inhibin B has also been proposed as a potential screening test for ovarian reserve. Inhibin B is produced by ovarian granulosa cells predominantly during the follicular phase of the menstrual cycle. Inhibin B suppresses the production of FSH by the pituitary gland. The normal rise in circulating levels of FSH associated with menopause is thought to be secondary to the decrease in inhibin B production accompanying the age-related depletion of functional ovarian follicles. In fact, in the CCCT, the main mechanism by which FSH is normally suppressed is via inhibin B production by granulosa cells. Women with decreased ovarian reserve have a lower rise in the day 10 serum inhibin B levels in response to the CCCT. In addition, women who have clinical evidence of diminished ovarian reserve and normal day 3 FSH levels have been found to have decreased day 3 inhibin B levels. This observation suggests that a decrease in day 3 serum inhibin B levels may precede detectable changes in day 3 FSH levels. However, basal inhibin B levels do not provide additional age-independent prognostic value for predicting pregnancy outcomes after ART. One possible reason for this is that levels of inhibin B may reflect granulosa cell function and thereby only forecast ovarian response in ART. Although granulosa cell competence is certainly associated with oocyte quality, clinical application of serum inhibin B testing will also depend on whether levels are predictive of normal meiotic division of the oocyte because foetal karyotype is an important determinant of pregnancy outcome.

CONCLUSION

Very few couples have absolute infertility, which can result from congenital or acquired irreversible loss of functional gametes in either partner or the absence of a uterus in the female. These specific couples should be counselled regarding their options of adoption, the use of donor gametes, or surrogacy. Rather, most couples who have difficulty conceiving have subfertility. According to this fundamental concept, most couples could conceive spontaneously in time, but because of known or unidentifiable causes, their spontaneous fecundity rate is so low that medical management is warranted. Another reason to seek medical attention, particularly amongst older women, is that as time passes during unsuccessful spontaneous attempts, fecundability will be further compromised by increasing age and concomitantly decreasing ovarian reserve. Although the identification of apparent causes of subfertility (such as anovulation or oligospermia) allows treatment to be targeted, effective empiric treatments greatly increase the chance of a pregnancy even when no distinct cause is identified. Overall, these treatments aim at increasing the probability of conception and implantation by optimising gamete (sperm and oocyte) and uterine factors. However, it is important to realise that the age of a woman is a factor to be considered and there should not be any delay in offering any form of treatment which is suitable for the couple. ART has changed the methodology of treatment and seems to be an effective method of infertility treatment.

SUGGESTED READING

1. Joshi N, Dmitry K, Anderson J. Trends and correlates of good perinatal outcomes in assisted reproductive technology. Obstet Gynecol. 2012;120(4):843-51.
2. Kushnir VA, Barad DH, Albertini DF. Systematic review of worldwide trends in assisted reproductive technology 2004-2013. Reprod Biol Endocrinol. 2017;15(1):6.
3. Luke B. Pregnancy and birth outcomes in couples with infertility with and without assisted reproductive technology: with an emphasis on US population-based studies. Am J Obstet Gynecol. 2017;217(3):270-81.

49

CHAPTER

Instruments in Gynaecological Procedures

Shripad Hebbar, Pooja HN, Muralidhar V Pai

Chapter Outline

- Instruments
- Gynaecological Procedures

INSTRUMENTS

Instruments in gynaecological surgery are both general and specific to gynaecological surgery. Many new modifications and variations in the instruments have come up, but a surgeon should insist on a broad range of high-quality functioning equipment that do not continually irritate by failing to work, whether it is a simple pair of scissors or the most sophisticated minimal access equipment.

In virtually all modern operation theatres, instruments and drapes are prepacked and sterilised in *sets* for individual or generic procedures in a central sterile supply department. This has a major advantage in terms of high standards of sterilisation over selecting instruments for a specific procedure and sterilising them immediately prior to an operation.

A wide range of prepacked and sterile disposable instruments of amazing complexity have been introduced in recent times, including much of the equipment used in minimal access surgery.

Besides the *set* and presterilised instruments, from time to time, an immediate sterilising facility is required so that, in many operation theatres, on-the-spot sterilisation is available for a number of specialised pieces of equipment.

The instruments can generally be divided into:

- A general operating set
- A minor procedure set
- Special instruments and laparoscopy instruments.

The general operating set commonly consists of:

- Sponge-holding forceps
- Towel clips
- Bard-Parker knife handle
- Lane's toothed dissecting forceps
- Nontoothed dissecting forceps
- Mayo's dissecting scissors
- Scissors—straight
- Lloyd-Davis needle holder
- A set of Grey-Turner Artery forceps—straight and curved
- A set of Allis forceps
- Kocher's clamps—straight and curved
- Hysterectomy clamps—straight and curved
- Vulsellum forceps
- Retractors—Czerny's, Deaver's, Richardson's, Doyen's and Langerhans'
- Babcock's forceps
- Needle holders
- Bulldog clamps

The minor procedure set consists of:

- Sponge holders
- Sims' vaginal speculum
- Anterior vaginal wall retractor
- Vulsellum forceps
- *Simpson* Uterine Sound
- Bladder sound
- One set of cervical dilators
- Blunt and sharp curettes
- Needle holders
- Artery forceps
- Scissors 6"

A minor vaginal set for dilatation and curettage (D&C) and suction evacuation is shown in **Figure 1**.

Some of the Instruments Mentioned Warrant Special Comments

Scissors

Often marketed as Mayo scissors **(Fig. 2)**, they are heavy but have a sureness about them, which allows accurate

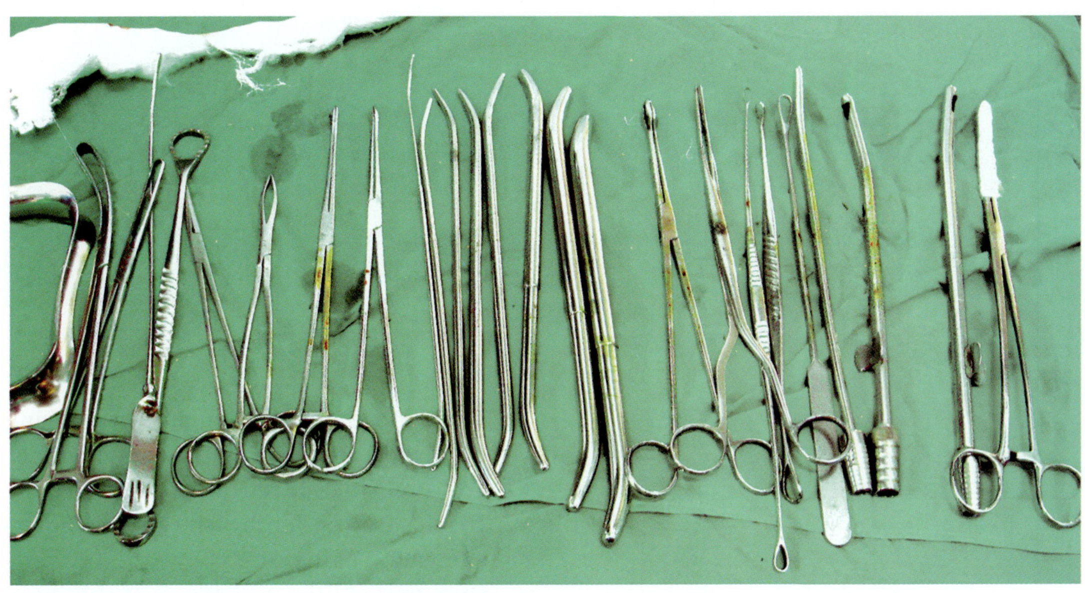

Fig. 1: Dilatation and curettage set.

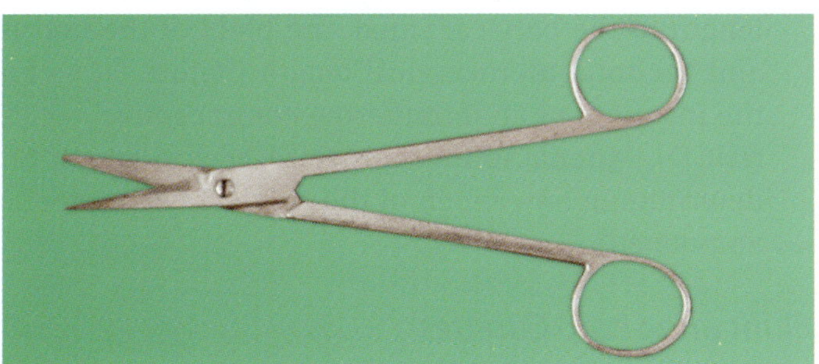

Fig. 2: Mayo scissors.

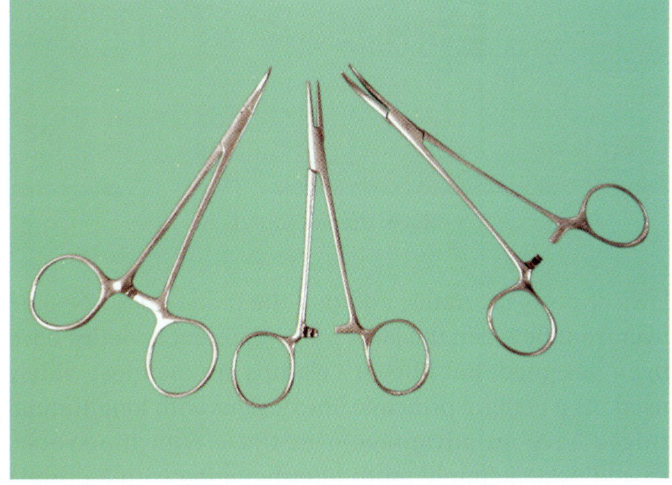

Fig. 3: Artery forceps.

gentle dissection, particularly of the *separate and cut* type. The ends of the scissors are relatively blunt and will do little damage when separating tissue, while the blades are powerful enough to cut when coupled with long levers of the handles. This latter characteristic is especially important in cancer work when operating on tissues previously treated with radiotherapy.

A lighter scissor with the same qualities, e.g. Monaghan's dissecting scissors, is also useful.

Artery Forceps (Fig. 3)

The forceps included in the set are almost all straight. Meig's right angle forceps are of great value in dealing with vessels deep into the pelvis. They are long and allow the suture to be placed around either the points or the heel of the forceps. These are straight or curved instruments with transverse serrations in the inner aspect of the blades for better grip. They are used to grasp the bleeding vessels as a haemostat, to hold the peritoneum while opening and closing and to hold the stay sutures and umbilical tapes (applied to the ureter during radical surgeries) and also the end of redundant thread attached to various stumps, for example, round ligament, vaginal angles.

Tissue Clamps

On many occasions in gynaecological surgery, it is necessary to clamp discrete blocks of tissues firmly and then suture the block to occlude the vessels contained with it. It is important that these clamps are strong, that the

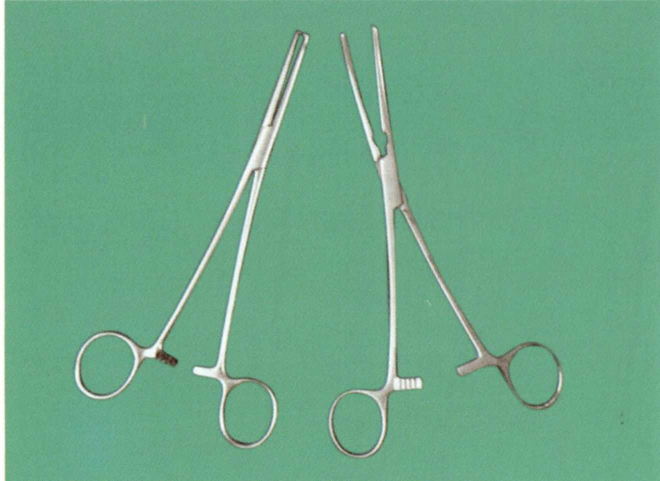

Fig. 4: Tissue clamps.

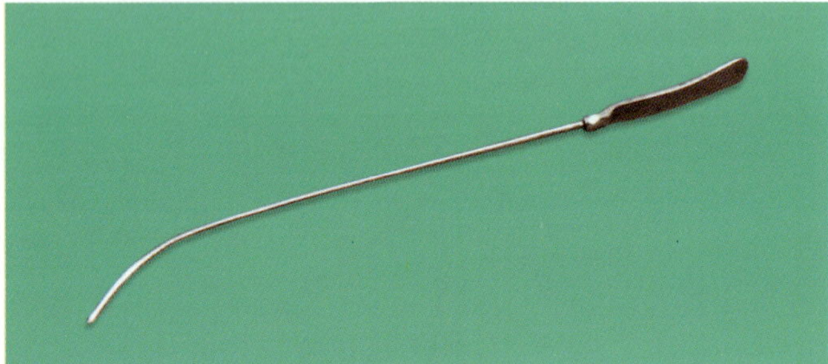

Fig. 5: Uterine sound.

jaws oppose accurately and that the tissue does not slide over from between the jaws. Many different varieties have been designed, but Kocher's clamps are the most widely used. As a general principle, the designs with longitudinal ridges have an advantage over those with transverse. In addition, a simple tooth interdigitating with a double tooth at the tips of the jaws assists in correct apposition so that the tissue does not slip. This instrument is used for holding pedicles in a hysterectomy. These clamps also allow correct transfixation of pedicles. The clamps can be straight or angled **(Fig. 4)**. Kocher's clamps can also be used for clamping the umbilical cord of the newborn at the time of delivery or for artificial low rupture of membranes.

Uterine Sound (Fig. 5)

Designed by Simpson, they are marked in inches and are 12" long. They have a blunt bounded tip. The uterine end is curved and angulated; the curve fits with the curvature of the cervix and measures around 2–3". They are used:

- To determine the length and direction of the uterus
- To diagnose and differentiate a polyp lying in the cervix
- To locate a misplaced intrauterine device
- To correct mobile retroversion of the uterus
- To measure the depth of the vaginal fornix in congenital elongation of the cervix
- One can feel the resistance of the internal os while passing the instrument through the cervical canal till the fundus and accordingly one can determine the length of the cervical canal, the body of the uterus and the total uterocervical length [before D&C, for the insertion of an intrauterine contraceptive device (IUCD), Mirena, to find the uterocervical length for determining how much of the cervical tissue can be amputated].

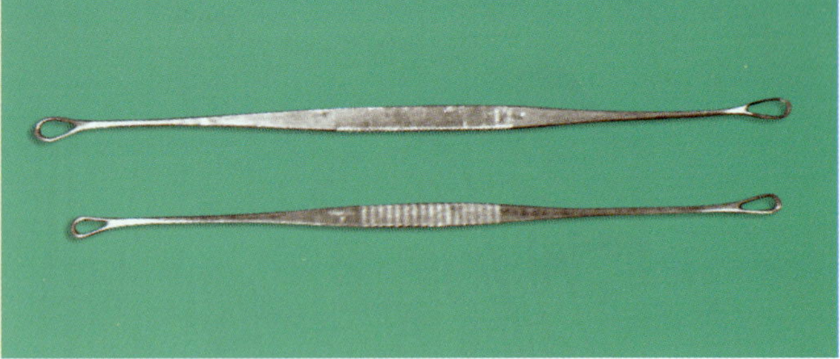

Fig. 6: Blunt and sharp curettage.

Blunt and Sharp Curettes

Designed by Blake, one end of the instrument is blunt, while the second end is sharp. It is used in D&C, dilatation and evacuation (D&E), infertility and dysfunctional uterine bleeding **(Fig. 6)**. Single-ended curettes are also available (Mathew-Duncan dilators) and are preferred by some gynaecologists. Each curette consists of three parts, i.e., the handle, the shank and the curetting end. The handle is corrugated on the aspect which corresponds to the direction of the bend at the tip so that its position in the uterus can be imagined, and the endometrium can be better curetted.

Sims' Double-bladed Posterior Vaginal Speculum (Fig. 7)

Designed by Marion Sims, the blades are of unequal breadth to fit different vaginas. It may be single-bladed also. It is used to visualise the cervix and inspect the lesions of the cervix and the anterior vaginal wall. It is also practically used for all vaginal operations, e.g. D&C, D&E and vaginal hysterectomies. The handle is slightly concave to collect

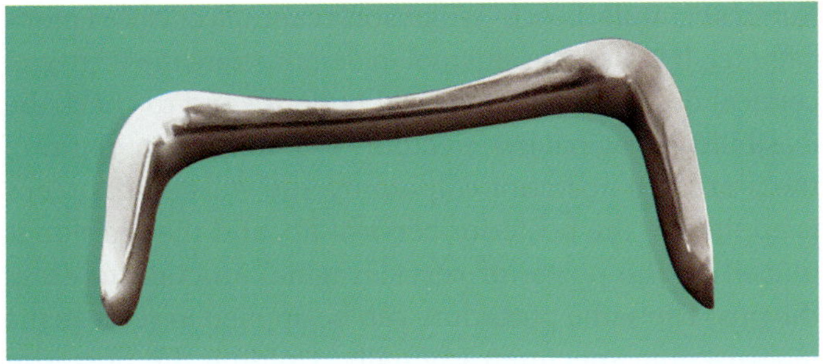

Fig. 7: Sims' speculum.

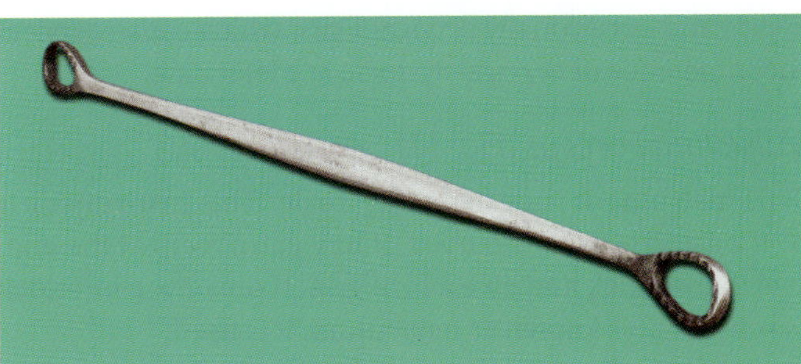

Fig. 9: Anterior vaginal wall retractor.

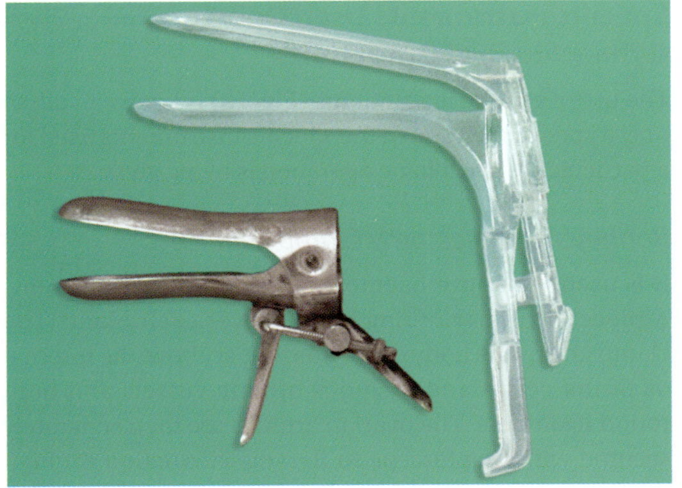

Fig. 8: Cusco's speculum.

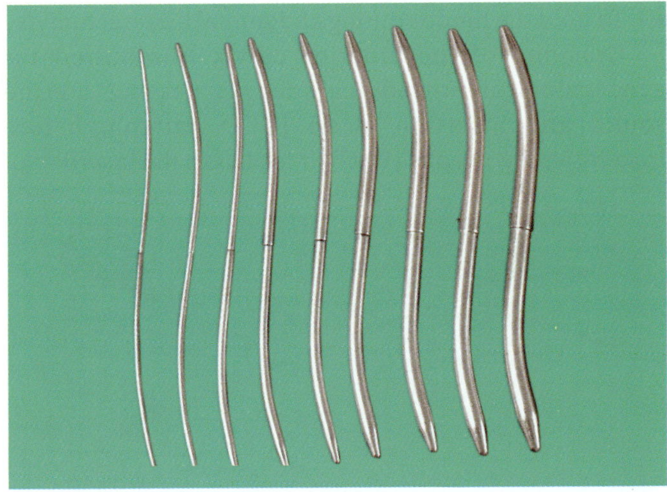

Fig. 10: Dilator set.

the drained blood and secretions. This instrument can be of limited value if assistance is required, especially when used to expose the cervix, for example, for taking Pap smear, as it is not self-retaining. As the instrument moves with the hand, it is not suitable for colposcopy. The patient also needs to be at the edge of the table.

Cusco's Bivalve Self-retaining Vaginal Speculum (Fig. 8)

The valves are to retract the anterior and posterior vaginal walls to have a good look at the cervix. It is used to:

- Visualise the cervix and vaginal fornices
- Collect vaginal pool materials and scrapings for cytologic study
- Perform minor operations on the cervix.

Compared to Sims' speculum, this instrument is easy to introduce in the vagina and is self-retaining; hence, there is no need for assistance and can be adjusted to the size of the vagina by separating the blades through a mechanism. However, it covers the anterior and posterior vaginal walls and limits the inspection, has decreased manoeuvrability and procedures like D&C are difficult to perform because of the less space available.

Anterior Vaginal Wall Retractor (Fig. 9)

This instrument has loop-shaped ends with transverse serrations on the loops. The loops are set at an angle of 15° to the shaft. It is used along with Sims' speculum to retract the sagging vaginal wall to have a good exposure of the cervix. Most of the indications are the same as that for Sims' speculum. It is very useful in demonstrating anterior vaginal wall prolapse.

Cervical Dilators (Fig. 10)

Many types are available, e.g., Hegar's, Das's and Hawkin-Ambler's. They are used to dilate the cervix before D&C, D&E, pyometra, haematometra, intracavitary radiation therapy, etc., where access to the uterine cavity is required through the cervical canal. However, if not used carefully, there can be uterine perforation, internal bleeding, sepsis and occasionally cervical tears, which cause cervical incompetence or cervical dystocia at a later date.

Vulsellum Forceps (Fig. 11)

This instrument is designed by Teale. This instrument is 8" long and is usually curved. It has sharp teeth at the end, which interlock and give a firm grip. If only 2 × 1 interlock is present, it is known as tenaculum. It is used:

- To grasp the anterior/posterior lip of the cervix and to make the cervix steady during cervical operations
- To remove polyps
- To hold the fundus during abdominal hysterectomy.

Grasping of the anterior cervix is required for gynaecological procedures such as passing uterine sound and insertion of an IUCD, Mirena, before hysterosalpingography (HSG). It facilitates the insertion of Rubin's cannula, Leech-Wilkinson's cannula or No. 8 Foley's catheter. It is also a useful tool to demonstrate the degree of cervical descent in uterovaginal prolapse and to check the feasibility of vaginal hysterectomy by noting the mobility of the uterus. In posterior colpotomy, the vulsellum forceps is applied to the posterior cervical lip, and the incision is placed on the posterior cervicovaginal junction to drain the pus. The same procedure can be applied to retrieve the laparoscopic specimen vaginally. Holding the posterior cervical lip is also applicable in culdocentesis.

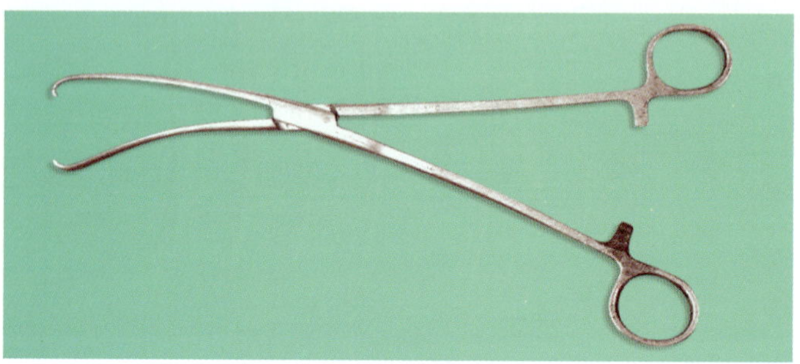

Fig. 11: Vulsellum forceps.

Specific Instruments Used Only for Gynaecological Operations

The use of general instruments **(Fig. 12)** is known to all, so only a special mention of the specific instruments used for a particular gynaecologic operation is being given.

Bonney's Myomectomy Clamp (Fig. 13)

It is used to control haemorrhage during myomectomy. A piece of rubber tubing is fixed over each blade. The clamp grasps the body of the uterus just above the internal os of the cervix and includes uterine vessels and both round ligaments. The ovarian arteries are then separately secured with ring forceps so that the circulation through the uterus is entirely arrested and the operation becomes bloodless.

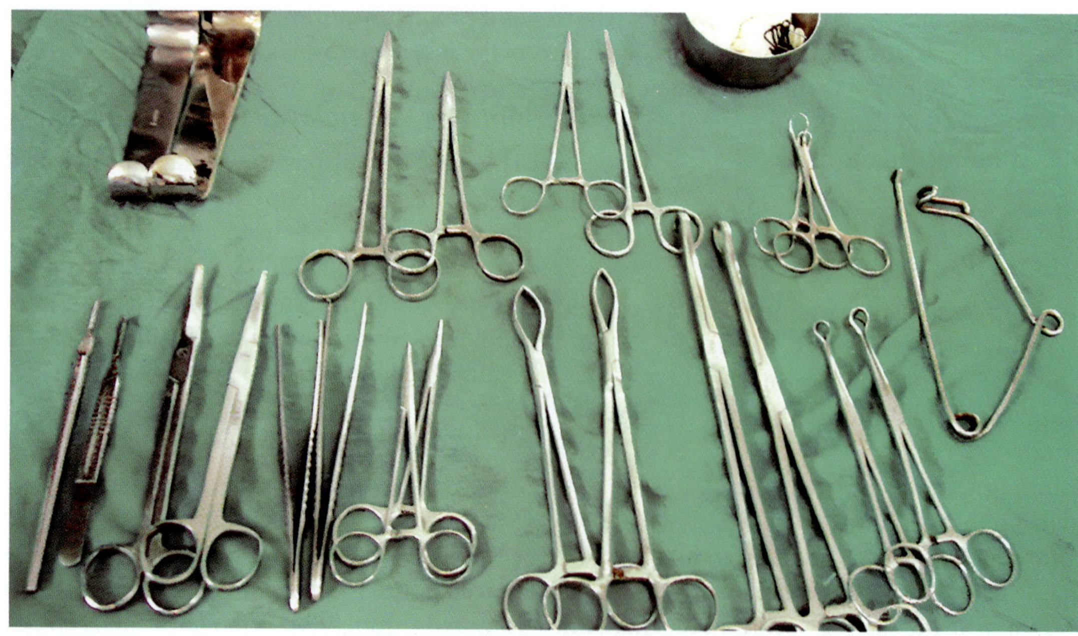

Fig. 12: Abdominal instrument set.

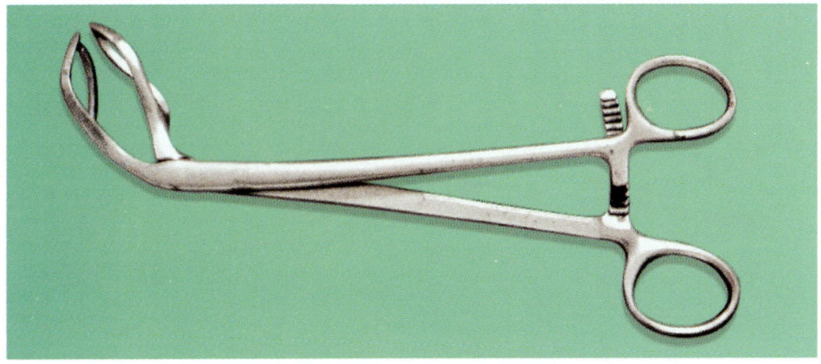

Fig. 13: Myomectomy clamp.

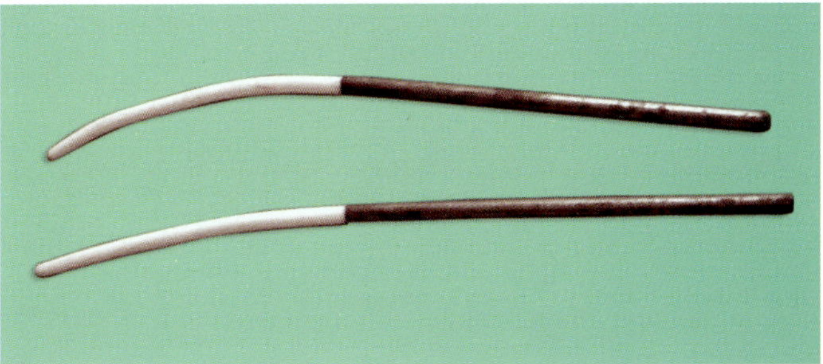

Fig. 15: Malleable probes.

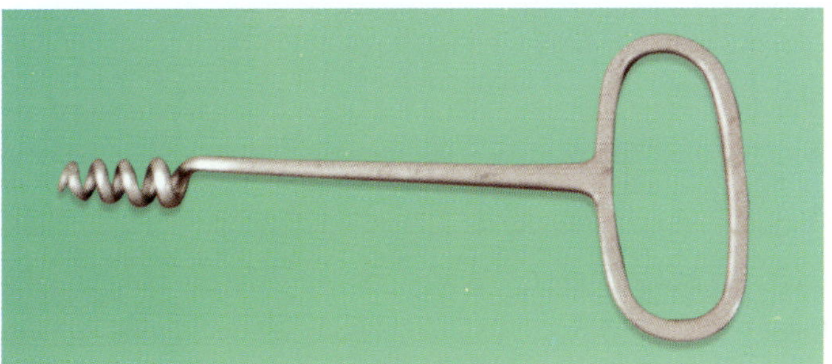

Fig. 14: Myoma screw.

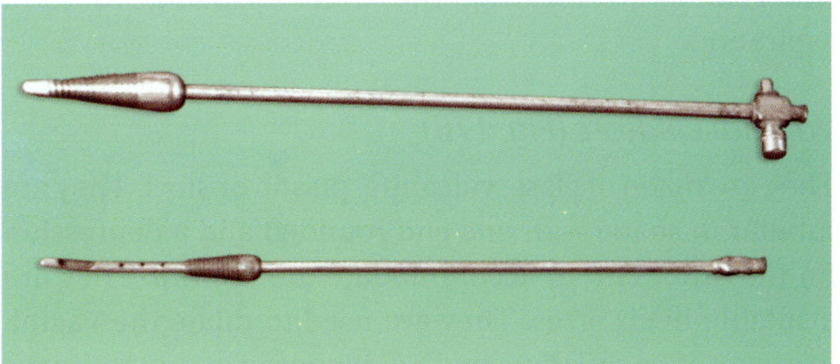

Fig. 16: Tubal patency testing cannulas.

Myoma Screw (Doyen's) (Fig. 14)

It is used to fix the myoma after the capsule is cut opened to give traction while the myoma is enucleated out of its bed. It is also used to give traction in a big uterus requiring a hysterectomy.

Malleable Probes (Fig. 15)

They are used in tubal recanalisation.

Rubin's Insufflation Cannula (Fig. 16)

It is used for tubal testing. With better diagnostic techniques available, it is not much in use now.

Leech–Wilkinson's Cannula (Fig. 16)

It is used for chromopertubation during laparoscopy and hysterosalpingography. A Leech-Wilkinson cannula is a surgical instrument used for manipulating the uterus and inserting fluid or gas. It has a wide end and an extended tip for precise uterine manipulation. A Leech-Wilkinson cannula has a thin shank for easy access through the cervix and smooth outer curves to prevent damage to the surrounding tissues. It is available in different working end sizes and can be sterilised and reused.

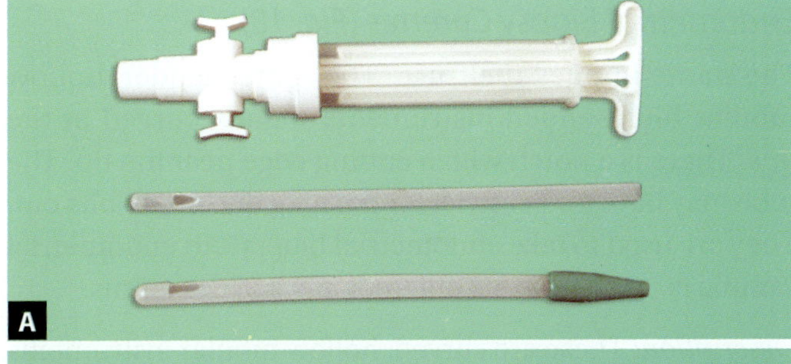

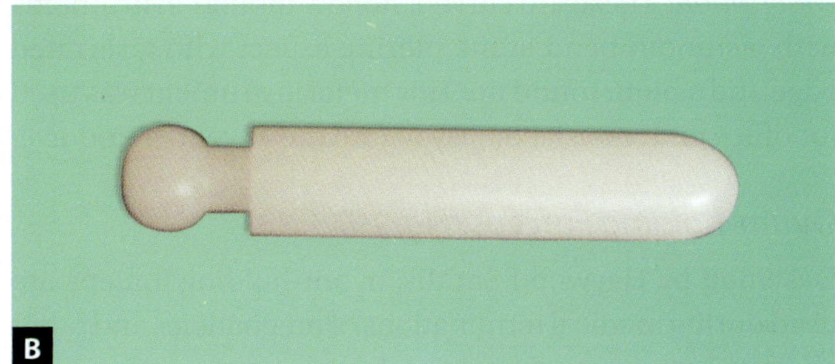

Figs. 17A and B: (A) Karman's syringe; (B) A vaginal dilator.

Karman's Syringe (Fig. 17A)

It is also known as a menstrual regulation syringe. It has a capacity of 50 mL. It is usually used for endometrial aspiration, especially when the patient has missed her periods. The flexibility of the Karman cannula reduces

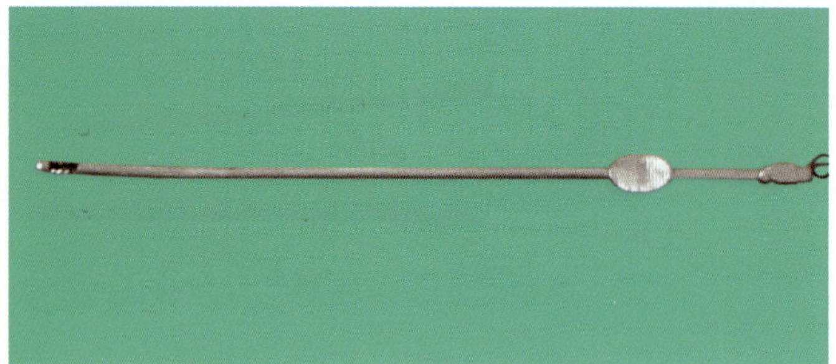

Fig. 18: An endometrial biopsy curette.

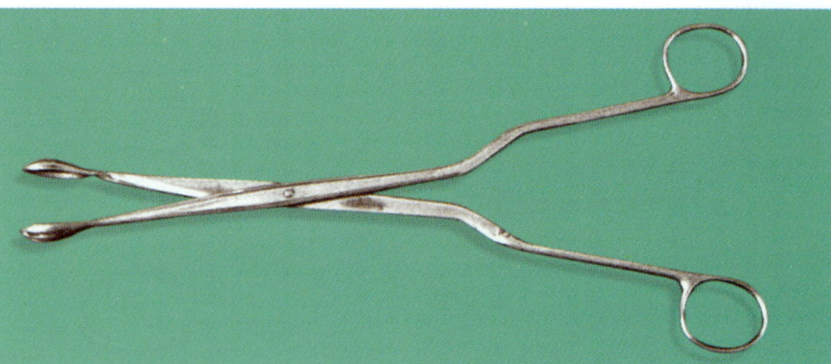

Fig. 19: Ovum-holding forceps.

the risk of perforating the uterus during vacuum aspiration.

Vaginal Dilators (Fig. 17B)

They are made of glass, vulcanite, plastic or steel. They are tubular in shape with one end rounded and a depression on the other end to accommodate the urethra. They are available in six sizes. They are used to dilate the vagina in cases of vaginismus and vaginal atresia due to burn/injuries/operations and artificial vagina in cases of congenital absence.

Endometrial Biopsy Curettes (Fig. 18)

The name implies their use. These are slender, hollow tubular blunt-ended instruments slightly curved at the tips. There is a notch with a cutting edge near the tip. The tube may have a steel stylet for pushing the biopsy bits out. They are used to take endometrial biopsy. An endometrial sample is taken from six different areas of the uterus.

Description: These are curved, hollow tubular instruments with a smooth bend at the uterine aspect with a serrated edge and a blunt round tip. This metal instrument was used for office endometrial biopsy before the advent of Endocel.

Ovum-holding Forceps (Fig. 19)

Designed by Haywood Smiths, ovum-holding forceps are used during medical terminations of pregnancies and other abortions to remove the retained products of conception or placenta. The blades of the instrument have spoon-shaped blunt fenestrated ends. Anything held in the blades is firmly caught but not nipped at its base. It has no catch.

Ayre's Spatula (Fig. 20)

It is used for taking cervical samples for Pap smears in suspected cases of cervical cancers. It is a wooden spatula

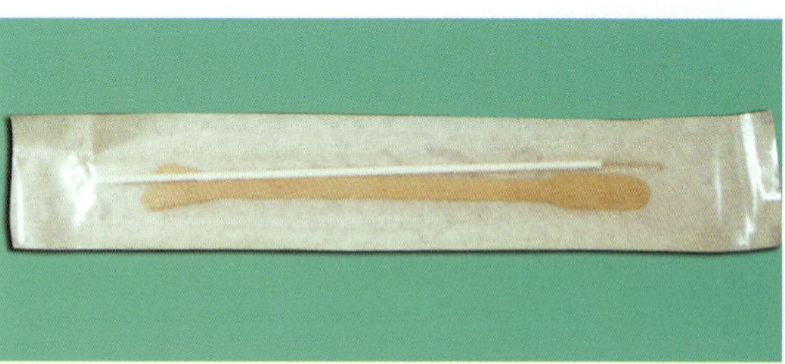

Fig. 20: Ayre's spatula.

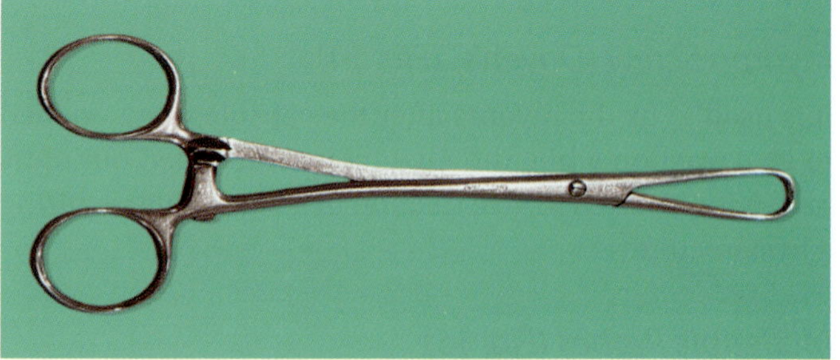

Fig. 21: Tenaculum.

with U-shaped openings on the one side and a flat surface on the other. The broad end is for vaginal sample collection and the narrow end is for cervical sample collection. It is rotated 360° in the vagina to obtain the cells to be sent for Pap smear examination.

Tenaculum (Jarcho's) (Fig. 21)

It is single-toothed and may be straight or curved. It is applied transversely just above the anterior lip of the cervix where airtight fitting of the cannula is required. It is used for tubal patency tests like hysterosalpingography and chromopertubation during laparoscopy and also to hold the cervical stump in subtotal hysterectomy while it is being sutured.

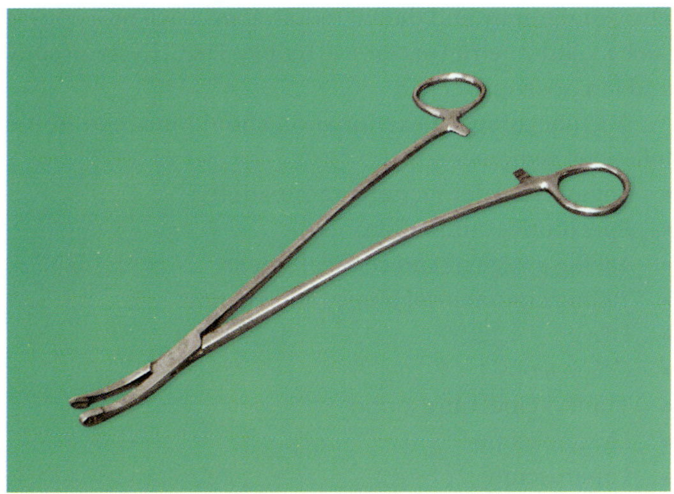

Fig. 22: Cervical punch biopsy forceps.

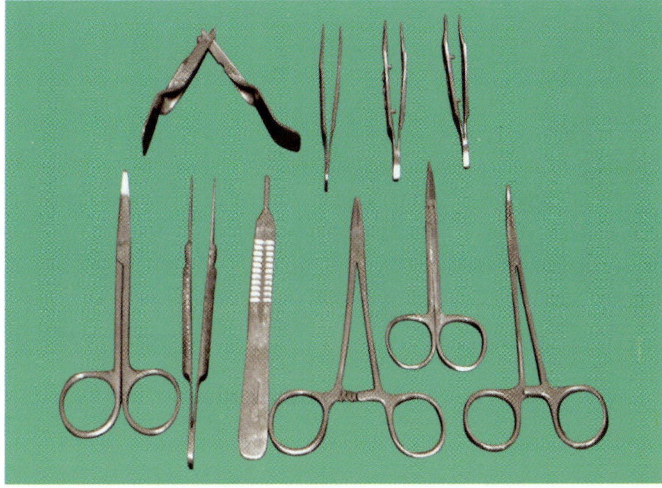

Fig. 23: Microsurgical instruments.

Cervical Punch Biopsy Forceps (Fig. 22)

They are used for taking cervical biopsy from any suspicious area on the cervix in cases of cervical malignancies. These are designed by Gellhorn. This instrument is 22.5 cm long and has punch-shaped ends inside the cup. On one end is a tiny pin to hold the specimen punched out. The instrument is made of stainless steel. It has cup-shaped sharp cutting ends, and one of the cups has a transverse groove that holds the biopsy specimen in place. There is no lock in the handle, which makes the instrument unique in the sense that an excessive force on the cervix can be applied, and hence cervical avulsion is avoided.

- Hysteroscopes, laparoscopes and other endoscopy instruments are now being widely used in gynaecologic practice. The era of minimally invasive surgery requires the surgeon to have special training in handling and using these instruments **(Fig. 22)**.
- Microsurgery instruments **(Fig. 23)** also require special training and care.

Uterine Manipulator (Fig. 24)

- It is a special instrument devised to manipulate the uterus from the vaginal route.
- It is used in laparoscopic sterilisation, for better visualisation of pelvic structures during laparoscopy.

Suture Materials

They may be organic, synthetic or metallic from a practical point of view. They may be classified as absorbable and nonabsorbable.

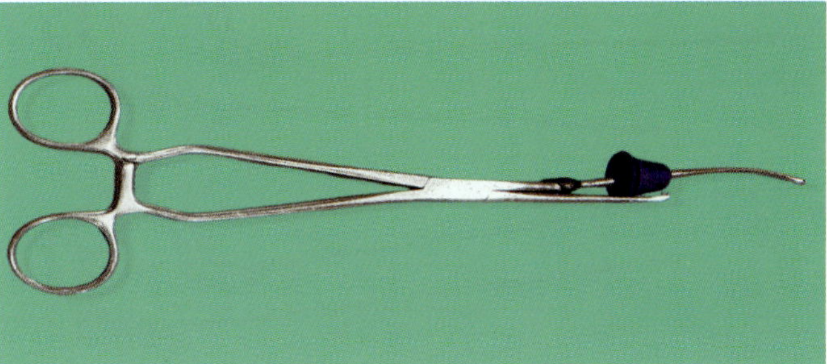

Fig. 24: Uterine manipulator.

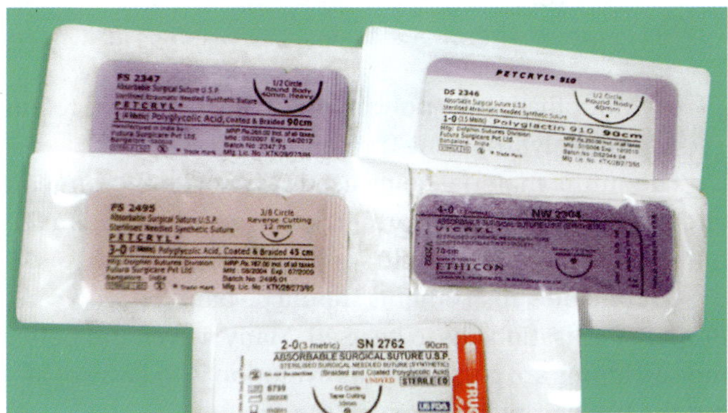

Fig. 25: Absorbable synthetic sutures.

- *Absorbable **(Fig. 25)**:*
  - Organic—Catgut
  - Synthetic—polyglycolic acid polyglactin (Vicryl)
- *Nonabsorbable **(Fig. 26)**:*
  - Braided/multifilament—silk, cotton, linen and mersilene

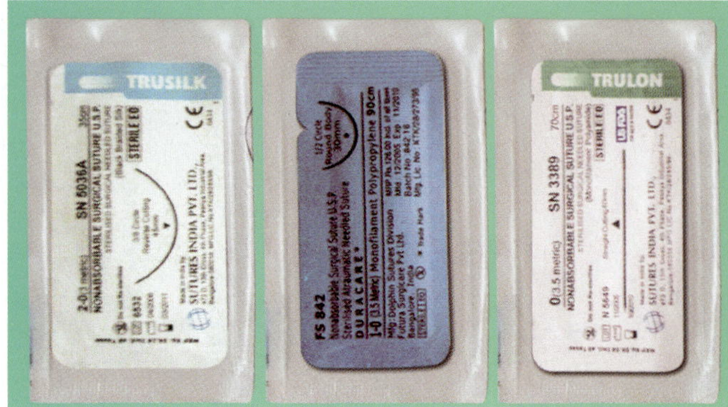

Fig. 26: Nonabsorbable sutures.

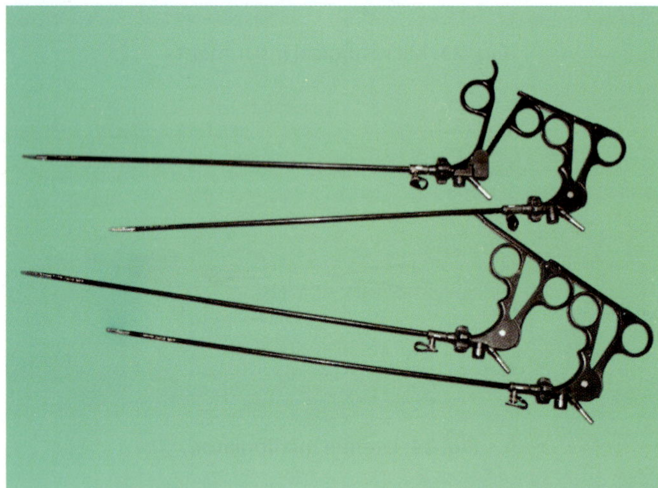

Fig. 27: Laparoscopic hand instruments.

- Monofilament—polyamide (nylon), dacron, teflon and polypropylene (prolene).

The suture material being used varies with the surgeon and availability, as with time it takes to get dissolved in the human body and the tensile strength is languid.

To conclude, instruments should be handled with care. Proper sterilisation has to be used. Many newer and better modifications are coming up as evolution is the way of life, but the basic principles remain the same.

GYNAECOLOGICAL PROCEDURES

Gynaecology today has evolved from the blind per a vaginal examination done in the Victorian era **(Fig. 27)** to modern gadgetry and equipment which aid us looking into the pelvis. Every gynaecological examination should be systematic and start with a per speculum and as per vaginal examination followed by colposcopy, ultrasonography and then if required invasive procedures such as endometrial or cervical biopsy, D&C, hysteroscopy and laparoscopy.

A gynaecological examination should proceed in the following sequence:

- Vaginal and per rectum examination
- Speculum examination
- Taking a vaginal and cervical smear
- Taking endometrial biopsy and cytology
- D&C
- Colposcopy
- Transvaginal ultrasound
- Hysteroscopy
- Laparoscopy

Speculum Examination

Speculum examination is done to view the structure of the vulva and vagina including the cervix and to obtain microbial and biopsy materials for laboratory examination. This procedure can be done in the outpatient department in a lithotomy position with no anaesthesia required.

Procedure

- Clean the external genitalia with 1% cetrimide using sponge-holding forceps.
- Introduce a lubricated speculum.
- Good light is necessary to visualise properly.

Instruments Used

- *Speculum:*
  - Sims' speculum
  - Cusco's self-retaining speculum
  - Fergusson's speculum
- Rampley's sponge-holding forceps

Other instruments that may be used include:

- Jayle's vaginal retractor
- Richter's vulva retractor
- Teale's vulsellum forceps
- Sims' anterior vaginal wall retractor

Vaginal Examination

The patient is examined in the lithotomy position. After separating the labia with the thumb and index fingers of the left hand, two fingers, usually the index and forefinger of the right hand, are gradually introduced beyond the introitus up to the fornices.

Uterus positioning and direction of the cervix can be noted. Consistency of the cervix is looked at. It is soft in pregnancy and firm in the nonpregnant state. The clinician should observe whether movement of the cervix causes pain. This is seen in ectopic pregnancy or pelvic inflammatory disease.

Now the left hand is placed over the abdomen and the uterus can be bimanually palpated for position, size, shape, mobility, tenderness and presence of any uterine pathology.

Swellings that can be identified are ovarian cysts, neoplasms, paraovarian cysts, tubo-ovarian masses and chronic ectopic pregnancy. Then, palpate posterior fornix, which enables the palpation of the contents of the pouch of Douglas. Common swellings felt can be due to a loaded rectum, uterine fibroids, ovarian neoplasms, chocolate cysts of the ovary and endometriotic nodules.

Dilatation of Cervix and Curettage

Dilatation and curettage is a gynaecological procedure, which has two components:

- To enlarge the cervical canal
- Removal of the endocervical or endometrial tissue for histologic study by scraping

Anaesthesia: Local/epidural/general

Position: Lithotomy

Procedure

Patient is explained the procedure:

- Lithotomy position.
- Empty the bladder.
- Clean the vulva, vagina and perineum.
- Drape with sterile towels.
- Sims' speculum is introduced with an anterior vaginal wall retractor.
- Vulsellum forceps are used for holding the anterior lip of the cervix.
- Pass uterine sound to determine the size and direction of the uterine cavity.
- Pass dilators steadily and gently.
- The cervix should be dilated enough to admit the curette easily.
- After dilatation, a sharp curette is passed in the axis of the cervicouterine canal till it touches the fundus.
- With a steady pressure, scrape down in all directions in a systematic way.
- A grating sensation is felt by the curette when the endometrium is satisfactorily removed.
- Collect the endometrium in saline or citrate solution.
- Gently massage the uterus between two hands to remove all blood.

Instruments Used

- Kidney dish
- Sponge forceps
- Sterile drapes
- Urinary catheter
- Antiseptic solution
- Sterile pads
- Sims' speculum
- Hegar's dilator
- Uterine curette—sharp and blunt
- Simpson's uterine sound
- Anterior vaginal wall retractor
- Vulsellum
- Sharman's biopsy curette

Contraindications

- Pregnancy
- Cervical and vaginal infections

Complications

- Perforation of the uterus
- Cervical tear
- Infection
- Asherman syndrome

Endometrial Biopsy

- Endometrial biopsy is done after giving a cervical block with a sedative.
- As per vaginal examination is done to determine the size and direction of the uterus.
- A uterine sound is passed to confirm the length and direction. A small dilator may be required prior to passing the curette.
- A specimen of the cervical canal or endometrium is obtained by using an endometrial biopsy curette.
- It is done for obtaining endometrial biopsy in cases of tuberculosis to confirm malignancy and in cases of infertility to confirm the act of ovulation.

Cervical Punch Biopsy

A cervical biopsy is taken in cases where there is a suspicious cervical lesion for malignancy. It may be taken

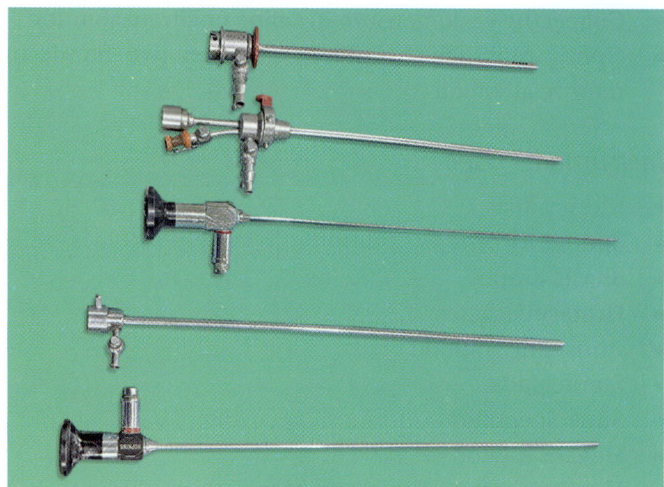

Fig. 28: Hysteroscopy set.

as a punch biopsy or by a knife as a wedge biopsy or a cone biopsy.

Steps

- Patient is put in a lithotomy position. A mild general anaesthesia or paracervical block is used.
- Biopsy is taken by the punch biopsy forceps at the junction of normal and abnormal cervical tissues. This may also be done under colposcopy guidance. Haemostasis is obtained by cauterising the raw area or by applying a stitch with a 2-0 absorbable suture material. Patient is given instructions for perineal hygiene and to avoid intercourse. The tissue obtained is sent for histopathological examination.

Hysteroscopy

Hysteroscopy is an endoscopic procedure of visualising the inside of a uterus by direct method **(Fig. 28)**.

Indications

- Evaluating the endocervical canal for any neoplastic extension
- Congenital malformation of the uterus
- *Abnormal bleeding:* It is easier to identify lesions like polyps, endometrial hyperplasia, vascular anomalies and endometrial carcinoma by hysteroscopy
- For locally lost intrauterine devices
- Pregnancy-related problems like retained molar tissues can be confirmed
- To see uterine synechiae and for the diagnosis of Asherman syndrome.

Technique

- *Position:* Lithotomy position
- The position of the uterus is confirmed by bimanual examination. A speculum is introduced, and the cervix is exposed. Clean the cervix with saline and betadine.
- Hold the anterior tip of the cervix with the vulsellum forceps and confirm the axis of the uterus with a uterine sound. The cervix is dilated up to 4 mm.
- A hysteroscope connected with a distension medium is advanced into the cavity under direct vision. The ostia, uterine walls and cavity are inspected, and the findings are documented.

Complications

- Infection
- *Perforation:* To avoid introducing the telescope under direct vision
- Bleeding diathesis
- Allergic reactions to the distension media
- Gas embolism can be reduced by using proper insufflating equipment.

Colposcopy

Colposcopy is used for obtaining a directed biopsy from suspicious areas on the cervix in women with positive Pap smears. Suspicious areas are seen as acetowhite areas, a mosaic pattern and punctuation with or without the presence of abnormal vessels.

Technique

Patient is placed in a lithotomy position, the cervix is exposed with a speculum, and a colposcope is introduced, focusing on the external os at a distance of about 20 cm.

The squamocolumnar junction is inspected before and after applying 3–5% aqueous acetic acid solution. Acetic acid precipitates proteins and the abnormal epithelium appears white.

For a clearer assessment of vascular architecture, a green light filter can be used. After this, the cervix is painted with Schiller's iodine, which differentiates darker glycogen-laden cells from paler glycogen-free cells. The neoplastic tissue is devoid of glycogen and it, therefore, does not take up iodine stain. The nonstained areas are then biopsied.

Indications

- Abnormal Pap smear cytology
- To obtain a directed biopsy
- To locate abnormal areas

- For conservative therapy under colposcopic guidance
- Follow-up cases

Colposcopy helps to reduce false-positive reports. Presently, exfoliative cytology and colposcopy are considered complimentary to each other and have contributed immensely in reducing the incidence of invasive cancers of the cervix.

Laparoscopy

Laparoscopy **(Fig. 27)** is discussed in detail in Chapter 54.

SUGGESTED READING

1. Obstetrics and Gynecology Instrumentation. (Instrument Continuing Education-ICE). [online] Available from https://www.studocu.com/in/document/indira-gandhi-national-open-university/community-health-nursing/obstetrics-and-gynecology-instrumentation-article-autor-anna-clarkson-and-deborah-bunn/66549990
2. Taşkın S, Şükür YE, Altın D, Turgay B, Varlı B, Baytaş V, et al. Bipolar energy instruments in laparoscopic uterine cancer surgery: a randomized study. J Laparoendosc Adv Surg Tech A. 2018;28(6):645-9.

50

CHAPTER

Ultrasonography in Gynaecology

Priti Venkatesh

Chapter Outline

- Indications for Ultrasound In Gynaecology
- Techniques
- Normal Female Pelvic Anatomy
- Uterus
- Myometrium
- Adenomyosis
- Endometrium
- Cervix
- Adnexa
- Polycystic Ovary
- Ovarian Malignant Lesions
- Fallopian Tubes
- Endometriosis
- Ultrasound Imaging in Gynaec Emergencies

Ultrasound is the third eye of the gynaecologist today giving true insight into the disease processes happening in the pelvis.

INTRODUCTION

Ultrasonography is the modality of choice for gynaecological imaging and diagnosis. In fact, ultrasound has become an integral part of the clinical evaluation of gynaec patients in the outpatient setting itself. In clinical evaluation, the gynaecologist palpates and feels the pelvic organs with his or her hands to determine the size and consistency of the organs, elicit tenderness and mobility. With ultrasound, one is able to image these internal organs and determine if they are normal or abnormal.

With the newer techniques in the field of ultrasonography (USG), it has become easier to diagnose even minor abnormalities without invasive procedures. It is highly cost effective and the sensitivity of diagnosis of gynaecological pathologies with skilled personnel has reached a level of >90% in the current era.

INDICATIONS FOR ULTRASOUND IN GYNAECOLOGY

Diagnostic Indications

Patients present to a gynaecologist with any of the following:

- Pelvic pain **(Flowchart 1)**
- Abnormal uterine bleeding (AUB)
- Discharge per vaginal
- Palpable mass
- Mass per vagina
- Infertility
- Family planning
- Intrauterine contraceptive device (IUCD) insertion, removal and localisation.

Most of these situations will require an ultrasound to complete the process of diagnosis and treatment.

Therapeutic indications:

- Cyst aspiration
- Abscess drainage
- Intrauterine device (IUD) placement
- Endometrial biopsy
- Intragestational instillation of methotrexate or KCl.

TECHNIQUES

Types of Ultrasounds

- Transabdominal sonography (TAS or TAUS)—3–5 MHz curvilinear probe with moderately full urinary bladder:
  - For pelvic overview prior to transvaginal sonography (TVS).
  - Where TVS is not feasible
  - For large pelvic and abdominopelvic masses
- TAS with high-frequency linear transducer—2.5–8.0 MHz:
  - For evaluation of abdominal wall lesions and sometimes even deeper lesions if possible
- Transvaginal (TVS or TVUS)—TVS probe: 9–12 MHz probe—scanning with empty bladder:

Flowchart 1: Ultrasound diagnosis of pelvic pain.

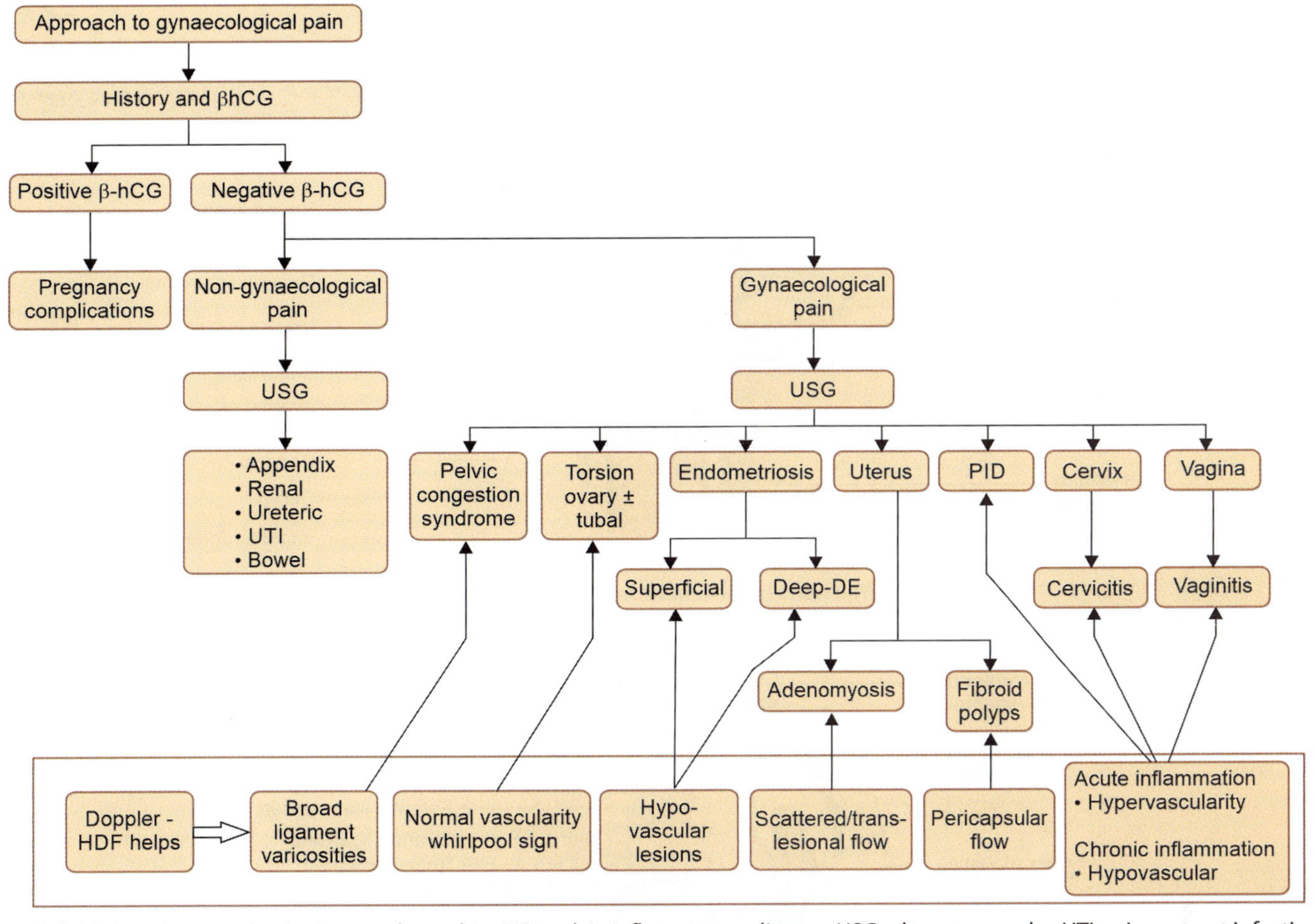

(β-hCG: beta human chorionic gonadotrophin; PID: pelvic inflammatory disease; USG: ultrasonography; UTI: urinary tract infection)

- It is a high-frequency transducer for high-resolution imaging with 3D/4D capability preferably.
- Preferred modality for most gynaecologic assessments of pelvic organs
- Close proximity to the organ of interest allows the use of higher frequency with better resolution

- Transrectal ultrasonography (TRUS):
  - When TVS is not feasible
- Translabial or transperineal ultrasonography:
  - Most useful for pelvic floor study
  - When TVS is not feasible
- 3D and 4D—volume transducers—transabdominal and transvaginal transducers—all these are capable of two-dimensional imaging with the added ability to scan a volume which can then be analised in multiple planes at any point of time
- Sonohysterography
- Sonohysterosalpingography
- Sonopodography

NORMAL FEMALE PELVIC ANATOMY (FIG. 1)

- *Internal organs:*
  - Uterus
  - Fallopian tubes
  - Ovaries
  - Vagina
  - Accessory glands
  - Skene's glands—paraurethral glands
  - Bartholin's glands—either side of the vagina
  - Urinary bladder
  - Rectum and anal canal
  - Ligaments
- *External structures:*
  - Labia minora
  - Labia majora
  - Clitoris

UTERUS (FIGS. 2 AND 3)

- *Perimetrium—outermost layer—serosa:* Composed of connective tissue

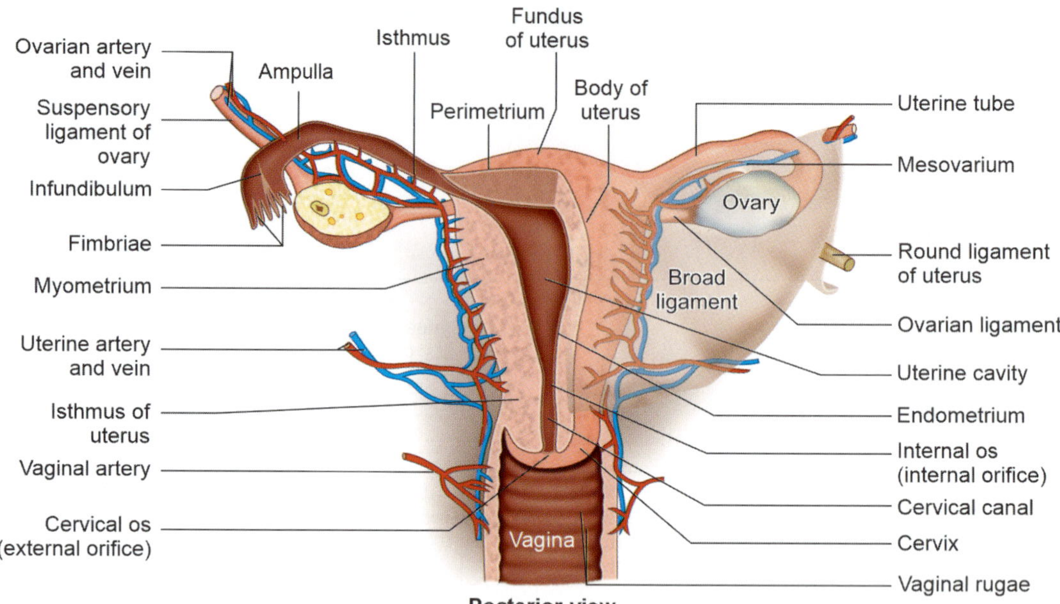

Fig. 1: The parts of the female reproductive system.

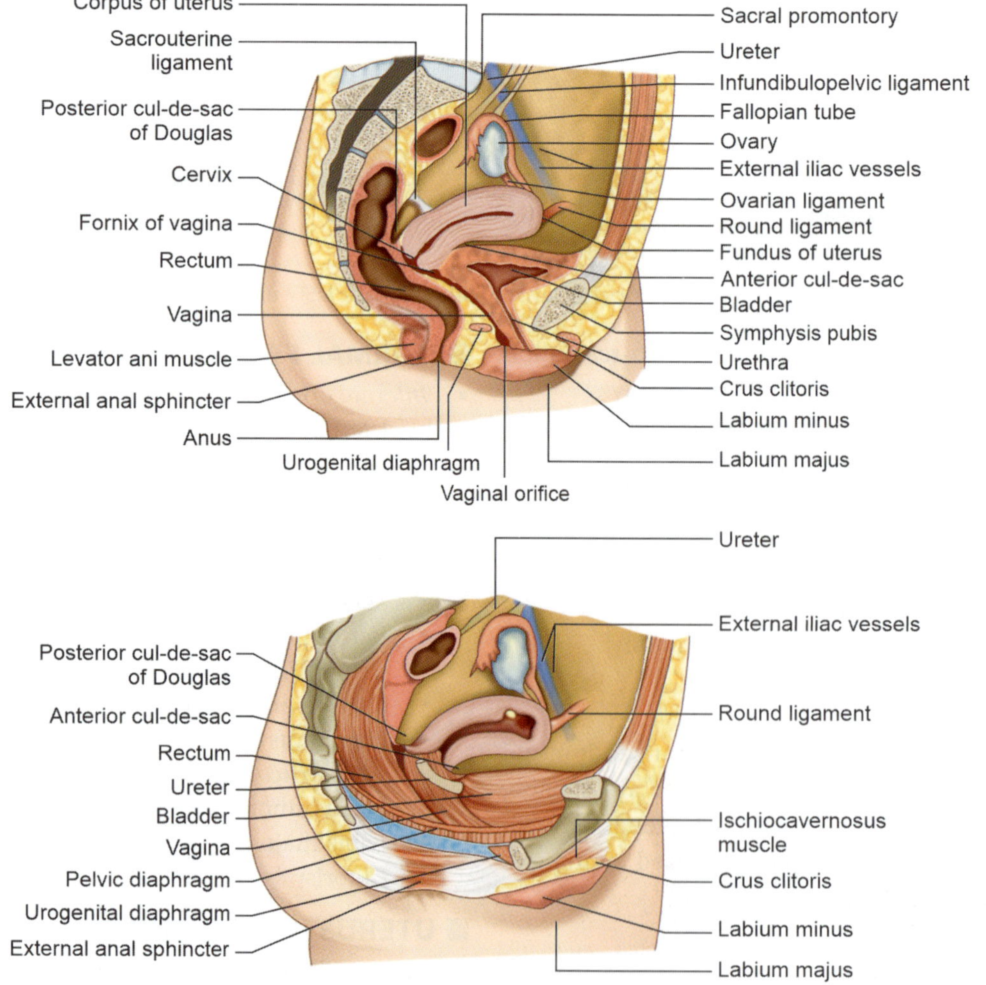

Fig. 2: Anatomy of pelvic viscera.

- *Myometrium—three layers* ***(Fig. 3)****:* Outer, middle layer which is the thickest layer and the inner layer—junctional zone (JZ) or the endomyometrial junction (EMJ) **(Figs. 4A and B)**
- *Endometrium—innermost layer—varies in thickness:* according to menstrual phase **(Figs. 5A to C)**
- Location—suspended by the round ligament, cardinal and uterosacral ligament in the pelvic cavity
- Posterior to the urinary bladder—separated by a fat plane
- Anterior to the rectum—separated by a fat plane
- Cervix—connects the uterine cavity with the vagina
- Size-shape—varies with age and physiologic status **(Figs. 6A and B) (Boxes 1 and 2)**

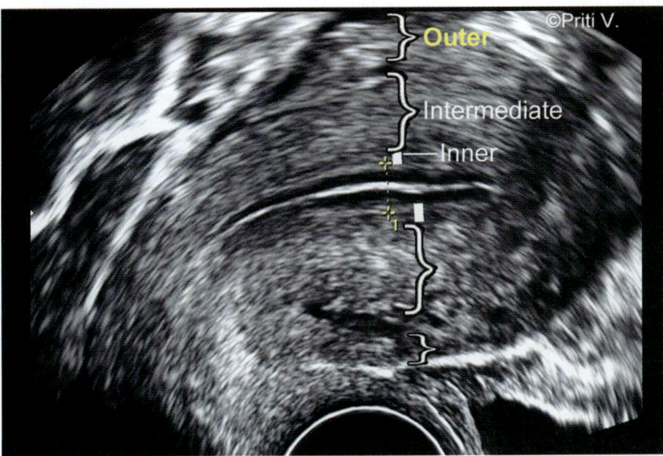

Fig. 3: Normal uterus. Three layers of myometrium.

Uterine Positions

- The most common position of the uterus is anteverted (cervix angles forward) and anteflexed (body is flexed forward).
- There is considerable variation in the position of the uterus in the adult, as shown in **Figure 7**.

Blood Supply (Fig. 8)

- *Arterial:* Uterine arteries—branches of the internal iliac arteries
- *Venous:* Uterine veins drain into the internal iliac veins.

Ultrasound Imaging of Pelvic Organs

Probe Orientation and Display of Image on the Ultrasound Screen

There are multiple ways to orient the transducer and display the image on the ultrasound monitor. Refer to **Figures 9A and B** for TAUS and **Figures 10A to C** for TVUS.

Two-dimensional Imaging

Any image, picture or display that you see on a screen or paper is a two-dimensional image with a *length* and a *breadth*. There is *no depth*.

Three-dimensional (3D) imaging has *depth* also. So, instead of a thin section of raw data, we have a volume of

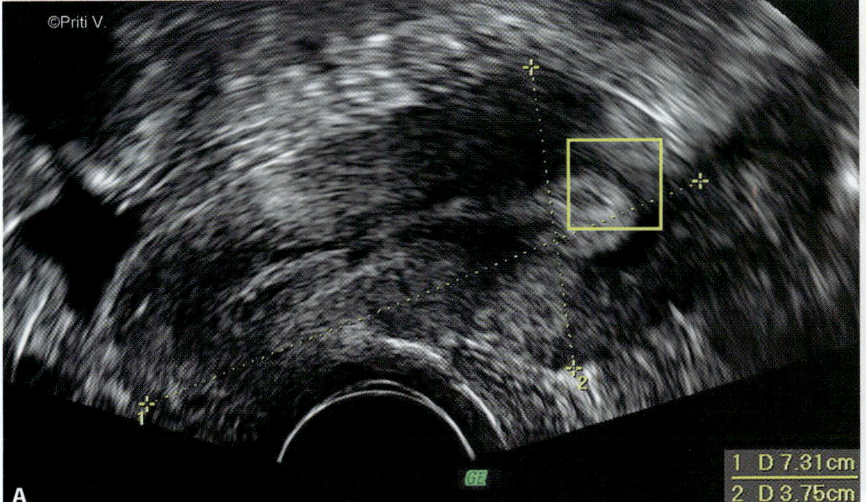

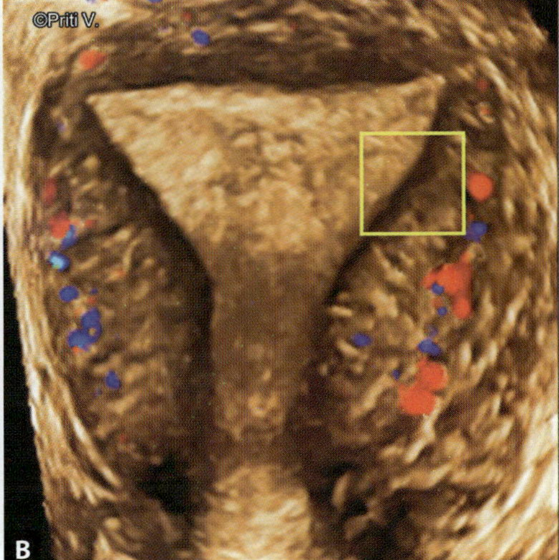

Figs. 4A and B: Normal uterus and endomyometrial junction (EMJ). EMJ—marked with yellow box—formed by the hypoechoic inner layer of the myometrium along with the sharp edge of the endometrium. Normally well-defined seen on 2D and 3D—better seen on 3D with volume contrast imaging (VCI).

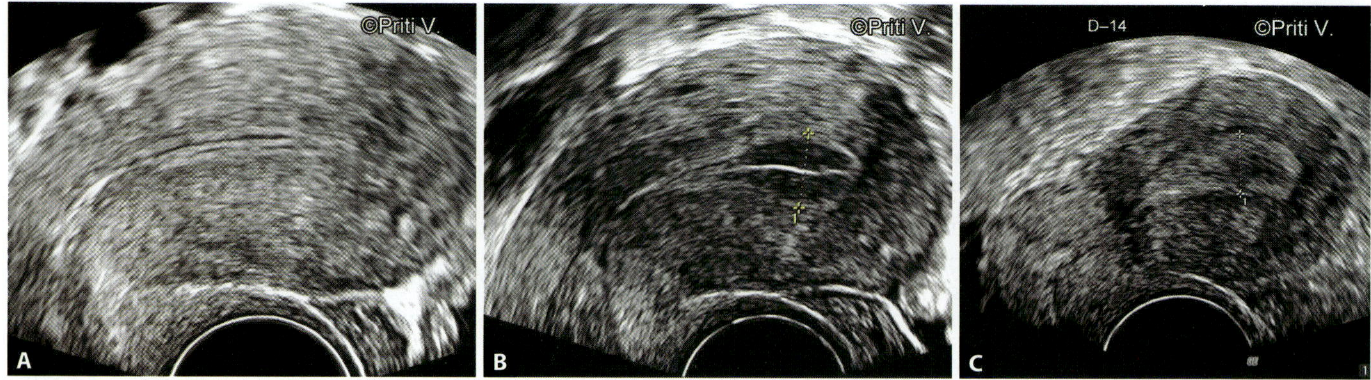

Figs. 5A to C: Endometrial changes during menstrual cycle—hormonal influence. (A) Inactive—postmenstrual; (B) Proliferative; (C) Secretory.

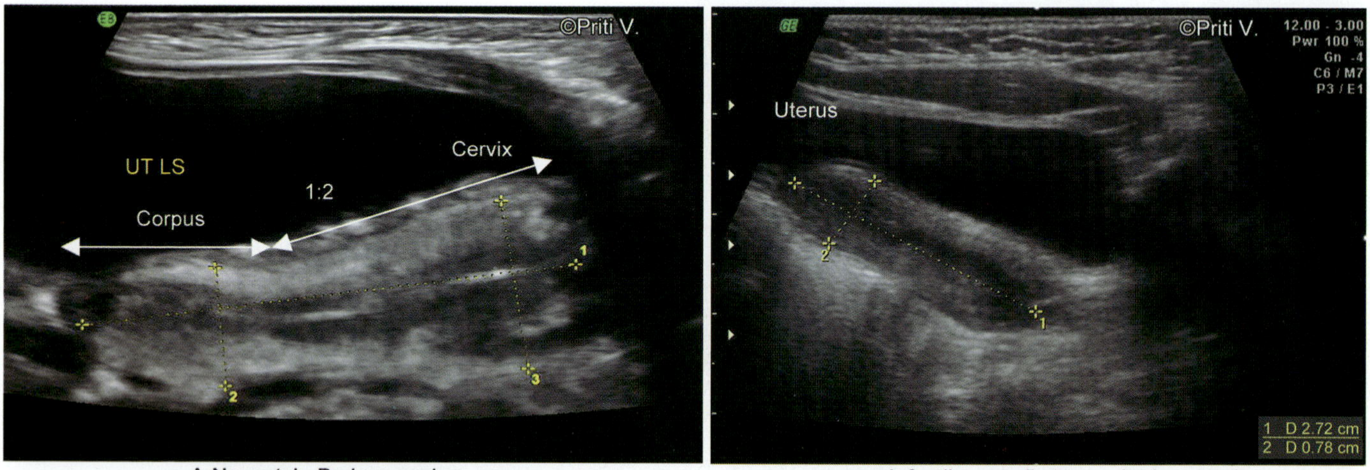

A-Neonatal - Body < cervix

Infantile - small uterus - body = cervix

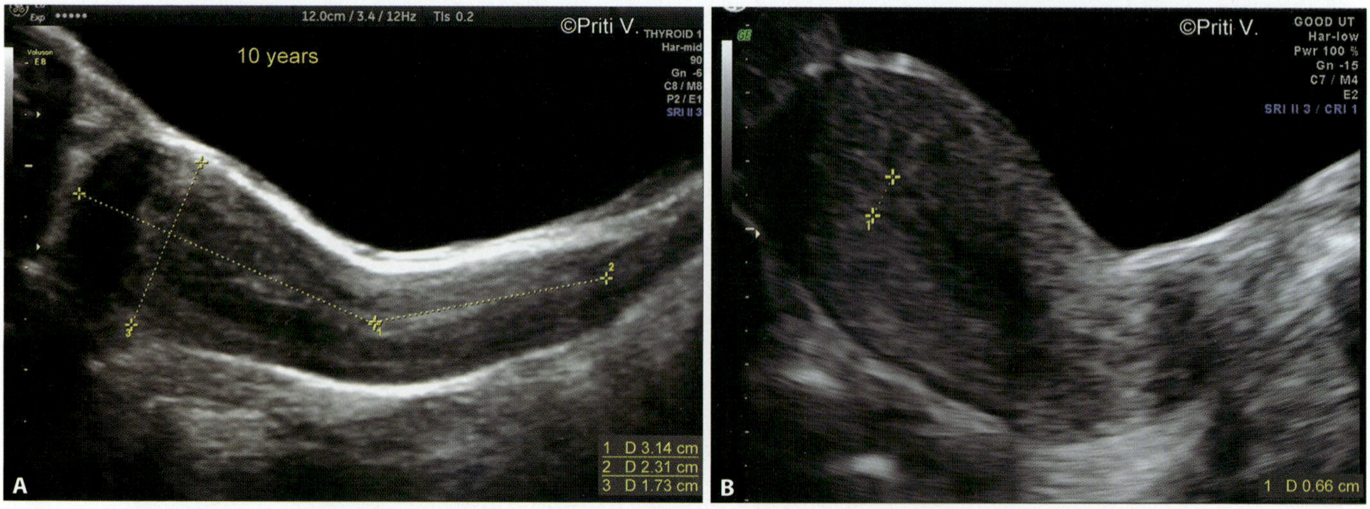

Prepubertal—corpus: Cx – 1.2:1 cervix

Postpubertal—corpus: Cx – 2:1 cervix

Figs. 6A and B: Change in uterine shape and size with physiologic state—hormonal influence.

BOX 1: Corpus: Cx ratio and size of uterus, size depends on physiologic state and parity rather than age.

- Neonatal—first month (1–3 months)—corpus: Cx : : 1:1—maternal pregnancy hormones
- Infant, child—1–6 years—corpus: Cx : : 1:2—smallest—paucity of female hormones
- Prepubertal girl—7–9/10 years
- Premenarcheal—10–13 years
- Reproductive age—corpus: Cx : :ss 2 :1

Uterine proportion gradually increases—1.2:1 to reach 2:1 by menarche

BOX 2: Uterine size in the reproductive age.

- Nulliparous uterus—length = 6.5–8.1 cm
- Parous uterus—length = 7.5–10 cm
- Uterine dimensions—normal range:
  - Length (L) = 6.5–9 cm
  - Width (TS) = 4.5–6 cm
  - Thickness (AP) = 2.5–4 cm
- Increases by about 1–1.5 cm in all dimensions after the first and second childbirth.
- No significant increase is noted after subsequent deliveries.
- Postmenopausal uterus—atrophic 5 years postmenopause

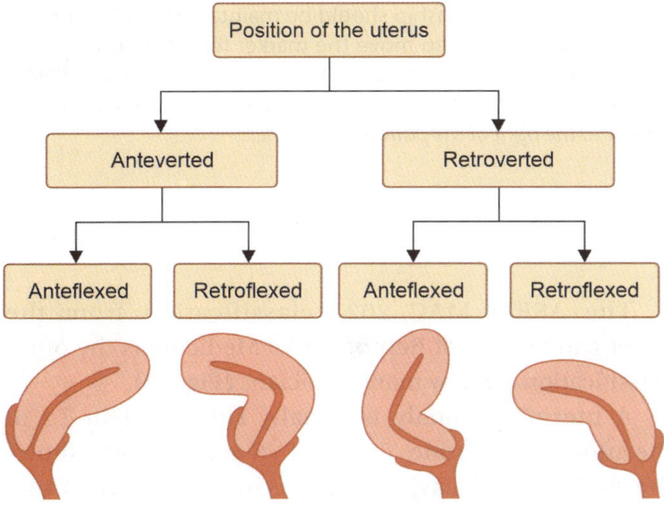

Fig. 7: Various positions of the uterus.

data. For this, the transducer has to have the capability of taking several such frames in front of and behind the frame of interest by using a motor-mounted moving piezoelectric crystal or a phased array arrangement of crystals that shoot waves in a sequence.

With two-dimensional imaging, one can see only the sagittal and transverse sections (TSs) of the uterus **(Figs. 11A and B)**.

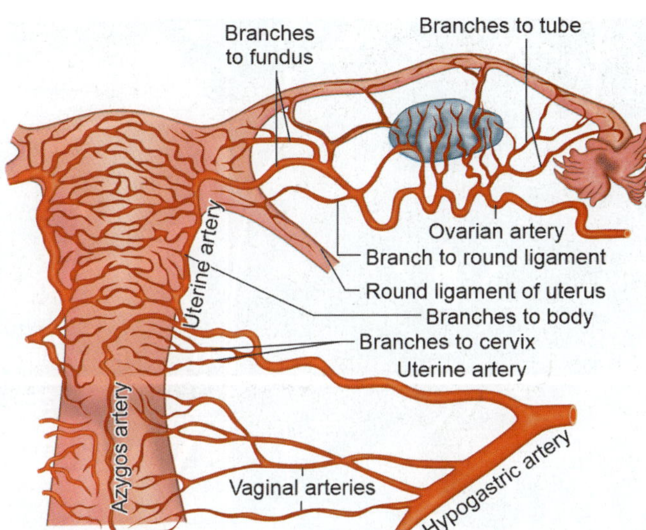

Fig. 8: Blood supply.

To get detailed information on the shape of the cavity, location of intracavitary lesions and lesions indenting or distorting the endometrial cavity, we should be able to examine the coronal plane of the uterus—all congenital or Müllerian uterine anomalies are described on the coronal section. We should also be able to rotate and turn the object to get the correct information from accurate sectional planes. All of this is possible with 3D imaging. **Figure 11C** is obtained by anticlockwise rotation of **Figure 11A**.

Application of Ultrasound in Various Gynaecological Conditions

Congenital anomalies/Müllerian anomalies: Congenital malformations of the female genital tract/Müllerian anomalies are defined as deviations from normal anatomy resulting from embryological maldevelopment of the Müllerian or paramesonephric ducts **(Flowchart 2)**.

The prevalence of Müllerian anomalies is 4–7% (Grimbizis et al. 2001; Saravelos et al. 2008; Chan et al. 2011).

Reproductive problems and symptoms depend on the type and the degree of anatomical distortion (Grimbizis et al., 2001, 2004; Joki-Erkkilä and Heinonen, 2003; Strawbridge et al., 2007; Mollo et al., 2009; Rock et al., 2010; Chan et al., 2011; Brucker et al., 2011; Gergolet et al., 2012).

Due to their prevalence and clinical importance, a reliable classification system seems to be extremely useful for their management. Effective categorisation enables more effective diagnosis and treatment as well as a better

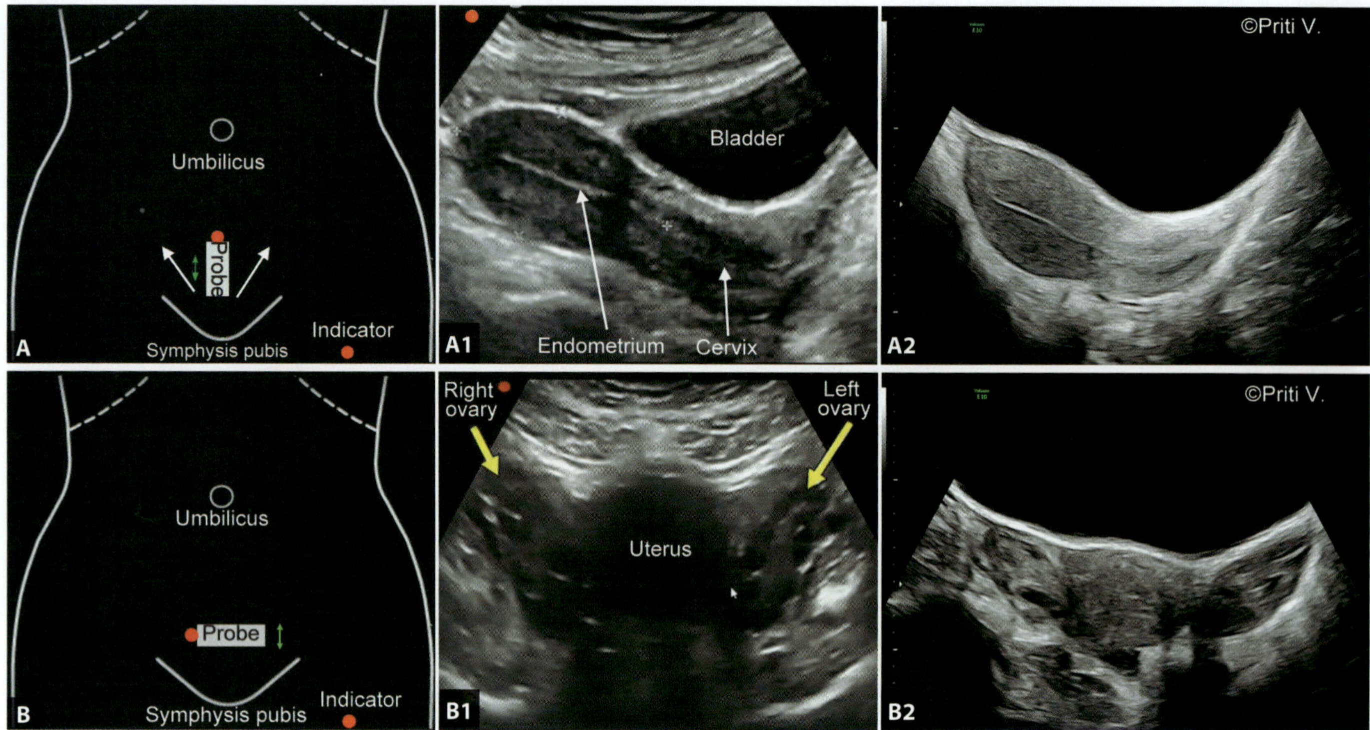

Figs. 9A and B: Probe orientation and image display. *The red dot* is the indicator on the transducer, and a similar dot is seen on the left side of the displayed images A1 & B1 and is replaced by a green company logo in images A2 & B2. These markers correspond to cranial end in sagittal images and to the right side of the patient in transverse images. This relationship should be maintained at all times. So, from the vertical position one needs to turn the transducer in the anticlockwise direction to move the marker form top to right. The upper row of images (A, A1, A2) show sagittal orientation. The lower row of images (B, B1, B2) show us the transverse orientation. *Rotate anticlockwise—red indicator dot* is to the *patient's right* and the red dot on the screen indicates the *right side of the pelvis. The red dot on the screen and the indicator on the transducer should be oriented either cranially or to the right of the patient at all times*.

understanding of their pathogenesis (Grimbizis and Campo, 2010).

The European Society of Human Reproduction and Embryology (ESHRE) and the European Society for Gynaecological Endoscopy (ESGE), recognising the clinical significance of female genital anomalies, established a common working group under the name Congenital Uterine Anomalies (CONUTA), with the goal of developing a new updated classification system **(Table 1 and Fig. 12)**. For this purpose, a scientific committee (SC) was appointed to run the project and look also for consensus within the scientists working in the field through the use of Delphi procedure (Grimbizis and Campo, 2010). The ESHRE/ESGE classification system of female genital anomalies **(Fig. 12)** was presented in this paper. Its design is clinically oriented and based on the anatomical variations of the female genital tract caused by failure in development at various stages.

The ASRM MAC 2021 classification from the American Society of Reproductive Medicine is the other classification used by many clinicians **(Fig. 13)**.

A uterine anomaly is usually suspected in TS of the uterus at routine TAS or TVS scan, which shows the endometrial cavity dividing into two **(Fig. 14A)**, indicating a septate or a bicornuate uterus, a narrow round or oval cavity **(Fig. 14B),** of a unicornuate uterus which does not widen at the fundus as in **Figure 14C,** which symmetrically widens on both sides resulting in a triangular cavity.

The next step in all such cases is to do a 3D evaluation to examine the coronal section of the uterus in detail to diagnose the type of defect **(Figs. 15 to 24)**.

Figures 15 to 24 show the various common congenital defects that can be diagnosed with 3D evaluation of the uterus.

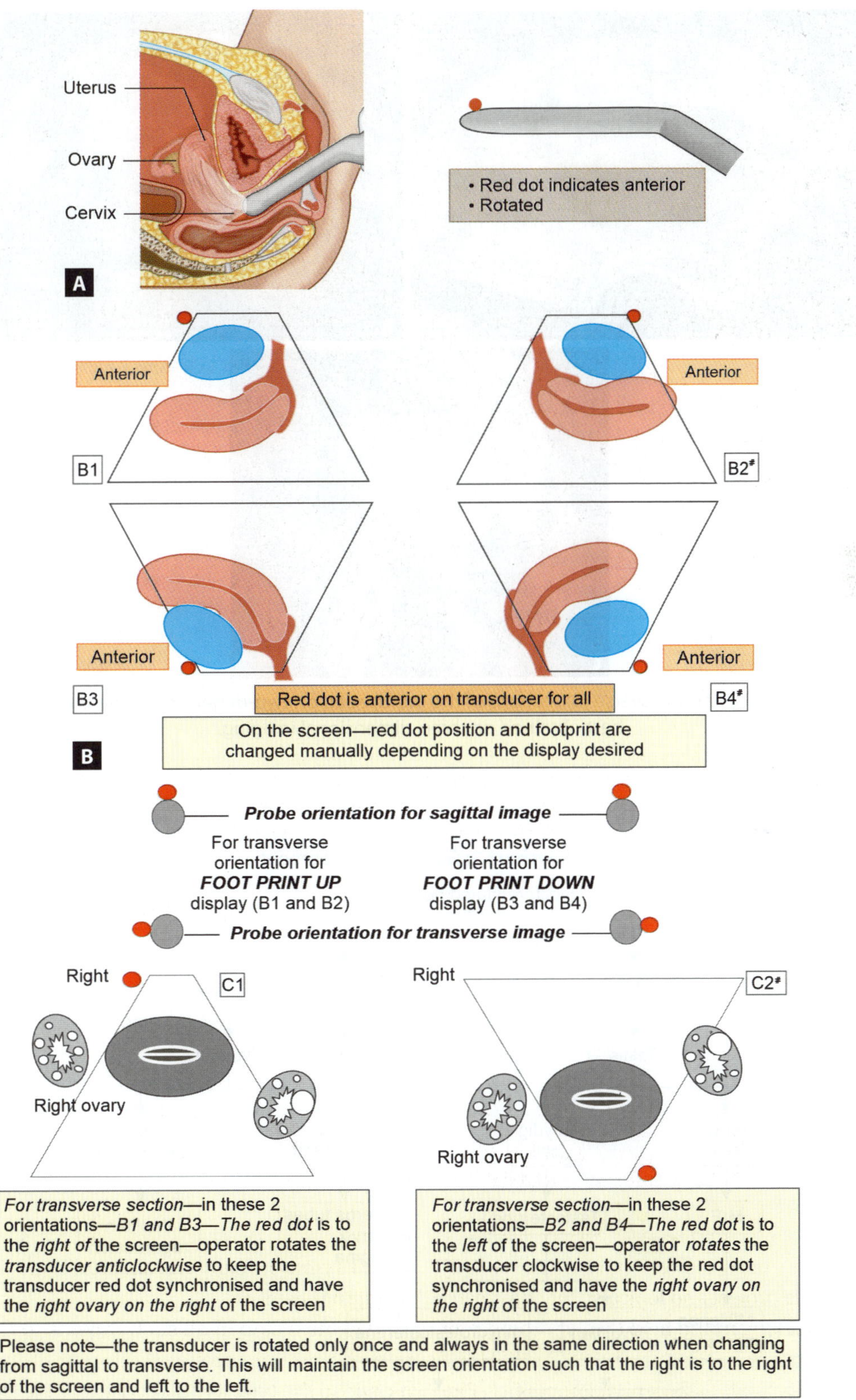

Figs. 10A to C: (A) Transducer orientation for TVS; (B) Corresponding sagittal view displays; (C) Corresponding transverse view displays. (TVS: transvaginal sonography)

#Indicates the orientation used in this chapter.

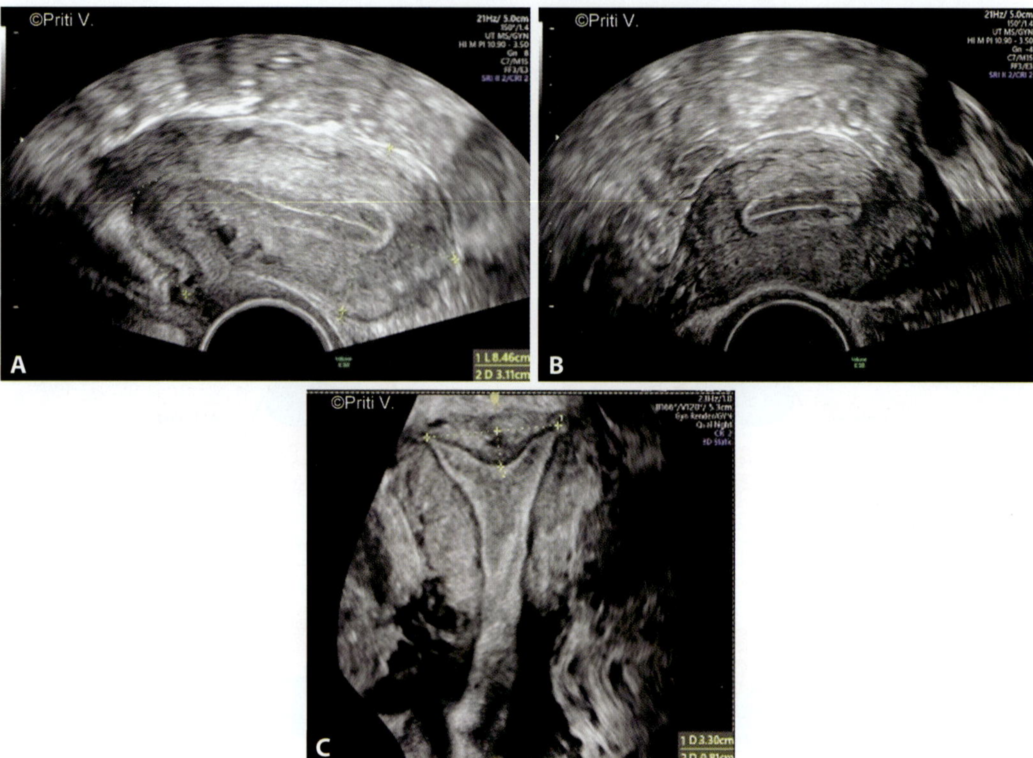

Figs. 11A to C: Sagittal (A) and transverse (B) sections of the uterus seen on two-dimensional imaging; (C) Coronal section, best obtained on three-dimensional imaging.

Flowchart 2: Gonadal development

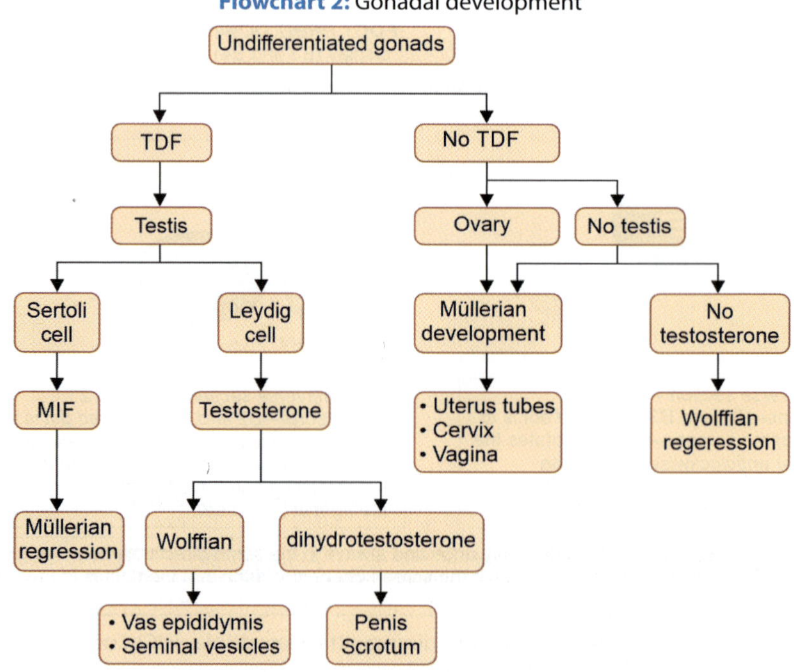

(TDF: testis-determining factor; MIF; Müllerian inhibiting factor)

TABLE 1: Development of the new classification system: CONUTA proposal for the classification of female genital tract malformations.

	Main class	***Main subclass***	***Coexistent subclass***
	Uterine anomaly		***Cervical/vaginal anomaly***
Class 0	Normal uterus		*Cervix:* • C0: Normal • C1: Septate • C2: Double 'normal' • C3: Unilateral aplasia/dysplasia • C4: Aplasia/dysplasia *Vagina:* • V0: Normal vagina • V1: Longitudinal nonobstructing vaginal septum • V2: Longitudinal obstructing vaginal septum • V3: Transverse vaginal septum/imperforate hymen • V4: Vaginal aplasia
Class I	Dysmorphic uterus	• T-shaped • Infantile	
Class II	Septate uterus	• Partial • Complete	
Class III	Dysfused uterus (including dysfused 'septate')	• Partial • Complete	
Class IV	Unilaterally formed uterus	• Rudimentary horn with cavity (communicating or not) • Rudimentary horn without cavity/aplasia (no horn)	
Class V	Aplastic/dysplastic	• Rudimentary horn with cavity (bilateral or unilateral) • Rudimentary horn without cavity (bilateral or unilateral)/ aplasia	
Class VI	Unclassified malformations		

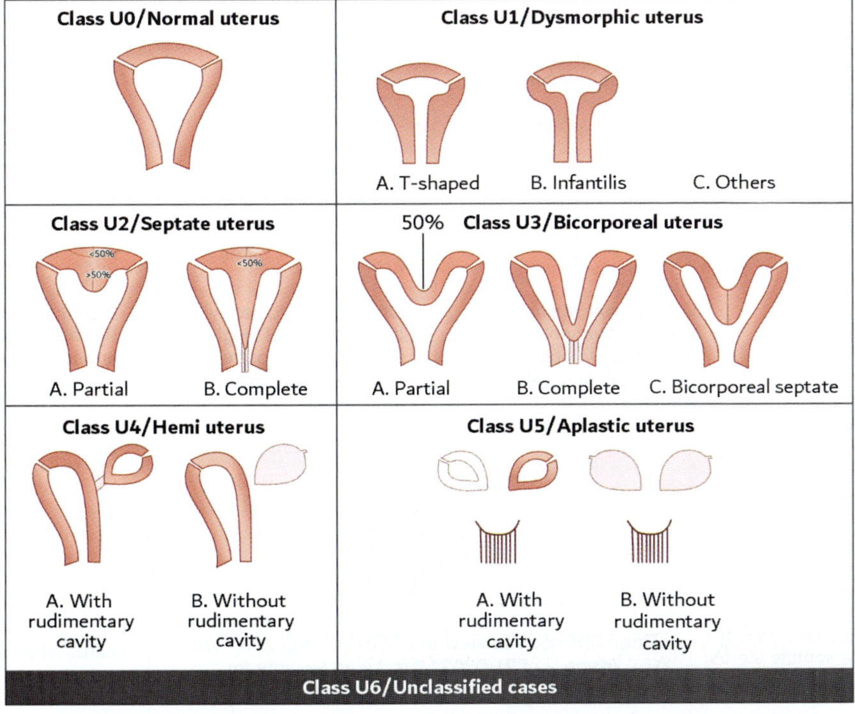

Fig. 12: ESHRE/ESGE classification of uterine anomalies (class U2: Internal indentation >50% of the uterine wall thickness and external contour straight or with indentation <50%; class U3: External indentation>50% of the uterine wall thickness; class U3b: Width of the fundal indentation at the midline >50% of the uterine wall thickness). (ESHRE: European Society of Human Reproduction and Embryology; ESGE: European Society for Gynaecological Endoscopy)

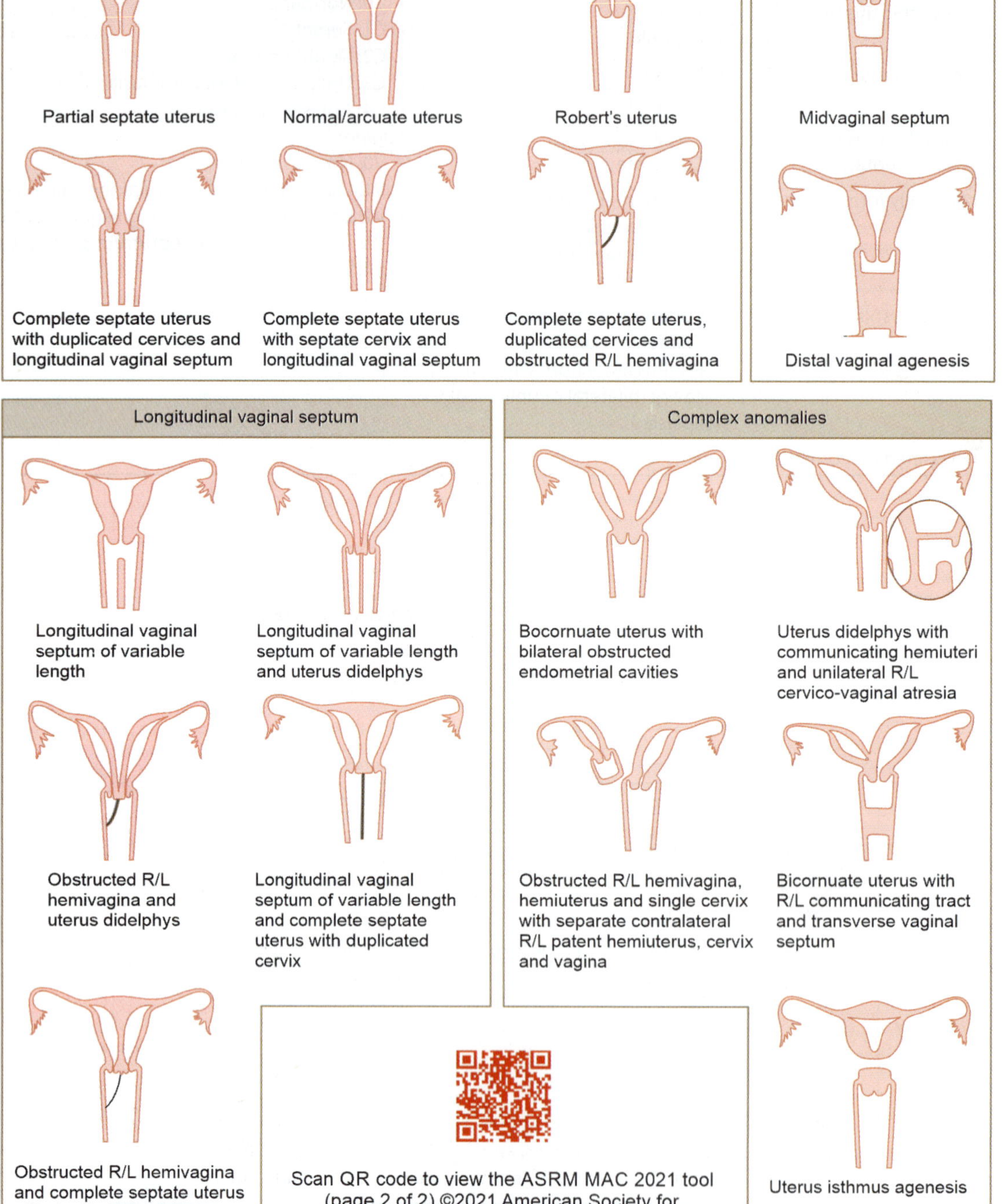

Fig. 13: The ASRM MAC 2021 classification from the American Society of Reproductive Medicine is the other classification used by many clinicians.

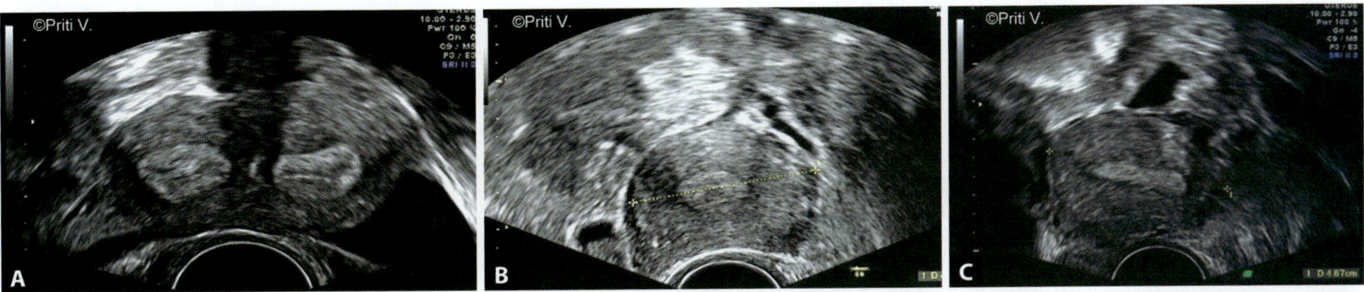

Figs. 14A to C: Transverse section of the uterus on 2D imaging—raises suspicion. (A) Septate or bicornuate uterus; (B) Unicornuate uterus; (C) Normal uterus.

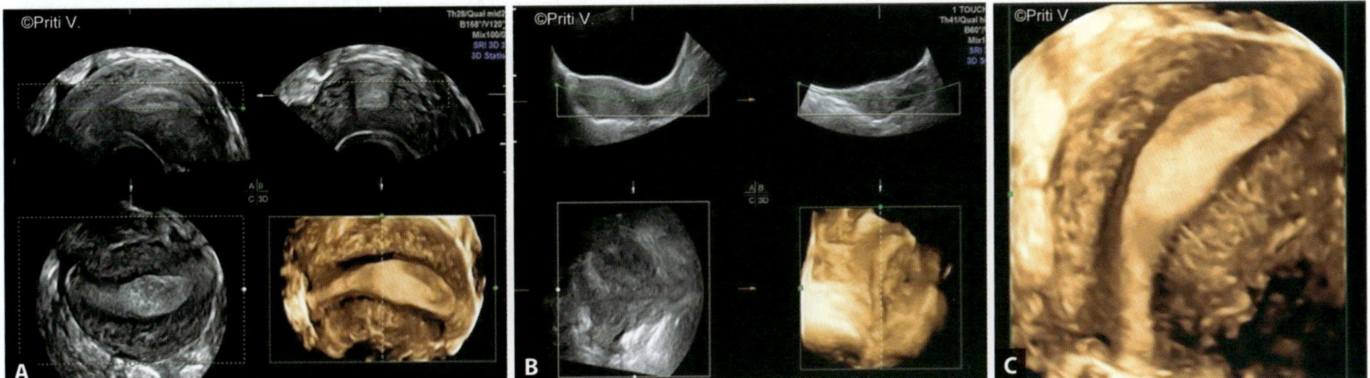

Figs. 15A to C: Unicornuate uterus—A and B are multiplanar images—A is TVS and B is TAS. Image C is a rendered TVS 3D image showing a coronal section of a unicornuate uterus with its typical banana shaped cavity.

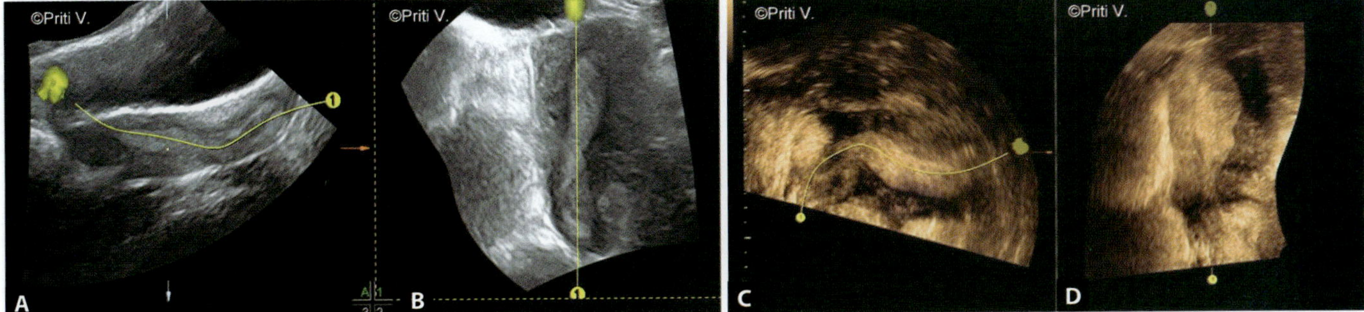

Figs. 16A to D: Unicornuate uterus—omniview —TAS (A) and (B) and TVS (C) and (D). Images A and C are 2D images with polyline marking the line of render and B and D are the corresponding coronal 3D images. (TAS: transabdominal sonography TVS: transvaginal sonography)

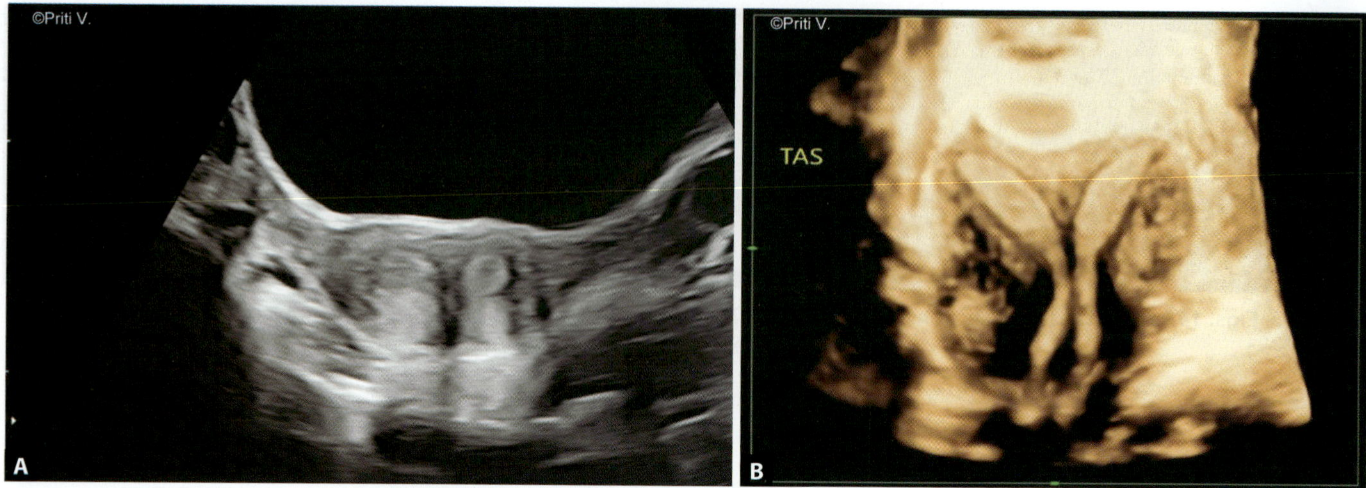

Figs. 17A and B: Septate uterus complete septum + cervical duplication—both are TAS images. (TAS: transabdominal sonography)

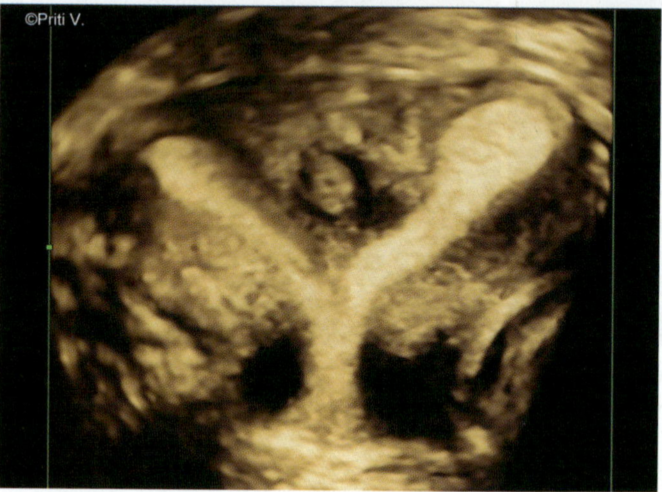

Fig. 18: Septate uterus complete septum—wide.

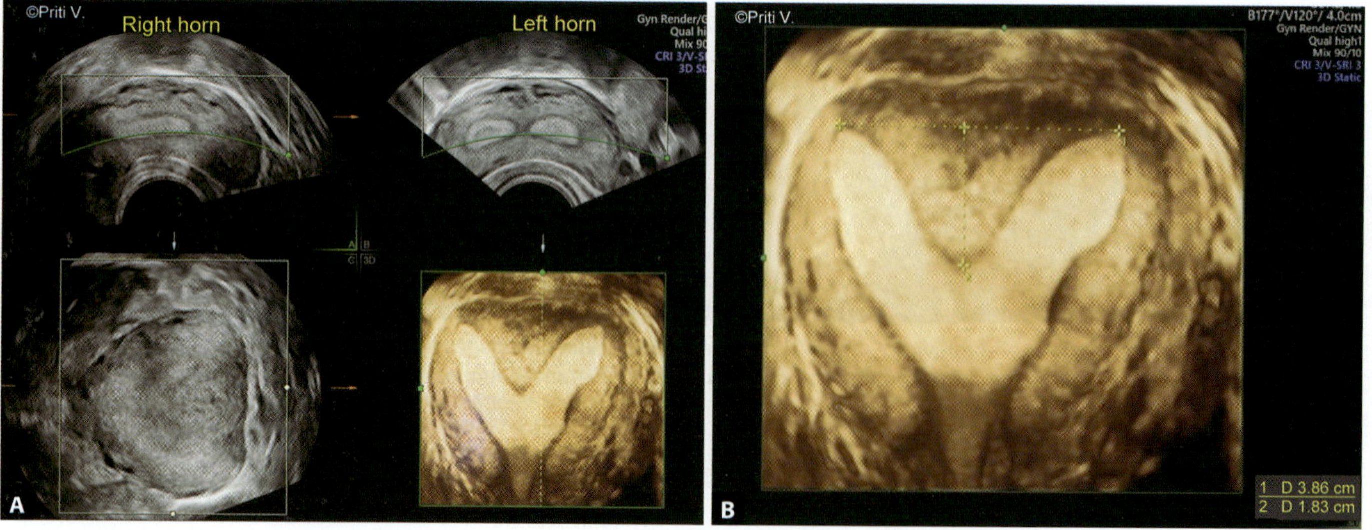

Figs. 19A and B: Septate uterus—partial septum—septal length—1.8 cm.

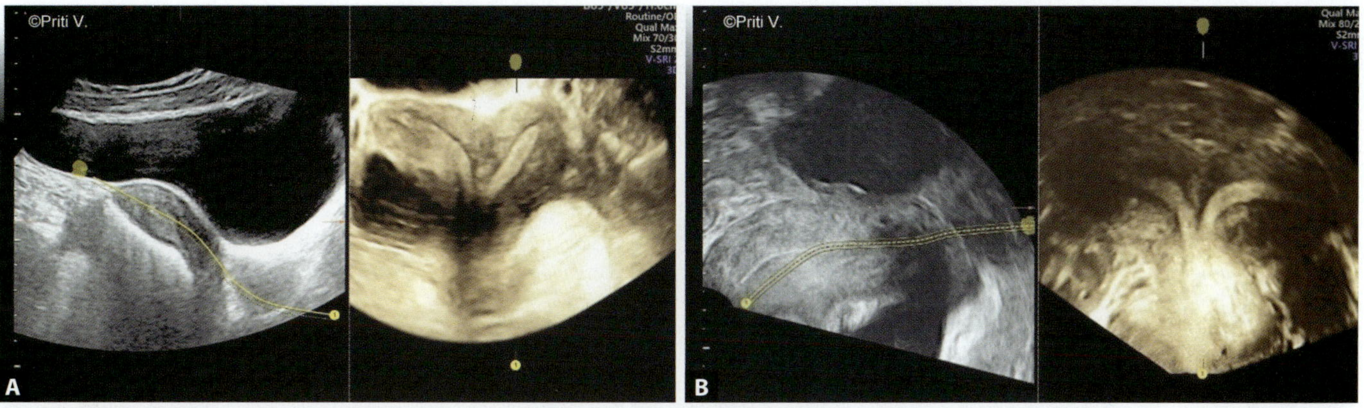

Figs. 20A and B: Bicornuate uterus—bicornis bicollis—TAS and TVS using omniview. (TAS: transabdominal sonography; TVS: transvaginal sonography)

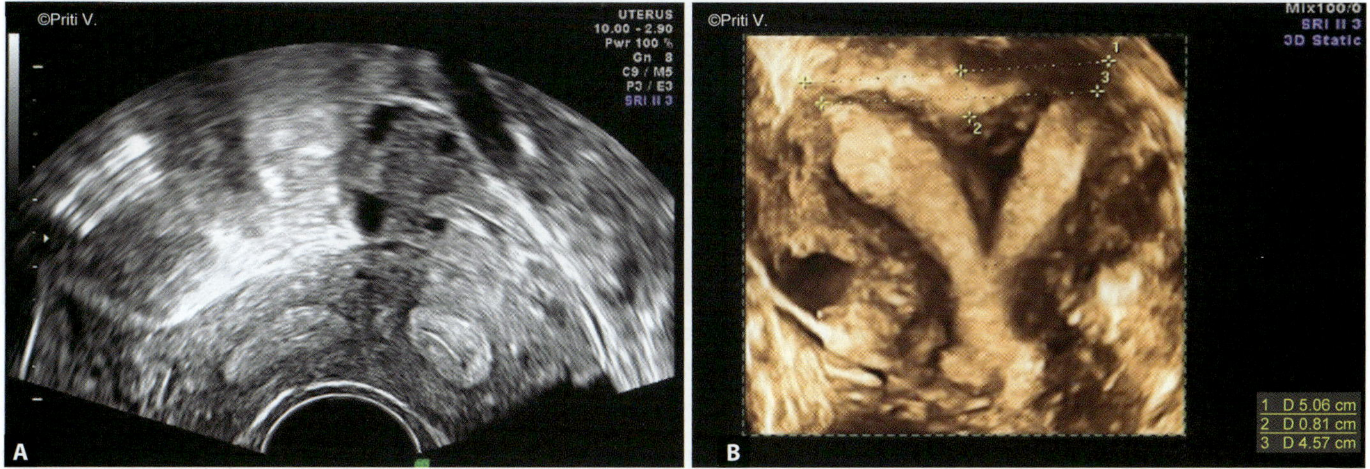

Figs. 21A and B: Bicornuate uterus—bicornis bicollis (A)—2D and (B)—3D.

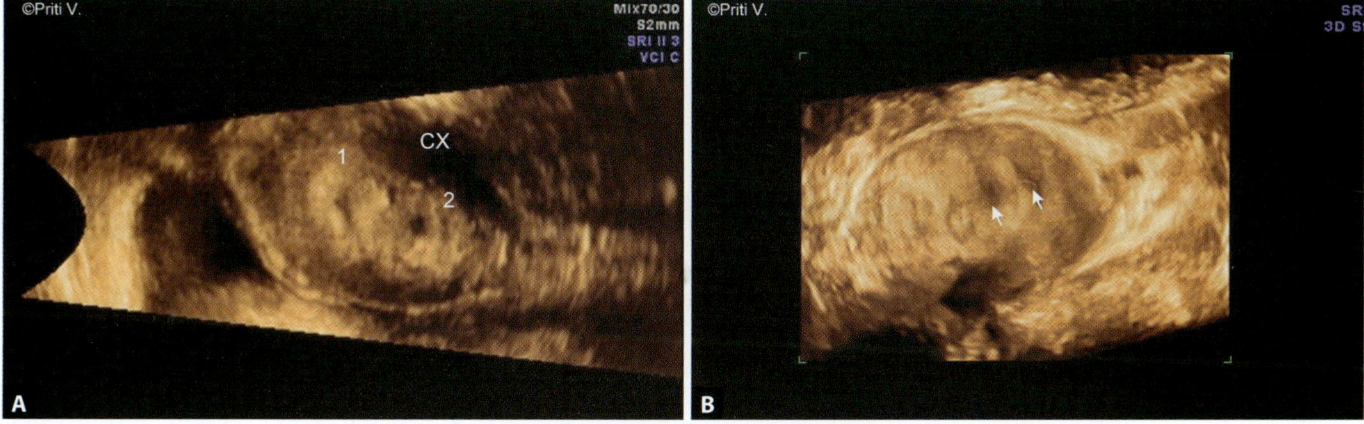

Figs. 22A and B: Double cervix or cervix bicollis (A) and septate cervix (B).

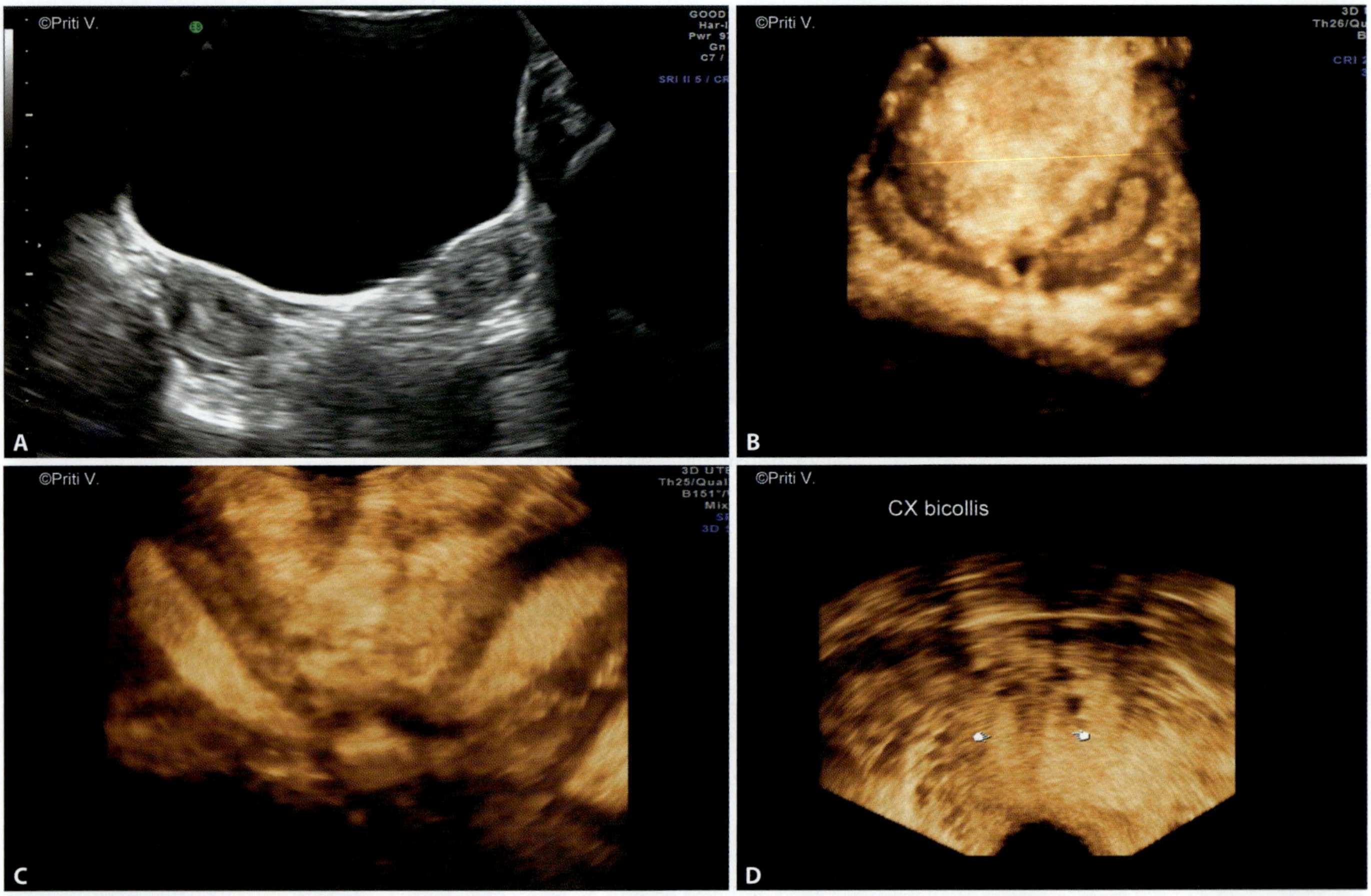

Figs. 23A to D: Didelphys uterus (A)—TAS transverse section of pelvis—two widely displaced cavities seen; (B) TAS-3D coronal view; (C) TVS-3D coronal view; (D) TVS-3D double cervix—coronal view. (TAS: transabdominal sonography; TVS: transvaginal sonography)

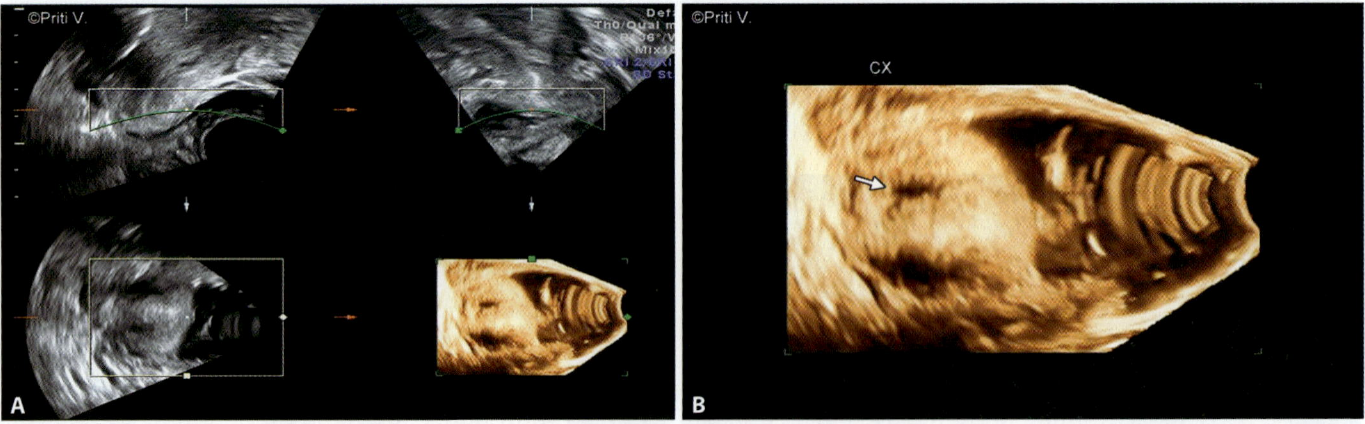

Figs. 24A and B: Single cervical canal confirmed by single external os on 3D. 3D can be used to confirm the number of external orifices—this can be done by speculum examination. Documentation, however, is easier on ultrasound 3D imaging.

Acquired Uterine Pathologies: Abnormal uterine bleeding and *pelvic pain* are the most common symptoms with which a patient presents to a gynaecologist. AUB is the most common symptom in the reproductive age group with a prevalence of heavy bleeding seen in 3–30% of these women and heavy + irregular, intermenstrual bleeding in 35%.

TABLE 2: Suggested "normal" limits for menstrual parameters in midreproductive years.

Clinical dimensions of menstruation and menstrual cycles				
Frequency of menses (in days)	Descriptive term	Frequent	Normal	Infrequent
	Definition	<24	24–38	>38
Regularity of menses cycle-to-cycle variation over 12 months (in days)	Descriptive term	Absent	Regular	Irregular
	Definition		Variation ±2–20	Variation >20
Duration of flow (in days)	Descriptive term	Prolonged	Normal	Shortened
	Definition	>8.0	4.5–8.0	<4.5
Volume of blood loss (in mL)	Descriptive term	Heavy	Normal	Light
	Definition	>80	5–80	<5

Note: Limits are based primarily on the data of Hallberg et al. (1966), and Belsey and Pinol (1997).

Source: Fraser. International definitions of abnormal menstrual bleeding. Fertil Steril. 2007.

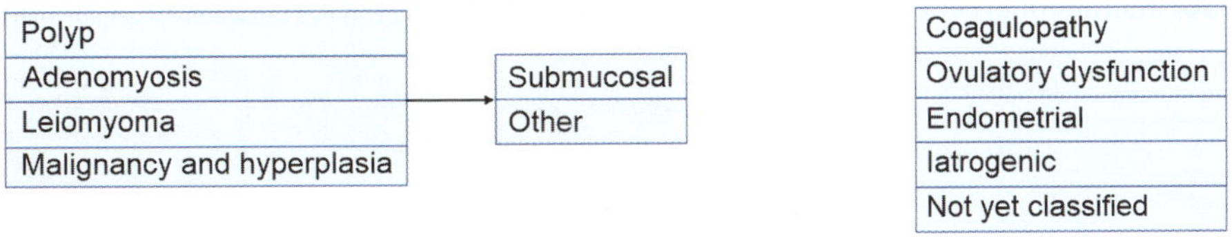

PALM		COEIN
Polyp		Coagulopathy
Adenomyosis	Submucosal	Ovulatory dysfunction
Leiomyoma →	Other	Endometrial
Malignancy and hyperplasia		Iatrogenic
		Not yet classified

Fig. 25: PALM—COEIN classification for causes of AUB—European Society of Gynaecological Endoscopy (ESGE). (AUB: abnormal uterine bleeding)

To standardise the terminology and definitions of AUB, International Federation of Gynecology and Obstetrics (FIGO) has proposed two classifications:

1. *FIGO AUB system 1*—classification of *symptoms* of AUB—gives description and definition for normal and AUB **(Table 2)**.

   To describe the causes of AUB, FIGO has proposed a classification system called the PALM-COEIN classification (FIGO AUB system 2).
2. *FIGO AUB system 2—the PALM-COEIN classification* for *causes* of AUB shown in **Figure 25**—PALM refers to the structural causes for AUB that can be imaged, and COEIN refers to functional and other causes.

   The FIGO classification for fibroids is given in **Figure 26**.

Consensus Opinions

Several consensus opinions have been published in the last 15-25 years in order to standardise the terminology, definitions and measurements we use to describe adnexal, myometrial and endometrial pathology. They are as follows:

- *The International Ovarian Tumour Analysis (IOTA)* group for *adnexal tumours* in 2000 (Timmerman D. Ultrasound Obstet Gynecol. 2000).
- *The International Endometrial Tumour Analysis (IETA)* group in 2010 for endometrial lesions (Leone F P G 2010 ultrasound Obstet Gynaecol 2010).
- *The Morphological Uterus Sonographic Assessment (MUSA)* group in 2015 (Van Den Bosch T, ultrasound Obstet Gynecol 2015) for myometrial and uterine masses.

All operators performing gynaecological ultrasound should use these terminologies when reporting. **All descriptions and measurements in this chapter will be based on these consensus statements**.

MYOMETRIUM

As pre-MUSA consensus statement, the evaluation of myometrial lesions begins with determining uterine size—enlarged or not, the uterine contour and the myometrium echotexture whether it is homogenous or not. **Figures 27 and 28** show how to describe these lesions using MUSA guidelines. When the myometrium is non-homogeneous or heterogeneous reason for the same should be elaborated. For example, the heterogenous echotexture could be because of focal or diffuse myometrial lesions such as fibroids, adenomyosis and accessory cavitated uterine malformation (ACUM). **Figure 29** shows

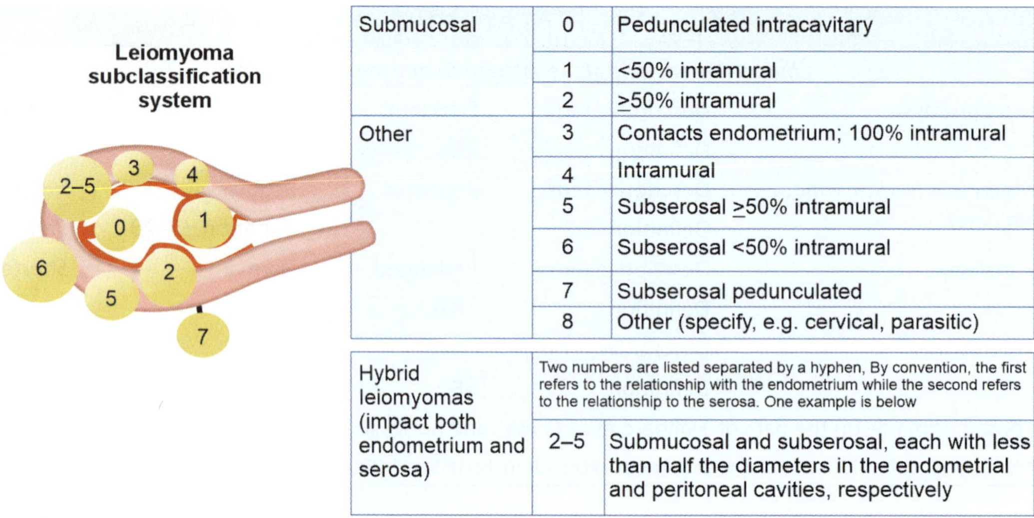

Submucosal	0	Pedunculated intracavitary
	1	<50% intramural
	2	≥50% intramural
Other	3	Contacts endometrium; 100% intramural
	4	Intramural
	5	Subserosal ≥50% intramural
	6	Subserosal <50% intramural
	7	Subserosal pedunculated
	8	Other (specify, e.g. cervical, parasitic)
Hybrid leiomyomas (impact both endometrium and serosa)	Two numbers are listed separated by a hyphen, By convention, the first refers to the relationship with the endometrium while the second refers to the relationship to the serosa. One example is below	
	2–5	Submucosal and subserosal, each with less than half the diameters in the endometrial and peritoneal cavities, respectively

Fig. 26: International Federation of Gynaecology and Obstetrics (FIGO) classification for fibroids.

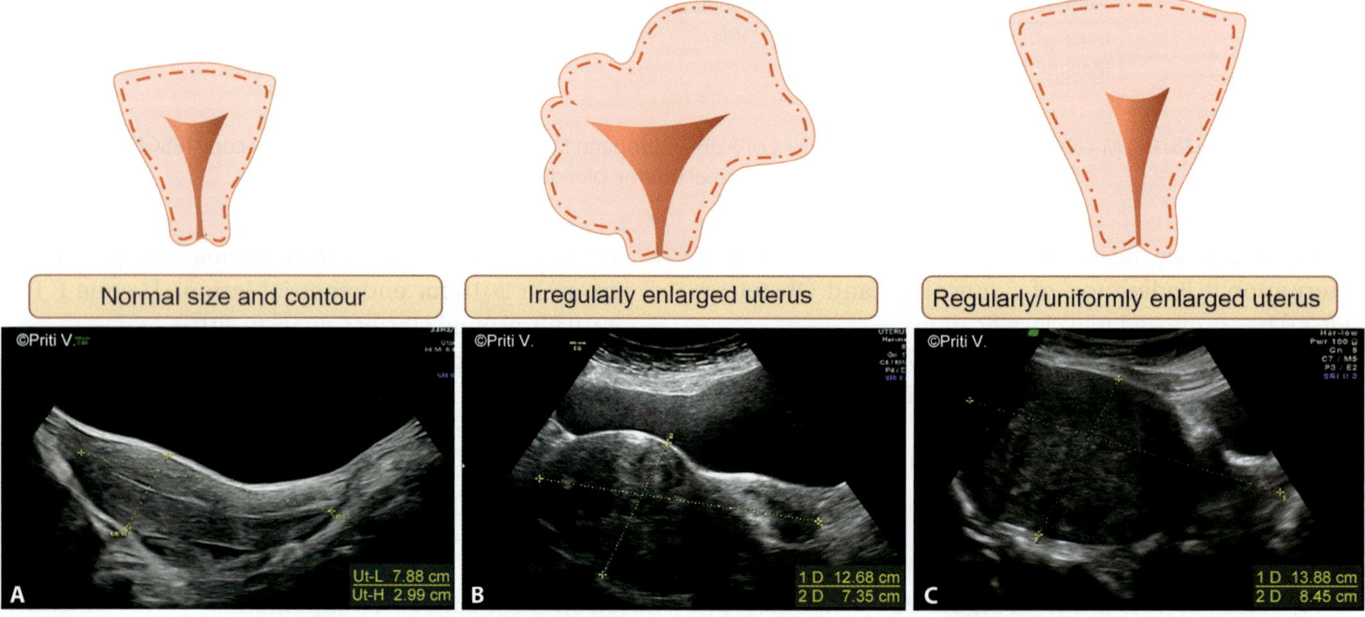

Figs. 27A to C: Assessment of the uterus—starts with—size and contour of the uterus.

diagrammatically the different types of shadows produced by various lesions, and **Figure 30** describes how to divide the uterus to help describe the location of these focal lesions in the myometrium. In the text that follows, the lesions recognised are mentioned and described in detail as per the MUSA consensus statement.

Leiomyomas

Leiomyomas: Uterine leiomyomas or fibroids are benign tumours of myometrial origin and are the most common solid benign uterine neoplasms.

Pathology (Figs. 31 and 32; Flowchart 3)

Leiomyomas are benign monoclonal tumours composed of smooth muscle cells with variable amounts of fibrous connective tissue. They are commonly *multiple (~85%)*, causing *irregular enlargement of the uterus* **(Figs. 31 and 32)** and vary significantly in size from a few millimetres to a large mass filling the entire abdomen.

Location of fibroids:

Intrauterine:

- *Intramural leiomyoma:* Most common **(Figs. 33A to F)**

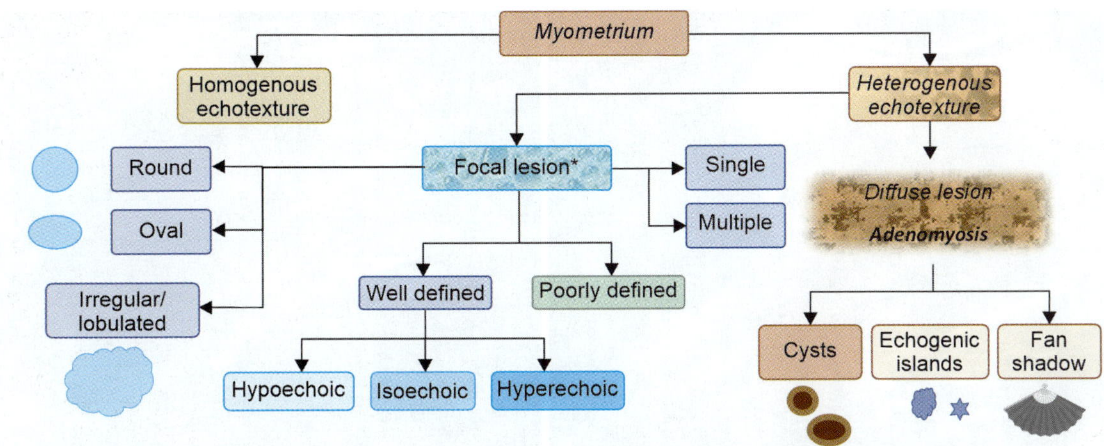

Fig. 28: MUSA consensus-based description of myometrial pathology using MUSA terminologies. (MUSA: Morphological Uterus Sonographic Assessment)

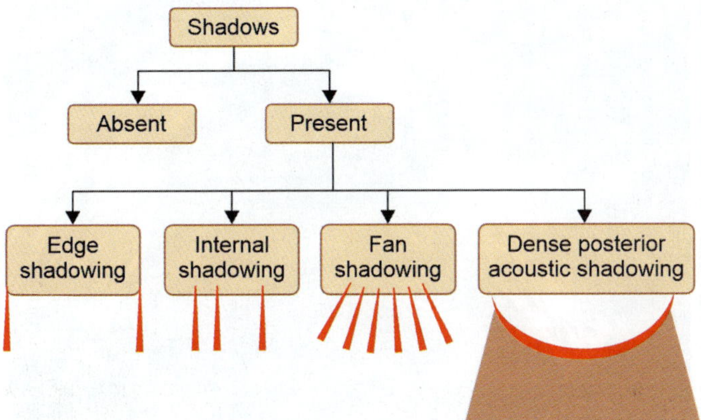

Fig. 29: Types of shadows.

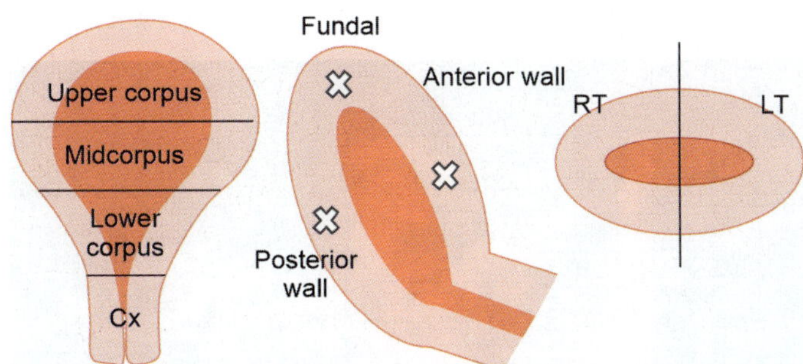

Fig. 30: Location of any focal lesion should be described in detail as per the parts of the uterus.

- *Subserosal leiomyoma*: Subserosal fibroids may be pedunculated and predominantly extrauterine—FIGO type 7, simulating an adnexal mass **(Figs. 34A to C)**. They may be partly intramural—FIGO types 5 and 6, causing only serosal irregularity **(Figs. 34B and D)**.
- *Submucosal leiomyoma:* Least common (10–15%) usually indenting the endometrium or protruding into it and may cause symptoms—infertility, pain or heavy bleeding **(Figs. 35 to 37)**.
- *Diffuse leiomyomatosis* is a rare condition characterised by the diffuse proliferation of smooth muscle and fibrous tissue resulting in uniform enlargement of the uterus. The myometrium appears to be studded with small, poorly defined hypoechoic fibroid-like lesions. Symptoms are similar to those of fibroids **(Figs. 38A and B)**.

Extrauterine:

- Broad ligament fibroid
- Cervical fibroid **(Fig. 39)**

Any fibroid may undergo atrophy, internal haemorrhage, degeneration, fibrosis or calcification.

Imaging—ultrasound features

Leiomyomas are usually well-defined solid and focal lesions of the myometrium.

- Predominantly *hypoechoic with a whorled pattern*—these are dense fibroids with more muscle tissue compared to myometrium.
- Isoechoic fibroids are less dense with muscle and fibrous tissue composition similar to that of the myometrium.
- Hyperechogenic fibroids are usually small fibroids with calcification, hyaline and fatty degeneration, making the fibroid appear echogenic.
- Usually, large and multiple fibroids cause enlargement of the uterus with irregular or lobulated outer contour.

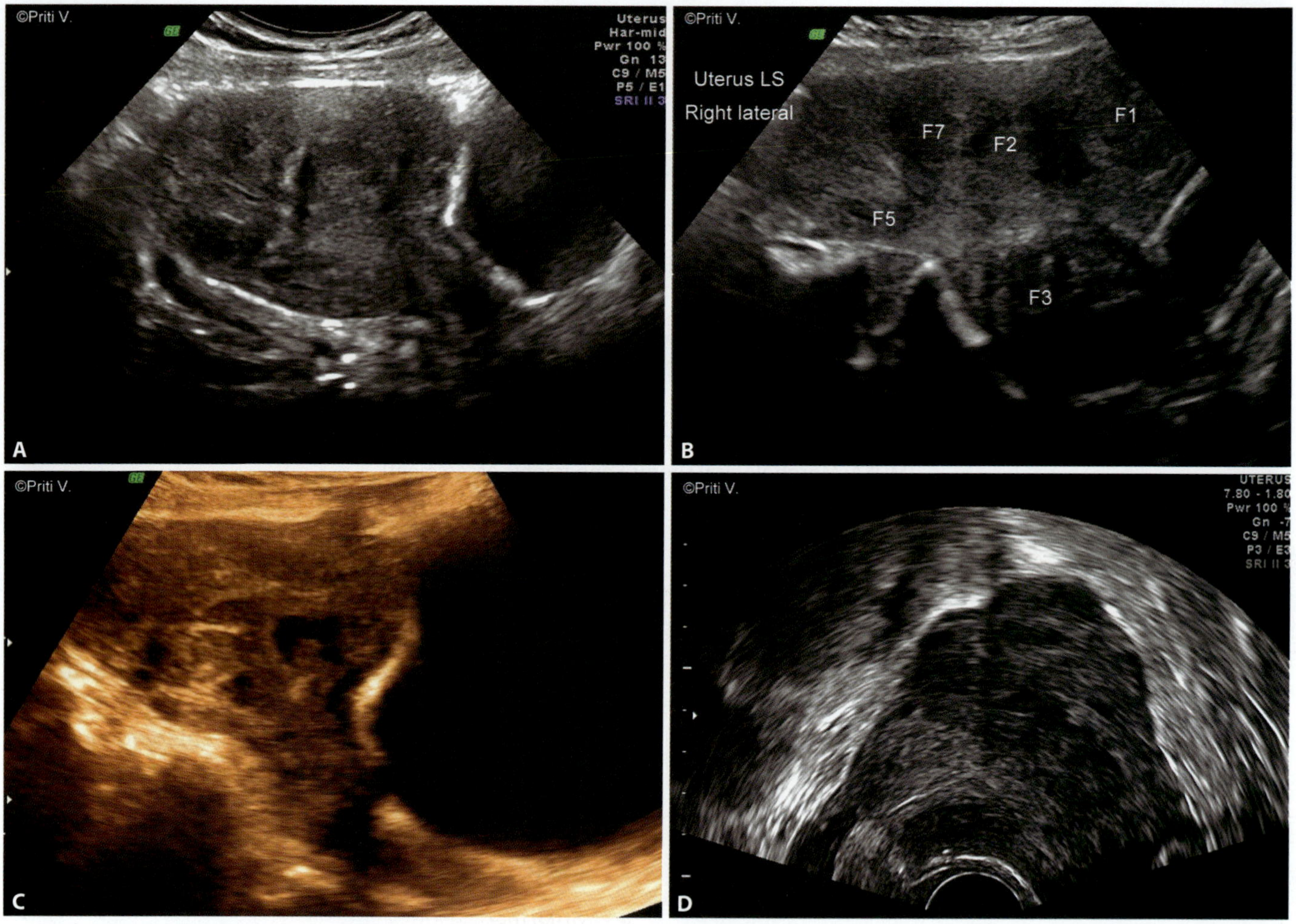

Figs. 31A to D: Irregularly enlarged uterus with multiple fibroids. (A) and (B) TAS images of patient 1; (C) TAS image of patient 2; (D) TVS image of patient 2. (TAS: transabdominal sonography; TVS: transvaginal sonography)

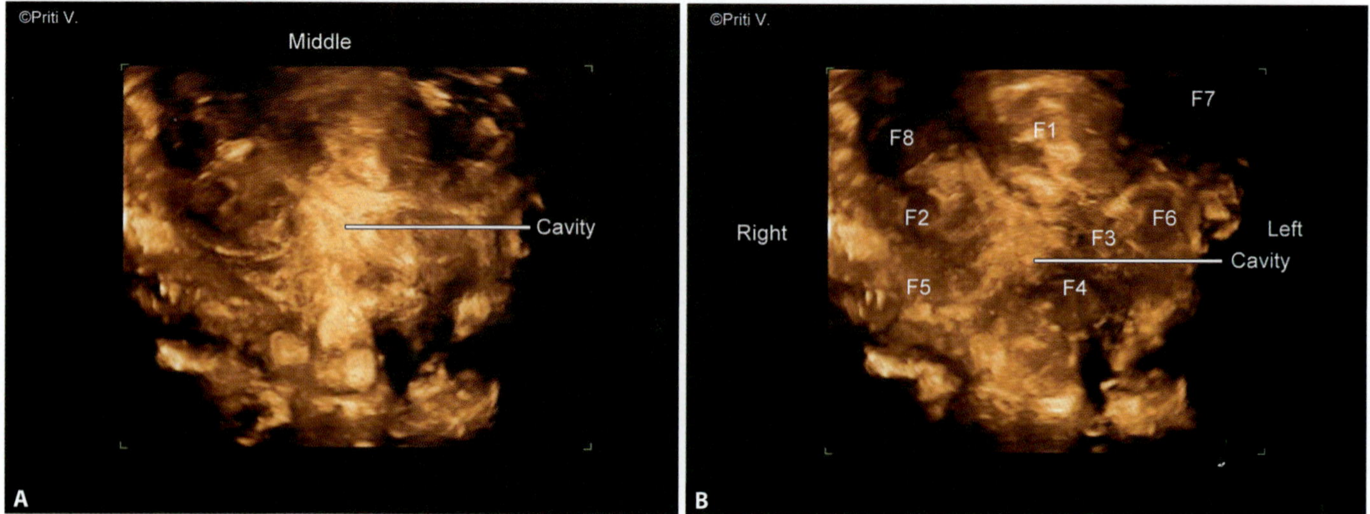

Figs. 32A and B: Multiple fibroids—in this patient, the fibroids are intramural, submucous and subserous, causing irregular enlargement of the uterus and distortion of the endometrial cavity.

Flowchart 3: Sonographic evaluation of fibroids.

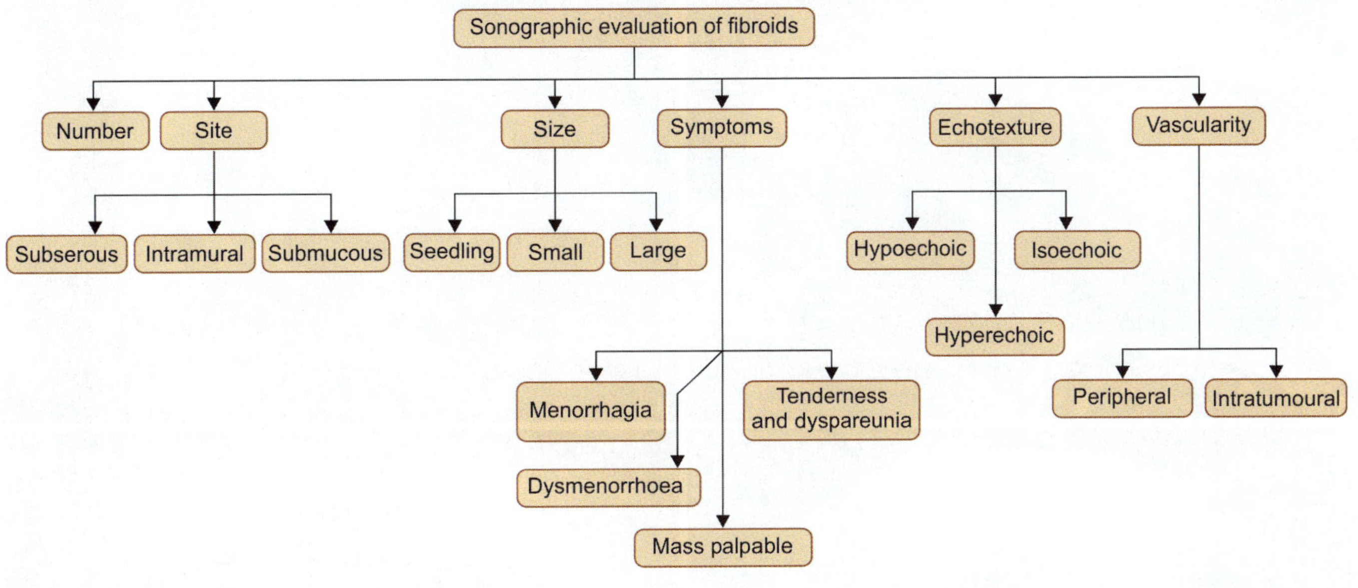

- *Shadowing* is another feature of fibroids.
  - Being well-circumscribed and dense lesions, fibroids produce *edge-shadowing.*
  - *Posterior acoustic shadowing* due to sound attenuation. Both these shadows are relatively more marked in calcified fibroids and subtle in non-calcified ones **(Figs. 40A and B)**.
  - Coarse internal shadows (in contrast to the fine internal shadows seen in adenomyosis) are produced by the whorled echotexture.
- *Degenerated fibroids* may have a complex heterogenous appearance, with cystic areas within and loss of posterior acoustic shadowing.
- *Colour Doppler* typically shows *circumferential vascularity* or *pericapsular flow.*
  - Fibroids which are necrotic or have undergone torsion will show absence of flow.
  - Submucous fibroids show a vascular pedicle with the vessels separating and coursing along the periphery of the polyp:
    - This vascular pattern and hypoechoic appearance help differentiate fibroid polyps from endometrial polyps. Because they are hypoechoic, they are better seen in the second half of the menstrual cycle when the endometrial lining is echogenic.
- Wandering fibroid is a fibroid that has lost its connection with the uterus and is getting its blood supply from elsewhere. They appear as fibroid-like adnexal masses but with no pedicle traceable to the uterus.

Transvaginal sonography is more sensitive for the imaging of small and moderate-size fibroids **(Flowchart 3 and Figs. 10A to C)**. However, in cases of large fibroids or retroverted uterus, the uterine fundus may be outside of the field of view on TVS. TAS is preferred for these cases, but views are often of limited value if the patient is obese.

Degenerated fibroids: Several types of degeneration are noted:

- Hyaline degeneration—focal or generalised—most common type of degeneration (seen in ~60% of cases). On ultrasound—appears hypoechoic—homogenous or nonhomogenous—loss of whorled appearance and reduced vascularity
- *Cystic degeneration:* ~5%, irregular cystic spaces with thin septa are seen within the fibroid **(Figs. 41A and B)**
- *Myxoid degeneration:* Uncommon, although reported as high as 50% by some authors
- *Red degeneration:* Due to haemorrhagic infarction which can occur particularly during pregnancy and may present with acute abdominal pain

Fibroid Mapping is a very important part of ultrasound evaluation of fibroids. Mapping involves describing the exact location of the fibroids and classifying their positioning in the uterus with respect to its relationship to the endometrial cavity, myometrium and the serosal surface as per the FIGO classification **(Fig. 26)**. Mapping helps accurate planning of treatment, surgeries and prognostication.

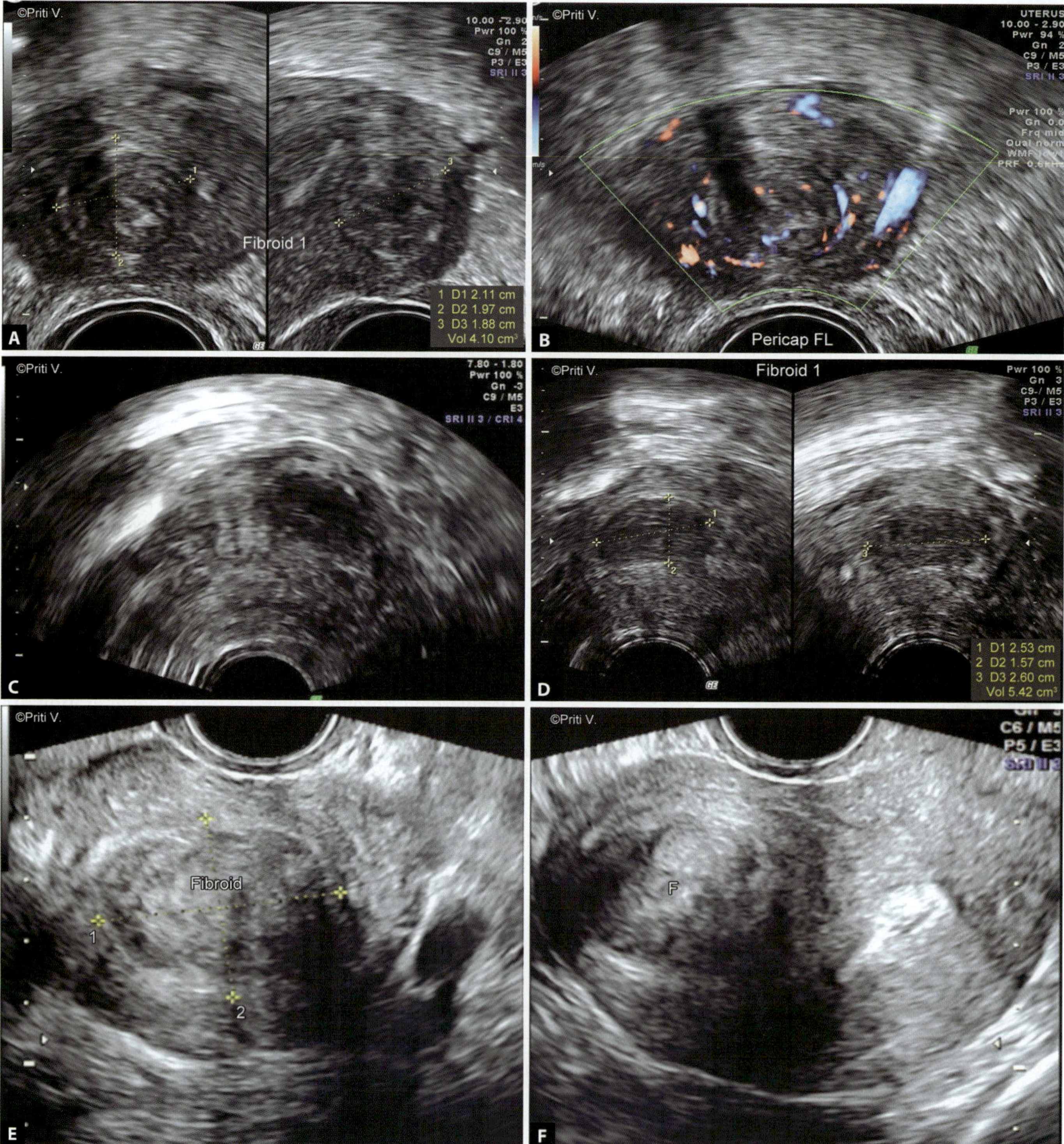

Figs. 33A to F: Intramural fibroid FIGO type 4 in three patients: 1—(A and B), 2—(C and D) and 3—(E and F). Note: Whorled appearance with classical pericapsular flow (A and B). (FIGO: International Federation of Gynaecology and Obstetrics)

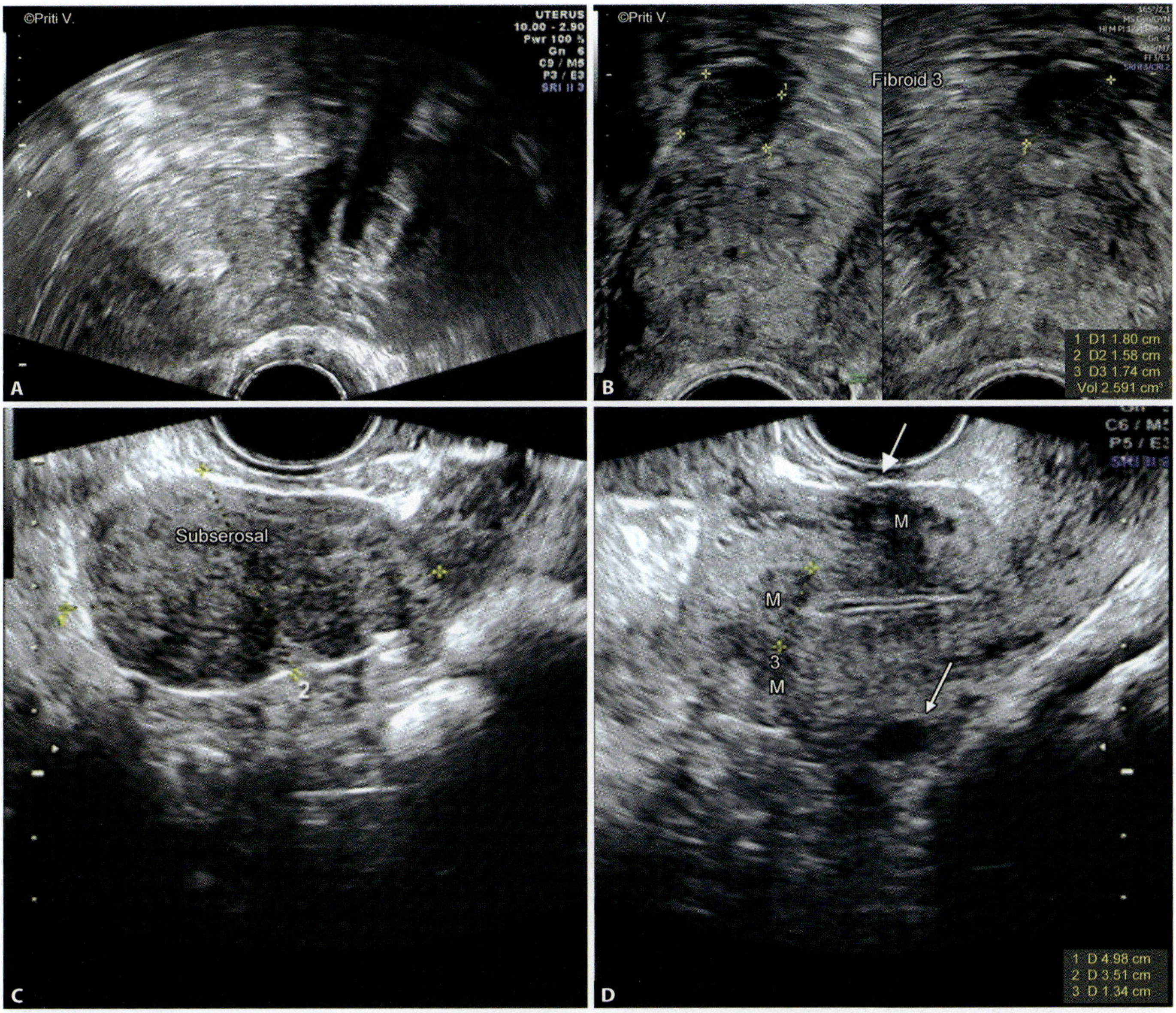

Figs. 34A to D: Subserous fibroid FIGO types 7, 6 and 5. Type 7—A and C. Type 6—B and Type 5—D (FIGO: International Federation of Gynaecology and Obstetrics)

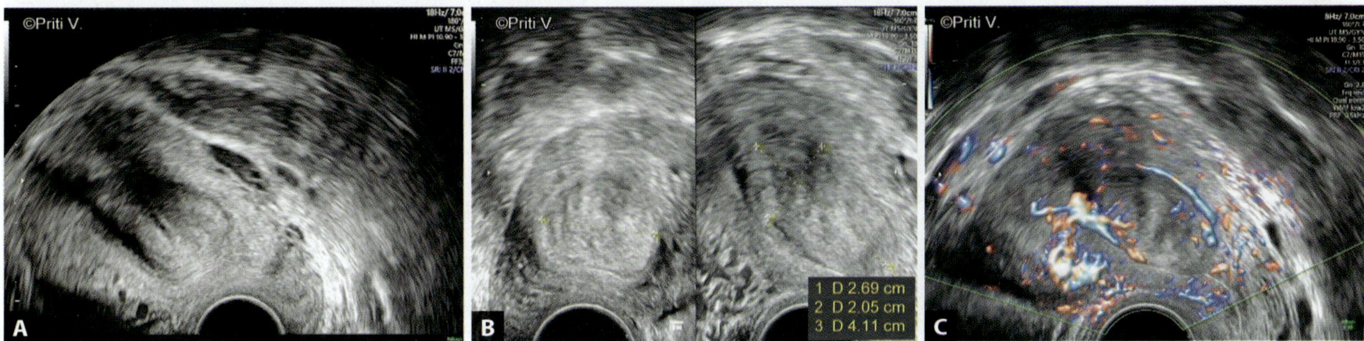

Figs. 35A to C: Submucous fibroid FIGO type 0 or fibroid polyp. Intracavitary. (FIGO: International Federation of Gynaecology and Obstetrics)

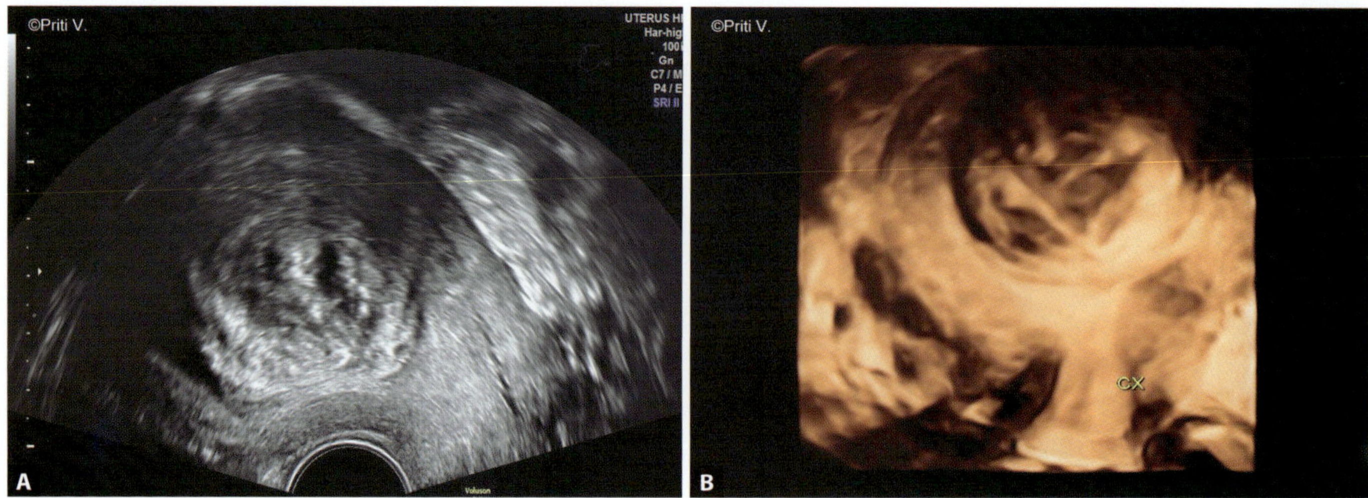

Figs. 36A and B: Submucous fibroid FIGO type 1. <50% intramural (FIGO: International Federation of Gynaecology and Obstetrics).

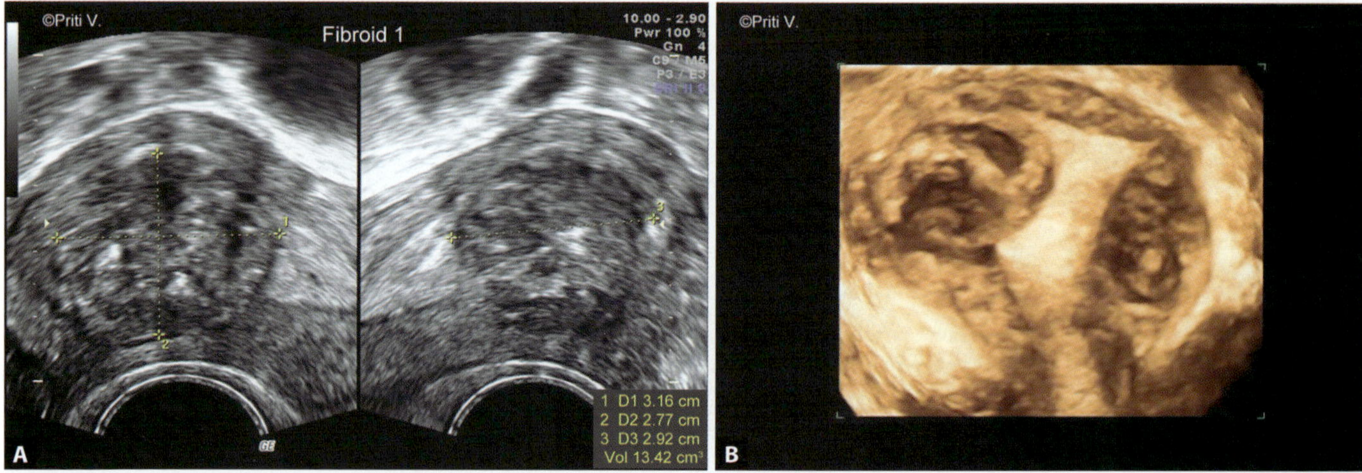

Figs. 37A and B: Submucous fibroid FIGO type 2. ≥50% intramural (FIGO: International Federation of Gynaecology and Obstetrics).

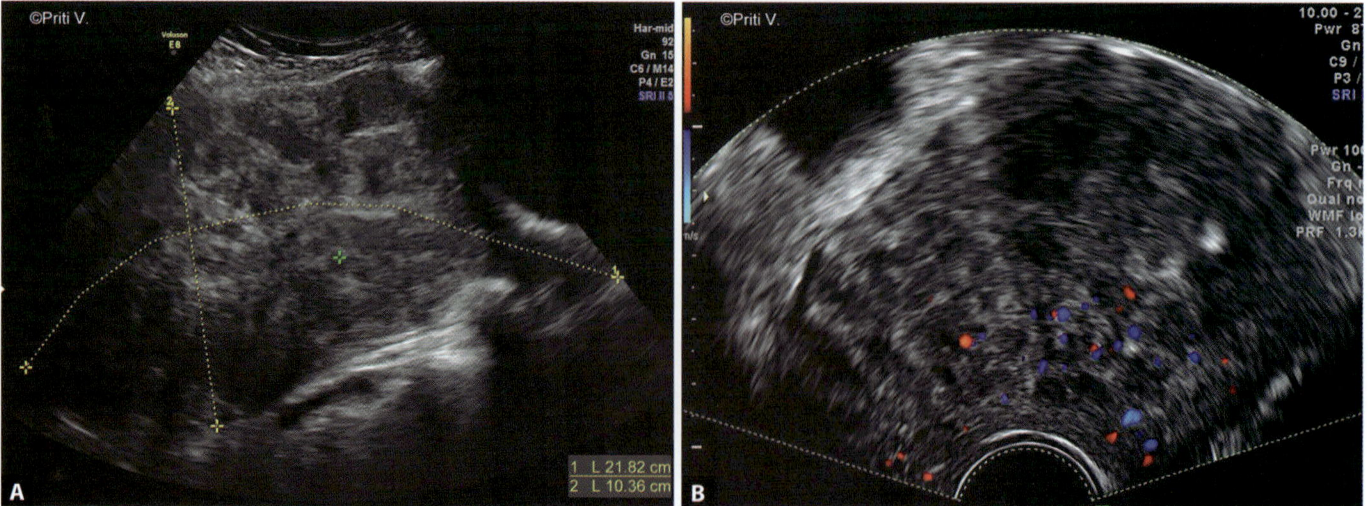

Figs. 38A and B: Diffuse fibromatosis.

ADENOMYOSIS (FLOWCHART 4)

Adenomyosis is a common non-neoplastic gynaecologic disease characterised by the presence of ectopic endometrium within the myometrium. Adenomyosis typically affects multiparous, premenopausal women >30 years of age and may cause dysmenorrhoea, and AUB.

Sonographic Findings (Figs. 42 to 47)

The sonographic findings of adenomyosis, best obtained by TVS, include the following:

- *Globular uterine enlargement*—uterine enlargement that is generally up to 12 cm in uterine length with a disproportionately larger anteroposterior diameter,

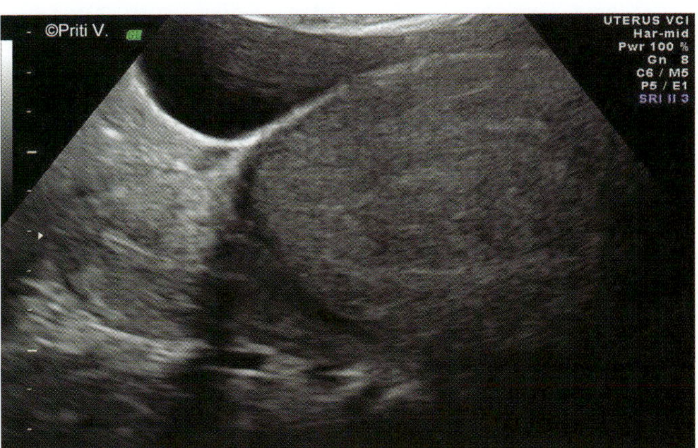

Fig. 39: Cervical fibroid.

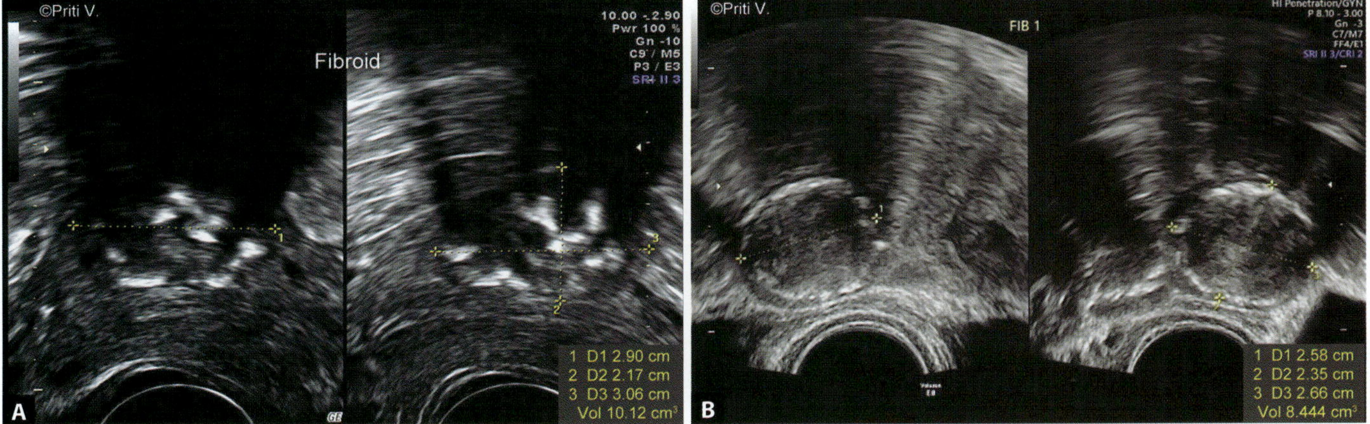

Figs. 40A and B: Calcification—intramural calcification and peripheral or eggshell calcification.

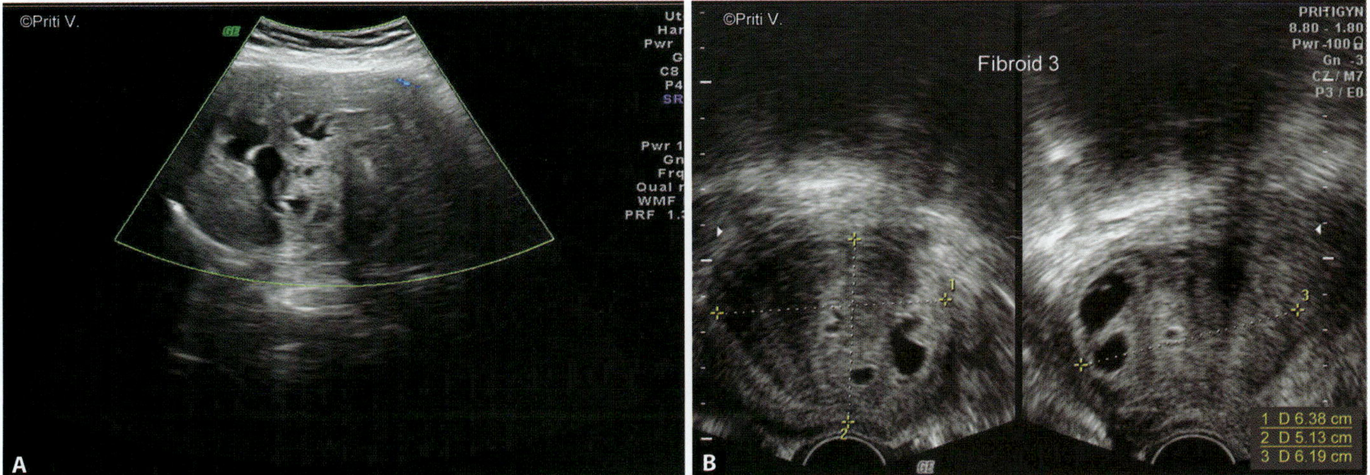

Figs. 41A and B: Cystic degeneration.

which is not explained by the presence of leiomyomata is a characteristic finding **(Figs. 42 and 43)**.

- *Heterogeneous echo texture*—there is a lack of homogeneity within the myometrium with evidence of architectural disturbance produced by echogenic islands of endometrial tissue composed of only stromal tissue or stroma + glands with little or no fluid collection within, alternating with foci of endometrial tissue with turbid collection within endometrium lined myometrial cysts of varying sizes. This appearance is *most predictive of adenomyosis* **(Figs. 42 to 44)**.
- Cystic and echoic spaces or lakes in the myometrium with echogenic rim and fluid containing low-level internal echoes—these are larger myometrial cysts of variable size seen throughout the myometrium, produced by a significant collection of menstrual blood, cyclically, within the foci of endometrial tissue. These lesions are pathognomonic of adenomyosis **(Figs. 44A to C)**.

The small arcuate vessels seen in the outer myometrium should not be confused with the cystic spaces of adenomyosis/adenomyomas **(Fig. 12)**. They do not have an echogenic rim and pick up colour on Doppler study at low-velocity scales with a PRF of 3–6 kHz.

- Uterine wall thickening—symmetric or asymmetric thickening of the anteroposterior diameter of the uterine wall due to the above changes **(Figs. 42 and 43)**
- Disruption of the EMJ or JZ by endometrial glands and stroma seen as endometrial lines and buds crossing the EMJ on ultrasound is the primary pathology in adenomyosis **(Figs. 47A to D)**.
- Thickening of the JZ—this zone is a layer that appears as a hypoechoic halo surrounding the endometrial margin. A thickness of 12 mm or greater on MRI has been shown to be associated with adenomyosis

Flowchart 4: Management of adenomyosis.

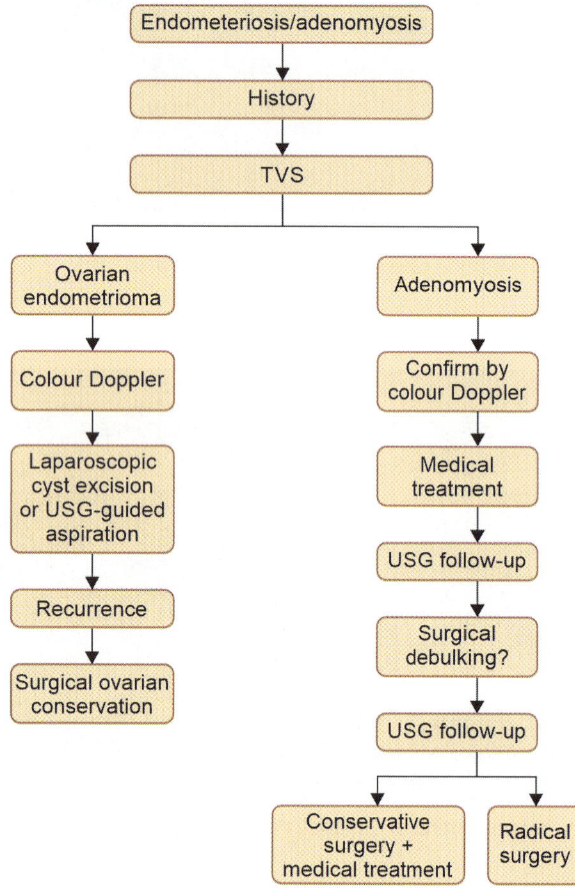

(TVS: transvaginal sonography; USG: ultrasonography).

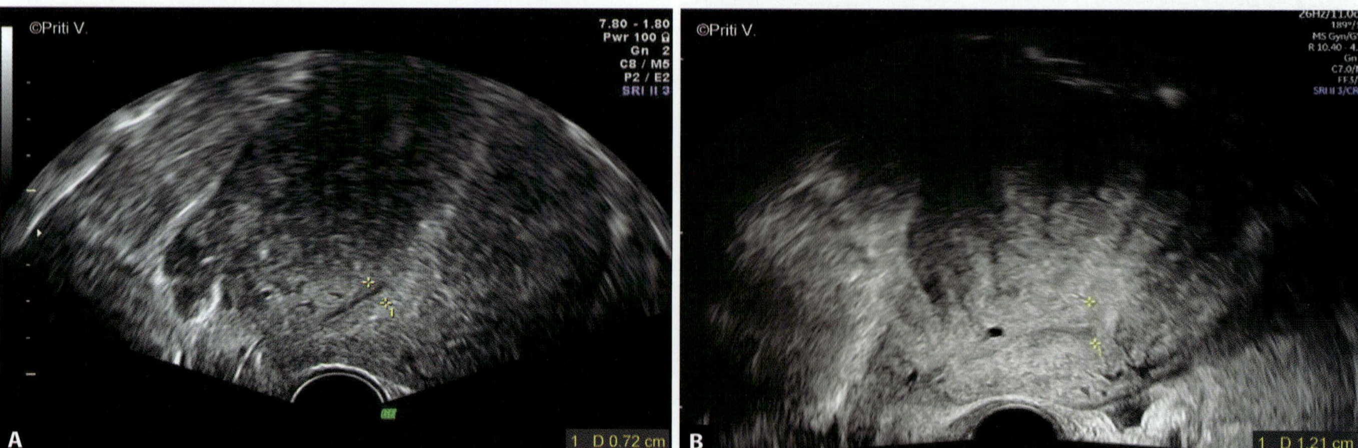

Figs. 42A and B: Globularly enlarged uteri with diffuse adenomyosis. (A) Symmetric enlargement; (B) Asymmetric enlargement.

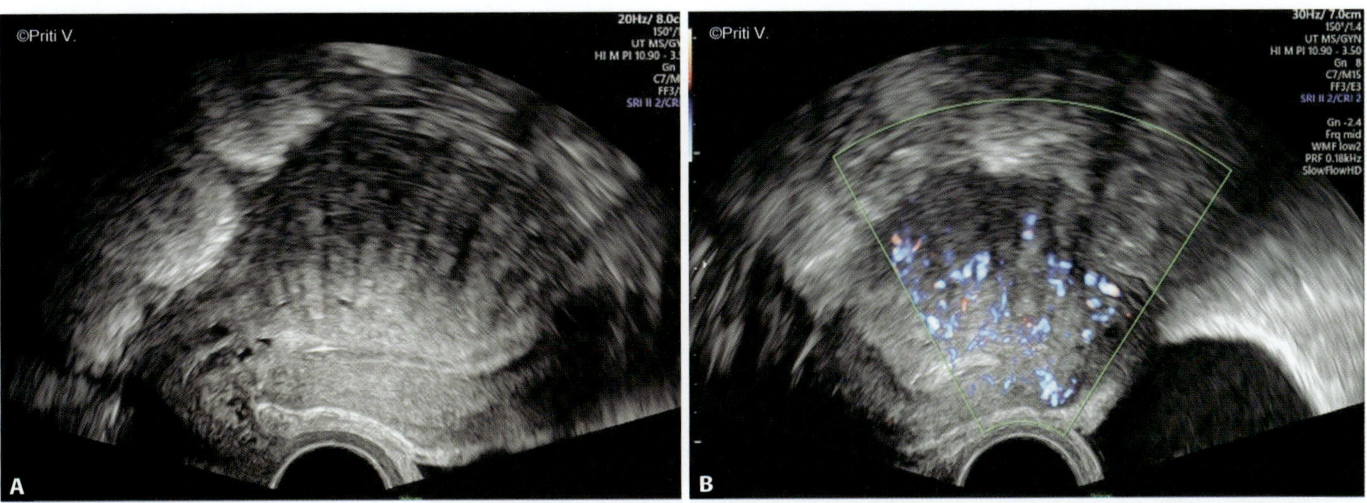

Figs. 43A and B: Diffuse adenomyosis—asymmetric involvement—more in the posterior wall. Note the scattered vascularity in **Figure B**.

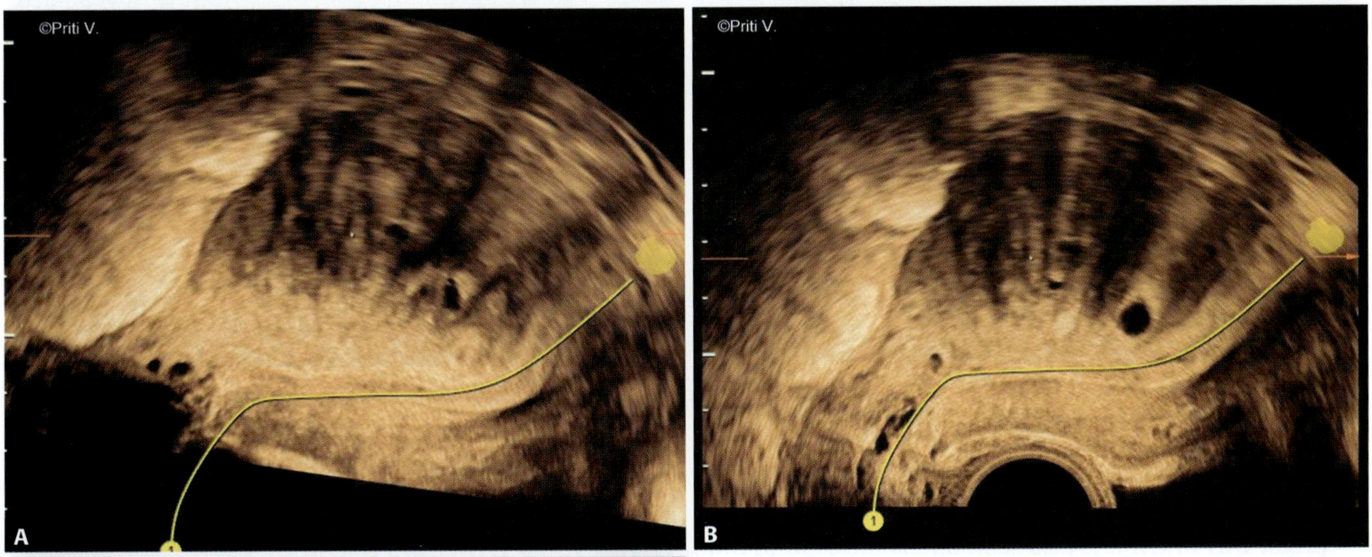

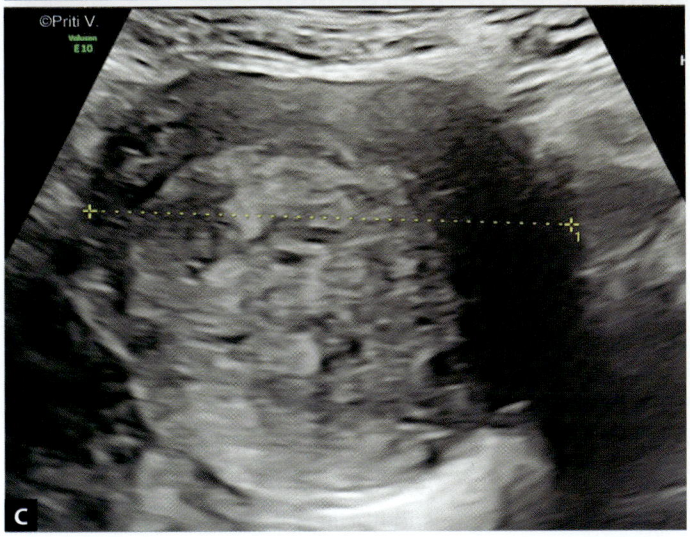

Figs. 44A to C: Characteristic echo texture of adenomyosis. Note that the echogenic islands and cystic space cause alternate shadowing and echo enhancement. The cystic spaces in adenomyosis–adenomyomatous cysts are thick-walled with thick echogenic margins. Compare this to the cystic spaces in fibroids with cystic degeneration in **Figure 40**, where the cysts are irregular with no echogenic rim.

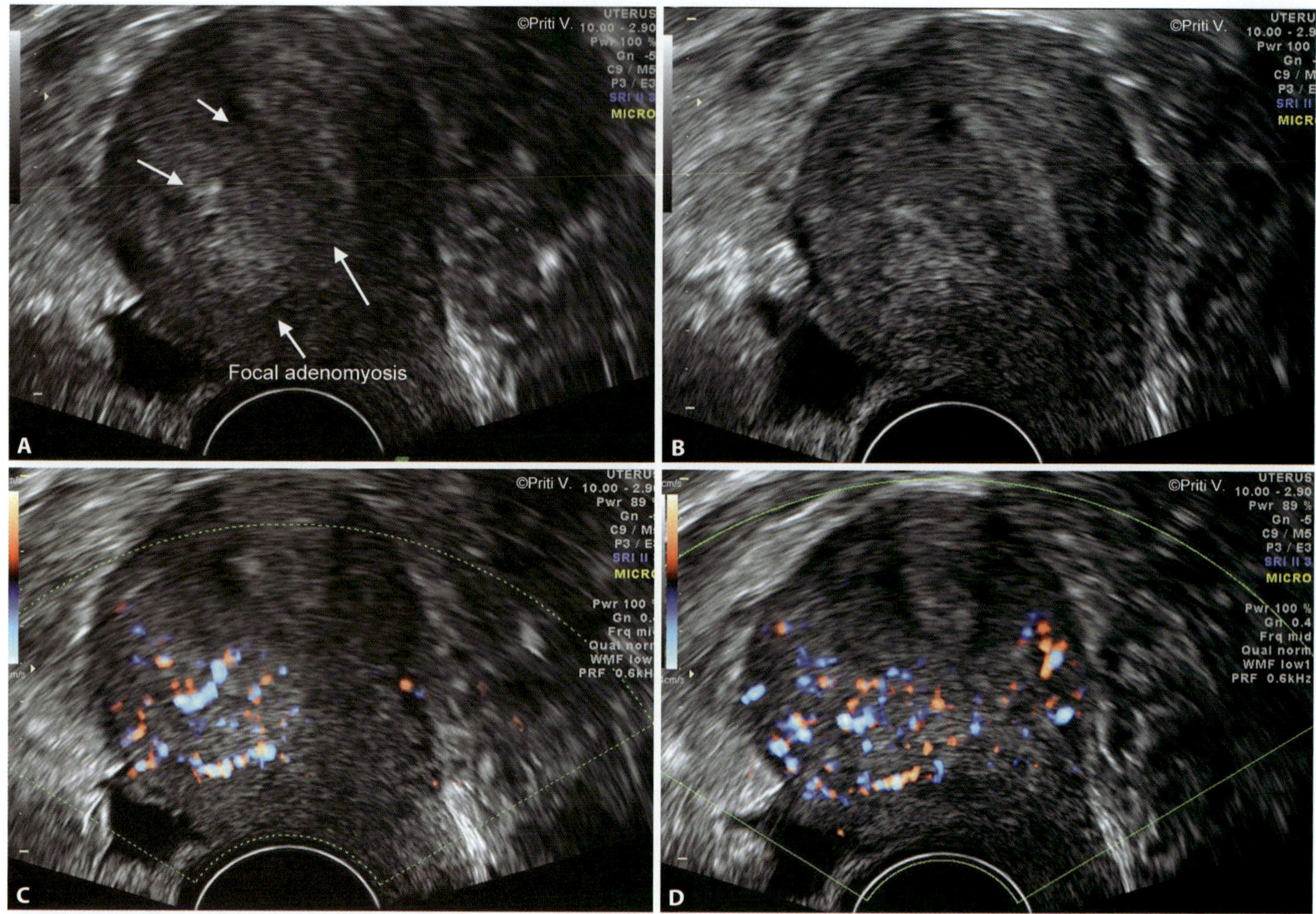

Figs. 45A to D: Focal adenomyosis—all images belong to the same patient. (A and B) 2D images showing focal adenomyosis in posterior wall at midcorpus level (arrows in image A); (C and D) Translesional and scattered flow, respectively, in slightly different sections of the same lesion.

(Figs. 14A to C). It is also seen on 2D ultrasound but is better appreciated on 3D using volume contrast imaging (VCI).

Thickening of the JZ is secondary to the disruption of the EMJ by endometrial infiltration which causes a series of changes in the JZ such as reactive hypertrophy and hyperplasia of myometrium, inflammation, fibrosis and increased vascularity.

On colour Doppler or high-definition (HD) flow images, adenomyosis and adenomyoma typically show irregular/serpiginous/tubular mesh of vasculature within the myometrium described as *scattered or translesional flow* **(Figs. 43B, 45C and D; 46B and C)**. The degree of vascularity is assessed by colour score which is usually around 3. On pulse wave Doppler, the flow is of high-resistance type.

Other Rare Uterine Lesions

Uterine Leiomyosarcomas (Figs. 48A to D)

Uterine sarcomas:

- *Uterine sarcomas are of two types*: Leiomyosarcomas (LMSs) which are rare, 0.5–7/100,000 women and endometrial stromal sarcomas (ESSs) which are even rarer, 1–2/1000,000 women
- Malignant transformation of leiomyomas into LMS is rare
- Leiomyomas and LMSs are different lesions pathologically and genetically:
    - Leiomyomas are monoclonal tumours arising from the uterine smooth muscles, rich in extracellular matrix with a large amount of collagen types I-III and disorganised fibril arrangement.

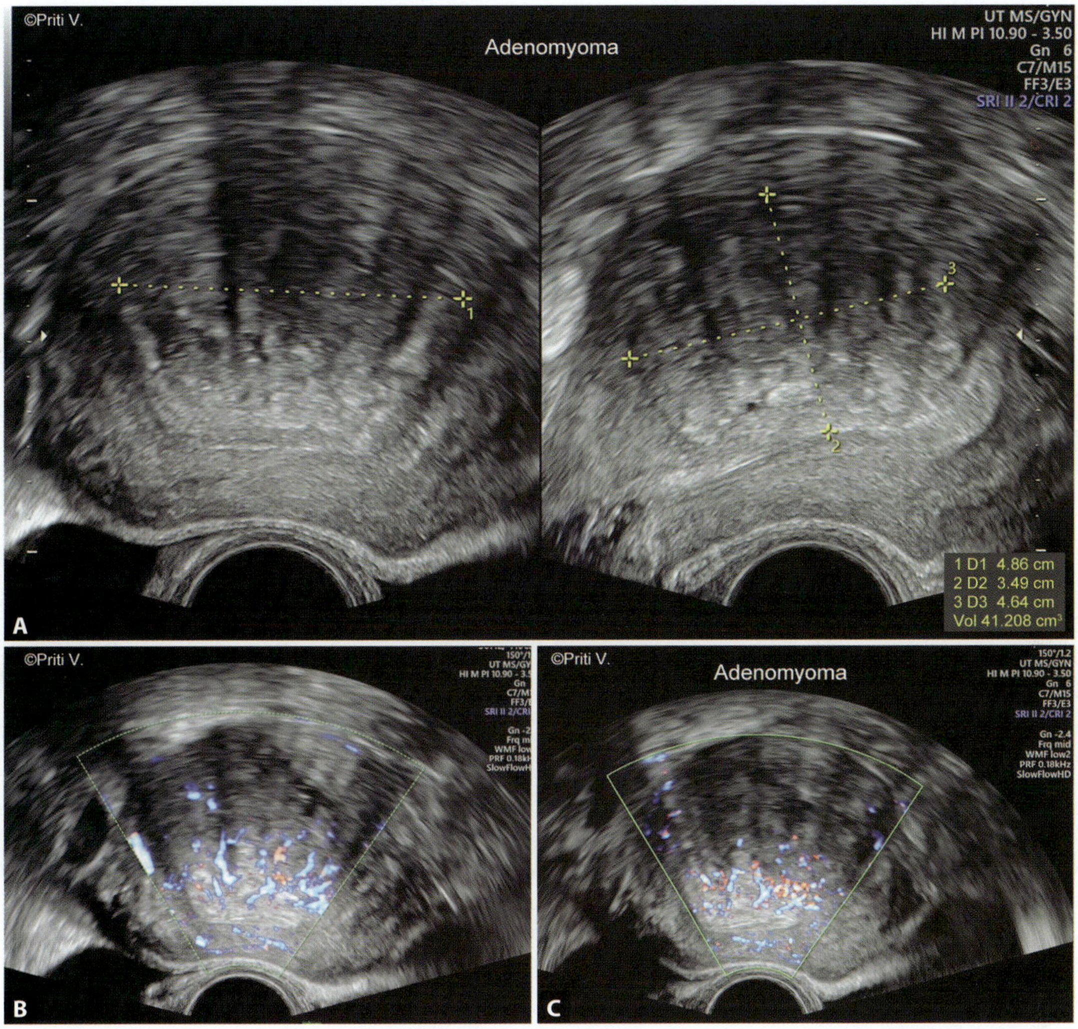

Figs. 46A to C: A posterior wall adenomyoma with vascular pattern. Note multiple cystic areas and steaky fan-shaped shadowing (A); (B and C) The vascular pattern in an adenomyoma, predominantly translesional flow, is shown in Figure B and scattered flow in Figure C.

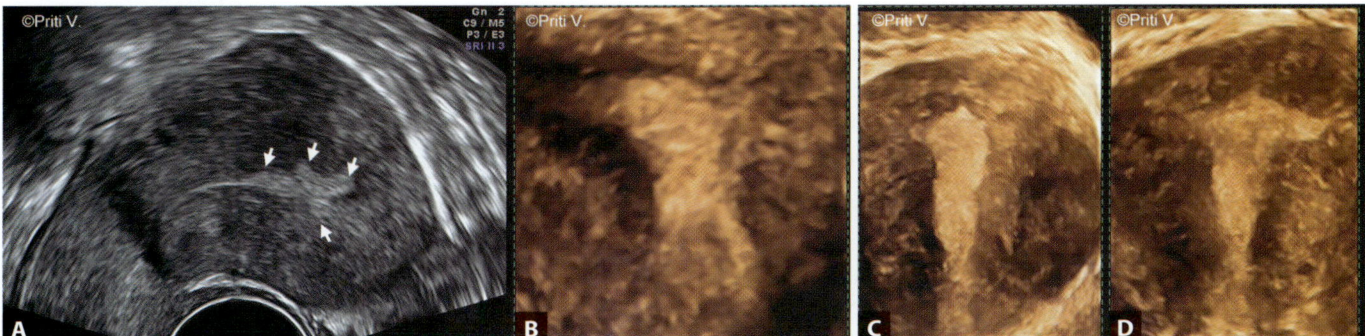

Figs. 47A to D: Irregular EMJ—these images are of two patients: 1—(A and B)—showing irregular EMJ in 2D sagittal view and B showing irregular EMJ in coronal view on 3D rendered image. Patient 2—(C and D) both are 3D rendered images in sagittal and coronal views showing irregular EMJ. Note the lines and buds from the endometrium cross the EMJ and enter the myometrium. (EMJ: endomyometrial junction)

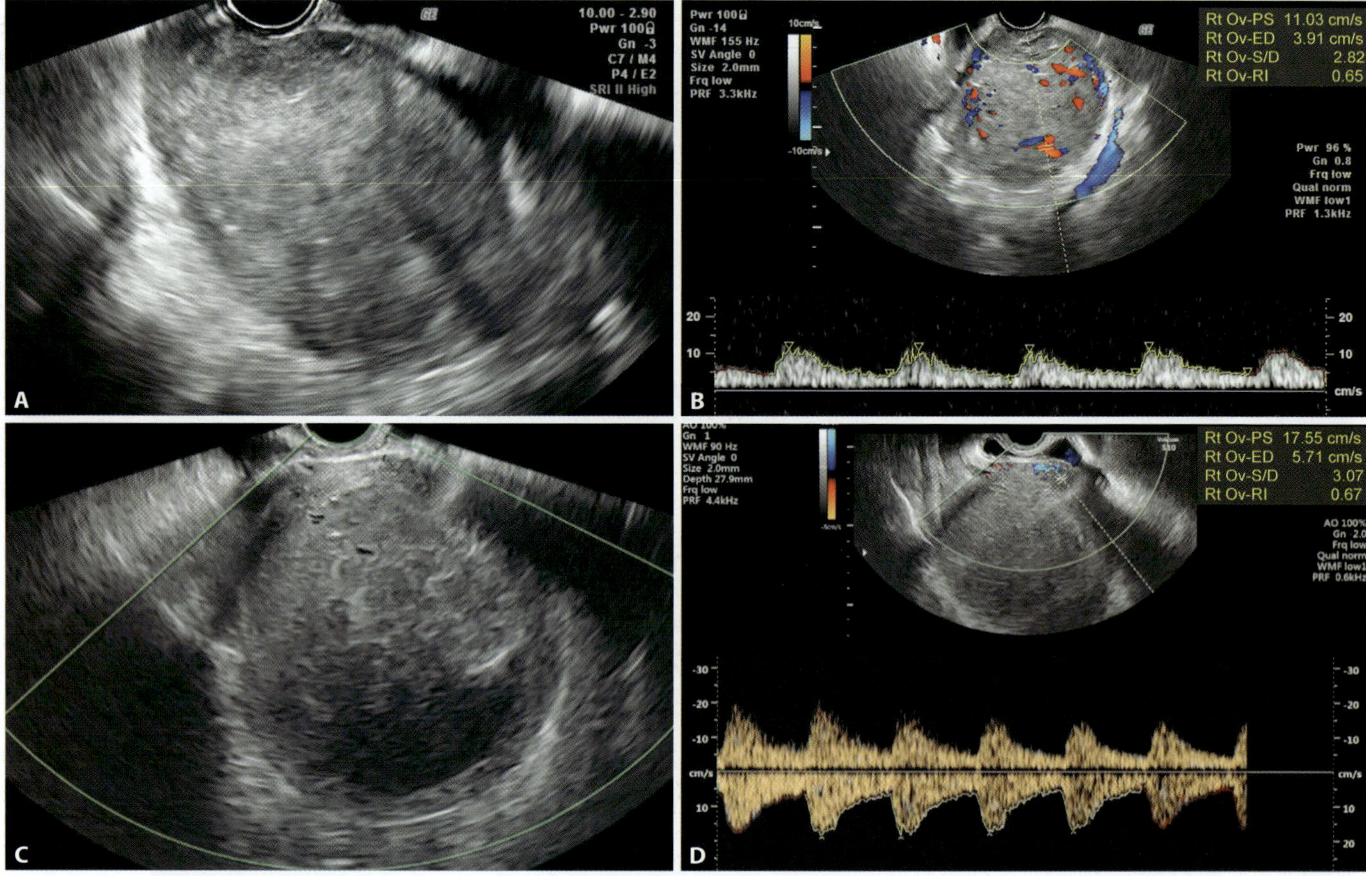

Figs. 48A to D: Two cases of uterine sarcoma—both 2D images show a circumscribed mass—reported as fibroid. Sarcoma was diagnosed on HPE. In 2D, the echotexture is very plain or bland—no whorled appearance, no coarse shadows. This is described as a 'cooked' or a 'washed-out' appearance. Vascularity has a colour score of 2–3 but flow is of low resistance type which is seen in fibroids very often. It is important to note that sarcomas are usually relatively large solitary lesions. (Images courtesy of Dr Nandini Devi)

- LMSs are of mesenchymal origin and chromosomally different from leiomyomas.

- Unfortunately, no imaging modality can reliably differentiate a benign leiomyoma from the rare LMS.
- Differentiation, is very important, because the management and prognosis of the two conditions are completely different. Leiomyosarcomas need to be treated much more aggressively than leiomyomas.
- *Possible differentiating features may be* ***(Figs. 48A to D)****:*
  - Large size >8 cms
  - Solitary lesion
  - Absence of a typical whorled appearance with no intenal or sharp edge shadowing
  - The echo-texture is typically 'bland', described as a 'washed out' or 'cooked appearance'
  - Increased vascularity - colour score 4, RI <0.5 high PSV is sometimes seen
  - More often the colour score is only 2-3 but the flow is of low resistance type
- **Figures 48** shows 2 cases of leiomyosarcomas dignosed as fibroids with no whorled appearance or classical shadowing typical of fibroids. Note the typical 'bland' or 'washed out' internal echo texture and the low resistance blood flow even though the color score was only 2-3.
- USG features my overlap with atypical fibroids but a combination of above features may help in the diagnosis.
- STUMP—uterine smooth muscle tumours of uncertain malignant potential—are rare.
- Uterine Lipoleiomyoma—greater fat content. The lesion is well-circumscribed and echogenic **(Fig. 49)** but with limited posterior shadowing compared to a calcified fibroid. (Sometimes considered a variant of a leiomyoma).

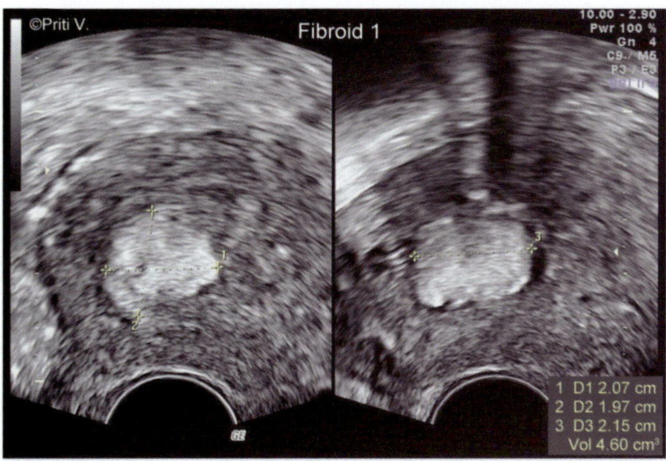

Fig. 49: A uterine lipoleiomyoma. A uniformly echogenic mass with relatively minimal shadowing.

Uterine Arteriovenous Malformations (Figs. 50 and 51)

- Uterine arteriovenous malformations (AVMs) *are rare lesions*—resulting from the formation of multiple arteriovenous abnormal fistulous connections within the uterus without an intervening capillary network. The AVMS can be congenital (rare) and acquired.

The acquired AVMs are associated with the following:

- Dilatation and curettage
- Surgical termination of pregnancy
- Molar pregnancies and GTD (gestational trophoblastic disease)
- Miscarriage
- Caesarean section.

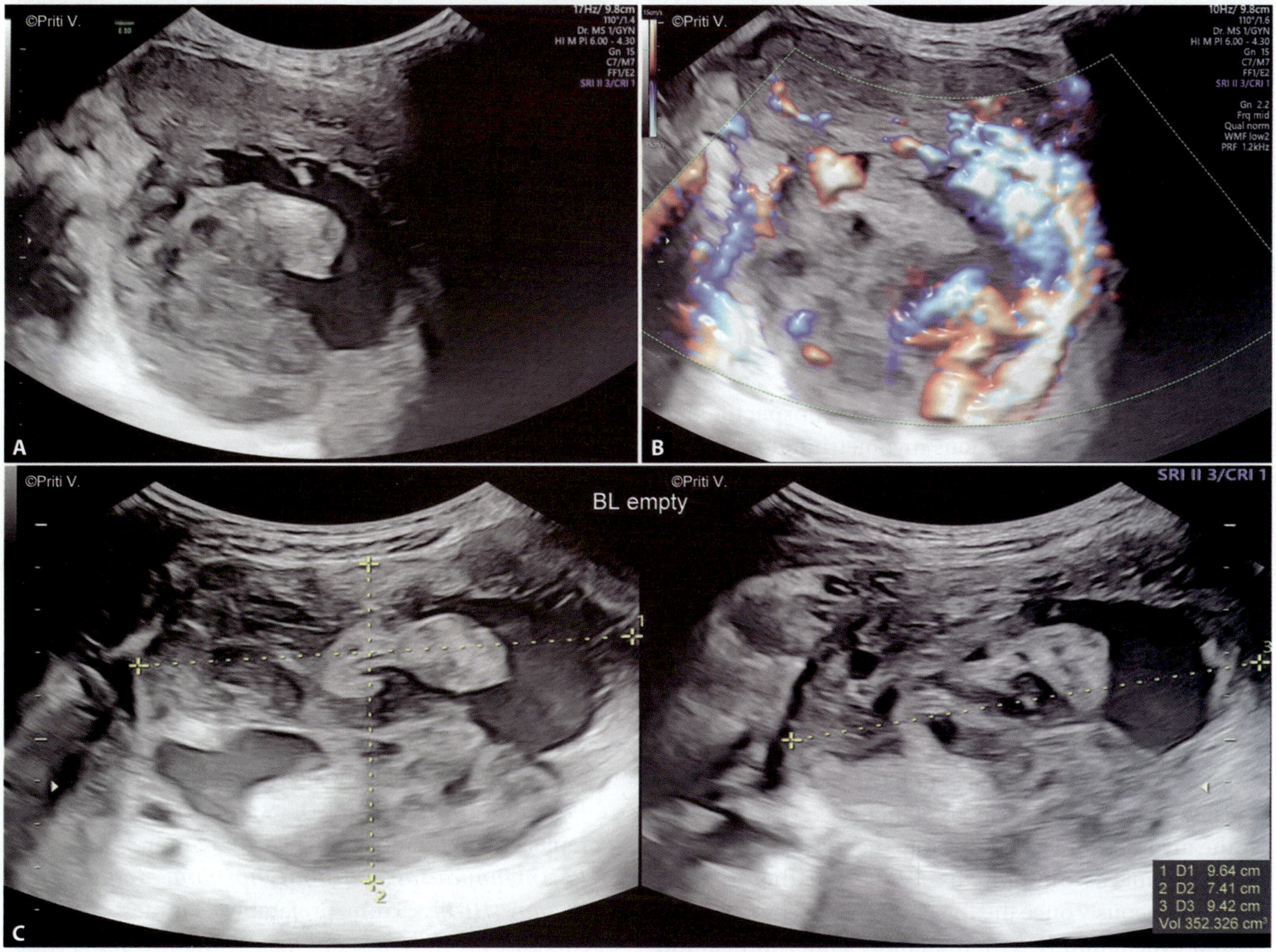

Figs. 50A to C: TAS images of an AVM. AVMs are rare. This was an AVM noted 2 years after the evacuation of a molar pregnancy. The patient presented with persistent bleeding PV. There was a posterior uterine wall mass which was highly vascular with large venous lakes and communicating with the parametrial vessels. (BL: bladder; AVM: arteriovenous malformation; TAS: transabdominal sonography)

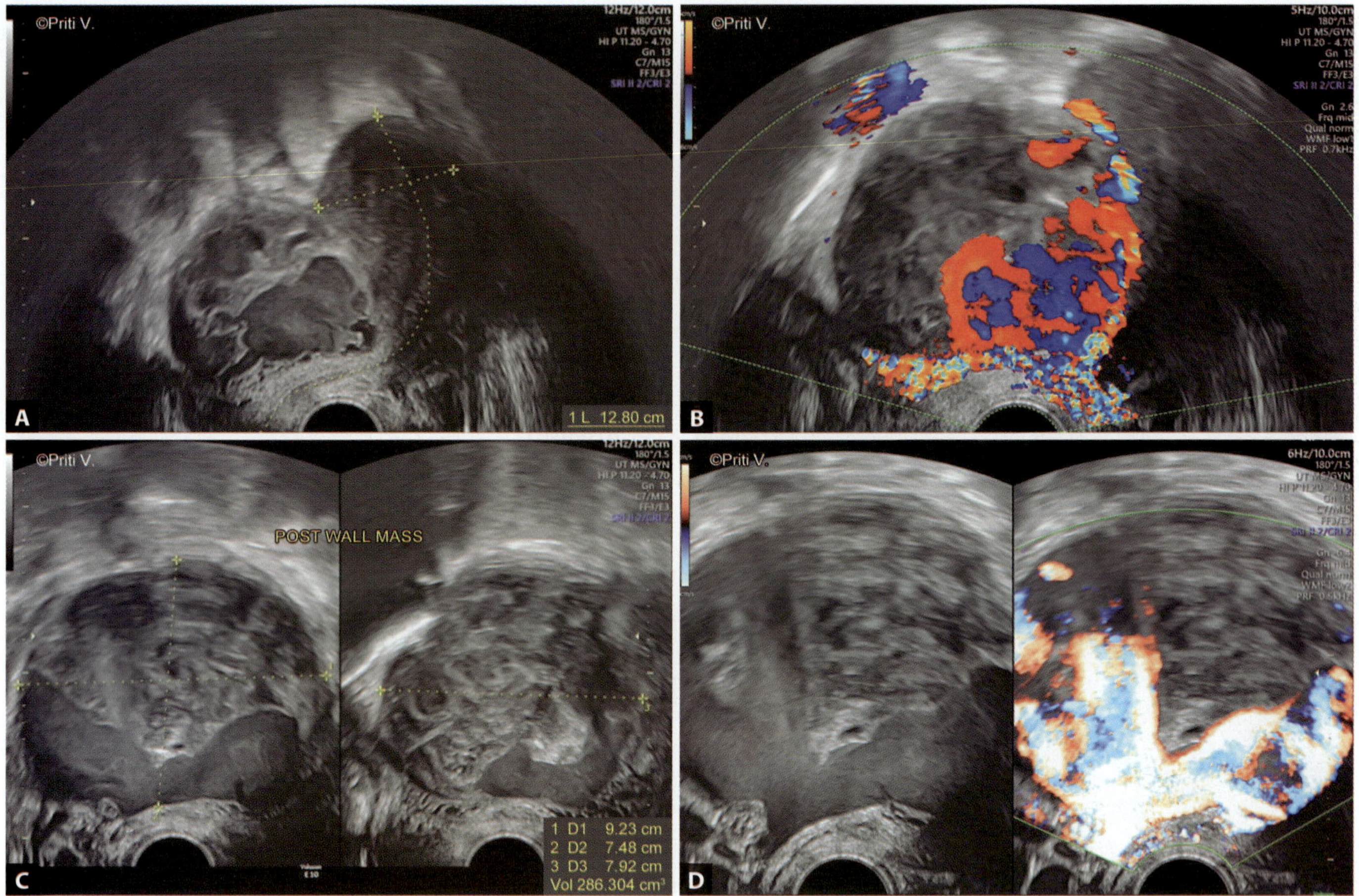

Figs. 51A to D: TVS images of the same AVM as in **Figure 50**. (AVM: arteriovenous malformation; TVS: transvaginal sonography)

Sonographic appearance is usually nonspecific and can range from a heterogenous myometrium to multiple tubular tortuous anechoic or hypoechoic cystic lesions within the myometrium showing a multicoloured mosaic pattern on color flow due to turbulent high velocity low ressistance flow. The vascularity may extend into the cavity. The lesion may resemble RPOC, GTD or a vascular tumor.

Enhanced Myometrial Vascularity (Figs. 52 and 53)

- These are *more common lesions* associated with retained products of conception (*RPOCs*).
- They are seen as focal areas of increased vascularity in the myometrium extending into the RPOC.
- They look as ominous as AVMs. But they regress spontaneously once the RPOC is removed by a dilation and evacuation (D&E), preferably under ultrasound guidance. **Figures 52 and 53** show images of EMV before and after evacuation of the RPOC.

ENDOMETRIUM

Normal Endometrium (Figs. 54 and 55)

The endometrial thickness (ET) and the appearance changes with age and the phase of the menstruation. *The accepted ET in asymptomatic women is:*

- *Premenopausal:* Should be between 1 and 14 mm, depending on the phase of menstruation
- *Postmenopausal:* With *continuous E-P HRT* (CERT)—<8 mm. Average thickness is 3 mm.
- *On tamoxifen—<8 mm* or even 12 mm because of estrogenic effect of tamoxifen and cystic changes.
- *Postmenopausal:* With *sequential* hormone replacement therapy (SERT): <10–12 mm.
- *Postmenopausal: Without hormone replacement therapy (HRT):* <5 mm, preferably <4 mm
- *Not only the thickness but the echotexture of the endometrium also changes with the menstrual cycle and the physiologic state of the woman and should beassessed.*

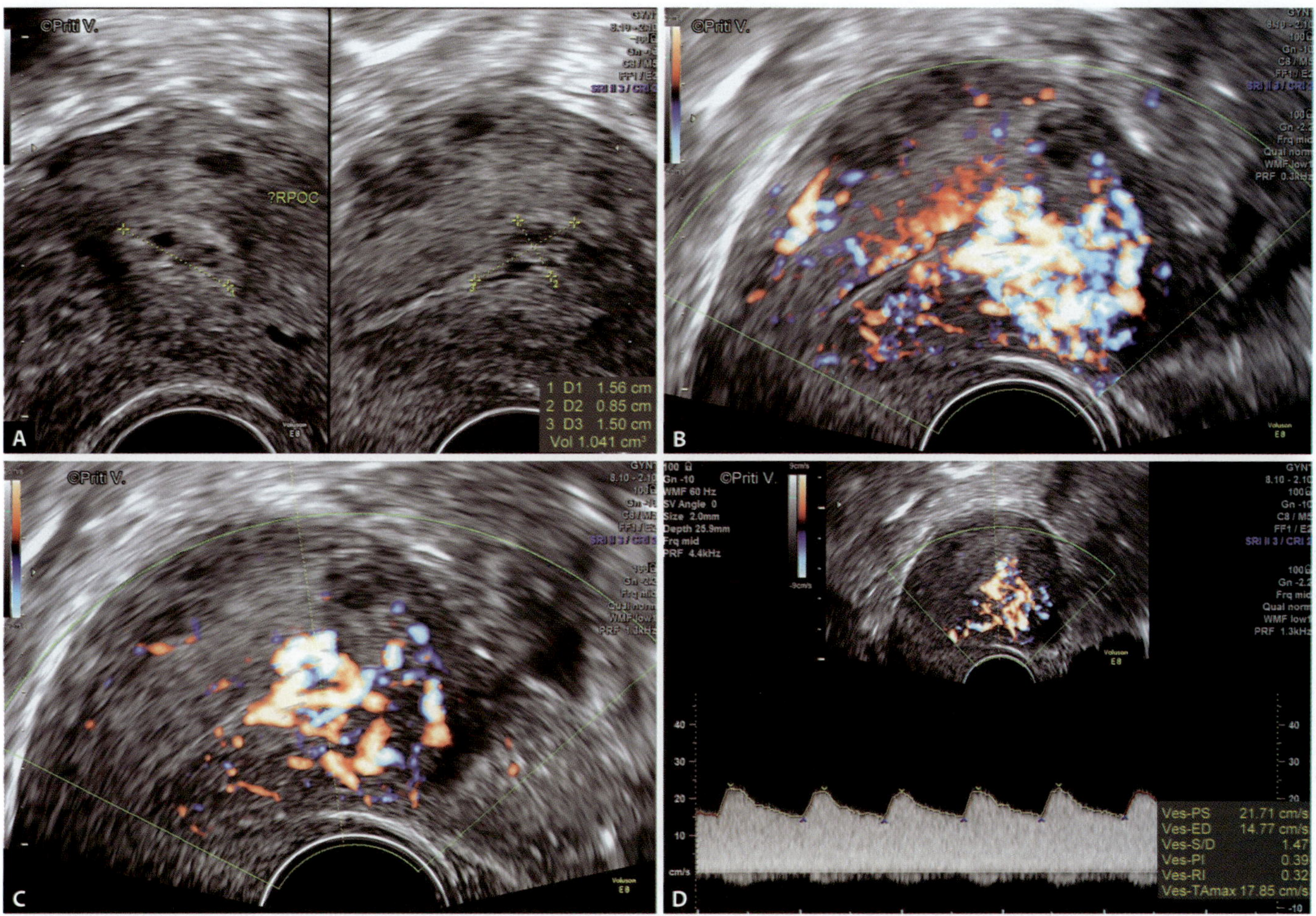

Figs. 52A to D: Patient I—EMV (enhanced endometrial vascularity)—(A)—RPOC present; (B and C) EMV in the anterior wall myometrium extends into the RPOC; (D) A very low resistance flow with PI = 0.39 and RI = 0.32. Complete resolution of the EMV noted after D&C for RPOC. (D&C: dilation and curettage; PI: pulsatility index; RI: resistive index; RPOC: retained products of conception)

- *In postmenopausal women any bleeding is abnormal and needs investigation. An ET of <4 mm and homogenous echotexture can be followed up. All others need endometrial sampling to rule out malignancy.*

Imaging the endometrium correctly is important for proper assessment. The endometrium is imaged in the sagittal plane with the endometrium being at 90° to the ultrasound beam, and it is measured from the outer edge of the basal layer anteriorly to the outer edge of the basal layer posteriorly. The endometrium should be measured where it is thickest.

Endometrial Cycle

Changes seen in the Endometrium (Figs. 54A to C)

- Days 1–5—menstrual phase—oestrogen and progesterone—lowest—ET <4 mm **(Fig. 5A)**.
- Days 6–13—proliferative phase **(Figs. 54A and B and 5B)**—increasing oestrogen in response to increasing FSH—results in endometrial proliferation and thickening up to 14 mm and a typical triple line appearance of a proliferative endometrium—ET <14 mm
- As LH peaks at midcycle, ovulation occurs and a corpus luteum is formed in the ovary which produces progesterone.
- Days 14–28 secretory phase **(Figs. 5C and 54C)**—under the influence of progesterone produced by the corpus luteum—endometrium undergoes secretary changes and on ultrasound, it progressively becomes echogenic from the periphery inwards.
- By midcycle—day 21, the endometrium is almost completely echogenic, with loss of the triple line and an ET of 9–16 mm **(Figs. 5C and 54C)**.

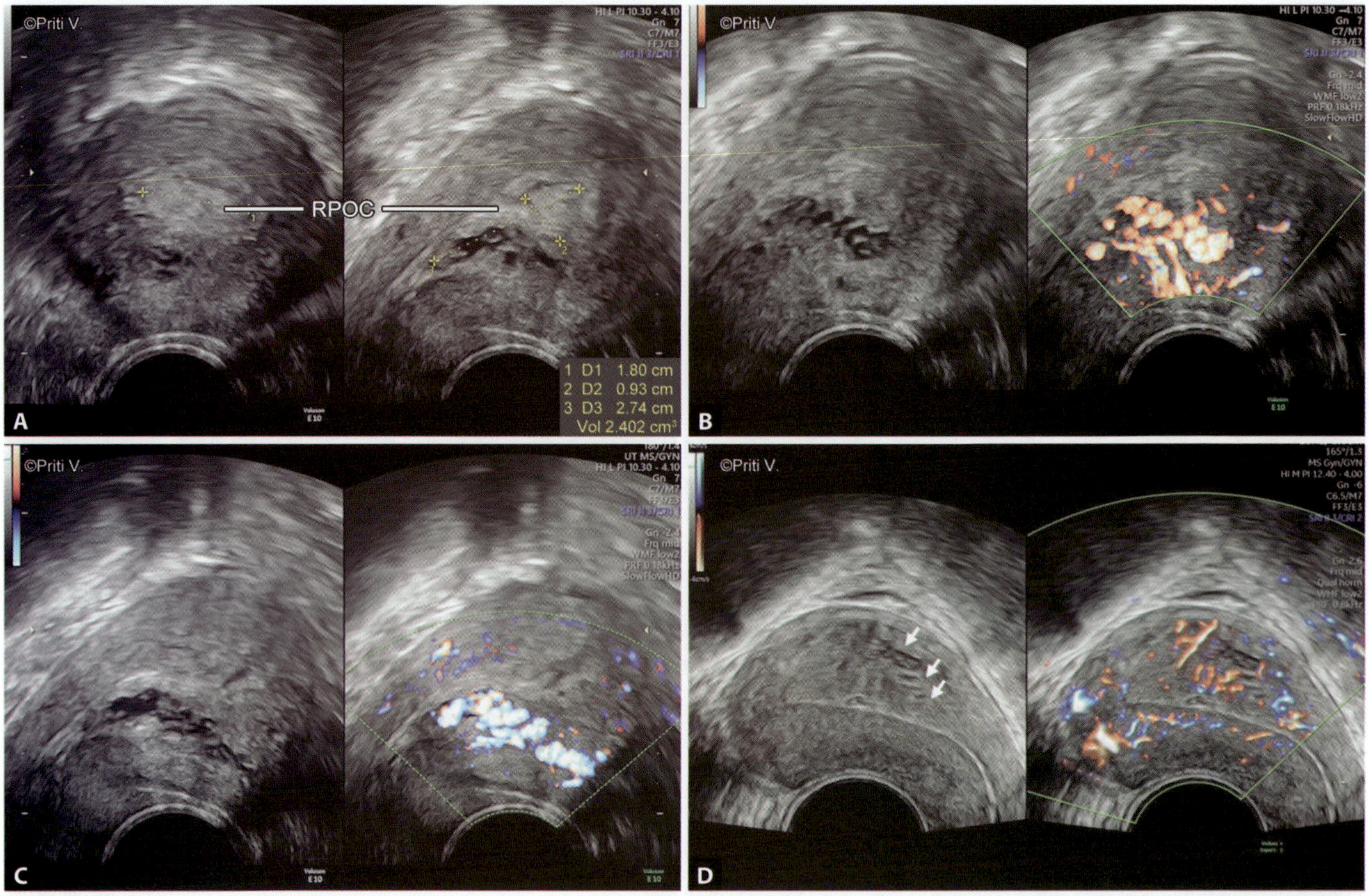

Figs. 53A to D: Patient II—EMV (enhanced endometrial vascularity)—(A)—anteverted uterus with RPOC seen in the cavity; (B and C) EMV in the anterior wall myometrium extends into the RPOC; (D) A retroverted uterus was found soon after the D&C for removal of the RPOC; Complete resolution post-D&C. Note the almost complete resolution of the EMV postsurgical removal of the RPOC. (D&C: dilation and curettage; RPOC: retained products of conception)

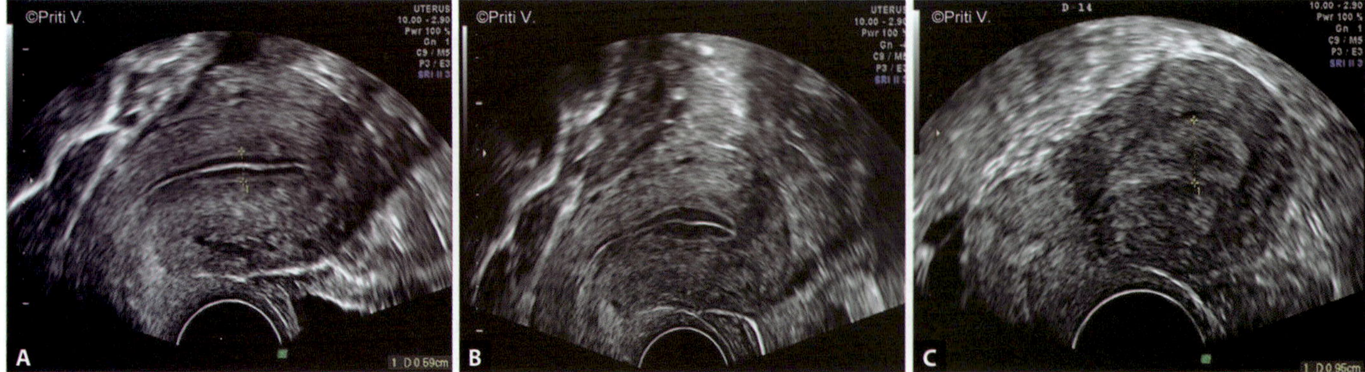

Figs. 54A to C: Cyclic endometrial changes—triple line early (A) and late (B) proliferative and echogenic secretary endometrium (C)—echogenicity extending from periphery inwards.

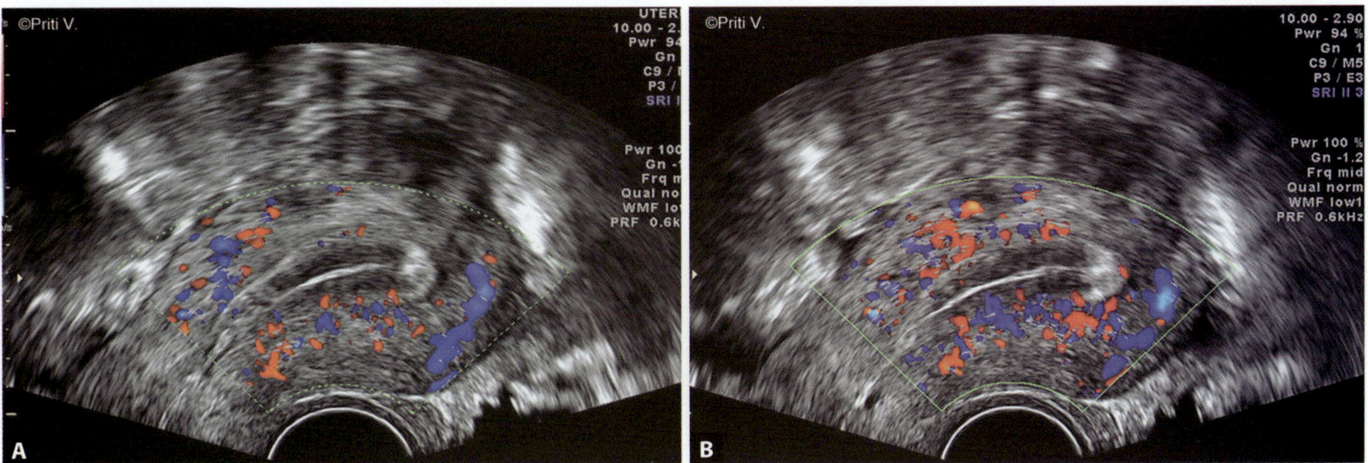

Figs. 55A and B: Late proliferative endometrium showing flow just reaching zone 3 (A) and reaching the midline stripe—zone 4 (B). Zone 1: 2 mm thick surrounding area the hyperechoic outer layer of the endometrium, zone 2: The hyperechoic outer layer of the endometrium, zone 3: The hypoechoic inner layer of the endometrium and zone 4: The endometrial cavity.

- With no fertilisation, progesterone reduces—the endometrium shrinks by 1–2 mm followed by menstruation.
- If fertilisation occurs, the endometrium continues to thicken and is called a decidualised endometrium.

Endometrial vascularity: The overall colour score of the endometrium is usually 3.

Michael Applebaum in his study with transvaginal colour Doppler divided the endometrium and periendometrial areas into four zones. In the study conducted by him, no pregnancy was reported in in vitro fertilisation (IVF) patients unless vascularity was demonstrated in zone 3 or within zone 3 or 4 prior to transfer **(Figs. 55A and B)**.

- *Zone 1:* 2 mm thick area surrounding the hyperechoic outer layer of the endometrium
- *Zone 2:* The hyperechoic outer layer of the endometrium
- *Zone 3:* The hypoechoic inner layer of the endometrium
- *Zone 4:* The endometrial cavity

Endometrial Hyperplasia (Figs. 56 to 60) (Flowchart 5)

Endometrial hyperplasia refers to an increased proliferation of the endometrial glands relative to the stroma in response to high oestrogen levels unopposed by progesterone. The differentiation between hyperplasia and carcinoma can be difficult.

Types of hyperplasia:

- Simple hyperplasia without atypia—or cystic endometrial hyperplasia
- Simple hyperplasia with atypia
- Complex hyperplasia without atypia
- Complex hyperplasia with atypia

Associations:

- Polycystic ovary syndrome (PCOS)
- Obesity
- Drug induced—tamoxifen therapy, Mifegest
- Oestrogen secreting tumours

Ultrasonography imaging:

Endometrial thickness—abnormal:

- Premenopausal >15 mm: Independent of the phase of the cycle
- Postmenopausal ≥5 mm is abnormal

Endometrial echotexture:

- Simple hyperplasia without atypia—also known as cystic endometrial hyperplasia appears as thick echogenic endometrium, often with small cystic areas distributed uniformly throughout the endometrium.
- The rest of the hyperplastic lesions show a uniformly echogenic appearance.
- Complex hyperplasia may show a polypoid or heterogenous appearance or focal lesions within.

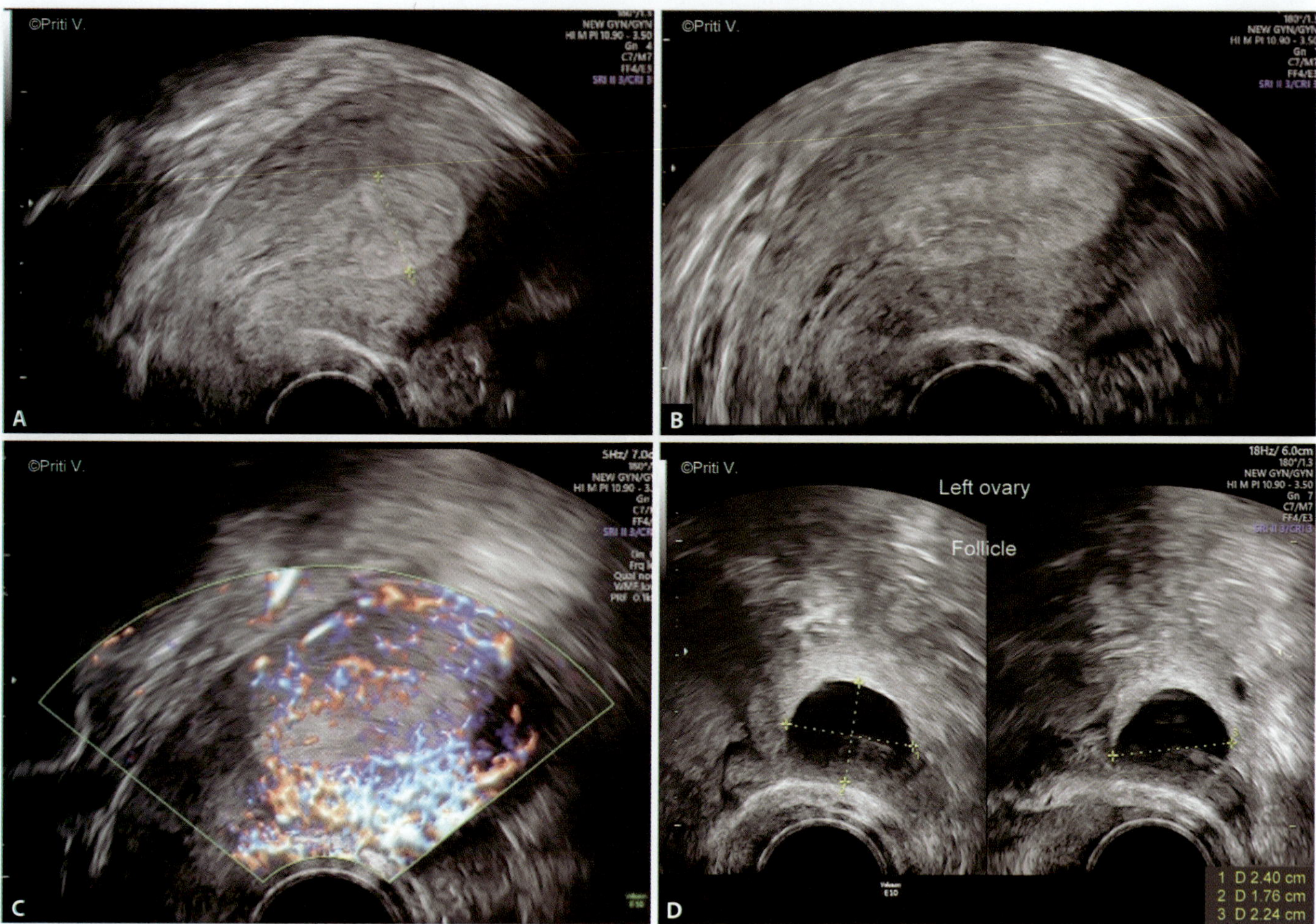

Figs. 56A to D: Simple hyperplasia without atypia: Thick uniformly echogenic endometrium of 17.8 mm (A) on day 19 of menstrual cycle with a persistent follicle in the left ovary. History of infertility present. Suggestive of an estrogenic endometrium due to anovulatory cycles. The central stripe is irregular; (B) because of the polypoidal nature of the endometrium. HDF shows multiple vessels crossing the EMJ ruling out a possible polyp within the cavity. (EMJ: endomyometrial junction; HDF: high definition flow)

Vascularity:

- Doppler imaging—it is advisable to use HD flow rather than the colour flow in gynaecology for better colour pick-up
- *In postmenopausal women:* Any abundance of flow or low impedance flow should raise a suspicion of underlying malignancy
- In hyperplasia, there is a diffuse increase in vascularity with colour score of 3 or 3–4:
  - Or there may be focal areas of increased vascularity
  - These vessels usually show low-impedance flow

Signs of malignancy in thick endometrium **(Figs. 61 to 63)**:

- Heterogenous echotexture
- Focal lesion
- Very thick endometrium with endometrial volume of 30 cc or more
- Increased vascularity with low impedance flow, disorganised vascular pattern and splashes of colour.

Endometrial Polyp (Figs. 64 and 65)

- Benign nodular proliferation of the endometrium at the surface
- It can be sessile or pedunculated
- Mostly asymptomatic even when relatively large
- Polyps <1 cm do not cause any symptoms
- May cause postmenopausal bleeding and intermenstrual bleeding in premenopausal women
- It is an important cause of infertility **(Flowchart 6)**
- Common locations—fundal and cornual regions
- Risk of malignancy in a polyp is the same as the risk of endometrial cancer in that woman based on her endometrial thickness.

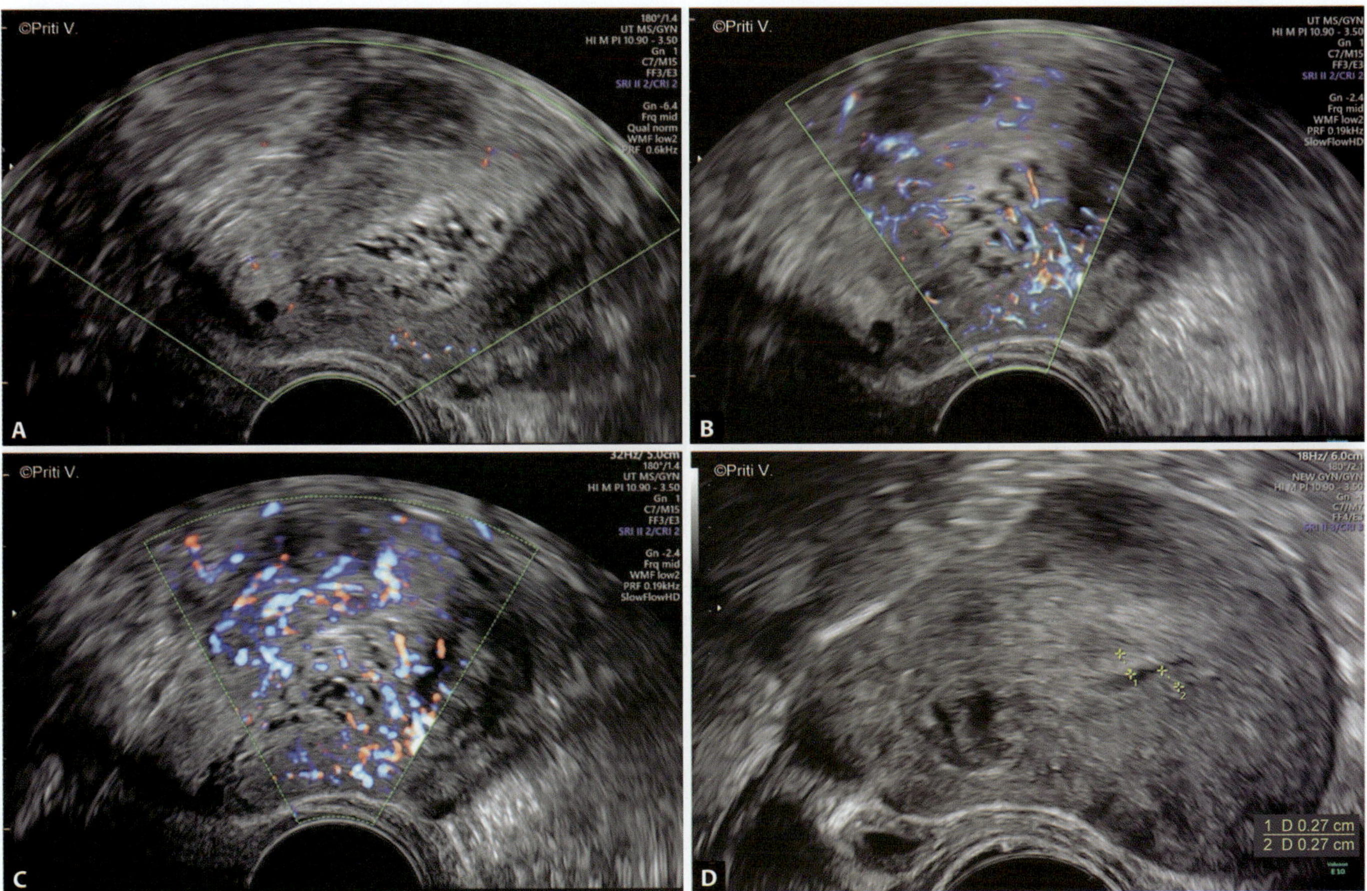

Figs. 57A to D: Thick endometrium of 12 mm with multiple cysts within in a 42-year-old P2L2 on Mifegest for 3 months for fibroid uterus, presented for a follow-up scan which showed a moderately thick endometrium of 12 mm with multiple cysts within. Multiple feeder vessels on HD flow ruled out a polyp filling the cavity. Mifegest was stopped. (D) On day 8, after the next period normal endometrium of 5.4 mm was seen (HD: high definition). This was drug induced hyperplasia which resolved with discontinuation of the drug.
Note: Because of minimal fluid collection in the cavity—maximum single layer endometrial thickness (SLT) was measured—anteriorly and posteriorly: 2.7 mm + 2.7 mm - ET = 5.4 mm.

Imaging:

- Focal well circumscribed echogenic lesion in endometrium interrupting the midline echo.
- Smaller ones are easier to recognise. Larger ones filling the cavity are more difficult to differentiate from diffuse endometrial lesions.
- Cystic spaces of varialble sizes within the polyp represent dilated glands and make identification of a polyp, especially in postmenopausal age easy.
- A 'white line' around the polyp demarcates it and marks the interphase between the polyp and the surrounding endometrial tissue.
- A small wedge of fluid collection between the tip of the polyp (mainly large ones) and the endometrial margins
- A single feeder vessel on Doppler image is diagnostic.

Sonohysterography:

- Echogenic, smooth and intracavitary masses outlined by fluid
- Complete visualisation of the stalk and origin of the polyp.

Endometritis (Figs. 66 and 67)

Inflammation or infection of the endometrium can be acute or chronic.

Associations:

- RPOC
- Premature rupture of membrane (PROM)
- Cervical stenosis
- Prolonged labour

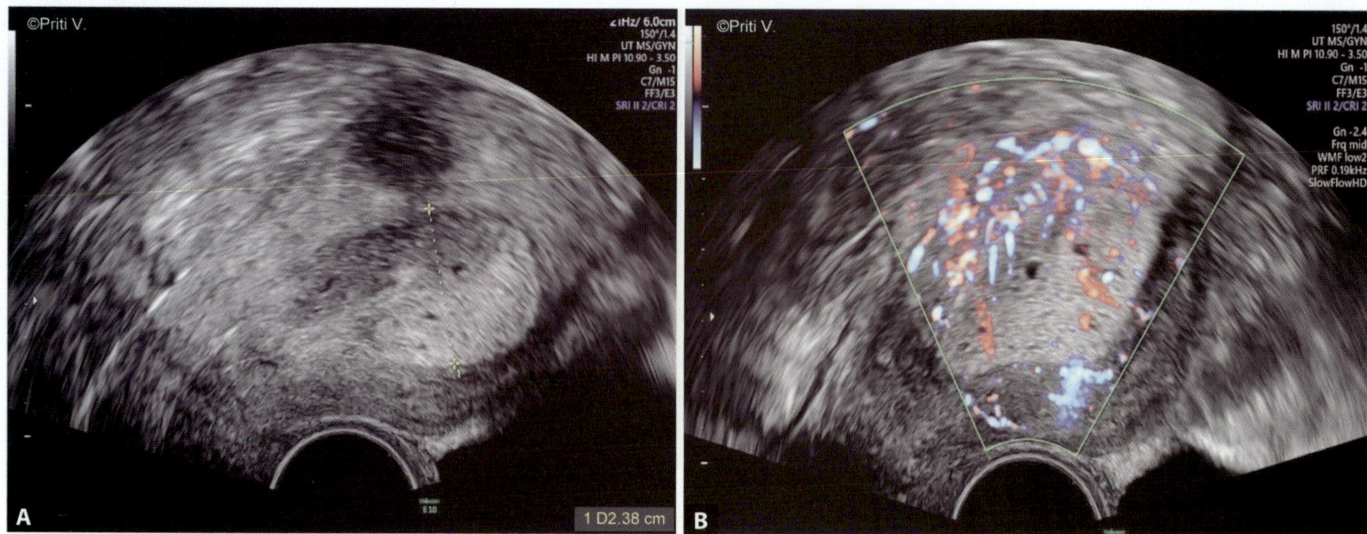

Figs. 58A and B: *Hyperplastic endometrium without atypia*: A 39-year-old P2L2 with AUB and a single posterior wall upper corpus intramural fibroid (FIGO-4) had a thick endometrium of 23.8 mm on D12 of MC and multiple feeder vessels entering the endometrium ruling out a polyp filling the cavity. HPE of this endometrium showed it to be a *hyperplastic endometrium without atypia*. (AUB: abnormal uterine bleeding; FIGO: International Federation of Gynaecology and Obstetrics)

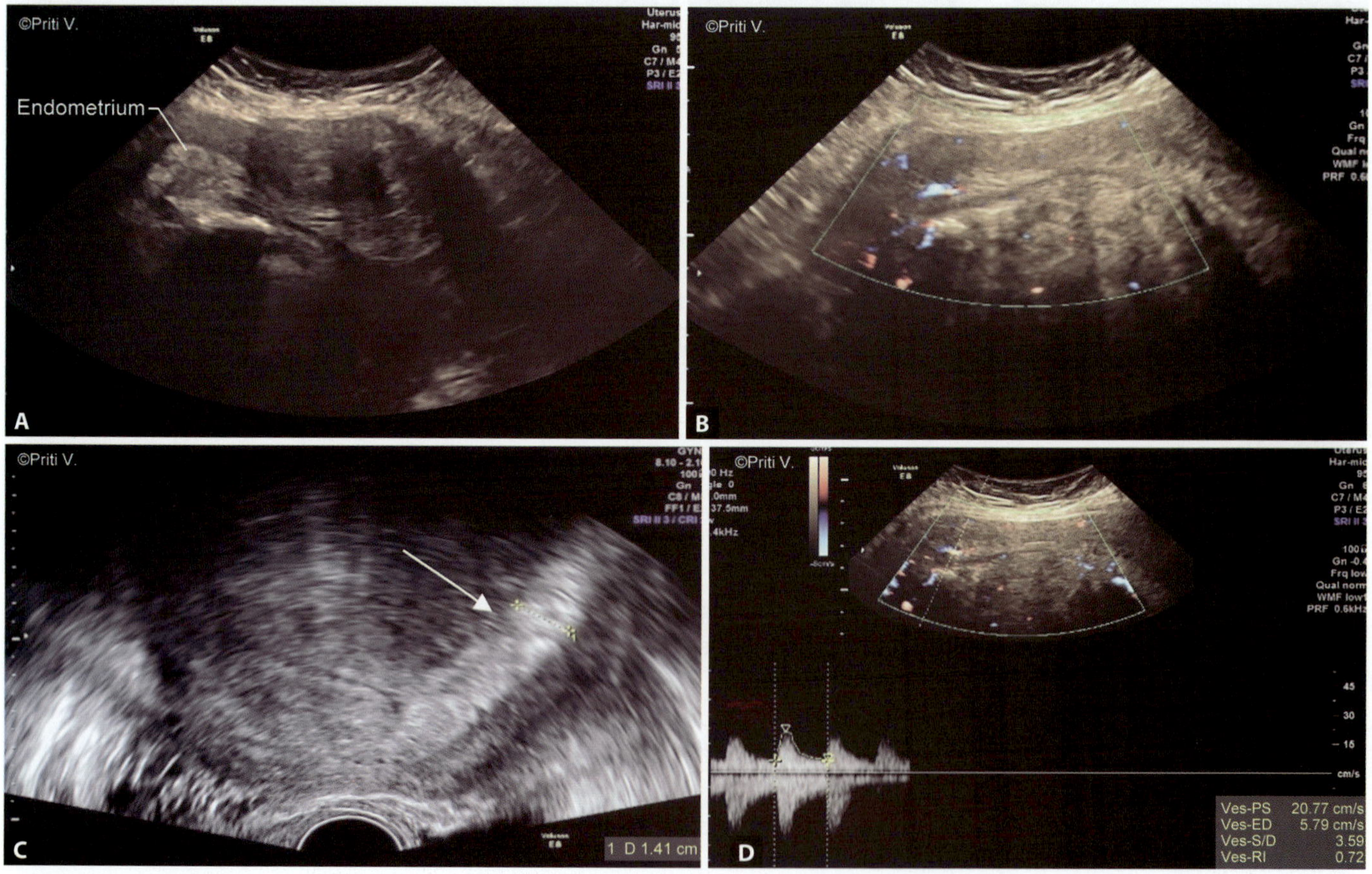

Figs. 59A to D: Thick endometrium in 60-year-old parous women with one episode of PMB of 4–5 days. She had an enlarged uterus with multiple fibroids, making endometrial assessment difficult. On TVS, ET was 14.1 mm. On TAS, moderate vascularity with PI = 1.04 and RI of 0.72. TAH+BSO done—HPE showed *endometrial hyperplasia without atypia*. (A) Thick endometrium TAS; (B and D) Minimal endometrial vascularity; (C) Thick endometrium TVS. (HPE: histopathological examination; PI: pulsatility index; PMB: postmenopausal bleeding; RI: resistive index; TAH+BSO: total abdominal hysterectomy with bilateral salpingo-oophorectomy; TAS: transabdominal sonography; TVS: transvaginal sonography)

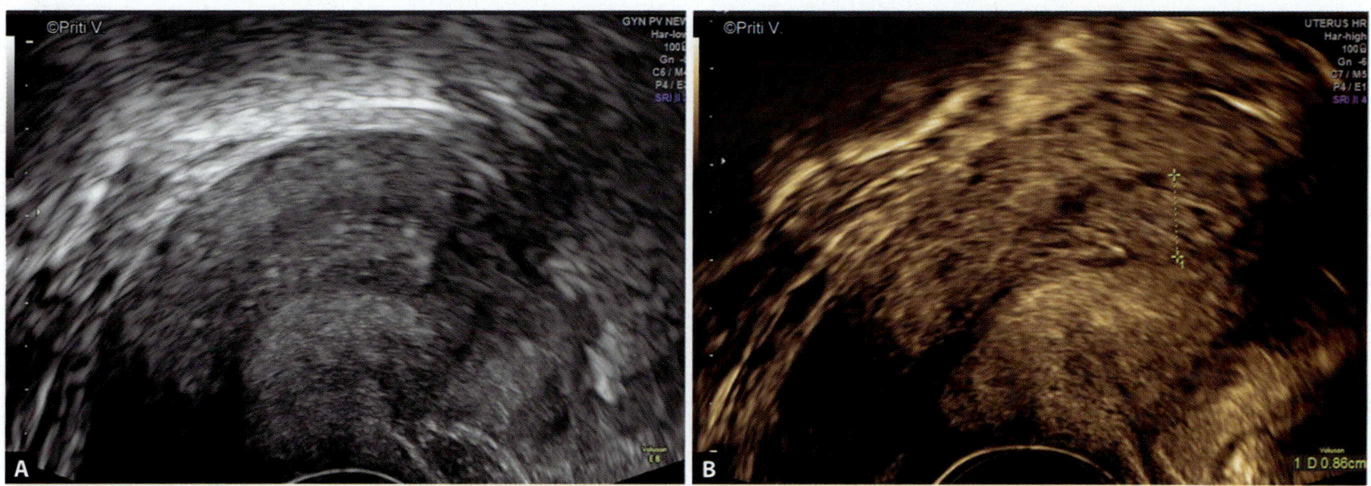

Figs. 60A and B: Thick endometrium on tamoxifen—2 years. A 46-year-old woman, P2L2, with a history of conservative surgery, chemotherapy and radiotherapy for breast cancer. Presented with spotting for 1 day. On USG, the endometrium was 8.6 mm, moderately echogenic with multiple small cystic areas within. (USG: ultrasonography)

Flowchart 5: Endometrial hyperplasia or thick endometrium.

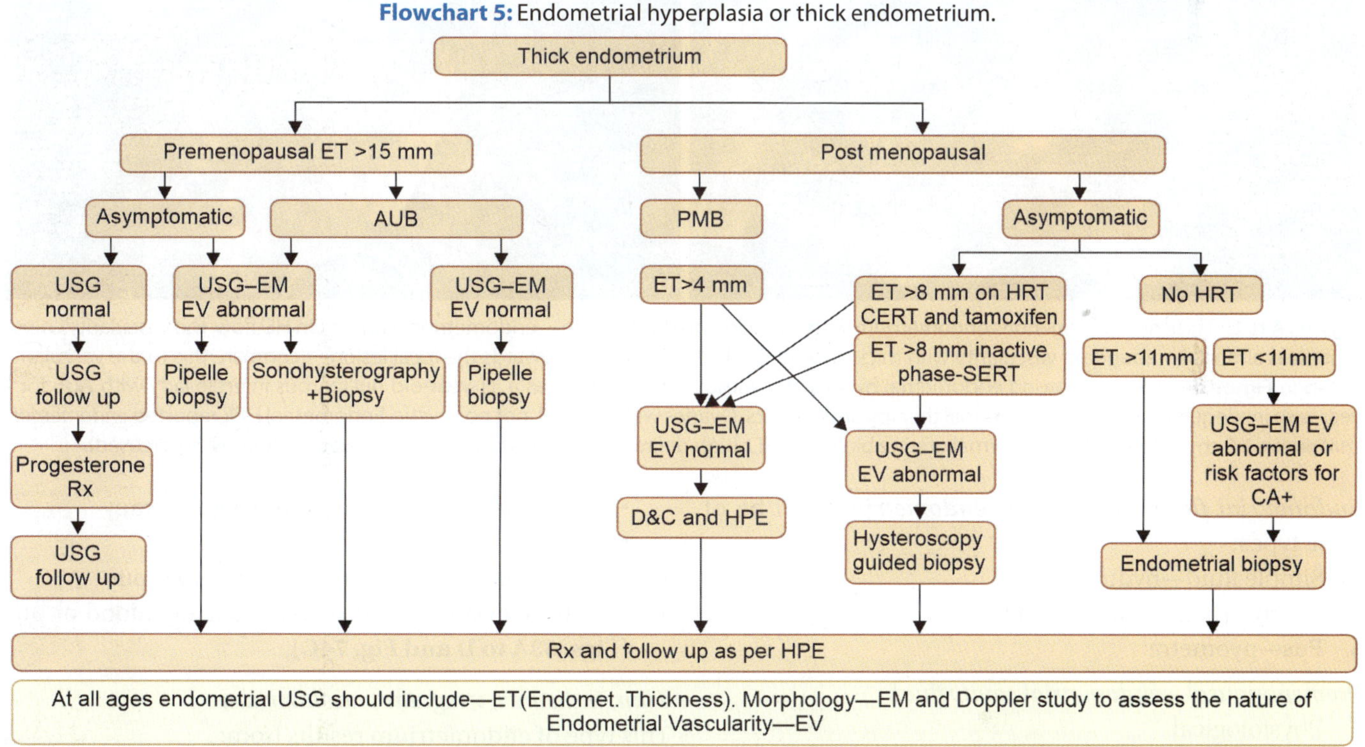

(CA: carcinoma; D&C: dilation and curettage; HPE: histopathological examination; HRT: hormone replacement therapy; OCP: oral contraceptive pill; PMB: postmenopausal bleeding; TVS: transvaginal sonography; USG: ultrasonography; r/o: rule out)

Imaging:

- Ultrasound findings are non-specific
- Thickened/irregularly thinned out or normal ET
- Heterogeneous echogenicity with echogenic foci or microcysts and calcification in tuberculous endometritis
- Fluid in endometrial cavity **(Figs. 22A and B)**

In acute endometritis in addition one can see:

- Air in endometrium
- RPOC
- Increased vascularity on Doppler imaging—up to zones 3 and 4

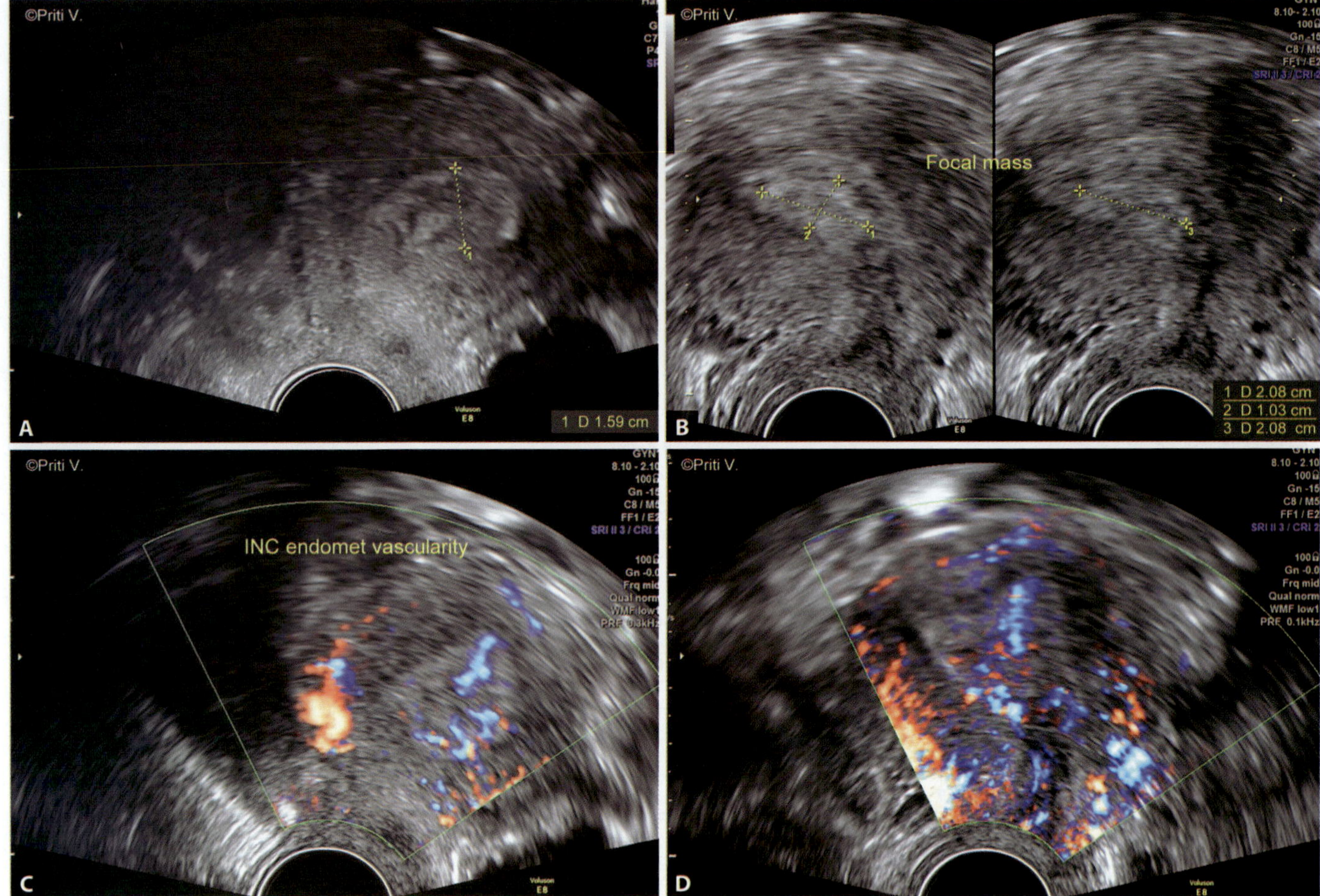

Figs. 61A to D: Thick nonhomogenous endometrium with suspicion of a focal lesion—endometrium cancer. On HD flow, the vascularity colour score was almost 4—abundant vascularity with thick disorganised vessels directed towards the focal lesion—(compare this to the vascularity noted in **Figures 55 to 57**), showing endometrial hyperplasia without atypia. This was a 31-year-old nulliparous infertile lady with AUB for 1 year with inadequate response to hormonal therapy and styptics. Ovaries were normal, not polycystic. Endometrial HPE reported *endometrioid carcinoma*, 1.5 cm pT1aN0. (AUB: abnormal uterine bleeding; HD: high definition; HPE: histopathological examination; INC: increased).

Endometrial fluid: Fluid in the endometrium can be of three types:

1. Simple fluid—hydrometra
2. Haemorrhage—haematometra
3. Pus—pyometra

Premenopausal—endometrial cavity fluid:

- Physiological
- Infective—endometritis
- Cervical stenosis and imperforate hymen

Postmenopausal—endometrial cavity fluid: Can be of any type depending on the cause. So, after assessing the nature of the fluid one needs to examine the endometrium carefully for thickness, echotexture and vascularity

- Fluid collection is usually clear in:
  - Incidental finding
  - Cervical stenosis
  - Hormone induced e.g., Tamoxifen therapy
  - Polyp
- Endometrial hyperplasia—clear, blood or pus
- Cancer of endometrium/cervix—usually blood or pus **(Figs. 63A to D and Fig. 74C)**.

Thin, indistinct, irregular endometrium

This type of endometrium results from:

- Hormonal deficiency—extremely low oestrogen levels occur in:
  - Postmenopausal uterus
  - Premature ovarian failure
  - Prepubertal uterus
- Destruction of the endometrial lining due to:
  - Infection, inflammation and healing:
    - Acute—postabortal, postpartum infection
    - Chronic infection as in tuberculosis

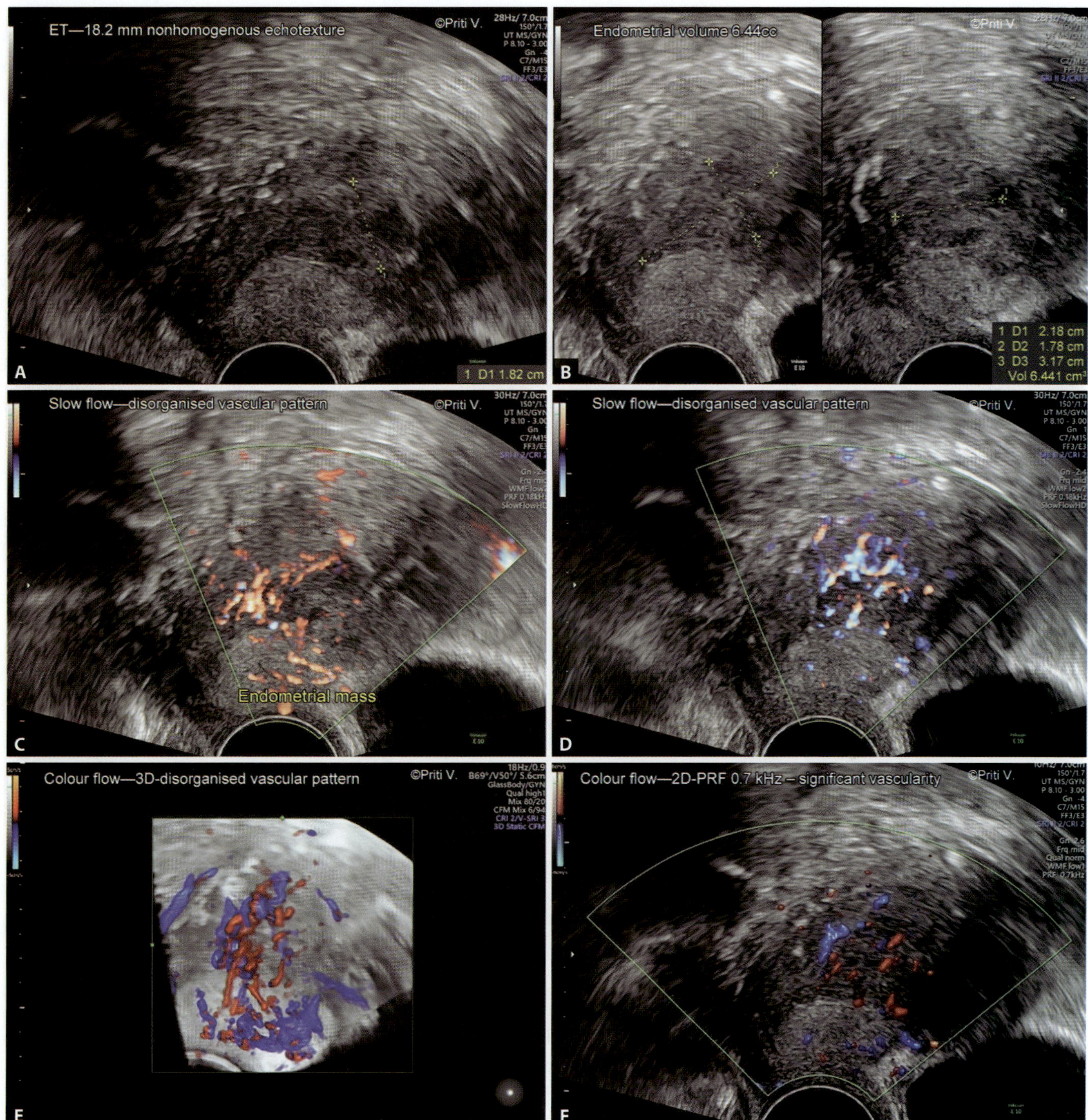

Figs. 62A to F: Endometrium cancer in 69-year-old woman, P2L2, with postmenopausal bleeding on and off for 5 months. Note the thick endometrium with a *nonhomogenous echotexture* (A and B)—almost isoechoic with the myometrium, with *abundant flow* with a colour score of 4, with *disorganized vascular pattern* (C to E); (E) 3D colour flow and image and (F) 2D colour flow at PFR of 0.7 kHz. There was significant flow in this postmenopausal endometrium. *TAH+BSO done. HPE—serous carcinoma, high grade, 3.0 cm, pT3N2a.* Also note that the endometrial vascularity is better evaluated on HD flow (C) than on colour flow (F). (ET: endometrial thickness; HPE: histopathological examination; PRF: pulse repetition frequency; TAH+BSO: total abdominal hysterectomy with bilateral salpingo-oophorectomy, HD: high definition).

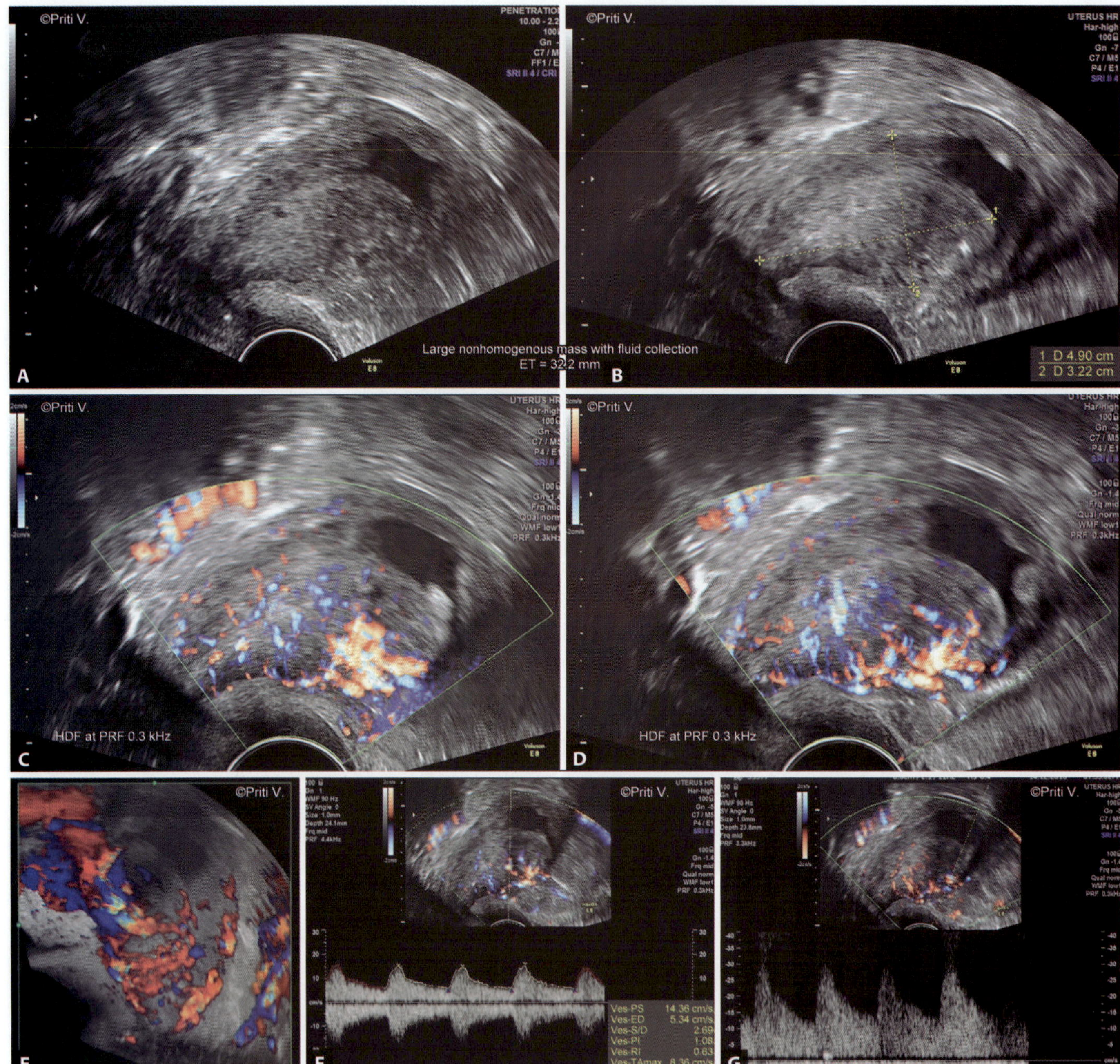

Figs. 63A to G: Endometrioid adenocarcinoma grade 2 >50% myometrial involvement-pT1bN0, seen in a 60-year-old, P4L4, 14 years postmenopausal lady with PMB 15 days. (A and B) Note the large endometrial mass with ET of 32.2 mm, fluid collection in the cavity and significant myometrial involvement along the anterior wall. Abundant and disorganized flow patterns are seen in the endometrium along the anterior wall on HDF 2D (C and D) and 3D colour flow (E). (F and G) PSV of up to 30 cm/s was noted in some areas, but PI and RI values are not different from other non-neoplastic gynaecologic lesions. (HDF: high definition flow; PMB: postmenopausal bleeding; PI: pulsatility index; PSV: peak systolic velocity; RI: resistive index)

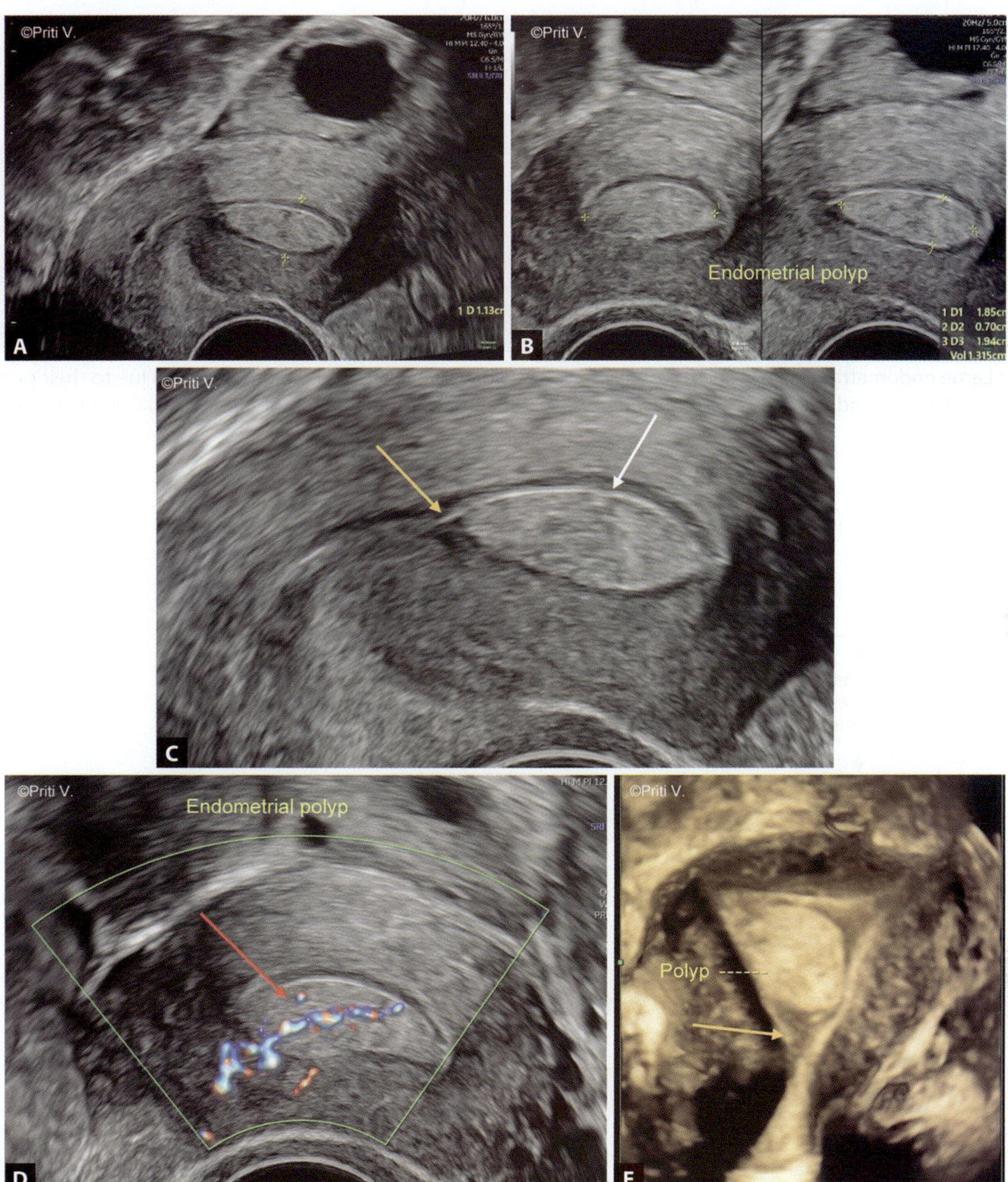

Figs. 64A to E: Endometrial polyp. (A) Shows how ET is measured in the case of endometrial polyp-at the widest point including the polyp; (B) The polyp is measured in three orthogonal planes; (C) The two important ultrasound findings in a polyp are the white line marking the interphase between the polyp and the endometrium—white arrow, and the 'V' sign or a wedge of fluid or seen between the polyp and the endometrial lining marked by a yellow arrow here and in image E. Image D and E give us the most conclusive findings - the single feeder vessel in D and the clearly defined echogenic polyp in the 3D image in E.

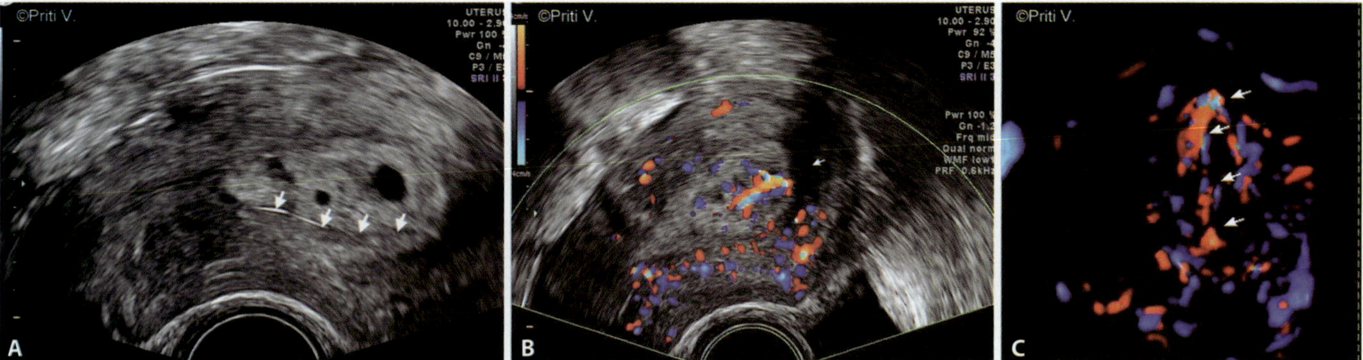

Figs. 65A to C: Large endometrial polyp—polyps usually have cysts of variable sizes which often give a clue to their presence. A white line along the periphery (A) and the presence of a feeder vessel (B) confirm the diagnosis of a polyp. (C) Colour Doppler 3D rendered image of the feeder vessel.

Flowchart 6: Postmenopausal bleeding.

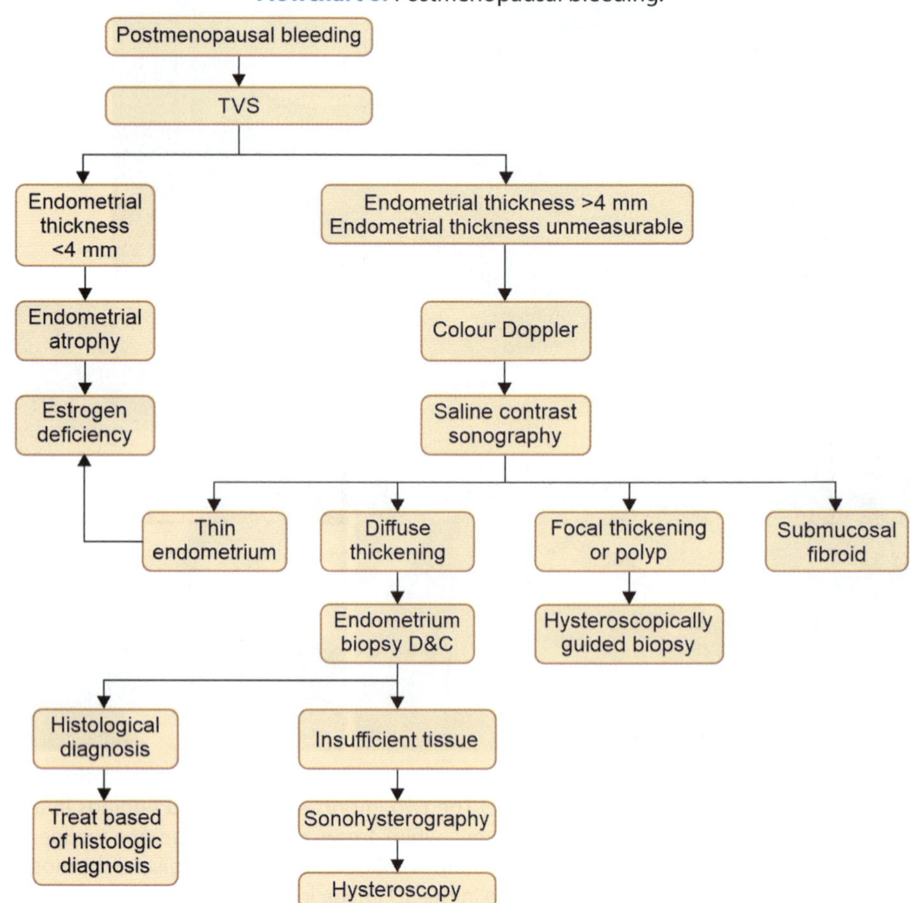

(D&C: dilation and curettage; TVS: transvaginal sonography)

- Excessive curettage especially in a gravid uterus
- Iatrogenic destruction of the endometrium with thermal balloons and cautery use within the endometrium.

Whenever there is destruction of the endometrium synechiae follow.

Uterine Synechiae (Figs. 68A and B)

- Are adhesions are developing within the endometrial cavity.
- 90% of synechiae occur after dilation and curettage (D&C) for pregnancy-related conditions.

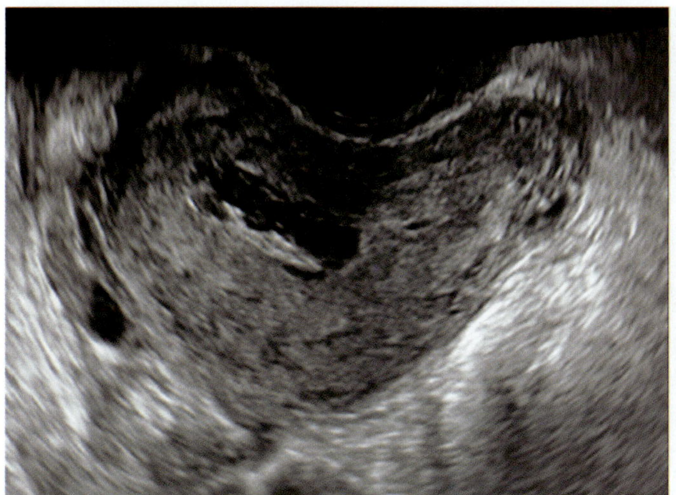

Fig. 66: Irregular fluid-filled endometrial cavity with diffusely thinned and irregular endometrium—case of infective endometritis with septations.

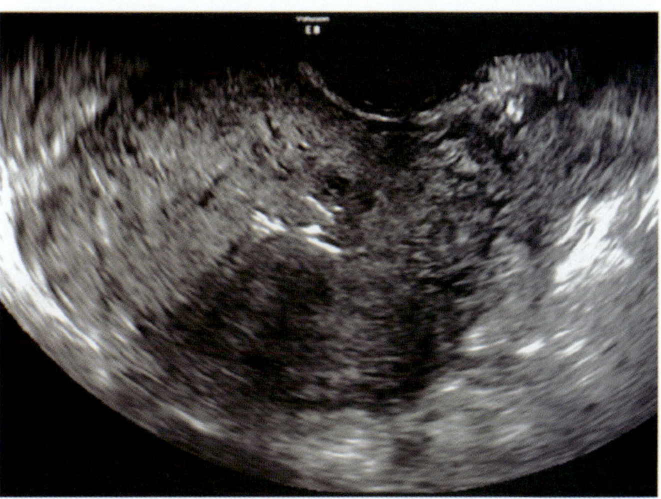

Fig. 67: Endometrium showing areas of calcification—the posterior shadowing—consistent with chronic endometritis—case of tuberculosis.

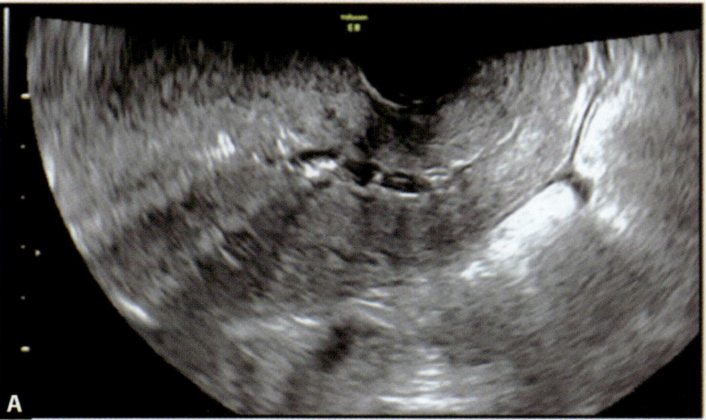

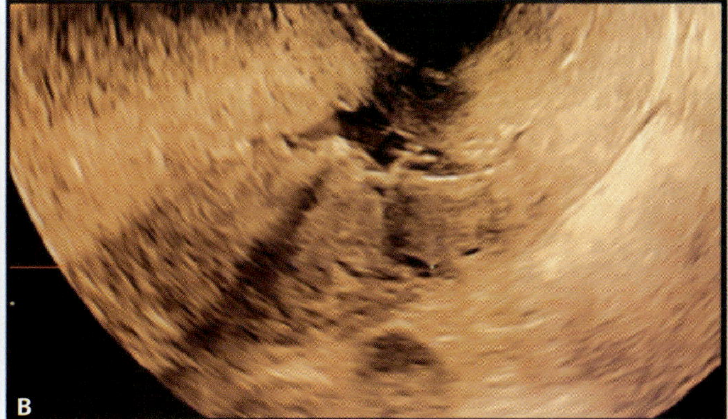

Figs. 68A and B: Irregular areas of fluid collection with septae and diffusely irregular endometrium s/o multiple synechiae—case of Asherman's syndrome.

- Prevalence is
  - 19% after D&C for miscarriage (Hooker et al., 2014),
  - 4% after endometrial tuberculosis and
  - 6–88% after hysteroscopic resections of myomas and septae.

Ultrasound appearance:

- Disruption of EMJ—irregular endometrial margins in the coronal plane
- Bands of myometrial tissue across endometrial cavity—interrupted endometrial stripe on sagittal view
- Irregular loss of endometrial echoes
- Pockets of fluid collection—hypoechoic areas with interruptions of endometrial layer (skip lesions—representing trapped menstrual blood)
- Hematometra—due to obliteration of the internal os (bands across these are rare because of atrophic endometrium unresponsive to oestrogen)
- Hyperechoic lesions with or without shadowing (fibrous and calcified synechiae)

CERVIX (FIGS. 69 TO 73)

Cervix is the narrow, lower part of the inverted pear-shaped uterus—which connects the uterus with the vagina and is freely movable like the uterus.

It is conical or cylindrical in shape and measures 3–5 cm in length.

Between the internal os and external os, the cervical canal is lined by the cervical mucosa-containing radially and obliquely arranged cervical mucous glands.

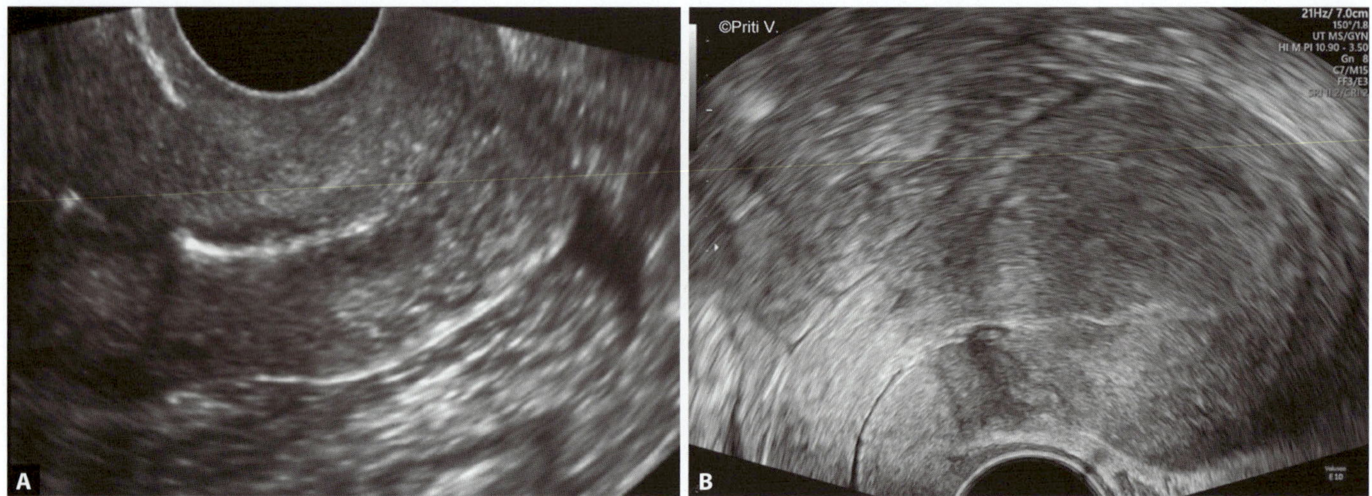

Figs. 69A and B: Normal cervix and & B—with central mucous layer seen in B.

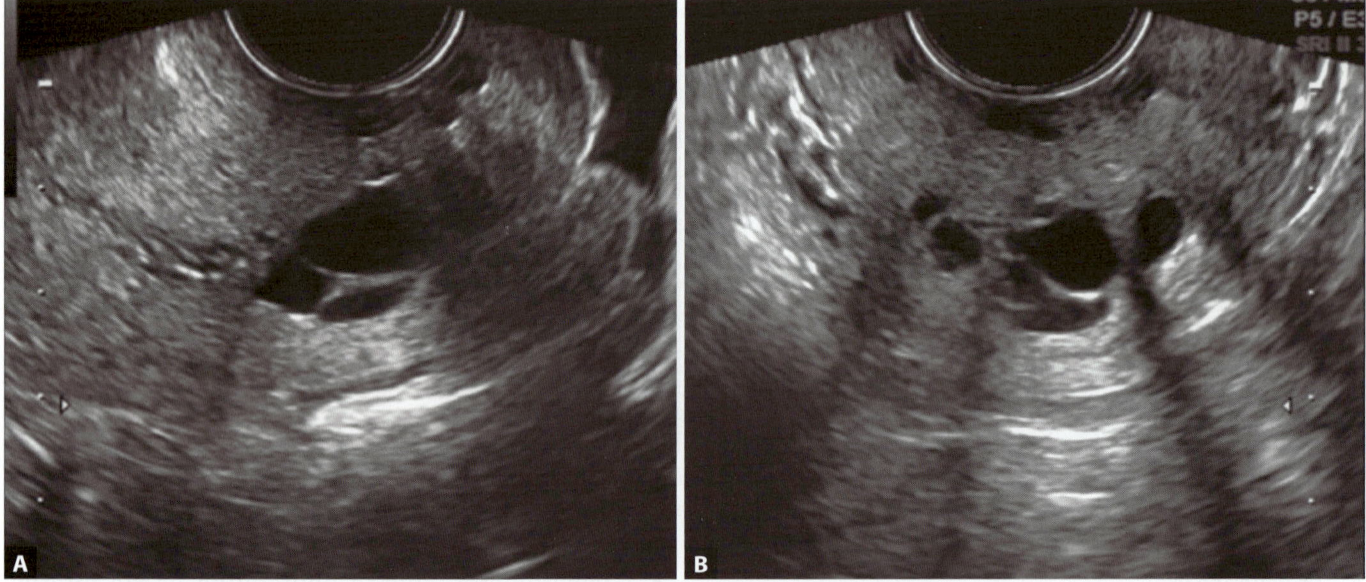

Figs. 70A and B: Enlarged cervix with multiple cystic spaces on both walls—case of cervicitis with multiple Nabothian cysts.

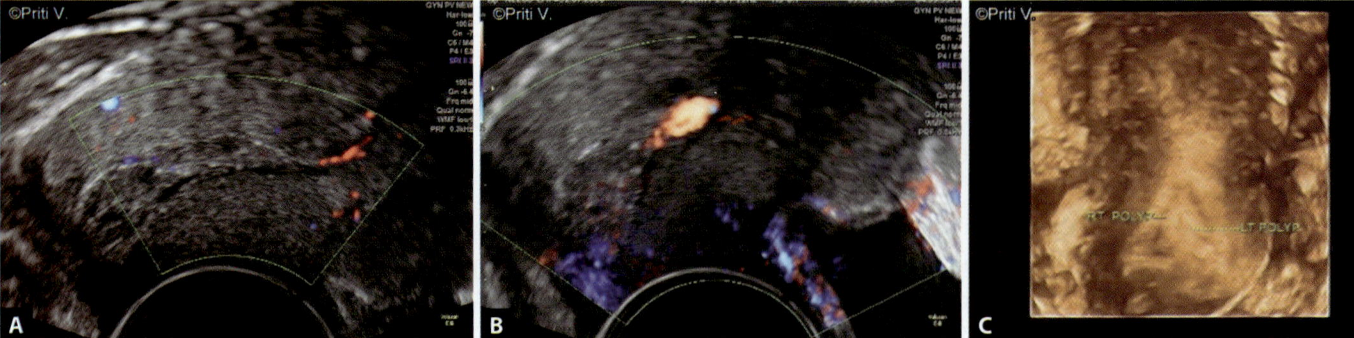

Figs. 71A to C: Cervical polyp clearly seen on 2D B-mode imaging and confirmed with a demonstration of a feeder vessel (A and B); (C) 3D rendered image of the cervical polyp.

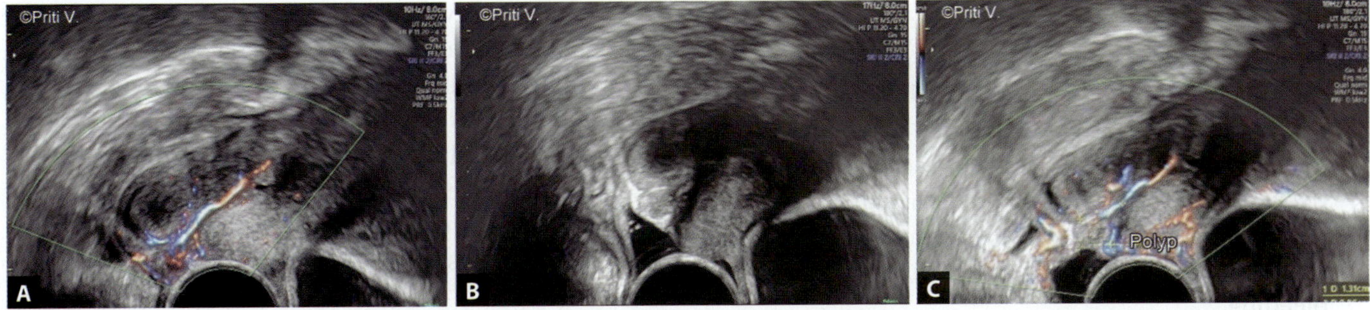

Figs. 72A to C: A very small cervical polyp is often suspected when a feeder vessel is seen, as in this case. The presence of polyp was confirmed by gel vaginal sonography and HD flow showing the pedicle. (HD: high definition)

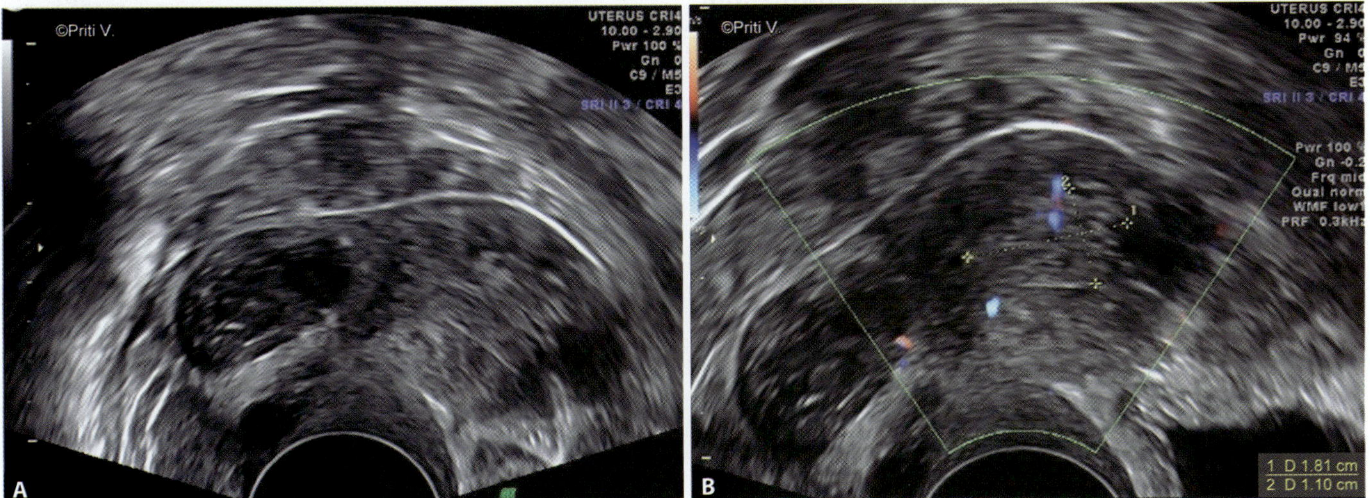

Figs. 73A and B: A posterior cervical fibroid is seen. This patient also had an endometrial polyp with a single feeder vessel.

It is attached to pubocervical ligament anteriorly, transverse cervical ligaments laterally, uterosacral ligaments posteriorly. These ligaments make the uterocervical junction relatively stable, so that the uterus and cervix can rotate about a horizontal axis traversing the uterocervical junction.

Anterior to the cervix is the base of the bladder—depending on the state of bladder filling (filled or empty) and the orientation of the uterus, the base and or the body are in contact with the cervix and uterus. An anteverted uterus rests on the body of the bladder.

Posteriorly is the rectum.

Imaging the cervix: On TVUS as the TV transducer approaches the uterus, the first structure seen is the cervix:

- The wall of the cervix has the same echotexture as the myometrium.
- The cervical canal is flanked by the cervical mucosa containing the glands.
- The cervical canal has a variable appearance depending on its contents:
  - A fully collapsed canal is seen as a white echogenic line **(Fig. 69A)**.
  - Thin clear secretions are seen as anechoic line **(Fig. 69B)** of variable thickness—maximum thickness is noted at midcycle due to high oestrogen levels.
  - After ovulation and during pregnancy, the cervical mucous is thick and echogenic.

Cervical Pathology

Congenital Abnormalities

- Failure of fusion during development—resulting in duplicated or septate cervix
- Congenital absence or hypoplasia may be associated with Müllerian abnormalities of the uterus.

Benign Lesion of Cervix

- *Polyps* **(Figs. 71 and 72)**: Endocervical polyps are the most common benign growths in the cervix, seen in 1.5–10% of women. They are hyperplastic endocervical folds with a core of vascular connective tissue stroma. Malignant transformation is rare. Endocervical polyps are usually asymptomatic with few perimenopausal women having vaginal discharge and bleeding.

  On ultrasound endocervical polyps appear like any uterine mucous polyps. They are pedunculated or sessile well-circumscribed polypoid growths with a feeder vessel arising from the wall of the cervix and extending into the pedicle and stromal core of the polyp which is a key to the diagnosis of these polyps. They are hyperechoic or isoechoic and may have small cystic areas within.

  Those arising close to external os may prolapse out and are best demonstrated using colour Doppler for feeder vessels and gel vaginal sonography help to outline the polyp.
- *Leiomyomas (fibroids)* **(Figs. 38 and 73)**: Uterine leiomyomas can involve the myometrium or the wall of the uterine cervix. Cervical leiomyomas account for 10% of all uterine leiomyomas.

  On ultrasound like uterine leiomyomas, they are usually hypoechoic or isoechoic, well-circumscribed lesions seen in intramural, subserous or submucous in location. They are hypovascular with pericapsular flow.

  Large cervical fibroid can push the uterine corpus cranially with significant stretching of the cervical canal **(Fig. 39)**. Demonstration of the cervical myoma and uterus in these cases requires very careful transabdominal as well as transvaginal evaluation.
- *Cervical endometriosis*: Cervix is a rare site for endometriosis. The lesion is seen as a well-circumscribed cyst with ground glass contents and small echogenic foci along the cyst wall.
- *Cervicitis* is a general term for inflammation of the cervical tissue. Inflammation may be acute or chronic, infectious or non-infectious. Acute inflammation is usually associated with infection and mucopurulent discharge.

  On ultrasound, acute cervicitis is seen as a heterogenous appearance of the cervix with the significant increase in vascularity.

  Chronic cervicitis presents as small groups of small bright dots in the endocervical canal. It may also show multiple Nabothian cysts with turbid contents.
- *Nabothian cysts* **(Figs. 70A and B)** are retention cysts.
- On ultrasound, they appear as well-defined cysts of variable size, number and appearance. They are usually anechoic or hypoechoic with low-grade internal echoes. Sometimes the fluid within is thick and echogenic. The larger ones may show a fluid level.
- *Tunnel clusters* are a type of Nabothian cyst with complex multicystic dilatation of the endocervical glands > common in multigravida >30 years of age.
- *Endocervical hyperplasia*
- This is a nonspecific diffuse hyperplasia of the endocervical epithelium. This may be associated with watery discharge. It is seen with women on oral progesterone-only contraception, in pregnant and postpartum women.

On ultrasound, the normal anatomy of the cervix is maintained with *diffuse thickening of the endocervical mucosa* with accentuation of the palm like branching mucosal folds.

Malignant Lesions (Figs. 74 to 76)

The cervix is highly prone to malignancy because of the presence of the transitional zone with high turnover of metaplastic cells, sexual exposure to trauma, infection and HPV virus and immune tolerance of this tissue. Malignant lesions seen in this area are:

- Squamous cell carcinoma
- Adenocarcinoma
- Adenoma malignum
- Other malignant tumours and endometrial cancer extending to the cervix **(Fig. 77)**
- *Squamous cell carcinoma:*
  - Accounts for *80–90%* cervical cancers
  - Ultrasound features include:
    - Distortion of normal cervical morphology with *heterogenous echotexture or a poorly defined hypoechoic lesion in the cervix*
    - *Increased vascularity* is seen on Doppler ultrasound (HD flow) in 95% of patients.
    - *Increased stiffness* noted on elastography
- *Adenocarcinoma:*
  - Account for 5–20% of primary cervical cancer
  - Ultrasound features include:
    - *Submucosal* in location

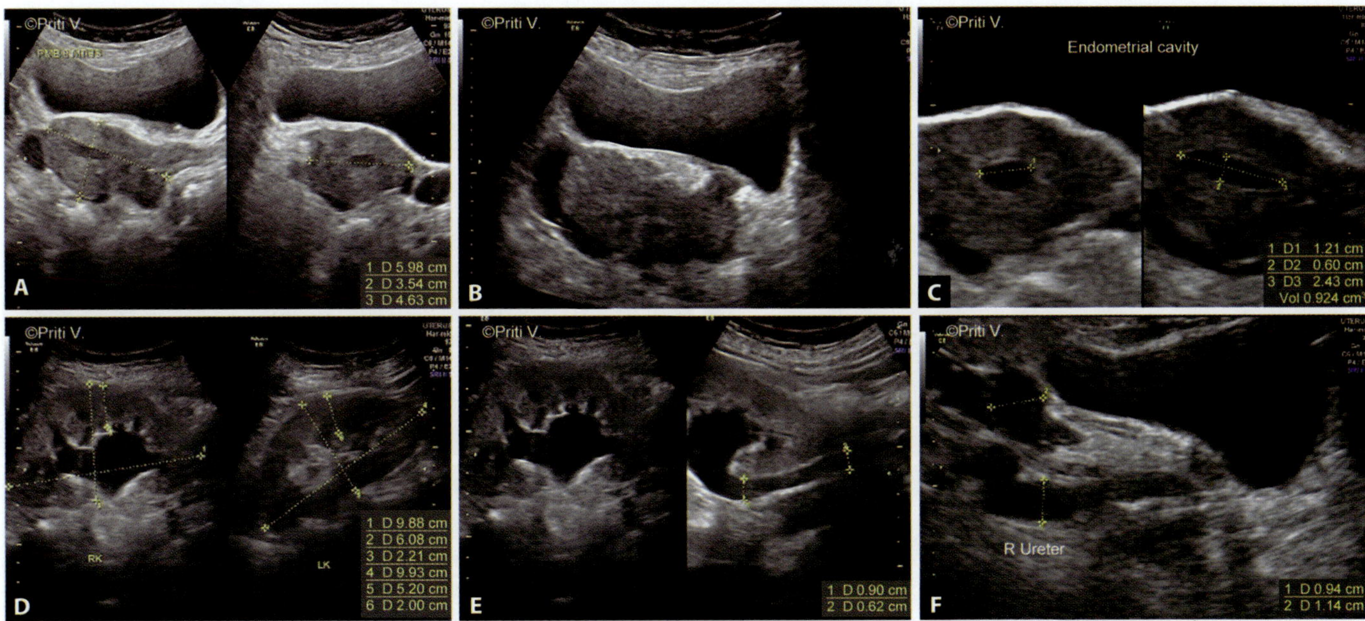

Figs. 74A to F: Case of cervical cancer with bladder, parametrial and right-sided ureteric obstruction. First 3 (A to C) are TAS images of the uterus in longitudinal and transverse sections. Fluid collection is seen in the endometrial cavity (A and C); (B) A cervical growth is seen extending to the bladder anteriorly; (D to F) Right-sided hydroureteronephrosis secondary to parametrial invasion of the cervical cancer. (F) Dilated lower one third of the ureter. (TAS: transabdominal sonography)

- Endocervical epithelium is, therefore, preserved.
- It usually appears as a *multilocular multicystic lesion in the wall of the cervix*, but can be *solid or mixed type*

- *Adenoma malignum:*
  - This is a special rare subtype of mucinous adenocarcinoma of the cervix
  - Presents with watery discharge per vagina
  - Ultrasound features include:
    - It usually appears as a *multilocular cystic lesion within the cervix*. Rarely, it may be solid in appearance.

Prognosis is controversial.

- *Other malignant tumours:* These are generally rare and are:
  - Extension from myometrial or endometrial tumours and rarely other pelvic tumours
  - Extension from extra pelvic tumours—extremely rare
  - Other malignancies such as melanoma, lymphoma, sarcoma and neuroendocrine tumours may develop—very rare.
  - Ultrasound features include:
    - Nonspecific appearance
    - Usually *heterogeneous* in nature with markedly increased vascularity on Doppler.
    - Few are *multilocular cystic lesion* as in adenocarcinoma, adenoma malignum and lymphomas. These resemble benign cystic lesion seen in cervicitis, hyperplasia, multiple Nabothian cyst and tunnel clusters.
- *Differentiation* from benign lesions on ultrasound is based on the *ill-defined, infiltrating* nature of malignant tumours and presence of *solid components.*
- Benign lesions are small, well-defined and cystic.

ADNEXA

Adnexa includes ovary + tubes + ligaments.

Ovarian Anatomy

- Intraperitoneal but only structure not covered by peritoneum
- Connected to uterus by the ovarian ligament
- Ureter, internal iliac artery and vein are posterior to the ovaries.

Both ovaries are placed *in ovarian fossa* **(Figs. 78A and B)**.

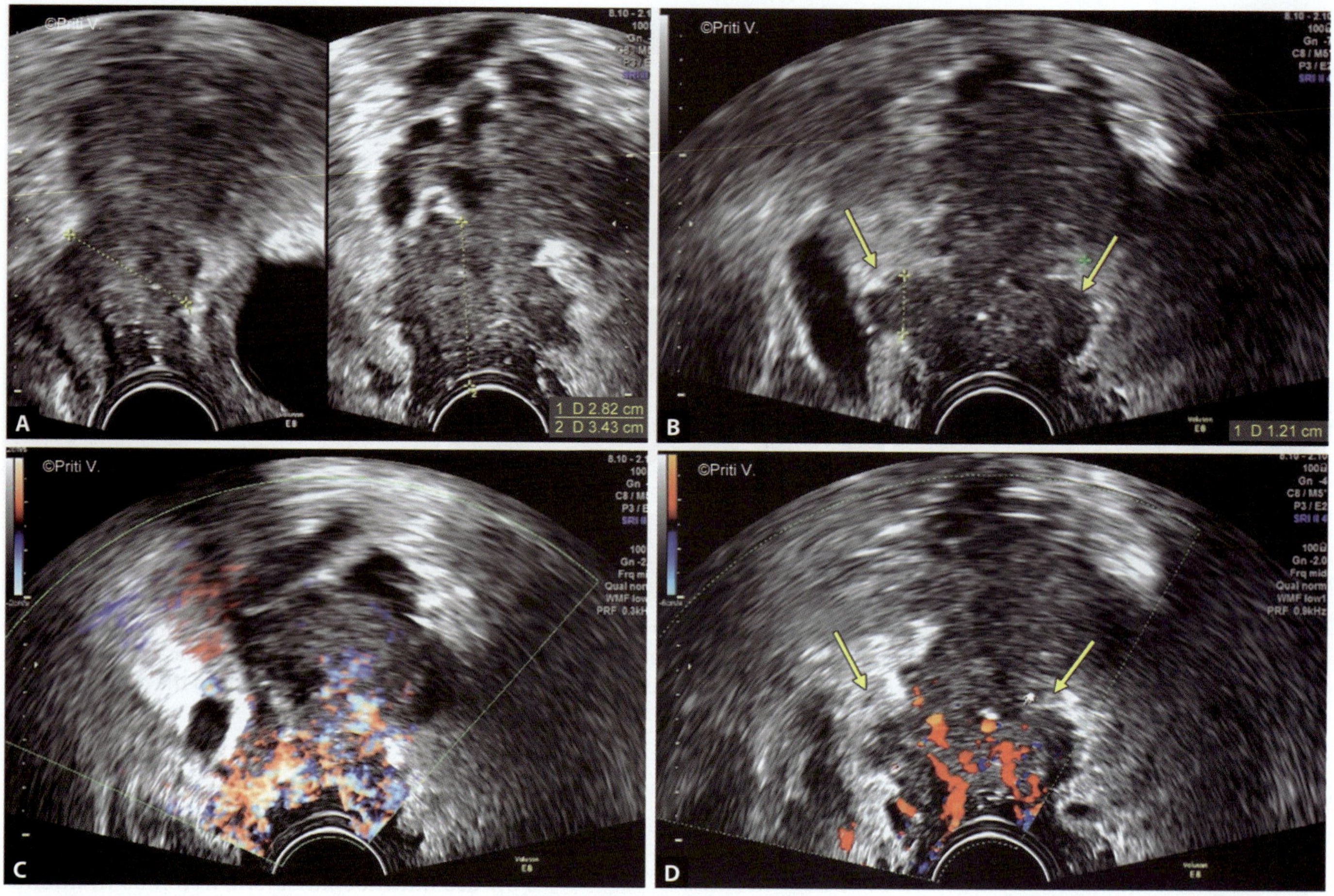

Figs. 75A to D: TVS images of the cervix and cervical lesion of the case of cervix cancer are shown in **Figure 74**. These are TVS images. The lesion is measured in Figure A. Yellow arrows show parametrial involvement in Figures B and D. The abundant colour flow and the dilated vessels are seen in HD flow and colour flow in Figures C and D. The patient was a 56-year-old P2L2 married at 16 years of age with PMB on and off for 6 months. More frequent and heavier for 3 months. Clinical diagnosis—a cervix stage 3B, and HPE—*squamous cell carcinoma, grade 3*. (HD: high definition; HPE: histopathological examination; TVS: transvaginal sonography)

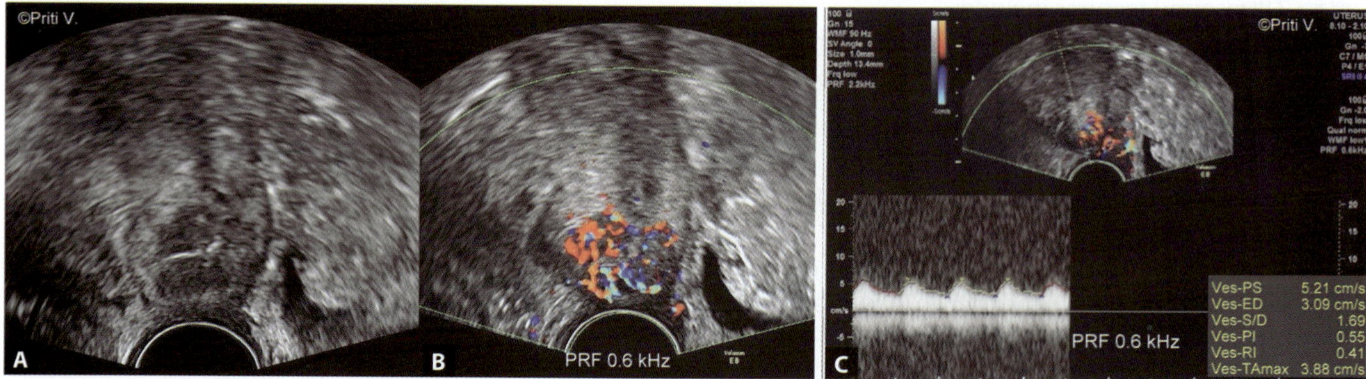

Figs. 76A to C: Case of cervix cancer in a 50-year-old perimenopausal lady—P5L5 with one episode of postcoital bleeding. On TVS, there was a focal hypoechoic lesion with abundant vascularity—colour score 4 at PRF of 0.6 kHz and very low resistance flow. HPE, *Squamous cell carcinoma*. (HPE: histopathological examination; TVS: transvaginal sonography)

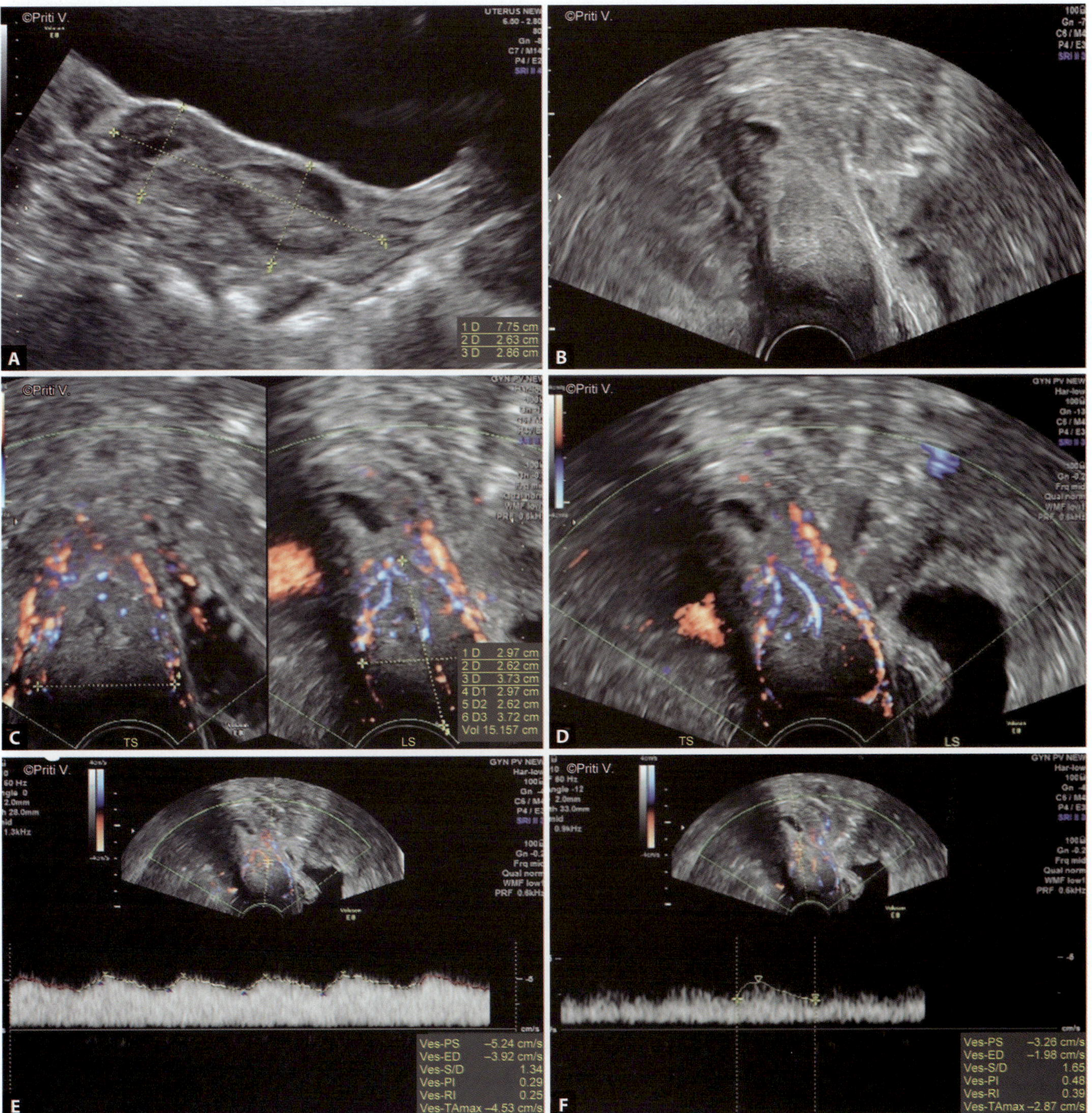

Figs. 77A to F: A large endocervical mass with hematometra was seen in a 70-year-old woman, P2L2. Vascularity was grade 3, but the flow within the mass was of very low resistance with RI 0.39–0.25. Clinical diagnosis was cervix cancer extending to uterus, but on HPE—endometrioid carcinoma, villoglandular variant, moderately differentiated, FIGO grade 2 with cervical stromal involvement and myometrial invasion of 57% found. (FIGO: International Federation of Gynaecology and Obstetrics; HPE: histopathological examination; RI: resistive index)

The *ovarian fossa* is bounded by:

- Anteriorly and superiorly by the external iliac vessels
- Medially by lateral border of uterus
- Posteriorly by the internal iliac vessels and the ureter
- Inferiorly the floor is formed by the obturator internus muscle and the broad ligament
- On ultrasound imaging, the ovary is seen inferomedial to the external iliac vessels.

Size and Structure (Figs. 79 to 81)

- Normal size—3 × 2 × 1 cm
- It has an outer cortex and an inner medulla
- Cortex contains:
  - Stroma and numerous primordial follicles
  - Few recruited follicles ranging in size from 2–10 mm in immature state, 18–25 in mature state
  - A corpus luteum is seen in the second half of the cycle. Irregular thick-walled cyst with crenated inner margins and low resistance peripheral vascularity is pathognomonic of a recent corpus luteum.
  - It also contains regressing and atretic follicles and corpora lutea.

Blood Supply

- *Arterial:* Ovarian arteries directly from the aorta via the suspensory or infundibulopelvic ligament
- *Venous:* Right ovarian vein into inferior vena cava (IVC)
  - *Left ovarian vein:* Into left renal vein

Ovarian Functions

- Secretion of hormones—oestrogen and progesterone
- Oogenesis

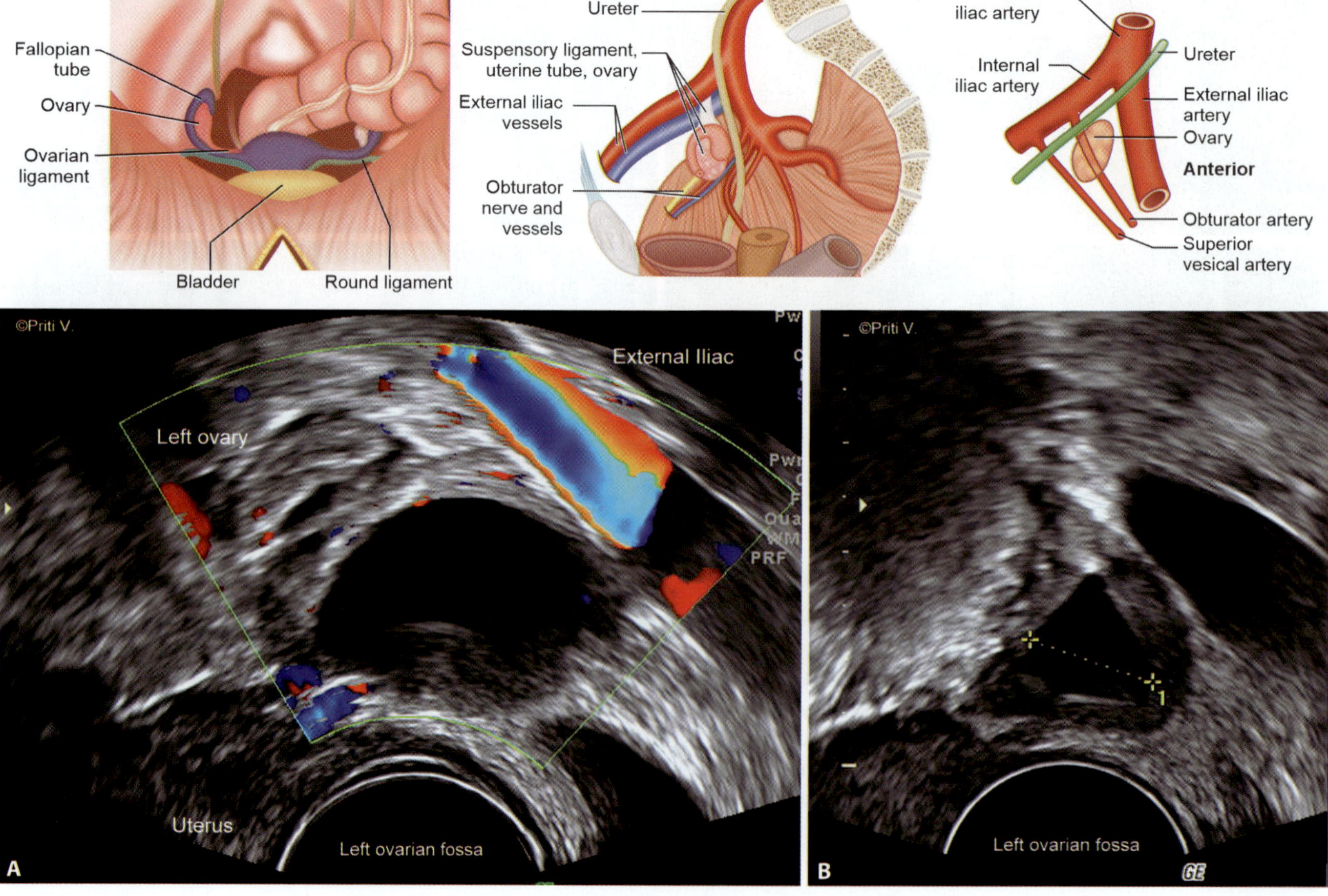

Figs. 78A and B: The ovarian fossa.

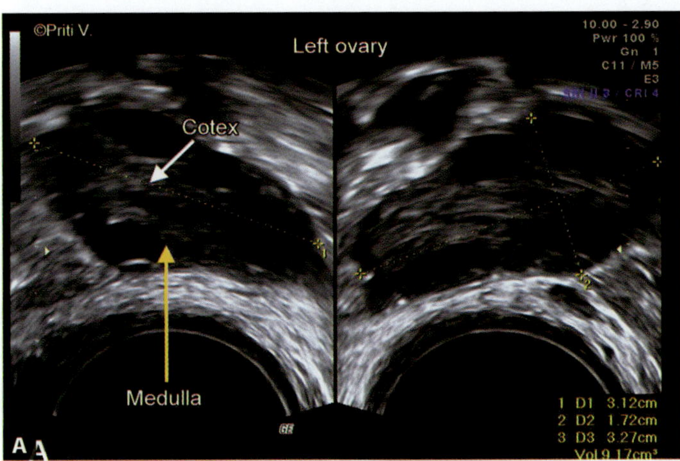

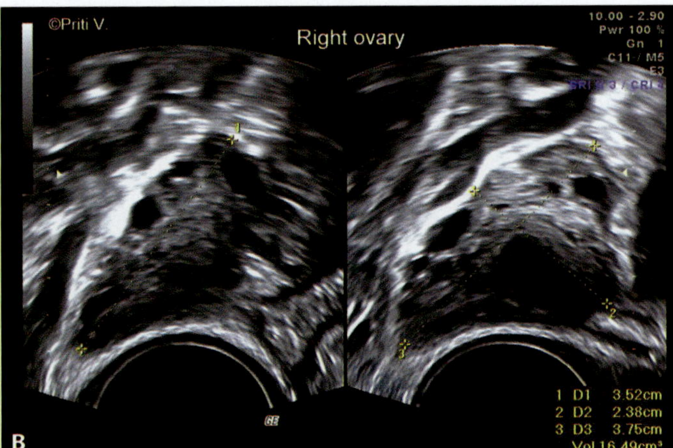

Figs. 79A and B: Normal ovarian structure as seen on ultrasound. Note the cortex and medulla. Follicles are seen in the cortex. The size of the ovary is approximately 3 × 2 × 1 cm. But the ovary that contains the dominant follicle or the corpus luteum will be larger, as seen in the right ovary here.

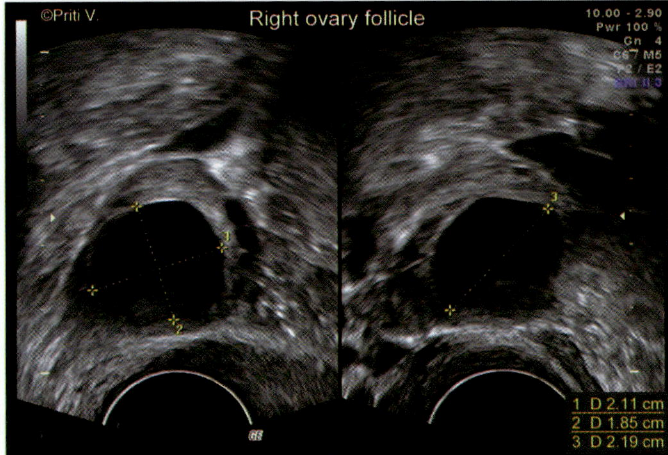

Fig. 80: Normal ovary with a dominant follicle of about 2.0 cm. Any follicle that crosses 1.0 cm in diameter is considered a dominant follicle. Normally, one dominant follicle develops in one of the ovaries during a menstrual cycle.

- Ovulation
- Provide support for the early-developing embryo

Imaging the Ovary and the Adnexa

- *Follicular cysts* **(Fig. 82 and Flowchart 7)**
  - Unilocular
  - Thin-walled with echoic contents
  - 3 cm or more in size (1.0–2.99 cm—dominant follicle) rarely exceeds 8–10 cm
  - Spontaneously resolves in 6 weeks
- *Corpus luteum cysts:*
  - Thick walled, hyperechoic
  - Peripheral circumferential blood flow
  - Spiderweb appearance
  - Blood clot within
  - Jelly-like wobbling movement of clot

Haemorrhagic Cyst (Figs. 83A and B)

- It results from haemorrhage into corpus luteal cyst **(Figs. 32A and B)** or other functional cysts
- Radiographic features are variable depending on the age of the haemorrhage
- *Most common appearance is lace-like reticular echoes or an intracystic solid clot:* A fluid—fluid level is possible.
- Thin walled, retracting clot may have sharp or concave borders, mural nodularity and does not have posterior acoustic enhancement
- *Doppler:* No colour flow within the nodule:
  - Circumferential blood flow in the cyst wall is typical and important differentiating feature between physiological cysts and other cysts, especially benign neoplastic cysts

Ultrasound Evaluation of Adnexal Masses

To evaluate and report ultrasound findings of the adnexa, it is necessary to use standard terminologies. Fortunately, this standardisation has been done by the IOTA group. Below are the terms and definitions that should be used when describing any adnexal mass.

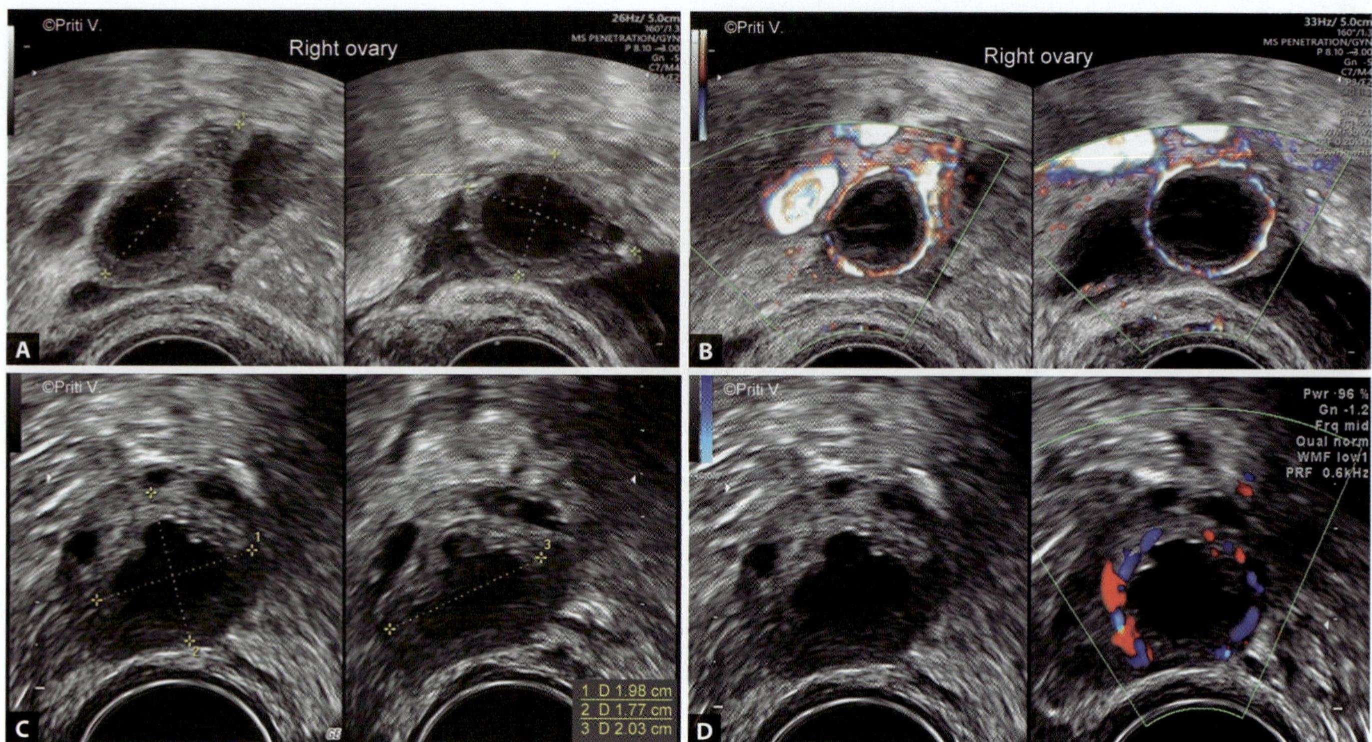

Figs. 81A to D: Vascular corpus luteum (VCL) is shown in these images. The left-sided images show grey-scale images of corpus luteum (CL)—it is thick-walled, usually irregular in shape with irregular inner margins (C and D), but can also have smooth regular walls (A). Most importantly, all recent corpora lutea are vascular with a complete ring of colour (B and D). The flow is of low-resistance type with a resistive index (RI) of 0.4–0.5 kHz.

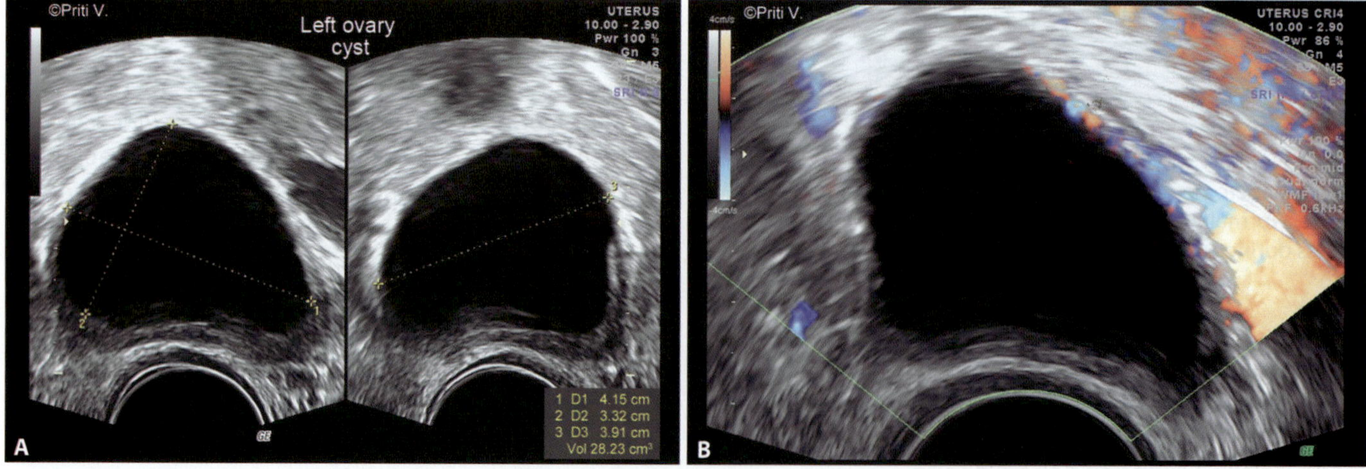

Figs. 82A and B: An anechoic unilocular cyst 4 cm in diameter—a follicular cyst which is a major differential diagnosis for a simple serous cyst or a benign serous cystadenoma. The HD flow showing good peripheral vascularity (Figure B) confirms the physiologic nature of the cyst—a follicular cyst. A follicle that grows beyond 3.0 cm is called a follicular cyst. It eventually regresses and needs no treatment. It usually takes 4–6 weeks or 1 or 2 menstrual cycle lengths to regress. (HD: high definition)

Flowchart 7: Simple ovarian cyst/unilocular ovarian cyst (D/D—follicular cyst, neoplastic and serous cystadenoma).

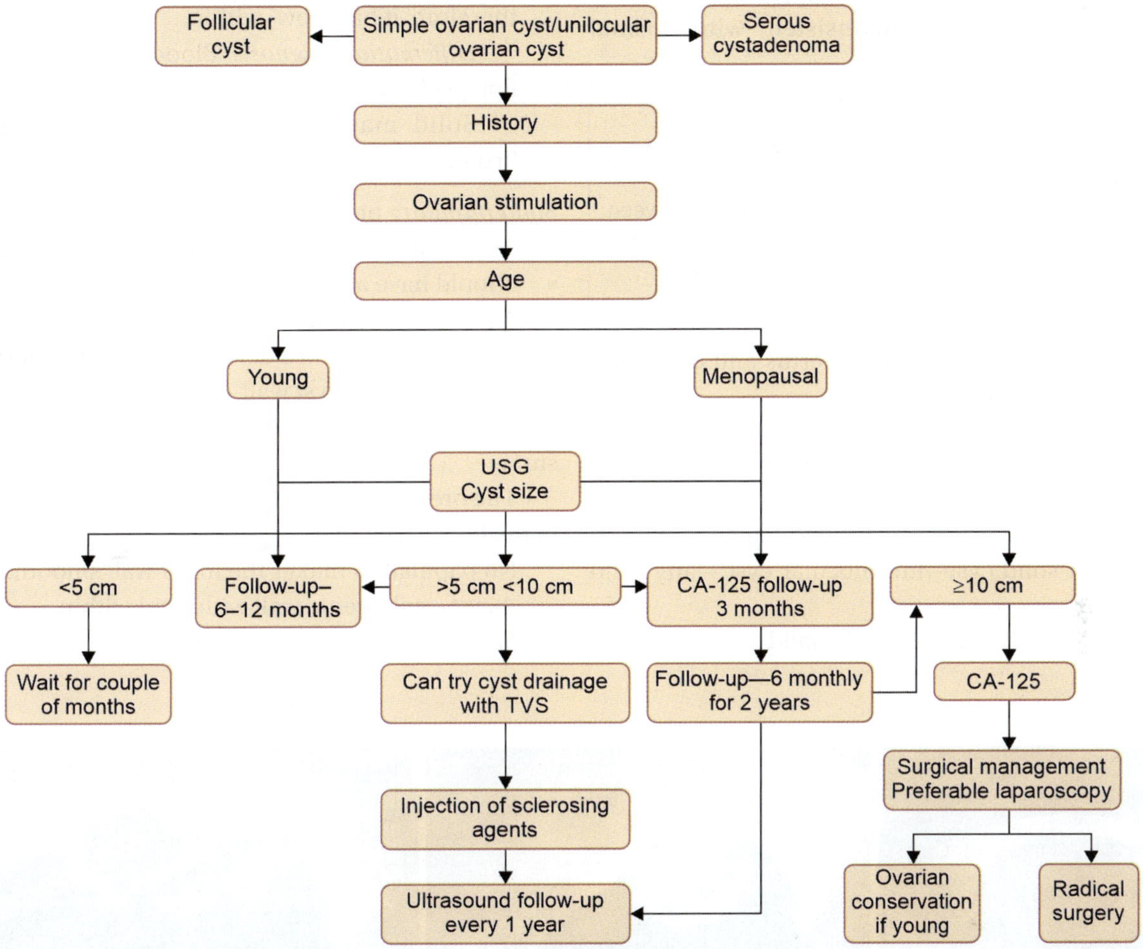

- Simple ovarian cyst/unilocular ovarian cyst
  - → Follicular cyst
  - → Serous cystadenoma
  - → History → Ovarian stimulation → Age
    - Young
    - Menopausal
    - USG Cyst size
      - <5 cm → Wait for couple of months
      - Young → Follow-up–6–12 months
      - >5 cm <10 cm
        - → Follow-up–6–12 months
        - → CA-125 follow-up 3 months → Follow-up—6 monthly for 2 years → ≥10 cm; → Ultrasound follow-up every 1 year
        - → Can try cyst drainage with TVS → Injection of sclerosing agents → Ultrasound follow-up every 1 year
      - Menopausal → CA-125 follow-up 3 months
      - ≥10 cm → CA-125 → Surgical management Preferable laparoscopy
        - → Ovarian conservation if young
        - → Radical surgery

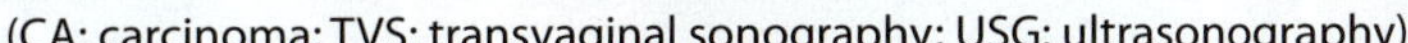
(CA: carcinoma; TVS: transvaginal sonography; USG: ultrasonography)

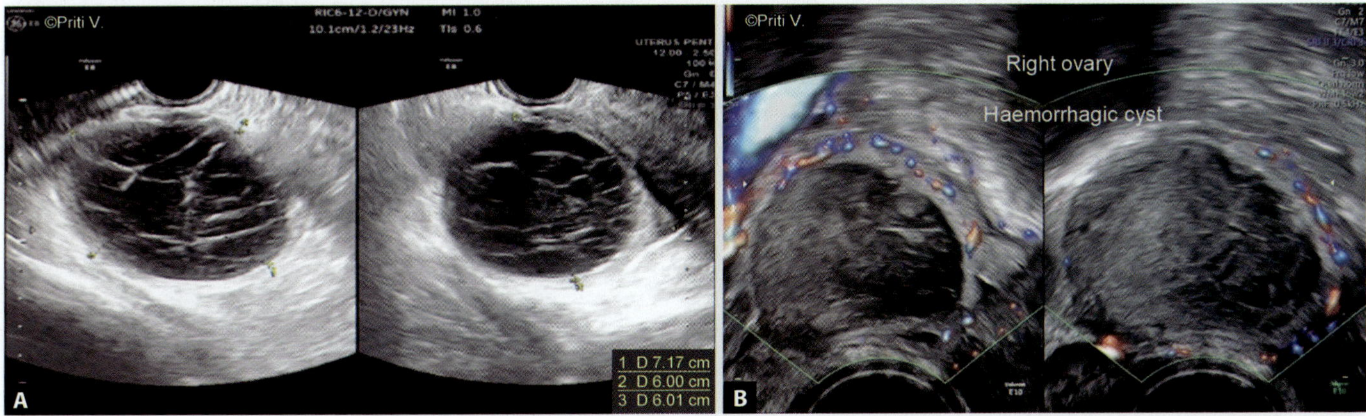

Figs. 83A and B: Haemorrhagic cysts. Physiologic cysts often become haemorrhagic. They eventually regress but because of a very variable appearance, they are confused with pathological cysts. The cyst in Figure A has a typical reticular or lace-like pattern. But the cyst in Figure B looks more solid and is often mistaken for a solid ovarian mass. However, looking at the vascularity helps—the clot inside a haemorrhagic cyst does not pick up colour (lower the PRF to almost 0.1 kHz). But it will show peripheral flow like the physiologic cyst. The degree of flow depends on how old or active the cyst is.

IOTA Terms and Definition

Lesion: Is anything that is inconsistent with normal physiology:

Image of normal ovary:	*Ovary with a 'lesion':*
• Follicle–anechoic unilocular cyst of 20–28 mm • > 3.0 mm—follicular cyst Haemorrhagic cysts and CL • These are physiologic structures *not lesions*	• A neoplastic cyst—is a lesion • Differentiation between a physiologic cyst and a *lesion* is important

Description of a lesion as per IOTA terms and definition **(Figs. 84A to E)**:

- Unilocular cyst—no septae, no solid areas
- Unilocular solid cyst—unilocular cyst + any solid component
- Multilocular cyst—cyst with multiple septae
- Multilocular solid cyst—multilocular cyst + any solid component
- Solid mass—>85% of the lesion in solid

Solid—means echogenic area representing 'tissue'; therefore, it has 'flow' within.

Differential diagnosis: Blood clot—not tissue, so no flow within.

Solid mass can have 'smooth' outer wall or 'irregular' outer wall.

Solid papillary projection or nodule:

- Any solid component protruding into the cystic area
- Should have a height of 3 mm or more

A papillary nodule is a tissue.

'Echogenic' area in a dermoid—not a papillary nodule.

'Sludge' on the cyst wall—not solid component

Papillary projection can be smooth or irregular on the surface.

The presence of papillary nodules makes the inner wall of the lesion irregular.

No papillation makes the inner wall smooth.

A cyst—echogenic wall with fluid within.

Septum or septae may be seen.

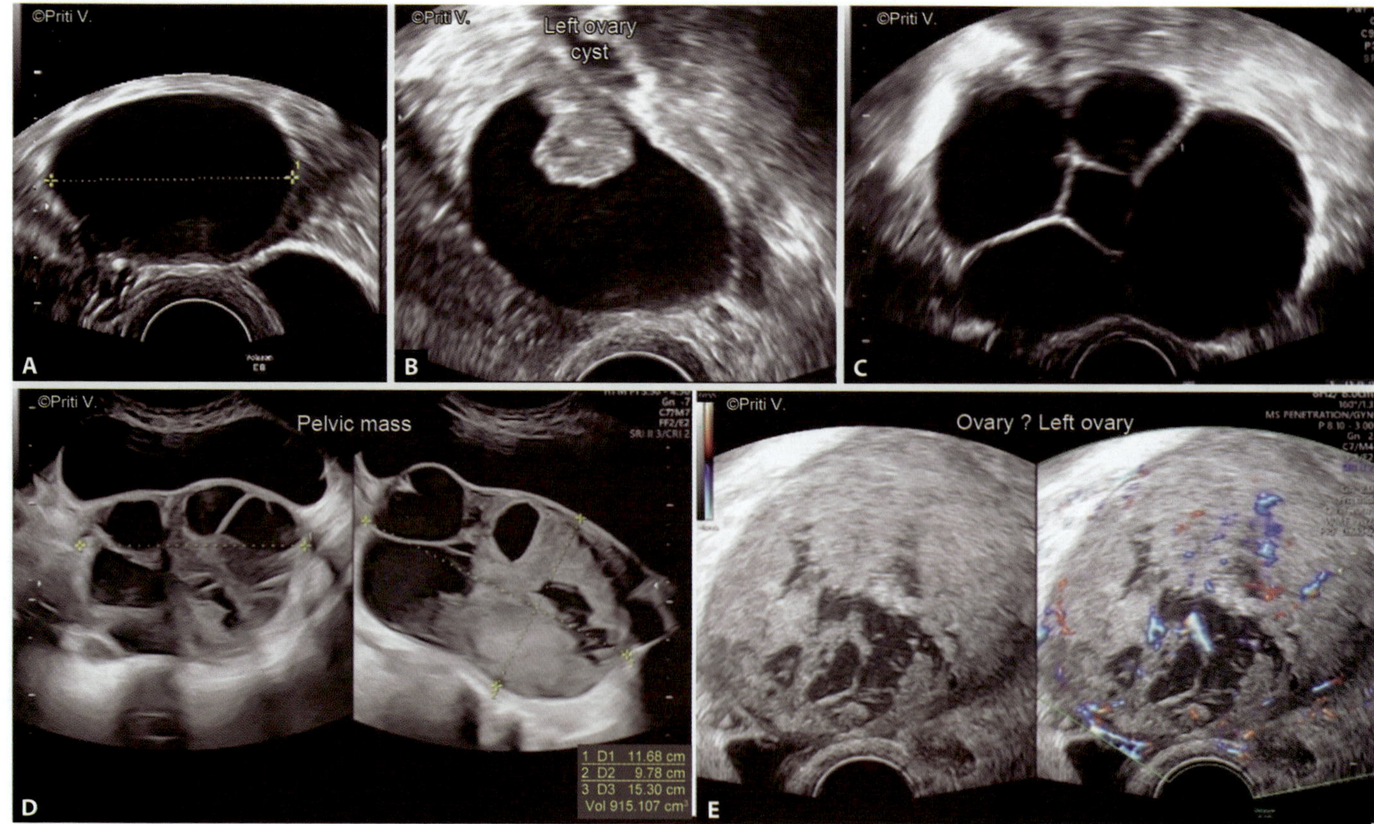

Figs. 84A to E: Description of a lesion as per IOTA terms and definition. (A) Unilocular cyst; (B) Unilocular solid cyst; (C) Multilocular cyst; (D) Multilocular solid cyst <80% of lesion is solid; (E) Solid mass >80% of the lesion is solid. (IOTA: International Ovarian Tumour Analysis)

A 'septum' is a strand of tissue extending from one internal surface to the contralateral (opposite) side.

A septum completely divides the cyst into two parts:

1. Multiple septae divide a cyst into multiple parts:
   - These parts or locules do not communicate with each other.
2. An '*incomplete septum*' is one that extends from one wall to another in one section but does not completely divide the cyst.

In some sections where it does not reach the opposite wall, it appears to end abruptly in the middle of the cyst.

Because the cyst is not divided completely a cyst with 'incomplete septum' is 'unilocular'.

Incomplete septae are typically seen in a hydrosalpinx; so, a hydrosalpinx is a unilocular elongated cyst with incomplete septae.

'*Fluid*' in the cyst should be described as follows:

- Anechoic if completely black
- Low-level internal echoes (homogeneous)
- Ground grass appearance if the content is uniformly echogenic

A haemorrhagic cyst has thin thread-like strands extending across the cyst forming:

- A star-shaped structure within the 'clot' showing concave margins
- A cobweb-like reticular pattern
- A jelly-like clot with convex or rounded margins floating in fluid with low-level echoes
- These are 'patterns' to be recognised

When describing a cyst that is not unilocular:

- Number of locules
- Number of papillary projections
- Height and length of the largest papilla should be measured.
- Largest solid component is measured in three dimensions.
- Sometimes the largest papillary projection is the largest solid component.

Common Ovarian Lesions Recognised by 'Pattern Recognition'

Endometrioma **(Figs. 85B and 86)**

- Pathological but non-neoplastic cysts
- Most commonly unilocular
- Sometimes multilocular
- *Diffuse low-level internal echoes*: Ground glass appearance seen in 82–95% of these cysts.
- Thick walls and nodularity along the cyst wall—these are brightly echogenic nodules indicating cholesterol deposits—height <3 mm—hence, it is wall nodularity *not* papillation.
- Low-level blood flow in the wall with a colour score of 2 or 2–3 only. Important differentiating point between endometriomas and physiologic haemorrhagic cysts (which are more vascular) that can sometimes present with uniform low-grade internal echoes and resemble endometriotic cysts.
- Atypical endometrioma scans have papillary projections; malignancy should be ruled out.

Malignant transformation occurs in 1–2% of endometriomas especially in larger endometriomas that are long-standing with prolonged unopposed oestrogen exposure particularly in low parity or nulliparous elderly (>40) and postmenopausal women (bleep—features of malignancy in endometriomas.

BLEEP—*acronym—features for diagnosis of malignancy in endometriotic cysts*

B: Bloody ascites or haemorrhagic acsites
L: Large cysts >9 cm - have a higher risk of being malignant
E: Endometriosis history - long-standing endometriotic cysts >10 years
E: Elevated tumour markers - CA125, CEA, CA 19-9
P: Post menopausal women with endometriotic that continue to grow.

Serous cyst adenoma **(Fig. 85A)**:

- Smooth thin-walled anechoic, fluid-filled neoplastic lesions
- They are bilateral in 15% of cases, mean size is 5–8 cm.
- Some contain fine septations and areas of haemorrhage appearing as small echogenic areas.

Dermoid cyst ***(Figs. 85D and 87A and B):***

- These are cystic benign teratomas seen in the reproductive age group.
- Ultrasound features include:
  - Typically, unilocular cysts with mixed echogenicity representing the different components such as fat, bone and fluid.
  - They often present with hyperechogenic masses within, with posterior shadowing resembling bowel gas, making them difficult to identify on ultrasound. They are often identified when imaging the ovary becomes difficult.

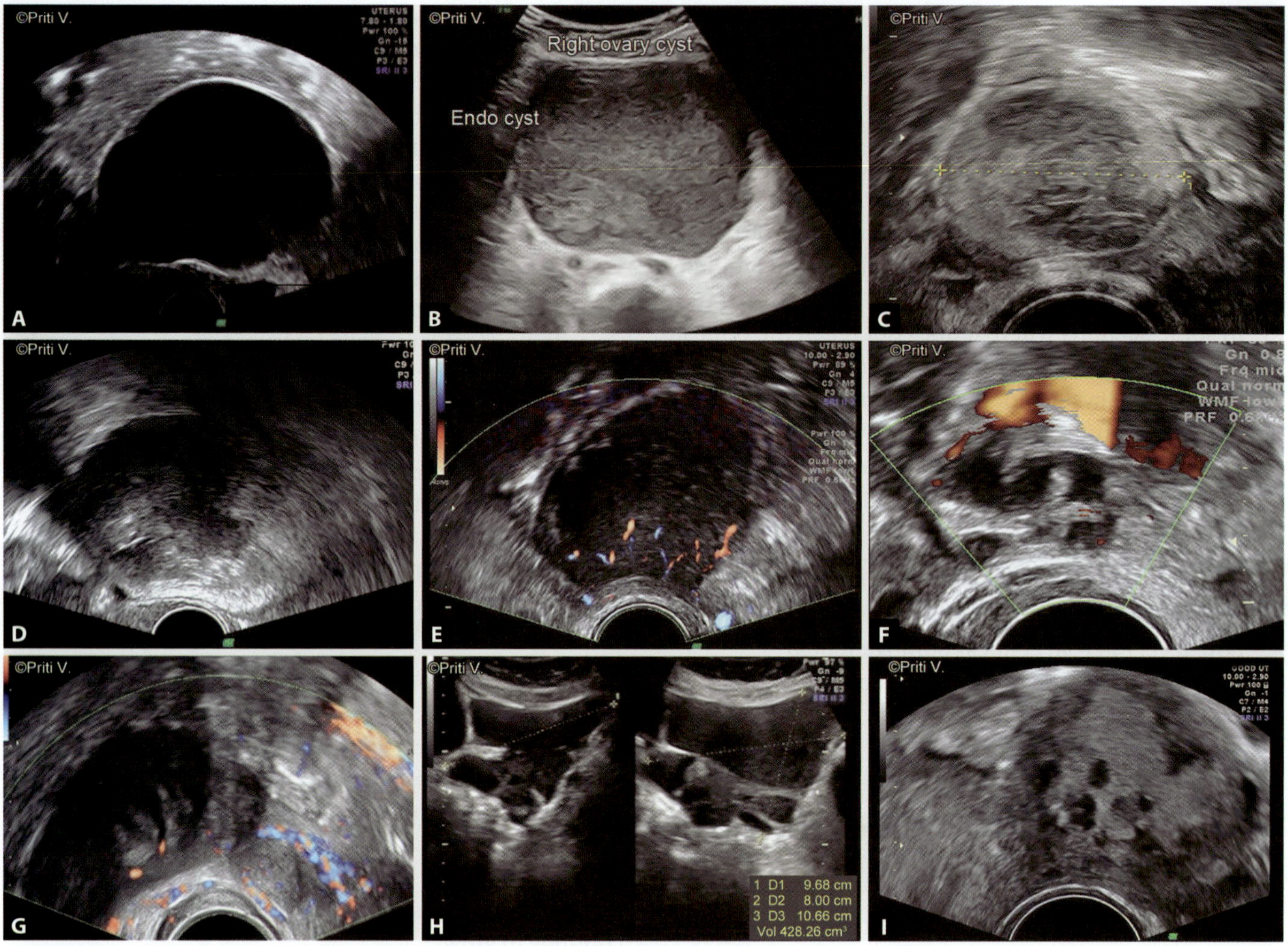

Figs. 85A to I: Some 'easy descriptors' which are lesions that can be diagnosed with simple pattern recognition. (A) Simple serous cyst; (B) Endometrioma; (C) Haemorrhagic cyst; (D) Dermoid; (E) Fibroma. (F) Hydrosalpinx; (G) Fibroid; (H) Peritoneal inclusion cyst; (I) Ovarian abscess.

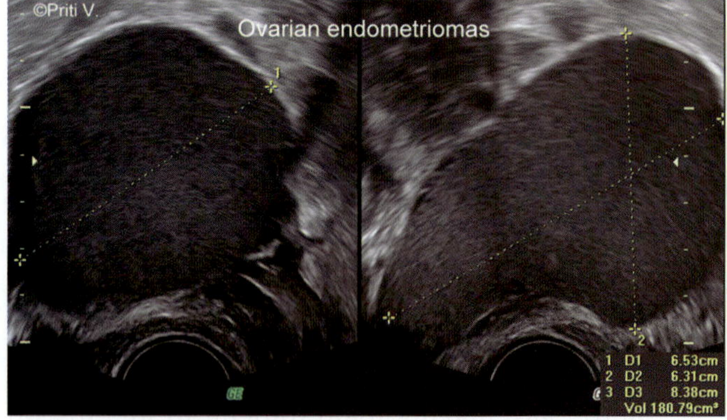

Fig. 86: Ovarian endometrioma with classic low-grade internal echoes giving it a ground glass appearance.

- The presence of cystic components with or without bright speckled echoes scattered within makes the identification of dermoid cysts easier.
- Pathognomonic of dermoid cysts is a Rokitansky nodule, a distinct hyperechoic mural nodule representing areas of floating hair in low-density fluid.
- There are often bright echoes and sharp acoustic shadows associated with hair or even teeth in the cyst.
- Ultrasound appearance of dermoids is very typical, and therefore, the diagnostic accuracy is very high based on 'pattern recognition'.

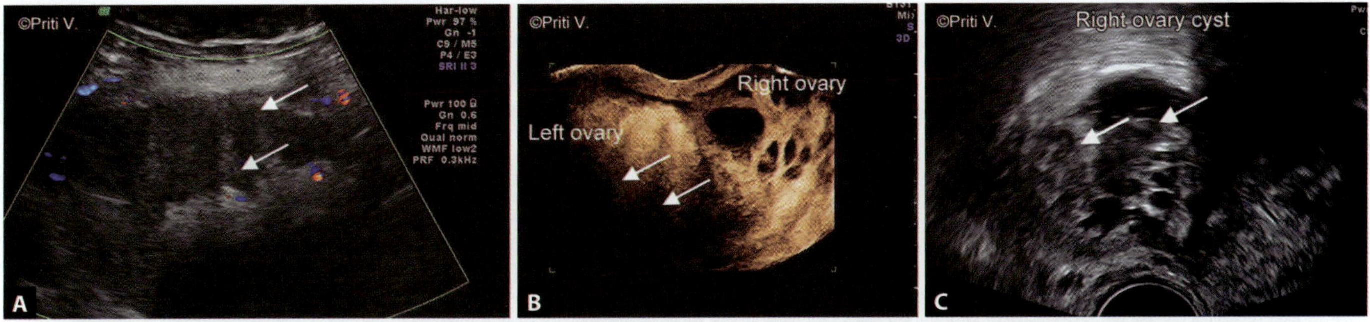

Figs. 87A to C: Important to look for acoustic shadowing as it goes in favour of benign neoplastic lesions. (A to C) Acoustic shadowing—(A and B) dermoids and (C) was a mucinous cystadenoma—recurrent.

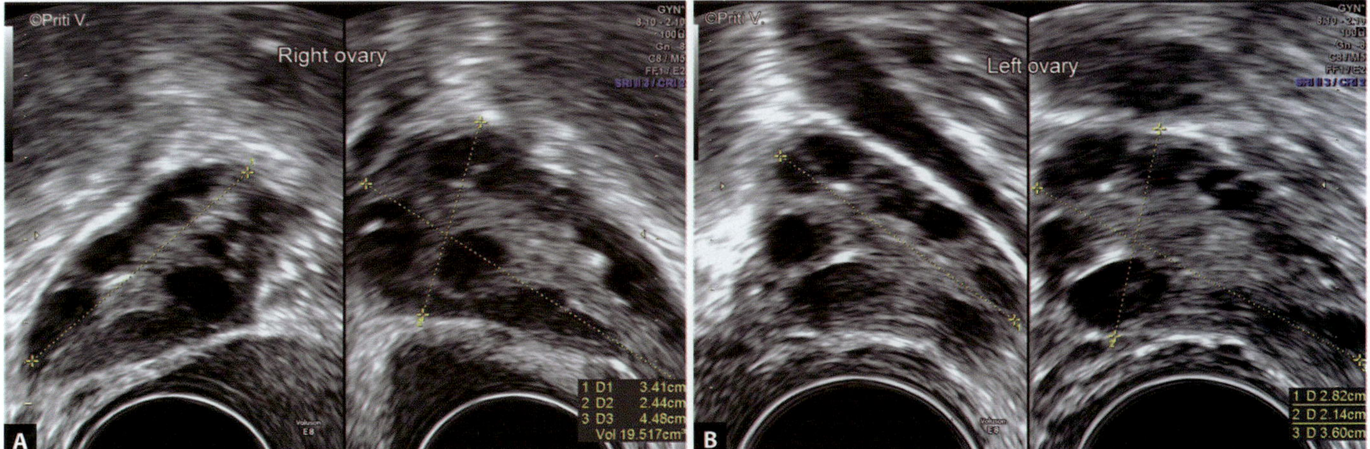

Figs. 88A and B: Bilateral polycystic ovaries are seen.

POLYCYSTIC OVARY (FIGS. 88A AND B)

Features can affects both ovaries or either one of the ovaries (unilateral PCO).

It is the commonest cause of anovulation and infertility, AUB and infrequent or absent periods.

It is familial and treated mainly symptomatically.

Ultrasonographic features include:

- More than 20 follicles per ovary (as compared to the previous Rotterdam criteria of 12 or more follicles)
- These follicles are generally similar in size and measures 2–9 mm in diameter
- Typical *string of pearls* appearance
- Ovarian enlargement (volume >10 cc)
- Central stromal brightness ± prominence, suggesting stromal hypertrophy.

Only one ovary fitting these criteria is sufficient to define PCO. If there is evidence of a dominant follicle (>10 mm) or a corpus luteum, the scan should be repeated during the next cycle because ovarian measurement becomes unreliable.

OVARIAN MALIGNANT LESIONS (FIGS. 89 TO 91)

Ultrasonography is important for assessing the likelihood of malignancy and planning the extent of surgery in cases of ovarian mass **(Figs. 84 to 91)**.

Common features of malignancy are as follows:

- Solid tumours
- Thick capsule
- Irregular outer surface
- Large multilocular cysts with:
  - Thick walls
  - Thick septae of 3–4 mm
  - Multiple papillary projections
- Ascites
- Abundant blood flow

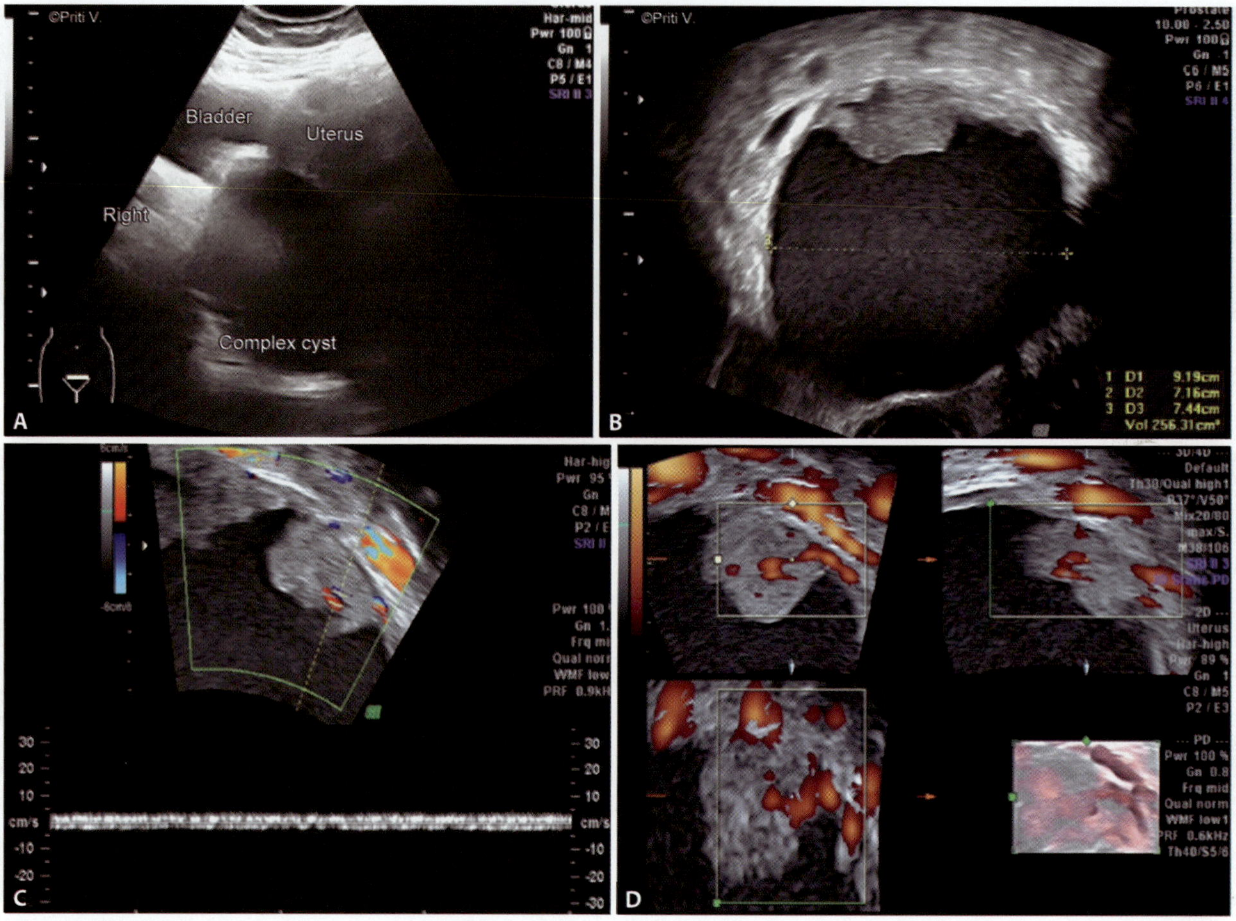

Figs. 89A and D: Ovarian carcinoma IA—transabdominal, transvaginal ultrasound, 3D power Doppler, colour Doppler and pulsed Doppler evaluation. (A) Ovarian carcinoma IA transabdominal ultrasound. The adnexal mass was not obtained due to shadowing and limited penetration/depth; (B) Transvaginal sonogram of ovarian cancer IA by B-mode. Note echogenic fluid and papillary intracystic projections. Sonographic finding was suggestive of ovarian carcinoma; (C) Colour Doppler and pulsed Doppler waveform analysis of ovarian carcinoma stage IA. Note continuous low resistance flow within the papillary projection; (D) Ovarian carcinoma IA by 3D power Doppler. Three-dimensional power Doppler ultrasound. Flow seen in the papilla and cyst wall demonstrated randomly dispersed vascular signals within the papillary protrusion.

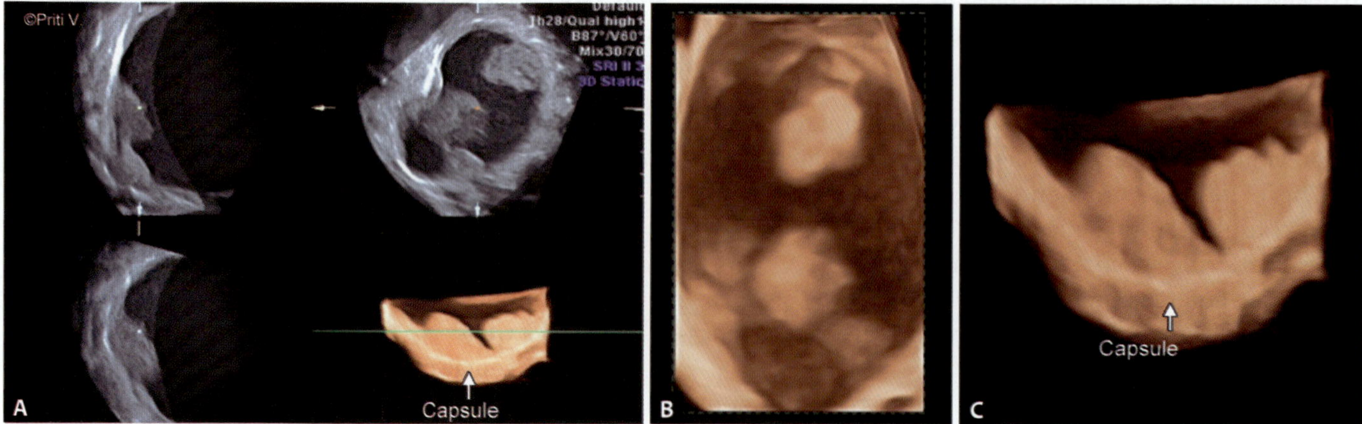

Figs. 90A to C: (A) 3D surface rendering and 'magic cut' through the basis of the papillary lesion of the same patient as in **Figure 89**. These modalities improve the depiction of infiltrative lesions; (B) 3D surface rendering of the lesion; (C) 3D surface rendering with 'magic cut' through the papillae demonstrates the continuity of the ovarian capsule. Note an echogenic band showing no interruptions.

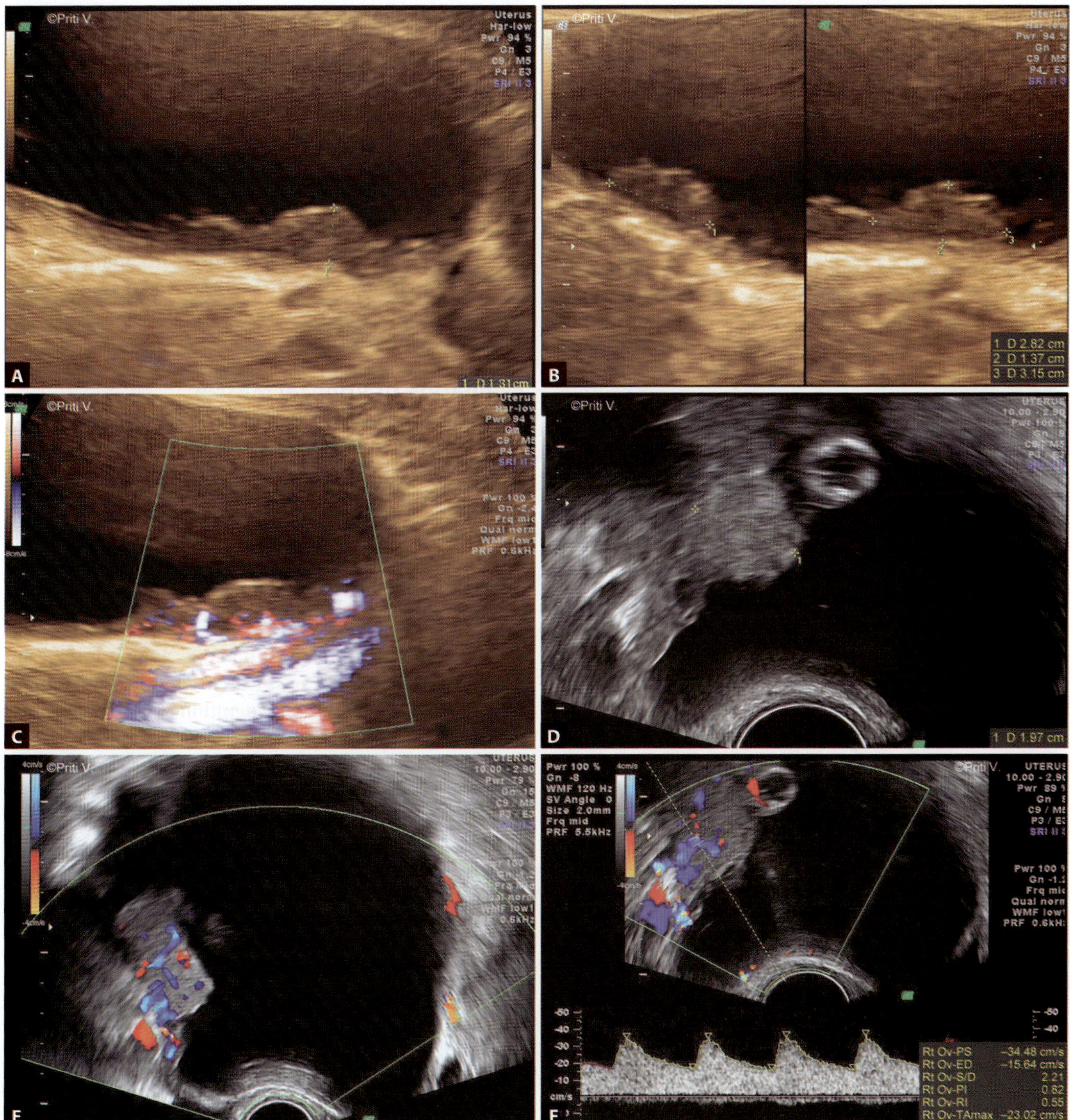

Figs. 91A to F: A large unilocular solid cystic with a small echogenic nodule of >13 mm in height clearly showing flow within the nodule with a colour score of 3 (image E) and a low resistance flow pattern with PI = 0.82 and RI = 0.55 (image F). The sepia images are TAS images. Note that the assessment was very good on TAS itself. The black and white images are TVS images. (PI: pulsatility index; RI: resistive index; TAS: transabdominal sonography; TVS: transvaginal sonography)

Ultrasound examination should not only include the assessment of pelvis but also of the kidneys and liver when malignancy is suspected. The possibility of a nonovarian primary cancer is increased in the presence of liver parenchymal metastasis. Significant hydronephrosis in the kidneys can also be identified on ultrasound examination, which is more relevant in cervical cancers.

Estimation of the Risk of Malignancy

An estimation of the risk of malignancy is an essential part of the assessment of an ovarian mass **(Table 3)**.

Risk of malignancy index (RMI) I was the most widely used index, for evaluation of malignancy in the past and is described in **Box 3**. It is not used anymore because of its lower sensitivity and availability of better methods today and a much higher reliance on ultrasound features.

Studies over the past two to three decades have shown that grey-scale morphology is the best parameter to differentiate benign from malignant lesions. The addition of CA-125 is of limited value, especially for diagnosis of borderline or stage I malignant lesions. Doppler at most increases the confidence with which a diagnosis is made.

In pattern recognition, differentiating between borderline and stage 1 ovarian masses is difficult. A recent study has reported the presence of microcysts in borderline malignant tumours seen in 98% of serous cystadenomas, 73% of mucinous cystadenomas and 60% of seromucinous borderline cystadenomas.

Over the last 20 years, the IOTA group and the American College of Radiologists have proposed several models for the differentiation of benign and malignant ovarian lesions **(Table 4)**.

In 2008, the IOTA group proposed the 'Simple Rules' (SRs).

In 2014, the ADNEX model (Van Calster et al., 2014).

In 2016, a risk calculation model based on SRs was published [simple rules risk (SRR)] (Timmerman et al., 2016).

Ovarian-Adnexal Reporting and Data System (O-RADS) to stratify the risk of malignancy with management recommendations in each O-RADS risk category was published by the American College of Radiology (ACR) in 2020 (Andreotti, 2020).

Evaluation of Adnexal Masses

The main purpose of the evaluation of adnexal masses is to differentiate between *benign* and *malignant*.

We do need to characterise every adnexal mass for proper diagnosis, treatment and management but the differentiation between benign and malignant is extremely important because of extremely poor prognosis and the urgent and radical nature of treatment needed for malignant lesions.

IOTA recommendations: Subjective evaluation by an expert examiner is the best way to identify a malignant lesion. They use 'pattern' recognition experience gained over a period of years. This is not always possible.

Hence, the IOTA group developed rules and models to characterise ovarian pathology that can be used to classify lesion as benign and malignant by examiners with

TABLE 3: Categorisation of ovarian masses based on ultrasound features.

Risk category	***Ultrasound features***	***Management options***
High risk	Features of malignancy, i.e. presence of solid components, nodules, thick septations (>2–3 mm) and size of lesion >10 cm	Surgical exploration
Intermediate risk	Not completely anechoic and/or unilocular, but there are no definite features of malignancy (e.g. a mass with thin septations or low-level echoes or size of the mass between 5 and 10 cm)	• Management must be based upon coexisting tumour marker levels, risk factors and symptoms • Many women may be managed with surveillance, but surgical exploration should be performed if clinically significant risk factors or symptoms are observed. Surgical exploration may be performed in women with a 5–10 cm mass who also have symptoms suggestive of ovarian cancer
Low risk	Anechoic unilocular fluid-filled cysts with thin walls	Surveillance rather than surgery is recommended in these cases because the risk of malignancy is less than the risk of complications associated with surgical exploration

BOX 3: Risk of malignancy index (RMI).

Definition:

- Combination of three presurgical features are used to calculate RMI:
  1. Serum CA-125 (CA-125)
  2. Menopausal status (M)
  3. Ultrasound score (U)

Calculation:

- RMI = U × M × CA-125
- *Note:* U = ultrasound score. The ultrasound result is scored 1-point for each of the following characteristics: multilocular cysts, solid areas, metastases, ascites and bilateral lesions. U = 0 (for an ultrasound score of 0), U = 1 (for an ultrasound score of 1) and U = 3 (for an ultrasound score of 2–5). The menopausal status is scored as 1 = premenopausal and 3 = postmenopausal; serum CA-125 is measured in international units per millilitre and can vary from 0 to 100 or even 1,000 of units

(RMI: Risk of Malignancy Index)

Source: National Institute for Health and Clinical Excellence. Ovarian cancer: the recognition and initial management of ovarian cancer.

TABLE 4: IOTA Group ultrasound 'rules' for classification of masses as benign or malignant.

Characteristics	***B-rules (benign)***	***M-rules (malignant)***
Consistency: Cystic/solid	Unilocular cysts	Irregular solid tumour
Presence of solid components—height >3 mm	The largest solid component <7 mm	Solid components >7 mm
Ascites	Absent	Present
Presence of acoustic shadowing	Present	Absent
Papillary structures	Less than four papillary structures	Four or more papillary structures
Surface: smooth/irregular	Smooth	Irregular
Tumour diameter	Largest diameter <100 mm	Largest diameter ≥100 mm
Blood flow	No blood flow	Very strong blood flow

(IOTA: International Ovarian Tumour Analysis)

Source: Timmerman D, Valentin L, Bourne TH, Collins WP, Verrelst H, Vergote I, et al. Terms, definitions and measurements to describe the sonographic features of adnexal tumors: a consensus opinion from the International Ovarian Tumor Analysis (IOTA) Group. Ultrasound Obstet Gynecol. 2000;16:500-5.

different levels of ultrasound experience and yet maintain similar degree of high accuracy.

Approach to Diagnosis of Adnexal Masses as Proposed by the International Ovarian Tumour Analysis Group

- *Easy descriptors* (**Figs. 85A to I**)*:* Certain masses have a characteristic appearance and grey-scale imaging. By using 'pattern' recognition, it is easy to identify these lesions with a high degree of accuracy even by an inexperienced operator. These include:
  - Endometriomas
  - Dermoid cyst
  - Haemorrhagic cyst
  - Paraovarian cyst
  - Hydro-, pyo- or haematosalphinx
  - Peritoneal inclusion cyst
  - Myomas
  - Ovarian fibroma/thecoma
  - Pelvic abscess

  The first step in the evaluation of adnexal masses is to use these easy descriptors to make a diagnosis.

  In the IOTA group, 42% of all tumours could be diagnosed in this way. No specific diagnoses were possible in 54%.

  Lesions that could not be diagnosed are then evaluated by SRs and ADNEX models in a sequential manner.
- *Simple Rules (SRs):* Where easy descriptors are not useful, SRs should be used. The IOTA group has identified 10 SRs to differentiate between benign and malignant tumours. There are five predictors of malignancy called the *M-rules* (M1–M5), which are ultrasound variables with the *highest positive predictive value (PPV) for malignancy.*

There are five predictors of benign lesion called the *B-rules* (B1–B5) which are ultrasound variables with the *lowest PPV for malignancy.* **Table 5** gives the 10 SRs.

When tested on 507 tumors, these 10 rules were applicable to 76% of all tumours and gave a sensitivity 93%, specificity of 90%, positive likelihood ratio (LR+) of 9.45 and negative likelihood ratio (LR–) of 0.08 for detection of malignant lesions.

Risk calculation is also possible using these SRs using this online calculator: https://www.mdcalc.com/calc/10517/international-ovarian-tumor-analysis-iota-simple-rules-risk-assessment.

TABLE 5: IOTA simple rules (SRs): **10 simple rules** for identifying a benign or malignant tumour.

Rules for predicting a malignant tumour (M-rules)		*Rules for predicting a benign tumour (B-rules)*	
M1	Irregular solid tumour	B1	Unilocular
M2	Presence of ascites	B2	Presence of solid components where the largest solid component has the largest diameter <7 mm
M3	At least four papillary structures	B3	Presence of acoustic shadows
M4	Irregular multilocular solid tumour with largest diameter ≥100 mm	B4	Smooth multilocular tumour with the largest diameter <100 mm
M5	Very strong blood flow (colour score 4)	B5	No blood flow (colour score 1)

How to use this table: 1. Presence of one or more M rules and no B rule classifies the lesion as malignant. 2. One or more B rules with no M rule classifies the lesion as benign. Both B or M rules noted—cannot be classified. No B or M rules noted—cannot be classified.
(IOTA: International Ovarian Tumour Analysis)

- *The ADNEX model* is applied to the rest of the tumours where easy descriptors and SRs do not apply. It can also be directly applied after the use of 'easy descriptors' to identify common benign masses such as endometriomas and haemorrhagic cysts.

The ADNEX model takes into account three clinical and six ultrasound parameters **(Table 6)**.

The three clinical parameters are as follows: (1) Age, (2) serum CA-125, and (3) type of centre.

The six ultrasound parameters are as follows: (1) Maximum diameter of the lesion in millimetre, (2) proportion of solid tissue (maximum diameter in mm), (3) number of papillary projections (0, 1, 2, 3 >3), (4) presence of >10 locules (yes/no), (5) acoustic shadows **(Figs. 87A to C)** (yes/no), and (6) presence or absence of ascites.

An example of risk calculation by ADNEX model using online calculator has been shown in **Table 7 and Fig. 92**.

The calculation can be done using ADNEX model calculators available online.

The final ADNEX model is available online and in mobile applications (www.iotagroup.org/adnexmodel/).

Table 8 has compared the various evaluation models developed for the adnexal masses.

TABLE 6: The information as needed to be entered in the ADNEX model risk calculator.

Parameters	*Information needed*
Age	Years
Type of centre—oncology centre	Yes/no
Maximum diameter of the lesion	mm
Maximum diameter of the largest solid component	mm
Number of papillary projections	0, 1, 2, 3, >3
Number of locules >10	Yes/no
Acoustic shadowing	Yes/no
Ascites	Yes/no
CA-125	U/mL
Submit	

TABLE 7: An example of risk calculation by ADNEX model. Hypothetical parameters are entered, and **Figure 104** shows the way in which the result is displayed.

Parameters	*Information needed*
Age	60 years
Type of centre—oncology centre	Yes
Maximum diameter of the lesion	139 mm
Maximum diameter of the largest solid component	52 mm
Number of papillary projections	0, 1, 2, 3, >3
Number of locules >10	Yes
Acoustic shadowing	No
Ascites	Yes
CA-125	80 U/mL
Submit	

TABLE 8: Comparison of sensitivity (SE) and specificity (SP) of ADNEX model, O-RADS and SRR at a threshold malignancy risk of >10%.

Evaluation model	*Sensitivity (SE) (%)*	*Specificity (SP) (%)*
RMI	72	92
SRR	88	84
ADNEX	92	88
O-RADS	93	89
SR + SRR	88	92
SR + ADNEX	90	93

(ADNEX: Assessment of Different NEoplasias in the adneXa; O-RADS: Ovarian-Adnexal Reporting and Data System; SRR: simple rules risk; and the two-step strategy based on the application of simple rules (SR)—SR + SRR or SR + ADNEX)
Source: Spagnol et al.

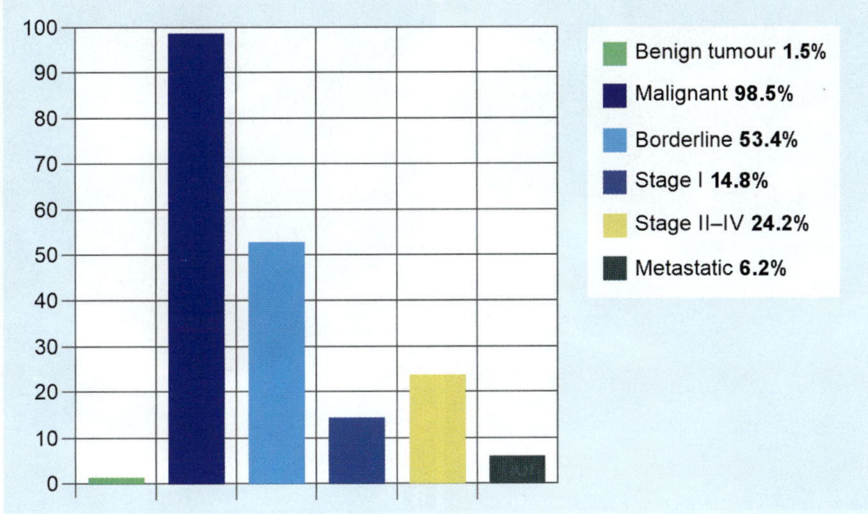

Fig. 92: Result.

FALLOPIAN TUBES (FIGS. 93 TO 96)

Also known as salpinges/oviducts or uterine tubes.

Funnel/trumpet shaped:
- 7–14 cm in length: Tortuous
- Extend from cornua to the superolateral aspect of the ovaries

Segments:
- Interstitial/cornual
- Isthmus—midportion
- Ampulla—widest and longest
- Fimbrial—distal funnel shaped with finger like projections for ovum pickup.

Functions:
- Ovum pick-up
- Acts as a path for the egg and sperm to meet, and the fertilised egg to reach the uterus.

The fallopian tube is a very dynamic organ.

The effect of the negative pressure and sucking action plays its best when the fimbrial end expands and covers the ovulation site of the ovary to effectively pick-up the ovum.

For these two important reproductive functions, the tube needs to be structurally healthy, freely mobile and free of adhesions.

Pathology affecting the fallopian tubes:
- Infection—most common
- Endometriosis—sometimes
- Malignancy—rare

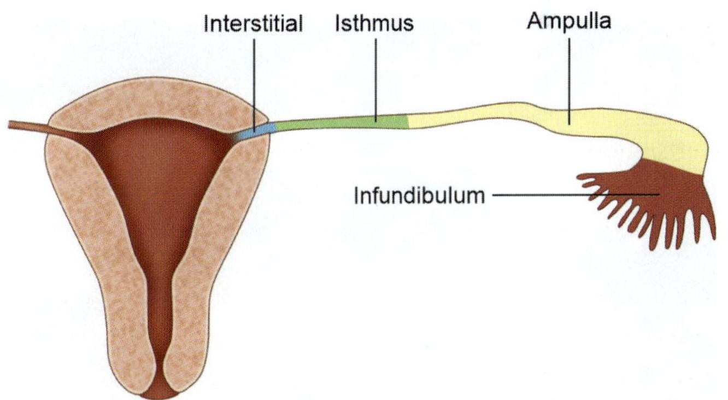

Fig. 93: Fallopian tube.

Ultrasonographic features of a diseased fallopian tube:
- Inflammation causes the fallopian tube to become:
  - Swollen—oedematous
  - Fluid filled—low-grade echoes followed by ground-glass appearance
  - Pyosalpinx in acute phase
  - *Hydrosalpinx after healing*

Hydrosalpinx (Figs. 94 and 95)

Fusiform or retort-shaped cystic lesion:
- Clear fluid
- Thin walls
- Incomplete septae
- Tiny fibrosed tubal folds—bead-on-string appearance

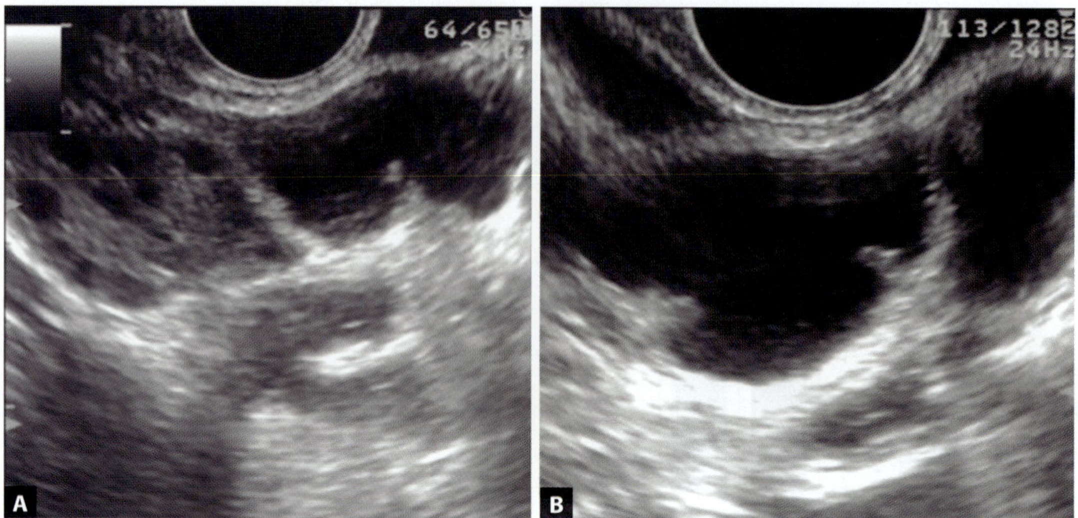

Figs. 94A and B: Dilated tubular structure in left adnexa with partial septae and anechoic contents—hydrosalpinx.

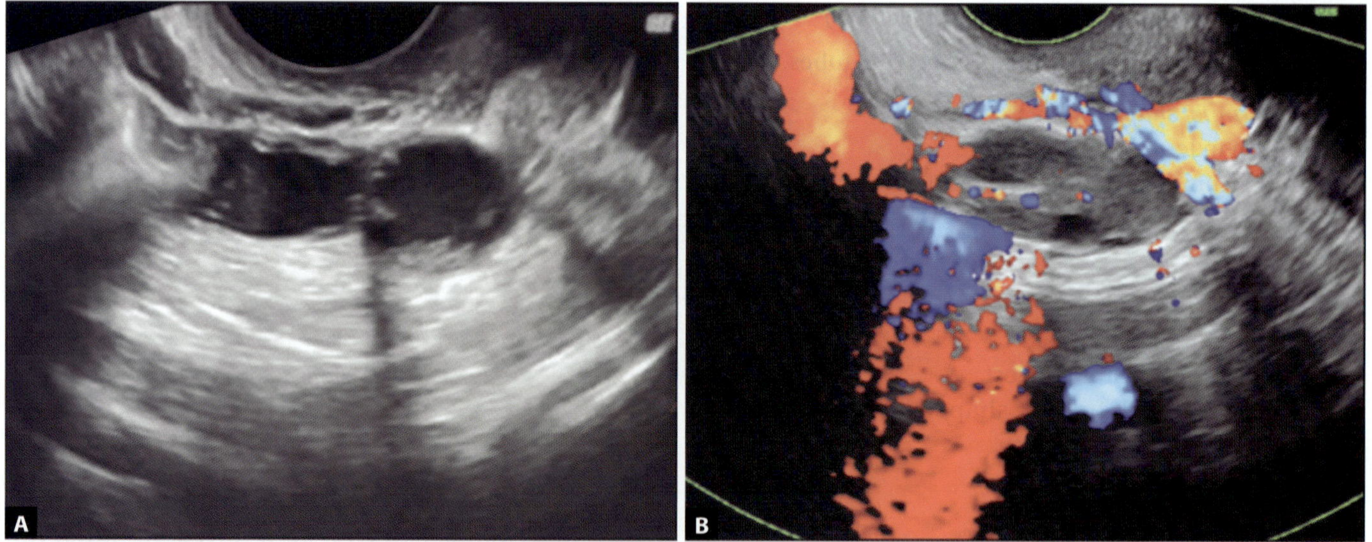

Figs. 95A and B: Elongated tortuous cystic structure with no flow within on colour Doppler confirms a non vascular structure - a fallopian tube filled with fluid with low internal echoes and good vascularity in the tubal walls—suggestive of a pyosalpinx.

Pyosalpinx ***(Fig. 96)****:*

- Due to acute inflammation
- Fusiform or convoluted tubular mass
- Thickened cyst wall
- Thick incomplete septae
- Purulent fluid showing low-level echoes
- Cogwheel sign due to peripherally arranged swollen tubal folds. In acute infection these folds are swollen and thick. After healing they become fibrosed and bead-like.

Haematosalpinx:

- Blood-filled tube
- From retrograde menstruation or fallopian tube endometriosis
- Similar appearance to hydrosalpinx but with particulate fluid within

ENDOMETRIOSIS (FIGS. 86 AND 97 TO 100)

Endometriosis ***(Figs. 86 and 97 to 100)***: Definition—ectopic functioning endometrial implants containing both

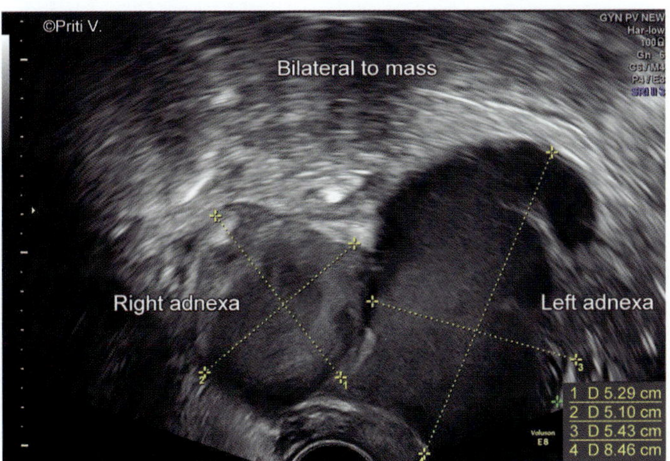

Fig. 96: Bilateral pyosalpinx in a case of severe acute pelvic inflammatory disease (PID). Tubes are predominantly the site for PID. Tubes take the brunt of PID.

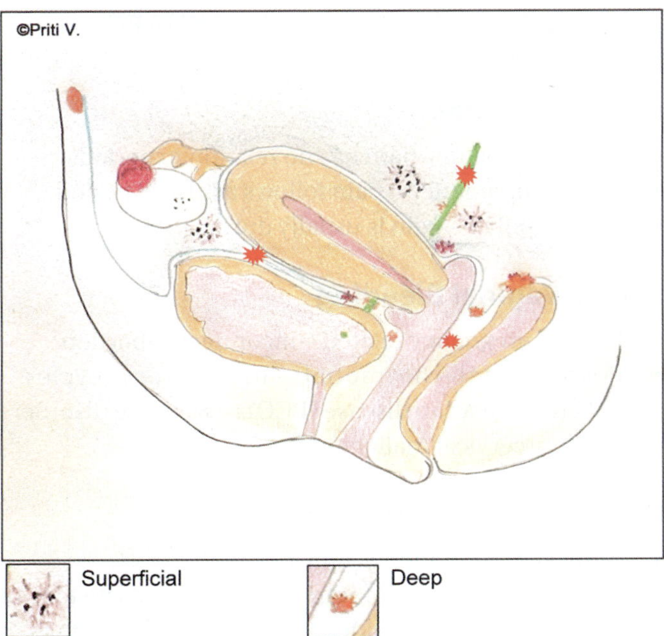

Fig. 97: Common sites of pelvic endometriosis—superficial and deep.

endometrial glands and stroma—seen outside the uterine cavity.

- Endometriosis can be *diffuse* or *focal*.
- Three types of endometriotic lesions are seen:
  1. Superficial endometriosis (SE)—involving the surface of the pelvic peritoneum **(Figs. 97 and 98)**
  2. Deep endometrioses (DE) are lesions that infiltrate >5 mm beneath the surface and affect surrounding organs such as the bowel, bladder and the ureter **(Fig. 100)**.
  3. Ovarian endometriosis—which is a focal cystic lesions **(Fig. 86)**

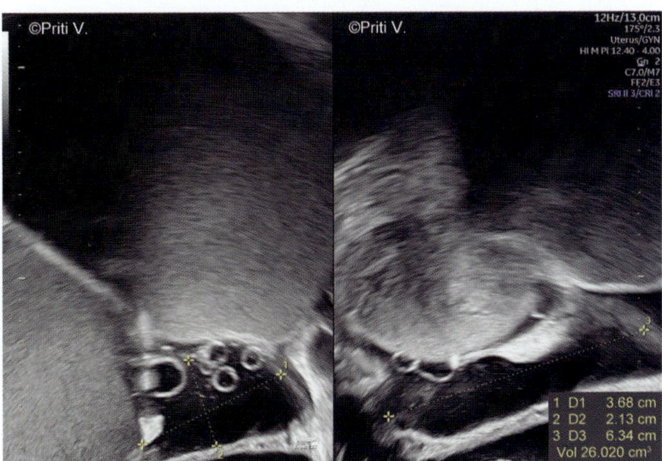

Fig. 98: Case of bilateral endometriomas with superficial peritoneal endometriosis with peritoneal blebs seen floating because of the presence of fluid in the pelvis. Thin bands and tags of tissue floating in the fluid are also pointers for superficial endometriosis.

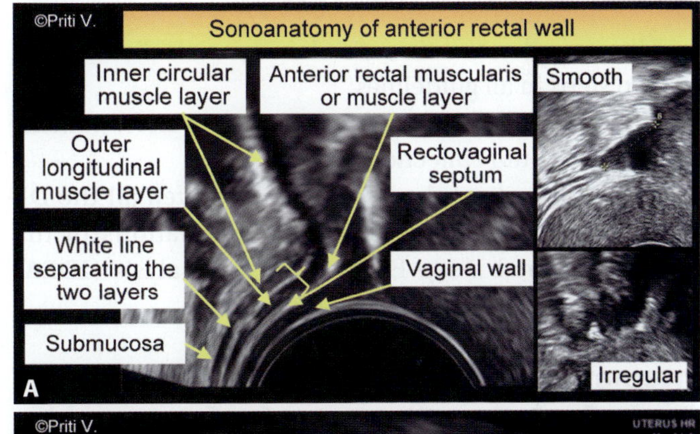

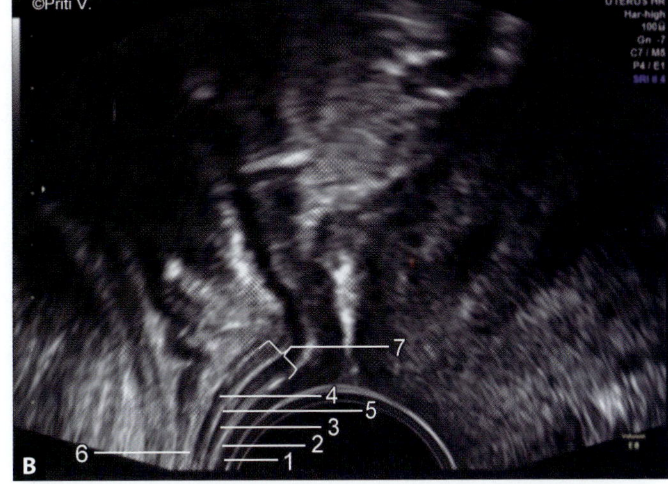

Figs. 99A and B: The anatomy of the posterior vaginal wall and the anterior rectal wall which are affected by deep endometriosis of the posterior compartment. Layers if the vaginal and anterior rectal wall: (1) Vaginal wall, (2) Rectovaginal septum, (3) Outer longitudinal muscle layer, (4) White line between the two muscle layers, (5) Inner circular muscle layer, (6) Submucosa and (7) entire muscularis.

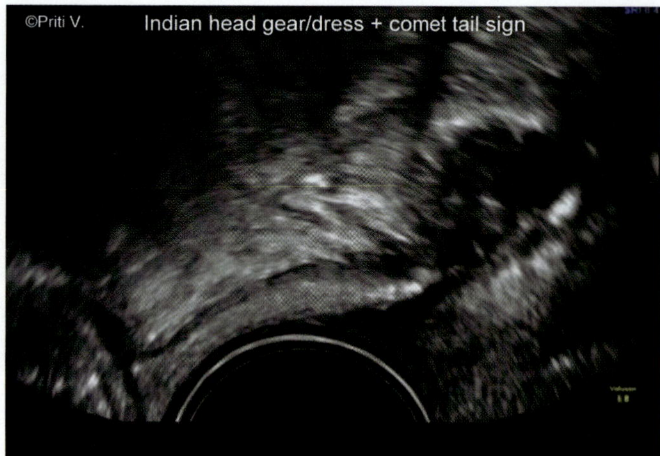

Fig. 100: Deep infiltrating endometriosis—DE lesion in the anterior rectal wall and adherent to the uterus, causing loss of the low sliding sign and probe tenderness on palpation of this area with the transducer. This is a sign of obliteration of the POD. (DE: deep endometriosis; POD: Pouch of Douglas)

- *Ultrasound evaluation of endometriosis* is divided into two steps in all guidelines:

1. *A basic standard ultrasound:* Uterus, ovaries, adnexa, and POD fluid collection
2. *An advanced pelvic ultrasound:* To unveil all the DE foci. Here we follow the recommendations of the International Deep Endometriosis Analysis (IDEA) group for the advance evaluation.

International Deep Endometriosis Analysis Group Consensus Statement for Sonographic Examination in Endometriosis

- *Step 1:*
  - Routine evaluation—uterus and adnexa
  - Look for USG signs of adenomyosis/endometrioma
- *Step 2:*
  - TVS for soft markers
  - Site-specific tenderness and ovarian mobility
- *Step 3:* Assessment of POD with dynamic testing—sliding sign
- *Step 4:* Assessment of deep infiltrating endometriosis (DIE) or DE nodules in anterior and posterior compartments—sliding sign helps identify areas of adhesions and tenderness, which will lead to the identification of DE lesions.

Positive findings in Step 1 increases the chances of finding more endometriotic or DE lesions. Soft signs like tenderness and absence of sliding sign leads one to the site of other dificult-to-identify lesions.

High and low sliding sign:

- With bimanual palpation, the uterus is gently pushed upwards while the abdominal hand provides steady counter pressure or downward push to make the bowel slide on the surface of the uterus:
  - With POD adhesions—low sliding sign is absent
  - With adhesions along the posterior surface of the uterus and fundus—high sliding sign is absent
- The 'sliding sign' specifically predicts *POD obliteration*
- A negative 'sliding sign' using TVS correlates well with obliteration of POD at laparoscopy
- The 'sliding sign' is simple to demonstrate and does not require advanced sonologic skills

ULTRASOUND IMAGING IN GYNAEC EMERGENCIES

Acute Pelvic Pain

- Ovarian torsion—pain has no relation to periods
- Ectopic pregnancy—pain follows a missed period
- Fibroid polyp—pain is usually during periods

Severe Vaginal Bleeding

- Usually pregnancy related—incomplete abortion
- Postpubertal—hormonal—anovulatory cycles—polycystic ovarian disease (PCOD)/bleeding disorders
- Uterine/cervical malignancies

Ovarian Torsion (Figs. 101 and 102)

- Clinical presentation is nonspecific:
  - Acute pain in abdomen—sometimes—history of pain following sudden physical activity, change in posture, emptying a full bladder can be elicited
  - Nausea and vomiting
- *Examination*:
  - Tenderness in right or left iliac fossa
  - *Unilateral* palpable tender mass

Ultrasound Findings

- TVUS is the most important diagnostic modality.
- TAUS is recommended in children and adolescents:
  - Unilateral enlarged oedematous ovary—in all studies—in all cases—100%, very constant finding

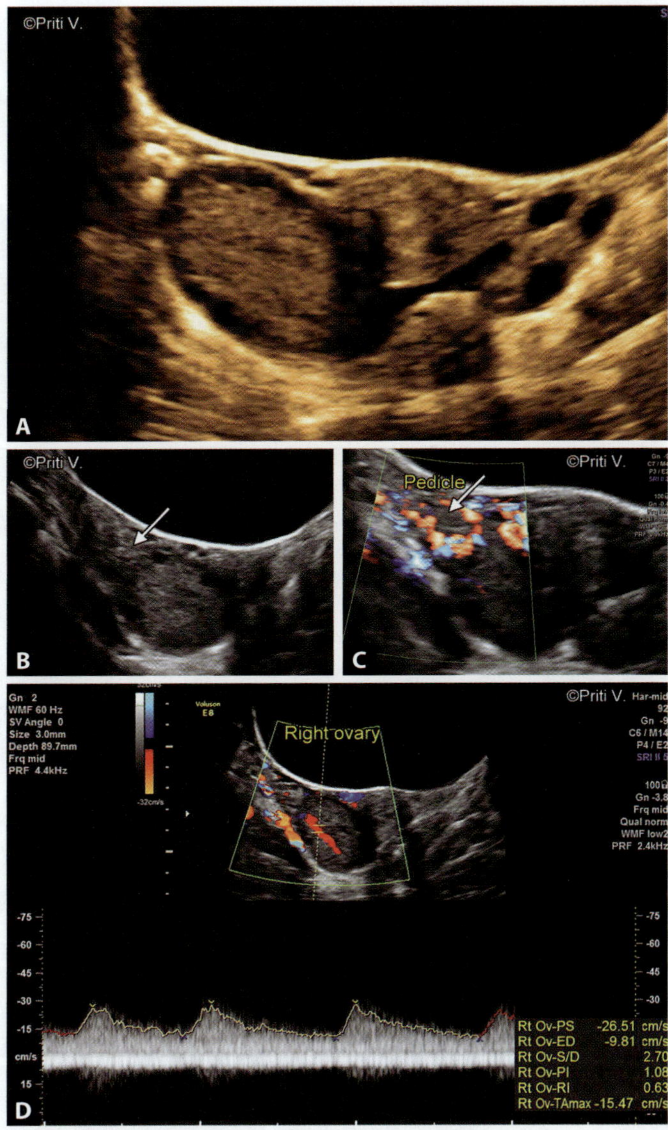

Figs. 101A to D: Ovarian torsion case diagnosed on TAS only. *Note:* (A) The grossly enlarged right ovary with peripherally arranged follicles in stark contrast to the normal left ovary—oedematous enlarged right ovary—the most consistent finding in ovarian torsion; (B and C) Pedicle of torsion is seen on grey-scale and colour flow images marked by a white arrow; (D) Persistence of vascularity in spite of torsion because of the dual blood supply of the ovary from the ovarian vessel and the branches of the uterine artery. (TAS: transabdominal sonography)

- Tenderness is always present
- Displaced ovaries—anterior to uterus or opposite side
- Stromal oedema with peripheral follicle arrangement—string of pearls—74%
- Pedicle of torsion seen as:
  - Target sign—on 2D
  - Whirlpool sign on real-time imaging on grey-scale (2D) imaging, as well as on colour flow demonstrated by to and fro movement of the transducer probe.
- *Follicular ring sign*—perifollicular or pericystic congestion rim of congestion surrounding follicles and other cystic structures.

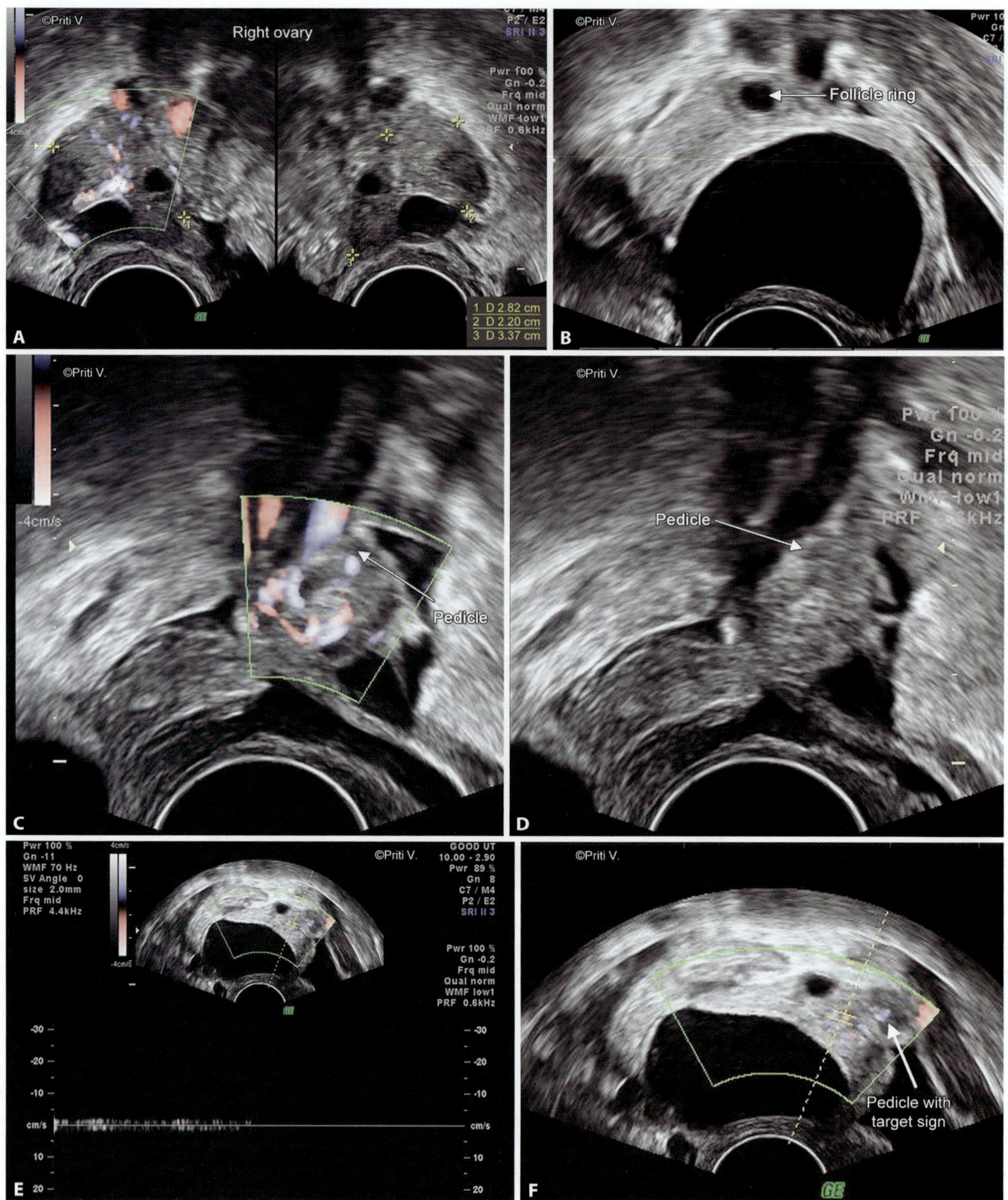

Figs. 102A to F: Ovarian torsion TVS. (A) Normal right ovary with normal thin-walled follicles; (B) An enlarged left ovary with a unilocular cyst and a follicle showing a thick rim—called the follicular ring sign—indicates perifollicular congestion; (C and D) Images show the pedicle of torsion with and without HDF; (E) Shows presence of flow in the ovarian stroma; (F) Showes stromal flow in left ovary using HDF and the white arrow is pointing at the echogenic dot in the centre of the pedicle giving it a target sign appearance pedicle. The position of the pedicle is posterolateral to the left ovary. (HDF: high definition flow; TVS: transvaginal sonography)

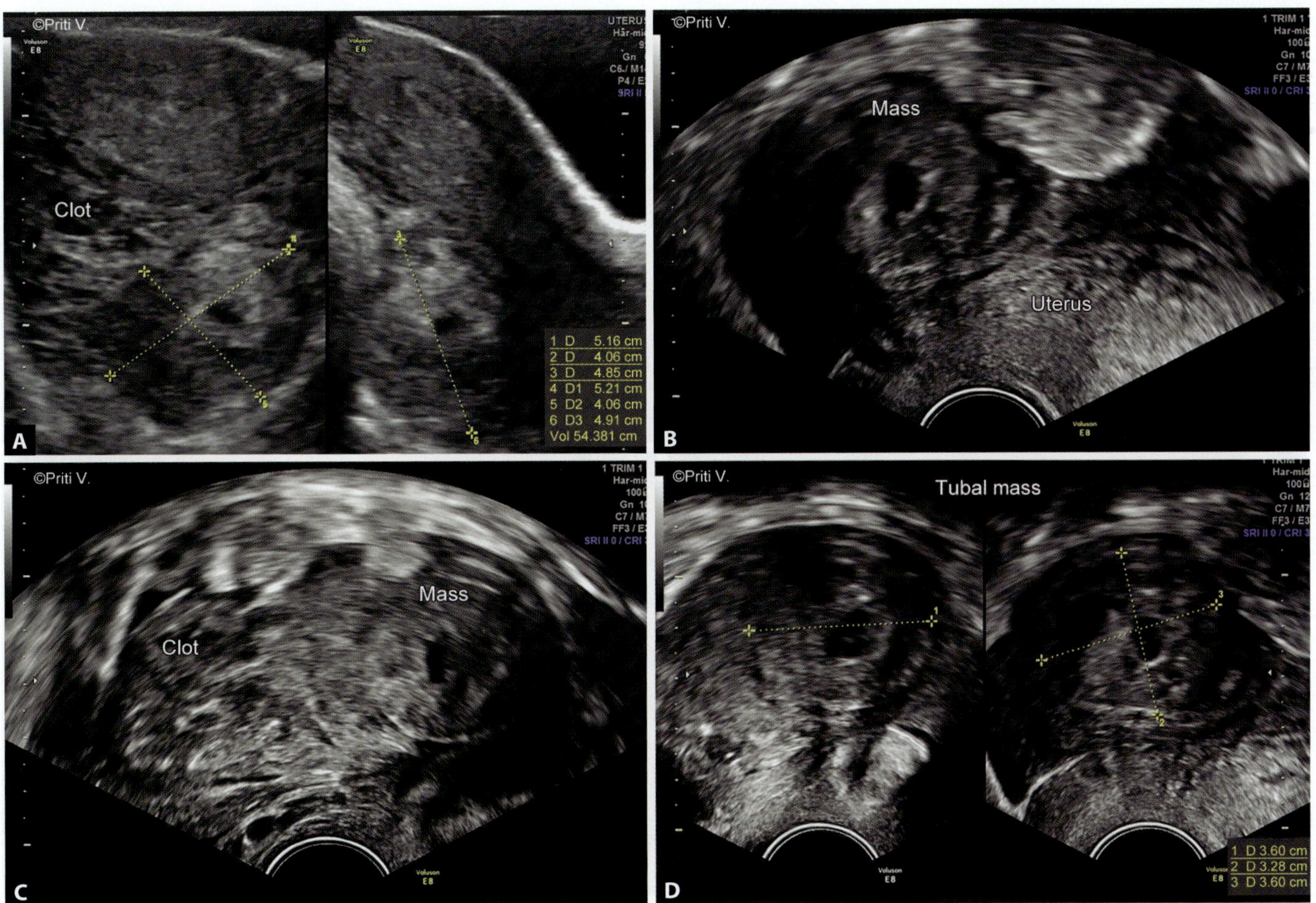

Figs. 103A to D: Tubal ectopic gestation: Tubal abortion with blood and clots in the pelvis. *Note:* (A) is a TAS image showing uterus and the POD. No intrauterine gestation seen. Tubal ectopic gestation mass is seen in the POD with clots seen superolateral to the mass; B, C and D are TVS images. (B) Ectopic gestation mass seen in POD on TVS; (C) Tubal ectopic gestation mass in POD with clots lateral to it; (D) The tubal mass is well circumscribed with all its components clearly—note from inside out—hypoechoic GS, echogenic trophoblastic rim which is thin and irregular here, a thick hypoechoic layer of oedematous tubal muscular layer and, finally, the thin serosal echogenic outline. (POD: pouch of Douglas; TVS: transvaginal sonography)

- A cystic or complex mass in the twisted ovary is seen in 46%.

(*Graif et al., 1988 AJR, ** Graif 1984 AJR; * Lee et al,1998 AJR; † Vijayaraghavan BS 2004, JUM; Sibal M, 2013, JUM)

Ectopic Pregnancy (Figs. 103 and 104)

- Presents with amenorrhoea followed by severe pain in the lower abdomen
- Urine pregnancy test (UPT) positive

Ultrasound on TVUS:

- No intrauterine gestational sac (GS) with beta-human chorionic gonadotropin (β-hCG) >discriminatory zone (DZ) (DZ: 1,000–2,000 IU/L)
- Thick decidualised endometrium with no GS
- Tubal mass with GS in the adnexal area—*tubal ring sign* **(Figs. 103A to D)**—ipsilateral to the location of corpus luteum.
- Exceptions to this are as follows:
  - Contralateral tubal ring—10–15%
  - Very early or failing gestation—IUP but GS not seen yet
  - Ruptured tubal ectopic gestation—GS not seen in adnexa. Complex mass is seen.
  - The *tubal ring* contains from into out—(1) The GS, (2) echogenic trophoblastic rim, (3) oedematous hypoechoic tubal muscle layer and (4) thin echogenic line of tubal serosa **(Figs. 103A to D)**.

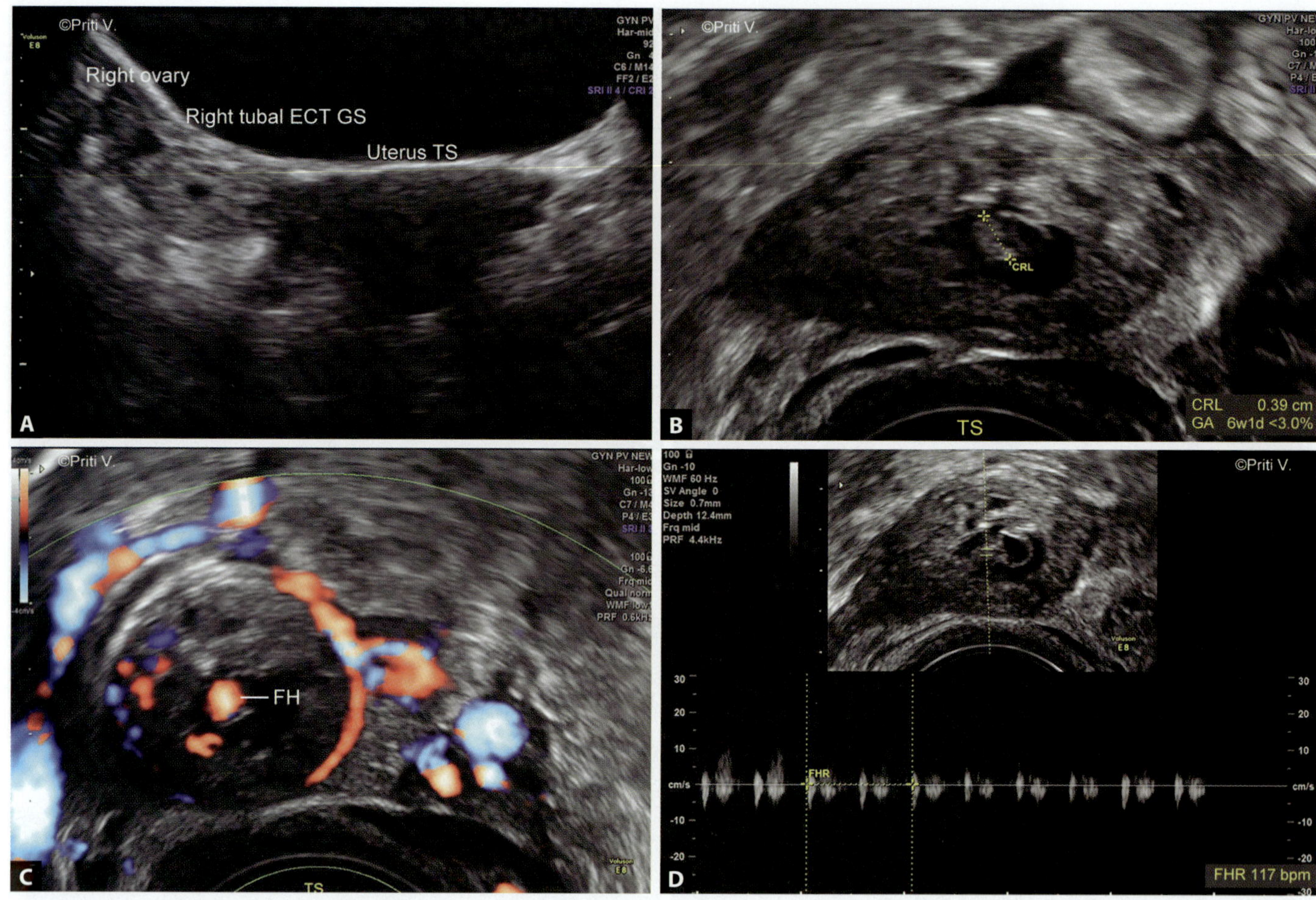

Figs. 104A to D: Live tubal ectopic gestation. (A) Is a TAS image with a panoramic view of the uterus, right ovary and the rigth tubal ectopic gestation between the two; (B, C and D) Are TVS images showing ectopic gestational sac with a live fetus—in (B) CRL is measured. In image (C) the HD color low around the tubal mass is well seen and the red dot in the centre of the tubal mass is the fetal heart picking the color. (D) Fetal heart rate recorded at 117bpm with pulse wave doppler.

Ectopic gestation is diagnosed with a combination of β-hCG and TV ultrasound; 90–95% are tubal.

Rare locations such as interstitial, cervical, cornual, abdominal, and heterotopic—in association with intrauterine gestation—can also be diagnosed with ultrasound. **Figures 103A to D** show a tubal abortion, and **Figures 104A to D** show a case of live tubal ectopic gestation.

SUGGESTED READING

1. Andreotti RF, Timmerman D, Strachowski LM, Froyman W, Benacerraf BR, Bennett GL, et al. O-RADS US risk stratification and management system: a consensus guideline from the ACR Ovarian-Adnexal Reporting and Data System Committee. Radiology. 2020;294(1):168-85.
2. Belsey EM, Pinol AP. Menstrual bleeding patterns in untreated women. Task force on long-acting systemic agents for fertility regulation. Contraception. 1997;55(2):57-65.
3. Berek JS, Matias-Guiu X, Creutzberg C, Fotopoulou C, Gaffney D, Kehoe S, et al.; Endometrial Cancer Staging Subcommittee, FIGO Women's Cancer Committee. Correction to FIGO staging of endometrial cancer. Int J Gynaecol Obstet. 2024;166(3):1374.
4. Berek JS, Matias-Guiu X, Creutzberg C, Fotopoulou C, Gaffney D, Kehoe S, et al.; Endometrial Cancer Staging Subcommittee, FIGO Women's Cancer Committee. FIGO staging of endometrial cancer: 2023. Int J Gynecol Obstet. 2023;162(2):383-94.
5. Brucker SY, Rall K, Campo R, Oppelt P, Isaacson K. Treatment of congenital malformations. Semin Reprod Med. 2011;29(02):101-12.
6. Chan YY, Jayaprakasan K, Zamora J, Thornton JG, Raine-Fenning N, Coomarasamy A. The prevalence of congenital uterine anomalies in unselected and high-risk populations: a systematic review. Hum Reprod Update. 2011;17(6):761-71.

7. Czekierdowski A. Re: Differences in ultrasound features of papillations in unilocular-solid adnexal cysts: a retrospective international multicenter study. C. Landolfo, L. Valentin, D. Franchi, C. Van Holsbeke, R. Fruscio, W. Froyman, P. Sladkevicius, J. Kaijser, L. Ameye, T. Bourne, L. Savelli, A. Coosemans, A. Testa and D. Timmerman. Ultrasound Obstet Gynecol 2018; 52: 269-278. Ultrasound Obstet Gynecol. 2018;52(2):157-8.
8. Dewilde K, Groszmann Y, Van Schoubroeck D, Grewal K, Huirne J, de Leeuw R, et al. Enhanced myometrial vascularity secondary to retained pregnancy tissue: time to stop misusing the term arteriovenous malformation. Ultrasound Obstet Gynecol. 2024;63(1):5-8.
9. Federation of Obstetric and Gynecological Societies of India. (2016). Management guidelines of Abnormal uterine bleeding in reproductive period. [Online] Available from https://www.fogsi.org/wp-content/uploads/2016/06/AUB-FOGSI-GCPR-Summary-of-recommendations.pdf [Last accessed July, 2025].
10. Fraser IS, Critchley HO, Munro MG, Broder M. Can we achieve international agreement on terminologies and definitions used to describe abnormalities of menstrual bleeding? Hum Reprod. 2007;22(3):635-43.
11. Fraser IS, Critchley HO, Munro MG, Broder M; Writing Group for this Menstrual Agreement Process. A process designed to lead to international agreement on terminologies and definitions used to describe abnormalities of menstrual bleeding. Fertil Steril. 2007;87(3):466-76.
12. Gergolet M, Campo R, Verdenik I, Šuster NK, Gordts S, Gianaroli L. No clinical relevance of the height of fundal indentation in subseptate or arcuate uterus: a prospective study. Reprod Biomed Online. 2012;24(5):576-82.
13. Graif M, Itzchak Y. Sonographic evaluation of ovarian torsion in childhood and adolescence. Am J Roentgenol. 1988;150(3):647-9.
14. Graif M, Shalev J, Strauss S, Engelberg S, Mashiach S, Itzchak Y. Torsion of the ovary: sonographic features. AJR Am J Roentgenol. 1984;143(6):1331-4.
15. Grewal K, Al-Memar M, Fourie H, Stalder C, Timmerman D, Bourne T. Natural history of pregnancy-related enhanced myometrial vascularity following miscarriage. Ultrasound Obstet Gynecol. 2020;55(5):676-82.
16. Grimbizis GF, Campo R. Congenital malformations of the female genital tract: the need for a new classification system. Fertil Steril. 2010;94(2):401-7.
17. Grimbizis GF, Camus M, Tarlatzis BC, Bontis JN, Devroey P. Clinical implications of uterine malformations and hysteroscopic treatment results. Hum Reprod Update. 2001;7(2):161-74.
18. Grimbizis GF, Tsalikis T, Mikos T, Papadopoulos N, Tarlatzis BC, Bontis JN. Successful end-to-end cervico-cervical anastomosis in a patient with congenital cervical fragmentation: Case report. Human Reprod. 2004;19(5):1204-10.
19. Groszmann YS, Healy Murphy AL, Benacerraf BR. Diagnosis and management of patients with enhanced myometrial vascularity associated with retained products of conception. Ultrasound Obstet Gynecol. 2018;52(3):396-9.
20. Hallberg L, Hôgdahl AM, Nilsson L, Rybo G. Menstrual blood loss–a population study: variation at different ages and attempts to define normality. Acta obstetricia et gynecologica Scandinavica. 1966;45(3):320-51.
21. Hooker AB, Lemmers M, Thurkow AL, Heymans MW, Opmeer BC, Brölmann HA, et al. Systematic review and meta-analysis of intrauterine adhesions after miscarriage: prevalence, risk factors and long-term reproductive outcome. Hum Reprod Update. 2014;20(2):262-78.
22. Hyunji Oh, Sung Bin Park, Hyun Jeong Park, Eun Sun Lee, Joonho Hur, Woosun Choi, et al. Ultrasonographic features of uterine cervical lesions. Br J Radiol. 2021;94(1121):20201242.
23. Jain K, Fogata M. Retained products of conception mimicking a large endometrial AVM: complete resolution following spontaneous abortion. J Clin Ultrasound. 2007;35(1):42-7.
24. Joki-Erkkilä MM, Heinonen PK. Presenting and long-term clinical implications and fecundity in females with obstructing vaginal malformations. J Pediatr Adolesc Gynecol. 2003;16(5):307-12.
25. Jokubkiene L, Sladkevicius P, Valentin L. Does three-dimensional power Doppler ultrasound help in discrimination between benign and malignant ovarian masses? Ultrasound Obstet Gynecol. 2007;29(2):215-25.
26. Kaijser J, Bourne T, Valentin L, Sayasneh A, Van Holsbeke C, Vergote I, et al. Improving strategies for diagnosing ovarian cancer: a summary of the International Ovarian Tumor Analysis (IOTA) studies. Ultrasound Obstet Gynecol. 2013;41(1):9-20.
27. Lee EJ, Kwon HC, Joo HJ, Suh JH, Fleischer AC. Diagnosis of ovarian torsion with color Doppler sonography: depiction of twisted vascular pedicle. J Ultrasound Med. 1998;17(2):83-9.
28. Leone FP, Timmerman D, Bourne T, Valentin L, Epstein E, Goldstein SR, et al. Terms, definitions and measurements to describe the sonographic features of the endometrium and intrauterine lesions: a consensus opinion from the International Endometrial Tumor Analysis (IETA) group. Ultrasound Obstet Gynecol. 2010;35(1):103-12.
29. Lin MY, Dobrotwir A, McNally O, Abu-Rustum NR, Narayan K. Role of imaging in the routine management of endometrial cancer. Int J Gynecol Obstet. 2018;143(Suppl 2):109-17.
30. Mollo A, De Franciscis P, Colacurci N, Cobellis L, Perino A, Venezia R, et al. Hysteroscopic resection of the septum improves the pregnancy rate of women with unexplained infertility: a prospective controlled trial. Fertil Steril. 2009;91(6):2628-31.

31. Moro F, Magoga G, Pasciuto T, Mascilini F, Moruzzi MC, Fischerova D, et al. Imaging in gynecological disease (13): clinical and ultrasound characteristics of endometrioid ovarian cancer. Ultrasound Obstet Gynecol. 2018;52(4):535-43.
32. Munro MG, Balen AH, Cho S, Critchley HO, Díaz I, Ferriani R, et al. The FIGO ovulatory disorders classification system. Hum Reprod. 2022;37(10):2446-64.
33. Munro MG, Critchley HO, Broder MS, Fraser IS; FIGO Working Group on Menstrual Disorders. FIGO classification system (PALM-COEIN) for causes of abnormal uterine bleeding in nongravid women of reproductive age. Int J Gynecol Obstet. 2011;113(1):3-13.
34. Munro MG, Critchley HO, Fraser IS; FIGO Menstrual Disorders Committee. The two FIGO systems for normal and abnormal uterine bleeding symptoms and classification of causes of abnormal uterine bleeding in the reproductive years: 2018 revisions. Int J Gynecol Obstet. 2018;143(3):393-408.
35. Nunes N, Ambler G, Foo X, Naftalin J, Widschwendter M, Jurkovic D. Use of IOTA simple rules for diagnosis of ovarian cancer: meta-analysis. Ultrasound Obstet Gynecol. 2014;44(5):503-14.
36. Oh H, Park SB, Park HJ, Lee ES, Hur J, Choi W, et al. Ultrasonographic features of uterine cervical lesions. Br J Radiol. 2021;94(1121):20201242.
37. Recker F, Gembruch U, Strizek B. Clinical ultrasound applications in obstetrics and gynecology in the year 2024. J Clin Med. 2024;13(5):1244.
38. Rock JA, Roberts CP, Jones Jr HW. Congenital anomalies of the uterine cervix: lessons from 30 cases managed clinically by a common protocol. Fertil Steril. 2010;94(5): 1858-63.
39. Rosen A, Chan WV, Matelski J, Walsh C, Murji A. Medical treatment of uterine arteriovenous malformation: a systematic review and meta-analysis. Fertil Steril. 2021;116(4):1107-16.
40. Saravelos SH, Cocksedge KA, Li TC. Prevalence and diagnosis of congenital uterine anomalies in women with reproductive failure: a critical appraisal. Hum Reprod Update. 2008;14(5):415-29.
41. Sibal M. Follicular ring sign: a simple sonographic sign for early diagnosis of ovarian torsion. J Ultrasound Med. 2012;31(11):1803-9.
42. Spagnol G, Marchetti M, De Tommasi O, Vitagliano A, Cavallin F, Tozzi R, et al. Simple rules, O-RADS, ADNEX and SRR model: Single oncologic center validation of diagnostic predictive models alone and combined (two-step strategy) to estimate the risk of malignancy in adnexal masses and ovarian tumors. Gynecol Oncol. 2023;177:109-16.
43. Strawbridge LC, Crouch NS, Cutner AS, Creighton SM. Obstructive Mullerian anomalies and modern laparoscopic management. J Pediatr Adolesc Gynecol. 2007;20(3):195-200.
44. Sun S, Bonaffini PA, Nougaret S, Fournier L, Dohan A, Chong J, et al. How to differentiate uterine leiomyosarcoma from leiomyoma with imaging. Diagnostic and interventional imaging. 2019;100(10):619-34.
45. Testa AC, Timmerman D, Van Holsbeke C, Zannoni GF, Fransis S, Moerman P, et al. Ovarian cancer arising in endometrioid cysts: ultrasound findings. Ultrasound Obstet Gynecol. 2011;38(1):99-106.
46. Testa AC. Malignant ovarian neoplasms: the sonographic voyage of discovery. Ultrasound Obstet Gynecol. 2008;31(6):611-4.
47. Timmerman D, Testa AC, Bourne T, Ameye L, Jurkovic D, Van Holsbeke C, et al. Simple ultrasound-based rules for the diagnosis of ovarian cancer. Ultrasound Obstet Gynecol. 2008;31(6):681-90.
48. Timmerman D, Valentin L, Bourne TH, Collins WP, Verrelst H, Vergote I; International Ovarian Tumor Analysis (IOTA) Group. Terms, definitions and measurements to describe the sonographic features of adnexal tumors: a consensus opinion from the International Ovarian Tumor Analysis (IOTA) Group. Ultrasound Obstet Gynecol. 2000;16(5):500-5.
49. Timmerman D, Van Calster B, Testa A, Savelli L, Fischerova D, Froyman W, et al. Predicting the risk of malignancy in adnexal masses based on the simple rules from the International Ovarian Tumor Analysis group. Am J Obstet Gynecol. 2016;214(4):424-37.
50. Timmerman D, Van Calster B, Testa AC, Guerriero S, Fischerova D, Lissoni AA, et al. Ovarian cancer prediction in adnexal masses using ultrasound-based logistic regression models: a temporal and external validation study by the IOTA group. Ultrasound Obstet Gynecol. 2010;36(2):226-34.
51. Timor-Tritsch IE, Foley CE, Brandon C, Yoon E, Ciaffarrano J, Monteagudo A, et al. New sonographic marker of borderline ovarian tumor: microcystic pattern of papillae and solid components. Ultrasound Obstet Gynecol. 2019;54(3):395-402.
52. Tingulstad S, Hagen B, Skjeldestad FE, Halvorsen T, Nustad K, Onsrud M. The risk-of-malignancy index to evaluate potential ovarian cancers in local hospitals. Obstet Gynecol. 1999;93(3):448-52.
53. Valentin L, Ameye L, Franchi D, Guerriero S, Jurkovic D, Savelli L, et al. Risk of malignancy in unilocular cysts: a study of 1148 adnexal masses classified as unilocular cysts at transvaginal ultrasound and review of the literature. Ultrasound Obstet Gynecol. 2013;41(1):80-9.
54. Valentin L, Ameye L, Savelli L, Fruscio R, Leone FP, Czekierdowski A, et al. Adnexal masses difficult to classify as benign or malignant using subjective assessment of gray-scale and Doppler ultrasound findings: logistic regression models do not help. Ultrasound Obstet Gynecol. 2011;38(4):456-65.
55. Valentin L, Ameye L, Savelli L, Fruscio R, Leone FP, Czekierdowski A, et al. Unilocular adnexal cysts with

papillary projections but no other solid components: is there a diagnostic method that can classify them reliably as benign or malignant before surgery? Ultrasound Obstet Gynecol. 2013;41(5):570-81.

56. Valentin L, Hagen B, Tingulstad S, Eik-Nes S. Comparison of 'pattern recognition' and logistic regression models for discrimination between benign and malignant pelvic masses: a prospective cross validation. Ultrasound Obstet Gynecol. 2001;18(4):357-65.
57. Valentin L. (2018). International Ovarian Tumor Analysis (IOTA) methods for discriminating between benign and malignant adnexal masses. [Online] Available from https://www.gynekologen.no/artikler/international-ovarian-tumor-analysis-iota [Last accessed July, 2025].
58. Valentin L. Comparison of Lerner score, Doppler ultrasound examination, and their combination for discrimination between benign and malignant adnexal masses. Ultrasound Obstet Gynecol. 2000;15(2):143-7.
59. Valentin L. Pattern recognition of pelvic masses by gray-scale ultrasound imaging: the contribution of Doppler ultrasound. Ultrasound Obstet Gynecol. 1999;14(5):338-47.
60. Valentin L. Prospective cross-validation of Doppler ultrasound examination and gray-scale ultrasound imaging for discrimination of benign and malignant pelvic masses. Ultrasound Obstet Gynecol. 1999;14(4):273-83.
61. Van Calster B, Timmerman D, Bourne T, Testa AC, Van Holsbeke C, Domali E, et al. Discrimination between benign and malignant adnexal masses by specialist ultrasound examination versus serum CA-125. J Natl Cancer Inst. 2007;99(22):1706-14.
62. Van Calster B, Van Hoorde K, Froyman W, Kaijser J, Wynants L, Landolfo C, et al. Practical guidance for applying the ADNEX model from the IOTA group to discriminate between different subtypes of adnexal tumors. Facts Views Vision ObGyn. 2015;7(1):32-41.
63. Van Calster B, Van Hoorde K, Valentin L, Testa AC, Fischerova D, Van Holsbeke C, et al. Evaluating the risk of ovarian cancer before surgery using the ADNEX model to differentiate between benign, borderline, early and advanced stage invasive, and secondary metastatic tumours: prospective multicentre diagnostic study. BMJ. 2014:349:g5920.
64. Van den Bosch T, Dueholm M, Leone FP, Valentin L, Rasmussen CK, Votino A, et al. Terms, definitions and measurements to describe sonographic features of myometrium and uterine masses: a consensus opinion from the Morphological Uterus Sonographic Assessment (MUSA) group. Ultrasound Obstet Gynecol. 2015;46(3):284-98.
65. Van Holsbeke C, Van Calster B, Guerriero S, Savelli L, Paladini D, Lissoni AA, et al. Endometriomas: their ultrasound characteristics. Ultrasound Obstet Gynecol. 2010;35(6):730-40.
66. Vijayaraghavan SB. Sonographic whirlpool sign in ovarian torsion. J Ultrasound Med. 2004;23(12):1643-9.
67. Xholli A, Scovazzi U, Londero AP, Paudice M, Vacca I, Schiaffino MG, et al.; Collaborators. Clinical and ultrasonographic characteristics of pregnancy-related enhanced myometrial vascularity: prospective cohort study. Ultrasound Obstet Gynecol. 2024;63(5):672-82.
68. Zappacosta R, Fanfani F, Zappacosta B, Sablone F, Pansa L, Liberati M, et al. Uterine Sarcomas: An Updated Overview. Part 1: Smooth Muscle Tumors. In: Shahzad HN (Ed). Neoplasm. IntechOpen; 2018.

51

CHAPTER

Ultrasound in Infertility

Vidyashree G Poojari, Muralidhar V Pai

Chapter Outline

- Method
- Uterine Abnormalities
- Cycle Assessment Consisting of Baseline Scan, Preovulatory Scan and Secretory Scan

INTRODUCTION

Ultrasound has been widely used for the assessment of infertile couples. It is used for the assessment of subfertile females as well as for the assessment of subfertile males. The female factors leading to fertility problems are abnormal ovulation, abnormal fallopian tubes and tubo-ovarian relationship, abnormal endometrium or intrauterine environment and non-sperm-friendly cervical environment and amongst the male factor, it is abnormal semen parameters, which may be in the form of abnormal count, motility or morphology.

Assessment of the female includes a detailed study of the uterus, fallopian tubes and ovaries, chiefly. Transabdominal and transvaginal are the two scan route options for the same. Usually, the assessment is started with the transabdominal scan. This allows the assessment of the abdominal and pelvic organs together. Among the assessment of the abdominal organs, the most important in the infertile females is the assessment of the kidneys. It is well known that abnormalities of the uterus are often associated with renal abnormalities. Abdominal scans appear to be easier to interpret and also to understand the orientation **(Figs. 1A and B)**.

But the disadvantage of transabdominal scan is lower resolution as the abdominal organs are placed far from the probe, so low-frequency probes are used, and this gives less resolution. Approximately 42% of ovarian details are missed by transabdominal scan.

Transvaginal or intracavitary probes are high-frequency probes (6–12 or 5–9 MHz) and therefore inherently have

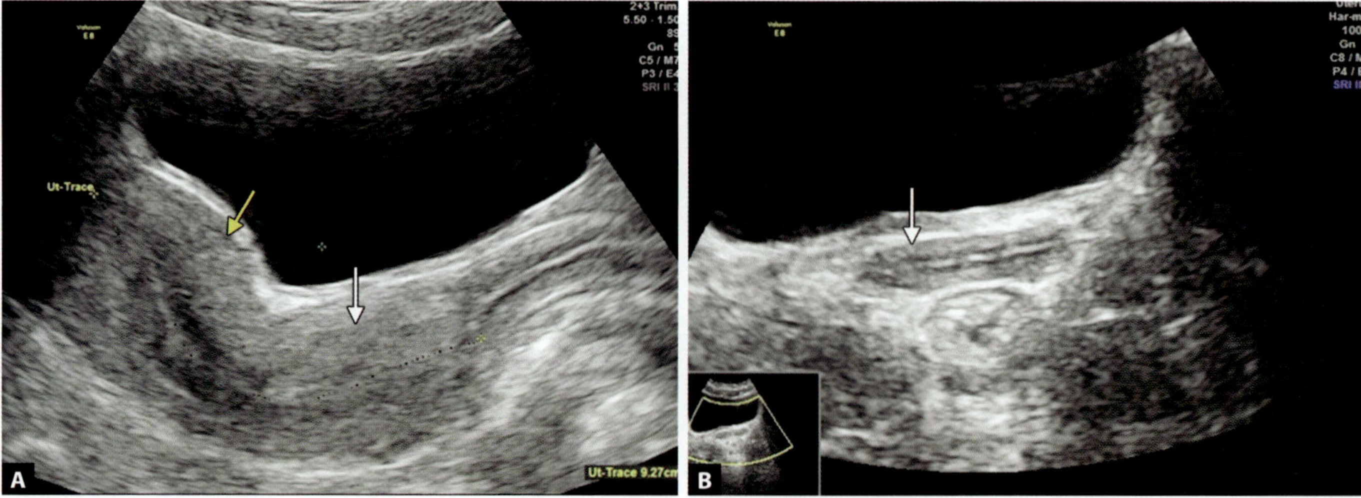

Figs. 1A and B: Longitudinal and transverse sections of the uterus as seen on transabdominal scan. Yellow arrow shows the body of the uterus and white arrow shows the cervix.

better resolution. Transvaginal ultrasound is therefore a primary investigation in these patients.

METHOD

For transvaginal scans, at least a verbal consent of the patient is essential. The patient is asked to empty the bladder. She is placed in lithotomy position on the gynaec couch in the same way as for per speculum or per vaginal examination. Gynaec couch is preferred to a simple bed as it allows free mobility of the probe. Ultrasound gel is placed on the head of the transvaginal probe, and then the probe is covered with the condom, not to allow any air between the probe and the condom. A small amount of gel is then placed over the condom on the probe head and the probe is gently slid into the patient's vagina. Counselling the patient before examination and explaining the whole procedure and ensuring adequate privacy help eliminate the anxiety and resistance. In case of difficulty in introduction of probe or patient's resistance to introduction, she is advised to take deep long breaths with open mouth, i.e. deep inspirations and long complete expirations. In spite of that if introduction of probe needs any force, the pressure should be exerted posteriorly towards the rectum which will make introduction of the probe into the vagina easier. Probe is introduced in the longitudinal position. That is the position in which the indicators on the probe remain up, facing the roof of the room that correlates with the anterior aspect of the patient **(Fig. 2)**.

These indicators on the probe match the indicator (logo of the company) **(Fig. 3)** on the screen. This means that if the indicator on the screen is on the right side of the screen, the structures anteriorly placed are on the right side of the screen and vice versa. Transverse section is achieved by 90° anticlockwise rotation of the probe. On this manoeuvre, the image achieved shows the right side of the patient on the right side of the screen and the left side of the patient on the left side of the screen.

Applications of transvaginal ultrasound and Doppler in an infertile female can be divided under two main headings:

1. Diagnosis of abnormalities causing subfertility
2. Cycle assessment

Diagnosis of abnormalities causing subfertility:

- *Uterine abnormalities:* Congenital and acquired
- Ovarian abnormalities
- Tubal lesions

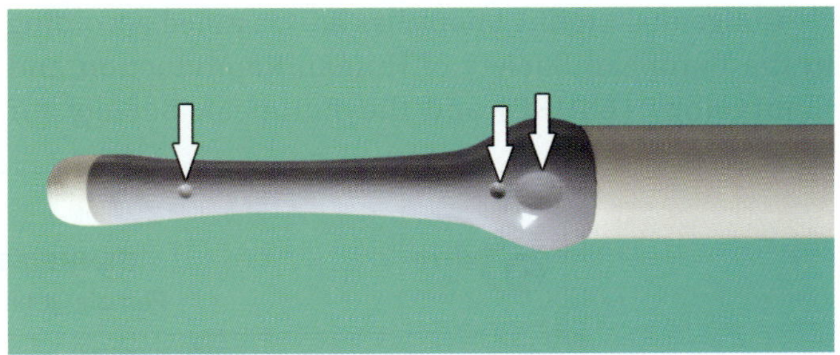

Fig. 2: Transvaginal volume probe with the markers shown by arrows.

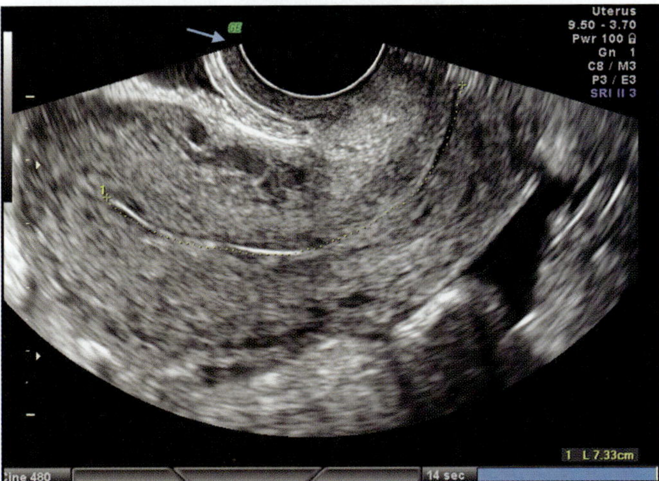

Fig. 3: Longitudinal section of the uterus showing the logo by arrow, corresponding with the anterior aspect of the patient.

TABLE 1: Sensitivity and specificity of various ultrasound methods.

Ultrasound	*Sensitivity (%)*	*Specificity (%)*
TVS	95.21	92.21
TVCD PD	99.29	97.23
Volume USG	98.38	100
Sonohysterography	98.18	100

(PD: power Doppler; TVCD: transvaginal colour Doppler; TVS: transvaginal sonography; USG: ultrasonography)

UTERINE ABNORMALITIES

Congenital Uterine Abnormalities

The incidence of congenital uterine abnormalities is 0.1–3.8% in normal fertile females but reaches 6.7% in infertile patients. Sensitivity and specificity of various ultrasound methods for the diagnosis of congenital uterine abnormalities are given in **Table 1**.

Congenital uterine anomalies are classified according to the European Society of Human Reproduction and Embryology (ESHRE) and the European Society for Gynaecological Endoscopy (ESGE) classification **(Figs. 4 and 5)**. This has been claimed to be more accurate, clear and correlated with clinical management and is

eshre | ESGE

ESHRE/ESGE classification
Female genital tract anomalies

	Uterine anomaly		
	Main class	***Subclass***
U0	Normal uterus	
U1	Dysmorphic uterus	a. T-shaped b. Infantilis c. Others
U2	Septate uterus	a. Partial b. Complete
U3	Bicorporeal uterus	a. Partial b. Complete c. Bicorporeal septate
U4	Haemi-uterus	a. With rudimentrary cavity (communicating or not horn) b. Without rudimentary cavity (horn without cavity/no horn)
U5	Aplastic	a. With rudimentrary cavity (bilateral or unilateral horn) b. Without rudimentary cavity (bilateral or unilateral uterine remnants/aplasia)
U6	Unclassified malformations	
U		

Cervical/vaginal anomaly	
Coexistent class	
C0	*Normal cervix*
C1	*Septate cervix*
C2	*Double 'normal' cervix*
C3	*Unilateral cervical aplasia*
C4	*Cervical aplasia*
V0	*Normal vagina*
V1	*Longitudinal non-obstructing vaginal septum*
V2	*Longitudinal obstructing vaginal septum*
V3	*Transverse vaginal septum and/or imperforate hymen*
V4	*Vaginal aplasia*
C	***V***

Fig. 4: European Society of Human Reproduction and Embryology (ESHRE)/European Society for Gynaecological Endoscopy (ESGE) classification described in tabular form.

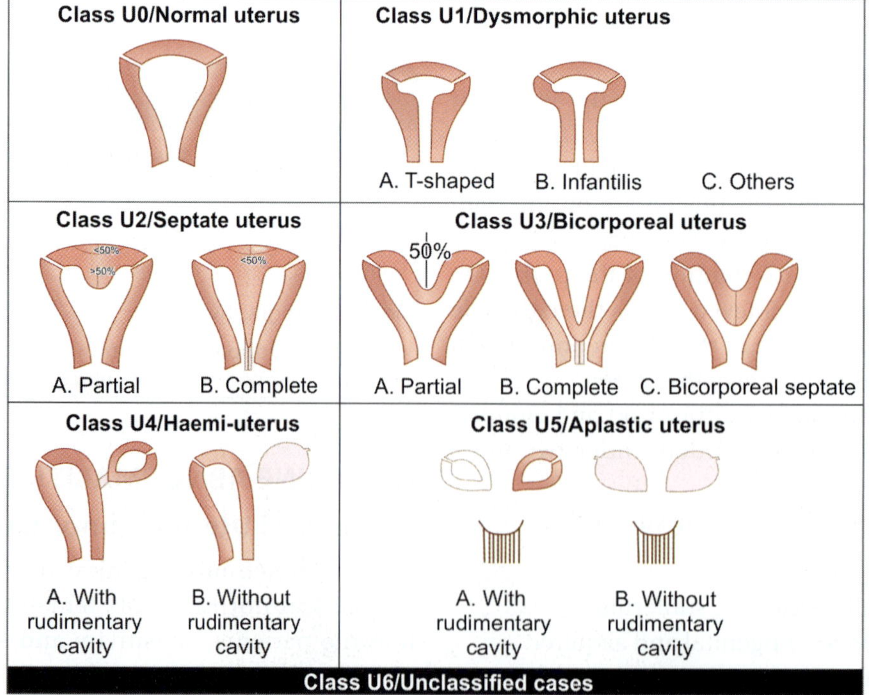

Fig. 5: Diagrammatic demonstration of congenital uterine abnormalities according to ESHRE/ESGE classification. (ESHRE: European Society of Human Reproduction and Embryology; ESGE: European Society for Gynaecological Endoscopy)

based on anatomy. It is a simple categorisation of female genital anomalies and also discusses cervical and vaginal anomalies and classifies these independently into subclasses. This system has been developed by a common working group under the name CONUTA (CONgenital UTerine Anomalies).

The details of the classification are given in the following text.

Class U0—Normal Uterus (Fig. 6)

Straight or curved interostial line but with an internal indentation at the fundal midline not exceeding 50% of the uterine wall thickness.

Class U1—Dysmorphic Uterus

Usually, dysmorphic uteri are smaller in size. Normal uterine fundal shape but with an abnormal shape of the endometrial cavity excluding septa:

- *Class U1a—T-shaped uterus* **(Fig. 7A)**: Narrow uterine cavity due to thickened lateral walls with normal uterocervical ratio (2:1)
- *Class U1b—uterus infantilis* **(Fig. 7B)**: Narrow uterine cavity without lateral wall thickening and an inverse uterocervical ratio
- *Class U1c—others* **(Fig. 8)**: Minor deformities of the uterine cavity, including those with an inner indentation at the fundal midline level of <50% of the uterine wall thickness

Class U2—Septate Uterus

- Normal fusion but abnormal absorption of the midline septum
- Shows normal fundal outline and an internal indentation at the fundal midline exceeding 50% of the uterine wall thickness
- The indentation may seep enough to divide partly or completely the uterine cavity, including in some cases of cervix and/or vagina

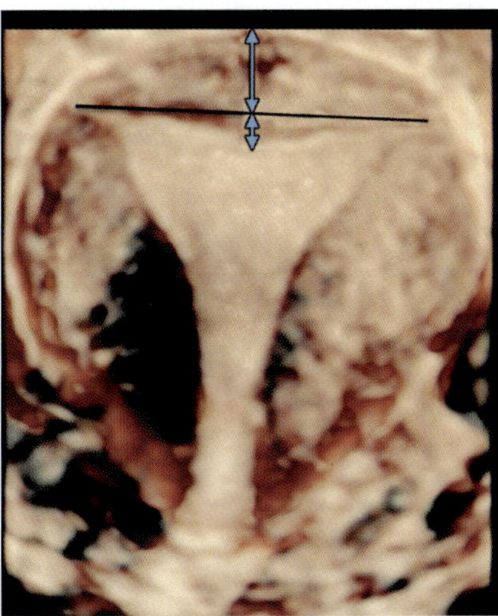

Fig. 6: 3D ultrasound image of the normal uterus, showing interostial line (black line) and the two blue arrow lines, the longer one indicating uterine wall thickness.

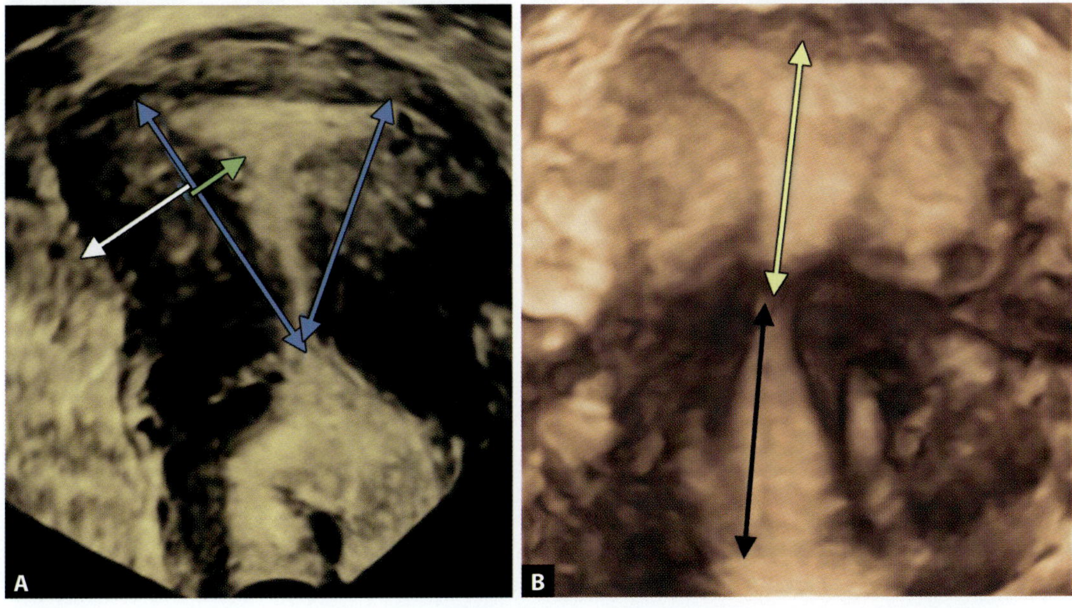

Figs. 7A and B: (A) Class U1a: T-shaped uterus; (B) Class U1b: hypoplastic uterus.

- *Class U2a* **(Fig. 9A)**—*partial septum:* Septum partially dividing the uterine cavity short of the internal cervical os
- *Class U2b* **(Fig. 9B)**—*complete septum:* Septum fully dividing the uterine cavity up to the level of the internal cervical os (may or may not have cervical and vaginal septum).

Class U3—Bicorporeal Uterus

External indentation at the fundal midline exceeding 50% of the uterine wall thickness and the inner indentation at the midline level that divides the cavity as happens also in case of septate uterus.

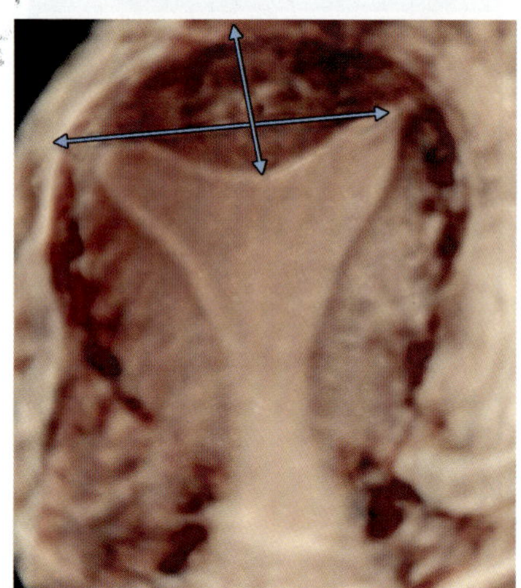

Fig. 8: Class U1c: Dysmorphic uterus.

- *Class U3a* **(Fig. 10A)**: Partial bicorporeal, where the external fundal indentation is partly dividing the uterine corpus above the level of the cervix.
- *Class U3b* **(Fig. 10B)**: Complete bicorporeal uterus, with external fundal indentation completely dividing the uterine corpus up to the level of the cervix.
- *Class U3c* **(Fig. 11)**: Bicorporeal septate uterus which is an absorption defect in addition to the main fusion defect. The width of the midline fundal indentation exceeds by 150% the uterine wall.

Class U4—Haemi-uterus

It is a formation defect. It is unilateral uterine development. The contralateral part could be either incompletely formed or absent. This group is further divided into two subclasses depending on the presence or not of a functional rudimentary cavity.

- Class U4a **(Figs. 12A and B)** or haemi-uterus with a rudimentary (functional) cavity which may be communicating or non-communicating with haemi-uterus
- Class U4b **(Figs. 12C)** or haemi-uterus without rudimentary (functional) cavity with non-functional contralateral uterine horn or by aplasia of the contralateral part.

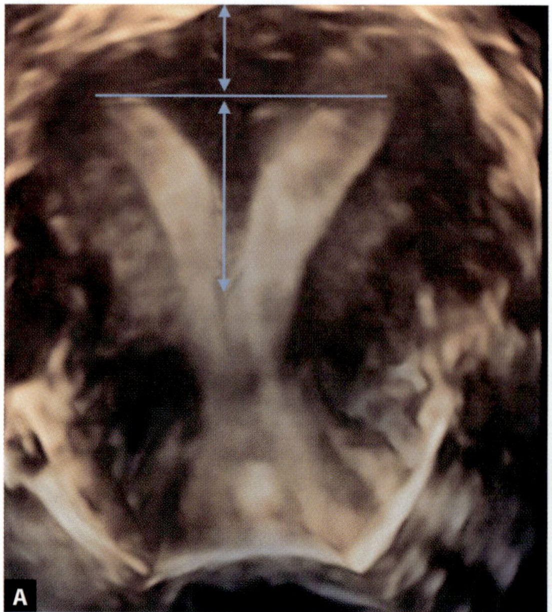

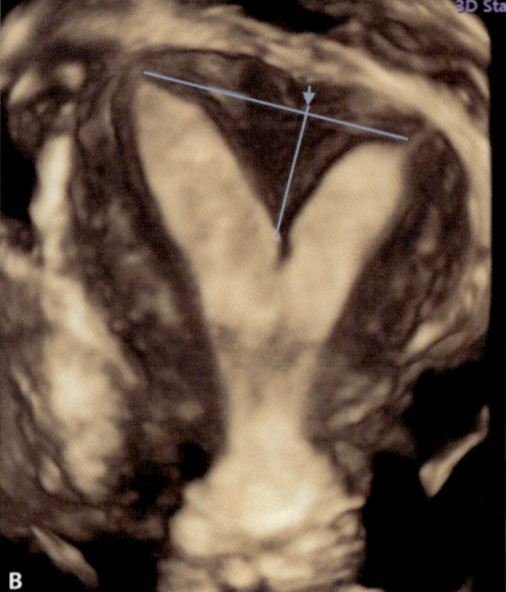

Figs. 9A and B: (A) Complete septum; (B) Partial septum.

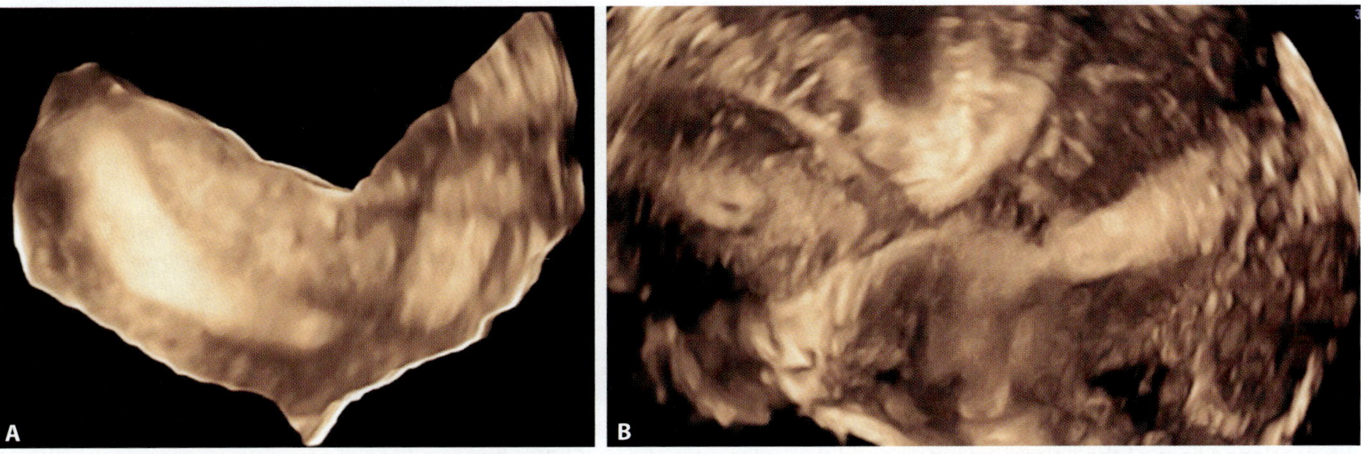

Figs. 10A and B: (A) Class U3a: Partial bicorporeal uterus; (B) Class U3b: Complete bicorporeal uterus.

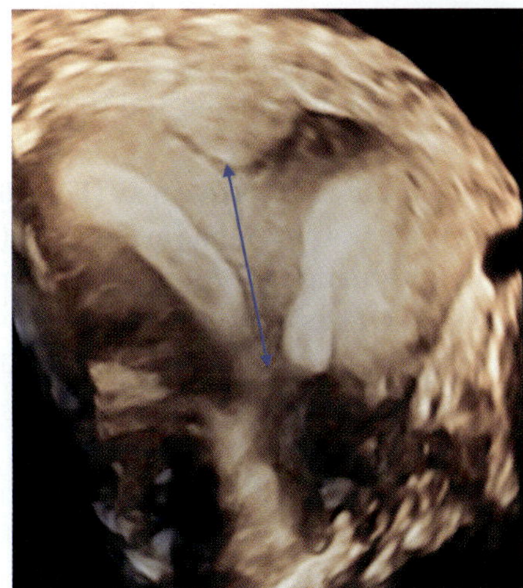

Fig. 11: Class U3c: Bicorporeal septate uterus.

Class U5—Aplastic Uterus–Uterus Aplasia

Absence of any fully or unilaterally developed uterine cavity **(Fig. 13)**. Unilateral or bilateral rudimentary horns with cavity may be seen in some, while in others there could be uterine remnants without cavity. Co-existent defects (e.g. vaginal aplasia/Mayer-Rokitansky-Küster-Hauser syndrome) are common with this group of abnormalities.

- *Class U5a:* Aplastic uterus with rudimentary (functional) bilateral or unilateral functional horn
- *Class U5b:* Aplastic uterus without rudimentary (functional) cavity.

Class U6—Unclassified Cases

- These are infrequent anomalies, subtle changes or combined pathologies that could not be allocated correctly to one of the six groups.
- The classification of cervical canal anomalies and vaginal anomalies also is an additional advantage.
    - C0—normal cervix **(Fig. 14A)**
    - C1—septate cervix **(Fig. 14B)**
    - C2—double normal cervix **(Fig. 14C)** can be confidently diagnosed by three-dimensional (3D) ultrasound. However, unilateral cervical aplasia which constitutes C3 class cannot be easily diagnosed on ultrasound. Cervical aplasia is rare.

Acquired Uterine Abnormalities

- Myometrial lesions
- Endometrial lesions
- Cervical lesions

Myometrium is normally homogeneously hypoechoic and the serosal surface is smooth and regular. Distortion in any of these two suggests myometrial lesion.

Myometrial lesions are fibroids, adenomyosis, adenomyomas and leiomyosarcomas.

Fibroid

Fibroids are found in 20–40% of women from age 30 years onwards and are more common in nulliparous women. These are well defined, hypoechoic, homogeneous, rounded, solid lesions, with peripheral hypoechoic rim due to displacement of myometrial fibres. Its echogenicity increases with the amount of fibrous tissue and vascularity. Fibroids may show calcification. Degeneration in fibroids causes heterogenicity of texture, or sometimes cystic degeneration may cause anechoic areas. Vascularity increases with degeneration or necrosis.

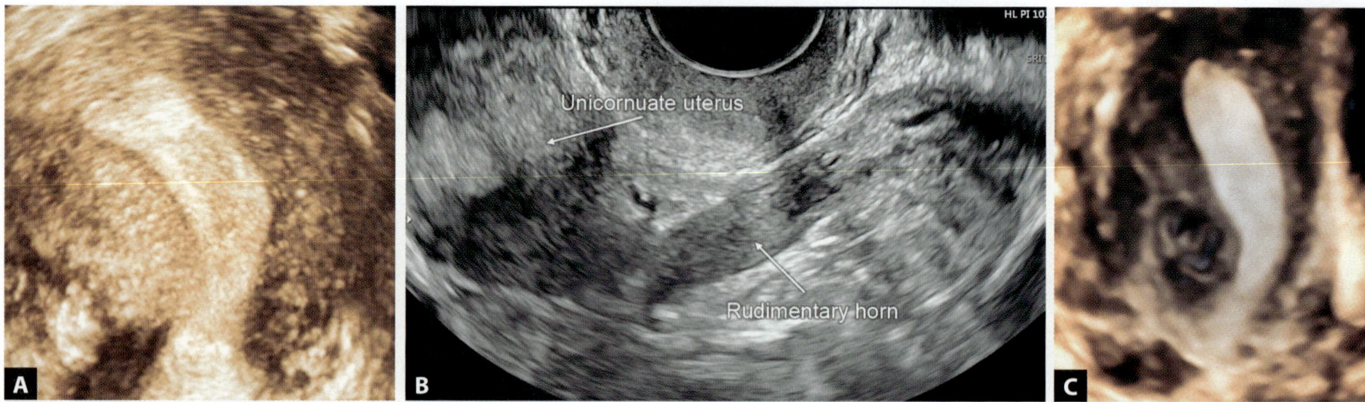

Figs. 12A to C: (A) 3D ultrasound image of the developed horn of unicornuate uterus; (B) B-mode image on transverse section showing the developed horn of the unicornuate uterus and the rudimentary horn; (C) 3D ultrasound image of a unicornuate uterus without rudimentary horn.

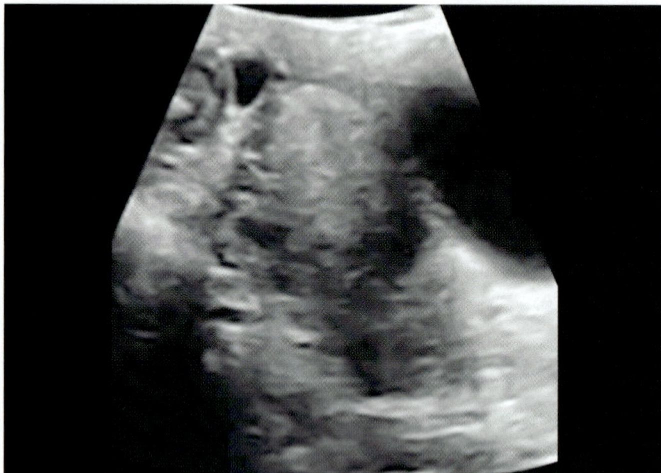

Fig. 13: B-mode image of the rudimentary horn of uterus.

Fibroids affect fertility because of:
- Distortion of endometrial cavity due to submucous fibroid
- Pressure of the fibroid and stretching of endometrium overlying it causing atrophy of endometrial glands and stroma
- Low flow due to stretching of vessels and less delivery of hormones.

Fibroids are classified according to their location as subserosal, intramural and submucosal **(Figs. 15A to C)**.

Subserosal and intramural fibroids are classified as:
- *Type 0:* Pedunculated subserosal fibroid
- *Type 1:* Involvement of <50% of the outer uterine wall
- *Type 2:* >50% of the myometrial wall
- *Type 3:* Fibroids extending from mucosa to serosa

Submucosal fibroids are classified as:
- *Type 0:* If they are pedunculated and 100% in the cavity **(Fig. 16A)**
- *Type 1:* If the fibroid is >50% in cavity **(Fig. 16B)**
- *Type 2:* If but if <50% is protruding in the cavity **(Fig. 16C)**.

But now the International Federation of Gynaecology and Obstetrics (FIGO) has developed a new classification system. This is a part of popularly known PALM-COEIN classification **(Fig. 17)**:
- *Class 0:* Intraendometrial pedunculated
- *Class 1:* Subendometrial with <50% of the fibroid intramural
- *Class 2:* Subendometrial with >50% of the fibroid intramural
- *Class 3:* 100% intramural fibroid, touching the endometrium
- *Class 4:* Intramural
- *Class 5:* Subserosal ≥50% intramural
- *Class 6:* Subserosal ≤50% intramural
- *Class 7:* Exophytic pedunculated subserosal fibroid
- *Class 8:* Others (cervical/parasitic, etc.)

For large fibroids, mention as two numbers where the first number indicates the relation to the endometrium and the second one to the serosa.

On colour Doppler: Peripheral vascularity is typical of a fibroid **(Fig. 18)**. These vessels are vessels of displaced muscle fibres and therefore show resistance similar to that of myometrium. Resistance is higher in submucosal fibroids and deep intramural fibroids and lower in subserosal fibroids. When degenerated, the fibroids show lower resistance with internal vascularity in addition to the

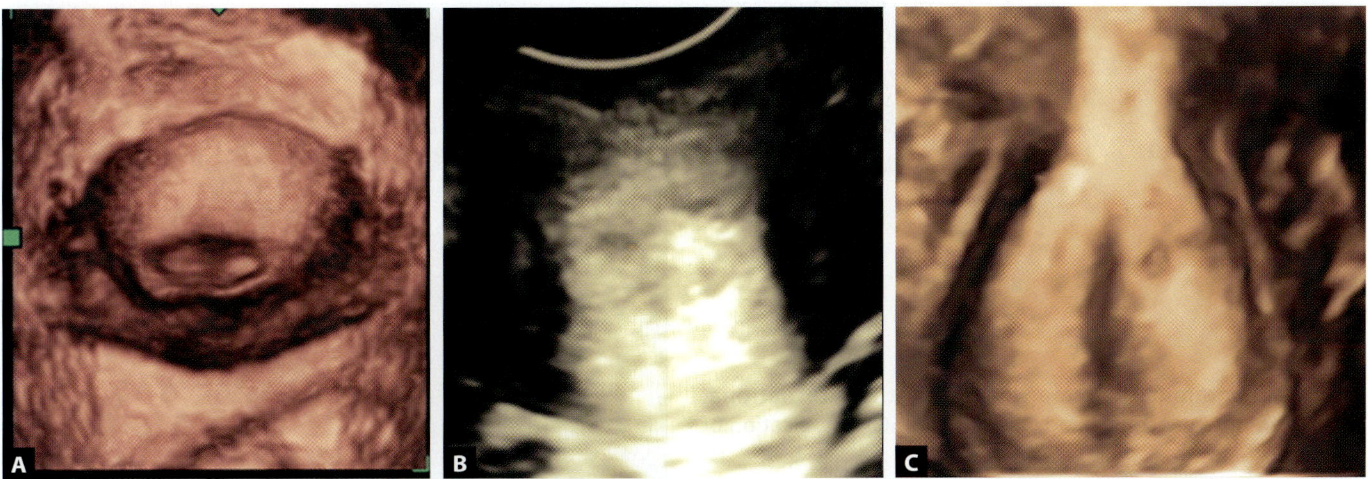

Figs. 14A to C: (A) Single normal cervix—C0; (B) Cervix with septum—C1; (C) Normal.

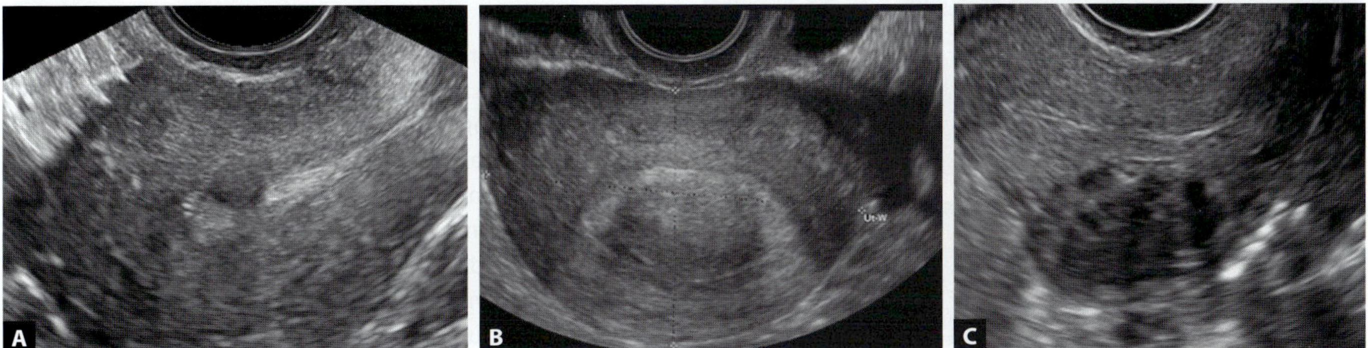

Figs. 15A to C: (A) Submucous; (B) Intramural; (C) Subserosal fibroid.

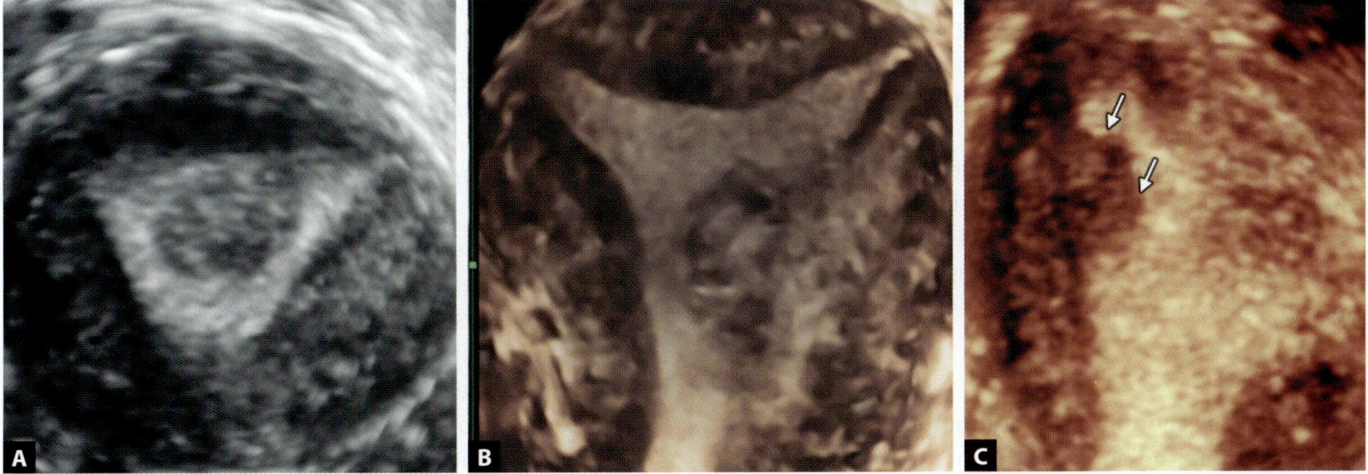

Figs. 16A to C: (A) Type 0; (B) Type 1; (C) Type 2 submucosal fibroids.

peripheral vascularity. The amount of vascularity decides the activity or growth potential of fibroid. Uteri with fibroids also show higher uterine artery peak velocity and lower resistance index (RI) (mean: 0.74 ± 0.09).

Volume ultrasound: Volume ultrasound is a perfect tool to assess the invasion or distortion of endometrial cavity. 3D power Doppler indices are especially useful for follow-up of fibroids in patients who are on gonadotrophin-releasing

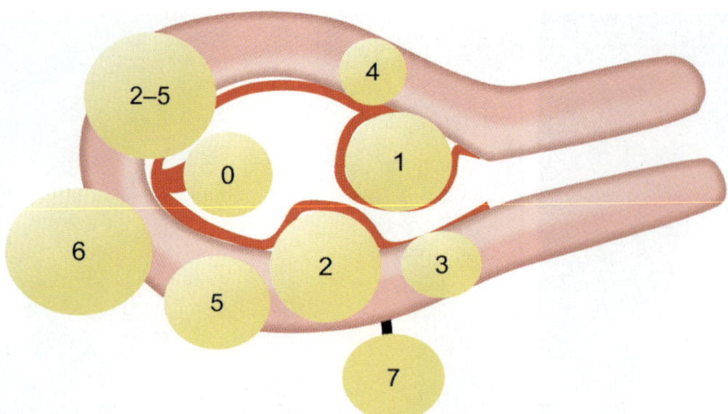

Fig. 17: Diagrammatic demonstration of the International Federation of Gynaecology and Obstetrics (FIGO) classification of fibroids.

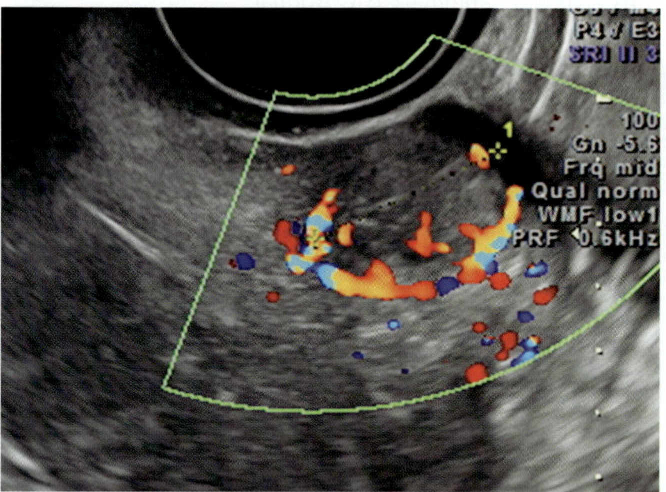

Fig. 18: Fibroid colour Doppler.

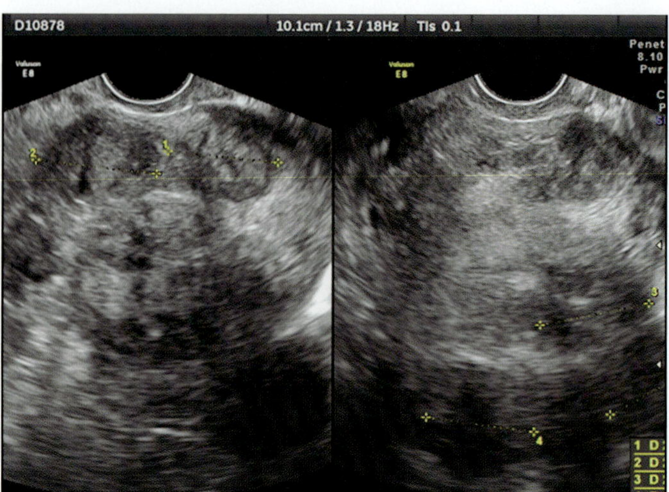

Fig. 19: Multiple fibroids—leiomyomatosis.

hormone analogue (GnRHa) therapy, menopausal or pregnant.

Diffuse leiomyomatosis is a rare condition in which there is diffuse and uniform involvement of the entire myometrium by multiple fibroids **(Fig. 19)**.

Fibroids are also seen arising from the cervix and show similar appearances to fibroid in the uterus.

Adenomyosis

Adenomyosis is common in multiparous women. It is an invasive lesion and so has indistinct margins. It may be generalised involving the whole uterus or localised to one wall or a part of one of the walls. When localised, it causes asymmetrical thickening of myometrium. These uteri are tender on probe pressure. On ultrasound, it shows heterogeneous echogenicity. Alternate hyperechoic and hypoechoic zones in myometrium are typically described as rain in forest appearance **(Fig. 20A)**. Echogenic spots and anechoic areas (myometrial cysts) are commonly seen typically known as salt-and-pepper appearance **(Fig. 20B)**. Echogenic flecks are seen close to junctional zone, and these are collapsed myometrial cysts **(Fig. 20A)**. Echogenic strands and areas are seen in relation to the endometrium. These are also commonly known as endometrial buds. Curvature of the fundal endometrial, commonly known as ear sign **(Fig. 20C)**, is also often seen in adenomyotic uteri.

Typically, the myometrium shows alteration in the echogenicity depending on the phase of the menstrual cycle. It is isoechoic in the follicular phase and hyperechoic in the secretory phase.

On colour Doppler, the affected myometrium shows markedly increased vascularity with vascular dilatation **(Fig. 20D)**. Decreased uterine artery resistance and increased velocity may be seen with large areas of adenomyosis.

The most difficult situation is the adenomyoma. This is a localised adenomyosis. When seen in the follicular phase, it appears hypoechoic like a fibroid, and if a fibroid is degenerated, it looks like adenomyoma. But like generalised adenomyosis, it alters its echogenicity with the phase of the cycle. The main differentiating point between the adenomyoma and the fibroid is the capsular vascularity that is seen in fibroid but is never seen in adenomyoma. When seen on 3D power Doppler also, a vascular fibroid shows circumferentially arranged vessels, while in adenomyoma, the vascular arrangement is radial or penetrating **(Figs. 21A and B)**. Endometrial strands extending into myometrium are also seen on 3D ultrasound **(Fig. 21C)**.

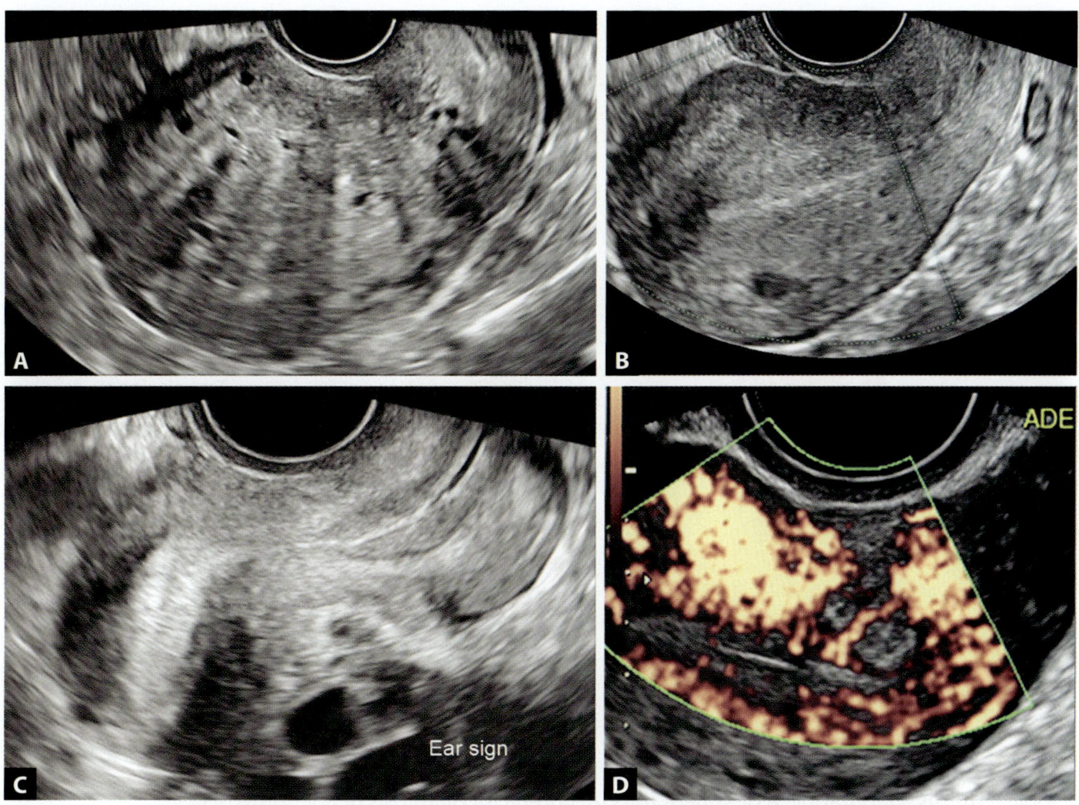

Figs. 20A to D: Adenomyosis uterus: (A) Swiss cheese and rain in forest appearance; (B) Heterogeneous echogenicity, salt-and-pepper appearance; (C) Ear sign; (D) Increased penetrating vascularity of adenomyosis.

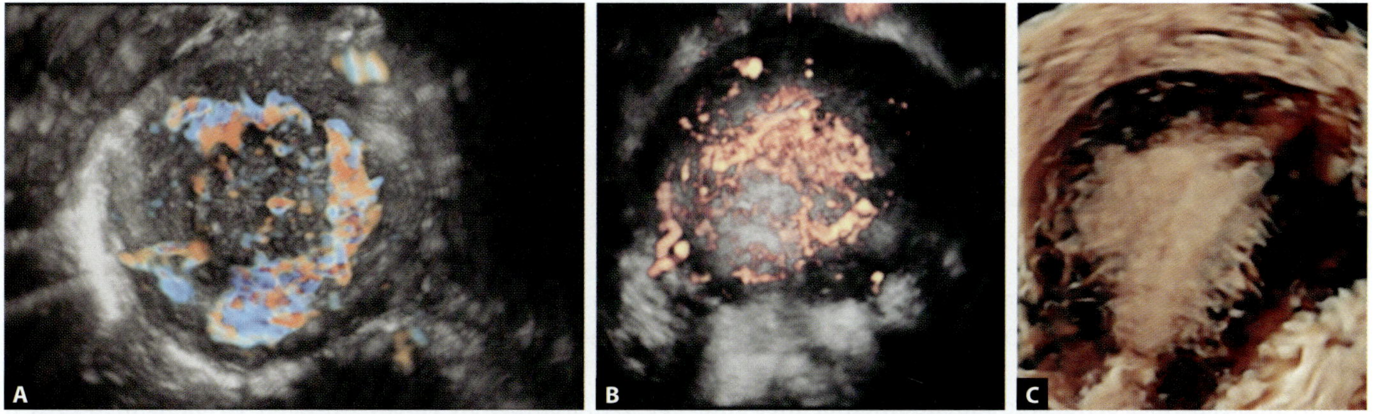

Figs. 21A to C: 3D power Doppler. (A) Degenerating fibroid; (B) Adenomyosis uterus; (C) Endometrial strands extending into the myometrium as seen on 3D ultrasound.

Morphological Uterus Sonographic Assessment (MUSA) criteria for the diagnosis of adenomyosis: Patient management is often based on ultrasound diagnosis alone. This highlights the importance of a uniform, reproducible and clinically relevant reporting system for ultrasound findings of adenomyosis. Uniform reporting system not only streamlines the assessment process but also enables comprehensive studies into adenomyosis prevalence, aetiology, clinical ramifications and treatment effectiveness. When evaluating a uterus for adenomyosis, attention should be given to seven key items for thorough examination and description:

1. *Presence:* Morphological Uterus Sonographic Assessment (MUSA) features typical of a uterus with adenomyosis include an enlarged globular uterus, asymmetrical thickening of the myometrium,

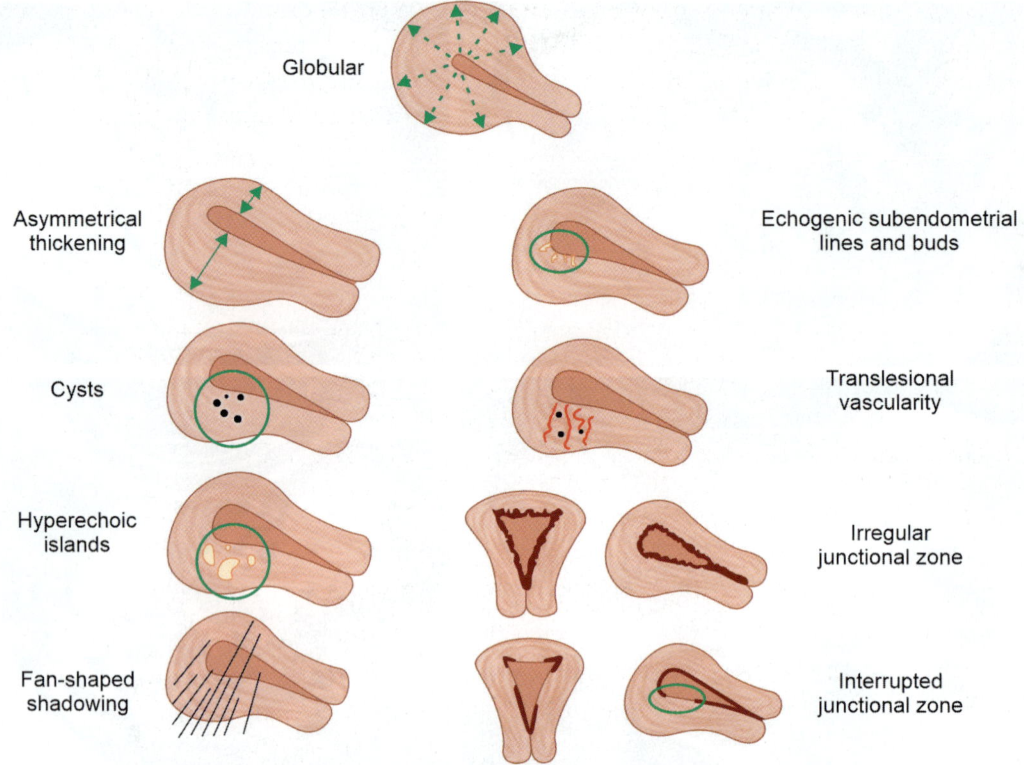

Fig. 22: Morphological Uterus Sonographic Assessment (MUSA) criteria for diagnosis of adenomyosis.
Source: Adapted from Van den Bosch T, Dueholm M, Leone FP, Valentin L, Rasmussen CK, Votino A, et al. Terms, definitions and measurements to describe sonographic features of myometrium and uterine masses: a consensus opinion from the Morphological Uterus Sonographic Assessment (MUSA) group. Ultrasound Obstet Gynecol. 2015;46:284-98.

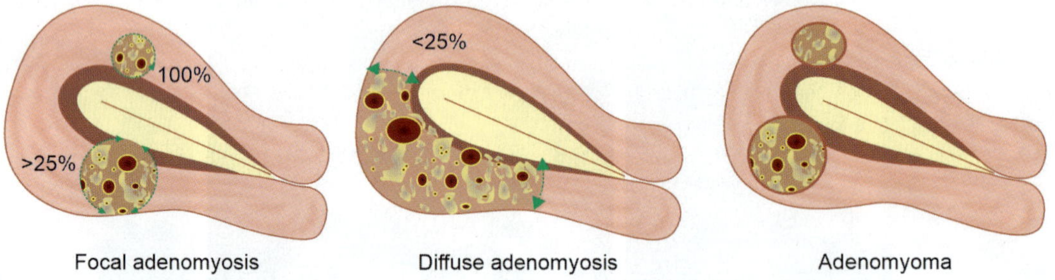

Fig. 23: Differentiation between focal and diffuse adenomyosis and adenomyoma.

myometrial cysts, echogenic subendometrial lines and buds, hyperechogenic islands, fan-shaped shadowing, an irregular or interrupted junctional zone and translesional vascularity on colour Doppler ultrasound examination **(Fig. 22)**.

2. *Location:* Describing the location of adenomyosis involves categorising it as anterior, posterior, lateral left, lateral right or fundal. To precisely identify its position, a comprehensive examination of the uterus should be conducted in both sagittal and transverse planes.
3. *Differentiation (focal/diffuse):* In each location, it should be determined whether the adenomyosis is focal or diffuse, by estimating the relative proportions of the lesion and the surrounding normal myometrium on a sagittal section through the uterus where the adenomyotic lesion appears to be at its largest **(Fig. 23)**.
4. *Cystic/non-cystic:* Adenomyosis should be classified as cystic or non-cystic. It is defined as cystic in the presence of measurable myometrial cysts, i.e., with largest diameter ≥2 mm **(Fig. 24)**.

5. *Uterine layer involvement:* Adenomyosis can affect any or all of the three layers of the uterus: (1) The junctional zone (inner myometrium, also known as the subendometrial layer, comprising tightly packed longitudinal and circular smooth muscle fibres), (2) the middle myometrium (situated between the vascular arcade and the junctional zone, composed of intersecting muscle fibres) and (3) the outer myometrium (subserosal layer, found between the serosa and the vascular arcade). Involvement of one of the three layers is recorded as type 1, 2 or 3, as appropriate. If more than one layer is involved, the type is recorded and described, e.g. as type 1–2, type 2–3 or type 1–3 **(Fig. 25)**.

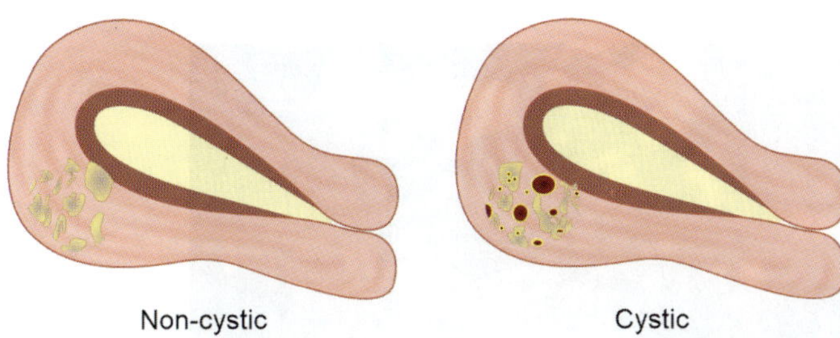

Fig. 24: Cystic and non-cystic focal adenomyosis.

6. *Extent:* The extent of the disease should be assessed subjectively, based on the estimated proportion of the uterine corpus that is affected by adenomyosis, and classified as: Mild (<25% affected), moderate (25–50% affected) or severe (>50% affected). If adenomyotic lesions are present in multiple locations, the sum of their volumes should be estimated to describe the overall extent of the disease.
7. *Size of lesion:* The largest diameter of the adenomyosis lesion(s) should be measured. In clinical situations, this should be done in the plane of the largest diameter of the largest lesion.

Endometrial Pathologies

Endometrium normally is pear-shaped and has an intact endometrio-myometrial junction (junctional zone) **(Fig. 26A)**. Distortion of endometrial contour and disruption of junctional zone are signs of endometrial pathologies.

Common endometrial pathologies are endometritis, polyps, endometrial hyperplasia, endometrial malignancies, synechia and other miscellaneous conditions with residual products of conception in endometrial cavity.

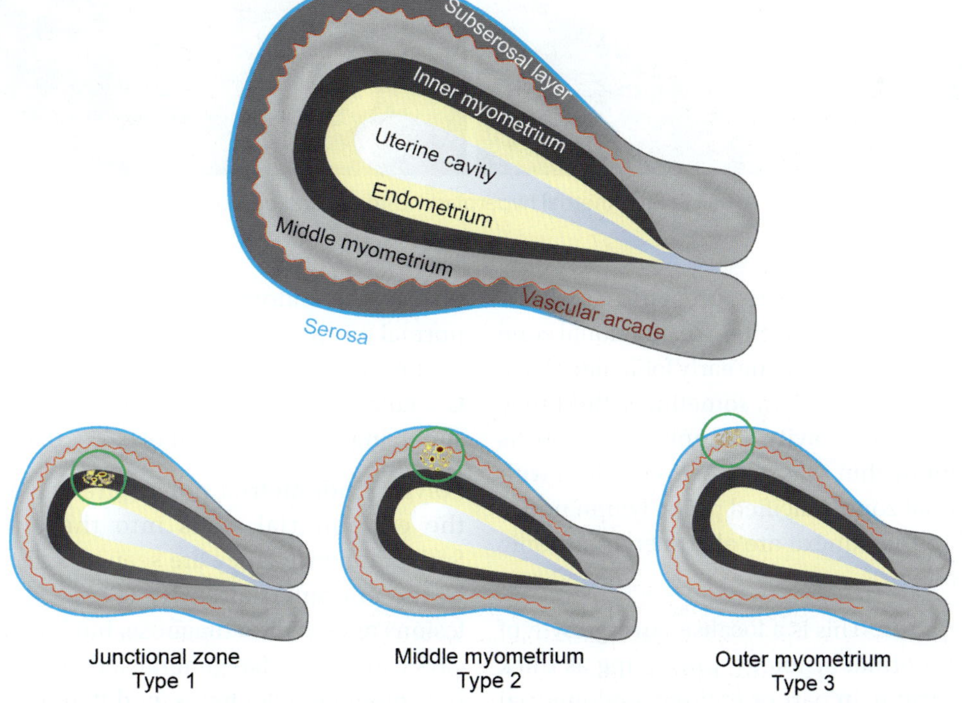

Fig. 25: Uterine layer infiltration. Diagrams are colour-coded as follows: Endometrium is yellow; junctional zone (inner myometrium) is dark grey; middle myometrium, located between vascular arcade (red) and junctional zone, is grey; outer myometrium (subserosa), located between vascular arcade and serosa, is also grey and serosa is blue.

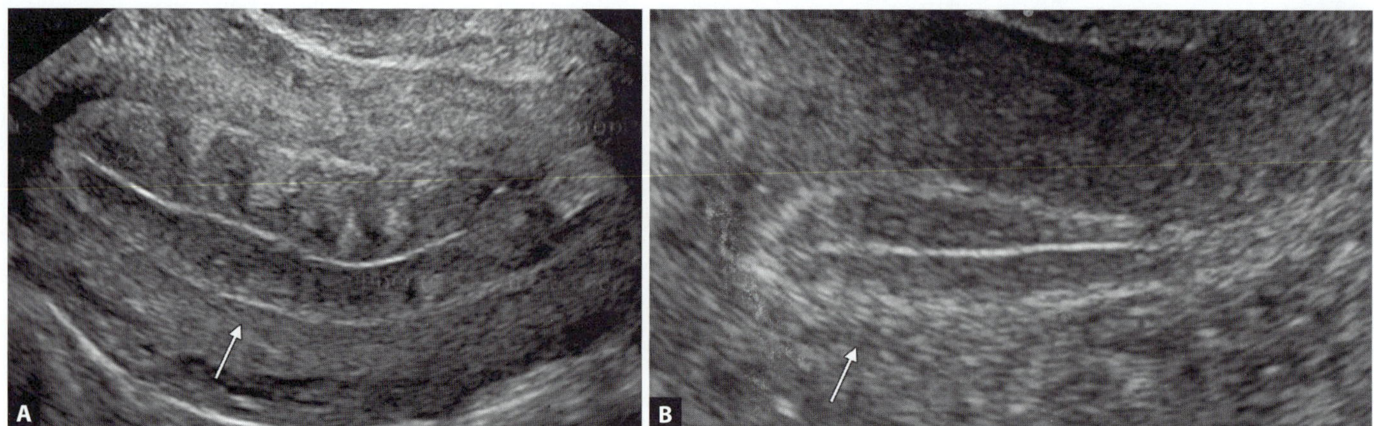

Figs. 26A and B: Endometritis. (A) Normal junctional zone; (B) Obliterated junctional zone.

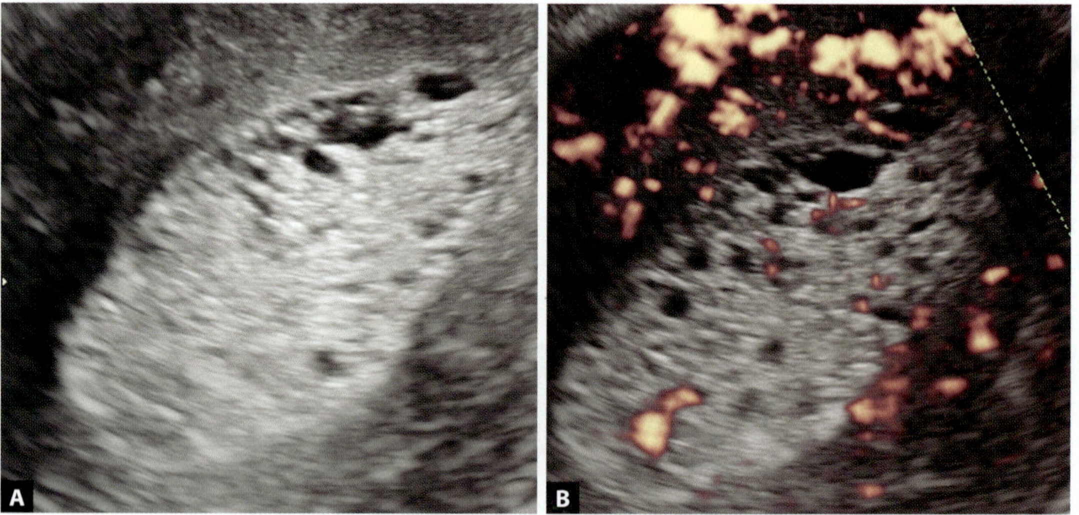

Figs. 27A and B: Endometrial hyperplasia: B-mode and power Doppler.

Endometritis: Acute endometritis presents as thick, isoechoic endometrium with disruption of junctional zone and increased vascularity, even in the early follicular phase **(Fig. 26B)**. In acute inflammation, sometimes, fluid may be seen in the endometrial cavity. Chronic endometritis presents as persistently thin avascular endometrium with a disrupted junctional zone. Calcified pelvic lymph nodes or calcified spots in the adnexa are also seen in chronic inflammatory lesions.

Endometrial hyperplasia: This is a localised overgrowth of endometrium with normal histology, presenting as thick echogenic endometrium, in part or entirely. Endometrial thickness >14 mm in a premenopausal patient and <5 mm in a postmenopausal patient is considered hypertrophic. But often in normal cycles in preovulatory or secretory phases, the endometrium may appear thicker than with normal morphology.

Endometrio-myometrial junction is well maintained. On colour Doppler, it shows regularly placed vessels supplying it with mean RI of 0.55 + 0.05 **(Figs. 27A and B)**.

Polyps: Endometrial polyps are projectile lesions from the endometrial walls into the endometrial cavity. Sonographically, they are seen as solid echogenic lesions in the endometrial cavity **(Figs. 28A and B)**. Smaller lesions are easier to diagnose, but larger lesions fill up the cavity and look like generalised endometrial thickening, but colour Doppler helps for differentiation.

On two-dimensional (2D) ultrasonography, the polyps are best visible in periovulatory phase or menstrual phase when there is fluid in the endometrial cavity. On Doppler,

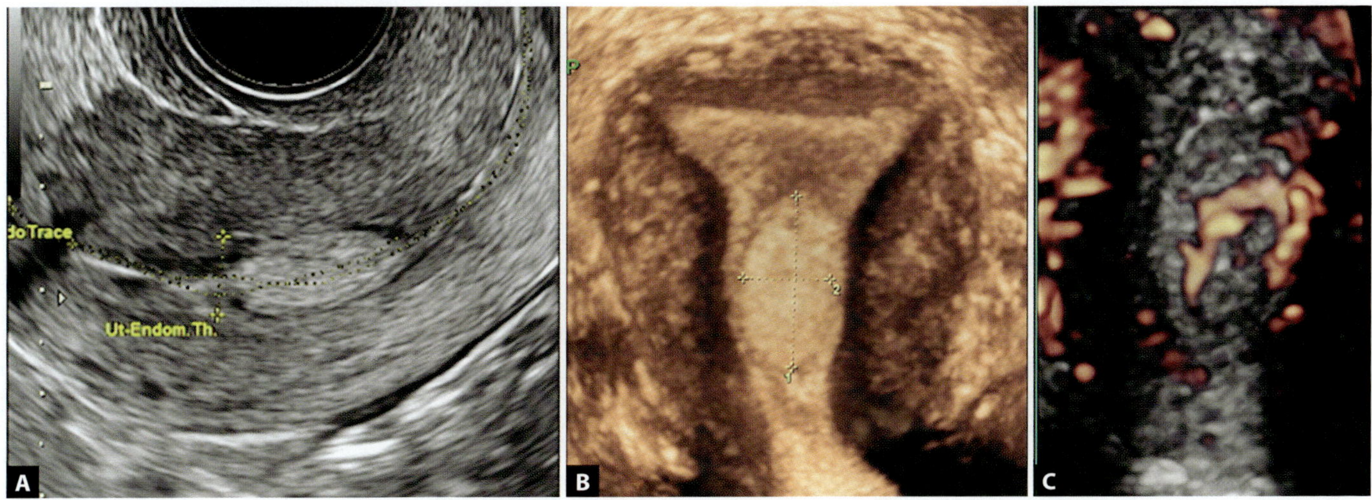

Figs. 28A to C: Endometrial polyp. (A) 2D ultrasonography; (B) 3D ultrasonography coronal view; (C) 3D colour Doppler showing two closely placed vessels in a pedicle of polyp.

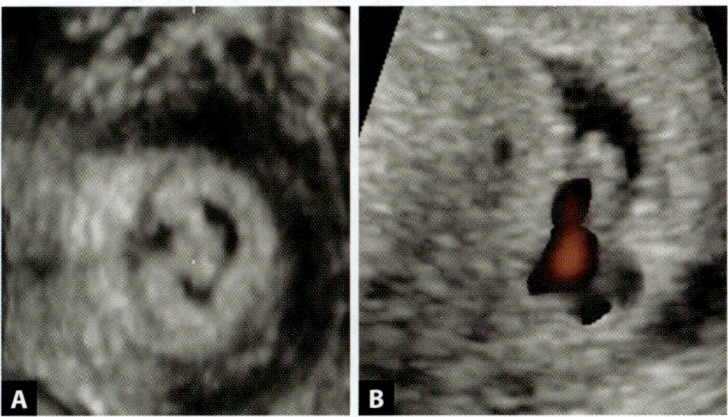

Figs. 29A and B: (A) 3D ultrasound showing cervical polyp; (B) 3D power Doppler of the same showing feeding vessel.

a polyp shows a single feeding vessel or maximum two vessels very closely placed (pedicular vessels) **(Fig. 28C)**. Infection, necrosis or atypia may show very low resistance. Vascular pattern has a high accuracy for differential diagnosis of endometrial lesions.

Polyps may arise in the cervix or may prolapse into cervix if these have long pedicle. Cervical polyps also show a single feeding vessel such as endometrial polyps **(Figs. 29A and B)**.

Single-vessel patterns for polyp:

- Sensitivity (81.2%)
- Specificity (88.2%)
- Positive predictive values (PPVs) (92.9%)
- Negative predictive values (NPVs) (71.4%).

Synechiae: When the endometrium is triple line or the cavity is distended with fluid, synechiae are seen as lines bridging between layers of endometrium **(Fig. 30A)**. In 3D ultrasonography, it helps in the exact assessment of restriction of cavity in case of bridging adhesions. Sonohysterography has 100% sensitivity for the differentiation of all endometrial pathologies **(Fig. 30B)**.

Sonohysterography is a simple procedure and can be done on outpatients. The patient is placed in a lithotomy position. A 6 French (external diameter: 1.6 mm, internal diameter: 1.1 mm) Foley catheter is placed in the cervix and the catheter balloon in the cervical canal. Distend balloon with 1.5–2 mL of fluid. Some may prefer a dedicated sonohysterography cannula. Remove all metal instruments and introduce the probe into the vagina with catheter in situ. Slowly inject 5 mL of normal saline with a 10-mL syringe to distend the uterine cavity. Ultrasound shows fluid-distended endometrial cavity. Endometrial lesions will be clearly seen **(Figs. 31A and B)**.

Other endometrial lesions are postcurettage endometrial collection, vesicular mole, missed abortion, incomplete abortion, etc. These are all avascular and show heterogeneous echogenicity. Clinical history guides to the diagnosis **(Figs. 32A and B)**.

Endometrial calcifications are common after curettage and medical termination of pregnancy **(Figs. 33A and B)**.

Whenever seen on B-mode ultrasound, 3D ultrasound is essential to find out the exact extent of the calcification.

Adnexal lesions can be categorised as:

- Ovarian lesions
- Tubal/tubo-ovarian lesions
- *Miscellaneous lesions:* Paraovarian cysts, peritoneal inclusion cyst and broad ligament fibroids.

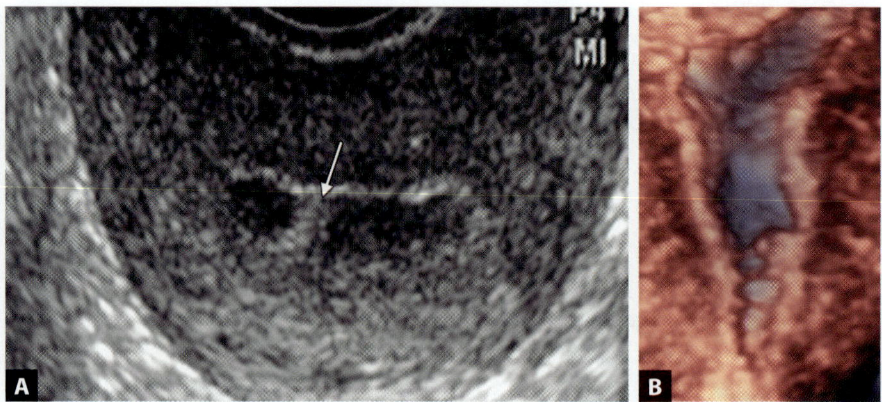

Figs. 30A and B: Synechiae. (A) 2D ultrasonography; (B) Synechiae on sonohysterography.

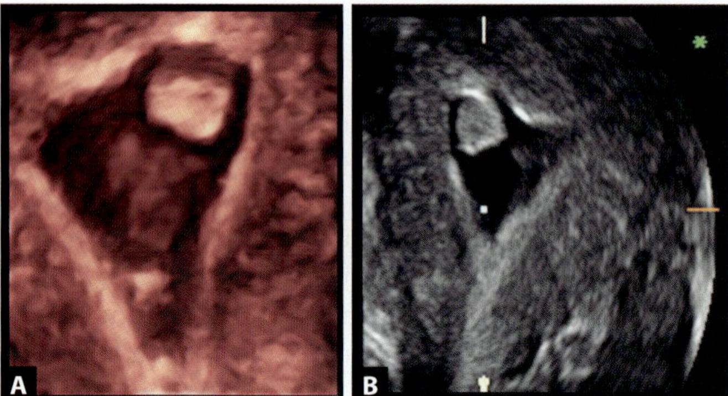

Figs. 31A and B: Sonohysterography showing polyp on (A) 3D rendering in coronal view and (B) 3D volume, tomographic ultrasound imaging in coronal view showing pedicle of the polyp.

Ovarian Lesions

Before describing a lesion, it is important to decide the origin of the lesion. To confirm its ovarian or extraovarian origin, place a probe in such a way that the lesion and the ovary are seen in the same frame on the screen. Apply pressure with the probe to separate the two. If probe pressure can displace the two away from each other, the lesion is not arising from the ovary. If the two cannot be separated, the lesion is either adherent to the ovary or is arising from the ovary. If the lesion is arising from the ovary, the lesion will be partially or completely covered by normal ovarian tissue and is typically described as a *rim sign* or *beak sign* **(Fig. 34)**.

Having confirmed the origin of the lesion from the ovary, the differential diagnosis of these lesions can be thought of. We would prefer to do this by dividing these lesions into different categories based on their ultrasound appearance.

Ultrasound-based classification of ovarian lesions:

- Nonseptated clear cysts
- Cysts with internal echogenicities and septae
- Solid lesions
- Complex lesions with cystic with solid areas.

Nonseptated clear cysts: These cysts are thin-walled and have no internal echogenicities, no septae or no solid areas in them. The lesions/structures in this category are:

- Follicular cyst
- Simple cyst of the ovary

Follicular cyst: Follicle starts growing in the early follicular phase. It grows till 18–24 mm in diameter before it ruptures due to the surge of luteinising hormone to release the ovum that it contains. If the surge is inadequate or does not occur, the follicle will not rupture and will result in a hormonally inactive/only minimally active structure. This is termed a follicular cyst when it grows beyond 25 mm and persists in the luteal phase of the cycle or even in the subsequent cycle. Contrary to the normal follicle, the follicular cyst shows scanty and high-resistance flow. But it is ultimately a physiological cyst and would resolve on its own.

Simple cyst of the ovary: It is a thin-walled intraovarian cystic structure usually >5 cm. Doppler shows no flow. It does not resolve on its own and may require ultrasound-guided aspiration usually.

Of course, follicles can be differentiated from these structures by their active low-resistance flow.

Cysts with internal echogenicities and septae: The most common lesions in these categories are:

- Corpus luteum
- Haemorrhagic cyst

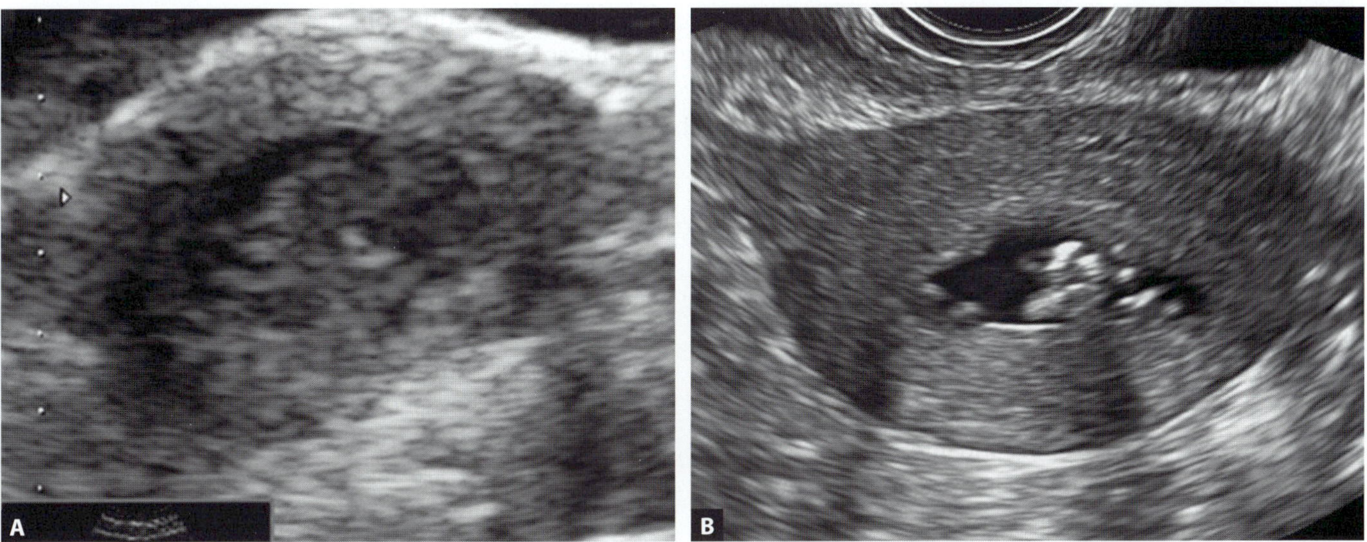

Figs. 32A and B: (A) Heterogeneous content in endometrial cavity: Postcurettage; (B) Incomplete abortion.

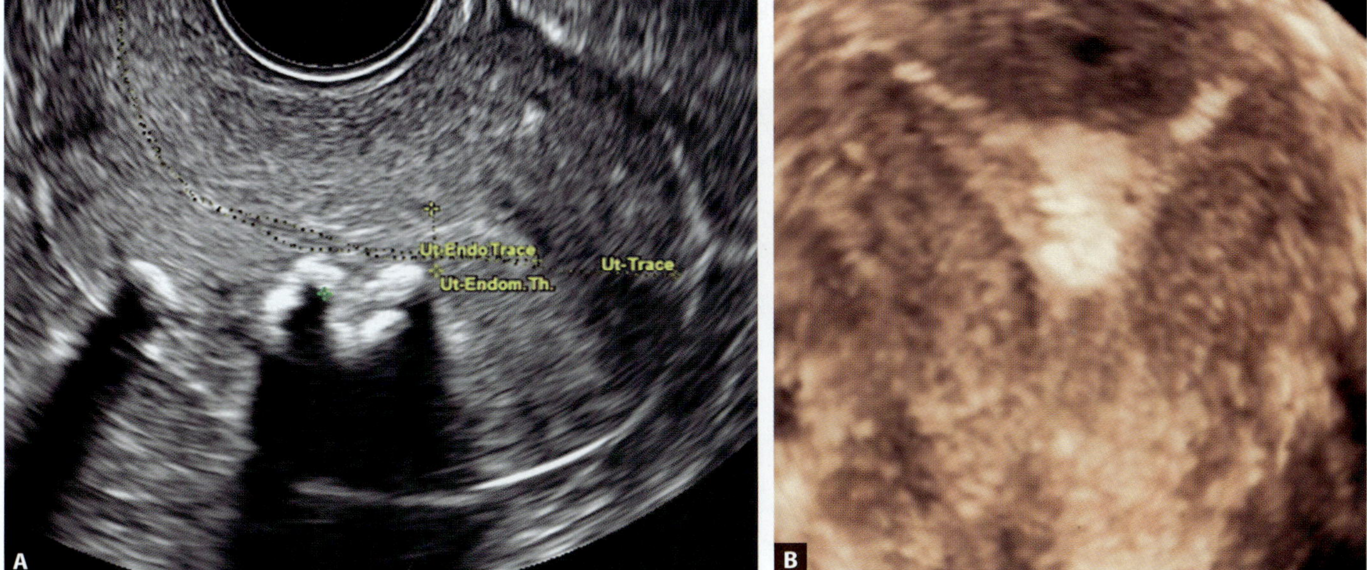

Figs. 33A and B: Endometrial calcification. (A) 2D; (B) 3D.

- Luteinised unruptured follicle (LUF)
- Endometrioma

All these structures have thick, shaggy walls, internal echogenicities and non-vascularised septae. The appearance may vary, namely absolutely isoechoic homogeneous, clear fluid, lace-like or cobweb pattern or ground-glass appearance.

Corpus luteum: It has thick, crenulated walls. Contents of the cyst show heterogeneous echogenicity with or without septae. The echogenicity and appearance of the contents may change at different times. Doppler gives almost a complete ring of colour with low resistance (RI <0.5). That is the most characteristic feature to separate it from other lesions with similar appearance on B-mode **(Figs. 35A to C)**.

Haemorrhagic cyst: It is a cyst containing blood. It is most of the times a result of an unresolved corpus luteum, but it is hormonally inactive and therefore shows very scanty and high-resistance blood flow. It changes echogenicity over time due to fibrinolysis of the clot **(Fig. 36)**.

Luteinised unruptured follicle: It has thick, hyperechoic but not very shaggy walls and does not contain blood or blood products. Therefore, it does show low-level internal echogenicity but not lace-like or cobweb echogenicity usually **(Fig. 37)**.

The three above-described lesions are physiologic ovarian cysts, and 53–89% of these show spontaneous regression on follow-up after 4–6 weeks. To avoid confusing these with other lesions, two examinations 2–3 weeks apart should be done so that assessment can be done in two different phases of the menstrual cycle, and complete or partial resolution of these lesions can be demonstrated.

Endometrioma: Endometriosis is detected in 15% of infertile women. It may cause acquired dysmenorrhoea, dyspareunia, irregular bleeding and infertility. One third to half of the ovarian endometriotic cysts are bilateral. Most endometriomas are positioned medially or retrouterine.

Features typical of endometriomas are thick shaggy walls with or without septae, internal echogenicities, ground-glass appearance, fluid levels, linear echogenic flecks in its walls and pain on pressure with the probe **(Figs. 38A to C)**. Adhesions are very common. Solid areas may be sometimes seen. Streaming sign is often seen. This is a slow downwards movement of small low-level echogenicities seen in endometrioma (chocolate cyst). This can be best appreciated on probe movement.

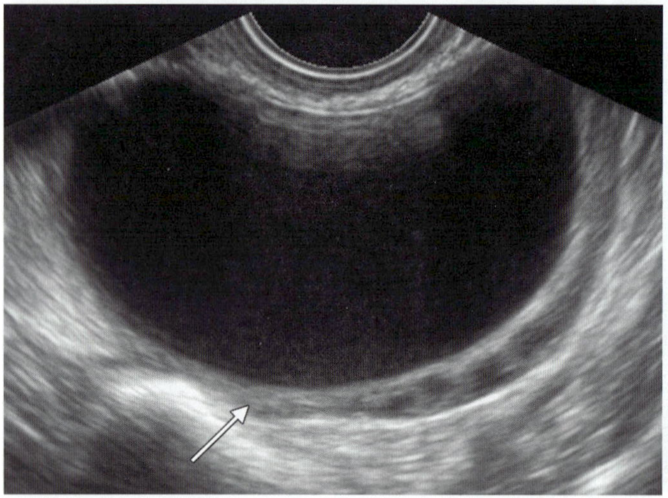

Fig. 34: Beak sign—intraovarian lesion.

On Doppler, endometriomas showing scattered vascularity at ovarian hilus with moderate vascular impedance have been described in the literature. Vascularity is higher during menstruation and in symptomatic patients. At the periphery of the endometrioma, short-coursed vessels are seen **(Fig. 39A)**. Vascularity can be used as a means to decide the mode of therapy for endometriomas. Avascular lesions indicate scarification and are less convenient for the delivery of medication and therefore should be considered for surgical therapy.

Three-dimensional ultrasound allows detection of surface of the endometrioma, visualisation of preserved ovarian tissue and assessment of the ovarian relationship with neighbouring pelvic structures. 3D power Doppler typically shows multiple short-coursed pericystic vessels giving a typical bird's nest appearance **(Fig. 39B)**.

Kurjak et al. have shown a sensitivity of 83.9%, specificity of 97.1%, PPV 82% and NPV 97.5% of vaginal sonography for characterisation of endometriomas. If CA 125 >35 IU/mL was added as a cutoff to these parameters, the sensitivity and specificity reached 99.04% and 99.64%, and PPV and NPV reached 98.10% and 99.82%. Similar results were also confirmed by several other workers.

Solid lesions: The most common lesion in this group is fibroma. It is a well-defined round/oval lesion with echogenicity like that of a fibroid—hypoechoic, homogeneous but sometimes may be heterogeneous and may also show calcifications **(Figs. 40A and B)**.

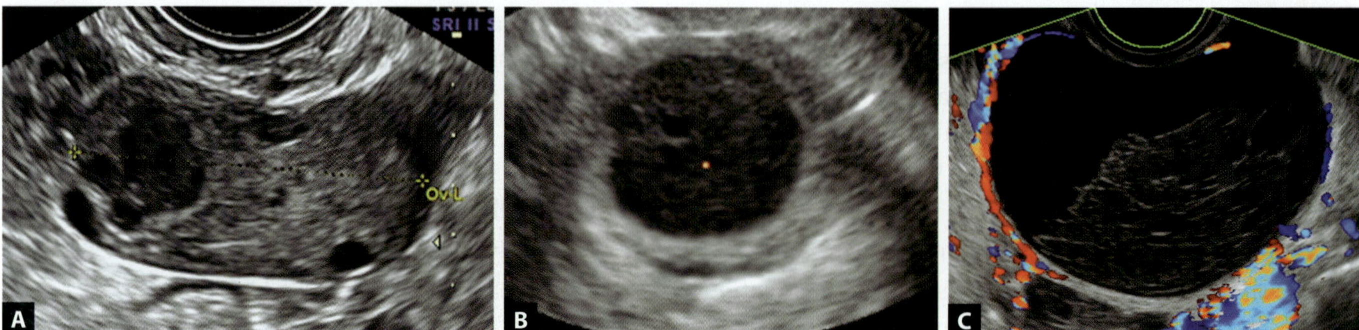

Figs. 35A to C: Different appearances of corpus luteum, also showing ring of colour in the last frame.

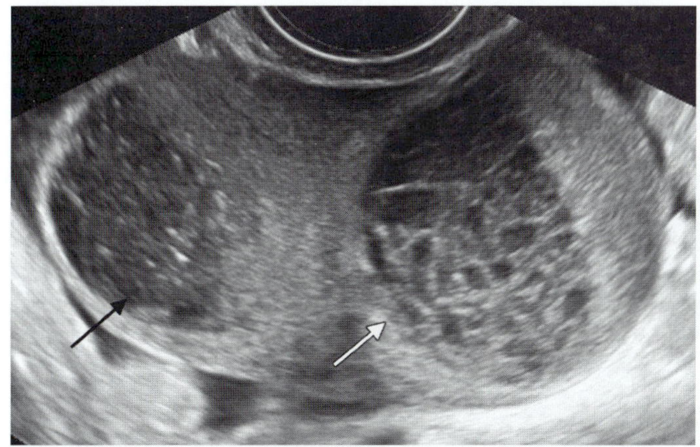
Fig. 36: Haemorrhagic cyst (white arrow) and endometrioma (black arrow).

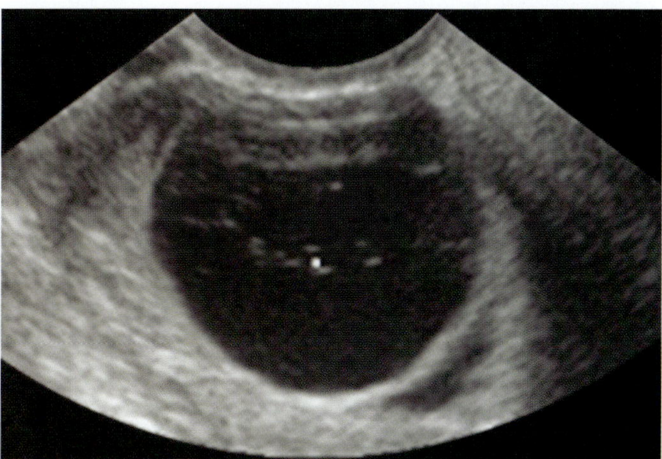
Fig. 37: Luteinised unruptured follicle: Echogenic margins and internal echogenicity.

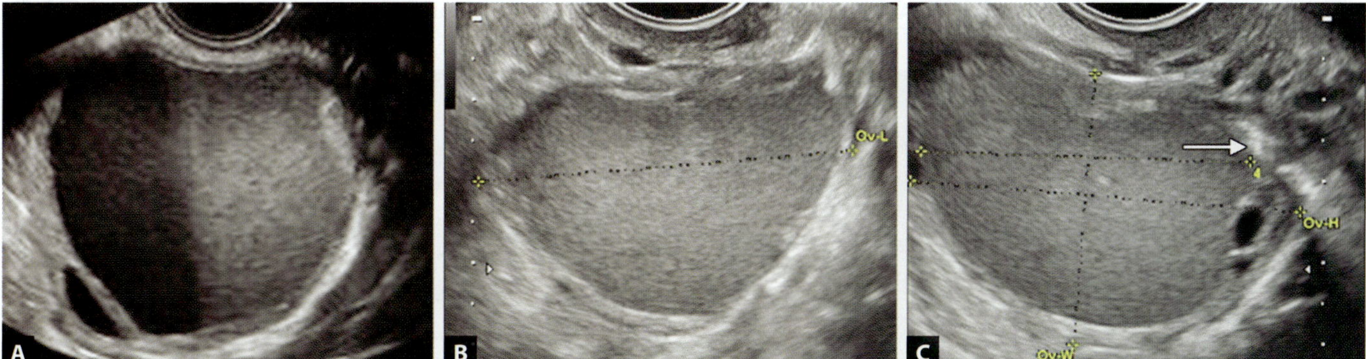

Figs. 38A to C: Endometrioma showing fluid–fluid level, ground-glass appearance and echogenic flecks in wall.

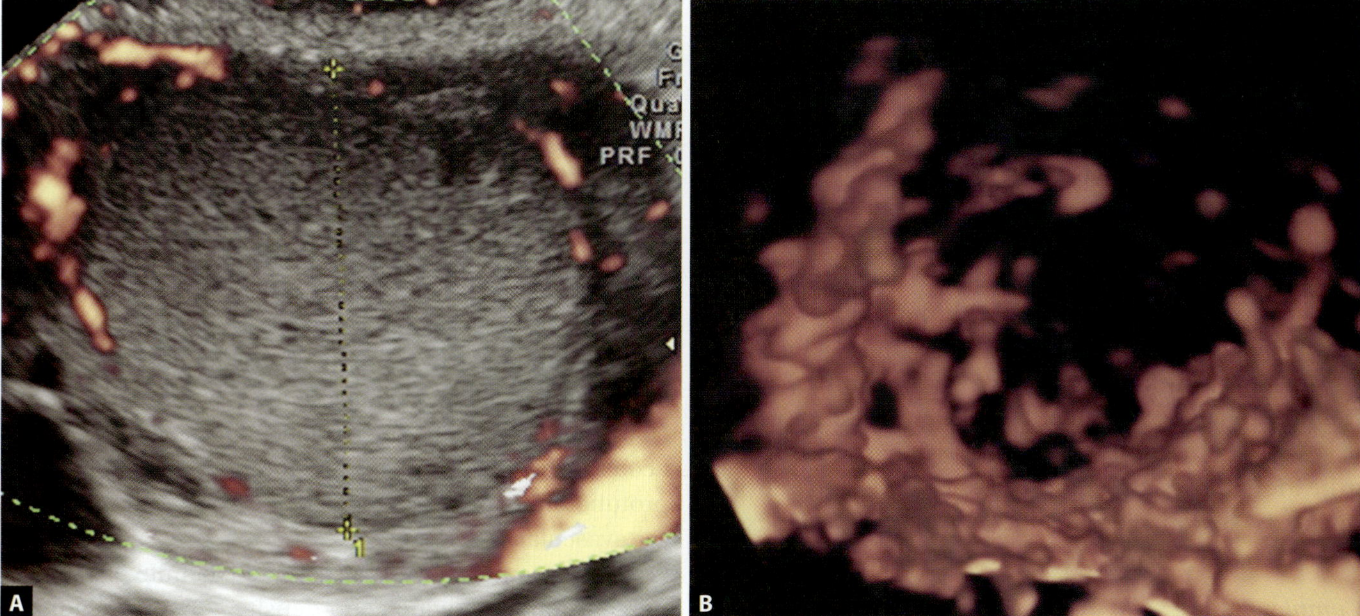

Figs. 39A and B: (A) Power Doppler showing short-coursed peripheral vessels; (B) 3D Power Doppler showing bird's nest appearance.

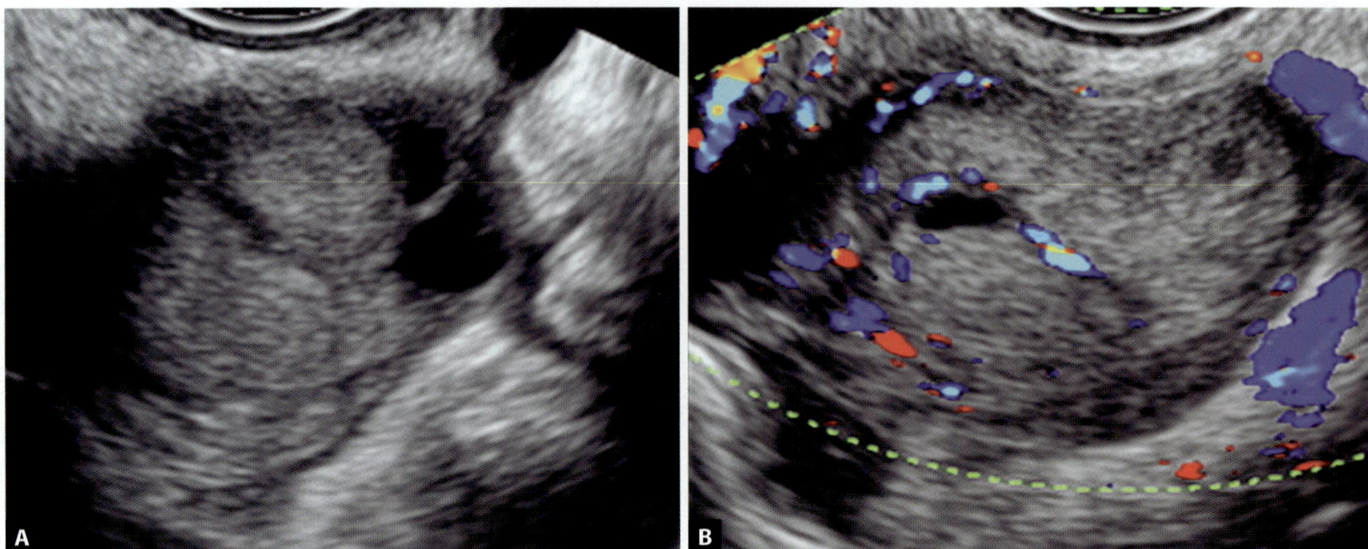

Figs. 40A and B: Ovarian fibroma with peripheral vascularity.

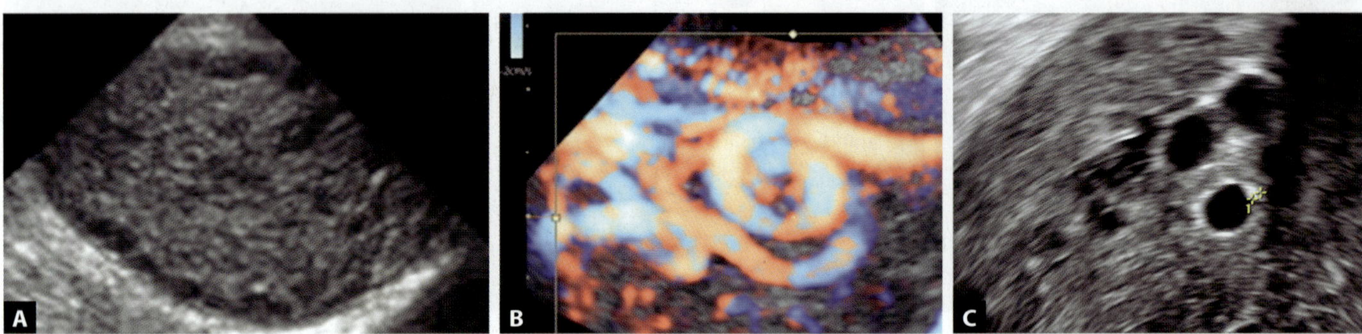

Figs. 41A to C: (A) Enlarged ovary with peripherally placed follicles; (B) Whirlpool sign; (C) Follicular ring sign.
Courtesy: Mala Sibal.

Fibromas can be differentiated from fibroids by tracing the blood supply. They are often bilateral and may also be associated with ascites and pleural effusion. This complication is known as Meigs' syndrome.

Other lesions in this group are very rare and may be thecoma, fibrothecoma, Brenner tumour, etc.

Solid-looking ovaries may also be seen in *ovarian torsion*. Stroma is hypoechoic with peripherally placed small follicles **(Fig. 41A)**. Vascularity may or may not be present and that decides the viability of the ovary. Definitive sign is a whirlpool sign in adnexa due to twisting of vessels **(Fig. 41B)**. Follicular ring sign has been claimed to be the earliest sign of ovarian torsion. But it is a transient sign and is seldom seen after the torsion is fully established **(Fig. 41C)**.

Complex lesions with cystic with solid areas: Lesions in this group have thick walls, with internal echogenicities and also solid projections arising from the walls. Lesions included in this group are:

- Dermoids
- Epithelial tumours
- Endometrioid tumours

Dermoids: These are often an incidental finding. Dermoids are well-defined lesions with thick walls, low-level echoes, fluid-fluid level (because of fat—sebaceous material floating and fluid), hyperechoic lines and dots due to hair, hyperechoic/calcified echoes such as teeth with posterior shadowing, regional diffuse bright echoes with or without acoustic shadowing due to hair clumps or fat in Rokitansky protuberance **(Figs. 42A to D)**. Majority of cystic teratomas are avascular.

These features have been assigned definite PPV. Eighty percent for shadowing echo density, 75% for regionally bright echoes, 50% for hyperechoic lines and dots and

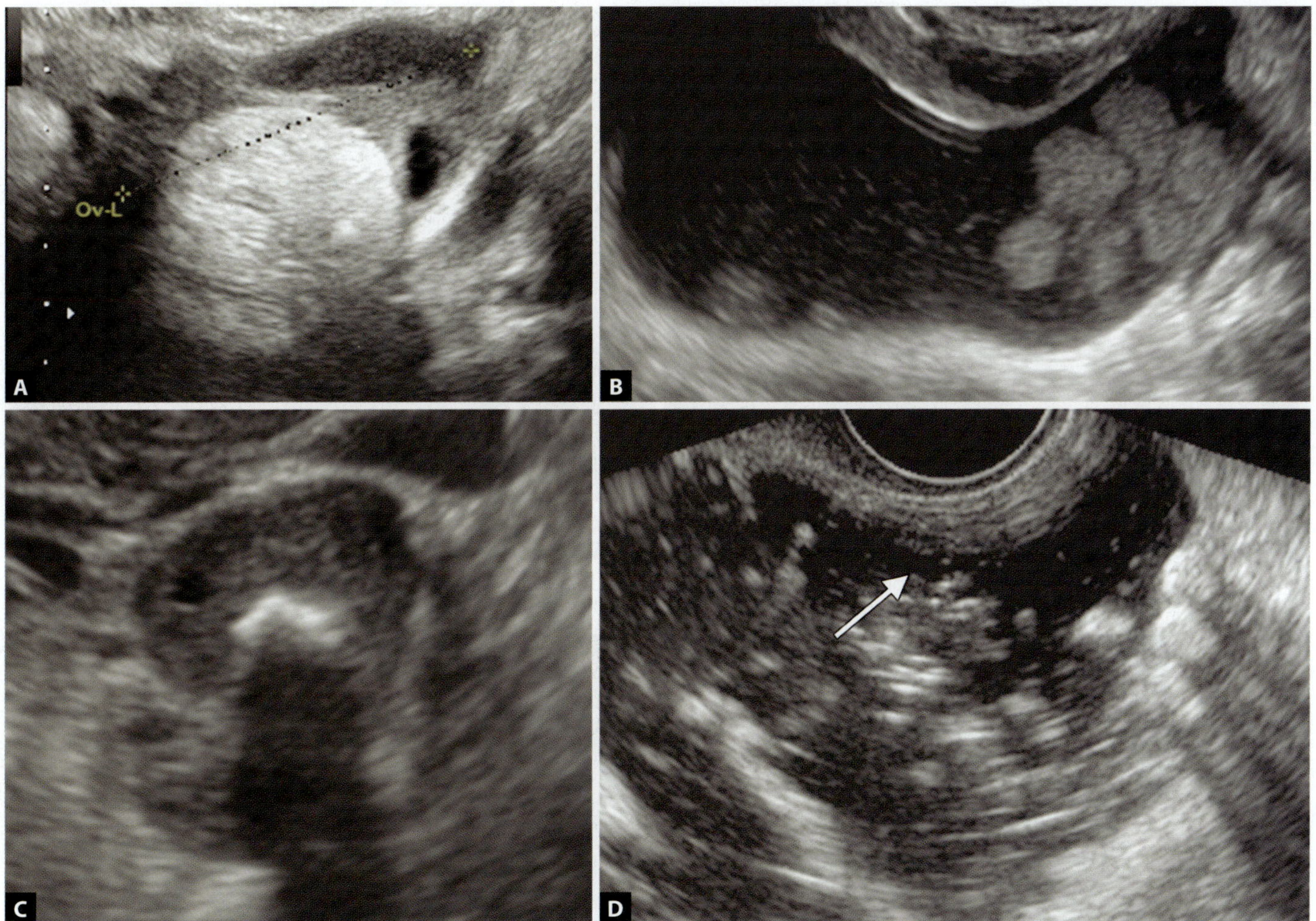

Figs. 42A to D: Dermoids. (A) Echogenic mass; (B) Hairballs in cyst; (C) Small hyperechoic area with posterior shadowing; (D) Teeth with posterior shadowing and echogenic lines and dots.

20% for fluid–fluid level. PPV for more than two features is 100%. Morphologic scoring system for dermoids by Kurjak et al. has a sensitivity of 93.1% and specificity of 99.4%. Including colour Doppler, sensitivity of 99% and specificity of 99.8% can be achieved.

Epithelial tumours: Surface epithelial–stromal tumours account for 60% of ovarian neoplasms and 80–90% of ovarian malignancies. Of all these, 46% are serous, 36.5% are mucinous and 7.5% are endometrioid. These tumours are chiefly complex with cystic and solid components, have septae, internal echogenicities and projections arising from its walls. Benign and malignant counterparts of these tumours have similar but overlapping ultrasound appearances. On ultrasound, therefore, it is not possible to give a histopathological diagnosis. One can only doubt its malignant nature by ultrasound, and this discussion is out of the scope of this chapter.

Tubal Lesions

Pelvic inflammatory disease: The most common of tubal lesions are inflammatory in origin. These lesions are usually a part of pelvic inflammatory disease (PID) and may also involve uterus and ovaries to a variable extent.

Inflammation of fallopian tubes is known as salpingitis. Like inflammation anywhere in the body, salpingitis leads to oedema and hyperaemia. On ultrasound, this is seen as a thickened adnexal soft-tissue band, >10 mm in transverse diameter, or thickened tube walls if there is fluid surrounding may be appreciated with central hyperechoic mucosa. Normally, blood vessels are seen in adnexa on colour Doppler and are parallel to the long axis of adnexa. But, in acute salpingitis, several small vessels are seen, and these are not parallel to the long axis of adnexa but the run across. On pulse Doppler, these vessels show low-resistance (RI <0.45) flow. Salpingitis is usually associated

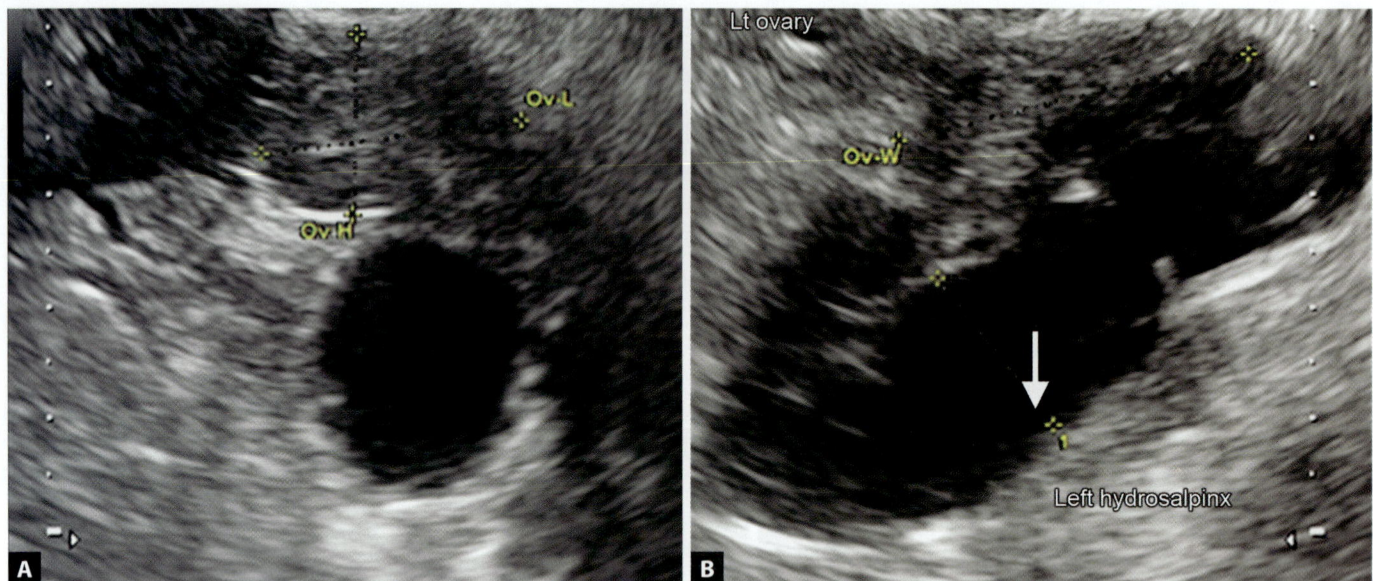

Figs. 43A and B: Hydrosalpinx: Cystic roundish lesion in adnexa change in shape on rotating the probe.

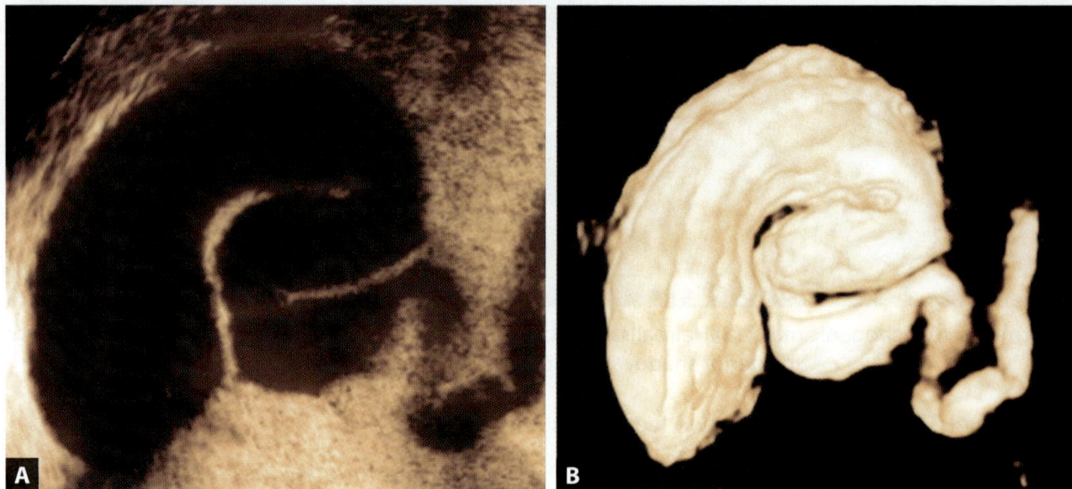

Figs. 44A and B: Hydrosalpinx: 3D ultrasonography, minimum mode rendering and inversion mode.

with oophoritis. This is characterised by enlarged ovaries with hypoechoic stroma and increased vascularity. In the early phase of PID, ovarian parenchymal blood flow also shows low-to-moderate RI 0.53 ± 0.09, but in chronic stage, it increases to 0.71 ± 0.09. Regression of the infection on its own or in response to antibiotic decreases the flow in tubes and ovaries. Salpingitis may lead to hydrosalpinx.

On ultrasound, an extraovarian cystic lesion is seen in adnexa. On rotating the probe 90°, it changes its shape and becomes elongated **(Figs. 43A and B)**. It may typically show a retort, sausage or serpiginous shape. It can be differentiated from bowel by lack of peristalsis and from a blood vessel by Doppler which shows no flow.

It may show incomplete septae that are due to tubal haustra (*see* **Fig. 43**, arrow). On transverse section, this tube gives a cogwheel appearance, due to fibrotic remnants of endosalpingeal tissue, or beads-on-a-string appearance on the long axis. The fluid may show low-level echoes if the collection becomes thicker and also at times purulent. 3D ultrasonography with inversion mode rendering is a very good tool to demonstrate such lesions **(Figs. 44A and B)**.

Extension of the inflammatory process further also may involve the ovary and also sometimes bowel or omentum in vicinity and forms a tubo-ovarian abscess **(Figs. 45A and B)**. It is seen as a complex lesion on ultrasound with

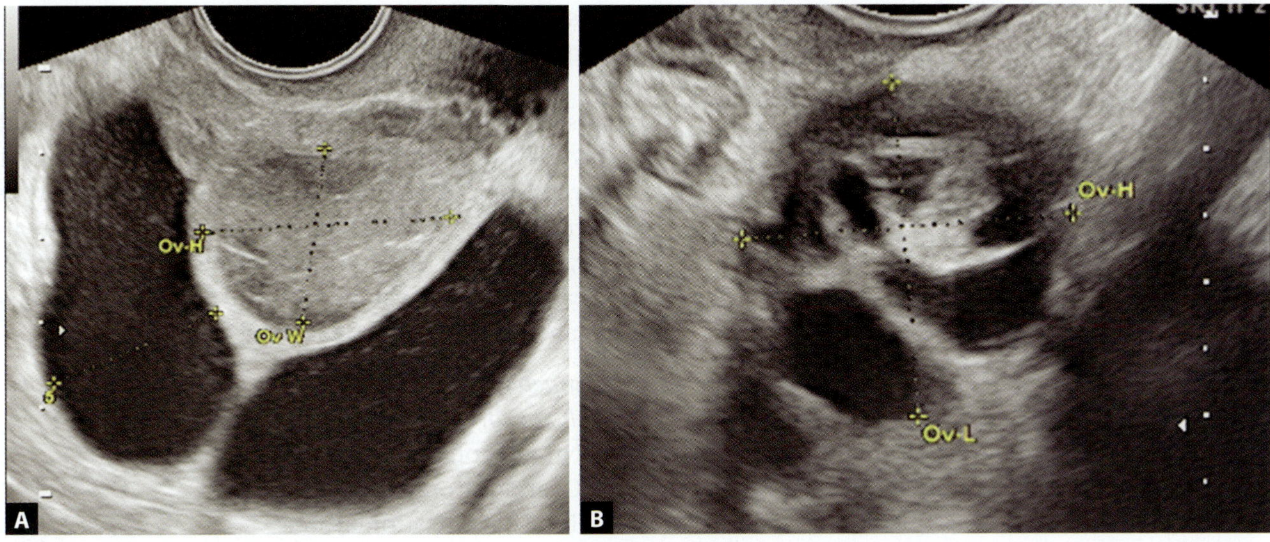

Figs. 45A and B: Pelvic inflammatory disease. (A) Adherent ovary and distended tube; (B) Tubo-ovarian abscess where tube and ovary cannot be separately identified.

TABLE 2: Sonographic markers for tubal inflammation.

	Acute (%)	*Chronic (%)*
Thickened tube wall ≥5 mm	100	3
Cogwheel sign	86	3
Incomplete septa (92%)		
Beads-on-a-string appearance	.00	57
Tubo-ovarian complex	36	2
Tubo-ovarian abscess		
Fluid in cul-de-sac	50	10

Note: Flattened/fibrotic endosalpingeal folds 2–3 mm hyperechoic nodules on cross-section of fluid-filled structure.

low resistance (RI 0.44 ± 0.04) vascularity in its solid areas and wall.

Free fluid may be seen in pelvis. Abscess when heals still leaves a cyst behind or causes fibrous scarring—tubo-ovarian adhesions—and then shows high-resistance vascularity (RI 0.75 ± 0.04).

Timor-Tritsch et al. defined the sonographic markers for the tubal inflammation **(Table 2)**.

Clinical correlation is very essential to differentiate inflammatory process from neoplastic process.

Miscellaneous Lesions

- *Broad ligament fibroid*: On ultrasound, it is a well-circumscribed, usually round, hypoechoic lesion. It can be separated from both uterus and ovary by probe pressure and shows peripheral vascularity.
- *Peritoneal inclusion cyst:* It is a fluid collection in the pelvic peritoneum with septations. It usually occurs as a result of a previous infection. This fluid collection is not under pressure and therefore changes shape on probe pressure and the septae inside, move with respiration, pressure or with pulsations of nearby vessels. These lesions typically do not show any vascularity **(Fig. 46)**.
- *Paraovarian cyst:* Up to 20% of adnexal masses may be paraovarian cysts. These are benign, avascular lesions with thin walls and anechoic contents. The shape does not change with pressure but can be easily separated from ovary **(Fig. 47A)**. Adhesions indicate infection, and solid projections in them may raise a possibility of malignancy. Paratubal cysts appear very similar to these cysts. Commonly seen fimbrial cysts are seen close to the fimbria **(Fig. 47B)**.

CYCLE ASSESSMENT CONSISTING OF BASELINE SCAN, PREOVULATORY SCAN AND SECRETORY SCAN

Hormonal changes occurring during the menstrual cycle are reflected as vascular changes, and therefore colour Doppler in this assessment is mandatory. 3D ultrasound is especially useful for volume measurements. 3D power Doppler has given promising results in initial studies.

Baseline Scan

Baseline scan is done on day 2–3 of the cycle. At this time of the cycle, oestrogen and progesterone are at the baseline and ovaries have no active follicles or residual corpus luteum. This scan consists of transvaginal sonography (TVS).

Transvaginal sonography, transvaginal colour Doppler (TVCD) and volume ultrasound of ovaries and uterus are done to assess the ovarian reserve and response that can guide to decide the stimulation protocols for assisted reproductive technology (ART).

Ovaries

Two-dimensional ultrasound assessment of the ovaries consists of assessment of ovarian diameters and volume and counting of antral follicles as quantitative assessment and qualitative assessment of stromal density. Colour or power Doppler is used to see the presence of vessels in the stroma. If vascularity is present, pulse Doppler is used for quantitative assessment of the flows. Intraovarian RI and peak systolic velocity (PSV) are the two parameters considered to be relevant **(Table 3)**. Then, 3D and 3D power Doppler volume of the ovary are acquired for ovarian volume and stromal volume, counting number of antral follicles. Global vascular indices vascularity index (VI), flow index (FI) and vascularity flow index (VSI) may be calculated; the values for these are not yet established but are likely to give promising results.

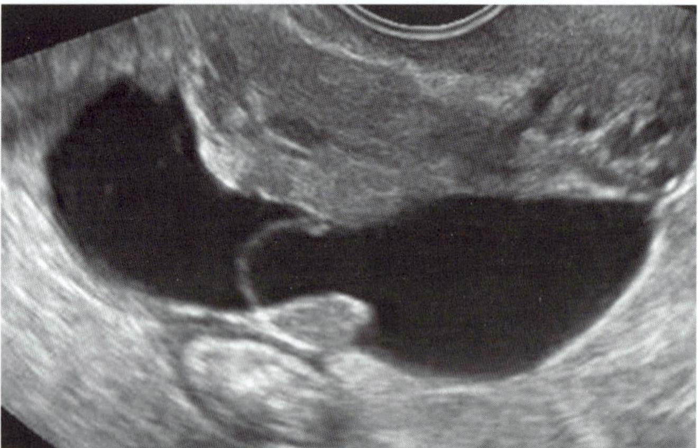

Fig. 46: Peritoneal inclusion cyst: Irregular shape and lax septum.

Parameters defining the reserve and response of the ovaries: Predictors of ovarian response:

- Number of antral follicles
- Ovarian stromal FI
- Total ovarian stromal area
- Total ovarian volume.

In that order of importance: Antral follicle count (AFC) and ovarian volume showed significant correlation with anti-Müllerian hormone (AMH), total testosterone and free androgen index. Number of antral follicles, measuring 2–10 mm in diameter, correlates well with the female's age, ovarian reserve and ovarian response to gonadotrophin stimulation. Normal AFC in one ovary ranging from 5 to 12 AFC <6 correlates well with reduced ovarian reserve and poor response to ovarian stimulation, with PPV of 75%. Total AFC >21 could lead to the decision to adjust the gonadotrophin dose in trying to prevent a hyper-response, leading to ovarian hyperstimulation syndrome (OHSS).

Precise calculation of AFC, therefore, can help in predicting the ovarian response. This can be done on 2D ultrasound by scanning across the whole ovary while

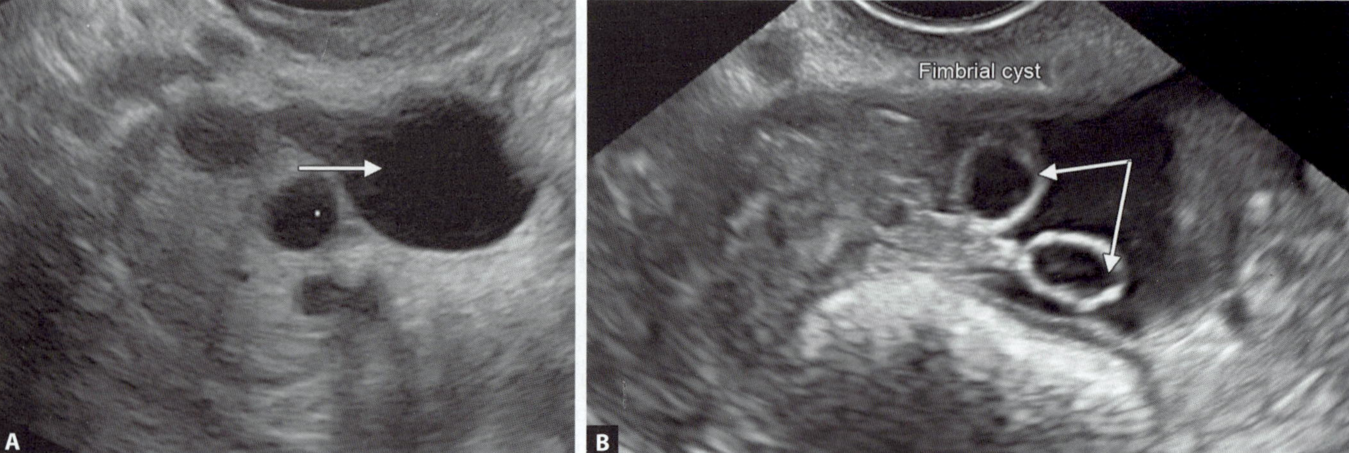

Figs. 47A and B: (A) Paraovarian cyst; (B) Fimbrial cyst.

TABLE 3: Parameters defining the reserve and response of the ovaries.

Ovarian parameters	*Normal reserve and response*	*High reserve–low response*	*Low reserve–low response*	*Low reserve–high response*	*High reserve–high response*
RI	0.6–0.7	>0.7	>0.7	<0.6	<0.6
PSV	5–10 c/s	<5 cc	<5 cc	>10 cc	>10 cc
FNPO	5–12	>12	<5	<5	>12
Ovarian volume	3–6.6 cc	>6.6 cc	<3 cc	<3 cc	>6.6 cc

(FNPO: follicle number per ovary; PSV: peak systolic velocity; RI: resistance index)

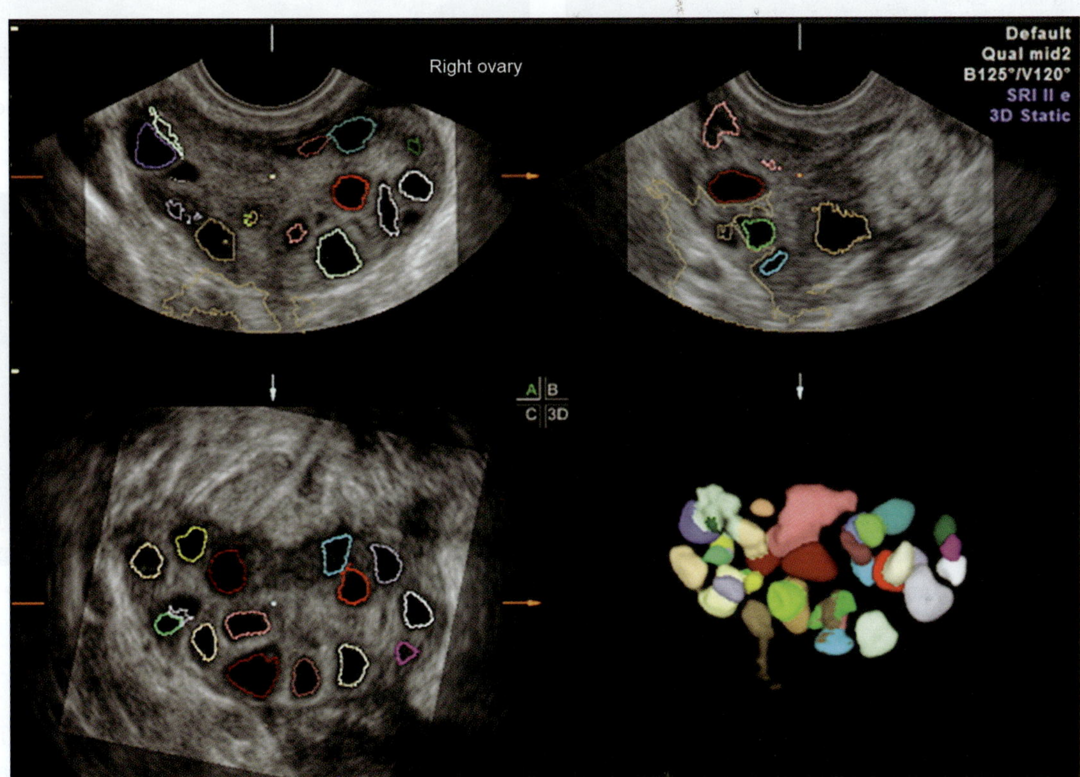

Fig. 48: 3D ultrasonography volume of polycystic ovary with sono AVC. (AVC: automated volume count)

counting the follicles. Both 2D and 3D can calculate the number of antral follicles correctly. But this has high chances of error when follicles are multiple as in polycystic ovaries. In these cases, counting the antral follicles by 3D US, using VOCAL, inversion mode or Sono AVC (GE Healthcare) is much more precise. Using this software, each follicle is coded by a different colour, and diameters and volumes of each are calculated separately. This is a more precise method as there is no overcounting of follicles. But to avoid undercounting, postprocessing is required **(Fig. 48)**.

The mean ovarian diameter significantly correlated with age, day 3 follicle-stimulating hormone (FSH), day 3 luteinising hormone (LH) and day 3 oestradiol. Another study has shown. A study by Lass et al. has shown that ovarian volume <3 cc was significantly predictive of higher in vitro fertilisation (IVF) cancellation rates >50%.

It has been shown by Zaidi et al. that stromal blood flow velocity after pituitary suppression was an independent predictor of ovarian response **(Fig. 49)**.

Kupesic has shown correlation between the ovarian stromal FI and number of mature oocytes retrieved in an IVF cycles and pregnancy rates.

These evidences justify the use of AFC, ovarian volume and stromal RI and PSV as predictors of ovarian response. The same parameters have been developed by another

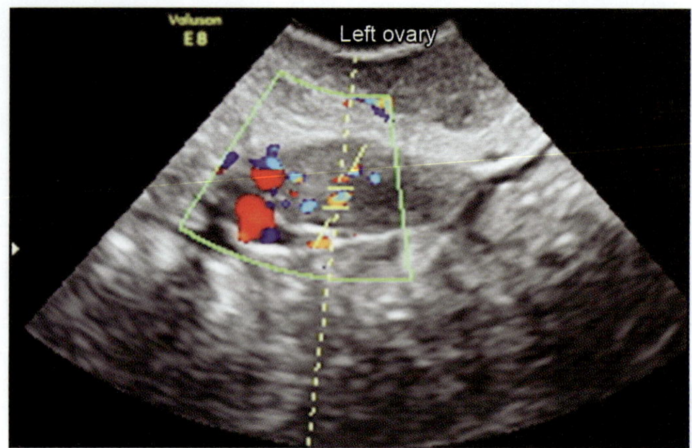

Fig. 49: Ovarian stromal flow as seen on colour Doppler.

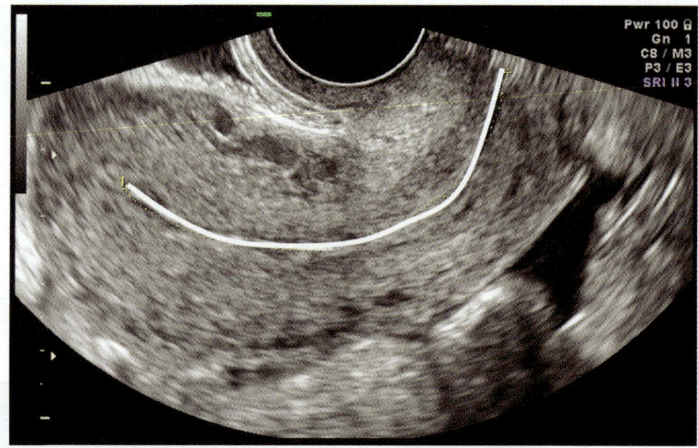

Fig. 50: Measuring functional uterocervical length.

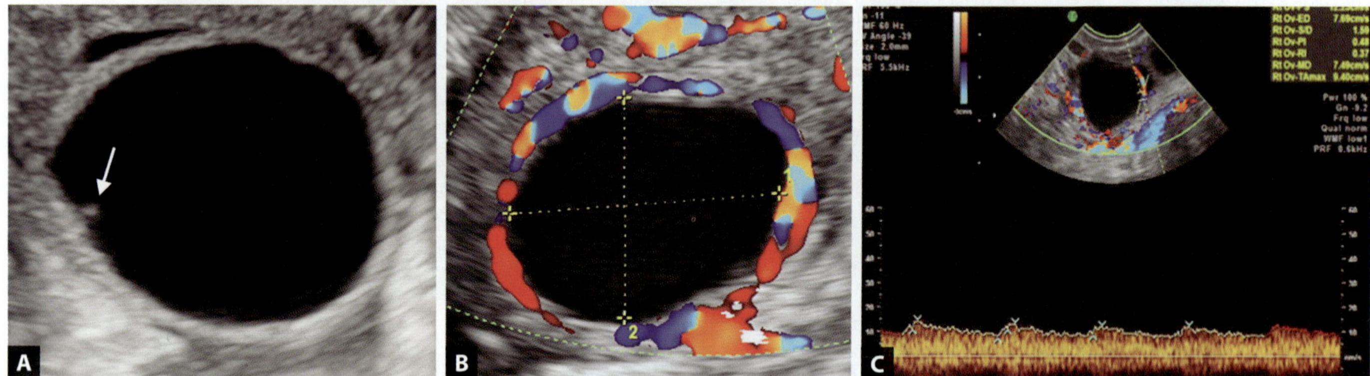

Figs. 51A to C: (A) Cumulus (arrow); (B) Perifollicular flow on power Doppler; (C) Spectral Doppler of perifollicular flow.

group to develop a scoring system to calculate the starting doses of gonadotrophins in intrauterine insemination (IUI) as well as IVF cycles.

Uterus

Baseline scan of the uterus is done to assess the uterocervical length by ultrasound. Midsagittal section of the uterus is imaged on the screen where the whole of the uterus is seen with endometrial cavity starting from the fundus to the internal os and external os. For all ART procedures, may it be IUI or embryo transfer (ET), the uterocervical length is measured from the fundal end of the endometrium to the external os and is known as functional/physiological uterocervical length **(Fig. 50)**. Doppler of the uterine artery is done. Uterine artery RI >0.79 indicates that high doses of stimulation will be required for endometrial maturation. Subendometrial flow on day 2, if present, indicates a low receptive endometrium for implantation.

Preovulatory Scan

A follicle that grows to 11–12 mm is a dominant follicle and grows at a rate of 2–3 mm/day and ovulation occurs at 18–24 mm size. Follicular flow can be first detected when the follicular size is 10 mm. A follicle is known to be mature when a rounded 16–18 mm sized follicle with thin walls and no internal echogenicity is seen. A sonolucent halo appears surrounding the follicle 24 hours prior to ovulation. Cumulus oophorus, a small solid projection from the wall in the follicular lumen, may be seen **(Fig. 51A)**.

Colour Doppler Assessment

Doppler settings for the optimum recording of these blood flows are set at low PRF (0.3–0.6) and low wall filters (30 Hz). On colour Doppler, vascularity is seen covering three fourths of the follicle. The conception was related to grade 3–4 vascularity **(Fig. 51B)**. On pulse Doppler, these vessels show RI 0.4–0.48, and PSV >10 cm/s **(Fig. 51C)**. This means that if the follicle is said to be functionally mature when PSV is at least 10 cm/s, that is the time when the LH surge starts and under the effect of that LH, the perifollicular PSV keeps rising constantly. A marked increase in the PSV around the follicle, in the presence of a relatively constant pulsatility index (PI), could be a sign of follicle maturity and impending ovulation. Based on these facts, we have done a study of 350 IUI cycles based on this. Single IUI was done between 36 and 38 hours and double IUI was done at 12–14 and 36–38 hours after human chorionic gonadotrophin (hCG) in all patients in whom perifollicular PSV >15 cm/s. When perifollicular PSV on the day of hCG was >20 cm/s, and perifollicular RI was within the normal range, double IUI has given higher pregnancy rates. It is important to make a note here that double IUI has not proved its role as a measure to improve pregnancy rates in a general infertile population undergoing IUI. However, in this small subgroup with high PSV on the day of ovulation trigger, it has a significant value.

Fertilisation of a follicle with a PSV of <10 cm/s has high chances of embryo with chromosomal abnormality. Rising PSV with steady low RI suggests that the follicle is close to rupture. Steady or decreasing PSV with rising RI suggests that the follicle is preceding towards LUF.

Application of 3D Ultrasound for Follicular Assessment

When there is multifollicular development as in polycystic ovary (PCO), the follicular shapes become polygonal and therefore follicular diameter may not be a reliable parameter of follicular size. Follicular volume by 3D is a more reliable parameter. Follicular volumes between 3 and 7 cc are optimum for oocyte retrieval. But in our experience, follicles with volumes of up to 1 cc on the day of ovulation trigger are likely to give fertilisable oocytes on oocyte retrieval. The limits of agreement between the volume of the follicular aspirate and 3D volume of the follicle were +0.96 to –0.43 with 3D and +3.47 to –2.42 by 2D volume estimation.

Cumulus can be seen in 80–90% of mature follicles using 3D ultrasonography rendering **(Fig. 52A)**. This is possible only in up to 30–40% follicles by 2D ultrasonography. On the day of ovulation trigger, if cumulus like echo is not seen in all three planes in the follicle, it is less likely to be mature fertilisable oocyte. This information is especially useful in ART cycles where very few follicles are available. If cumulus is seen in the follicle and ovum is not retrieved, flushing of follicle may be recommended only in this small subgroup. 3D power Doppler gives an idea about the global vascularity of the follicle **(Fig. 52B)**. We have done a large study taking this into consideration. Based on a study of >1,000 cycles, follicular volume of 3–7.5 cc, VI >6–20 and FI >35 if used as additional features of a mature follicle apart from the follicular features mentioned earlier in this chapter increased the pregnancy rates significantly **(Fig. 52C)**.

Assessment of Preovulatory Endometrium

On 2D ultrasound, endometrium should be 6 mm or more in thickness, preferably 8–10 mm. It should have an intact uniform endometrio-myometrial junction and should be multilayered. But its morphological assessment is essential.

Endometrial grading:

- *Grade A endometrium*: Multilayered with intervening area more echogenic than myometrium **(Fig. 53A)**

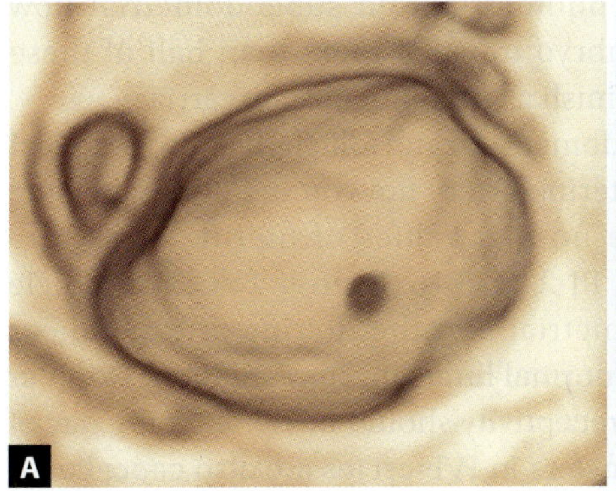

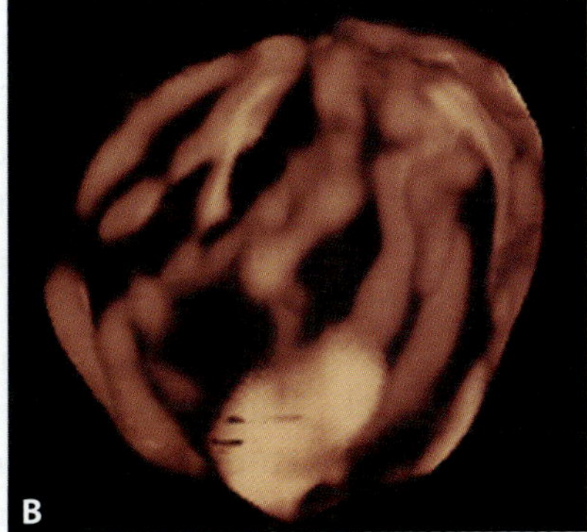

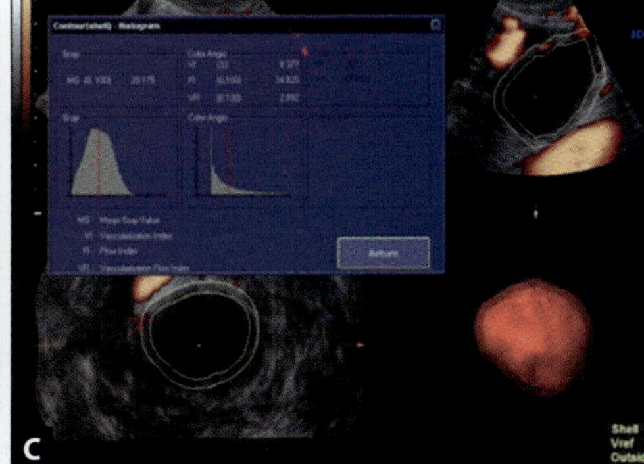

Figs. 52A to C: (A) Cumulus oophorus in follicle on 3D ultrasonography of follicle rendered view; (B) 3D power angiography of perifollicular flow; (C) Calculation of 3D power Doppler vascular indices (volume histogram) after VOCAL and shell volume for perifollicular flow.

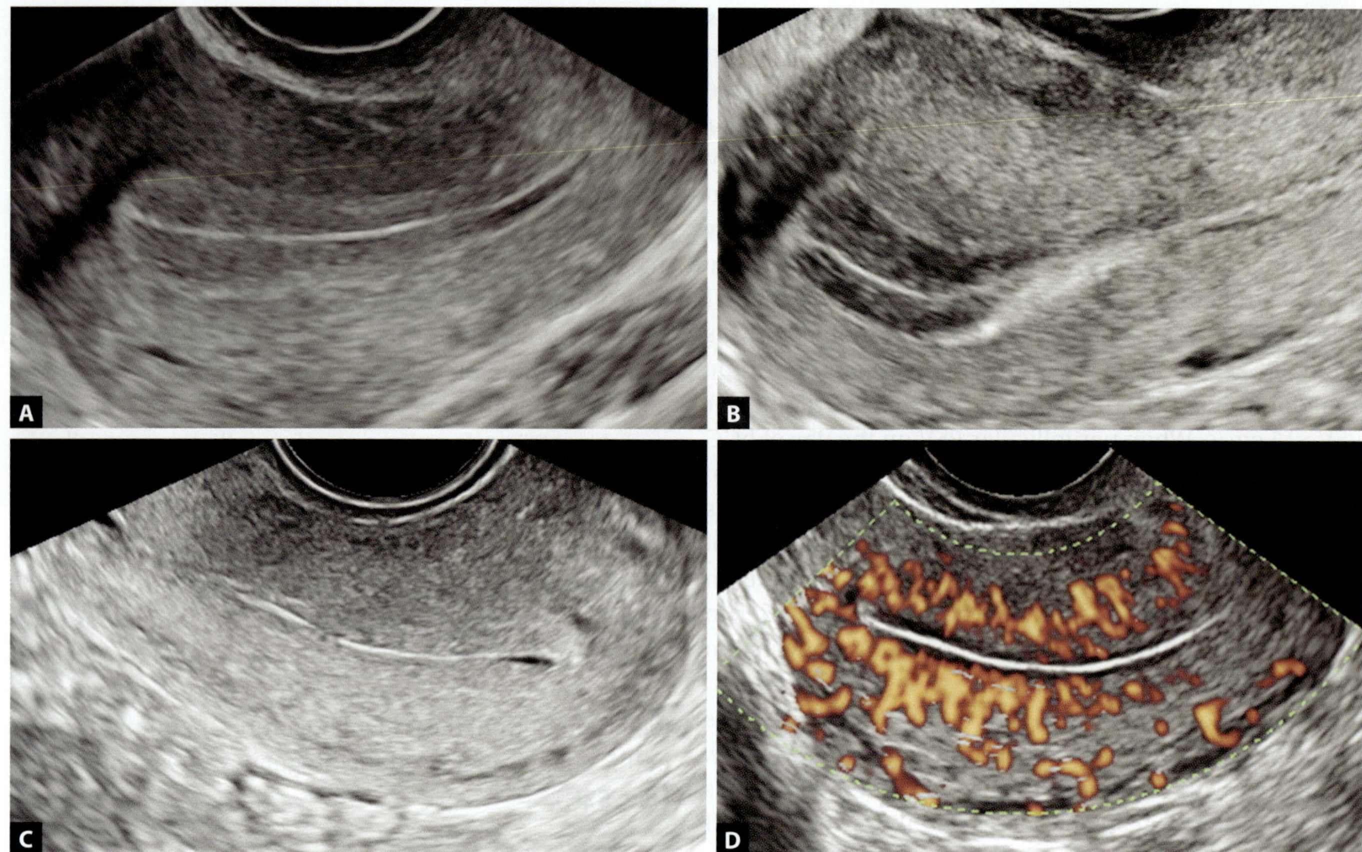

Figs. 53A to D: (A) Grade A endometrium on B mode; (B) Grade B endometrium on B-mode; (C) Grade C endometrium on B-mode; (D) Zone 4 vascularity seen in endometrium on power Doppler.

- *Grade B endometrium:* Multilayered with intervening area hypoechoic to myometrium **(Fig. 53B)**
- *Grade C endometrium:* Homogeneous isoechoic endometrium **(Fig. 53C)**.

2D ultrasound assesses the anatomy of the endometrium, but its functional maturity can be assessed by Doppler of spiral arteries.

On colour Doppler, the vascularity is classified by Applebaum as follows:

- *Zone I:* Blood vessels reaching the endometrio-myometrial junction surrounding the endometrium **(Fig. 53D)**
- *Zone II:* Blood vessels reaching hyperechoic endometrial edge
- *Zone III:* Blood vessels reaching internal endometrial hypoechoic zone
- *Zone IV:* Blood vessels reaching endometrial cavity. On pulse Doppler, these blood vessels should show RI 0.49–0.59 and PI 1.1–2.3.

Even if TVCD of follicle is normal, endometrial and the uterine artery indices should be within normal limits for implantation. Absent subendometrial and intraendometrial vascularisation on the day of hCG appears to be a useful predictor of failure of implantation in IVF, irrespective of morphological appearance. It has also been observed that when pregnancy is achieved in the absence of endometrial and subendometrial flow on the day of embryo transfer, more than half of these pregnancies will finish as spontaneous miscarriage.

Apart from endometrium and follicle, it is also essential to evaluate the uterine artery flow on the dominant side before hCG. The normal values of uterine artery are RI 0.60–0.80 and PI 2.22–3.16. Even if TVCD of follicle is normal, endometrial and the uterine artery indices should be within normal limits for implantation. Doppler study for uterine receptivity should be done on the day of hCG. Embryo transfers in IVF cycles are also cancelled if the uterine artery PI >3.2. hCG administration induces a significant increase in the resistance of uterine artery for

48 hours and can affect its evaluation on the day of follicular aspiration/rupture; therefore, Doppler study for uterine receptivity should be done on the day of hCG.

As for the follicle, the endometrium, also if evaluated by 3D and 3D power Doppler, is more reliable. It gives endometrium volume instead of endometrial thickness. When we measure endometrial thickness, we measure it at the thickest part, and this thickness might not be uniform in the whole endometrium. Moreover, sometimes in spite of normal thickness, the length of the endometrial cavity may be so little that the total endometrial volume is not enough for implantation. Moreover, 3D power Doppler gives an idea about the global vascularity of the endometrium not only in terms of quality but also in terms of quantity, which should be a more useful parameter than 2D Doppler where we can see vessels only in one plane at a time and also interrogate a few vessels not all. In our study, 3D power Doppler studies that we have found reliable are endometrial volume >3 cc, FI >20 and VFI >5 **(Figs. 54A and B)**. There are several other people who have also worked on endometrial receptivity assessment by 3D and 3D power Doppler. A study by Merce et al. of 40 IVF cycles has shown endometrial volume of 3–7 mL as most favourable for conception. Median values for a favourable endometrium are 4.28 ± 1.9 mL. Endometrial volume of >2.0 mL has a significantly higher pregnancy rates, and no pregnancies were recorded with endometrial volume of <1 mL.

No pregnancy was documented when endometrial volume <3 mL and VI <10. Exceptionally, better pregnancy rates were achieved with endometrial volume >7 mL and subendometrial VI between 10% and 35%.

A study by Kupesic et al. shows lower RI of 0.49–0.57 in subendometrial vessels and FI of 11.0–15.4 in conception cycles compared to 9.5–13.3 otherwise. VFI on the day of hCG is more sensitive than volume, VI and FI for the prediction of pregnancy. VFI >0.24 has sensitivity of 83.3%, specificity of 88.9%, PPV 93.8% and NPV 72.3% for prediction of pregnancy with 33% pregnancy rate.

A scoring system has also been developed for endometrial receptivity, which apart from the endometrial thickness, morphology and vascularity, and uterine artery Doppler also includes uterine contraction count. Calculating contractions/min >5 contractions/min is considered bad for implantation, and 3 contractions/min is considered good for implantation. This is purely based on the fact that a uterus which is highly contractile will not allow implantation. Though this scoring system is not practically applicable, as even with full scores pregnancy might not occur.

Secretory Scan

With the rupture of the follicle, corpus luteum is formed and secretory changes are seen in the endometrium in the form of echogenicity of the endometrium that starts from outside, proceeding to the central line, making a ring sign of the endometrium.

Assessment of the corpus luteum, endometrium and uterine artery by Doppler gives information about the luteal phase normalcy and progesterone levels. A clear correlation between RI of corpus luteum and plasma progesterone levels has been seen in natural cycle. RI of the corpus luteum can, therefore, be used as an adjunct to plasma progesterone assay as an index of luteal

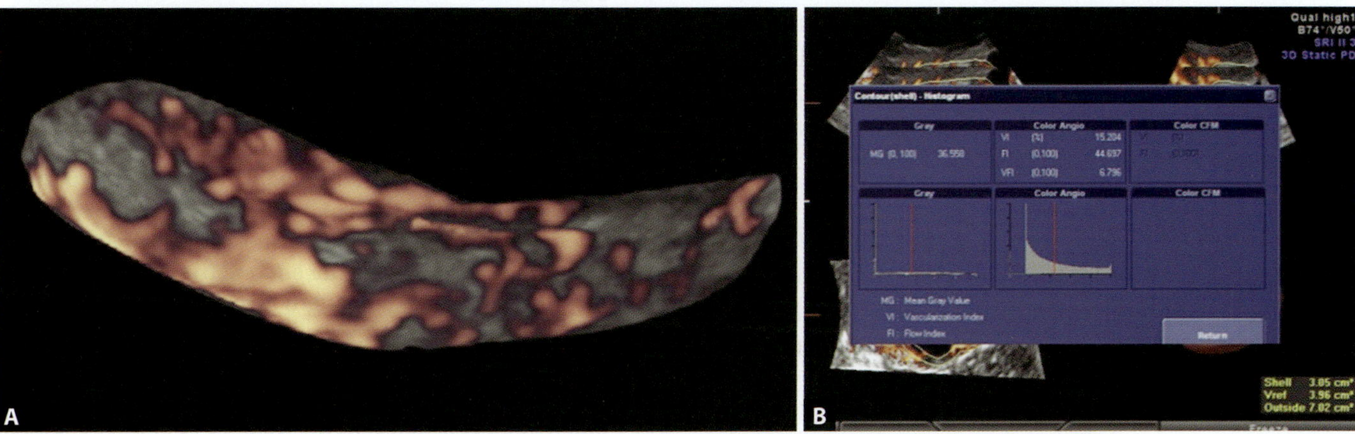

Figs. 54A and B: (A) 3D power angiography; (B) Volume histogram of endometrium.

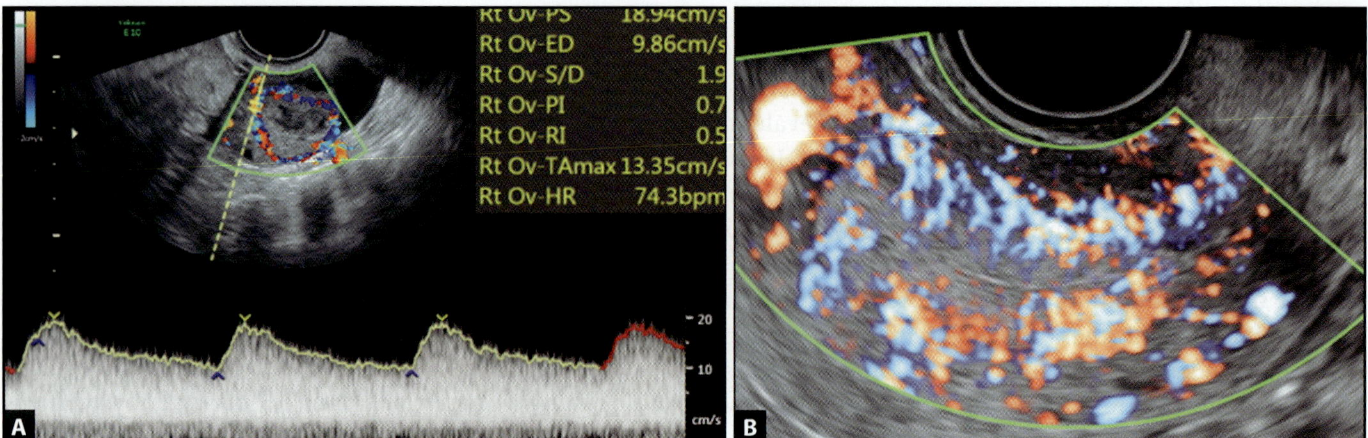

Figs. 55A and B: (A) Corpus luteum on colour Doppler; (B) Endometrial Doppler in secretory phase.

function. A healthy corpus luteum will show a vascular ring surrounding itself on colour Doppler and on power Doppler, these vessels show RI 0.35–0.50, PI 0.70–0.80 and PSV 10–15 cm/s **(Fig. 55A)**. This resistance starts increasing on day 23 of the cycle in a nonconception cycle. Endometrial Doppler shows branches of spiral arteries piercing the outer echogenic margins of the endometrium and better if vascularity reaches the central line with RI 0.48–0.52 **(Fig. 55B)**. Uterine artery at this time of the cycle is 2.0–2.5 and PSV is 15–20 cm/s.

Based on these values, abnormal parameters indicate luteal phase problems such as LUF or luteal phase defect.

Luteinised Unruptured Follicle

On 2D ultrasound, LUF is seen as persistent follicle with thick walls and progressive loss of cystic appearance which is difficult to differentiate from corpus luteum. Endometrium is thick and echogenic, and no fluid is seen in pouch of Douglas (POD). On Doppler, perifollicular RI is 0.51–0.59, which is higher than normal and remains almost steady till the end of the cycle. Nondominant ovary also shows similar Doppler indices. Endometrial flow is also absent.

Luteal Phase Defect

On Doppler, corpus luteum shows high resistance RI 0.58 ± 0.04. Bilateral ovarian RI shows no difference. Increased resistance is also seen in spiral arteries RI 0.72 ± 0.06.

Increased resistance to uterine blood flow in the mid-luteal phase may be an important contributing factor to some causes of infertility and the cause of some previously *unexplained* infertility. Segmental uterine and ovarian artery perfusion demonstrates a significant correlation with histological and hormonal markers of uterine receptivity and may aid in assessment of luteal phase defect.

As quoted by Golan et al., Shoham et al. and Tan et al., *in the hands of experienced operators, ultrasound alone suffices for cycle monitoring, with no necessity for additional hormonal estimations.*

SUGGESTED READING

1. Applebaum M. The 'steel' and 'teflon' endometrium-ultrasound visualization of endometrial vascularity in IVF patients and outcome. Presented at the Third World Congress of Ultrasound in Obstetrics and Gynecology. Ultrasound Obstet Gynecol. 1993;3(Suppl 2):10.
2. Bald R, Hackeloer BJ. Ultraschall-darstellung verschiendener endometrium for men. In Otto R, Jan FX (Eds). Ultraschalldiagnostik 1982. Stuttgart: Thieme; 1983. p. 187.
3. Bassil S, Magritte JP, Roth J, Nisolle M, Donnez J, Gordts S. Uterine vascularity during stimulation and its correlation with implantation in in vitro fertilization. Hum Reprod. 1995;10(6):1497-501.
4. Bourne T, Jurkovic D, Waterstone J, Campbell S, Collins WP. Intrafollicular blood flow during human ovulation. Ultrasound Obstet Gynecol. 1991;1(1):53-9.
5. Chein LW, Au HK, Chen PL, Xiao J, Tzeng CR. Assessment of uterine receptivity by the endometrial-subendometrial blood flow distribution pattern in women undergoing IVF-ET. Fertil Steril. 2002;78(2):245-51.
6. Chen MJ, Yang WS, Chen CL, Wu MY, Yang YS, Ho HN. The relationship between anti-mullerian hormones, androgen and insulin resistance on the number of antral follicles in women with polycystic ovarian syndrome. Hum Reprod. 2008;23(4):952-7.

7. Chui KC, Pugh ND, Walker SM, Gregory L, Shaw RW. Follicular vascularity—the predictive value of transvaginal power Doppler ultrasonography in an in vitro fertilization program: a preliminary study. Hum Reprod. 1997;12(1):191-6.
8. Coulam CB, Stern JJ, Soenksen DM, Britten S, Bustillo M. Comparison of pulsatility indexes on the day of oocyte retrieval and embryo transfer. Hum Reprod. 1995;10(1):82-4.
9. Di Donato N, Bertoldo V, Montanari G, Zannoni L, Caprara G, Seracchioli R. Question mark form of uterus: a simple sonographic sign associated with presence of adenomyosis. Ultrasound Obstet Gynecol. 2015,46(1):126-8.
10. Feichtinger W. Transvaginal three-dimensional imaging for evaluation and treatment of infertility. In: Merz E (Ed). 3D Ultrasound in Obstetrics and Gynecology. Philadelphia: Lippincott Williams and Wilkins; 1998. pp. 37-43.
11. Fratelli JL, Levi AJ, Miller BT. A prospective novel method of determining ovarian size during in vitro fertilization cycles. J Assist Reprod Genet. 2002;19(1):39-41.
12. Glock JL, Brumsted JR. Colour flow pulsed Doppler ultrasound in diagnosing luteal phase defect. Fertil Steril. 1995,64(3):500-4.
13. Gonen Y, Caspers RF. Prediction of implantation by the sonographic appearance of the endometrium during controlled ovarian stimulation for IVF. J In Vitro Fertil Embryo Transf. 1990;7(3):146-52.
14. Grimbizis GF, Gordts S, Di Spiezio Sardo A, Brucker S, De Angelis C, Gergolet M, et al. The ESHRE/ESGE consensus on the classification of female genital tract congenital anomalies. Human Reprod. 2013;28(8):2032-44.
15. Grimbizis GF, Tsalikis T, Mikos T, Papadopoulos N, Tarlatzis BC, Bontis JN. Successful end-to-end cervico-cervical anastomosis in a patient with congenital cervical fragmentation: case report. Hum Reprod. 2004;19(5):1204-10.
16. Hull MGR. Polycystic ovarian disease: clinical aspects and prevalence. Res Clin Forums. 1989;11:21-34.
17. Jayaprakasan K, Hilwah N, Kendall NR, Hopkisson JF, Campbell BK, Johnson IR, et al. Does 3D ultrasound offer any advantage in the pre-treatment assessment of ovarian reserve and prediction of outcome after assisted reproduction treatment? Hum Reprod. 2007;22(7):1932-41.
18. Kupesic S, Bekavac I, Bjelos D, Kurjak A. Assessment of endometrial receptivity by transvaginal colour Doppler and three-dimensional power Doppler ultrasonography in patients undergoing in vitro fertilization procedures. J Ultrasound Med. 2001;20(2):125-34.
19. Kupesic S, Kurjak A, Pasalic L, Benic S, Ilijas M. The value of transvaginal colour Doppler in the assessment of pelvic inflammatory disease. Ultrasound Med Biol. 1995;21(6):733-8.
20. Kupesic S, Kurjak A, Vujisic S, Petrović Z. Luteal phase defect: comparison between Doppler velocimetry, histological and hormonal markers. Ultrasound Obstet Gynecol. 1997;9(2):105-12.
21. Kupesic S, Kurjak A. Predictors of in vitro fertilization outcome by three-dimensional ultrasound. Hum Reprod. 2002;17(4):950-55.
22. Kupesic S, Kurjak A. The assessment of normal and abnormal luteal function by transvaginal colour Doppler sonography. Eur J Obstet Gynecol. 1997;72(1):83-7.
23. Kupesic S, Kurjak A. Uterine and ovarian perfusion during the periovulatory period assessed by transvaginal colour Doppler. Fertil Steril. 1993;60(3):439-43.
24. Kurjak A, Kupesic S, Babic MM, Goldenberg M, Illijas M, Kosuta D. Preoperative evaluation of cystic teratoma: What does colour Doppler add? J Clin Ultrasound 1997;25(6):309-16.
25. Kurjak A, Kupesic S, Miric D. The assessment of benign uterine tumour vascularization by transvaginal colour Doppler. Ultrasound Med Biol. 1992;18(6-7):645-9.
26. Kurjak A, Kupesic S. Scoring system for prediction of ovarian endometriosis based on transvaginal colour and pulse Doppler sonography. Fertil Steril. 1994;62(1):81-8.
27. Kwee J, Elting ME, Schats R, McDonnell J, Lambalk CB. Ovarian volume and antral follicle count for the prediction of low and hyper-responders with in vitro fertilization. Reprod Biol Endocrinol. 2007;5:9.
28. Kyei-Mensah A, Zaidi J, Pittrof R, Shaker A, Campbell S, Tan SL. Transvaginal three-dimensional ultrasound: accuracy of follicular volume measurements. Fertil Steril. 1996;65(2):371-6.
29. Lass A, Skull J, McVeigh E, Margara R, Winston RM. Measurement of ovarian volume by transvaginal sonography before ovulation induction with human menopausal gonadotrophin for in-vitro fertilization can predict poor response. Hum Reprod. 1992,12(2):294-7.
30. Nagori CB, Panchal SY. Double IUI in cases with high pre-hCG perifollicular PSV for better pregnancy rates: a randomized study of 350 IUI cycles. Presented at 16th World Congress on Ultrasound in Obstetrics and Gynaecology, 2006, London. J Ultrasound Obstet Gynecol. 2006;28(4):612.
31. Nargund G, Doyle PE, Bourne TH, Parsons JH, Cheng WC, Campbell S, et al. Ultrasound-device indices of follicular blood flow before hCG administration and prediction of oocyte recovery and pre-implantation embryo quality. Hum Reprod. 1996;11:2512-7.
32. Osmers R. Sonographic evaluation of ovarian masses and its therapeutic implications. Ultrasound Obstet Gynecol. 1996;8(4):217-22.
33. Panchal S, Nagori C. Ultrasound-based decision making on stimulation protocol for superovulated IUI cycles. IJIFM. 2016;7(1):7-13.
34. Panchal S, Nagori CB. Ultrasound based decision making on stimulation protocol in IVF. DSJUOG. 2016;10(3):330-7.
35. Panchal SY, Nagori CB. Can 3D PD be a better tool for assessing the pre-hCG follicle and endometrium? A randomized study of 500 cases. Presented at 16th World Congress on Ultrasound in Obstetrics and Gynecology, 2006, London. J Ultrasound Obstet Gynecol. 2006;28(4):504.

36. Patel MD, Feldstein VA, Lipson SD, Chen DC, Filly RA. Cystic teratomas of the ovary: diagnostic value of sonography. AJR Am J Roentgenol. 1998;171(4):1061-5.
37. Raga F, Bonilla-Mosules F, Blanes J, Osborne NG. Congenital mullerian anomalies: diagnostic accuracy of three-dimensional ultrasound. Fertil Steril. 1996;65(3):523-8.
38. Raga F, Bonilla-Musoles F, Casan EM, Klein O, Bonilla F. Assessment of endometrial volume by three-dimensional ultrasound prior to embryo transfer: clues to endometrial receptivity. Hum Reprod. 1999;14(11):2851-4.
39. Raine-Fenning N, Jayaprakasan K, Deb S. Three-dimensional ultrasonographic characteristics of endometriomata. Ultrasound Obstet Gynecol. 2008;31(6):718-24.
40. Richman TS, Viscomi GN, Cherney AD, Polan ML, Alcebo LO. Fallopian tubal patency assessment by ultrasound following fluid injection. Radiology. 1984;152:507-10.
41. Rock JA, Roberts CP, Jones HW. Congenital anomalies of the uterine cervix: lessons from 30 cases managed clinically by a common protocol. Fertil Steril. 2010;94(5):1858-63.
42. Salim A, Kurjak A, Zalud I. Ovarian Luteal flow in normal and abnormal early pregnancies. J Matern Foetal Invest. 1992;2:119.
43. Scheffer GJ, Broekmans FJ, Looman CW, Blankenstein M, Fauser BC, Te Jong FH, et al. The number of antral follicles in normal women with proven fertility is best reflection of reproductive age. Hum Reprod. 2003;18(4):700-6.
44. Sibal M. Follicular ring sign: a simple sonographic sign for early diagnosis of ovarian torsion. J Ultrasound Med. 2012;31(11):1803-9.
45. Steer CV, Tan SL, Mason BA, Campbell S. Mid-luteal phase vaginal colour Doppler assessment of uterine artery impedence in subfertile population. Fertil Steril. 1994;61(1):53-8.
46. Timor-Tritsch IE, Lerner JP, Monteagudo A, Murphy KE, Heller DS. Transvaginal sonographic markers of tubal inflammatory disease. Ultrasound Obstet Gynecol. 1998; 12(1):56-66.
47. Timor-Tritsch IE, Rottem S, Lewitt N. The fallopian tube. In: Timor-Tritsch IE, Rottem S (Eds). Transvaginal Sonography, 2nd edition. New York: Chapman and Hall; 1991. pp. 131-44.
48. Van Blerkom, Antczak M, Schrader R. The developmental potential of human oocyte is related to the dissolved oxygen content of follicular fluid: association with vascular endothelial growth factor levels and perifollicular blood flow characteristics. Hum Reprod. 1997;12(5):1047-55.
49. Van den Bosch T, Dueholm M, Leone FP, Valentin L, Rasmussen CK, Votino A, et al. Terms, definitions and measurements to describe sonographic features of myometrium and uterine masses: a consensus opinion from the Morphological Uterus Sonographic Assessment (MUSA) group. Ultrasound Obstet Gynecol. 2015;46:284-98.
50. Wamsteker K, de Blok S. Resection of intrauterine fibroids. In: Lewis BV, Magos AL (Eds). Endometrial Ablation. Edinburgh, UK: Churchill Livingstone; 1993.
51. Wamsteker K, Emanuel MH, de Kruif JH. Transcervical hysteroscopic resection of submucous fibroids for abnormal uterine bleeding: results regarding the degree of intramural extension. Obstet Gynecol. 1993;82(5): 736-40.
52. Wu HM, Chiang CH, Huang HY, Chao AS, Wang HS, Soong YK. Detection of subendometrial vascularization blood flow by three-dimensional ultrasound may be useful for predicting pregnancy rate for patients undergoing in vitro fertilisation-embryo transfer. Fertil Steril. 2003;79(3): 507-11.
53. Zaidi J, Barber J, Kyei-Mensah A, Bekir J, Campbell S, Tan SL. Relationship of ovarian stromal blood flow at baseline ultrasound to subsequent follicular response in an in vitro fertilization program. Obstet Gynecol. 1996;88(5):779-84.
54. Zaidi J, Campbell S, Pittrof R, Tan S. Endometrial thickness, morphology, vascular penetration and velocimetry in predicting implantation in an in vitro fertilization program. Ultrasound Obstet Gynecol. 1995;6(3):191-8.
55. Zalel Y, Soriano D, Lipitz S, Mashiach S, Achiron R. Contribution of colour Doppler flow to the ultrasonographic diagnosis of tubal abnormalities. J Ultrasound Med. 2000; 19(9):645-9.

52

CHAPTER

Ultrasound in Menopause

Priti Venkatesh

Chapter Outline

- Normal Uterus in Menopause
- Ultrasound Evaluation of the Endometrium in Postmenopausal Women
- Postmenopausal Bleeding
- Hormone Replacement Therapy and Tamoxifen
- Incidental Finding of Thick Endometrium
- Normal Atrophic Ovary
- Fluid In Pouch of Douglas
- Ovary and Ovarian Cancer Screening

INTRODUCTION

Menopause represents the beginning of the non-reproductive phase of a women's life cycle. It is a retrospective diagnosis made after menstruation has ceased for 12 months. With aging, the number of ovarian follicles decreases, follicular recruitment fails and there is reduced production of oestrogen and progesterone, which leads to anovulatory cycles, inadequate endometrium stimulation and growth, resulting in infrequent irregular and scanty menstruation. In the perimenopausal period, irregularity of menstruation occurs both in frequency and amount. Sometimes bleeding may be heavy too. This transition can take a decade to attain menopause and affects the body physically and psychologically.

At this stage of life, changes in hormones have an effect on morphology of reproductive organs too. This is the period when cancers may develop and women require a regular pelvic examination. Many a times, due to hormonal fluctuation irregular heavy bleeding causes an anxiety of cancer development in both women and their gynaecologists.

With the increasing life expectancy, the menopausal population is on the rise. The ultrasound technology, which is presently available, offers a unique insight into the anatomical, physiological and pathological states of the women in the menopausal age group.

Imaging the uterus and ovary and evaluating the pelvis from close proximity using ultrasound has revolutionised treatment protocols in gynaecology. Being noninvasive it can be used frequently to evaluate the cause of irregular bleeding and various adnexal masses. To begin with, it is necessary to understand the normal physiological changes of menopause to enable the ultrasonologist to have a suspicion of the pathological entities.

Transabdominal ultrasound (TAUS or TAS) and transvaginal ultrasound (TVUS or TVS) with high-frequency probes, colour flow mapping, duplex Doppler studies and three-dimensional (3D) reconstruction have changed the approach to clinical problems in the perimenopausal and menopausal phase. A normal endovaginal sonogram in a postmenopausal patient has a high negative predictive value and high overall accuracy rate for excluding major disorders of the uterus and ovaries, with excellent pathologic correlation. Because TVUS can be used to accurately assess the endometrium, sequential ultrasound examinations can be of value for close monitoring of endometrial thickness (ET).

As a result of hormonal fluctuations, ultrasonographic appearance of uterus and ovaries changes in the lifespan of a woman. The sonologist must understand these normal physiological changes in order to be able to identify pathological changes accurately.

Transvaginal ultrasonography (USG) is the most popular imaging modality used for the initial assessment of possible gynaecologic abnormalities in patients of all ages and may be the only examination needed for diagnostic evaluation of the uterus, ovaries and adnexa.

NORMAL UTERUS IN MENOPAUSE

- The atrophic endometrium appears as a thin pencil-line echogenicity or an ecogenic line with average endometrial thickness (ET) of 3.0 mm **(Figs. 1 and 2)**.

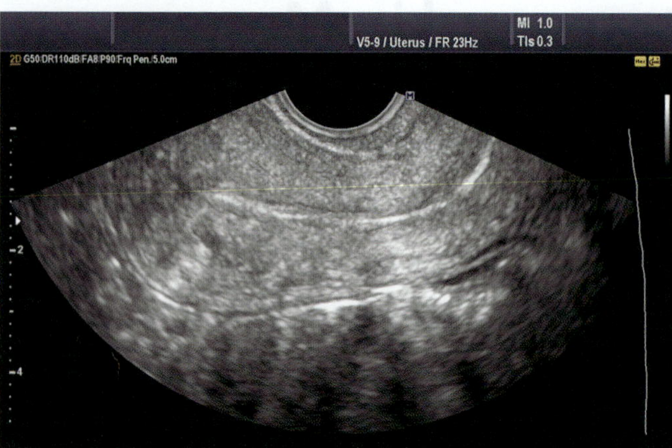

Fig. 1: Atrophic thin endometrium.

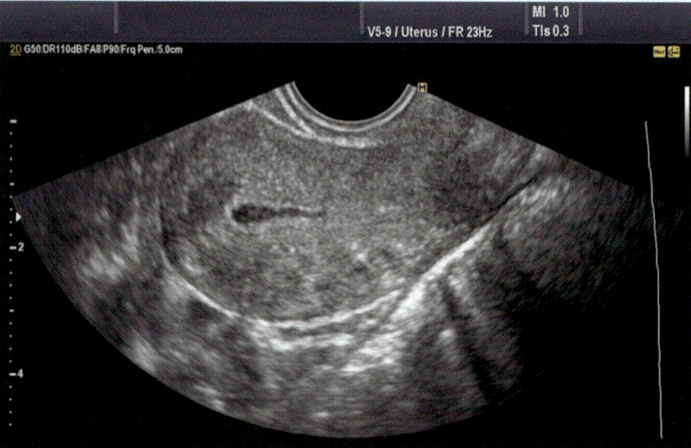

Fig. 2: Thin endometrium with collection.

- The measurement on scanning should definitely include the maximum anteroposterior thickness in the sagittal long-axis view.
- The cutoff level of the ET for detection of endometrial disease should also be based on the length of time since menopause.
- Myometrium is heterogeneous and sometimes calcified uterine vessels are seen along the outer one third of the myometrium. Morphology also depends upon pre-existing diseases such as fibroids or adenomyosis too.

ULTRASOUND EVALUATION OF THE ENDOMETRIUM IN POSTMENOPAUSAL WOMEN (FLOWCHART 1)

Transvaginal ultrasound is recommended for evaluation of the endometrium of postmenopausal women for accurate assessment of ET **(Figs. 3A and B)**. When evaluating the endometrium, the following steps should be followed:

- ET—two layers, in millimeters.
- If there is fluid in the cavity—single layer thickness—maximum anterior layer and maximum posterior layer thickness are measured and the sum of the two measurements is taken as the ET.
- Morphology should be next evaluated in all cases. Nonhomogenous echotexture is abnormal.
- Zoom and evaluate the echotexture for focal lesions, diffuse hyperplasia and polyps.
- Doppler: Use high-definition flow (HDF) (more sensitive for low velocity flows than colour flow). Slow flows in newer machines are also useful but may lead to overdiagnosis of colour scores.

Always keep PRF very low, 0.6 kHz or lower when assessing blood flow in gynaecology.

POSTMENOPAUSAL BLEEDING

Postmenopausal bleeding (PMB) is the presenting complaint in >90% of women with endometrial cancer. But PMB usually occurs due to atrophic changes in the endometrium and vagina. Endometrial cancer is found in 1–14% of women with PMB. The higher percentage is in older women with other risk factors.

A TVUS evaluation of the endometrium is a good initial step for the evaluation of women with PMB, because an ET of ≤4 mm has a negative predictive value of >99%, which means that the risk of missing an endometrial malignancy with this cutoff is extremely low.

In a woman with PMB, if TVUS shows an ET of ≤4 mm, no further test is needed.

Endometrial thickness of >4 mm is a good cutoff for offering further testing to rule out malignancy.

However, if the woman has any of the following high-risk factors—advance age, obesity and use of unopposed oestrogen for hormone replacement therapy (HRT), polycystic ovary syndrome (PCOS), type 2 diabetes mellitus (DM) and atypical glandular cells on screening cervical smear or family history of cervical cancer—then endometrial sampling should be added.

ET of >4 mm and ≤4 mm + abnormal endometrial morphology on TVUS or high-risk factors requires endometrial biopsy.

Abnormal endometrial morphology ***(Figs. 4 to 10)*** other than confirmed benign polyp with a single feeder vessel **(Fig. 11)** requires endometrial biopsy.

Office cervical biopsy can also be done under ultrasound guidance to ensure proper sampling.

If the blind/office biopsy is negative or if there is recurrent PMB, then hysteroscopy and dilation

Flowchart 1: Evaluation of postmenopausal endometrium.

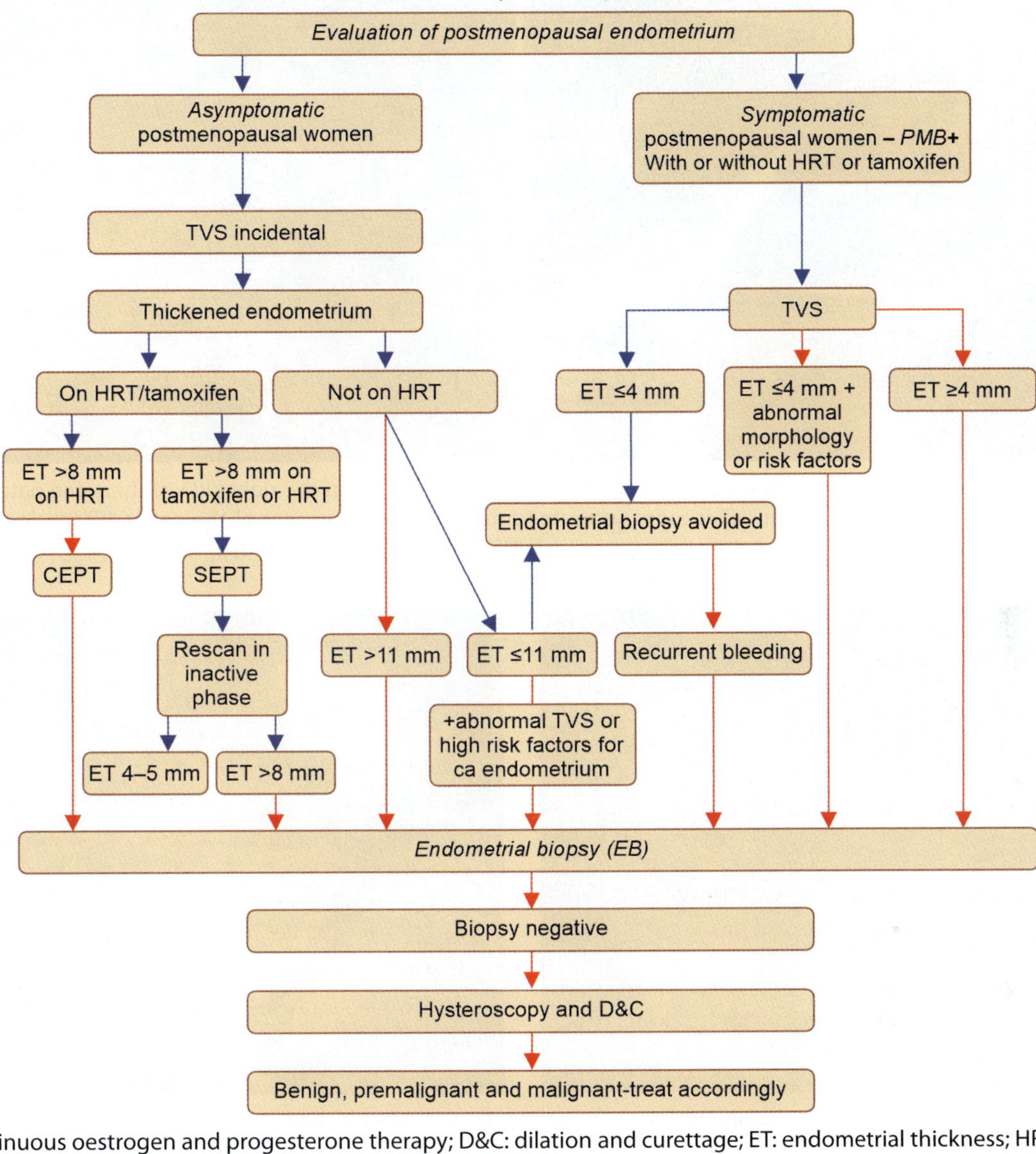

(CEPT: continuous oestrogen and progesterone therapy; D&C: dilation and curettage; ET: endometrial thickness; HRT: hormone replacement therapy; SEPT: sequential oestrogen and progesterone therapy; TVS: transvaginal sonography)

and curettage (D&C) are recommended. This is not recommended as a primary procedure because of the very low risk of malignancy at an ET cutoff of 4 mm and the relatively high complication risk of hysteroscopy and D&C in postmenopausal women.

Ultrasound is an important tool to evaluate endometrial diseases in asymptomatic postmenopausal women too.

Endometrial thickness <4 mm is usually associated with benign histopathologic findings in majority of the postmenopausal women.

HORMONE REPLACEMENT THERAPY AND TAMOXIFEN

One has to remember special considerations in those women who are on HRT or tamoxifen therapy.

Hormone replacement therapy: Definition of normal ET depends on the type of HRT.

Continuous oestrogen and progesterone therapy (CEPT) leads to endometrium atrophy. The average ET in continuous E/P HRT is 3.5 mm versus 5.5 mm in sequential HRT.

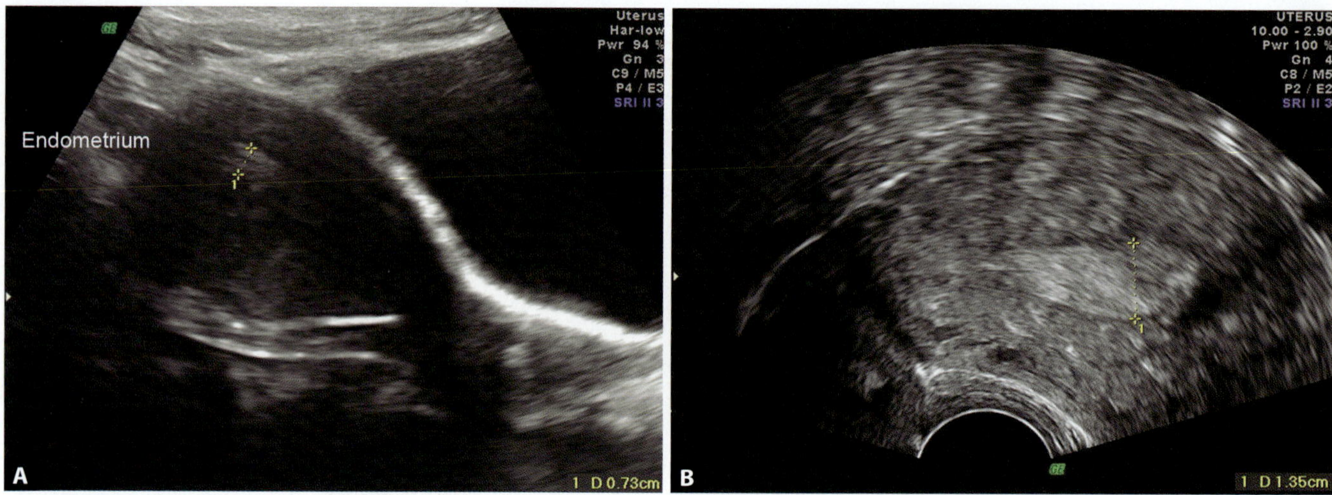

Figs. 3A and B: TAUS on the left (A) shows an ET of 7.3 mm and a TVUS image (B) on the right side of the same patient shows an ET of 13.5 mm. This demonstrates clearly that TVS is more accurate for ultrasound assessment of the pelvis. (ET: endometrial thickness; TAUS: transabdominal ultrasound; TVS: transvaginal sonography; TVUS: transvaginal ultrasound)

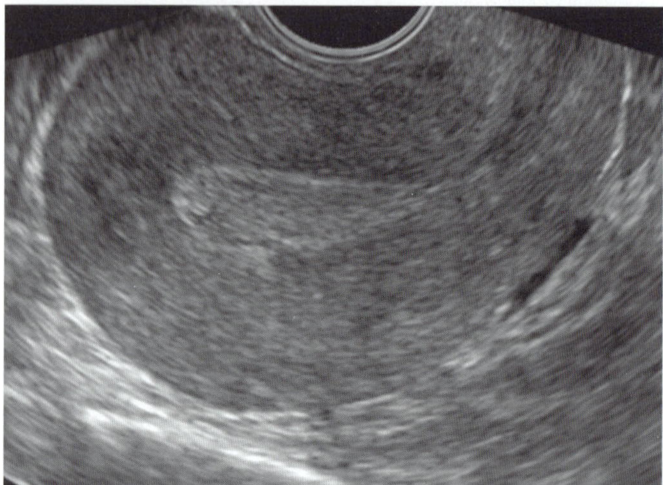

Fig. 4: Thick in-homogeneous endometrium.

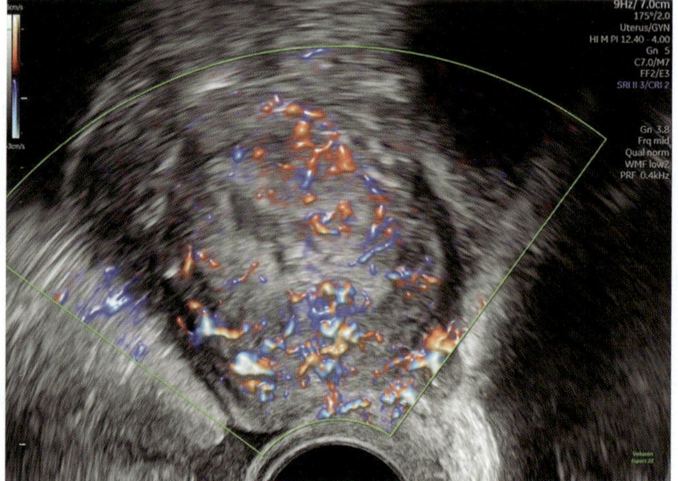

Fig. 5: TVUS showing thick nonhomogenous endometrium with collection in the cavity indicating a high risk of endometrial carcinoma in a 70-year-old postmenopausal woman. (TVUS: transvaginal ultrasound)

Sequential oestrogen and progesterone therapy (SEPT) causes similar endometrial changes as in normal periods and is associated with:

- Proliferative, secretory and inactive patterns corresponding to oestrogen, progesterone and bleeding phases of the cycle, respectively.
- ET can increase to 10–12 mm in proliferative phase but should be <5 mm after withdrawal bleeding.
- Endometrial polyps—seen in 16–24% of women on SERT. More than 50% become symptomatic at sometime.
- Endometrial hyperplasia—low risk <1% after 3–5 years if progesterone dose is adequate.

Tamoxifen: Many patients of breast cancer are kept on tamoxifen which has an effect on endometrium and can lead to endometrial hyperplasia. Nearly half of all postmenopausal women undergoing tamoxifen therapy have an ET >8 mm, and most are asymptomatic, without abnormal vaginal bleeding. The most common histopathologic findings, including hyperplasia and polyps, are benign, with an approximate 1% risk of endometrial carcinoma. This group of patients also require a biopsy if they become symptomatic. Refer to **Flowchart 1** on the evaluation of PMB.

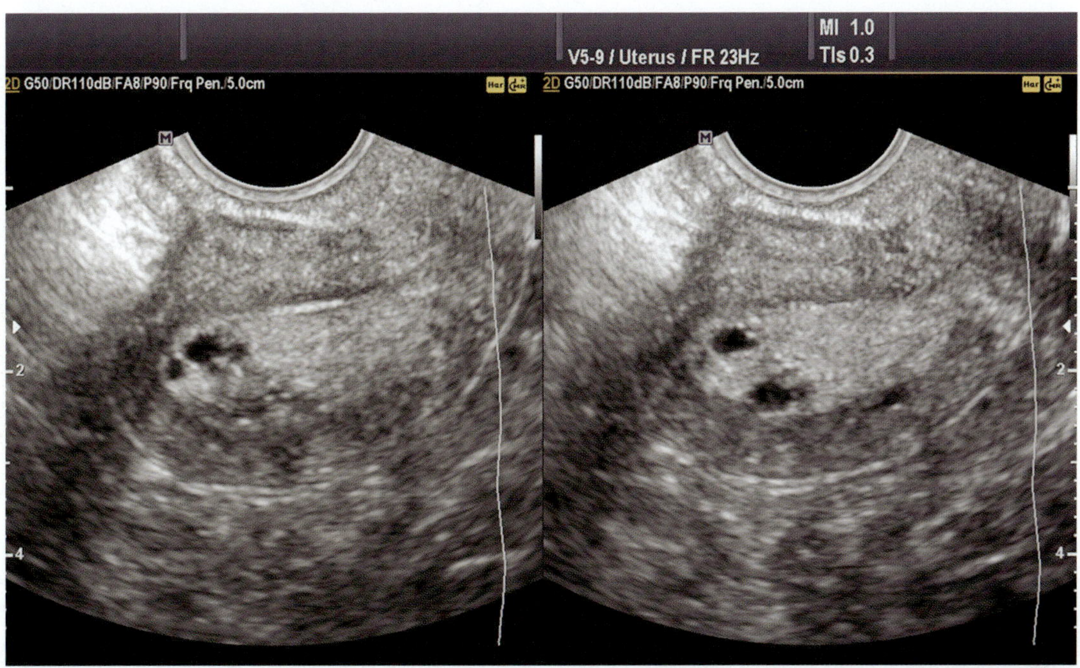

Fig. 6: Thick nonhomogenous endometrium with cystic spaces. Could be an endometrial polyp filling the cavity—needs confirmation with Doppler—HDF or PD (Power Doppler).

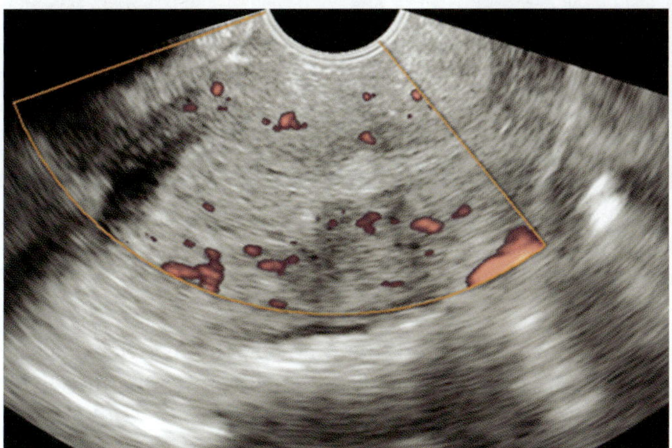

Fig. 7: Thick non-homogeneous, irregularly thickened endometrium always raises a suspicion of malignancy.

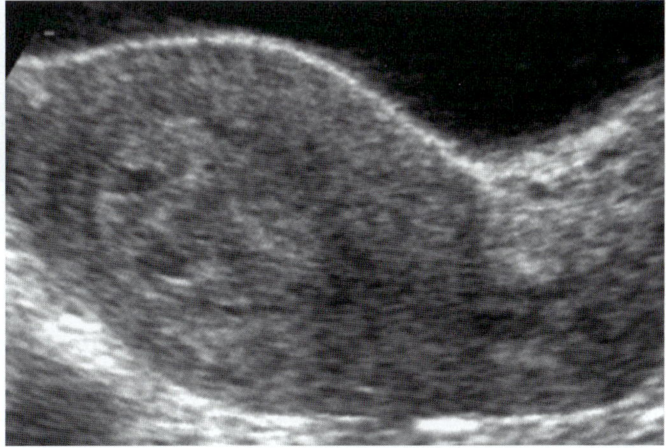

Fig. 8: Transabdominal scan with a thick endometrium in a case of postmenopausal bleeding.

INCIDENTAL FINDING OF THICK ENDOMETRIUM

Since >90% of patients with endometrial carcinoma present with bleeding prevagina, and there is no difference in outcome between patients diagnosed after PMB or after an incidental finding of thick endometrium in asymptomatic women—routine screening for ET is not recommended. However, incidental detection of thick endometrium may occur. Evaluation of these women should include:

- A TVUS
- Assessment of ET
- Detail morphologic assessment
- Endometrial biopsy is needed for:
    - ET ≥11 mm
    - ET <11 mm with abnormal morphology or with risk factors.

The 8 mm threshold has no formal backing in asymptomatic women unless other concerns exist.

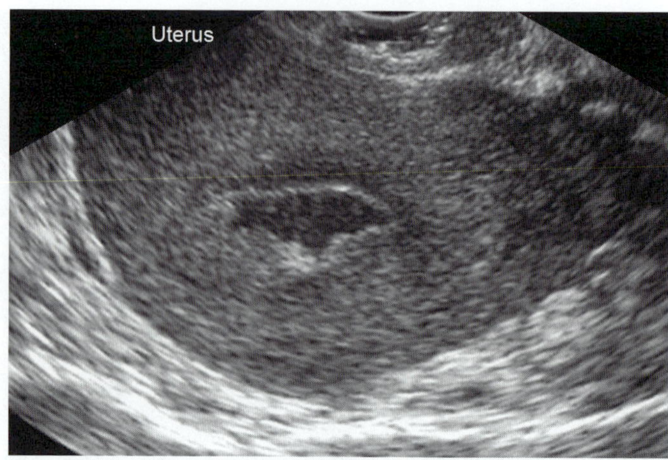

Fig. 9: Thickened endometrium with non-homogeneous fluid collection and loss of endometrial–myometrial interface in the posterior aspect.

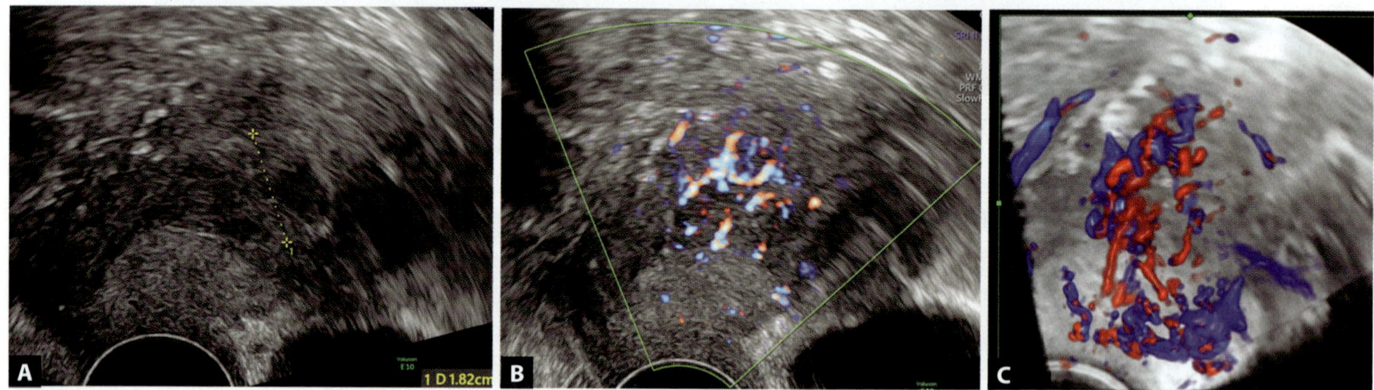

Figs. 10A to C: 69-year-old, menopause 15 years back with PMB: (A) A thick endometrium 18.2 mm; (B) Abundant vascularity with HDF on 2D imaging—colour score 4 for her post menopausal status. (C) Abundant vascularity and colour score 4 with colour Doppler on 3D. HPE after surgery—High grade serous carcinoma of the endometrium with >75% myometrial invasion.

ET ≤4 mm reassure, no further action. ET of 5–10 mm—individualise based on endometrial morphology on TVUS and presence of other risk factors to endometrial cancer.

NORMAL ATROPHIC OVARY

The ovary lacks follicles after menopause and, therefore, looks like an area of nonspecific solid echoes, making it more difficult to identify on both transabdominal and transvaginal scans. The normal postmenopausal ovary is less echogenic, is smaller and generally has fewer or no follicles than the normal ovary during the reproductive years **(Fig. 12)**. Sometimes a small follicle-like thin-walled cyst with no septa or nodules is seen, especially in the first 5 years after menopause **(Fig. 13)**. This may be physiological but needs Ca 125 and follow-up scans. Some authors have suggested that an ovary that is twice as large as the contralateral ovary, regardless of absolute size, should be considered abnormal.

FLUID IN POUCH OF DOUGLAS

In early menopause, a small amount of free peritoneal fluid is occasionally seen in postmenopausal women and is not necessarily pathologic if it is simple in appearance. Free fluid in late menopause is abnormal and could be related to a variety of conditions, including intraperitoneal malignancy and ascites due to cardiac, renal and liver disease.

OVARY AND OVARIAN CANCER SCREENING

More than two thirds of the cases of ovarian cancer are diagnosed when they reach stage III or IV.

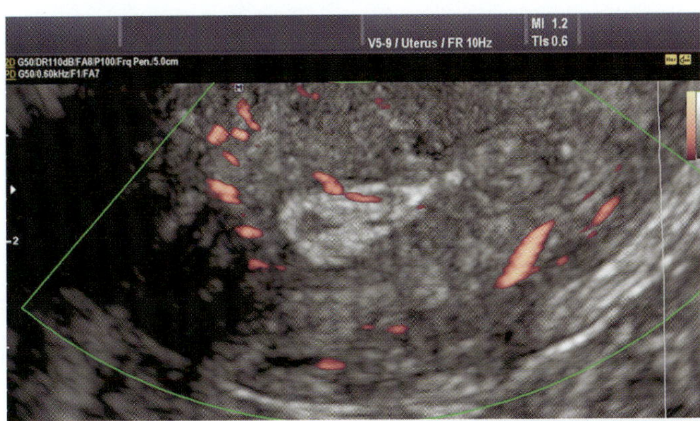

Fig. 11: Thick endometrium with polyp and single feeder vessel. Treat this as a benign polyp—ET ≤11 mm—no PMB no risk factor— follow up—+PMB or + risk factors—do EB.

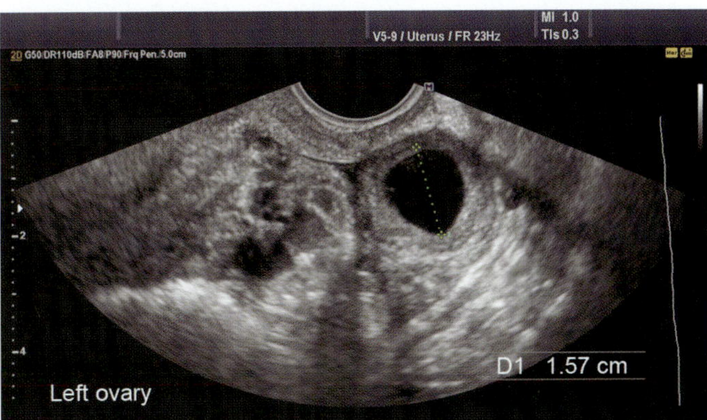

Fig. 13: Thin-walled clear cyst with no features suggesting malignancy a follow-up is required but no invasive procedures are needed.

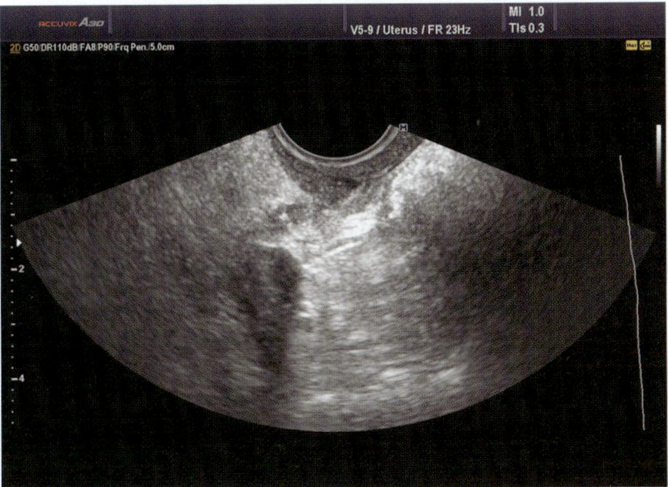

Fig. 12: Atrophic ovary in a postmenopausal lady.

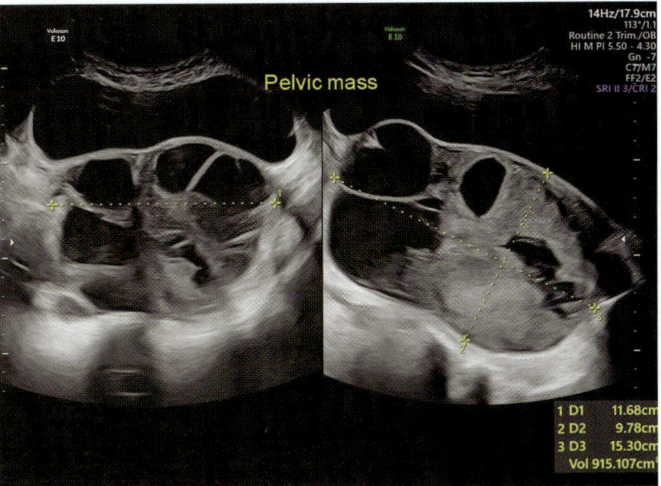

Fig. 14: Multiloculated mass with thick septa and solid areas.

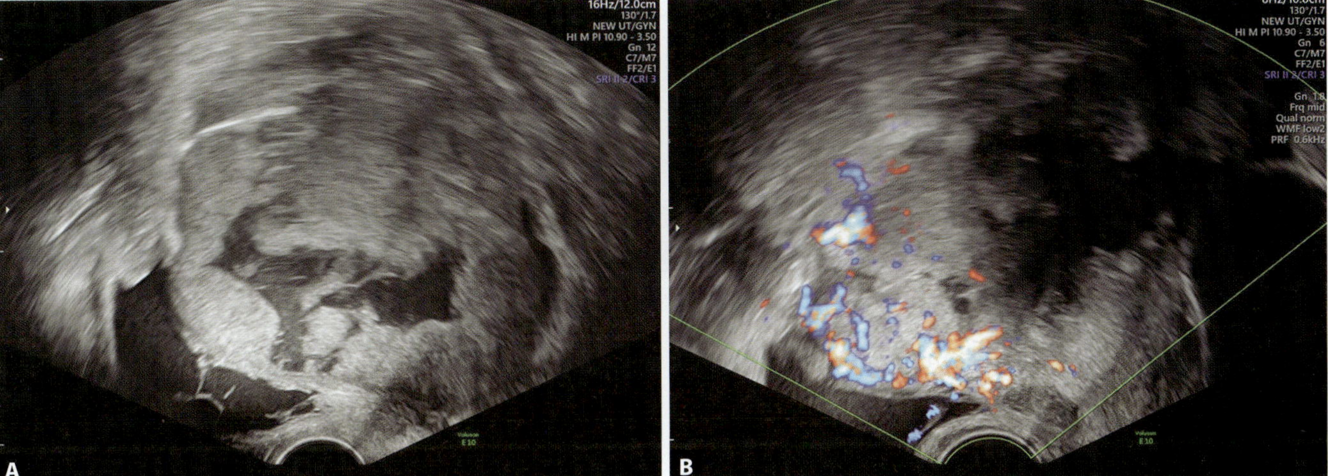

Figs. 15A and B: Predominantly solid mass with abundant vascularity. Colour score is only 3, but the vessels are thick and disorganised and there are splashes of colour.

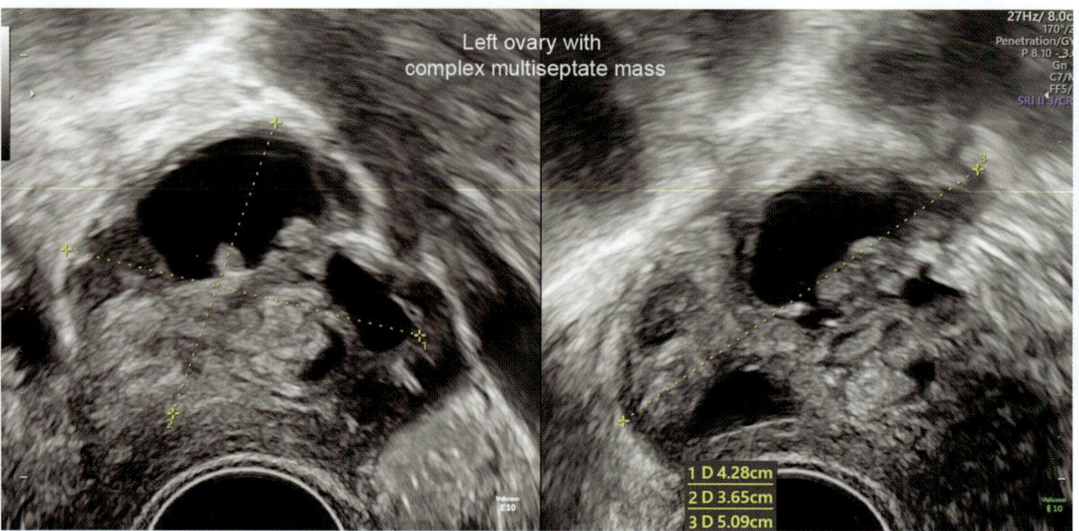

Fig. 16: Ovarian cyst with irregular thick-walls and mural nodules – Serous cystadenocaecinoma.

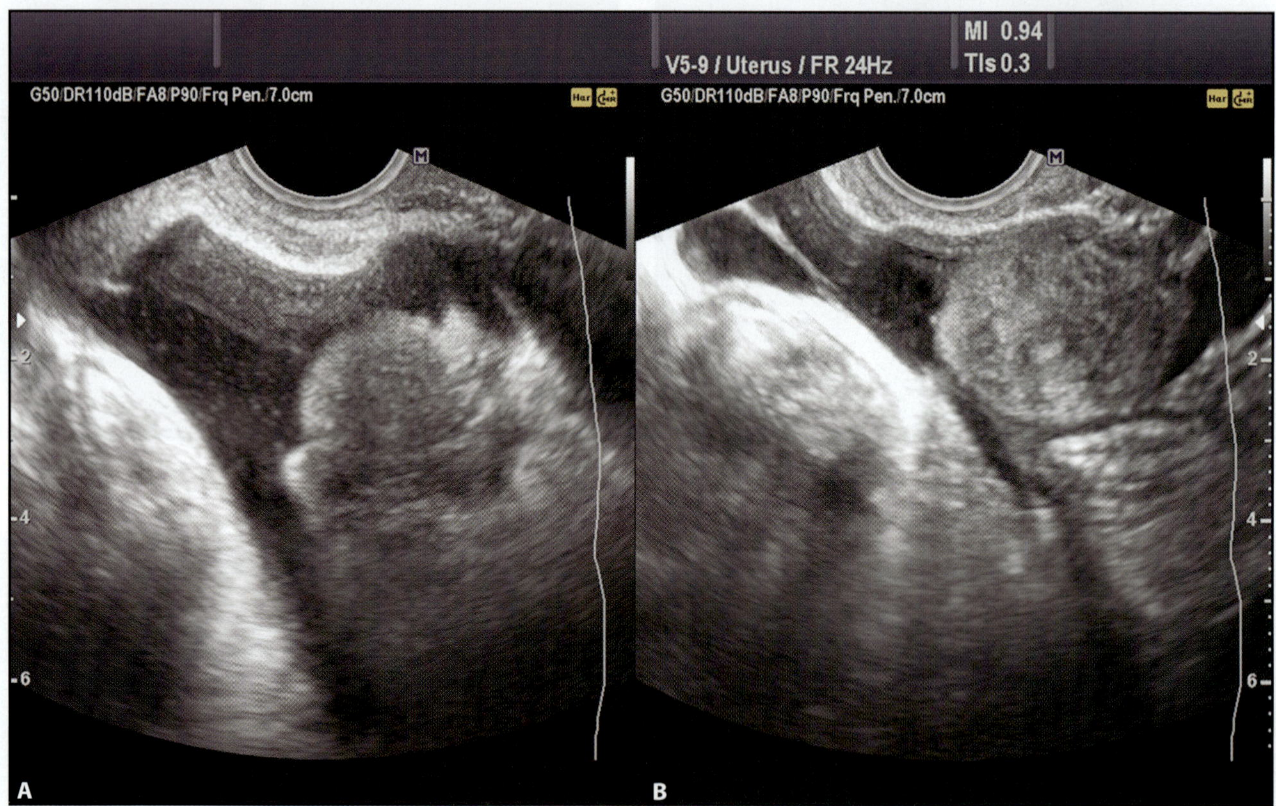

Figs. 17A and B: Ascites noted. Carefully assess the uterus and ovaries.

An annual pelvic examination, tumour marker levels and grey-scale USG with colour Doppler and 3D reconstruction of tumour vascularity have emerged as reliable ovarian cancer screening tools when used together.

The criteria for diagnosis remain the same as in the premenopausal age group (refer Chapter 50). These include grey-scale observations of a solid mass, a cystic mass with solid areas, focal or diffusely thick walls or septations, mural nodules and heterogeneous internal echoes **(Figs. 14 to 17)**.

Pelvic and para-aortic lymph node enlargement, ascites **(Figs. 17A and B)**, suprarenal and liver metastases and pleural effusions can be elucidated by transabdominal scanning.

SUGGESTED READING

1. ACOG Committee Opinion No. 724. (2018). "The Role of Transvaginal Ultrasonography in Evaluating the Endometrium of Women With Postmenopausal Bleeding." This opinion replaced Committee Opinion No. 440 (2009).
2. Andreotti RF, Bennett GL, Lee SI, Dejesus Allison SO, Brown DL, Dubinsky T, et al. ACR appropriateness criteria® on abnormal vaginal bleeding. J Am Coll Radiol. 2011;8(7):460-8.
3. Epstein E, Valentin L. Gray-scale ultrasound morphology in the presence or absence of intrauterine fluid and vascularity as assessed by color Doppler for discrimination between benign and malignant endometrium in women with postmenopausal bleeding. Ultrasound in Obstetrics and Gynecology: The Official Journal of the International Society of Ultrasound in Obstetrics and Gynecology. 2006;28(1):89-95.
4. Feeley KM, Wells M. Hormone replacement therapy and the endometrium. J Clin Pathol. 2001;54(6):435-40.
5. Franchi M, Ghezzi F, Donadello N, Zanaboni F, Beretta P, Bolis P. Endometrial thickness in tamoxifen-treated patients: an independent predictor of endometrial disease. Obstet Gynecol. 1999;93(6):1004-8.
6. Giri SK, Nayak BL, Mohapatra J. Thickened endometrium: when to intervene? A clinical conundrum. The Journal of Obstetrics and Gynecology of India. 2021;71(3):216-25.
7. Goldstein SR, Khafaga A. Ability to successfully image endometrium on transvaginal ultrasound in asymptomatic postmenopausal women. Ultrasound Obstet Gynecol. 2021;58(4).
8. Goldstein SR. The role of transvaginal ultrasound or endometrial biopsy in the evaluation of the menopausal endometrium. Am J Obstet Gynaecol. 2009;201(1):5-11.
9. Hall DA, McCarthy KA, Kopans DB. Sonographic visualisation of the normal post-menopausal ovary. J Ultrasound Med. 1986;5(1): 9-11.
10. Imaoka I, Sugimura K, Masui T, Takehara Y, Ichijo K, Naito M. Abnormal uterine cavity: differential diagnosis with MR imaging. Magn Reson Imaging. 1999;17(10):1445-55.
11. Jill E, Langer MD, Edward R. Imaging of the Female Pelvis through the life cycle. RSNA. 2012; 3,(6).
12. Jokubkiene L, Sladkevicius P, Valentin L. Transvaginal ultrasound examination of the endometrium in postmenopausal women without vaginal bleeding. Ultrasound Obstet Gynecol. 2016;48(3):390-6.
13. Karlsson B, Granberg S, Wikland M, Ylöstalo P, Torvid K, Marsal K, Valentin L. Transvaginal ultrasonography of the endometrium in women with postmenopausal bleeding—a Nordic multicenter study. Am J Obstet Gynecol. 1995;172(5):1488-94.
14. Markovitch O, Tepper R, Fishman A, Shapira J, Aviram R, Cohen I. The value of transvaginal ultrasonography in the prediction of endometrial pathologies in asymptomatic postmenopausal breast cancer tamoxifen-treated patients. Gynecol Oncol. 2004;95(3):456-62.
15. Merz E, Miric-Tesanic D, Bahlmann F, Weber G, Wellek S. Sonographic size of uterus and ovaries in pre-and postmenopausal women. Ultrasound in Obstetrics and Gynecology: The Official Journal of the International Society of Ultrasound in Obstetrics and Gynecology. 1996;7(1):38-42.
16. Mossa B, Imperato F, Marziani R, Perniola F, Melluso J, Perniola G, Napolitano C. Hormonal replacement therapy and evaluation of intrauterine pathology in postmenopausal women: a ten-year study. Eur J Gynaecol Oncol. 2003;24(6):507-12.
17. Omodei U, Ferrazzi E, Ramazzotto F, Becorpi A, Grimaldi E, Scarselli G, Spagnolo D, Spagnolo L, Torri W. Endometrial evaluation with transvaginal ultrasound during hormone therapy: a prospective multicenter study. Fertility and sterility. 2004;81(6):1632-7.
18. Salem S. Diagnostic ultrasound. In: Rumack CM, Wilson SR, Charboneau JW, Levine DL (Eds) Gynaecology, 4th edition. Philadelphia, Pa: Mosby; 2011. pp. 547-612.
19. Sladkevicius P, Valentin L, Maršál K. Transvaginal gray-scale and Doppler ultrasound examinations of the uterus and ovaries in healthy postmenopausal women. Ultrasound in Obstetrics and Gynecology: The Official Journal of the International Society of Ultrasound in Obstetrics and Gynecology. 1995;6(2):81-90.
20. Smith-Bindman R, Kerlikowske K, Feldstein VA, Subak L, Scheidler J, Segal M, Brand R, Grady D. Endovaginal ultrasound to exclude endometrial cancer and other endometrial abnormalities. JAMA. 1998;280(17):1510-7.
21. Smith-Bindman R, Weiss E, Feldstein V. How thick is too thick? When endometrial thickness should prompt biopsy in postmenopausal women without vaginal bleeding. Ultrasound Obstet Gynaecol. 2004;24(5):558-65.
22. Smith-Bindman R, Weiss E, Feldstein V. How thick is too thick? When endometrial thickness should prompt biopsy in postmenopausal women without vaginal bleeding. Ultrasound in Obstetrics and Gynecology: The Official Journal of the International Society of Ultrasound in Obstetrics and Gynecology. 2004;24(5):558-65.
23. Smith-Bindman R, Weiss E, Feldstein V. How thick is too thick? When endometrial thickness should prompt biopsy in postmenopausal women without vaginal bleeding. Ultrasound in Obstetrics and Gynecology: The Official Journal of the International Society of Ultrasound in Obstetrics and Gynecology. 2004;24(5):558-65.
24. Sokalska A, Valentin L. Changes in ultrasound morphology of the uterus and ovaries during the menopausal transition and early postmenopause: a 4-year longitudinal study. Ultrasound Obstet Gynaecol. 2008;31(2):210-7.

25. The role of transvaginal ultrasonography in evaluating the endome trium of women with postmenopausal bleeding. ACOG Committee Opinion No. 734. American College of Obstetricians and Gynecologists. Obstet Gynecol 2018; 131:e124–9.
26. Thierry Van den Bosch, Leuven UZ. Use of pelvic ultrasound screening in post-menopausal women. BMS. 2010:13.
27. Timmermans A, Opmeer BC, Khan KS, Bachmann LM, Epstein E, Clark TJ, Gupta JK, Bakour SH, Van Den Bosch T, Van Doorn HC, Cameron ST. Endometrial thickness measurement for detecting endometrial cancer in women with postmenopausal bleeding: a systematic review and meta-analysis. Obstet Gynecol. 2010;116(1):160-7.
28. Van den Bosch T, Van Schoubroeck D, Ameye L, De Brabanter J, Van Huffel S, Timmerman D. Ultrasound assessment of endometrial thickness and endometrial polyps in women on hormonal replacement therapy. Am J Obstet Gynecol. 2003;188(5):1249-53.
29. Van Den Bosch T, Verbakel JY, Valentin L, Wynants L, De Cock B, Pascual MA, Leone FP, Sladkevicius P, Alcazar JL, Votino A, Fruscio R. Typical ultrasound features of various endometrial pathologies described using International Endometrial Tumor Analysis (IETA) terminology in women with abnormal uterine bleeding. Ultrasound Obstet Gynecol. 2021;57(1): 164-72.

53

CHAPTER

Robotic Surgery

Rani Akhil Bhat

Chapter Outline

- About da Vinci Surgical System
- Distinguishing Laparoscopy from Robotic Surgery: Unveiling Contrasts in Minimally Invasive Techniques
- Robotic Surgery Considerations for Patients
- Robotic Surgery Considerations for Doctors
- Introduction of da Vinci Robotic in Gynaecology
- Revolutionising Medicine: The Future Horizons of Robotic Surgery Innovation

INTRODUCTION

The advent of da Vinci robotic surgery has revolutionised the medical field, offering unparalleled precision and minimally invasive techniques. This chapter explores the introduction of da Vinci robotic surgery in the medical field and its specific applications in gynaecological procedures. It covers the distinctive features of the da Vinci robot, its indications, drawbacks and a detailed examination of its role in managing various gynaecological conditions. Additionally, the chapter discusses the latest advances in robotic surgery, shaping the future of surgical interventions.

ABOUT da VINCI SURGICAL SYSTEM

The da Vinci Surgical System is a revolutionary robotic surgical platform designed to enhance minimally invasive surgery. It was developed by Intuitive Surgical, Inc., a company founded in 1995 by Frederic Moll, John Freund and Robert Younge. The da Vinci system was named after Leonardo da Vinci, the renowned Italian polymath, reflecting the system's aim to combine advanced technology with the art of surgery.

The development of the da Vinci Surgical System began in the late 1980s and early 1990s. The initial idea was to create a system that could enable surgeons to perform complex surgeries with enhanced precision, dexterity and minimally invasive techniques. The system went through several prototypes and iterations before reaching its current form.

The da Vinci Surgical System received its initial clearance from the United States Food and Drug Administration (FDA) in 2000 for general laparoscopic surgery. Since then, the system has received additional clearances for various surgical procedures, making it one of the most widely used robotic surgical platforms globally.

da Vinci® Surgical System (Fig. 1)

The da Vinci Surgical System is composed of three main components, each playing a crucial role in facilitating minimally invasive robotic-assisted surgeries. These components work together seamlessly to provide surgeons with enhanced precision, dexterity and visualisation. The three main components are discussed here.

Surgeon's Console (Fig. 2)

Design and functionality: This is where the surgeon sits during the procedure, viewing a three-dimensional (3D), high-definition image of the surgical site. The surgeon's console is the command centre of the da Vinci System. It typically resembles a workstation with a computer, ergonomic controls and a viewing interface. The design is meant to provide comfort to the surgeon during long procedures while offering easy access to controls. The surgical console comprises various components that exhibit similarities across the two most recent iterations of the robotic system (Si/Xi): Stereo viewer, master controllers, touchpad and the footswitch panel. This console is furnished with both hand and foot controls, enabling the surgeon to skilfully operate the robotic arms and instruments. The hand controls function akin to master manipulators, translating the surgeon's hand

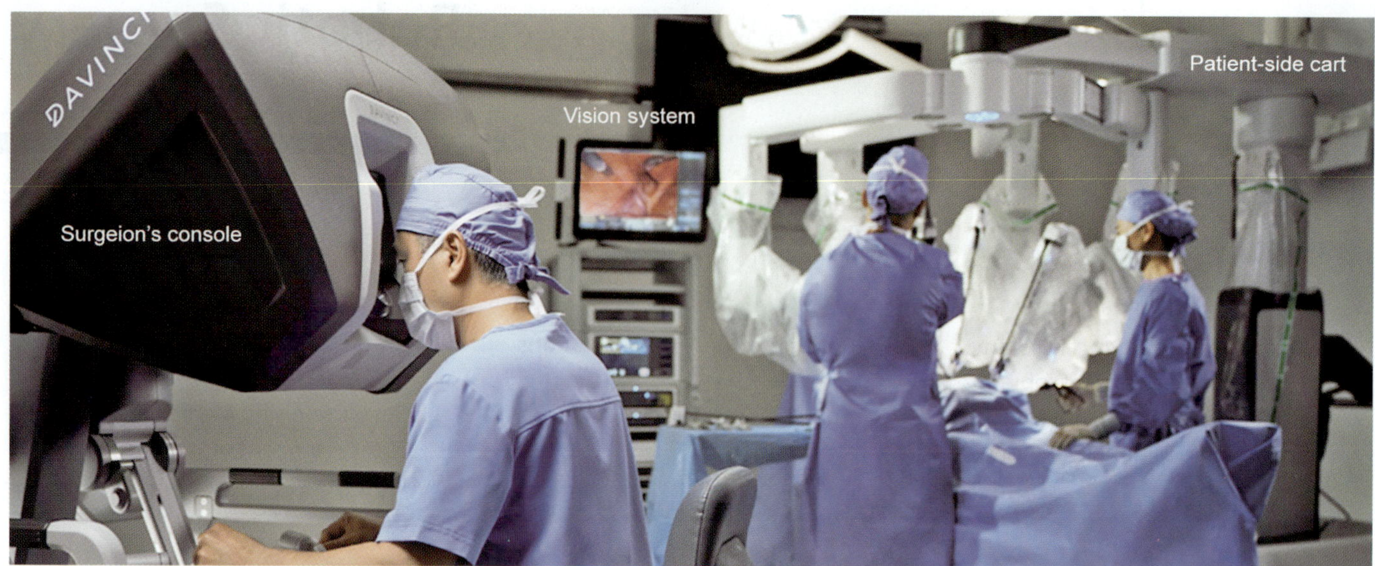

Fig. 1: da Vinci® Surgical System.

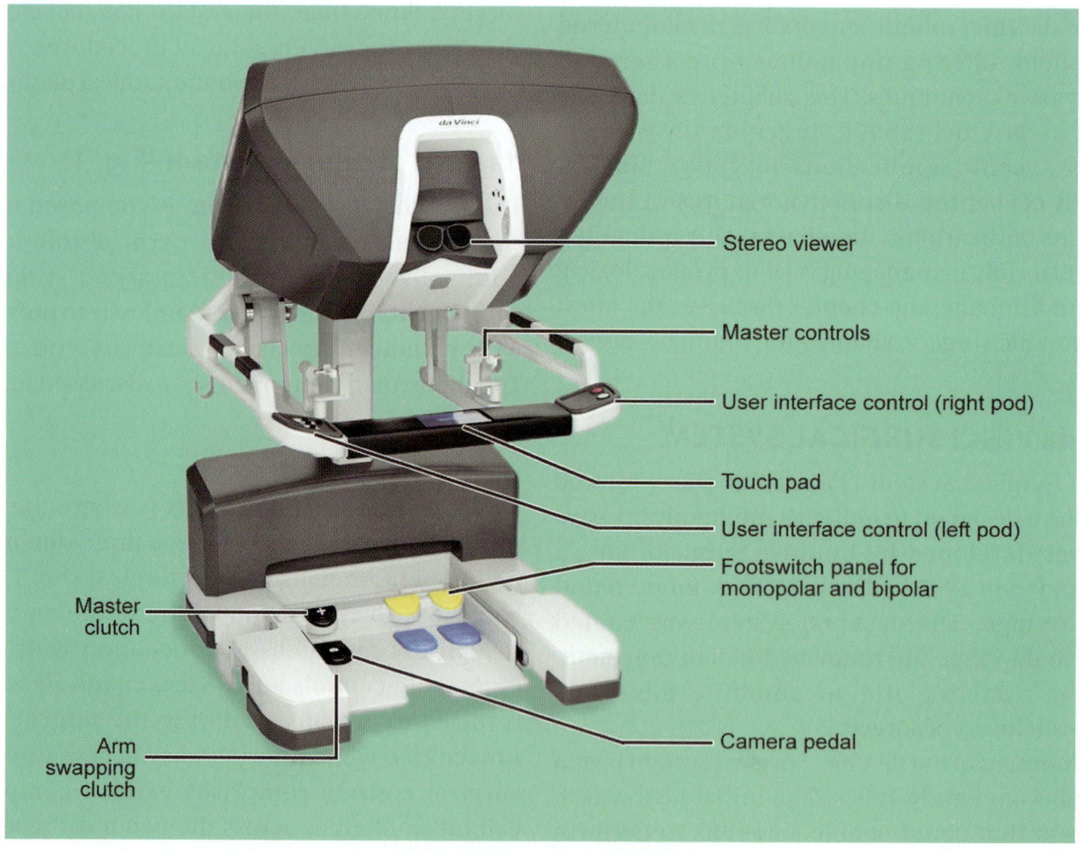

Fig. 2: Surgeon console.

movements into precise motions executed by the robotic arms. Additionally, foot pedals are employed to manage functions such as camera adjustments and energy sources for surgical instruments.

Stereo viewer ***(Fig. 3)***:

- The stereo viewer delivers a high-definition 3D perspective of the surgical field, offering magnification capabilities of up to 10×. Ergonomically crafted, the

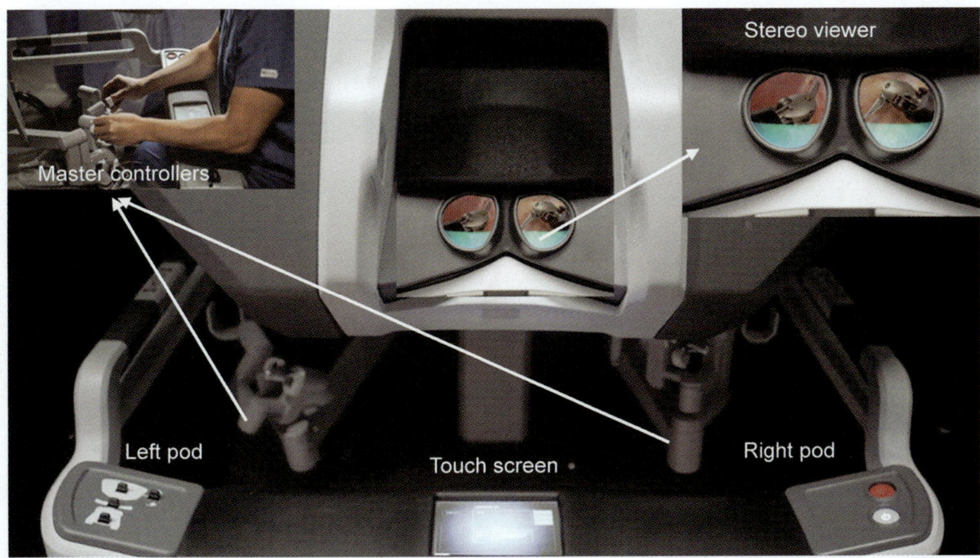

Fig. 3: Stereo viewer and master controllers.

stereo viewer provides support for the surgeon's head and neck during surgical procedures. Moreover, it serves as a platform to relay system status messages and icons to the user.

- Functioning as a 'stereo viewer', it interprets the image captured by the endoscope, presenting it in front of the surgeon's eyes to create a sense of surgical immersion. In the stereo viewer, instrument tips align with the surgeon's hands on the master controllers, mirroring the natural eye, hand and instrument alignment observed in open surgery. This intentional design aims to replicate the familiar alignment, optimising hand-eye coordination and allowing the surgeon to maintain dexterity comparable to open surgery while operating in a minimally invasive environment.
- *Three-dimensional visualisation:* The console features a 3D, high-definition display that provides the surgeon with a magnified and immersive view of the surgical site. This enhances depth perception and helps the surgeon navigate intricate anatomical structures with greater accuracy.
- To enhance control, the system incorporates features such as motion scaling and tremor reduction, minimising the impact of natural hand tremors or unintentional movements during surgical procedures.

Master controllers: The surgeon console features control pods on both sides. The left pod adjusts stereo viewer, armrest and footswitch panel. User settings are saved and automatically recalled. The right pod has power and emergency stop buttons. The centre touchpad lets surgeons save preferences and access controls. Tabs at the bottom of the screen offer video, audio and utility settings. Footswitch panel controls robotic arm swapping, master clutching, camera and instrument activation. Left pedals enable arm control and camera adjustments. Right pedals activate instrument functions such as coagulation and cutting.

Ergonomics: The console is designed to minimise surgeon fatigue during lengthy procedures, with adjustable settings to accommodate individual preferences.

Patient-side Cart (Fig. 4)

The patient cart, an integral part of the da Vinci System, serves as the slave unit supporting instrument and stereo endoscopic camera arms. Remote centre technology allows the arms to move around a fixed point in space, minimising force on the patient's body. These instruments work within the sterile field, while the surgeon and console stay outside. The computerised control system extends the surgeon's presence by transmitting video images to the console and replicating hand motions from master interfaces to the slave manipulators. The assistant surgeon manages the patient cart, handling instrument and endoscope exchanges and other patient-side tasks. An optional touchscreen monitor on patient-side cart provides a view of the operative site. For patient safety, actions of the assistant surgeon take precedence over the surgeon console operator.

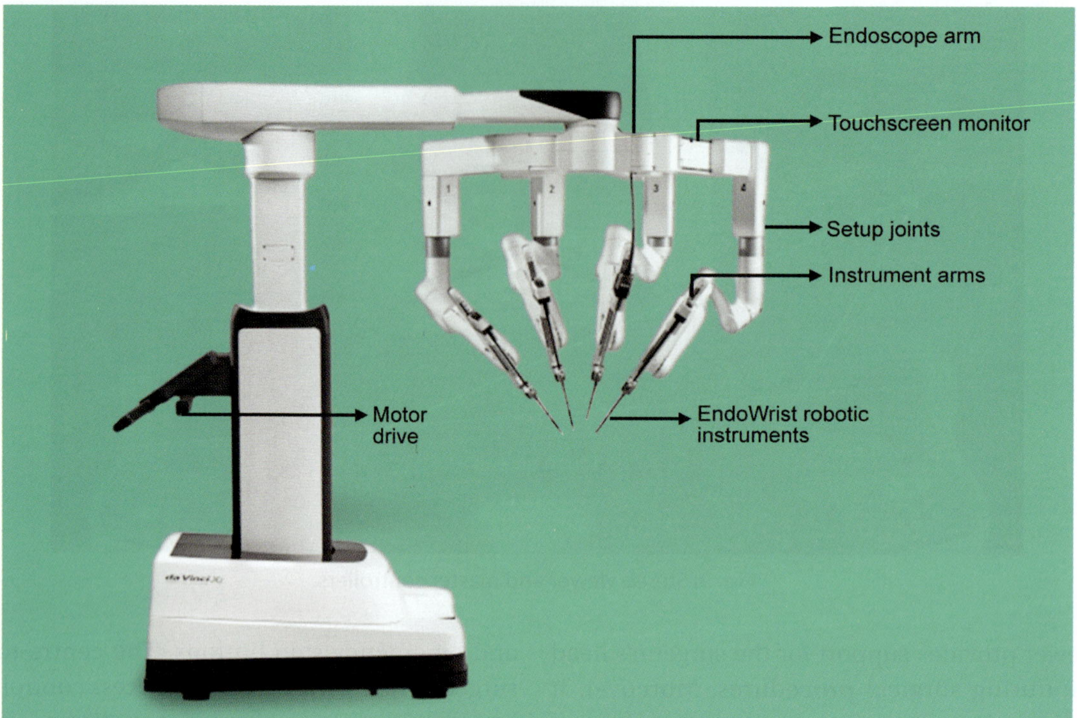

Fig. 4: Patient-side cart.

Key components include:

- Setup joints
- Instrument arms
- Camera arm
- Touchscreen monitor
- Motor drive and
- EndoWrist robotic instruments

EndoWrist instruments ***(Fig. 5)****:* Intuitive surgical's exclusive EndoWrist instruments emulate the natural dexterity and full range of motion of the human hand, surpassing its capabilities. Modelled after the human wrist, these instruments offer even greater flexibility. Internal cables, akin to human tendons, ensure maximum responsiveness, enabling rapid and precise suturing, dissection and tissue manipulation. With 7° of freedom, 90° of articulation, intuitive motion and fingertip control, as well as features such as motion scaling and tremor reduction, EndoWrist instruments enhance surgeons' dexterity, precision and control. The da Vinci EndoWrist end effector offers a diverse range of motions mirroring those of the human hand. This includes flexion and extension, allowing for bending and straightening movements; adduction and abduction, facilitating lateral motions; and grasping capabilities, providing a comprehensive spectrum of dexterous actions.

Vision System

- *Three-dimensional vision technology:* The da Vinci Surgical System's vision system delivers a 3D perspective of the surgical field, enhancing depth perception and providing the surgeon with a clearer visualisation of anatomical structures.
- *Image processing:* The system is equipped with advanced image processing capabilities to guarantee a clear and sharp image throughout the procedure. This feature is crucial for precise navigation and manipulation of instruments.
- *Illumination:* The vision system includes powerful lighting to effectively illuminate the surgical site, ensuring optimal visibility, particularly in complex and deep-seated areas.

DISTINGUISHING LAPAROSCOPY FROM ROBOTIC SURGERY: UNVEILING CONTRASTS IN MINIMALLY INVASIVE TECHNIQUES

Table 1 shows the comparison of laparoscopic and robotic surgery.

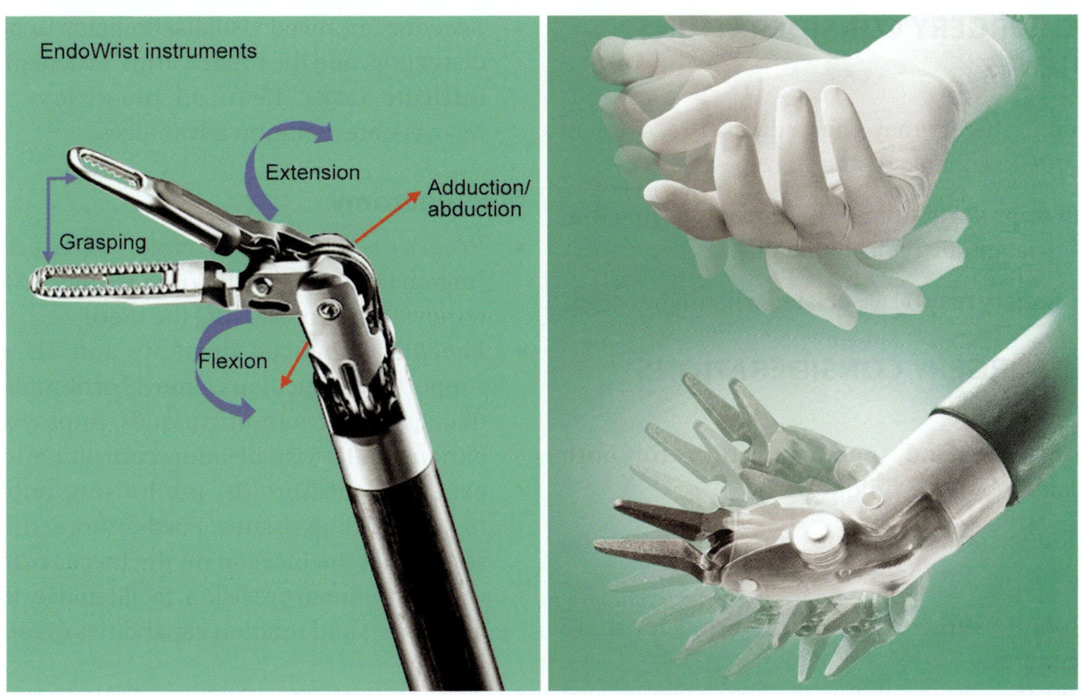

Fig. 5: EndoWrist instrument.

TABLE 1: Comparison of laparoscopic and robotic surgery.

	Laparoscopy surgery	***Robotic surgery***
Procedure		
Technique	Laparoscopic surgery, also known as minimally invasive or keyhole surgery, involves making small incisions through which a laparoscope and specialised instruments are inserted	Robotic surgery involves the use of a robotic surgical system, such as the da Vinci System, where the surgeon controls robotic arms equipped with instruments from a console
Control	*Direct control:* Surgeons directly manipulate the instruments, and the movements are translated onto a video monitor	*Remote control:* The surgeon operates the system from a console, and the robotic arms replicate their hand movements with enhanced precision
Patient benefits	• *Recovery time:* Generally, shorter recovery time compared to traditional open surgery • *Scarring:* Smaller incisions lead to reduced scarring • *Hospital stay:* Often results in a shorter hospital stay • *Cost:* May be cost-effective compared to robotic surgery	• *Precision:* Improved precision and dexterity due to the robotic system's capabilities • *3D Visualisation:* Enhanced 3D visualisation of the surgical site • *Versatility:* Allows for a wider range of motion with robotic arms • *Complex procedures:* Enables complex procedures that may be challenging with traditional laparoscopy
Challenges	• *Limited range of motion:* Laparoscopic instruments have limited degrees of freedom • *Hand-eye coordination:* Requires precise hand-eye coordination due to the lack of robotic assistance • *Tactile feedback:* Limited or no tactile feedback for the surgeon	• *Cost:* Generally more expensive compared to laparoscopic surgery • *Training:* Requires specialised training for surgeons to operate the robotic system effectively • *Setup time:* Longer setup time due to the complexity of the system • *Instrument size:* Robotic instruments may be bulkier than laparoscopic instruments

ROBOTIC SURGERY CONSIDERATIONS FOR PATIENTS

Recovery: Robotic surgery may offer a quicker recovery in certain cases due to enhanced precision.

Scarring: Both approaches aim to minimise scarring, but laparoscopic incisions are typically smaller.

Cost: Robotic surgery may be associated with higher costs.

ROBOTIC SURGERY CONSIDERATIONS FOR DOCTORS

Training: Surgeons need specific training for both laparoscopic and robotic techniques.

Precision: Robotic surgery provides improved precision and dexterity.

Versatility: Robotic surgery may be preferred for more complex procedures.

Ultimately, the choice between laparoscopic and robotic surgery depends on the specific case, the surgeon's expertise and available resources. Each approach has its advantages and limitations, and the decision is often made collaboratively between the surgeon and the patient based on individual circumstances.

INTRODUCTION OF da VINCI ROBOTIC IN GYNAECOLOGY

The da Vinci Surgical System was first used in gynaecological surgery in the late 1990s. The initial procedures were primarily focused on hysterectomy and other gynaecological surgeries. The system received clearance from the US FDA for general laparoscopic surgery in 2000, and its application in gynaecological procedures has since expanded to include a wide range of surgeries, as discussed in the previous response. The adoption of the da Vinci System in gynaecology marked a significant advancement in minimally invasive surgical techniques in this medical specialty. Here is an overview of its use in specific gynaecological conditions.

Hysterectomy

- *Procedure:* The da Vinci System is commonly employed for total hysterectomies. It allows for smaller incisions compared to traditional open surgery, reducing scarring and promoting faster recovery.
- *Benefits:* Improved visualisation aids in delicate tissue dissection, and the robotic arms' articulation facilitates intricate tasks. Reduced blood loss and quicker recovery are common advantages.

Myomectomy

- *Procedure:* In the removal of uterine fibroids (myomectomy), the da Vinci System enables precise removal while preserving the uterus.
- *Benefits:* Enhanced dexterity and 3D visualisation support the meticulous removal of fibroids, minimising damage to surrounding tissues. Improved agility and enhanced 3D visualisation contribute to the precise extraction of fibroids, minimising potential injury to surrounding tissues. Furthermore, the meticulous suturing of the incision on the uterus can be achieved with exceptional precision, facilitated by the controlled movement and rotation capabilities of robotic arms.

Endometriosis Resection

- *Procedure:* In the realm of deep endometriosis surgery, the da Vinci Surgical System stands out with its unparalleled advantages in performing intricate and fine dissections of deep infiltrating endometriosis lesions.
- *Benefits:* The system's robotic arms offer superior dexterity and precision, allowing surgeons to navigate complex anatomical structures with heightened accuracy. The 3D visualisation provided by the da Vinci System enhances the surgeon's ability to discern and delicately remove deep-seated endometriotic tissue while minimising damage to surrounding structures. This level of precision is particularly crucial in deep endometriosis cases, where meticulous dissection is required to ensure thorough lesion removal while preserving vital organs and tissues. The robotic approach not only facilitates a more thorough and precise procedure but also contributes to reduced postoperative pain and faster recovery for patients undergoing deep endometriosis surgery.

Ovarian Cystectomy

- *Procedure:* Removal of ovarian cysts, whether benign or cancerous, can be performed using the da Vinci System. This allows for a more precise approach while minimising damage to healthy ovarian tissue.

- *Benefits:* The robotic platform facilitates meticulous dissection, minimising the risk of damage to surrounding ovarian tissue and preserving follicles.

Pelvic Organ Prolapse Repair

- *Procedure:* The da Vinci System is employed to address pelvic organ prolapse (POP) by repositioning organs such as the bladder, uterus or rectum.
- *Advantages:* The robotic arms offer superior suturing capabilities, leading to a more resilient repair. Enhanced visualisation facilitates the precise placement of mesh or other supportive materials. The robotic arm with EndoWrist allows for ease of operation in navigating deep pelvic spaces.

Gynaecologic Cancer Surgery

- *Procedure:* The da Vinci System is employed in surgeries for gynaecologic cancers, such as cervical, endometrial or ovarian cancers.
- *Benefits:* The da Vinci robot has revolutionised the approach to treating gynaecological malignancies, providing a minimally invasive and highly precise surgical option. Its utilisation in procedures such as hysterectomy, lymph node dissection and tumour removal allows for smaller incisions, reduced blood loss and faster recovery times compared to traditional methods. The robot's advanced technology enhances the surgeon's dexterity and provides a 3D, high-definition view of the surgical site, enabling precise manoeuvres in complex gynaecological oncology surgeries. Overall, the da Vinci robot plays a crucial role in improving outcomes and patient experiences in the management of gynaecological malignancies.

The incorporation of indocyanine green (ICG) fluorescence imaging further elevates the da Vinci robot's efficacy in gynaecological malignancy surgeries, specifically in sentinel lymph node dissection **(Fig. 6)**. By utilising ICG, surgeons can visualise and distinguish the lymphatic drainage pathways in real-time, aiding in the identification of sentinel lymph nodes with exceptional precision. This targeted approach not only ensures the removal of the most relevant lymph nodes but also minimises the risk of unnecessary node excision, reducing the likelihood of complications such as lymphoedema. The combination of da Vinci robot technology and ICG fluorescence imaging enhances the overall safety and accuracy of sentinel lymph node dissection in gynaecological malignancies, contributing to improved patient outcomes and quality of care.

The da Vinci Surgical System has emerged as a pivotal tool in the realm of gynaecological surgery, ushering in a new era of improved patient care. Its multifaceted advantages, including diminished invasiveness, heightened precision and accelerated recovery, have significantly impacted the landscape of surgical interventions for various gynaecological conditions. The system's ability to adapt to the intricacies of each procedure, coupled with its advanced technological features, allows for a tailored

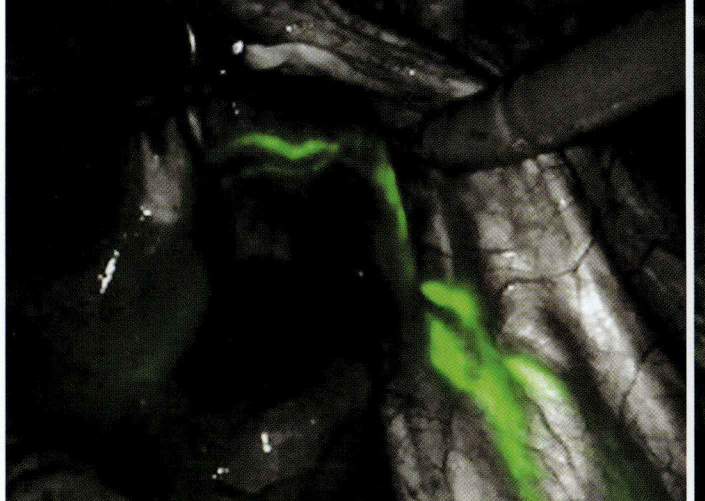

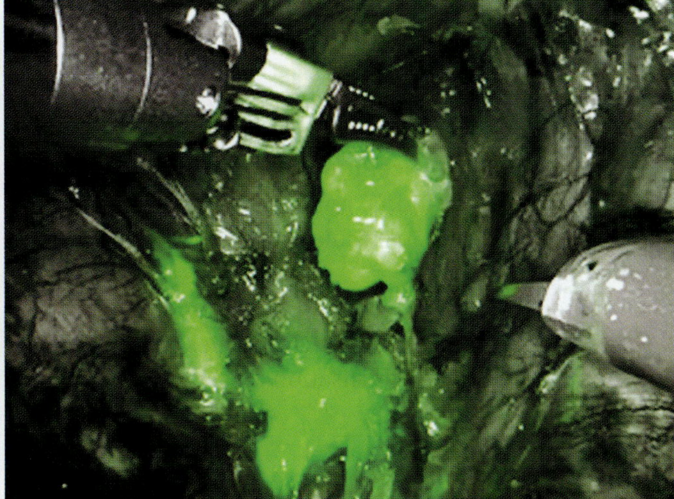

Fig. 6: Indocyanine green (ICG) fluorescence imaging-guided sentinel lymph node dissection in endometrial cancer.

approach that caters to the unique characteristics of both the surgical task and the individual patient. Whether performing complex surgeries such as hysterectomies or delicate procedures such as lymph node dissection, the da Vinci System consistently demonstrates its versatility in optimising outcomes. Ultimately, its integration into gynaecological surgery underscores a commitment to patient well-being, offering a comprehensive set of benefits that collectively contribute to enhanced surgical experiences and improved overall healthcare.

REVOLUTIONISING MEDICINE: THE FUTURE HORIZONS OF ROBOTIC SURGERY INNOVATION

The future of robotic surgery is marked by transformative potential, propelled by technological advancements and an evolving comprehension of its benefits. Key trends are poised to shape this trajectory.

- *Enhanced robotic platforms:* Ongoing refinement of robotic platforms, encompassing improved robotic arms, imaging systems and overall system ergonomics, promises heightened precision and versatility in various surgical procedures.
- *Artificial intelligence (AI) integration:* The integration of AI and machine learning is anticipated to play a pivotal role. AI's real-time analytics, predictive modelling and decision support stand to significantly enhance surgical outcomes, offering surgeons intelligent insights.
- *Miniaturisation and microbotics:* Advances in miniaturisation and microbot development open avenues for minimally invasive surgeries on a smaller scale, particularly in delicate or hard-to-reach areas of the body.
- *Remote surgery and teleoperation:* The prospect of remote surgery or teleoperation holds promise for performing procedures on patients in different geographical locations, potentially improving access to specialised care, particularly in regions with limited medical resources.
- *Augmented reality (AR) and virtual reality (VR):* Integration of AR and VR technologies is expected to enhance surgeons' visualisation and spatial awareness during robotic procedures, fostering improved navigation and accuracy in complex surgeries.
- *Surgical training and simulation:* Advancements in realistic surgical training and simulation programs on robotic platforms contribute to shaping the proficiency of the next generation of robotic surgeons, ensuring competence in utilising advanced technologies.
- *Expanded applications:* Robotic surgery is anticipated to extend beyond its current focus on urology, gynaecology and general surgery. Neurosurgery, orthopaedics and cardiovascular procedures are potential areas for increased adoption of robotic assistance.
- *Cost reduction and accessibility:* Efforts to reduce the overall cost of robotic systems and associated procedures, as technology matures and gains wider acceptance, may enhance accessibility, allowing more medical facilities to embrace the transformative potential of robotic surgery technology.

CONCLUSION

The future of robotic surgery innovation is poised to bring about transformative changes in surgical practices, making procedures more precise, less invasive and potentially more accessible to a broader population. Ongoing research and collaboration between medical professionals, engineers and technology experts will continue to drive these advancements.

SUGGESTED READING

1. Ballantyne GH, Moll F. The da Vinci telerobotic surgical system: the virtual operative field and telepresence surgery. Surg Clin North Am. 2003;83(6):1293-304.
2. Fairag M, Almahdi RH, Siddiqi AA, Alharthi FK, Alqurashi BS, Alzahrani NG, et al. Robotic revolution in surgery: diverse applications across specialties and future prospects review article. Cureus. 2024;16(1):e52148.
3. George EI, Brand TC, LaPorta A, Marescaux J, Satava RM. Origins of robotic surgery: from skepticism to standard of care. JSLS. 2018;22(4):e2018.00039.
4. Rivas-López R, Sandoval-García-Travesí FA. Robotic surgery in gynecology: review of literature. Cir Cir. 2020;88(1):107-16.

54

CHAPTER

Endoscopic Surgery in Gynaecology

Vidya Bhat, Mythreyi Kadambi

Chapter Outline

Laparoscopic Surgery
- Surgical Equipment
- Indications
- Contraindications to Laparoscopy
- Preoperative Preparation
- Surgical Steps
- Postoperative Care
- Advantages
- Disadvantages
- Complications

Hysteroscopic Surgery
- Surgical Equipment
- Indications
- Preoperative Preparation
- Surgical Steps
- Postoperative Care
- Advantages
- Disadvantages
- Complications
- Hysteroscopic Resectoscope
- Slim Resectoscope
- Hysteroscopic Morcellator

Laparoendoscopic Single-site Surgery
- Surgical Equipment
- Indications
- Laparoendoscopic Single-site Surgical Techniques
- Advantages
- Complications
- Robotic Surgery

LAPAROSCOPIC SURGERY

INTRODUCTION

Laparoscopy is a type of endoscopy, which helps in the visualisation of the peritoneal cavity. The earliest description of the use of endoscopy for visualising the interior of the body organs can be attributed to Philipp Bozzini, who attempted to visualise the interior of the urethra in 1805. However, it was only in the past three decades that the potential applications of laparoscopy in the field of operative laparoscopy have been recognised. During the last 35 years, gynaecologic laparoscopy has evolved from a limited surgical procedure used only for diagnosis and tubal ligations to a major surgical tool used for the treatment of a large number of gynaecological indications.

Today, laparoscopy has become one of the most common surgical procedures performed by gynaecologists. It is a hybrid surgical approach that shares characteristics of both minor and major surgery. To patients, laparoscopic procedures often seem to be minor surgery because of the small incisions, reduced hospital stay, reduced amount of postoperative pain and other complications, and shortened convalescence period.

However, at its core, laparoscopy remains an intra-abdominal procedure. Therefore, it can be associated with various intraoperative and postoperative complications of laparotomy, such as infection and injury to adjacent intra-abdominal structures. Since laparoscopy requires a small incision, the postoperative pain and morbidity is significantly less in comparison to that associated with laparotomy. Besides this, laparoscopic procedures are associated with unique risks and complications related to the methods used for creating pneumoperitoneum and the placement of abdominal wall ports.

Some of the areas where laparoscopic surgery has become the treatment of choice include ectopic pregnancy, treatment of endometriosis, or a benign ovarian cyst. Compared with laparotomy, laparoscopy is a form of minimally invasive surgery which is associated with a low complication rate, reduced pain, better cosmetic result, reduced rate of adhesion formation, shorter recovery time and reduced duration of hospital stay.

SURGICAL EQUIPMENT

The first step in any laparoscopic surgery comprises the placement of a Veress needle and a primary trocar. Placement of both Veress needle and primary trocar can be particularly dangerous because this is the time when uncontrolled axial penetrating forces may be applied blindly to the sharp instruments.

Veress Needle

The Veress needle is used for creating a pneumoperitoneum, which can be considered the first step of most laparoscopic surgeries. This helps in separating the internal organs and tissues from the abdominal wall, so that the trocar can be inserted safely without causing any injury to the surrounding structures. The Veress needle is available in three sizes depending on its length:

1. 80 mm
2. 100 mm
3. 120 mm.

It has an inner blunt tip, which springs out when the needle enters the peritoneal cavity **(Fig. 1)**.

The most commonly used gas for insufflation is CO_2. It is a noncombustible gas, which is rapidly absorbed by the blood where it gets converted to carbonic acid after combination with water. A CO_2 gas insufflator **(Fig. 2)** must provide a continuous flow rate of gas in order to maintain the intra-abdominal pressure (IAP) between 10 and 15 mm Hg. A high IAP facilitates the introduction of the trocar as well as helps in increasing the distance between the trocar and the retroperitoneal vessels. The insufflator display must always remain within the surgeon's vision because it helps in providing important information regarding the patient's IAP, flow rate and total volume of CO_2 which has been insufflated.

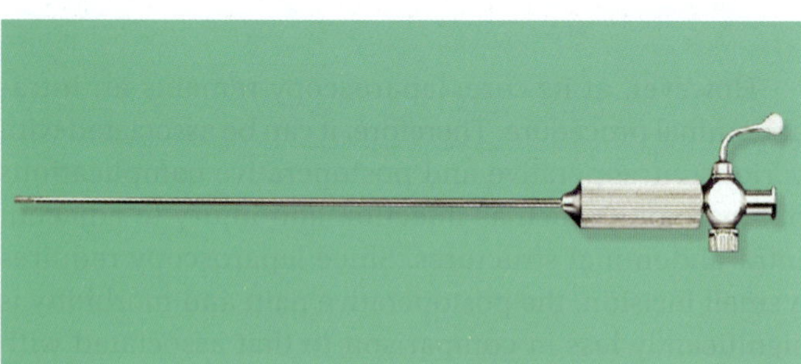

Fig. 1: Veress needle.

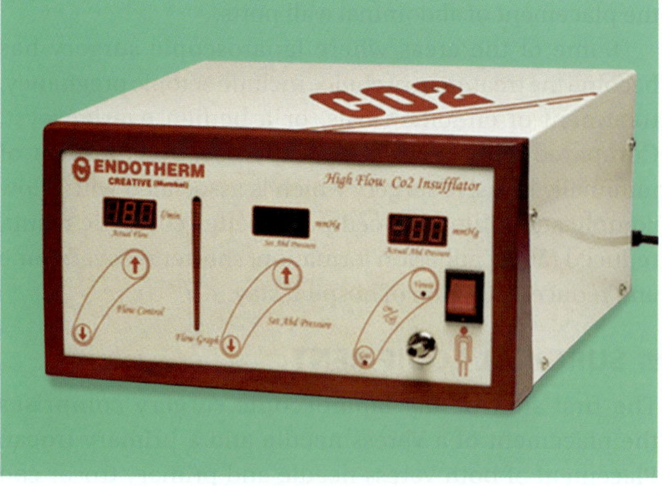

Fig. 2: High-flow electronic insufflator.

Laparoscopic Access Equipment (Trocars)

There are two types of laparoscopic access equipment:

1. First-generation equipment (with a central trocar and an encasing outer sheath or cannula)
2. Second-generation equipment (based on visual access method)

First-generation Laparoscopic Access Instruments

First-generation laparoscopic access instruments consist of two parts:

1. A removable central trocar
2. An encasing outer cannula **(Figs. 3 and 4)**.

Once this access instrument is placed inside the body's cavity, the central trocar is removed in order to place the laparoscope and other operating instruments. The proximal end of the primary trocar is designed to accommodate the palm of the surgeon's dominant hand.

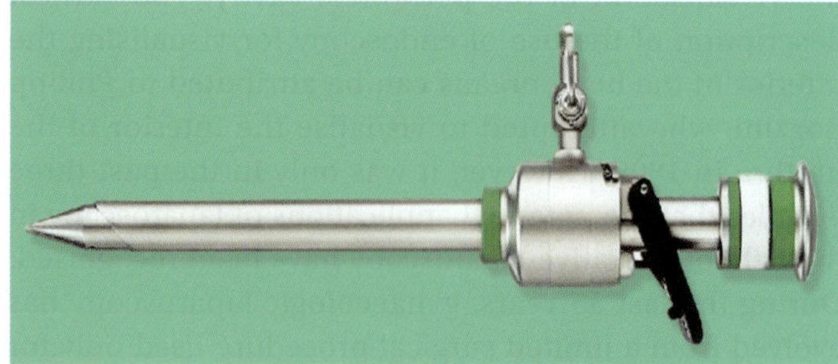

Fig. 3: Primary trocar and cannula.

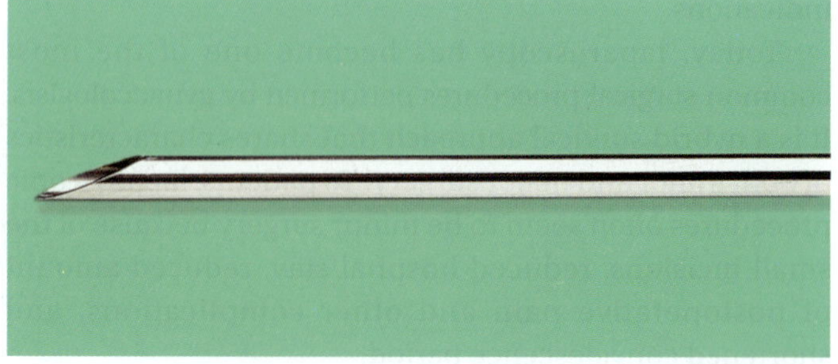

Fig. 4: Cannula tip shown separately without the trocar.

The distal end of the trocar could have a pointed, sharp, conical or bevelled pyramidal cutting blade tip. Conical trocars have pointed, nonbladed, sharp tips with no cutting edges. These types of trocars require considerably more penetrating force because the various tissue layers are not resected, but rather parted radially in order to accommodate the outer diameter of the cannula. Disposable trocars are also available, which have the advantage of being safe, transparent, stable, and both surgeon- and patient-friendly **(Fig. 5)**.

The sharp edges of the trocars may sometimes cause damage to the small blood vessels and other organs. With the blunt trocar tips, the chances of injury are relatively low because the blood vessels are pushed aside at the time of insertion and are thereby protected to a large degree. Optical access trocars, which help in visualising the layers of the abdominal wall during placement, are also available. A spring mechanism similar to that in the Veress needle is present on most disposable trocars, which helps in increasing their safety.

The actual trocar is a stylet which is introduced through the cannula. The cannula allows the insertion of laparoscopic instruments inside the abdominal cavity. The most commonly used trocars vary between the sizes of 5 and 10 mm. Trocars usually have two types of valves to prevent the escape of gas. These include the flap valve and trumpet valve. The trumpet valves protect the telescope from contamination by tissue and blood particles at the time of insertion. These valves have to be pressed at the time of insertion. However, the main disadvantage associated with their use is that they are likely to grip the instruments, thereby preventing their smooth movement. Hence, the flap valve trocars are generally preferred.

Second-generation Laparoscopic Access Instruments

Second-generation laparoscopic access instruments with a visual access method are also sometimes used. These include the optical access trocars, which help in visualising the layers of the abdominal wall during placement. The endoscopic threaded imaging port (Endo Tip), a sheath with screw threading, is a new second-generation instrument, which allows safe peritoneal entry under direct vision **(Fig. 6)**. In this method, the sheath which has screw thread tip is inserted with the telescope inside so that as the sheath is screwed in, the tissue layers can be visualised and therefore inadvertent injury to the internal organs may be avoided. This technique may especially prove to be safe in cases where dense adhesions are expected, especially in cases where the patient had a previous laparotomy. The screwed Endo Tip prevents it from slipping out of the intraperitoneal space.

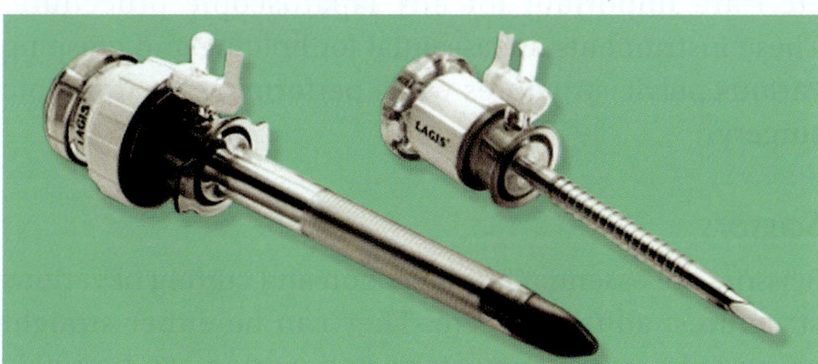

Fig. 5: Disposable trocar.

Laparoscopic Telescope

Following the removal of the primary trocar, the laparoscopic or operative telescopes **(Figs. 7 and 8)** are inserted through the cannula in order to visualise the abdominal cavity. Laparoscopic telescopes are available in various

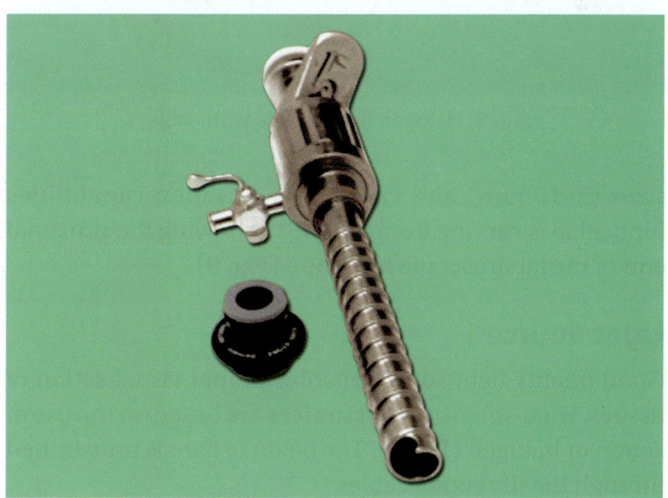
Fig. 6: Endo Tip reusable visual access cannula.

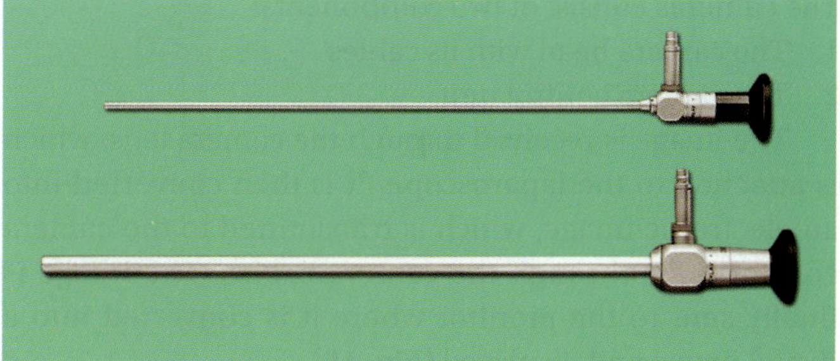
Fig. 7: Laparoscopic telescope.

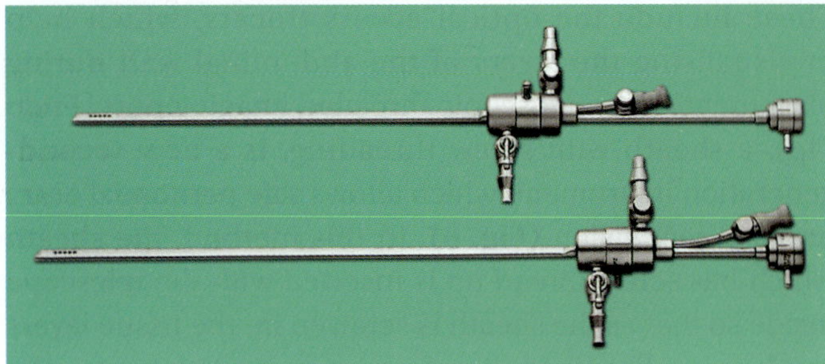

Fig. 8: Operative telescope.

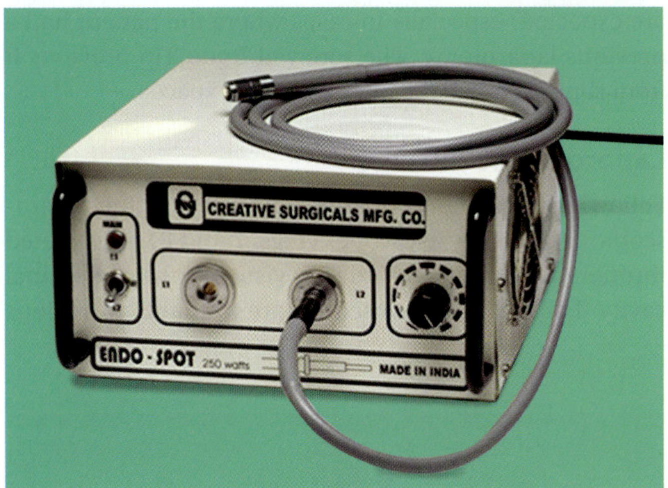

Fig. 9: Halogen light source with cable.

sizes (2–10 mm) and various visualisation capabilities (optical axis varying from 0° to 45°), showing the proximal end of the laparoscopic telescope **(Fig. 9)**.

Light Source

Good quality light source enables proper visualisation of tissues. High-intensity light sources are based on the use of xenon or halogen **(Fig. 9)**. The beam of light is transmitted through the fibreoptic cables.

Cameras

The cameras consist of two components:

1. The camera head with its cables
2. The camera control unit.

The image is received through the camera lens, which is attached to the laparoscope. It is then converted into an electronic image, which is transmitted to the camera control units through the camera cables. The image is finally sent to the monitor where it is converted into a digital image and displayed **(Fig. 10)**.

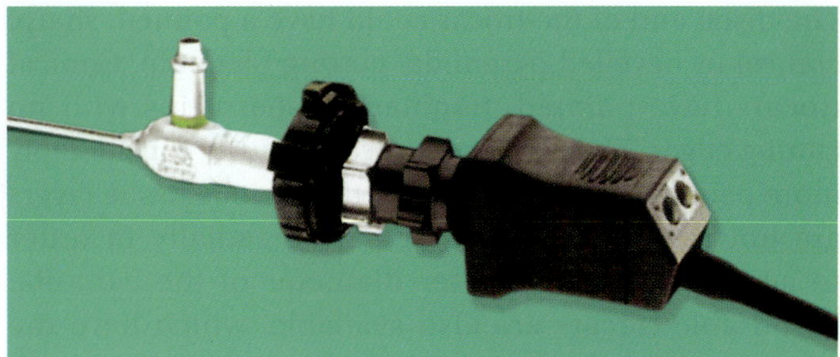

Fig. 10: Charged-coupled device camera.

Ancillary Instruments

Various other ancillary instruments, which are used to facilitate laparoscopic surgery, include the following **(Figs. 11 to 13)**:

Blunt Probe

This is one of the simplest instruments and is used for stabilising or manipulating the organs, especially the uterus. Some of these manipulators also facilitate the instillation of an inert coloured solution (such as sterile saline with indigo carmine dye) into the uterine cavity to determine the patency of the fallopian tubes **(Figs. 14A and B)**.

Electromechanical Morcellator

Many laparoscopic surgeries involve the removal of large sections of tissues such as in uterine myomectomy or removal of large ovarian masses. This can be achieved with help of electromechanical morcellator **(Fig. 15)**. The morcellator comprises of a motor-driven cutting tube, which can be inserted directly into the abdomen without using an additional trocar cannula. A cylindrical block of tissue can be cut out and removed.

Graspers

Graspers with different sizes and designs (claw forceps, Allis-type forceps, spoon forceps, atraumatic forceps, etc.) are important for any laparoscopic procedure. These instruments are essential for holding and grasping various pelvic structures while performing laparoscopic surgery.

Scissors

Scissors are essential for dissection and cutting of various structures, adhesions, etc. They can be either straight or curved types. Haemostasis and cutting can be safely

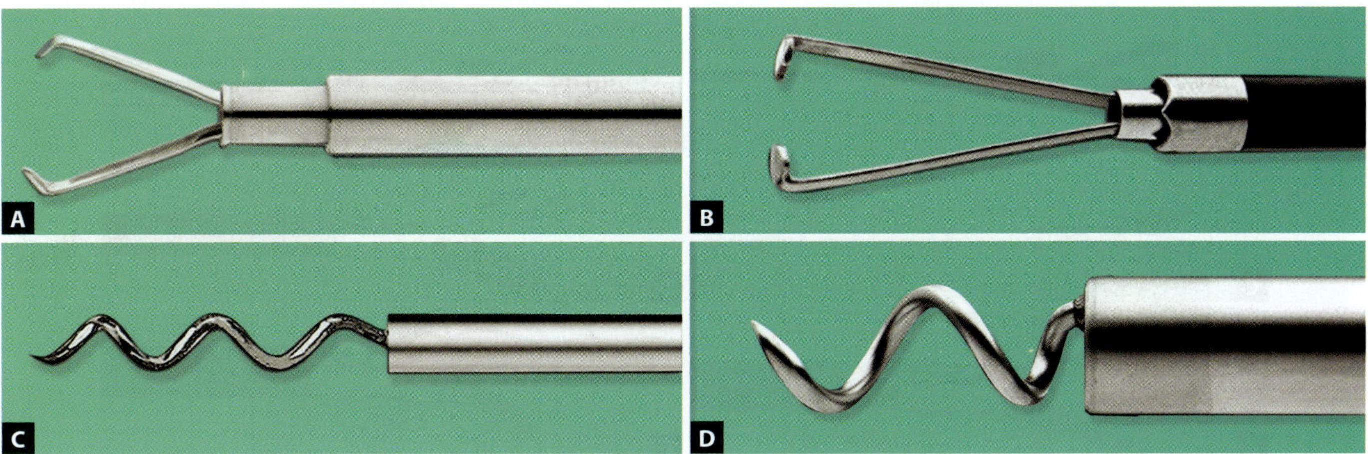

Figs. 11A to D: Grasping and holding equipment.

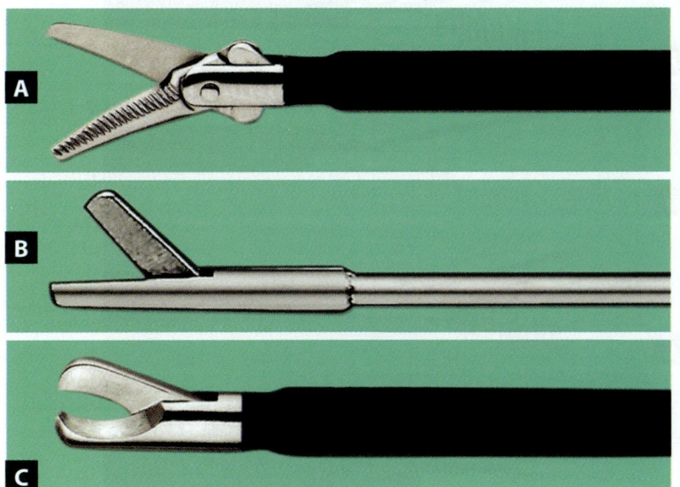

Figs. 12A to C: Straight and curved blade scissors.

achieved using simple instrumentation, provided that the surgeon has a sound understanding of both pelvic anatomy and the techniques or energy modalities and their impact on the tissues. There can be two types of electrosurgical units:

1. Unipolar
2. Bipolar

Haemostatic Instruments and Electrosurgery

The ability to achieve haemostasis is integral to any endoscopic procedure. Modern generators offer two types of modes: (1) Unipolar and (2) bipolar. The generator can be connected through cables to various instruments such as scissors, graspers, hooks, spatulas and bipolar forceps.

In a unipolar system, current passes from the instrument to the tissue to a ground plate and then back to the generator **(Fig. 16).** Depending on the instrument used and current configuration (cutting or coagulation), various different tissue effects can be achieved including cutting, desiccation, coagulation and fulguration.

The bipolar system uses two insulated jaws of the instrument to carry the current. The tissue between the jaws completes the circuit, and the tissue is heated (coagulated) by the passage of current **(Fig. 17)**. Bipolar forceps of various types (1 mm, 3 mm, 5 mm, Kleppinger) are available **(Fig. 18)**.

All the above-explained instruments are arranged in a mobile cart **(Fig. 19)**.

New technologies have been developed in electro-surgery; they are:

- *Harmonic scalpel:* The harmonic scalpel is a surgical instrument used to simultaneously cut and cauterise tissue. Ultrasonic energy is famously used in the harmonic scalpel where ultrasonic energy is newly converted to mechanical energy at the active blade **(Fig. 20)**. Sealing of the vessels is achieved through denatured protein coagulum, which occurs due to tamponade and coaptation.
- *Enseal:* Designed for use in open and laparoscopic surgical procedures, ENSEAL™ X1 curved jaw tissue sealer is one of the latest innovations in the advanced bipolar ENSEAL™ portfolio that provides secure sealing. This device has a curved, tapered tip and offers simplified steps for use with one-handed 360° rotation, separate seal and cut buttons and an efficient, ergonomic handle.
- *Ligasure:* LigaSure™ 5-mm blunt tip laparoscopic instrument is the latest sealer/divider from Medtronic. LigaSure™ uses a combination of pressure and

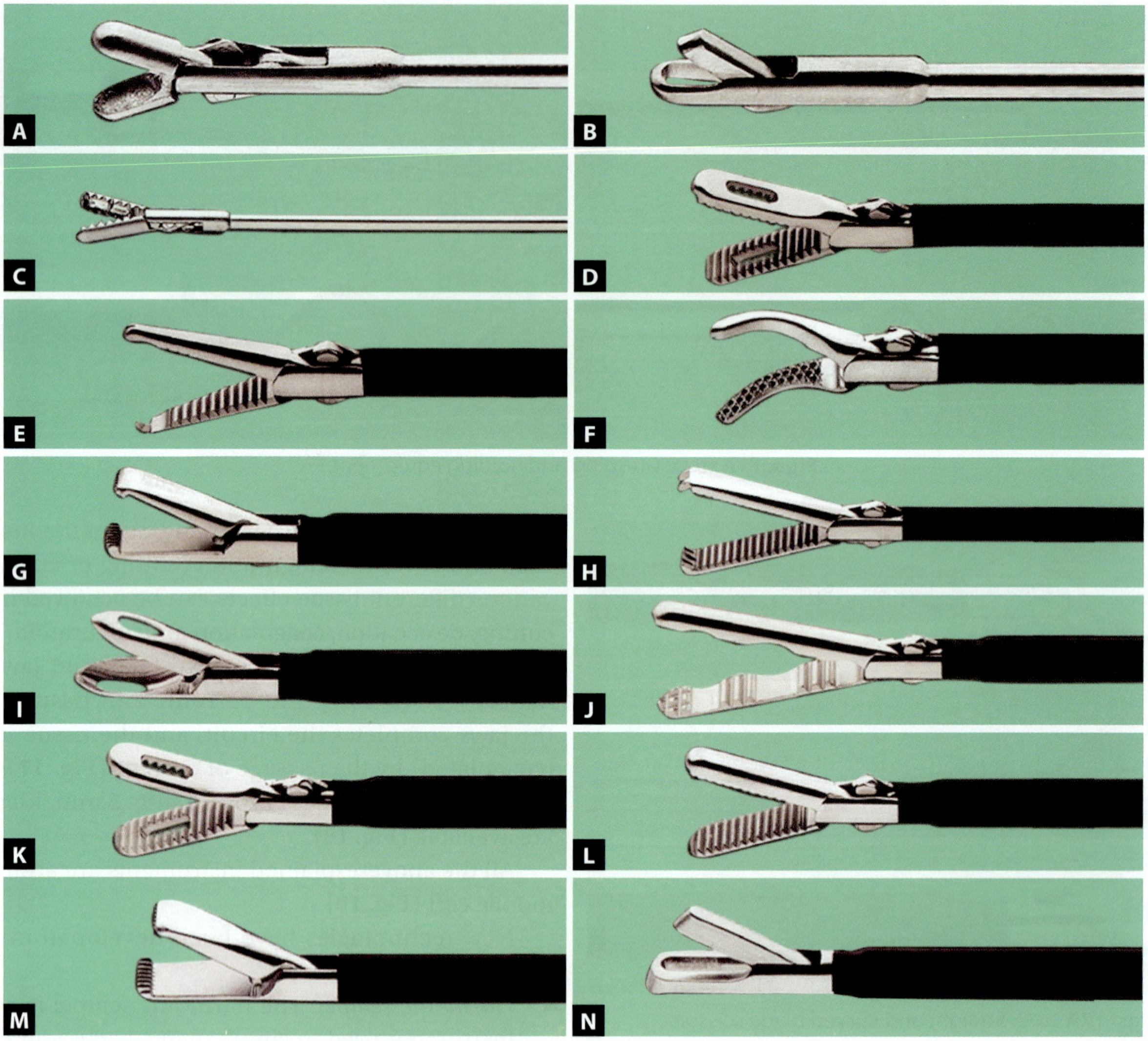

Figs. 13A to N: Various types of laparoscopic bipolar forceps.

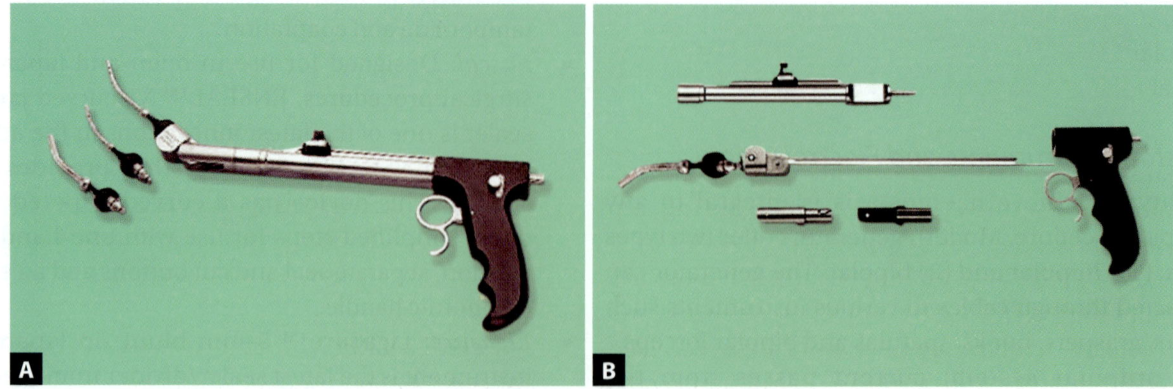

Figs. 14A and B: Uterine manipulator.

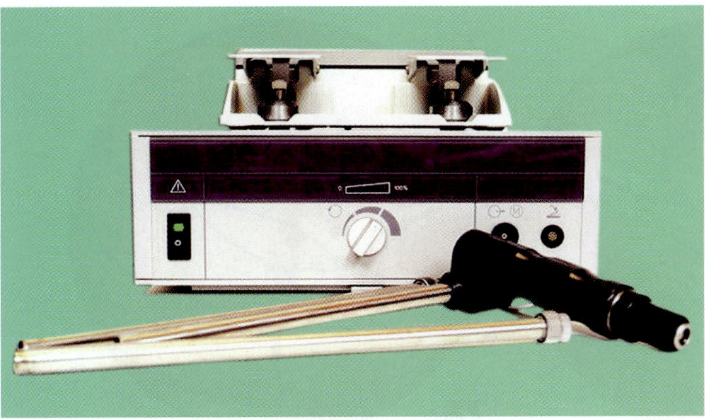

Fig. 15: Electromechanical morcellator.

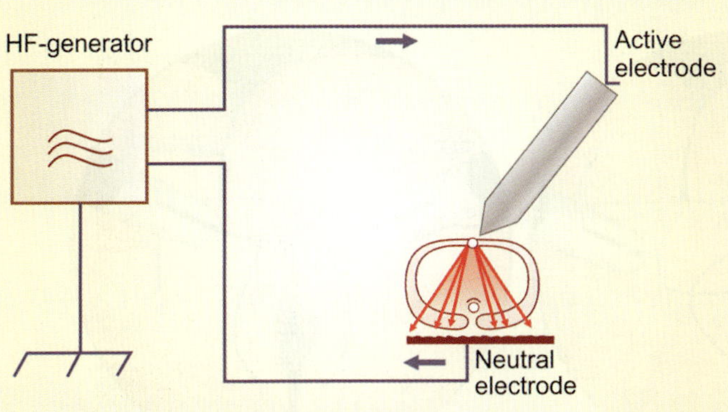

Fig. 16: Monopolar circuit. (HF: high-frequency)

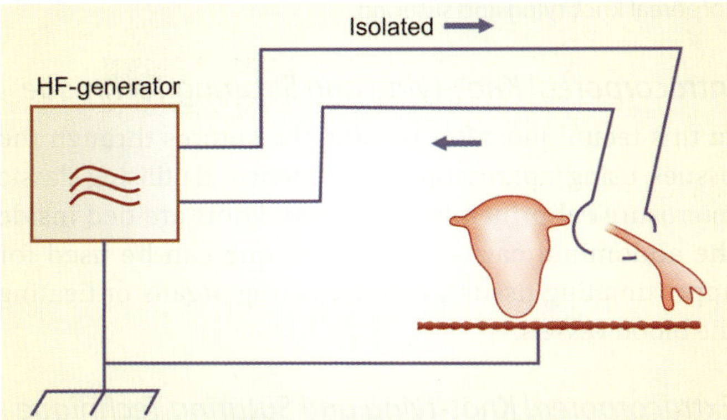

Fig. 17: Bipolar circuit. (HF: high-frequency)

continuous bipolar energy to create vessel fusion. LigaSure™ seals vessels by applying high, uniform mechanical compression while monitoring and adjusting energy delivery to the tissue.

- *THUNDERBEAT:* The THUNDERBEAT portfolio combines high performance and efficiency with 7 mm vessel sealing, significantly faster tissue dissection and the versatility to replace multiple instruments with a single handpiece.

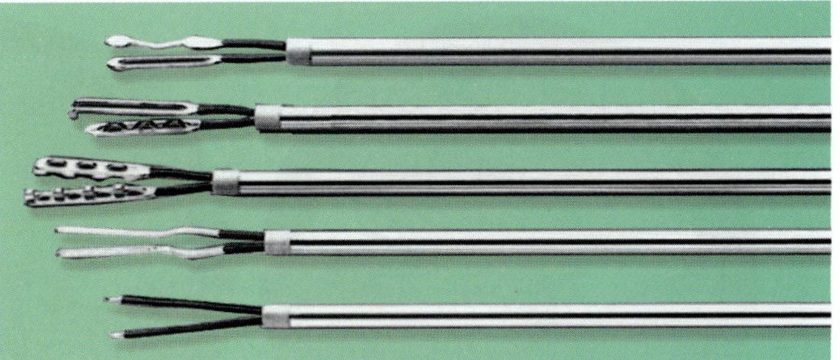

Fig. 18: Bipolar forceps.

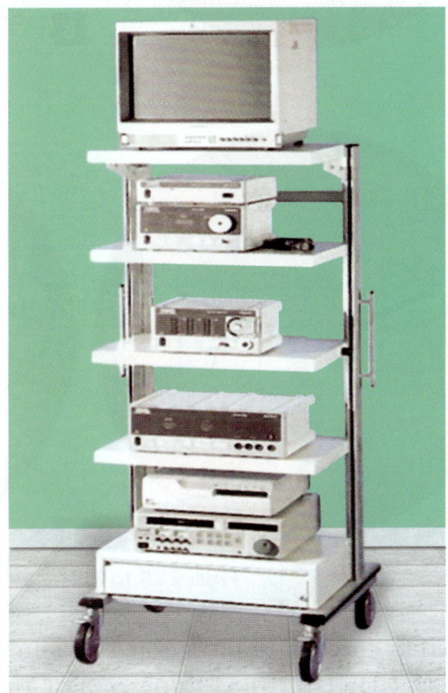

Fig. 19: Endoscopy cart.

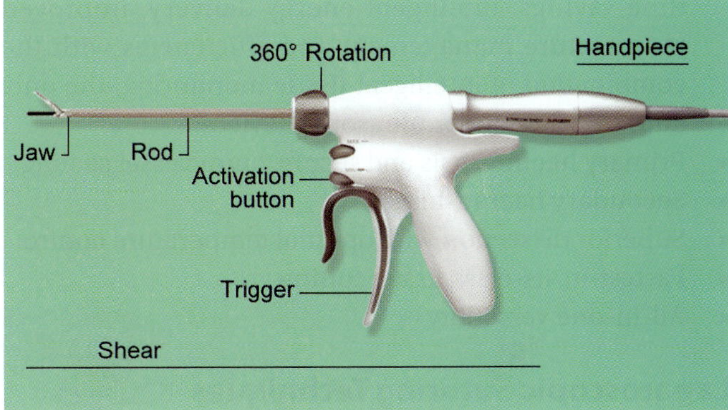

Fig. 20: Ultrasonic scalpel tool.

THUNDERBEAT type S enables reliable sealing of vessels ≤7 mm through hybrid energy combined with more consistent pressure and energy distribution

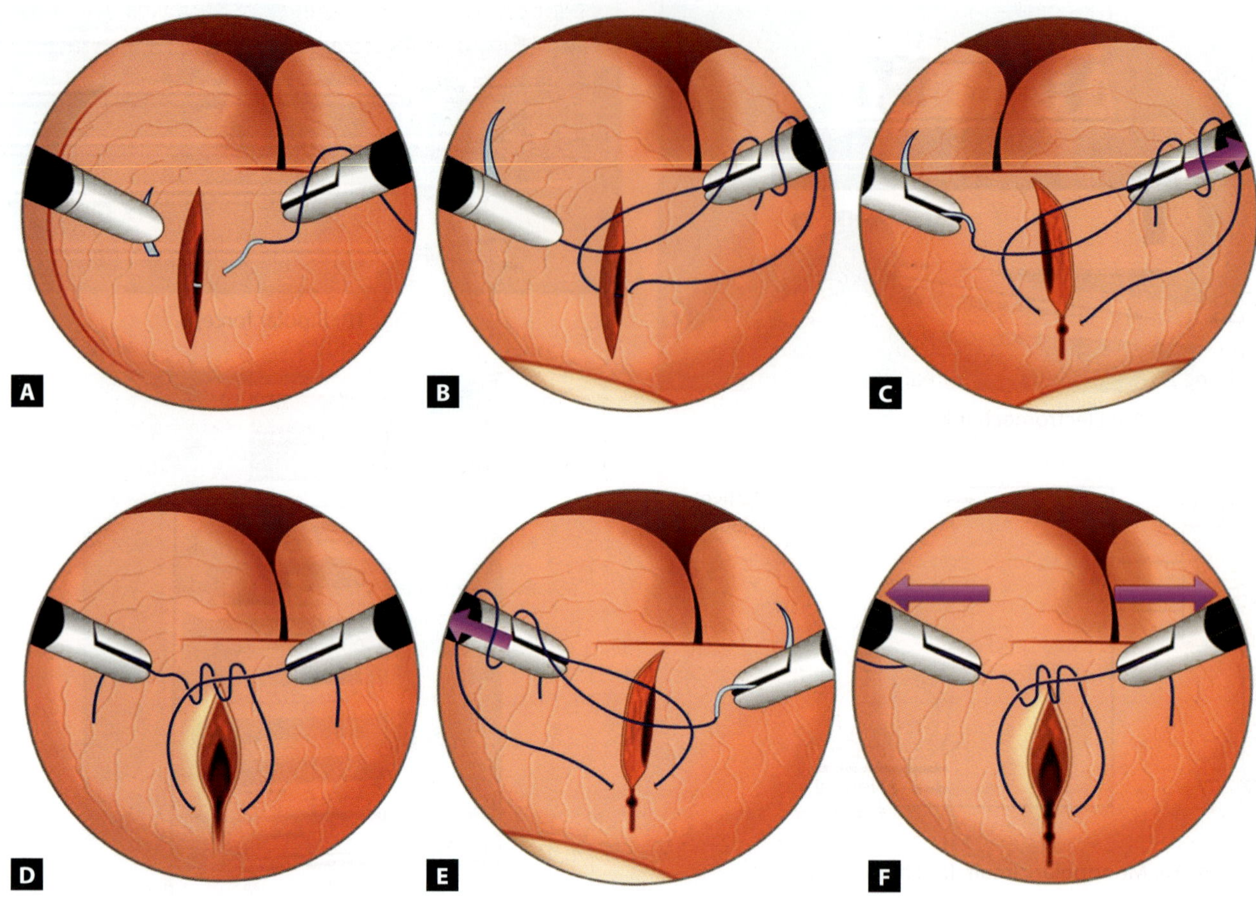

Figs. 21A to F: The technique of intracorporeal knot tying and suturing.

provided by the centre-pivot wiper jaw. In preclinical testing, THUNDERBEAT type S had the highest average burst pressure. Efficiency through up to 79% faster cutting speeds, which can contribute to OR time savings, intelligent energy delivery, improved temperature management and efficiencies with the combination of intelligent tissue monitoring, the only auto stop system for ultrasonic devices.

- Primary haemostasis and secure 7 mm vessel sealing
- Secondary haemostasis
- Superior dissection with optimal temperature control
- Fastest-in-its-class tissue cutting
- All-in-one versatility

Laparoscopic Suturing Techniques

There are two types of laparoscopic suturing techniques: (1) Intracorporeal suturing **(Figs. 21A to F)** and (2) extracorporeal suturing **(Figs. 22A to C)**. Both techniques are safe and reliable and can be performed in different clinical situations.

Intracorporeal Knot-tying and Suturing Technique

In this technique, after passing the sutures through the tissues, using laparoscopic equipment and utilising classic microsurgical principles, surgeons' knots are tied inside the abdominal cavity. This technique can be used for approximating tissues, reconstructing organs or ligating the blood vessels.

Extracorporeal Knot-tying and Suturing Technique

In this technique, after passing the suture through the tissues, both ends are brought back out of the peritoneal cavity. Extracorporeal knots are formed outside of the body and pushed into the peritoneal cavity through the cannula sleeve using a knot pusher.

INDICATIONS

Diagnostic Laparoscopy

Diagnostic laparoscopy helps in the direct visualisation of the abdominal and pelvic organs and helps in the

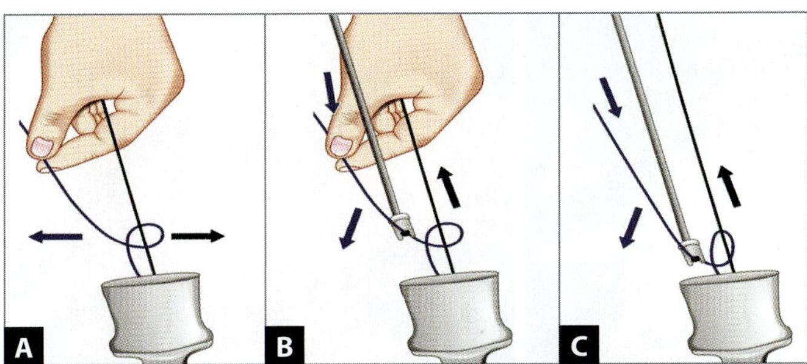

Figs. 22A to C: The technique of extracorporeal knot tying and suturing. (A) The ends of the suture are brought back out of the peritoneal cavity; (B) Extracorporeal knots are formed outside of the body; (C) A hollow plastic rod is used to push down the extracorporeal knot into the peritoneal cavity.

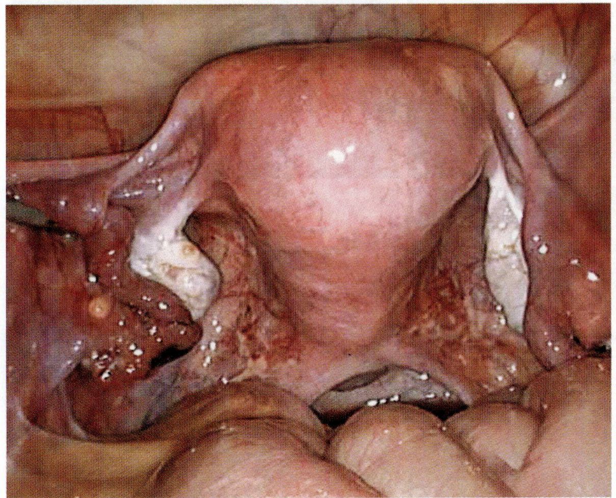

Fig. 23: Normal laparoscopic view of the pelvis.

establishment of definitive diagnosis in cases where the diagnosis could not be made on the basis of findings of clinical and radiological investigations. **Figure 23** shows a normal laparoscopic view of the pelvis. The most common indications for diagnostic laparoscopy are as follows:

- Assessment of the pelvis in cases of acute or chronic pelvic pain, adnexal masses, ectopic pregnancy, endometriosis, adnexal torsion or other pelvic pathology **(Figs. 24A to I)**.
- Determination of tubal patency through transcervical dye instillation (chromopertubation) **(Figs. 25A to C)**.
- A biopsy specimen can be obtained, if required, to aid in the diagnosis of endometriosis or malignancy.

At the time of diagnostic laparoscopy, the patient must be placed in a 20° Trendelenburg position in order to displace the bowel and omentum so as to obtain a clear view of the abdominal and pelvic organs. After insertion of the laparoscope, the surgeon must perform a panoramic view of the abdomen to ensure that no inadvertent damage has been caused by the needle or trocar. The inspection of the abdominal and pelvic cavity must be performed in a clockwise manner so as to visualise all the abdominal and pelvic organs such as the caecum, ascending colon, liver, stomach, transverse colon and descending colon. The presence of any adhesions must also be noted. After visualisation of the pelvic organs, such as uterus, both the ovaries and cul-de-sac, patency of both the tubes is checked through chromopertubation by injecting methylene blue inside the tubes via a uterine cannula. The tubes can be considered patent if the dye passes out of the fimbrial ends.

Therapeutic Laparoscopy

Various surgeries performed through the laparoscopic route are listed in **Box 1** and are described next in detail.

Tubal Sterilisation

Trocar placement is similar to diagnostic laparoscopy. Bipolar electrosurgery, clips or silastic bands may be used to occlude the tubes at the midisthmic portion, approximately 2–3 cm from the cornua.

Lysis of Adhesion

Adhesions may be present as a result of pelvic inflammatory disease, endometriosis or previous surgery. Adhesions may be lysed by blunt or sharp dissection. Unfortunately, the results of laparoscopic lysis of adhesions have been disappointing in terms of improving pain relief or future fertility. Adhesions may reform after lysis, although this can be reduced by observing precautions such as maintenance of good haemostasis and minimal use of electrocautery.

Treatment of Endometriosis

Laparoscopy is the most common procedure used for the diagnosis and treatment of endometriosis. Endometriotic lesions may be resected or ablated using any of the power instruments under laparoscopic visualisation. There is good evidence to show that this technique helps in improving fertility and reducing pelvic pain.

Treatment of Ectopic Pregnancy

Presently, the laparoscopic approach has become the surgical approach of choice for most cases of ectopic

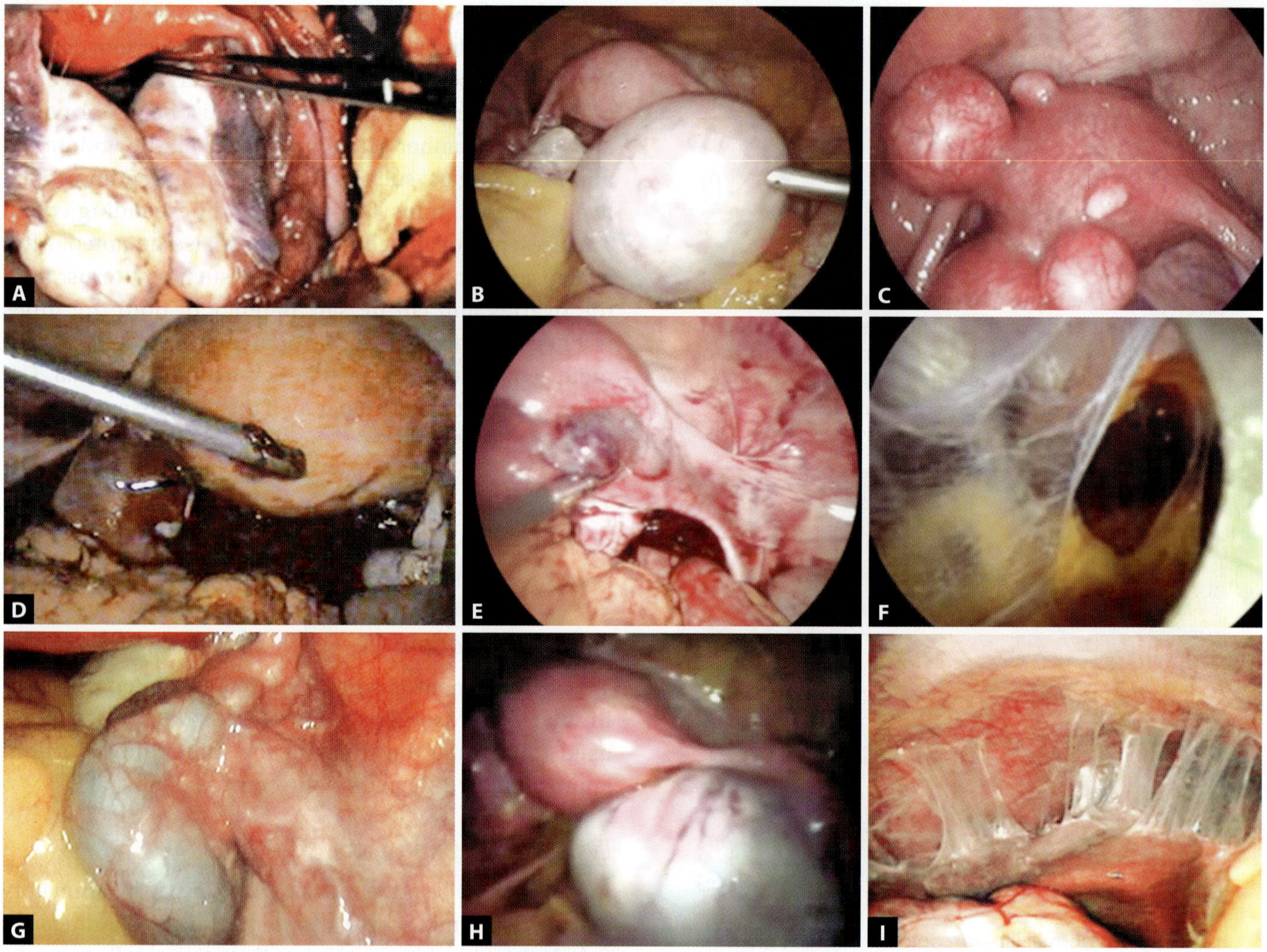

Figs. 24A to I: Laparoscopic diagnosis of various gynaecological pathologies: (A) Polycystic ovaries as observed on laparoscopic examination; (B) Large dermoid cyst on the left side; (C) Multiple uterine subserosal fibroids; (D) Collection of blood in the pelvic cavity with tubal ectopic on the right side; (E) Tubal ectopic on the left side; (F) Adhesions between the omentum and pelvic organs as visualised on laparoscopic examination; (G) Right-sided hydrosalpinx; (H) A large endometrioma on the right side; (I) Fitz-Hugh-Curtis syndrome.

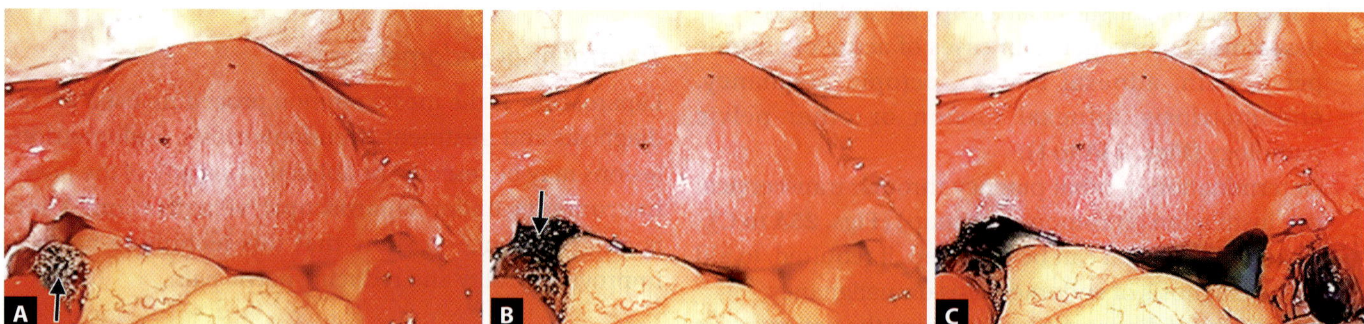

Figs. 25A to C: Process of laparoscopic chromopertubation: (A) Slight spillage of dye from right-sided tube (indicated by arrow); (B) Spillage of dye more pronounced on right side (indicated by arrow); (C) Bilateral spillage of dye on both sides.

BOX 1: Operations performed through a laparoscopic approach.

Operation on uterus:

Correction of Müllerian anomalies (rudimentary horn excision)
- Myomectomy (subserous/intramural)
- Hysterectomy for benign indications (laparoscopic assisted vaginal hysterectomy, total laparoscopic hysterectomy)
- Hysterectomy for malignant conditions

Operations on adnexa (conservative):
- Ovariolysis/fimbriolysis/salpingolysis
- Puncture of ovarian cysts
- Polycystic ovarian disease drilling
- Ovarian cystectomy
- Fimbrioplasty
- Cuff salpingostomy/salpingoneostomy
- Linear salpingostomy in ectopic pregnancy
- End-to-end anastomosis (reversal)
- Removal of paraovarian cysts

Operations on adnexa (radical):
- Oophorectomy
- Salpingectomy (partial/total)
- Tubal sterilisation
- Adnexectomy

Laparoscopy in endometriosis:
- *Peritoneal deposits:* Coagulation/excision/laser vaporisation
- Endometrioma drainage/fulguration of lining/cystectomy
- Adhesiolysis (salpingolysis/ovariolysis/omental adhesiolysis)

Laparoscopy for genital suspension operations:
- Burch colposuspension
- Sacrofixation of vagina (vault prolapse)
- Correction of cystocele/rectocele/enterocele
- McCall culdoplasty

Other indications:
- Appendectomy
- Evaluation in ascites
- Laparoscopy during pregnancy
- Second-look laparoscopy

pregnancies. In these cases, either salpingostomy or salpingectomy may be performed under laparoscopic guidance to remove the embryo and the gestational sac.

Ovarian Cystectomy

Laparoscopic approach can be used for the removal of ovarian cysts in cases where simple cysts having a size of 6 cm or more persist for two or more cycles in premenopausal, nonpregnant woman. In case the cyst appears to be complex, malignancy must be ruled out first before proceeding with cyst removal using clinical and diagnostic tests. Laparoscopic cyst removal should be undertaken only in cases where the cyst has been shown to be benign. If any doubt exists, the cyst wall should be sent for frozen section to confirm its nature through histopathological examination. If malignancy is found, a laparotomy should be performed.

Oophorectomy

An oophorectomy may be more appropriate in postmenopausal women or those with a cyst, which is persistent or is progressively increasing in size, or in cases where there is a higher risk of malignancy.

Myomectomy

For subserosal and intramural fibroids, laparoscopic myomectomy is preferred. For submucosal fibroids of size <4 cm, hysteroscopic myomectomy is preferred.

Hysterectomy

Presently, three basic laparoscopic approaches for hysterectomy are used, which include laparoscopic-assisted vaginal hysterectomy (LAVH), laparoscopic hysterectomy (LH) and laparoscopic supracervical hysterectomy. Controversy exists over the risks, benefits and most appropriate indications of each. For details regarding LAVH, kindly refer to Chapter 60: Hysterectomy and Its Aftermath.

Oncologic Procedures

Laparoscopy has long been used in oncology for second-look procedures following surgical and chemical treatment of malignancy. More recently, laparoscopy has also been used for staging, including obtaining peritoneal washes with biopsy, partial omentectomy, pelvic and periaortic lymphadenectomy, etc.

Ovarian Drilling

Laparoscopic ovarian drilling can be considered as the procedure of choice in patients with polycystic ovarian disease who are resistant to medical treatment such as clomiphene citrate and letrozole.

Laparoscopic Tubal Ligation

Laparoscopic tubal ligation can be carried out using techniques such as mechanical blockage of tubes using Falope rings or Filshie clips **(Figs. 26A to D)**.

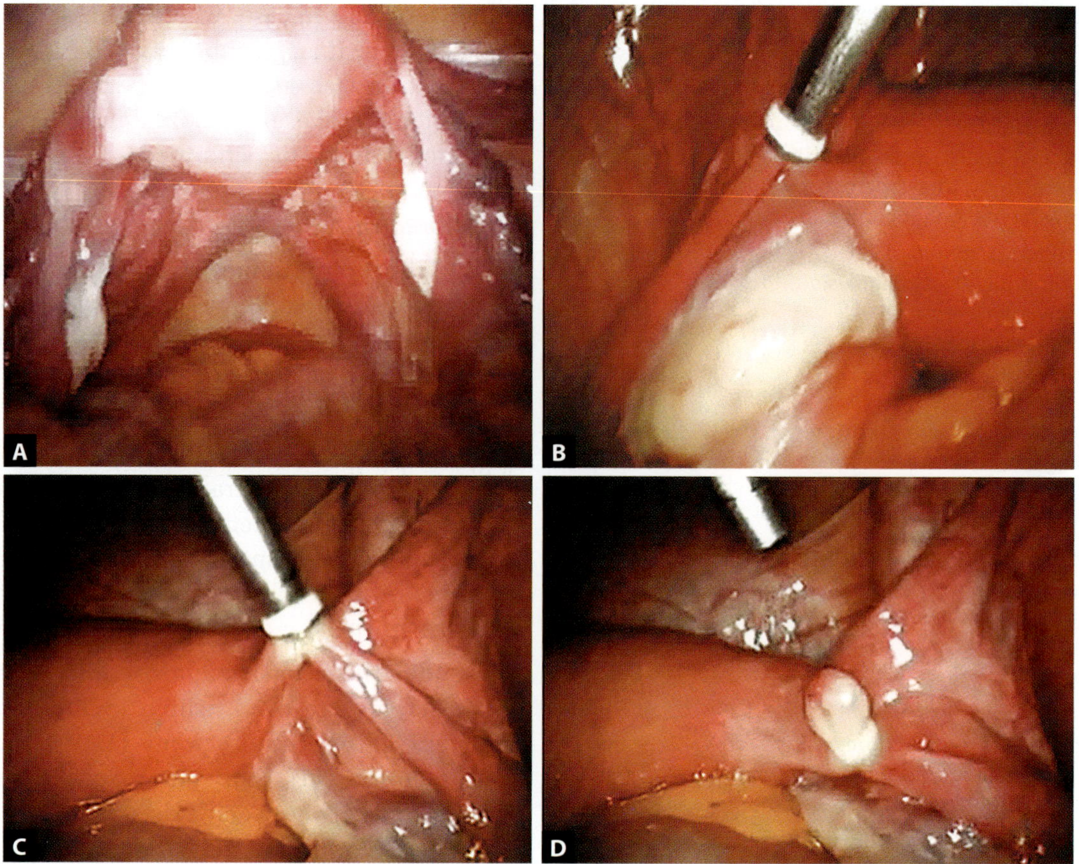

Figs. 26A to D: Steps of laparoscopic sterilisation: (A) Laparoscopic visualisation of the fallopian tubes of both sides; (B) Application of Falope rings; (C) Applicator being withdrawn after ring application; (D) Ligated tube with the Falope ring in place.

CONTRAINDICATIONS TO LAPAROSCOPY

Absolute

- Mechanical or paralytic ileus
- Large abdominal mass (>24 weeks of gestation size)
- Shock
- *Medical conditions precluding surgery:*
  - Severe obstructive airway disease
  - Cardiorespiratory failure
- Irreducible external hernia

Relative

- Multiple abdominal incisions
- Generalised peritonitis
- Hiatus or diaphragmatic hernia
- Blood dyscrasias and coagulopathy
- Extreme obesity
- Advanced pregnancy

PREOPERATIVE PREPARATION

The following steps must be taken preoperatively.

Investigative Studies

The laboratory studies which must be performed prior to the surgery are a complete blood cell count, pregnancy test (to rule out pregnancy), and urine analysis (to rule out any urinary infection). In patients with known health problems, other laboratory tests, such as liver function tests/kidney function tests or evaluation of electrolyte levels, may also be indicated. An alternative to performing routine pregnancy tests prior to surgery is to schedule all elective surgeries during the follicular phase (i.e. within 2 weeks of the last menstrual period). Imaging tests such as a preoperative chest radiograph are not indicated for patients with no risk factors. In patients with coexisting bronchopulmonary conditions or abnormal clinical cardiopulmonary findings, a preoperative chest

X-ray is important. Imaging studies are also part of the basic work-up for anyone who may have a gynaecologic malignancy. Intravenous pyelograph or kidney ultrasound may be performed in women with uterine anomalies, who are at risk for concomitant urologic anomalies, e.g. in some cases of severe endometriosis. A preoperative electrocardiogram may be considered in all women older than 50 years, because the risk of heart disease increases at this age. It is also indicated in women with risk factors (e.g. diabetes mellitus, hypertension, thromboembolic diseases, stroke, etc.), which put them at an increased risk of cardiovascular disease.

Informed Consent

Informed consent must be taken from the patient after explaining the nature of the procedure, the risks, complications and alternatives. The patient should also be counselled regarding the likelihood of a possible laparotomy.

Preoperative Medications

Gonadotrophin-releasing Hormone Agonists

Some women may benefit from the use of gonadotrophin-releasing hormone (GnRH) agonists prior to the surgery. These agents are commonly used in the presence of a large leiomyoma when the large size of the myoma is likely to make surgery difficult. In general, uterine volume can be decreased by up to 50% with 2–3 months of administration of a long-acting GnRH agonist.

Prophylactic Antibiotics

The use of prophylactic antibiotics help in reducing the risk of postoperative infections after gynaecological surgery.

Preoperative Gastrointestinal Preparation

Bowel Preparation

In case the surgeon is planning a significant surgical division of intestines or removal of intestinal adhesions, and either endometriosis or pelvic adhesions are suspected of being present, preoperative bowel preparation is commonly used with the aim of reducing the risk of serious postoperative sequelae. The most commonly used method of bowel preparation includes the use of an oral agent such as magnesium citrate. The patient must be instructed to remain Nulla per os (NPO) after midnight (i.e. after 12:00 am) to avoid the risk of aspiration in case she is scheduled for surgery in the early next morning. In patients whose cases are scheduled later, clear liquids until 6 hours prior to surgery may be allowed, especially in the summer months in order to reduce the degree of preoperative dehydration.

Other Preoperative Considerations

Intravenous Access

In case the surgeon suspects a major blood loss during laparoscopy and establishment of intravenous access may be required prior to starting the case. For this, an intravenous catheter of at least 18 gauge is usually inserted and through this, a balanced salt solution is administered at a moderate rate.

Bladder Catheterisation

Ideally, prior to the placement of the Veress needle or the primary trocar, the bladder must be catheterised to minimise the risk of bladder injury.

Deep Vein Thrombosis Prophylaxis

This helps in preventing the risk of thromboembolism. The American College of Chest Physicians (ACCP) has recommended thromboprophylaxis for patients based on their stratification into low, medium, high and highest risk. For details regarding the ACCP guidelines, refer to **Table 1**.

Patient Positioning

Gynaecologic laparoscopy procedures are usually performed with the patient in the low dorsal lithotomy position, with the buttocks extended over the end of the table. This allows the surgeon to obtain adequate vaginal access for uterine manipulation. Most laparoscopists now use pneumatic boot stirrups specially designed for laparoscopy. In case of prolonged procedures, the legs should be given a compression bandage in order to reduce the incidence of thromboembolism. The patient is positioned in a semilithotomy position with sequential stockings and arm pads, pressure point pads and abduction of the arms to her sides. Modern stirrups are sufficiently padded and have gel inserts, which help in minimising injury at the time of surgery.

Once the primary trocar is placed, the patient is usually placed in no more than a 25° Trendelenburg position to help keep the bowel out of the pelvis. Both the patient's arms should be either abducted or tucked in by the

TABLE 1: The American College of Chest Physicians (ACCP) guidelines for thromboprophylaxis.

Risk stratification	*Thromboprophylaxis*
Low-risk patients (Those younger than 40 years with no additional risk factors, and the duration of surgery is <30 minutes)	No need for prophylaxis
Moderate-risk patients (Those aged 40–60 years with no additional risk factors, undergoing surgery of any duration)	Thromboprophylaxis with sequential compression devices (external pneumatic compression devices) or unfractionated heparin 5,000 units BD or low-molecular-weight heparin (e.g. enoxaparin 40 mg daily)
High-risk patients (Those aged 40–60 years with one additional risk factor, such as prior deep vein thrombosis, varicose veins, infection, malignancy, obesity, oestrogen therapy or surgery lasting longer than 5 hours)	More frequent heparin dose of 5,000 units TDS
Highest-risk patients (same as the high-risk group, but with more than one risk factor	Combination of both sequential compression devices and heparin

patient's side. This allows restriction of movement at the time of manipulation of instruments.

Skin Preparation

Shaving of abdominal and pubic hair is not routinely advocated. In case the hair extends to the intended site of ancillary trocar placement, clipping the pubic hair above the symphysis may be required. The site of surgery is prepared by cleaning and draping the abdominal skin with antiseptic solutions. Following this, specially designed fenestrated laparoscopy drapes are placed over the site of surgery. After changing gloves in order to avoid contamination, vaginal dilators are then inserted inside the uterine cavity for the purpose of uterine manipulation. The vagina is then draped separately to keep the abdominal field separate from the lower vaginal field.

Anaesthesia

Though general anaesthesia with endotracheal intubation is most commonly used for laparoscopy, other anaesthetic techniques, including regional blocks and local infiltration, can also be used.

SURGICAL STEPS

Numerous techniques are available for placing a laparoscopic port into the abdomen. Some of these techniques include the following:

- Veress needle insertion followed by a primary trocar insertion
- Direct trocar insertion
- Open laparoscopy
- Expanding-access cannulas

Open Laparoscopy

In the open technique (Hasson's technique), the peritoneal cavity is entered through a mini-laparotomy incision, which may be transverse or vertical in the subumbilical region after incising the anterior rectus fascia. The primary trocar can also be introduced through Palmer's point, which is about two finger breadths below the left costal margin in the midclavicular line. After making a small incision about 1 cm wide at any of the previously mentioned locations, a blunt-tipped trocar with a sleeve is placed vertically through the incision. Following the insertion of the cannula, it is then sutured to the peritoneum and fascia. The obturator is withdrawn, and CO_2 is attached to the cannula to establish a pneumoperitoneum. The laparoscope is then inserted. In these cases, intra-abdominal CO_2 insufflation is not performed prior to the insertion of the trocar. Also, the chance of injury to various intra-abdominal structures is reduced because the Veress needle and trocar are not inserted blindly. The technique of open laparoscopy was initially developed to reduce the risk of complications associated with the blind insertion of the Veress needle.

Expanding-access Cannulas

This is a relatively new technique for the placement of laparoscopic trocars. In this technique, after insufflation of the peritoneal cavity with CO_2, the Veress needle is removed and reinserted after it is placed into an expandable sleeve. Once the needle, along with the expandable sleeve, is placed inside the peritoneal cavity, the needle is removed, with the sleeve left in place. Following this, the sleeve is dilated to a diameter of about 5–10 mm. This helps in accommodating a laparoscopic lens.

Veress Needle Insertion Followed by a Primary Trocar Insertion

This technique of laparoscope insertion is a closed one, where the peritoneal cavity is initially distended with CO_2, and the trocar is blindly introduced into the peritoneal cavity. The primary cannula with the stylet is usually inserted through the umbilical port, and then the laparoscopic telescope is introduced through the primary cannula. Since this technique of laparoscope insertion is most commonly used, it would be described in detail and comprises the following steps:

Veress Needle Insertion

Prior to the insertion of the Veress needle, a small subumbilical incision about 3–4 mm in size, just adequate for the introduction of the needle, is made. Before inserting the needle, the abdomen is maximally lifted by grasping the middle of the abdomen below the umbilicus. In order to avoid injury to the surrounding structures, the needle should be held by the shaft in the form of a dart. It should be directed towards the centre of the pelvic cavity at an angle of 45° to the horizontal. In a very thin patient, the vital structures are much closer to the abdominal wall, with sometimes the distance between the skin and large retroperitoneal vessels being as little as 4 cm. In such cases, it is important to insert the needle at an angle of 45° rather than adopting a more vertical approach. On the other hand, in obese patients [body mass index (BMI) of 30 kg/m^2 or more], a more vertical approach, approximately 70–80°, is required because of the increased thickness of the abdominal wall. Without using the vertical insertion, the needle or trocar would not be long enough to penetrate the layers and enter the peritoneal cavity. At the time of insertion of the Veress needle, two distinct pops are usually felt. The first one occurs when the needle punctures through the anterior rectus fascia, and the second occurs when the needle passes through the posterior fascia and peritoneum. Once the second pop is felt, the insertion of the needle is stopped. Some common sites of Veress needle placement are as follows:

- Intraumbilical placement
- *Palmer's point:* Left subcostal margin in the midclavicular line
- McBurney's point
- *Transvaginal approach:* Insertion of the needle is performed through the posterior cul-de-sac. This technique may prove useful in patients in whom previous attempts at needle insertion were unsuccessful. Since some of the most dangerous complications at the time of laparoscopic surgery can occur at the time of insertion of the Veress needle and the sharp primary trocar, the operator must observe utmost precaution at the time of insertion of either the Veress needle or the primary trocar. The entry of the needle into the peritoneal cavity and its proper placement can be ascertained with the help of the following signs:

- *Sound of air:* As the needle enters the peritoneal cavity, there would be a hissing sound of air being sucked inside.
- *Palmer's test:* A 20-mL syringe is half-filled with saline and is attached to the hub of the Veress needle. The plunger is first drawn back. Aspiration of blood or bowel contents implies that the needle is in a major splanchnic structure, such as a bowel or blood vessel. If no blood or bowel contents are aspirated back, then 10 mL of saline contained inside the syringe can be flushed back into the peritoneal cavity. This can occur easily without resistance if the needle is positioned properly inside the peritoneal cavity. As the saline enters the peritoneal cavity, it cannot be aspirated back. The last phase of this test comprises withdrawing the plunger again.

  When the needle is positioned properly, no fluid would be sucked back into the syringe. However, if the needle tip is lying within the adhesions or in the abdominal wall, the saline is likely to have collected in the form of a pool and can be drawn back.
- *Hanging drop test:* This test is done by placing a drop of saline at the open end of the Veress needle. The abdominal wall is then elevated, while observing if the saline drop disappears into the shaft or not. The drop of saline instilled into the needle will be sucked in if the needle is inside the peritoneal cavity. However, if the needle is extraperitoneal, the saline drop would remain there.
- *Measurement of IAP with carbon dioxide insufflation:* The Veress needle may be attached to the insufflator with the valve in the off position (with the gas off). The valve is then opened so that the gas starts distending the abdomen. If a negative pressure reading is observed on the insufflation instrument, it is indicative of correct needle placement. Only when the needle has been securely placed intraperitoneally and the pressure reading is <10 mm Hg, the insufflation rate is increased.
- *Loss of liver dullness:* The intraperitoneal placement of the needle can also be confirmed by visualising uniform distension of the abdomen and

obliteration of the liver dullness. If the needle has been correctly placed, following the insufflation of gas, four-quadrant percussion in the hepatic area produces a tympanic note, with the loss of liver dullness. If the needle is extraperitoneal, distension would be confined to the hypogastrium, and the pressure recorded would be high.

If results from one of the above-mentioned tests indicate malposition of the needle, it needs to be repositioned.

Carbon Dioxide Insufflation

After confirming the position of the Veress needle, CO_2 insufflation can begin at the rate of 3 L/min. The purpose of CO_2 insufflation is to raise the abdominal wall away from the underlying structures, so that the surgeon can safely insert the sharp trocar into the gas-filled abdominal cavity without causing any harm to the underlying structures. The amount of gas to be insufflated is measured in terms of IAP produced by the gas. In an average-built woman, 3 litres of insufflated gas is likely to produce an IAP of 10 mm Hg. Trocar insertion usually requires a force of 4–5 kg. When the IAP of approximately 22 mm Hg has been obtained, the force of 4–5 kg applied for trocar insertion indents the abdominal wall in such a way that there is still a gas barrier of at least 5 cm between the abdominal wall and the bowel.

Insertion of Primary Trocar and Cannula

After an adequate amount of IAP has been created, the trocar and cannula (most commonly 5 mm or 10 mm in diameter) are placed at an angle similar to that of the Veress needle, aiming at the hollow of the sacrum. Following this, the laparoscope is inserted. Once the primary trocar is in position, the IAP is reduced to 14 mm Hg. While introducing the primary cannula and trocar through the umbilical port, the patient should be made to lie in the supine horizontal position without Trendelenburg tilt. This is important because placing the patient in Trendelenburg position is likely to bring the aortic bifurcation more anteriorly, and therefore it is more likely to get injured.

Placement of Secondary Trocars

Barring the diagnostic laparoscopies, secondary trocars are required for most operative gynaecologic laparoscopy procedures. Additional ports are placed lateral to the inferior epigastric vessels on both sides **(Fig. 27)**. After identifying the epigastric vessels by transillumination and

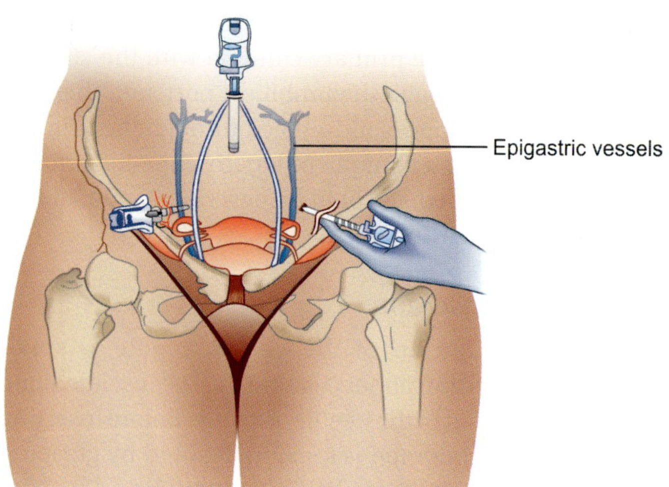

Fig. 27: Additional ports inserted under vision lateral to inferior epigastric vessels.

intraperitoneal observation, secondary trocars are placed. The trocars are placed either in the midline, 3 cm above the pubic symphysis, or approximately 8 cm lateral to the midline and 8 cm above the pubic symphysis to avoid injury to the epigastric (inferior and superficial) and the superficial circumflex iliac vessels.

Introduction of the Laparoscopic Telescope

The trocar is removed from its sleeve (cannula) and the laparoscopic telescope then inserted inside through the cannula. The flapper valve of the trocar allows the surgeon to insert the laparoscope and other instruments without the loss of gas. Prior to insertion, the telescope must be examined to ensure that lenses are clear and bright and may be cleaned if they appear dirty.

Performance of Laparoscopic Procedures

Depending on the indication of laparoscopic surgery, diagnostic or operative procedures are performed next.

POSTOPERATIVE CARE

Following the performance of a major gynaecologic laparoscopic procedure, the bowel function may take several days to normalise. The pain may be worse on the day following the procedure, but generally improves after that. Also, the postoperative incision usually becomes healthy within the first week. Patients should be counselled about this course of events, which usually occurs postoperatively. The patients should be instructed to contact their physician if any variation from this course occurs or they experience extensive pain or bleeding at any point.

In the absence of complications, in most of the cases, the patient is able to return to full activity within 72 hours after most gynaecologic laparoscopic procedures. Recovery from LH can be expected within 2–3 weeks.

ADVANTAGES

Laparoscopic surgery is associated with several advantages over laparotomy, such as:

- Reduced duration of hospital stay and earlier discharge from the hospital
- Reduced postoperative pain
- Reduced blood loss

DISADVANTAGES

In gynaecology, the most commonly suggested contraindication for laparoscopic surgery is haemodynamic instability resulting from a ruptured ectopic pregnancy. However, following appropriate fluid resuscitation, laparoscopy can be considered a safe approach. Another traditional contraindication was pregnancy. In the last few years, several large series have documented the safety of using an open technique for laparoscopy during pregnancy. Several risk factors for laparoscopic surgery are as follows:

Patient Risk Factors

Obesity

- Obesity is a well-recognised factor that increases the risk of any abdominal surgery. Women with a BMI >25 kg/m^2 are classified as overweight, and those with a BMI >30 kg/m^2 are considered obese. In an average-sized woman of approximately 160 cm, these cut-off points correspond roughly to weights of 73 kg (160 lbs) and 91 kg (200 lbs), respectively.
- In women who are overweight, and even more so in those who are obese, every aspect of laparoscopy becomes more difficult and potentially more risky. Placement of laparoscopic instruments becomes much more difficult and often requires special techniques. Bleeding from abdominal wall vessels may be more common, because these vessels become difficult to locate. Many intra-abdominal procedures become increasingly difficult because of a restricted operative field secondary to retroperitoneal fat deposits in the pelvic sidewalls and increased bowel excursion into the operative field.

Age

- Another well-described surgical risk factor is age. Older patients are at an increased risk of having concomitant disease processes that affect their perioperative morbidity and mortality.
- Probably, the single most important consideration is an age-associated increase in cardiovascular disease. Risk is increased even greater in women who have not taken replacement hormones after menopause. Intraoperative cardiac stress related to anaesthesia and the surgery itself may result in sudden cardiac decompensation based on arrhythmia, ischaemia or infarction.
- Of special importance is the increased susceptibility of elderly persons to hypothermia, because the vast majority of patients experience some degree of hypothermia during laparoscopy. In older patients, even mild degrees of hypothermia may increase the risk of cardiac arrhythmias and prolong recovery time.

Previous Abdominal Surgery

As far as laparoscopic complications are concerned, one of the most important risk factors is the history of previous abdominal surgery. The risk of adhesions of omentum and/or bowel to the anterior abdominal wall after previous abdominal surgery is >20% of sharp instruments into the abdominal cavity and a reasonable assumption is that previous surgery would increase the risk of bowel injury.

COMPLICATIONS

Besides causing the long-established complications related to surgery, such as infection and generalised bleeding, laparoscopic surgery can result in some unique complications related to the procedure itself. Some of these are described next in detail.

Gas Embolism

Since carbon dioxide is used to create the pneumoperitoneum during laparoscopic procedures, gas embolisation is an uncommon but very serious complication, which can occur. Embolisation is usually caused by inadvertent placement of the Veress needle into a major vessel during attempts to insufflate the abdominal cavity with carbon dioxide. To avoid this complication, the operator must verify intraperitoneal placement of the Veress needle prior to insufflation.

Retroperitoneal Vessel Injury

Although laceration of a major abdominal blood vessel is one of the least common complications, it is one of the most life-threatening complications in laparoscopy. This may occur during insertion of the Veress needle or the primary trocar. Since the umbilicus usually lies over the bifurcation of the aorta at L4, the aorta and inferior vena cava are avoided if one inserts the Veress needle or trocar through the umbilicus towards the hollow of the pelvis. At times, there may be a variation in the level of aortic bifurcation. Patients who are thin are at an additional risk, because the distance from the umbilicus to the retroperitoneal vessels may be as short as 2–3 cm. When placing the Veress needle, the patient must be in the horizontal position (not Trendelenburg), and the angle of entry must vary depending on the patient's weight.

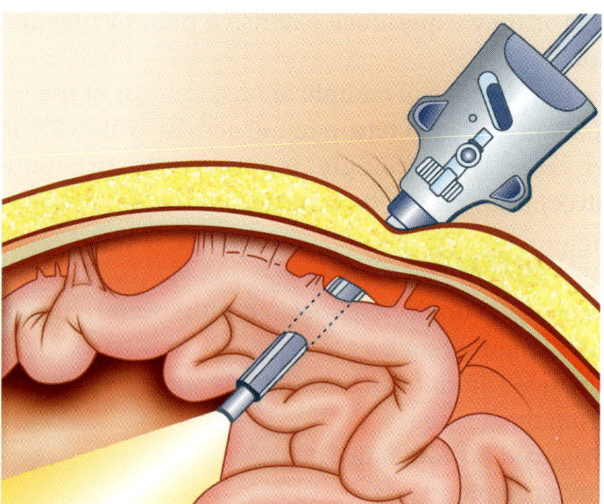

Fig. 28: Bowel injury during trocar insertion in a patient with bowel adhesions.

Abdominal Wall Vessel Injury

Placement of numerous and large accessory trocars lateral to the rectus muscles at the time of laparoscopic surgery has increased the risk of abdominal wall vessel injury. Injury to the epigastric vessels (inferior and superficial) and the superficial circumflex iliac vessel may occur during the placement of secondary ports. The superficial epigastric vessels originate from the femoral artery, while the inferior (deep) epigastric vessels originate from the external iliac arteries. These arteries are accompanied by corresponding veins in most cases. Damage to these vessels can cause significant blood loss, resulting in a haematoma formation or postoperative haemorrhage.

This risk can be reduced by using techniques such as direct laparoscopic visualisation of the inferior epigastric vessels. Very often, the superficial abdominal wall vessels can be visualised by transilluminating the abdominal wall with the laparoscope. The inferior epigastric artery cannot be transilluminated but may be seen intraperitoneally beneath the peritoneum. Prior to insertion of the lateral trocars, the operator should make an effort to identify and avoid these vessels. Another way of avoiding such injuries is the insertion of trocars lateral to the edge of the rectus muscle or at least 8 cm lateral to the midline. The use of conical trocars, in contrast to the pyramidal-tipped trocars, can also help reduce the risk of injury to these vessels.

Intestinal Injury

Both the small and large intestines can be injured during laparoscopy, which can act as a life-threatening situation, if it remains unrecognised **(Fig. 28)**. Recently, disposable trocars have been introduced, which have a safety shield to help reduce the occurrence of bowel injury with entry of the trocar into the peritoneal cavity. Moreover, there is a risk of thermal injury to the bowel, especially when using electrocautery, particularly monopolar electrosurgery. This injury can cause peritonitis if it remains unrecognised. This is a potentially life-threatening situation if not treated immediately.

Urologic Injuries

Injury to the bladder or ureters can occur during trocar placement or during the use of power instruments, and stapling or suturing devices. The greatest challenge is recognising that the injury has occurred, so that treatment can be performed in a timely manner. One important step for avoiding injuries to the bladder is catheterising the bladder before starting the laparoscopic surgery. Ureteral injuries can occur with any procedure involving instrumentation near the ureters.

Incisional Hernia

Incisional hernias were rare in those days when small-sized ports were used. However, with the use of larger ports (>5 mm), the incidence of incisional hernias has increased.

Nerve Injuries

Patient positioning during laparoscopic surgery is associated with a low risk of potentially serious nerve injury to either the lower or upper extremities (e.g. brachial plexus injury). To minimise the risk of brachial plexus injuries during laparoscopy, the arms should be tucked at the side of the patient whenever possible. Arms extended on arm boards should be abducted at <90° angle. On the other hand, lithotomy position for prolonged periods of time can result in injuries to nerves of the lower extremity, including the femoral, lateral femoral cutaneous, obturator, sciatic and common peroneal nerves. Entrapment of the peroneal nerve can occur when there is undue pressing of the knees against some structure. In order to prevent any nerve-related injury, some important things which must be kept in mind while placing the patient in lithotomy position include maintaining hip flexion of 60–170° and knee flexion of 90–120°. Hip abduction should be maintained at no more than 90°, and there should be minimal external rotation of the hip joint. Extrinsic pressure on the legs should be avoided.

Anaesthetic Complications

Complications related to anaesthetic medications can also occur.

Reducing Laparoscopic-related Complications

Steps to be taken to reduce the complications related to laparoscopic surgery are as follows:

- The patient should be lying flat at the time of surgery.
- The bladder must be empty.
- The abdomen must be palpated to rule out the presence of any abdominal mass.
- The primary incision should be either subumbilical or at the base of the umbilicus.

CONCLUSION

This minimally invasive procedure has become a preferred method of choice for the diagnosis and treatment of several gynaecological surgical conditions. Laparoscopic surgery is associated with numerous advantages such as reduced duration of hospital stay, reduced recovery time and reduced incidence of postoperative complications such as pain. Furthermore, the advent of robotic laparoscopic surgery appears to be changing the approach to many gynaecological surgery cases. The robotic system allows surgeons to perform procedures that previously would have been performed via laparotomy using modified laparoscopic procedures.

HYSTEROSCOPIC SURGERY

INTRODUCTION

Hysteroscopy is a minimally invasive procedure, involving the direct inspection of the cervical canal and endometrial cavity through a rigid, flexible or contact hysteroscope **(Figs. 29A to C)**. The procedure allows for the diagnosis of intrauterine pathology and serves as a method for surgical intervention (operative hysteroscopy). Hysteroscopy has the benefit of allowing direct visualisation of the uterus, thereby avoiding or reducing iatrogenic trauma to delicate reproductive tissues. Not only does hysteroscopy allow direct observation of the intrauterine or endometrial pathology (presence of submucous fibroids, endometrial cancer, etc.), but also it acts as a way of sampling the endometrium under direct visualisation.

Both diagnostic and operative hysteroscopy have now become a standard part of routine gynaecological practice. Besides diagnosing certain uterine pathologies and aiding in the biopsy, hysteroscopy has now also become the method of choice for the treatment of intrauterine pathology.

SURGICAL EQUIPMENT

Hysteroscope

The hysteroscopic system comprises a rigid telescope that is used together with an outer sheath for instillation of the distension media.

Telescope

Telescopes of different diameters (2–4 mm) and a variety of viewing capabilities are available (0°, 12°, 30°, 70°). The most popular hysteroscope is a 4 mm, 30° telescope with a 5.5 mm outer sheath for diagnostic as well as operative hysteroscopy. A sharp and clear image can be obtained with the help of a 4 mm telescope **(Fig. 30)**. This is also associated with the smallest outside diameter. The most desirable optics provides a large field that subtends an angle of approximately 105°. The telescopes are available with a 0° straight-on or a 30° fore-oblique view. The major advantage of the 0° lens is that it allows the operator to see the operative devices as a relatively distant panorama, whereas this view is lost when the 30° lens is used. The telescope has three parts:

1. The eyepiece
2. The barrel
3. The objective lens

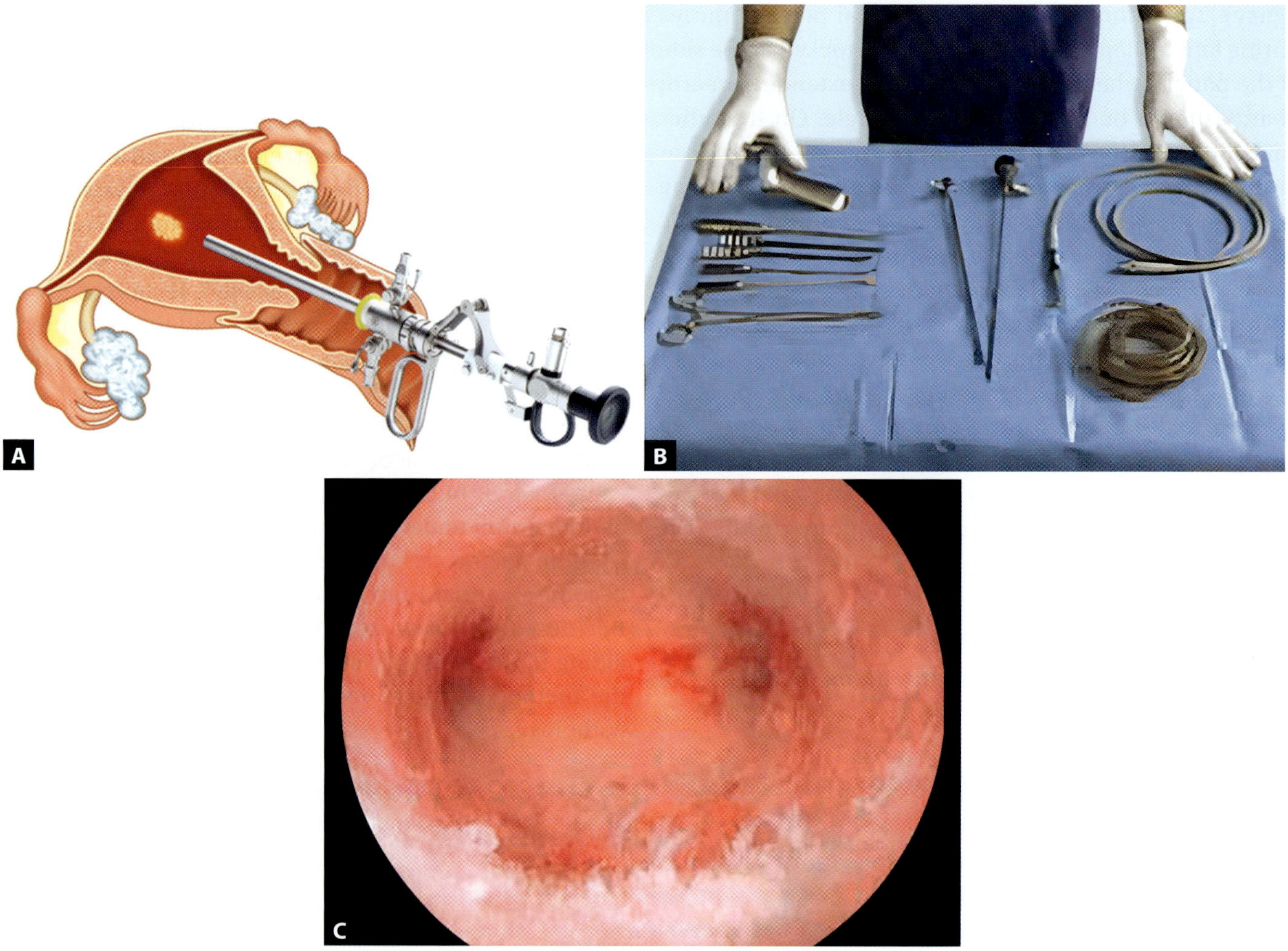

Figs. 29A to C: (A) Diagrammatic view of a hysteroscope inside the uterine cavity; (B) Instruments used at the time of diagnostic hysteroscopy; (C) Hysteroscopy—normal cavity.

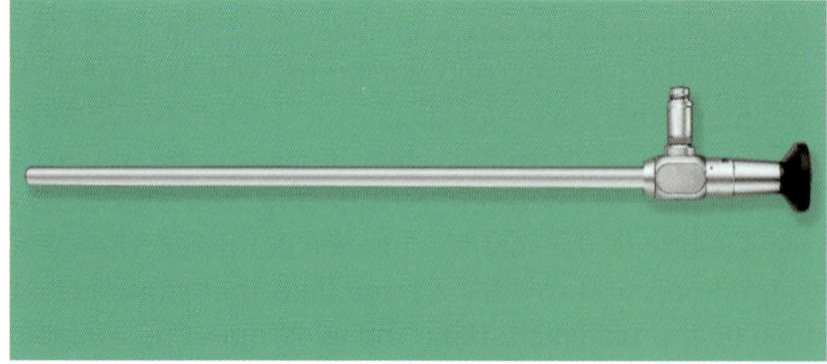

Fig. 30: Telescope.

Light generators act as a source of light for the hysteroscope. Three types of light generators are available:
1. Tungsten
2. Metal halide
3. Xenon

Diagnostic and Operative Sheath

The diagnostic sheath helps in the delivery of the distension media inside the uterine cavity. The diagnostic sheath commonly used is 5 mm and allows 1 mm clearance space between its inner wall and the telescope, through which the distending medium is delivered. A 6.5-mm double-channel continuous-flow sheath is available and is useful when the uterine cavity is bleeding **(Fig. 31)**. The same telescope can be used with an operative hysteroscopy sheath and resectoscope.

The diameter of the operative sheath is usually greater than that of the diagnostic sheath and ranges from 7 to 10 mm **(Fig. 32)**. The operative sheath has space for instillation of the distension medium for the 4 mm telescope and for the insertion of operating devices. The resectoscope is a specialised electrosurgical endoscope comprising an inner and outer sheath. In the inner sheath, there is a common channel for the telescope, medium and electrode **(Figs. 33A and B)**. There is a trigger device which pushes the electrode out beyond the sheath and pulls it back within the sheath. The operating tool comprises two basic electrodes:

1. A 4-mm ball
2. A 5-mm cutting loop

The internal lumen of the sheath must be of adequate size to allow the passage of the telescope and operative instruments, e.g. scissors, biopsy forceps, catheters and coagulation electrodes. The external sheath diameter ranges from 3.7 to 7 mm to allow the passage of the telescope, operative instruments and liquid distension medium. Resectoscope has been used by urologists to perform operative procedures such as excision of submucous myomas, polypectomy, division of uterine septa and endometrial ablation or resection. The main characteristics of the widely used Karl Storz resectoscope are described in **Table 2**.

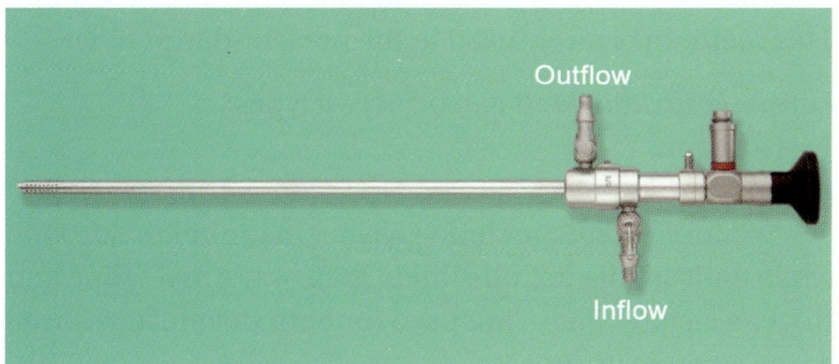

Fig. 31: Continuous-flow examination sheath.

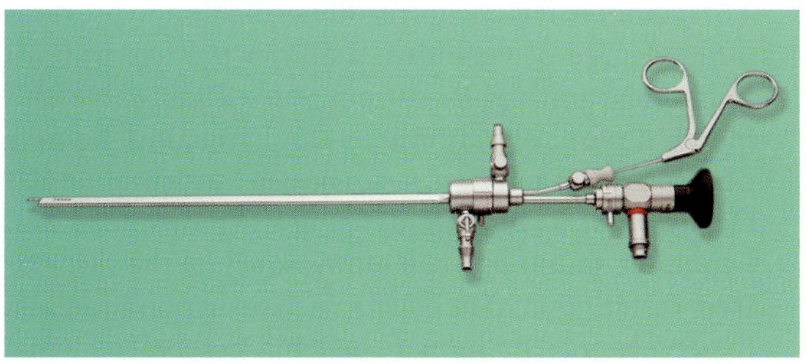
Fig. 32: Operative hysteroscope with instruments through the operative channel.

A diagnostic sheath is required to deliver the distending medium into the uterine cavity. The telescope fits into the sheath and is secured by means of a water-tight seal that locks into place. The hysteroscope must be inserted under direct vision, and the axis of the cervical and uterine canal must be carefully followed until the uterine corpus has been reached. This way, the chances of uterine perforation can be minimised. Improper coupling between the telescope and sheath is likely to result in leakage of the medium at that interface. Operative sheaths have a larger diameter, varying between 7 and 10 mm (average 8 mm).

Distension Medium

Various types of distension media are used at the time of hysteroscopic surgery. Distension media used at the time of hysteroscopy can be either gaseous or liquid. Water is usually not used as a distension medium due to its hypo-osmolar nature. Also, once it is absorbed, it can cause haemolysis.

Gaseous distension medium: The most commonly used gaseous medium for diagnostic hysteroscopy is CO_2. It is inexpensive, does not produce any mess, is readily

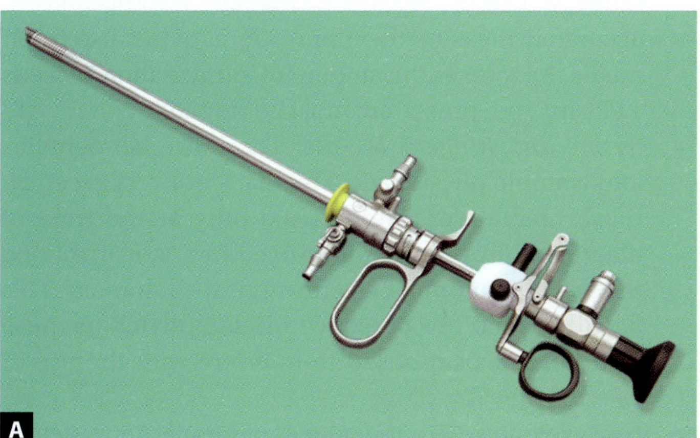

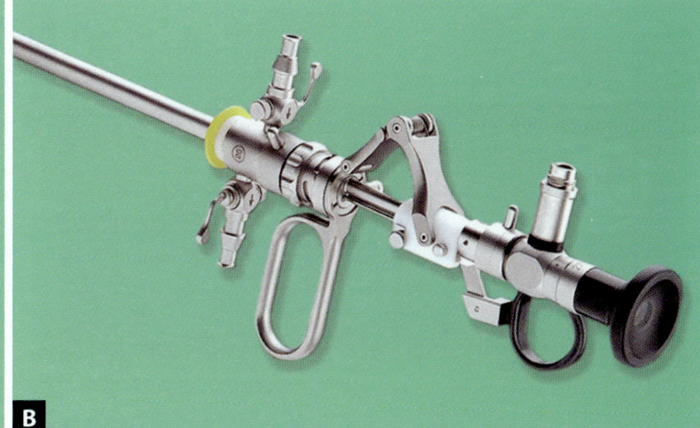

Figs. 33A and B: (A) Resectoscope (Karl Storz); (B) Resectoscope sheath including connecting tube for inflow and outflow for continuous irrigation and suction with bipolar electrode.

available and helps in providing a clear view. However, in the presence of blood or mucus, it can produce a distorted view. CO_2 is rapidly absorbed by the blood and speedily cleared by the lungs. If proper flow rate and pressure are maintained, the incidence of intoxication or embolism due to CO_2 can be considerably reduced. However, CO_2 can sometimes leak around the hysteroscope, making diagnosis very difficult. Mild contamination of the lens by the mucus or blood can result in the formation of troublesome bubbles with the use of CO_2. This may result in the obscuration of the picture quality. With the use of CO_2 as the distension medium, the pressure should be maintained in the range of 100–120 mm Hg, with a flow rate of 30–60 mL/min. This corresponds to the final intrauterine working pressure of 40–80 mm Hg. With office hysteroscopy, it is best to use fluid distension media rather than CO_2 gas distension media for the visualisation of the uterine cavity.

One requires the use of a dedicated gas hysteroflator, which helps in maintaining the IAP and adjustment of CO_2 insufflation flow rate **(Fig. 34)**. Laparoscopic insufflators having high flow rates must not be used. Inadvertent use of these laparoscopic insufflators can lead to CO_2 embolism and even death.

Liquid media: Fluid distension media can be used for both diagnostic and operative purposes. This involves the use of high viscosity or high molecular weight media such as Hyskon, or the low viscosity, low-molecular-weight media such as saline or glycine.

TABLE 2: Main characteristics of the widely used Karl Storz resectoscope.

Diameter	*Telescope*	*Electrosurgical system*
26 Fr	0°, 12°, 30°	Monopolar

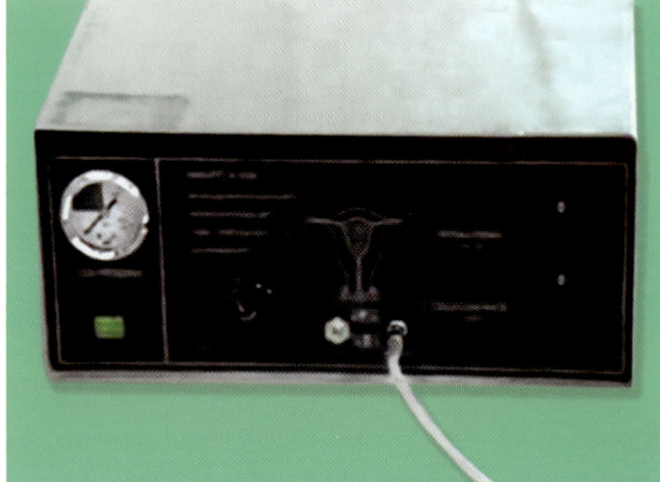

Fig. 34: Carbon dioxide insufflator.

High viscosity media/high-molecular-weight dextran: It has been used in the past as the distension media for hysteroscopy. The main disadvantage of this medium is that it is viscous, messy and inconsistent and has the potential to immobilise the moving parts of the hysteroscope, if not properly cleaned. There is a risk of causing complications, such as pulmonary oedema, disseminated intravascular coagulation or anaphylaxis, if its amount exceeds 500 mL. This medium is rarely used in the present-day practice.

Low viscosity media: It can be of two types:

1. Nonionic
2. Ionic

Nonionic media include glycine, mannitol or sorbitol, while ionic media include fluids such as normal saline and ringer's lactate. These are used for both diagnostic as well as therapeutic purposes.

- *Glycine:* It is a simple amino acid, which is used as a distension medium after mixing it with water to form a 1.5% solution. It is cheap, readily available and provides a fair degree of visibility. It allows the use of both monopolar and bipolar current. Since it is miscible with blood, it requires continuous-flow irrigation. Being a nonelectrolyte solution, it can be used with monopolar electrosurgical equipment. Being a hypo-osmolar and hypotonic solution, it can intravasate into the vascular tree, resulting in side effects such as hyponatraemia, hypervolaemia, pulmonary oedema, cerebral oedema, heart failure and death. Water intoxication and fluid overload especially occur if the fluid (800–1,000 mL) intravasates into the patient. Therefore, it is important to accurately measure the input/output of the distension media. As soon as the amount of intravasation exceeds 1,000 mL, the procedure must be stopped.
- *Saline and Ringer's lactate:* These are iso-osmolar and isotonic physiological media. Until very recently, these media were being used only at the time of diagnostic hysteroscopic procedures, not involving the use of monopolar electrosurgical equipment. This is so because the presence of electrolytes in these solutions was supposed to interfere with the use of electrosurgical systems.

However, now with the advent of bipolar intrauterine surgery, the use of electrolyte-free solutions can be avoided at the time of surgery. This has encouraged the use of solutions such as normal saline for hysteroscopic surgery.

Electrolyte-free Distension Media (Sorbitol-Mannitol Solution)

Sorbitol is commonly used as a distension medium for operative hysteroscopy. It is a hypo-osmolar solution, absorption of which poses a risk for the development of cerebral oedema. Absorption of the hypo-osmolar solution by the brain causes the brain to pump out the cations. This cation-pumping mechanism in the brain may be deficient in women under the effect of the hormone, progesterone. Therefore, women are at a higher risk of developing cerebral oedema.

Distension Machines

The various types of distension machines which can be used include:

- Gravity
- Pressure cuff
- Hysteromat **(Fig. 35)**
- Total input-output system

The hysteromat can be considered as the ideal system of all, because it helps in maintaining intrauterine pressure of approximately 70 mm Hg.

Hysteroscopic Operating Equipment

Various types of hysteroscopic scissors and grasping forceps are shown in **Figures 36 and 37**, respectively.

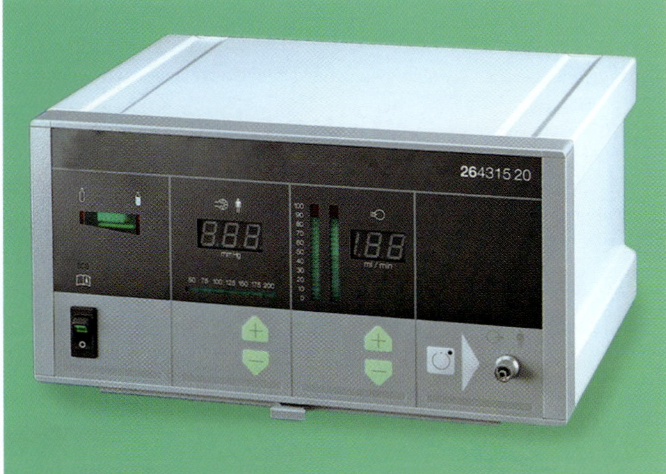

Fig. 35: Hysteromat of Hamou helps in providing a constant flow of low viscosity fluid, which helps in maintaining sufficient pressure to keep the uterine walls distended.

There are various types of unipolar cutting thermal loops and electrodes with different shapes and sizes **(Figs. 38A to E)**, which can be used with resectoscope sheaths.

INDICATIONS

Hysteroscopy is useful in numerous diagnostic as well as operative procedures.

Diagnostic Indications

- Diagnosis of causes of infertility [abnormalities on hysterosalpingography such as filling defects, intrauterine synechiae **(Fig. 39)**, adhesions **(Fig. 40)** and Asherman's syndrome].
- Diagnosis of cases of recurrent miscarriage
- Diagnosis of causes of abnormal bleeding such as menorrhagia, irregular bleeding, abnormal uterine bleeding (AUB) and postmenopausal bleeding. This could be related to causes such as the presence of

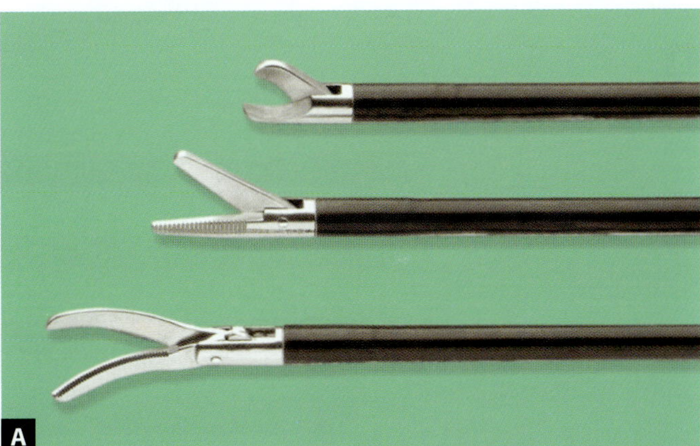

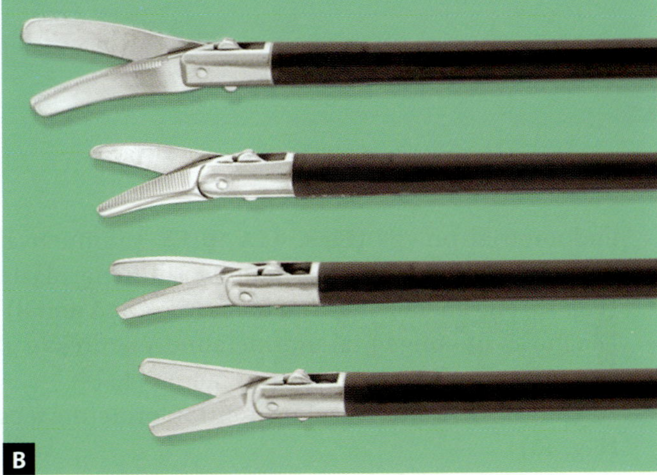

Figs. 36A and B: Various types of scissors.

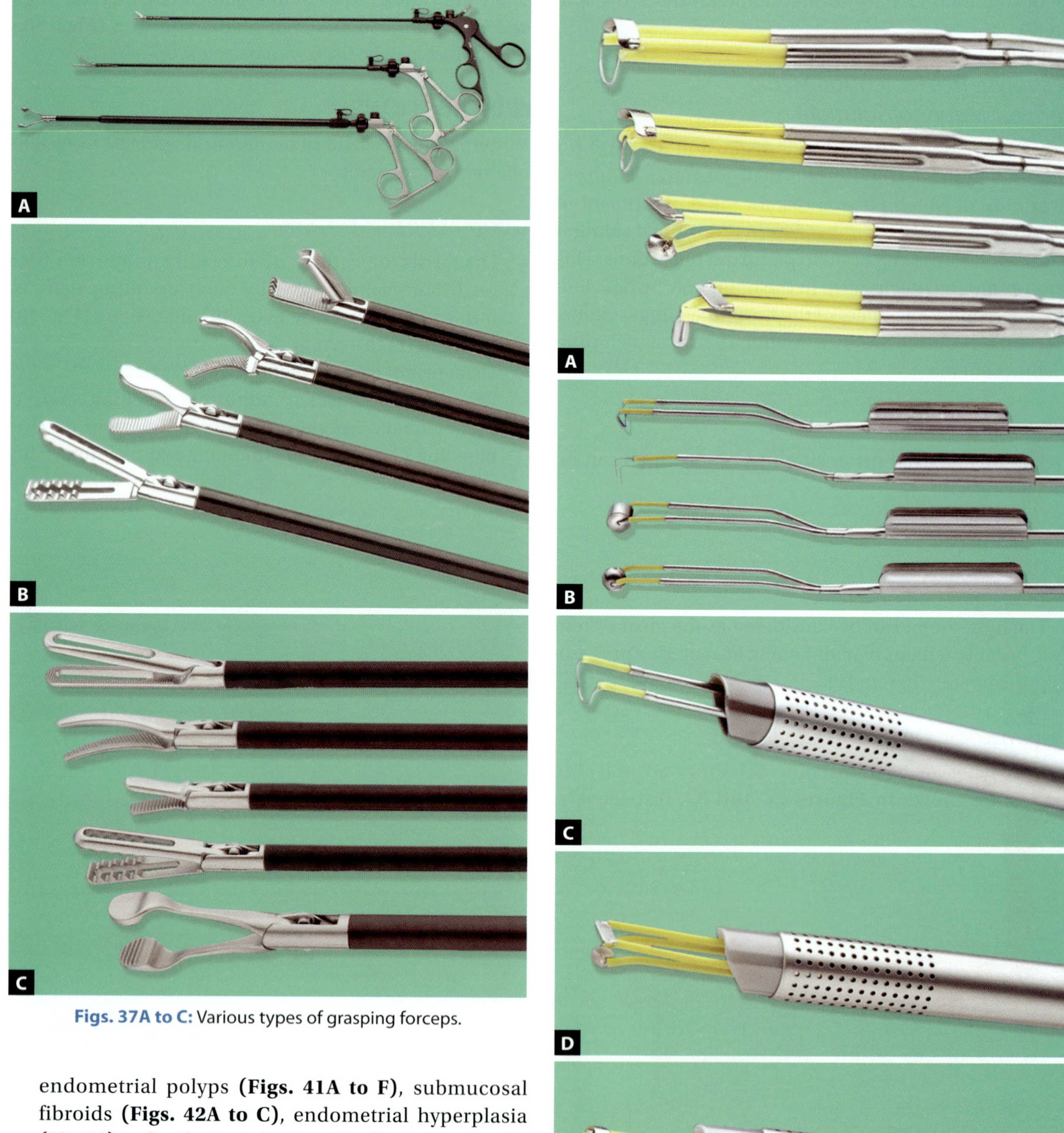

Figs. 37A to C: Various types of grasping forceps.

Figs. 38A to E: Unipolar cutting loops and electrodes (for use with resectoscope sheaths).

endometrial polyps **(Figs. 41A to F)**, submucosal fibroids **(Figs. 42A to C)**, endometrial hyperplasia **(Fig. 43)** and endometrial carcinoma **(Figs. 44A and B)**.

- Diagnosis of congenital uterine abnormalities [e.g. septate uterus **(Fig. 45)**, T-shaped uterus, etc.]
- Diagnosis of lost or misplaced intrauterine devices **(Fig. 46)**
- Examination of endocervical mucosa **(Figs. 47 and 48)**
- Assessment of tubal-ostia **(Fig. 49)**

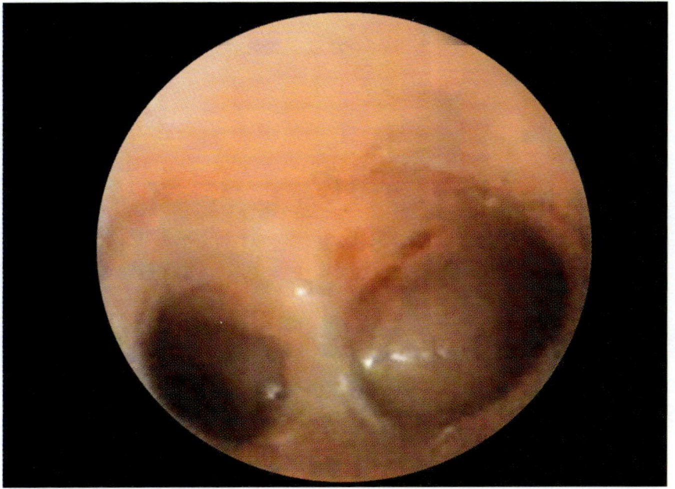
Fig. 39: Intrauterine synechiae.

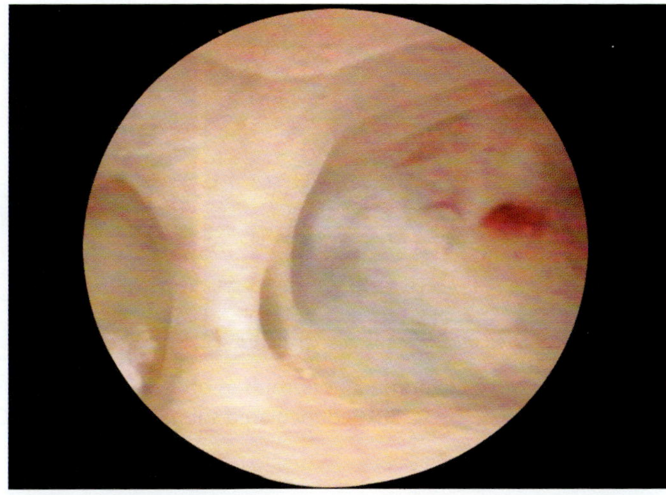
Fig. 40: Hysteroscopy—adhesions.

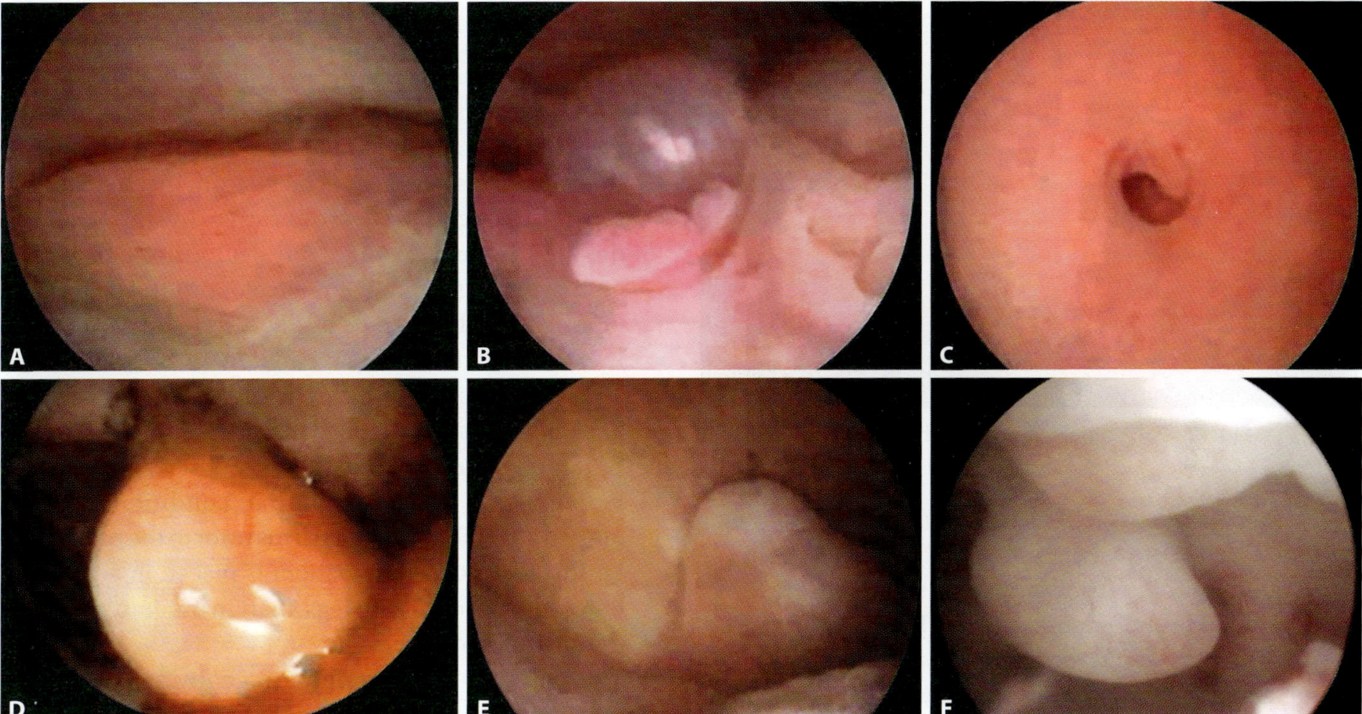
Figs. 41A to F: Various polyps as observed on hysteroscopic examination: (A) A large cervical polyp; (B) Cervical mucosal polyp; (C) Cornual polyp; (D) Endometrial polyp; (E) Endometrial polyp in another patient; (F) Large fundal polyp.

Operative Indications

The indications of operative hysteroscopy are as follows:

- Treatment of AUB [endometrial ablation **(Figs. 50A to F)**, transcervical resection of endometrium (TCRE) **(Figs. 51A to C)**]
- *Polypectomy:* Removal of endometrial polyps
- *Adhesiolysis:* Hysteroscopic resection of adhesions is achieved either using microscissors or thermal energy modalities. This method is also used in case of the presence of intrauterine adhesions (e.g. Asherman's syndrome).
- Myomectomy for submucosal fibroids
- Hysteroscopic resection of the uterine septum **(Figs. 52A to H)**
- Removal of misplaced/embedded intrauterine contraceptive device (IUCD)

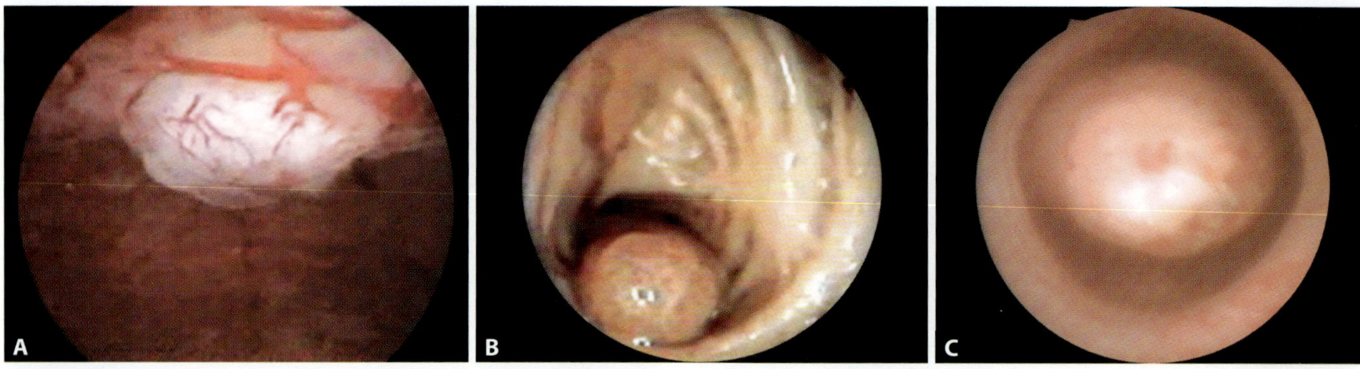

Figs. 42A to C: Submucous fibroids as observed on hysteroscopic examination: (A) Intramural fibroid in the fundal region; (B) Pedunculated submucosal fibroid; (C) Submucosal fibroid arising from fundus.

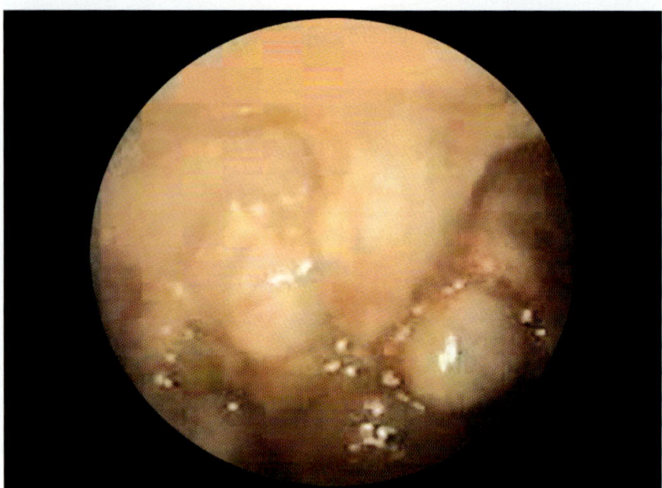

Fig. 43: Polypoidal endometrial hyperplasia.

- Sterilisation [use of electrocoagulation or tubal plugs to block the cornual ends of the tubes **(Fig. 53)**]
- Targeted endometrial biopsy in suspected cases of tuberculosis, endometrial cancer **(Figs. 54A and B)**.
- *Hysteroscopy allows access to the uterotubal junction for entry into the fallopian tube:* This is useful for tubal occlusion procedures for sterilisation and for falloposcopy.
- *Management of cornual and interstitial tubal blockage:* Tubal cannulation can be useful in cases of cornual or interstitial blocks. The whole procedure of hysteroscopic tubal cannulation is described in **Figures 55A to G**.

PREOPERATIVE PREPARATION

- Hysteroscopy has been done in the hospital, surgical centres and offices.
- Hysteroscopy is best done in the immediate postmenstrual phase when the endometrium is relatively thin which facilitates intracavitary viewing.
- Paracervical block using 1% lidocaine is usually sufficient for diagnostic hysteroscopy procedures. Operative hysteroscopic interventions are usually performed under general endotracheal anaesthesia.
- Informed consent must be taken from the patient.
- Prior to diagnostic or operative hysteroscopy, a detailed patient history, physical examination and discussion regarding the choice of procedure and the type of anaesthesia to be used needs to be performed.
- In order to reduce the pain and discomfort associated with the procedure, mild sedatives or nonsteroidal anti-inflammatory drugs (ibuprofen, 600–800 mg) can be administered prior to the procedure.
- Patients with high-risk cardiac conditions may be offered an antibiotic prophylaxis prior to the procedure.
- For the procedure, the patient is placed in a standard lithotomy position with legs apart in order to maximise the vaginal access.
- The perineum and vagina are gently swabbed with povidone-iodine or another suitable antiseptic solution.

SURGICAL STEPS

Diagnostic Hysteroscopy

The steps of diagnostic hysteroscopy are as follows:

- The posterior vaginal wall is retracted using Sims' speculum.
- The anterior edge of the cervix is grasped with the help of a single-toothed tenaculum.
- Most diagnostic hysteroscopic procedures using a 5 mm diagnostic sheath can be performed without

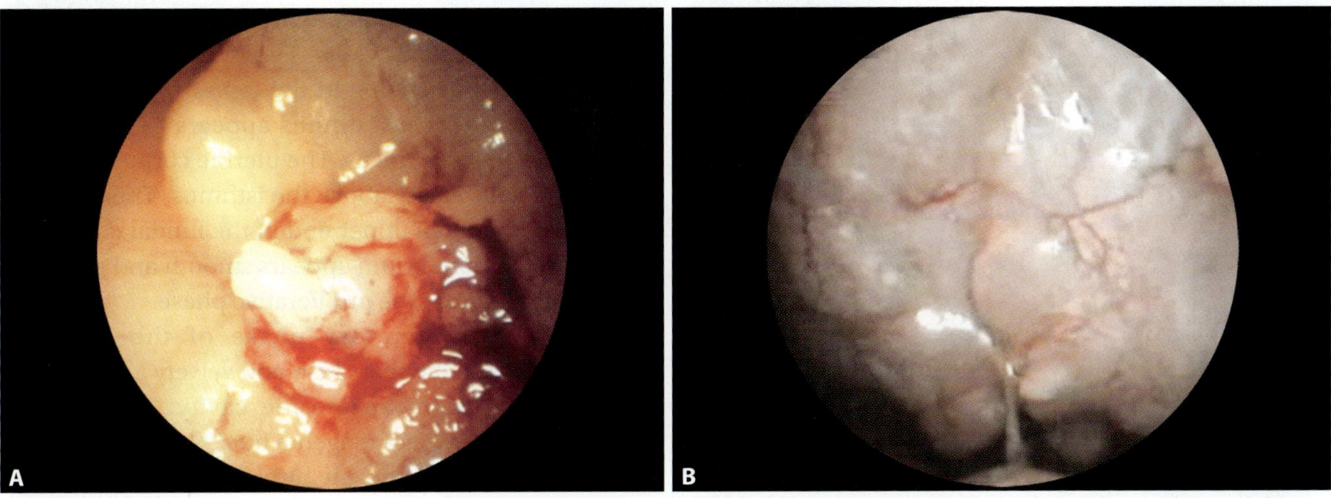

Figs. 44A and B: Endometrial cancer: (A) Necrotic haemorrhagic growth as observed on hysteroscopic examination; (B) Polypoidal growth showing abnormal proliferation of blood vessels. Biopsy revealed the diagnosis of malignancy.

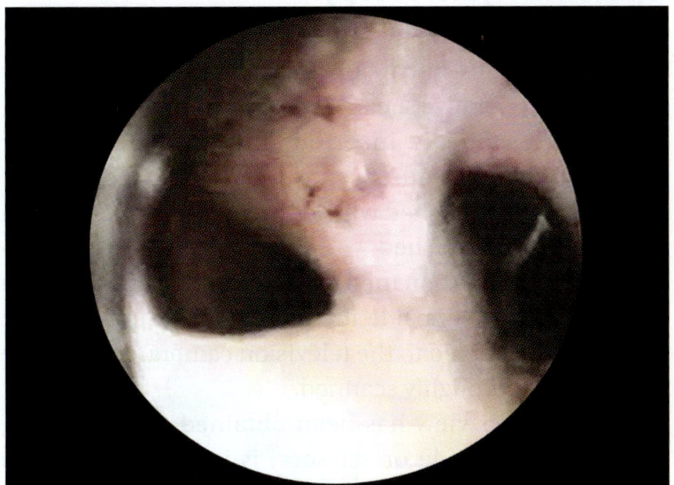

Fig. 45: Uterine septum as observed on hysteroscopic examination.

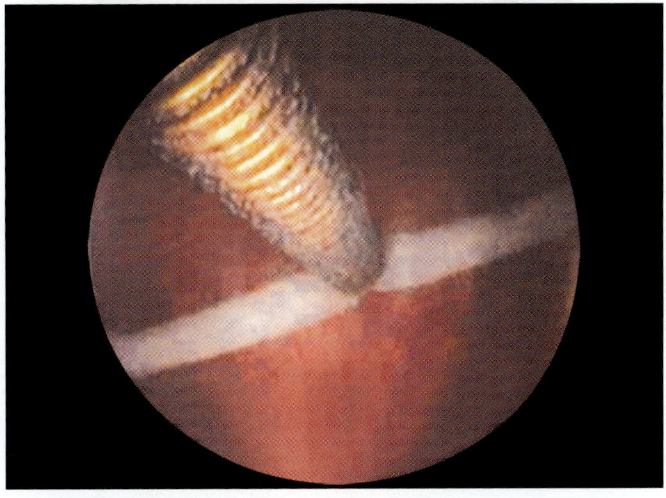

Fig. 46: Intrauterine contraceptive device in the endometrial cavity as observed on hysteroscopic examination.

cervical canal dilatation. The newer operative sheaths measure at least 8 mm in diameter and require cervical dilatation prior to insertion.

- Surgeon then selects a suitable telescope and checks its eyepiece for proper clarity. If required, the lens is cleansed with the help of a saline or water-soaked sponge.
- The light generator is switched on and the fibreoptic cable is attached to the telescope.
- The telescope is inserted into the diagnostic sheath.
- The selected distension medium is flushed through the sheath to expel any air.
- Before introducing the hysteroscope, the irrigation system is connected and the fluid is let in, so that it starts filling the tubing.
- The hysteroscope is engaged into the external cervical os, following which it is gently advanced inside the endocervical canal into the uterine cavity.
- As the hysteroscope engages into the external os, the flow of distension medium must be started.
- The hysteroscope is gently moved forward, keeping the endocervical canal at the 6 o'clock position eccentrically. This position is especially required to keep the telescope in the centre when a 30° telescope is used.

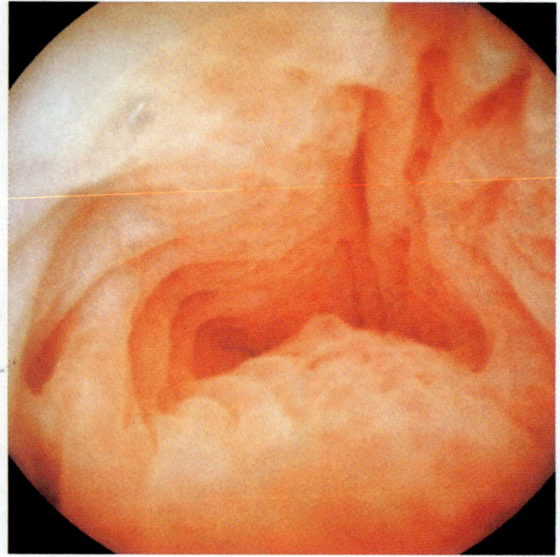

Fig. 47: Endocervical mucosa.

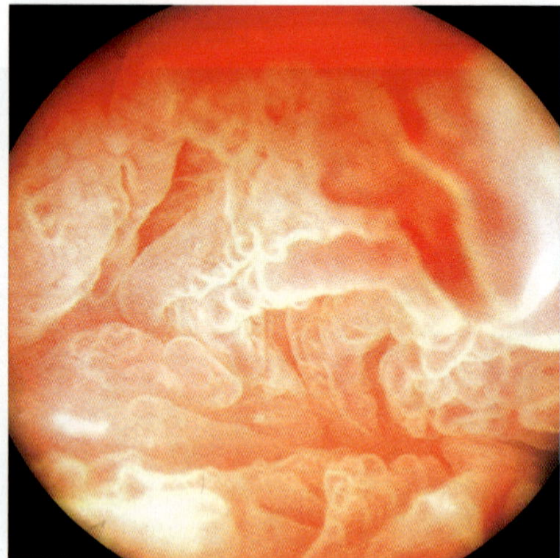

Fig. 48: Endocervical polyp.

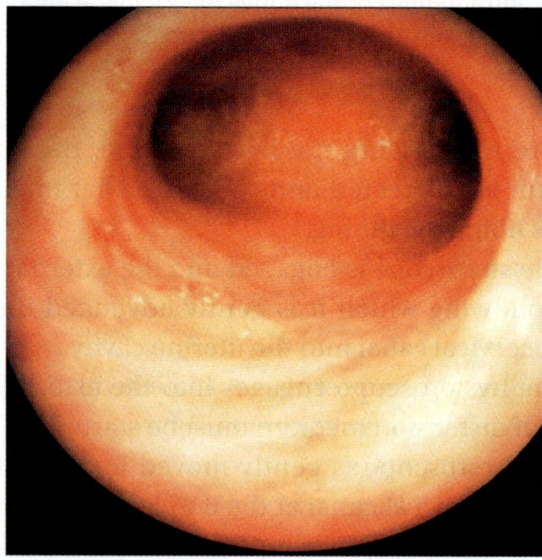

Fig. 49: Panoramic view of bilateral tubal ostia.

- The endocervical canal typically shows longitudinal folds, papillae and clefts. The internal os appears as a narrow constriction at the top of the endocervical canal. The uterine isthmus appears as a cylindrical extension above the os. The uterine corpus appears as a capacious cavity above the isthmus. The tubal ostia are visible at the upper end of the fundal cornua. The uterine endometrium appears smooth and pink-white in colour during the proliferative phase.
- During the secretory phase of the cycle, the endometrium appears lush and velvety and protrudes irregularly into the uterine cavity. The secretory endometrium has a magenta hue.
- There should be no air bubbles when using liquid distension media; air bubbles can be sucked out using VersaPoint™.

Operative Hysteroscopy

The steps of operative hysteroscopy are as follows:

- The cervix must be carefully dilated with a Hegar's dilator until the operative sheath negotiates through the cervix.
- The telescope is inserted into the operative or resectoscope sheath.
- The sheath is flushed with a distending medium, and a light cable is attached.
- With the distension medium flowing, the hysteroscope can be inserted inside the uterine cavity under direct vision or coupled to the television camera. The uterine cavity is thoroughly scanned.
- After a clear view has been obtained, the operating device (electrode or scissors) is inserted inside the uterine cavity and slowly advanced in order to make contact with the endometrium.
- In some cases, it may be advantageous to perform a laparoscopy simultaneously (e.g. lysis of uterine adhesions, excision of large submucous myomas and cutting of uterine septa). Digital cameras and recorders can be employed to record the surgery.

POSTOPERATIVE CARE

Following the procedure, especially operative hysteroscopy, the patient must be observed for at least 6–12 hours for the signs of any potential complications. The presence of bowel injury could be associated with signs and symptoms such as worsening of postoperative pain, fever, nausea and abdominal distension. On the other hand, signs such as diminished urinary output, fever

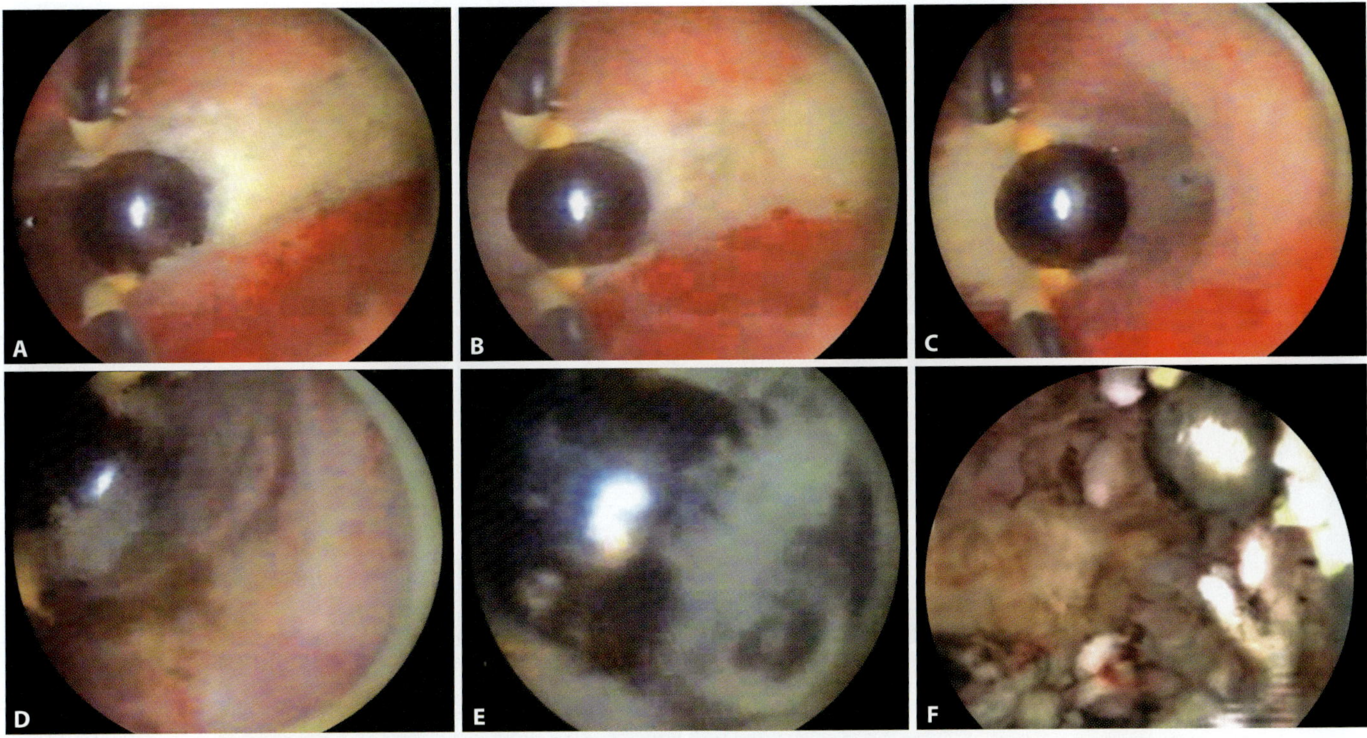

Figs. 50A to F: Roller ball ablation of endometrium: (A and B) Roller ball ablation of the fundal region; (C) Roller ball ablation of the cornual region; (D and E) Progression of the ablation process; (F) Process of ablation is complete.

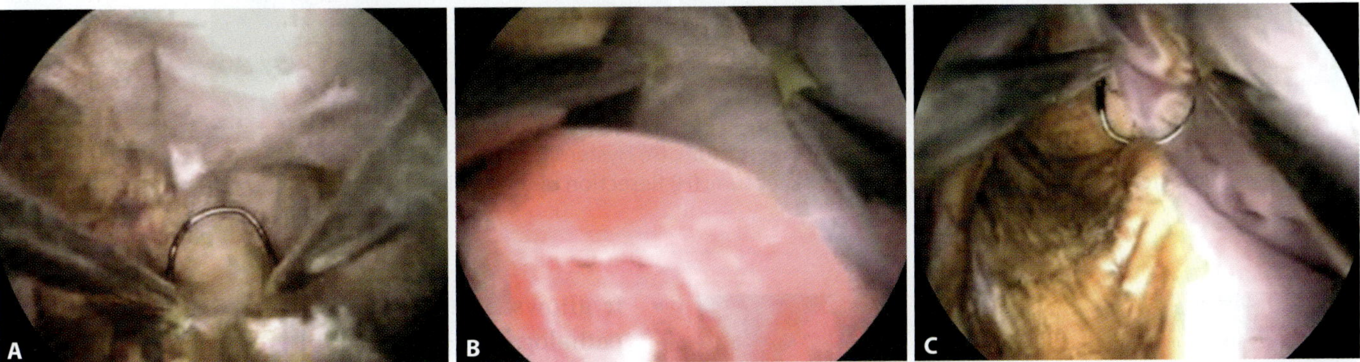

Figs. 51A to C: Transcervical resection of endometrium: (A) Beginning of resection; (B) Process of resection in progress; (C) Resection is complete.

and abdominal distension could be suggestive of bladder or urethral trauma and/or injection. Tachycardia and/or hypotension could be suggestive of continuing third-space haemorrhage.

ADVANTAGES

Hysteroscopy is associated with the following advantages:

- *Minimally invasive procedure:* Hysteroscopy is the least invasive form of surgery, which uses the endocervical canal to gain entry into the uterine cavity.
- It is associated with shortened hospital stay and reduced recovery time.
- No scar tissue remains on the abdominal or uterine walls.
- Hysteroscopic surgery is associated with a lower rate of intra- and postoperative morbidity in comparison with traditional surgery.
- Allows ablation or endometrial resection, which has become an acceptable alternative to hysterectomy for the management of AUB.

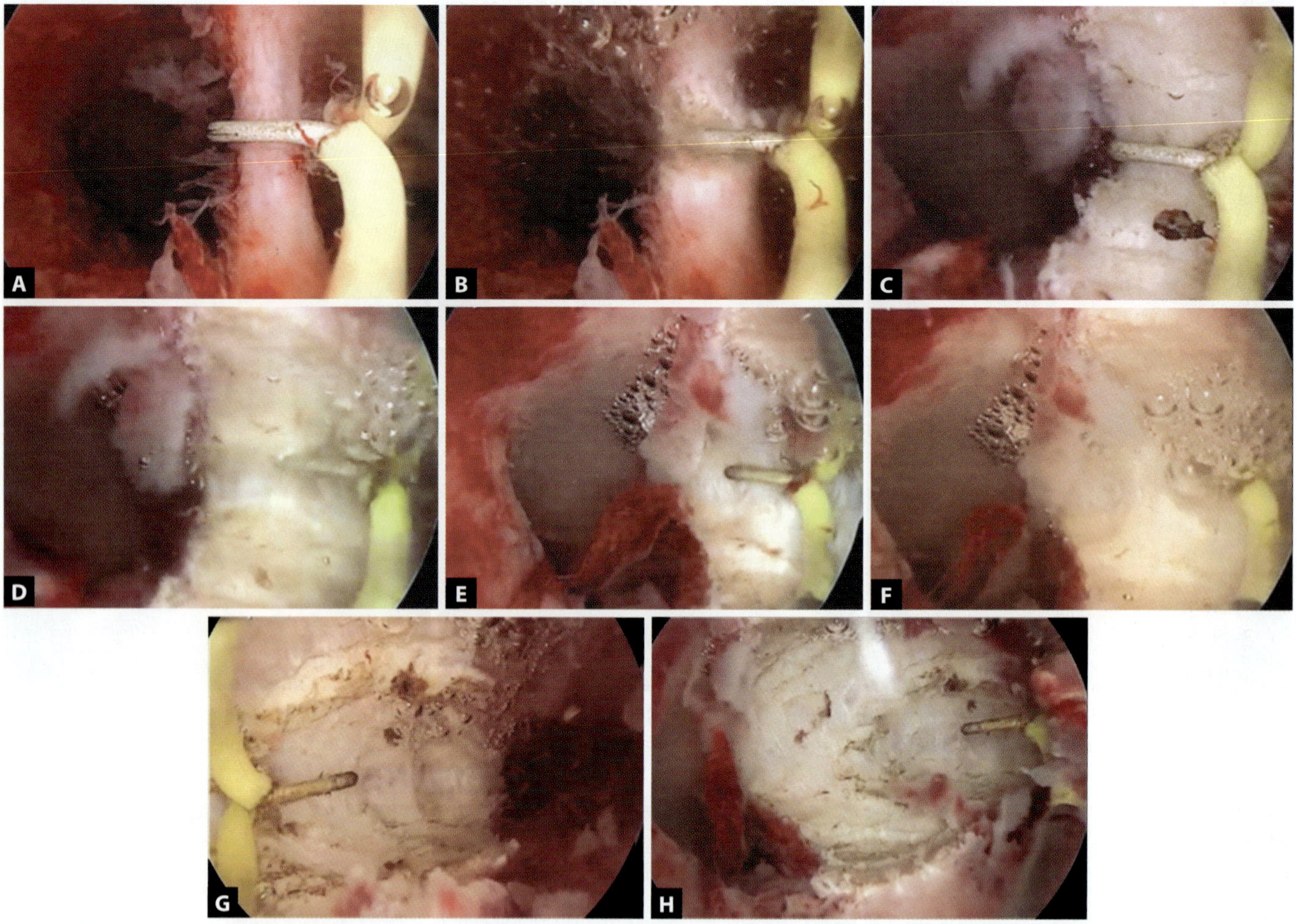

Figs. 52A to H: Hysteroscopic resection of the uterine septum: (A) Hysteroscopic appearance of the uterine septum; (B to G) Resectoscope loop transecting the uterine septum; (H) Resection of the uterine septum is almost complete.

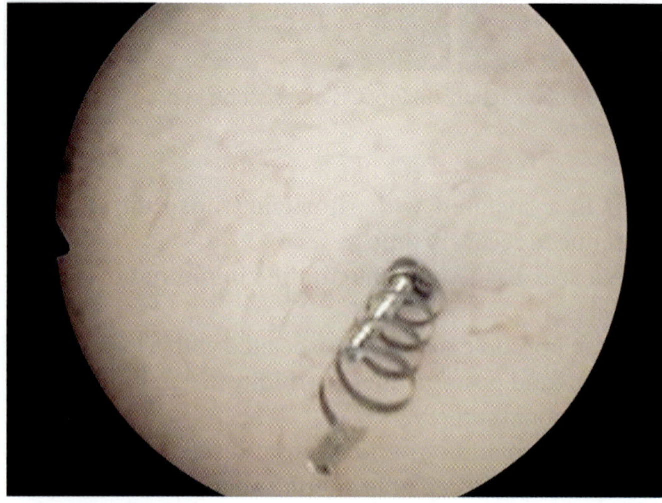

Fig. 53: Hysteroscopic sterilisation using Essure™.

- It allows direct visualisation of any intrauterine pathology.
- A biopsy can be taken under direct vision.

DISADVANTAGES

Some contraindications related to hysteroscopy are listed in **Box 2.**

COMPLICATIONS

The overall complication rate for diagnostic and operative hysteroscopy is 2%, with serious complications occurring in <1% of cases. Operator's experience and exclusion of any contraindication for hysteroscopy before performance of the procedure are two important prerequisites for preventing the occurrence of complications. Various

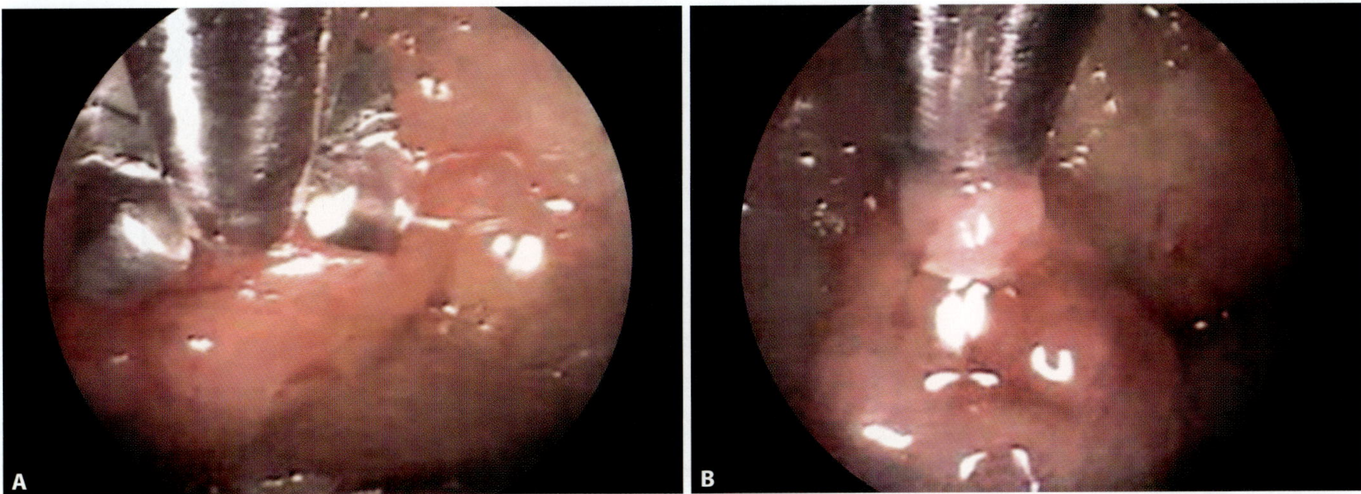

Figs. 54A and B: Targeted endometrial biopsy: (A) Biopsy forceps with its jaws opened approaching the area of suspected malignancy; (B) A small bit of tissue gripped by the forceps to be sent for biopsy.

complications related to hysteroscopy are summarised in **Box 3**. Previously, there had been concerns that hysteroscopy performed as a routine office procedure in cases of AUB might cause undiagnosed endometrial cancer to spread transtubally. However, there is absence of any strong evidence to prove this point. Now, hysteroscopy has nearly replaced blind dilation and curettage as the procedure of choice for the diagnosis of intrauterine pathology.

Intraoperative Complications

Traumatic Injury

Intraoperative complications, which can occur during the procedure, include traumatic injury to the cervix and, rarely uterus as well. At times, injury to the bowel and bladder can also occur.

Perforation

A possible problem associated with the procedure is uterine perforation, which commonly occurs when either the hysteroscope itself or one of its operative instruments breaches the uterine wall. A small perforation may be symptomless and heal on its own. A large perforation, however, can cause considerable bleeding and damage to other organs. Damage to organs such as the bladder or bowel can result in spilling of the intestinal contents inside the peritoneal cavity, producing peritonitis and sepsis, which may even prove to be fatal. The operative hysteroscopic procedures, such as resection of the uterine septum, myomectomy procedures, and adhesiolysis, are associated with a high risk of uterine perforation. The best way to prevent the occurrence of uterine perforations is simultaneous laparoscopy. Moreover, the hysteroscope must be inserted inside the cervix and uterine canal under direct vision.

Poor Visibility of the Operative Field

Inability to properly visualise the operative field may commonly be associated with deep insertion of a hysteroscope or over-dilatation of cervix. Over-dilatation of cervix may result in excessive leakage of the distending medium, thereby resulting in an inability to maintain distension within the uterine cavity. Moreover, the presence of blood and debris may cloud the operative field.

Intraoperative and Postoperative Bleeding

A common complication associated with the procedure is the occurrence of bleeding during and after the procedure. The bleeding occurring during the procedure can be controlled in the following ways:

- Aspiration of the blood
- Increasing the pressure of the distending medium so that it compresses the wall of the uterus, thereby stopping the bleeding.
- Electrocoagulation of a bleeding vessel with an electrode.
- Insertion of an intrauterine balloon inflated to about 5–10 mL. In case of continuous bleeding, uterine

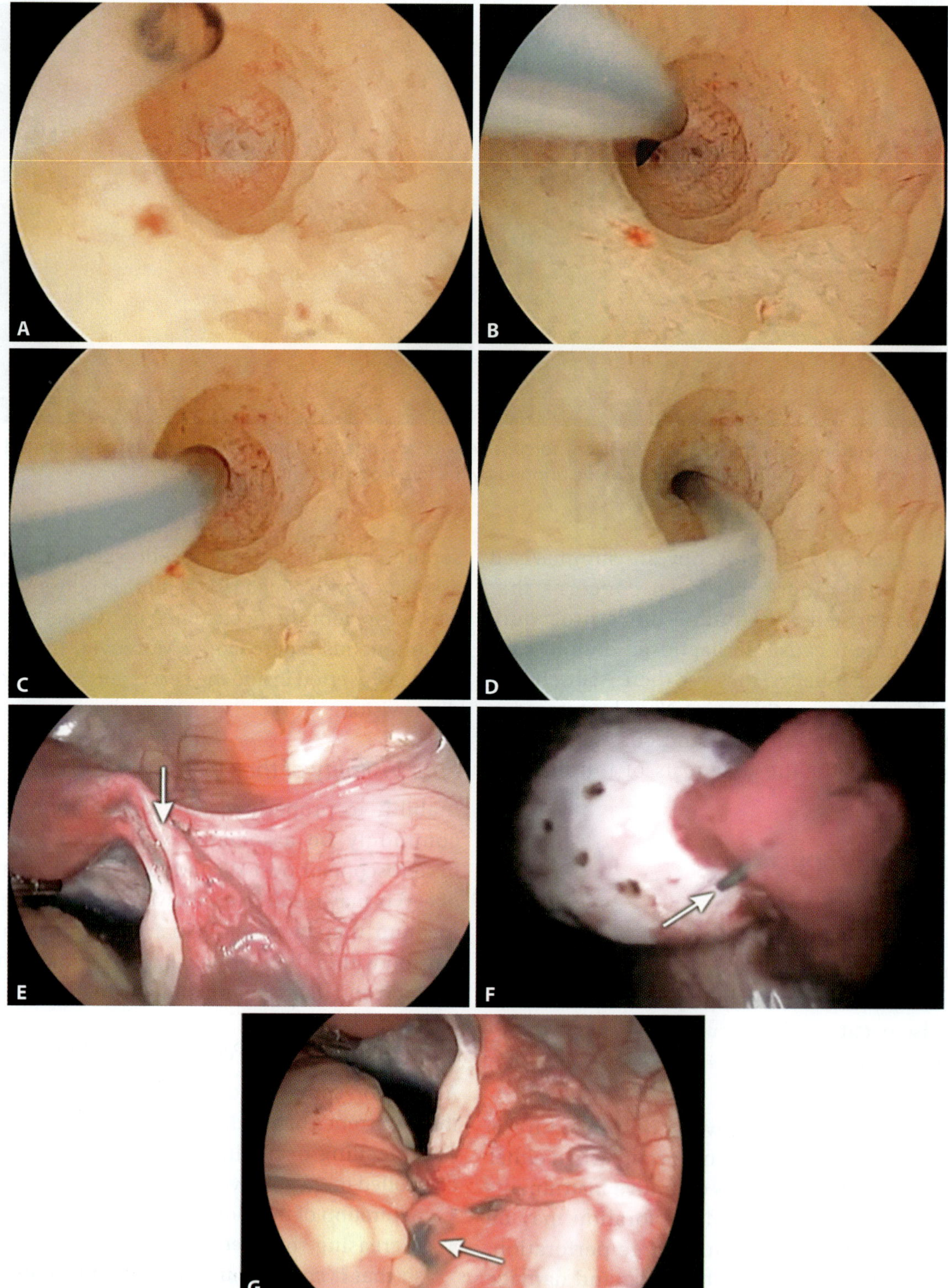

Figs. 55A to G: Hysteroscopic tubal cannulation: (A) Right-sided tubal ostium is identified with the help of hysteroscope; (B) A simple cannula with the guidewire inside is introduced through the operating channel; (C) The tip of the cannula is then advanced near the ostium under constant hysteroscopic visualisation; (D) Guidewire is advanced into the ostium to negotiate the intramural portion of the tube; (E and F) The appearance of the tube and adnexa under laparoscopic visualisation showing the advancement of hysteroscopically directed catheter via the fallopian tube out through the fimbrial end of the tube; (G) Dye seen ejecting out from the fimbrial end of the tube.

BOX 2: Contraindications for diagnostic hysteroscopy.

Absolute contraindications:
- Intrauterine pregnancy
- Known cervical or uterine infection (recent or active pelvic inflammatory disease, acute cervicovaginal infections, etc.)
- Cancer of cervix
- Profuse/active uterine bleeding (which might obscure the operative field)

Relative contraindications:
- Cervical stenosis
- Endometrial cancer

BOX 3: Complications of hysteroscopy.

Instrument-related complications:
- Cervical trauma
- Uterine perforation
- Bleeding
- Infection

Complications related to the use of distension media:
- *CO_2:* Hypercarbia resulting in arrhythmias and shoulder pain
- *Glycine (1.5%):* Dilutional hyponatraemia and pulmonary oedema
- *Dextran:* Anaphylactic shock, ascites
- *Dextrose (5%):* Dilutional hyponatraemia and pulmonary oedema
- *Sorbitol:* Cerebral oedema

tamponade can be performed by inserting a Foley's catheter inside the uterine cavity and inflating its bulb. The catheter can be removed after 4–5 hours, once the bleeding has ceased to occur.

- Injection of a vasoconstrictor drug, such as vasopressin, can also help to control bleeding.

Infection

Infection rarely occurs if the procedure is performed using strict aseptic precautions. Moreover, the uterine endometrium is usually resistant to various micro-organisms; therefore, infection is an unlikely complication. Nevertheless, hysteroscopy must be avoided in the presence of gross cervical infections, sexually transmitted diseases, uterine infection or salpingitis. Prophylactic antibiotics need to be administered only in high-risk cases such as patient with the history of rheumatic carditis, congenital heart disease, prolapsed mitral valves, etc.

Gas Embolism

Gas embolism is a rare but devastating complication of hysteroscopy. It can result in clinical signs and symptoms such as reduction in end-tidal CO_2, hypoxia, tachycardia, hypotension, followed by bradycardia and cardiovascular collapse.

Electrical and Laser Injuries

Uterine perforation caused by either laser fibre or electrode is likely to be more serious than the injury caused by mechanical devices, such as scissors, because thermal injury is likely to inflict greater damage to the surrounding tissues. Moreover, the injury due to thermal damage may not manifest itself until 2–3 days after surgery. Therefore, in these cases, laparoscopy or laparotomy must be done to determine the exact extent of injury.

Complications Caused by the Distension Media

The use of insufflation media can result in serious and even fatal complications due to embolism or fluid overload with electrolyte imbalances. Furthermore, the use of CO_2 as a distension medium can result in the formation of gas emboli.

Fluid absorption: Fluid overload can occur with the use of distension media such as normal saline.

This can be corrected by the use of diuretics, oxygen and central venous pressure monitoring. An important precaution which helps in preventing fluid overload is to restrict intrauterine pressure from increasing above 100 mm Hg at the time of procedure. Fluid overload with media, such as glycine, can present with symptoms such as nausea, vertigo, hyponatraemia, confusion and disorientation. With excessive fluid overload, sometimes the blood ammonium levels may rise, resulting in encephalopathy. As previously mentioned, fluid overload with sorbitol can result in development of cerebral oedema.

Endometrial Cancer

Since clusters of viable endometrial tissues can persist in women who have undergone TCRE; it has been hypothesised that there is a risk of development of endometrial cancer from the remnant tissues in future. Such patients must be followed-up with transvaginal sonography (TVS) to detect abnormal changes in the residual endometrium. Abnormal bleeding in these patients must be duly investigated to rule out the risk of endometrial cancer.

Haematometra

Haematometra may occur due to the development of intrauterine adhesions in the area of active endometrium, which continues to undergo active cyclical bleeding. Patients may present with cyclical pain, and the condition may be diagnosed on TVS. Drainage may be performed by a repeat hysteroscopy.

Uterine Rupture

Uterine rupture during pregnancy has been reported in cases where women have become pregnant following endoscopic procedures such as myoma or septum resection.

Operator Inexperience

The most likely complications with hysteroscopy commonly occur in the presence of the operator's inexperience. If the surgeon is properly acquainted with hysteroscopic techniques, the rate of complications would be much less.

CONCLUSION

Hysteroscopic-guided surgery has now become an important tool for the gynaecological surgeon. Hysteroscope can be used both for diagnostic and therapeutic purposes. It is a form of minimally invasive surgery which helps in avoiding giving a scar on the patient's abdomen and sometimes also helps in preventing the removal of the uterus. With the help of a hysteroscope, the surgeon gains entry into the endometrial cavity via the cervix. Since the procedure does not require opening up the patient's abdomen or peritoneal cavity, it is associated with minimal postoperative morbidity and mortality in comparison to that associated with laparotomy. During the past two decades, due to major advances in the field of science and technology, hysteroscopic myomectomy has acquired great importance amongst the various gynaecologic surgical techniques.

HYSTEROSCOPIC RESECTOSCOPE

The gynaecological resectoscope, born from its urological equivalent, is commonly used in gynaecological practice to resect or remove intracavitary pathology and also to perform endometrial ablation. The resectoscope consists of a telescope (2.9 and 4 mm, preferably with a 12° angle of view to always keep the loop within the viewing field), an electrical loop to perform passive cuts and two sheaths for continuous flow suction and irrigation of liquid distension medium. Besides the cutting loop, other instruments such as microknives or series of coagulation or vaporisation electrodes of various shapes can be connected to the resectoscope. Both monopolar and bipolar sources can be used. There are essentially two types of resectoscopes, which differ in outer diameter: 7.5 and 9.2 mm. The 7.5 mm resectoscope should be used in case of narrow cervical canal or difficult dilatation; the 9.2 mm resectoscope allows to perform major surgery.

SLIM RESECTOSCOPE

The extremely thin Princess resectoscope (7 mm) from Richard Wolf ensures a low resistance to insertion and minimal dilation effort, and also considerably reduces trauma to the cervical channel. It is therefore especially suitable for a stenotic cervical canal, and in addition works well for patients undergoing fertility and sterility treatment. One of the main advantages of the Princess resectoscope is that it can be used for both monopolar and bipolar resection, depending on the user's requirement **(Fig. 56)**.

HYSTEROSCOPIC MORCELLATOR

Although hysteroscopic loop electrode resectoscopy provided a reliable method for removing intrauterine pathology for many years, the distension media issues, and the risk of perforation, and visual field limitation created by resected chips all combine to encourage the development of alternate treatment methods. US FDA

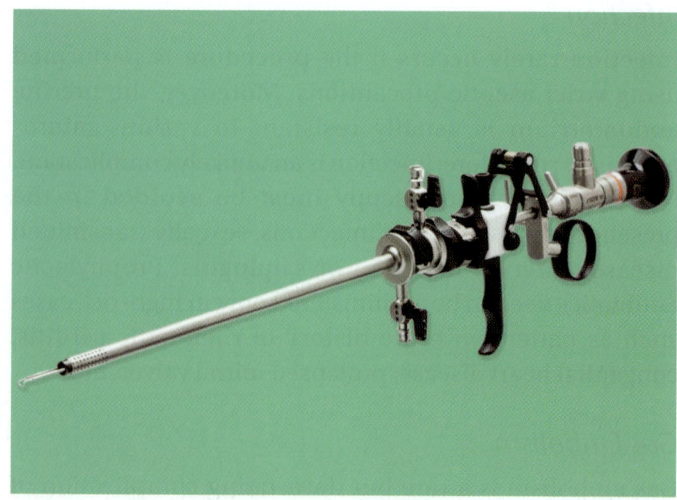

Fig. 56: Slim resectoscope.

(United States Food and Drug Administration) approved the first generation Truclear hysteroscopic morcellator as the first mechanical morcellator for intrauterine pathology. Later second generation Myosure system was developed. In patients with polyps and type 1 submucosal myomas, hysteroscopic morcellation allows for the use of smaller diameter hysteroscopes that require less cervical dilatation and less anaesthesia.

LAPAROENDOSCOPIC SINGLE-SITE SURGERY

INTRODUCTION

Operative laparoscopy was introduced in the field of gynaecology nearly five decades back. By the early 1980s, the laser and electric energy technology had been incorporated into laparoscopic surgery. As a result, operative laparoscopy extended to include complicated gynaecologic procedures such as hysterectomy, adnexal surgery and uterine myomectomy. Presently, laparoscopic surgery has become an integral part of surgical treatment for various gynaecologic diseases. Since the introduction of laparoscopic surgery in the 1970s, there have been several innovations in this field, especially robotic surgery, laparoendoscopic single-site surgery (LESS), natural orifice transluminal endoscopic surgery (NOTES), hand-assisted laparoscopic surgery, etc.

Laparoendoscopic single-site surgery can be considered the most recent innovation in minimally invasive laparoscopic surgery. The single-port laparoscopic approach had already been widely applied in gynaecology. The principal idea of LESS involves placing all the laparoscopic working ports through the same incision. The first single-incision tubal ligation in 1969 was performed by Wheeless. Soon thereafter, total hysterectomy with bilateral salpingo-oophorectomy using the single puncture technique was performed by Pelosi in 1991. However, hysterectomy using LESS did not gain extensive usage due to many technical difficulties. Nevertheless, nowadays this technique is been widely employed for hysterectomy and various adnexal surgeries.

SURGICAL EQUIPMENT

As previously described, LESS involves placing all the laparoscopic working ports through the same incision. However, this may result in the collision of hands outside the abdomen and the clashing of instruments within the abdomen. Nowadays, various devices have been introduced to overcome these technical challenges. These devices include laparoscopic ports designed in such a way that multiple instruments can be introduced through a single incision. Moreover, flexible/long endoscopes and articulating instruments of variable lengths have also been introduced. Additionally, the da Vinci® robotic platforms with articulating instruments can also be integrated into single-port laparoscopic surgery (SPLS) for performing surgeries such as hysterectomy or salpingo-oophorectomy.

Port Devices

The various port devices which can be employed for LESS are as follows **(Figs. 57A to J)**:

- *Conventional laparoscopic ports:* The technique was first developed by Paul Curcillo, Jeffrey Caddedu
- *R-Port™:* Tri Port **(Fig. 57G)** and Quad Port **(Fig. 57I)**
- Uni-X (P-Navel)
- SILS™ Port, Covidien **(Fig. 57J)**
- SITRACC®, single trocar access platform, Edlo **(Fig. 57D)**
- Gel Point® and Gel Port®, Applied medical **(Fig. 57E)**
- SSLAS, Ethicon
- X-CONE® **(Figs. 57A and B)** and ENDOCONE® **(Fig. 57C)**, Karl Storz
- AirSeal®, SurgiQuest **(Fig. 57H)**
- Alexis wound retractor **(Fig. 57F)**

Instruments

The various instruments which could be inserted through these access devices include articulating instruments **(Figs. 58A to C)**, prebent instruments **(Fig. 59)**, operative laparoscope **(Fig. 60A)** and laparocator for laparoscopic tubal ligation with Falope rings **(Figs. 60B and C)**. Straight instruments have a significant role to play in LESS. Articulating/bent instruments should be available in case of need in specific situations.

Familiarity with articulating instruments during standard laparoscopy increases its usefulness during the LESS procedure.

Prebent Instruments

The prebent instruments offer the following advantages:

- Provides internal triangulation and external separation
- Has rigidity similar to straight instruments
- Lower cost (reusable)

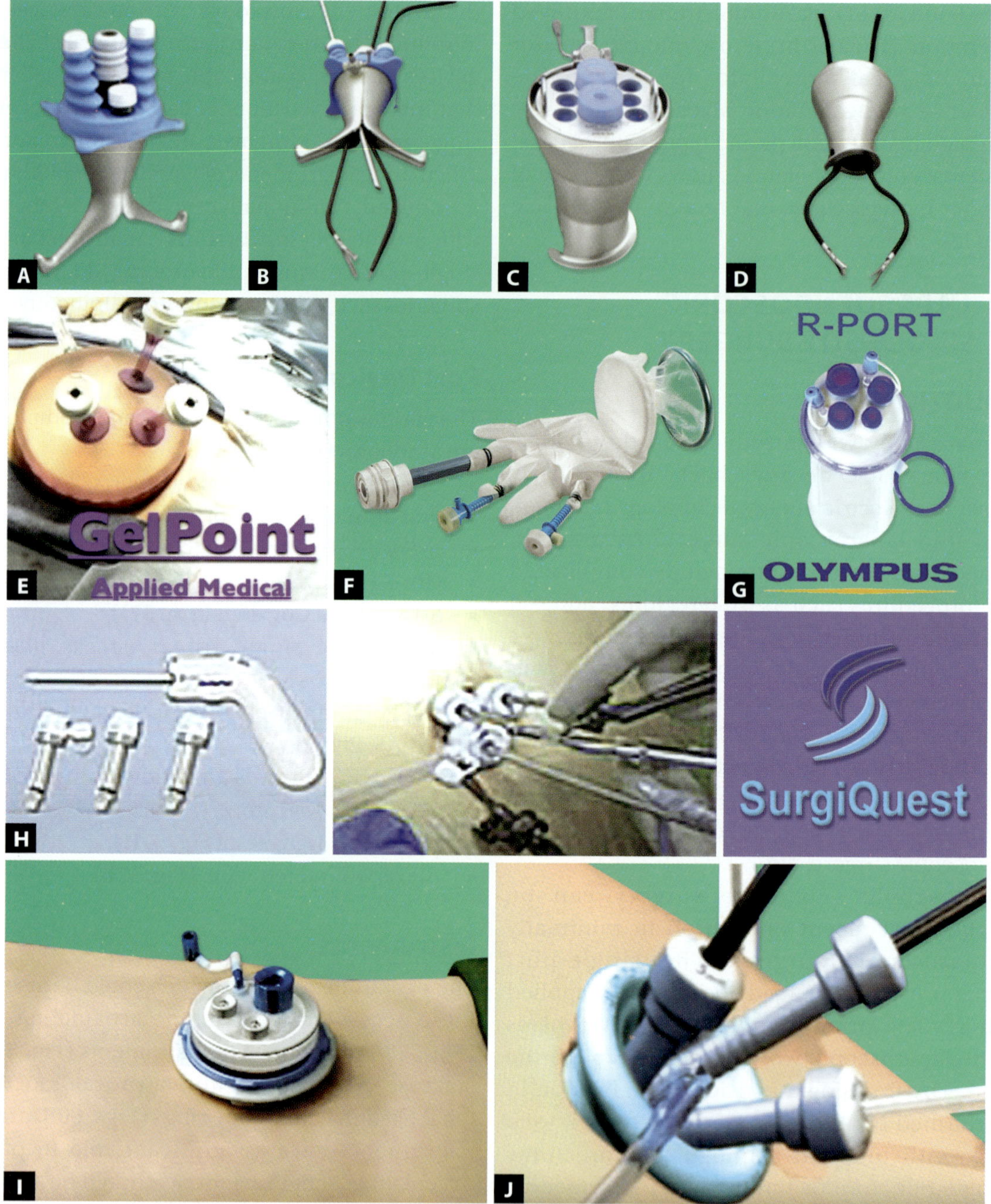

Figs. 57A to J: Various port devices for single incision laparoscopic surgery. (A and B) X-CONE® of Karl Storz; (C) ENDOCONE® of Karl Storz; (D) SITRACC®, single trocar access platform; Edlo; (E) GelPoint®, Applied Medical; (F) Alexis wound retractor with the globe inserted into the rim of the retractor. Fingers of the glove function as multiple channels for instruments; (G) R-Port Olympus®; (H) AirSeal®, SurgiQuest; (I) OctoPort; (J) SILSTM Port, Covidien.

The prebent instruments are associated with the following limitations:

- Long learning curve
- Requirement of a specialised access trocar for insertion.

Articulating Instruments

These instruments are associated with the following advantages:

- Increased freedom of movement
- Better triangulation

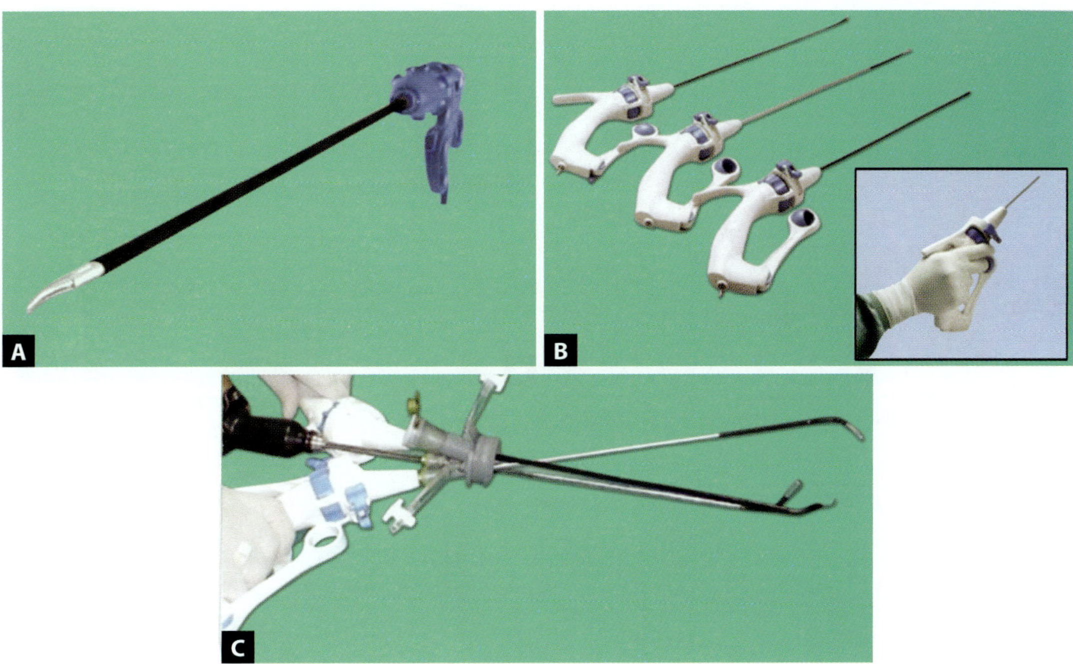

Figs. 58A to C: Articulating instruments: (A) Real Hand™, Novare®; (B) Cambridge Endo®; (C) Passing the articulating instruments through the port.

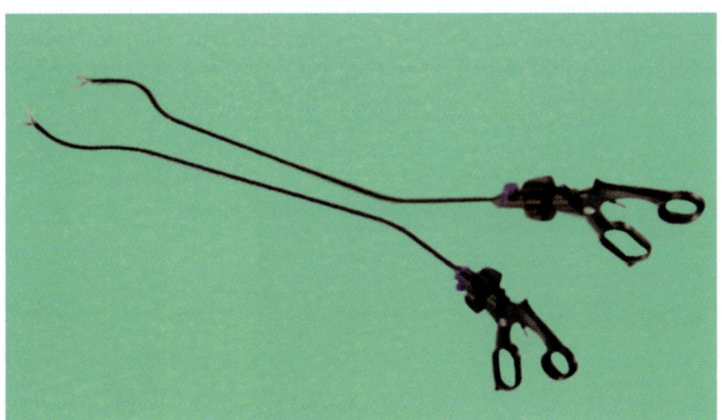

Fig. 59: Prebent instrument.

These instruments have following limitations:
- Longer learning curve
- Low strength for retraction
- External ergonomics
- High-cost factor

Various technical nuances associated with actively articulating instruments:
- If both the instruments are straight, there is a need to cross the instrument.
- If the right instrument is straight and left is articulating, dissection is easier with right, whereas the retraction is less robust on the left side.
- If the right instrument is articulating and left is straight, retraction is more robust on the right side, whereas the dissection is difficult.

INDICATIONS

Some of the indications for SPLS are explained in **Box 4**.

LAPAROENDOSCOPIC SINGLE-SITE SURGICAL TECHNIQUES

The access though a single incision defines LESS surgery. The site of access is the umbilicus, and the anatomical configuration of the umbilicus should be maintained during incision and closure. The type of incision depends on shape and size of umbilicus and surgeon's preference. Local infiltration of anaesthetics preoperatively provides enhanced postoperative pain relief. The preoperative and postoperative steps are similar to that in laparoscopic surgery described previously in the text. The various techniques of LESS are described here.

Single-incision But Multi-port Technique

This technique is also termed as single incision, multiple ports laparoendoscopic surgery (SIMPLE) by some authors. In their technique, a single skin incision is given at the umbilicus. Once a flap of the umbilicus is raised,

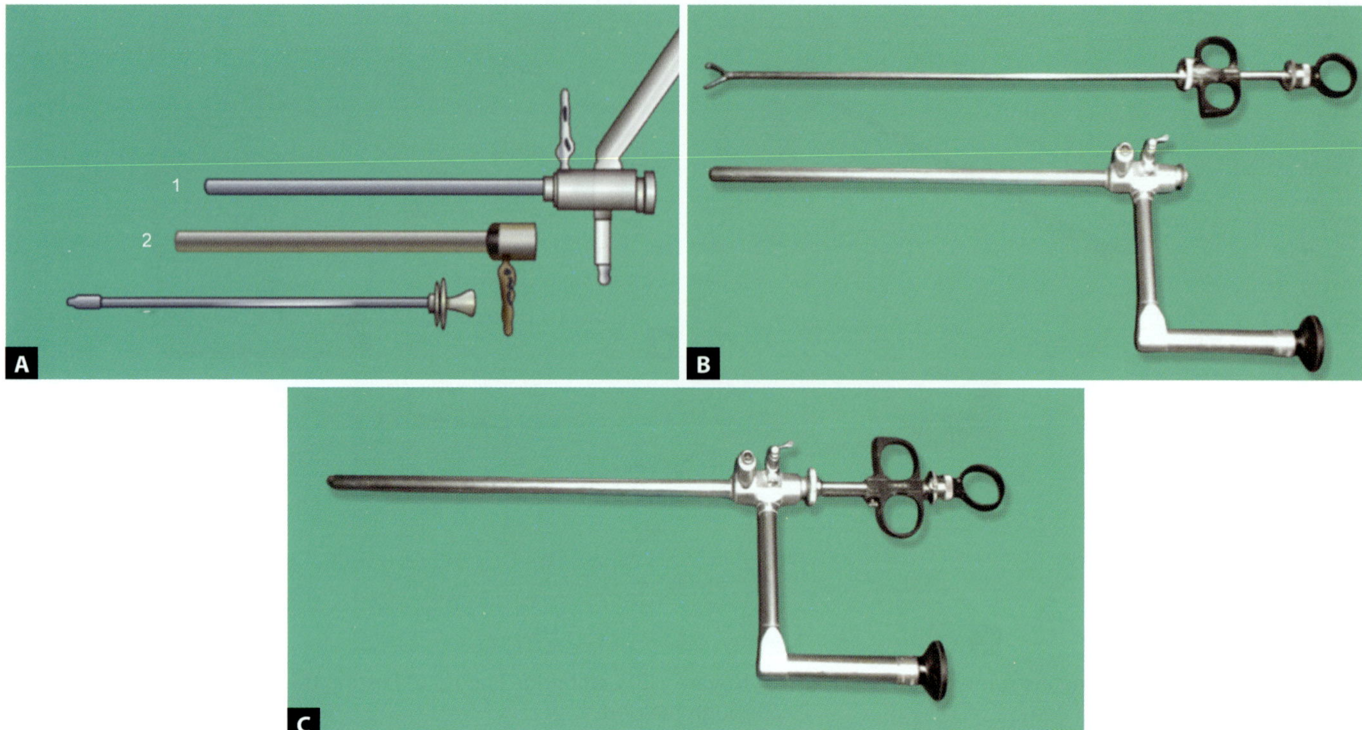

Figs. 60A to C: Operative laparoscope: (A) The Frazee operative laparoscope (Karl Storz, Tuttlingen, Germany) is an 8-mm straight viewing Hopkins laparoscope, 30-cm length, with a 5-mm working channel; (B) Laparocator channel (Operative laparoscope) with offset eyepiece and operating channel. The ring applicator for application of Falope channel rings is seen with prongs at the distal end (top); (C) The ring applicator has been inserted through the operating channel.

BOX 4: Indications of laparoendoscopic single-site surgery in gynaecology.

- Hysterectomy—total laparoscopic hysterectomy/subtotal hysterectomy/laparoscopic-assisted vaginal hysterectomy
- Myomectomy
- Tubal ligation
- Surgery for ectopic pregnancy—salpingectomy/salpingostomy
- Benign adnexal disease—salpingo-oophorectomy/oophorectomy/ovarian cystectomy
- Adnexal tumours
- Adhesiolysis
- Early endometrial cancer
- Pelvic and/or para-aortic lymph node sampling or lymphadenectomy (early-stage gynaecologic malignancies)
- Abdominal sacral colpopexy
- Endometriosis
- Concomitant gynaecologic and surgical procedures: Appendectomy/cholecystectomy with hysterectomy/adnexal procedures

three to four separate incisions are made in the sheath at a distance of 2–3 cm from each other in the *Mickey Mouse* configuration **(Fig. 61)**. This makes it possible

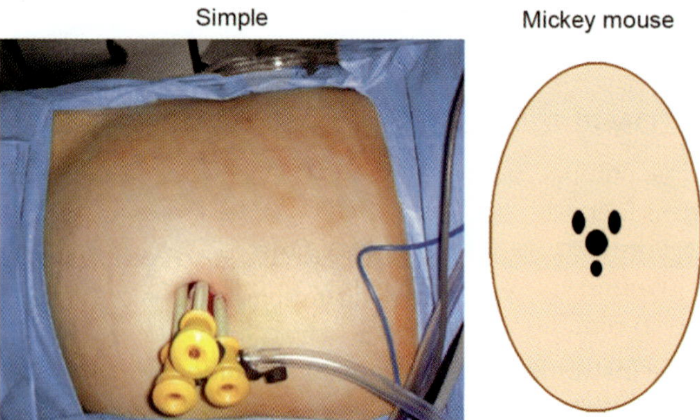

Fig. 61: Single incision technique having *Mickey mouse* configuration.

for the surgeon to insert three or even four low profile trocars. Through these trocars, one optic and two working instruments can be inserted.

Use of a Singular Access Device

This second technique involves the use of a singular access device, which allows the insertion of three or four instruments through a single opening in the umbilicus into which the device is first inserted. The first of these devices to be available was the R-Port™ (Advanced Surgical Concepts, Wicklow, United Kingdom). Presently, many such devices are available [SILS™ port by Covidien, SSLAS by Ethicon, AirSeal® by SurgiQuest, OctoPort™ by Daikin Surgical, Korea, X-CONE® by Karl Storz and Alexis wound retractor **(Figs. 57A to J)**]. These ports were inserted through an incision measuring anywhere between 17 and 50 mm, depending on the port and the organ to be accessed or removed.

ADVANTAGES

Laparoendoscopic single-site surgery provides the following advantages:

- Improved cosmesis
- Ease of tissue retrieval due to a large umbilical incision
- Improved patient acceptance
- Overall improved quality of life
- *Reduced postoperative complications associated with trocar insertion:* Complications such as epigastric vessel injury, visceral organ herniation, wound infection, and damage to the visceral organs are likely to be reduced in cases of single-port laparoscopic surger (SPLS) due to no requirement for insertion of ancillary ports.
- *Reduced postoperative pain:* This is probably related to a single skin incision resulting in reduced penetration of skin, muscle and fascia.

COMPLICATIONS

Some complications which can occur as a result of LESS are as follows:

- Formation of incisional hernias
- Wound complications
- No reduction in postoperative pain in comparison to the conventional laparoscopic methods
- *Technical problems:* Despite the availability of novel devices for LESS, clashing of laparoscopic instruments and limited vision of in-line view are still present as potential disadvantages of LESS. This may be associated with longer operative times, longer learning curves and difficulty in training the new surgeons.

CONCLUSION

Presently, there is minimal or no literature available examining the potential benefits of LESS in gynaecology in comparison to the conventional laparoscopic approach. Therefore, there is a requirement of multicentric randomised controlled trials in future for the evaluation of the advantages of a single-port approach in comparison to the conventional laparoscopy. Presently, all the available ports for LESS are associated with their own pros and cons. The surgeon must aim to have familiarity with more than one system and develop expertise with at least one. Some ports are better suited for certain indications than others.

Laparoendoscopic single-site surgery currently has a long way to go. In the armamentarium of minimal access surgery, at the present time, LESS stands between standard laparoscopy and NOTES. With more good quality evidence being available in future regarding the success and effectiveness of LESS, this surgery may occupy an important place in gynaecological surgery. Furthermore, the indications of single-port surgeries in gynaecology are expanding, and the performance of complex procedures depends on the skill of the surgeon.

ROBOTIC SURGERY

The birth of robotic surgery took place when there is an increasing demand for greater surgical precision and safe operation in era where surgeons were increasingly adapting minimal invasive surgical (MIS) technologies to enhance their outcome **(Fig. 62)**.

Technical advantage for the surgeon:

- Better visualisation as there is higher magnification
- Elimination of hand tremor allowing greater precision
- Allows up to 7° of freedom
- Allows 360° of movement

Advantages over conventional laparoscopy:

- Complex pelvic and urological procedures where greater precision is needed robotic surgery has replaced laparoscopy.
- Robotic keyhole surgery compared with conventional keyhole surgery improves surgical performance without increasing operation time and minimises blood loss and intra/postoperative complications
- Instrument movement replicates movements of the surgeon's hand, which is in contrast to conventional laparoscopy where hand and instrument movements are counter intuitive.

Disadvantages:

- Increase in cost of surgery
- Long duration of surgery

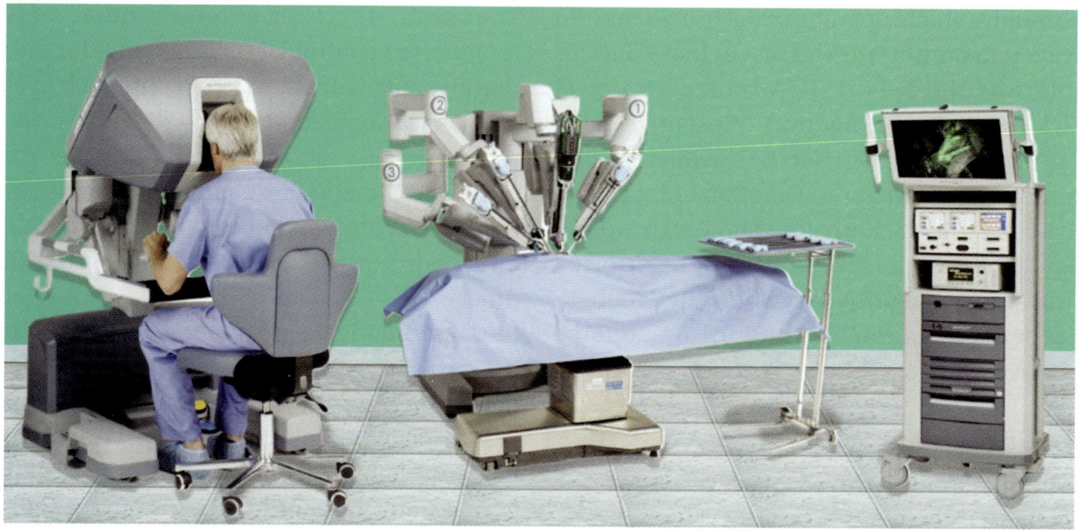

Fig. 62: Robotic-assisted laparoscopy.

Uses of robotic-assisted laparoscopy (RAL):

- RAL is well established in benign gynaecological surgeries, especially tubal reconstructive surgeries, myomectomies and hysterectomy.
- It helps the surgeon to perform excision earlier and more safely in endometriosis, especially as nerve-sparing surgery, as there is better improvement with 3D (three-dimensional) vision
- RAL sacrocolpopexy compared with laparoscopy is associated with improved voiding symptoms and sexual function
- RAL decreases the number of open surgeries in women with endometrial cancer.

SUGGESTED READING

1. Agostini A, Cravello L, Bretelle F, Shojai R, Roger V, Blanc B. Risk of uterine perforation during hysteroscopic surgery. J Am Assoc Gynecol Laparosc. 2002;9(3):264-7.
2. Aydeniz B, Gruber IV, Schauf B, Kurek R, Meyer A, Wallwiener D. A multi-centre survey of complications associated with 21,676 operative hysteroscopies. Eur J Obstet Gynecol Reprod Biol. 2002;104(2):160-4.
3. Baggish MS, Brill AI, Rosenweig B, Barbot JE, Indman PD. Fatal acute glycine and sorbitol toxicity during operative hysteroscopy. J Gynecol Surg. 1993;9:137-43.
4. Baggish MS. Contact hysteroscopy: a new technique to explore the uterine cavity. Obstet Gynecol. 1979;54(3):350-4.
5. Baggish MS. Hysteroscopic media: a two-edged sword. J Gynaecol Surg. Winter 1992;8(4):197.
6. Barakat EE, Bedaiwy MA, Zimberg S, Nutter B, Nosseir M, Falcone T. Robotic-assisted, laparoscopic, and abdominal myomectomy: a comparison of surgical outcomes. Obstet Gynecol. 2011;117(2 Pt 1):256-65.
7. Barnett JC, Hurd WW, Rogers RM Jr, Williams NL, Shapiro SA. Laparoscopic positioning and nerve injuries. J Minim Invasive Gynecol. 2007;14(5):664-72.
8. Baumann R, Magos AL, Kay JD, Turnbull AC. Absorption of glycine irrigating solution during transcervical resection of endometrium. BMJ. 1990;300(6720):304-5.
9. Bell MC, Torgerson J, Seshadri-Kreaden U, Suttle AW, Hunt S. Comparison of outcomes and cost for endometrial cancer staging via traditional laparotomy, standard laparoscopy and robotic techniques. Gynecol Oncol. 2008;111(3):407-11.
10. Bettocchi S, Ceci O, Nappi L, Di Venere R, Masciopinto V, Pansini V, et al. Operative office hysteroscopy without anesthesia: analysis of 4863 cases performed with mechanical instruments. J Am Assoc Gynecol Laparosc. 2004;11(1):59-61.
11. Bettocchi S, Nappi L, Ceci O, Selvaggi L. What does 'diagnostic hysteroscopy' mean today? The role of the new techniques. Curr Opin Obstet Gynecol. 2003;15(4):303-8.
12. Bhattee GA, Rahman J, Rahman MS. Bowel injury in gynaecologic operations: analysis of 110 cases. Int Surg. 2006;91(6):336-40.
13. Boggess JF, Gehrig PA, Cantrell L, Shafer A, Ridgway M, Skinner EN, et al. A comparative study of 3 surgical methods for hysterectomy with staging for endometrial cancer: robotic assistance, laparoscopy, laparotomy. Am J Obstet Gynecol. 2008;199(4):360.e1-9.
14. Boggess JF. Robotic surgery in gynaecologic oncology: evolution of a new surgical paradigm. J Rob Surg. 2007;1(1):31-3.
15. Bosteels J, Van Herendael B, Weyers S, D'Hooghe T. The position of diagnostic laparoscopy in current fertility practice. Hum Reprod Update. 2007;13(5):477-85.
16. Böttger TC, Hermeneit S, Müller M, Terzic A, Rodehorst A, Elad L, et al. Modifiable surgical and anesthesiologic risk factors for the development of cardiac and pulmonary

complications after laparoscopic colorectal surgery. Surg Endosc. 2009;23(9):2016-25.
17. Bradley LD. Complications in hysteroscopy: prevention, treatment and legal risk. Curr Opin Obstet Gynecol. 2002;14(4):409-15.
18. Canes D, Desai MM, Aron M, Haber GP, Goel RK, Stein RJ, et al. Transumbilical single-port surgery: evolution and current status. Eur Urol. 2008;54:1020-9.
19. Cheong Y, Ledger WL. Hysteroscopy and hysteroscopic surgery. Obstet Gynecol Reprod Med. 2007;17(4):99-104.
20. Chung SM, Jung YW, Lee SH, et al. Cost-effectiveness analysis of hysterectomy via laparotomy, laparoscopy and robotic assisted laparoscopy. J Gynecol Oncol. 2009;20(Suppl 1):150S.
21. Clarke-Pearson DL. Prevention of venous thromboembolism in gynaecologic surgery patients. Curr Opin Obstet Gynecol. 1993;5(1):73-9.
22. Cohen S, Greenberg JA. Hysteroscopic morcellation for treating intrauterine pathology. Rev Obstet Gynecol. 2011;4(2):73-80.
23. Da Vinci Surgery. (2013). Da Vinci. Changing the Experience of Surgery. [online] Available from www.davinci surgery. [Accessed March 2018]
24. Di Spiezio Sardo A, Mazzon I, Bramante S, Bettocchi S, Bifulco G, Guida M, et al. Hysteroscopic myomectomy: a comprehensive review of surgical techniques. Hum Reprod Update. 2008;14(2):101-19.
25. Dulemba JF, Pelzel C, Hubert HB. Retrospective analysis of robot-assisted versus standard laparoscopy in the treatment of pelvic pain indicative of endometriosis. J Robot Surg. 2013;7(2):163-9.
26. Emanuel MH, Wamsteker K. Uterine leiomymas. In: Brosens I, Wamsteker K (Eds). Diagnostic Imaging and Endoscopy in Gynaecology. London: WB Saunders; 1997. pp. 185-98.
27. Estape R, Lambrou N, Diaz R, Estape E, Dunkin N, Rivera A. A case matched analysis of robotic radical hysterectomy with lymphadenectomy compared with laparoscopy and laparotomy. Gynecol Oncol. 2009;113(3):357-61.
28. Fanning J, Fenton B, Purohit M. Robotic radical hysterectomy. Am J Obstet Gynecol. 2008;198(6):649.e1-4.
29. Ghezzi F, Cromi A, Fasola M, Bolis P. One-trocar salpingectomy for the treatment of tubal pregnancy: a 'marionette-like' technique. BJOG. 2005;112(10):1417-9.
30. Ghezzi F, Cromi A, Uccella S, Siesto G, Zefiro F, Bolis P. Incorporating laparoscopy in the practice of a gynaecologic oncology service: actual impact beyond clinical trials data. Ann Surg Oncol. 2009;16(8):2305-14.
31. Gill IS, Advincula AP, Aron M, Caddedu J, Canes D, Curcillo PG II, et al. Consensus statement of the consortium for laparoendoscopic single-site surgery. Surg Endosc. 2009;24(12):762-8.
32. Godfrey C, Wahle GR, Schilder JM, Rothenberg JM, Hurd WW. Occult bladder injury during laparoscopy: report of two cases. J Laparoendosc Adv Surg Tech A. 1999;9(4):341-5.
33. Hirvonen EA, Nuutinen LS, Kauko M. Hemodynamic changes due to Trendelenburg positioning and pneumoperitoneum during laparoscopic hysterectomy. Acta Anaesthesiol Scand. 1995;39(7):949-55.
34. Hirvonen EA, Poikolainen EO, Pääkkönen ME, Nuutinen LS. The adverse hemodynamic effects of anesthesia, head-up tilt, and carbon dioxide pneumoperitoneum during laparoscopic cholecystectomy. Surg Endosc. 2000;14(3):272-7.
35. Hoyte L, Rabbanifard R, Mezzich J, Bassaly R, Downes K. Cost analysis of open versus robotic-assisted sacrocolpopexy. Female Pelvic Med Reconstr Surg. 2012;18(6):335-9.
36. Hurd WW, Amesse LS, Gruber JS, Horowitz GM, Cha GM, Hurteau JA. Visualisation of the epigastric vessels and bladder before laparoscopic trocar placement. Fertil Steril. 2003;80(1):209-12.
37. Hurd WW, Pearl ML, DeLancey JO, Quint EH, Garnett B, Bude RO. Laparoscopic injury of abdominal wall blood vessels: a report of three cases. Obstet Gynecol. 1993;82(4 Pt 2 Suppl):673-6.
38. Intuitive Surgical. (2013). Da Vinci surgery. [online] Available from www.intuitivesurgical.com/company/clinical-evidence [Accessed May 2025].
39. Jansen FW, Vredevoogd CB, van Ulzen K, Hermans J, Trimbos JB, Trimbos-Kemper TC. Complications of hysteroscopy: a prospective, multi-center study. Obstet Gynecol. 2000;96(2):266-70.
40. Johnson N, Barlow D, Lethaby A, Tavender E, Curr L, Garry R. Methods of hysterectomy: systematic review and meta-analysis of randomised controlled trials. BMJ. 2005;330(7506):1478.
41. Jung YW, Kim SW, Kim YT. Recent advances of robotic surgery and single port laparoscopy in gynaecologic oncology. J Gynecol Oncol. 2009;20(3):137-44.
42. Kaali SG, Barad DH. Incidence of bowel injury due to dense adhesions at the sight of direct trocar insertion. J Reprod Med. 1992;37(7):617-8.
43. Karande VC. LigaSureTM 5-mm blunt tip laparoscopic instrument. J Obstet Gynaecol India. 2015;65(5):350-2.
44. Kim AH, Adamson GD. Surgical treatment options for endometriosis. Clin Obstet Gynecol. 1999;42(3):633-44.
45. Kosumi T, Kubota A, Usui N, Yamauchi K, Yamasaki M, Oyanagi H. Laparoscopic ovarian cystectomy using a single umbilical puncture method. Surg Laparosc Endosc Percutan Tech. 2001;11(1):63-5.
46. Lau S, Vaknin Z, Ramana-Kumar AV, Halliday D, Franco EL, Gotlieb WH. Outcomes and cost comparisons after introducing a robotics program for endometrial cancer surgery. Obstet Gynecol. 2012;119(4):717-24.
47. Litynski GS. Laparoscopy—the early attempts: spotlighting Georg Kelling and Hans Christian Jacobaeus. JSLS. 1997;1(1):83-5.
48. Loffer FD. Preliminary experience with the Versa Point bipolar resectoscope using a vaporising electrode in a saline distending medium. J Am Assoc Gynecol Laparosc. 2000;7(4):498-502.

49. Lowe MP, Chamberlain DH, Kamelle SA, Johnson PR, Tillmanns TD. A multi-institutional experience with robotic-assisted radical hysterectomy for early stage cervical cancer. Gynecol Oncol. 2009;113(2):191-4.
50. Maggioni A, Minig L, Zanagnolo V, Peiretti M, Sanguineti F, Bocciolone L, et al. Robotic approach for cervical cancer—comparison with laparotomy: a case control study. Gynecol Oncol. 2009;115(1):60-4.
51. Magrina JF, Kho RM, Weaver AL, Montero RP, Magtibay PM. Robotic radical hysterectomy: comparison with laparoscopy and laparotomy. Gynecol Oncol. 2008;109(1):86-91.
52. Meeks GR, Harris RL. Surgical approach to hysterectomy: abdominal, laparoscopy-assisted, or vaginal. Clin Obstet Gynecol. 1997;40(4):886-94.
53. Mencaglia L, Lugo E, Consigli S, Barbosa C. Bipolar resectoscope: the future perspective of hysteroscopic surgery. Gynecol Surg. 2009;6:15-20.
54. Mintz M. Risks and prophylaxis in laparoscopy: a survey of 100,000 cases. J Reprod Med. 1977;18(5):269-72.
55. Modlin IM, Kidd M, Lye KD. From the lumen to the laparoscope. Arch Surg. 2004;139(10):1110-26.
56. Munoz JL, Jimenez JS, Hernandez C, Vaquero G, Pérez Sagaseta C, Noguero R, et al. Hysteroscopic myomectomy: our experience and review. JSLS. 2003;7(1):39-48.
57. Murray H, Baakdah H, Bardell T, Tulandi T. Diagnosis and treatment of ectopic pregnancy. CMAJ. 2005;173(8):905-12.
58. Palmer R. Safety in laparoscopy. J Reprod Med. 1974;13(1):1-5.
59. Papadopoulos NP, Magos A. First-generation endometrial ablation: roller-ball vs. loop vs. laser. Best Pract Res Clin Obstet Gynaecol. 2007;21(6):915-29.
60. Payne TN, Dauterive FR, Pitter MC, Giep HN, Giep BN, Grogg TW, et al. Robotically assisted hysterectomy in patients with large uteri: outcomes in five community practices. Obstet Gynecol. 2010;115(3):535-42.
61. Payne TN, Dauterive FR. A comparison of total laparoscopic hysterectomy to robotically assisted hysterectomy: surgical outcomes in a community practice. J Minim Invasive Gynecol. 2008;15(3):286-91.
62. Pelosi MA, Pelosi MA 3rd. Laparoscopic hysterectomy with bilateral salpingo-oophorectomy using a single umbilical puncture. N J Med. 1991;88(10):721-6.
63. Pelosi MA, Pelosi MA 3rd. Laparoscopic supra-cervical hysterectomy using a single-umbilical puncture (mini-laparoscopy). J Reprod Med. 1992;37(9):777-84.
64. Persson J, Reynisson P, Borgfeldt C, Kannisto P, Lindahl B, Bossmar T. Robot assisted laparoscopic radical hysterectomy and pelvic lymphadenectomy with short and long term morbidity data. Gynecol Oncol. 2009;113(2):185-90.
65. Propst AM, Liberman RF, Harlow BL, Ginsburg ES. Complications of hysteroscopic surgery: predicting patients at risk. Obstet Gynecol. 2000;96(4):517-20.
66. Rao PP, Rao PP, Bhagwat S. Single-incision laparoscopic surgery-current status and controversies. J Minim Access Surg. 2011;7(1):6-16.
67. Scandola M, Grespan L, Vicentini M, Fiorini P. Robot-assisted laparoscopic hysterectomy vs traditional laparoscopic hysterectomy: five meta-analyses. J Minim Invasive Gynecol. 2011;18(6):705-15.
68. Siddiqui NY, Geller EJ, Visco AG. Symptomatic and anatomic 1-year outcomes after robotic and abdominal sacrocolpopexy. Am J Obstet Gynecol. 2012;206(5):435.e1-5.
69. Siegler AM, Kemmann E. Location and removal of misplaced or embedded intrauterine devices by hysteroscopy. J Reprod Med. 1976;16(3):139-44.
70. Sinha R, Sanjay M, Rupa B, Kumari S. Robotic surgery in gynecology. J Minim Access Surg. 2015;11(1):50-9.
71. Smorgick N, Barel O, Halperin R, Schneider D, Pansky M. Laparoscopic removal of adnexal cysts: is it possible to decrease inadvertent intraoperative rupture rate? Am J Obstet Gynecol. 2009;200(3):237.e1-3.
72. Stamatellos I, Bontis J. Hysteroscopic myomectomy. Eur Clinics Obstet Gynecol. 2007;3:17-23.
73. Talamini MA, Chapman S, Horgan S, Melvin WS. A prospective analysis of 211 robotic-assisted surgical procedures. Surg Endosc. 2003;17(10):1521-4.
74. Trew GH. Hysteroscopy and hysteroscopic surgery. Curr Obstet Gynaecol. 2004;14:183-90.
75. Tulandi T, Saleh A. Surgical management of ectopic pregnancy. Clin Obstet Gynecol. 1999;42(1):31-8.
76. Tulandi T. Modern surgical approaches to female reproductive tract. Hum Reprod Update. 1996;2(5):419-27.
77. Van Kruchten PM, Vermelis JM, Herold I, Van Zundert AA. Hypotonic and isotonic fluid overload as a complication of hysteroscopic procedures: two case reports. Minerva Anestesiol. 2010;76(5):373-7.
78. Vecchio R, MacFayden BV, Palazzo F. History of laparoscopic surgery. Panminerva Med. 2000;42(1):87-90.
79. Vilos GA, Abu-Rafea B. New developments in ambulatory hysteroscopic surgery. Best Pract Res Clin Obstet Gynaecol. 2005;19(5):727-42.
80. West JH, Robinson DA. Endometrial resection and fluid absorption. Lancet. 1989;2(8676):1387-8.
81. Wheeless CR Jr. A rapid, inexpensive and effective method of surgical sterilisation by laparoscopy. J Reprod Med. 1969;3(5):65-9.
82. White W, Goel R, Kaouk J. Single-port laparoscopic retroperitoneal surgery: initial operative experience and comparative outcomes. Urology. 2009;73(6):1279-82.
83. Wieser F, Tempfer C, Kurz C, Nagele F. Hysteroscopy in 2001: a comprehensive review. Acta Obstet Gynecol Scand. 2001;80(9):773-83.
84. Wortman M, Dagget A. Hysteroscopy myomectomy. J Am Assoc Gynecol Laparosc. 1995;3(1):39-46.
85. Yu D, Wong YM, Cheong Y, Xia E, Li TC. Asherman's syndrome—one century later. Fertil Steril. 2008;89(4):759-79.
86. Yuzpe AA. Pneumoperitoneum needle and trocar injuries in laparoscopy. A survey on possible contributing factors and prevention. J Reprod Med. 1990;35(5):485-90.

55

CHAPTER

Contraception

Shobha N Gudi

Chapter Outline

- General Consideration
- Epidemiology
- Impact of Contraception Throughout the World
- Efficacy of Contraception
- Indications for Contraception
- Criteria for the Use of Various Contraceptive Methods
- Contraceptive Methods
- Natural Family Planning Method
- Barrier Methods
- Intrauterine Contraceptive Devices
- Hormonal Contraception Methods
- Progestogen-only Contraception
- Emergency Postcoital Contraception (Morning after Pills)
- Other Methods of Contraception
- Choice of Methods
- Contraception Choice for Older Women
- Contraception and Litigation

GENERAL CONSIDERATION

Contraception is the prevention of conception by means and methods other than abstinence from coitus. It is useful to limit the size and age structure of a family in family planning. Contraceptive advice is an essential component of good preventive health care. The role of a clinician is to provide the information necessary for the patient to make proper choices through the 'Cafeteria approach'. The approach in principle involves a structured counselling session offering a basket of choices of contraceptives with an emphasis on safety and benefits, and that will have a major impact on contraceptive uptake and adherence to the method. The major reasons for adverse maternal and perinatal outcome are high-risk pregnancies with medical comorbidities conceived without planning, unintended pregnancies ending in unsafe abortions and decreased spacing between pregnancies. There is no doubt that family planning and contraception save maternal lives. It also provides a better quality of life by helping families to use their limited resources for better outcomes.

EPIDEMIOLOGY

The National Survey of Family Growth is conducted by the National Centre for Health Statistics of the Centers for Disease Control and Prevention. **Figure 1** shows the graph of the increase in the world population, which is expected to touch 11.5 billion by 2150.

- According to the data available from 2015 to 2016, Asia accounts for 60% of the world population, while India contributes about 16%.
- The percentage of married couples using sterilisation as a method of contraception more than doubled from 1972 to 1988 and has remained stable since then.
- The use of oral contraception reached a peak in 1992 and then decreased in 1995, especially among Hispanic and black Americans.
- Among newer married women, oral contraception has been the leading method of birth control, but

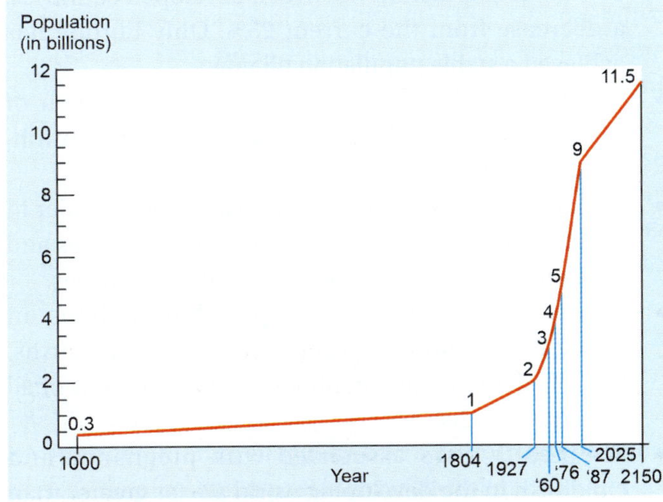

Fig. 1: Increase in the World Population by 2150.

from 1988 to 1995, oral contraceptive use decreased in women younger than 25 years and rose among women aged 30–44 years. This may be due to the availability and use of implants and injectable methods.

- The recent increase in overall contraceptive use is due to the increase in condom use, which rose from 5.1 million in 1988 (15%) to 7.9 million in 1995 (20%). This increase occurred in all races and ethnic groups. These changes reflect the concern regarding sexually transmitted disease (STD), including human immunodeficiency virus (HIV).
- In 1982, 56% of US women, aged 15–44 years, were using contraception, and this increased in 1995 to 64%.
- The number of reproductive age group women using intrauterine contraceptive device (IUCD) has decreased from 2 million in 1982 to only 0.3 million in 1995 in the US.
- The oral contraceptive is the most popular method among teenagers.
- During the years of maximum fertility, oral contraceptives are the most common method, peaking at the age of 20–24 years. The use of condoms is the second most widely used method of reversible contraception, rising from 15% to 20% in 1995.

IMPACT OF CONTRACEPTION THROUGHOUT THE WORLD

- World population is expected to stabilise at between 11 and 12 billion around 2150, with a fertility rate of 2.1 children per woman. Approximately 95% of the growth will occur in developing countries, so that by 2100, only 13% of the population will live in developed countries, a decrease from the current 25%. Only Europe has achieved a stable population till now.
- Throughout the world, 45% of married women of reproductive age (MWRA) practice contraception, while 69% in East Asia and only 11% in Africa.
- Female sterilisation and the IUCD are most popular in developing countries, whereas oral contraceptives and condoms are most popular in developed countries.
- Nearly 76% of the world's population living in developing countries account for 85% of all births, 95% of all infant and childhood deaths, and 99% of all maternal deaths.
- The health risks associated with pregnancy and childbirth in the developing world are far greater than risks secondary to the use of modern contraception.
- The interaction between clinician and patient for the purpose of contraception also provides an opportunity to control STDs. If an infection is symptomatic, it can be treated during the same visit in which contraception is requested.
- The impact of contraception can be measured in terms of both morbidity and mortality.

National Family Health Survey (NFHS)-5 (2019–20) data for India: Available for 22 states/union territories (UTs) and 342 districts, which includes 104 indicators (at district-level), 12 indicators on family planning, and 17 indicators on maternal/delivery care, amongst others. The outcomes show promising results for family planning data. The mean Contraception prevalence rate (mCPR) change from NFHS-4 to NFHS-5 has been very encouraging in some districts/states/UTs. The total fertility rate (TFR) is already ≤2.1 in 19 out of 22 states/UTs. A shift to reversible modern methods and a good method mix is evident at the district/state level. These are important facts as family planning (FP) program coverage variables will have a continuing role to play in the socioeconomic and developmental determinants of the country.

EFFICACY OF CONTRACEPTION

Contraceptive efficacy is generally assessed by measuring the number of unplanned pregnancies that occur during a specified period of exposure and use of a contraceptive method. The two methods that have been used to measure contraceptive efficacy are the Pearl index and life table analysis.

Pearl Index

The Pearl index is defined as the number of failures per 100 women years (HWY) of exposure multiplied by 1,200, if the denominator consists of months or by 1,300 if the denominator consists of cycles.

Pearl index = Number of pregnancies/Total months or cycle of exposure from the onset of method × 1,200

With most methods of contraception, failure rates decline with duration of use. Pearl index is usually based on a specific exposure (usually 1 year) and therefore fails to accurately compare methods at various durations of exposure. This limitation is overcome by using the method of life table analysis. Nevertheless, the Pearl index remains the most common tool for evaluating and comparing efficacy between methods.

Life Table Analysis

Life table analysis calculates a failure rate per month of use. A cumulative failure rate can then compare methods for any specific length of exposure. Women who leave a study for any reason other than unintended pregnancy are removed from the analysis, and contributing their exposure until the time of the exit.

Contraceptive failure occurs for many reasons. Thus, method effectiveness and use effectiveness have been used to designate efficacy with correct and incorrect use of a method. It is less confusing to simply compare the very best performance (perfect use—the lowest expected failure rate) with the usual experience (typical use—typical failure rate). The lowest expected failure rates are determined in clinical trials.

INDICATIONS FOR CONTRACEPTION

- *The commonest reason in India is to prevent unintended pregnancy:* Almost 50% of all pregnancies are unintended, and more than half of them end in safe and unsafe abortions. The resultant increase in maternal mortality and morbidity can be prevented by the optimal use of the spacing method.
- *Limiting the population*: This suits the economic interest of the community. Population control is now a pressing problem throughout the world. This is because the advancements in medicine and civilisation have resulted in death control. The world population has doubled in the last 50 years, increasing from approximately 8 million in 8,000 BC, the world population is expected to be 11–12 billion around 2150. India and China have both crossed the 1 billion mark. The factors concerned in birth rate, family size and population increase include climate, nutrition, fertility, age of marriage, custom and fashion, desire for sons, law of inheritance, religion, political warfare, education and the infant death rate. It is said that a decreasing infant death rate, which makes a mother with only a small family feel more secure, inevitably results in a falling birth rate. This is not so far manifest in all countries, which means there is an urgent need for a widespread distribution of contraceptive devices and instructions on their use. To ensure a zero-population growth rate, the average number of children per family should not exceed 2.2. The most important time to intervene for ensuring uptake of contraception through structured counselling is in the postabortal and postpartum period.
- *Early marriage*: It is often wise for a couple to practice contraception during the early part of marriage, but this does not apply when the partners are no longer young, when they are already well adjusted by a long engagement or when their circumstances are propitious. Indeed, many young brides decide to have a limited number of children as soon as is reasonable with the object of completing their childbearing within a few years and returning to their work of profession as soon as their maternal responsibilities allow.
- *Birth spacing:* If a woman has children too frequently, she has no time to recover from one before she is faced with another one. She is then prone to anaemia, muscle and ligament strains, postural defects, and nervous exhaustion. She is unable to cope with her domestic responsibilities, allows the home to become dirty and cheerless, neglects her children, and as a result, the whole family suffers.
- *Previous obstetrical complications:* Recurrent pregnancy hypertension, repeat caesarean section, repaired obstetrical injuries such as vesicovaginal fistula and a previous operation for prolapse can justify the avoidance or deferment of further childbearing.
- Family limitation
- *Chronic systemic diseases in the woman*: These include nephritis, hypertension, cardiac disease, pulmonary insufficiency, psychoses, neurosis, blood disorders and any disease which makes a woman less able to withstand the strain of pregnancy and labour or which makes her unfit to cope with the rearing of another child.
- Temporary ill health in either partner.
- *Later years of marriage*: When the family is complete, contraception can be used in place of permanent sterilisation.
- *On request*: There is much to be said for giving contraceptive advice to any girl or woman, or man who asks for it, irrespective of their circumstances. If they have decided to be sexually active and if consultation makes it clear that they appreciate the implications, they should be protected from having an unwanted child or an induced abortion.
- *Emergency contraception (EC)*: Occasionally, a couple may have unprotected coitus or there may be a problem with the contraceptive method used, e.g. condom rupture, displaced IUCD or irregular hormonal contraception; an EC may be required. However, it is not a substitute for a regular contraceptive method.

TABLE 1: World Health Organization eligibility criteria for the use of various contraceptive methods.

Category	*Description*
1	A condition where there is no restriction on the use of the contraceptive method
2	A condition where the advantages of using the method generally outweigh the theoretical or proven risks
3	A condition where the theoretical or proven risks usually outweigh the advantages of using the method
4	A condition that represents an unacceptable health risk if the contraceptive method is used

CRITERIA FOR THE USE OF VARIOUS CONTRACEPTIVE METHODS

The World Health Organization (WHO) eligibility criteria for the use of various contraceptive methods have been described in **Table 1**.

CONTRACEPTIVE METHODS

Various contraceptive methods available are enumerated in **Box 1.**

BOX 1: Various methods of contraception.

Temporary methods:
- Natural regulation of fertility
- Barrier methods
- *Hormonal contraception:*
  - Combined hormonal contraception (CHC)
  - Combined oral contraceptive pills (COCPs):
    - Monophasic pills (each tablet containing a fixed amount of oestrogen and progestogen)
    - Biphasic pills (each tablet containing a fixed amount of oestrogen, while the amount of progestogen increases in the luteal phase of the cycle)
    - Triphasic pills (the amount of oestrogen may be fixed or variable, while the amount of progestogen increases over three equally divided phases of the cycle)
      - ◊ Evra® patch
      - ◊ NuvaRing®
  - Progestogen-only contraception:
    - Progestin-only pill (POP)
    - Injections (DepoProvera®), Intramuscular and subcutaneous
    - Implants (Norplant® I and II), Implanon-NXT, the etonogestrel implant
    - Patches
    - Vaginal rings
- IUCDs
- Emergency (postcoital) contraception

Permanent methods:
- Sterilisation
- Female sterilisation—tubal ligation
- Male sterilisation—vasectomy

(IUCD: intrauterine contraceptive device)

NATURAL FAMILY PLANNING METHOD

Fertility Awareness-based Method or Traditional Methods

This method refers to methods for planning and preventing pregnancies by observation of the naturally occurring signs and symptoms of the fertile and infertile phases of the menstrual cycle, with the avoidance of sexual intercourse during the fertile phase (WHO, 1982).

The fertile phase is calculated by the following methods.

Rhythm Method or Safe Period or Calendar Method (Fig. 2)

It is based on the fact that most women ovulate approximately 2 weeks or 14 days before each menstruation, regardless of the length of their menstrual cycle. A couple avoids intercourse during the fertile period.

The woman records the number of days in each menstrual cycle for at least 6 months. The first day of the menstrual cycle bleeding is always counted as day 1. The woman subtracts 18 from the length of her shortest recorded cycle. This tells her the estimated first day of her fertile period. Then she subtracts 11 days from the length of her longest recorded cycle. This tells her the last day of her fertile period. The couple avoids sex or uses a barrier method or withdrawal during the fertile period.

For example, if her recorded cycles vary from 26 days to 32 days, then 26 – 18 = 8th day, so the couple start avoiding unprotected sex on day 8, 32 – 11 = 21st day, while they continue avoiding unprotected sex till day 21 of the cycle.

Disadvantage: A woman with irregular cycles cannot use this method.

Cervical Mucus Method or 'Billings' Method Change (Figs. 3A to C)

The cervical mucus method is one of the natural fertility awareness methods. This method is based on the fact that as the fertile time approaches, the cervical mucus

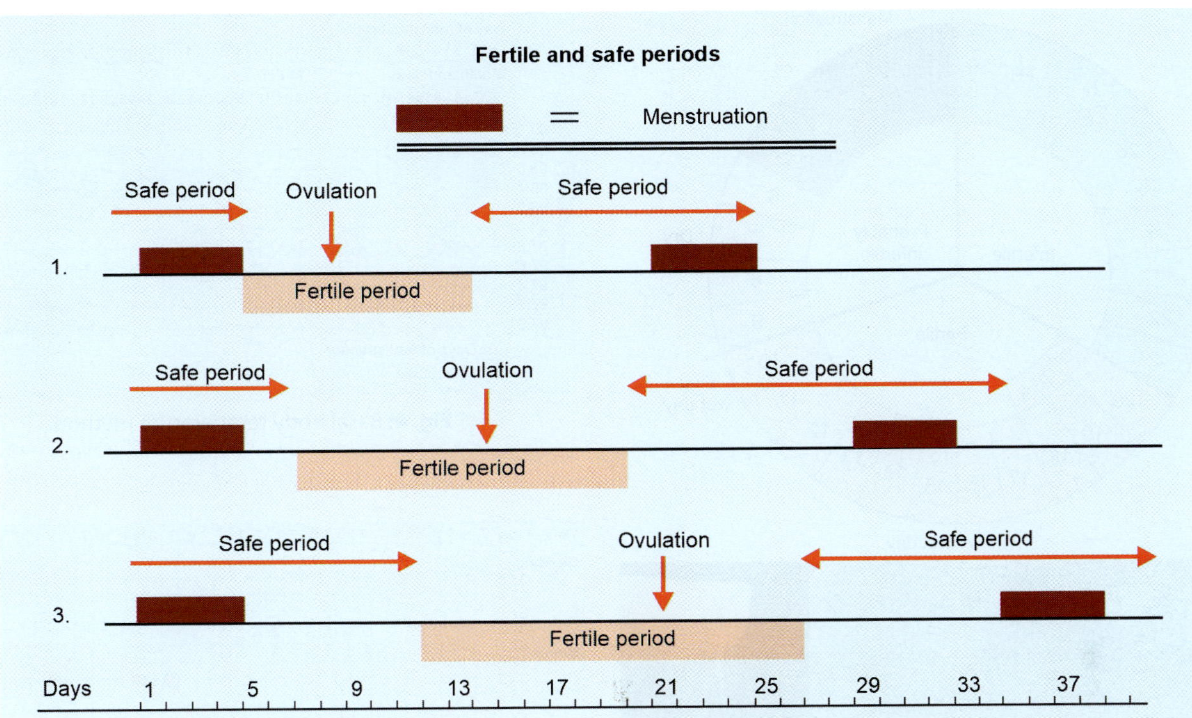

Fig. 2: The fertile and 'safe' periods during (1) 21-day cycle, (2) 28-day cycle and (3) 35-day cycle.

increases in amount and becomes clearer in colour, wetter, stretchy, and slippery. Following ovulation, the mucus usually becomes sticky, thicker, and pasty in character and reduces in amount. This method is safe, and there are no side effects. Sexual intercourse is considered safe during the days immediately following the menses until the cervical mucus attains the previously described characteristics. Thereafter, the couple must abstain from having sexual intercourse until the 4th day after the 'peak mucus day'.

Under the effect of oestrogens, cervical mucus becomes thin, watery, clear and profuse. It has a high content of sodium chloride in it due to which it forms a characteristic pattern of ferning when dried on a glass slide. It has great elasticity and is able to withstand stretching up to 10 cm. This is also known as the spinnbarkeit or the thread test, which is evidence of oestrogenic activity.

On the other hand, under the effect of progesterone, the mucus becomes thick, tenacious, and highly viscous. It loses its property of spinnbarkeit and easily fractures when put under tension. This property is known as tack. **Figure 3D** shows typical pattern of progesterone-dominant cervical mucus when smeared on a glass slide and observed under a microscope.

This method is associated with a high failure rate of approximately 20–25 pregnancies per HWY of use, which commonly results due to irregular ovulation or irregular menstrual cycles.

Basal Body Temperature Method

Basal body temperature (BBT) is the temperature of body at rest. It is taken when the patient is in bed, after getting up from sleep, without taking anything from mouth. The BBT rises from a lower level to a higher level of at least 0.5°C or 1°F. This occurs shortly after ovulation. It remains at a higher level until she begins to menstruate again **(Fig. 4)**. It can only be used to tell when the late infertile phase begins, but not the end of it. The couple avoids sex from first day of menses until the woman's temperature has risen above her regular temperature and stayed up for 3 full days.

Symptothermal Method (Fig. 5)

This is a combined method in which a woman identifies fertile and infertile days by combining BBT, cervical mucus changes and other signs and symptoms of ovulation such as abdominal pain, breast tenderness. The failure rate of

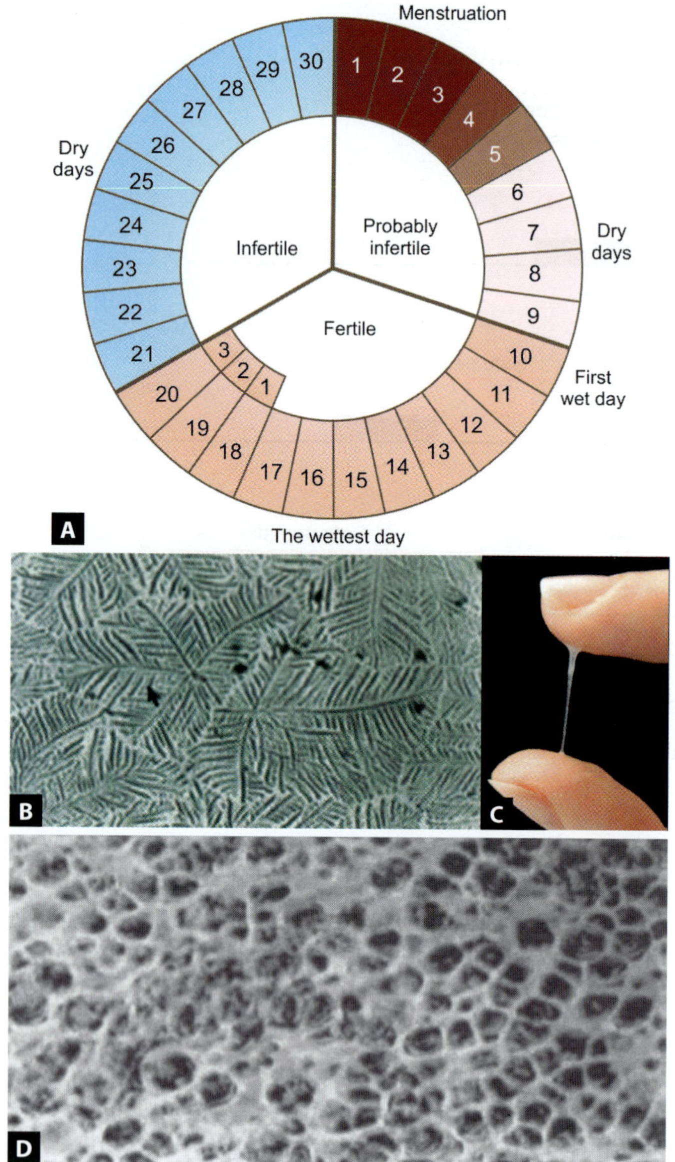

Figs. 3A to D: (A) Cervical mucus method; (B and C) Oestrogen-dominant cervical mucus: (B) Ferning pattern; (C) Spinnbarkeit test; (D) Progesterone-dominant cervical mucus.

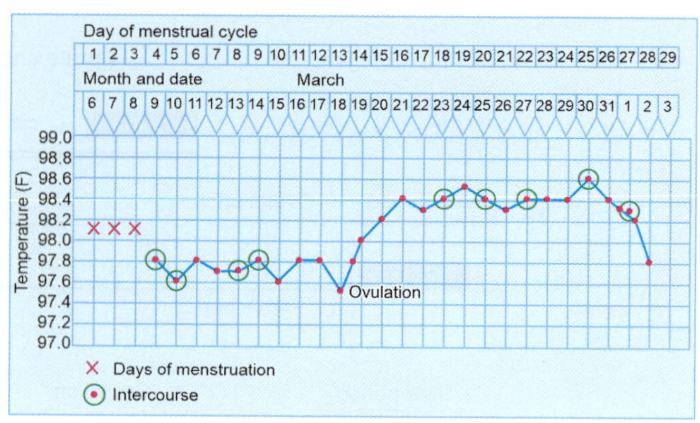

Fig. 4: Basal body temperature method.

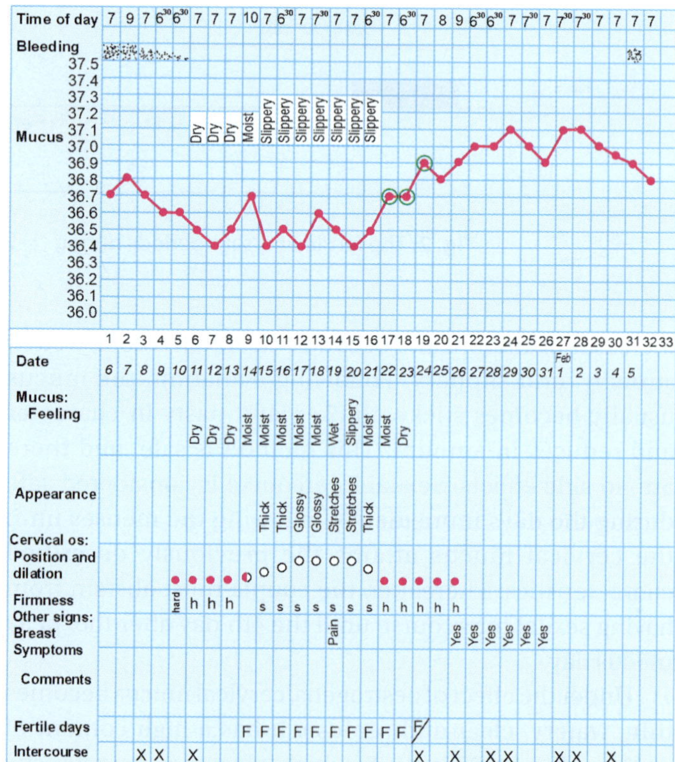

Fig. 5: Symptothermal methods.

natural family planning method is 18–25 pregnancies per HWY. This is because the time of ovulation varies even in regularly menstruating women.

CycleBeads

This is a natural family planning method, which is designed for women with cycles between 26 days and 32 days **(Fig. 6)**. The fertile period in these women lasts from 8th to 19th day, which can be identified by the presence of white beads. Brown beads mark the 'safe days' or the period during which the woman is likely to be least fertile. During this time, the couple can have unprotected intercourse. A rubber band is moved head-to-head every day to track the cycle. This method helps in preventing unwanted pregnancies, using the 'standard days method'. The users are instructed to avoid unprotected sex by using a condom or abstaining during days 8–19 of the cycle (identified by the white beads).

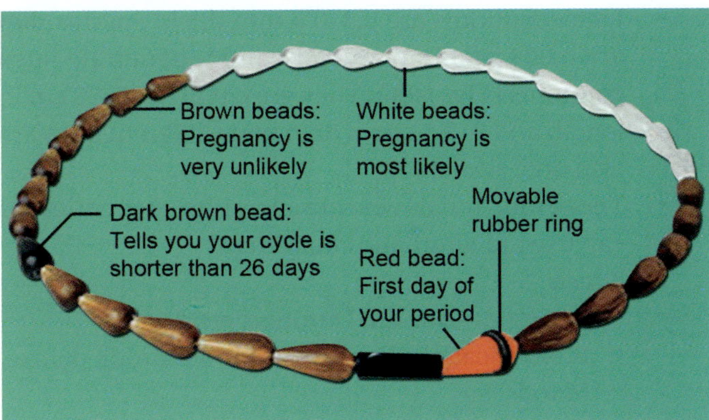

Fig. 6: CycleBeads.

Flowchart 1: Use of lactational amenorrhoea method (LAM algorithm).

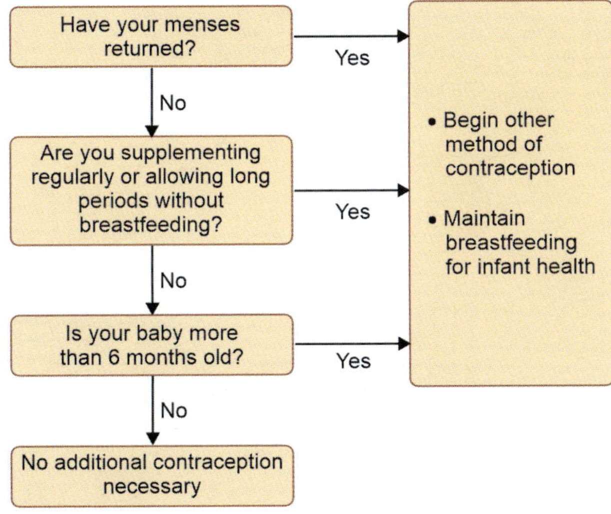

Lactational Amenorrhoea Method

It is described as:

- Lactational amenorrhoea method (LAM) is based on the physiology of breastfeeding **(Flowchart 1)**.
- There is only a 1–2% chance of becoming pregnant in a lactating woman who fulfils the following three conditions (The Bellagio's Criteria):
  1. She is breastfeeding her baby on demand, both day and night and not feeding him or her other foods or liquids regularly.
  2. Menses have not yet returned.
  3. The baby is <6 months of age.

Women who fulfil these three conditions are naturally protected against pregnancy. Hence, this method is also considered a natural family planning method.

- Rule of 3's for postpartum initiation of contraception, i.e. full breastfeeding, begins in the third postpartum month and partial or no breastfeeding begins in the third postpartum week.
- Elevated levels of prolactin inhibit the pulsatile release of gonadotrophin-releasing hormone (GnRH), leading to erratic or anovulatory cycles, with a short luteal phase and interference with implantation owing to suckling-induced release of oxytocin.

Personal Fertility Monitors

Persona® monitor (Swiss Precision Diagnostics GmbH, Switzerland) is a handheld device, which measures the woman's urine levels of oestrone-3-glucuronide and luteinising hormone (LH) at home to determine the fertile period. As a contraceptive device, Persona® displays a green light during the infertile phase and a red light during the fertile phase. A symbol is also displayed in this device during the fertile phase, which indicates the surge in LH and impending ovulation. Women may use these devices to prevent pregnancy by avoiding intercourse (or using backup methods of contraception) during the phase when the red light is displayed.

Coitus Interruptus (Withdrawal Method)

It is described as:

- It means the discharge of semen outside the female genitalia at the end of intercourse.
- This method needs great motivation and self-control in the male partner, and the female partner may develop sex neurosis, pelvic congestion syndrome, but there is no definite evidence regarding this.
- The typical average failure rate is 18–20 per 100 women users. The failure is mostly due to a lack of male self-control, pre-ejaculating discharge and sometimes ascent of sperm from the external genitalia.

Advantages of Natural Family Planning Method

The advantages are:

- No physical side effects
- No financial cost
- It increases self-awareness and knowledge
- It can be provided by a trained natural family planning teacher and not necessarily by highly skilled medical personnel.

Disadvantages of Natural Family Planning Method

The disadvantages are:

- It does not provide protection against HIV and STDs.
- There may be emotional stress due to abstinence of 10–12 days/cycle.
- Involvement of both partners is essential.
- High failure rate.

BARRIER METHODS

The barrier methods are described as:

- Barrier contraceptives are family planning methods, which act as barriers and prevent the union of sperm and ovum necessary for pregnancy.
- Recently, barrier methods of contraception have gained much more importance in view of the fact that they prevent precancerous lesions, cancer of the cervix, and the spread of acquired immunodeficiency syndrome (AIDS). Only condoms have been proven to prevent HIV infection. STD protection has a beneficial impact on the risk of tubal infertility and ectopic pregnancy.
- The risk of toxic shock syndrome (TSS) is increased with female barrier methods, but the actual incidence is so rare that this is not a significant clinical consideration.

Different kinds of barrier methods are available, which are discussed here.

Condoms

Male Condom

- It is the only contraceptive proven to prevent HIV infection **(Figs. 7 to 9)**.
  The following are the specific goals:
  - Correct use
  - Consistent use
  - Affordable and easy availability
- Various types of condoms are available:
  - Most are made of latex. Polyurethane and silicone rubber condoms are also now manufactured.
  - Latex condoms are 0.3–0.8 mm thick. Sperms that are 0.003 mm in diameter cannot penetrate latex condoms **(Fig. 10A)**. They are circular, 15–20 cm in length and 3–3.5 cm in diameter (different sizes are also now available).
  - Those individuals who are allergic to latex condoms can use polyurethane condoms.
  - *Types*:
    - Dry type—Nirodh, Duropac, etc.
    - Prelubricated—Durex, Kohinoor, Nirodh deluxe, Moods, etc.
    - Medicated—coated with nonoxynol-9, e.g. Share, Ramses, Dean, etc. These are names of Indian brands of condoms.

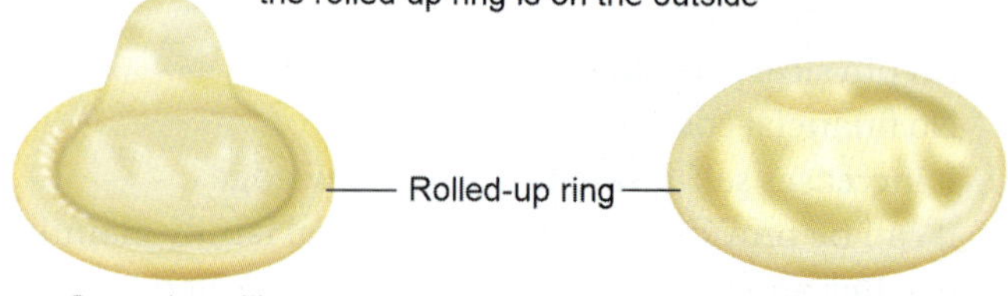

Fig. 7: Correct position of applying a male condom.

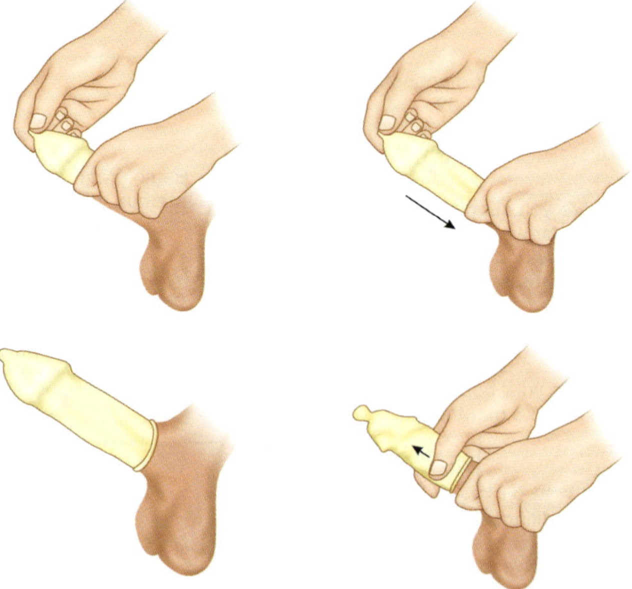

Fig. 8: Application of a male condom.

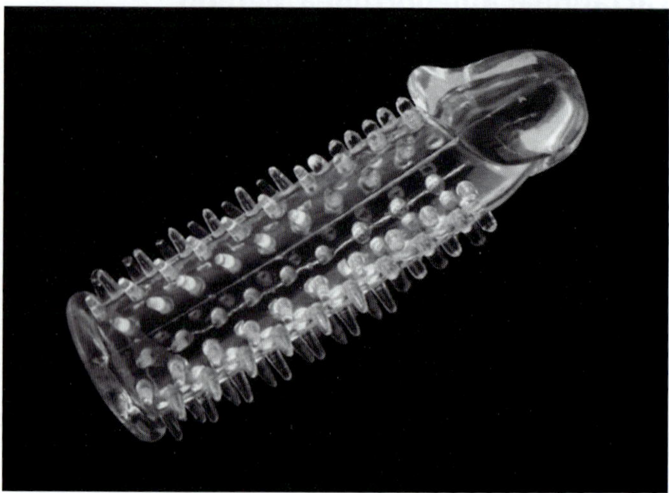

Fig. 9: Silicone rubber condom.

- Average lifespan is 5 years from the date of manufacturing.
- Should be kept in cool and dry places.

Acceptability and usage: Condom use is more common in the developed countries, where 12% of MWRA are protected by condoms, against 4% in the developing countries. Condoms are used worldwide, particularly as a preventive measure against HIV and STDs.

Effectiveness: Typical average failure rate of condom as commonly used is 12% (WHO, 1994). When used correctly and consistently failure rate is only 3%.

Advantages:
- Condoms need no prescription and no medical help for use.
- An easily available and harmless method of contraception.
- It gives very good protection against STDs, HIV and hepatitis B virus.
- They are suitable for any age group, during lactation, and for those who cannot tolerate oral pills and IUCDs.
- Barrier methods reduce the chance of developing severe cervical dysplasia and cervical cancer.

Disadvantages:
- Breakage is a greater problem for couples at risk of STDs
- Rarely, they produce hypersensitisation
- No major disadvantage
- Storage and disposal problems.

How to use: A condom must be placed on the penis before it touches a partner. An uncircumcised man should pull the foreskin back. Prior to unrolling the condom to the base of the penis, air should be squeezed out of the reservoir tip with a thumb and forefinger. The tip of condom should extend beyond the end of the penis to provide a reservoir to collect the ejaculate. If lubricants are used, they must be water-based. Oil-based lubricants will weaken the latex. After intercourse, the condom should be held at the base as the still erect penis is withdrawn. Semen must not be allowed to spill or leak. It should be handled very gently.

If there is evidence of any spillage or leakage, or when a condom breaks:
- Spermicidal agents should be quickly inserted into the vagina.
- A woman should contact a clinician within 72 hours. EC should be provided.

Newer developments: Some of the latest forms of male condoms include synthetic nonlatex condoms, which most men prefer.
- New condom materials, such as polyurethane and styrene-ethylene-butylene-styrene (SEBS)—a synthetic material known commercially as Tactylon—have been developed, and this will prove to be beneficial for men who are sensitive or allergic to latex.
- Over latex condoms, these polyurethane and SEBS condoms have two advantages—they have a longer shelf life and can be used with oil-based lubricants, which can damage the latex condoms.

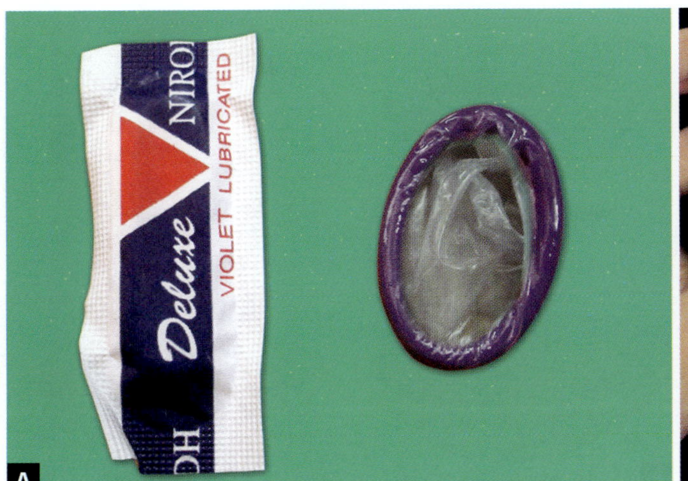

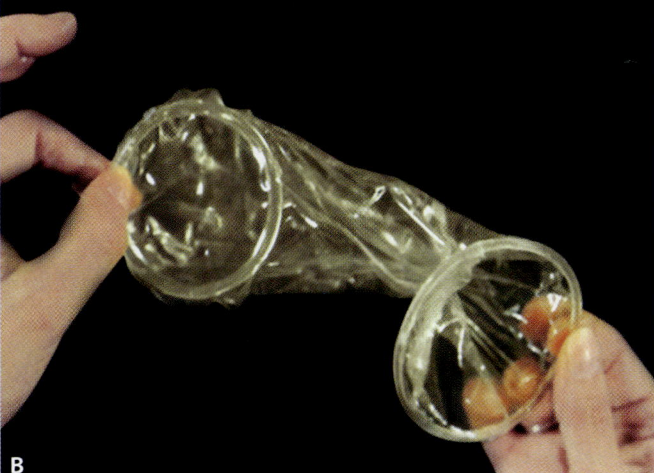

Figs. 10A and B: (A) A male condom; (B) A female condom.

- Some users also found that nonlatex condoms have less odour, fit more comfortably, and are less constricting and transfer body heat better than latex condoms.

Silicone condoms: Currently, there is also a patented silicone condom [Origami male condom (OMC)] that is in the process and presently undergoing clinical trials. It is still awaiting approval from the Food and Drug Administration (FDA) **(Fig. 9)**.

The Origami condom™ is the first nonrolled and engineered condom, which does not require unrolling and is likely to improve the consumer's acceptability, safety, comfort, and compliance.

Female Condom (Fig. 10B)

- The female condom is a pouch made of polyurethane, which lines the vagina.
- An internal ring in the closed end of the pouch covers the cervix and an external ring remains outside the vagina, partially covering the perineum.
- It is prelubricated with silicone; no need to use spermicidal agents.
- These devices are more cumbersome than male condoms and have high rates of problems, such as slippage.
- Efficacy rate similar to diaphragm: 5–20/HWY

Diaphragm (Dutch Cap)

The first effective barrier contraceptive method under a woman's control was the vaginal diaphragm. The vaginal diaphragm or Dutch cap consists of a saucer-shaped rubber diaphragm with a metal coil spring in its rim, which fits snugly across the upper vagina **(Fig. 11A)**. There are three types of diaphragms and most manufacturers produce them in sizes ranging from 50 to 105 mm diameter, in increments of 2.5–5 mm. Most women use sizes between 65 and 80 mm. The three types of diaphragms **(Fig. 11B)** available are as follows:

1. Diaphragm with flat spring
2. Diaphragm with arcing spring
3. Diaphragm with hinged spring.

The latex arcing spring diaphragm has a firm rim, which makes its insertion in the posterior fornix easier. The rim of a coil spring diaphragm is soft and flexible, which does not form an arc when folded. This is usually used in women with moderate tone of vaginal muscles. The flat spring diaphragm is similar to a coil spring, but has a thinner and more delicate rim. It may be used in women with good tone of vaginal muscles. The diaphragm **(Figs. 11A and B)**, made with a flat metal spring or a coil spring, remains in a straight line when pinched at the edges. This type is suitable for woman with good vaginal muscle tone and an adequate recess behind the pubic arch. Arcing diaphragms are easier to use for most women.

They come in two types. The all-flex type bends into an arc, no matter where around the rim the edges are pinched together. The arcing diaphragms allow the posterior edge of the diaphragm to slip more easily past the cervix and into the posterior cul-de-sac. *Women with poor vaginal muscle tone, cystocele, rectocele, a long cervix, or an anterior cervix of a retroverted uterus use arcing diaphragms more successfully.*

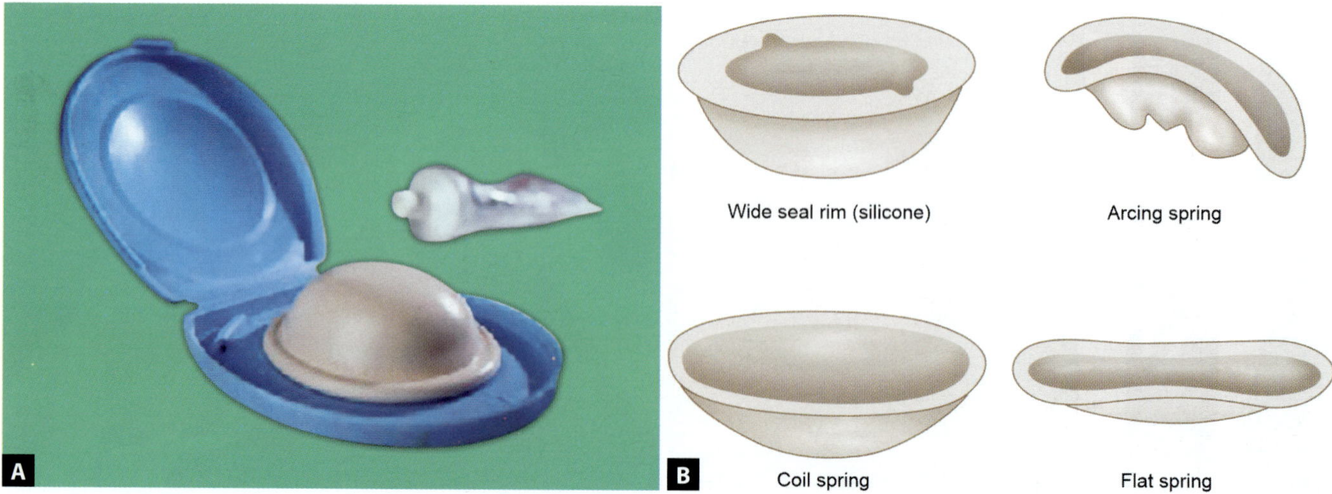

Figs. 11A and B: Types of diaphragms used. (A) Cervical diaphragm; (B) Different types of cervical diaphragms.

The hinged type of diaphragm must be pinched between the hinges in order to form a symmetrical arc. It forms a narrower shape when pinched together and thus may be easier for some women to insert.

Fitting: The successful use of the diaphragm depends on proper fitting. The clinician must have available aseptic fitting rings or diaphragms themselves in all diameters. These devices should be disinfected by soaking in a bleach solution. At the time of pelvic examination, the middle finger is placed against the vaginal wall and posterior cul-de-sac, while the hand is lifted anteriorly until the pubic symphysis abuts the index finger. This point is marked with the examiner's thumb to approximate the diameter of the diaphragm. The corresponding fitting ring is inserted, and the fit is to be assessed by both clinician and patient. If the diaphragm is too tightly pressed against the pubic symphysis, a smaller size is selected. After a good fit is obtained, the diaphragm is removed by hooking the index finger under the rim behind the symphysis and pulling. It is important to instruct the patient in these procedures during and after fitting. The patient should then insert the diaphragm, practice checking for proper placement, and attempt removal.

There should be reasonably firm apposition, particularly in the posterior fornix, and the lower rim should be at least one fingerbreadth above the external urethral meatus.

The diaphragm is compressed with the cavity facing upward and then it is pushed into the vagina as far as it will go. The leading edge is behind the cervix. The front edge is behind the symphysis pubis. Move the finger around the rim; find the bulge of the cervix in the middle, and it should be snug. For removal, insert the index finger under the front rim and pull downwards and outwards **(Figs. 12A to C)**.

Timing: The diaphragm should be inserted no longer than 6 hours prior to sexual intercourse. About a tablespoonful of spermicidal cream or jelly should be placed in the dome of the diaphragm prior to insertion, and the source of the spermicide spread around the rim of the diaphragm.

- The diaphragm should be left in place for approximately 6 hours (but not more than 24 hours) after intercourse.
- Additional spermicide should be placed in the vagina before each episode of sexual intercourse while the diaphragm is in place.

Reassessment: The fit of a diaphragm should be assessed every year at the time of regular examination. Weight loss, gain, vaginal delivery and even sexual intercourse can change vaginal calibre.

Care of the diaphragm: After removal, the diaphragm should be washed with soap and water, rinsed and dried. It should be stored in a cool and dark location. It is wise to use water to periodically check for leaks. The diaphragms need replacement every 6 months to 2 years (depending on their care). The woman should be warned against constipation, because a loaded rectum can prevent the diaphragm from fitting accurately.

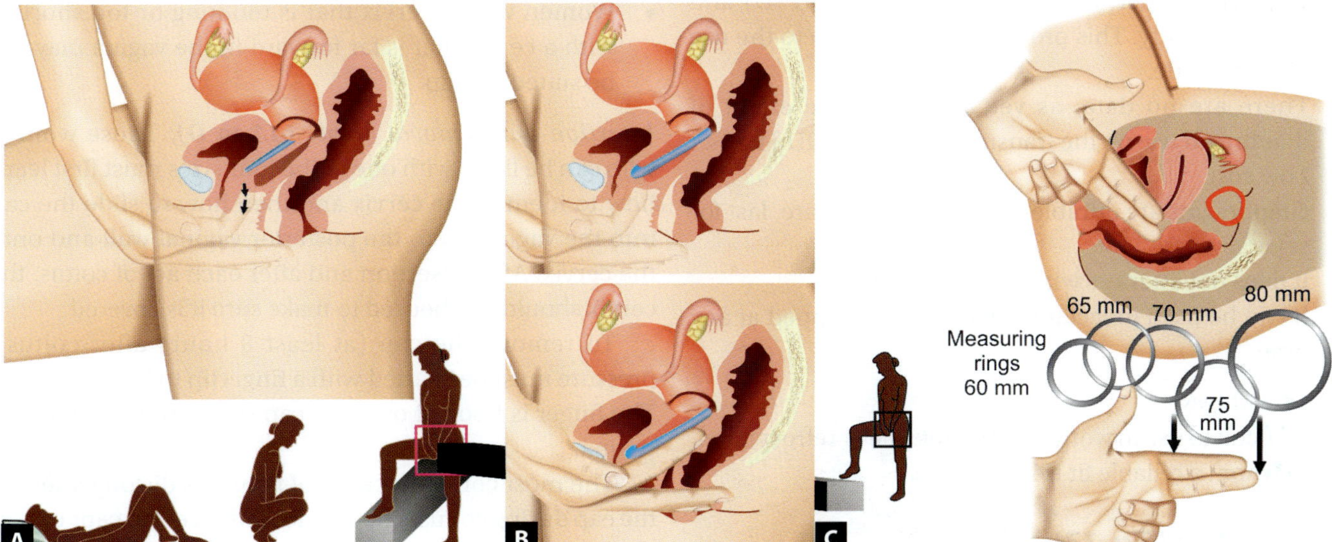

Figs. 12A to C: How to use a diaphragm. (A) Removal of diaphragm; (B) Checking diaphragm position; (C) Fitting of diaphragm (assessment of diameter).

Efficacy: Failure rates vary from as low as 2% per year of use to as high as 23% per year. The typical use failure rate after 1 year of use is 12.1%. Young and literate woman can use diaphragms very successfully, if they are properly encouraged and counselled.

Side effects:
- <1% of women discontinue it because of vaginal irritation caused by latex rubber or spermicidal jelly or cream.
- Urinary tract infections are twofold to threefold more common among diaphragm users than among women using oral pills. Possibly, the rim of the diaphragm presses against the urethra and causes irritation, which is perceived as infection or true infection sometimes occurs from touching the perineal area or incomplete voiding of the bladder. Clinical experience suggests that voiding after sexual intercourse is helpful, and if necessary, a single postcoital prophylactic antibiotic can be recommended (cephalexin 250 mg, nitrofurantoin 100 mg or trimethoprim-sulphamethoxazole one tablet postcoitus).
- Improper fitting or prolonged retention can cause vaginal abrasion or mucosal irritation.
- There is no link between the normal use of diaphragms and TSS. It makes sense, however, to minimise the risk of TSS by removing the diaphragm after 24 hours and during menses.

Advantages:
- Diaphragm use reduces the incidence of cervical gonorrhoea, pelvic inflammatory disease (PID) and tubal infertility. This protection may be due to the use of spermicide.
- There are no data, as yet, regarding the effect of diaphragm use on the transmission of the AIDS virus.
- Low cost
- Diaphragms are durable and, with proper care, last for several years.
- It does not interfere with natural coitus.
- It can be used in lactating women and stopped at any time.

Disadvantages:
- Difficult to use in women with prolapse or retroversion, in whom a reliable fit is impossible.

Cervical Cap (Fig. 13)

The cervical cap was popular in Europe long before its reintroduction into the United States. The cervical cap is a small and firm cap-shaped device, which fits over the cervix. It is available in four sizes—22, 25, 28 and 31 mm.

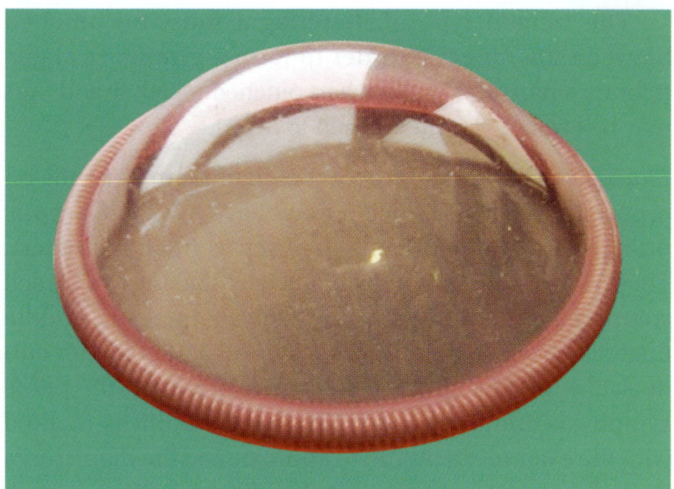

Fig. 13: Cervical cap.

Advantages over the diaphragm:
- It can be left in place for a longer time (up to 48 hours).
- It need not be used with spermicide. However, a tablespoonful of spermicide placed in the cap before application is reported to increase efficacy.
- Women with pelvic relaxation can use a cap.

Disadvantages over the diaphragm:
- Somewhat harder to fit, as it comes in only four sizes.
- More difficult to insert, as it must be placed precisely over the cervix.
- Efficacy is significantly reduced in parous women.
- Women with a cervix that is too long or too short or with a cervix that is far forward in the vagina may not be suited for cap.

Insertion and removal ***(Figs. 14A to D)****:* Those women who can be fitted with one of the four sizes must first learn how to identify the cervix and then how to slide the cap into the vagina up to the posterior vaginal wall and onto the cervix. After insertion and after each act of coitus, the cervix should be checked to make sure it is covered.

To remove the cap (at least 8 hours after coitus), pressure must be exerted with a fingertip to break the seal. The finger is hooked over the cap rim to pull it out of the vagina.

The most common cause of failure is dislodgement of the cap during coitus. There is no evidence that caps causes TSS or dysplastic changes in the cervical mucosa. They also provide protection from STDs, such as diaphragms, but not from HIV. The cervical caps can be left in place for

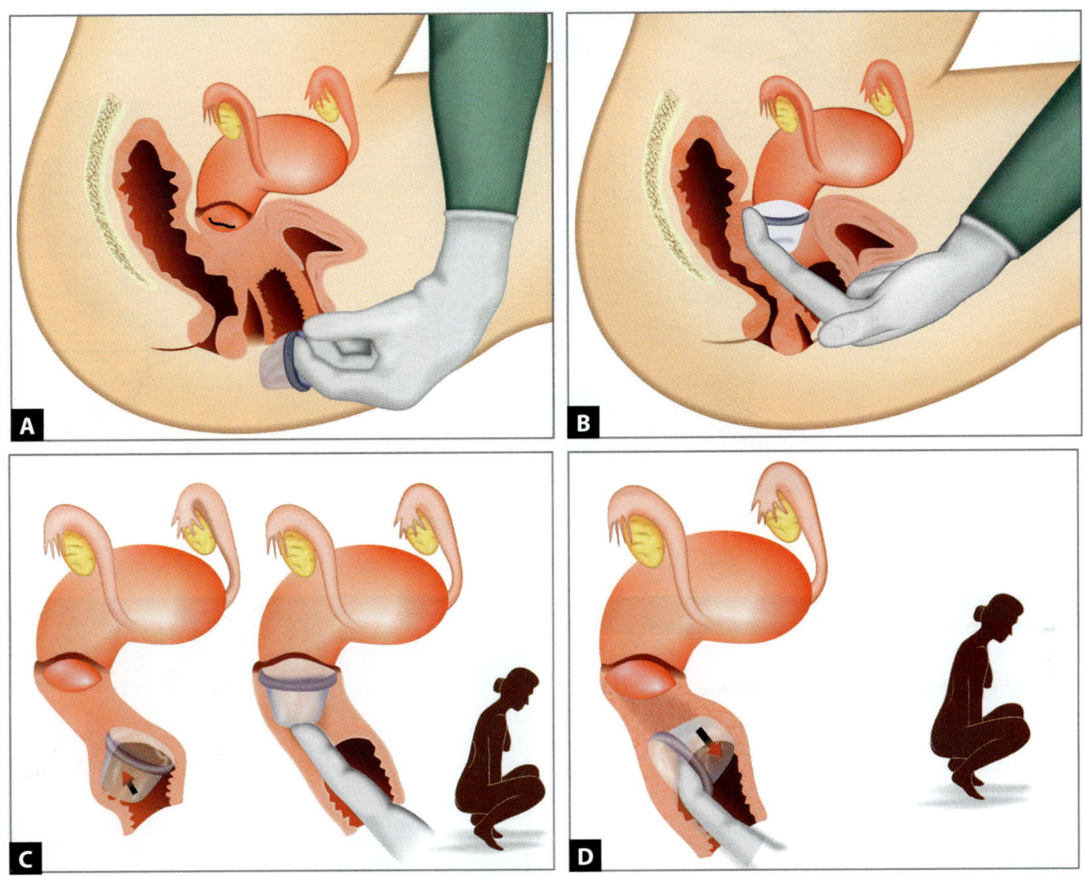

Figs. 14A to D: Insertion and removal of cervical cap.

2 days, but some women develop a foul-smelling discharge by then.

Efficacy: Failure rate: 2–20 per HWY of use.

Fem Cap

The fem cap, made of nonallergic silicone rubber, is shaped like a sailor's hat, a design that allows a better fit over the cervix and in the vaginal fornices and provides a rim for easier removal. This cap may be easier to fit and use. There are two sizes, one for nulliparous women and a larger size for multiparous women. Because some women experience difficulty in removing fem cap, a modified fem cap (with removal strap) is being evaluated.

Contraceptive Sponge or Today Sponge (Figs. 15A and B)

Sponge is a safe and nonhormonal form of contraception, which provides protection for nearly 24 hours. The contraceptive sponge is marketed under the brand name of Today's sponge in the United States, and the brand names of Protectaid and Pharmatex sponges in the United Kingdom (UK). Besides acting as a physical barrier, it also contains a spermicidal agent (nonoxynol-9). The sponges provide contraceptive action in two ways. One is by preventing the sperm from moving inside the cervix. Second is the presence of spermicide in the sponge, which causes immobilisation of the sperm. Success rates with the use of Today's sponge have been found to vary between 77% and 91%. Though Today's sponge was first launched in 1983, it was withdrawn from the market in 1994 due to the probable risk of TSS and again launched in 2009 because the linkage with TSS remained unproven.

Method of application: Before insertion, the sponge is soaked in water, so that it gets completely wet. This causes activation of the spermicidal agent. Then it is inserted inside the vagina so that it covers the cervix.

It can be inserted up to 24 hours before the sexual intercourse. It should be inserted about 6 hours following sexual intercourse. However, it should not be worn for >30 hours in one go.

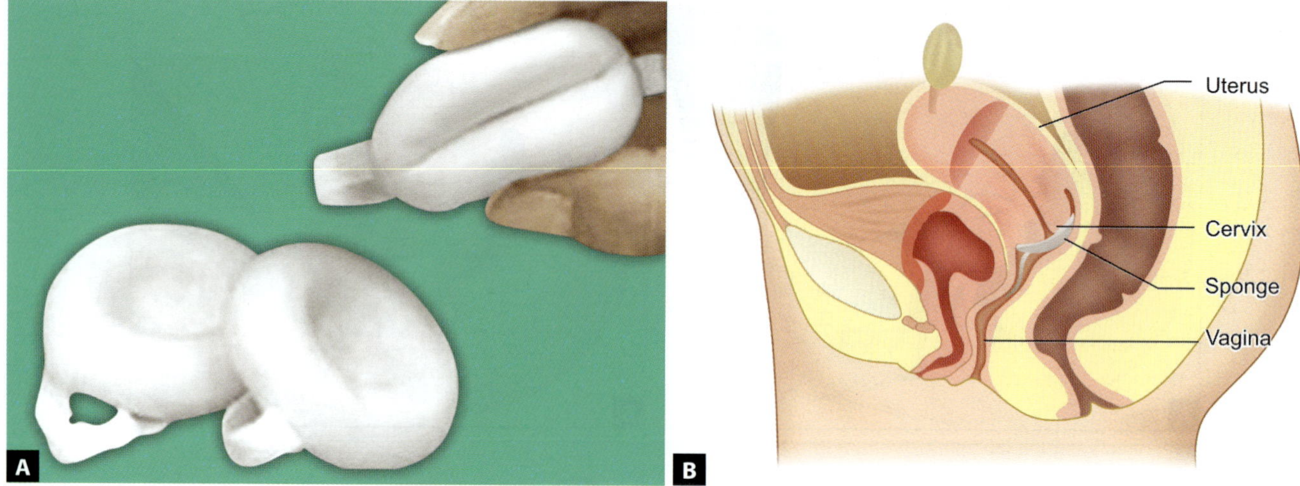

Figs. 15A and B: (A) Today's sponge; (B) Application of Today's sponge.

TABLE 2: Timings of various methods.

	Diaphragm	*Cap*	*Sponge*	*Female condom*
Insertion before coitus, no longer than	6 hours	6 hours	24 hours	8 hours
After coitus, it should be left in place for	6 hours	8 hours	6 hours	—
Maximal wear time	24 hours	48 hours	30 hours	8 hours

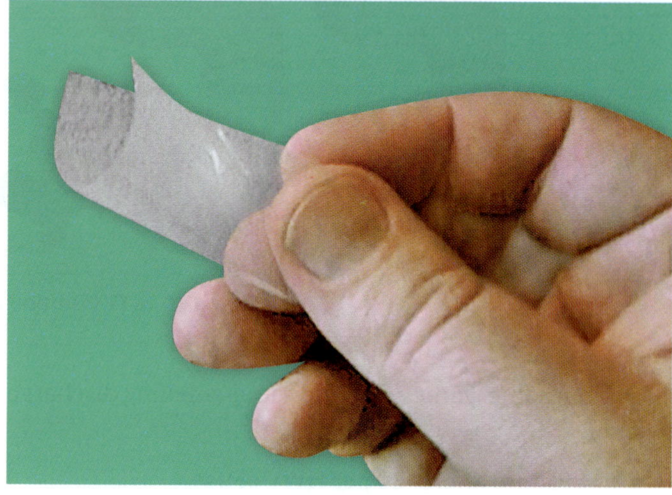

Fig. 16: Vaginal contraceptive film.

According to different timings, various female barrier methods are used. **Table 2** compares usage timings of various female barrier methods.

Vaginal Contraceptive Film (Fig. 16)

Vaginal contraceptive film (VCF) is a nonhormonal, safe and effective form of barrier contraception, which is in form of a plastic film containing a spermicidal agent. It provides protection within 15 minutes of use and remains active up to 3 hours. It can be used several times a day. However, it is less effective than other barrier methods of contraception.

The VCF can be inserted deep inside the vagina by either of the partners. First the VCF is held between the index finger and thumb, and then using the fingertip, it is inserted deep inside the vagina over the cervix. Once inside the vagina, it dissolves to form gel-like substance, containing a spermicidal agent.

Spermicides

- Various chemicals and wide variety of vehicles have been used vaginally as contraceptives for centuries.
- Modern spermicidal agents, introduced in 1950s, contain surface active agents that damage the sperm cell membranes; this same action occurs with bacteria and viruses, explaining the protection against STDs.
- The agents currently used are:
  - Nonoxynol-9
  - Octoxynol-9
  - Benzalkonium chloride
  - Menfegol
- Most preparations contain 60–100 mg of these agents in each vaginal application with concentration ranging from 2% to 12.5%.

- Available in the form of foam, jellies, creams, VCF and suppositories.
- 'Advantage 24' is a contraceptive gel that adheres to the vaginal mucosa and provide longer availability of nonoxynol-9 effective for 24 hours.

Efficacy: Failure rate of approximately 20–25/HWY during a year of use is most typical.

- The principal minor problem is allergy that occurs in 1–5% of users.
- Spermicide users who have an altered vaginal flora, providing the colonisation of *Escherichia coli*, leads to greater susceptibility of urinary tract infections.
- Spermicides should not be used without condoms if the primary objective is to prevent infection with HIV, gonorrhoea and chlamydia.

INTRAUTERINE CONTRACEPTIVE DEVICES

- Intrauterine contraceptive devices are made of plastic or metal, or a combination of these materials, meant for insertion into the uterine cavity for contraception.
- The IUCD is the second most commonly used family planning method, after voluntary female sterilisation (WHO, 1997).
- IUCDs are an effective, safe, and convenient contraceptive method. They are particularly suitable for a woman who:
  - Wants to delay pregnancy for some years
  - Is breastfeeding
  - Prefers a method that does not require supervision or action before sexual intercourse.

History

The first widely used IUCD was introduced in Germany by Gräfenberg in the late 1920s known as the Gräfenberg ring. Ota rings were developed in Japan. These are composed of relatively nonirritant metals such as silver, gold and alloys of copper (Cu). The addition of Cu was suggested by Zipper. The Progestasert was developed by Alza Corporation. The progesterone diminishes the account of cramping and the amount of blood loss. The short lifespan has been solved by using more potent progesterone, such as levonorgestrel (LNG). The IUCDs of the future will possibly be medicated and frameless.

Types of Intrauterine Contraceptive Devices (Figs. 17 to 31)

Various types of IUCDs are enumerated further and are described in detail next.

- Unmedicated or inert IUCDs, e.g. Lippes loop, Saf-T-coil, Ota ring and Mahua ring
- Medicated IUCDs, e.g. Cu-releasing IUCDs—Cu 7, CuT 200, Multiload Cu 250, Multiload Cu 375, Nova T, CuT 380Ag and CuT 380A.

  Hormone-releasing IUCDs—Progestasert, LNG IUCD.

As previously described, IUCDs are flexible plastic devices,

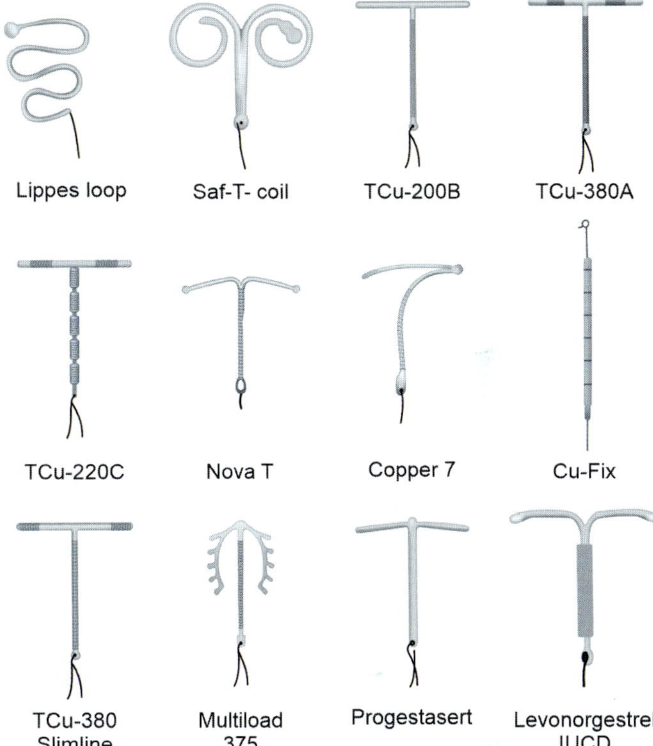

Fig. 17: Types of intrauterine contraceptive devices (IUCDs).

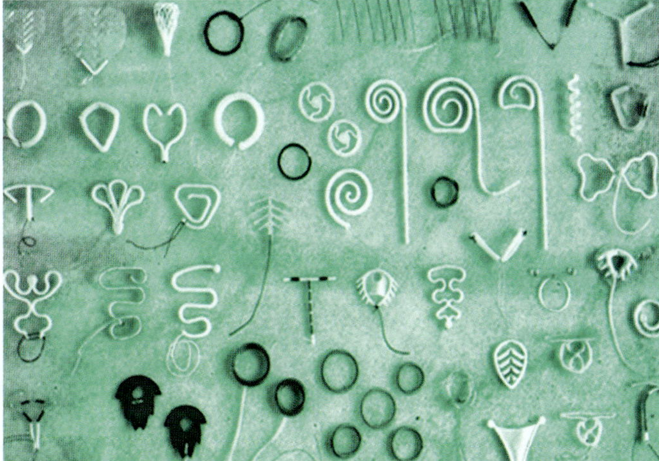

Fig. 18: Varieties of intrauterine contraceptive device (IUCD) seen in the ortho intrauterine device (IUD) collection. The history of the contraceptive museum.

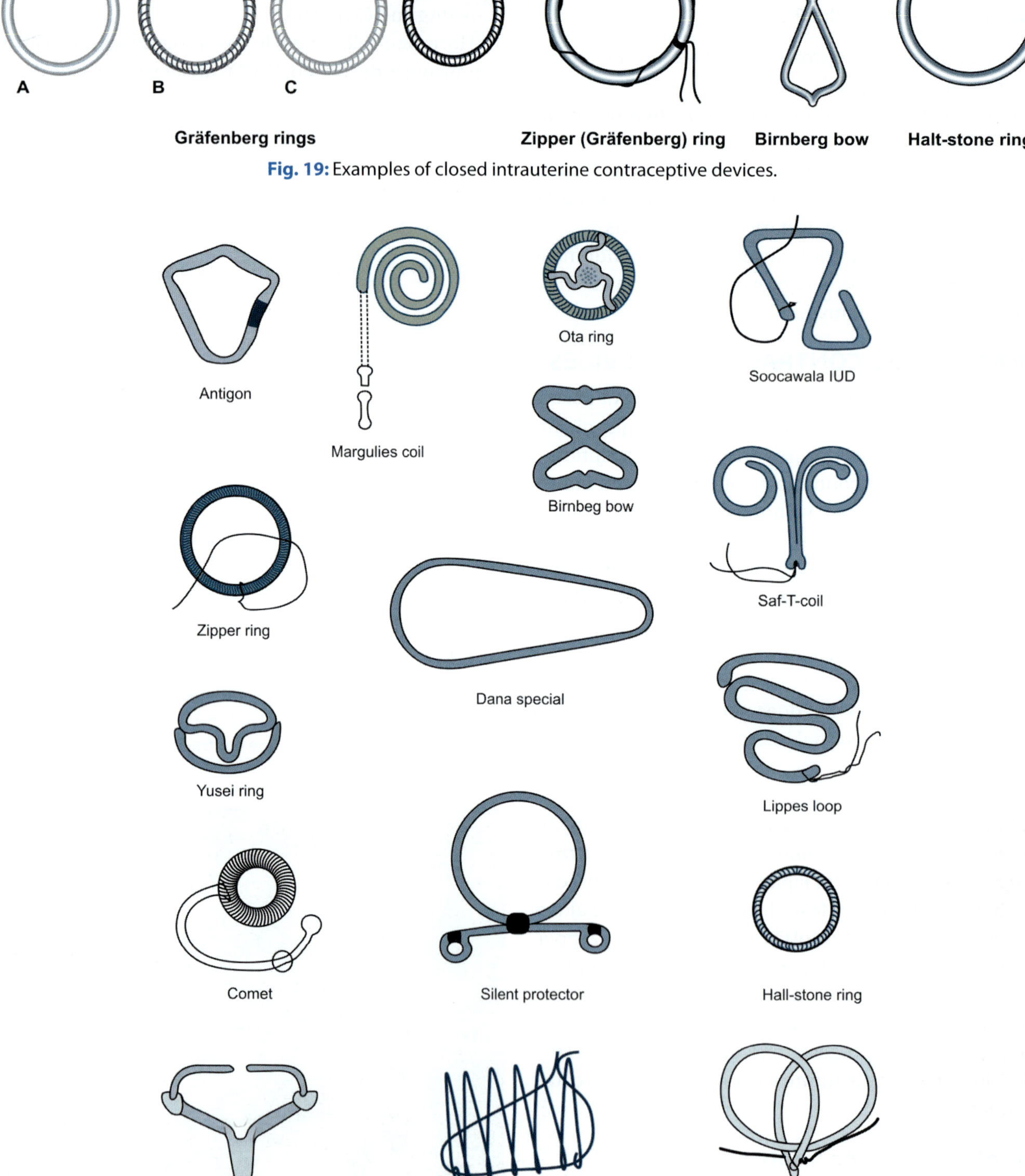

Fig. 19: Examples of closed intrauterine contraceptive devices.

Fig. 20: Other varieties of closed types of intrauterine contraceptive devices (IUCDs).

made up of polyethylene, which are inserted inside the uterine cavity for the purpose of contraception. Each device has a nylon thread, which protrudes through the cervical canal into the vagina, where it can be felt by the patient or the doctor. Initially, biologically inert devices such as Lippes loop and saf-T-coil were introduced, which have now been withdrawn from the market. Newer devices are medicated and contain substances such as Cu and progestogens. Cu-carrying devices include CuT 200, Cu 7, multiload Cu 250, CuT 380, CuT 220 and Nova T. Their effective life varies from 3 to 5 years. T-shaped IUCDs (CuT 380A or Paraguard), which have Cu on their arms,

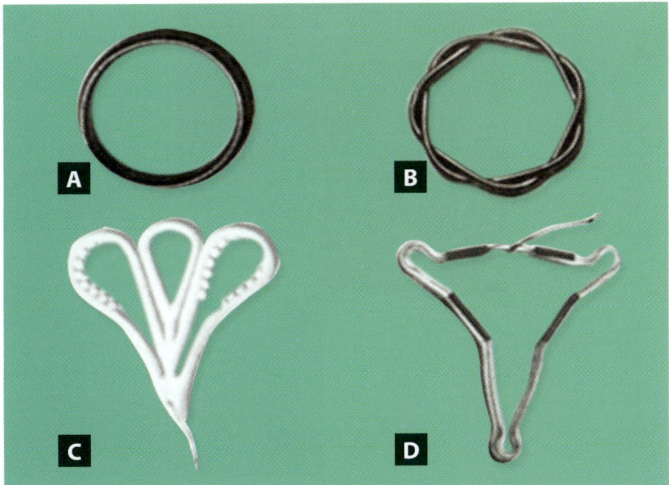

Figs. 21A to D: Commonly used and popular intrauterine contraceptive devices (IUCDs), used in China; (A) Single stainless steel; (B) Double-coiled mahua ring; (C) Canton flower with flexible plastic petals; (D) Shanghai copper V 200.

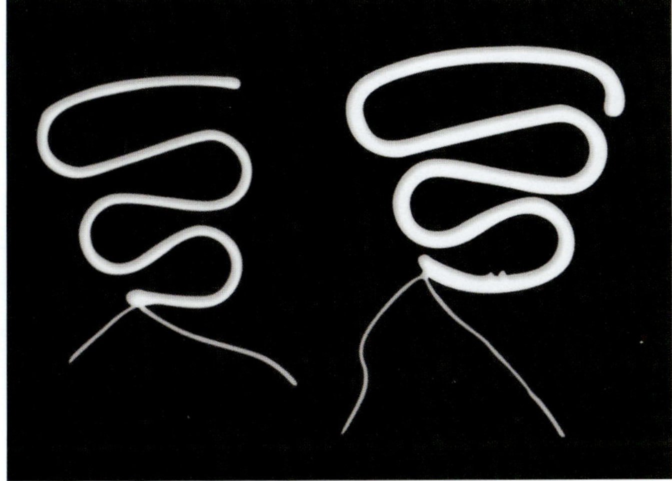

Fig. 22: Lippes loop.

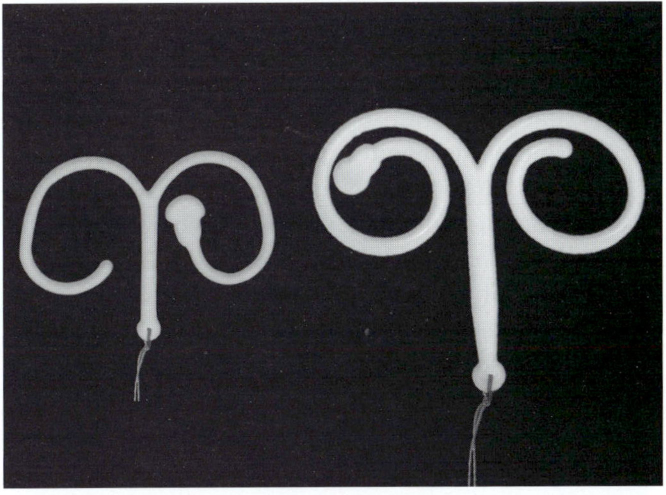

Fig. 23: Saf-T-coil.

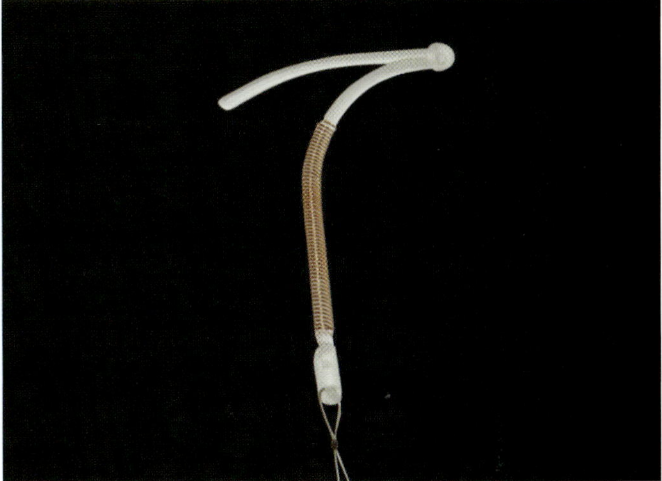

Fig. 24: Copper 7 or Gravigard.

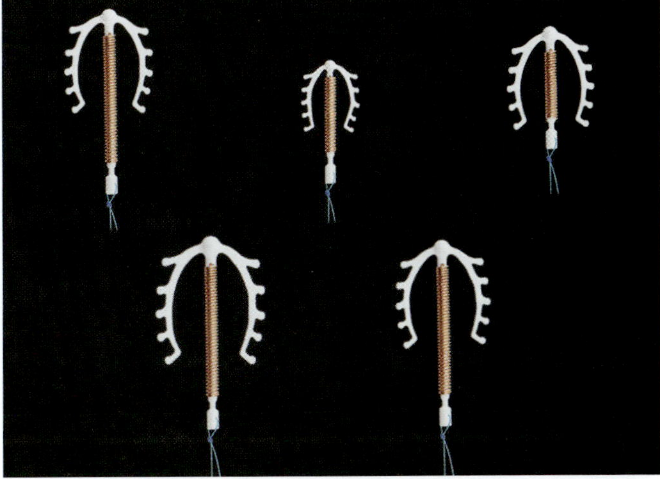

Fig. 25: Multiload intrauterine contraceptive device (IUCD) available in different sizes.

containing at least 380 mm^2 of Cu, can be considered as the IUCD of choice. They are likely to be most effective and have the longest duration of action (approximately 10–12 years). A state-of-the-art recent advance in intrauterine contraception has been the development of the SCu300A intrauterine ball (IUB). This is 3D (3-dimensional), spherical Cu IUCD, which is inserted and removed in a manner similar to the 2D T-shaped IUCDs. It is spherical in shape, which helps in reducing the likelihood of complications such as perforation, malposition and expulsion.

Intrauterine contraceptive devices containing progestogen include Progestasert, Levosert and Mirena®.

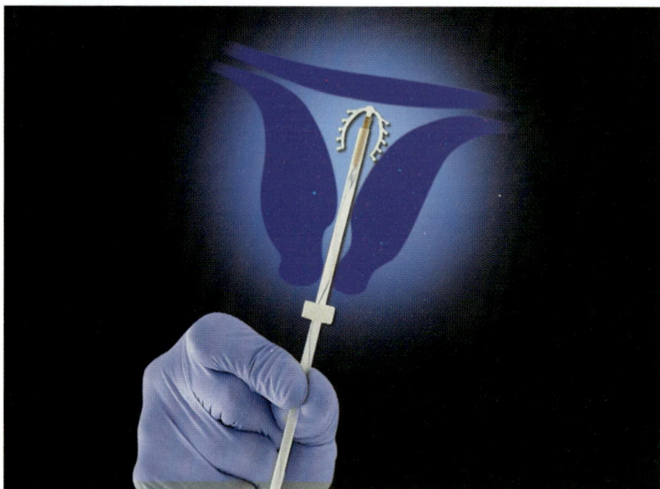

Fig. 26: Multiload with intrauterine contraceptive device (IUCD) inserter.

These devices are known as an intrauterine system (IUS). Mirena® is a type of progestogen-containing IUCD, having 52 mg of LNG, which is released at the rate of 20 µg/day. The effects of Mirena® last for about 5 years. It is sometimes also known as levonorgestrel intrauterine system (LNG IUS). Using 90 consecutive days with no bleeding or spotting as criteria for amenorrhoea, 20% of

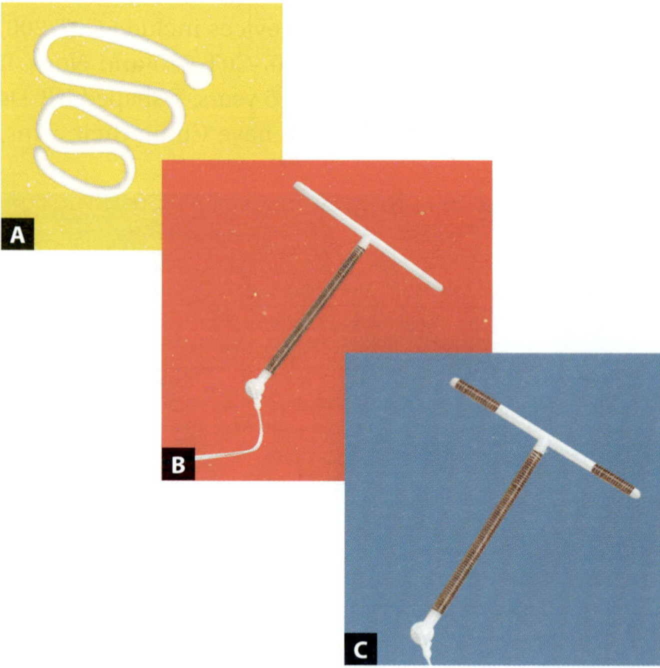

Figs. 28A to C: (A) First-generation intrauterine contraceptive device (IUCD) is Lippes loop; (B) Second-generation IUCD is copper T200; (C) Third-generation IUCD is Gyne T380 with 4 years of intrauterine life.

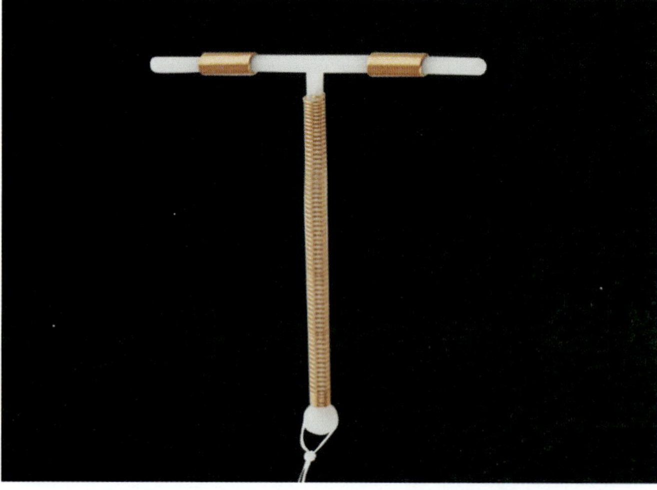

Fig. 27: Copper (Cu) T 380A and CuT 380 Ag.

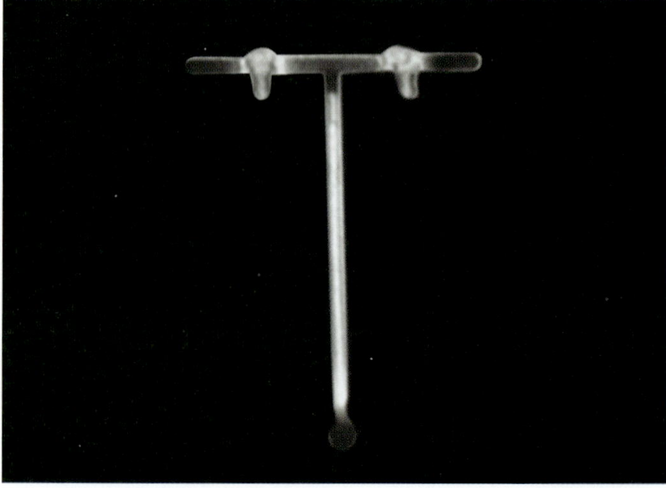

Fig. 29: Intrauterine contraceptive device (IUCD) for postpartum insertion.

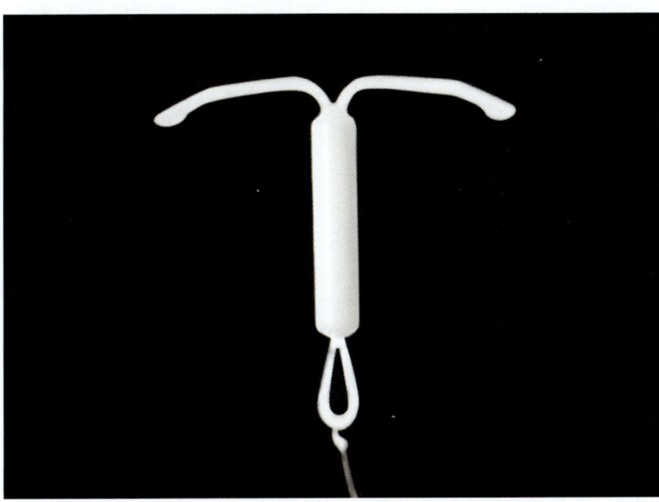

Fig. 30: Fourth-generation intrauterine contraceptive device (IUCD).

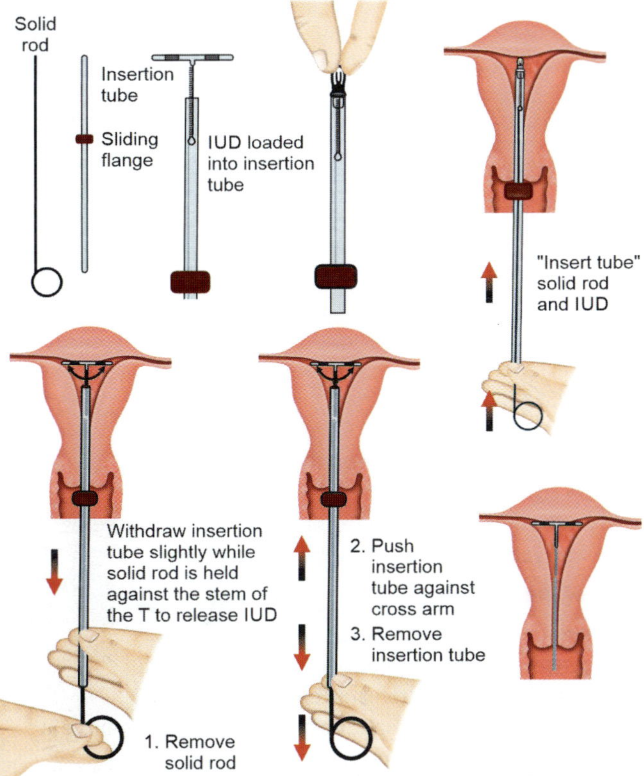

Fig. 31: Techniques of insertion.

LNG IUS users are amenorrhoeic after 1 year of use. The WHO medical eligibility criteria for the use of LNG IUS are elucidated in **Table 3**.

Another LNG IUS, which has been recently introduced in the UK, is Jaydess®, also known as Skyla® (Bayer). It is slightly smaller in size in comparison to Mirena® **(Table 4)**. As a result, this device can be used in younger and even nulliparous women. Jaydess® contains 13.5 mg of LNG, which is released at the rate of 6–10 μg/day. It is licensed for use for a period of 3 years. It has a silver ring, which differentiates it from Mirena® on ultrasound and enables its visualisation by X-ray. Initial placement of Jaydess® is easier and less painful for women in comparison to Mirena®. However, the bleeding profiles of both are similar. The advantages of the LNG IUS are explained in **Box 2**.

Progestasert is a T-shaped IUCD made of ethylene vinyl acetate copolymer-containing titanium oxide. The vertical stem contains a reservoir of 38 mg progesterone together with barium sulphate dispersed in silicone fluid. The horizontal arms are solid and made of the same copolymer. Two blue-black monofilament strings are attached at a hole in the base of the stem. The progesterone is released at a rate of 65 μg/day. Its effective lifespan is only 1 year.

New Types of Intrauterine Contraceptive Devices

Introduction of the hormone-containing IUS has been the latest addition to the IUCDs. The first LNG IUS to be introduced was Mirena (LNG IUS 20) in the year 2000; and Mirena has been discussed in detail previously in the text. It is a highly effective method of contraception. However, its use may be associated with several side effects such as systemic exposure to higher concentration of LNG, difficulty in insertion, risk of perforation, pain, risk of expulsion, bleeding irregularities, PID, and fear of subsequent infertility. This has led to a demand for further improvement of the currently available IUS.

A new, smaller version of LNG-releasing IUS (IUS-12) has been introduced since the year 2013 and is being marketed as 'Skyla' in the US and 'Jaydess' elsewhere. Skyla and Jaydess have been previously described in the text. Due to their smaller size and lower LNG content, these IUS are able to better address the needs of nulliparous women. On March 2, 2015, the FDA approved another new intrauterine device (IUD), Liletta, which was designed keeping in mind the concept of affordability. Liletta is already available in Europe.

Liletta

Liletta is a novel 52 mg LNG-releasing IUD from Actavis with a T-shaped polyethylene frame packaged with a

TABLE 3: The World Health Organization (WHO) medical eligibility criteria for use of levonorgestrel intrauterine system [LNG IUS (Mirena®)].

UKMEC category I:

- Postpartum is between 0 hours and 48 hours and ≥4 weeks
- Age >20 years
- *Thyroid disorders*: Simple goitre, hyperthyroid and hypothyroid
- Obesity ≥30 kg/m^2 BMI and menarche to <18 years and ≥30 kg/m^2 BMI
- Endometriosis
- *Anaemias:* Thalassaemia, sickle cell disease and iron-deficiency anaemia
- *Diabetes:* History of gestational disease
- Irregular pattern without heavy bleeding and heavy or prolonged bleeding (includes regular and irregular patterns)
- *Schistosomiasis:*
  - Uncomplicated, fibrosis of the liver (if severe, cirrhosis)
- *Neurological conditions*:
  - Idiopathic intracranial hypertension
  - Epilepsy
  - Depressive disorders
- *Cardiovascular disease*:
  - Cardiomyopathy—normal cardiac function
  - Cardiac arrhythmias—known as long QT syndrome—continuation
- *Breast and reproductive tract conditions*:
  - Gestational trophoblastic disease (GTD)—undetectable hCG levels

UKMEC category II:

- *Age*: Menarche to <20 years
- *Gastrointestinal conditions*: Gallbladder disease, history of cholestasis
- *Cardiovascular disease*:
  - Known dyslipidaemias
  - Cardiomyopathy—impaired cardiac function
  - Cardiac arrhythmias—atrial fibrillation
- *Breast and reproductive tract conditions*:
  - Breast conditions—undiagnosed mass/breast symptoms
  - Carriers of known gene mutations associated with breast cancer (e.g. *BRCA1/BRCA2*)
- Systemic lupus erythematosus (SLE)—severe thrombocytopaenia
- *Diabetes*: Nonvascular disease—noninsulin dependent, insulin dependent, nephropathy/retinopathy/neuropathy, etc.
- *Human immunodeficiency virus infection*: High risk of HIV infection and CD4 count ≥200 cells/mm^3
- *Rheumatic diseases*: Rheumatoid arthritis, SLE with no antiphospholipid antibodies and positive antiphospholipid antibodies
- *Neurological conditions*: Migraine without aura at age <35 years and age >35 years, with aura, at any age

Initiation of method	***Continuation of the method***
	• *Breast and reproductive tract conditions*: – Cervical cancer—awaiting treatment – *Ovarian cancer*—Sexually transmitted infections (STIs)—asymptomatic and symptomatic chlamydial infection, purulent cervicitis or gonorrhoea (current), etc. • *HIV infection*: CD4 count <200 cells/mm^3

UKMEC category III:

- SLE—unknown or positive antiphospholipid antibodies
- *Neurological conditions*: Migraine with aura at any age
- *Breast and reproductive tract conditions*:
  - Gestational trophoblastic disease (GTD)—decreasing hCG levels
  - Cervical cancer—radical trachelectomy

Contd...

Contd...

Initiation of method	***Continuation of the method***

• Postpartum is between 48 hours and <4 weeks
• Cirrhosis—severe, decompensated
• Liver tumours—malignant hepatoma and hepatocellular adenoma
• AIDS
• Organ transplant
  – *Complicated*: Graft failure (acute or chronic), rejection, and cardiac allograft vasculopathy
  – *Cardiac arrhythmias*: Known long QT syndrome
• *HIV infection*: CD4 count <200 cells/mm^3
	• Past and present history of ischaemic heart disease
	• Stroke
	• Pelvic tuberculosis

UKMEC category IV:	
• Breast and reproductive tract conditions: Gestational trophoblastic disease (GTD)—persistently elevated hCG levels or malignant disease	
Initiation of method	***Continuation of the method***
• Puerperal sepsis • Postseptic abortion • Unexplained vaginal bleeding • GTD—malignant disease or persistently elevated β-hCG levels • Cervical cancer in women awaiting treatment • Endometrial cancer • Ovarian cancer • Breast cancer—current • Current pelvic inflammatory disease (PID), purulent cervicitis, or symptomatic and asymptomatic chlamydial infection • Pelvic tuberculosis • *Breast and reproductive tract conditions*: – Cervical cancer—awaiting treatment	

(AIDS: acquired immunodeficiency syndrome; BMI: body mass index; hCG: human chorionic gonadotrophin; UKMEC: UK Medical Eligibility for Contraceptive Use)

Source: WHO. Medical eligibility criteria for contraceptive use, 5th edition. Switzerland: WHO Press, WHO; 2015.

TABLE 4: Comparison of size between Mirena® and Jaydess®.

Type of IUS	*Height (mm)*	*Breadth (mm)*
Mirena®	32	32
Jaydess® (Skyla)®	30	28

(IUS: intrauterine system)

sterilised inserter. Initially, the release rate of LNG is 18.6 µg daily, and it drops progressively to 16.3 µg/day at 1 year, 14.3 µg/day at 2 years, and 12.6 µg/day at 3 years. In the clinical trials, the most common adverse reactions were vaginal infections (13.6%), vulvovaginal infections (13.3%), acne (12.3%), headache or migraine (99.8%), nausea or vomiting (7.8%), dyspareunia (7%), abdominal pain or discomfort (96.8%), breast tenderness or pain (6.7%), pelvic pain (6.1%), depression (5.4%) and mood changes (5.2%).

Liletta will be the fourth IUD currently available in the United States, whenever it will be released. It joins ParaGard (also called the CuT), which began being sold to women in the United States in 1988. **Table 5 and Figure 32** describe contrasts amongst the three most effective hormonal IUDs.

Future Intrauterine Contraceptive Devices

These include Flexiguard, GyneFix, CuFix and Fibroplant for the perimenopausal women.

GyneFix

GyneFix is a frameless Cu IUD containing several Cu cylinders strung together, which is then anchored into the uterus. Development of the string-shaped and flexible design of the GyneFix device aimed at a significant

BOX 2: Advantages of the levonorgestrel intrauterine system.

Contraceptive advantages:
- *Safe:* Associated mortality is estimated to be <1 in 500,000
- High efficacy
- Low accidental pregnancies
- Can be used in the interval period or after an abortion
- Sexually convenient
- Better compliance compared to oral contraceptives
- Long acting
- Continuation rates are high—can be used for a longer duration
- Reversible
- Immediate return of fertility after removal

Other health benefits like:
- Lessening of menstrual blood loss and duration of loss
- Better iron balance
- Better life quality
- Reduction of dysmenorrhoea
- Lower risk of PID and endometritis
- Lower risk of ectopic pregnancy
- Less abortions
- Less endometriosis

(PID: pelvic inflammatory disease)

TABLE 5: Comparison between three intrauterine systems (IUS).

Characteristic	*Mirena*	*Skyla*	*Liletta*
Hormone	Levo-norgestrel	Levo-norgestrel	Levo-norgestrel
Efficacy	99%	99%	99%
String colour	Black	Black	Blue
Size	32 mm × 32 mm	29 mm × 30 mm	32 mm × 32 mm
Commercial cost	$810.51	$650.32	$625.00
340B cost	$322.25	$497.18	$50.00
Evidence-based duration	7 years	3 years	7 years
Dose of levonorgestrel	52 mg	13.5 mg	52 mg

enhancement of the acceptability of the method and a significant reduction of side effects commonly seen with conventional IUDs, such as pain and bleeding.

GyneFix is a newly developed nonhormonal intrauterine contraceptive. It is made up of a small and flexible chain with four (GyneFix mini) or six (GyneFix standard) Cu sleeves, each 5 mm in length and 2.2 mm in diameter **(Figs. 33A and B)**. The six Cu sleeves are threaded, and the uppermost and lowest sleeves are crimped onto polypropylene suture thread.

A single knot is made in the upper portion of the thread, which serves as a small retention body when inserted in the myometrium of the uterine fundus at a controlled depth of 1.0 cm. The weight of the six Cu cylinders is 420 mg, and the total surface of Cu, including the inner and outer surfaces, is approximately 330 mm^2. Notably, the GyneFix lacks a plastic frame and this accounts for its flexibility. The anchoring system is essential for the retention of the frameless device.

Its flexibility means that the Cu IUD can adapt to all movements and cannot be felt either during physical activity or throughout the menstrual cycle. It is fixed in the upper part of the uterus using a small hook to prevent slippage. The GyneFix Cu chain is also known as an intrauterine implant (IUI).

Mode of action: The Cu ions that are released from the Cu sleeves in small quantities reduce the mobility of the sperm and prevent any fertilised egg cells from implanting in the uterus. The balance of hormones is not affected. The natural menstrual cycle is retained, and ovulation occurs as usual.

Duration of use: It is effective for up to 5 years of use.

Effectiveness: It can be considered to be highly effective with a Pearl index of 0.1–0.9.

Insertion: The GyneFix Cu IUD is inserted into the uterus through the cervix with the help of an insertion sleeve. If possible, the GyneFix should be inserted during a woman's period when the cervix is slightly open.

During the procedure, the woman may experience a pulling pain, but this is generally well tolerated. If desired, the Cu IUD may be inserted under general anaesthetic. The insertion instrument to anchor the GyneFix IUD in the fundal wall of the uterus consists of two parts. The 3.8 mm wide tube is semirigid to avoid reduction of the inner diameter of the tube during bending.

The plunger has a stainless steel stylet, the pointed end of which is especially shaped with a 'shoulder' or notch that carries the anchoring knot. The proximal end of the plunger is a handle. The IUD is preloaded into the inserter and packed in a peel pack. The units are ethylene oxide—sterilised, ready for use. The flexible Cu chain adjusts to the individual size of the uterus, so women who have not had any children can also use it.

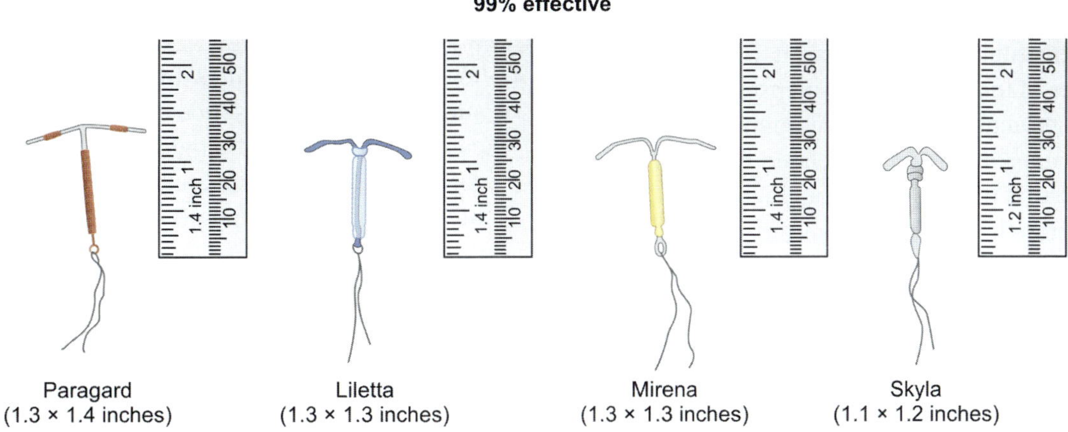

Fig. 32: Different types of intrauterine contraceptive devices (IUCDs).

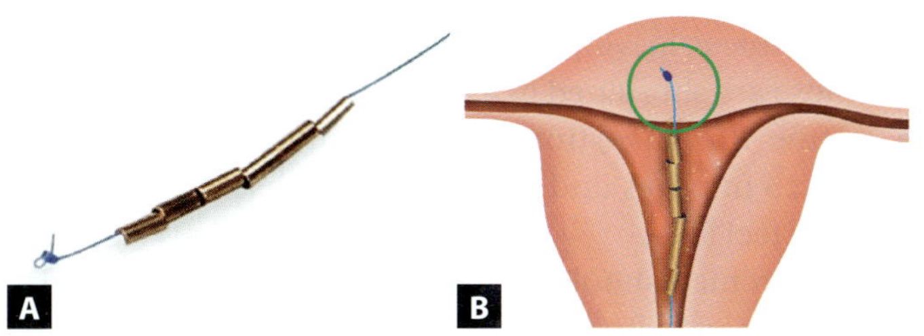

Figs. 33A and B: (A) GyneFix and (B) Insertion of GyneFix into the uterus.

Position check: The position of the GyneFix can be checked at any time using the retrieval thread that protrudes from the cervix. Regular ultrasound examinations every 6 months are also recommended to confirm that the contraceptive is working properly. It is particularly important to check after the first period.

The Cu IUD can be easily and painlessly removed at any time using the retrieval thread. Fertility rapidly returns to normal after removal of the IUD. It is possible to become pregnant immediately.

Complications: The mobility of the Cu chain means that GyneFix is well tolerated. However, there may be lower abdominal pain, heavier menstrual bleeding, breakthrough bleeding or spotting in the early stages. After a period of adjustment, these side effects generally disappear.

The GyneFix Cu chain is suitable for all women who would like a long-term and nonhormonal contraceptive. GyneFix can remain inserted up to 5 years, which means it is a good alternative to sterilisation once family planning is complete.

Mechanism of Action

- The contraceptive action of all IUCDs is mainly in the uterine cavity.
- *Nonmedicated IUCDs*: It depends for contraception on the general reaction of the uterus to a foreign body, a sterile inflammatory response sufficient enough to be spermicidal. So very few, if any, sperm reach to the ovum in the fallopian tube. Inflammatory response would also prevent implantation.
- *Copper IUCDs*: The Cu IUCDs release free Cu and Cu salts that have both a biochemical and morphological impact on the endometrium and also produce alteration in cervical mucus and endometrial secretions. The Cu IUCD is associated with an enhanced inflammatory response, marked by production in the endometrium of cytokine peptides breakdown, and enhanced prostaglandin production.
- *The progesterone-releasing IUCDs*: They add the endometrial action of progesterone to the foreign body reaction. The endometrium becomes decidualised with atrophy of glands. It causes inhibition of implantation and inhibition of sperm capacitation and survival. Progesterone IUCD thickens the cervical mucus, creating a barrier to sperm penetration. They decrease menstrual blood loss (by about 40–50%) and dysmenorrhoea.
- *LNG IUCD*: It produces serum concentration of the progestin about half that of Norplant, so that ovarian follicular development and ovulation are also partially inhibited. Bleeding can be reduced by 90%, 1 year after insertion.

Time of Insertion

- During menstruation or on the last day of menstruation. Advantages of insertion during menses or shortly after are—(1) Cervical canal is more open, so insertion is easier, (2) masking insertion-related bleeding and (3) knowledge that the patient is not pregnant.
- After childbirth, it can be inserted anytime within 48 hours or as early as 4–6 weeks after delivery. The disadvantages of immediate postpartum insertion are a higher expulsion rate and uterine perforation.
- Postcoital insertion should be done within 5 days of unprotected intercourse.
- Postabortal insertion of IUCD can be done safely immediately after evacuation of the uterus. Postabortion insertion has a high acceptance rate.
- Insertion in a lactating woman is safe, as it does not affect the quantity and quality of breast milk.

Insertion Technique (Figs. 34A to C)

- Before any IUCD is inserted, the patient should be informed, preferably in writing, of the principles involved in the method, its possible side effects, management and failure rate. She should give written consent for the insertion.
- Prior to the operation, a complete history and a complete pelvic examination should be carried out to exclude any abnormality and a cervical smear taken for cytology.
- All the plastic IUCDs have their own introducer as well as attached nylon tails, which hang through the cervix into the vagina. These permit the woman and her medical attendant a means of confirming that the device is in place and also of removing it by simple traction.
- The plastic material is impregnated with barium sulphate, so the presence and position of the device can be confirmed radiologically.
- After the application of an antiseptic, the length of the uterine cavity is measured by a uterine sound and its direction confirmed.
- An appropriate device is then chosen and loaded into its introducer, which is passed into the uterus up to its flange or another marker. The method of insertion now depends on the device used. When the Lippes loop plunger is pressed to release the device, it resumes its inherent shape to lie in the uterus. With CuT, the loaded applicator is passed up to the fundus and the sheath is withdrawn to release the device.
- The plunger is then withdrawn together with the introducer, leaving the nylon threads in the vagina, and these are shortened to a reasonable length.
- After the insertion, the patient should rest for 10–15 minutes and remain under observation as she may feel faint.
- The woman should be taught to feel for and recognise the threads. She should also be fully aware of the shape of the IUCD inserted.
- If at any time during the procedure, the woman experiences significant pain or she collapses, the procedure should be abandoned. Difficulty in inserting the sound or introducer through the cervix calls for the greatest caution, because it is easy to make a false track and perforate the tissues **(Figs. 35 and 36)**.
- Localisation of misplaced IUCD is depicted in **Figures 37 to 62**.

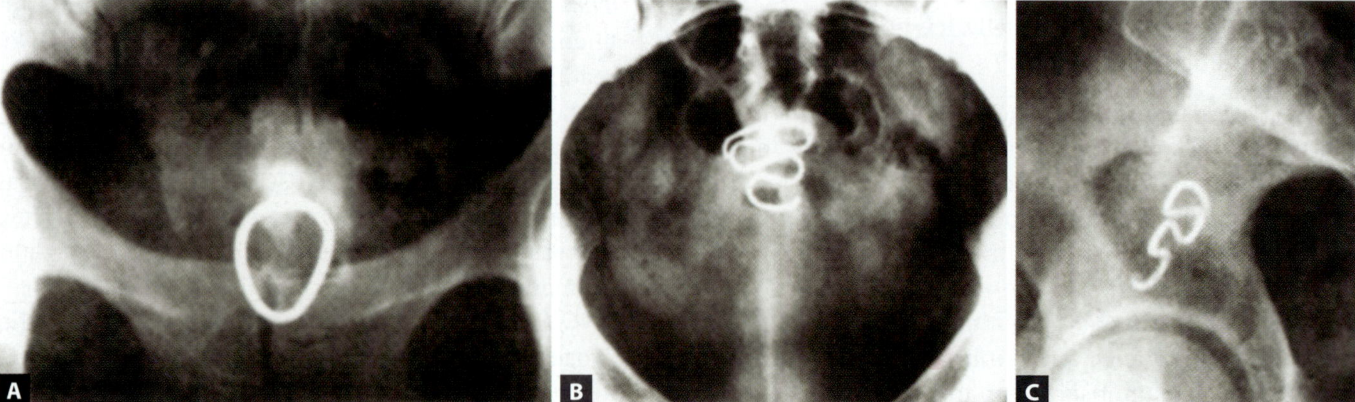

Figs. 34A to C: Devices in proper position in the uterus as shown by radiography. (A) Gräfenberg ring; (B) Lippes loop—anteroposterior view; (C) Lippes loop—lateral view.

Further Supervision and Management

- Before or at the time the IUCD is introduced, the patient should be warned of possible initial reactions such as uterine bleeding and colic, and be told to report any significant reactions immediately.
- In any case, she should have a routine follow-up visit immediately after her next menstrual period, so that the retention of the device can be checked and any adverse side effects discussed.
- Next follow-up after 3–6 months is desirable; thereafter, the woman is seen at yearly intervals, if necessary, the device can be removed and a new one inserted.
- There is no time limit for leaving inert devices in place, and one can remain for several years without any harmful result. Sometimes after a year or two, they do get embedded in the endometrium and cause bleeding and discharge. This is an indication for taking out the device and inserting a new one after the next menses.
- Copper devices need to be replaced at intervals specified by the manufacturers. CuT 200 is recommended for 3 years, multiload 250 for 3 years, multiload 375 for 5 years and CuT 380 lasts for 10 years.

Intrauterine contraceptive device is removed permanently, once the menopause is established or if, at

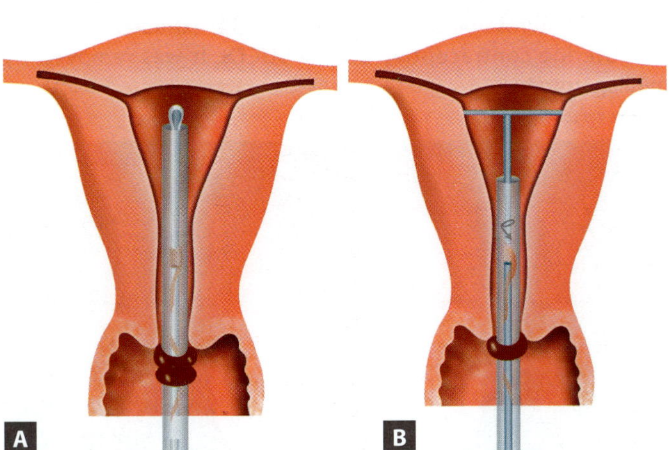

Figs. 35A and B: The principle governing the insertion of a Copper T. (A) The loaded introducer is inserted up to the fundus of the uterus; (B) Insertion is by withdrawal of the introducer over the plunger. The device is removed by pulling out the 'tail'.

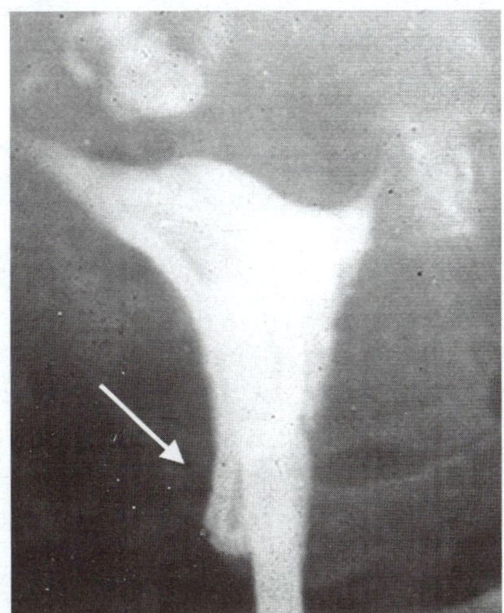

Fig. 37: Intrauterine position of Gräfenberg ring confirmed by doing hysterosalpingography. Gräfenberg ring is partly seen at the lower part of the uterus, as shown by arrow. Both Gräfenberg ring and contrast are radio-opaque.

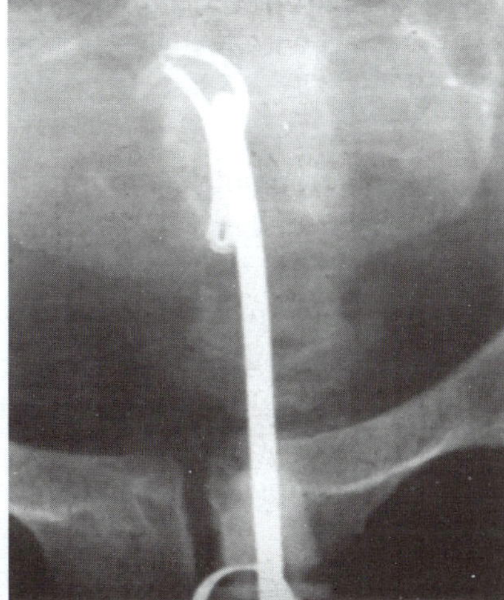

Fig. 36: Intrauterine position of Gräfenberg ring confirmed by putting a uterine sound. Both are in the same line and together.

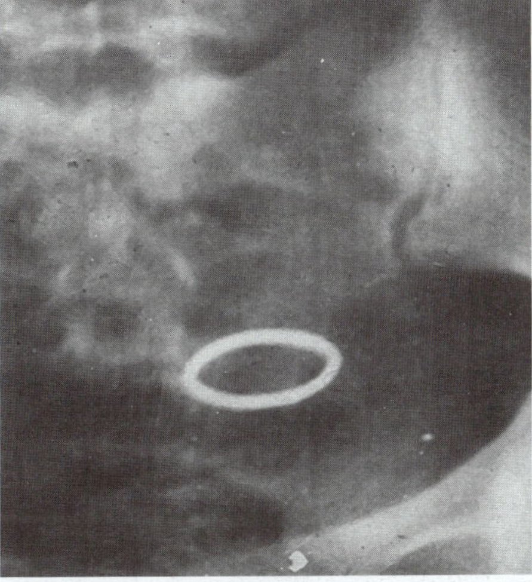

Fig. 38: X-ray showing Gräfenberg ring in the pelvis.

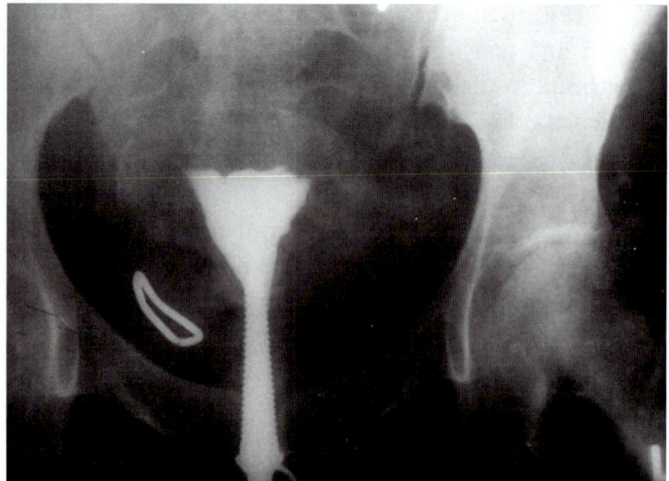

Fig. 39: Extrauterine Gräfenberg ring.

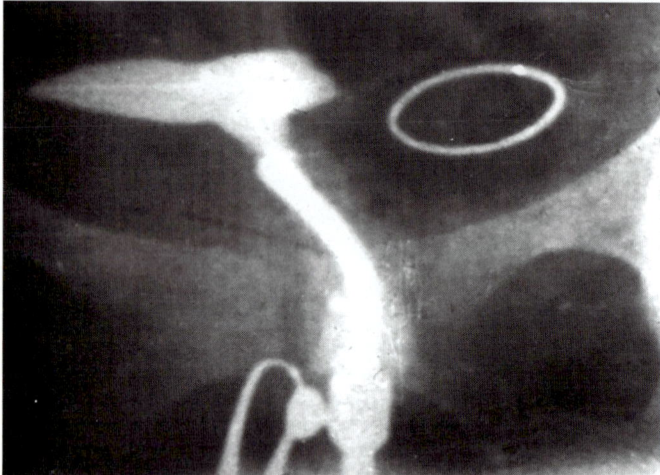

Fig. 40: Hysterosalpingography shows extrauterine position of Gräfenberg ring.

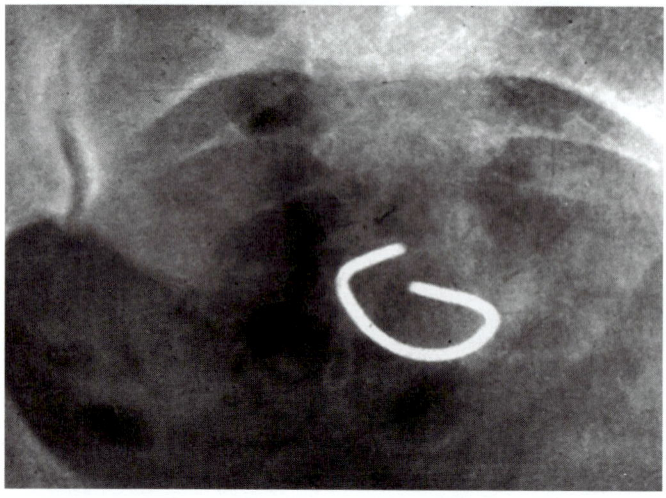

Fig. 41: Broken Gräfenberg ring inserted before 12 years.

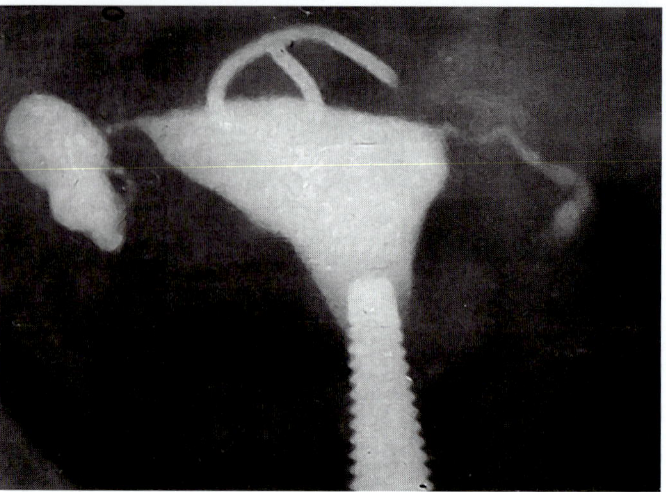

Fig. 42: Hysterosalpingography showing the extrauterine broken intrauterine contraceptive device (IUCD). It was removed by minilaparotomy.

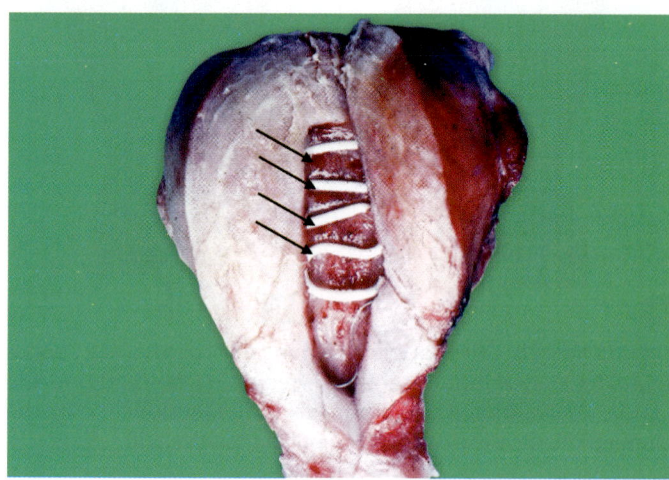

Fig. 43: The position of Lippes loop in the uterus. Please note that each spiral is in contact with another spiral. Lippes loop, when expanded, means extrauterine.

any time, it causes unacceptable symptoms. If the device originally chosen is extruded, it is necessary to replace it with one of a different size or shape.

- Prospective IUCD users should be aware of the following important possibilities:
  - Protection against unwanted pregnancy begins immediately after insertion.
  - Menses can be longer and heavier except for hormonal IUCD.
  - Slightly increased risk of pelvic infection in the first few months after insertion.
  - Protection against STDs requires the use of condoms.

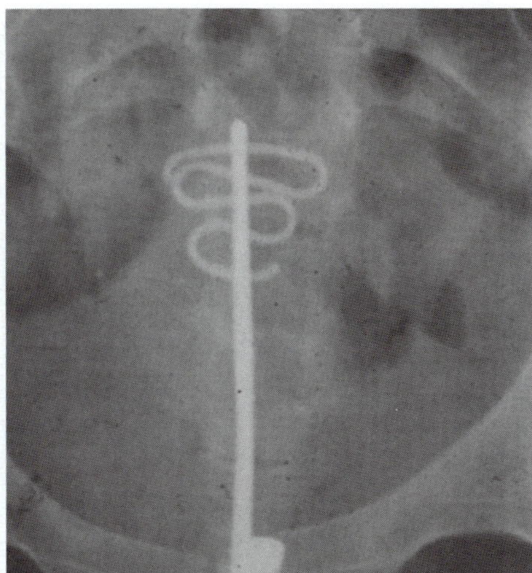

Fig. 44: Lippes loop and uterine sound are in the same line.

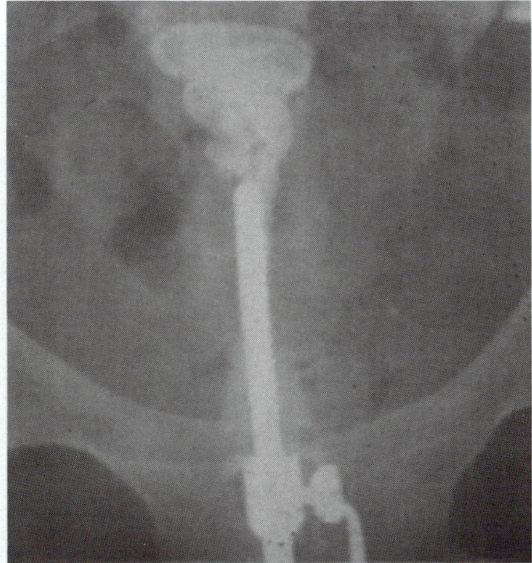

Fig. 45: Intrauterine position of Lippes loop confirmed by injecting contrast medium in uterine cavity. Lippes loop is faintly visible due to contrast, as both are radio-opaque.

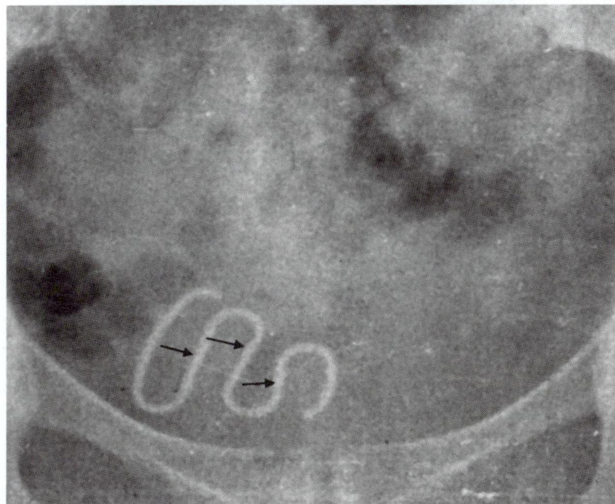

Fig. 46: Extrauterine Lippes loop.

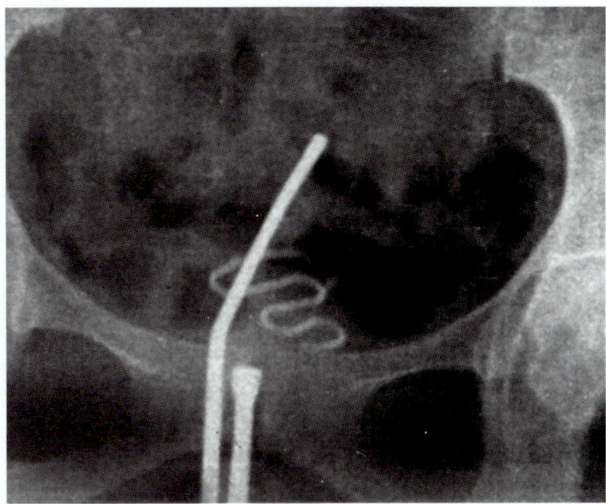

Fig. 47: Extrauterine Lippes loop in pelvis.

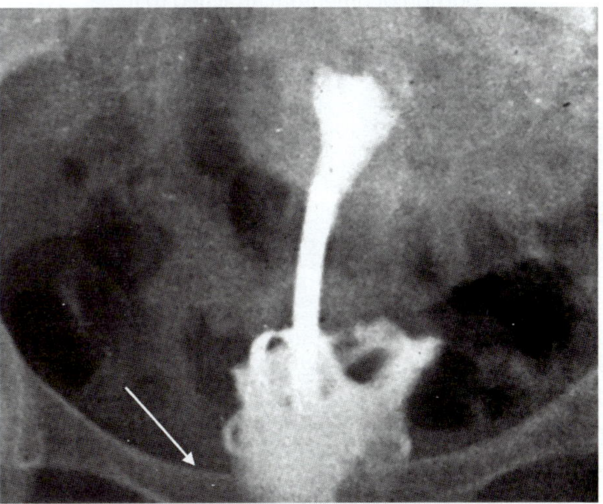

Fig. 48: Lippes loop is near the cervix. Because of contrast, loop is seen only partly as shown by arrow pointer.

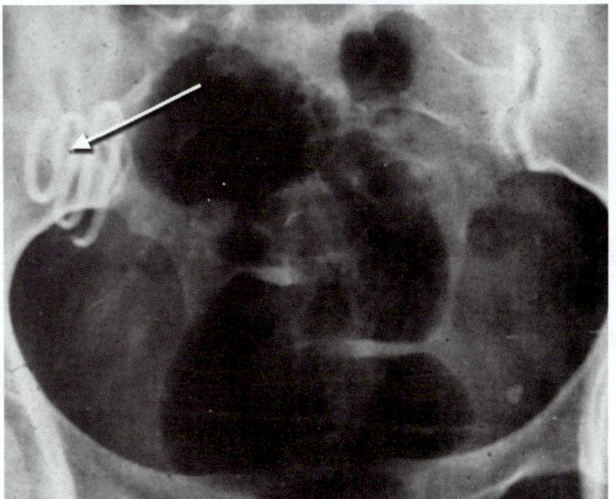

Fig. 49: X-ray pelvis showing Lippes loop in right iliac fossa. Expanded loops indicating extrauterine, as shown by arrow.

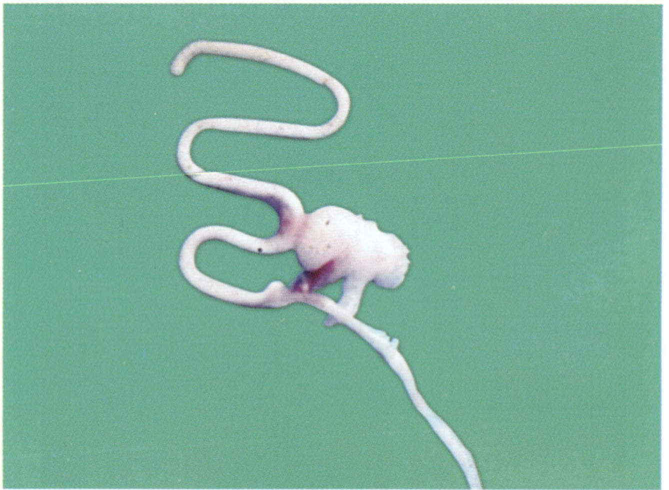

Fig. 50: Lippes loop removed from abdominal cavity. Please note portion of omentum attached to it.

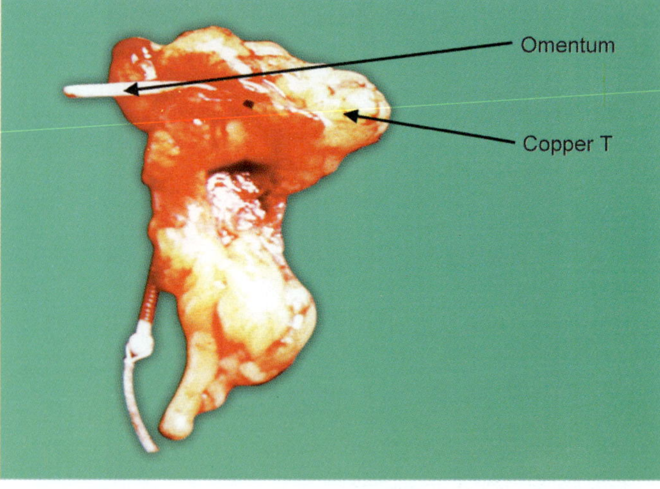

Fig. 53: Copper T entangled in omentum. It was removed by laparotomy.

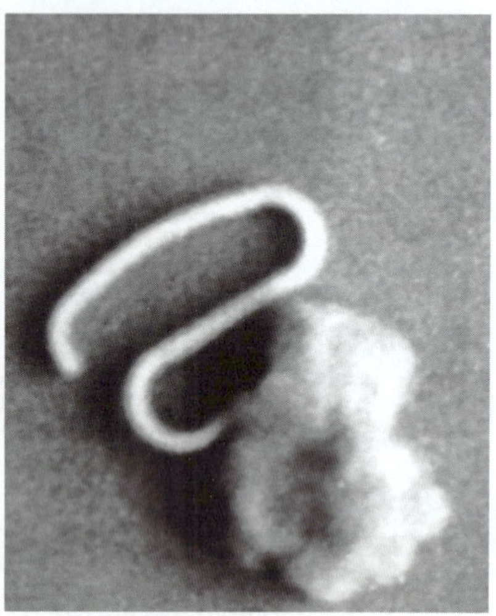

Fig. 51: Slide showing Lippes loop with a piece of omentum. It was removed by laparotomy.

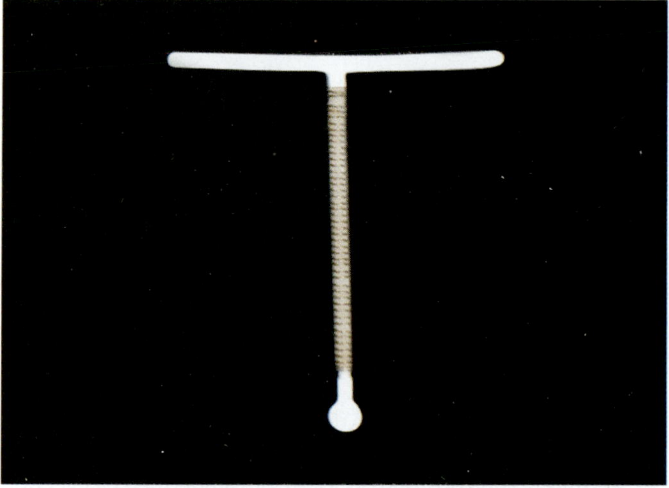

Fig. 54: Copper T (CuT 200).

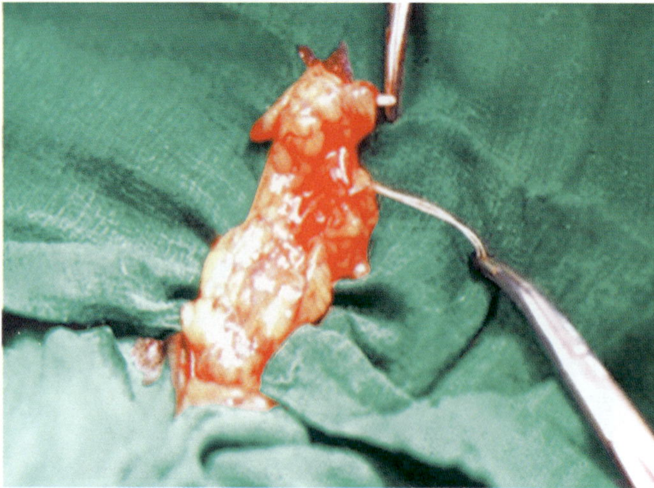

Fig. 52: Copper T embedded in omentum. It was removed by minilaparotomy.

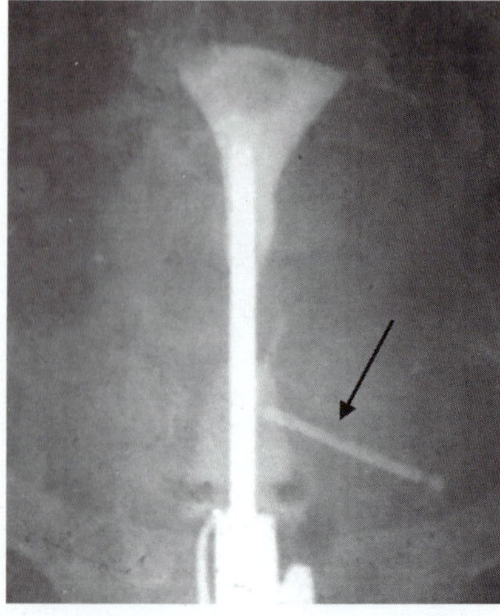

Fig. 55: Hysterosalpingography showing Copper T, extrauterine arrow shows Copper T. It was removed by laparoscopy.

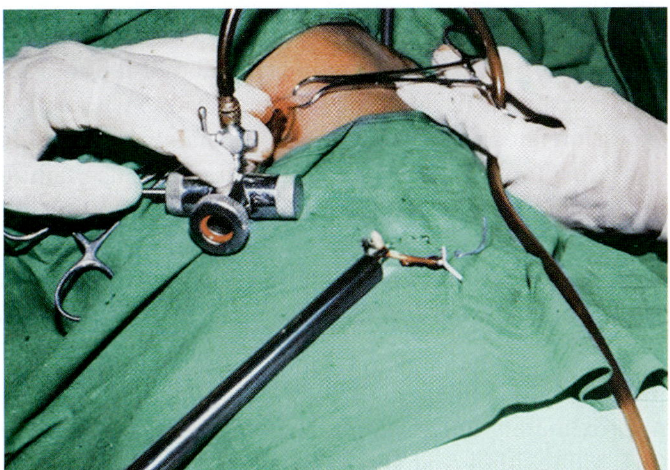

Fig. 56: Copper T was removed in this case by laparoscopy. T is seen being held in the single-puncture laparocator.

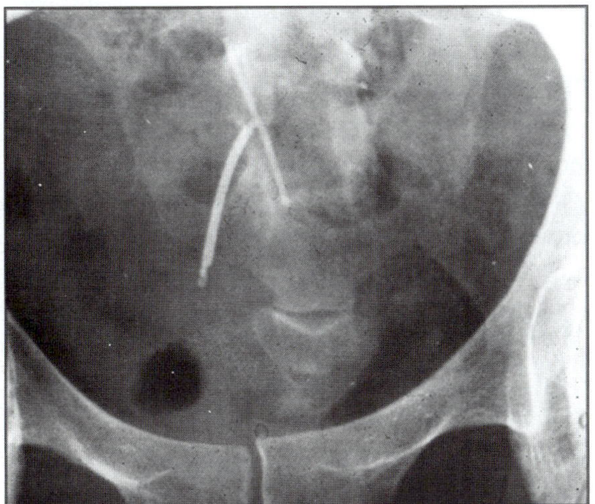

Fig. 57: Copper T seen in pelvis at X-ray.

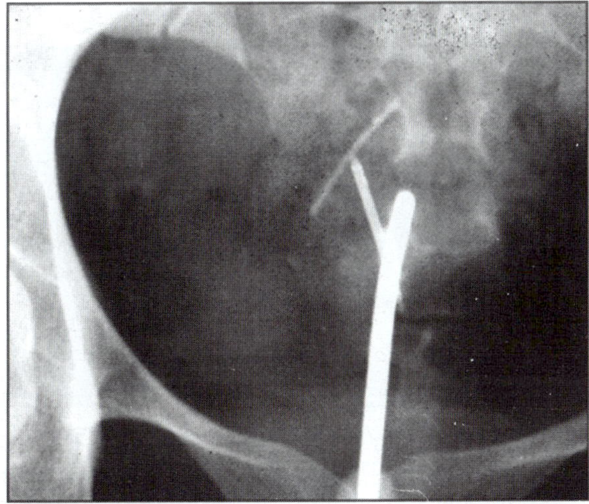

Fig. 58: X-ray taken after introducing uterine sound.

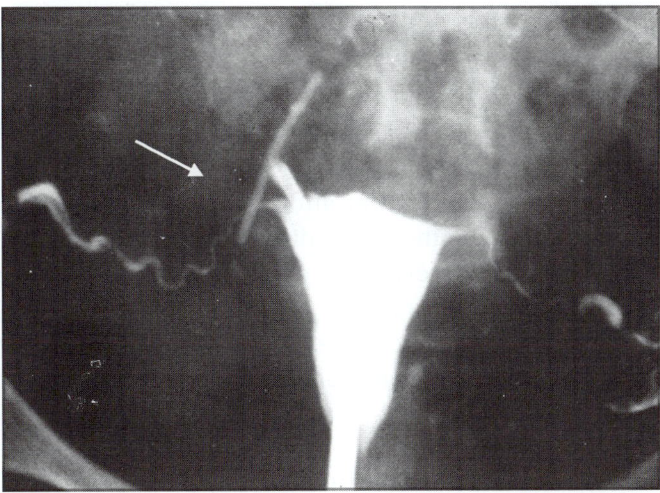

Fig. 59: Hysterosalpingography done in the same patient. Part of Copper T is seen outside of uterine cavity. Patient was multiparous and keen for hysterectomy.

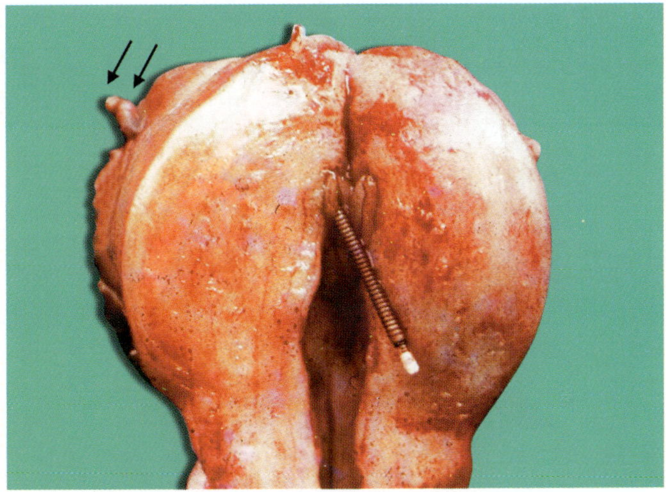

Fig. 60: Copper T embedded in the myometrium, the arrow pointer shows a part right arm of Copper T, coming out of myometrium on right side of uterus.

- Ectopic pregnancies can still occur.
- The IUCD can be spontaneously expelled; monthly palpation of the IUCD strings is important to avoid unwanted pregnancies. If the strings are not felt, a clinician should be notified immediately.

Indications

- Those who want that one-time insertion last for many years.
- The method required is the one which is independent of the act of coitus.
- The IUCDs are especially valuable for an irresponsible woman or for the mentally challenged.

- In whom oral contraceptive pills are contraindicated and who do not want to use other methods.
- As an EC

Contraindications

- Woman with irregular and heavy periods, uterine leiomyoma or other pelvic disease
- When there is evidence of present or past pelvic infection of any kind.
- If the uterus is bicornuate. In this, pregnancy in one horn may be protected, and a conceptus can implant in the other.
- Nulliparous woman
- Diabetes and heart disease
- A history of previous ectopic pregnancy (doubtful)

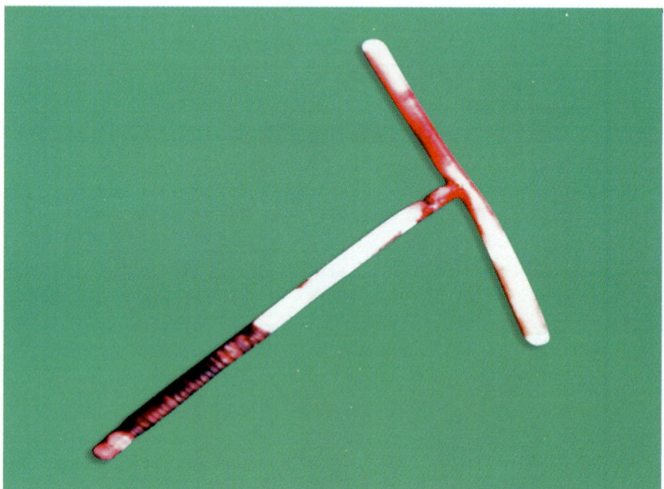

Fig. 61: Copper T as seen after removal by minilaparotomy.

Efficacy of Intrauterine Contraceptive Device

Considering all IUCDs together, the actual failure rate in the first year of use is approximately 3%, with a 10% expulsion rate and 15% rate of removal mainly for bleeding and pain **(Table 6)**. With increasing duration of use, failure rate decreases. The performance of CuT 380A in recent years has proved to be superior.

Failure rates with CuT 380A and other new Cu IUCDs are less than one per HWY.

Expulsion

Approximately 5% of patients spontaneously expel the CuT 380A within first year. This event can be associated with cramping, vaginal discharge or uterine bleeding or sometimes lengthening, or absence of IUCD string. The patient should be cautioned to request immediate attention if expulsion is suspected.

Ectopic Pregnancy

The previous use of an IUCD does not increase the risk of subsequent ectopic pregnancy. The current use of IUCD, other than the Progestasert, offers some protection against ectopic pregnancy. Therefore, when an IUCD user becomes pregnant, the pregnancy is more likely to be ectopic. However, the actual occurrence of an ectopic pregnancy in an IUCD user is a rare event. The lowest ectopic pregnancy rates are seen with the most effective IUCDs, such as CuT 380A = 0.20%, LNG IUCD 0.20 per 1,000 women year (90% less likely compared with noncontraceptors).

Progestasert has a higher rate, 6.8 per 1,000 women year, because its action is limited to a local effect on the endometrium.

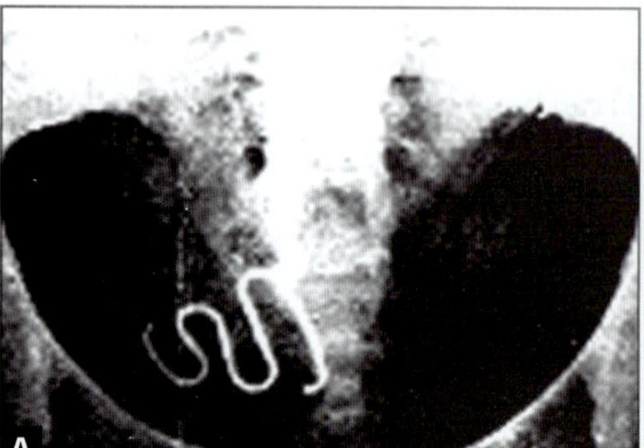

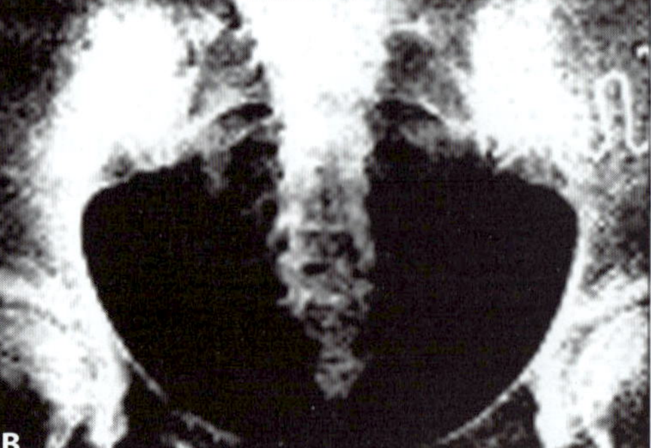

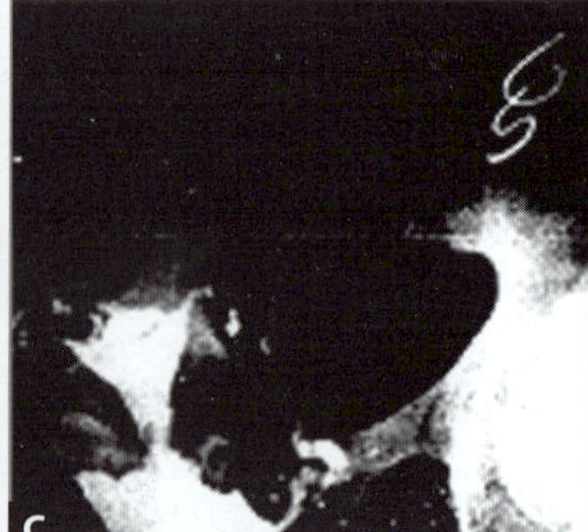

Figs. 62A to C: Intraperitoneal translocation of intrauterine contraceptive device (IUCD). (A) Radiograph taken after 2 months of insertion, because nylon tail was no longer projecting through cervix; (B) Radiograph 18 months later showing loop in peritoneal cavity; (C) Extrauterine site of IUCD.

TABLE 6: First-year clinical trial results in parous women.

Device	Pregnancy rate (%)	Expulsion rate (%)	Removal rate (%)
Lippes loop	3	12–20	12–15
CuT 200	3	8	11
CuT 380A	0.5–0.8	5	14
Progestasert	1.3–1.6	2.7	9.3
Mirena	0.2	6	17

So, the protection against ectopic pregnancies provided by CuT 380A and LNG IUCD makes these IUCDs acceptable choices for contraception in women with previous ectopic pregnancies.

Adverse Effects and Complications of Intrauterine Contraceptive Devices

- Fainting or collapse of the patient at the time of insertion of the IUCD
- Intermenstrual spotting or menorrhagia occurs in about 55% of women. They are mostly seen during the first few days and months and tend to disappear later. Nevertheless, a tendency of anaemia can result.
- *Dysmenorrhoea or intermenstrual pain due to uterine colic*: These subside as the patient becomes tolerant, or the patient can be treated with nonsteroidal anti-inflammatory agents during the first few cycles for 3–5 days.
- Amenorrhoea can develop sometimes with Progestasert and LNG IUCDs due to decidualising atrophic impact on the endometrium with LNG IUCD; 70% of patients are oligomenorrhoeic and 30% amenorrhoeic within 2 years.
- *Endometritis*: IUCD always cause local foreign body reactions in the endometrium; aseptic endometritis, pressure atrophy, glandular hyperplasia, oedema and leucocytic infiltration. Such reactions disappear quickly, once the device is removed, probably because of the natural monthly shedding of the endometrium.
- *Cervical injury*: Sometimes, devices can cause ulceration of the cervical tissues. Abnormal cervical smears are found, but it is very rare.
- Acute and chronic salpingo-oophoritis occurs in 1% of women per year. This happens mostly when the infection has been present already and has passed unrecognised, or when it is inserted too soon after delivery or abortion. The presence of the IUCD may also encourage exposure to a new STD, and if the infection is contracted, it is more likely to spread to the tubes if an IUCD is in place. If infection does occur, antibiotic therapy should be given and the device removed. The previous presence of infection with IUCD does not alter the treatment of PID. IUCD-associated pelvic infection is more likely to be caused by non-STD organisms. HIV-infected women who utilise IUCDs for contraception do not have a greater incidence of complications, including PID.
- *Actinomyces*: The significance of actinomycosis infection in IUCD users is unclear. There has been some evidence of actinomycosis in cervical smears from IUCD users (around 30%). The rate is much lower (<1%) with Cu devices and varies with the duration of use. The clinician must decide whether to remove the IUCD and treat the patient or treat with IUCD in place, or simply remove the IUCD. If uterine tenderness or pelvic mass is present, then IUCD should always be removed after the initiation of oral penicillin G 500 mg QID that should continue for a month. Timely detection and treatment prevent the development of pelvic actinomycotic masses.
- *Perforation of uterus*: Sometimes, the IUCD penetrates the uterine wall and escapes into the peritoneal cavity and causes adhesions and intestinal obstruction. It is nearly always the result of the uterine wall being perforated or deeply injured at the time of the insertion. Once in the peritoneal cavity, IUCD travels to any site. Without X-ray screening, it can sometimes be very difficult to find the device at laparoscopy or laparotomy. If it is an inert device, there is often no need to remove it. In case of Cu IUCD, removal is always indicated as there is a risk of pelvic adhesions due to continuous release of Cu. Removal is often possible by laparoscopy rather than by laparotomy.
- *Embedded IUCDs*: If removal of the IUCD is not easily accomplished, direct visualisation of the IUCD with sonography or hysteroscopy can be helpful. Sonography is safer and less expensive. Under abdominal ultrasound guidance, we can remove it by forceps. If this method fails, then hysteroscopy is indicated.
- *Displaced IUCD*: When an IUCD cannot be found on expulsion, one has to consider perforation in the abdominal cavity or embedment into the myometrium. A quick and real-time sonography is the best method to locate a lost IUCD, whether or not removal is desired.

If the IUCD cannot be visualised by ultrasound, abdominal X-rays are necessary because the IUCDs is radio-opaque and can be high and hidden. If the IUCD is identified perforating the myometrium or in the abdominal cavity, it should be removed using operative laparoscopy under general anaesthesia. If it is located in the uterine cavity, first try to remove it under ultrasound guidance; otherwise, hysteroscopy is the best approach **(Figs. 62A to C)**.

- Spontaneous expulsion occurs during the first year in 2–10% of cases, particularly common, if it is introduced in the early puerperium while the cervix is still atonic and sometimes the IUCD tail gets entangled with a vaginal tampon and pulled out inadvertently.
- *Pregnancy with an IUCD in situ*: The incidence of pregnancy with an IUCD in place is 2% during the first year after insertion; thereafter, the rate increases to 3%. Associated complications are:
    - *Spontaneous miscarriage*: It occurs in approximately 40–50% of cases. After the removal of an IUCD with visible strings, the spontaneous miscarriage rate is approximately 30%. So, if the IUCD is easily removed without trauma or expelled during the first trimester, the risk of spontaneous miscarriage is not increased.
    - *Septic abortion*: There is no evidence that there is an increased risk of septic abortion if pregnancy occurs with an IUCD in situ, except the Dalkon shield. If a patient plans to terminate a pregnancy, the IUCD should be removed in a clinic if there is no evidence of infection. If an IUCD is in an infected pregnant uterus, removal of the device should be undertaken only after antibiotic therapy has been initiated and equipment for cardiovascular support and resuscitation is immediately available, as removal in an infected uterus can lead to septic shock.
    - *Preterm labour and births*: The incidence is increased approximately fourfold when the IUCD is left in place during pregnancy.
    - *Congenital anomalies*: There is no evidence that exposure of the foetus to medicated IUCD is harmful. The risk of congenital malformation is increased among infants born to women with an IUCD in place during pregnancy.
    - *Other complications*: Obstetrical complications at delivery (e.g. haemorrhage, stillbirth and difficulties with place of removal) have been reported only with the Dalkon shield in situ.

Advantages

- They offer a cheap and practical means of considerably lowering fertility for a reasonably long period without the woman needing to pay any heed.
- No serious side effects, if any, disappear immediately after the device is removed.
- This method does not require privacy or toilet facilities, as does the use of the diaphragm.
- It does not lower fertility.
- It can be used as EC within 5 days of unprotected intercourse.
- No interaction with any medicine.
- No hormonal side effects.
- No effect on the amount or quality of breast milk.

HORMONAL CONTRACEPTION METHODS

Combined Hormonal Contraception (Flowchart 2)

There are two main types of hormonal contraception, the first being the combined hormonal contraception (CHC) (containing both oestrogen and progestogen), commonly available as combined oral contraceptive pills (COCPs), patch and an intravaginal ring, and the second being the formulations containing progestogen only. Three types of COCPs formulations are available: (1) Monophasic pills, (2) biphasic pills and (3) triphasic pills. The dosage of oestrogen and progestogen is changed during the various phases of the cycle in biphasic and triphasic pills, thereby imitating the body's cyclical variation in the hormonal levels. Most traditional COCPs are contained in a compact package of 21 active pills and seven inactive pills (or no pills) and are taken as 21/7 regimens. Some COCPs formulations, which are not consumed as 21/7 regimens, have been introduced in the world. Some such newly available contraceptive pills include Zoely® and Qlaira®.

Combined Oral Contraceptive Pills

Combined hormonal oral contraceptive pills contain both oestrogen [usually ethinyl oestradiol (EE)] and a progestogen.

Oestrogen

Ethinyl oestradiol is a very potent oral oestrogen used in oral contraceptives. The dose of oestrogen used in the combined pill ranges from 15 to 50 µg. Low-dose oral pills containing 20–35 µg of oestrogen are also available. Low-dose pills are safe, because cardiovascular risk and risk

Flowchart 2: Oral contraceptives and its doses.

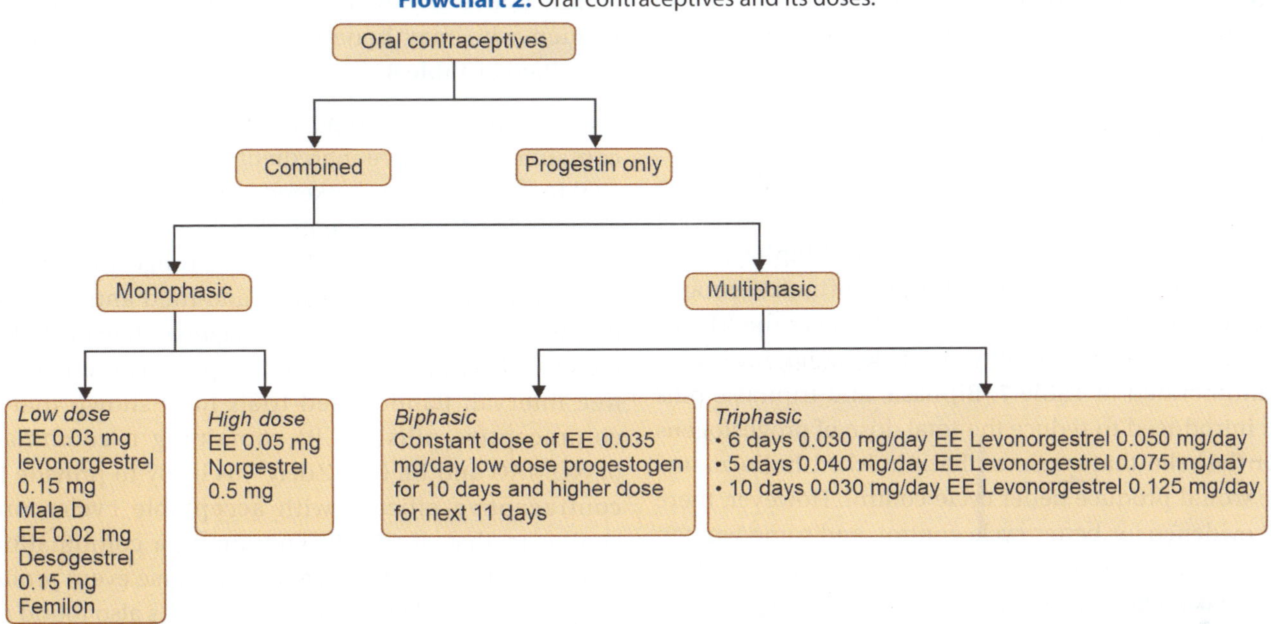

Note: Oestrogens used—ethinyl oestradiol (EE), mestranol; progesterones—(1) norethindrone, (2) norgestrel, (3) gestodene, desogestrel and (4) drospirenone.

of thrombosis are mainly from oestrogen content of pill and are dose-related. Therefore, the dose of oestrogen is a critical issue in selecting an oral contraceptive.

Progesterone

The progestational derivatives of testosterone were designated as 19-nortestosterones (denoting the missing 19-carbon). The androgenic properties of these compounds were not totally eliminated, and minimal anabolic and androgenic potential remains within the structure.

Progestogens used in currently available pills are divided into four groups:

1. First-generation progestogens = Norethindrone group
2. Second-generation progestogens = Norgestrel group. 0.05–0.25 μg of LNG, which is an active isomer of norgestrel.
3. Third-generation progestogens = Gestodene 0.075 μg, desogestrel 0.15 μg, norgestimate 0.25 μg.
4. Newest progestogens—some of the newest progestogens, which have been synthesised, include dienogest, drospirenone, nestorone, nomegestrol and trimegestone. These newly designed progestogens have no androgenic or oestrogenic actions.

Different progestogens have different potencies, and so contraceptive effectiveness is achieved at different doses. The main function of progestogens is to counteract undesirable side effects of oestrogen, such as endometrial hyperplasia and heavy withdrawal bleeding. The third-generation progestogens have a higher affinity for the progesterone receptor and therefore have a role in inhibiting ovulation. For this reason, comparable contraceptive efficacy is obtained even when low-dose formulations with 20 μg of EE are used, although these may be associated with poorer cycle control.

New progestins, because of their reduced androgenicity, predictably do not adversely affect the cholesterol lipoprotein profile and may be of greater clinical value in the treatment of acne and hirsutism.

Definitions Used in Epidemiological Studies

- Low-dose oral contraceptives—products containing <50 μg EE.
- First-generation oral contraceptives—products containing 50 μg or more of the EE.
- Second-generation oral contraceptives—products containing LNG, norgestimate and the other members of the norethindrone family and 30 or 35 μg EE.
- Third-generation oral contraceptives—products containing desogestrel or gestodene with 20 or 30 μg EE.
- Fourth-generation oral contraceptives—products containing drospirenone, dienogest and nomegestrol acetate (NOMAC).

- Newer combined oral contraceptives (COCs)—these contain oestradiol valerate (E2V) in combination with fourth-generation progestins.

Formulations

Combined oral contraceptive pills are available in monophasic preparation (in which every pill in the packet contains the same dose of steroids) and biphasic and triphasic preparations (in which the dose of both oestrogen and progestogen changes once or twice over the 21-day period). Some of the currently available monophasic pills are enumerated in **Table 7**. Biphasic and triphasic pills were introduced to reduce the total dose of progestogens and in the belief that a regimen that mimicked the hormonal cycle would produce better cycle control. However, there is no evidence for better cycle control, and some women find such preparations confusing, particularly when they want to take two packets of pills consecutively to postpone menstruation. As previously mentioned, certain COCP formulations have been introduced in the world, which are not consumed as 21/7 regimens. Zoely® and Qlaira® are some examples of such newly available contraceptive pills, which are available in the UK.

Minesse® is another 24/4 formulation available in India, which contains 15 µg of EE and 60 µg of gestodene. It is an ultra-low-dose contraceptive formulation. Possible advantages and disadvantages of ultra-low-dose contraceptive formulations are described in **Box 3,** and women who may benefit with such formulations are described in **Table 8**.

Zoely®: Zoely® is a type of hormonal contraception containing two active ingredients: 1.5 mg EE and 2.5 mg NOMAC. It has been marketed in the UK since May 2013. EE present in Zoely® is identical to the endogenous human 17β-oestradiol, while NOMAC is a progestogenic agent with strong antigonadotrophic and mild antiandrogenic properties. It is taken as a 24/4 regimen, having 24 active tablets followed by four inactive pills. There is no pill-free interval. Randomised trials have shown that oral contraceptive pills (OCP) containing a combination of NOMAC and EE (e.g. Zoely®) is likely to provide high contraceptive efficacy with acceptable cycle control similar to that of COCPs containing a combination of drospirenone and EE. The overall adverse event profile of these two types of OCP formulations was also found to be similar. Some women taking Zoely® may experience side

TABLE 7: Commercially available monophasic pills.

Pill (COC)	*Ethinyl oestradiol*	*Progestin*
Minesse 24/4	20 µg	0.6 mg gestodene
Femilon 21/7	20 µg	0.15 mg desogestrel
Loette/Locon/Combee 21/7	20 µg	0.10 mg levonorgestrel
Novelon 21/7	30 µg	0.15 mg desogestrel
Ovral G 21/7	50 µg	0.5 mg norgestrel
Duoluton L/Ovral 21/7	50 µg	0.25 mg levonorgestrel
Ovral L/Choice/Mala D 21/7	30 µg	0.15 mg levonorgestrel
Yasmin/Tarana 21/7	30 µg	3 mg drospirenone
Diane/Krimson 21/7	35 µg	2 mg cyproterone acetate
Yaz 24/4	20 µg	3 mg drospirenone
Zoely®	1.5 mg	2.5 mg nomegestrol acetate

(COC: combined oral contraceptive)

BOX 3: Various advantages and disadvantages of ultra-low-dose oral contraceptives.

Advantages:
- Ultra-low-dose oral contraceptives efficacy is similar to low-dose OCPs
- Probably less oestrogen-related side effects
- *Greater safety*: Less occurrence of thrombotic stroke and myocardial infarction

Disadvantages:
- Higher rates of bleeding pattern disruptions
- More breakthrough bleeding
- Reduced vaginal lubrication

(OCPs: oral contraceptive pills)

TABLE 8: Who may benefit from ultra-low-dose oral contraceptives?

Women with side effects associated with oestrogen dose	• Nausea • Breast tenderness • Bloating and fluid retention • Headache
Women at risk for thrombotic stroke and myocardial infarction	• Heavy smokes • Obese • History of thrombophilia
	• History of nausea, oedema, or hypertension in pregnancy • Uterine fibroids • Fibrocystic breasts • Heavy menses • Migraines

effects such as weight gain and acne. Withdrawal bleeding associated with Zoely® is shorter and lighter in comparison to other hormonal agents. Withdrawal bleeding may be sometimes completely absent with Zoely®.

Qlaira®: Qlaira® is a COCP containing E2V and dienogest (DNG) in the dosage as described in **Table 9**. This pill delivers 17β-oestradiol, which is similar to that released in the body. It is taken as 26/2 regimen, further reducing the pill-free interval to 2 days. Reduction in the pill-free interval is likely to result in a decline in the oestrogen withdrawal symptoms such as mood changes, headache, menstrual loss, pelvic pain, etc.

Qlaira® (E2V and DNG) has proven to be safe, effective, and well-tolerated in three large-scale clinical trials conducted across Europe and North America. Qlaira® is associated with a failure rate of 0.4 per HWY, which is similar to that reported with the conventional COCP. The majority of women using Qlaira® are satisfied with its use. Use of Qlaira® is likely to result in a bleeding profile similar to that of an EE-based COC. Qlaira® is well tolerated and associated with a low incidence of adverse events and serious adverse events similar to other low-dose oral contraceptives.

Women treated with Qlaira® are likely to experience a shorter and lighter episode of withdrawal bleeding. Withdrawal bleeding may be frequently absent. Some women may be concerned about the absence of withdrawal bleeding, so they need to be counselled regarding the fact that the presence or absence of withdrawal bleeding with Qlaira® treatment may not always be an indicator of contraceptive efficacy. Qlaira® has proven to be useful for the treatment of heavy menstrual bleeding (HMB). Clinical trials have shown that use of Qlaira® serves as an oral, noninvasive, reversible and fertility-conserving treatment, which helps in causing a significant, rapid, and sustained reduction in the menstrual blood loss by approximately 90% after 6 months of treatment in comparison with baseline data.

TABLE 9: Dosage of various hormones in Qlaira®.

No. of pills	*Colour*	*Dosage of oestradiol valerate*	*Dosage of dienogest*
First two pills	Dark yellow	3 mg oestradiol	—
3rd–7th pill	Medium red	2 mg oestradiol	2 mg dienogest
8th–24th pill	Light yellow	2 mg oestradiol	3 mg dienogest
25th–26th pill	Dark red	1 mg oestradiol	—
27th–28th pill	White (placebo pills)	—	—

Evra® Patch: This is the first transdermal patch contraceptive releasing 20 µg of oestradiol and 150 µg of norelgestromin every 24 hours. It is applied weekly for 3 weeks, followed by a patch-free interval. Its efficacy, cycle control and side effects profile are similar to that of other COCPs. A randomised controlled trial (RCT) has shown that extended use of the Evra® transdermal patches (weekly application for 12 consecutive weeks, 1 patch-free week, and three more consecutive weekly applications) is likely to delay menses and results in fewer bleeding days in comparison to the cyclical use (four consecutive cycles of 3 weekly applications and 1 patch-free week) of these patches. This regimen may represent a useful alternative for women who prefer fewer episodes of withdrawal bleeding. Therefore, extended use of Evra® patches may represent a useful alternative for women preferring fewer episodes of withdrawal bleeding.

NuvaRing®: NuvaRing® is a combined hormonal contraceptive vaginal ring made up of flexible plastic material (ethylene vinyl acetate copolymer) manufactured by Merck and is available on prescription **(Fig. 63)**. It releases 120 µg of etonogestrel and 15 µg of EE daily. It is 54 mm in diameter and 4 mm in thickness. Contraceptive efficacy, cycle control, and compliance of NuvaRing® have been found to be higher in comparison to COCPs.

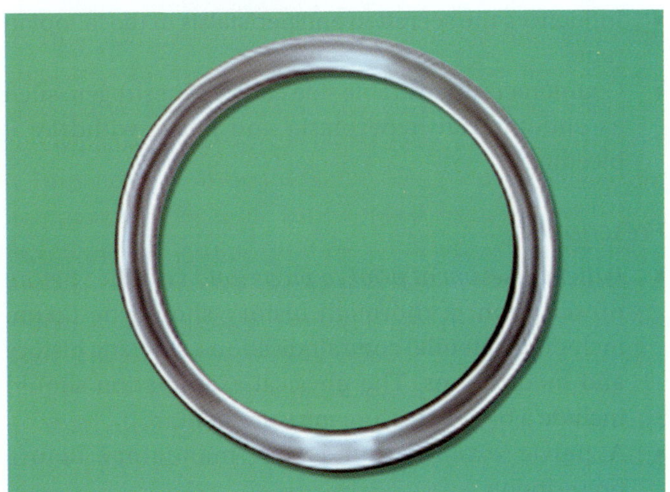

Fig. 63: Contraceptive vaginal ring.

The incidence of side effects such as breast tenderness, headache and nausea is comparable to the conventional COCPs containing 30 µg of EE. However, women using NuvaRing® are likely to experience a higher rate of local complications such as vaginitis, leucorrhoea, foreign body sensation and expulsion.

Mode of Action

- Inhibition of ovulation
- Alteration of the endometrium
- Changes in cervical mucus that interfere with sperm transport
- Tubal motility may be altered.
- Atrophy of the endometrium
- Uterine receptivity, essential for successful implantation, may be impaired.

Action of oestrogen:

- Decreased follicle-stimulating hormone (FSH) release.
- Prevents the emergence and selection of a dominant follicle.
- Provides stability to the endometrium.
- Prevents irregular shedding and unwanted breakthrough bleeding
- Potentiates the action of progestational agents.

Action of progestogens:

- Prevent LH surge necessary for ovulation.
- Cervical mucus becomes thick and impervious to sperm transport.
- Produces an endometrium not receptive for implantation (decidualised bed with exhausted and atrophic glands)
- Influences the secretion and peristalsis of the fallopian tube.
- Counteracts undesirable side effects of oestrogen, such as endometrial hyperplasia and heavy withdrawal bleeding.

Prescription

- *Patient assessment prior to prescription of CHC*: Before prescription, a thorough history should be taken, including potential contraindications, smoking history and medications. The physical examination should include a blood pressure measurement.
- A pelvic examination is not mandatory before prescription.
- Adequate counselling prior to initiation of CHCs may help to improve compliance and adherence.

Yasmin®: Yasmin®, one of the commonly used OCP formulations, which is taken in form of 21/7 regimen, contains 3 mg drospirenone and 0.03 mg EE.

- Conventionally, the COCPs must be started during the first day of the menstrual cycle.
- Once a woman has started taking a COCPs, it is important for her to be consistent and take the pill regularly at the same time each day.
- Women who use a 21-day preparation need to take the pills for 21 days, followed by a 7-day pill-free interval. She should be cautioned not to exceed the 7-day pill-free interval between packs.
  - If the woman forgets to take one or two tablets of 21-day preparation, e.g. Yasmin®, she should take the most recent pill as soon as she remembers and then continue to take the remaining pills as usual. This may mean taking two pills on the same day (one at the time of remembering and the other at the regular time) or even both at the same time.
  - If the woman forgets to take three or more tablets, she should take the most recent pill as soon as she remembers and then continue to take the remaining pills as usual. She should be advised to use condoms or abstain from sexual activities until she takes the pills for 7 days continuously.
  - Additionally, if the woman misses taking a pill in week 1 (first 7 days), the pill-free interval has been extended. EC should be considered if she had unprotected sexual activity during the pill-free interval in week 1. Also, if the woman misses taking the pills in week 3, it is important to avoid extending the pill-free interval. In these cases, she should be counselled to finish all the remaining active pills in the pack, omit the pill-free interval and start the new pack from the next day.
  - Backup method of contraception (e.g. condoms, foam) may be required in case the woman exceeds the pill-free interval of 7 days; experiences a serious adverse effect; or requires protection from STDs.

Zoely®:

- If the woman has not been using any hormonal contraceptive method in the past month, she should start taking Zoely® on first day of her menstrual bleeding. When doing so, no additional contraceptive measures are necessary. She needs to take one pill every day for a period of 28 days (24 active pills + 4 placebo pills). The successive pack must be started immediately after finishing the previous pack without having a break in the daily tablet intake and irrespective of the presence or absence of withdrawal bleeding.

- If the woman has been using any of the hormonal contraceptive methods (ring, patch or COCP) in the past month, she should start with Zoely® preferably on the day after the last active tablet (of her previous COC). At the latest, Zoely® must be started on the day following the usual tablet-free or placebo tablet interval of her previous COC. In case a vaginal ring or transdermal patch has been used, the woman should start using Zoely® preferably on the day of removal, but at the latest when the next application would have been due.
- The missed pill guidelines for Zoely® are as follows:
  - *Pill missed on days 1–7*: The missed pill must be taken as soon as possible, and extra precautions must be observed for the next 1 week.
  - *Pill missed on days 8–17*: The last missed pill must be consumed as soon as possible. The rest of the pack must be finished in a similar manner.
  - *Pill missed on days 18–24*: In these cases, the four inactive pills must be omitted and the next packet must be started straight away.

Qlaira®: If the woman has not been previously taking hormonal contraceptive agents in the past month, she should start taking Qlaira® from the first day of her menstrual bleeding. If she had been previously taking some form of combined hormonal contraceptive (COCP, vaginal ring or transdermal patch), she should start with Qlaira® on the day after the last active tablet of her previous COC. In case a vaginal ring or transdermal patch has been used, the woman should start using Qlaira® on the day of removal. In case the woman forgets to take a pill for >12 hours, the missed pill regimen is as follows:

- *Pill missed on days 1–17*: The missed pill must be taken immediately as soon as the woman remembers it. The subsequent pill must be taken at the usual time, even if it means taking two pills at the same time. The rest of the packet must be consumed in a similar manner. Use of an additional contraceptive method or abstinence must be practised for 9 days rather than 7 days, as in the case of the conventional 21/7 regimen COCPs.
- *Pill missed on days 18–24*: Rest of the packet must be discarded. The woman must start taking the first pill from a new packet, and this packet must be consumed in a usual manner. Use of an additional contraceptive method or abstinence must be practised for 9 days.
- *Pill missed on days 25 and 26*: The missed tablet must be taken immediately. The next tablet must be taken at the usual time, even if it means taking two tablets on the same day. Additional contraceptive protection is not required in these cases.
- *Pill missed on days 27 and 28*: The forgotten tablets must be discarded, and the rest of the tablets continued in a normal way. No additional contraception is required.

Evra® patch: As previously described, an Evra patch must be applied weekly for 3 weeks, followed by a patch-free interval. In case the woman forgets to apply a patch for >12 hours, the missed patch regimen is as follows:

- If the woman applies the patch late during week 1, she should apply a new patch as soon as she remembers. If she is >48 hours late in the application of the new patch, new patch must be applied as soon as she remembers. However, a backup method for contraception must be used for a week following the application of the new patch. If during this period, the patient has a sexual intercourse without using a backup method, she should use EC.
- If the woman applies the patch late during week 2 or 3:
  - If she is <48 hours late in changing her patch, she should be advised to change it as soon as she remembers. She should change to her next patch as she would have normally done.
  - If she is >48 hours late in changing her patch, she should change it as soon as she remembers it and then wear it for 1 week. She should then continue to change to the next patch on the same day of the next week.
  - A backup method for contraception must be used for a week following the application of the new patch. If during this period, the patient has sexual intercourse without using a backup method, she should use EC.
- If the woman forgets to apply the patch on time during the fourth week, she should be advised to remove the patch when she remembers. A new patch must be applied on her regular patch change day.

NuvaRing®: The ring is placed inside the vagina for every 3 weeks followed by a ring-free interval of 1 week.

Subsequently, a new ring must be inserted.

The WHO eligibility criteria for use of conventional COCPs are enumerated in **Table 10**, whereas those for the use of low-dose COCPs are enumerated in **Table 11**. Some of the factors to consider in starting or switching OCPs are explained in **Table 12**.

TABLE 10: World Health Organization (WHO) eligibility criteria for use of conventional combined oral contraceptive pills.

WHO category I	*WHO category II*
• Menarche to 40 years • Postabortion • Smoking • History of preeclampsia • History of ectopic pregnancy • Postpartum 21 days, ectopic feeding • Breastfeeding >6 weeks postpartum • Irregular menstrual bleeding/dysmenorrhoea • Obesity • History of gestational diabetes • Cervical erosion • Fibroids • Endometrial or ovarian cancer • Pelvic inflammatory diseases • Gestational trophoblastic disease • Varicose veins • Thyroid disease • Epilepsy • Hepatitis (not active or carrier) • Schistosomiasis • Malaria • Iron deficiency anaemia • Tuberculosis • Increased risk of HIV • Past history or existing sexually transmitted diseases (STDs) or acquired immunodeficiency syndrome (AIDS)	• Age >40 years • Uncomplicated valvular heart disease • Smokers <35 years, light smoker >35 years • Headache without neurological symptoms • Breastfeeding >6 months postpartum • History of jaundice • Undiagnosed breast disease • Unexplained vaginal bleeding • Cancer cervix or precancerous lesions • Mild hypertension • Thalassaemia • Sickle cell disease • Diabetes uncomplicated • Gallbladder disease • Mild cirrhosis
WHO category III	*WHO category IV*
• Breastfeeding—breastfeeding between 6 weeks and 6 months postpartum, and fully or almost fully breastfeeding • Postpartum—<21 days postpartum • Smoking—aged ≥35 years and smoking <15 cigarettes per day, or stopped smoking <1 year ago • Obesity—BMI >35 kg/m^2 • Cardiovascular disease—multiple risk factors for arterial cardiovascular disease • Hypertension—elevated blood pressure – >140–159 mm Hg systolic or – >90–94 mm Hg diastolic; also adequately controlled hypertension • Family history of venous thromboembolism (VTE) in a first-degree relative aged <45 years • Immobility (unrelated to surgery)—wheelchair use, debilitating illness • Known hyperlipidaemias—familial hypercholesterolaemia • Migraine without aura, at any age—continuation of the method • Past history (>5 years ago) of migraine with aura at any age • Undiagnosed breast mass—initiation of the method • Past history of breast cancer and no evidence of recurrence for 5 years; carriers of known gene mutations associated with breast cancer (e.g. *BRCA1*) • Diabetes—with nephropathy/retinopathy/neuropathy, or vascular disease • Gallbladder disease—symptomatic, medically treated, or current • History of cholestasis—past COC-related • Viral hepatitis—acute or flare • HIV—on antiretroviral therapy (drug interactions) • Drugs, which induce liver enzymes—rifampicin, rifabutin, ritonavir, St John's Wort and certain anticonvulsants (i.e. phenytoin, carbamazepine, barbiturates, primidone, topiramate, oxcarbazepine) and lamotrigine	• Breastfeeding—<6 weeks postpartum • Smoking—aged ≥35 years and smoking ≥15 cigarettes per day • Cardiovascular disease—multiple risk factors for arterial cardiovascular disease • Hypertension—blood pressure ≥160 mm Hg systolic and/or ≥95 mm Hg diastolic; or vascular disease • VTE—current (on anticoagulants) or past history • Major surgery with prolonged immobilisation • Known thrombogenic mutations • Current and history of ischaemic heart disease • Stroke • Valvular and congenital heart disease—complicated by pulmonary hypertension, atrial fibrillation, history of subacute bacterial endocarditis • Migraine headaches—with aura at any age • Breast disease—current breast cancer • Diabetes—with nephropathy, retinopathy, neuropathy, or vascular disease • Viral hepatitis—active or flare • Cirrhosis—severe decompensated disease • Liver tumours—benign hepatocellular adenoma and malignant hepatoma • Systemic lupus erythematosus (SLE)—positive or unknown antiphospholipid antibodies

(BMI: body mass index; COC: combined oral contraceptive; HIV: human immunodeficiency virus)

TABLE 11: World Health Organization (WHO) precautions for the use of low-dose oral contraceptive pills.

Category 4 (refrain from use)	*Category 3 (exercise caution)*	*Category 2 (advantages outweigh risks)*	*Category 1 (no restrictions)*
• Venous thromboembolism • Cerebrovascular or coronary artery disease • Structural heart disease • Diabetes with complications • Breast cancer • Pregnancy • Lactation (<6 weeks postpartum) • Liver disease • Headaches with focal neurologic symptoms • Major surgery with prolonged immobilisation • Age >35 years and smoke 20 cigarettes or more per day • Hypertension (blood pressure of >160/100 mm Hg or with concomitant vascular disease)	• Postpartum <21 days • Lactation (6 weeks to 6 months) • Undiagnosed vaginal or uterine bleeding • Age >35 years and smoke fewer than 20 cigarettes/day • History of breast cancer but no recurrence in the past 5 years • Interacting drugs • Gallbladder disease	• Severe headaches after initiation of oral contraceptive pills • Diabetes mellitus • Major surgery without prolonged immobilisation • Sickle-cell disease or sickle-cell haemoglobin C disease • Blood pressure of 140/100–150/109 mm Hg • Undiagnosed breast mass • Cervical cancer • Age >50 years • Conditions predisposing to medication noncompliance • Family history of lipid disorders • Family history of premature myocardial infarction	• Postpartum ≥21 days • Postabortion, with abortion performed in the first or second trimester • History of gestational diabetes • Varicose veins • Mild headaches • Irregular vaginal bleeding patterns without anaemia • Past history of PID • Current or recent history of PID • Current or recent history of STD • Vaginitis without purulent cervicitis • Increased risk of STD • HIV-positive or at high risk for HIV infection or AIDS • Benign breast disease • Family history of breast cancer or endometrial or ovarian cancer • Cervical ectropion • Viral hepatitis carrier • Uterine fibroids • Past ectopic pregnancy • Obesity • Thyroid conditions

(AIDS: acquired immunodeficiency syndrome; HIV: human immunodeficiency virus; PID: pelvic inflammatory disease; STD: sexually transmitted disease)

TABLE 12: Factors to consider in starting or switching oral contraceptive pills.

Objective	*Action*
To reduce the high risk of thrombosis	Choose a product with a lower dosage of oestrogen
To minimise nausea, breast tenderness or vascular headaches	
To decrease spotting or breakthrough bleeding	Select a product with a higher dosage of oestrogen or a progestin with greater potency
To minimise androgenic effects	Choose a product containing a third-generation progestin, low-dose norethindrone or ethynodiol diacetate
To avoid dyslipidaemia	

Follow-up

Follow-up visit in cases of CHC is required after 6 weeks to check patient compliance and well-being.

Extended and Continuous Regimens of Combined Oral Contraceptive Pills

The efficacy of COCPs may be reduced if the pills are missed at the beginning of the pack, in this manner extending the days without the active pills. This increases the risk of ovulation, thereby increasing the failure rate of the pills. Continuous or extended use of OCPs is likely to reduce this risk of ovulation by reducing the number of active pills, which are missed when the pack is delayed. Continuous or extended use of COCPs, respectively, involves continuous intake of active contraceptive pills without any period of inactive pills or greatly increasing the interval at which inactive pills are taken. Some OCP products, which have been approved for extended or continuous contraception, include Seasonale®, Seasonique® and Lybrel®. Seasonale® contains 84 days of active pills and 7 days of inactive pills. Seasonique® contains 84 days of active pills and 7 days of low-dose oestrogen pills. Lybrel® contains a full year of active pills with no inactive pills. A Cochrane review has shown that the bleeding pattern with extended or continuous regimens is similar to that of cyclic regimens.

The available evidence demonstrates that extended and continuous cycle OCPs are likely to have efficacy similar to that of classic 21 + 7 cyclic OCPs. Nevertheless, the women with extended or continuous regimens may at times experience bothersome uterine bleeding. Extended or continuous use regimens are also likely to reduce menstrual symptoms, including dysmenorrhoea and premenstrual symptoms.

Efficacy

When used correctly, combined hormonal contraceptives are almost 100% effective. The failure rate during perfect use is 0.1%. Because of errors in pill taking, failure rate associated with typical use of pills is about 8%.

Advantages

- If instructions are followed and the pill is taken regularly, the pregnancy rate is as low as 0.1 per HWY, though in actual use, it may be 6–8 per HWY.
- Once the pill habit is acquired, the method is simple, divorced from single act of intercourse and aesthetically attractive.
- The woman enjoys a self-controlled regular 'menstrual' cycle, which is usually lighter and without dysmenorrhoea.
- The incidence of anaemia is decreased.
- If the woman decides to have more children, discontinuation of the medication is usually quickly followed by conception. Regular ovulation returns within 3 months in 98% of cases.
- It protects against ectopic pregnancy, benign breast disease, PID, ovarian cysts, and ovarian and endometrial cancer.
- This is one of the best methods of contraception, especially true for women <35 years of age and even after, if they do not smoke.

Complications

Combined hormonal contraception has an effect on almost every system in the body. Most side effects such as nausea, vomiting, mood change, weight gain or fluid retention, headache, loss of libido, mastalgia, breast enlargement and greasy skin, are minor common complaints, which also occur in the absence of contraceptive use. Many improve or disappear within 3–6 months of starting the method, but side effects often lead to discontinuation. Some side effects may be alleviated by changing to a different delivery system. For example, the patch is associated with less nausea. Among pill users, the dose of oestrogen or type of progestogen can be altered by changing to a different brand of pill, and it is worth trying this if time alone does not solve the problem. Chloasma is much less common and is definitely related to steroid hormones. It can also occur with progestogen-only methods.

Serious side effects involve mainly the cardiovascular system (CVS). COC affects both the venous [venous thromboembolism (VTE)] and arterial (myocardial infarction, cerebrovascular accidents) circulations. In both cases, the increased risk appears to be related to an increased thrombotic tendency.

Side Effects

- *Nausea and vomiting:* These subside within a few months and are less troublesome if the pill is taken with milk.
- *Headache and dizziness:* Except for the rare development of migraine, such symptoms are not significantly associated with treatment.
- *Mastalgia:* This is temporary and can be disregarded.
- Chloasma is rarely a nuisance.
- Depression and lassitude are often present before treatment is commenced. If they are a result of the pill, then they may be prevented by giving pyridoxine 50 mg daily.
- Acne and greasy scalp, low-dose pills improve.
- *Loss of libido:* This may be caused by dryness of the vagina and emotional changes but is rarely experienced by women.
- Muscle cramps in the legs.
- Breakthrough uterine spotting is common in the early months and rarely needs treatment. If it does, a more oestrogenic preparation is indicated.
- *Menstrual upsets:* Scanty menstruation is of no importance. Menorrhagia calls for a preparation, which

is more progestogenic. Amenorrhoea, with or without galactorrhoea, is an indication for stopping treatment. When this is done, menstruation usually returns, but amenorrhoea can be persistent. This is more likely in women whose original menstrual cycle is irregular and infrequent, and is a sequel to oral contraceptive in <1% of cases.

- Candida vulvitis and vaginitis are encouraged by the environment, which mimics that of pregnancy.
- *Increase in weight:* This occurs temporarily as a result of fluid retention. A persistent increase in weight is caused by deposition of fat, as in pregnancy and is related to a change in appetite.

Other Side Effects

- *Venous thromboembolism*: The combined pill is associated with a threefold increase in the relative risk of VTE. Risk is unaffected by age, smoking and duration of pill use, but is higher in obese women [body mass index (BMI) >30 mg/m^2] and in women with a history of pregnancy-induced hypertension. Combined pills containing the third-generation progestogens, gestodene or desogestrel have about twofold increased risk of VTE compared with pills containing LNG. Although the reason for this difference is unclear, it is known that oral contraceptive use reduces the efficiency with which activated protein C downregulates in vitro thrombin formation, and this phenomenon is more pronounced in women using a pill containing desogestrel rather than LNG.
- The absolute risk of VTE in COC users is very low (15/10,000 women years). The risk returns to normal within 3 months of stopping the pill. The committee on safety of medicines warns that women should be informed of the increased risk of VTE, if third-generation pills are prescribed. The risk of VTE is the same with other routes of administration of CHC (patch, ring or injectable).
- Women with inherited thrombophilias (e.g. factor V Leiden) are at increased risk of VTE, and a family history of VTE is an indication for testing for various thrombophilias.
- Smoking has no effect on the risk of venous thrombosis.

Arterial thrombosis: Arterial disease in pill users is much more serious than venous disease; however, the absolute risk of myocardial infarction and stroke in young women is less. Stroke is the most important possible side effect.

Myocardial infarction: While there is widespread agreement that there is an increased risk of myocardial infarction among women who take the pill and smoke or have hypertension, the relationship between myocardial infarction and COC use is controversial among women with no other risk factors.

- A recent meta-analysis of 23 studies concluded that the risk of myocardial infarction was increased among current COC users compared with newer users.
- The risk among past users was not increased, nor was the risk for women using third-generation pills or pills containing 20 µg EE. The risk for myocardial infarction was increased for women using second-generation pills and for smokers (by nine times) and women with hypertension (tenfold).
- Thus, smoking and oestrogen have an additive effect on the risk of arterial thrombosis.
- Low-dose oral contraception (<50 µg EE) does not increase the risk of myocardial infarction or stroke in healthy and nonsmoking women regardless of age.
- Almost all myocardial infarctions and strokes in oral contraceptive users occur in users of high-dose products or users with cardiovascular risk factors over the age of 35 years.

Stroke: The risk of stroke attributable to COC use is small. The relative risk of haemorrhagic stroke is not increased in women under 35 years and only slightly increased in older women. The risk of ischaemic stroke is slightly increased (relative risk 1.5) and is also slightly higher in women over the age of 35 years. Smoking and hypertension increase the risk of stroke by tenfold and threefold, respectively.

Hypertension: A very slight rise in blood pressure is not uncommon and matters little. In 1% of cases, there can be a sharp rise but this is more likely in women with past history of hypertension in pregnancy. Stopping the pill, which is necessary, results in return of the blood pressure to its original level within 3 months.

Combined oral contraceptives are contraindicated in women who have a history of idiopathic VTE and also in women who have a close family history (parents and siblings) of idiopathic VTE. By effectively screening for the presence of smoking and cardiovascular risk factors, especially hypertension in older women, we can limit any increased risk for arterial thrombosis associated with low-dose pills, so low-dose oral contraceptives are very safe for healthy young women with no increased risk of cardiovascular events on long-term use.

Other Metabolic Effects

- A lowered tolerance to carbohydrate can result in glycosuria, and this is a warning to stop medication.
- Hyperlipidaemia is rarely seen, only in women who are prone to it. The newer progestogens such as desogestrel, are lipid-friendly.
- Sometimes increase in the blood level of protein-bound iodine, but oral contraceptives do not affect intrinsic thyroid function, and they may be used in patients who are hypothyroid or hyperthyroid.
- Sometimes change in liver function, which is not revealed by ordinary tests and is of no consequence. Occasionally, cholestatic jaundice develops, and this is a contraindication for continuing the treatment.
- Oestrogen increases the cortisol-binding globulin. Free and active cortisol both are increased, because oestrogen decreases the ability of the liver to metabolise cortisol.

Risk of Cancer

Endometrial cancer: The use of COC protects against endometrial cancer. Use for at least 12 months reduces the risk of developing endometrial cancer by 50%, with the greatest protective effect gained by use for >3 years. This protection persists for 20 or more years after discontinuation and is greatest in women at highest risk, such as nulliparous and low-parity women. Protection is seen with all monophasic formulations of oral contraceptives, including pills with <50 µg oestrogen.

Ovarian cancer: Protection against ovarian cancer, the most lethal of female reproductive tract cancers, is one of the most important benefits of oral contraception. The risk of developing epithelial ovarian cancer of all the histologic types in users of oral contraceptives is reduced by 40% compared with that of nonusers. This protection is seen in women who use oral contraception for as little as 3–6 months and increases with duration of use and continues for at least 10–15 years after stopping the medication. The protective effect of oral contraceptives is especially observed in women at high risk of ovarian cancer.

Cancer of cervix: Some studies have indicated that the risk for dysplasia and carcinoma in situ of uterine cervix increases with the use of COCs for >1 year. It is well recognised that the number of partners a woman has had and age at first coitus are the most important risk factors for cervical neoplasia. Other confounding factors are exposure to human papillomavirus, smoking and use of barrier contraception (protective). These are difficult to control, so conclusions regarding cervical cancer are not definitive.

Centers for Disease Control and Prevention concluded through a study that there is no increased risk of invasive carcinoma in COCs users and an apparent increased risk of carcinoma in situ is due to enhanced detection of disease (more frequent Pap smear in COCs users).

In the WHO study of neoplasia and steroid contraceptives, a Pap smear screening bias was identified, nevertheless, the evidence still suggested an increased risk of *cervical intraepithelial neoplasia* (CIN) with long-term oral contraceptive use. It is reasonable to perform a Pap smear every 6 months in women using oral contraception for 5 or more years.

Breast cancer: Current and recent use of oral contraceptives may be associated with about a 20% increased risk of early premenopausal breast cancer, essentially limited to localised disease and a very small increase in the actual number of cases. This finding may be due to detection or surveillance bias and accelerated growth of already present malignancies, a situation similar to the effect of pregnancy and postmenopausal hormone therapy on the risk of breast cancer.

- Previous oral contraceptive use may be associated with a reduced risk of metastatic breast cancer later in life and possibly with a reduced risk of postmenopausal breast cancer.
- Oral contraceptives do not further increase the risk of breast cancer in women with positive family histories of breast cancer or in women with proven benign breast disease.

Oral contraceptives and risk of breast cancer:

- *Current users*: Relative risk (RR) = 1.24; 95% confidence interval (CI): 1.15–1.33
- 1–4 years after stopping: RR = 1.16; 95% CI: 1.08–1.23
- 5–9 years after stopping RR = 1.07; 95% CI: 1.02–1.13.

Even though the data indicated that young women who begin use before the age of 20 years have higher relative risks of breast cancer during current use and in the 5 years after stopping, this is a time period when breast cancer is very rare and thus, there would be little impact on actual number of breast cancers.

Liver adenomas and liver cancer: Hepatocellular adenomas can be produced by steroids, both the oestrogen and androgen families. The adenomas are not malignant, and their significance lies in the potential for haemorrhage. The most common presentation is acute right upper quadrant or epigastric pain. This may be asymptomatic or may present suddenly with haemoperitoneum. The risk appears to be related to the duration of oral contraceptive use and to the steroid dose in the pills. This is reinforced by the rarity of the condition ever since low-dose pills became available.

No reliable screening test or procedure is currently available. Routine liver tests are normal. Palpation of the liver should be a part of the periodic evaluation in oral contraceptive users. If an enlarged liver is found, oral contraception should be stopped, and regression should be evaluated, followed by imaging.

There is no evidence of an increased risk of liver cancer in oral contraceptive users.

Fertility and Oral Contraception

There is no evidence that infertility is increased by the use of oral contraception. In fact, in young women, previous oral contraceptive use is associated with a lowered risk of primary infertility. Ovulation returns to normal within 3–6 months of stopping the oral contraceptive pill, and 90% become pregnant by 24 months.

Women who become pregnant while taking oral contraceptives or inadvertently take birth control pills early in pregnancy should be advised that the risk of a significant congenital anomaly is no greater than the general rate of 2–3%.

Breastfeeding

Oral contraception has been demonstrated to diminish the quantity and quality of lactation in the postpartum period. Also of concern is the potential hazard of transfer of contraceptive steroids to the infants; however, no adverse effects have thus far been identified.

Breakthrough Bleeding

- A major continuation problem is breakthrough bleeding. At the start of oral contraceptives, a patient needs to be fully informed about breakthrough bleeding.
- The most frequently encountered breakthrough bleeding occurs in the first few months of use (1–3 months), ranging from 10% to 30% in the first month to <10% in the third. It is higher with the lowest dose oral contraceptive pills (with formulations containing 20 µg of EE) and smoking.
- It is best managed by encouragement and reassurance; this bleeding usually disappears by the third cycle in the majority of women. It is helpful to explain to the patient that this bleeding represents tissue breakdown as the endometrium adjusts from its usual thick state to a relatively thin state allowed by oral contraceptives.
- Breakthrough bleeding that occurs after many months of oral contraceptive use is a consequence of the progestin-induced decidualisation; this endometrium and blood vessels tend to be fragile and prone to breakdown and asynchronous bleeding.
- Cervical infection can be another cause of breakthrough bleeding; the prevalence of cervical chlamydial infections is higher among oral contraceptive users who report breakthrough bleeding.
- If breakthrough bleeding is prolonged or if it is aggravating for the patient, regardless of the point in the cycle, control of the bleeding can be achieved with a short course of exogenous oestrogen, conjugated oestrogen 1.25 mg, or oestradiol 2 mg daily for 7 days, no matter where the patient is in her pill cycle. The patient continues to adhere to the normal schedule of pill taking. If recurrence does occur (usually does not occur), a repeat course of oestrogen for 7 days can be given.
- The addition of extra oestrogen while keeping the progesterone dose unchanged is logical and effective. This allows the patient to remain on the low-dose formulation with its advantage of greater safety. Any bleeding that is not handled by this routine requires investigation for the presence of pathology.

Amenorrhoea

The incidence of amenorrhoea in the first year of use with low-dose contraception is <2%. This incidence increases with duration, up to 5% after several years of use. It is important to give information to the patient upon starting oral contraception that diminished bleeding or no bleeding may ensue on using oral combined pills.

This is more with low-dose oral contraceptives, oestrogen content is not sufficient in some women to stimulate endometrial growth. The progestational effect dominates to such a degree that a shallow atrophic endometrium is produced, lacking sufficient tissue to yield withdrawal bleeding.

It should be emphasised that permanent atrophy does not occur and resumption of normal ovarian function, which restores endometrial growth and development occurs within few months.

Management: Management comprises the following steps:
1. Reassurance to the pill user
2. A pregnancy test for the presence of pregnancy, even at this early stage
3. Assess BBT during the end of pill-free week. BBT <98°F is not consistent with pregnancy.
4. Sometimes, the addition of extra oestrogen for 1 month (1.25 mg conjugated oestrogen or 2 mg EE for 21 days) while taking the oral contraceptive pills. It will rejuvenate the endometrium, and withdrawal bleeding will resume.

Migraine Headaches

Oral contraceptives should be avoided in women who have migraine with complex or prolonged aura or if additional stroke factors are present (older age, smoking and hypertension).

Prior studies with high-dose pills indicated that migraine was linked with a risk of stroke, but recent studies with low-dose pills yield mixed results.
- So, if the patient is on a higher dose, a change to low-dose formulations may relieve the headache.
- Women who experience an exacerbation of their headache with oral combined pills should consider one of the progestin-only methods.

Severe vascular headache is identified if:
- Headache lasts for a long time
- Headache with nausea, vomiting and dizziness
- With blurred vision or scotomata
- Episodes of blindness
- Unilateral, unremitting headaches
- Headache that continues despite medication.

Drugs that Affect Efficacy

Drugs, which stimulate the liver's metabolic capacity, can affect oral contraceptive efficacy. Patients on medications that affect liver metabolism should choose an alternative contraceptive. These drugs are as follows:
- Rifampicin
- Phenobarbital
- Phenytoin
- Primidone
- Carbamazepine

Possibly:
- Ethosuximide
- Griseofulvin
- Troglitazone

Benefits of Low-dose Oral Contraceptive Pills

- *Effective contraception*:
  - Less need for induced abortion
  - Less need for surgical sterilisation
- Less endometrial cancer
- Less ovarian cancer
- Fewer ectopic pregnancies
- *More regular menstrual flow*:
  - Less dysmenorrhoea
  - Less anaemia
  - Less flow
- Less salpingitis
- Less anaemia
- *Probably less endometriosis*:
  - Less benign breast disease
  - Less rheumatoid arthritis
  - Fewer fibroids
  - Fewer ovarian cysts
  - Protection against atherosclerosis

Other Uses

Oral contraceptives are frequently utilised to manage the following problems and disorders:
- Dysfunctional uterine bleeding
- Dysmenorrhoea
- Mittelschmerz
- Endometriosis prophylaxis
- Acne and hirsutism
- Hypothalamic amenorrhoea
- Prevention of menstrual porphyria
- Control of bleeding (dyscrasias, anovulation)
- *Sometimes used for*:
  - Functional ovarian cyst
  - Premenstrual syndrome

For patients having anovulatory dysfunctional uterine bleeding and who need effective contraception, oral contraceptives are a good choice. Oral contraceptives are also a good choice to provide prophylaxis against the recurrence of endometriosis. To protect against endometriosis, oral contraceptives should be taken daily with no break and no withdrawal bleeding.

Oral contraceptives have long been used to speed the resolution of ovarian cysts, but the efficacy of this treatment has not been established.

Clinical Pearls

- The use of COCPs provides a protective effect against the development of ovarian and endometrial cancer and probably even colorectal cancer.
- Use of COCPs is a highly effective method of reversible contraception, with the failure rate being approximately 0.1 per HWYs of use.
- The COCPs do not provide any protection against STDs or HIV infection.
- Normal menstrual cycles are likely to occur in 99% of women within 6 months of stopping the pills. However, the return of fertility may be slightly late due to the delayed return of ovulation.
- Combined hormonal contraceptive agents such as Zoely® and Qlaira® are nonenzyme-inducing agents. Therefore, antibiotics can be easily used in patients using these hormonal contraceptive agents.
- Women may or may not experience withdrawal bleeding while using hormonal methods of contraception.

PROGESTOGEN-ONLY CONTRACEPTION

Progestogen-only contraceptives are now available with the active hormone administered as oral preparations, injectable, implants or intrauterine systems. Progestogen-only containing contraceptive methods are available in various formulations:

- Progestogen-only pill (POP) or minipill
- Subdermal contraceptive implants (Norplant® I, II and Implanon)
- Progestogen-only injectables (POI), e.g. depot medroxyprogesterone acetate (DMPA)
- Intrauterine system (Mirena® and Progestasert).

Progestogen-only Pill

Progestogen-only pills (POPs) shall be discussed here. Other types of progestogen-only contraceptive methods have been subsequently discussed in the chapter. There are two different types of POP:

1. *Three-hour POP*: These are traditional POPs, which must be taken within 3 hours of the same time each day. The POPs may contain 350 µg of norethisterone or 75 µg of norgestrel, or 30 µg of LNG. Some examples of POPs include Femulen®, MicroNor®, Norgeston® and Noriday®. Types of progestogen contained in POPs are indicated in **Table 13**.
2. *12-hour POP*: These include desogestrel pills, such as Cerazette®, which must be taken within 12 hours of the same time each day. Cerazette® contains 75 µg of desogestrel.

TABLE 13: Types of progestogen contained in minipill.

Types of progestogen	*Dose*	*Commercial name*
Desogestrel	75 µg	Cerazette®
Levonorgestrel	75 µg	Ovrette, Neogest
Norgestrel	30 µg	Microval, Microlut
Norethisterone	350 µg	Noriday, Micronor
Lynestrenol	500 µg	Exluton
Ethynodiol diacetate	500 µg	Femulen

The available evidence suggests that the failure rates of the traditional POP and the desogestrel pill are similar. Amongst the breastfeeding women, the difference in efficacy between the traditional POPs and desogestrel is likely to be insignificant. Desogestrel, however, may be more effective than LNG in women who are not breastfeeding. The potential for better efficacy of desogestrel is counterbalanced by its higher incidence of adverse events (e.g. irregular bleeding patterns) in comparison to LNG.

Minipills are recommended over COCPs in women who are breastfeeding, because they do not affect milk production. These pills can also be safely used in women of any age group with a history of migraine (with or without aura).

Effectiveness of POPs may vary between 0.3 and 8.0 per HWY. The efficacy of POPs is likely to be lower in older women (>40 years) in comparison to the younger women.

Mode of Action

Progestogen-only pills act through the following mechanisms:

- Thickening of cervical mucus, thereby reducing sperm viability and penetration
- Making the endometrium unfavourable to implantation
- *Inhibition of follicular development and ovulation*: This effect of POP is variable and may only occur in about 60% of cases. However, in the case of Cerazette®, desogestrel-only pill, the main mode of action is inhibition of ovulation.

Prescription

Progestogen-only pills must be started on the first day of the menstrual cycle. Unlike the COCPs, these pills must be taken on a continuous basis without any breaks between packets. These must be consumed in accordance with a strict time schedule every day (within 3 hours for traditional POPs vs. 12 hours for Cerazette®). If a woman is >3 hours late taking a dose, she should take another pill as soon as she remembers. The next pill must be taken at the usual time. If the woman missed taking more than one pill, she just needs to take one pill as soon as she remembers. The next pill must be taken at the usual time. A backup method should be used for 2 days if a woman is >3 hours late taking a dose. Backup contraception should be considered during the first month when the woman first starts taking minipills and then at midcycle every month thereafter (the time when ovulation is likely to occur).

Complications

Unlike the COCPs, minipills are not associated with an increased risk of complications such as VTE, myocardial infarction, stroke, heart disease or breast cancer.

- *Changes in the bleeding pattern*: Irregular bleeding, spotting, breakthrough bleeding, amenorrhoea, etc.
- Depression, headache and migraine
- Weight gain and ectopic pregnancy
- Mastalgia (breast tenderness)
- Mood swings
- Abdominal cramps

Injectable Contraceptives

These comprise delivering certain hormonal drugs in the form of deep intramuscular injections into the muscles of the arms or buttocks. Two types of injectable contraceptives are available: (1) Progestogen-only formulations and (2) combined formulations **(Table 14)**. The POIs contain only the hormone—progestogen. Two main types of POIs are (1) DMPA and (2) norethisterone enanthate (NET-EN). Combined formulations (e.g. Mesigyna and Cyclofem), on the other hand, contain both progestogen and oestrogen.

Injectable contraceptive provides women with safe, highly effective and reversible contraceptive protection, with the failure rate being 0.1–0.4%. They overcome the inconvenience of daily compliance required with POPs or COCP. This is a suitable method for women in whom oestrogens present health risks. POIs can be used by breastfeeding women at 6 weeks postpartum without adverse effects on nursing infants. Fertility is not impaired after discontinuation of DMPA or NET-EN, although its return may be delayed. They do not provide protection against HIV and STDs.

TABLE 14: Common injectable contraceptives.

Name	***Active ingredients***	***Duration of effect***
Progestogen-only injectables (POIs)		
DMPA (progestogen-only): Available as DepoProvera	150 mg medroxy-progesterone acetate in an aqueous micro-crystalline suspension	90 days
DMPA (progestogen-only)	300 mg	180 days
NET-EN (progestogen-only): Available as Noristerat	200 mg NET-EN in an oily preparation	60 days
Combined injectable contraceptives (CICs)		
Mesigyna	50 mg NET-EN and 5 mg E2V	30 days
Cyclofem	25 mg DMPA and 5 mg of oestradiol cypionate	
Marvelon	150 μg of desogestrel and 30 μg of ethinyl oestradiol	
Femovan	75 μg of gestodene and 35 μg of ethinyl oestradiol	

(DMPA: depot medroxyprogesterone acetate; NET-EN: norethisterone enanthate)

Mode of Action

- DepoProvera is not a sustained-release system; it relies on higher peaks of progestins to inhibit ovulation and thicken cervical mucus.
- It inhibits ovulation by effectively suppressing LH surge. FSH suppression is not as intense as with COC, therefore, follicular growth is maintained sufficiently to produce oestrogen levels comparable to the early phase of the normal menstrual cycle. So, symptoms of oestrogen deficiency such as vaginal atrophy or decrease in breast size do not occur.
- The injection should be given within the first 7 days of the current menstrual cycle; otherwise, a backup method is necessary for 1 week. It should be given deeply into the muscle by the Z-track technique and not massaged.

Indications

- Breastfeeding mothers
- Sickle cell disease

- Seizure disorder
- Oestrogen-free contraception needed
- Coitally independent method desired

The WHO eligibility criteria for the use of progestogen-only contraception are enumerated in **Box 4**.

Efficacy

Depot medroxyprogesterone acetate and NET-EN are almost as effective as COCs. Pregnancy rates at 1 year for DMPA are around 0.3 per HWY, and for NET-EN, it is 0.4 per HWY of use on the usual regimen.

BOX 4: World Health Organization (WHO) eligibility criteria for the use of progestogen-only contraception.

Category 1—unrestricted use:
Can be used without restriction in the presence of:
- Age over 16 years
- Smoking
- Obesity >30 kg/m^2 BMI
- Obstetric or gynaecological conditions:
  - Past history of preeclampsia
  - Pregnancy-induced jaundice
  - Uterine fibromyomas
  - Carcinoma endometrium
  - Carcinoma ovary
  - Postinduced or spontaneous abortion
- Postpartum use:
  - Nonbreastfeeding (<21 to ≥42 days)
  - Breastfeeding [≥6 weeks to <6 months (primarily breastfeeding) and ≥6 months postpartum]
- Chronic diseases and other conditions:
  - Valvular heart disease
  - Nonactive hepatitis
  - Thyroid disease
  - Iron deficiency anaemia
  - Thalassaemia and sickle cell disease
  - Epilepsy
  - Malaria
  - Depressive disorders
  - Tuberculosis
  - Risk of sexually transmitted disease
- *Superficial venous disorders*: Varicose veins and superficial venous thrombosis
- *HIV/AIDS*: High risk of HIV
  - *Antiretroviral therapy*: Nucleoside reverse transcriptase inhibitors (NRTIs) such as abacavir, tenofovir and zidovudine
  - *Non-nucleoside reverse transcriptase inhibitors (NNRTIs)*: Efavirenz (EFV), nevirapine (NVP) and protease inhibitors (PIs) such as ritonavir-boosted atazanavir.
  - Integrase inhibitors such as raltegravir (RAL)
- Cervical ectropion, cervical intraepithelial neoplasia and cervical cancer (awaiting treatment)
- Gestational trophoblastic disease (GTD)—decreasing or undetectable β-hCG levels and persistently elevated β-hCG levels or malignant disease
- Pelvic inflammatory disease

Category 2—other conditions:
Can generally be used with precautions in the presence of:
- Age under 16 years
- Obstetric or gynaecological conditions:
  - Previous ectopic pregnancy
  - Irregular, heavy or prolonged bleeding
  - Undiagnosed breast mass

Contd...

Contd...

- Chronic diseases and other conditions:
  - Cerebrovascular or coronary artery disease
  - Hypertension with BP ≥ 160/110 mm Hg
  - Hypertension with vascular disease
  - Migraine with focal neurological symptoms
  - Diabetes
  - History of deep vein thrombosis or pulmonary embolism
  - Mild compensated cirrhosis
  - Gallbladder disease
  - Known hyperlipidaemias
- Use of griseofulvin and antiretroviral drugs
- Rheumatic diseases—systemic lupus erythematosus (SLE) (severe thrombocytopaenia)

Category 3–requires careful consideration:
Should generally not be used in the presence of:
- Current deep vein thrombosis or pulmonary embolism
- Acute liver disease
- Liver tumour (benign or malignant)
- Severe decompensated cirrhosis
- History of breast cancer with no evidence of disease for the last 5 years
- Breastfeeding and 4 weeks postpartum
- Use of rifampicin or anticonvulsants such as phenytoin, carbamazepine and barbiturates
- *Rheumatic diseases*: Systemic lupus erythematosus (SLE)—positive (or unknown) antiphospholipid antibodies

Category 4—contraindications:
Should not be used in the presence of:
- Breast cancer within the past 5 years.

(BMI: body mass index; hCG: human chorionic gonadotrophin)
Source: World Health Organization. (2015). Medical eligibility criteria for contraceptive use. [online] Available from https://www.who.int/publications/i/item/9789241549158. [Last accessed May, 2025].

Prescription

The medicine must be injected into the thigh, buttocks or deltoid muscle four times a year (every 11–13 weeks) and provides pregnancy protection starting a week after the first injection. The injection site should not be massaged afterwards, since this may accelerate absorption of the drug.

Since DMPA is an aqueous suspension, a DMPA vial must be shaken vigorously before it is loaded into the syringe to resuspend any active ingredient at the bottom of the vial. The syringe should then be checked to ensure that it contains the correct dosage. Any leakage from the syringe should be checked and kept under control.

Complications

- *Menstrual irregularities*: Disruptions of the menstrual cycle, including amenorrhoea, prolonged menses, spotting between periods and heavy or prolonged bleeding
- *Other side effects*: These include adverse effects such as weight gain, headache, dizziness and low bone mass.

Progestogen-only Implants

The contraceptive implant is a method of birth control, where the device is inserted under the skin. Available subdermal implants are as follows:
- Norplant I and Jadelle (Norplant II)
- Implanon
- Sinoimplant II marketed as Zarin, Femplant and Trust
- Uniplant
- Biodegradable implants
- These implants ensure slow and sustained release of progestogens. It is a long-acting form of contraception, which is associated with minimal side effects.
- *Norplant I:* This contains six silastic capsules made up of siloxane of the size 34 × 2.4 mm, with each containing about 36 mg of LNG **(Fig. 64)**. Its effect lasts for approximately 5 years. The implants release 85 mg of LNG/day in the first 3 months; 50 mg/day for the

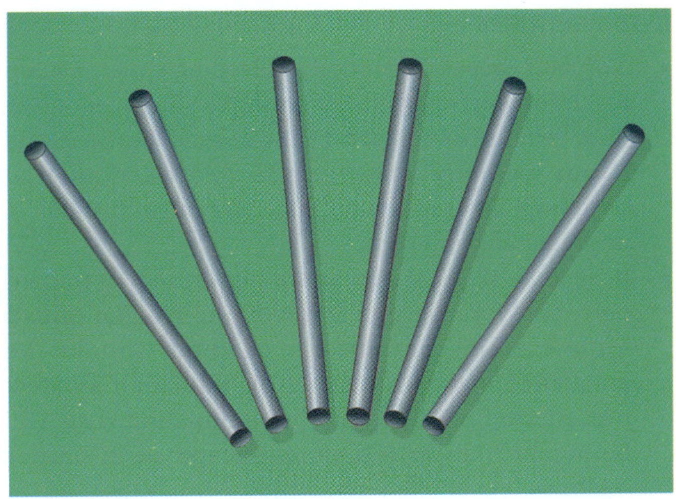

Fig. 64: Norplant I.

next 18 months, and then gradually level to about 30 mg/day.

- *Norplant II*: This comprises two rods, each containing about 70 mg of LNG. The daily release of the hormone is about 50 mg, and it provides protection for 3–5 years.
- *Implanon*: This is a single rod, having dimensions 4 cm × 2 mm, containing 67 mg of a progestogen, desogestrel, and usually remains effective for a period of 3 years. Approximately, 30 µg of hormone is released daily.
- *Uniplant*: Uniplant is single-implant contraceptive containing 38 mg NOMAC in a 4 cm silastic tube with a 100 µg/day release rate. It provides contraception for 1 year.
- *Biodegradable implant contraception*: It delivers sustained levels of progestins for a variable period of time from a vehicle that dissolves in body tissues. The utility of this implant would be improved by the elimination of the need for surgical removal.

Two types are under evaluation:

1. Capronor
2. Norethindrone pellets.

1. *Capronor*: It is a single capsule, biodegradable and LNG-releasing subdermal implant composed of the polymer ε-caprolactone. Implants measure 0.24 cm in diameter and either 2.5 or 4 cm in length, providing contraception for 1 year. The capsule remains intact for the first 12 months of use, allowing easy removal. After 12 months, the capsule begins to disappear.

   Capronor shares the advantage of Norplant with the convenience of use and few metabolic side effects. Its removal is easier and quicker.

   Biodegradable implants could continue to release a small noncontraceptive amount of hormone after their period of use as a contraceptive has expired. Although it is unlikely that such a low serum level of progestin would be harmful to users or their pregnancies, this question needs to be solved.
2. *Norethindrone pellet or annuelle*: It is injected subdermally and maintains a circulating contraceptive level of progestin for up to 3 years. This pellet is composed of 10% pure cholesterol and 90% norethindrone and is about the size of a grain of rice. This method is currently under development.

   Return of fertility is almost immediate, following the removal of these capsules. It does not harm the quality and quantity of the breast milk and can be used by nursing mothers starting 6 weeks after childbirth. These capsules do not provide protection against STDs.

Mode of Action

The LNG diffuses through the wall of the tubing into the surrounding tissues, where it is absorbed by the circulating system and distributed systemically, avoiding an initial high level in circulation as with oral or injectable steroids. Within 24 hours of insertion, the plasma concentration of LNG ranges from 0.4 to 0.5 µg/mL and high enough to prevent conception.

Body weight affects the circulating levels of LNG. The greater the weight of the user, the lower the LNG concentrations at any time during Norplant use. But even for heavy women, the release rate is high enough to prevent pregnancy at least as reliably as oral contraceptives.

Norplants work in a similar way to the other progestogen-only contraceptives.

- The LNG suppresses both the hypothalamus and the pituitary. The LH surge necessary for ovulation is suppressed in approximately 50% of cycles. In those cycles that are ovulatory, there is a high incidence of luteal insufficiency.
- The cervical mucus thickens and decreases in amount, forming a barrier to sperm penetration.
- The LNG suppresses the oestradiol-induced cyclic maturation of endometrium and causes atrophy. These changes prevent implantation.

Insertion

The implants are inserted subdermally on the inner aspect of the left upper arm under local anaesthesia

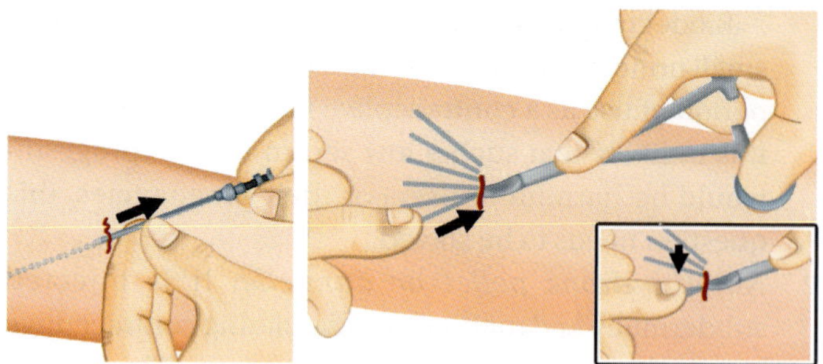

Fig. 65: Subdermal insertion of Norplant I.

after proper counselling and written consent. The implants are inserted on the first day of the menstrual cycle. Following application of a local anaesthetic over the upper arm, a needle-like applicator is used to insert the Norplant capsules under the skin **(Fig. 65)**. They are inserted subdermally on the medial aspect of the upper arm. Since the capsules are nonbiodegradable, they need to be removed at the end of use or earlier, if the side effects are intolerable. Both insertion and removal of these implants require local anaesthesia and a small incision.

Efficacy

- The overall pregnancy rate after 5 years of use is 1.1/HWY and 0.2/HWY after 2 years of use.
- Heavier women (>70 kg) may experience slightly higher pregnancy rates in the fourth and fifth years of use compared with lighter women.

Advantages

- It is a sustained-release method with a high degree of efficacy.
- There are no forgotten pills, broken condoms or lost diaphragms. It is not a coitus-related method.
- It is an excellent choice for breastfeeding women and can be inserted immediately postpartum, but at least a 3-day postpartum delay is recommended to allow the decline in pregnancy levels of oestrogen and progesterone and the establishment of lactation.
- Norplant use has not been associated with changes in carbohydrate or lipid metabolism, coagulation, liver and kidney function or immunoglobulin level.
- It allows women to plan their pregnancies precisely; return of fertility after removal is prompt, in contrast to 18-month delay in ovulation that can follow DepoProvera injection.

Disadvantages

- Norplant causes disruption of bleeding patterns in up to 80% of uterus, especially during the first year of use. Endogenous oestrogen is nearly normal, but progestin is not regularly withdrawn to allow endometrial shedding. Consequently, the endometrium sheds at unpredictable intervals.
- It needs a surgical procedure performed by trained personnel for insertion and removal. Women cannot initiate or discontinue the method without the assistance of a clinician. As it requires a surgical procedure, initiation and discontinuation costs will be higher than with oral contraceptives or barrier methods.
- It can be visible under the skin; this may be unacceptable by some women.
- It does not protect against STDs, users at risk should use barrier methods to prevent infection.

Indications

- Desire a highly effective, long-term method of contraception
- Experience serious or minor side effects with OCs
- Have completed childbearing but do not desire permanent sterilisation
- Those who do not want to use other methods
- Women with chronic illnesses
- Have a history of anaemia with HMB.

Contraindications

- Active thrombophlebitis
- Undiagnosed genital bleeding
- Acute liver disease
- Benign or malignant liver tumour
- Known or suspected breast cancer.

Complications

The occurrence of serious side effects is very rare.

- The most common side effect experienced by users is headache; approximately 20% of women who discontinue use, do so because of headache.
- *Weight change*: Women more frequently complain of weight gain than weight loss. Counselling for weight changes should include dietary review and focus on dietary changes.
- Bilateral mastalgia occurring premenstrually is usually associated with complaints of fluid retention. After

pregnancy has been ruled out, reassurance and therapy aimed at symptomatic relief are indicated.

- Galactorrhoea is more common among women who have had insertion of the implants after discontinuation of lactation. The patient should be reassured after ruling out pregnancy, and a thorough breast examination should be done. If amenorrhoea accompanies galactorrhoea, then a prolactin level should be obtained.
- Acne is the most common skin complaint. It is caused by the androgenic activity of the LNG. Proper counselling, reassurance and dietary changes to maintain good skin hygiene with the use of soaps or skin cleansers and application of 1% clindamycin creams or erythromycin ointment are required.
- Menstrual effect is highly variable; some alteration of menstrual pattern will occur during the first year in approximately 80% of users, later decreasing to about 40%.
- *Ovarian cyst*: Adnexal masses are approximately eight times more frequent in Norplant users compared with normally cycling women. Unlike OCs, low-serum progesterone levels maintained by Norplant do not suppress FSH, which continues to stimulate ovarian follicular growth, while LH peaks are usually abolished, so that these patients do not ovulate. However, some continue to grow and cause pain or are palpated at the time of examination. Because these are simple cyst most regress spontaneously within 1 month of detection; they need not be evaluated sonographically or laparoscopically.
- *Ectopic pregnancy*: The rate of ectopic pregnancy during Norplant use has been 0.28 per 1,000 women year. Although the risk is low but if pregnancy does occur, ectopic pregnancy should be suspected, as 30% of Norplant pregnancies are ectopic.

Etonogestrel Implant

Features of Implanon NXT: It is a single rod, 4 cm long and 2 mm in diameter (size of a matchstick), made of ethinyl vinyl acetate—causes less fibrosis, easy to remove. It is impregnated with barium sulphate to render radio-opaque and is in a preloaded sterile disposable applicator, which makes subdermal insertion easy **(Figs. 66A and B)**.

FAQs on Implanon NXT:

1. *What is it?*
   It is the currently available subdermal contraceptive implant, the size of a matchstick, inserted beneath the skin in the upper arm of the woman. Contains 68 mg of Etonogestrel (Progestin-only-contraceptive) with the addition of barium sulphate, that makes it radio-opaque. It is approved by DCGI.
2. *How does it act as a contraceptive?*
   The etonogestrel inhibits ovulation consistently during the first two years and for most of the third year, and also thickens the cervical mucus, thereby preventing access of sperm to the uterine cavity.
3. *What is the period of use?*
   Approved for a period of three years.
4. *What is the clinical effectiveness?*
   Highly effective. Best among long-acting reversible contraceptives. 0.05% of Implanon users would have an unintended pregnancy during the first year of use.
5. *How safe is it?*
   It is a safe method with no major adverse effects. Side effects can be rarely troublesome, such as menstrual disturbances. About one in five women will experience amenorrhea of varying duration, and one in five will

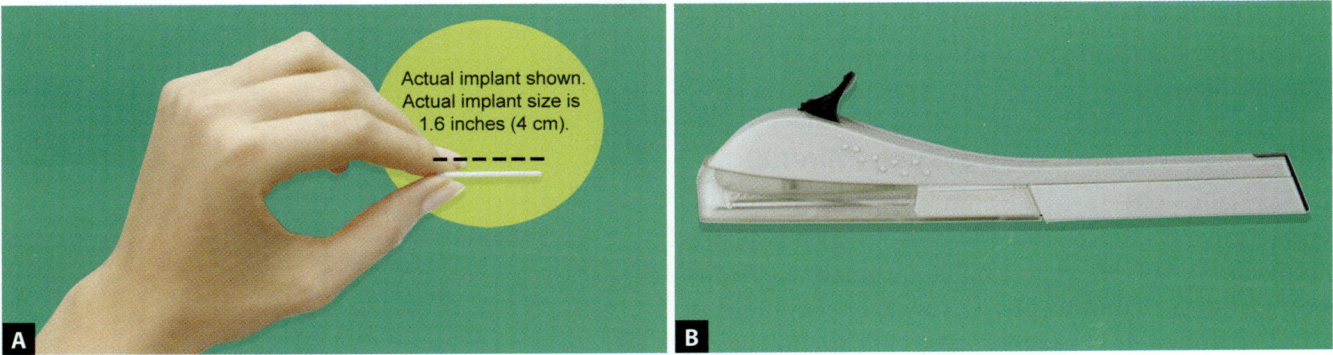

Figs. 66A and B: (A) Implanon NXT size; (B) Implanon NXT preloaded applicator.

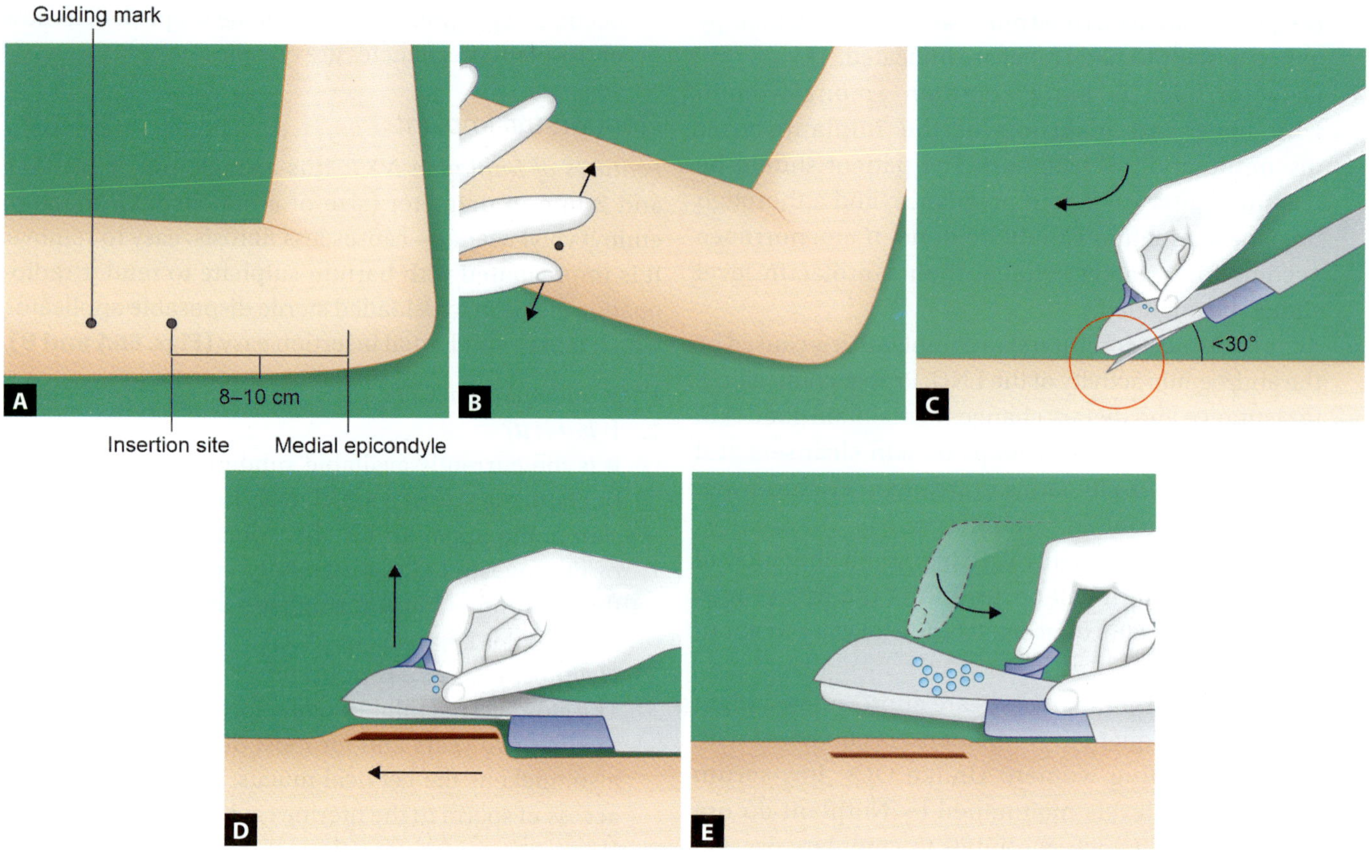

Fig. 67A to E: Insertion steps.

develop irregular or heavy periods. Headache, acne and weight gain are other reported side effects in <5% of users. There is no significant impact on bone mineral density.

6. *What about return to fertility?*
   Within 1 month of removal.
7. *Is insertion/removal difficult/painful?*
   Requires doctors who are trained in the procedure of insertion (**Figs. 67A to E**) and removal (**Figs. 68A to D**). Removal involves a small incision in the upper arm under local anaesthetic. Insertion needs only a local anaesthetic.

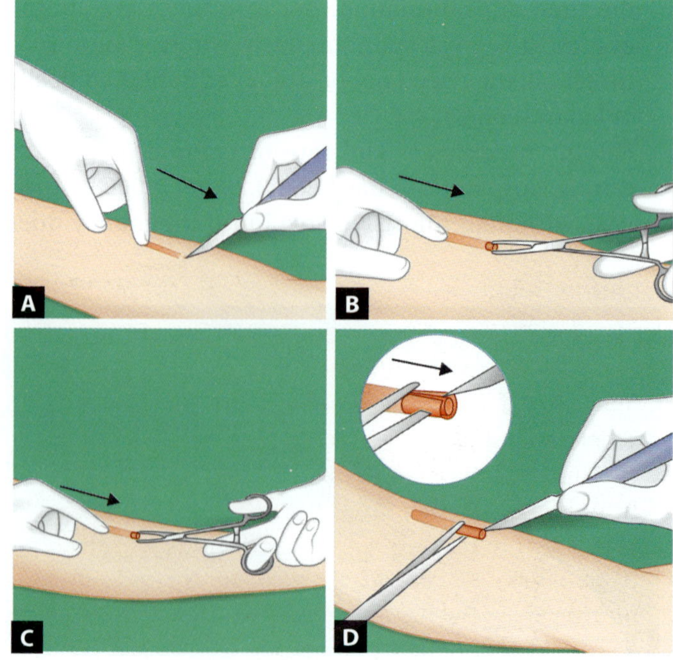

Figs. 68A to D: Removal steps.

Progestogen Intrauterine System (Mirena)

Mirena (**Fig. 69**) is a new intrauterine hormonal contraceptive system releasing LNG. It has been available worldwide since 1995, and >6 million women worldwide have used it for contraception. Nowadays, in addition to contraception, it is used for idiopathic menorrhagia, for therapeutic benefits in fibroids, adenomyosis,

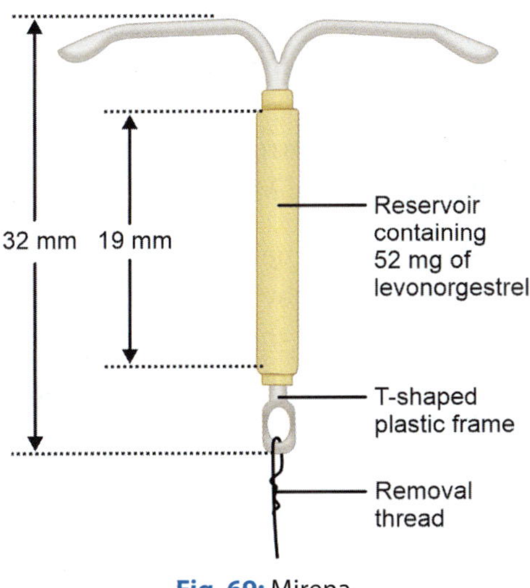

Fig. 69: Mirena.

endometriosis, and more recently as the progestogen component of hormone replacement therapy.

Structure

Mirena consists of a plain plastic T-shaped frame with a steroid reservoir around the vertical stem. This reservoir consists of a cylinder, made of LNG and polydimethylsiloxane mixture, containing a total of 52 mg of LNG. The total length of the system is 32 mm. The reservoir forms a 19 mm long sleeve around the vertical arm of the plastic body and is covered by a polydimethylsiloxane membrane, which regulates the minimal intrauterine release of LNG. T-shaped frame is impregnated with barium sulphate to make it radio-opaque. With Mirena, only 20 µg/day of LNG is released.

The recommended duration of use for Mirena is 5 years. Thereafter, it should be removed and replaced by a new system, if needed.

Mechanism of Action

The contraceptive effect of the LNG IUS intrauterine system—Mirena is based on local effects of LNG in the uterine cavity. These are as follows:

- Thickening of cervical mucus, so that the passage of sperm and their migration is inhibited.
- Inhibition of sperm motility and function inside the uterus and the fallopian tubes, preventing fertilisation.
- It causes endometrial atrophy by making the uterine mucosa thin, stroma swollen, endometrial glands atrophic and epithelial cells inactive. So, the endometrium becomes unresponsive to oestrogen and does not undergo menstrual shedding. After removal of Mirena, the endometrium returns to normal, and within 30 days, menstruation begins.
- *Ovarian function*: During the first year of use, some women experience changes in ovarian function. After the first year, most cycles are ovulatory (around 85%).
- Serum oestradiol (E_2) level remains normal during the use of Mirena.
- Oligoamenorrhoea or amenorrhoea develops despite normal ovarian function due to endometrial atrophy.

Time of Insertion

It should be inserted within the first 7 days of the menstrual cycle when bleeding is not heavy.

Efficacy

With Mirena, 1-year and 5-years pregnancy rates are 0.1% and 0.5%, respectively, and it has a very high continuation rate with around 82% of women using it after 3 years.

Indications

- *Contraception*: Mirena is a highly effective contraceptive. It provides fertility control comparable to female sterilisation. Nulliparity is not a contraindication. Ideally, the uterus should be between 6 and 9 cm. Uterine anomalies can compromise success by increasing expulsion rates and risk of perforation.
- *Idiopathic menorrhagia*: It also markedly reduces menstrual blood flow by 86% at 3 months and 97% at 6 months and alleviates dysmenorrhoea. Anaemia parameters such as haematocrit and ferritin are improved.
- *It has been compared with endometrial ablation for reduction of blood loss in many RCTs and was found to be comparable at 2 years of follow-up.* It is an alternative to hysterectomy for women with menorrhagia.
- For the regression of *endometrial hyperplasia.*
- In endometriosis LNG IUS, there is a reduction in recurrence of pelvic pain, bleeding rates, and increased rate of satisfaction compared with GnRH analogues.
- It can prevent endometrial proliferation and reduce the uterine bleeding associated with oral or transdermal oestradiol.
- Mirena may be effective for long-term prevention of fibroids and also regulates the growth of fibroids. Role of LNG IUS for reduction of menorrhagia due to fibroids is now an established fact.

- Studies have not been consistent regarding the effect of LNG IUS on leiomyoma size. Grigorieva found decreased uterine size from 6 to 12 months of use. Other studies failed to show a decrease in fibroid size. Further evidence is awaited. Progesterone may have both stimulatory and inhibitory effects on myometrial cells.

Adverse Effects

- During the first few months after insertion of Mirena, the recipient may experience transient hormonal side effects including oedema, headache, breast tenderness, acne or other skin problems.
- Irregular bleeding and cramping are the most frequently noted side effects noted due to the intrauterine location of device and endometrial atrophy.
- Sometimes, lower abdominal or back pain, vaginal discharge and nausea.

Changes in bleeding pattern: A fairly predictable bleeding pattern follows insertion of Mirena. The first few months are characterised by an increase in total bleeding days, intermenstrual spotting also sometimes occur. After the first 3 months, however, the menstrual blood loss decreases and the number of bleeding days decline. Thorough counselling and discussion before insertion will result in high continuation rate and user satisfaction.

Some 20% of women end up having no monthly bleeding at all within the first year of use. Women should be reassured that the absence of bleeding is most unlikely to signify pregnancy and neither indicative of hormonal abnormality. They can be assured that a normal menstrual bleeding will return within the first month of Mirena being removed.

Risk of pelvic inflammatory disease: The incidence of PID with Mirena is low, at 5 years—the rate is <1/HWY. Some studies suggest that this system offers protection against PID and may be related to the thickening of cervical mucus, endometrial suppression and reduction in the amount of bleeding.

Risk of ectopic pregnancy: The ectopic pregnancy rate is among the lowest of the intrauterine contraceptive methods. At 5 years, the ectopic pregnancy rate is around 0.02/HWY. Indeed, for women aged 25–34 years and using no contraception, the expected ectopic pregnancy rate is around 7.5–10.6/1,000 women years.

Return to fertility:

- Cyclical ovarian function is immediately restored after removal of Mirena.
- Conception rates are normal, as high as 96 per 100 at 12 months after removal of Mirena.

Expulsion: This system can be expelled without the woman noticing it or sometimes having bleeding or pain. Partial expulsion may decrease the effectiveness of Mirena. Increase in menstrual blood flow may be indicative of expulsion. The women should be advised how to check Mirena thread.

Perforation: It is very rare with Mirena and may occur rarely, most often during insertion. Then it must be removed.

Lost threads: If the retrieval threads are not visible at the cervix on follow-up examination, pregnancy must be excluded. Then the thread may usually be located by gently probing with a suitable instrument. X-ray may be used to locate it. Ultrasound diagnosis may be used to ascertain the correct position of the system.

Delayed follicular atresia: Since the contraceptive effect of Mirena is mainly due to its local effect, ovulatory cycles with follicular rupture usually occur in women of fertile age. Sometimes atresia of the follicle is delayed and folliculogenesis may continue. These enlarged follicles cannot be distinguished clinically from ovarian cysts. Enlarged follicles have been diagnosed in about 12% of subjects. Most of these follicles are asymptomatic, sometimes accompanied by pelvic pain or dyspareunia. In most cases, the enlarged follicles disappear spontaneously during next 2–3 months, ultrasound monitoring is recommended to review.

Insertion and Removal

- Before insertion, a woman must be informed of the efficacy, side effects and risks. Proper counselling should be done.
- A physical examination, including pelvic examination, examination of breasts and a cervical smear, should be performed.
- Pregnancy and STDs must be excluded and have to be treated.
- The position and size of uterine cavity should be determined.

- Fundal positioning of Mirena is particularly important in order to ensure uniform exposure of the endometrium to the progestogen, to prevent expulsion and maximise efficacy.
- After insertion, woman should be re-examined 4–12 weeks after and once a year thereafter.
- It is inserted within 7 days of the onset of menstruation and can be replaced by a new system at any time in the cycle. It can also be inserted immediately after first-trimester abortion. Postpartum insertion should be delayed until 6 weeks after delivery.
- Mirena may not be suitable for use as a postcoital contraceptive.
- Mirena is removed by gently pulling the thread with a forceps. If the thread is not visible then it may be removed using a narrow tenaculum.
- Insertion and removal may be associated with some bleeding and pain. It may precipitate fainting as a vasovagal reaction or a seizure in epileptic patients.

EMERGENCY POSTCOITAL CONTRACEPTION (MORNING AFTER PILLS)

Emergency contraception, also known as 'postcoital contraception' or the 'morning after pill', is a method of contraception, which is used after intercourse and before the potential time of implantation. It prevents pregnancy and does not interrupt previously established pregnancy. ECs are not a good option for providing long-term contraception and do not protect against STDs. EC provides women with a safe means of preventing pregnancy following unprotected sexual intercourse (UPSI) or potential contraceptive failure. EC cannot be considered an abortifacient. EC is a backup method for occasional use, and should not be used as a regular method of birth control.

The various methods used for EC are enumerated next.

- *Progestogen-only EC:* This comprises the administration of a single dose of 1.5 mg LNG (levonelle 1500 or levonelle one-step or the morning after pill) as soon as possible after UPSI. It can be administered up to 96 hours outside the product license. The mode of action of LNG for the prevention of pregnancy is not fully understood. It probably acts through inhibition of ovulation and fertilisation, and also through the alteration of the endometrial lining.
- *Ulipristal acetate*: Ulipristal acetate (EllaOne®) is a selective progesterone receptor modulator. One tablet containing 30 mg of ulipristal acetate must be taken as soon as possible following UPSI or contraceptive failure, but no later than 120 hours. In case vomiting occurs within 3 hours, another tablet must be taken.
- *Nonhormonal method*: This comprises of postcoital insertion of a Cu-containing IUCD.
- *Use of COCPs, containing both oestrogen and progestin (Yuzpe's regimen)*: This method comprises the oral administration of two doses of 100 µg EE and 500 µg LNG taken 12 hours apart. This can be considered as the least effective method for EC.

It is also to be taken into consideration that while LNG can be taken more than once in a cycle, use of ulipristal acetate for more than once in the cycle is not recommended. The uses of ECs do not increase the risk of ectopic pregnancy, nor do they affect future fertility. Also, presence of pregnancy (either confirmed or suspected) is a contraindication for the use of EC, because it would not be effective in these cases.

Indications

Indications for the use of EC are as follows:

- Unwanted pregnancy
- Failure to use a contraceptive method
- Condom breakage or leakage
- Dislodgement of a diaphragm or cervical cap
- Two or more missed birth control pills
- Injection of DepoProvera® is late by 1 week or more.
- Sexual assault when the woman had not been using reliable contraception

Advantages

- Saves the couple from unwanted pregnancies
- From unnecessary operative interferences for fear of pregnancy
- From the agony of waiting for the next menstrual cycle
- Prevents adolescent pregnancies
- Helps to reduce unsafe abortion

Two methods of EC are available now—hormonal and mechanical

Management

Prerequisites

- A pelvic examination is not a prerequisite to providing EC.
- There should be no history of recent PID and vaginal or cervical infection. According to the current

recommendations by WHO, IUCDs must not be preferably inserted in women currently having PID, purulent cervicitis, active gonorrhoea or chlamydial infection.

- Prior to IUCD insertion for EC, women considered to be at the risk of STIs should be at least offered testing for *Chlamydia trachomatis* at the minimum. In case the results for STI testing are not immediately available at the time of IUCD insertion, prophylactic antibiotics (particularly against chlamydia) are recommended.

Method of Administration

Hormonal EC (LNG and ulipristal acetate) should be considered for any woman wishing to avoid pregnancy who presents within 5 days of unprotected or inadequately protected sexual intercourse. The dosages in which these hormonal preparations must be used have been previously described in the text. Although they have generally been used only up to 72 hours after intercourse, hormonal method of EC is effective when taken between 72 and 120 hours after unprotected intercourse.

A postcoital IUCD insertion can be considered up to 5 days after ovulation (in case the timing of ovulation can be determined). It is effective immediately after insertion. IUCDs containing at least 380 mm2 of Cu have the lowest failure rates and should be the first line of choice, particularly if the woman intends to continue the IUCD as long-term contraception.

The available evidence indicates that ulipristal acetate is the most effective hormonal emergency contraceptive pill (ECP). The available evidence has indicated the failure rate of ulipristal acetate ranges between 0.9% and 2.1%, while that following the use of LNG ranges from 0.6% to 3.1%. The greater efficacy of ulipristal is probably due to the fact that it disrupts ovulation even after the beginning of the LH surge. On the other hand, LNG is ineffective after the beginning of the LH surge. Presently, there is no study comparing the efficacy of ulipristal acetate to IUCD (used for EC).

While some research studies have shown that LNG ECPs may be effective up to 4 days after sexual intercourse, other studies have suggested that LNG ECPs are likely to be effective for up to 5 days after sexual activity. However, the efficacy may be reduced.

The available evidence points towards the use of Cu IUCD as the most effective option for EC. It is likely to be associated with a pregnancy rate of <0.1%, indicating that it helps in preventing almost all expected pregnancies. Furthermore, the Cu IUCD is associated with an additional benefit of providing highly effective ongoing contraception, if left in situ after placement for EC.

Drug Interactions and Their Consequences on the Efficacy of Emergency Contraception

- Drugs inducing the liver enzymes (e.g. rifampin, griseofulvin, certain anticonvulsant drugs, Saint John's wort, and certain antiretroviral drugs), which are likely to reduce the efficacy of OCPs, may also reduce the efficacy of ECPs such as LNG, ulipristal acetate and combined ECPs. However, the efficacy of Cu IUCDs remains unaffected by these drugs. Therefore, Cu IUCDs can be offered to women who are using these medications and also desire EC. If women using these medications still choose to use LNG EC (or if it is the only most easily available method), she should be advised to take the double dose of 3 mg. Use of ulipristal is not recommended in women using enzyme-inducing drugs.
- Ulipristal, being a progesterone receptor modulator, is likely to block the action of progestin, thereby reducing the efficacy of other hormonal contraceptives containing progestin. A study demonstrating this relationship is presently underway, but results have not yet been published. Presently, the use of a backup method (abstinence or a barrier method) for 14 days following use of ulipristal is recommended amongst women continuing or starting progestin-only methods after use of ulipristal.
- Use of ulipristal acetate with drugs, which increase gastric pH (e.g. antacids, H_2 receptor and proton pump inhibitors), may reduce the absorption of ulipristal, thereby reducing its efficacy.

Repeated Use of Emergency Contraceptive Pills

Clinician should make sure that ECPs must not be repeatedly used as a routine method of contraception because of the availability of far more clinically effective and cost-effective methods for contraception. Women who present for EC and do not desire pregnancy in the near future must be counselled to use a Cu IUCD or another ongoing method of contraception of their choice.

Complications

- Emergency contraceptive pills are associated with an excellent safety profile. No deaths or serious complications have been causally linked to any ECP regimen. Minor adverse effects have been commonly reported.

- The common side effects of hormonal EC are gastrointestinal and mainly include nausea, vomiting, dizziness and fatigue. Antiemetics such as meclizine can be used for controlling these side effects.
- Less common side effects of hormonal methods include headache, bloating, abdominal cramps and spotting or bleeding.
- Ulipristal acetate can cause side effects such as abdominal pain and menstrual disorders (e.g. irregular vaginal bleeding, premenstrual syndrome and uterine cramps).
- Possible complications of postcoital IUCD insertion include—pelvic pain, abnormal bleeding, pelvic infection, perforation and expulsion.

The WHO criteria for use of IUCD are explained in **Table 15**.

OTHER METHODS OF CONTRACEPTION

Hormone Agonist and Antagonist

There is an ongoing search for methods of suppressing ovulation without using oestrogens. One possible development in this field is the synthesis of GnRH agonist and antagonists. GnRH agonists prevent FSH and LH surges. However, suppression of ovarian activity has undesirable side effects on the bone, CVS, etc. and incomplete suppression lead to the consequences of unopposed oestrogen action. At the present time, they may have a place in short-term contraception, e.g. in the breastfeeding mother.

Mifepristone (Progesterone Antagonist)

Progesterone antagonist have a greater potential for fertility regulation, mifepristone blocks the action of progesterone on the endometrium and is used in EC. Daily doses of 2 mg and weekly doses of 100 mg are effective in inhibiting ovulation. Development of once a month pill given in luteal phase is also under consideration (WHO, 1994).

Centchroman

A novel nonsteroidal selective oestrogen receptor modulator known as Centchroman (Ormeloxifene—C30H35NO3) is produced by the Central Drug Research Institute, Lucknow, India. It was initially marketed around 1992 as a nonsteroidal once-a-week oral contraceptive and was included in the National Family Welfare Programme in 1995.

Mechanism of action: As ormeloxifene is a selective oestrogen receptor modulator (SERM), it acts on oestrogen receptors differently. It has a weak oestrogen agonistic activity in some tissues such as bones, and a potent antiestrogenic action in uterus and breast. It does not possess any progesterone, androgenic and antiandrogenic properties.

The contraceptive action of Centchroman appears to mainly rely on the ability to prevent embryonic implantation in the uterine wall by suppressing endometrial proliferation and decidualisation.

Advantages: Users of Centchroman do not complain of any side effects such as nausea, vomiting, weight gain and dizziness. Any delay in return of fertility after stopping does not occur, as it does not interrupt ovulation. It maintains normal ovulatory cycles. No adverse effects on endocrine, haematologic, liver and lipid function have been noted. It has many advantages as a contraceptive including once weekly administration, a long serum half-life, few to no side effects since it does not affect ovulation or the levels of the female hormones in the body and effective and efficient reversal of fertility upon discontinuation of the drug.

Contraceptive action: The standard dose of centchroman is 30 mg twice weekly for the first 3 months followed by once weekly. The pregnancy rates get reduce by 38%, if the loading dose is 60 mg. The efficacy of the drug in the first month of use is uncertain and some form of backup protection has often been suggested. With ideal use, the failure rate of this drug is about 1–2%, which is slightly less effective in comparison with COCPs. In lactating women, the dose of the medication in breast milk is unlikely to cause any adverse effect in babies. It has also been observed that children born of method and user failure pregnancies were congenitally normal with normal milestones.

Immunological Method

- Efforts to make a woman infertile by vaccinating her with semen to produce antibodies have so far failed. A vaccine against part of the β-subunit of LNG has been developed, which can be effective for 6–12 months but has a significant local reaction. In India, a vaccine against the whole β-subunit has been developed.

TABLE 15: World Health Organization (WHO) medical eligibility criteria for use of intrauterine contraceptive device (IUCD).

UKMEC category I:	
• Postpartum between 0 to <48 hours and ≥4 weeks • *Cardiovascular disease*: Multiple risk factors for arterial cardiovascular disease (such as older age, smoking, diabetes, hypertension and known dyslipidaemias), deep vein thrombosis/pulmonary embolism, cardiomyopathy (normal cardiac function), cardiac arrhythmias (atrial fibrillation) and uncomplicated valvular heart disease • *Neurological conditions*: Headaches [nonmigrainous (mild or severe) and migraine] idiopathic intracranial hypertension (IIH), epilepsy • Depressive disorders • *Breast and reproductive tract conditions*: Gestational trophoblastic disease (GTD)—undetectable hCG levels, irregular pattern without heavy bleeding, cervical ectropion • Superficial venous disorders—varicose veins and superficial venous thrombosis • *Rheumatic diseases*: Systemic lupus erythematosus—positive (or unknown) antiphospholipid antibodies • Schistosomiasis—uncomplicated and fibrosis of the liver • Malaria • Diabetes and thyroid disorders • *Therapies*: Antimicrobial and anticonvulsant	
UKMEC category II:	
• Heavy or prolonged bleeding (includes regular and irregular patterns) • Systemic lupus erythematosus—immunosuppressive treatment • Endometriosis • High risk of HIV, asymptomatic or mild HIV clinical disease (WHO stage 1 or 2) • Anaemias—thalassaemia, sickle cell disease and iron-deficiency anaemia	
Initiation of method	***Continuation of the method***
	• Unexplained vaginal bleeding before evaluation • Cervical cancer (awaiting treatment)
UKMEC category III:	
Initiation of method	***Continuation of the method***
• Postpartum is between 48 hours and <4 weeks • Organ transplant • *Complicated*: Graft failure (acute or chronic), rejection, cardiac allograft vasculopathy • Venous thromboembolism (VTE)—current (on anticoagulants) • Ovarian cancer • Acquired immunodeficiency syndrome • Systemic lupus erythematosus in women with extreme thrombocytopaenia • *Cardiovascular disease*: Cardiac arrhythmias (known as long QT syndrome) • GTD—decreasing hCG levels • Severe or advanced HIV clinical disease (WHO stage 3 or 4)	• Pelvic tuberculosis
UKMEC category IV:	
Initiation of method	***Continuation of the method***
• Pregnancy, immediate postseptic abortion and puerperal sepsis • Unexplained vaginal bleeding • Gestational trophoblastic disease—persistently elevated β-hCG levels • Cervical cancer (awaiting treatment) • Endometrial cancer • Ovarian cancer • Current pelvic inflammatory disease, symptomatic and asymptomatic chlamydial infection or purulent cervicitis or gonorrhoea • Pelvic tuberculosis	

(hCG: human chorionic gonadotrophin)
Source: World Health Organization. (2015). Medical eligibility criteria for contraceptive use. [online] Available from https://www.who.int/publications/i/item/9789241549158. [Last accessed May, 2025].

It cross reacts with LH, but there is no significant menstrual disturbance. However, the duration of effectiveness and long-term safety have not yet been established.

- Vaccines against the zona pellucida are effective in animal studies, but in animals they lead to permanent ovarian dysfunction, sterility and premature menopause.

Male Contraceptive Pill

A reversible method of contraception for men has been sought for years. Hormonal contraception for men is inherently a difficult physiological problem because, unlike cyclic ovulation in women, spermatogenesis is continuous, dependent upon gonadotrophin and high levels of intratesticular testosterone. Investigational approaches to inhibit production of sperm include the administration of gossypol, a derivative of cotton seed oil, sex steroids and the use of GnRH analogues.

The sex steroids reduce testosterone synthesis, which leads to loss of libido and development of female secondary sexual characteristics. Furthermore, despite the use of large doses, sperm counts are not adequately reduced in all subjects. LNG, cyproterone acetate and medroxyprogesterone acetate all have been studied, combined with testosterone, given intramuscularly to provide the desired systemic androgen effects.

Gonadotrophin-releasing hormone analogues also decrease the endogenous synthesis of testosterone and supplemental testosterone must be provided. The overall metabolic and health consequences of these approaches have not been assessed and frequent injections are required. Gossypol effectively decreases sperm counts to contraceptive levels, apparently by incapacitating the sperm producing cells. Gossypol pills are taken daily for 2 months until sperms are no longer observed in the ejaculate and then the pills are taken weekly. Fertility returns to normal 3 months after discontinuation. Although the experience in China has been largely positive, animal studies in the UK indicate that gossypol or contaminants of the preparation are toxic. Analogues of gossypol may offer potential, but are years away from development.

Choice of Contraception

The choice of contraceptive method depends on the circumstances in which it is applied and on its acceptance by the patient. The acronym 'GATHER' is used to refer to the process of counselling for contraceptive use:

- G—Greet the client
- A—Ask the client about herself
- T—Tell the client about the choices available
- H—Help the client to make an informed choice
- E—Explain fully how to use the chosen method
- R—Return visit should be encouraged

Eventually, the choice of a contraceptive is a very personal one.

Postpartum Choice of Contraception

Additional contraception is necessary during lactation for most women. After 3 months, the first ovulation can precede the first menstrual bleed. Contraception is usually on the mind of both clinician and patient at the first postpartum visit.

Rules of 3's

- In the presence of full breastfeeding, a contraceptive method should be used beginning in the third postpartum month.
- With partial and no breastfeeding, a contraceptive method should begin during the third postpartum week.
- After the termination of pregnancy of <12 weeks, oral contraception can be started immediately.
- After a pregnancy of 12 or more weeks, the third postpartum week rule should be followed. This delay has been based on a theoretical concern over an increased risk of thrombosis early in postpartum period.

Oral Contraception

In the postpartum period, because of the concerns regarding the impact of COCs on breastfeeding, a useful alternative is to combine the contraceptive effect of lactation with the progestogen-only minipill, as there is no evidence of any adverse effect on breastfeeding as measured by milk volume and infant growth and development. Progestin-only minipill even provides a modest boost to milk production and helps to breastfeed longer. In addition, the minipill can protect against the bone loss associated with lactation.

Because of the slight positive impact on lactation, the minipill can be started soon after delivery, but at least a 3-day postpartum delay is recommended to allow the decline in pregnancy levels of oestrogen and progesterone and the establishment of lactation.

- Those who insist on low-dose OC pills, the full breast feeder should begin during the third postpartum month, all others during the third postpartum week.
- DepoProvera can be administered immediately postpartum and certainly should be utilised no later than the third postpartum week. It should be used with caution in all women with previous gestational diabetes.
- *Barrier methods*: Barrier methods have no impact on breastfeeding, and they are an excellent choice for motivated couples. Condoms, spermicides and foam should be used in the immediate postpartum period, and use of the sponge, cap or diaphragm can be started around the sixth postpartum week.

Postpartum Intrauterine Contraceptive Device

Immediate postpartum insertion of IUCDs has been practised in China since 1975. Providing postpartum contraceptive services avoids overcrowded outpatient facilities allowing more women to be served, eliminates transportation costs and service fees paid by women for making an additional visit for IUCD insertion, if that visit does not coincide with infant care service. There is no effect on breast milk quantity or quality.

A 2010 Cochrane review concluded that postpartum intrauterine contraceptive devices (PPIUCDs) were a safe and effective contraceptive method. The women are accessible to PPIUCDs following facility births.

Counselling

Choices of methods should be discussed during routine prenatal visits, allowing women to choose the most appropriate method.

A woman who presents in early labour or prior to caesarean can be counselled for an immediate PPIUCD.

A woman could decide after delivery to have an IUCD inserted. Counselling should be done once the emotional and physical stresses of labour have ended.

Postpartum Uterus and Postpartum Intrauterine Contraceptive Device Insertion (Fig. 70)

Immediately after expulsion of the placenta, the fundus of the uterus is just below the umbilicus and is approximately 30 cm in length thus requiring a longer instrument for fundal placement of IUCD.

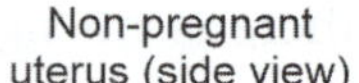

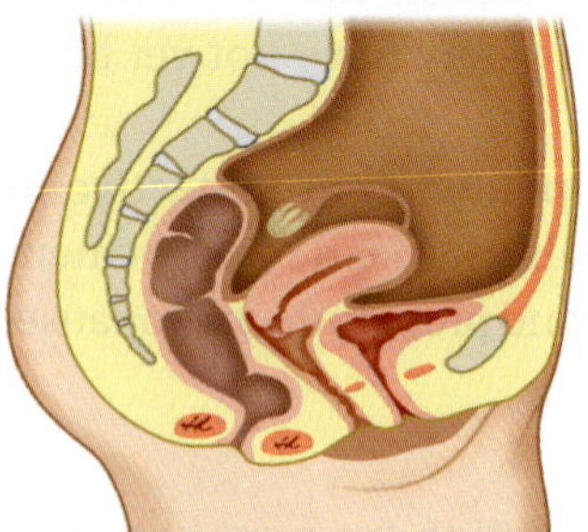
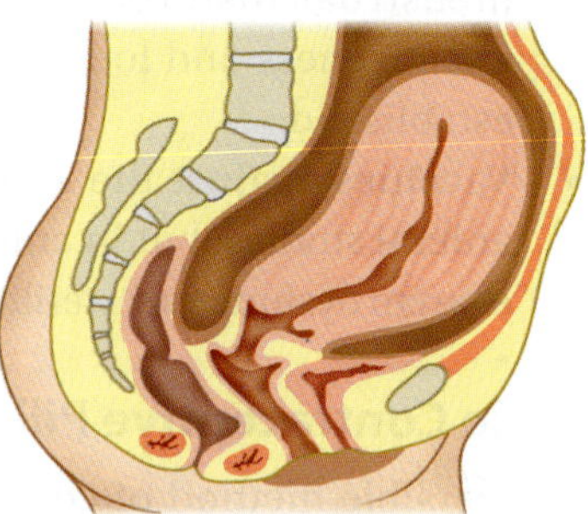

Fig. 70: Postpartum uterus and postpartum intrauterine contraceptive device (PPIUCD) insertion.

The anterior and posterior walls of the body of the uterus are about 4–5 cm each in thickness, making chances of perforation very rare.

This disparity in consistency and weight between the heavy and thickened body of the uterus and the stretched and folded lower uterine segment contributes to the extreme curvature, which can be noted upon bimanual examination. Immediately following delivery—the uterus contracts and is slightly tilted forwards in the lower abdominal cavity. The axis of the uterine cavity is at right angle to the axis of the postpartum vagina. During insertion of the immediate PPIUCD, this sharp angle can make insertion difficult. Manual correction of this angle is very important for correct fundal placement.

Long placental forceps (Kelley's forceps) is required for insertion of PPIUCD. A common error is to mistake the posterior wall of the uterus for the fundus. Careful confirmation of fundal placement by manual palpation minimises this error, which can lead to an increased risk of expulsion.

Clinical Assessment

- *First assessment* of women should be done during antenatal visits and if women has presented for the first time only at delivery and had no prior assessment. The following conditions should be assessed:
  - Known distorted uterine cavity fibroid, uterine septum
  - Acute purulent discharge
  - Malignant or benign trophoblastic disease
  - Suffering from AIDS and neither clinically ill nor on ART.

- *Second assessment should be done immediately prior to insertion to rule out following conditions*:
    - Chorioamnionitis
    - Postpartum endometritis/puerperal sepsis
    - More than 18 hours from the rupture of membranes to delivery of baby
    - Unresolved postpartum haemorrhage
    - Extensive genital trauma

Precautions before Postpartum Intrauterine Contraceptive Device Insertion

Asepsis and proper infection prevention measures should be taken. Before insertion, a water-based antiseptic is applied to the cervix and vagina two or more times. No touch technique should be used.

The IUCD should not touch the perineum, the vaginal walls or any surface that may contaminate it. Ideally, the IUCD should not be passed through the cervical OS more than once. Visible strings after removing the forceps during immediate postplacental insertion indicate that IUCD is placed lower than the fundus. In such cases, the IUCD may be removed and tried once more for fundal placement.

Appropriate Times for Postpartum Intrauterine Contraceptive Device Insertion

- *Postplacental insertion*: Immediately within 10 minutes of delivery of the placenta
- *Intracaesarean insertion*
- *Immediate postpartum insertion*: Within 48 hours of delivery
- *Interval insertion*: 6 weeks after delivery or after an abortion.

Intracaesarean Insertion

This is done manually or using a regular ring forceps, followed by closure of uterine incision. There is no need to fix the IUCD with a ligature, not to attempt to pass the strings of the IUCD through the cervical OS before closure of the uterus.

These periods are recommended as the cervix is open and limp, and an IUCD can easily be placed high in the fundus. After 48 hours postpartum, the cervix is not open enough to allow for an easy and relatively painless instrument insertion.

The PPIUCD should not be inserted between 48 hours and 6 weeks after birth, because the uterus is softer and more vascular than in its nonpregnant state. Therefore, an increase in perforation and infection has been observed.

Immediate Postpartum Intrauterine Contraceptive Device Insertion and

Active Management of Third-stage Labour

No aspect of active management of third-stage labour (AMTSL) should be modified to accommodate immediate PPIUCD insertion. Immediate PPIUCD does not increase the risk of uterine atony.

Postinsertion Care

The patient should report any increase in more than expected vaginal bleeding or uterine cramping.

If severe uterine cramping occurs and persists after immediate PPIUCD insertion, a speculum examination should be performed to check for expulsion.

At 6 weeks postpartum, the IUCD strings can be felt by some women. It is not necessary for her to check the strings.

Problems Encountered after Postpartum Intrauterine Contraceptive Device Insertion

Changes in menstrual bleeding patterns: A slight increase in the amount and duration of menstrual bleeding, more than what is expected in the postpartum period or intermenstrual bleeding, requires just reassurance.

Heavy and prolonged bleeding or associated with severe anaemia may require removal with the patient's consent.

Cramping or pain: Mild intermittent cramping in the first weeks after IUCD insertion is generally masked by the usual cramping associated with uterine involution postpartum. Nonsteroidal anti-inflammatory drugs (NSAIDs) help to reduce menstrual pain and cramping. If cramping or pain is severe, remove the IUCD.

Infection: No increased risk of pelvic infection occurs with postpartum IUCD insertion.

The risk of upper genital tract infection is <1%. This risk is highest within the first 20 days after PPUICD insertion, and is related either to lack of proper infection (prevention practices) and or preexisting infection rather than to the IUCD itself. Lower abdominal pain, fever, painful intercourse, bleeding after intercourse or between periods once resumption of normal monthly periods has occurred postpartum, new onset of pain associated with periods, abnormal vaginal discharge, nausea and vomiting are the symptoms suggestive of infection.

Rule out PID, endometritis, appendicitis, partial IUCD expulsion, uterine perforation, pregnancy/ectopic pregnancy, or urinary tract infection. Antibiotics for reproductive tract infection/sexually transmitted infection (RTI/STI) can be given. Remove the IUCD, if symptoms persist >72 hours.

The IUCD can be removed 2–3 days after antibiotic treatment has begun, if the patient does not want to continue. Pelvic pain in most of the women gets relieved by analgesics, and persisted in only 4.4% at 12 months. According to an Indian Council of Medical Research (ICMR) study on urban women, pelvic pain is a common symptom reported in 25% users following interval IUCD insertion.

String problems: Reassure the women that the string is not very harmful. If they are bothersome to the women, the strings can be cut short if they are long. If the strings are too short and bother the partner, a new IUCD may be inserted.

Missing thread: Visibility of strings is important, as it assures both the IUCD user and the healthcare worker about proper placement of the device, and provides ease of removal. In intracaesarean insertion, though at the time of insertion threads are not outside cervical OS, involution of uterus makes them visible in most cases at the first visit; in a few cases, threads may get curled up and not be seen at external OS. This may cause apprehension as missing strings and may indicate expulsion, malpositioning, or perforation.

The IUCD strings were visible in 61.87% women at first visit and visibility increased to 84.62% at 12 months.

Bhutta et al. reported string visibility of 92% and 96% at 6 months after intracaesarean and interval insertion, respectively.

Follow-up Care and Counselling

Client should be advised to come for a checkup at 6 weeks and thereafter as and when necessary. A speculum examination on the first visit to assess the strings have descended into the vagina is a must. Thereafter, a pelvic examination is not required if the patient has no problems. If the woman does not have any complaints, even an additional follow-up is not required.

Complications

The risk of uterine perforation for postpartum IUCD insertion is low. In addition, insertion complaints caused by lochial blood and cramping are masked.

One multisite study found that after 6 months, the cumulative expulsion rate was 9% for immediate postplacental insertion. Expulsion rates can vary extensively depending on the timing of insertion, the technique used, skill of the person doing the insertion and the type of IUCD used.

In general, the expulsion rate is between 10% and 14%, it is still an acceptable expulsion rate, because it can provide 86–90% of retention of IUCD.

Maximal expulsions in previous studies have been detected during the first follow-up visit. The rate of expulsion of IUCD was 3.6% by 6 weeks of follow-up. In Mali, the expulsion rates for immediate postpartum insertions were skewed by the high rates for one of the three providers, who had far less training and experience than the other two.

High fundal placement of the IUCD, elevation of the uterus, keeping the forceps closed while going in and open while coming out of the uterine cavity by an experienced and trained provider are the tips for reducing expulsion. Infection prevention practices including aseptic and no touch technique may influence expulsion rates.

Postplacental and intracaesarean insertions have lowest expulsion rates.

The IUCDs inserted postplacentally and in the immediate postpartum period are more likely to be expelled than those inserted in the interval period. Immediate postpartum IUCD insertion has a higher retention rate than if the IUCD is inserted postplacentally.

After birth, as the uterine contractions expel retained placental tissues and blood clots, this may have a similar effect on any foreign body introduced into the uterus. IUCDs inserted postplacentally have a lower expulsion risk than immediate postpartum insertions. After a partial or complete IUCD expulsion, a pelvic examination is conducted to rule out infection and pregnancy.

Perforation: The perforation risk at 1 month for immediate postpartum insertions was no greater than that associated with interval insertion, about 1 per 2,000 insertions. In a study in Paraguay by VB Araujo et al. no perforation was documented out of 3,029 insertions. The cumulative 6 month PID rate was 1.4 to 2 per 100 women.

Infection: Most cases of PID occur within 3 months of insertion, and some were the result of endometritis associated with delivery rather than with the IUCD. Wekovic et al. found no increased incidence of endometritis and increased haemorrhage with PPIUCD in women using PPIUCD versus women who did not use PPIUCD.

What new is being tried?

Recently, LNG intrauterine system has been successfully tried as an immediate postpartum contraception. Lopez Farfan compared intracaesarean insertion of Mirena and IUCD and found an expulsion rate of 4.5% in both groups at 1-year follow-up. Menstruation was lighter with less dysmenorrhoea in Mirena group versus IUCD group. Continuation rate of approximately 91% in both the groups was seen at the end of 1 year. Main reason for discontinuation was prolonged bleeding (35%) in CuT group and amenorrhoea 11.7% in Mirena group.

The clinical advantage of MIRENA at the time of caesarean includes improvement of uterine involution, decreasing lochia and dysfunctional bleeding.

- Copper IUCDs can be inserted between 4 and 8 weeks postpartum without an increase in pregnancy rates, expulsion, uterine perforation or removal for bleeding and/or pain. Expulsion rate is less with new IUCDs.
- Insertion can even occur immediately after a vaginal delivery, if no intrauterine infection is present or suspected. A slightly higher rate of expulsion is to be expected, compared to insertion 4–8 weeks postpartum.
- Insertion of an IUCD in breastfeeding women is relatively easier and is associated with a lower removal rate for bleeding or pains, perforation rate is not more.
- An IUCD can be inserted immediately after a first trimester abortion but after a second-trimester abortion, it is recommended to wait until uterine involution occurs.

Adolescent's Choice of Contraception

Providing contraception or information about contraception for young people under the age of 20 years is an important factor. Teenage girls carry the burdens of unprotected sexual activity such as unwanted pregnancy, undetected STDs, and PID. Rates of HIV infection are rising faster in young women than in any other group. Premature parenthood and the STDs are the risks of sexual experimentation.

Contraceptive education must be combined with an emphasis on overall life issues and interventions including decision to become sexually active, no single message or approach by itself will be broadly effective for all adolescents.

- Our goals are to promote abstinence among teenagers who are not yet ready to cope with sex and its consequences and to promote behaviour that will prevent pregnancy and STDs in sexually active adolescents.
- Building trust and good communication are requirements for a successful interaction between clinician and adolescents.

CHOICE OF METHODS

Oral Contraception

The COC is the most popular and requested method of contraception by teenagers. OCs are almost never medically contraindicated in healthy adolescents. Thus, the high efficacy of COC is an excellent choice for teenagers.

- Because younger women change partners more frequently than older ones, a dual approach is recommended, COCs combined with the use of barrier methods, so that they can prevent PID, STDs and HIV.

Barrier Methods

After oral contraception, the condom use with a spermicide is the next best choice for young women, obviously this is the only choice for male adolescents. The diaphragm and cervical caps should be reserved for very motivated and young people.

Intrauterine Device

The IUCDs have not been recommended for nulligravid women and those who have a high risk of STDs. It can be considered for young parous woman who is in stable monogamous relationship. It is also a good choice for patients with chronic illness, such as diabetes mellitus or systemic lupus erythematosus (SLE).

- The creams, foams, suppositories and jellies are not ideal for adolescents. They require proper timing, careful placement and consistent use to achieve good efficacy.
- There are special candidates to consider for long-acting contraception (DepoProvera or Norplant), teens who have failed oral contraception and who are mentally retarded or have chronic illnesses.

- Because adolescents often have unplanned sexual intercourse, access to emergency postcoital contraception is very important. The failure rate is approximately 2% using OCPs and 1% using LNG pills.

CONTRACEPTION CHOICE FOR OLDER WOMEN

Oral Contraception

Oral contraceptive benefits to be emphasised with older women.

- Less endometrial cancer
- Less ovarian cancer
- More regular menses
- Increase in bone density and others mentioned before
- In all women >35 years of age, nonsmoker, lowest dose oestrogen (20 μg) combined pills should be used.
- The progestin-only minipill is a good choice for older woman, especially in whom combined pills are contraindicated.
- The oral contraceptives that contain 20 μg oestrogen provide effective contraception, improve cycle regularity, diminish bleeding and relieve menopausal symptoms.
- *Transition from oral contraception to postmenopausal hormone therapy*: It is very important to change because even with lowest oestrogen dose oral contraceptive available, the oestrogen dose is fourfold greater than the standard postmenopausal dose. With increasing age, dose-related risks with oestrogen become significant.

  To establish the onset of postmenopausal years, FSH level is measured yearly beginning at the age of 50 years, sample is taken on day 6 or 7 of a pill-free week. When FSH is >20 IU/L, it is time to change to a postmenopausal hormonal therapy.
- Long-acting methods are especially advantageous for smokers and for women with a history of thromboembolic disease.
- The IUCDs (Cu and LNG IUCDs) are amongst the most effective contraceptive for older women, as they are more likely to be mutually monogamous and less likely to develop PID, as they have already had their children.

CONTRACEPTION AND LITIGATION

- Clinicians are concerned about the prospect of bad outcomes associated with contraceptive use, leading to litigation. Actually, these events are very unusual compared with the widespread use of contraception. Patients who sue usually claim there were contraindications or risks that were not conveyed by clinician. The best way to avoid litigation is good patient communication and keeping good records.
- Document that the risks and benefits of all methods were discussed.
- Document a plan for follow-up.
- Document all interactions with the patient, including phone calls.

SUGGESTED READING

1. Adams K, Beal MW. Implanon: a review of the literature with recommendations for clinical management. J Midwifery Womens Health. 2009;54(2):142-9.
2. Ahrendt HJ, Makalová D, Parke S, Mellinger U, Mansour D. Bleeding pattern and cycle control with an estradiolbased oral contraceptive: a seven-cycle, randomized comparative trial of estradiol valerate/dienogest and ethinyl estradiol/levonorgestrel. Contraception. 2009;80(5):436-44
3. Anderson FD, Hait H. A multicenter, randomized study of an extended cycle oral contraceptive. Contraception. 2003;68(2):89-96.
4. Apter D, GemzellDanielsson K, Hauck B, Rosen K, Zurth C. Pharmacokinetics of two low-dose levonorgestrel-releasing intrauterine systems and effects on ovulation rate and cervical function: pooled analyses of phase II and III studies. Fertil Steril. 2014;101:1656-62.
5. Archer DF, Jensen JT, Johnson JV, Borisute H, Grubb GS, Constantine GD. Evaluation of a continuous regimen of levonorgestrel/ethinyl estradiol: phase 3 study results. Contraception. 2006;74(6):439-45.
6. Baram I, Weinstein A, Trussell J. The IUB, a newly invented IUD: a brief report. Contraception. 2014;89(2):139-41.
7. Bonnar J, Flynn A, Freundl G, Kirkman R, Royston R, Snowden R. Personal hormone monitoring for contraception. Br J Fam Plann. 1999;24(4):128-34.
8. Çelen Ş, Sucak A, Yıldız Y, Danışman N. Immediate postplacental insertion of an intrauterine contraceptive device during cesarean section in Turkey. Contraception. 2011;84:240-3.
9. Chen BA, Hayes JL, Hohmann HL, Perriera LK, Reeves MF, Creinin MD. A randomized trial of postplacental compared to delayed insertion of levonorgestrol releasing intrauterine device after vaginal delivery. Contraception. 2009;80(2):205.
10. Chil C, Zhou SW, Balogh S, NG K. Post caesarean insertion of intrauterine devices. Am J Public Health. 1984:74(11):1281-2.
11. Cleland K, Zhu H, Goldstuck N, Cheng L, Trussell J. The efficacy of intrauterine devices for emergency contraception: A systematic review of 35 years of experience. Hum Reprod. 2012;27(7):1994-2000.

12. Creinin MD, Schlaff W, Archer DF, Wan L, Frezieres R, Thomas M, et al. Progesterone receptor modulator for emergency contraception: A randomized controlled trial. Obstet Gynecol. 2006;108(5):1089-97.
13. Dorflinger. Family Health International Contraceptive Development. 2004;71:23.
14. Edelman A, Micks E, Gallo MF, Jensen JT, Grimes DA. Continuous or extended cycle vs. cyclic use of combined hormonal contraceptives for contraception. Cochrane Database Syst Rev. 2014;(7):CD004695.
15. Etonogestrel implant (Implanon) for contraception. Drug Ther Bull. 2001;39(8):579.
16. Faculty of Sexual and Reproductive Health (FSRH). Progestogen-only injectable contraception clinical effectiveness unit. London: FSRH; 2014.
17. Faculty of Sexual and Reproductive Health (FSRH). UK medical eligibility criteria for contraceptive use. London: FSRH; 2009.
18. Fine P, Mathe H, Ginde S, Cullins V, Morfesis J, Gainer E. Ulipristal acetate taken 48–120 hours after intercourse for emergency contraception. Obstet Gynecol. 2010;115(2):257-63.
19. Fraser IS, Parke S, Mellinger U, Machlitt A, Serrani M, Jensen J. Effective treatment of heavy and/or prolonged menstrual bleeding without organic cause: pooled analysis of two multinational, randomised, double-blind, placebo-controlled trials of oestradiol valerate and dienogest. Eur J Contracept Reprod Health Care. 2011;16(4):258-69.
20. Gallo MF, Grimes DA, Scholz KF. Nonlatex versus latex male condom. Cochrane Database of systemic review. Contraception. 2003;36(5):319-26.
21. GemzellDanielsson K, Schellschmidt I, Apter D. A randomized, phase II study describing the efficacy, bleeding profile, and safety of two low dose levonorgestrel-releasing intrauterine contraceptive systems and Mirena®. Fertil Steril. 2012;97(3):61622.
22. Glasier AF, Cameron S, Fine PM, Logan SJ, Casale W, Van Horn J, et al. Ulipristal acetate versus levonorgestrel for emergency contraception: A randomised non inferiority trial and metaanalysis. Lancet. 2010;375(9714):555-62.
23. Goa KL, Warner GT, Easthope SE. Transdermal ethinylestradiol/norelgestromin: a review of its use in hormonal contraception. Treat Endocrinol. 2003;2(3):191-206.
24. Goujard J, RumeauRouquette C. First trimester exposure to progestogen/estrogen and congenital malformations. Lancet. 1977;1(8009):482-3.
25. Grimes DA, Lopez LM, Schulz KF, Van Vliet HA, Stanwood NL. Immediate postpartum insertion of intrauterine devices. Cochrane Database Syst Rev. 2010;12(5):CD003036.
26. Guida M, Bramante S, Acunzo G, Pellicano M, Cirillo D, Nappi C. Diagnosis of fertility with a personal hormonal evaluation test. Minerva Ginecol. 2003;55(2):167-73.
27. Gujju RLB, Prasad U, Prasad U. Study on the acceptance, complications and continuation rate of postpartum family planning using the Postplacental Intrauterine Contraceptive device among women delivering at a tertiary care hospital. Int J Reprod Contracept Obstet Gynecol. 2015;4(2):388-91.
28. Harlap S, Prywes R, Davies AM. Birth defects and oestrogens and progesterones in pregnancy. Lancet. 1975;1(7908):682-3.
29. Harlap S, Shiono PH, Ramcharan S. Congenital abnormalities in the offspring of women who used oral and other contraceptives around the time of conception. Int J Fertil. 1985;30(2):394-7.
30. Hatcher RA, Warner DL. New condoms for men and women, diaphragms, cervical caps, and spermicides: overcoming barriers to barriers and spermicides. Curr Opin Obstet Gynecol. 1992;4(4):513-21.
31. Heads of Medicines Agencies. (2010). Qlaira® EU Summary of Product Characteristics. [online] Available from www.hma.eu/ mri. Html. [Last accessed May, 2025].
32. Hook EB. Cardiovascular birth defects and prenatal exposure to female sex hormones: a reevaluation of data from a large prospective study. Teratology. 1994;49(3):162-6.
33. Irving S, Janet S, Soledad D. Rates and outcomes of planned pregnancy after use of levonorgestrel-releasing or copper T 380Ag intrauterine contraceptive devices. Am J Obstet Gynecol. 1992;166(4);1208-13.
34. Jain J, Jakimiuk AJ, Bode FR, Ross D, Kaunitz AM. Contraceptive efficacy and safety of DMPASC. Contraception. 2004;70(4):269-75.
35. Jensen JT, Parke S, Mellinger U, Machlitt A, Fraser IS. Effective treatment of heavy menstrual bleeding with estradiol valerate and dienogest: a randomized controlled trial. Obstet Gynecol. 2011;117(4):777-87.
36. Jishabai CP. A Study on the Complications of Immediate PostPartum IUCD Insertion. J Evid Based Med Healthcare. 2015;2(9):1246-51.
37. Kapp N, Curtis KM. Intrauterine device insertion during the postpartum period: A Systematic Review. Contraception. 2009;80(4):327-36.
38. Kaunitz AM, Darney PD, Ross D, Wolter KD, Speroff L. Subcutaneous DMPA vs. intramuscular DMPA: a 2-year randomized study of contraceptive efficacy and bone mineral density. Contraception. 2009;80(1):7-17.
39. Kerin JF, Cooper JM, Price T, Herendael BJ, Cayuela-Font E, Cher D, et al. Hysteroscopic sterilization using a microinsert device: results of a multicentre Phase II study. Hum Reprod. 2003;18(6):122330.
40. Kerin JF, Munday DN, Ritossa MG, Pesce A, Rosen D. Essure hysteroscopic sterilization: results based on utilizing a new coil catheter delivery system. J Am Assoc Gynecol Laparosc. 2004;11(3):388-93.
41. Khatun HA. Postpartum IUCDA New Method in Postpartum Contraception. Int J Gynecol Obstet. 2009;107(2):620.

42. Kulier R, O'Brien PA, Helmerhorst FM, Usher-Patel M, D'Arcangues C. Copper containing, framed intrauterine devices for contraception. Cochrane Database Syst Rev. 2007;(4):CD005347.
43. Kumar S, Sethi R, Balasubramaniam S, Charurat E, Lalchandani K, Semba R, et al. Women's experience with postpartum intrauterine contraceptive device use in India. Reproductive Health. 2014;11:32.
44. Letti Müller AL, Lopes Ramos JG, MartinsCosta SH, Palma Dias RS, Valério EG, Hammes LS, et al. Transvaginal Ultrasonographic Assessment of the Expulsion of Intrauterine Devices inserted in the Immediate Postpartum period: A pilot study. Contraception. 2009;72(3):192-5.
45. Levi E, Cantillo E, Ades V, Banks E, Murthy A. Immediate Postplacental IUD insertion at Caesarean delivery. Contraception. 2012;86(2):102-5.
46. Levie MD, Chudnoff SG. Prospective analysis of office-based hysteroscopic sterilization. J Minim Invasive Gynecol. 2006;13(2):98-101.
47. Lidegaard O, Hougaard NL, Skovlund CW, Løkkegaard E. Venous thrombosis in users of nonoral hormonal contraception: followup study, Denmark 200110. BMJ. 2012;344:e2990.
48. Long-term reversible contraception. Twelve years of experience with the TCu380A and TCu220C. Contraception. 1997;56:341-52.
49. LopezFarfan JA, MacielMartínez M, VelezMachorro IJ, et al. Application of MIRENA® during Caesarean Section. Eur J Contracept Reprod Health Care. 2010;15(Suppl. 1):165-6.
50. Mansour D, Verhoeven C, Sommer W, Weisberg E, Taneepanichskul S, Melis GB, et al. Efficacy and tolerability of a monophasic combined oral contraceptive containing nomegestrol acetate and 17β-oestradiol in a 24/4 regimen, in comparison to an oral contraceptive containing ethinylestradiol and drospirenone in a 21/7 regimen. Eur J Contracept Reprod Health Care. 2011;16(6):430-43.
51. Miller L, Hughes JP. Continuous combination oral contraceptive pills to eliminate withdrawal bleeding: a randomized trial. Obstet Gynecol. 2003;101(4):653-61.
52. Mills A. Barrier contraception. Clin Obstet Gynaecol. 1984;11(3): 64160.
53. Mishra S. Evaluation of Safety, Efficacy, and Expulsion of Post Placental and IntraCesarean Insertion of Intrauterine Contraceptive Devices (PPIUCD). J Obstet Gynaecol India. 2014;64(5):337-43.
54. Mohamed SA, Kamel MA, Shaaban OM, Salem HT. Acceptability for the use of postpartum intrauterine contraceptive devices: Assiut experience. Med Princ Pract. 2003;12(3):170-5.
55. National Institute for Health and Clinical Excellence Guidelines. Postpartum Contraception the effective and appropriate use of long-acting reversible contraception. London: RCOG Press; 2005.
56. Nelson A, Apter D, Hauck B, Schmelter T, Rybowski S, Rosen K, et al. Two low-dose levonorgestrel intrauterine contraceptive systems: a randomized controlled trial. Obstet Gynecol. 2013;122(6):1205-13.
57. Nelson AL, Sampson Landers C, Parke S, et al. Efficacy of estradiol valerate/dienogest OC: results of 3 large studies in North America and Europe. Abstract plus poster presentation at 57th Annual Clinical Meeting of the American College of Obstetricians and Gynecologists. Chicago, IL: American College of Obstetricians; 2009.
58. Novikova N, Weisberg E, Stanczyk FZ, Croxatto HB, Fraser IS. Effectiveness of levonorgestrel emergency contraception given before or after ovulation—a pilot study. Contraception. 2007;75(2):112-8.
59. Noé G, Croxatto HB, Salvatierra AM, Reyes V, Villarroel C, Muñoz C, et al. Contraceptive efficacy of emergency contraception with levonorgestrel given before or after ovulation. Contraception. 2011;84:486-92.
60. Ogburn JA, Espey E, Stonehocker J. Barriers to Intrauterine device insertion in post partum women. Contraception. 2005;72(6):426-9.
61. Palacios S, Wildt L, Parke S, Machlitt A, Römer T, Bitzer J. Efficacy and safety of a novel oral contraceptive based on oestradiol (oestradiol valerate/dienogest): A Phase III trial. Eur J Obstet Gynecol. 2010;149(1):57-62.
62. Parke S, Makalová D, Ahrendt HJ, Mansour D. Bleeding patterns and cycle control with a novel four-phasic combined oral contraceptive containing estradiol valerate and dienogest. Eur J Contracept Reprod Health Care. 2008;13(1):94-5.
63. Piaggio G, Kapp N, von Hertzen H. Effect on pregnancy rates of the delay in the administration of levonorgestrel for emergency contraception: a combined analysis of four WHO trials. Contraception. 2011;84:359.
64. Pongsatha S, Ekmahachai M, Suntornlimsiri N, Morakote N, Chaovisitsaree S. Bone mineral density in women using the subdermal contraceptive implant Implanon for at least 2 years. Int J Gynaecol Obstet. 2010;109(3):223-5.
65. RCOG and Faculty of Sexual and Reproductive Healthc[a]re Clinical Guidance. Male and female sterilisation. London: Faculty of Sexual and Reproductive Healthcare; 2014.
66. Rosen DM. Learning curve for hysteroscopic sterilisation: lessons from the first 80 cases. Aust N Z J Obstet Gynaecol. 2004;44(1):624.
67. Roumen FJ. Review of the combined contraceptive vaginal ring, NuvaRing®. Ther Clin Risk Manag. 2008;4(2):441-51.
68. Sahaja K, Kabadi YM. Enhancing contraceptive usage by post-placental intrauterine contraceptive devices (PPIUCD) insertion with evaluation of safety, efficacy, and expulsion. Int J Reprod Contracept Obste Gyneco. 2012:1(1):26-32.
69. Singal S, Bharti R, Dewan R. clinical outcome of postplacental copper T 380A insertion in women delivering by caesarean section. J CIin Diagn Res. 2014;8(9):OC01OC04.

70. Steiner MJ, Dominik R, Rountree RW, Nanda K, Dorflinger LJ. Contraceptive effectiveness of polyurethane condom and Latex Condom. Obstet and Gynaecol. 2003;101(3):539-47.
71. Stewart FH, Kaunitz AM, Laguardia KD, Karvois DL, Fisher AC, Friedman AJ. Extended use of transdermal norelgestromin/ethinyl estradiol: a randomized trial. Obstet Gynecol. 2005;105(6):1389-96.
72. Stuart GS, Bryant AG. Feasibility of Postpartum placement of the levonorgestrel intrauterine system more than 6 hour after vaginal birth. Contraception. 2011;85(4):359-62.
73. Sunita S, Rekha B, Rupali D. Clinical outcome of postplacental copper T 380A insertion in women delivering by caesarean section. J Clin Diagn Research. 2014; 8(9): OC01OC04.
74. Tatum HJ, Beltran RS, Ramos R, Van Kets H, Sivin I, Schmidt FH. Immediate postplacental insertion of GYNET 380 and GYNET 380 postpartum intrauterine contraceptive devices: a randomized study. Am J Obstet Gynecol. 1996;175(5):1231-5.
75. Welkovic S, Costa LO, Faundes A, de Alencar Ximenes R, Costa CF. Postpartum bleeding and Infection after Postplacental IUD insertion. Contraception. 2011;63(3): 155-8.
76. Westhoff C, Kaunitz AM, Korver T, Sommer W, Bahamondes L, Darney P, et al. Efficacy, safety, and tolerability of a monophasic oral contraceptive containing nomegestrol acetate and 17bestradiol: a randomized controlled trial. Obstet Gynecol. 2012;119(5):989-99.
77. Whiteman Mk, Cox S, Tepper NK. Postpartum intrauterine device and postpartum tubal sterilization in the united states. Am J Obstet Gnecol. 2011;206(2):127.
78. World Health Organisation (WHO). Medical Eligibility Criteria for Contraception Use, 3rd edition. Geneva: WHO; 2008.

56

CHAPTER

Sterilisation and Termination of Pregnancy

Priya Ballal K, Nikil Shetty, Ektha M Shetty

Chapter Outline

- Sterilisation
- Female Sterilisation
- Male Sterilisation
- Termination of Pregnancy

STERILISATION

Definition

Sterilisation is a procedure that can permanently block procreative function. It can prevent a woman or a man from bearing further children. In other words, destruction of reproductive function is the primary purpose of any sterilisation procedure. Although procedures such as a hysterectomy for any benign or malignant condition or bilateral salpingectomy or oophorectomy done along with or without hysterectomy could incidentally result in loss of reproductive function, the term sterilisation is restricted to those procedures whose primary aim is to prevent further pregnancies. Many procedures have been described for the purpose of sterilisation; however, a perfect method of sterilisation with zero failure rate and acceptable reversibility is yet to be designed. Hence, various choices of surgeries are performed by different surgeons to achieve the same goal. Sterilisation procedures can be performed both on male and female patients.

Legality

- *Consent*: Since this procedure is one of the choice of the patient to choose not to conceive a child permanently, it is one that needs serious deliberation. Adequate information with regard to the permanency, risks involved with the procedure as well as anaesthesia needs to be placed before the patient. His or her options for long-term contraception must also be made aware to the patient. The awareness that major surgery may be required for the reversal of tubal ligation or need for in vitro fertilisation (IVF) treatment in case the patient changes her mind later is to be provided to the patient. Although there is no age limit to sterilisation procedures, certain countries include this in their guidelines. In India, the Ministry of Health and Family Welfare suggests an age limit of 22–49 years. Consent of a spouse is not mandatory, as marital status is not of consideration if a woman wants to undergo sterilisation procedure. In a situation regarding intellectual disability, the patient's consent may require validation from the judicial court.

Indications

The strict medical indications are like those for contraception. To justify sterilisation, however, the condition should be one which is permanent and unlikely ever to be cured or improved sufficiently to allow pregnancy with safety. As medical knowledge and skills grow, the place of sterilisation changes. As one indication disappears, heart disease amenable to surgery for example, another takes its place, high parity for example.

The indications for sterilisation cannot be defined exactly; each case must be judged on its merits, and it is necessary to take cognisance of mental as well as physical health.

Nevertheless, the procedure should not be recommended or undertaken lightly, because it may be irreversible, and the woman or man may later change their mind. Tubal ligation with a third caesarean section may seem reasonable at the time but what if the woman later remarries or if her children die? The woman who is sensitised to the Rhesus factor and has had a series of stillbirths may be glad to be sterilised, until she finds herself a widow and about to marry a Rhesus-negative man. In any case, some women (and their husbands) like to know that they could have more children if they wished, even if they regard their family as complete **(Box 1)**.

BOX 1: Indications for sterilisation.

- Permanent ill health of the potential mother
- Permanent ill health of the potential father
- Transmissible genetic defects
- Previous obstetric complications and operations—rupture uterus
- Family limitation
- Population control

Incidence of Tubal Occlusion

Worldwide, there is a decreasing trend in sterilisation rates and an increase in the use of long-acting reversible contraception (LARC) with most countries showing a 30% decline. In the USA, there is a rise in the incidence of bilateral salpingectomy from 4.6% to 13.2% and a decline in tubal ligation procedure from 11.3% to 2.4%. The rise in salpingectomy rates is attributable to a recommendation from the American College of Obstetricians and Gynaecologists (ACOG) to consider bilateral salpingectomy as an option for permanent contraception along with a reduction in risk for epithelial ovarian cancer. In contrast to global trends, in India, there has been a steady increase in the incidence of contraception, with female sterilisation being the most preferred method according to the Centre for Economic Data and Analysis in 2024. An increase was noted from 26.8% in 1992 to 37.9% in 2021.

FEMALE STERILISATION

Techniques

Permanent sterilisation in the female can be achieved by blocking the path (fallopian tube) for the sperm to fertilise the egg. This can be achieved by:

- *Tubal resection:* Wherein the tube is ligated and resected like Pomeroy technique or even salpingectomy.
- *Tubal occlusion:* The tube can be occluded by banding (Falope ring), clipping (Hulka–Clemens clip, Filshie clip) or cauterising (bipolar/unipolar coagulation). Techniques of occluding the ostia through the hysteroscopic insertion of gel foams or titanium devices have been tried.

Timing

The decision on the timing of the sterilisation is based on the patient's preference, previous pregnancy and associated comorbid conditions **(Table 1)**.

In lower resource settings, postpartum sterilisation is the most preferred, due to the advantage of convenience of recuperating for both postpartum recovery and surgical sterilisation simultaneously. The feeling of regret for performing a permanent method is higher among postpartum women compared to those opting for it in interval sterilisation.

TABLE 1: Timing of sterilisation.

Timing	*Description*	*Preferred method*
Interval sterilisation	Sterilisation is performed outside the postpartum period and before ovulation of that cycle (usually before postmenstrual day 7)	Laparoscopic methods/mini-laparotomy
Postabortal sterilisation	Sterilisation is performed immediately after surgical evacuation	Laparoscopic methods
Postpartum sterilisation (PPS)	Sterilisation is performed 2nd to 4th day postpartum	Laparotomy

Routes of Sterilisation

The permanent method can be achieved by performing the resection or occlusion techniques on the tube through the following approaches such as abdominal, laparoscopic, vaginal or hysteroscopic.

Surgical Techniques

Of the simpler operations on the fallopian tubes, the best is the Pomeroy procedure in which a loop of the tube is excised and the cut ends secured with a ligature **(Figs. 1A and B)**. This method requires only limited access and is quick, with failure rate of <0.05%. The technique of crushing and ligation of the tubes without excising any part of them (Madlener operation) is unreliable, with the failure rate being 3.0%; it is rarely practised.

Whatever technique is used for dividing the tubes, it is important to ligate their cut ends with plain catgut. This is much more likely to result in the cut ends of the tubes falling apart than with the use of delayed absorbable material. It is important to select the site of tubal ligation carefully which should ideally be done at the tubal isthmus. This is because in the event of the patient desiring a tubal recanalisation procedure, the isthmo-isthmic anastomosis carries the best chances of success.

Resection of the tubes is usually carried out by laparotomy and is particularly easy to perform 2–4 days

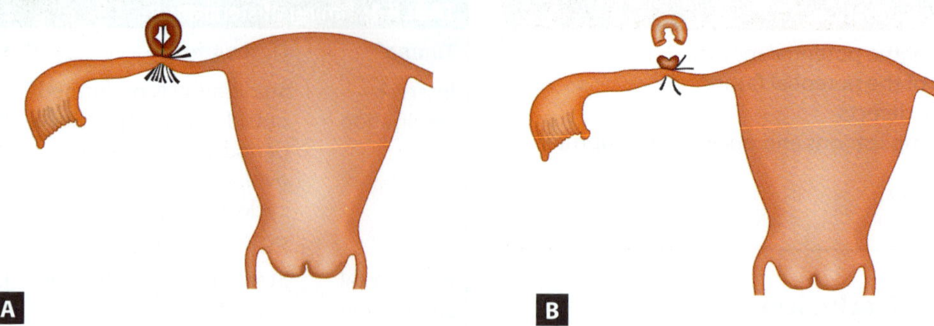

Figs. 1A and B: Types of tubal resection (ligation) sterilisation procedures. (A) Madlener operation in which the tube is tied and not resected; this is most unreliable; (B) Pomeroy operation, for which an absorbable suture material should be used.

after delivery when the uterus is an abdominal organ, and the tubes are readily accessible. Incision may be a midline vertical or transverse incision two finger breadths below the palpable fundus of uterus. Procedure can be carried out under local anaesthesia, general anaesthesia or regional anaesthesia. This technique can also be used at the time of caesarean section. Interval sterilisation or postabortal sterilisation can be performed through a suprapubic mini-laparotomy incision where vaginal packing may be used to raise the uterus to the abdominal incision. Tubal resection can also be performed vaginally during the course of another operation, e.g. Fothergill's operation. However, the vaginal operation usually results in the tubes being divided lateral to the isthmus which may pose a problem if the patient later desires recanalisation.

The portions removed from the tubes, either abdominally or vaginally, should always be submitted for histological examination. This is to provide evidence that, in the event of the patient subsequently conceiving, the operation was properly performed. This precaution may be the first indication to a gynaecologist that a piece of round ligament was removed and not the tube on one side, in time to warn the patient before the operation 'fails.'

Several techniques of sterilisation such as Irving, Uchida, Parkland, Kronig's, Aldrich and Shirodkar methods have been described, but these are not commonly practised **(Table 2)**.

Laparoscopic Sterilisation

Destruction of the isthmic portions of the tubes under laparoscopic control is in vogue, because the method avoids making surgical incisions which are longer than 1–2 cm and normally cause the patient such little discomfort that she can return home the same day. Its sterilising effect is nearly as certain as surgical resection of the tubes, and it appeals to women who think they are avoiding an operation.

It can be performed under local anaesthesia or general anaesthesia. The uterus and tubes are manipulated into convenient positions by a uterine elevator through the cervix or by a probe from above. A portion of each tube, with its inner margin 1 cm from the cornu of the uterus, is coagulated with diathermy and divided or clips or rings applied. Diathermy involves the destruction of a large segment of the tube, and this can pose a problem if subsequent recanalisation is desired. There are also increased chances of ectopic pregnancy if the procedure fails. The preference nowadays is for the use of silastic Yoon rings which are placed over a loop of tube. This can be done through a single port and obviates the need for diathermy, but the rings may be difficult to apply if the tube is fat or rigid. The Hulka clip (stainless steel and polycarbonate) and the Filshie clip (titanium lined with silicone rubber) are commonly used in the United Kingdom. The laparoscopic method enjoys wide popularity and has much to be said in its favour.

Noncontraceptive Benefits of Tubal Resection/Occlusion

- *Lower incidence of pelvic inflammatory disease*: Although tubal ligation does not prevent the acquisition of sexually transmitted diseases (STDs), sterilisation has been demonstrated to reduce the spread of organisms from the lower genital tract.
- *Lower incidence of epithelial ovarian cancer*: Several studies report the protective effect of sterilisation against ovarian cancer. Protection is hypothesised to result from reduced exposure from ovaries to

TABLE 2: Techniques of female sterilisation.

Route	*Name*	*Procedure*
Abdominal	Pomeroy procedure	A loop of tube is created and ligated using chromic catgut, and a 1–1.5 cm length of tube is resected
	Bilateral salpingectomy	This method has the advantage of no failure rate and reduced chances of hydrosalpinx and has a role as prophylaxis in preventing epithelial ovarian cancers
	Madlener operation	A loop of tube created, ligated with absorbable sutures, crushed using a haemostat and cut. This had a higher incidence of recanalisation and failure
	Irving method	The tube was ligated, and the proximal part of the tube was buried into the myometrium ensuring no chance of failure
	Parkland method	A window is created in the mesosalpinx, the tube is ligated using absorbable sutures at the proximal and distal ends and the tube is cut in between the sutures
	Uchida method	Saline was injected subserosally in the ampullary part of the tube, and the peritoneum opened longitudinally. A length of tube was resected, and the proximal part of the tube was buried in the subserosa, leaving the distal part of the tube outside the serosa. This ensured 100% efficacy
	Kroner method	The fimbrial end of the tube is ligated and cut usually with nonabsorbable sutures
	Aldrich method	The fimbrial end of the tube was buried in the leaves of the broad ligament using nonabsorbable suture materials
	Shirodkar method	The ligated end of the fallopian tube after ligation is folded on itself and religated, so that the two ends do not meet
Laparoscopy	Diathermy	Bipolar coagulation is preferred, and coagulation needs to be done to ensure that the lumen is completely occluded
	Silastic rings––Yoon and Falope	Done laparoscopically and use specific applicators to either band or occlude the lumen of the fallopian tube
	Clips––Hulka and Filshie	
Uterine	Quinacrine pellets	Not recommended at present
	FEMCEPT	
	Essure	

environmental carcinogens. Salpingectomy as a method of sterilisation is a prophylactic measure to reduce epithelial ovarian cancer in women.

Contraindications

There are no absolute contraindications for sterilisation procedures. However intrapartum or postdelivery complications on the mother or neonate would be a relative contraindication. Also, the relative contraindications for the laparoscopic approach such as severe cardiopulmonary dysfunction, severe obesity and multiple abdominal surgeries with adhesion may apply to sterilisation procedures also.

Complications (Table 3)

Overall, contraceptive failure for sterilisation procedures is 0.5. According to the CREST study, the largest study of contraceptive methods in USA, the overall failure rate is 18.5/1,000 procedures.

MALE STERILISATION

Sterilisation of the male partner, even in the interests of the female, is being practised increasingly on the grounds that it involves a much simpler and less hazardous operation. It can have an important part to play in family planning and in population control. Despite the present enthusiasm for male rather than female sterilisation and its growing popularity, there is a need for caution in its application. The man must be convinced that he wishes it and not be persuaded by his wife. Moreover, it is to be avoided in young men. If a woman is sterilised on the grounds of parity, the objection to her having more children remains in any subsequent marriage. If, however, a man is

TABLE 3: Complications of female sterilisation.

Immediate complications	Anaesthesia-related complications
	Surgical complications such as: • Haemorrhage from mesosalpinx vessels due to inadvertent transaction of tubes or injury to the major vessels • Injury to internal organs such as bowel, bladder, ureters and blood vessels
	Blood transfusion
	Conversion from laparoscopy to laparotomy
	Rarely death (1 in 100,000 procedures)
Delayed complications	Contraception failure
	Ectopic pregnancy—the incidence of ectopic pregnancy in sterilised women is 7.3 per 1,000 procedures
	Regret—the risk of patients feeling regret for a permanent procedure is more likely if they are younger at the time of procedure (20–30 years) and more common if the sterilisation procedure was performed postpartum
	Postligation syndrome
	Does not protect against STDs

(STDs: sexually transmitted diseases)

sterilised because of his wife's parity, his position becomes untenable if he later marries a nulliparous woman whose concern is to have a family.

Techniques

Vasectomy

Vasectomy is the removal of a portion of each vas, not the complete structure as the term suggests. This is a minor surgical procedure, which for reasons of economy is often performed under local anaesthesia without hospitalisation of the subject. Several methods of dealing with the vasa are described, sometimes with the object of making it easier to anastomose the cut ends if the need arises in the future. Reliable sterilisation, however, calls for removal of 3–4 cm of each vas, care of the suture and separation of the remaining cut ends.

Following vasectomy, active spermatozoa still appear in the ejaculate for 2–3 months and sometimes for much longer. So, the man must be warned to practise contraception until two successive specimens of semen are shown to be free from spermatozoa. During this time, frequent coitus with consequent many (about 20) ejaculations tends to clear the reservoir; so long as any spermatozoa are found, even isolated nonmotile ones, pregnancy is still possible.

There are reports of the finding, in centrifuged semen, of a few nonmotile spermatozoa in 40% of cases at 6 months, and in 15% of cases at 12–18 months, after operation. This can happen, it is said, in men pronounced sterile at 3 months, the spermatozoa have been lurking in the ampulla of the vas or the seminal vesicles.

Contraindications

Vasectomy is not recommended in the presence of active STD, scrotal skin infection, scrotal mass, filariasis or infection in the genital tract. If there is a hernia, it should be repaired concurrently.

Reliability of Vasectomy

Once the semen becomes clear of spermatozoa, the man is usually permanently sterile, but recanalisation and junction of the segments of the vas can occur. For this and other reasons, and despite observation of the above rules, 0.2–0.4% of vasectomised men subsequently father a pregnancy.

Adverse Effects of Vasectomy

Immediate complications are not common, but, even in the hands of competent surgeons, scrotal haematoma, scrotal abscess and epididymitis can follow the operation.

Later, there are no physical ill effects, and coitus with ejaculation continues normally. There is some evidence that the retention and dissolution of spermatozoa can result in the development of sperm agglutinins and other antibodies in the circulation. Such a happening may explain why, when the vasa are subsequently reanastomosed, the man sometimes remains sterile although not azoospermic. Sperm granulomas may form at the cut ends of the vas. These are inflammatory swellings consequent to sperm leakage. They may need excision if they are painful. A higher failure rate has been associated with the presence of granulomas.

There may be psychological repercussions for the man or his wife or both. Many women, whilst not wanting more children, dislike the idea that their menfolk are sterile.

The husband may subconsciously feel that he has lost his manhood. Frigidity, impotence and failure to achieve orgasm are described in either or both partners. But, again, if the cases are well chosen, such sequelae are rare, and studies show that only 1–2% of wives and husbands have any sort of adverse reaction.

No-scalpel Vasectomy

The technique of no-scalpel vasectomy, first developed in China, is gaining immensely in popularity. As the name suggests, no scalpel is used. A stab incision is made with a specially designed instrument, the vas is isolated, delivered through the scrotum and ligated; the procedure is repeated on the other side. No suture is required, and the patient can return home the same day. This procedure has been found to be highly acceptable.

Other Methods

Percutaneous injection of sclerosants has been tried in China. Silicone plugs have been injected into the vas which can be removed if recanalisation is desired.

TERMINATION OF PREGNANCY

Induced abortion is the purposeful expulsion of products of conception before the period of viability. Globally, termination of pregnancy (TOP), or induced abortion, is a common and essential component of reproductive health care. When it is performed according to clinical standards using the World Health Organization (WHO) recommended methods, appropriate to the gestational age, and by trained healthcare providers, it is a safe medical procedure associated with minimal risks.

Unsafe abortion has become a critical public health and human rights concern affecting developing countries and populations in vulnerable situations, where access to skilled healthcare providers, safe abortion methods and accurate information may be limited. Around 45% of all abortions are unsafe, including 14.4% categorised as 'least safe'. These unsafe procedures frequently result in severe morbidity and mortality, with long-term consequences for individuals and the healthcare system alike **(Table 4)**.

It is estimated that between 4.7% and 13.2% of all maternal deaths are due to complications from unsafe abortions, which is alarming. Around 97% of all unsafe abortions occur in developing countries, wherein 53.8% occur in Asia, 24.8% occur in Africa and Latin America and the Caribbean contributes 19.4% of unsafe abortions, thus highlighting the urgent need for universal access to safe, legal and affordable abortion services.

Given the above scenario, it is imperative for healthcare providers to be well versed with safe abortion practices, including indication, contraindication, various medical and surgical methods, various protocols and postabortion care.

TABLE 4: Contributing factors for unsafe abortions.

Social stigma	Lack of awareness, gender inequality and limited decision-making power for women
Policy-level issues	Shortage of trained healthcare providers, inadequate infrastructure and coercion regarding contraceptive choices
Economic barriers	High private sector costs and wage loss deter women from seeking care
Poor physical access	Especially in underserved areas, judgmental attitudes of providers further restrict safe abortion access

BOX 2: Indication for termination of pregnancy.

- Risk to life of women or injury to physical or mental health
- Pregnancy caused by rape or incest
- Failure of contraception
- There is a significant risk that the child, if born, would have severe physical or mental disabilities
- Minors
- Women who suffer from mental illness
- Pregnancy in humanitarian settings/disaster/emergency situations as may be declared by the Government

Indication for Termination of Pregnancy (Box 2)

Termination of pregnancy as a method of abortion is governed by the laws of the land, and different countries across the globe have various opinions and laws in this context, some being as rigid as totally prohibiting induced abortion, while others allow it in governed settings.

Ethical and Legal Considerations

After it is viable, the foetus in utero is protected by law in most countries and accorded the rights of an individual human being. Whether it has such rights before viability is a subject of dispute and opinion, but the courts have already upheld a claim for damages brought by a child who was alleged to suffer disability because of an accident sustained by his mother when only 8–10 weeks' pregnant. In any case, the embryo or foetus of any age is protected by the Hippocratic code.

The World Medical Association laid down some principles in the Declaration of Geneva and stated that 'abortion should only be performed as a therapeutic measure' and that doctors should be advised always to act on the principle 'I will maintain the utmost respect for human life from the time of conception'.

Through the ages, the laws governing the induction of abortion have changed from time to time and from country to country, but those enacted in the 19th century generally aimed to make TOP an offence unless it was definitely needed to save the life or health of the mother. In recent years, however, there has been a remarkable shift in world opinion with consequent liberalisation of the abortion laws in many countries and states; in some, they even provide for abortion on socio-economic grounds alone or on the request of the woman concerned **(Table 5)**. Indeed, there is no doubt that more has been learned about TOP as a medical procedure and as a social phenomenon during the past 30 years than at any other time.

The changes are motivated by a need to eliminate the practice of criminal abortion; avoid the economic and other stresses which the birth of a baby imposes on an unmarried mother; remove unwanted pregnancies which result in unwanted and, therefore, neglected children—here there was, and is, confusion with 'unplanned' pregnancies, in the sense that there was no deliberate attempt to conceive and they represent 20–30% of all pregnancies; abolish illegitimate offspring and provide an additional means for family planning and population control.

It has long since been well established that the widespread practice of abortion does not solve these problems. With increasing emancipation, it is the right, it is said, of any woman to decide whether her pregnancy be removed, even though she is ignorant of what this involves and of the attendant risks to her life and health. There remain, however, religious groups who regard TOP as being morally unacceptable in any circumstances, even if the life of the mother is seriously threatened. There also remain countries in which the law either forbids abortion or allows it only for strict medical indications. So, the world is divided into three parts, one in which only narrowly defined medical indications permit abortion, a second in which abortion remains therapeutic but with very liberal views on the interpretation of 'therapeutic' and a third where pregnancy can be terminated on socio-economic grounds alone and this means on request or demand. Gynaecologists working under the first of these conditions meet few cases in which abortion is indicated or permissible, and their actions need to be guided by the following rules:

- The need for terminating pregnancy must be determined for each case and must be strong enough to be accepted, if the position arises, by a Court of Law.
- The need must be agreed to by not less than two doctors of high professional standing.
- The operation should only be performed in a reputable hospital by a specialist gynaecologist who is convinced of its propriety.
- Those advising therapeutic abortion should satisfy themselves that the physical and mental hazards of the procedure are less than those of allowing the pregnancy to proceed.

Doctors working in areas where the abortion laws, although liberalised, still recognise only medical and medico-social indications for terminating pregnancy have to observe the regulations which apply to their particular community. These, sometimes, rule out an abortion after the 20th to 24th weeks (400–500 g foetus); in many places, each case has to be judged by a special tribunal, set up by a hospital or the government, and not by individual doctors.

A liberal abortion policy has important consequences for society as a whole. The outcome includes:

- The outlook on abortion changes among the public, medical and nursing professions, criminal abortionists and Court of Law.
- The practice of criminal abortion, although not eliminated, is considerably reduced.
- The number of maternal deaths from abortion of all kinds is reduced.

TABLE 5: Global abortion laws for termination of pregnancy.

Categories	*Laws*	*Example of countries*
I	Prohibit abortion entirely or permit it only to save a woman's life	Egypt and Haiti
II	Permit abortion to protect a woman's life and health on therapeutic grounds	Ghana, Columbia, Monaco and Zimbabwe
III	Permit abortion for socio-economic reasons	Great Britain, Belize and Zambia
IV	Most liberal laws—abortion without restriction and woman has the right to choose	United States, Canada, South Africa and Denmark

- There is a lowering of moral standards with an increase in sexual freedom in the expectation that any resulting conception can be removed.
- There is an increase in STDs.
- The last two consequences are seen particularly among young girls, <16 years of age, in whom pregnancy creates a special problem because it is often not diagnosed until it is so far advanced that it cannot be interrupted or can only be interrupted at great risk. This is because, in young girls, the occurrence of amenorrhoea is often dismissed (by them and their parents) as being of no significance.
- The practice of contraception is discouraged as being unnecessary, and this is particularly true of the young who, having had one pregnancy terminated, become heedless if not promiscuous and soon come back with another. In some countries, 50% of those who have had one abortion return for another within 2 years.
- The illegitimacy rate is not reduced, although this may reflect a change in the views of the modern generation regarding marriage.

Techniques of Termination of Pregnancy

Termination of pregnancy can be achieved by medical and surgical methods with preferences depending on gestational age **(Table 6)**.

TABLE 6: Methods for termination of pregnancy.

Trimester	*Medical*	*Surgical*
First	Mifepristone and a prostaglandin (sulprostone, gemeprost and misoprostol)	Suction evacuation—manual or electrical methods
	Methotrexate and misoprostol	Dilatation and evacuation
	Tamoxifen and misoprostol	
	Misoprostol alone	
	Prostaglandins (PGE1, PGE2 and PGF2α)	Dilatation and evacuation
Second	Intra-amniotic and extra-amniotic injections (sodium chloride and ethacridine lactate)	Hysterotomy
	Intravaginal prostaglandins (gemeprost, dinoprostone and misoprostol)	

(PGE1: prostaglandin E1; PGE2: prostaglandin E2; PGF2α: prostaglandin F2α)

Medical Methods of Termination in First-trimester Abortion

Medical methods of abortion (MMA) can be tried up to 9 weeks of gestation. Mifepristone (RU 486), a synthetic steroid, is a derivative of norethindrone with antiprogestin action. It binds to the progesterone receptor in endometrium and decidua, resulting in necrosis and detachment of products of conception. Misoprostol is a prostaglandin E1 (PGE1) analogue that binds to myometrial cells, causing myometrial contractions with softening and dilatation of the cervix. Mifepristone, used alone in a single oral dose of 600 mg, brings about complete abortion in 60% of pregnancies; this success rate is increased to 95% if a prostaglandin [sulprostone (PGE2), 0.25–0.5 mg intramuscularly (IM), or gemeprost (PGE1), 1 mg vaginal pessary, or most commonly, misoprostol (PGE1) 800 μg buccal or vaginally] is administered 36–48 hours later. Abortion occurs 4 hours later with pain and bleeding and is usually likened to a heavy period. If it does not, the dose of prostaglandin is repeated. Bleeding may occur for 10–20 days. Patients are re-evaluated after 2 weeks to assess whether suction evacuation is required. There are no significant adverse effects with the mifepristone–misoprostol combination. Heavy bleeding causing collapse is seen in <1% of patients, while severe pain is seen in 10–20%. Some women are averse to the two-stage nature of the procedure.

A combination of methotrexate–misoprostol has also been used. Methotrexate 50 mg/m^2 is administered IM on day 1 followed by 800 μg misoprostol vaginally on day 7, repeated, if required, on day 8. Complete abortion occurs in 92% of cases. Compared with the mifepristone–misoprostol combination, it is slightly less effective and takes longer for abortion with a longer interval of vaginal bleeding but is cheaper. Tamoxifen 20 mg BD for 4 days followed by misoprostol has also been tried, and the results have been found to be comparable to methotrexate–misoprostol.

Medical Methods of Termination in Mid-trimester Abortion

Medical methods: Intra-amniotic instillation of various solutions was a popular method for terminating pregnancies in the second trimester after the 14th week. The materials used were 40 g sodium chloride in 200 mL of water, a 25% solution of mannitol, 80 g of urea in 100 mL of 0.9% saline or a solution containing prostaglandins (see further).

The presence of renal disease or hypertension is a contraindication for the use of saline or urea, and, before the last is given, blood urea estimation is always essential. When saline is used, 50% is absorbed and can cause some blood electrolyte changes; another consequence is a minor degree of disseminated intravascular coagulation in four out of five cases. This can usually only be detected by haematological studies but, rarely, is the full and dangerous clinical picture seen. If saline enters the bloodstream by accident, death of the woman occurs; the significant findings at autopsy are multiple foci of oedema and haemorrhagic necrosis in the brain.

It may take the uterus 2–4 days to expel its contents, and the mean induction to abortion interval is 20–46 hours, varying with the agent employed.

Because of the serious nature of the side effects, this method of TOP has been superseded by the use of prostaglandins.

Prostaglandins: These are acidic lipids which have a capacity to stimulate smooth muscle. In minute amounts, they have a wide distribution in the body, but, for therapeutic purposes, they are manufactured biosynthetically.

In obstetrics and for inducing an abortion, the ones in current use are mainly PGE2 and prostaglandin F2α (PGF2α). In general, PGE2 is used to produce cervical dilatation (although dinoprostone has been used successfully for mid-trimester abortion), and PGF2α is used to stimulate the uterine myometrium to contract.

Gemeprost is a PGE1 analogue used for mid-trimester abortion. Prostaglandins such as these cannot be administered orally in doses sufficient to terminate a pregnancy without causing severe vomiting, diarrhoea and other systemic upset. So, they are applied in other ways such as vaginal suppositories.

Misoprostol is a PGE1 analogue, which is administered by buccal, sublingual or vaginal route and is effective in inducing an abortion in both the first and second trimesters.

By themselves, they are less efficient at an earlier stage. Prostaglandins are also used to promote the expulsion of a missed abortion.

Intramuscular injection: Intramuscular injections of 15-methyl PGF2α (carboprost, tromethamine) 250 μg are administered every 2–3 hours up to a maximum of 10 doses. The mean induction to abortion interval is 16 hours, and 87% of patients abort successfully within 24 hours. Pretreatment with laminaria tents or PGE2 gel has been shown to increase the success rate to 95% while decreasing the mean induction to abortion interval to 8 hours. It also decreases the incidence of bucket-handle tears in the cervix.

In 40% of cases, abortion with intramuscular prostaglandin is incomplete and needs to be completed with curettage. There is a high incidence of nausea, vomiting, diarrhoea and cramping abdominal pain. So, prophylactic antiemetics and intestinal motility inhibitors are often recommended. Bronchospasm and mild fever may occur. Prostaglandins should not be used in asthmatics or in patients with a compromised cardiovascular status. Sulprostone, a PGE2 analogue used IM, was as effective as intramuscular PGF2α in inducing abortion but was withdrawn following reports of cardiovascular deaths.

Intra-amniotic injection: Prostaglandins injected into the amniotic sac by way of abdominal amniocentesis are safer than 20% saline and other solutions. After withdrawing 10 mL of liquor under aseptic precautions, 2.5 mg (10 mL) 15-methyl PGF2α is instilled intra-amniotically. This procedure is not to be necessarily done under ultrasound guidance, but units equipped with the facility prefer to use it to avoid penetrating the placenta. The mean induction to abortion interval is 12–14 hours. In general, there are few adverse effects, certainly fewer than those seen with the parenteral administration of the drug; however, vasovagal collapse, or more usually transient hypotension, can be an immediate reaction; occasional cases of cardiovascular collapse and death have been reported. Pyrexia, vomiting and diarrhoea may occur.

Intravaginal applications: Vaginal pessaries containing 1 mg gemeprost are applied 6 hourly (up to four doses) between 12 and 16 weeks of gestation. In 82% of patients, abortion is reported within 24 hours with a mean induction to abortion interval of about 15 hours. However, the placenta is expelled in only 7–40% of cases, and the rest require surgical intervention. Nausea, vomiting and diarrhoea are seen in 20–40% of patients. Rarely, cardiac arrhythmias have been reported even with the vaginal route.

Dinoprostone, a PGE2 derivative, has been used as a 2.0-mg vaginal suppository every 3 hours. The mean induction to abortion interval in mid-trimester patients is 12 hours, and 90% abort within 24 hours. However, it is expensive, needs refrigeration and is not suitable for use in developing countries. It is contraindicated in patients with glaucoma and bronchial asthma.

Misoprostol has been used both vaginally and orally. A 400-µg oral dose 3 hourly up to five doses is successful for inducing a mid-trimester abortion with a mean induction to abortion interval of 12 hours. A 200-µg dose used vaginally can produce the same effect. At 24 hours, 89% of patients, and at 38 hours, all patients receiving misoprostol are reported to abort. Adverse effects of nausea, vomiting and diarrhoea are seen with the same frequency as with gemeprost when the drug is administered by the oral route but are seen in only 4% of women in whom the drug is used intravaginally.

Misoprostol works well in pregnancies complicated by intrauterine foetal demise. It is effective from the mid-trimester up to 41 weeks. 3-hourly oral doses of 400 µg have been used in these patients. The induction to abortion interval in those with mid-trimester pregnancies has been found to be shorter in those with intrauterine foetal death (10.4 hours) than in those with a live foetus (15.4 hours).

Misoprostol is cheap, stable at room temperature and has a low incidence of side effects.

Considering various available data on dosage, routes of administration and intervals between doses, the International Federation of Gynaecology and Obstetrics (FIGO) has recommended guidelines for the use of prostaglandins for termination appropriate for gestational age. Revised in 2023, the recommendations can be found at https://www.figo.org/figo-mifepristone-misoprostol-and-misoprostol-only-dosing-charts-2023.

Ethacridine lactate: Ethacridine lactate (Emcredil) is an acridine derivative with uterotonic and antiseptic properties. The exact mechanism of action is unknown. A 16-F Foley catheter is used to introduce 0.1% ethacridine into the extra-amniotic space in a dose of 10 mL/week of gestation to a maximum of 150 mL. The bulb of the catheter is inflated with 10–15 mL of saline to seal the internal os. The catheter is removed after 6 hours, and an oxytocin infusion of 50 mIU/min is started to expedite the procedure. Alternatively, the catheter is left in place until it is expelled on its own once cervical dilatation occurs. The mean induction to abortion interval varies from 24 to 36 hours with ethacridine alone; with oxytocin supplementation, it is about 18 hours.

Extra-amniotic 15-methyl PGF2α has also been used instead of oxytocin.

Ethacridine once widely used because of the advantages of low cost, widespread availability has taken a backseat with a more effective and easy to administer widespread use of misoprostol.

BOX 3: Relative contraindication for the medical management of termination.

- Confirmed or suspected ectopic pregnancy or undiagnosed adnexal mass
- Anaemia (haemoglobin <8 g%)
- Chronic adrenal failure
- Uncontrolled hypertension
- Uncontrolled seizure disorder
- Severe renal, liver or respiratory
- Glaucoma
- Inherited porphyria
- Allergy to drugs used for TOP

(TOP: termination of pregnancy)

Note: Additional consideration may be required for patients on long-term steroid therapy, on anticoagulants and patients with intrauterine device.

Several alternative agents used to induce uterine contractions and facilitate abortion beyond 12 weeks of gestation include intra-amniotic injections of hypertonic saline or hyperosmolar urea, intra- or extra-amniotic administration of ethacridine lactate, parenteral or intra-amniotic use of prostaglandin analogues and intravenous or intramuscular administration of oxytocin that are generally more invasive, associated with increased risks and are considered less safe compared to modern regimens. Additionally, the time required to achieve complete abortion using these agents is typically longer when compared to evidence-based protocols involving a combination of mifepristone and misoprostol, which are currently recommended by the WHO for their higher efficacy and safety profile (WHO, 2012). The relative contraindications for medical management for TOP are highlighted in **Box 3**.

Surgical Methods

The techniques used are vacuum aspiration (manual or electric) before 12–14 weeks and dilatation and evacuation after 14 weeks of gestation. These procedures require a high level of skill, sterile technique, follow-up care and efficacious management of complications.

Vacuum for uterine aspiration can be produced with either an electric pump or a handheld syringe (manual vacuum). Manual vacuum aspiration (MVA) cannula which accommodates cannulas with a 12-mm base which will attach 14- and 16-mm cannulas provides adequate uterine evacuation throughout the first trimester and even the early second trimester.

With the advent of the medical methods, dilatation and evacuation is rarely used these days for the termination in second trimester; it should be reserved for gestational age <15 weeks.

Vacuum aspiration (<12–14 weeks): Vacuum aspiration is a two-step process involving cervical preparation/ dilatation and evacuation. Dilatation is done by either pharmacological dilators such as mifepristone, misoprostol or mechanical dilatation. It should be sufficient to allow the insertion of the proper sized vacuum cannula. The diameter of the cannula is determined by the gestational age. It should be 1–2 mm smaller than the gestational age. For uterine evacuation, 60–80 mm Hg of negative pressure is used for an electric pump and a full vacuum for a 60-cc manual syringe. The aspirator/vacuum is connected to cannula. When the cannula is mid-uterus, the suction is initiated. The contents are evacuated by gently rotating the cannula by 180° in each direction to evacuate the uterus.

Dilatation and evacuation (14–16 weeks): Ultrasound-guided approach is usually preferred beyond 14 weeks of gestation to enhance safety and precision. MTP cannula (Karman) is introduced through the cervical canal. It is connected to a vacuum source or aspirator and advanced carefully only up till mid-uterine level to minimise the risk of uterine perforation. With a gentle rotational technique, suction is applied to facilitate effective evacuation. The cannula may be withdrawn, cleaned and reinserted. Products of conception (POC) is aspirated from the lower uterine cavity, and evacuation is completed using atraumatic ovum forceps. The completion of procedure is confirmed by the appearance of red/pink foam, absence of tissue passing in the cannula and gripping effect of uterus on the cannula.

Pain management for surgical methods: Non-narcotic analgesics, such as ibuprofen, are commonly used to manage pain during and after the procedure. Anxiolytics such as diazepam may be administered to help reduce anxiety and promote muscle relaxation. For additional comfort, sedation may be provided through an intravenous injection of pentazocine 30 mg and promethazine 25 mg. Depending on the individual case and clinical requirements, local or general anaesthesia may also be administered to ensure effective pain relief throughout the procedure.

Hysterotomy: Abdominal hysterotomy was performed for the removal of a second-trimester pregnancy and for terminating pregnancy at any stage if there was a need to sterilise the woman as well, but it is now infrequently used. In seriously ill women, it can be performed under local infiltration anaesthesia without difficulty. The incision in the uterus should be a vertical one, placed as low as possible after reflection of the bladder and covered, in part at least, by the bladder subsequently. Some prefer lower segment hysterotomy with a transverse incision, but this is technically difficult; the lower segment is not of sufficient width at this stage in pregnancy. This method has the advantage that it permits safe and complete removal of the POC without any injury other than that of the incision. Its disadvantage is that, being an abdominal procedure, it carries a slightly higher mortality rate (mostly from embolism) and leaves a scar in the uterus which is liable to rupture during later pregnancy and labour. The danger of this is just as great as that following caesarean section at term, and subsequent pregnancies should generally be delivered abdominally. If the woman is sterilised simultaneously, this problem does not arise. There is a greater incidence of scar endometriosis following hysterotomy than caesarean section.

Complications of Induced Abortions

Immediate: Significant operative and postoperative complications occur in 10% of cases when the pregnancy is <12 weeks advanced. The figure rises to 15% for 12–13 weeks pregnancies and 30–40% for later ones. The overall morbidity rate for all gestations is 12%.

The complications include:

- *Haemorrhage and shock:* These are always likely and can be severe. A loss of >500 mL of blood from the uterus occurs in 3–5% of cases, and a need for blood transfusion is reported in 2–5%. This applies even when prostaglandins are used. The risk of haemorrhage is decreased if the procedure is carried out under local anaesthesia and if the cervix is prepared with prostaglandins.
- *Retained POC:* This complicates 10% of procedures other than abdominal hysterotomy and necessitates conventional curettage.
- *Cervical injury:* Tearing of the cervix during surgical dilatation is common, especially in young primigravidae whose tissues are resistant. Gross injury is recognisable at the time in 1–2% of cases and can cause haemorrhage and shock. Deep tearing of the undilated cervix can also result from violent uterine contractions induced by

oxytocics, especially combinations of prostaglandins and oxytocin. Lateral tearing of the cervix or expulsion of the conceptus through its posterior wall to leave a cervicovaginal fistula has been reported. In most of these cases, an oxytocin infusion was supplemented by an intra-amniotic injection of prostaglandin. This accident is least likely when the cervix has been primed, or the drug administered extra-amniotically, possibly because the balloon of the Foley catheter protects and opens the cervix.

- *Perforation of the uterus:* This occurs during not <0.3% of evacuations by the vaginal route and in some cases, the figure is as high as 2%. This accident occurs even when the operators are skilled and when suction techniques are used; a sound, dilator, curette or suction tube can be the responsible instrument, and the risk is particularly high when the uterus is retroverted. If the accident is not immediately recognised, intestines and other abdominal and pelvic viscera can be damaged. Management depends on the stage of the procedure at the time of occurrence (whether completed or not); the instrument causing the damage and the consequent size of the perforation and damage to the abdominal viscera, chiefly the intestines, although vascular injury can also occur.
- *Infection:* Significant pyrexia follows TOP in 5–10% of cases, and, in 1–2%, this is caused by such severe endometritis, salpingitis and peritonitis as to leave the pelvic organs permanently damaged. Prophylactic doxycycline therapy reduces the risk.
- *Thrombosis and embolism:* Deep venous thrombosis and pulmonary embolism are more likely after abdominal operations than after vaginal procedures. Chemical and air embolism can complicate certain techniques.

Remote Psychological

Maternal instinct may be so strong that permanent regret and remorse are left in the minds of some women who demand or agree to TOP. When the indications are flimsy from the standpoint of health, the incidence of psychological reactions of some degree appears to be like that for pregnant women, being higher in divorced, separated or widowed women. Aborted and pregnant women are most at risk of admission to a psychiatric unit during the first 3 months after an abortion or delivery. For the vast majority of women, feelings of guilt and depression are mild and transitory, followed by a sense of relief associated with the resolution of a crisis.

Remote Physical

The late overall permanent physical disability rate is probably not <5% comprising disorders listed further. The exact incidence of each or all is unknown, because late follow-up studies are impracticable. Most women, and especially unmarried ones, do not wish to be reminded of the event some years later, by which time their circumstances are likely to have changed.

- *Menstrual disturbances* include menorrhagia, polymenorrhoea, dysmenorrhoea, menstrual tension and, occasionally, amenorrhoea (Asherman's syndrome). Some of these are the outcome of chronic pelvic infection and can give rise to a need for hysterectomy.
- *Infertility* is the result in 1–2% of cases, being mostly caused by tubal obstruction secondary to salpingitis.
- *Abortion and premature labour* in subsequent pregnancies are 10 times more likely than expected in women who have had a pregnancy terminated, especially if they were primigravid at the time. The cause may be related to cervical insufficiency.
- *Rupture of the uterus* during a later pregnancy or labour. This may represent the dehiscence of a hysterotomy or cervical scar, with or without extension. Often, however, it occurs in an unsuspected weak area of the uterine wall; this being the result of an undiagnosed instrumental injury at the time of the evacuation.
- *Rhesus isoimmunisation:* Unless Rhesus-negative women are routinely protected with anti-D gamma globulin at the time their pregnancy is terminated, 5–10% develop antibodies which threaten their future reproductive life.
- *Ectopic pregnancy:* When tubes are damaged by infection but not closed, there is a risk of tubal pregnancy in the future.
- *Cervical conditions:* These include ectropion, chronic cervicitis and cervicovaginal fistulas.
- *Endometriosis of the cervix and vagina* can develop after vaginal procedures; pelvic and scar endometriosis may follow abdominal hysterotomy.

57

CHAPTER

Urinary Incontinence

Shripad Hebbar, Muralidhar V Pai, Chandra Mithila

Chapter Outline

- Bladder Dysfunction
- Urethral Sphincter Dysfunction
- Investigation of Urinary Problems
- Treatment of Urinary Problems
- Incontinence of Urine
- Management
- Overview of Surgical Management
- Enuresis
- Urinary Retention and Difficulty in Micturition

INTRODUCTION

Urinary incontinence (UI) deals with those disturbances of bladder and urethral function, which are commonly present to the gynaecologist. To understand them, the knowledge of the physiology of micturition and its control is necessary (*refer to* Chapter 2: Anatomy). This knowledge has been considerably enhanced in recent years by the development of urodynamics. Urodynamic studies enable the delineation between bladder dysfunction and urethral dysfunction, which aids the management of patients with urinary symptoms, and in particular, of women who present with UI. This chapter initially describes the symptoms and signs of bladder and urethral dysfunction, and then, the investigation and management of these problems are discussed. Following that, UI is described in greater detail, and finally, difficulties with micturition including urinary retention are discussed.

BLADDER DYSFUNCTION

Bladder Irritability and Instability

Irritability of the bladder can be caused by local disease, which directly stimulates the detrusor muscle or heightens the sensitivity of the stretch receptors in the bladder wall. The bladder muscle then becomes so insensitive that the central nervous system may fail to control it, producing detrusor instability.

Alternatively, irritability and/or instability may be the result of a primary error in the nervous inhibition of an essentially normal bladder muscle.

Irrespective of the mechanism behind detrusor irritability, the sphincter mechanism is normal, and the fault lies in the bladder which becomes intolerant of even moderate amounts of fluid. The clinical effects are frequency, urgency and nocturia. If detrusor instability develops, then either urge incontinence or enuresis may occur. Moreover, if the bladder wall goes into spasm, then pain and dysuria are added.

Dysuria can also be explained by any disease, making the urethra or vulva sensitive to the passage of the urinary stream. Certain local causes of bladder irritability—those characterised by congestion and ulceration—also result in haematuria.

Causes of Bladder Dysfunction

Polyuria

A complaint of frequency, diurnal and/or nocturnal is sometimes explained merely by an increased excretion of urine. This can be caused by the following:

- A cold environment, causing a reduction in the excretion of fluid by the body's surface
- A habit of drinking large quantities of tea, coffee or other fluids. Such a habit can have a background of nervous tension, loneliness and unhappiness.

  The woman drinks to console herself or for want of something to do. This type of patient tends to have urgency as well as polyuria.
- *Pregnancy:* Except in the later weeks, when the presenting part crowds the pelvic organs and makes the bladder intolerant to large volumes, frequency in pregnancy may be explained by polyuria.
- Diabetes mellitus and diabetes insipidus

- Impaired renal function results in the output of large quantities of unconcentrated urine. This is mostly seen in old age.
- *Insomnia:* Women often attribute insomnia to a nocturnal desire to void. An alternative explanation is more likely.

Because they are wakeful, their kidneys continue to secrete. This, as well as the need for something to do, causes frequency and urgency.

Mechanical Factors

Displacement of the Bladder

Any displacement which stimulates the stretch receptors can cause a frequent desire to void. This is seen typically in cystocele, when the frequency is only diurnal because the displacement disappears on rest.

Pelvic and Lower Abdominal Tumours

These may cause direct pressure on the bladder wall and result in diurnal frequency, if they are mobile, or diurnal and nocturnal frequency, if they are impacted in the pelvis.

Adhesions and Bands in the Uterovesical Pouch

These may result from operations, infections and endometriosis. They act mainly by opposing enlargement of the bladder, but unless the causal disease is active and progressive, the bladder can learn to accommodate itself to the new anatomy.

Incomplete Emptying of the Bladder

This is a common feature of cystocele and the patient, having voided, has an almost immediate urge to void again. Incomplete emptying is a common sequel to postoperative retention and is deceptive in that the patient complains of frequency and not of difficulty in voiding.

Diseases of Organs Adjacent to the Trigone

Diseases of the anterior vaginal wall and the cervix, by causing congestion and irritation of the trigone, or by interfering with the nerve supply to the bladder, can be the basis for frequency and dysuria. They include the following:

- Any pelvic operation which disturbs the bladder base. Wertheim's and other radical operations often result in permanent detrusor dysfunction because they damage the innervation of the bladder as well as disturb the anatomy. Occasionally, detrusor dysfunction follows pelvic surgery for benign disease but is usually less severe and may be temporary.
- Endometriosis of the anterior lip of the cervix, of the anterior vaginal wall, or of the bladder wall itself
- *Carcinoma of the cervix:* By the time, this disease irritates the base of the bladder, the forward extension is usually serious and there is a threat of fistula formation.
- Chronic cervicitis is not a cause of bladder irritability but may be associated with urethritis which may produce bladder irritability (described later).

Diseases of the Renal Pelvis and Ureter

These include especially pyelonephritis and ureteric calculus.

Diseases of the Bladder

All these are likely to cause dysuria, and sometimes haematuria, as well as frequency and urgency.

Cystitis: The susceptibility of women to cystitis is commonly blamed on the shortness of the female urethra and the close proximity of the bacteria-infested vagina and anus. Approximately 8% of women of childbearing age and 20–25% of women over 60 years of age have significant bacilluria (100,000 or more organisms per mL in at least two separate specimens). It requires little to change from a carrier to an infectious state. Precipitating factors include pregnancy, labour, operations, urinary retention and incomplete emptying of the bladder. In many cases, however, cystitis is traceable to catheterisation. Few women escape this procedure, requiring it at some time in life, in association with childbirth or operations.

The bacilluria of the apparently normal adult woman probably dates back to childhood when there may not have been overt attacks of cystitis. Recurrent cystitis in young girls can be associated with ureteric reflux which causes urinary stasis.

Recurrent attacks of acute cystitis in women are sometimes explained by an underlying nidus of low-grade infection in a hydronephrosis, diverticulum or other anatomical fault; but in many cases, there is no evidence of these. When investigated, a number of women who suffer from recurrent cystitis are found to have lower urinary tract dysfunction—incomplete bladder emptying. The attacks of frequency and dysuria may occur without evidence of any infection in the bladder. Often they represent exacerbations of chronic urethritis (described later). Otherwise, a condition of allergic cystitis and urethritis is not uncommon. Attacks can be attributable to reactions to toilet preparations, antiseptics, drugs and chemical contraceptives.

Diverticula: These cause problems mainly because the urine residing within them becomes infected or because of calculus formation. Bladder diverticula, except possibly multiple tiny ones, are uncommon in women.

Vesical calculus and foreign bodies: Except when it forms in a diverticulum or an incarcerated cystocele, or around a foreign body, a vesical calculus is rare in women. This is because any stone which negotiates the ureter is easily passed through the short straight urethra **(Fig. 1)**. Occasionally, mineral deposits are found in the bladder in severe chronic cystitis.

Papilloma and carcinoma of the bladder: These generally cause haematuria as well as bladder irritability.

Trigonitis

In many women with long-standing bladder irritability, the only positive finding on investigation is slight injection of the vessels on the trigone. This leads to a diagnosis of 'trigonitis', despite the fact that urinalysis does not usually reveal any evidence of infection.

Diseases of the Urethra

Urethral conditions can reflexly cause bladder irritability or can account for dysuria, which is mistakenly attributed to cystitis. They include the following:

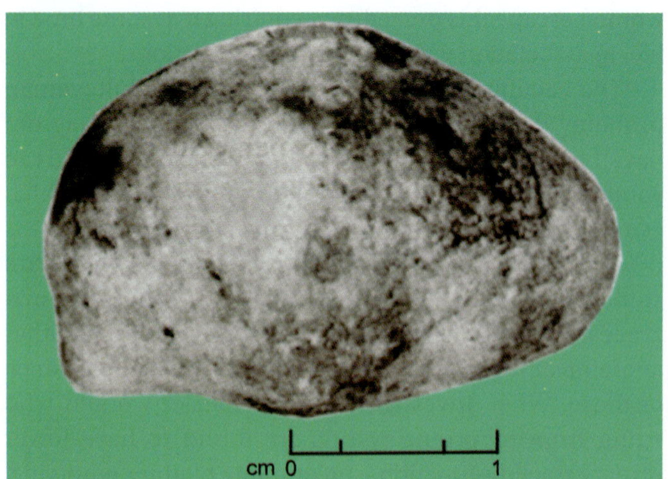

Fig. 1: A urinary calculus passed spontaneously per urethra. Its size illustrates the distensibility of the female urethra.

- *Trauma:* Urethral injury may be sustained during catheterisation, operation and childbirth. Coitus too can irritate the urethra and commonly causes a desire to void. Honeymoon cystitis is mostly attributable to trauma of the external urethral meatus.
- *Urethral prolapse: Refer to* Chapter 28: Tumours of the Vulva
- *Urethritis:* Bacterial and viral organisms have been implicated in the aetiology of acute and chronic urethritis. In addition to bacterial pathogens isolated from the urine, chlamydia, candida and trichomonas may result in infection of the urethra, producing symptoms similar to cystitis. Urine examination is generally unhelpful. The term urethral syndrome is used to describe the symptoms of frequency, dysuria and urgency produced by chronic urethritis. Atrophic urethritis commonly presents 2 or 3 years after the menopause and is an inflammatory mucosal reaction to oestrogen deficiency which often parallels changes in vaginal epithelium.
- *Urethral tumours:* These include caruncle, papilloma, diverticulum, paraurethral cysts and carcinoma (*refer to* Chapter 28: Tumours of the Vulva)

Diseases of the Vulva and Vagina

Any painful and tender lesion of the introitus or vulva can give rise to a complaint of dysuria as the urine passes over it.

Diseases of the Central Nervous System

Frequency of micturition and urgency are common manifestations of organic disease in the central nervous system. Examples include multiple sclerosis, previous vascular accidents and disc lesions of the spine which may be asymptomatic. Among sufferers of multiple sclerosis, 60% have urgency, 50% frequency and 35% urge incontinence at some stage of the disease. Moreover, such symptoms are the first manifestations of multiple sclerosis in 2% and amongst the first in 12% of cases.

Neurological disease may produce a hyperactive or a hypoactive detrusor. The former is associated with urgency and urge incontinence and the latter with an atonic bladder, producing urinary retention and overflow incontinence. If the neurological deficiency affects both sensory and motor pathways, an 'automatic bladder' results. This fills and empties without the woman being aware of it, the control being the basic spinal reflex.

Senility can result in loss of central inhibition and this, as well as incomplete emptying of an atonic bladder, causes frequency and urge incontinence.

Functional: The Psychogenic Bladder

In some women suffering from chronic and resistant frequency and urgency, investigation fails to reveal an organic cause. At most, cystoscopic examination reveals what is labelled 'trigonitis'. These may represent, in part, unknown pathology but often the cause of the bladder irritability is essentially a bad habit, or failure of the central nervous system to inhibit the detrusor reflex.

The habit of voiding frequently may develop in childhood, being acquired from another member of the family. Sometimes, there is a history of enuresis in adolescence. Occasionally, the dysfunction starts with true cystitis, or urethral injury during catheterisation, and persists when the primary lesion is cured. More often, the onset dates from psychological trauma such as death of the husband or a friend, a child sustaining a serious accident or illness, or a marital quarrel.

Sufferers of this functional disorder are generally women, sometimes girls, of anxious and tense disposition, nail biters, often lonely or unhappy with an insecure home life, fearful of cancer and full of complaints. They usually have had many operations, investigations and treatments, all with only temporary improvement in symptoms. Common associated conditions are irritable bowel syndrome, headache, depression, nervous exhaustion and obesity (from seeking consolation in food). A history of frank psychosis in the patient or a close relative is not uncommon. Indeed, psychotherapy and hypnosis may be modes of treatment.

With this background, the patient not only loses her inhibitory control of the bladder but also the stretch receptors become more sensitive, and the detrusor muscle itself is 'on edge' ready to contract at the slightest provocation. The provocation may be the thought of a full bladder, the sound of running water or even physical movement. The escape of urine on changing position can give rise to a false diagnosis of stress incontinence.

When urge incontinence occurs, the woman loses confidence in her bladder and then voids more and more frequently in the hope of avoiding an accident. The bladder, therefore, is never allowed to fill and becomes intolerant of fluid. In severe cases, even 50 mL of fluid may be enough to excite detrusor contraction, but the bladder never becomes organically contracted. Under general anaesthesia, its capacity is always normal. Colicky action of the hypertonic detrusor can also cause intense pain and dysuria.

It is characteristic for the frequency and urgency to occur only by day. When severe, however, bladder spasms can wake the patient or lead to nocturnal enuresis.

Hypotonic Bladder

This is generally associated with neurological disease (as described above) but may follow pelvic surgery. If the motor denervation is accompanied by a sensory denervation, the woman will be unaware of the urinary retention until overflow incontinence develops. It is a far less common clinical problem than the hypertonic irritable bladder.

URETHRAL SPHINCTER DYSFUNCTION

The urethral sphincter is designed to permit bladder emptying when required and to prevent the escape of urine from the bladder at rest and when the intravesical pressure is increased secondary to raised intra-abdominal pressure (IAP). Urinary loss which occurs with sudden elevations of the IAP without detrusor contraction is called stress incontinence.

Stress Urinary Incontinence

Stress urinary incontinence (SUI) could result from anatomic hypermobility of the urethra, which produces defective urethral closure pressure under stress and intrinsic sphincter weakness or deficiency.

During conditions of increased IAP, the urethra remains well supported by:

- Integrity of endopelvic fascia which connects vagina to pelvic side walls and white line
- Strength of levator ani muscle complex and its connection to endopelvic fascia
- Co-ordination of levator ani muscle contraction with coughing

When these urethral supports are damaged, the result is urethral hypermobility (prevents effective urethral closure).

Intrinsic sphincter deficiency (ISD) is end result of damage to external and internal urethral sphincter mechanisms due to various reasons such as trauma, nerve injuries and prior surgeries.

Anatomical Classification (Blaivas and Olsson, 1998) (Figs. 2A to E)

- *Type O:* Typical history of stress incontinence but no urinary leak is demonstrable during clinical examination
- *Type I:* Vesical neck is closed at rest and situated above the inferior margin of symphysis during stress—vesical neck and proximal urethra open and descend <2 cm and UI is apparent during periods of increased IAP.
- *Type IIA:* During stress—vesical neck and proximal urethra open, and there is rotational descent characteristic of cystourethrocele. UI is apparent in increasing IAP.
- *Type IIB:* Vesical neck closed at rest and situated below the inferior margin of symphysis. During stress, proximal urethra opens and incontinence occurs.
- *Type III:* Vesical neck and proximal urethra open at rest in the absence of detrusor contraction

Grading of Stress Urinary Incontinence

- 0: Incontinence without leakage
- I: Incontinence with stress and with little descent

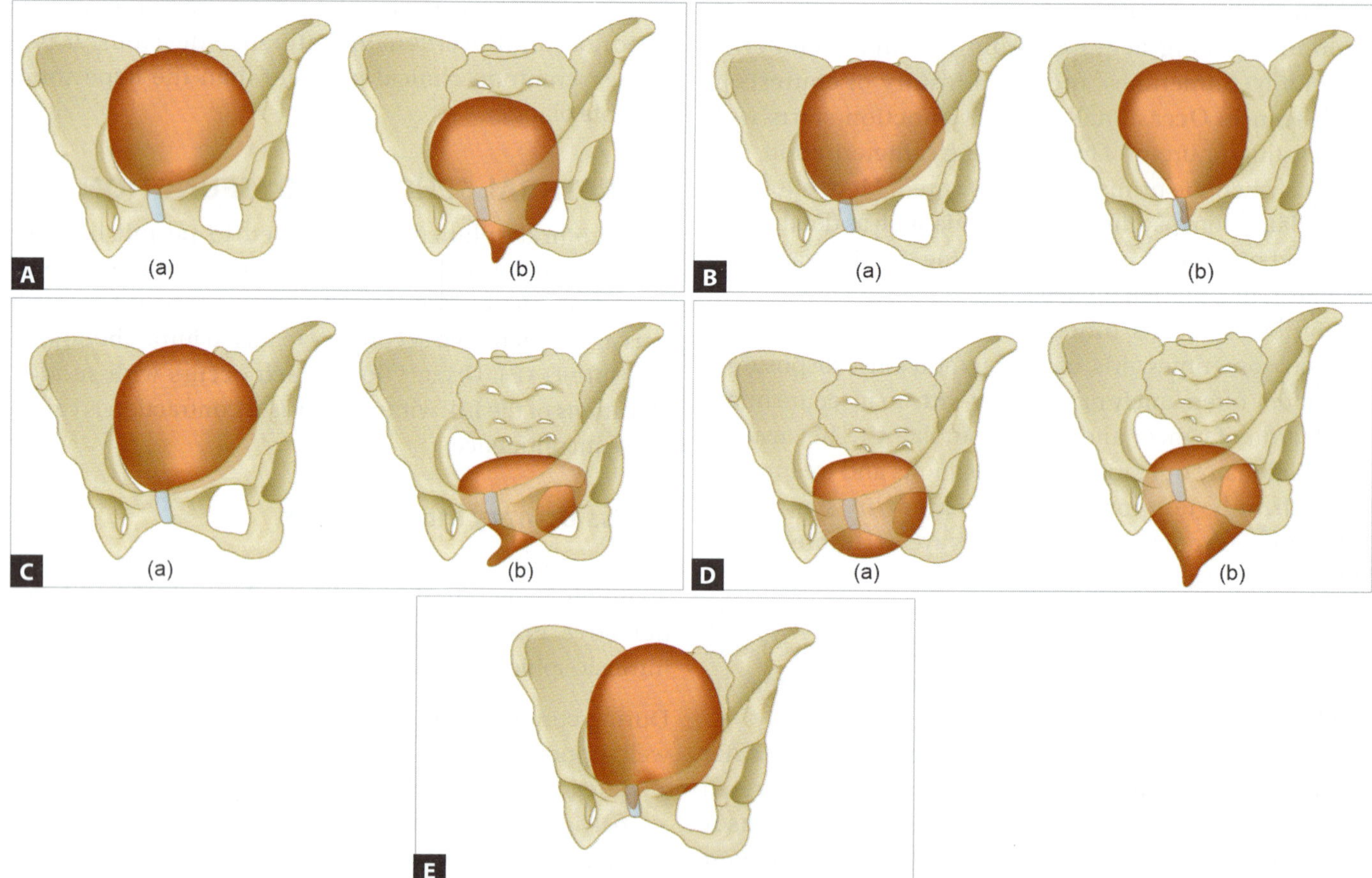

Figs. 2A to E: Blaivas and Olsson classification. (A) Type 0 stress incontinence. (a) At rest, base of bladder is flat and situated above the superior margin of symphysis pubis (solid line). (b) During cough, there is rotational descent of urethra and bladder base. Vesical neck opens, but urinary leakage is not visualised; (B) Type I stress incontinence. (a) At rest, base of bladder is flat and situated at superior margin of symphysis pubis (solid line). (b) During Valsalva's manoeuvre, bladder base descends approximately 1 cm, vesical neck and urethra open, and leakage occurs; (C) Type IIA stress incontinence. (a) During bladder filling, base of bladder is flat and situated at the level of superior margin of symphysis pubis. (b) During cough, there are marked descent and rotation of bladder and urethra well below inferior margin of pubis. Urethra opens widely and leakage occurs; (D) Type IIB stress incontinence. (a) During filling, base of bladder is flat but it is situated below the level of inferior margin of pubis. (b) During cough, there is further descent and opening of urethra with visible leakage; (E) Type III stress incontinence. During bladder filling, base of bladder is just below superior margin of symphysis pubis. Indentation on either side of vesical neck is from two prior Marshall–Marchetti–Krantz operations. The proximal urethra and vesical neck are open despite intravesical pressure of only 6 cm water.

- II: Incontinence with stress and with 2 cm descent
- III: Neck and urethra wide open even without bladder contraction

Stress incontinence is reported as an occasional event in up to 50% of young nulliparous women, but sometimes may be more frequent. It occurs more commonly during pregnancy, but frequently it first presents immediately after delivery. Thus, pregnancy and delivery are implicated in the aetiology of the condition. In some women, it first presents many years after pregnancy, inferring an age-related aetiology. Several factors contribute towards UI with stress.

Urethral Sphincter

The internal smooth muscle and external striated muscle sphincter combine to provide a considerable functional reserve of urethral closure pressure (described later). Women with stress incontinence have a reduced maximum urethral closure pressure, which reduces the capacity to resist urinary leakage under pressure. In urethral sphincter weakness, both the smooth and striated muscle components of the sphincter are invariably weakened.

Urethral Length

Weakness of the urethral muscle wall tends to result in funnelling of the proximal urethra, resulting in a shortening of the functional urethral length. It is unlikely that urethral shortening itself is a primary factor in the aetiology of stress incontinence.

Pelvic Floor

The pubococcygeus muscle of the pelvic floor lies lateral to the urethra on each side. Contraction of the pelvic floor elevates and lengthens the urethra and maintains the posterior urethrovesical angle due to the fascial attachment to the urethra. This position of the urethra is important for the sudden elevation of IAP to be transmitted to the proximal urethra (encouraging closure) as well as to the bladder (encouraging urethral opening). The improvement in posterior urethrovesical angle produced by urethral elevation aids continence with stress by preventing proximal urethral funnelling. Different types of posterior urethrovesical angles are shown in **Figure 3**. Women with significant stress incontinence usually have pelvic floor weakness which may be sufficiently severe to allow genitourinary prolapse. A surgical cure of stress incontinence necessitates elevation of the proximal urethra to an intra-abdominal position to improve pressure transmission and improve the posterior urethrovesical angle.

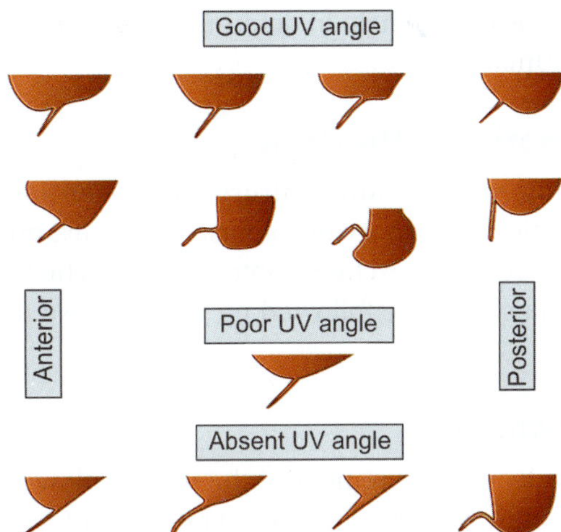

Fig. 3: Types of 'posterior urethrovesical angles' seen on lateral urethrocystography. The presence or absence of the angle is merely a radiological sign of a good or incompetent internal urethral sphincter. (UV: ureterovesical)

Current research suggests that the pelvic floor and urethral sphincter muscle weakness is due to muscle denervation. This denervation is a normal accompaniment of ageing and appears to be increased by pregnancy and parturition.

Any factors which produce an acute or chronic rise in IAP may precipitate stress incontinence. Intra-abdominal tumours should not be overlooked. Obesity and a chronic smoker's cough are common associations with stress incontinence.

Detrusor Sphincter Dyssynergia

This represents a small proportion of the sphincter dysfunction group. Detrusor contraction is accompanied by urethral sphincter contraction instead of relaxation, resulting in voiding difficulty. The cause of this is generally neurogenic.

INVESTIGATION OF URINARY PROBLEMS

History and Examination

A careful history is necessary in the investigation of urinary problems. Examination of the patient should include a full neurological examination, particularly, if bladder dysfunction is suspected. Vaginal atrophy or infection should be noted. History and examination may, however, be of little help in determining the precise cause of incontinence.

Examination of the Urine

Urine microscopy and culture are essential in the investigation of urinary problems. Repeat examinations may be required to exclude contamination. The finding of glycosuria should be followed up by a glucose tolerance test.

Uroflowmetry

This involves measurement of the urinary flow rate. The normal adult voids at a maximum rate >20 mL/s resulting in complete bladder emptying. Reduced urinary flow and incomplete bladder emptying indicate detrusor and/or sphincter dysfunction. A patient with incomplete bladder emptying will probably complain of frequency rather than voiding difficulty.

Cystometry

In its simplest form, cystometry employs a fluid-filled manometry system to record intravesical pressure during bladder filling. Isotonic saline at body temperature is infused into the bladder at 50 mL/min through a urethral catheter. In the normal bladder, the first sensation of the desire to void is recorded at 100–250 mL. Capacity is generally recorded at 450–750 mL. The intravesical pressure rise during filling to capacity is not normally >10 cm of water. Detrusor instability is defined as a pressure rise of at least 15 cm of water during filling cystometry when the patient is trying to inhibit micturition. The intravesical pressure recorded clearly represents the cumulative recording of detrusor-generated pressure and IAP. To establish the intrinsic detrusor muscle pressure, a balloon catheter is placed in the rectum to record IAP and a graphic recording of intravesical, intra-abdominal and detrusor pressures (intravesical minus IAP) is made. Thus, any pressure rise recorded by the detrusor muscle recorder will represent detrusor muscle activity.

Microtip pressure transducers are now available. These allow more provocative manoeuvres to be performed by the patient during cystometry (e.g. walking) than is possible with a fluid-filled system.

Radiological screening of filling cystometry and micturition has been developed and may be recorded on videotape [videocystourethrography (VCU)]. Inevitably, greater sophistication involves greater expense and technical expertise. Examples of filling cystometrograms are shown in **Figures 4A to C**.

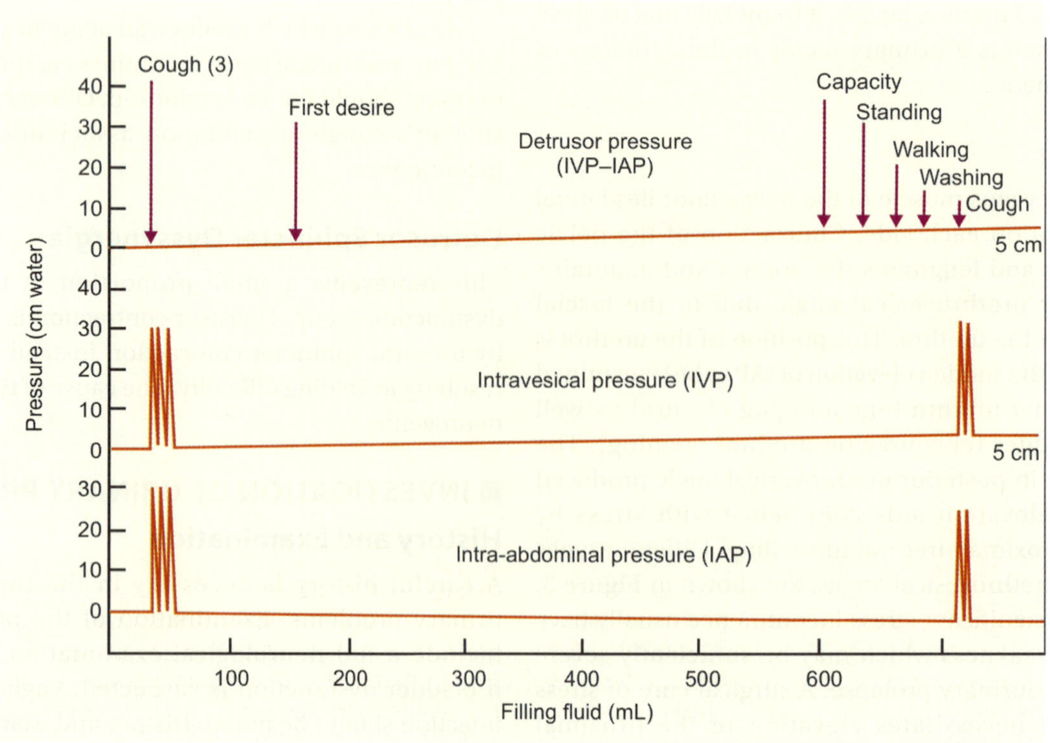

Fig. 4A

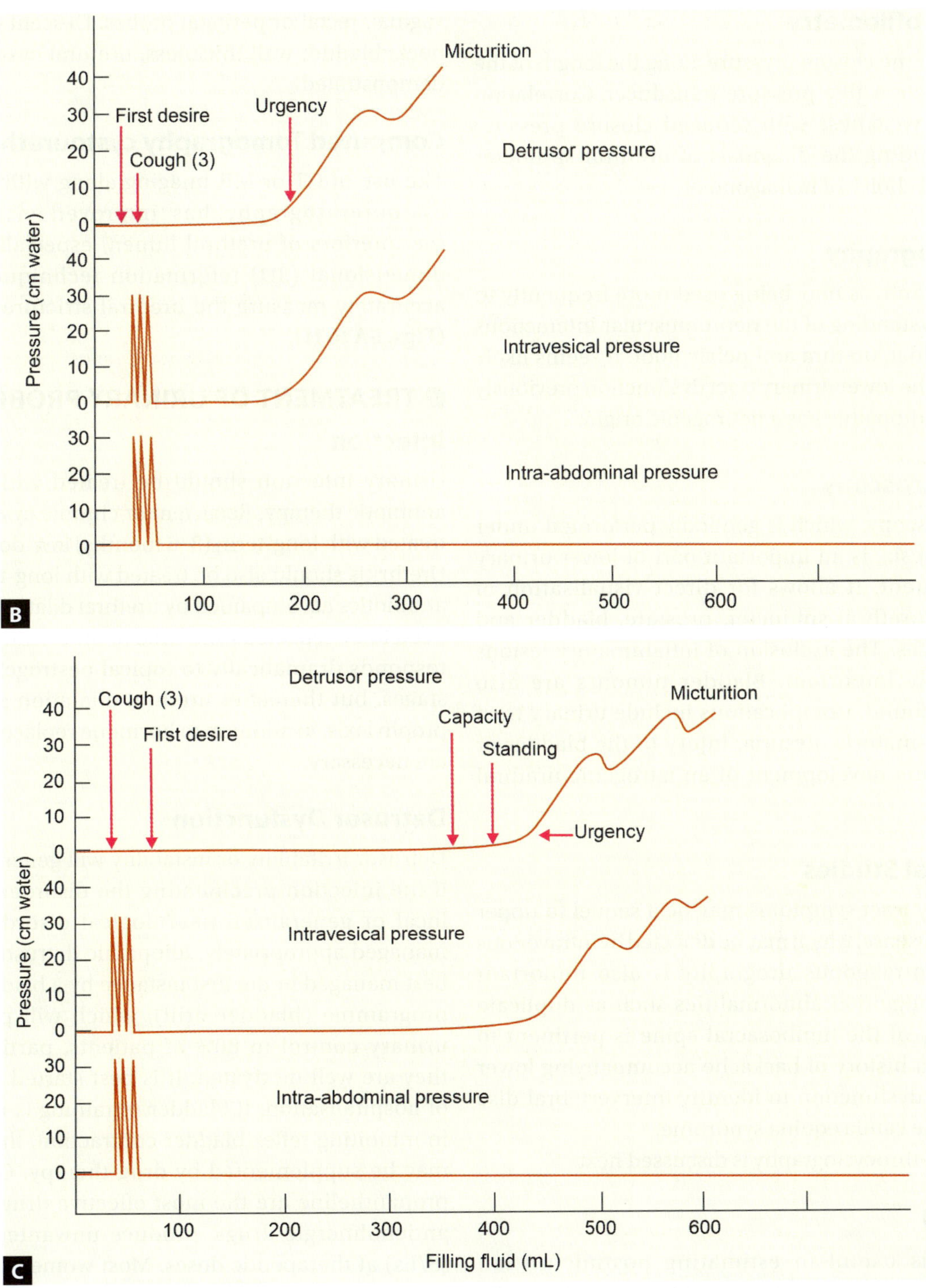

Figs. 4B and C

Figs. 4A to C: (A) Normal cystometry. The diagram illustrates a recording of a three-channel filling cystometry. Fluid is infused at 50 mL/min. Three coughs are recorded by the rectal catheter (intra-abdominal pressure) and the intravesical catheter recorders, but there is no increase in the detrusor pressure. The 'first desire' to void is noted here after infusion of 175 mL which is normal. There is no significant rise in detrusor pressure on filling to capacity (5 cm water). No detrusor contractions are recorded when provocative actions (standing and hand washing) are performed; (B) Detrusor instability. In this recording, the 'first desire' to void is noted early (30 mL). After infusion of <200 mL into the bladder, the detrusor pressure rises and is followed by involuntary micturition; (C) Detrusor instability with provocation. In this recording, the detrusor muscle is stable to a reduced capacity of 375 mL in the supine position. However, on standing detrusor instability is demonstrated with involuntary micturition.

Urethral Profilometry

A recording of the closure pressure along the length of the urethra is made with a pressure transducer. Correlation of sphincter weakness with reduced closure pressure is possible, aiding the diagnosis of urethral sphincter weakness and choice of management.

Electromyography

Electromyography is now being used more frequently to gain an understanding of the neuromuscular interactions between bladder, urethra and pelvic floor. It seems likely that much of the lower urinary tract dysfunction previously described as idiopathic has a neurogenic origin.

Cystourethroscopy

Cystourethroscopy, which is generally performed under local anaesthesia, is an important part of lower urinary tract assessment. It allows for direct visualisation of the urethra, urethral sphincter, prostate, bladder and ureteral orifices. The exclusion of inflammatory lesions is particularly important. Bladder tumours are also occasionally found. Complications include urinary tract infection, haematuria, dysuria, injury to the bladder or urethra and the development of an iatrogenic urethral stricture.

Radiological Studies

Lower urinary tract symptoms may be a sequel to upper urinary tract disease, which may be detected by intravenous urography. Intravenous urography is also important to exclude congenital abnormalities such as duplicate ureters. X-ray of the lumbosacral spine is pertinent to women with a history of backache accompanying lower urinary tract dysfunction to identify intervertebral disc lesions and the cauda equina syndrome.

Lateral urethrocystography is discussed next.

Ultrasound

Ultrasound is useful in estimating postmicturition residual volume and in assessing the bladder neck and the surrounding areas.

Estimation of residual urinary volume is done by measuring the three diameters in two perpendicular planes and multiplying the product of the three by a correction factor of 0.625, since the bladder is not spherical until full. The bladder neck can be evaluated by abdominal, vaginal, rectal or perineal probes. Descent of the bladder neck, bladder wall thickness, urethral cysts, etc., can be demonstrated.

Computed Tomography cystourethrography

The use of CT or MR imaging along with conventional cystourethrography has improved visualisation of the interiors of urethral lumen, especially with three-dimensional (3D) reformation technique, and it can accurately measure the urethral stricture length if any **(Figs. 5A to H)**.

TREATMENT OF URINARY PROBLEMS

Infection

Urinary infection should be treated with appropriate antibiotic therapy. Recurrent or chronic cystitis should be treated with long-term (3–6 months) low-dose antibiotics. Urethritis should also be treated with long-term low-dose antibiotics accompanied by urethral dilatation which may need to be repeated from time to time. Atrophic urethritis responds dramatically to topical oestrogens in its early stages, but thereafter urethral dilatation and antibiotic prophylaxis, in addition to hormone replacement therapy, are necessary.

Detrusor Dysfunction

Detrusor irritability or instability will generally disappear if the infection precipitating the disorder is treated. A local or generalised neurological disorder should be managed appropriately. Idiopathic detrusor instability is best managed in the first instance by a bladder retraining programme (bladder drill), which will produce good urinary control in 80% of patients, particularly when they are well motivated. It is best started with a period of hospitalisation. If bladder retraining is not successful in inhibiting reflex bladder contraction, the programme may be supplemented by drug therapy. Oxybutynin or propantheline are the most effective drugs but, like all anticholinergic drugs, produce unwanted side effects (S/Es) at therapeutic doses. Most women tolerate the S/Es if the therapy is effective. Antidepressant agents such as imipramine may also be useful in decreasing bladder contractility.

Hypotonic detrusor dysfunction may be treated with distigmine bromide. Cholinergic S/Es may, however, be intolerable and self-catheterisation may have to be used intermittently.

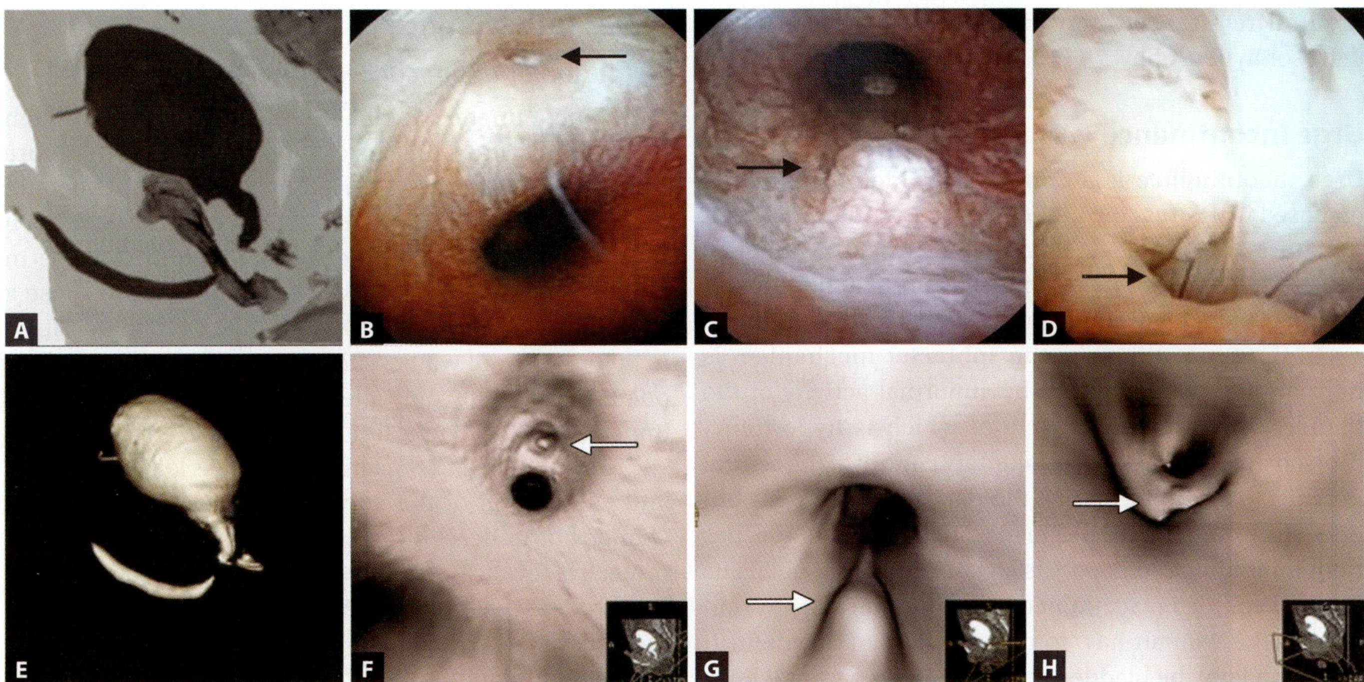

Figs. 5A to H: (A and E) CT cystourethrography and 3D reformatted image demonstrated posterior urethral defection associated with obvious urethrorectal fistula; (B) Small pit was noticed near the bladder neck (solid arrow-headed, conventional cystourethroscopy); (C) Verumotanum was found in the urethral lumen (solid arrow-headed, conventional cystourethroscopy); (D) Urethrorectal fistula was found at the end of the distal urethra (solid arrow-headed, conventional cystourethroscopy); (F) Small pit was noticed near the bladder neck (white arrow-headed, virtual cystourethroscopy); (G) Verumotanum was found in the urethral lumen (white arrow-headed, virtual cystourethroscopy); (H) Urethrorectal fistula was found at the end of the distal urethra (white arrow-headed, virtual cystourethroscopy). (3D: three-dimensional)

Occasionally, bladder dysfunction is refractory to treatment. Urinary diversion is the choice of a few women who are prepared to undergo the major surgery involved and the inconvenience of a stoma bag thereafter.

Sphincter Dysfunction

A large proportion of women who leak urine with stress are unable to adequately contract their pelvic floor and voluntary urethral sphincter muscles. Pelvic floor physiotherapy is designed to strengthen these muscles by voluntary contraction (Kegel's exercises), often with the aid of electrical stimulation. This treatment produces satisfactory control in many women, particularly when the stress incontinence is not severe and precludes the need for surgery.

Surgery for stress incontinence essentially provides an increased resistance to urinary outflow by producing a mechanical obstruction in the urethra under stress conditions. It cannot replace the muscular weakness, which will remain forever. Surgery may be undertaken by the vaginal or abdominal approach (described later).

INCONTINENCE OF URINE

A woman, who complains of an uncontrollable escape of urine, or of feeling constantly wet, sometimes confuses vaginal discharge with urine. The characteristic odour of the latter is one of the guides in distinguishing the two. There are four types of UI: (1) Continual (true), (2) overflow, (3) urge and (4) stress.

Continual Incontinence

This is also described as true incontinence. In this condition, the urine flows continuously day and night. It is caused by some form of urinary tract fistula, either acquired or developmental, the latter including ectopia vesicae and aberrant ureter.

Overflow Incontinence

This occurs as the sequel to prolonged and neglected retention. Its mechanism is not certain but incontinence occurs when the pressure in the bladder overcomes the urethral resistance; there may also be compensatory detrusor hypertrophy.

Urge Incontinence

Urge incontinence is a common problem, frequently confused with stress incontinence but essentially different in nature and aetiology. In genuine stress incontinence (GSI), bladder function is completely normal, but there is urethral sphincter dysfunction (described previously).

In urge incontinence, the sphincter mechanism is normal but is overpowered by abnormal activity of the bladder, the detrusor muscle of which is hypertonic, oversensitive or outside the voluntary control of the central nervous system. Ordinarily, the patient is continent but once she experiences a desire to void, the bladder escapes from inhibition and contracts so strongly that it opens its urethral sphincter. So, immediately after the urge to void occurs, the woman has 'to run to avoid an accident'. If she is too late, the bladder empties itself in part or whole. Diurnal frequency is an inevitable accompaniment and sometimes there is nocturnal frequency as well, especially, if the woman has insomnia.

The problem is one of 'bladder irritability', the causes and treatment of which are described next.

The diagnosis of urge incontinence rests primarily on the fact that the leakage of urine occurs in relatively large amounts (not drops) and is heralded by a desire to void. However, it can be extremely difficult to assess because the woman's description is often muddled. Moreover, a bladder detrusor which is hypertonic, unlike the normal one, is stimulated to activity by movement of the body. So, when a patient says that the urine escapes on changing position on rising from a chair, e.g. it is easy to assume that she has stress incontinence.

In long-standing cases, bladder sensation may also be lost, so the subject is unaware of fullness or emptiness and may suffer a constant involuntary escape of urine. This can then be mistaken for stress incontinence or incontinence from a fistula.

The assessment is made more difficult by the fact that it is not uncommon for a woman to have a mixture of stress incontinence and urge incontinence, the latter sometimes developing from a habit of frequent voiding adopted to limit the former. For these mixed types, it is generally best to re-educate the bladder and to cure the urgency first. The stress incontinence is then treated surgically, and bladder discipline is continued postoperatively.

Stress Incontinence

Definition and Clinical Features

Stress incontinence means the escape of urine through the urethra when the intra-abdominal (and therefore intravesical) pressure is raised by a sudden movement, coughing, laughing, walking or, in certain cases, even turning in bed. In extreme cases, it requires a rise in bladder pressure to only 20 or 30 cm of water to cause a leak; in the mildest, the pressure may have to be raised to 70 or 80 cm of water. The amount of urine lost at any one time is usually only a few drops, and this is a feature important in the diagnosis **(Table 1)**.

The frequent and repeated small leaks lead to soreness and excoriation of the vulva, and necessitate frequent changes of underclothing or the constant wearing of a protective towel. In severe cases, the woman's life becomes a misery; she feels like a social outcast and avoids leaving the house.

Even more important, she ceases to buy new clothing and wears dark colours, which will not show any stains. All those things which matter most in preserving youth and health become unattainable so the woman sits at home, eats to comfort herself, and becomes fat. It is noticeable that many women with stress incontinence are overweight but, as suggested here, this may be the result rather than the cause of the complaint.

In an effort to keep dry, most patients resort to emptying the bladder frequently. This, however, does not prevent stress incontinence and a few drops often escape when the bladder is apparently empty. It is indeed a feature of stress incontinence that it occurs irrespective of the degree

TABLE 1: Medications that affect urinary tract.

Medications	***Effect on urinary tract***
Alcohol	Impairs mobility and causes diuresis
Sedatives	Cause confusion and 2° incontinence
Anticholinergics	Impair detrusor contractility
α-Agonists	Increase outlet resistance and lead to voiding difficulties
α-Blockers	Decrease urethral closure pressure and cause SUI
Calcium-channel blockers	Reduce smooth muscle contractility and cause voiding problems
ACE inhibitors	Result in chronic cough that can result in SUI

(ACE: angiotensin-converting enzyme; SUI: stress urinary incontinence)

of fullness of the bladder; although it causes leakage when the volume of urine is low, rather higher intravesical pressures are required.

Demonstration of Stress Incontinence

Before accepting that a woman suffers from stress incontinence, it is essential to see the escape of urine when the patient coughs or strains. In this respect, it should be noted that some women find it impossible to demonstrate incontinence except when they stand. It is, therefore, imperative that all women complaining of incontinence are examined both supine and erect. The character and timing of an observed urethral leakage also deserve analysis.

Bonney's test: This clinical test, illustrated in **Figure 6**, is often said to have the object of seeing whether an uplift of the urethrovesical junction will stop the incontinence during coughing, so giving a guide as to the operation required. Victor Bonney himself, however, described the application of pressure, not uplift. A positive test merely shows that closure of the internal sphincter by pressure from the vagina controls the leak. It, therefore, has limited value in the assessment of UI.

Bonney's test, standing position, is done by placing two fingers at the ureterovesical (UV) junction. The uplift of the UV junction will stop. The incontinence during coughing—light pressure to be applied immediately to the side of the upper urethra and is directed forward such pressure merely tightens or closes the internal sphincter and will of course, control any form of urethral incontinence.

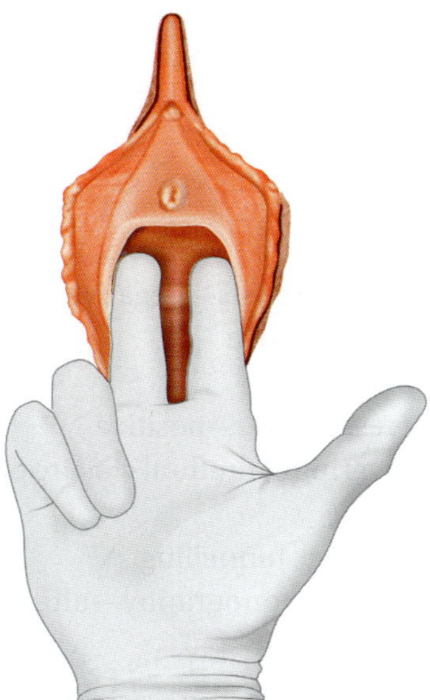

Fig. 6: Bonney's test for stress incontinence as described by the late Victor Bonney. Light pressure is applied immediately to the sides of the upper urethra and is directed forwards. There is no suggestion that the test involves 'uplift'. The effect of such pressure merely tightens or closes the internal sphincter and will, of course, control any form of urethral incontinence.

Q-tip test: The Q-tip test detects urethral hypermobility and assesses the likelihood of response to surgery.

The patient is placed in the lithotomy position. A lubricated sterile cotton-tipped swab is passed through the urethra into the bladder and then withdrawn to the level of the urethrovesical junction. The axis of the urethrovesical junction at rest and after straining using a Valsalva's manoeuvre is measured. If the cotton-tipped swab moves upward by >30° after straining, it indicates urethral hypermobility. A negative Q-tip test in a patient with previous failed surgery suggests GSI.

Investigation of Urinary Incontinence

This has been discussed under the investigation of urinary problems **(Table 2)**; the management of UI is summarised in **Flowchart 1**.

Radiological findings: Lateral urethrocystography (micturating cystourethrogram or micturating cystogram) may be used to demonstrate urethral sphincter weakness in cases of suspected or proven stress incontinence. A radio-opaque medium is introduced into the bladder through a urethral catheter, and lateral radiographs are taken at rest, under strain, and with micturition.

During normal voiding, the posterior urethrovesical angle is lost so that the floor of the urethra and trigone come into line and the bladder neck opens **(Fig. 7A)**. In women who have an incompetent internal urethral sphincter,

TABLE 2: Urinary incontinence.

Stress incontinence	***Urge incontinence***	***Detrusor incontinence***
Leakage of urine coincides with stress	Unable to control escape of urine, once there is urge to void	Incontinence may occur abruptly even without a full bladder
No prior urge to void	Large amount	Large amount
Small amount	Patient aware	Patient not aware
Patient fully aware of micturition	Urgency and frequency	Frequency and nocturia
Negative micturition		

Flowchart 1: Management of urinary incontinence.

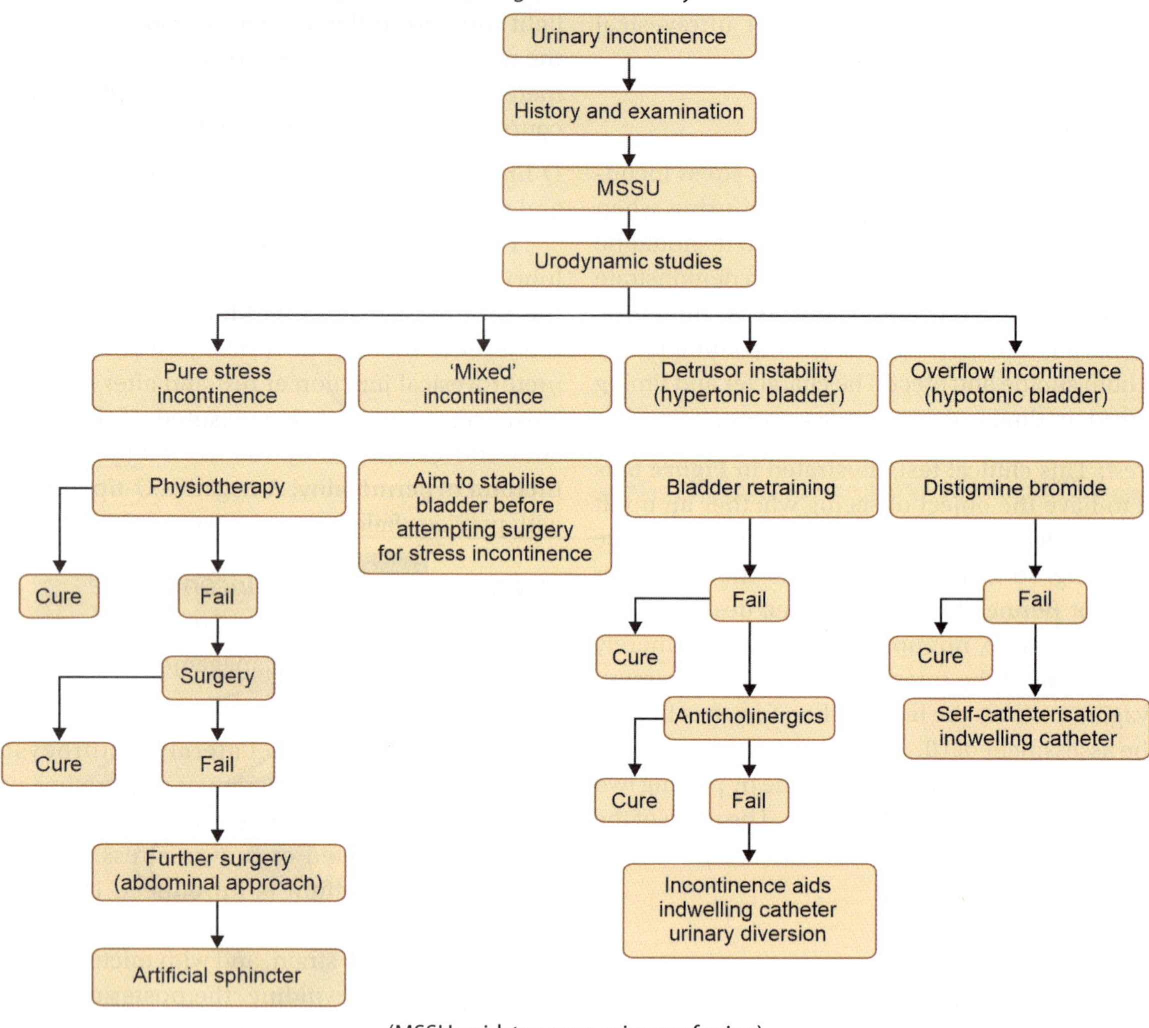

(MSSU: midstream specimen of urine)

the posterior urethrovesical angle is also lost **(Figs. 7B and C)**. In severe cases, this feature is apparent even when the woman is sitting or standing quietly; in others, it appears only with straining. After successful urethrocystopexy, the anatomy of the urethrovaginal junction is restored, resulting in a more competent internal sphincter **(Fig. 7D)**.

The lateral urethrocystograph is also useful in the assessment of the woman in whom surgery for stress incontinence was unsatisfactory. **Figures 8 and 9** illustrate problems encountered after surgery and their recognition by cystourethrography.

Diagnosis of Genuine Stress Incontinence

- Clinical stress test—positive
- Pad test—positive, increase in per gram is significant
- Midstream urine analysis—negative
- Uroflowmetry—negative
- Cystometry—negative
- Leak-point pressure test—positive
- Significant lowering of urethral closure pressure during strain
- VCU—bladder neck funnelling
- Transvaginal endosonography—altered anatomical relationship

Selection of patients for detailed urodynamic studies: A detailed history and examination, including urinalysis, of women complaining of UI will not always determine the precise cause of the incontinence.

Invasive urodynamics may be omitted before surgery in women with uncomplicated SUI and before initiating

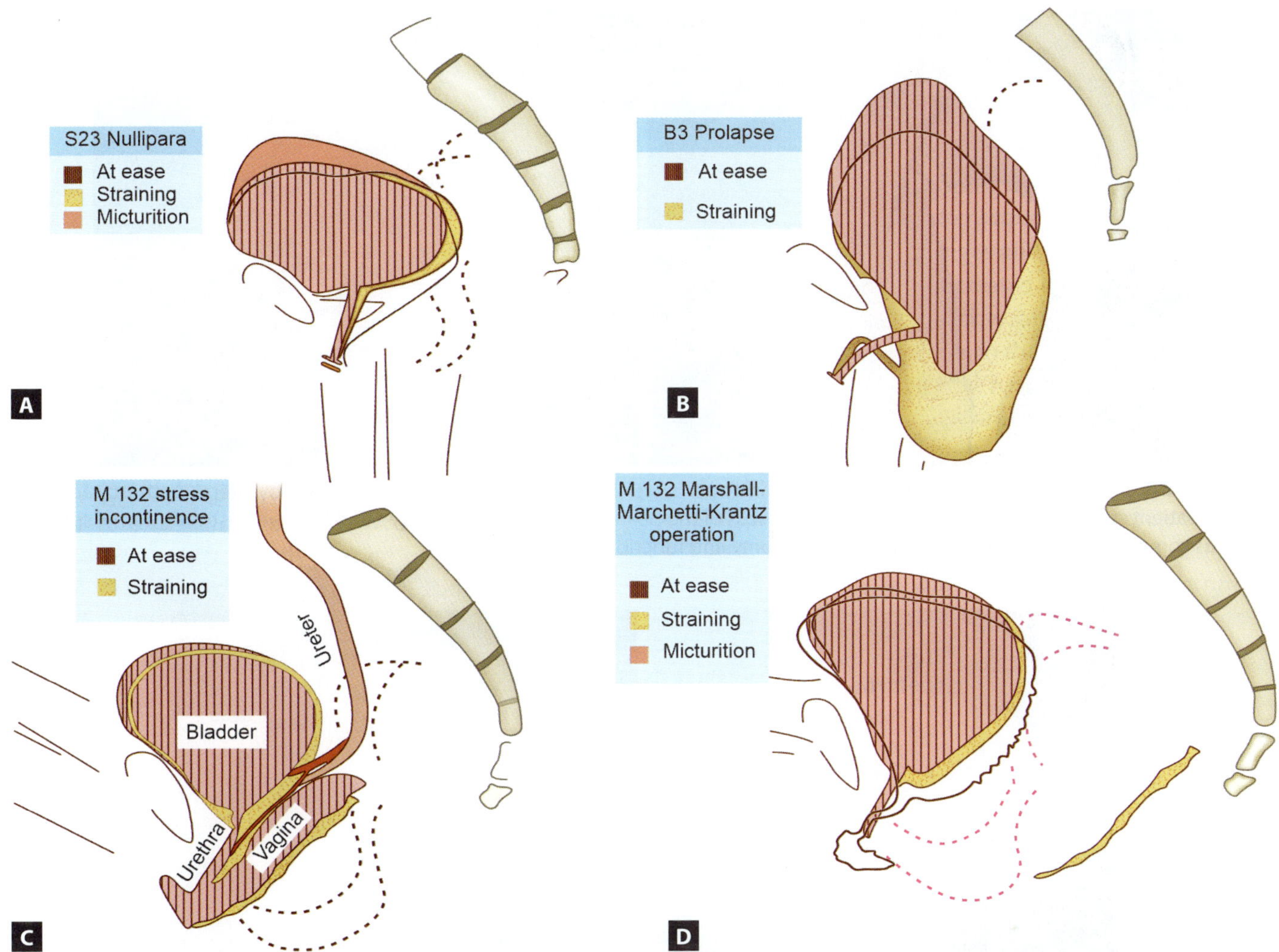

Figs. 7A to D: Tracings of urethrocystograms to help in the interpretation of others. (A) Nulliparous woman with normal bladder function; (B) Multiparous woman with prolapse but not stress incontinence. The anatomy of the urethrovesical junction remains normal even when the patient bears down; (C) A case of urinary stress incontinence. A poor posterior urethrovesical angle is present when the patient is at ease but disappears when she strains; (D) The situation after a successful urethrocystopexy carried out in case (C). The anatomy of the urethrovesical junction is restored, meaning a competent internal sphincter; even on voiding the posterior angle does not fall away completely—a characteristic of successful operations of this type.

noninvasive treatment. All other women should undergo urodynamics before SUI surgery.

Urodynamic studies should ideally be performed on all incontinent women, but this is not always possible that diagnostic cystoscopy is not recommended in the evaluation of UI in women.

The clinician must select those patients who would benefit from detailed urodynamic studies, if limited facilities are available, otherwise they would be overburdened. In general, surgery should not be performed without urodynamic studies when there are any symptoms suggestive of bladder dysfunction.

MANAGEMENT

Medical Management

This should always be tried as the first line of therapy. Kegel's exercises (*refer* Chapter 63: Nutrition and Exercise in Women) strengthen the pubococcygeal and periurethral muscles producing an objective response in 21–80% of patients. Biofeedback aids the response. Patient counselling regarding lifestyle modification as moderation of caffeine consumption, modification of fluid intake, treatment of constipation and reduction of obesity can benefit patients with urge incontinence. Pelvic floor

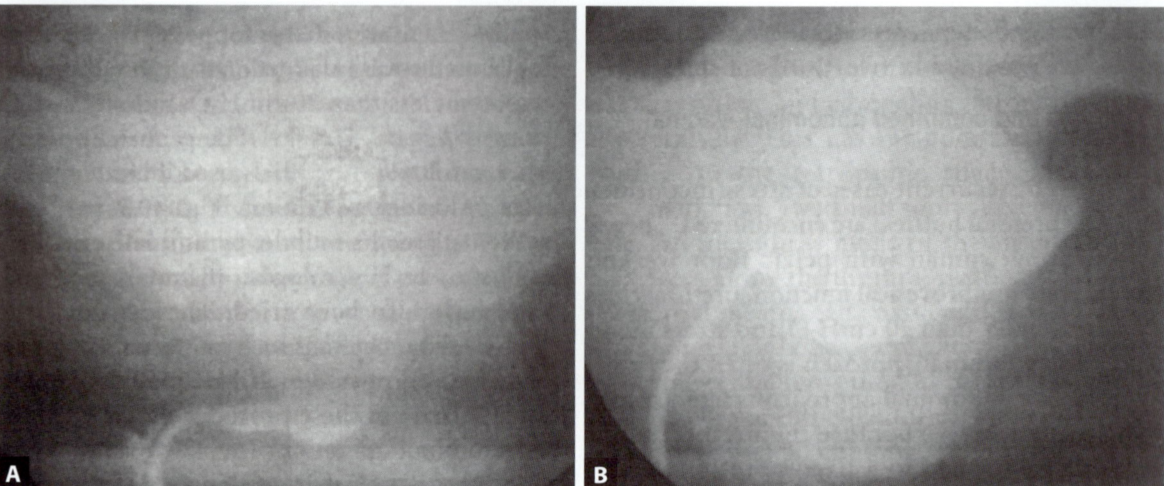

Figs. 8A and B: The effect of a successful urethroplasty and internal sphincter plication operation as shown by lateral urethrocystography with the patient straining. (A) Before operation, there is loss of the posterior urethrovesical angle and leakage past the internal sphincter as well as some cystocele; (B) After operation, the anatomy and function restored to normal.

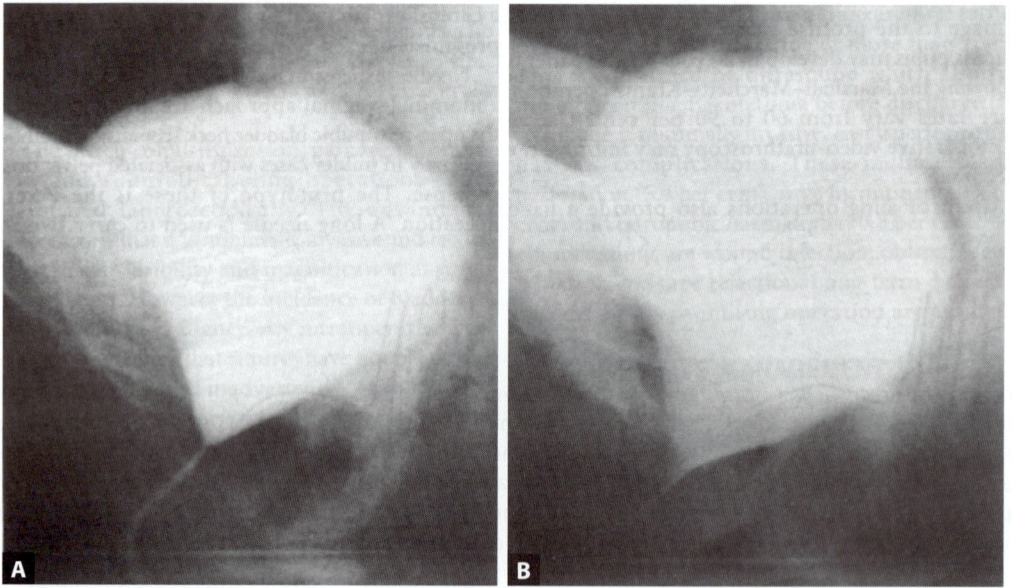

Figs. 9A and B: A failed Aldridge sling operation. The patient concerned, aged 75 years, had two previous urethroplasty operations, and prospects for cure by a sling seemed good until it was noted at operation that the abdominal fascia was very weak. The stress incontinence recurred within 1 month, and these radiographs were taken 3 months after operation. (A) When the woman bears down the posterior angle, very poor at ease, and virtually disappears; (B) During voiding, there is no sign of the slight kink just below the urethrovesical junction which is a feature of successful operations.

muscle training (PFMT) is effective in the prevention and treatment of UI during pregnancy and postpartum.

Pharmacological therapy often produces disappointing results and has significant S/Es on the autonomic nervous system, but should be tried, especially in patients with mixed incontinence. Imipramine 25–150 mg/day increases the tone and may improve mild-to-moderate incontinence. Other drugs which have been used are adrenergic stimulators such as phenylpropanolamine 25–150 mg/day.

The use of topical oestrogens thrice a week for 6–12 weeks has been associated with a subjective response.

Pharmacological Management

Stress incontinence: The tone of urethra and bladder neck is maintained in large part by adrenergic activity from sympathetic nervous system:

- Drugs:
    - Imipramine (relaxing effect on detrusors) 10–25 mg BD, S/Es—orthostatic hypotension
    - Ephedrine 15–30 mg BD
    - Norepinephrine
    - Duloxetine
- Oestrogen—improves urethral closure pressure (2 mg/day)

Urge incontinence:

- Beta-3 receptor agonists such as mirabegron, upcoming drug vibegron, side effects include dry mouth, constipation and cognitive dysfunction in elderly patients.
- Anticholinergics such as solifenacin, fesoterodin and tolterodin, trospium and propiverine —blocking activity of acetylcholine at muscarinic receptor sites. Combination of mirabegron with antimuscarinics is more efficacious than either drug alone.
  Newer—darifenacin and oxybutynin (lesser side effects).
- *Paraurethral implants*: Implants using Teflon increasing functional length of urethra.
- Periurethral bulking injections of glutaraldehyde cross-linked (GAX) collagen is effective (Contigen), other examples include polyacrylamide hydrogel injection (PAHG), carbon beads (Durasphere). It prevents premature bladder neck opening, however they require multiple doses and are less effective than transvaginal tape (TVT).
- Intravesical Botulinum toxin injections (BoNT - A) is reserved for patients not responding to conservative or pharmacological methods. These injections are administered via cystoscopy.
- Neuromodulation methods such as percutaneous tibial nerve stimulation (PTNS), sacral neuromodulation (SNM) wherein a device is implanted near sacral nerve.
- Electrical stimulation devices
- SUI electrical chairs
- Vaginal cones inserted

Mechanical Devices

- *Vaginal:* Intriol and continence guard
- *Urethral:* Urethral plugs, Reliance 7M urinary control insert, Autocath 100 device and continence control pad

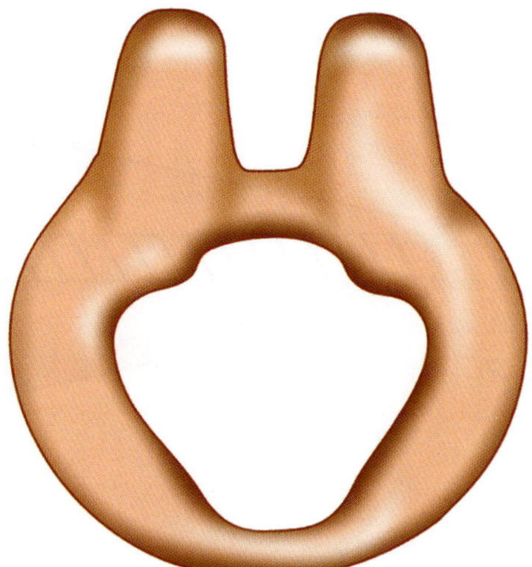

Fig. 10: Intriol.

- *Intriol*:
    - This pessary consists of silicone rubber flexible bag with two blunt prongs located at one end **(Fig. 10)**.
    - When placed in vagina, prongs elevate UV angle in a manner like bunch colposuspension.
    - S/Es—vaginal abrasions, cystitis
- *Continence guard*: Intravaginal device made of hydrophilic polyurethane foam, when saturated with water increases in size by 30% **(Fig. 11)**.
- *Urethral plug*:
    - Made of thermoplastic elastomer
    - Nielson 1990
    - Consists of metal plate, soft stalk and either one or two prongs
    - Midpoint of proximal sphere is placed at bladder neck while distal sphere is placed at maximal urethral pressure point.
    - Proximal sphere reduces amount of urine pushed into the proximal urethra during increased IAP.
- *Autocath 100*:
    - Consists of a cylinder constructed of surgical steel coated with silver
    - Within cylinder, there is spring loaded plunger which regulates the flow of urine.

OVERVIEW OF SURGICAL MANAGEMENT

Surgery forms the mainstay of treatment for cases of stress incontinence. The vaginal surgery for stress incontinence involves the following:

- Suburethral slings (bladder neck slings and midurethral sling)

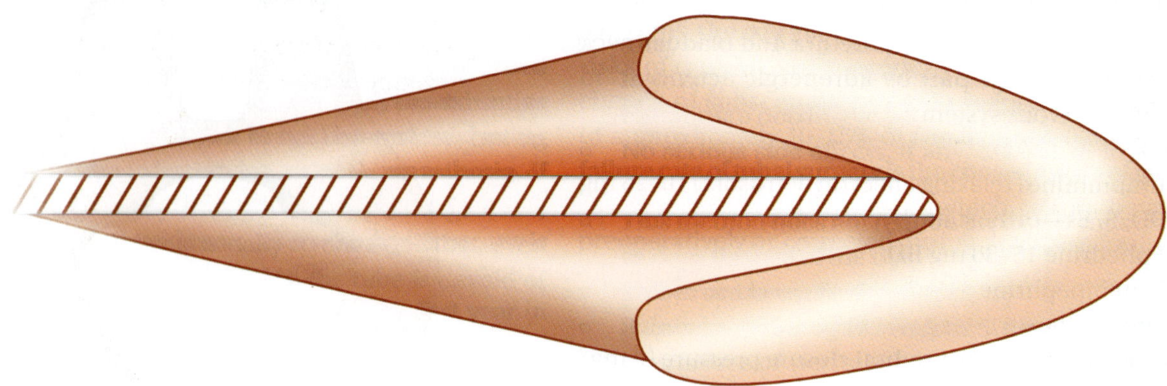

Fig. 11: Continence guard.

- Retropubic bladder neck colposuspension (especially Burch colposuspension)
- Injection of urethral bulking agents.

The advent of synthetic tapes, especially that of tension-free vaginal tapes (TVTs) has further revolutionised the surgery for stress incontinence. Several newer modifications of these tapes are available nowadays, such as transobturator tapes (TOTs) and crossover tapes. The advantage, which the sling surgery has over the previously used surgeries (especially Burch procedure), is the potential of sling surgery to treat ISD in addition to the urethral hypermobility. Since some element of ISD seems to be mandatory for a leak, it is nearly always present in cases of stress incontinence and is commonly the cause of long-term recurrence. As a result, nowadays, most surgeons favour sling surgery over Burch colposuspension.

Surgery for Urge Incontinence

Surgical therapy should be considered only in severe and refractory cases of urge incontinence and include bladder augmentation procedures, denervation procedures, urinary diversion and sacral neuromodulation.

Aims of Surgery

Various procedures for stress incontinence share the common goal of stabilising the bladder neck and proximal urethra.

Indications for Surgery

Indications for sling surgery are as follows:

- Various forms of stress incontinence, especially those with ISD
- Stress incontinence with concomitant pelvic organ prolapse
- Failed procedures such as needle suspension or Burch colposuspension
- Women with a urethral diverticulectomy or urethral loss such as after a urethra-vaginal fistula repair (an autologous sling is preferred over synthetic sling in these cases).

Preoperative Preparation

Preoperative evaluation involves taking the complete history from the patient and performing a complete general physical examination, focusing on the following parameters:

- *The type of incontinence*: Whether the symptoms are suggestive of stress incontinence, urge incontinence or mixed (both the types).
- *Performance of tests for confirmation of stress incontinence*:
  - *Cough stress test or urinary stress test:* In this test, the patient with stress incontinence is asked to perform a Valsalva's manoeuvre (the patient is asked to tense her abdominal muscles) or cough. Instantaneous leakage of urine with cough or Valsalva's manoeuvre is suggestive of SUI. Delayed leakage of urine is usually suggestive of incontinence due to detrusor overactivity.
  - *Measurement of the postvoidal residual volume:* In this test, the patient with a full bladder is asked to void as she normally would, without the requirement of an additional effort to fully empty the bladder. Following voiding, the residual urine

in the bladder is measured either by catheterisation or bladder sonography. Generally, a postvoidal residual volume of >200 cm^3 may be suggestive of voiding dysfunction or detrusor weakness.

- The patient must be asked to maintain a complete voiding diary.
- The clinician must assess the pelvic anatomy including strength of the muscles of pelvic floor.
- The surgeon also needs to determine if there is any associated voiding dysfunction suggestive of ISD. This might have an impact on the surgical management plan to be followed as well as the future prognosis because the patients with ISD do not have as good a long-term outcome with any procedure in comparison to those patients having predominant hypermobility. A patient with an underactive detrusor may be associated with the likelihood of voiding difficulty following surgical treatment of incontinence.
- The surgeon must also determine if there is any associated pelvic floor dysfunction such as cystocele, enterocele, rectocele, anal sphincter incompetence or vault prolapse. In case any such dysfunction is present, it must be taken care of at the time of surgery.
- The performance of urodynamic studies may provide important diagnostic and prognostic information and must be performed prior to any invasive therapy. Urodynamic evaluation is not necessary for many women with uncomplicated SUI. Urodynamic testing may prove to be useful in cases where the symptoms are not consistent with physical examination findings or in women having mixed/complicated incontinence situations.
- Oestrogen replacement therapy prior to surgery may enhance urethral, bladder and vaginal tissue integrity.
- Treatment of various underlying medical disorders such as asthma, chronic obstructive pulmonary disease (COPD), diabetes and chronic constipation must be undertaken prior to surgery.
- Good nutrition helps to maximise tissue integrity and to support good healing.
- *Patient counselling*: This must comprise of a thorough discussion of risks, benefits, anticipated success rates and potential common complications related to the procedure.
- Patient is placed in the lithotomy position under general or spinal anaesthesia.

Intraoperative Details

The various types of surgeries which can be performed for stress incontinence are discussed further.

Suburethral Sling

A suburethral sling is a sling that is inserted through a small vaginal incision and placed either at the bladder neck, midurethra or proximal urethra for the purpose of supporting the urethra in women with SUI. There are two types of suburethral slings: (1) Bladder neck slings and (2) midurethral slings.

Bladder neck sling: Also known as a proximal urethral sling, this sling is placed at the level of the proximal urethra and bladder neck. This procedure is usually performed using both a vaginal and abdominal incision. These slings can be made of either biological materials (including the patient's own tissue) or synthetic mesh. The bladder neck slings are also referred to as pubovaginal slings when the arms of the sling material are affixed to the anterior rectus fascia rather than the pubic bone or Cooper's ligament. Pubovaginal slings involve the use of autologous fascia, which can be harvested from the patient's rectus sheath or alternatively from the patient's thigh (fascia lata).

Midurethral sling: This is a suburethral sling that is inserted via a small vaginal incision and placed at the level of the midurethra in a tension-free manner. This surgery involves the interplay of three structures: (1) Pubourethral ligaments, (2) suburethral vaginal tissues and (3) the pubococcygeus muscle. Though there can be several variations of these procedures, all involve the placement of a synthetic mesh. Based on the route of placement, i.e. whether a retropubic or a transobturator approach is used, these procedures can be classified as follows:

- Retropubic method: TVT
- Transobturator approach: TOT

Retropubic approach: There are several commercially available kits and one commonly used technique is the TVT. In this technique, one trocar is placed through a vaginal suburethral incision lateral to the urethra and brought out suprapubically through a skin incision **(Figs. 12A to E)**. The TVT devices are associated with a 71% cure rate at 11.5 years.

Transobturator approach: This approach was introduced to reduce the risks related to injury to the lower urinary tract and vascular structures, which can be associated

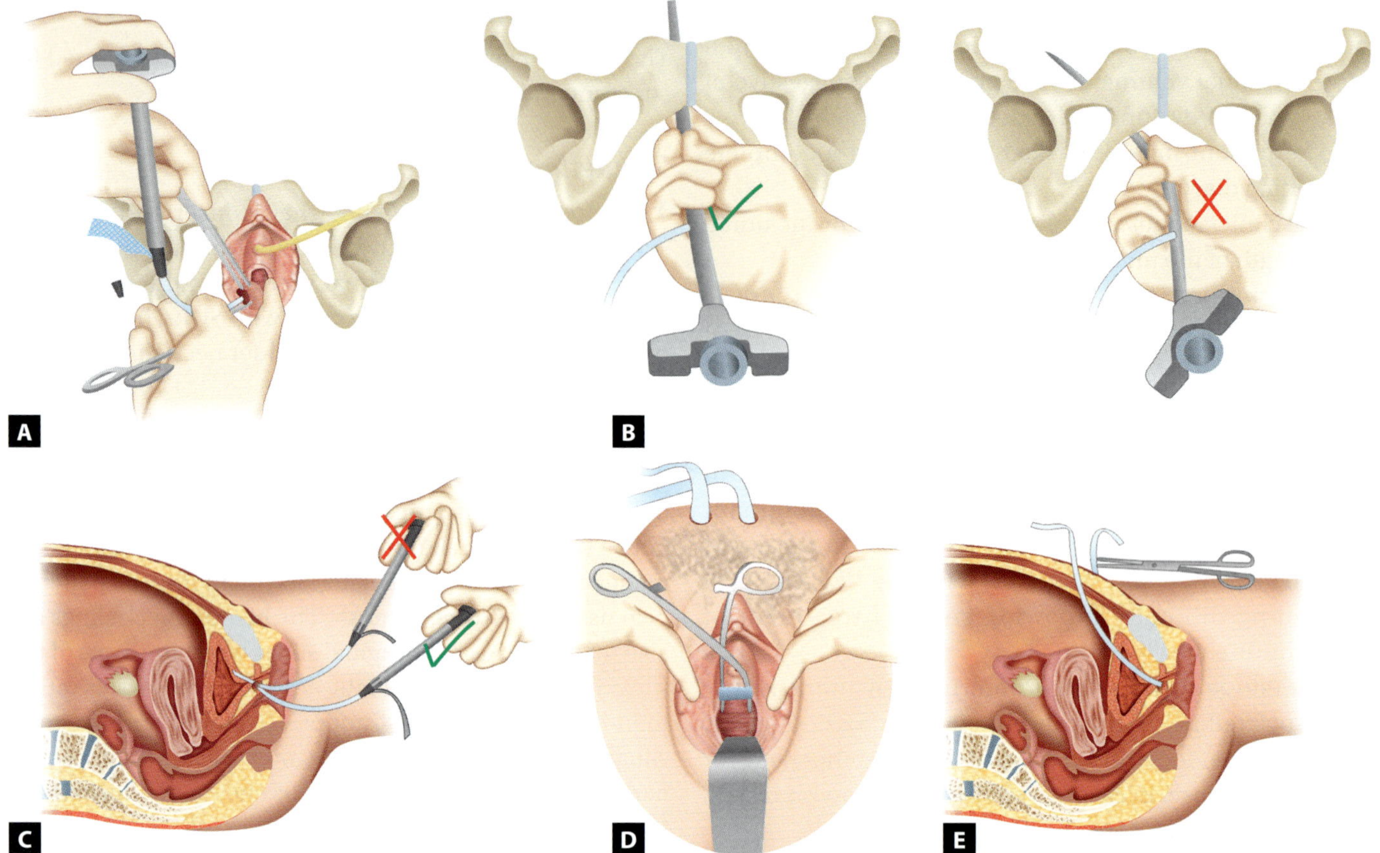

Figs. 12A to E: Tension-free vaginal tape surgery. (A) Placing the needle through the submucosal tunnel; (B) Correct and incorrect positioning of the transducer; (C) Correct and incorrect positioning of the hand and the transducer; (D) Setting mesh tension; (E) Bringing the tape out through the suprapubic abdominal incision and trimming the tape.

with traversing the retropubic space. Various kits for this approach are available, each containing a needle and a mesh design sling material made up of polypropylene. In this surgery, the sling material is directed bilaterally through the obturator foramen underneath the midurethra **(Figs. 13A to D)**. The point of entry overlies the proximal tendon of adductor longus muscle. Based on the method of needle placement, the transobturator procedures can be of two types:

1. *An 'in-to-out' approach:* Needle placement begins inside the vagina and is directed outwards.
2. *An 'out-to-in' approach:* Needle placement begins outside the vagina and is directed inwards.

Initially, when the transobturator sling procedure was introduced, an 'out-to-in' approach was used. However, this approach was associated with several complications such as injury to the bladder and urethra. The 'in-toout' approach was then introduced with the aim of reducing injury to the lower urinary tract.

However, in this approach, the needle travels to the obturator neurovascular bundle. Though each method has theoretical advantages, the possibility of injury cannot be completely excluded. Nevertheless, the transobturator approach serves as an effective day surgery technique with potentially lower rate of bladder injury. However, some retrospective studies have shown that it may show limited effectiveness in patients having urodynamic criteria for ISD.

Pubovaginal Sling Surgery

This surgery comprises the following steps **(Figs. 14A to G)**:

- *Harvesting the strip of rectus fascia:* In this surgery, first, a strip of rectus fascia is harvested by making a 3-inch-long transverse incision just above the pubis below the pubic hairline down to the surface of the rectus fascia. The rectus fascia is dissected free of subcutaneous

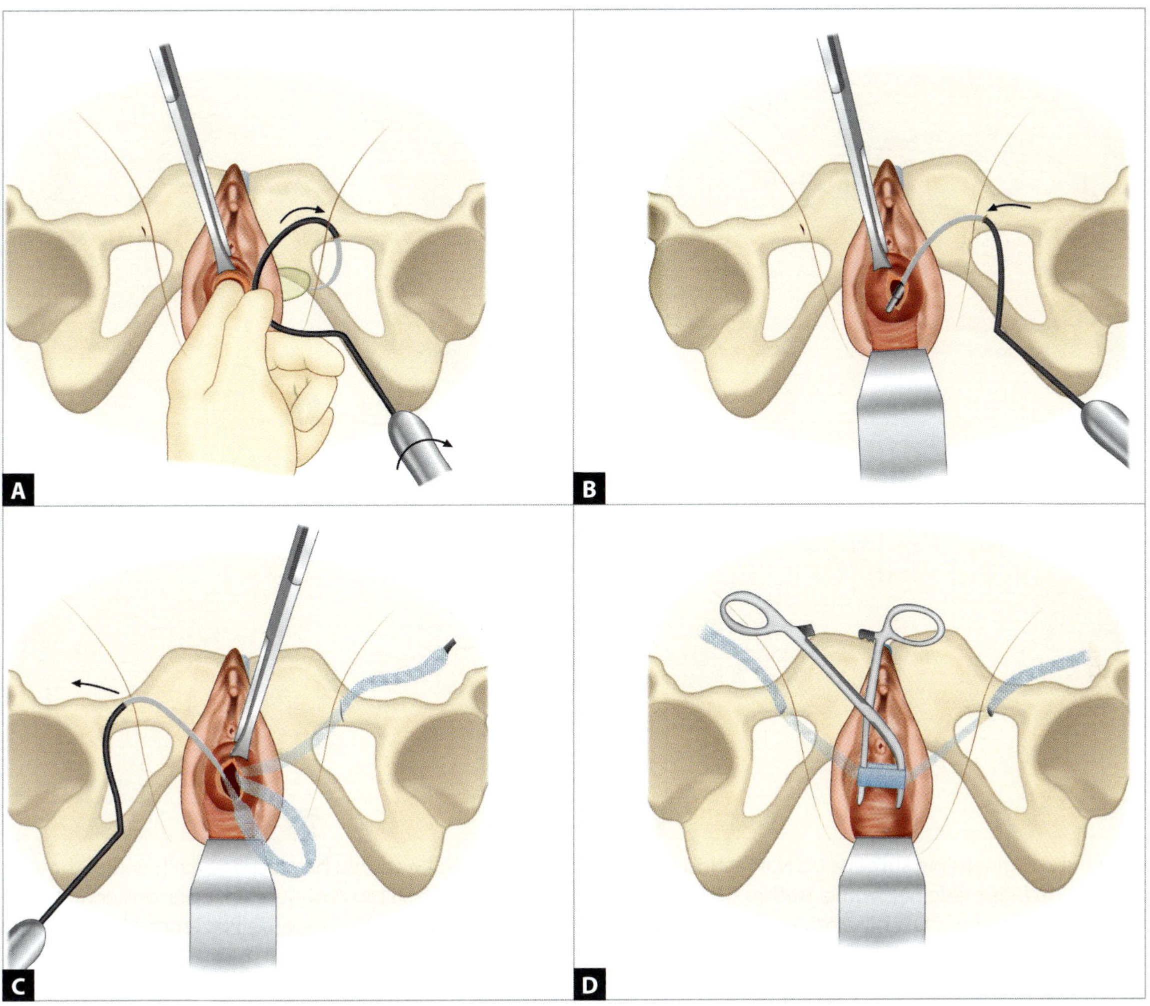

Figs. 13A to D: Tension-free obturator tape. (A) Introduction of the needle; (B) Passage of the needle; (C) Placing the tape; (D) Setting mesh tension.

tissue from the above and freed from the muscles below to fashion out a rectus fascia sling, which is about 12–16 cm long and 2 cm in width. Once the entire dissection is complete, the fascial strip is excised and placed in a basin of saline. A helical stitch is placed using a 0-gauge delayed-absorbable polypropylene sutures at each end of the fascial strip. The abdominal wound is packed temporarily and the vaginal surgery is begun.

- *Identification of bladder neck:* A Foley catheter is inserted into the bladder. The bladder neck can be identified by inserting a Foley catheter inside the urethra. Applying gentle traction on the Foley catheter and palpation of the balloon would help in delineation of bladder neck.
- *Vaginal dissection to reach the pubic bone:* A vertical incision or a gently curved horizontal incision (about 5-6 cm long) is made about 2 cm below the urethral meatus on the anterior vaginal wall superficial to the pubocervical fascia **(Fig. 14B)**. The edges of the incision are held using Allis forceps, and a combination of sharp and blunt dissection is used to lift the vaginal epithelium off the underlying fibromuscular layer. The plane corresponding to the undersurface of the anterior vaginal wall is identified by noting the characteristic shiny white appearance. Blunt dissection is then performed to create a space up to the pubic bone by entering the space of Retzius. The dissection is carried out using the dissecting scissors, pointing laterally until the pubic bone is reached. A combination of sharp

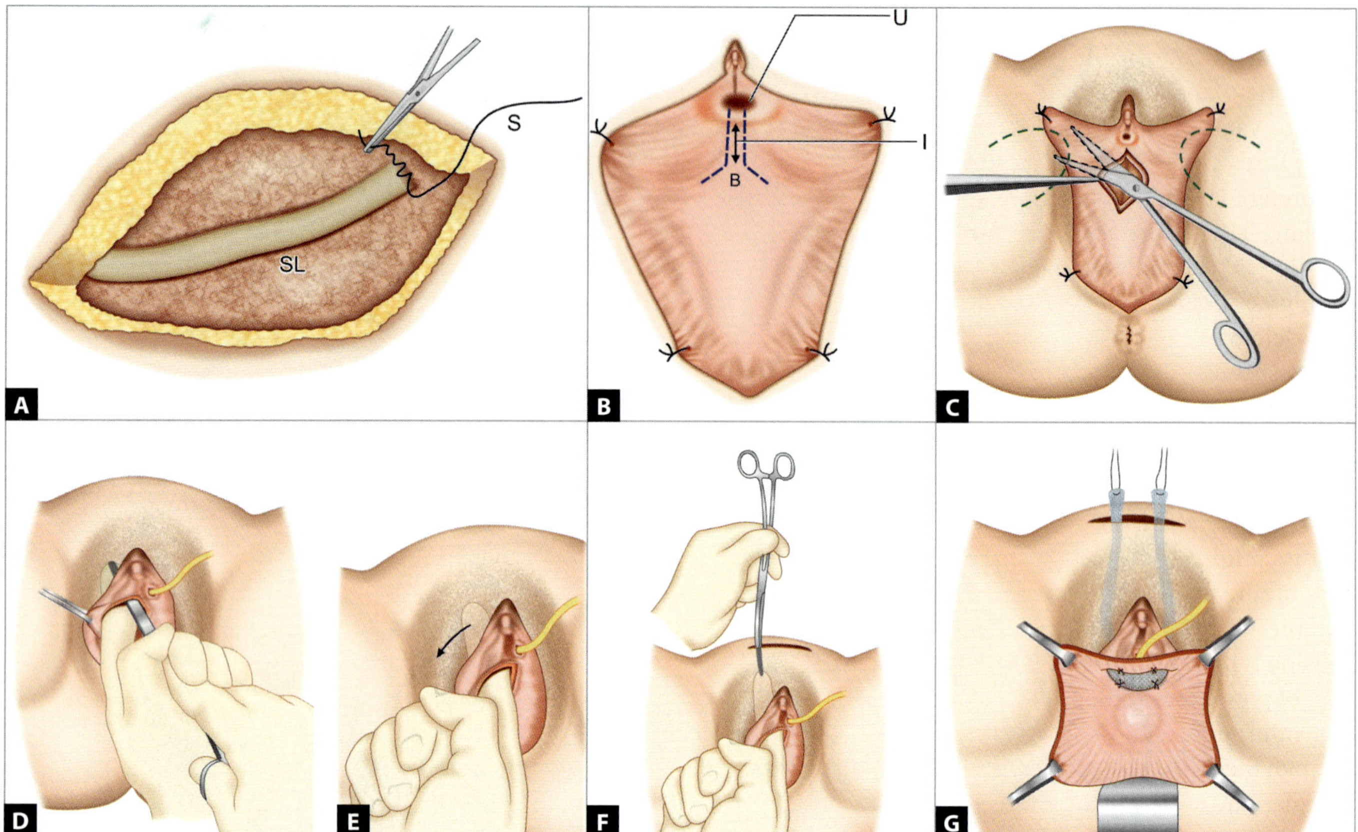

Figs. 14A to G: Pubovaginal sling surgery. (A) Harvesting the strip of rectus fascia: (S) should be placed at each end of the sling (SL); (B) A short vertical incision (I) is made below the urethra (U); (C) A combination of sharp and blunt dissection is performed until the finger can palpate the ischiopubic ramus; (D) Entry into the space of Retzius; (E) Palpation of the pubic bone; (F) Placement of the strip of fascia; (G) Suturing the fascial sling in place.

and blunt dissection is performed until the finger can palpate the ischiopubic ramus. During this part of the dissection, the surgeon must try to stay as far lateral as possible to avoid injury to the urethra, bladder and ureters.

- *Placing the urethral sling*: Using the surgeon's right hand, a long dressing or packing forceps or needle ligature carrier is used from the abdominal side to perforate the rectus sheath caudal to the prior harvest incision. Simultaneously, the surgeon's left index finger is placed in the vagina to bluntly retract the bladder neck medially. The forceps is placed against the back of pubic bone and advanced towards the vagina. Concurrently, the surgeon guides the instrument using his fingers within the space of Retzius. The suture at one end of the harvested rectus fascial strip is grasped with the penetrating forceps and threaded up through the abdominal incision on the side of urethra. A similar procedure is repeated on the other side with the other end of the sling. As a result, the fascial sling lies positioned beneath the bladder neck. The sling is fixed beneath the bladder neck using 3–4 delayed absorbable sutures. Two small stab wounds are made in the rectus fascia just above the pubis, and the sling is brought through them on either side.
- *Placing the sling in a tension-free manner*: Sutures attached to the sling are then tied together above the rectus sheath. While tying the knot, a space of two- or three-finger breadth is left between the knot and the fascia to prevent future complications such as bladder neck obstruction and urinary retention. Once the knot has been secured, there should be no upward angulation of the urethra or bladder. The sling is placed in a tension-free manner, just like the TVT. One should be able to place a heavy pair of scissors between the sling and the urethra to ensure that the sling is not under tension.

- *Closure of the vaginal incision*: Cystoscopy is performed to ensure that the urinary tract is safe, and there has been no bladder perforation or obstruction of urethra. The vagina is then closed using 2-0 chromic catgut sutures in a running fashion. Some surgeons may prefer to close the vagina before the sling has been tied since adequate access may become difficult once the sling is tied and the bladder neck has moved up to a higher and a less accessible location. A Foley catheter is left in place.
- *Closure of the abdominal incision*: At the end of surgery, the abdominal incision is closed using interrupted silk sutures.

Minimally Invasive Slings

Modification of TVT and TOT procedures is observed with minimally invasive slings, sometimes also known as the microslings or minislings. In this technique, a small incision is made in the vagina, through which an 8-cm long strip of polypropylene synthetic mesh is placed across and beneath the midurethra. Since the mesh is not threaded through the retropubic space, it helps in avoiding potential vascular injury.

Retropubic Bladder Neck Colposuspension

All these procedures are performed through a lower abdominal incision and involve the attachment of periurethral and perivesical endopelvic fascia (vaginal wall adjacent to midurethra and bladder neck) to some other supporting structure in the anterior pelvis **(Table 3 and Fig. 15)**. These procedures are also referred to as retropubic urethropexy. Nowadays, some of these procedures are performed through laparoscopic and robotic surgery. These procedures had been long considered as the gold standard for the surgical treatment of stress incontinence, with 1-year continence rates varying between 85% and 90%. Some complications commonly associated with retropubic urethropexy include detrusor overactivity, urinary retention, and in the case of Marshall-Marchetti-Krantz procedure, osteitis pubis.

Injection of Urethral Bulking Agents

Periurethral injections are performed under local anaesthesia and involve the administration of various types of materials around the periurethral tissues to facilitate their coaptation under conditions of increased IAP. Various bulking agents have been used including collagen, carbon-coated zirconium, ethylene vinyl alcohol, polydimethylsiloxane, polytetrafluoroethylene and glutaraldehyde cross-linked bovine collagen (Contigen). The use of periurethral bulking agents is employed in those cases who are unable to tolerate surgery or those who want to avoid it. It can also be used in patients with recurrent or refractory incontinence or those in whom sling surgery for stress incontinence had previously been performed.

TABLE 3: Various supporting structures in different types of retropubic procedures.

Name of surgical procedure	*Supporting structure in the anterior pelvis*
Paravaginal procedure	Arcus tendineus
Modified Marshall–Marchetti–Krantz procedure	Back of pubic symphysis
Burch colposuspension	Iliopectineal ligament (Cooper's ligament)
Turner–Warwick vaginal obturator shelf procedure	Fascia over obturator internus

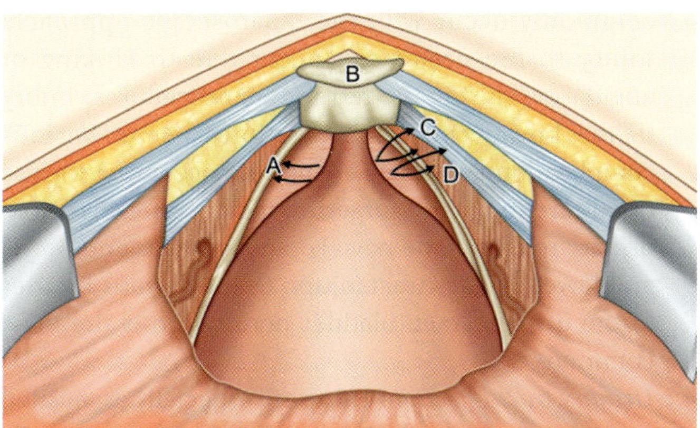

Fig. 15: Point of attachment of endopelvic fascia during bladder neck suspension procedures: (A) Arcus tendineus; (B) Periosteum of the pubic symphysis; (C) Iliopectineal ligaments (Cooper's ligaments); (D) Obturator internus fascia.

Postoperative Care

- Voiding trials are begun as soon as the patient is comfortable, usually on the first or second postoperative day.
- Bladder drainage is an essential aspect of postoperative care. Most patients are able to void spontaneously in 3–7 days.
- Measures must be taken to control chronic cough and to avoid or treat constipation.

- The patient should avoid lifting anything heavier than 10 pounds for 12 weeks.
- The patient must be instructed to avoid smoking and other activities that may repetitively stress the pelvic floor, resulting in long-term failure of the procedure.

Complications

- *Haemorrhage*: Bleeding is usually from the perivesical venous plexus. Haemorrhage can occur in nearly 2% cases undergoing retropubic procedures.
- *Urinary tract and visceral injury*: Bladder injuries can commonly occur with the laparoscopic approach. Injury to the ureter can occur due to kinking or angulation during the retropubic procedures. Injury to the bowel can also sometimes occur. Various complications, which may especially occur with the use of midurethral sling surgeries, include mesh erosion, urinary retention, de novo UI and vascular and bowel and lower urinary tract injury. Of the various injuries to the urinary tract, bladder perforation is the most common.
- *Urinary tract infection*: These are especially associated with postoperative voiding difficulties, resulting in prolonged catheterisation.
- *Wound infection*: Prophylactic antibiotics in the form of a single dose of a broad-spectrum agent are usually effective.
- *Osteitis pubis*: This is a self-limited inflammation of the pubic bone related to the placement of foreign body material such as sutures. Osteomyelitis can rarely occur.
- *Urogenital fistula*: This is also a rare complication.
- *Nerve injuries*: Injuries to various nerves such as common peroneal, sciatic, obturator, femoral, saphenous and ilioinguinal nerves have been reported.
- *Voiding dysfunction*: This may manifest in the form of a slow or poor urinary stream or in the inability to void.
- *Detrusor overactivity*: De novo detrusor overactivity may at times develop postoperatively
- *Pelvic organ prolapse*: Enterocele formation may be as high as 8% following surgery. The rate of rectocele formation also may be increased.
- *Other complications*: These may include complications such as dyspareunia, chronic suprapubic pain and sinus tract formation.

Discussion

Nowadays, midurethral sling procedures are commonly used. Midurethral slings are as effective as other surgical treatments for SUI, but with a shorter operative duration and a lower risk of certain postoperative complications.

Midurethral slings are associated with considerably reduced morbidity and voiding dysfunction in comparison to the bladder neck slings. Therefore, bladder neck slings are used only in those women where the midurethral slings are contraindicated or unsuccessful. Moreover, midurethral slings are associated with several advantages such as high short-term cure rate and better quality of life. Of the two approaches (retropubic and transobturator approach) commonly used in cases of midurethal sling surgeries, both the approaches appear to offer comparable results.

Despite these favourable comparisons, abundant long-term data regarding the efficacy of transobturator approach are lacking. Pubovaginal rectus fascia slings have excellent long-term results with >80% of the patients remaining continent beyond 5 years of surgery.

Some surgical procedures which were commonly used previously but are rarely used nowadays for the treatment of incontinence include anterior colporrhaphy with Kelly's plication, transabdominal paravaginal repair and transvaginal needle suspension procedures. Transvaginal urethropexies/needle suspension procedures/Pereyra-Raz's/Stamey's procedure involves the passage of sutures between the vagina and anterior abdominal wall using an especially designed long needle carrier, which is inserted through the vaginal incision made at the level of the bladder neck. The other end of the suture passes through a small abdominal incision, which is made transversely just above the pubic bone and is carried down to the rectus fascia. These surgeries, therefore, relied on the strength and integrity of the periurethral tissue and the abdominal wall.

Before undertaking any surgery, the following factors need to be considered by the surgeon:

- *ISD versus hypermobility*: If hypermobility predominates, both pubovaginal sling and Burch colposuspension are equally effective. However, if ISD predominates, a pubovaginal sling is more effective.
- *Findings of the urodynamic studies*: If the urodynamic findings are suggestive of underactive detrusor, the surgeon must take extra caution in order to avoid urethral obstruction during the procedure. It might

also require the surgeon to counsel the patient regarding a possible postoperative clean intermittent catheterisation.

- *Patient's lifestyle*: A sling surgery may be better suited to a young and very active patient, whereas an old patient, with an underlying medical condition, unfit for surgery may benefit from the use of minimal therapy, such as a collagen injection.

ENURESIS

Aetiology

Nocturnal incontinence of urine (bed-wetting) is the rule in children, until they have learned to inhibit the automatic action of the bladder during sleep as well as during consciousness. It continues for a variable number of years and can persist in the adolescent and the adult. Sometimes it is 'secondary' in that it represents the breakdown of an acquired control, usually under stress. It is then closely related to functional urge incontinence. Many bedwetters have diurnal urgency.

In children, the complaint is more often seen in boys than girls; in either sex, it tends to be familial and its causes are discussed further.

Natural Variability in Age

There is a natural variability in the age at which control is developed; this is dependent on the time of maturation of the nervous system. Enuresis persists until the age of 5 years in 10% of children and to puberty in 1%.

Organic Disease

Conditions which may underlie or contribute to enuresis include lesions of the central nervous system, urinary tract infection and diseases causing polyuria. These are more often found in adults than in children. In the latter, an organic basis is found in <1% of cases. In girls, an intermittent leak from an accessory ureter can be mistaken for enuresis.

Psychological Disturbances

These are the most important of all causes, and primary enuresis is nearly always the result of a combination of delayed maturation with a variety of psychological and environmental factors. The latter include an unhappy and insecure home background and lack of parental care and guidance in the conditioning of the bladder reflex.

Once established, and depending on its handling, enuresis can persist as a means of attracting attention or avoiding unwanted occupations and responsibilities.

Subnormal Bladder Capacity

Although it is sometimes alleged, the capacity of the bladder is never organically small; the detrusor muscle is merely intolerant of large volumes and behaves in exactly the same manner as is described for the irritable bladder.

Management and Treatment

The investigation and treatment of enuresis in the adult are the same as for the irritable bladder already described. What follows applies mainly to enuresis in childhood and adolescence, although some of the measures and drugs mentioned can be useful in adults. When enuresis in a child persists for an unreasonable time and despite treatment, full investigation is indicated to exclude an organic basis. Otherwise, it is best avoided lest it exaggerate the problem in the mind of the sufferer. If urinalysis and physical examination revealed no abnormalities, the symptoms should be treated on the assumption that their cause lies in the psyche. The fact that it is psychological makes treatment difficult and explains why 30% of 'cures' are followed by relapse.

- *General approach*: It is best not to worry the child, for if the problem can be disregarded a spontaneous cure is encouraged. The fact that spontaneous cure is always likely makes it extremely difficult to claim success for any remedy. It is reckoned that when general measures and drugs (not including the bed buzzer) fail, 50% of enuretic children cure themselves by the age of 9 years and at least another 25–30% by the age of 14 years. It is most exceptional for the complaint to persist after the age of 19 years. So, exhortation at night and scolding in the morning are to be avoided. Some say there should be no comment on whether the bed is wet or dry; others say that comment on success gives encouragement to a child who is probably losing confidence and becoming distressed inwardly.

  Children and their parents certainly deserve help and support and, as time goes by, it is not enough to give an assurance that the girl will 'grow out of the habit'.
- Correction of the background of unhappiness, insecurity and nervous stress
- Bladder discipline during the day

- Avoidance of drinking any fluid for 3 hours before retiring
- *Drugs:* Desmopressin is the drug of choice. Propantheline, amitriptyline and imipramine are also used. However, the benefits of drug therapy are often not sustained over a period of time after discontinuation. Great caution is necessary in increasing the dose or in continuing medication for a long time because imipramine can cause fatal poisoning, and there is no specific antidote to it.
- Waking the child to empty the bladder every 3–4 hours. The resentment to interruption of sleep can also have a good disciplinary effect.
- Electric bed buzzers act in a similar way and are activated by the initial escape of water. They should not be used for children <7 years of age and need to be put in place regularly for not <3 months. The results are good (a 75% cure rate is claimed) and long-lasting, but care is necessary to avoid their producing burns or shocks.
- Specialist psychiatric treatment

URINARY RETENTION AND DIFFICULTY IN MICTURITION

For an understanding of the causes and mechanisms whereby a woman develops retention of urine, the reader is advised first to review the physiology of voiding.

The classical gynaecological cause of urinary retention is an impacted pelvic tumour. In such a case, the diagnosis is usually made clear by attention to associated symptoms, as indicated in **Table 4**.

TABLE 4: Differential diagnosis of urinary retention.

Retention	+	Primary amenorrhoea	=	Haematocolpos
	+	Secondary amenorrhoea	=	Retroverted gravid uterus
	+	Menorrhagia	=	Uterine leiomyoma
	+	No menstrual upset	=	Ovarian or broad ligament tumour
	+	Irregular bleeding	=	Threatened abortion from a retroverted gravid uterus, pelvic haematocele or pelvic abscess

Causes and Mechanisms of Retention

Acute retention occurring under the above circumstances has long been explained by assuming that the tumour elevates the bladder base into the lower abdomen, thus elongating and stretching the urethra. Attenuation of the urethra, rather than direct compression, is, thus, held accountable for difficulty in outflow of urine. How did this concept arise?

Schatz in 1870 and Halliday Groom in 1890 studied the pelvic anatomy of women dying from an impacted gravid uterus. Both emphasised that the urethra is not elongated in this condition and that the urethrovesical junction remains at its normal level in the pelvis **(Fig. 16)**. Despite careful documentation by these authors, their illustrations were misinterpreted by subsequent writers who, without any anatomical evidence, fostered the notion that retention is caused by attenuation of the urethra.

Lateral urethrocystography in women suffering from retention caused by an impacted gravid uterus or other pelvic tumours **(Figs. 17A and B)** confirms the accuracy of the observation by Groom and Schatz and also demonstrates the reason for retention. The urethrovesical junction remains in its normal pelvic position, and the urethra is not elongated. The patient fails to void

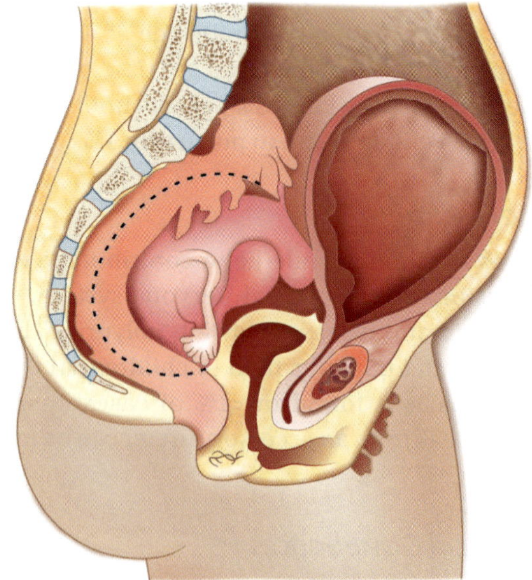

Fig. 16: Drawings from a frozen section of the trunk of a woman who died as a result of acute urinary retention caused by impaction of retroverted gravid uterus. Although the appearances at first suggest elongation of the urethra, it is the collapsed lower compartment of the bladder. The urethrovesical junction is not elevated and is in its normal position behind the symphysis pubis.

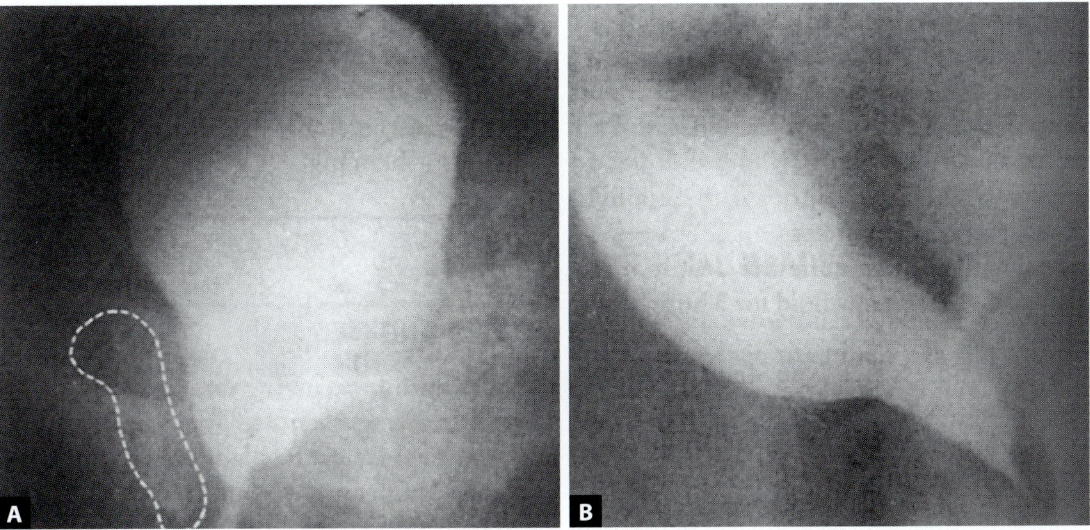

Figs. 17A and B: Retention of urine caused by tumours impacted in the pelvis. The mechanism is not elongation of the urethra. Although the fundus of the bladder rises into the lower abdomen, the urethrovesical junction is at its normal level behind the symphysis pubis. Voiding fails because, despite contraction of the bladder detrusor muscle, the internal sphincter cannot open properly—because of the pressure of the tumour from behind. (A) Retroverted gravid uterus (14 weeks of amenorrhoea); the urethra is marked by a catheter, but the patient is trying to void; (B) Uterine leiomyomas impacted in the pelvis. The patient is trying to void but has only succeeded in getting a few drops of fluid into the upper urethra. The posterior urethrovesical angle is still present to some degree.

in these cases because the tumour interferes with the opening of the internal urethral sphincter, and this shows radiographically by persistence of the posterior urethrovesical angle. Incidentally, retention of urine by this mechanism can be reproduced experimentally merely by packing the vagina tightly with gauze to produce an artificial tumour.

Retention of urine in the female can always be explained by one of four mechanisms.

The bladder detrusor muscle may fail to contract and thus open the upper urethra: This is the usual mechanism for retention after lower abdominal operations, but happens whenever:

- The woman fails to contract the abdominal muscles as an initial trigger to voiding
- There is inhibition of the detrusor muscle by emotional upsets such as hysteria, excessive modesty and fear.
- The excitatory nerves to the bladder are paralysed by disease of the central nervous system or are injured during extensive pelvic operations (e.g. radical hysterectomy).
- The bladder muscle becomes atonic from overstretching; this may result from neglect of retention of any kind.

Interference with the Opening of the Internal Sphincter

This mechanism for retention is seen in the following circumstances:

- When a tumour such as the retroverted gravid uterus, a cervical leiomyoma, an impacted ovarian cyst or the foetal head late in labour, crowds the pelvic space. It is still too commonly stated that, in labour, the bladder is lifted up into the lower abdomen, and that this elongates and attenuates the urethra to cause retention. Radiography during labour shows that, although the fundus of the bladder does rise as the presenting part descends, the urethrovesical junction always remains at its normal level behind the symphysis pubis, and the urethra is not lengthened. This is true no matter how long labour lasts and even when it is obstructed. This is the reason that obstetrical fistulas resulting from prolonged labour and pressure are always sited in the trigone of the bladder and not in the urethra:
- When the vagina is tightly packed for any therapeutic reason
- After operations which buttress the tissues behind the urethrovesical junction with the object of curing stress incontinence of urine

- When these tissues are made inelastic by disease, such as cancer extending from the cervix and vagina
- When a urethral sling is made too tight or urethrocystopexy is performed too enthusiastically **(Fig. 18)**.

Spasm of the Voluntary External Urethral Sphincter

Despite the proper contraction of the bladder detrusor and proper opening of the upper urethra, retention can still occur as a result of failure of the voluntary external sphincter to relax **(Figs. 19A and B)**.

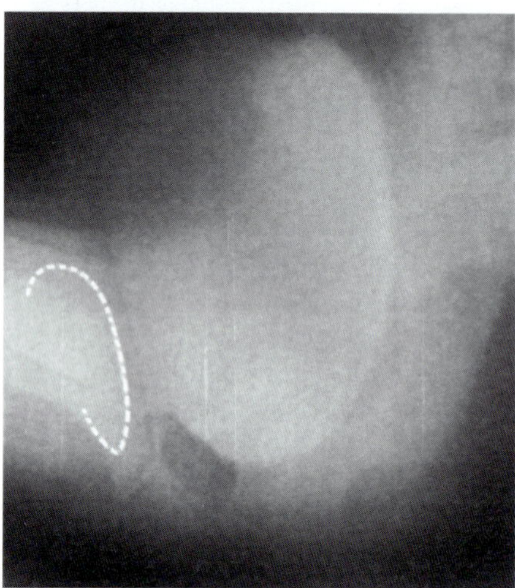

Fig. 18: The effect of urethrocystopexy in which the tissues were stitched too high behind the symphysis pubis. The urethrocystogram taken during attempts to void shows that the detrusor muscle is contracting, but the posterior urethrovesical angle cannot fall away to open the internal sphincter fully. A very tiny stream of urine escapes with difficulty.

This produces a typical radiological appearance which is identical to that seen during the wilful arrest of the normal voiding act. Failure of the external sphincter to relax occurs in the following circumstances: (1) Nervousness and embarrassment of the woman; (2) perineal injuries during childbirth; (3) operations on the perineum and perianal tissues; (4) urethritis; and (5) neurological disease.

Moreover, the base of the bladder forms a pouch below the level of the outflow and cannot be emptied. The patient in this case suffered postoperative retention for several weeks and thereafter had incomplete emptying.

It appears that the compressor urethrae and the levator ani muscles act in unison, and lesions which cause the latter to go into spasm tend to have the same effect on the external urethral sphincter. This explains why vaginal operations rarely cause retention of urine unless posterior colpoperineorrhaphy is included.

Obstruction of the Urethra

This is the rarest mechanism of urinary retention and its causes include the following:

- Congenital atresia, valves or functional closure can cause gross distension of the bladder and ureters of the foetus in utero.
- Foreign bodies and calculi are rare, because the urethra is so distensible.

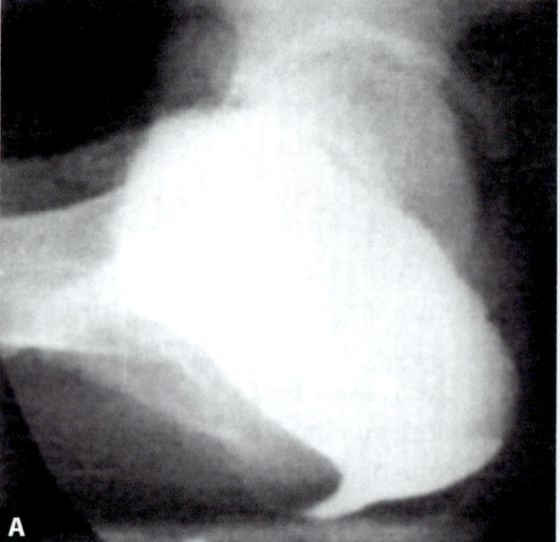

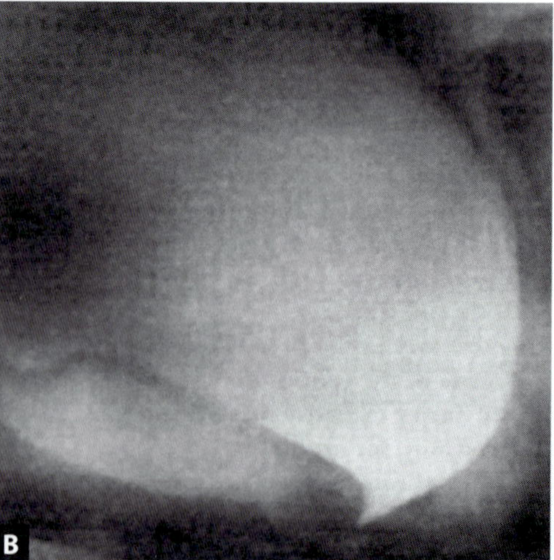

Figs. 19A and B: Retention of urine caused by spasm of the voluntary external sphincter of the urethra. (A) Deliberate contraction of the external sphincter by a normal woman instructed to stop voiding; she arrests the stream despite the fact that the detrusor has not stopped contracting; (B) An identical appearance in the case of a woman who suffered retention following perineorrhaphy; she is contracting the bladder which opens the upper urethra, but she cannot relax the external sphincter.

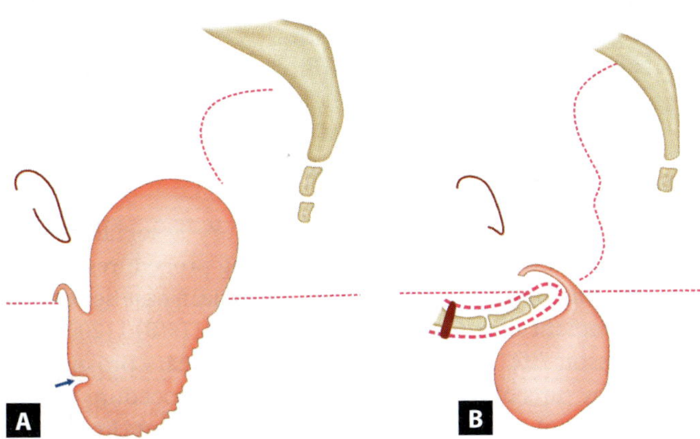

Figs. 20A and B: Tracings of lateral urethrocystograms which show retention of urine caused by angulation of the urethra associated with procidentia. (A) During voiding the stream has to pass upwards and attempt to negotiate a sharp bend in the urethra. The arrow marks the hypertrophied interureteric bar; (B) In order to avoid the difficulty, the patient has learned to insert a finger in such a position as to lessen the angulation of the urethra.

- Stenosis of the urethra following injury or infection is rare.
- Stenosis of the vulva
- Paraurethral cysts and abscesses
- Carcinoma of the urethra, vulva or vagina
- *Angulation of the urethra*: This occurs in cases of gross prolapse of the uterus and anterior vaginal wall **(Fig. 20A)**. The more the patient strains, the more the angulation, so she learns to lift up the prolapsed tissue and thus straighten the urethra in order to void **(Fig. 20B)**.

Treatment

The treatment of urinary retention and incomplete emptying of the bladder is primarily by catheterisation and then by dealing with the cause. Pelvic tumours require removal; management in the case of an impacted gravid uterus is described in Chapter 18: Other Displacements of the Uterus. The treatment of postoperative retention, in which any of the first three causal mechanisms may be concerned, is described in Chapter 62: Preoperative and Postoperative Management and Postoperative Complications. When the bladder is temporarily or permanently paralysed, the possible treatments are as follows:

- Continuous drainage to keep the bladder empty and to allow its walls to recover tone. Clamping the catheter with intermittent release does not hasten or facilitate the recovery.
- For residual urine, a catheter is passed once daily until the amount is <50 mL.
- Cholinergic drugs are most uncertain in their effects on the bladder detrusor muscle. If they stimulate it at all, they often cause incomplete emptying and thus deceive the attendants.
- *Change of posture:* This may be the only way to ensure evacuation of the bladder in women suffering from diseases of the central nervous system.
- *Expression:* Women can be taught to express urine by manual pressure over the lower abdomen. This is appropriate for certain cases of bladder paralysis.
- Dilatation of the urethra and the urethrovesical junction may compensate for a weak detrusor action, or correct an operative overtightening.
- *Resection of the bladder neck:* This operation, sometimes recommended for idiopathic 'atony' of the bladder as well as for persistent retention, is rarely justified in women. It is usually unnecessary and carries a real risk of damaging the all-important internal sphincter. Idiopathic atony is generally the effect of nothing more than a habit of voiding too infrequently. It can be cured by disciplinary measures. Resection of the internal sphincter may, however, sometimes be indicated in the management of chronic retention in senile women suffering from true detrusor atrophy.
- *Intermittent self-catheterisation:* Some women are able to ensure adequate bladder emptying by self-catheterisation on a once- or twice-daily basis. Infection is rarely a problem with reasonable hygienic measures.
- An ileal loop bladder may be an option.

SUGGESTED READING

1. Anger JT, Weinberg AE, Smith AL, Albo ME, Kim J-H, Rodríguez LV, et al. Trends in surgical management of stress urinary incontinence among female Medicare beneficiaries. Urology. 2009;74(2):283-7.
2. Benson JT, Lucente V, McClellan E. Vaginal versus abdominal reconstructive surgery for the treatment of pelvic support defects: a prospective randomized study with long-term outcome evaluation. Am J Obstet Gynecol. 1996;175(6):1418-21.
3. Carlson K, Andrews M, Bascom A, Baverstock R, Campeau L, Dumoulin C, et al. 2024 Canadian Urological Association guideline: female stress urinary incontinence. Can Urol Assoc J. 2024;18(4):83-102.

4. Cody J, Wyness L, Wallace S, Glazener C, Kilonzo M, Stearns S, et al. Systematic review of the clinical effectiveness and cost-effectiveness of tension-free vaginal tape for treatment of urinary stress incontinence. Health Technol Assess. 2003;7(21):1-189.
5. deTayrac R, Deffieux X, Droupy S, Chauveaud-Lambling A, Calvanèse-Benamour L, Fernandez H. A prospective randomized trial comparing tension-free vaginal tape and transobturator suburethral tape for surgical treatment of stress urinary incontinence. Am J Obstet Gynecol. 2004;190(3):602-8.
6. Dmochowski RR, Blaivas JM, Gormley EA, Juma S, Karram MM, Lightner DJ, et al. Update of AUA guideline on the surgical management of female stress urinary incontinence. J Urol. 2010;183(5):1906-14.
7. Glazener CM, Cooper K. Bladder neck needle suspension for urinary incontinence in women. Cochrane Database Syst Rev. 2004;(2):CD003636.
8. Goktolga U, Atay V, Tahmaz L. Tension-free vaginal tape for surgical relief of intrinsic sphincter deficiency: results of 5-year follow-up. J Minim Invasive Gynecol. 2008;15(1):78-81.
9. Jha S. What's new in guidance? Urinary incontinence and pelvic organ prolapse (NICE guideline NG 123). Obstet Gynecol. 2024;26:95-6.
10. Jonsson Funk M, Levin PJ, Wu JM. Trends in the surgical management of stress urinary incontinence. Obstet Gynecol. 2012;119(4): 845-51.
11. Kane AR, Nager CW. Midurethral slings for stress urinary incontinence. Clin Obstet Gynecol. 2008;51(1):12435.
12. Lapitan MC, Cody JD, Grant A. Open retropubic colposuspension for urinary incontinence in women. Cochrane Database Syst Rev. 2009;(2):CD002912.
13. Laurikainen E, Valpas A, Kivelä A, Kalliola T, Rinne K, Takala T, et al. Retropubic compared with transobturator tape placement in treatment of urinary incontinence: a randomized controlled trial. Obstet Gynecol. 2007;109(1):4-11.
14. Leach GE, Dmochowski RR, Appell RA, Blaivas JG, Hadley HR, Luber KM, et al. Female Stress Urinary Incontinence Clinical Guidelines Panel summary report on surgical management of female stress urinary incontinence. The American Urological Association. J Urol. 1997;158(3):875-80.
15. Lim HS, Kim JM, Song PH. Impact of the midurethral sling procedure on quality of life in women with urinary incontinence. Korean J Urol. 2010;51(2):122-7.
16. Meschia M, Pifarotti P, Buonaguidi A. Tension-free vaginal tape (TVT) for treatment of stress urinary incontinence in women with low-pressure urethra. Eur J Obstet Gynecol Reprod Biol. 2005;122(1):118-21.
17. Miller JJ, Botros SM, Akl MN, Aschkenazi SO, Beaumont JL, Goldberg RP, et al. Is transobturator tape as effective as tension-free vaginal tape in patients with borderline maximum urethral closure pressure? Am J Obstet Gynecol. 2006;195(6):1799-804.
18. Morey AF, Medendorp AR, Noller MW, Mora RV, Shandera KC, Foley JP, et al. Transobturator versus transabdominal mid urethral slings: a multi-institutional comparison of obstructive voiding complications. J Urol. 2006;175(3):1014-7.
19. Morton HC, Hilton P. Urethral injury associated with minimally invasive mid-urethral sling procedures for the treatment of stress urinary incontinence: a case series and systematic literature search. BJOG. 2009;116(8):11206.
20. Nilsson CG, Palva K, Rezapour M. 11 years prospective follow-ups of tension free vaginal tape procedure for the treatment of stress of urinary incontinence. Int Urogynecol J Pelvic Floor Dysfunct. 2008;19(8):1043-7.
21. Ogah J, Cody JD, Rogerson L. Minimally invasive synthetic suburethral sling operations for stress urinary incontinence in women. Cochrane Database Syst Rev. 2009;(4):CD006375.
22. O'Connor RC, Nanigian DK, Lyon MB. Early outcomes of mid-urethral slings for female stress urinary incontinence stratified by Valsalva leak point pressure. Neurourol Urodyn. 2006;25(7):685-8.
23. Paick JS, Ku JH, Kim SW, Oh S-J, Son H, Shin JW. Tension-free vaginal tape procedure for the treatment of mixed urinary incontinence: significance of maximal urethral closure pressure. J Urol. 2004;172(3):1001-5.
24. Paick JS, Ku JH, Shin JW. Tension-free vaginal tape procedure for urinary incontinence with low Valsalva leak point pressure. J Urol. 2004;172(4):1370-3.
25. Rezapour M, Ulmsten U. Tension-free vaginal tape (TVT) in women with mixed urinary incontinenc—a long-term follow-up. Int Urogynecol J Pelvic Floor Dysfunct. 2001;12 (Suppl 2):S15-8.
26. Richter HE, Albo ME, Zyczynski HM, Kenton K, Norton PA, Sirls LT, et al. Retropubic versus transobturator midurethral slings for stress incontinence. N Eng J Med. 2010;362(22):2066-76.
27. Schimpf MO, Rahn DD, Wheeler TL, Patel M, White AB, Orejuela FJ, et al. Sling surgery for stress urinary incontinence in women: a systematic review and metaanalysis. Am J Obstet Gynecol. 2014;211(1):71.e1-e27.
28. Sinha D, Blackwell A, Moran PA. Outcome measures after TVT for mixed urinary incontinence. Int Urogynecol J Pelvic Floor Dysfunct. 2008;19(7):927-31.
29. Sinha S, Agarwal MM, Vasudeva P, Khattar N, Madduri VKS, Yande S, et al. The Urological Society of India Guidelines for the evaluation and management of nonneurogenic urinary incontinence in adults (executive summary). Indian J Urol. 2019;35(3):185188.
30. Smith AR, Dmochowski R, Hilton P. Surgery for urinary incontinence. In: Abrams P, Cardozo L, Khoury S, Wein A (Eds). Incontinence. Plymouth: Health Publication Ltd; 2009.

31. Stav K, Dwyer PL, Rosamilia A. Risk factors of treatment failure of midurethral sling procedures for women with urinary stress incontinence. Int Urogynecol J. 2010;21(2):149-55.
32. Thaweekul Y, Bunyavejchevin S, Wisawasukmongchol W, Santingamkun A. Long-term results of anterior colporrhaphy with Kelly plication for the treatment of stress urinary incontinence. J Med Assoc Thai. 2004;87(4):357-60.
33. Trabuco EC, Klingele CJ, Weaver AL, McGree ME, Lightner DJ, Gebhart JB. Preoperative and postoperative predictors of satisfaction after surgical treatment of stress urinary incontinence. Am J Obstet Gynecol. 2011;204(5):444. e1-6.
34. Walters MD, Karram MM. Sling procedures for stress urinary incontinence. In: Walters MD, Karram MM (Eds). Urogynecology and Reconstructive Pelvic Surgery, 3rd edition. Philadelphia: Mosby Elsevier; 2007. p. 197.
35. Ward KL, Hilton P, UK and Ireland TVT Trial Group. Tension-free vaginal tape versus colposuspension for primary urodynamic stress incontinence: 5-year follow up. BJOG. 2008;115(2):226-33.
36. Witte LPW, Engberts MK, Smits MAC, Steures P, van der Meer AC, van Balken MR. 2024 Revised Dutch guidelines for urinary incontinence: addressing clinical bottlenecks through a modular approach. Continence. 2024;12:101699.

58

CHAPTER

Urinary Tract Infection

Shripad Hebbar, Chandra Mithila, Muralidhar V Pai

Chapter Outline

- Aetiology
- Diagnosis
- Investigations
- Management
- Treatment
- Complications
- Clinical Pearls
- Evidence-based Medicine

INTRODUCTION

Urinary tract infections (UTIs) involve a spectrum of infections ranging from asymptomatic bacteriuria to severe pyelonephritis. UTI can be classified as complicated or uncomplicated. Uncomplicated UTI can be defined as UTI in which infection occurs without any underlying structural or functional abnormality of the urinary tract (kidneys, ureter, bladder and urethra). Complicated UTI, on the other hand, occurs in the presence of an underlying anatomical or functional abnormality of the urinary tract. As a result, the outcome of a complicated UTI is more serious than expected in comparison to its occurrence in individuals not having any identified risk factors (i.e. uncomplicated UTI) **(Flowchart 1)**.

Symptomatic UTIs are classified as cystitis, pyelonephritis and urosepsis **(Table 1)**, with infections in males e.g. prostatitis, penile urethritis must be considered separately, given the great diversity of clinical presentations, and male accessory gland.

Symptoms on presentation are as follows:

The classification system for UTI by the European Association of Urology (EAU), also known as ORENUC, is based on the clinical presentation of the UTI and its associated host risk factors **(Table 2)**. The various categories are as follows:

- *O:* No known or associated risk factor, e.g. healthy premenopausal women

Flowchart 1: Prevalence of urinary tract infection (UTI) among different groups of people over the last few years.

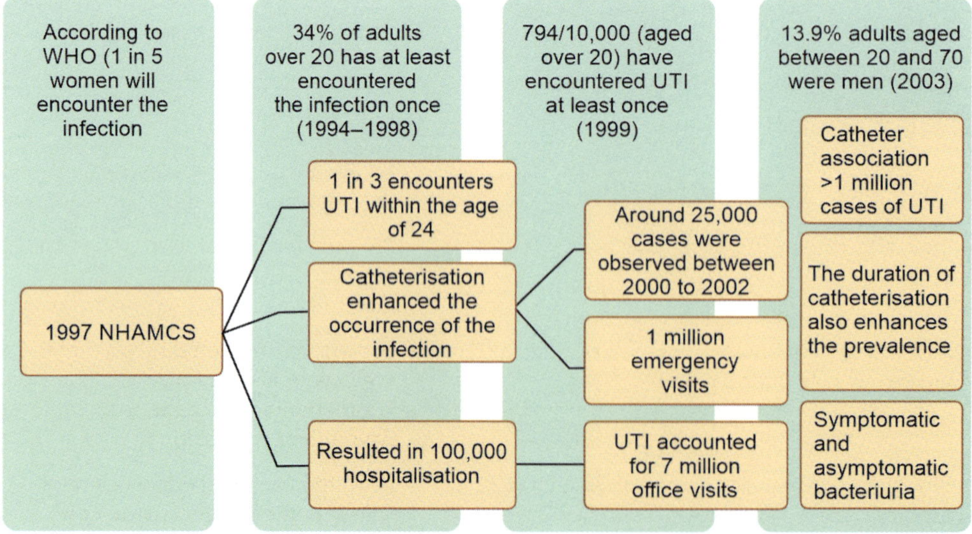

(NHAMCS: National Hospital Ambulatory Medical Care Survey; UTI: urinary tract infections)

TABLE 1: Clinical presentation of cystitis, pyelonephritis and urosepsis and grading of severity.

Acronym	*Clinical diagnosis*	*Clinical symptoms*	*Grade of severity*
CY-1	Cystitis	Dysuria, frequency, urgency, suprapubic pain; sometimes unspecific symptoms (see **Table 4**)	1
PN-2	Mild and moderate pyelonephritis	Fever, flank pain, CVA tenderness; sometimes unspecific symptoms with or without symptoms of CY	2
PN-3	Severe pyelonephritis	As PN-2, but in addition, nausea and vomiting with or without symptoms of CY	3
US-4	Urosepsis (simple)	Temperature >38°C or <36°C; heart rate >90 beats/min; respiratory rate >20 breaths/min or $PaCO_2$ < 32 mm Hg (<4.3 kPa); WBC >12,000 cells/mm^3 or <4,000 cells/mm^3 or ≥10% immature (band) forms; with or without symptoms of CY or PN	4
US-5	Severe urosepsis	As US-4, but in addition, associated with organ dysfunction, hypoperfusion or hypotension. Hypoperfusion and perfusion abnormalities may include, but are not limited to lactic acidosis, oliguria or an acute alteration of mental status	5
US-6	Uroseptic shock	As US-4 or US-5, but in addition, with hypotension despite adequate fluid resuscitation along with the presence of perfusion abnormalities that may include but are not limited to lactic acidosis, oliguria or an acute alteration in mental status. Patients who are on inotropic or vasopressor agents may not be hypotensive at the time of perfusion	6

(CY: cystitis; PN: pyelonephritis; US: urosepsis; WBCs: white blood cells)

TABLE 2: Host risk factors in urinary tract infections categorised according to the ORENUC system.

Phenotype	*Category of risk factor*	*Examples of risk factors*
O	No known risk factor	Otherwise, healthy premenopausal women
R	Risk factors for recurrent urinary tract infection, but no risk of more severe outcome	• Sexual behaviour (frequency, spermicide) • Hormonal deficiency in postmenopause • Secretor type of certain blood groups • Well-controlled diabetes mellitus
E	Extraurogenital risk factors with risk of more severe outcome	• Prematurity, newborn • Pregnancy • Male gender • Badly controlled diabetes mellitus • Relevant immunosuppression (not well defined)
N	Nephropathic diseases with risk of more severe outcomes	• Relevant renal insufficiency (not well defined) • Polycystic nephropathy • Interstitial nephritis (e.g. due to analgesics)
U	Urologic risk factors with risk of more severe outcome, which can be resolved during therapy	• Ureteral obstruction due to a ureteral stone • Well-controlled neurogenic bladder disturbances • Transient short-term external urinary catheter • Asymptomatic bacteriuria
C	Permanent urinary catheter and unresolvable urologic risk factors with risk of more severe outcomes	• Long-term external urinary catheter • Unresolvable urinary obstruction • Badly controlled neurogenic bladder disturbances

- *R:* Recurrent risk factor for UTI, but there is no risk of severe outcome, e.g. promiscuous sexual behaviour, use of contraceptive devices and controlled diabetes mellitus.
- *E:* Extra-urogenital risk factor, with risk of more severe outcome, e.g. pregnancy and poorly controlled diabetes mellitus
- *N:* Nephropathic disease, with risk of more severe outcome, e.g. relevant renal insufficiency and polycystic nephropathy
- *U:* Urological risk factor, with risk of more severe outcome, which can be resolved with therapy, e.g. ureteral obstruction due to stone and stricture, and temporary short-term urinary tract catheter, etc.
- *C:* Permanent urinary catheterisation and nonresolvable urological risk factor, with risk of more severe outcome, e.g. nonresolvable urinary obstruction and poorly controlled neurogenic bladder.

In adults, uncomplicated UTIs fall under categories O, R and partially E, while complicated UTIs mainly fall in categories N, U and C.

A modified view of this UTI classification was proposed in the EAU guidelines on urological infections in 2015 **(Fig. 1)**. The current guidelines cover both UTIs and accessory gland infections and are based on the best features of current definitions and classifications, and are more suitable to strategise management options.

Other entities commonly related to UTIs in clinical practice include recurrent UTI and asymptomatic bacteriuria. Recurrent UTI can be defined as presence of three or more episodes of UTI during a period of 1 year or two episodes of infection within a 6-month period. If the recurrent episodes of UTI are caused by the same organism following adequate therapy, this is known as relapse.

Asymptomatic bacteriuria, on the other hand, refers to the presence of bacteria in the urine of asymptomatic

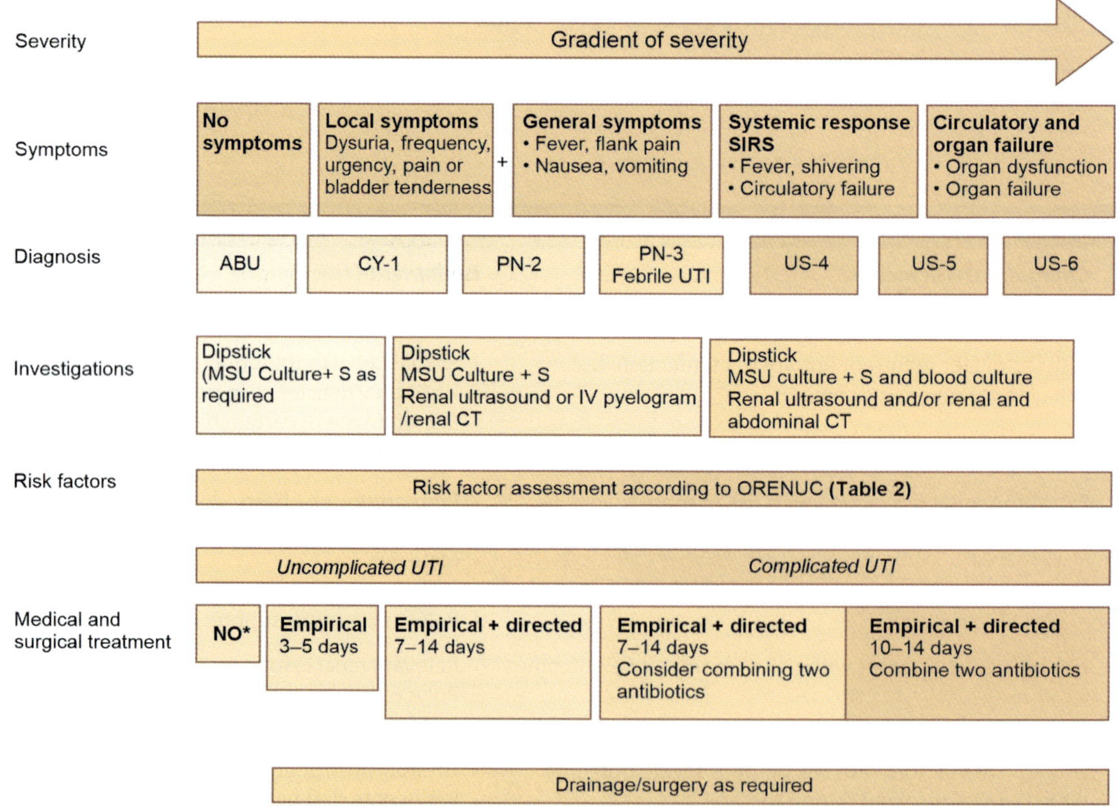

Fig. 1: Synoptic view of the classification of urinary tract infection as proposed by the European Association of Urology Section of Infection in Urology and including the basic principles of diagnosis and treatment.
**Two presently accepted exceptions:* During pregnancy and prior to urological surgery.
(ABU: asymptomatic bacteriuria; CT: computed tomography; CY: cystitis; IV: intravenous; MSU: midstream sample of urine; PN: pyelonephritis; SIRS: systemic inflammatory response syndrome; US: urosepsis; UTI: urinary tract infection)
Source: Reproduced with permission from the European Association of Urology.

women. Bacteria must be present in the quantities of at least 100,000 CFU/mL of urine in at least two consecutive voided specimens. Asymptomatic bacteriuria does not usually cause renal disease or damage. Treatment for asymptomatic bacteriuria is likely to increase the risk of subsequent symptomatic UTIs, hence, it is not usually recommended.

AETIOLOGY

Urinary tract infections occur when the urinary tract becomes infected by bacteria. In most cases, bacteria enter the urinary tract via the urethra. The majority of uncomplicated UTIs are caused by *Escherichia coli* (causing 70–95% of cases), with organisms such as *Proteus mirabilis, Klebsiella* species, *Staphylococcus saprophyticus, Pseudomonas, Serratia* and *enterococci* accounting for rest of the cases. Possible risk factors for the development of recurrent UTI are tabulated in **Table 3**.

TABLE 3: Possible risk factors for recurrent urinary tract infections (UTIs) in women.

Young and premenopausal women	*Postmenopausal and elderly women*
• Sexual intercourse • Use of spermicide with condoms or contraceptive diaphragms • A new sexual partner • Maternal history of UTI • History of UTI during childhood • Medical conditions such as diabetes, obstruction of the urinary tract as a result of calculi, etc.	• History of UTI before menopause • Urinary incontinence • Atrophic vaginitis due to oestrogen deficiency • Cystocele • Increased postvoid residual urine volume • Blood group antigen, urine secretory status • Weakened immune system • Urine catheterisation and functional status • Deterioration in elderly women

DIAGNOSIS

Clinical signs and symptoms consistent with uncomplicated UTI are described as follows:

- Dysuria
- Increased frequency or urgency of micturition
- Back pain or costovertebral angle tenderness
- Cloudy or foul-smelling urine
- Presence of red blood cells (RBCs) in the urine
- General malaise, lower abdominal pain and tiredness
- Usually, there is no accompanying vaginal discharge or irritation in cases of uncomplicated UTI. In presence of vaginal discharge, alternative diagnoses such as sexually transmitted diseases (STDs) and vulvovaginitis, usually due to *Candida*, must be considered.

The symptoms, which may occur in the presence of upper UTIs, include the following:

- High temperature of 38°C (100.4°F) or above
- Pain on the sides or back
- Shivering and chills
- General malaise, nausea and tiredness
- Confusion
- Agitation or restlessness

There is usually no requirement for investigations in uncomplicated UTI. Empirical treatment with an antibiotic must be commenced in otherwise healthy women aged <65 years presenting with severe or greater than or equal to three symptoms of UTI **(Table 4)**.

TABLE 4: Symptoms occur in different types of urinary tract infection (UTI).

Asymptomatic bacteriuria	*Lower UTI/cystitis*	*Upper UTI/ pyelonephritis*
No clinical signs or symptoms	Frequency	Pyrexia
	Dysuria	Loin pain
	Low-grade fever	Dysuria
	Suprapubic pain	Rigours
		Clinical signs of septic shock

INVESTIGATIONS (FLOWCHART 2)

Urine Routine or Microscopy

Parameters, which can be assessed at the time of urine routine or microscopic examination, include its colour, appearance and smell, presence of ions and trace elements, proteins, enzymes, blood cells, white blood cells (WBCs), small molecules (glucose, ketone bodies, bilirubin, etc.).

Urine Culture and Sensitivity

Urine culture helps in isolating the causative organism and providing antibiotic sensitivity for guiding antimicrobial treatment. Conventional laboratory practice in the UK determines aerobic bacteria in the urine at a value of $\geq 10^4$ CFU/mL. Urine cultures are recommended in

Flowchart 2: Evaluation of recurrent urinary tract infection.

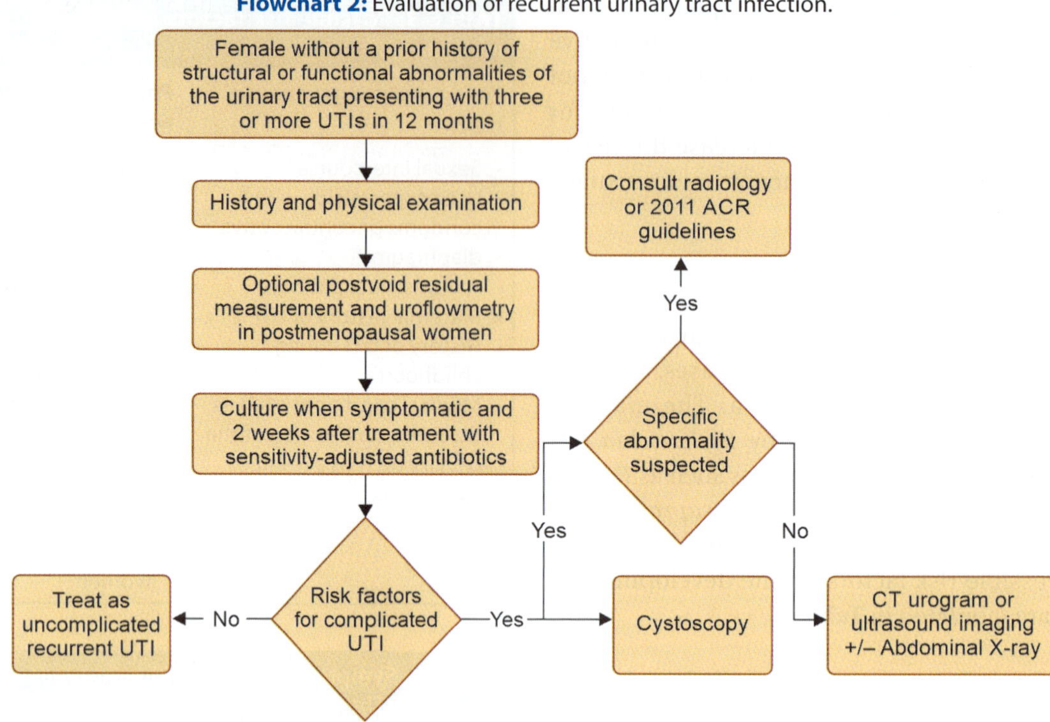

(ACR: American College of Rheumatology; CT: computed tomography; UTI: urinary tract infection)

patients having risk factors for complicated UTIs and in the following situations:

- Suspected acute pyelonephritis
- Symptoms not resolving within 2–4 weeks after completion of antibiotic treatment
- Women presenting with atypical symptoms
- Pregnant women
- Male patients with suspected UTI.

Dipstick Test

Urine dipstick test for detecting the presence of nitrites and leucocytes can be used for diagnosing UTI. The probability of having UTI is particularly high if the dipstick test is positive for both. Urine dipstick analysis serves as a reasonable alternative to urine culture for diagnosing cases of acute, uncomplicated cystitis. Urine dipstick tests can be used for guiding treatment in otherwise healthy women under 65 years of age presenting with mild or less than or equal to two symptoms of UTI.

MANAGEMENT

Many other factors have been thought to predispose women to recurrent UTIs, such as voiding patterns pre- and postcoitus, wiping technique, wearing tight undergarments, deferred voiding habits and vaginal douching; nevertheless, there has been no proven association. In order to prevent the development of UTI, the patient should be asked to observe the following precautions:

- Avoiding the use of perfumed bubble bath, soap or talcum powder, especially around the genitals.
- Emptying her bladder as soon as possible after having sexual intercourse or as soon as she has an urge to micturate, and taking care to always empty her bladder fully.
- *Staying adequately hydrated*: Drinking plenty of fluids is likely to help the patient feel better.
- Using another method of contraception rather than using a contraceptive diaphragm or condoms with spermicidal lubricant
- Wearing underwear made from cotton, rather than synthetic material such as nylon, and avoiding tight-fitting jeans and trousers.
- Use of methenamine hippurate must be considered in women without any known abnormalities of the upper renal tract to prevent the development of symptomatic UTI.

TREATMENT

Complicated Urinary Tract Infections

The treatment strategy for complicated UTIs depends upon the severity of the illness. Hospitalisation is often necessary in these cases. Numerous intravenous (IV) and oral antimicrobial treatment options are available. Majority of patients with serious UTIs require initial IV therapy due to the likelihood of bacteraemia or sepsis or impaired gastrointestinal absorption. While there are no contemporary guidelines for treatment of these infections and targeted therapy should be initiated once susceptibility data for the causative organisms are known. Agents commonly prescribed include aminoglycosides, beta-lactam or beta-lactamase inhibitor combinations, imipenem, advanced-generation cephalosporins and fluoroquinolones.

Fluoroquinolones are often recommended when conventional agents have failed or are not appropriate due to concerns related to toxicity or hypersensitivity, or in cases of high resistance. Many experts agree that empirical therapy for the institutionalised or hospitalised patient with a serious UTI should include an IV antipseudomonal agent due to an increased risk of urosepsis.

Uncomplicated Urinary Tract Infections

- *Painkillers*: Over-the-counter painkillers such as paracetamol or ibuprofen can help to reduce the pain. However, there is no evidence demonstrating the efficacy of over-the-counter painkillers in such women.
- *Antibiotics:* Uncomplicated UTIs are normally treated with a short course of antibiotics. An appropriate antibiotic should be selected either empirically or based on the results of culture and sensitivity. The drug should also be able to reach an appropriate concentration within the urinary tract. The recommended treatment of first choice in cases of uncomplicated UTI is nitrofurantoin in the dosage of 50 mg every 6 hourly or 100 mg every 12 hourly for 5 days. Scottish Intercollegiate Guidelines Network (SIGN) and Health Protection Agency (HPA) recommend the use of nitrofurantoin or a 3-day course of trimethoprim sulphamethoxazole [160/800 mg (1 double-strength tablet) twice-daily for 3 days] (first-line therapy) for empirical treatment of uncomplicated UTI among nonpregnant women of any age group. In case of the failure of first-line therapy, the second-line treatment comprises of performing urine culture and prescribing against the urine culture results. Particular care should be taken when prescribing nitrofurantoin to elderly patients, who may be at an increased risk of toxicity. Nonpregnant women with symptoms or signs of acute uncomplicated UTI can be treated with a course of ciprofloxacin for 7 days or co-amoxiclav for 14 days (second-line therapy). Use of broad-spectrum antibiotics (e.g. co-amoxiclav, quinolones and cephalosporins) should be preferably avoided due to an increased risk of development of antibiotic resistance, *Clostridium difficile* infection, methicillin-resistant *Staphylococcus aureus* (MRSA), resistant UTIs, etc. Women with lower UTI, who are prescribed nitrofurantoin, must not be simultaneously advised to take alkalinising agents (such as potassium citrate) because the minimum inhibitory concentration (MIC) of this drug rises with an increase in pH. There is no need to treat nonpregnant women (of any age) having asymptomatic bacteriuria with an antibiotic.

In a few regions, the uropathogen resistance rates to the fluoroquinolones have exceeded 10–25%. This has made empirical therapy with fluoroquinolones difficult. beta-lactams are not recommended because of suboptimal clinical and bacteriological results compared with those of non-beta-lactams. If a beta-lactam is chosen, it should be administered for at least 7 days. Among all urinary isolates collected over a year, fosfomycin resistance was documented in 1% of *Escherichia coli* versus 19% of *Klebsiella* species, and fosfomycin was found to be safe and effective for use in patients with complex comorbidities and over prolonged time periods. **Table 5** shows the various regimens for uncomplicated acute bacterial cystitis.

Treatment of Urinary Tract Infections in Pregnancy

In case of a pregnant woman presenting with the symptoms of UTI, a standard quantitative urine culture should be routinely performed during the first antenatal visit. The presence of bacteriuria in urine must be confirmed with a second urine culture. Testing with a dipstick should not be used for screening for bacterial UTI during the first or subsequent antenatal visits during pregnancy. Pregnant women with symptomatic UTI should be treated with an antibiotic. Choice of antibiotic therapy must be based on the results of culture and sensitivity and the local guidelines. A 7-day course of treatment is usually

TABLE 5: Various regimens for uncomplicated acute bacterial cystitis.

Antimicrobial agent	*Dose*	*Adverse events*
Trimethoprim-sulphamethoxazole	One tablet (160 mg trimethoprim, 800 mg sulphamethoxazole), twice daily for 3 days	Fever, rash, photosensitivity, neutropaenia, thrombocytopaenia, anorexia, nausea and vomiting, pruritus, headache, urticaria, Stevens–Johnson syndrome and toxic epidermal necrosis
Trimethoprim	100 mg, twice daily for 3 days	Rash, pruritus, photosensitivity, exfoliative dermatitis, Stevens–Johnson syndrome, toxic epidermal necrosis and aseptic meningitis
Ciprofloxacin	250 mg, twice daily for 3 days	Rash, confusion, seizures, restlessness, headache, severe hypersensitivity, hypoglycaemia, hyperglycaemia and Achilles tendon rupture (in patients older than 60 years)
Levofloxacin	250 mg, once daily for 3 days	Same as for ciprofloxacin
Norfloxacin	400 mg, twice daily for 3 days	Same as for ciprofloxacin
Gatifloxacin	200 mg, once daily for 3 days	Same as for ciprofloxacin
Nitrofurantoin macrocrystals	50–100 mg, four times daily for 7 days	Anorexia, nausea, vomiting, hypersensitivity, peripheral neuropathy, hepatitis, haemolytic anaemia and pulmonary reactions
Nitrofurantoin monohydrate	100 mg, twice daily for 7 days	Same as for nitrofurantoin macrocrystals
Fosfomycin tromethamine	3 g dose (powder single dose)	Diarrhoea, nausea, vomiting, rash and hypersensitivity

adequate. A urine culture should preferably be performed after 7 days, following the completion of antibiotic therapy, to confirm bacteriological cure.

Asymptomatic bacteriuria detected during pregnancy must also be treated with a 3–7-day course of antibiotic because such treatment is likely to reduce the risk of complications such as preterm deliveries and low-birth weight babies. Antibiotics such as penicillin or cephalosporins or nitrofurantoin are unlikely to have any toxic effects or an increased risk of congenital malformations in pregnant women during the first or second trimester. However, nitrofurantoin may be associated with a very low risk of haemolysis in women with glucose-6-phosphate dehydrogenase deficiency. Therefore, its use must be avoided in the third trimester. Sulphonamides should also be avoided during the third trimester due to the risk of hyperbilirubinaemia and kernicterus. Fosfomycin is an effective drug, which has newly been introduced into the market, administered in a single dose, and is very effective against resistant *Escherichia coli* infections.

Moreover, trimethoprim must not be prescribed to pregnant women during the first trimester or to women with established folate deficiency, low-dietary folate intake, or women taking other folate antagonists because trimethoprim may cause adverse effects in the presence of folate deficiency. Similarly, use of fluoroquinolones should also be avoided during early pregnancy due to their adverse effect on the foetal cartilage **(Table 6)**.

Group B Streptococcal Infection in Pregnancy

Group B streptococcal (GBS) vaginal colonisation is known to be a cause of neonatal sepsis and is associated with preterm rupture of membranes, and preterm labour and delivery. GBS is found to be the causative organism in UTIs in approximately 5% of patients. Evidence that GBS bacteriuria increases patient risk of preterm rupture of membranes and premature delivery is mixed.

A randomised controlled trial compared the treatment of GBS bacteriuria with penicillin to treatment with a placebo. Results indicated a significant reduction in rates of premature rupture of membranes and preterm delivery in the women who received antibiotics. It is unclear, if GBS bacteriuria is equivalent to GBS vaginal colonisation, but pregnant women with GBS bacteriuria should be treated as GBS carriers and should receive a prophylactic antibiotic during labour.

TABLE 6: Various antibiotics for different categories of pregnancy.

Antibiotic	*Pregnancy category*	*Dosage*	*Comments*
Cephalexin (Keflex)	B	250 mg two or four times daily	
Erythromycin	B	250–500 mg four times daily	
Nitrofurantoin (Macrodantin)	B	50–100 mg four times daily	Can be used during the first and second trimesters. Avoid use in the last trimester due to the risk of haemolytic anaemia in the newborn
Amoxicillin-clavulanic acid (Augmentin)	B	250 mg four times daily	Recommended for use in pregnancy
Fosfomycin (Monurol)	B	One 3-g sachet	Can be used
Trimethoprim-sulphamethoxazole (Bactrim)	C → D	160 or 180 mg twice daily	Avoid use if there are alternatives. Use in the first trimester is associated with an increased risk of foetal neural tube defects. In the third trimester, there is an increased risk of hyperbilirubinaemia and kernicterus. If necessary for use, the second trimester would be the safest window
Fluoroquinolones (e.g. ciprofloxacin)	C	500 mg twice daily	Avoid use if there are alternatives

Treatment of Recurrent Urinary Tract Infection

Various strategies for the prevention of recurrent UTI infection have been previously described in the text. Use of cranberry juice or probiotics is often advised for the prevention of recurrent UTI. However, there is currently little evidence to suggest that drinking cranberry juice or using probiotics is likely to significantly reduce a woman's chances of developing UTI. A Cochrane review by Albert et al. (2004) has shown that continuous antibiotic prophylaxis for 6–12 months is likely to reduce the rate of UTI during prophylaxis in comparison to placebo. However, no difference in the incidence of UTI is observed following the discontinuation of the antibiotic therapy. Moreover, the women who received antibiotic therapy were associated with a high risk of adverse events.

The risk-benefit balance needs to be assessed with the use of any medication in individual patients. Consider involving their obstetrician if there are any concerns.

FDA pregnancy risk categories include:

- *Category A*: No risk in human studies.
- *Category B*: No risk in animal studies
- *Category C*: Risk cannot be ruled out. There are no satisfactory studies in pregnant women, but animal studies demonstrated a risk to the foetus; potential benefits of the drug may outweigh the risks.
- *Category D*: Evidence of risk. Studies in pregnant women have demonstrated a risk to the foetus; potential benefits of the drug may outweigh the risks.
- *Category X*: Contraindicated. Studies in pregnant women have demonstrated a risk to the foetus, and/or human or animal studies have shown foetal abnormalities. Risks of the drug outweigh the potential benefits.

The available evidence also shows that long-term use of antibiotics in individuals with recurrent UTI is associated with little benefit. On the other hand, its use may be associated with an increased risk of microbial resistance. Therefore, this strategy is best avoided. The available evidence also shows that the use of vaginal oestrogen preparations (vaginal cream, tablets or ring) can be considered in the postmenopausal women with urogenital atrophy suffering from recurrent UTI **(Flowchart 3)**.

COMPLICATIONS

Renal Scarring

Though the outcome of UTI is usually benign, infection in early childhood may sometimes result in renal scarring, which may lead to several complications in adulthood, including hypertension, proteinuria, renal damage and sometimes even chronic renal failure, requiring treatment with dialysis.

Flowchart 3: Treatment options for a nonpregnant female patient with suspected uncomplicated recurrent urinary tract infection (UTI).

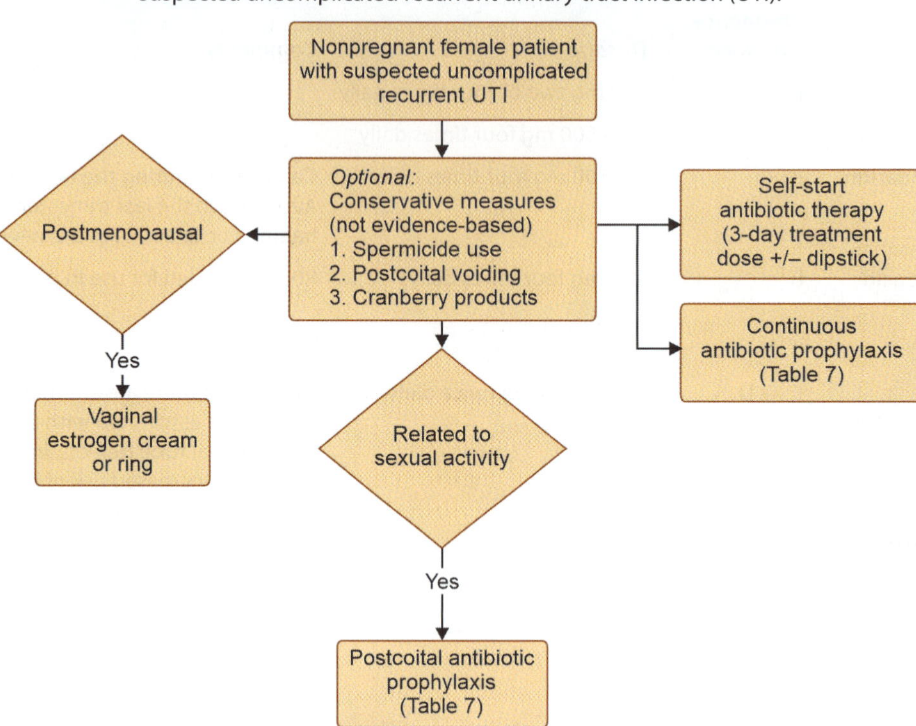

TABLE 7: Suggested antibiotic prophylaxis.

Continuous	*Postcoital (within 2 hours of coitus)*
Trimethoprim/sulfamethoxazole (TMP/SMX) (40 mg/200 mg daily or thrice weekly)	TMP/SMX (40 mg/200–80 mg/400 mg)
Trimethoprim (100 mg daily)	
Ciprofloxacin (125 mg daily)	Ciprofloxacin (125 mg)
• Cephalexin (125–250 mg daily) • Cefaclor (250 mg daily)	Cephalexin (250 mg)
Nitrofurantoin (50–100 mg)	Nitrofurantoin (50–100 mg daily)
Norfloxacin (200 mg daily)	Norfloxacin (200 mg)
Fosfomycin (3 g every 10 days)	
	Ofloxacin (100 mg)

Spread of Infection

Lower UTIs are usually not a cause for major concern. Upper UTIs, on the other hand, can be serious if left untreated, as they could damage the kidneys or spread to the bloodstream, respectively, resulting in the development of pyelonephritis and septicaemia.

Adverse Effects of Urinary Tract Infection on Pregnancy

Urinary tract infection in pregnancy can result in adverse outcomes such as preterm births, low-birth weight infants, foetal growth restriction and increased perinatal mortality. UTI in pregnancy can also be associated with maternal adverse outcomes such as chorioamnionitis and endometritis.

CLINICAL PEARLS

- Uncomplicated lower UTI remains one of the most commonly treated infections among women in primary care. UTIs are most commonly seen in sexually active young women.
- Treatment of patients with serious complicated UTIs presently remains challenging.
- Women may be more likely to acquire UTIs because they have a shorter urethra, which is closer to anus, in comparison to men.

- It is important to rule out the diagnosis of urogenital tuberculosis and/or malignancy in patients presenting with persistent, nonresolving symptoms of UTI.
- *Escherichia coli* remains the chief uropathogen in acute cases of community-acquired uncomplicated UTIs.
- Use of antimicrobial therapy must be based on the results of culture and sensitivity.

EVIDENCE-BASED MEDICINE

- There is currently little evidence to suggest that drinking cranberry juice or using probiotics is likely to significantly reduce a woman's chances of developing UTI. A recent Cochrane review has indicated that the use of cranberry juice is less effective in the treatment of UTI than was indicated by previous studies. Women should be advised that intake of cranberry capsules may be more convenient than juice, and high-strength capsules are likely to be most effective.
- Despite the lack of adequate evidence showing a reduction in UTI using probiotics, the use of probiotics is likely to be useful for the prevention of recurrent UTI in women. Larger, well-designed randomised trials are required in the future to demonstrate the beneficial effect of probiotics in comparison to antibiotics in cases of UTI.
- The available evidence shows that the clinical outcomes for UTIs treated with antibiotics are better in comparison to those treated with a placebo.
- The available evidence supports the use of fluoroquinolones for serious UTIs. Presently, the most commonly used fluoroquinolone is ciprofloxacin. Recently, its once-daily extended-release tablet formulation has been introduced.
- The available evidence indicates that 3 days of treatment with antibiotics is as effective as 5–10 days of antibiotic therapy for attaining symptomatic cure in cases of uncomplicated UTI treatment. However, a longer duration of therapy is more effective in obtaining bacteriological cure. Longer duration of antibiotic therapy is also associated with an increased risk of adverse effects.

SUGGESTED READING

1. Albert X, Huertas I, Pereiró II, Sanfélix J, Gosalbes V, Perrota C. Antibiotics for preventing recurrent urinary tract infection in non-pregnant women. Cochrane Database Syst Rev. 2004;(3):CD001209.
2. Al Lawati H, Blair BM, Larnard J. Urinary tract infections: Core curriculum 2024. Am J Kidney Dis. 2024;83(1):90-100.
3. Carson C, Naber KG. Role of fluoroquinolones in the treatment of serious bacterial urinary tract infections. Drugs. 2004;64(12):1359-73.
4. Flores-Mireles AL, Walker JN, Caparon M, Hultgren SJ. Urinary tract infections: epidemiology, mechanisms of infection and treatment options. Nat Rev Microbiol. 2015;13(5):269-84.
5. Foxman B. Epidemiology of urinary tract infections: incidence, morbidity, and economic costs. Am J Med. 2002;113(Suppl 1A):5S-13S.
6. Grabe M, Bartoletti R, Bjerklund Johansen TE, et al. (2015). Guidelines on Urological Infections. [online] Available from uroweb.org/wp-content/uploads/19-Urological-infections_LR2.pdf. [Accessed March, 2018].
7. Guay DR. Contemporary management of uncomplicated urinary tract infections. Drugs. 2008;68(9):1169-205.
8. Gupta K, Hooton TM, Naber KG, Wullt B, Colgan R, Miller LG, et al. International clinical practice guidelines for the treatment of acute uncomplicated cystitis and pyelonephritis in women: A 2010 update by the Infectious Diseases Society of America and the European Society for microbiology and infectious diseases. Clin Infect Dis. 2011;52(5):e103-20.
9. Health Protection Agency, British Infection Association. Management of infection guidance for primary care for consultation and local adaptation. London: Health Protection Agency; 2010.
10. Jepson RG, Williams G, Craig JC. Cranberries for preventing urinary tract infections. Cochrane Database Syst Rev. 2012;10: CD001321.
11. Kranz J, Bartoletti R, Bruyère F, Cai T, Geerlings S, Köves B, et al. European Association of Urology Guidelines on Urological Infections: Summary of the 2024 Guidelines. Eur Urol. 2024;86(1):27-41.
12. Lee BS, Simpson JM, Craig JC, Bhuta T. Methenamine hippurate for preventing urinary tract infections (Cochrane Review). Cochrane Database Syst Rev. 2012;10(10):CD003265.
13. Matthews PC, Barrett LK, Warren S, Stoesser N, Snelling M, Scarborough M, et al. Oral fosfomycin for treatment of urinary tract infection: a retrospective cohort study. BMC Infect Dis. 2016;16(1):556.
14. Miller LG, Tang AW. Treatment of uncomplicated urinary tract infections in an era of increasing antimicrobial resistance. Mayo Clin Proc. 2004;79(8):1048-53.
15. Milo G, Katchman EA, Paul M, Christiaens T, Baerheim A, Leibovici L. Duration of antibacterial treatment for uncomplicated urinary tract infection in women. Cochrane Database Syst Rev. 2005;18(2):CD004682.

16. Nelson Z, Aslan AT, Beahm NP, Blyth M, Cappiello M, Casaus D, et al. Guidelines for the Prevention, Diagnosis, and Management of Urinary Tract Infections in Pediatrics and Adults: A WikiGuidelines Group Consensus Statement. JAMA Netw Open. 2024;7(11):e2444495.
17. Perrotta C, Aznar M, Mejia R, Albert X, Ng CW. Oestrogens for preventing recurrent urinary tract infection in postmenopausal women. Cochrane Database Syst Rev. 2008;(2):CD005131.
18. Salvatore S, Salvatore S, Cattoni E, Siesto G, Serati M, Sorice P, et al. Urinary tract infections in women. Eur J Obstet Gynecol Reprod Biol. 2011;156(2):131-6.
19. Schwenger EM, Tejani AM, Loewen PS. Probiotics for preventing urinary tract infections in adults and children. Cochrane Database Syst Rev. 2015;(12):CD008772.
20. Scottish Intercollegiate Guidelines Network (SIGN). Management of suspected bacterial urinary tract infection in adults. Edinburgh: SIGN; 2012.
21. Smaill FM, Vazquez JC. Antibiotics for asymptomatic bacteriuria in pregnancy. Cochrane Database Syst Rev. 2007;(8):CD000490.
22. Smelov V, Naber K, Bjerklund Johansen TE. Improved classification of urinary tract infection: future considerations. Eur Urol Suppl. 2016;15(4):71-80.
23. Wagenlehner FM, Naber KG. Current challenges in the treatment of complicated urinary tract infections and prostatitis. Clin Microbiol Infect. 2006;12(Suppl 3):67-80.
24. Williams G, Craig JC. Long-term antibiotics for preventing recurrent urinary tract infection in children. Cochrane Database Syst Rev. 2011;(3):CD001534.

59

CHAPTER

Menopause

Shyjus P

Chapter Outline

- History
- Definitions and Staging of Menopause
- Physiology of Menopause
- Problems Associated with Menopause
- Effect of Oestrogen Deficiency
- Menstrual Problems
- Management of Menopause
- Symptoms of Menopause
- Various Types of Hormonal and Nonhormonal Pharmacological Agents Available
- Use of Progesterones in Menopausal Hormone Therapy
- Hormone Therapy in Special Circumstances
- Androgens in Menopause

INTRODUCTION

As the life expectancy around the globe is increasing, women will have to spend almost one-third of their lives in menopausal years. In comparison to the Western world, menopause occurs about 6 years earlier among the Asians. The Indian data comes from the study done by the Indian Menopause Society (2012–2013) published in 2016 which showed the average age of menopause to be 45.59 ± 5.59 years. Considering the life expectancy in India to be around 68 years, that would mean 20 plus menopausal years, and hence, an understanding of menopause and its related problems is much needed.

HISTORY

Not much was known about menopause till the mid-60s. Studies on menopause got initiated, and our understanding of the relationship between a fall in ovarian hormone levels and resulting symptoms got better. The International Menopause Society was formed in the year 1978. Research on menopause has picked up pace since then. In spite of all that, gaps in knowledge and understanding of menopause still exist. Rather than the number of years, what matters is the quality of life for our menopausal women. Thus, there is a need to focus on the preventive aspects and lifestyle management as well, which ideally should start earlier in life.

DEFINITIONS AND STAGING OF MENOPAUSE

Menopause is defined as the permanent cessation of menses. By convention, the diagnosis of menopause is not made until the individual has had 12 months of amenorrhoea.

Menopause is not just the cessation of menstruation; it is depletion of ovarian follicles, leading to a fall in ovarian hormone levels.

Menopause is thus characterised by the menstrual changes that reflect oocyte depletion and subsequent reduction in ovarian hormone production. However, the manifestations that occur around the time of menopause are caused by the underlying ovarian changes, rather than by the cessation of menstruation itself. Therefore, a woman who has undergone a hysterectomy but has her ovaries retained will not experience menopausal symptoms till her ovaries are functioning. But remember that depletion of oocytes and symptoms of menopause tend to occur earlier in these women, in comparison to those women with an intact uterus and ovaries. Natural menopause can occur at any time beyond 45 years of age and has no underlying pathologic cause.

Induced menopause may occur after:

- Chemotherapy
- Pelvic radiation

- Surgical removal of both ovaries
- Menopause is termed early when it occurs before 45 years of age, and is termed premature when it occurs before 40 years of age.
    - *The climacteric*, a term though now used infrequently, refers to the time of waning ovarian function manifesting with menstrual irregularity and vasomotor symptoms.
    - *Perimenopause* is the time between the onset of the climacteric till a year after the last menses.
- *Premenopause* is the entire reproductive span before the onset of the menopausal transition, and postmenopause is the span of life after menopause.

Menopausal Transition

Menopausal transition is the preferred term to describe the phase of physiological changes that happen around the cessation of ovarian function. This is the stage, which precedes menopause, has an average duration of 4 years, with a range of 0–10 years. The mean age at which menopause occurs in developed countries is 51 years and may be increasing. The standard deviation around this mean is about 2 years. Approximately 95% of women experience menopause by 55 years of age.

Postmenopause

According to the World Health Organization (WHO), the term postmenopause is defined as the phase commencing from the time of menopause, which can only be ascertained after 12 months of amenorrhoea.

The postmenopause lasts for about 10–15 years and is followed by senescence from about 65 years of age to the end of life. This phase of life is marked by the successive occurrence of cardiovascular, orthopaedic and oncologic diseases. Beyond this age, even oestrogen replacement may be risky due to higher vascular and oncologic risks

Senescence

Senescence is defined as the phase after the age of 60 years, some use 65 years as the cut-off. The STRAW (Stages of Reproductive Aging Workshop) staging defined seven stages of an adult woman's life into three broad categories: (1) Reproductive, (2) menopausal transition and (3) postmenopause. Each of the seven stages were broken down by the length of the stage, description of menstrual cycles and follicle-stimulating hormone (FSH) levels.

The 'first ever' Staging of Menopause by Dr Behram Anklesaria in 1997 ***(Table 1)****:* He divided menopausal transition and menopause into three stages, each with a duration line, an events line and an action line.

1. *Stage I:* From the earliest perimenopausal symptom (usually vasomotor instability or menstrual irregularity) to cessation of menses (menopause). The stage can last for 3–5 years before menopause.
2. *Stage II:* Up to 5 years after menopause. This stage is further subdivided into Stage IIA and Stage IIB.
    a. *Stage IIA:* From the cessation of menstruation up to 1 year (i.e. up to confirmation at menopause, as per WHO definition). The main symptoms of menopause during this stage are vasomotor instability and urethral syndrome.
    b. *Stage IIB:* From the end of stage IIA up to 4 years. The usual symptoms here are:
        - Atrophic symptoms, vaginitis and dyspareunia
        - Urinary symptoms
        - Weight gain + abnormal weight distribution
        - Skin and hair changes
        - Genital prolapses
        - Late psychological symptoms
        - Sexual disorders.
3. *Stage III:* From 5 years after menopause up to an indefinite period; probably her lifetime. These are divided into the following:

TABLE 1: Stages of menopause by Dr Behram Anklesaria.

Stage I	*Stage IIA*	*Stage IIB*	*Stage III*
• Roughly 3–5 years before the menopause • Early (Premenopausal) symptoms • IA: Menstrual irregularity • IB: Vasomotor instability • IC: Early psychosomatic symptoms • Establish communication	1 year	• Up to 5 years after the menopause • Local atrophic changes • Late psychosomatic symptoms • Treat	• From 5 years after menopause up to her lifetime • IIIA: Late atrophic changes • IIIB: Ischaemic heart disease • IIIC: Osteoporosis • IIID: Very late complications such as cerebrovascular accidents and Alzheimer's disease • Prevent

- *IIIA:* Late atrophic symptoms
- *IIIB:* Ischaemic heart disease
- *IIIC:* Osteoporosis
- *IIID:* Very late complications such as cerebrovascular accidents and Alzheimer's disease.

In the United States, in 2003, the survey percentage of menopausal women was as under:

- At years, 89%
- At 40–50 years, 6.9%
- Under 40 years, 0.5%
- Surgical 4%

The average age of menopause of an Indian woman is 46.2 years, which is much less than that of their western counterparts (51 years). With better facilities and increasing life expectancy, the projected figure of women 45 years or older by 2026 in India is a staggering 401 million. As per the National Family Health Survey (2019–2021), the estimated prevalence of early menopause (before 45 years) was 16.2%, and premature menopause (before 40 years) was 2.2%. Thus, in the years to come, the quality of life of this population will assume more and more significance, and every clinician will have to update themselves on understanding and managing menopause.

Factors Influencing Age of Menopause

Several factors appear to influence the age at which women have their last menses and experience menopausal symptoms.

- Menopause occurs approximately 1 year earlier in women who smoke
- Menopause occurs earlier in nulliparous women
- Menopause may also occur earlier in women who have had surgeries involving the ovary, cystectomies/oophorectomies or ovarian drilling done for polycystic ovarian disease (PCOD)
- Women who receive pelvic radiotherapy or chemotherapy
- Indian women have an earlier menopause compared to their Western counterparts, with genetic or racial factors contributing to it.

PHYSIOLOGY OF MENOPAUSE

In females, throughout the reproductive life, ovarian follicles undergo depletion by a degenerative process called atresia. In fact, this process starts much earlier in foetal life itself. At 5 months of foetal age, the ovaries contain their peak number of primordial follicles, totalling approximately 2 million. At birth, girls have 1 million primordial follicles, approximately 25% of which remain at puberty. During the reproductive years, though multiple follicles begin to develop during each ovulatory cycle, all except the dominant follicle, will become atretic. As the atretic process continues, only around 1,000 follicles remain in the ovaries of a woman at 50 years of age. Some follicles do persist in the ovaries for a few more years after menopause, but these are poorly responsive. This progressive loss of follicles that goes on with ageing is characteristic of all mammals studied to date; however, what factors control this process have not yet been well-defined.

Beginning as early as 10–15 years before menopause, there is shortening of the follicular phase of the cycle, and thus the length of the menstrual cycle starts decreasing. This decrease in cycle length continues until the onset of the menopausal transition, when both the average cycle length and the standard deviation of cycle length begin to increase, as follicles are depleted and ovulation occurs less frequently. Insufficient follicular development results in inadequate oestrogen production. With little oestrogen available to stimulate the endometrium, amenorrhoea results **(Flowchart 1)**. There is good evidence that the timing of natural menopause is genetically programmed, but the specific genes involved are yet to be defined. Common allelic variants of the oestrogen receptor gene (oestrogen receptor—*ER*-α and *ER*-β] contribute to the variability in the timing of menopause. In addition, all of the steroid receptors, as well as the proteins and enzymes involved in steroid biosynthesis and metabolism, are known to be coded by polymorphic sites (genetic changes found in at least 1% of the population). Because of this variability, the type and appearance of menopausal symptoms, its intensity and duration, all seem to vary.

Hormonal Changes

A subtle rise in the concentration of FSH is the earliest and most consistent clinically measurable hormonal change noted in studies of reproductive ageing. An FSH level measured during the early follicular stage of the menstrual cycle that is >2 standard deviations (SD) above the mean level in women of reproductive age is a marker of impending menopausal transition.

In the premenopausal years, ovarian granulosa cells under the influence of FSH produce oestrogens. As more follicles undergo atresia closer to menopausal transition,

Flowchart 1: Chronology of age-related oestrogen production.

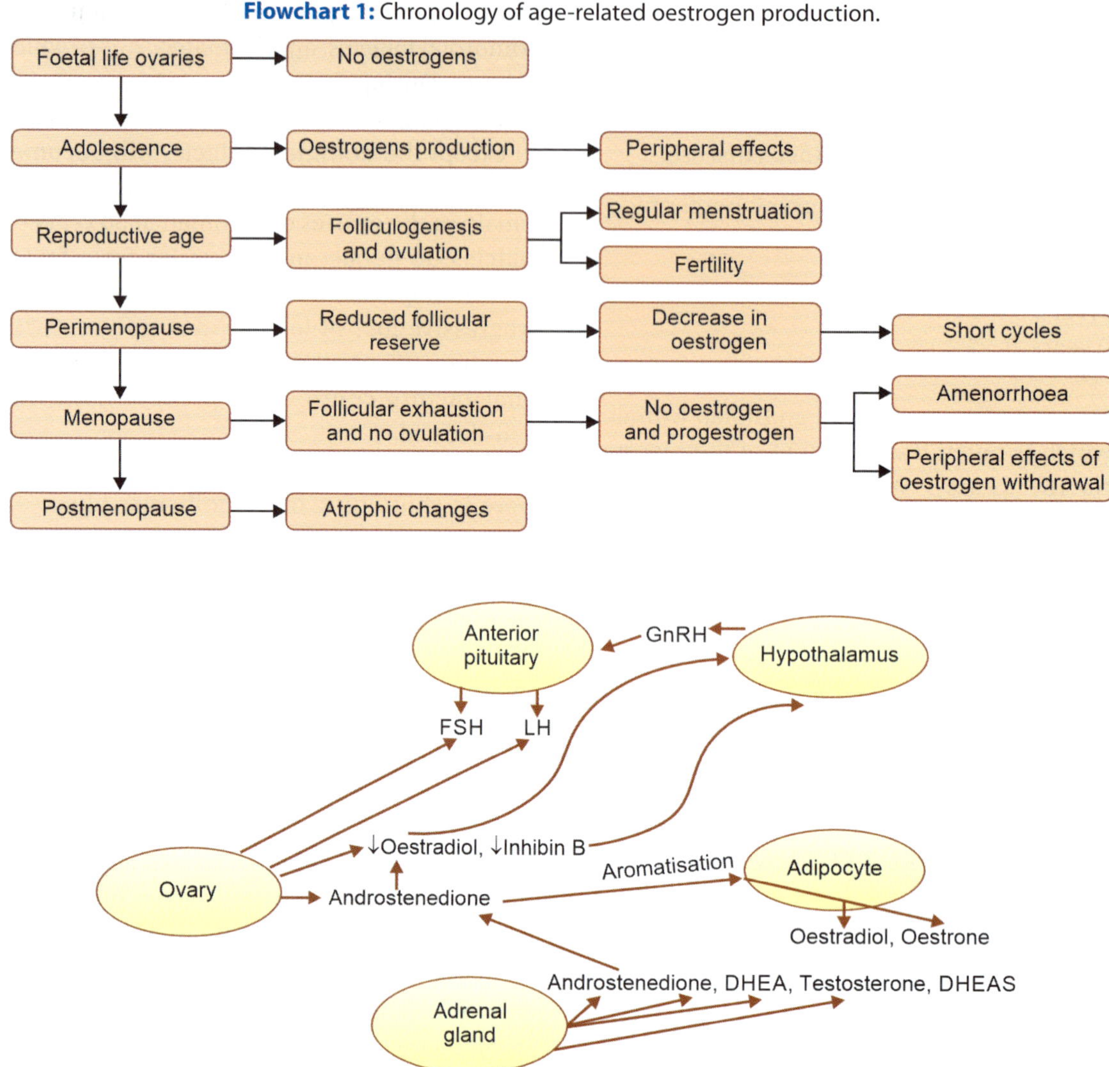

Fig. 1: Cycle of hormonal changes in menopause. (DHEA: dehydroepiandrosterone; DHEAS: dehydroepiandrosterone sulphate; FSH: follicle-stimulating hormone; GnRH: gonadotrophin-releasing hormone; LH: luteinising hormone).

there is first a fall in oestradiol levels and inhibin B levels, which leads to an increase in levels of FSH. Levels of oestradiol further drop, and thus oestrone becomes the dominant hormone, because of the peripheral conversion of testosterone to oestrone.

A slow rise in FSH occurs first, followed by a rise in luteinising hormone (LH) and a decline in oestradiol and oestrone levels. There are no abrupt changes in testosterone levels, but a gradual continuous decline occurs. This begins before menopausal transition because of an ageing adrenal cortex. But ovaries continue to produce androgens and so at menopause, there is not much fall in testosterone levels.

Luteinising hormone levels remain normal initially, but it also gets elevated as ovarian steroid secretion falls and gonadotrophin-releasing hormone (GnRH) rises in response to follicular atresia. Inhibin B levels fall leading to an early selective increase in FSH. Inhibin A and B hormones which are involved in directing follicular development suppress pituitary FSH production. So, as follicle development and ovulation fail to happen in the perimenopausal phase, FSH and LH remain chronically elevated **(Fig. 1)**.

There is a 10-fold to 20-fold increase in the FSH levels and a 3-fold to 5-fold increase in the LH levels, with oestradiol levels falling below 50 pg/mL.

Even in menopause, ovarian theca cells continue to produce androstenedione and testosterone under the influence of increased levels of LH. They are the source of androgens in menopausal women and the sudden fall in androgens noticed in oophorectomised women is because of loss of this source of androgens. By aromatisation, adipocytes produce oestrone from testosterone and thus in menopausal women, oestrone becomes the dominant hormone. Hormonal synthesis by the adrenal gland remains fairly constant, undergoing changes associated with ageing, not menopause per se. Because of ageing of adrenal gland, levels of androgens fall up to 50% at 60 years of age as compared with women at 40. After the age of 70 years, levels of dehydroepiandrosterone (DHEA) and dehydroepiandrosterone sulphate (DHEAS) levels are 20% or less.

Final Hormonal Changes with Established Menopause

Compared with the typical hormonal changes in the early follicular phase of ovulatory women, in postmenopausal women, the most significant findings are marked reductions in oestradiol (E2) and oestrone (E1) levels. The serum E2 level is lower than the serum E1 level. Serum E1 is produced primarily by peripheral aromatisation of androgens, which are not as dramatically affected by menopause. Postmenopausal levels of E2 average 15 pg/mL and range from 10 to 25 pg/mL. In oophorectomised women, levels are usually 10 pg/mL or lower. Serum E1 values average 30 pg/mL but may be higher in obese women, because aromatisation increases because of increased mass of adipose tissue. Oestrone sulphate (E1S), an oestrogen conjugate that serves as a stable circulating reservoir of oestrogen, has the highest levels of any oestrogen. In premenopausal women, E1S is usually above 1,000 pg/mL; in postmenopausal women, levels average 350 pg/mL.

- Androgens produced by adrenals are androstenedione, DHEA, DHEAS, testosterone and dihydrotestosterone (DHT). However, androstenedione, DHEA and DHEAS are considered proandrogens, because they must be converted to testosterone, in order to be effective. Androgen biosynthesis occurs in the ovary and the adrenals under stimulation by LH and adrenocorticotrophic hormone (ACTH), respectively, along with intraglandular paracrine and autocrine regulatory mechanisms. Starting from the third decade of life, independent of menopausal transition, circulating Δ-5 androgen levels fall linearly with age. After natural menopause, theca cells of the ovary continue producing androgen, under the influence of LH. In contrast, after surgical menopause by an oophorectomy, there is a sudden fall of androgens to about 50% of preoperative values, be it in perimenopause or postmenopause.
- Women in the transition from pre to postmenopause have some changes in the type and levels of androgens. Specifically, both androstenedione and testosterone start to decline 3 years before menopause, and some fluctuations in the testosterone levels occur even after menopause. However, immediately after menopause, it is the decline in androstenedione, which is greater than that of testosterone. Thus, in early postmenopause, testosterone levels may be indistinguishable from those in premenopausal women. During postmenopause, virtually 100% of active sex steroids derive from the peripheral conversion of precursors, mainly DHEA and DHEAS, to oestrogens and androgens. Ultimately, several years after menopause, the levels of androstenedione and testosterone are significantly lower than levels measured in premenopausal women.

PROBLEMS ASSOCIATED WITH MENOPAUSE

Two oestrogen receptors exist: ER-α and ER-β. Although the DNA-binding domains of the two receptors are almost identical (about 97% homology), the ligand-binding domains are different and have only 60% homology. Various oestrogens have different affinities for ER-α and ER-β, which, in turn, have different tissue distributions in the body. For example, preliminary evidence suggests that in certain regions of the brain (e.g. frontal cortex), ER-β predominates over ER-α. In the cerebellum, only ER-β is expressed.

Because ERs are abundant throughout the body, the menopausal decline of oestrogen potentially affects virtually all organ systems.

Though most problems of menopause are associated with oestrogen deficiency, deficiency of other hormones like testosterone too may cause problems.

So far, 35 symptoms have been found to be associated with menopause:

1. Hot flashes, flushes, night sweats and/or cold flashes, clammy feeling
2. Bouts of rapid heartbeat

3. Irritability, mood swings
4. Sudden tears
5. Trouble sleeping through the night (with or without night sweats)
6. Irregular periods; shorter, lighter periods; heavier periods, flooding; phantom periods, shorter cycles, longer cycles
7. Loss of libido
8. Dry vagina
9. Crashing fatigue
10. Anxiety, feeling ill at ease
11. Feelings of dread, apprehension, doom
12. Difficulty concentrating, disorientation, mental confusion
13. Disturbing memory lapses
14. Incontinence, especially upon sneezing, laughing, urge incontinence
15. Itchy, crawly skin
16. Aching, sore joints, muscles and tendons
17. Increased tension in muscles
18. Breast tenderness
19. Headache change: Increase or decrease
20. Gastrointestinal (GI) distress, indigestion, flatulence, gas pain, nausea
21. Sudden bouts of bloat
22. Depression
23. Exacerbation of existing conditions
24. Increase in allergies
25. Weight gain
26. Hair loss or thinning, head, pubic, or whole body; increase in facial hair
27. Dizziness, light-headedness, episodes of loss of balance
28. Changes in body odour
29. Electric shock sensation under the skin and in the head
30. Tingling in the extremities
31. Gum problems, increased bleeding
32. Burning tongue, burning roof of mouth, bad taste in mouth, change in breath odour
33. Osteoporosis
34. Changes in fingernails: Softer, crack or break easier
35. Tinnitus: Ringing in ears, bells, 'whooshing' buzzing, etc.

EFFECT OF OESTROGEN DEFICIENCY

Brain and Central Nervous System

Oestrogen receptors are abundant in the brain. Oestrogen is known to have a role in many brain processes, and the absence of oestrogen can result in deficiency symptoms. Oestrogen is important for cerebral blood flow, cerebral glucose metabolism, synaptic activity, neuronal growth, the survival of cholinergic neurons as well as such complex functions as cognition.

Hot Flushes

Hot flushes are an early and acute symptom of oestrogen deficiency. They often begin in the perimenopause when oestrogen levels fluctuate widely. It is the rapid fall in oestrogen levels that precipitates the symptoms. Hot flushes typically last from 0.5 to 5 years after natural menopause but may persist as long as 15 years. They tend to last longer and be more severe with surgically induced menopause.

Night sweats can be more upsetting than daytime flushes because they disrupt sleep. Hot flushes can lead to insomnia, which can result in:

- Irritability
- Tiredness
- Forgetfulness

However, psychological changes due to chronic sleep disturbances may be more disturbing than the above effects of hot flushes. A direct effect of changing hormonal status may also play a role.

But these symptoms are not universally experienced, and high prevalence in western societies (58–93% in the first two menopausal years) is not found in other societies, elsewhere. Japanese women report very few hot flushes and Mayan women from Mexico do not report any symptoms of menopause. Among Indians too, the symptoms are not very common. Thus, the prevalence of vasomotor symptoms varies widely across populations and is strongly influenced by culture and ethnicity.

Physiology of Hot Flushes

Although the proximate cause of flushes remains elusive, the episodes result from a hypothalamic response (probably mediated by catecholamines) induced by a change in oestrogen status. The flush has been well-characterised physiologically: heat dissipation occurs through an increase in peripheral temperature (e.g. in the fingers and toes); a decrease in skin resistance, associated with diaphoresis; and a reduction in core body temperature. Heart rate and skin blood flow peak within approximately 3 minutes of hot flush onset, which leads to vasodilatation and a decrease in internal temperature

(0.1–0.9°C), leads to a feeling of chill. Skin temperature returns to normal usually within 30 minutes. No significant change in blood pressure is associated with hot flashes.

There are hormonal correlates of flush activity, such as an increase in serum LH and plasma proopiomelanocortin peptides (ACTH, β-endorphin) at the time of the flush; however, these occurrences are thought to be epiphenomena that result as a consequence of the flush and are not related to its aetiology.

Diagnostic or Metabolic Workup for Differential Diagnosis of Hot Flushes

- Levels of FSH indicate ovarian reserve. FSH values of >10 IU/L are indicative of declining ovarian function. FSH values >20 IU/L are diagnostic of ovarian failure in women in the perimenopausal age group with hot flushes, even in the absence of cessation of menstruation.
- Serum-pooled prolactin levels are useful in differentiating hyperprolactinaemia from menopause. After 1–3 years of cessation of menstruation (menopause), LH levels reach over 30 IU/L.
- Although multiple different aetiologies could cause hot flushes apart from menopause, carcinoid syndrome is one that is essential to be suspected and excluded given the underlying association with a malignancy. This is associated with systemic symptoms and elevated levels of urinary 5-hydroxyindoleacetic acid (5-HIAA).

Management

Counselling the woman is most important.

- *Pharmacological preparations:* The gold standard of treatment for menopausal hot flushes is oestrogen therapy. Hormone therapy (HT) is given with either oestrogens alone (in hysterectomised women) or in combination with progestogen (in women with an intact uterus) at the lowest dosage, for the shortest period of time. Oestrogens can be given by the oral, transdermal or transvaginal route. Other than oestrogen, no other therapy has been approved by the US Food and Drug Administration (FDA) for the treatment of hot flushes. However, some women may be unsuitable for menopausal hormone therapy (MHT) due to contraindications, unwilling to take MHT or unable to continue MHT due to intolerable side effects.
- Tibolone is another drug, found to be effective in hot flushes. The various nonpharmacological options for managing hot flushes are as follows:
- *Lifestyle modifications:*
    - Adopting certain lifestyle measures can decrease the intensity and frequency of hot flushes. It is recommended that all women with hot flushes be counselled regarding these options and encouraged to use them.
    - Avoidance of triggering factors like stress, caffeine, alcohol, spicy foods and beverages
    - Avoiding smoking
    - Reduction of stress—practice meditation, yoga, massage, paced breathing
    - Staying in a cold environment, avoiding warm places
    - Keeping cool and the ambient temperature low, drinking cold drinks, bathing in cool water, using fans, using cotton sheets, wearing appropriate breathable cotton clothing and dressing in layers
    - Exercise—undertake aerobic and weight-bearing exercises (Exercise reduces hot flushes in 50% of cases)
    - Weight loss.
- *Placebo:* Placebo use may lead to 20–50% reduction in hot flushes with 4 weeks of treatment.
- *Non-hormonal* medications used for the control of hot flashes are :
    - Antidepressants-Venlafaxine (serotonin and norepinephrine reuptake inhibitors), paroxetine, fluoxetine
    - Propranolol
    - Gabapentin-A, γ-aminobutyric acid (GABA) analogue used for seizure disorders as an anticonvulsant
    - Evening primrose oil
    - Veralipride
    - Herbal remedies—black cohosh, red clover, dong quai
    - Clonidine—α-adrenergic agonist, commonly used as an antihypertensive
    - Cetirizine
    - Nutraceuticals-like vitamins—B complex, C and E
    - Dietary phytoestrogens
- *Behavioural interventions:*
    - Paced respiration (slow deep abdominal breathing)
    - Relaxation training

- Cognitive behavioural intervention and diversion techniques
- Progressive muscle relaxation or biofeedback or applied relaxation
- Hypnosis
- Acupuncture

Among the nonpharmacological therapeutic options, antidepressants *venlafaxine, paroxetine and fluoxetine* have better results.

Mood Changes and Cognitive Function

- In general, oestrogen has a positive effect on mood and contributes to a sense of well-being.
- Exercise like aerobic training, dance, meditation, yoga and swimming may also help in some cases.
- The role of oestrogen deficiency in postmenopausal depression, declining cognitive function, dementia, and Alzheimer's disease is not clear and is an area of intensive debate and research.

Migraines

Oestrogens and progestins affect central serotoninergic and opioid neurons.

Alterations in the level and cycling of these hormones may cause a change in the prevalence or intensity of headaches. Because the orderly pattern of oestrogen and progesterone secretion is lost as menopause approaches, perimenopausal women with a history of menstrual migraines may experience an exacerbation.

Vision

There is an increased incidence of some vision-threatening conditions in postmenopausal women. For example, idiopathic full-thickness macular degeneration predominantly affects women over 60 years. There appears to be a hormonal component, because symptoms become more severe with menopause. Changes in hormonal status may thus affect the physiology of the eye.

There are gender and age differences in ER-α expression in the retina. ER-α was detected in the retina and retinal pigment of young female eyes but not in the eye tissues of postmenopausal women.

Collagen

Oestrogen has a positive effect on collagen, which is important for bone and skin. Both oestrogen and androgen receptors have been identified in skin fibroblasts. The loss of collagen is more rapid in the first few years after menopause, and 30% of skin collagen is lost within the first 5 years after menopause. The rate of collagen reduction is approximately 2% per year for the first 10 years after menopause. This statistics, which is similar to that of bone loss after menopause, strongly suggests a link between skin thickness, bone loss and the risk of osteoporosis. In addition, reductions in collagen support and atrophy of the vaginal and urethral mucosa have been associated with a variety of symptoms, including uterine prolapse and urinary incontinence.

Urogenital Syndrome of Menopause

Oestrogen deficiency has deleterious effects on the urogenital system. It has been reported that as many as one-third of women aged 50 years and older experience urogenital problems. Oestrogen deficiency results in a:

- Thin and paler vaginal mucosa
- Loss of normal rugosities
- Low moisture content
- The pH increases (usually pH is <5).
- It may exhibit inflammation and small petechiae.
- Cytology reveals a loss of superficial cells and an increase of basal and parabasal cells.
- In reproductive age women, the vaginal flora is dominated by lactobacilli. In postmenopausal women, the vagina is gradually repopulated with diverse flora, including pathogenic organisms commonly found in urinary tract infections (UTI) (e.g. coliform bacteria), as a result of the reduced acidity. The decrease in lactobacilli, yeast and bacterial vaginosis-associated bacteria may also explain the lower incidence of bacterial vaginosis and yeast vaginitis in postmenopausal women than in women of reproductive age **(Fig. 2)**.
- The lower urinary tract and the genital tract in females have a common embryological origin. Oestrogen receptors have been reported in the trigone of the bladder and the proximal and distal urethra.

Functional changes which have been noted include the following:

- Elderly women have lower flow rates.
- Higher bladder volume at the first sensation to void
- Increasing urinary residue
- Similarly, changes in collagen in the endopelvic fascia and periurethral tissue account for the hypermobility and reduced urethral closure pressure and may thus explain the prevalence of stress incontinence.

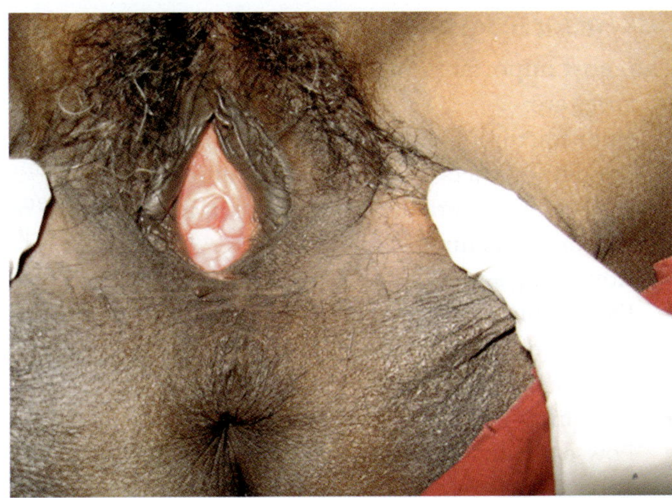

Fig. 2: Vaginal atrophy, loss of rugosities and pale epithelium.

Dry and atrophic vaginal and urethral epithelium can cause:

- Vaginal discomfort
- Itching
- Dyspareunia
- Recurrent vaginitis.

International Society for Study of Women's Sexual Health and North American Menopause Society came to a consensus to replace atrophic vaginitis or urogenital atrophy, with anew terminology of GSM—genitourinary syndrome of menopause.

Genitourinary syndrome of menopause is defined as a collection of symptoms and signs associated with a decrease in oestrogen and other sex steroids involving changes to the labia majora/minora, clitoris, vestibule/introitus, vagina, urethra and bladder. The syndrome may include but is not limited to genital symptoms of dryness, but lubrication, discomfort or pain and impaired function; and urinary symptoms of urgency, dysuria and recurrent urinary tract infections. Women may present with some or all of the signs and symptoms, which must be bothersome and should not be better accounted for by another diagnosis.

Urinary Symptoms at Menopause

Common urinary symptoms encountered around or after menopause are:

- Increased frequency during daytime and nocturia
- Urgency with varying degrees of urge incontinence
- Stress incontinence
- Dysuria
- Incomplete voiding of varying degrees to frank urinary retention with overflow incontinence
- Recurrent UTI and asymptomatic bacteriuria
- Enuresis

Recommendation

All women presenting with urinary symptoms should be evaluated with a detailed history and the following tests, as appropriate to the individual:

- Urine routine and culture
- Cytology (where indicated)
- Ultrasonography
- Urodynamic study
- Hormonal profile
- Bladder diary

Treatment

Treatment includes:

- Antibiotics for UTI
- Local oestrogens are the first-line treatment and mostly the only treatment needed for atrophic vaginitis or GSM
- Systemic oestrogen therapy ± progesterone therapy is needed only rarely
- Appropriate surgical intervention, when needed, mostly for stress urinary incontinence (SUI)/cystocele
- Bladder training.

Weight Gain and Loss of Muscle Mass (Sarcopenia)

- The prevalence of obesity in adult women rises significantly with each decade, until it begins tapering off late in life.
- About 20% gain weight of about 4.5 kg in the 3 years surrounding menopause, while only 3% lose that amount of weight.

Changes in Fat Distribution

Although weight changes may be more strongly associated with ageing than with menopause:

- Women who have undergone menopause may have higher levels of body fat and a more central fat distribution than age-matched controls.
- Women lose more of lean muscle mass and gain more of fat.

From a clinical standpoint, the effect of menopause on abdominal obesity is of major concern, since abdominal obesity has been shown to be an independent predictor of type 2 diabetes, dyslipidaemia, hypertension, certain cancers and cardiovascular disease (CVD).

Causative factors for these changes:

- The age-related decline in resting metabolic rate (RMR) and decreased physical activity, with or without increased caloric intake, could easily result in weight gain.
- Changes in RMR have been observed, which may be due in part to a decline in fat-free mass or sarcopenia.
- Loss of ovarian function and loss of interleukin in the luteal phase of the menstrual cycle may also contribute to decreased RMR.
- Oestrogen has been found to influence eating behaviour, and its loss causes weight gain in animals.

Prevention of Weight Gain

Lifestyle modifications are the mainstay of prevention and control.

Currently, the most effective behavioural approach for management of overweight and obesity is a combination that includes:

- Reduced caloric intake (typically 1,000–1,200 kcal/day for women)
- Dietary fat reduction (30% of calories)
- Increased physical activity (at least 30–45 minutes of moderate-intensity activity on most days of the week) when losing weight, along with aerobic activity. Resistance and strength-building exercises should also be started to counteract the loss of lean muscle mass.
- Behavioural guidance.

Bone Loss (Osteoporosis) and Fracture Risk

In women, peak bone mass is achieved by the second decade and begins to decrease thereafter, especially beyond 35 years of age.

In industrialised western countries, more than one-third of women older than 65 years suffer from symptoms of osteopenia/osteoporosis, a disorder characterised by low-bone mass **(Table 2)**.

TABLE 2: Projected prevalence of osteoporosis and/or low-bone mass of the hip in the US women ≥50 years.

	2002	*2010*	*2020*
Women			
Osteoporosis	7,800,000	9,100,000	10,500,000
Low bone mass	21,800,000	26,000,000	30,400,000

Risk Factor Assessment

The most important risk factors for osteoporosis-related fractures are:

- Prior fracture(s) with trivial trauma as an adult, which strongly predicts the potential for future fractures
- Low-bone mineral density (BMD) in an adult with or without a fracture
- Advancing age
- Family history of osteoporosis or fractures in first-degree relatives
- Loss of >1.5 inches in height
- Vitamin D deficiency (very common in India)
- Low-calcium intake (<300 mg/day)
- Tobacco use
- Alcohol intake >7 oz per week
- Weight loss and low body weight
- Any condition that increases the risk of falling
- Other secondary causes of bone loss (which may be present in up to one-third of women)
- Activity level and lifestyle
- Extremely important is the total amount of bone a woman has at the time of menopause.

Definition: Postmenopausal osteoporosis is characterised by low-bone mass and microarchitectural deterioration of bone tissue leading to enhanced bone fragility and increased fracture risk.

According to the WHO, osteoporosis is defined based on the following bone density levels:

- BMD is compared to two norms—healthy young adults (T-score) and age-matched (Z-score) **(Fig. 3)**.

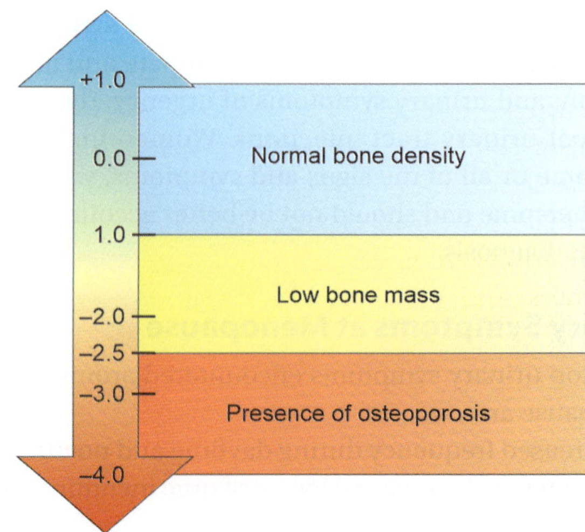

Fig. 3: T-score normal, osteopenia and osteoporosis.

BOX 1: Bone mineral density (BMD)—measures solidness and mass of the bone.

Types:
- *DEXA:* Dual X-ray absorptiometry measures spine, hip or total body
- *QUS:* Quantitative USG measures density at calcareous, tibia and patella
- *QCT:* Quantitative computed tomography measures spine

(USG: ultrasonography).

A T-score within 1 SD (+1 or –1) of the young adult mean indicates normal bone density **(Box 1)**.

- A T-score of 1–2.5 SD below the young adult mean (–1 to –2.5 SD) indicates low bone mass.
- A T-score of 2.5 SD or more below the young adult mean (> –2.5 SD) indicates the presence of osteoporosis.

Oestrogen deficiency is a dominant pathogenic factor in bone loss. This can be noted for the first time during perimenopause. From 1.5 years before menopause to 1.5 years after menopause, spine BMD decreases by 2.5% per year, compared with a premenopausal loss rate of 0.13% per year.

At menopause, an accelerated loss of bone occurs, which results in a 3% reduction in bone mass per year for the first 5 years. Thereafter, the rate of loss of bone ranges from 1% to 2% per year. Dramatic changes in bone architecture accompany this loss of bone, significantly increasing the risk of fracture. Every SD of reduction in bone mass results in a 1.5- to 2-fold or greater risk of fracture **(Fig. 4)**.

Role of Oestrogen in Osteoporosis

Oestrogen action on bone is mediated by direct effects through the oestrogen receptor and by its effects on collagen. The accelerated decline in bone mass that occurs with oestrogen deficiency is mediated by a variety of mechanisms, but the primary event is increased resorption (osteoclastic activity), which becomes uncoupled from bone formation (osteoblastic activity).

- There are also indirect effects mediated by parathyroid hormone and cytokines, which oppose the resorptive effects.
- Osteoprotegerin (OPG), e.g. a member of the TNF-receptor (tumour necrosis factor receptor) family, is a soluble protein that inhibits osteoclastic bone resorption. OPG is secreted by osteoblasts and binds to OPG ligand, a factor necessary for osteoclastogenesis. Serum levels of OPG appear to be significantly elevated in postmenopausal women with osteoporosis. In addition, oestrogen enhances OPG secretion by osteoblasts in vitro, suggesting that OPG may have an important role in the antiresorptive action of oestrogen on bone.
- In postmenopause, the positive effects of oestrogen on growth factors, calcitonin, vitamin D metabolism and calcium absorption are also diminished.

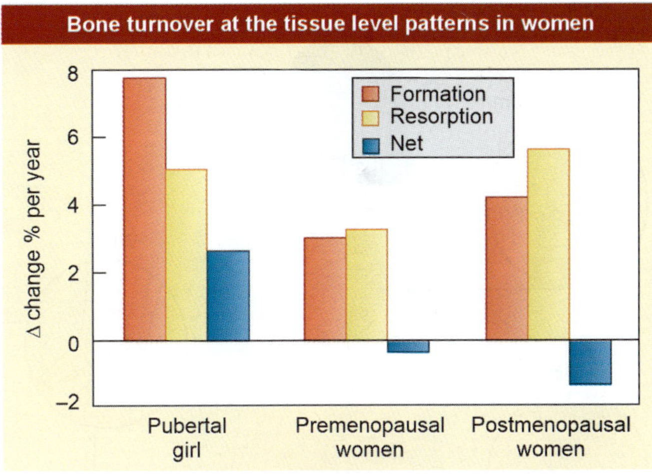

Fig. 4: Bone turnover from puberty to menopause.

Biochemical Markers of Bone Turnover

- Biochemical markers of bone turnover could reflect primarily formation (serum bone-specific alkaline phosphatase enzyme, serum osteocalcin), or resorption (urinary C or N-telopeptides-collagen breakdown products). These biochemical markers are not useful in the diagnosis of postmenopausal osteoporosis, because the values in normal and in those with osteoporosis show a substantial overlap. However, they may be useful in the following situations.
- Assessing response to antiresorptive therapy
- Assessing compliance to medications.

The three main sites of increased risk of fracture in postmenopausal women are **(Fig. 5)**:

1. Wrist
2. Hip
3. Spine (30% of spine fractures, unfortunately go unnoticed)

Spinal Complications of Osteoporosis

- Kyphosis
- Vertebral wedging
- Compression fractures

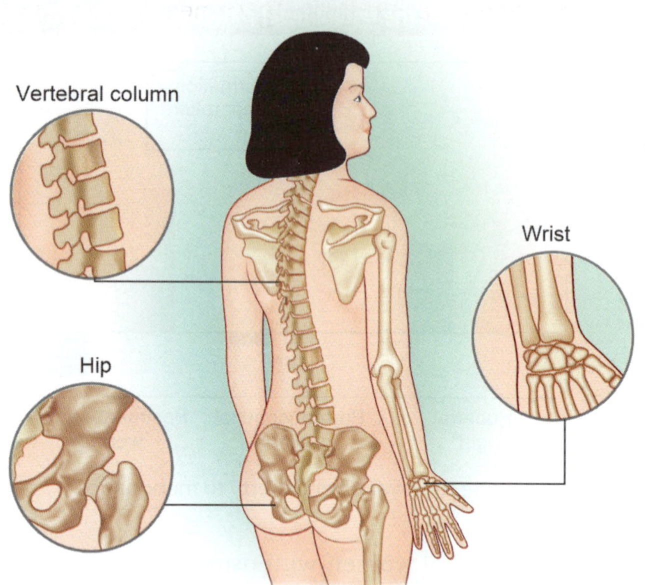

Fig. 5: Common sites of fracture.

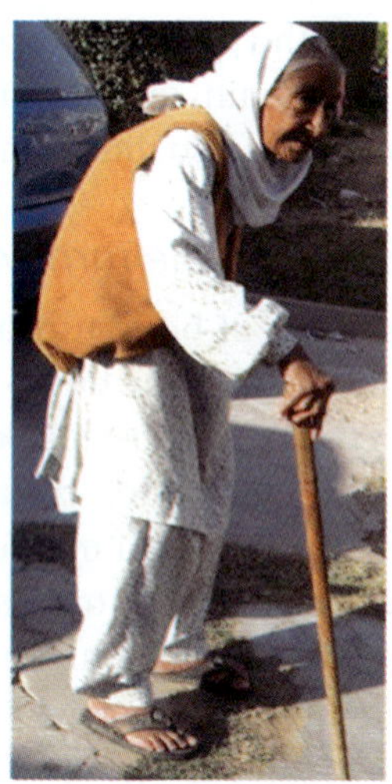

Fig. 6: Kyphosis in menopause.

The most common fractures due to osteoporosis are vertebral fractures, and yet, only less than a third of all vertebral fractures get clinically diagnosed **(Fig. 6)**.

These complications lead to poor quality of life for these women, and they have problems in walking and in carrying out their routine activities.

Back Exercises for Kyphosis

The thoracic kyphosis of oestrogen-deficient women has been found to be directly correlated with weakness of the back extensor muscles, and thus, increasing the back extensor strength has been shown to decrease the kyphosis. In this instance, when the torso is carried flexed forward, the patient will need to retrain the extensor muscles of the spine with isotonic resistance exercises. This is most effective when done in an upright and weight-bearing position. So from 35 years onwards, all women should do resistance exercises to strengthen their back muscles.

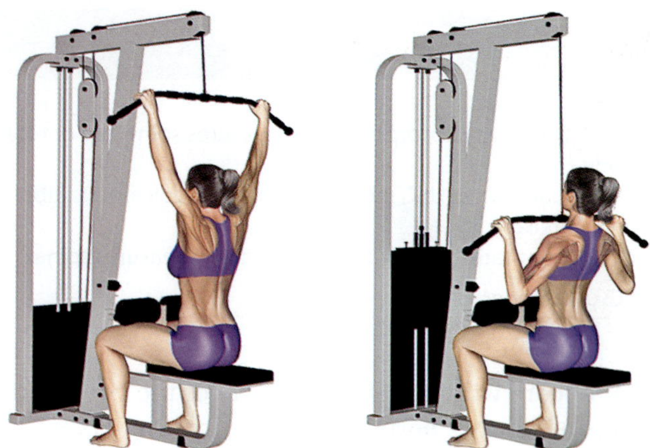

Fig. 7: Wide grip pulley press for upper back muscles. *Source:* homegymreview.co.uk.

Prevention and Management of Osteoporosis

A management strategy focused on lifestyle approaches may be all that is needed for women who are at low risk for osteoporotic fracture.

These lifestyle modifications are:
- No smoking
- Calcium 1,200–1,500 mg/day
- Vitamin D 800–1,000 IU/day

But mainstay is exercise, and these have to be weight-bearing and resistance exercises, especially for back muscles to prevent kyphosis **(Figs. 7 and 8)**, wrist muscles, to prevent fractures of wrist, to strengthen thigh and buttock muscles, and to prevent fractures of hip bone. Quadriceps muscles weakness causes buckling of knees in old women, and hence these muscles have to be strengthened. These exercises, along with proper calcium and nutrition, should be started at the adolescent level itself, so that they do not end up with a negative BMD at midlife. Exercise, especially weight-bearing and resistance exercises, has no age bar and can be started at any age, even at 80–90 years. They do increase functional independence, increase in strength and bone density.

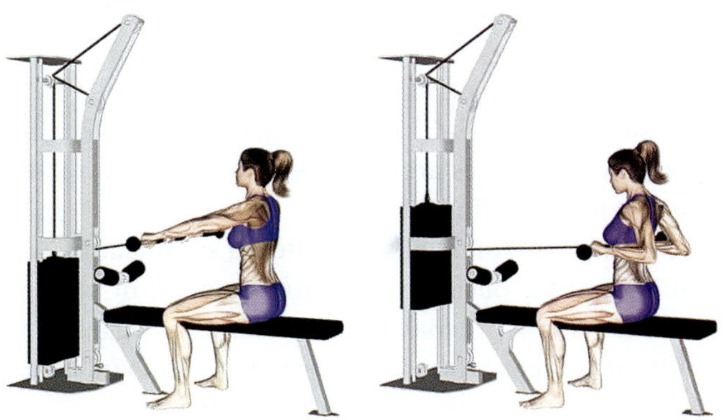

Fig. 8: Back-strengthening exercises for menopausal women. *Source:* homegymreview.co.uk.

Recommendations for Pharmacological Treatment

- All postmenopausal women with total hip or spine *T* scores worse than –2.5
- All postmenopausal women with total hip or spine *T* scores from –2.0 to –2.5 and at least one additional risk factor for fracture
- All postmenopausal women with an osteoporotic vertebral fracture (no BMD is needed).
  - *In premature menopause:* MHT is recommended for prevention of osteoporosis till the time of her natural menopause, and then it can be substituted by other pharmacological agents along with lifestyle modifications and exercise.

  Several other agents are as effective as HT in preventing fractures due to osteoporosis:
- *Bisphosphonates:* Alendronate, risedronate and ibandronate are commonly used for both prevention and treatment of osteoporosis. For prevention, alendronate is given at a daily dose of 5 mg and a weekly dose of 35 mg. For treatment of postmenopausal osteoporosis, the doses are 10 mg daily and 70 mg weekly. For maximal GI absorption and to reduce the incidence of oesophageal irritation, alendronate must be taken in the morning on an empty stomach (½ an hour before breakfast) with about 240 mL of plain water, and the patient must remain upright for ½ an hour after ingestion.
- Bisphosphonates in combination with oestrogen are more effective than either agent alone.
- *Selective oestrogen receptor modulators (SERMs):* SERMs like Raloxifene are indicated for the prevention and treatment of osteoporosis. They are not indicated for treating menopausal symptoms and may even aggravate hot flashes in some women. They also do not help vaginal atrophy. As with oestrogen, a past history of venous thrombosis is a contraindication to their use. Current venous thrombosis is an absolute contraindication. They have a favourable effect on lipid profile and are cardioprotective. They are used at a dose of 60 mg/day for prevention as well as for treatment.
- *Calcitonin:* The nasal spray used for osteoporosis treatment that inhibits bone resorption and reduces fracture rates. Nasal irritation and cost limit its use. Calcitonin is available as a subcutaneous injection (about 100 IU/day) and as a nasal spray (about 200 IU/day) for the treatment of postmenopausal osteoporosis.
- *Parathyroid hormone (PTH, e.g. teriparatide):* Daily subcutaneous injections of PTH are used for osteoporosis treatment. PTH is FDA-approved but carries a black box warning about the possible risk for osteosarcoma based on rat studies.
- *Combinations of Bazedoxifene (BZA) and conjugated equine oestrogen (CEE):* This tissue-selective oestrogen complex (TSEC) has recently entered the market for the treatment of postmenopausal osteoporosis, and is particularly targeted to women with significant vasomotor symptoms. It decreases breast density, and its risk of venous thromboembolism (VTE) is equal to that of placebo. BZA 20 mg/CE 0.45 mg and BZA 20 mg/CE 0.625 mg have both shown efficacy in reducing the frequency and severity of hot flushes, relieving symptoms of VVA, and maintaining bone mass while protecting the endometrium and breast. These BZA/CE doses have been associated with a favourable safety/tolerability profile, with higher rates of cumulative amenorrhea and lower incidences of breast pain than those reported for oestrogen-progestin therapy (EPT). Thus, BZA/CE may be a promising alternative to conventional EPT for treating non-hysterectomised, postmenopausal women.
  - Oestrogens are also advocates for the prevention of osteoporosis, when indicated for other symptoms. In cases of premature ovarian failure, oestrogens are in fact given as replacement therapy for the prevention of osteoporosis.
  - *Tibolone:* It is a STEAR (selective tissue oestrogen activity regulator)
    - 2.5 mg single daily dose orally
    - 1.25 mg may be equally effective
    - Adverse effects are nausea and weight gain

- No change in high-density lipoprotein (HDL) level
- Increases risk of recurrence in a breast cancer survivor.
- *Contraindications for prescribing tibolone:*
  - Undiagnosed genital bleeding
  - Women over 60 years, women with risk factors for stroke like those with hypertension, smoking, diabetes and atrial fibrillation
  - Known or suspected breast cancer, known or suspected oestrogen-dependent malignant tumour, endometrial hyperplasia
  - Previous or current VTE (DVT, pulmonary embolism), known thrombophilic disorders (e.g. protein C, protein S or antithrombin deficiency)
  - History of arterial thromboembolic disease [e.g. angina, myocardial infarction, stroke or transient ischaemic attack (TIA)], acute liver disease or with abnormal liver function tests, porphyria.

- *Osteoprotegerin:* This is a new drug, a naturally occurring protein and a negative regulator of osteoclast formation showing promise as a potential treatment for osteoporosis.

Zoledronic acid is a new drug approved by FDA. A single intravenous infusion of Zoledronic acid 5 mg over a 15-minute period once in a year decreases bone turnover and improves bone density and is effective in reducing hip, vertebral and other fractures.

Cardiovascular Effects

The degree to which oestrogen deficiency increases the risk of CVD in women has not been definitively established and is a subject of intense debate and research.

Various studies have found increased incidence of CAD in menopausal women. Globally, it is also the leading cause of morbidity and mortality in women (54% in women vs. 43% in men).

Although the death rate has fallen in men, it has increased in women because of the rising prevalence of hypertension, diabetes mellitus, sedentary habits, obesity and a lesser decline in smoking.

- The most prevalent finding is that total cholesterol rises at an accelerated rate after menopause.
- This increase in total cholesterol results from an increase in levels of low-density lipoprotein cholesterol (LDL-C).
- Increase in lipoprotein a [LP(a)] levels has also been noted.
- The oxidation of LDL-C is also enhanced. HDL-cholesterol (HDL-C) levels may decrease over time, but these changes are small and insignificant relative to the increases in LDL-C.
- Coagulation balance is not altered significantly with menopause, because a counterbalance of changes occurs; some procoagulation factors increase (factor VII, fibrinogen), but so do certain fibrinolytic factors such as antithrombin III and plasminogen.
- Blood flow in all vascular beds decreases after menopause.
- Prostacyclin production decreases.
- Endothelin levels increase.
- Vasomotor responses to acetylcholine challenges are constrictive.
- Further, circulating plasma levels of nitric oxide increase.
- Levels of angiotensin-converting enzyme decrease.
- Oestrogen and progesterone receptors have been found in vascular tissues, including coronary arteries. Overall, the direct vascular effects that occur after menopause are considered as important as, or more important than, the changes in lipid and lipoproteins in terms of CVD risk.

The Women's Health Initiative (WHI) study showed some possible initial adverse cardiovascular effects, perhaps due to the dose of oestrogen being too high, but was suggestive of an eventful benefit. The benefit appeared to be greater in those women on oestrogen alone than in those on combined hormonal therapy, suggesting a possible adverse effect due to medroxyprogesterone acetate (MPA). Age of patient when oestrogen is started is of importance. *If oestrogen is started earlier then cardioprotective effect is seen; but at present, MHT is not indicated for prevention of CVD.*

Randomised clinical trials have shown no benefit, and some trials have suggested an increased risk of coronary heart disease (CHD) during the first year after randomisation by HT.

Present Recommendations

Specific recommendations from several sources currently include the following:

- Identify and treat all risk factors for CHD.
- Do not initiate MHT for the prevention of CHD.

- Do not initiate MHT in patients with known CHD.
- If CHD develops while on MHT, consider other alternatives.
- For prevention of CHD and to increase cardiorespiratory endurance, 30 min/day of moderate aerobic activity is recommended such as walking at a brisk pace, or swimming, cycling, yoga, tai chi, lawn mowing, or any other activity which causes repetitive movement of large muscles, along with a proper diet.

MENSTRUAL PROBLEMS

The perimenopausal phase begins 2–5 years before the final menstrual period and lasts for 1 year thereafter. It is complex and unpredictable, and abnormal uterine bleeding (AUB) is one such complexity. Contrary to popular belief, *oestradiol levels do not gradually wane in the years before menopause but remain slightly elevated until 6 months to 1 year before follicular growth and development cease.*

The greatest concern about AUB in this age group is the relative oestrogen excess with endometrial hyperplasia/neoplasia, although the usual finding is one of a non-neoplastic tissue with oestrogenic effects unopposed by progesterone. The menstrual cycle becomes irregular and unpredictable with both short and long follicular phases, defective ovulation/anovulation and highly erratic cycles. This pattern of irregularity should be distinguished from regular menstrual cycles interspersed with intermenstrual bleeding. Intermenstrual bleeding is associated with genital tract pathology and the gynaecologist should not overlook this. Anovulatory menorrhagia is frequent in this period, but age-related and pathology-related changes in the uterus and ovaries may also be responsible. Experience and sensitivity are required to distinguish 'normal' perimenstrual patterns from pelvic pathology.

Similarly, serious pathology may be present in 10–20% of women with postmenopausal bleeding, and it should be diagnosed and treated accordingly.

- The endometrium is normal in 50%
- Atrophic in 20%
- Endometrial hyperplasia is seen in 15%
- Polyps in 3% and endometrial cancer in 2%
- In India, cervical malignancies, genital tuberculosis (cervix and endometrium), genital prolapse with decubitus ulcers are common causes of postmenopausal bleeding.
- 10% of women with benign findings at initial evaluation will subsequently develop pathology in 2 years. Persistence of abnormal bleeding requires re-evaluation.
- Approach for patients with perimenopausal and postmenopausal bleeding
  - *History and examination:*
    - Careful history with menstrual pattern over the past 2–3 years is essential. A complete physical examination including breast must be done. Local examination of vulva, urethra for caruncles and anal region for fissures/piles to rule out other causes of bleeding. A Pap smear should be taken before a pelvic examination. At pelvic examination, vagina and cervix must be thoroughly inspected for polyps, growths, ectropion, etc. Finally, a bimanual pelvic examination is done and uterine and adnexal pathology are assessed.
  - *Transvaginal sonography:*
    - Transvaginal sonography is the next step, and endometrial thickness, fibroids, adenomyosis as well as ovarian pathology are evaluated. In a postmenopausal woman, endometrial thickness >4 mm mandates an endometrial biopsy.
  - *Endometrial sampling:*
    - An outpatient or office biopsy with a plastic endometrial suction device using a 3–4 mm cannula is now recommended. No traditional Dilation and Curettage (D & C) is needed as the first step.
  - *Colposcopy, cervical biopsy, fractional curettage and hysteroscopy*:
    - Additional procedures would be colposcopy, cervical biopsy and endocervical curettage for abnormal cytology or obvious lesions. Hysteroscopy and saline infusion sonography may be done in problematic cases with persistent bleeding to rule out polyps, any focal lesions or submucous fibroids.
    - Management
    - Perimenopausal AUB
    - In the absence of organic disease, management will depend on the age of patient and endometrial histopathology. In women with a proliferative endometrium or hyperplasia without atypia, oral progestins for 10–14 days of a month for 3 cycles are given. Hyperplasia with atypia does not respond to progestins. Progestin therapy reverses hyperplasia in majority of patients and

is continued till withdrawal bleeding ceases. Stoppage of withdrawal bleeding reliably indicates oestrogen deficiency and oestrogen can be added then on or the combined MHT started.

- If contraception is required, a low-dose pill will provide contraception, prophylaxis against irregular, heavy anovulatory bleeding and neoplasia, regularise cycles and relieve menopausal symptoms.

Postmenopausal Bleeding

- Any organic pathology: Appropriate management
- Staging laparotomy for endometrial cancer
- Radical Wertheim's hysterectomy in invasive cancer cervix
- Total abdominal hysterectomy with bilateral salpingo-oophorectomy in fibroids, adenomyosis, etc. and MHT thereafter, for women showing menopausal symptoms

Management of Bleeding in Women on Menopausal Hormone Therapy

- *Counselling* prior to initiating MHT is a must. With sequential MHT, a regular withdrawal bleed is seen in 80–90% of women. In a continuous combined regime, irregular breakthrough bleeding may be seen in the first 6 months, but majority of them achieve amenorrhoea by the end of 1 year. Persistence of breakthrough bleeding need to be treated. Increasing the oestrogen or progestin dosage, patient education, and support, will help.
- Persistent bleeding needs to be re-evaluated by TVS and endometrial sampling/hysteroscopy, if needed. Levonorgestrel intrauterine device (LNG-IUD), endometrial ablation, or switching over to a more predictable sequential regime are other strategies.

Cancer Screening in Menopause

The leading cancers in women are:

- Breast cancer
- Cervical cancer
- Endometrial cancer.

Recommendations for screening for breast cancer: Early diagnosis of breast cancer is important. The 5-year survival rate depends on the stage at the time of diagnosis and ranges from 100% for stage 0 to just 16% for stage IV. Other concomitant medical conditions also influence the survival rate.

- All women should be told by the age of 20 years, about the benefits and limitations of breast self-examination (BSE). Monthly BSEs should be supplemented with a clinical breast examination by a health professional every 1–3 years, until the age of 40 years. After the age of 40 years, women should have a clinical breast examination every year and a mammogram every 1–2 years.
- In some instances, physicians may recommend to begin screening mammography even before the age of 40 years. In woman with a family history of breast and ovarian cancer, annual mammogram should start by 35 years of age. In women belonging to proven breast and ovarian cancer families (those with genetic mutations) or those who have multiple first or second-degree relatives with breast or ovarian cancers, an annual mammogram must start as early as 25 years.

MANAGEMENT OF MENOPAUSE

Women can present as:

- *Asymptomatic with no risk factors:* Counsel about lifestyle modifications and call again for follow-up
- Symptomatic without risk factors: Treat them
- Symptomatic with risk factors for osteoporosis, CHD, or metabolic syndrome: Treat, Counsel and Assess
- *Symptomatic with comorbidities:* Assess and Advise

SYMPTOMS OF MENOPAUSE

Symptoms can be classified into early symptoms and delayed manifestations, seen after 5 years of menopause.

- Vasomotor symptoms and sleep disturbances
- Musculoskeletal symptoms
- GSM
- Sex-related problems
- Depression and mood changes
- AUB
- CHD risk, Alzheimer's, osteoporosis and metabolic syndrome.

In all patients, do basic history taking, family/personal/past-regarding osteoporosis/CHD/ diabetes/hypertension.

Indications for Menopausal Hormone Therapy

- Vasomotor symptoms—moderate to severe hot flashes/night sweats
- Symptoms of GUSM
- Prevention and treatment of osteoporosis

Additional benefits of Menopausal Hormone Therapy

- Improved sleep
- Lesser muscle and joint pains
- Improvement in mood disorders
- Sexual dysfunction and quality of life improves
- Decrease in colon cancer risk
- Decrease in diabetes and metabolic syndrome
- Possible benefit in CVD and cognition

Assessment before Starting Menopausal Hormone Therapy

- Menstrual history, menarche and age of menopause
- Physical examination
- Height, weight, BMI, BP, chest auscultation, WHR, rule out Breast/Thyroid swelling
- *Local examination:* P/S, P/V, VIA (if not done in the past) for cervical cancer screening and a TVS
- *Do basic investigations of:*
  - Complete blood count (CBC)
  - *Blood sugars:* Fasting (FBS) and postprandial (PPBS)
  - TSH
  - Lipid profile

This is a physiological phenomenon, and most women breeze through menopause without having any problems. But remember that they can develop problems later too, which might influence her quality of life. She could also develop other medical problems which can be diagnosed and effectively treated.

So, when a woman come to us in menopausal transition, assess her for any high-risk factors, which could influence her quality of life later on and these include the following:

- Assess her weight/height and calculate her BMI, which should be between 19 and 23 for Asians and between 20 and 25 for others.
- If she is overweight, advise her regarding lifestyle modifications such as weight-bearing exercises, regular aerobic exercises and a proper diet.
- Take a family history of osteoporosis or fragility fractures or other risk factors for osteoporosis.
- History of diabetes and hypertension
- History of previous fracture
- History of any drug intake
- Family or past history of chronic heart disease
- Any history of breast cancer in the family
- Pap smear, if not already done and then every year till the age of 50 years
- TVS, if not already done or if there is AUB
- There is no need to do FSH or hormonal levels for diagnosis of menopause.
- Advise BSE once a month
- Clinical breast examination (CBE) once a year
- Mammography 1–2 years after 40 years and every year after the age of 50 years.

Creating Awareness

The first step is creating awareness about the prevalence of problems related to menopause and their prevention, in women/in society as a whole. Awareness initiatives should focus on vasomotor symptoms, genitourinary symptoms, loss of muscle mass and bone mass, screening for the common cancers and the guidelines to be followed. Dedicated menopause clinics are the way forward.

Lifestyle Modifications

- Avoid smoking
- Avoid alcohol
- Calcium 1,200–1,500 mg/day, preferably from dietary sources
- Vitamin D 600 IU/day
- Exercise routines, including aerobic for cardio-respiratory/general fitness and weight-bearing/resistance training for sarcopenia and loss of BMD.

Prescription of Exercise

Exercise should be advised to all women to prevent osteoporosis/sarcopenia, for weight loss, for mood elevation and for better quality of sleep. By exercising regularly, flexibility and range of movement of joints are increased, with an added advantage of prevention of metabolic diseases such as diabetes, hypertension and CVD, adding to overall health benefits. Resistance and weight-bearing exercises under the care of a trainer initially and then by integrating into lifestyle modifications would go a long way in preventing osteoporosis and sarcopenia **(Fig. 9)**.

Exercise can be:

- Aerobic exercises such as walking, dancing, cycling and treadmill every day for cardiorespiratory benefits
- Strength training and resistance training two to three times a week

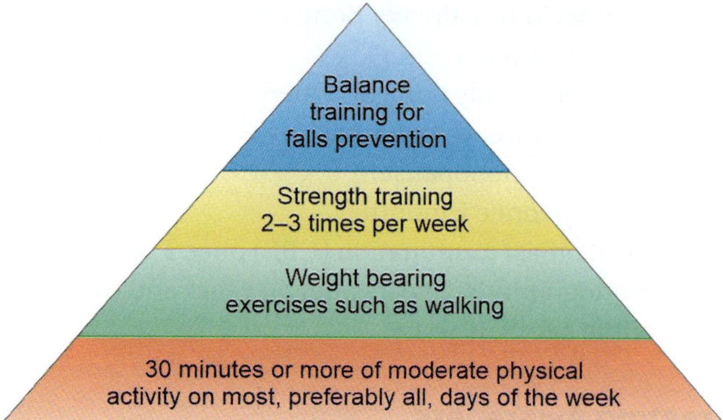

Fig. 9: Global recommendations: physical activity in middle-aged and older adults (50+ years of age).

- Balance training like Tai Chi
- Flexibility and endurance with yoga.

Informed Consent for Menopausal Hormone Therapy

This is an era of informed choice by the patient. They deserve to know the benefits and the uncertainties regarding any form of therapy. The clinician's role is to provide the necessary facts based on available evidence, so as to help them decide for or against it.

Before initiating therapy, women should undergo a complete health evaluation, including a comprehensive history, physical examination and mammography. Other specific examinations, such as bone densitometry, should be considered on an individual basis.

Women should be informed about the concerns regarding MHT in the light of various studies such as Women's Health Initiative (WHI), HERS and Million Women Study.

Advantages of Menopausal Hormone Therapy

Women must also be informed about the benefits of MHT. Documented benefits of MHT not directly related to menopausal symptoms include the following:

- Significant reductions in hip, vertebral and total fractures with CEE/MPA
- Significant increases in spine and hip BMD with CEE/MPA
- Prevention of osteoporosis
- Cardioprotective effect, if started early
- Reductions in the risk of colorectal cancer
- Possible reduced risk of Alzheimer's disease/dementia.

VARIOUS TYPES OF HORMONAL AND NONHORMONAL PHARMACOLOGICAL AGENTS AVAILABLE

Natural Oestrogens

Numerous natural oestrogen preparations are available, the principle products being oestradiol, oestrone and oestriol in that order of potency.

- Oestradiol is the most physiological oestrogen, since it is the predominant circulating oestrogen in the premenopausal reproductive age grouped women.
- Oestrone is less potent than oestradiol. Both oestradiol and oestrone have been demonstrated to be cardioprotective and osteoprotective.
- Oestriol is a least potent natural oestrogen that has not yet been shown to be cardioprotective and osteoprotective but has a good local action on genitourinary structures and also controls vasomotor symptoms.

Semisynthetic Oestrogens

Because native steroids are relatively water insoluble, modifications of oestrogens for oral administration and GI absorption includes conjugated oestrogens (oestrone sulphate, oestradiol valerate and conjugated equine oestrogen) and micronised oestrogens (micronised oestradiol).

- *Oestradiol valerate:* It is a natural human source of oestrogen, which is chemically synthesised, provides rapid relief from climacteric symptoms, prevents postmenopausal osteoporosis, and cardiovascular risks. Bioavailability is good. Only 3% is sufficient to exert effect on target organ.
- Micronisation of oestradiol results in good levels of systemic oestrogens, although it is rapidly metabolised to oestrone and conjugated to oestrone-3-glucuronide in the liver.

Synthetic Oestrogens

Ethinyl oestradiol, quinestrol and diethylstilbestrol, although used in contraceptives and other indications are not used in MHT because of their increased potency and extended half-life. A regimen for hormone administration is given in **Table 3**.

- Oral and nonoral MHT regimens (such as transdermal oestradiol) have an equivalent effect on relieving symptoms of oestrogen deficiency, such as hot flashes, vulvovaginal atrophy and loss of BMD.

TABLE 3: Method of hormone administration.

Regimen	*Oestrogen*	*Progestogen*
Oestrogen only	Everyday	Not used
Combined sequential	Everyday	1st–14th day or 13th–25th of every month
Continuous combined	Everyday	Everyday
Seasonal	Everyday	Last 14 days/every 3rd month

- Combination of CEE 0.625 mg (conjugated equine oestrogen) with MPA 2.5 mg is as effective as CEE 0.3 mg/MPA 1.5 mg.
- Now combined patches of oestrogen and progestogen are available for women with intact uterus, and there is no need to supplement oral progestogens. A combined transdermal patch containing norethisterone acetate 0.25 mg/day and 17 beta oestradiol 50 µg/day is available. Transdermal MHT has favourable effect on total HDL cholesterol and triglycerides and no potentially adverse effect on glucose and insulin levels, in contrast to oral therapy. The efficacy of low dose of oestrogens has been well studied.

Some new preparations are also available in the market with oestradiol as the oestrogenic component. The dosage could be 2 mg/day to as low as 0.5 mg/day. If patient is hysterectomised, then there is no need to add a progestogen. But if patient has an intact uterus, then progestogens should be added for endometrial protection.

Disadvantages of oral route are:
- Increased VTE risk
- Adverse lipid changes
- Hepatic side effects
- Gastrointestinal irritation
- Peaks and troughs in plasma levels of hormones

Dosage of Oestrogens for Hot Flushes

Conjugated equine or synthesised conjugated oestrogens (0.3–0.625 mg)
- Micronised 17β-oestradiol for oral administration (0.5–1 mg) or injection
- Transdermal oestradiol (25–100 µg)
- Ethinyl oestradiol (0.01–0.02 mg)
- Topically applied oestradiol emulsion, gel and spray
- Vaginal oestrogenic preparations, including a vaginal oestradiol ring and creams of CEE and oestradiol.

Hormone Delivery System

Additional investigations are required to clarify differences between various hormone delivery systems.

Since transdermal oestrogen bypasses first-pass metabolism in the liver, the transdermal delivery system achieves therapeutic concentrations in a steadier and smoother manner.

Transdermal route also facilitates the use of lower doses than are required with oral route, with the benefit of reducing the potential for adverse effects.

Transdermal delivery system is available as patches, gels, creams and now as spray too.

Transdermal gels and sprays do not cause irritation as with transdermal patch.

Intranasal oestradiol preparations are also available

Subcutaneous oestrogen pellets too are an option, except that they require an office visit every 3–6 months.

Transvaginal Route

Drugs available as:
- *Vaginal creams*: Creams are available and does provide local benefits at the site of application.
- Oestradiol ring releases 8 mg oestradiol per 24 hours, at a constant rate. The ring is easy to insert and remove, as it is soft and flexible. Each ring is to be used continuously for 90 days and is well-tolerated giving significant relief from vaginal dryness, itching, dyspareunia and dysuria.
- Vaginal tablets of oestradiol are also available.
- All low-dose vaginal oestrogen preparations available are equally effective. The choice of treatment should therefore be individualised based on clinical experience and patient preference.
- Oestrogen cream is usually applied at a dose of 2–4 g/day for 2 weeks, and the dose is lowered to the minimum needed to give symptomatic relief.
- The sustained-release oestradiol ring needs to be replaced every 90 days.
- The oestradiol tablet is usually inserted into the posterior fornix once daily for 2 weeks, and the dose is then decreased to twice weekly.

Local oestrogen therapy is extremely effective and is the preferred mode of therapy for symptoms of vaginal atrophy, though it is not of use in vasomotor symptoms and for bone health.

Vaginal oestrogen therapy reduces vaginal pH by restoring lactobacilli.

Vaginal atrophy due to drugs such as gonadotrophin-releasing agonists/antagonists, aromatase inhibitors and selective oestrogen receptor modulators can also be managed with vaginal oestrogens. Local oestrogen therapy should be considered immediately following pelvic irradiation to stimulate epithelial regeneration.

When low-dose oestrogen is administered locally for vaginal atrophy, progestogens are generally not indicated. Data are insufficient to recommend annual endometrial surveillance in asymptomatic women using vaginal oestrogen therapy.

Vaginal oestrogen therapy should be continued as long as women continue to have distressing symptoms. Management of vaginal atrophy is similar for the group of women without a cancer history and for women treated for nonhormone-dependent cancers. However, for women with a history of hormone-dependent cancer, management recommendations are individualised and vary based on the patient's preference, in consultation with her oncologist.

Overall, subjective improvement occurs in 80–90% of women treated with local vaginal oestrogens.

USE OF PROGESTERONES IN MENOPAUSAL HORMONE THERAPY

Progesterone generation by the ovaries comes to a stop at menopause. Hence, the need to replace progesterone, along with oestrogen. Currently, progesterones are viewed as endometrial protective agents. They are also used as progesterone-only pills in perimenopause and for control of AUB in anovulatory cycles. As per the current evidence, progesterone has to be co-prescribed along with oestrogen in MHT, in all women with an intact uterus.

Issues related to progesterone use are patient's intolerance and the adverse effects on lipid profile and the breast. With the advent of natural progesterones and newer drug delivery systems, we are able to bypass the first-pass effect on the liver and reduce the rates of intolerance. We propose here a novel scoring system to help the gynaecologist tailor MHT to the individual woman's need.

The currently available compounds are:

- *Natural progesterones:* Natural micronised progesterone
- *Progesterone analogues:*
  - Dydrogesterone
  - Hydroxyprogesterone
  - Medroxyprogesterone acetate
- *Testosterone analogues:*
  - Norethisterone
  - Norgestrel
  - Levonorgestrel IUD
- *Newer synthetic:*
  - Desogestrel
  - Norgestimate
  - Gestodene
  - Halogenated progesterone
  - Cyproterone acetate (with antiandrogenic property)
  - Drospirenone (with antimineralocorticoid property)

Regimes of Progesterone Therapy

It has been given along with oestrogen regime **(Table 4)**.

The two main concerns are intolerance and adverse effects. Intolerance can be circumvented by assessing the

TABLE 4: Comparative doses of progesterone.

Types of progesterone	*mg available*	*Sequential minimum effective dose/day × 12 days/month*	*Combined continuous*
Dydrogesterone	10 mg	10 mg	5 mg
MPA	10 mg, 5 mg, 2.5 mg	5 mg	2.5 mg
Norethisterone	5 mg	1 mg	0.3 mg
Norethindrone	5 mg, 1 mg	2.5 mg	0.50 mg
Neogest	0.075 mg	0.150 mg	0.075 mg
Vaginal micronised	100, 200, 400 mg	200 mg	100 mg
Oral micronised	100, 200, 400 mg	300 mg	200 mg
Cyproterone acetate	50 mg, 1 mg	1 mg	—

(MPA: medroxyprogesterone acetate)

individual patient's symptoms, altering the preparation, tailoring the dose and choosing a nonoral route of administration.

Present Scenario of Hormone Therapy: Risks and Contraindications

Key Points

- There may be a small increase in breast cancer risk after several years of HT, although this continues to be debated.
- Progestogens added to the MHT regimen largely eliminate any increased risk of endometrial cancer. If hysterectomy has been done, then oestrogen can be given alone.
- The risk for VTE is increased approximately twofold in current, but not former users of MHT, although the absolute risk is still very low.
- Hormone therapy should be given for the shortest period of time, in the smallest dosage possible, for providing symptomatic relief only.

HORMONE THERAPY IN SPECIAL CIRCUMSTANCES

- *Gallbladder disease:* The risk of gallbladder disease (cholelithiasis and cholecystitis) and cholecystectomy is increased in women taking MHT. This effect was seen in women taking oestrogen only as well as oestrogen/progestin combination therapy. But after cholecystectomy, MHT can be safely taken.
- *Ovarian cancer:* There may be a weak association between the prolonged use of oestrogen and ovarian cancer, but no epidemiological evidence has been established.
- *Myocardial infarction:* There does not appear to be an overall effect on the rate of fatal myocardial infarction (MI) associated with an MHT regimen, although the EPT arm of the WHI trial noted an increase in the rate of nonfatal MI. The oestrogen-only arm did not show an increase in MI. MHT should not be used in known cases of MI, and if MI occurs in women on MHT, it should be stopped.
- *Alzheimer's disease and dementia:* An MHT initiated early seems significantly protective against development of Alzheimer's disease. A delayed start makes it less effective. Combined oestrogen and progestin and oral oestrogen alone increase the risk of Non-AD dementia, while transdermal oestrogen is not associated with dementia risk.
- *Colorectal cancer:* The WHI EPT arm confirmed that HT lowers the risk of developing colon cancer. The oestrogen-only arm did not show a reduction in colon cancer. However, HT should not be used solely for colon cancer prevention, and women taking HT still need colorectal cancer screening at the recommended intervals.

Contraindications to Hormone Therapy

- *Unexplained vaginal bleeding and pregnancy:* These are temporary but absolute contraindications to HT.
- *Past history of breast cancer or endometrial cancer:* While usually considered contraindications to MHT, short-term use for severe menopausal symptoms may be considered with proper precautions.

  An increasing number of younger women are being cured of breast cancer, and some of these women may require treatment for severe vasomotor symptoms or GSM. Short-term oral or transdermal MHT or vaginal oestrogens may be considered after consultation with an oncologist.

  Most oncologists agree that women with past history of stage I endometrial cancer that has been successfully treated may safely use MHT, if it is otherwise indicated.
- *Women with a past history of venous thrombosis* are at increased risk for recurrence; however, taking OCPs or MHT confers an overall low increase to this risk of recurrence.
- *Family history of premenopausal breast cancer*: In the Iowa Women's Health Study, there was no increased incidence of breast cancer in HT users with a family history of breast cancer, relative to those HT users without a family history of cancer.
- *Hypertriglyceridaemia*: Oral oestrogens are contraindicated in them because of the danger of precipitating pancreatitis. Transdermal oestrogens or vaginal oestrogens, which avoid the first-pass hepatic effect, do not carry this risk.
- *Chronic liver disease*: Oral MHT is a relative contraindication. Again, transdermal and vaginal oestrogens avoid the first-pass hepatic effect of oral HT.
- *HT is not contraindicated* in those clinical settings where many practitioners have often been reluctant (often unjustifiably so) to recommend oral contraceptives.

(Remember that OCPs have much more potent oestrogenic effects than MHT and thus MHT is much safer). These conditions include:

- Endometriosis
- Fibrocystic breast changes
- Hypertension
- Mastalgia
- Migraine headache
- Obesity
- Tobacco use
- Uterine leiomyomata (fibroids).

Gonadomimetic Agents

A widely acting gonadomimetic hormone (with a combination of all oestrogenic, progestogenic and androgenic actions) known as tibolone is also included as a form of MHT. The pharmacological agent is not an oestrogen, progestogen or androgen. It is called STEAR (Selective Tissue Estrogen Activity Regulator).

Temporal Implications of Menopausal Hormone Therapy Use

The temporal implications of MHT use may be differentiated into the following patterns of use:

- Short-term MHT implies use for 2–3 years
- Long-term MHT implies use for >5 years (This is to be differentiated from long-cycle therapy)
- And now to add a multifocal aspect is:
  - *MHT relayed placement*: Where changes of the MHT types and forms are made over a period of time, shifting from the initial use of EPT to gonadomimetic use, to raloxifene and finally in some handing over to the nonhormonal agents or to vaginal oestriol.
- This placement of various therapies in a woman's postmenopausal lifespan with a view to maximising benefits and minimising risks of individual groups of hormones gives the women a reason to want to continue it over the long term.
- *Concomitant multiple hormone therapy*: Where simultaneous administration of some form of MHT takes place along with another MHT form (e.g. oestrogen) progestogen combined with raloxifene, oestradiol combined with oestriol or another route [e.g. oral estrogen-progestogen replacement therapy (EPRT) with vaginal oestriol].
- *Concomitant multimodal therapy*: When MHT is variably combined with another therapeutic modality (e.g. MHT with bisphosphonates and calcium, MHT with antioxidants, micronutrients, multivitamins and calcium). These combinations may need to be considered for maximal therapeutic outcomes. Hence, their duration of use would vary along with the risk-benefit connotations and choice of the individual woman.
- *Long-term intermittent therapeutic MHT*: Implies the use of 6–12 weekly EPRT or local vaginal ERT intermittently for recurring urogenital symptoms.

ANDROGENS IN MENOPAUSE

While no testosterone products have received FDA approval for treating symptoms of sexual dysfunction in women, some women may benefit from testosterone therapy. Now it is recommended that postmenopausal women may be candidates for testosterone therapy, if they complain of symptoms of decreased sexual desire associated with personal distress and are unable to identify another cause for their sexual concerns.

Foremost, other physical, psychological and emotional relationship factors that may influence sexual function must be ruled out.

Once other factors have been ruled out, the primary candidates for testosterone therapy are women with significant, near-total androgen depletion.

- These include women with loss of adrenal or ovarian function, which may be caused by Addison's disease or bilateral oophorectomy
- Women with premature ovarian failure of autoimmune origin and
- Women with Turner's syndrome who may also have abnormally low-androgen levels.

Testosterone is readily absorbed through the skin. While transdermal patches are currently available for use in men, these patches are not appropriately dosed for use in women. Patches delivering lower doses of testosterone ranging from 150 to 300 mg per day are currently being studied for use in women. Transdermal testosterone gels, creams and ointments have been approved in the United States for use in men. However, because these products deliver high doses, women may experience masculinising effects with their use. These formulations have not undergone rigorous trials and quality-control testing. Yet they are still not approved by FDA, for use in women. Since no testosterone preparations specifically meant for women are available in the market, transdermal gels used in men, are the ones which are being used in women too.

There is limited value in giving DHEA to healthy women. However, the potential of DHEA therapy given at a dose, which re-establishes levels found in the serum of normal young women to improve quality of life in premenopausal or postmenopausal women needs further exploration. This is particularly significant in light of the commercial availability of DHEA over the counter.

Phytoestrogens and isoflavones: Soy products or isoflavones, either through diet or supplementation, may not reduce the incidence of hot flashes. Inconsistencies among studies to date may be explained by different doses, products, sources and processing.

Herbal preparations and dietary supplements: Black cohosh, dong quai, evening primrose oil, flaxseed, ginseng, red clover and wild yam extract are commonly used but poorly studied.

So, to conclude, MHT is to be tailor-made according to the needs of perimenopausal or postmenopausal women and with informed consent and follow-up of these patients is must.

SUGGESTED READING

1. Ahuja, M. Age of menopause and determinants of menopause age: A PAN India survey by IMS. J. Midlife Health. 2016;7:126-31.
2. Chester RC, Kling JM, Manson JE. What the Women's Health Initiative has taught us about menopausal hormone therapy. Clin Cardiol. 2018;41(2):247-52.
3. Meeta M, Digumarti L, Agarwal N, Vaze N, Shah R, Malik S. Clinical Practice Guidelines on Menopause: *An Executive Summary and Recommendations: Indian Menopause Society 2019–2020. J Midlife Health. 2020;11(2):55-95.
4. Meher T, Sahoo H. Premature menopause among women in India: evidence from National Family Health Survey-IV. J Obstet Gynaecol Res. 2021;47:4426-39.
5. National Comprehensive Cancer Network (NCCN) guidelines for Screening in Breast Cancer (Updated in June 2024).
6. Sarri G, Pedder H, Dias S, Guo Y, Lumsden MA. Vasomotor symptoms resulting from natural menopause: a systematic review and network meta-analysis of treatment effects from the National Institute for Health and Care Excellence guideline on menopause. BJOG. 2017;124:1514-23.
7. The NAMS 2017 Hormone Therapy Position Statement Advisory Panel. The 2017 hormone therapy position statement of The North American Menopause Society. Menopause. 2017;24:728-53.
8. Zhu D, Chung HF, Dobson AJ, Pandeya N, Brunner EJ, Kuh D, et al. Type of menopause, age of menopause and variations in the risk of incident cardiovascular disease: pooled analysis of individual data from 10 international studies. Hum Reprod. 2020;35:1933-43.

60

CHAPTER

Hysterectomy and its Aftermath

Shashikala K Bhat, Muralidhar V Pai

Chapter Outline

- History
- Types of Hysterectomy
- Preoperative Preparation
- Abdominal Hysterectomy—Operative Steps
- Minimally Invasive Hysterectomy Procedures
- Total Laparoscopic Hysterectomy in Special Situations
- Vaginal Hysterectomy
- Complications of Hysterectomy

INTRODUCTION

Hysterectomy is one of the most frequently performed gynaecological surgeries, with over 90% of cases conducted for benign conditions and approximately 9.8% for malignancies. The primary indications include fibroids, menorrhagia and prolapse, accounting for nearly 70% of cases. It varies between countries ranging from 11.35% in India to 21.1% in the United States. However, in recent times, the incidence of emergency peripartum hysterectomy was 1.1 cases per 1,000 births. With the increasing adoption of minimally invasive techniques, the abdominal approach is now predominantly reserved for more complex cases or when complications are anticipated. Compared to traditional open surgeries, minimally invasive hysterectomies offer significant benefits, including reduced postoperative pain, faster recovery and shorter hospital stays.

HISTORY

In the early days, hysterectomy was considered a hazardous procedure, with a high mortality rate among patients. However, advancements in anaesthesia, antibiotics, blood transfusion and antisepsis transformed it into a much safer operation. From 1900 to 1940, subtotal hysterectomy, which involved leaving the cervix intact, was the most commonly performed technique. In 1929, Richardson performed the first total abdominal hysterectomy, marking a significant milestone. By the early 1950s, total hysterectomy had gained popularity, gradually replacing the subtotal approach.

TYPES OF HYSTERECTOMY

Hysterectomy is primarily performed for gynaecological reasons, though it is occasionally indicated for obstetric conditions as well. The procedure can be executed through various approaches: Abdominal, vaginal, laparoscopic or robotic. Abdominal hysterectomy is done by opening the abdomen, which may take a few weeks to heal. Removing the uterus through the vagina has fewer complications and early recovery from surgery. Keyhole laparoscopic surgeries are aesthetic with less postoperative pain. The choice between a simple or radical hysterectomy depends on whether the condition is benign or malignant. A subtotal hysterectomy involves removing only the uterine corpus while retaining the cervix, whereas a total hysterectomy entails the removal of both the uterine corpus and cervix. In premenopausal women, bilateral salpingectomy is often performed alongside hysterectomy, while bilateral oophorectomy is more common in postmenopausal women or when the ovaries are diseased in premenopausal women. Classic intrafascial supracervical hysterectomy (CISH) is preferred in those without malignancy and provides better support for the vaginal stump by preserving the endopelvic fascia. In intrafascial hysterectomy too, less urinary tract and bowel injury occur, and the anatomic relationship between the endopelvic fascia and vagina is preserved. In contrast, the extent of extrafascial hysterectomy varies by class (I, II, III, IVand V) or degree of dissection of the ureters, uterine artery and resection of the uterosacral and cardinal ligaments, as well as the upper portion of the vagina (Piver–Rutledge–Smith classification). The Querleu–Morrow classification is based on the lateral extent of resection of paracervix and dorsal and ventral parametrium. The extent of radical hysterectomy must, therefore, justify the curative surgery and is more commonly associated with complications of bladder and bowel dysfunction.

There are many types of hysterectomy based on the extent of tissues removed, as shown in **Figure 1**.

Based on the structures dissected and excised in onco-hysterectomies, the classification is shown in **Table 1**.

PREOPERATIVE PREPARATION

Patients should be counselled regarding the indication for hysterectomy after thorough clinical evaluation and investigations. Alternatives to hysterectomy should always be discussed, and the merits and demerits of each option

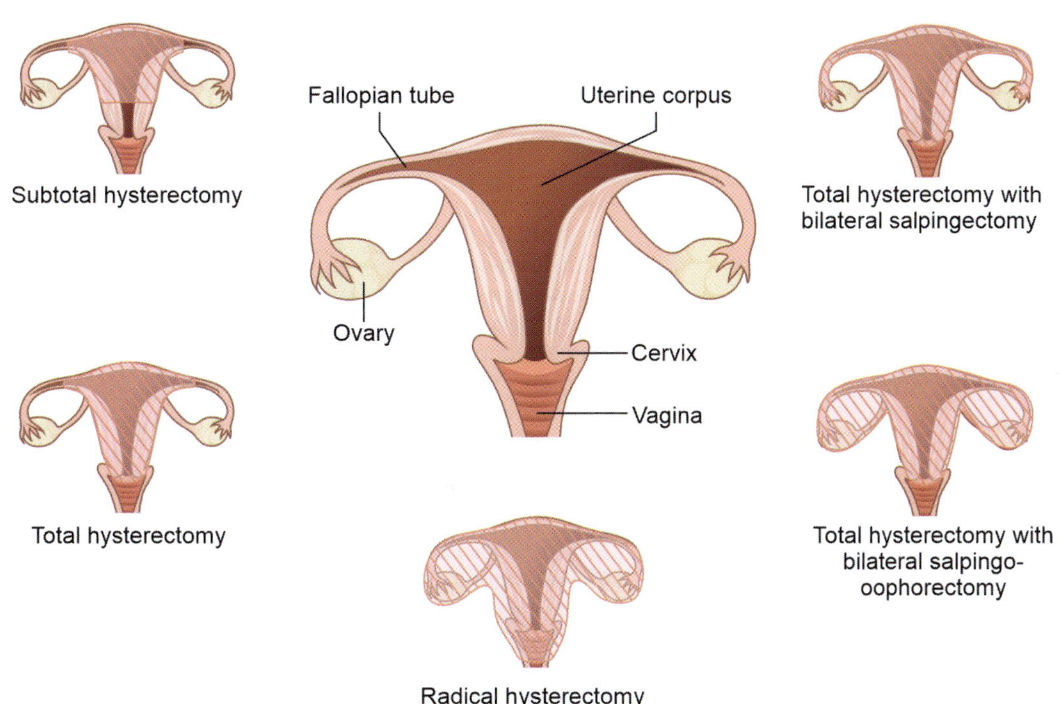

Fig. 1: Types of hysterectomy.

TABLE 1: Classes of hysterectomy.

	Piver–Rutledge–Smith		***EORTC-GCG***		***Querleu and Morrow***
Class I	*Extrafascial hysterectomy* The identification of the ureters is accomplished by maintaining transparency and preventing injury, thereby keeping them outside the operator's field without the need for dissection. The uterine artery is laterally sectioned and ligated. The uterosacral and cardinal ligaments remain intact, and no part of the vagina is excised	Type I	*Simple hysterectomy*	Type A	*Extrafascial hysterectomy* The ureters should be identified and palpated without dissecting the ureteral layer. The uterine arteries, uterosacral ligaments and cardinal ligaments should be resected as close to the uterus as possible. Additionally, a vaginal portion as small as possible (<10 mm) should be removed

Contd...

Contd...

	Piver–Rutledge–Smith		***EORTC-GCG***			***Querleu and Morrow***
Class II	*Modified radical hysterectomy (Wertheim)* The ureters are carefully dissected in the paracervical region without resecting them from the pubovesical ligament. The uterine arteries are meticulously sectioned beside and medial to the ureter. The uterosacral ligaments are excised midway from their sacral insertion. The cardinal ligaments are resected up to their medial half. Subsequently, the upper third of the vagina is removed, followed by a pelvic lymphadenectomy	Type II	*Modified radical hysterectomy* The ureters are carefully dissected up to the point at which they enter the bladder. The uterine arteries are precisely sectioned and ligated at the medial half of the parametrium. The proximal uterosacral ligament is resected, and the medial half of the cardinal ligaments is excised. Additionally, 1–2 cm from the upper portion of the vagina is removed	Type B	B1	The procedure involves deperitonising the ureters and rolling them to the lateral side. Additionally, there is partial resection of the uterosacral and vesicouterine ligaments. The paracervical tissue is sectioned at the ureteral tunnel level. A minimum of 10 mm of the vagina is measured from the cervix or the tumour *without the removal of the lateral paracervical lymph nodes*
					B2	The surgical procedure involves deperitonising the ureters and rolling them to the lateral side. It also includes a partial resection of the uterosacral and vesicouterine ligaments, as well as the sectioning of paracervical tissue at the level of the ureteral tunnel. The measurement of at least 10 mm of the vagina from the cervix or the tumour is taken, and the *lateral paracervical lymph nodes are removed*
Class III	*Classical radical hysterectomy (Meigs)* The following procedures were performed: • Complete dissection of the ureters and pubovesical ligaments, except for a small part where the umbilical bladder artery is situated, to the level of their penetration into the bladder • The uterine arteries were cutoff at the origin of the hypogastric region (umbilical bladder) • The uterosacral ligaments were excised at their sacral insertion • The cardinal ligaments were resected as close to the pelvic wall as possible • Removal of the upper half of the vagina • Routine pelvic lymphadenectomy	Type III	*Radical hysterectomy* The procedure involves extensive removal of the uterosacral ligaments, resection of the parametrium in close proximity to the pelvic wall, ligation of the uterine vessels at their origin, and removal of one-third of the upper vagina	Type C	C1	The surgical procedure involves the following steps: • Complete mobilisation of the ureters • Cutting the uterosacral ligaments at the level of the rectum • Cutting the vesicouterine ligaments at the level of the bladder • Complete removal of paracervical tissue • Resection of 15–20 mm of tissue from the vagina towards the cervix or tumour, including the corresponding paracolpos • *Preservation of the autonomic nerves*
					C2	The surgical procedure involves the following steps: • Full mobilisation of the ureters • Cutting of the uterosacral ligaments at the level of the rectum

Contd...

Contd...

	Piver–Rutledge–Smith		***EORTC-GCG***		***Querleu and Morrow***	
						• Cutting of the vesicouterine ligaments at the level of the bladder • Complete removal of paracervical tissue • Resection of 15–20 mm from the vagina towards the cervix or tumour and the corresponding paracolpos • *No preservation of the autonomic nerves*
Class IV	It differs from the previous class in the following aspects, which make it more radical: Complete dissection of the ureter from the pubovesical ligament, sacrifice of the umbilical-vesical artery, and removal of 3/4 of the upper vagina	Type IV	*Extended radical hysterectomy* Similar to type III but with the removal of ¾ of the vagina and paravaginal tissue counterpart	Type D	D1	*The paracervical tissue will be completely resected up to the pelvic bone wall, inclusive of the hypogastric vessels, with the exposure of the sciatic nerve roots. The ureter is fully mobile*
					D2	*Full resection of the paracervical tissue up to the pelvic bone wall, along with the hypogastric vessels, exposing the sciatic nerve roots; ureter fully mobile; resection of muscles and adjacent fascia*
Class V	The procedure is more radical than other methods, as it involves the excision of a portion of the ureter or bladder that is invaded, followed by the reimplantation of the ureter into the bladder	Type V	• Partial pelvectomy • Terminal ureter, bladder or rectum is resected with the uterus and parametrium (supralevatorial)			

(EORTC: European Organisation for Research and Treatment of Cancer; GCG: Gynaecological Cancer Group)

should be explained. After the decision of surgery is taken, preoperative blood and urine tests, chest X-ray, serology, etc. are done. Cardiac and preanaesthetic evaluations are done, and associated illnesses such as diabetes mellitus are appropriately treated. Anaemia should be corrected too. As most hysterectomies are elective procedures, adequate preoperative management of comorbid illnesses results in better surgical outcomes.

ABDOMINAL HYSTERECTOMY—OPERATIVE STEPS

The patient is placed in the dorsal lithotomy position, and pelvic examination is performed with the patient under anaesthesia. A Foley catheter is inserted in the bladder for drainage. The patient is then placed in dorsal supine position for the procedure. The choice of incision is determined by the need of exposure, potential need to enlarge the incision, location of previous surgical scars, cosmesis of the healed incision and surgery for gynaecological malignancies.

Midline incisions are preferred for malignant disease; for benign diseases, the Pfannenstiel incision is an adequate alternative to the midline incision **(Fig. 2)**. Reported advantages include better cosmetic results, less pain and low incidence of hernia formation. On the other hand, transverse incision limits exploration of the upper

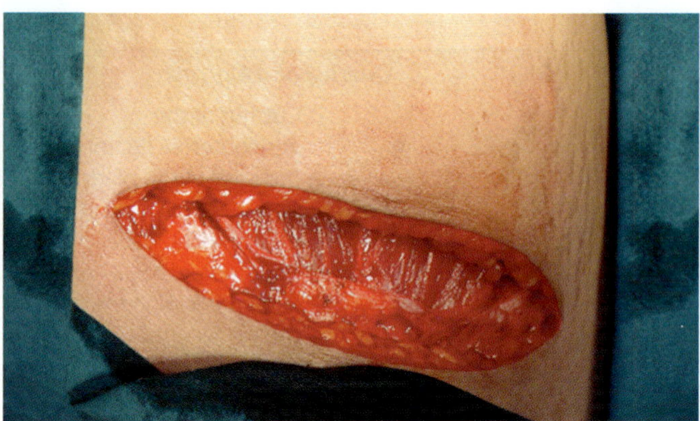

Fig. 2: Pfannenstiel incision.

abdomen. Also, they are associated with a risk of greater blood loss and haematoma formation when compared with a midline incision. Nerve injury, which can result in paraesthesia of the overlying skin, is more frequent in a transverse incision compared with a midline incision.

When the bowel has been packed away and exposure to the pelvis is satisfactory, the round ligaments and utero-ovarian ligaments are grasped with a clamp on each side. The uterus is deviated towards left side; this puts right round ligament on stretch. They are clamped, cut and ligated. The small artery of Sampson's runs under the round ligament and in many cases, transilluminating the area allows the surgeon to easily visualise the artery and be sure that the suture is passed under it, so that the artery will be ligated. The same is repeated on other side. This separates anterior and posterior leaves of broad ligament.

By extending the incision cephalad on the posterior leaf of broad ligament, ureters are traced. The ureter is identified crossing the common iliac artery, which should be left attached to the medial leaf of broad ligament to protect its blood supply.

If the ovary and tubes are to be left in situ, a window in the peritoneum beneath the fallopian tube between the uterus and ovary is created. The tube and the utero-ovarian ligament are divided, and the pedicle ligated as previously noted with a free tie is followed by a suture ligature. If ovaries are to be removed, the peritoneal opening is enlarged extended superiorly lateral to the ovary and parallel with the infundibulopelvic ligament. A hole in the peritoneum is created between the ureter and ovarian vessels superior to the ovary under direct vision. The infundibulopelvic ligament on each side is clamped, divided and doubly ligated using delayed absorbable sutures.

The next step is a dissection of bladder from anterior cervix. The vesicoperitoneal fold is opened, and the fine filmy attachments of the bladder to the pubovesicocervical fascia are visible. The bladder can be dissected from the lower uterine segment of the uterus and cervix by either blunt or sharp dissection. Once the bladder has been freed from the anterior cervix, the uterine vessels are skeletonised.

Heaney clamp is placed perpendicular to the uterine artery at the junction of the cervix and body of uterus. The vessels are ligated and cut. The same procedure is repeated on the opposite side.

Once the bladder anteriorly and rectum posteriorly have been freed from the cervix, the uterus is placed on tension exposing the deeper portion of broad ligament and pulling the lower uterine segment away from the ureter. The cardinal and uterosacral ligaments are clamped and cut inside the vaginal cuff and ligated. Usually, the vault of the vagina is opened at one angle while cutting these pedicles off or if not, it is deliberately opened, extended on both sides, and uterus is removed. The angles of vagina are closed with 'figure-of-eight' sutures, which include the fascial cuff. The vaginal vault is closed by interrupted sutures or can be left open to heal secondarily where a running locking suture is used for haemostasis along the cuff edge. In the classic Richardson technique, the peritoneum over the posterior cervix is divided, the peritoneum is dissected off the cul-de-sac and the uterosacral ligaments are also clamped separately and subsequently attached to the vaginal cuff for support.

MINIMALLY INVASIVE HYSTERECTOMY PROCEDURES

Kurt Semm, from Germany, first described the use of laparoscopy for performing hysterectomy in 1984. However, the first laparoscopic hysterectomy was performed by Harry Reich in Pennsylvania in 1984 using bipolar and scissors. Thereafter, the technique got refined with the availability of modern gadgets.

Classification and nomenclature of laparoscopic hysterectomy is inconsistent, and literature describes a wide range of spectrum, including laparoscopically assisted vaginal hysterectomy and total laparoscopic hysterectomy. Laparoscopic subtotal or supracervical hysterectomy such as CISH, laparoscopic-assisted vaginal hysterectomy (LAVH), total laparoscopic hysterectomy (TLH), transvaginal natural orifice transluminal endoscopic surgery (V-NOTES) and robotic-assisted total hysterectomy (RAH) is some types of minimally invasive hysterectomy. One of the classifications designed by Munro and Parker was based on the degree of dissection of structures done laparoscopically.

Operative Steps

The first and most important step in laparoscopic hysterectomy is the port placement either by creating pneumoperitoneum or direct trocar insertion into the peritoneal cavity without pneumoperitoneum. Pneumoperitoneum can be created by various techniques using a Veress needle. The present evidence, however, supports direct trocar entry over using a Veress needle. The use of Veress needle was associated with an increased incidence of failed entry, extraperitoneal insufflation and omental injury. Direct trocar entry is, therefore, a safer closed-entry technique. A recent Cochrane review also advocates a direct trocar entry against Veress entry. Hasson's open method of accessing technique is very useful in patients with previous abdominal surgeries.

In case of previous abdominal surgery with suspected adhesions, Lee–Huang point or Palmer point can be utilised for entry. If Veress needle is utilised, correct placement can be checked by aspiration test, bubble test or checking the pressures, which should be <10 mm Hg.

Port Placement

- Usually, one primary part of 10 mm for the optical trocar and three secondary ports of 5 mm are used. The primary port is usually insufflated at the umbilicus in normal size uterus. If the uterus is large, then primary camera port is inserted supraumbilically. While introducing the primary port, the patient should be straight and table should be at the lowest height for perfect control.
- The second port is placed 2 cm above and medial to anterosuperior spine on the left side.
- The third port is placed to a palm distance from the second port on the left midclavicular line.
- The fourth port is a mirror image of the third port.

Uterine Manipulator

After the patient is put in position, anterior lip of the cervix is held, and the uterine is sounded to determine the length and direction of the uterine cavity. The uterine manipulator is placed to aid the mobility of the uterus and traction, thereby providing better visibility of the structures within the abdominal cavity.

Division of Round Ligament

The round ligament is held 2–3 cm medial to the pelvic attachment, cauterised, and cut **(Figs. 3A to C)**.

Opening of the Anterior Leaf of Broad Ligament and Vesicouterine Fold of Peritoneum

Both the leaflets of broad ligament are separated, and the anterior leaf of the board ligament is coagulated and cut on both sides from the round ligament till vesicouterine peritoneal reflection.

Opening Posterior Leaf of Broad Ligament

The posterior leaf of broad ligament is dissected and cut towards the uterosacral ligament. The uterine pedicles are, thus, skeletonised. The same is repeated on the opposite side.

Division of Tubo-ovarian Ligament

When ovaries are to be preserved, the tubo-ovarian ligament is coagulated and cut. It is prudent to stay at least 2 cm away from the uterus to avoid medial oozing.

Separation of Uterovesical Fold of Peritoneum and Dissecting Vesicovaginal Space

The uterus is pushed cephalad and by using atraumatic forceps, the peritoneum and bladder are held in the middle. The uterovesical fold of peritoneum is then cut perpendicular to the uterus and dissected down to create a clear vesicovaginal space **(Figs. 4A and B)**. This is called central technique. But in case of previous caesarean section, where the bladder is densely adherent to the uterus, the lateral technique is employed by identifying the space of Sethe.

Ligating the Uterine Vessels

The uterus is pushed to the opposite side, and the uterine vessels are cauterised and cut perpendicular to the vessels **(Figs. 5A to C)**. Alternatively, uterine artery ligation can be done **(Figs. 6A and B)**. In malignancies, uterine artery is clipped at its origin **(Figs. 7A to C)**. The pericervical space at the level of coagulated uterine vessel is incised, and clear intrafascial plane is created. The bladder anteriorly and rectum posteriorly should be separated from the cervix.

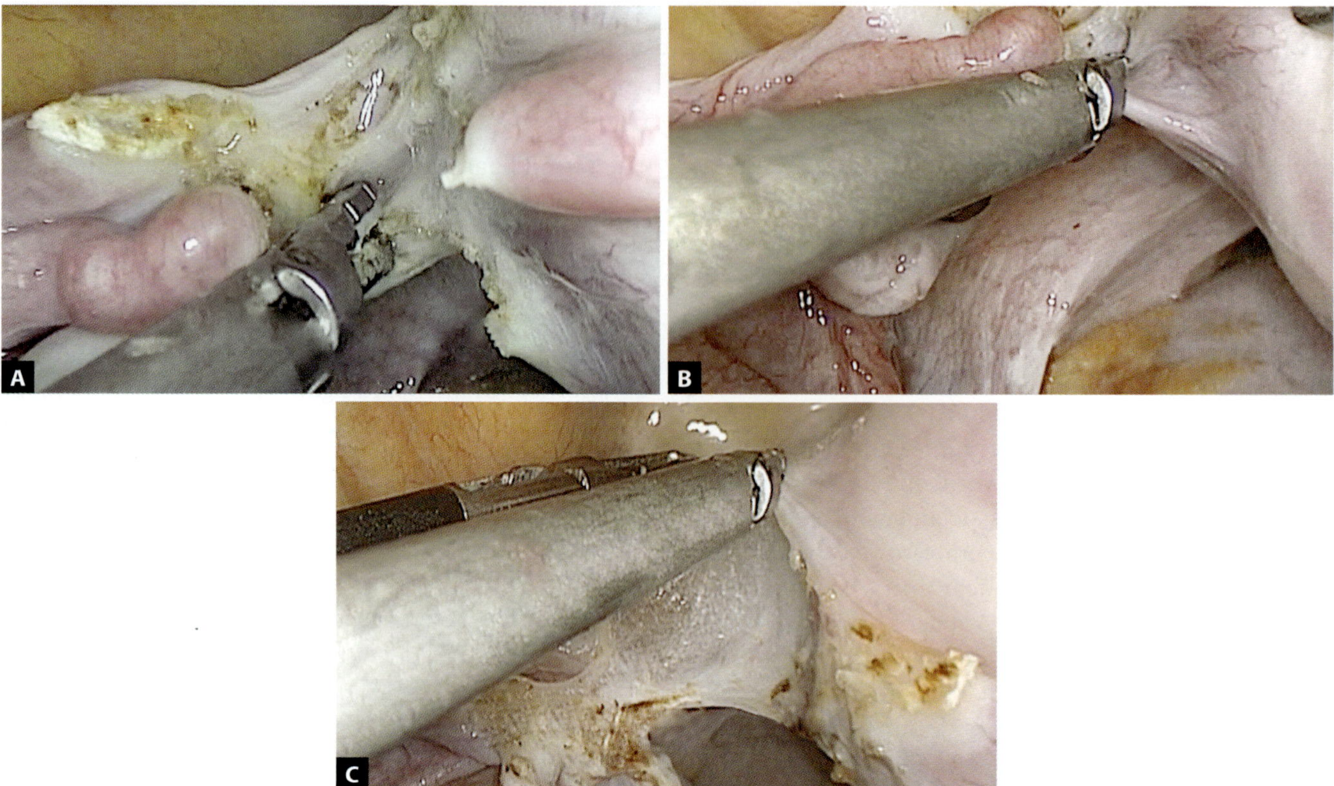

Figs. 3A to C: Division of round ligament and opening of anterior and posterior leaves of broad ligament.

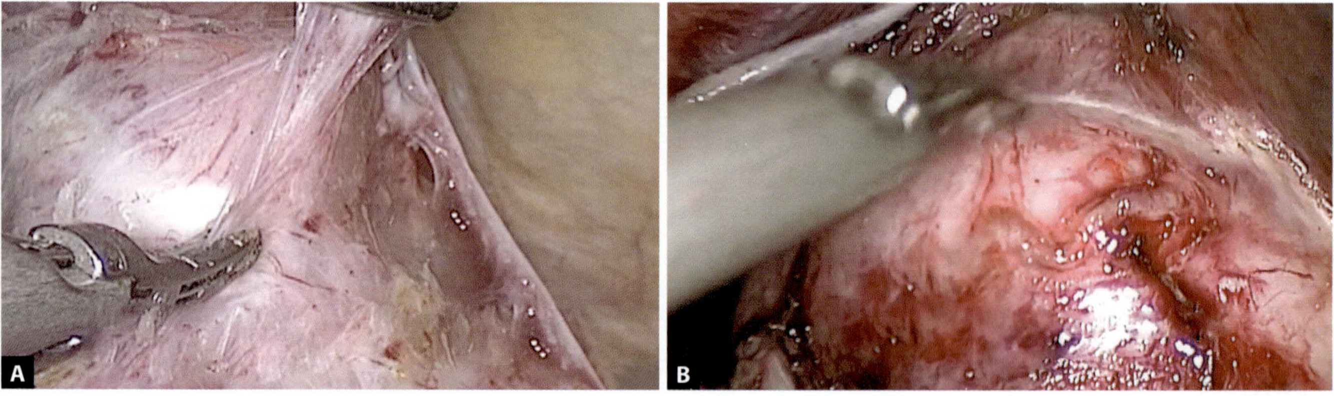

Figs. 4A and B: (A) Uterovesical fold separation by central approach; (B) Bladder dissection from the lower uterine segment.

The uterus is placed on tension to expose the ureter clearly **(Fig. 8)**. The cervicovaginal ligament and uterosacral ligament are coagulated and sectioned.

Opening the Vault

The uterus is pushed cephalad; the cup of the uterine manipulator is pushed up, which will demarcate the fornices and using either a monopolar hook or harmonic scalpel, the vault is opened along the rim of the cup **(Figs. 9A to C)**. The incision is extended laterally and posteriorly by manipulating the uterus. The uterosacral ligament is separated at its attachment to the uterus, thereby maintaining the integrity of the vault.

Separation of Infundibulopelvic Ligament

If the ovaries are to be removed, the infundibulopelvic ligament is cauterised and cut at the end of the surgery to prevent dangling of the tissues and interfering during the

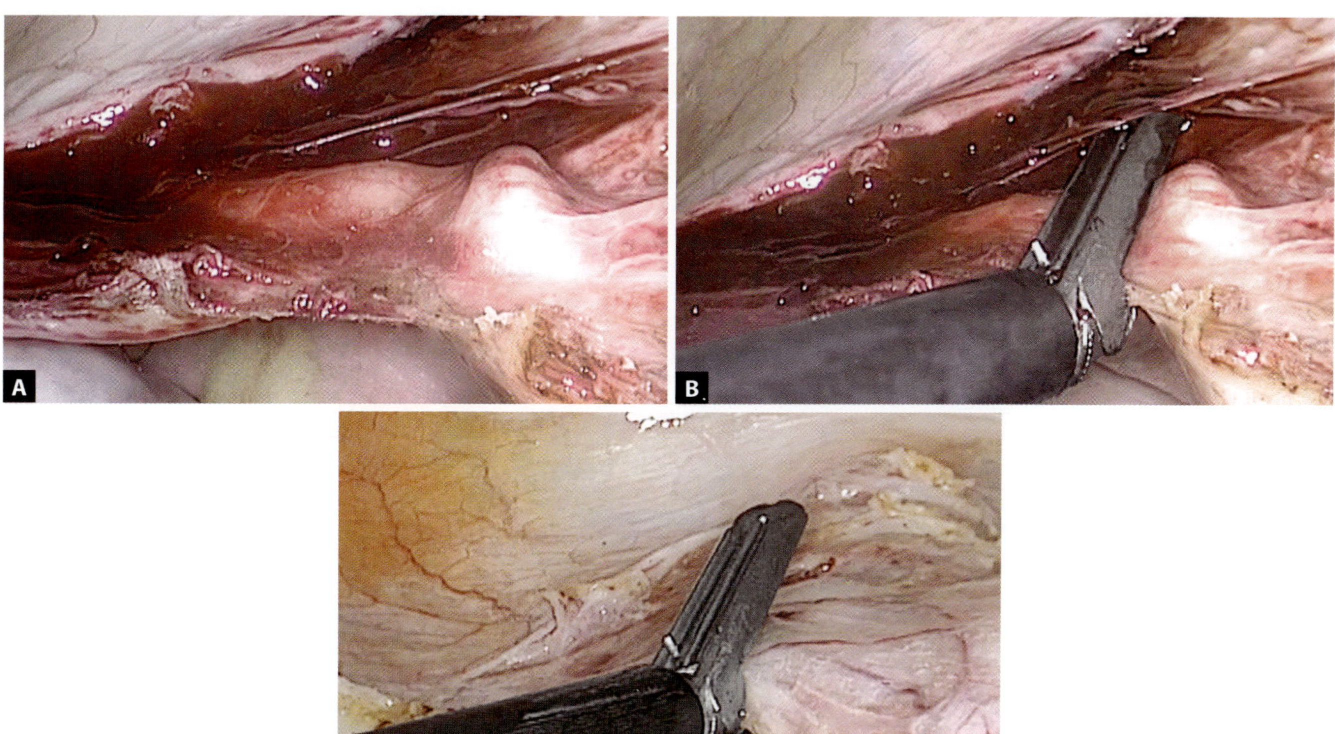

Figs. 5A to C: Skeletonisation of uterine artery and cautery.

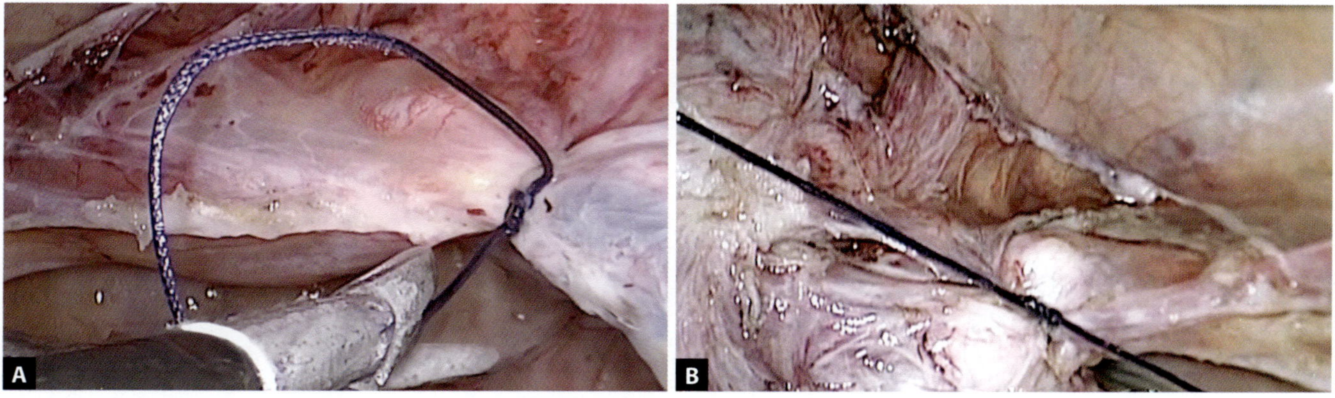

Figs. 6A and B: Uterine artery ligation.

procedure. The ligament is cauterised and cut close to the ovary by giving gentle traction on the ovary medially.

Extraction of Specimen

The entire specimen is now pushed vaginally. In case the uterus is very large, then either morcellation of the uterus using a morcellator or reducing the bulk of the uterus by bisecting or lateral coring technique can be performed to deliver the specimen.

Closure of Vault

Vault can be sutured either by interrupted suture as single or double layers using Vicryl (polyglactin 910) or barbed sutures **(Fig. 10)**. The initial step on the vault should incorporate the uterosacral ligament to prevent vault prolapse. A thorough suction and irrigation are done to check for any bleeding.

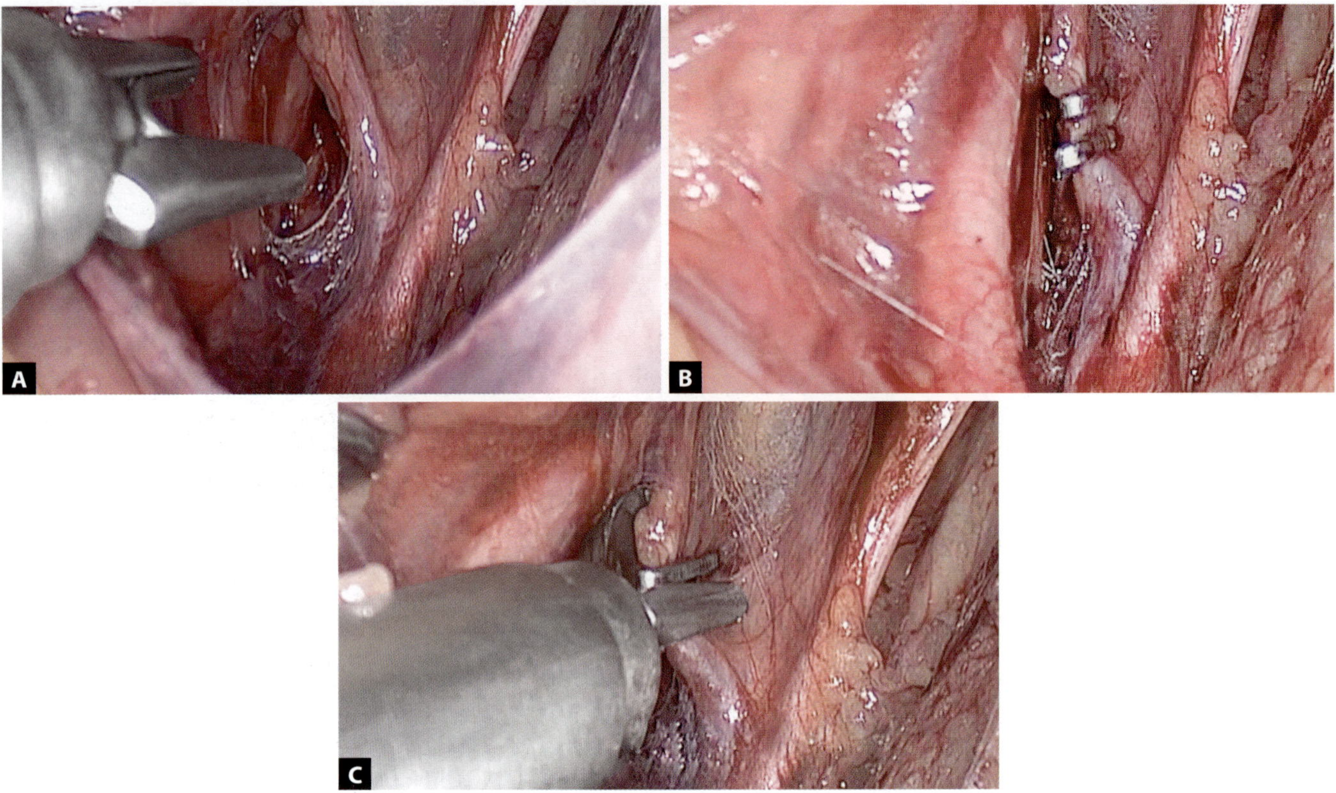

Figs. 7A to C: Clipping the uterine artery at origin.

Port Closure

Finally, pneumoperitoneum is let out, and port sites are closed. All ports should be closed. A 5-mm port can be closed with simple sutures or tissue adhesives. Those ports sized >5 mm may require additional suturing of rectus sheath to prevent complications.

TOTAL LAPAROSCOPIC HYSTERECTOMY IN SPECIAL SITUATIONS

Indications

- Large uterus
- Previous multiple abdominal surgeries
- Endometriosis
- Obese women

Special steps to be taken:

- Preoperative ureteric stenting can be done in frozen pelvis due to endometriosis.
- Certain technical modifications need to be done such as placement of the port at Lee-Huang point or Palmer point.
- Ligation of uterine artery at the origin can be done.

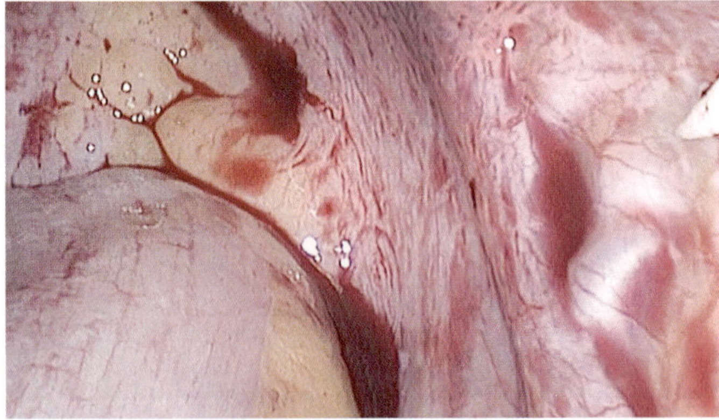
Fig. 8: Placing the uterus under tension to expose the ureter.

- Using lateral window technique in case of previous caesarean section with dense bladder adhesions
- Using both the myoma screw and the uterine manipulator with long tip for retractions

VAGINAL HYSTERECTOMY

Vaginal hysterectomy has been proved and accepted to be superior to the abdominal route, and the surgical

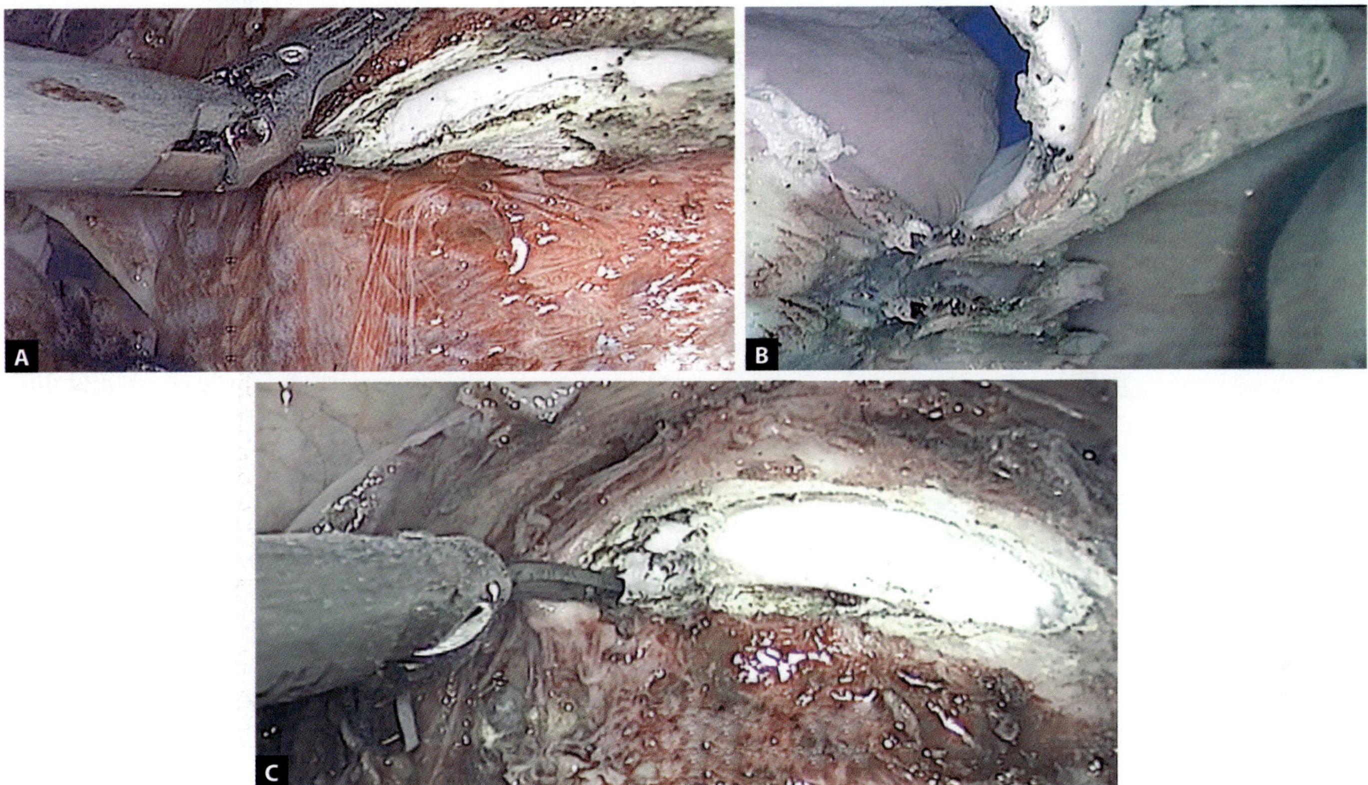

Figs. 9A to C: Colpotomy.

art and skill of vaginal hysterectomy is the hallmark of a gynaecologist. The first vaginal hysterectomy was performed by Langenbeck in 1813.

Operative Steps

The anterior and posterior lips of the cervix are held with two tenaculi; a circular incision is given around the cervix about 5 mm away from the os. Infiltration of saline beneath the cervicovaginal junction aids in hydrodissection and minimising the blood loss. The right place of dissection is identified, and the vaginal wall is separated from cervix. In case of prolapse uterus, circular incision is made around the cervix and extended upwards and towards the external urethral orifice. The vaginal flaps are then mobilised laterally away from the bladder in absence of prolapse.

The lower limit of the bladder is identified and separated from the underlying cervix using sharp dissection with curved scissors. The right plane is extended, and the bladder is pushed up close to the uterus, till the anterior peritoneum is visible. Next, the uterus is lifted anteriorly, and the posterior peritoneum in the pouch of Douglas is opened and extended laterally. The lower supports of the uterus, uterosacral ligaments and cardinal ligaments are then divided and transfixed. The same procedure is repeated on the opposite side. It is very important to open the uterovesical fold of peritoneum anteriorly before the uterine arteries are clamped, cut and ligated on both the sides. Next, the upper pedicles, broad ligament, ovarian ligament and round ligament are clamped, cut and ligated, and the same is repeated on the opposite side. If there is no prolapse, the uterosacral with cardinal ligaments is transfixed for vault suspension. If enterocele is present, McCall's culdoplasty **(Fig. 11)** is done. This is followed by repair of anterior compartment. In case of uterovaginal prolapse, a vertical incision is made on the anterior vaginal wall after saline infiltration, anterior vaginal flaps are held away laterally, and the pubovesicocervical fascia is plicated in the midline with sutures. The plication is done until the entire cystourethrocele is reduced. The excess vaginal tissue is trimmed, and the edges are approximated with absorbable sutures. This is followed by vault suspension. Rectocele repair is done with posterior colpoperineorrhaphy.

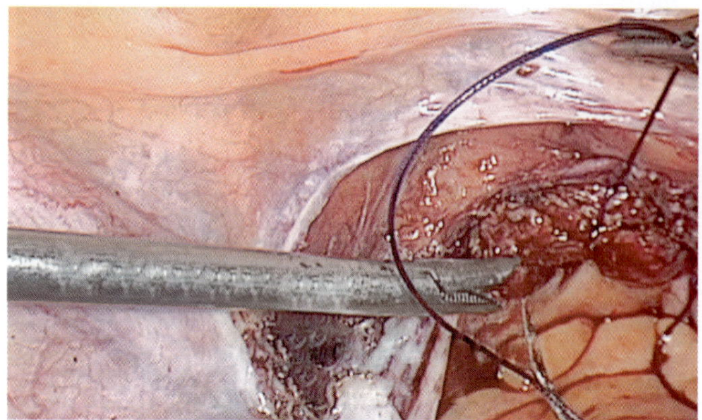

Fig. 10: Vault suturing.

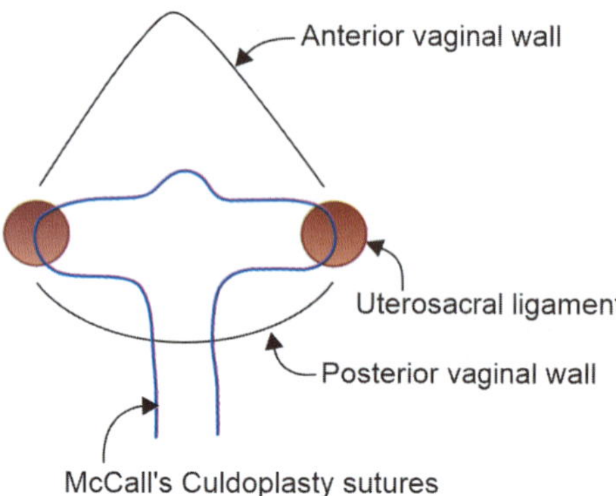

Fig. 11: McCall's culdoplasty.

Perform Opportunistic Salpingectomy (or) Salpingo-oophorectomy

Recent evidence suggests that the risk of ovarian malignancy is probably from the fallopian tubes. Hence, it is advised to remove the fallopian tubes even if ovarian preservation is required. There are studies to suggest a decreased risk of adnexal mass formation if the fallopian tubes are removed during hysterectomy. At the same time, there is an associated increased risk of early degeneration of ovaries associated with salpingectomy.

In general, removal of the ovaries at the time of hysterectomy is usually not recommended before the age of 45 years unless there is an increased risk of breast cancer or ovarian cancer. Oestrogen deficiency occurs after removal of ovaries in both pre- and postmenopausal women. The risks of cardiovascular and cerebrovascular events along with declining bone mineral density due to oestrogen deficiency must be kept in mind before considering the removal of normal ovaries at the time of hysterectomy for benign indications.

COMPLICATIONS OF HYSTERECTOMY

Numerous operative, immediate and late complications can occur following hysterectomy. Haemorrhage, need for transfusion, bladder, ureteral, intestinal injury or large blood vessel injury can occur. Intraoperative complications (10% vs. 3.4%) and reoperations (3.6% vs. 1.9%) are, however, more in oncosurgeries than those done for benign indications. Women with more pelvic vascularity, large fibroids, dense adhesions and frozen pelvis due to endometriosis have higher risk of complications. During the postoperative period, febrile morbidity due to surgical site infections, urinary tract infections and thromboembolic complications may contribute to longer hospital stays.

The eVALuate study compared abdominal hysterectomy, vaginal hysterectomy and laparoscopic hysterectomy. LAVH, though had longer operating time, had fewer perioperative complications and faster return to normal activities. Apart from conversion to laparotomy, other complications were comparable in open, vaginal and laparoscopy groups. In some studies, women returned to normal activities sooner after vaginal compared to abdominal hysterectomy and had lesser wound infections, urinary tract infections and febrile episodes. Compared to LAVH or TLH, vaginal hysterectomy has shorter operating time, hospital stay and cost. However, complications occur in 5% of surgeries; the most common complications being cuff infection/abscess (1.2%) and dissection cystotomy (0.5%). While inadequate training is a challenge for vaginal hysterectomy, longer learning curves and higher operating costs pose challenges for laparoscopic and robotic hysterectomies. Total laparoscopic hysterectomy is a less invasive and safe alternative to total abdominal hysterectomy, offering the benefits of minimally invasive surgery, especially for those unsuitable for vaginal hysterectomy.

Hysterectomy has a strong effect on women's sexuality, with poor body image and other factors, which lead to depression. However, meta-analysis of depression following hysterectomy varies. Some studies reported increase in depression in women who underwent hysterectomy compared to the control group.

Emphasising on preoperative self-care by reducing weight, quitting smoking and drinking and taking iron to correct anaemia significantly improved health status among women who underwent hysterectomy. Adhering to the enhanced recovery after surgery (ERAS) protocol immediately postsurgery resulted in fewer complications, early recovery and faster discharge from hospital. Postsurgery, self-care by early ambulation, avoiding heavy lifting, proper diet avoiding constipation, using optimal painkillers and refraining from sexual activity for up to 8 weeks after surgery improve surgical outcomes. Preoperative psychological intervention could effectively improve the mental condition of women undergoing hysterectomy, thereby facilitating good postoperative recovery. Though hysterectomy increases the risk of psychiatric ailments compared to uterus-conserving procedures in women, an appropriate psychosocial support before and after the procedure may help to reduce psychological distress.

SUGGESTED READING

1. Agarwal M, Sinha S, Haripriya H, Kokkayil P, Singh S. Surgical site infection in laparoscopic hysterectomy versus abdominal hysterectomy in gynecological disease(s): an overview. Gynecol Minim Invasive Ther. 2023;13(1):25-9.
2. Aitchison LP, Chen AZL, Toms C, Sandroussi C, Yeo DA, Steffens D. To stitch or not to stitch: the skin closure of laparoscopic port sites, a meta-analysis. Surg Endosc. 2022;36(10):7140-59..
3. Alliende RI, Carrasco AM, Levancini M, Kovoor E, Guzmán-Rojas RA, Miranda-Mendoza I. 5,926 hysterectomies: complications described by Clavien–Dindo classification. J Obstet Gynaecol. 2021;41(7):1102-6.
4. Badakhsh MH, Taftachi F, Mehrabi F, Derakhshan A. The effect of hysterectomy in securing sexual desire and satisfaction. Iran J Surg. 2009;17(1):75-80.
5. Begüm Ö. Vaginal hysterectomy: indications avoiding complications. In: Shoupe D (Ed). Handbook of Gynecology. Switzerland: Springer; 2023. pp. 834-47.
6. Choi HG, Rhim CC, Yoon JY, Lee SW. Association between hysterectomy and depression: a longitudinal follow-up study using a national sample cohort. Menopause. 2020;27(5):543-9.
7. Darwish M, Atlantis E, Mohamed TT. Psychological outcomes after hysterectomy for benign conditions: a systematic review and meta-analysis. Eur J Obstet Gynecol Reprod Biol. 2014;174:5-19.
8. Evans EC, Matteson KA, Orejuela FJ, Alperin M, Balk EM, El-Nashar S, et al. Salpingo-oophorectomy at the time of benign hysterectomy: a systematic review. Obstet Gynecol. 2016;128(3):476-85.
9. Garry R, Fountain J, Mason SU, Hawe J, Napp V, Abbott J, et al. The eVALuate study: two parallel randomised trials, one comparing laparoscopic with abdominal hysterectomy, the other comparing laparoscopic with vaginal hysterectomy. BMJ. 2004;328(7432):129.
10. Gottlieb AS, Sivasubramanian N, Chilka PR, Mahalakshmi B, Daminiben BP, Gopal R. Pre and post-operative self-care management among women undergoing hysterectomy. Bioinformation. 2023;19(6):721-4.
11. Harvey SV, Pfeiffer RM, Landy R, Wentzensen N, Clarke MA. Trends and predictors of hysterectomy prevalence among women in the United States. Am J Obstet Gynecol. 2022;227(4):611.e1-12.
12. Jeyamani B, Reddy SC. Enhanced recovery after surgery in patients undergoing total abdominal hysterectomy. Obstet Gynaecol Forum. 2024;34(3):2435-40.
13. Kallianidis AF, Rijntjes D, Brobbel C, Dekkers OM, Bloemenkamp KWM, van den Akker T. Incidence, indications, risk factors, and outcomes of emergency peripartum hysterectomy worldwide: a systematic review and meta-analysis. Obstet Gynecol. 2023;141(1):35-48.
14. Kotsopoulos J, Narod SA. Prophylactic salpingectomy for the prevention of ovarian cancer: Who should we target? Int J Cancer. 2020;147(5):1245-51.
15. Lee HJ, Kim SJ, Park EC. Psychiatric outcomes after hysterectomy in women with uterine myoma: a population-based retrospective cohort study. Arch Womens Ment Health. 2017;20(4):487-94.
16. Marin F, Plesca M, Bordea CI, Moga MA, Blidaru A. Types of radical hysterectomies: from Thoma Ionescu and Wertheim to present day. J Med Life. 2014;7(2):172-6.
17. McPherson K, Metcalfe MA, Herbert A, Maresh M, Casbard A, Hargreaves J, et al. Severe complication of hysterectomy: the VALUE study. BJOG. 2004;111(7):688-94.
18. Morrison JE, Jacobs VR. Classic intrafascial supracervical hysterectomy (CISH): 10-year experience. JSLS. 2006;10(1):26-9.
19. Pande B, Pradhan P, Pradhan SK, Mansingh S, Mishra SK. Complications of total laparoscopic hysterectomy in a tertiary care center. Cureus. 2023;15(3):e36510.
20. Rout D, Sinha A, Palo SK, Kanungo S, Pati S. Prevalence and determinants of hysterectomy in India. Sci Rep. 2023;13:14569.
21. Sutton CJG. Hysterectomy: a historical perspective. In: Wood C, Maher P (Eds). Baillière's Clinical Obstetrics and Gynaecology. London: Bailliere Tindall; 1997. pp. 1-23.
22. van Lieshout LAM, Steenbeek MP, De Hullu JA, Vos MC, Houterman S, Wilkinson J, et al. Hysterectomy with opportunistic salpingectomy versus hysterectomy alone. Cochrane Database Syst Rev. 2019;8(8):CD012858.
23. Yi YX, Zhang CO, Zhou Q, Guo WR, Su Y. Laparoscopic-assisted vaginal hysterectomy vs abdominal hysterectomy for benign disease: a meta-analysis of randomized controlled trials. Eur J Obstet Gynecol Reprod Biol. 2011;159(1):1-18.

61

CHAPTER

Conditions of the Lower Intestinal Tract

Srirama Bhat M

Chapter Outline

- Rectal Prolapse
- Incontinence of Faeces and Flatus
- Diarrhoea
- Difficult Evacuation
- Irritable Bowel Syndrome
- Pruritus ANI
- Pilonidal Sinus (Jeep Bottom; Driver's Bottom) Pilus—Hair; Nidus—Nest
- Rectal and Anal Pain
- External Pile/Haemorrhoids
- Anorectal Abscess
- Fistula-in-Ano
- Proctitis
- Endometriosis
- Neoplasm of the Anal Canal

INTRODUCTION

The close anatomical relationship between the lower gastrointestinal and the genital tract brings certain anal and rectal conditions within the purview of the gynaecologist; the following comments represent this particular view and do not aim to be all-embracing or comprehensive. Rectal prolapse, fissure in ano, piles and incontinence are commonly associated with gynaecological conditions and pregnancies. It is important that all practicing obstetricians and gynaecologists should have proper knowledge about these conditions and management policies **(Fig. 1)**.

RECTAL PROLAPSE

It is circumferential descent of rectum or rectosigmoid across anorectum; it could be partial thickness or complete. It is red/pink in colour. It is common in females (6:1) and common in infants, children and elderly. Faecal incontinence, discharge and associated vault/uterine prolapse are common in females (>20%); urinary incontinence is also known to occur (>35%).

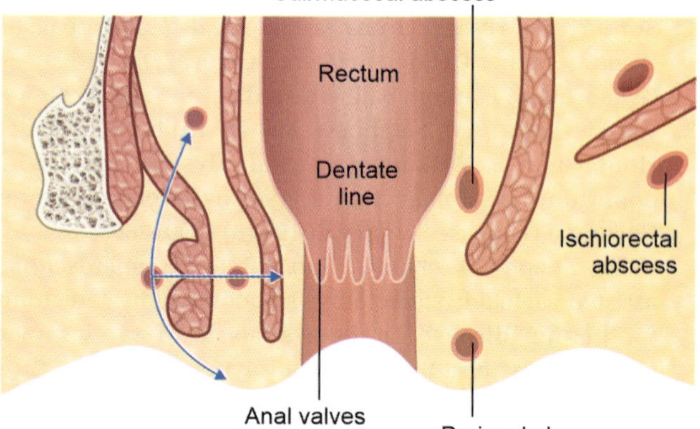

Fig. 1: Surgical anatomy of anal canal.

Aetiology

It is said to be the sliding herniation of the pouch of Douglas through the pelvic floor fascia across anorectum mainly into the anterior wall of the rectum.

It is also proposed as procidentia due to rectal wall intussusception across the anorectum beginning at 7.5 cm above the dentate line.

Other causes: Other causes include chronic constipation, diarrhoea, weakness of pelvic musculature, chronic cough, repeated pregnancies with birth injuries, altered sacral curvature, reduced anorectal muscle and sphincter tone, pudendal nerve damage, old age, neurological and spinal causes, levator ani muscle weakness, malnutrition, diabetes mellitus and obesity.

Types (Figs. 2A and B)

- *Partial:* It is <3.75 cm; only mucosal prolapse with submucosa (but not muscular layer); common in children and young individuals **(Fig. 3)**.
- *Complete:* It is >3.75 cm and contains a muscular layer of the rectum also along with mucosa and submucosa, often associated with uterine prolapse (procidentia).

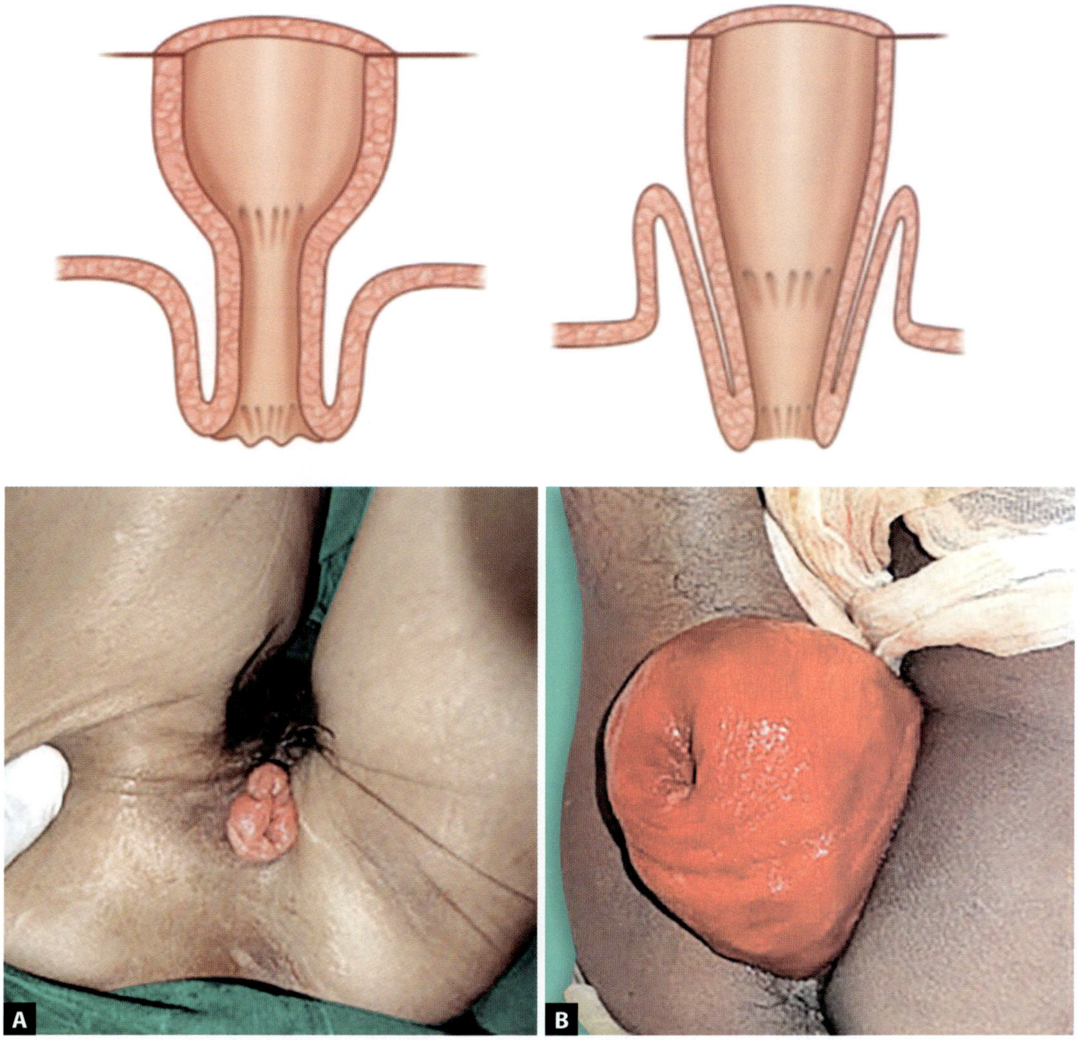

Figs. 2A and B: Types of rectal prolapse. (A) Partial; (B) Complete.

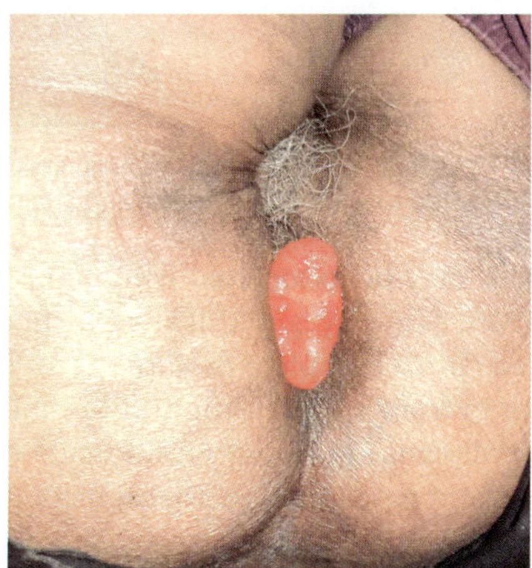

Fig. 3: Partial rectal prolapse.

- *Hidden/concealed:* It is internal intussusception of the sigmoid usually of mucosa and submucosa across the rectum but not coming out of the anal canal.

Partial Rectal Prolapse

Features

It is common in infants and children. It is mucosal and submucosal; <3.75 cm. It is due to decreased sacral curvature and reduced anal tone.

Mass per anum, more while the child is straining with occasional bleeding and discharge. Discomfort and pain are also not uncommon. Constipation or diarrhoea is common. Improper bowel regulation, sensation of incomplete evacuation and tenesmus are other features.

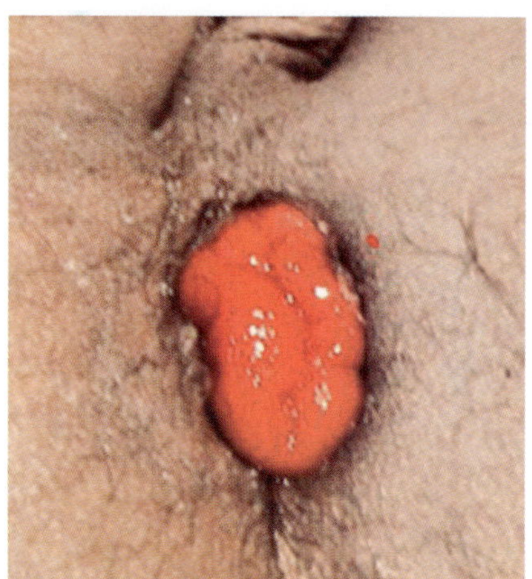

Fig. 4: Partial rectal prolapse.

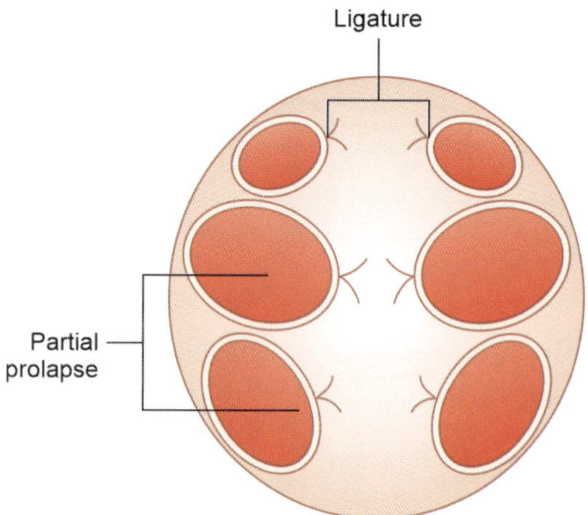

Fig. 5: Goodsall's ligature.

On examination, circumferential protruded red or pink coloured mass with faecal staining. Digital rectal examination (DRE) may show lax sphincter tone; repositioning can be done easily **(Fig. 4)**.

Evaluation: In children, the condition is clinically diagnosed. Assessment is needed in relation to nutrition and haematocrit.

Treatment of Partial Rectal Prolapse

In infants and early childhood, digital repositioning using lignociane gel local application at regular intervals, correction of constipation and improvement in nutrition are quite useful.

Submucosal injection of 10 mL 5% phenol in almond oil or ethanolamine oleate into the apex or base or both of the prolapse mass at various points (four sites) which leads to aseptic inflammation thereby causing tethering and fixing of the mucosa into the muscular layer of the rectum. 30% of tetracycline or oxytetracycline or hypertonic saline can also be used.

Goodall's ligature: It is ligation of the mucosa at its base at three sites on each side using nonabsorbable (silk) or delayed absorbable (polyglactin) suture material which fixes the mucosa into a deeper plane due to inflammation and fibrosis. Stapled transnational rectal resection (STARR) surgery is also beneficial **(Fig. 5)**.

Complete Rectal Prolapse

It is called as procidentia. It is full-thickness prolapse including the rectal muscular layer; it is >3.75 cm. All layers of the wall are involved. It is common in females; common in elderly. Often, it becomes irreducible with ulceration.

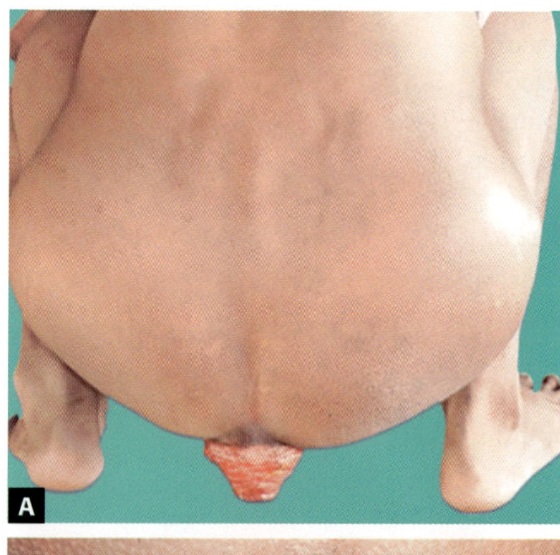

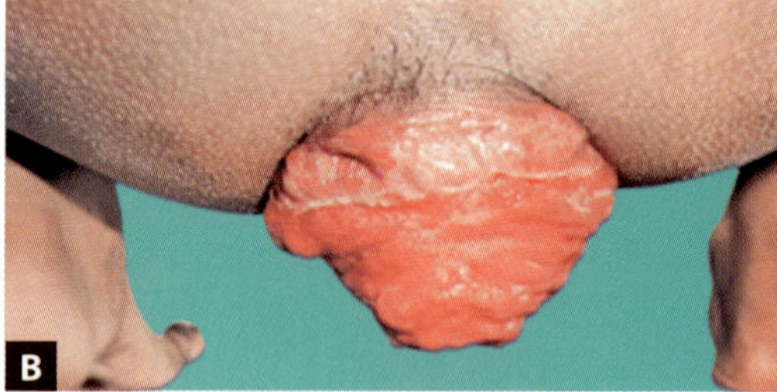

Figs. 6A and B: Complete rectal prolapse which will be clinically appreciated in squatting position and straining.

In females, it may be associated with complete uterine prolapse. Mucosa may get thickened, ulcerated and incarcerated. Once complete prolapse is >5 cm, it drags peritoneum in front with intestine within the peritoneal sac which will cause gurgling sound while doing rectal examination and repositioning. Faecal incontinence with lax anorectum is observed with mucus discharge with an abnormally mobile rectum with descent and obliterated anorectal angle **(Figs. 6 and 7)**.

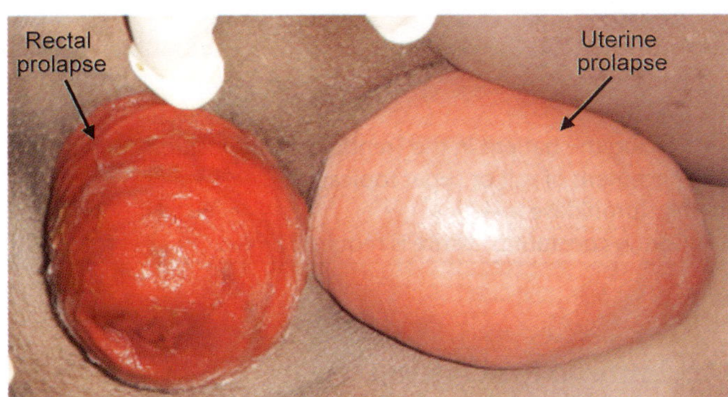

Fig. 7: Rectal and uterine prolapse.

Symptoms

- Difficulty in bowel regulation—constipation (67%) or diarrhoea (15%); sensation of incomplete evacuation
- Discomfort, tenesmus
- Blood and mucus discharge; faecal incontinence (70%)
- Associated uterine prolapse is common in females
- Mass is reducible and painless; but when incarcerated or infected, it will be painful and with fever.
- *Floridiform:* Permanently extruded rectum

Signs

- Circumferentially protruding rectum across anal canal which is red or pink in colour
- Superficial ulceration in the mucosa
- Patulous anal sphincter with reduced sphincter tone and diminished squeeze pressure
- Mucosa—superficial ulceration
- Anaemia, elevated temperature
- Anteriorly peritoneal sac will come down as pouch which contains a small bowel.
- Diminished sphincter tone, diminished squeeze pressures
- Examination

Grades of Prolapse

- First degree (high or early, 'concealed' and 'invisible')
- Second degree (externally visible on straining, sulcus evident between rectal wall and anal canal)
- Third degree (externally visible)

Differential Diagnosis

- *Third-degree piles:* Rectal prolapse is circumferential, red or pink in colour, folds are concentric; piles are radial, nonconcentric haemorrhoidal cushions which are plum coloured with cutaneous component **(Fig. 8)**.

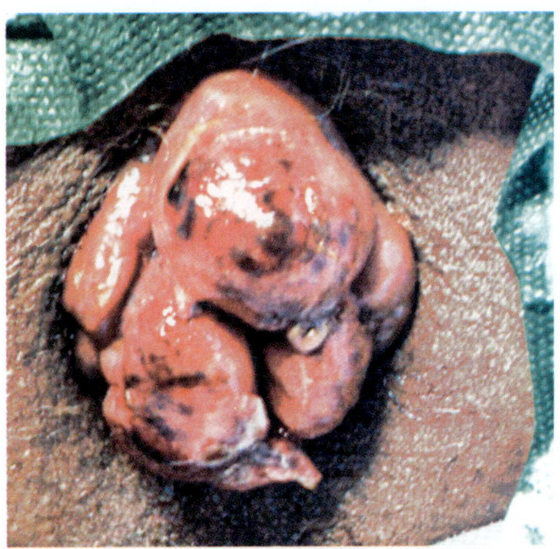

Fig. 8: Typical look of prolapsed grade IV piles.

- *Rectosigmoid intussusception* differs from rectal prolapse with inability to get the invigilation edge even though often it is difficult to assess.
- *Rectal polyp:* It comes out as localised pedunculated lesion with an often warty surface at the summit.

Complications of Rectal Prolapse

- Anaemia, sepsis, bleeding and proctitis
- Incarceration, gangrene, rupture and evisceration

Diagnostic Workup

Grade 1 or 2 prolapse:

- *Daefecography:* Cine/magnetic resonance defaecography
- *Cinedefaecography:* It is a useful modality when the diagnosis of procidentia is suspected but cannot be demonstrated. Among patients with clinical rectocoeles and defaecatory dysfunction, there is a 33% incidence of occult rectal prolapse **(Figs. 9 and 10)**.

Defecographic grading of rectal prolapse:

- N—normal rectal fixation, sphincter relaxation and rectal emptying
- (1)—nonrelaxed puborectalis
- (2)—mild intussusception
- (3)—moderate intussusception
- (4)—severe intussusception
- (5)—prolapse
- (6)—rectocele

Note: Preprolapse is funnel-shaped rectum with a lack of fixation, excessive rectosigmoid mobility, ring pocket

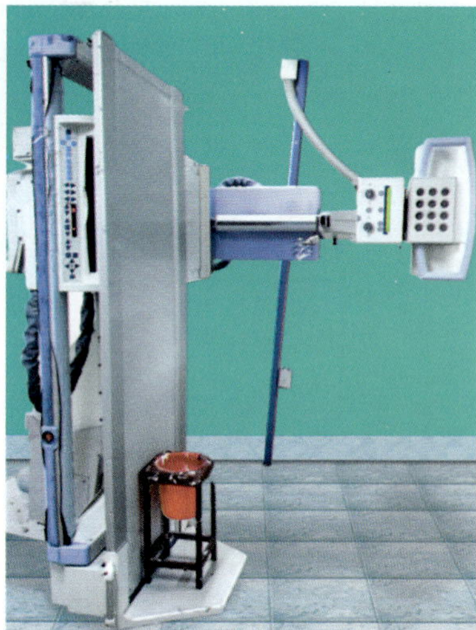

Fig. 9: Cinedefaecography suite where imaging of simulated defaecation with a radiocontrast is performed.

formation and intussusception. There is no clear-cut clinically demonstrable descent of the rectum across the anus but funnelling and lax sphincter can be appreciated.

- *Incontinent patients:* Anorectal physiology testing: Manometry, endorectal ultrasound and pudendal nerve terminal motor latency (PNTML)
- *Constipated patients:* Colonic transit studies
- *Elderly patients:* Colonoscopy, sigmoidoscopy, prevalence of rectosigmoid carcinoma with prolapse was 5.7% as opposed to 1.4%
- *Anal manometry:* Resting pressure of the internal sphincter (40 mm Hg) and squeeze pressure of the external sphincter (80 mm Hg) is measured by placing water-filled balloons attached to catheters with transducers.
- *PNTML study:* It is done by wearing a glove-like device which contains specialised transducer; this gloved finger is inserted into the rectum and directed over the right and left of the levator ani complex. The electrode in the finger glove measures the PNTML which is normally 1.8–2.2 msec. It is prolonged in pudendal nerve damage.
- *Electromyography study* of the puborectalis muscle tone is also very useful in assessing muscle laxity.

Surgical Management (Table 1)

The advances in laparoscopic surgery have meant that all the abdominal procedures for rectal prolapse can be safely accomplished laparoscopically.

Acute management of rectal prolapse.

- Early reduction
- Sedation
- Placing the patient in the Trendelenburg position
- Placement of salt or sugar topically
- Hyaluronidase injection
- Gentle constant pressure is required

Abdominal Procedures

Abdominal procedures are usually preferred in younger patients, but older patients with good functional status and adequate cardiopulmonary reserve may also derive benefits from minimal access surgery.

Principles

- Procedures incorporating transabdominal rectal fixation are typically the procedures of choice for the treatment of prolapse.
- Division of the lateral stalks during rectal dissection may worsen symptoms of constipation postoperatively, but it is associated with decreased recurrence rates.
- Rectopexy is a key component of all these repairs.
- A sigmoid resection may be added to rectopexy in patients with prolapse and preoperative constipation.
- Anterior resection alone is associated with higher recurrence rates and morbidity; it should not be considered as a first-line treatment.

Note: Laparoscopic posterior mesh rectopexy is the standard procedure currently; however, choices are made based on the individual patients as so many procedures are in practice. Ports are placed with patient head down and low lithotomy position. Peritoneum on the right side is cut and presacral avascular plane is reached and dissected adequately. Care should be taken not to injure the hypogastric nerves and ureters. Lateral ligaments are left or dissected depending on need. Anterior mobilisation and Dsenonvillier's fascia are done for 5 cm below. 10 × 6 cm mesh is placed posteriorly in presacral space and is sutured to sacral promontary; mesh is wrapped partially and sutured to lateral wall of the rectum also. When sigmoid is very redundant, sigmoid resection is required; in such situation, the mesh is not used; only posterior and lateral fixation of the rectum is done using polypropylene sutures.

Perineal Procedures

Elderly/debilitated patients with significant comorbidities may have acceptable outcomes with perineal procedures.

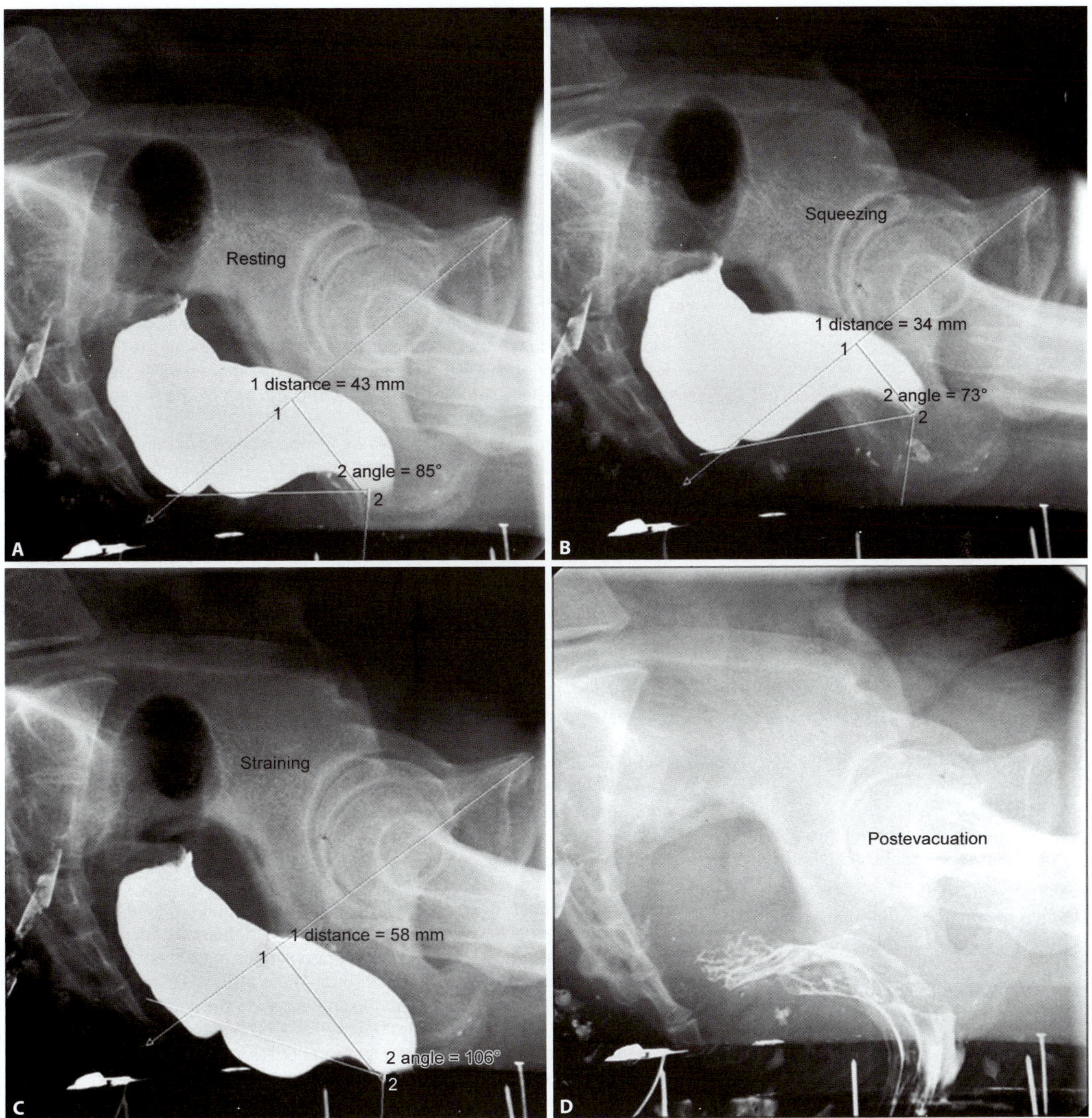

Figs. 10A to D: Cinedefaecography films taken at rest, maximum squeeze, strain and postevacuation phase.

However, young men who may prefer to accept a high recurrence rate of a perineal procedure (over impotence/infertility) can also be offered these procedures.

Altemeier Perineal Rectosigmoidectomy

Indications: Intermediate surgical risk patients, adults opting for a perineal procedure and long segment prolapse.

Steps: Circumferential incision of rectum proximal to dentate line, delivery of redundant rectum and sigmoid colon, ligation of blood supply to rectum, placement of purse-string suture on proximal bowel and excision of redundant colon and rectum, proximal purse-string suture secured around a central shaft, proximal bowel advanced through anus and distal purse-string tied, approximation

TABLE 1: Aim and different procedures for rectal prolapse.

<table>
<tr><td>Aim of the treatment:
• To correct prolapse
• To restore continence
• To prevent constipation
• To prevent recurrence</td><td>Abdominal procedures:
• Laparoscopic rectopexy with mesh or polypropylene sutures to sacral promontory and sacrum (fascia)
• Resection of redundant sigmoid and anastomosis and suture rectopexy without mesh (Frykman–Goldberg procedure). It is indicated in young individuals, redundant sigmoid, constipation and concomitant pathology
• Well's operation: Polyvinyl alcohol sponge wrapping around the mobilised rectum; but infection and fistula formation and constipation are higher; so polypropylene mesh is used
• Ripstein operation: Placement of 5 cm width Teflon (polytetrafluoroethylene) mesh sling around the rectum to fix it to sacral promontory, sacrum and in front after complete posterior mobilisation of the rectum up to the coccyx. It has shown good results with a recurrence rate 2.6% and morbidity (16%)
• Suture rectopexy alone: Here, after complete mobilisation, sutures are placed using polypropylene sutures to fix the rectum and to increase the anorectal angle
• Lahaut's operation: Mobilised rectosigmoid loop is passed in front through posterior rectus sheath behind the rectus muscle as extraperitoneally to pull the rectosigmoid forward—not done now
• Other procedures: Goligher's operation (low mobilisation up to anorectal ring and fixing into presacral fascia using interrupted polypropylene sutures); Devdhar's rectal plication using silk sutures considering it as intussusception; Roscoe Graham's rectal fixation (suturing using vicryl to anal canal and rectum to sacral fascia); Muir low anterior resection</td></tr>
<tr><td>Principles:
• Adequate rectal mobilisation posteriorly as well as anteriorly
• Avoid injuries to hypogastric nerves which may cause impotence (in males specifically)
• Avoid injury to ureters
• Avoid perforating rectosigmoid!
• Absolute haemostasis
• Fixation of rectum to sacrum through mesh or polypropylene nonabsorbable sutures
Complications:
• Injuries to urinary bladder, ureter, small bowel; bleeding from sacral vessels/rectal wall
• Sepsis, abscess formation, discharge, infertility/impotence
• Constipation, diarrhoea, anorectal pain and discomfort
• Recurrence
• Faecal incontinence</td><td>Perineal procedures:
• Delorme's sleeve mucosal resection and rectopexy (see further)
• Perineal posterior fixation of the rectum of Lockhart–Mummery: After creating retrorectal space through perineal approach, posterior rectal wall is sutured to sacrum and coccyx
• Wyatt operation: Here, after retrorectal space dissection through perineal transanal approach, Marlex mesh is placed in the space and sutured to sacral promontory, sacrum and rectal wall
• Altemeier's rectosigmoidectomy (see further)
• Mikulicz–Miles perineal transanal rectosigmoidectomy (amputation of prolapse) and suturing of the sigmoid to the anal margin
• Thiersch (1891) anal encircling—indications: Elderly people who are bedridden with short life expectancy, multiple comorbidities, dementia patients. Here under local anaesthesia, two small incisions are made in front and posteriorly midline sites; silver wire is encircled through these incisions to one complete round; assistant puts his finger into the anorectum (it prevents complete closure by purse string effect) and wire is tightened around the assistant finger which prevents the descent of the rectum temporarily. Now, polypropylene/nylon/ thick vicryl is used. Silver wire causes often severe pain, erosions, bleeding and discomfort. Since it is temporary, it can be repeated when the rectum descends again as outpatient procedure</td></tr>
</table>

of anvil to cartridge and activation of stapler and anastomosis completed. Here the pelvic floor is supported by suturing puborectalis muscle in front of the rectum using nonabsorbable sutures.

Complications: Anastomotic dehiscence, postoperative bleeding, anastomotic stricture, small bowel injury (after the peritoneal sac has been opened) and perforation of posterior vaginal wall.

Delorme Procedure

Indications: Elderly with comorbidities, complete rectal prolapse, in young where infertility risks are to be avoided.

Steps: Under spinal anaesthesia, after passing number 16 urinary Foley's catheter, in lithotomy or jackknife position, prolapsed rectum is held with Babcock's forceps at its apex; submucosa is infiltrated with 1 in 200,000 adrenaline solution with or without 0.5 xylocaine to reduce oozing during submucosal sleeve resection; circular incision is made just below the prolapsed dentate line (but rectal wall is so much congested and oedematous often it is difficult to dissect such as tubular mucosal sleeve from above downwards towards apex and in such situations like many times longitudinal multiple incisions can be made to complete the submucosal resection from dentate line to apex); haemostasis is achieved by sutures using vicryl or bipolar cautery; concentric rectal musculature is visible; care should be taken not to perforate rectal wall; anteriorly urinary bladder and peritoneal pouch with small bowel may be there which should not be injured or opened; rectal muscular tube is plicated by series of zero vicryl interrupted sutures from just below the dentate line up to apex of the prolapse in circumferential pattern; first all suture bites should be taken (around 20); then knot tying is done one after other to complete the plication; once plication is done bleeding will not occur; apex mucosa is sutured to the dentate line area circumferentially using 2-zero vicryl interrupted sutures; mass is reduced into the rectal area; often for short period until plication sutures fix the rectum into deeper plane number one vicryl encircling (such as Thiersch wiring) can be added upon. Catheter is removed in 24 hours.

Complications: Wound dehiscence; injury to the rectum, urinary bladder, small bowel; sepsis; sphincter injury and incontinence; anal stricture; constipation; discharge and respiratory complications.

Descending Perineal Syndrome

When a healthy person increases the intra-abdominal pressure and relaxes the pelvic floor muscles, there will not be any changes in the concavity of the perineum. In chronic ill patients, malnourished and people with preprolapse, perineal descent can occur with obliteration of the normal concavity of the perineum. It is called descending perineal syndrome.

Levators got injured directly or indirectly causing weakening of the pelvic floor. Anal canal is situated many centimetres below the pubococcygeal line. Usually 3–4 cm low during straining.

Presentations are tenesmus, incomplete evacuation and incontinence.

Defecography is ideal for evaluating such patients. Perineometer is also used.

Treatment is diet, laxatives, avoiding straining, and suppositories. Restoration of pelvic floor by various surgical methods may be needed often with rectal resection and suspension. Total pelvic Marlex mesh repair; transcoccygeal posterior hitching of the rectum (Kraske); and correction of cystocele, rectocele and enterocele may be needed. Results are not very good as recurrence or residual problems may persist.

INCONTINENCE OF FAECES AND FLATUS

Faecal incontinence is more common in women than in men. *Minor faecal incontinence* is the inadvertent passage of flatus or soiling in the presence of diarrhoea. Incontinence of flatus is generally more embarrassing and troublesome than faecal incontinence. The latter, unlike the former, can be controlled to a large extent by the woman learning to keep the stools well-formed and by using muscles such as the levator ani in place of damaged anal sphincters. The escape of flatus *per vagina* has to be distinguished from the escape of air which enters a relaxed introitus. *Major faecal incontinence* is the inadvertent passage of formed stools at least twice weekly.

In this syndrome, the perineum balloons down below the level of the bony pelvis, especially on straining. The pudendal nerves are stretched, and the pelvic muscles are denervated. This leads to a constant perineal aching pain in the upright position, anal incontinence and a feeling of incomplete emptying caused by prolapse of the anterior rectal wall mucosa into the anal canal. There may also be a solitary midrectal ulcer caused by prolapse of the anterior rectal wall mucosa into the anal canal. There may also be a solitary midrectal ulcer caused by the excessive straining which may bleed and is sometimes painful.

Continence of anal canal is maintained by two factors: (1) Normal rectal and colonic pressure; (2) normal stable pelvic floor function.

Incontinence may be—(1) *Urge:* Here rectal and colonic pressure is raised but normal pelvic floor; (2) *true:* Here rectal and colonic pressures are normal but there is defective pelvic floor; (3) *full:* Here rectal and colonic pressure is reduced and also there is defective pelvic floor; (4) *temporary:* It is due to temporary causes such as postsurgery; treated by reassurance and (5) *permanent:* It needs definitive surgical therapy as all components are defective including a reduction in pressures.

Causes

Refer **Table 2** below.

Evaluation

- *DRE*
- *Evaluation for specific causes:* Colonoscopy, imaging [contrast-enhanced computed tomography (CECT) abdomen and pelvis/MRI spine/pelvis], blood parameters and neurological assessment
- *Others:* Anorectal manometry, electromyography, defaecography, perineometer to assess the level and angle of anorectal junction.

Treatment

Injured or inherently defective anal sphincters can usually be reconstituted sufficiently well to restore continence; fistulas can be closed. Rings of fascia, or unabsorbable material, can be inserted subcutaneously around the anus to replace sphincters. The tendon of the gracilis muscle has also been used.

Faecal incontinence due to senility or a nerve lesion calls for a low-residue diet and good nursing rather than surgery.

The anterior rectal mucosal prolapse in the descending perineum syndrome can be treated by sclerotherapy or by surgical excision. Perineal body descent can be corrected surgically. The solitary rectal ulcer syndrome may require rectopexy if associated with rectal prolapse.

Electrical stimulation of puborectalis is effective in many patients.

SECCA therapy (SECCA device; USA): Temperature-controlled radiofrequency energy in the anal canal and distal rectum to create scarring and fibrosis of internal sphincter and adjacent tissues.

DIARRHOEA

Diarrhoea has many possible causes, but it is necessary to emphasise that this symptom can be caused by pelvic lesions which irritate and 'hurry' the bowel. These are pelvic peritonitis, pelvic abscess, pelvic haematocoele or antibiotic therapy—conditions which should always be suspected when a woman develops diarrhoea following a gynaecological operation.

TABLE 2: The causes of incontinence of faeces and flatus.

Category	*Mechanism*	*Causes*
(A) Sensory loss	*Afferent nerve injury:* Unable to detect rectal filling	Diabetic neuropathy, spinal cord injury and multiple sclerosis
(B) Sphincter weakness	Sphincter muscle injury	Obstetric trauma, motor vehicle accident and foreign body trauma
	Pudendal nerve injury	Obstetric trauma, diabetic peripheral neuropathy, multiple sclerosis and idiopathic
	Central nervous system injury	Spina bifida, traumatic spinal cord injury, cerebrovascular accident and multiple sclerosis
(C) Functional	Faecal impaction; dilated internal anal sphincter	Pelvic floor dyssynergia (difficulty relaxing sphincter when defaecating), drug side effects, idiopathic and spinal cord injury
	Diarrhoea; rapid transit and/or large volume	Irritable bowel syndrome; infectious and metabolic causes of diarrhoea
	Cognitive, psychological; social in difference	Dementia, psychosis and willful soiling

Note: Causes may be denervation (spinal injury, spina bifida), damage (childbirth, wounds and surgeries), descent (rectal prolapse, perineal descent), debility (old age, diseases), destruction (radiotherapy, malignancy), dementia (senility, psychosis), and deficiency (congenital anomalies).

DIFFICULT EVACUATION

Constipation

It is sometimes said that all women are constipated. This is not true but many women think they are. They develop a phobia about bowel action and encourage the same in their daughters. Their habit of taking laxatives regularly is good for manufacturing chemists but bad for the physiology of the lower bowel. These women think that constipation causes headaches, lethargy and all manner of ills. In fact, it is without any ill effect, as is shown when bowel action is deliberately suppressed for 5–10 days after certain operations. Nevertheless, the accumulation of large masses of hard faeces in the rectum can cause dyspareunia; their passage is painful and can result in fissures.

Pregnancy and Puerperium

Constipation is common in pregnancy; difficulty in evacuation for 1 or 2 weeks after delivery is almost the rule and can cause considerable distress, even collapse from straining. In both circumstances, the factors responsible are as follows: Atony of the bowel, stretching of the muscles of expulsion and physical inactivity. An acute episode in the puerperium is treated by a simple enema or stimulant suppository. Thereafter, the situation is corrected by muscle exercises, fluids and mild laxatives, if necessary.

Rectocoele

The ballooning forward of the rectum into a rectocoele causes difficulty in evacuation unless the posterior vaginal wall is pressed back digitally.

Constriction of the Rectum and Anus

Stricture Following Infection

The main causes under this heading are lymphogranuloma venereum (LGV) and granuloma inguinale. Drugs are doxycycline 100 mg twice daily orally for 3 weeks, erythromycin 500 mg four times daily for 3 weeks or azithromycin 1 g weekly once for 3 weeks. Later, regular dilatation or stricturoplasty may be needed.

Stricture Following Operation or Radiotherapy

Overenthusiastic treatment for haemorrhoids can sometimes lead to anal stricture requiring anal dilatation or the use of advancement flaps. Postradiation rectal strictures may occur in cases of carcinoma of the cervix

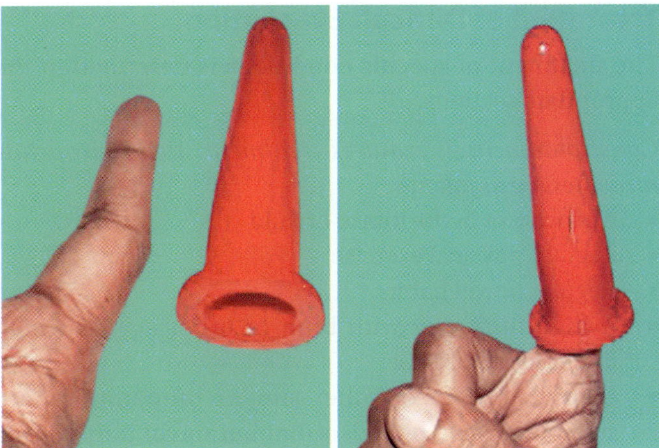

Fig. 11: Anal dilator.

and may develop several months or years after treatment. After proper assessment, regular anal dilatation using an appropriate dilator is very useful; dilatation is done once a day wherein the dilator is passed into the anal canal gently with lignocaine gel application and kept for few minutes; repeated daily for 2–3 months **(Fig. 11)**. Anoplasty is needed if regular dilatation fails.

Pelvic Tumours

Benign tumours such as cysts and leiomyomas rarely cause difficulty in emptying the bowel, even when they are so impacted as to result in retention of urine. The same applies to a retroverted gravid uterus. A retroverted nonpregnant uterus never causes bowel symptoms. A tumour which causes dyschezia is usually malignant and may arise from the vagina, uterus or ovary.

Endometriosis

When this disease involves the rectum, some narrowing may result but the main complaint of the patient is pain on defaecation. Treatment specifically for endometrium should be undertaken.

Carcinoma of the Rectum

While this may be associated with a change in bowel habits, there is also likely to be some rectal bleeding.

Faulty Powers of Expulsion

Neurological disorders, old age, debilitating disease and physical inactivity lead to constipation by causing atony of the voluntary muscles of expulsion and the involuntary muscles of the bowel.

Treatment of Difficult Evacuation

The treatment of specific conditions is described in the appropriate sections.

Constipation itself requires treatment; the appropriate measures are as follows:

- An increase in the intake of fluid
- Regular physical exercise
- Regular bowel habits.
- A high-fibre diet with bran or other agents which increases stool bulk
- Liquid paraffin or other similar preparations are suitable for short periods of time but are contraindicated for regular use, because they may interfere with the capacity of the bowel to absorb vitamins, have carcinogenic potential, and can cause pruritus ani.
- Saline laxatives and preparations containing mucilage or senna are more suitable for prolonged usage.
- Stimulant laxatives which act by increasing intestinal motility, such as bisacodyl, are often used but prolonged use should be avoided as they can eventually precipitate the onset of an atonic nonfunctioning colon and hypokalaemia.
- Enemas and stimulating rectal suppositories should not be used repeatedly, only as isolated procedures for clearing the lower bowel for specific indications.

IRRITABLE BOWEL SYNDROME

The irritable bowel syndrome is a functional disorder, which is twice as common in women as in men. It is mostly seen between the ages of 20 and 60 years and is usually more troublesome during the week preceding menstruation to form part of the premenstrual syndrome. The resulting pain is therefore often mistaken for dysmenorrhoea. The patient suffers considerable discomfort over the course of the descending colon, which is usually palpable as a cord in the left iliac fossa. Associated symptoms are constipation (which is the *result* and not the *cause* of the spasm), alternating constipation and diarrhoea, flatulence and sometimes attacks of diarrhoea alone. With or without allied spasm of the rectum, colonic spasm can also be the basis of dyspareunia.

Caecal distension is commonly present as well; it causes similar symptoms, but the pain is right sided. The caecum is palpably distended and tender.

The condition persists for many years with intermittent exacerbations related mainly to periods of nervous stress. The clinical picture is also described as the spastic colon.

The syndrome frequently leads to unnecessary appendicectomy, laparotomy for 'adhesions' and even hysterectomy for 'pelvic pain'.

Causes

The underlying cause in a high proportion of cases, but not exclusively, is a state of nervous tension and neurosis. The resulting instability of the autonomic nervous system makes the colon irritable and 'on edge', ready to react to any stimulus or circumstance.

Affected women may be of anxious or emotional disposition, sometimes spoiled by mother or husband and always looking for sympathy. Domestic stresses, family illness and bereavement, financial worries, fear of cancer and similar factors are of 10%. Given such a background, specific factors which precipitate attacks of discomfort are the abuse of purgatives—women themselves, in the belief that the pain is due to constipation, often make matters worse by taking laxatives which have an irritant effect on the colon, certain foods which cause flatulence, a domestic crisis or other sources of worry, the death of a relative or friend from cancer and premenstrual tension.

Diagnosis

The diagnosis of irritable bowel syndrome is readily made on the basis of the clinical features. Barium enema radiography confirms the spasmodic action of the bowel wall in 75% of cases and excludes the presence of other lesions. This investigation is important, as is sigmoidoscopy in some cases, because this is such a common syndrome that it is easy to overlook the occasional presence of some organic lesion in the bowel which gives rise to similar clinical features. Diseases such as diverticulitis and carcinoma of the colon must therefore be excluded.

Treatment

Once an organic lesion of the bowel is excluded, treatment is always on medical lines and never by surgery. In this respect, the important measures are as follows:

- Reassurance and explanation of the situation to the patient and relatives; teach the woman to live with her symptoms.
- Attention to the psychological and environmental factors which are nearly always present in the background
- A high-fibre diet and bran supplements
- Avoidance of laxatives which excite the gut. The pain is not caused by constipation but by muscle spasm of

which constipation is merely a sign. Purgatives make the spasm worse. Saline laxatives, senna, or one of the mucilage preparations, which make the stools big and soft, are helpful if taken regularly.

- Antispasmodics with anticholinergic effects or those that have a direct effect on smooth muscle may be used when the pain is severe.

Results

When the case is handled well, the results are good, although complete elimination of the discomfort is unusual and the symptoms tend to reappear during periods of stress; the woman should be warned of this and told to avoid surgery.

PRURITUS ANI

This complaint is nearly as common as pruritus vulvae and is equally distressing; the two sometimes occur together. The perianal skin may be pink or red but, in the chronic case, is usually white, thickened and keratinised. It shows epithelial changes similar to those found in the vulva and these have sometimes been as described lichen sclerosis or leukoplakia. The affected skin frequently cracks, not only at the anal margin but also in the natal cleft. It very rarely undergoes malignant change.

Causes of Anal Pruritus

The causes of anal pruritus have been shown in **Table 3**.

Treatment

Pruritus ani can last for years, and there is a widespread idea that it is incurable. This is a pessimistic view, and the results are good provided treatment is sufficiently conscientious and persistent. Any obvious cause must be eliminated but, if none is found, pruritus ani is best treated on the assumption that it represents a chronic fungus or other infection with a nidus elsewhere.

- Careful anal hygiene is of utmost importance as prolonged contact with faeces can be detrimental to personal hygiene. In some cases, use of stool-bulking agents may also be necessary.
- If further treatment is necessary, a fungicidal ointment or powder should be applied regularly after washing, as described above.
- If these measures fail, oral antifungals should be tried.
- Steroid ointments and suppositories may give temporary symptomatic relief.

TABLE 3: The causes of anal pruritus.

Personal hygiene	Chronic exposure to residual irritating faeces; conversely, overmeticulous cleansing leading to 'polishing the anus syndrome'
Diet	Intake of large volumes of coffee (caffeinated and decaffeinated products), chocolate, citrus, spicy foods, tea, beer and foods high in milk content; vitamins A and D deficiencies, and fat substitutes
Anatomic compromise	Obesity, deep anal clefts, excessive hair, tight-fitting clothing (tight clothing or clothing that impairs adequate ventilation), fistula, fissure, skin tags, prolapsing papilla or mucosal prolapse
Gynaecologic conditions	Pruritus vulvae and vaginal discharge (endocervicitis and vaginitis)
Neoplasms	Bowen's disease, extramammary Paget's disease, squamous cell carcinoma, cloacogenic carcinoma and anorectal polypoid lesions
Systemic disease	Jaundice, diabetes mellitus, chronic renal failure, iron deficiency, thyrotoxicosis, myxoedema, Hodgkin's lymphoma and polycythaemia vera
Diarrhoeal status	Irritable bowel syndrome, Crohn's disease and chronic ulcerative colitis
Radiation	Postirradiation changes
Psychogenic	Anxiety, neuroses and psychoses
Drugs	Quinidine, colchicine, antibiotics (tetracycline), intravenous hydrocortisone phosphate, ointments or creams that contain 'caine' drugs and non-prescription medications for personal hygiene such as perfumed soaps and ointments that may contain alcohol, witch hazel or other astringents
Dermatologic conditions	Psoriasis, seborrhoeic dermatitis, atopic dermatitis, lichen simplex and lichen sclerosis
Infections	• *Viruses*: Herpes simplex, cytomegalovirus and papillomavirus • *Bacteria*: *Staphylococcus aureus*, erythrasma, mixed infections and syphilis • *Fungi*: Dermatophytosis and candidiasis • *Parasites*: Pinworms, scabies and pediculosis

- There is another 'over-achiever group' who have anal pruritus secondary to their personal hygiene practice of compulsively cleaning the perianal area. Abrasive rubbing and the use of irritating alkaline soaps have been described in the literature as 'polishing the anus syndrome'. Adoption of a less traumatic perianal hygiene program leads to immediate relief.
- Surgical treatment may be required to correct the anatomic deformities leading to anal pruritus.

PILONIDAL SINUS (JEEP BOTTOM; DRIVER'S BOTTOM) PILUS—HAIR; NIDUS—NEST

It is epithelium lined tract, situated a short distance behind the anus, containing hairs and unhealthy diseased granulation tissue. It is due to the penetration of hairs through the skin into subcutaneous tissue. It forms granuloma/unhealthy granulation tissue in the deeper plane. It is of infective origin and occurs in sacral region between the buttocks, umbilicus and axilla **(Fig. 12)**.

It is common in hairdressers (seen in interdigital clefts), jeep drivers. It is common in 20–30 years of age. It is common in males and mostly affects hairy men. Causative factors are: Male preponderance—74%; male sex hormone effect, hairy body, more sweat and maceration; occurs in young—20–29 years, who have active pilosebaceous glands; dark-haired—stiff hairs; obese and overweight—deep natal cleft; prolonged sitting—are typical.

Primary sinus occurs in the midline. Secondary sinus occurs laterally (paramedian). Always disease spreads upwards; multiple secondary sinuses can occur.

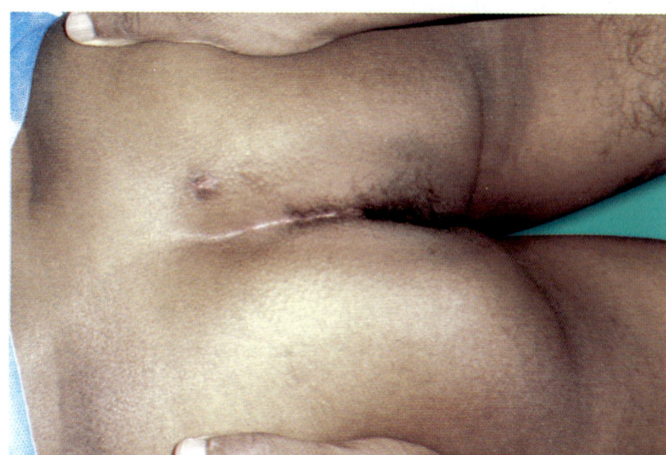

Fig. 12: Pilonidal sinus.

Features

Discharge—either serosanguinous or purulent, pain—throbbing and persistent type, a tender swelling seen just above the coccyx in the midline (primary sinus) and on either side of the midline (secondary sinus).

Tuft of hairs may be seen in the opening of the sinus.

Presentation may be as an acute exacerbation (abscess), or as a chronic one. It causes recurrent infection, abscess formation which bursts open forming recurrent sinus with pain, discharge and discomfort.

Complications and problems: Rarely sacral osteomyelitis, necrotising fasciitis. Recurrent abscess and discharge causing discomfort.

Differential diagnoses: Boil, infected sebaceous cyst, carbuncle in sacral region and buttock.

Management

Pilonidal sinus is a clinical diagnosis; ultrasound of sacral region or MRI are confirmative.

Treatment is wide excision, which includes diseased skin and all sinus tracts, unhealthy granulation tissues, tuft of hairs up to the sacral none is a must. Later wound coverage is done by different procedures such as rhomboid Limberg flap, Z-plasty and advancement flap. Laser treatment is also used for pilonidal sinus. After removing all diseased tissues, wound is left open to allow healthy granulation tissue to form and epithelialisation. In spite of all this, recurrence rate is high >30%. Hair removal using laser at a later period is essential to reduce recurrence.

RECTAL AND ANAL PAIN

Fissure in Ano

Definition

It is a longitudinal ulcer in lower anal canal, usually in posterior midline but can occur in anterior midline or lateral locations. More than 90% are posterior; anterior one is common in females.

Causes

- Chronic constipation
- Altered sacral curvature
- Hard stool, previous surgery such as haemorrhoid-ectomy
- Crohn's disease, ulcerative colitis, tuberculosis and human immunodeficiency virus (HIV)

Types

Acute

Features: It starts suddenly causing a deep acute tear/ulcer in the lower anal canal usually on posterior aspect with acute inflammation and oedema of the surrounding tissues. There is a severe sphincter spasm in the anal canal. Chronic fissures occasionally can cause fibrosis due to repeated inflammation leading to stricture in ano. DRE should be avoided in acute fissures in ano as pain is severe with sphincter spasm.

Treatment: It is treated with local applications, analgesics, stool softeners such as lactulose, bulk laxatives, more liquid intake, fibre-rich diet and sitz bath **(Fig. 13)** three times a day. Local applicants such as nitroglycerine (0.2%) or diltiazem 2% or injection of botulinum toxin (25 units) relax the internal sphincter, thereby promoting the healing of the acute fissure in ano. Often requires if pain persists, lateral sphincterotomy or anal stretching (four-finger stretching of the sphincter). Either open or closed method is used for lateral sphincterotomy. Lateral sphincterotomy is an ideal method with 96% cure rate for acute fissure in ano. Closed method is done under local or general anaesthesia; using 11 numbered blade intersphincteric groove is felt; upper internal sphincter part is firmly pressed to make it prominent; blade is turned upwards facing the lower one third of the internal sphincter and is cut; sphincter release and relaxation can be felt instantly. The area is pressed with saline-soaked gauze for 10 minutes to avoid oozing and haematoma formation.

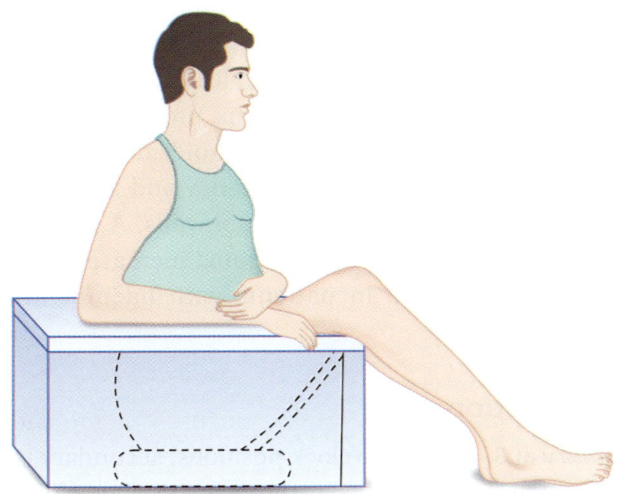

Fig. 13: Sitz bath.

Chronic

It is chronic indolent ulcer in posterior or anterior part of the lower anal canal. It is common in posterior midline; often can occur anterior midline and occasionally lateral too **(Figs. 14 and 15)**.

It is chronic ulcer with distal sentinel pile and proximal hypertrophied papilla. DRE and proctoscopy are possible here as it is less painful compared to acute fissure in ano. Associated haemorrhoids should be confirmed through proctoscopy as more bleeding if present, it could be due to haemorrhoids also.

Evaluation: Crohn's disease and ulcerative colitis must be ruled out. Colonoscopy, blood assessment such as haematocrit, carcinoembryonic antigen (CEA) and imaging of the abdomen and chest whenever needed should be done.

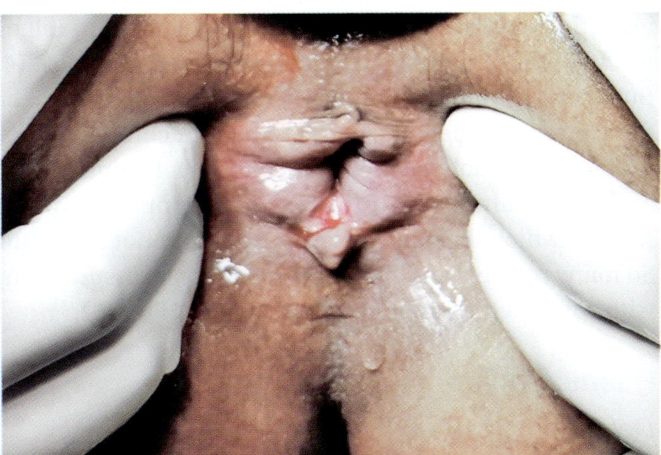

Fig. 14: Chronic anal fissure with sentinel pile.

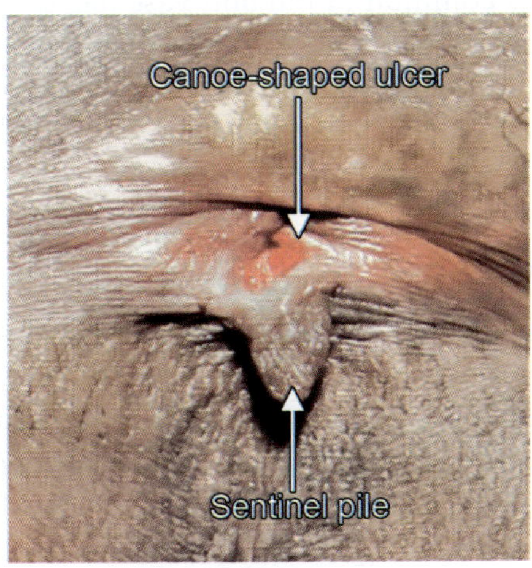

Fig. 15: Chronic fissure in ano.

Treatment: (1) Dorsal fissurectomy with lateral sphincterotomy is a good procedure wherein the ulcer with sentinel pile and hypertrophic papilla is excised using scissor or cautery, i.e. entire pathological part is excised; together lateral sphincterotomy is done by cutting the lower one third or half of the internal sphincter. It is achieved by feeling the intersphincteric groove through which a small incision is made; internal sphincter is felt like a firm cord and seen like whitish collar fibers; using number 11 blade sphincter part is cut at its lower margin; one can feel the relaxation immediately through the palpating finger. Tissue should be sent for histology. Problem here is delayed wound healing, pain and discharge. (2) If piles are present, they should be treated accordingly—haemorrhoidectomy/laser/high ligation or any hybrid procedures. (3) Lord's eight-finger dilatation once earlier popular is no longer practised as trauma to sphincter complex including puborectalis is higher with chances of incontinence. However, four-finger anal stretching still be useful with minimum damage to sphincter complex. (4) But lateral sphincterotomy has become standard. It can be done as either open or closed method. In chronic fissure, problem with only lateral sphincterotomy is sentinel pile and to certain extent proximal hypertrophic papillae persists which the patient feels treatment is not adequate. So many patients and surgeons prefer dorsal fissurectomy with sphincterotomy as accepted therapy **(Fig. 16)**.

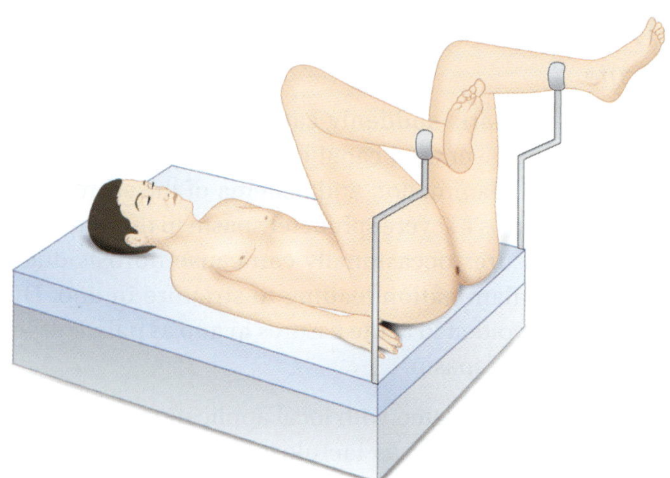

Fig. 16: Lithotomy is the position which is commonly used for perianal surgeries; however, many procedures are preferably done often in jackknife prone position also.

Haemorrhoids

Definition

Haemorrhoids are descent of anal cushions as a pathological entity, which may be mucosal or vascular; mucosal is common in old and vascular is common in young (haemorrhoids—Greek word means blood to ooze; piles in Latin means ball). So, many causes have been postulated.

Causes

Hereditary

Morphological: Superior rectal veins have no valves hence congestion occurs and anal cushions descend. Superior rectal artery divides into right and left; right divides into anterior and posterior; hence, there are two piles on the right side (right anterior at 11 o'clock position; right posterior at 7 o'clock position) and one on the left side (at 3 o'clock position). Suspensory ligament of Park's which supports the anal cushions which get damaged leading to piles.

Other causes: Other causes include chronic constipation, diarrhoea, straining, hard stool, low-fibre diet, pregnancy, carcinoma rectum (in old age recent onset of piles means one should suspect carcinoma rectum and sigmoidoscopy/colonoscopy should be done and DRE is a must) and bulging of haemorrhoidal venous plexus.

Pathology

Haemorrhoidal cushions appear predictably in all individuals at right anterior, right posterior and left lateral positions with secondary haemorrhoidal complexes in between **(Figs. 17A and B)**. Excessive straining, chronic constipation or low-fibre diet can lead to damage to the connective tissue of these cushions, producing bleeding with or without prolapse. Haemorrhoids develop as part of the pelvic congestion of pregnancy and are probably encouraged by atony of the vessel walls. A number of investigators have also demonstrated increased internal anal sphincter tone in patients with haemorrhoidal disease.

Classification

Primary at 3, 7 and 11 o'clock positions; secondary is the one which occurs between the primary sites **(Figs. 18 and 19)**.

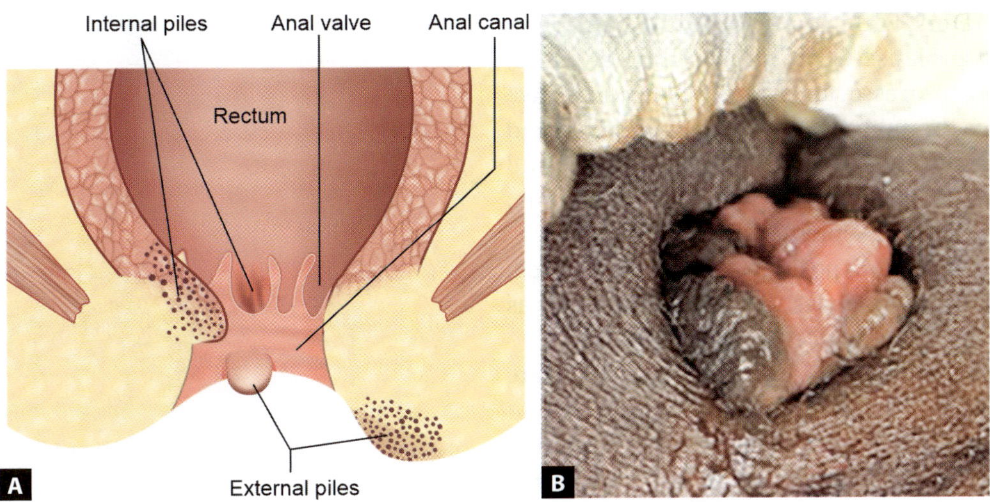

Figs. 17A and B: Typical location of internal piles.

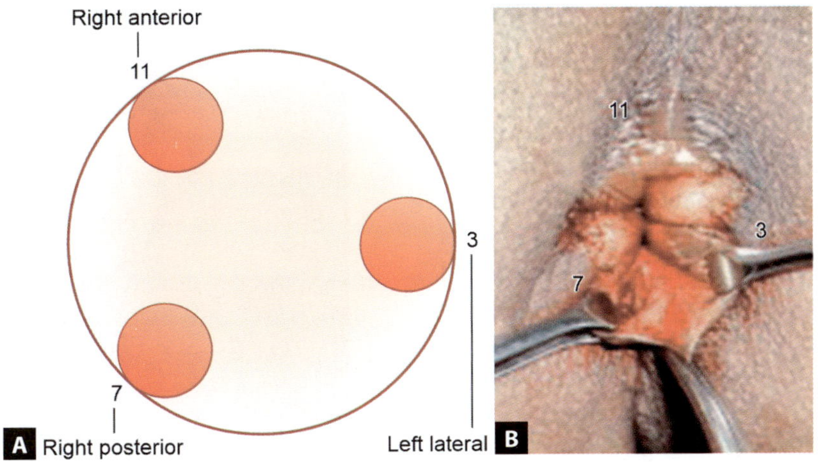

Figs. 18A and B: Position of piles.

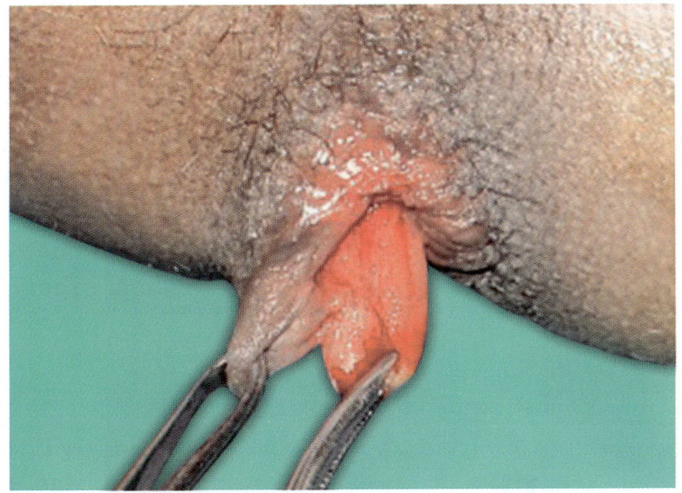

Fig. 19: Parts of piles—internal and external.

Degrees of haemorrhoids: First degree—pile within bleeds but does not come out, diagnosis is confirmed by proctoscopy; *second degree*—pile prolapses during defaecation but returns spontaneously inside; *third degree*—pile prolapses during defaecation and can be replaced back manually only and *fourth degree*—pile that is permanently prolapsed.

Features

The typical symptom associated with haemorrhoidal disease is *painless bleeding* at the time of defaecation. It is usually described as bright red blood either on the toilet paper or into the commode (splash in the pan) after bowel movements. In some patients, the bleeding may be sufficient to lead to iron deficiency anaemia.

Pain associated with haemorrhoids can be a consequence of prolapse of the haemorrhoidal tissue, thrombosis or due to an associated anorectal condition like anal fissure. Once thrombosed, they remain extruded and patients present become swollen, tense, oedematous and tender haemorrhoids with systemic signs of inflammation; a condition which requires emergency treatment.

Mass per anum at various positions often needs manual repositioning. Eventually, mass may not be reduced as such—a feature of prolapsed piles **(Figs. 20 and 21)**.

Mucoid discharge, pruritus, discomfort in sitting are common.

Pile mass is not felt on DRE but associated condition such as carcinoma may be diagnosed. Thrombosed pile mass can be felt and is firm, tender mass.

Proctoscopy is a must; number of piles and positions can be seen properly. Associated chronic fissure if present should be noted down.

Differential diagnoses such as carcinoma rectum/anal canal or rectal prolapse or rectal polyp should be kept in mind. Mass may itself be carcinoma with hard, proliferative and induration features. Rectal prolapse is circumferential, red/pink, without any specific skin component, whereas pile mass is noncircumferential, plum coloured and with cutaneous component. Other causes of bleeding per anum should be kept in mind such as ulcerative colitis, polyps, vascular anomaly and mesenteric ischaemia **(Figs. 22A and B)**.

Complications of haemorrhoids are profuse haemorrhage which will become an emergency with need for blood transfusion, urgent surgical intervention, thrombosis, ulceration, gangrene, suppuration,

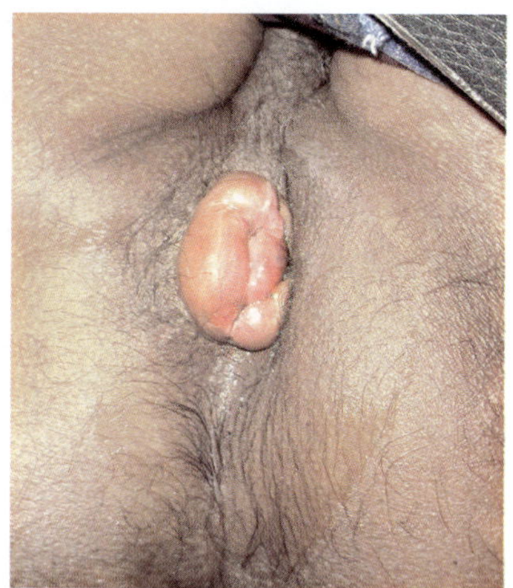

Fig. 20: Prolapsed piles.

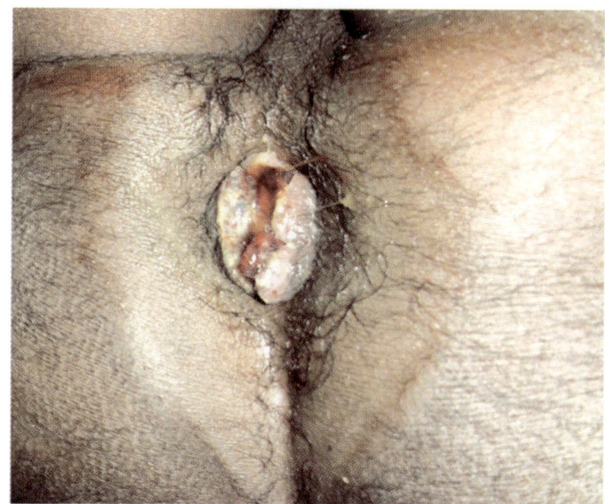

Fig. 21: Strangulated piles.

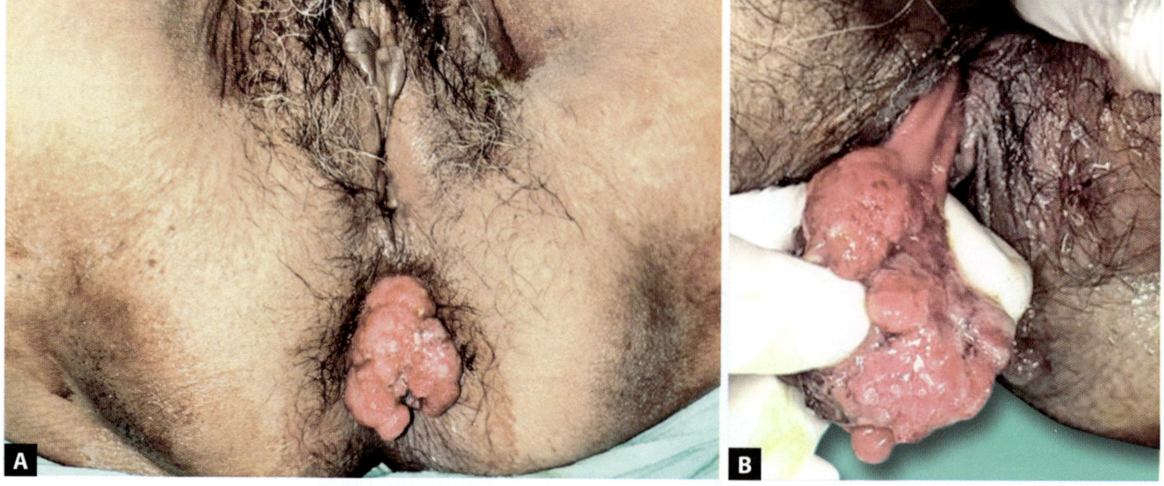

Figs. 22A and B: Rectal polyp—differential diagnosis for piles.

rarely septicaemia or portal pyaemia in old age and immunosuppressed individuals.

Prevalence is 4.4% in the world, equal in both sexes, and occurs between 30 and 70 years of age commonly.

Evaluation: Blood parameters such as haematocrit, sigmoidoscopy/colonoscopy in elderly, CEA if carcinoma is suspected and specific relevant evaluation methods for identifying the cause and to plan the treatment.

Treatment

Nonoperative—sitz bath daily two to three times a day as sitting in warm water bath with the anus dipping in it for 10–15 minutes. It reduces oedema and pain. Analgesics, anti-inflammatory drugs, fibre diet, laxatives, bulk-forming agents, local applications to reduce oedema and to smoothen the anal canal but better one should avoid steroid local applicants. In infected/gangrenous haemorrhoids antibiotics should be started orally or intravenously.

Dilatation or stretching of the anal canal in prolapsed, inflamed oedematous piles. Four-finger stretching is done. Lord's eight-finger dilatation even though helps in reducing the content well and the chances of incontinence are high; ideally stretching should be done under general anaesthesia.

Office procedures: (1) Injection sclerosant therapy using phenol in almond oil or sodium tetradecyl sulphate (STS) or ethanolamine oleate using a strong Gabriel syringe is useful in first and early second-degree piles. (2) Barron's banding—it is useful in second-degree piles using specialised devices; done under local anaesthesia; band is placed to pile mass 2 cm above the dentate line. (3) Cryotherapy—it is done using (-98°) nitrous oxide or liquid nitrogen (-196°) and done under local anaesthesia, with a specialised cryo device pile mass is frozen for 2 minutes, and then defrost is done. It is not used now due to discharge. (4) Infrared coagulation—using a handheld applicator infrared radiation is used to burn the pile mass; probe is placed over the pedicle above the dentate line. (5) Doppler-guided haemorrhoidal artery ligation (DGHAL).

Surgery: Milligan Morgan haemorrhoidectomy is ideal treatment for third- and fourth-degree haemorrhoids. Stapled haemorrhoidopexy is a painless procedure, useful for prolapsed piles **(Figs. 23 and 24) (Table 4)**.

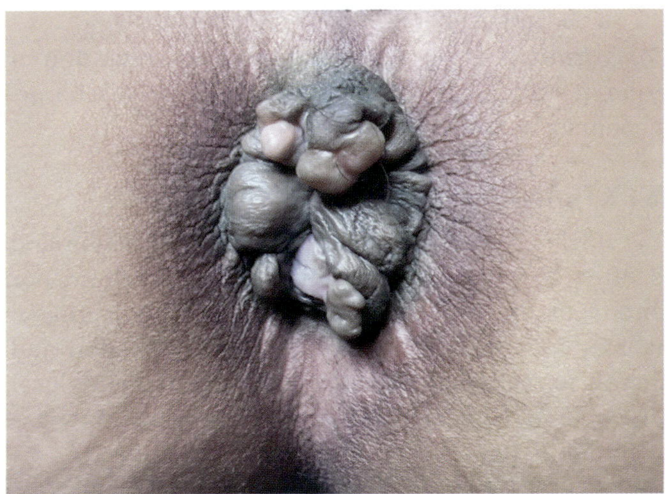

Fig. 23: Internoexternal haemorrhoids.

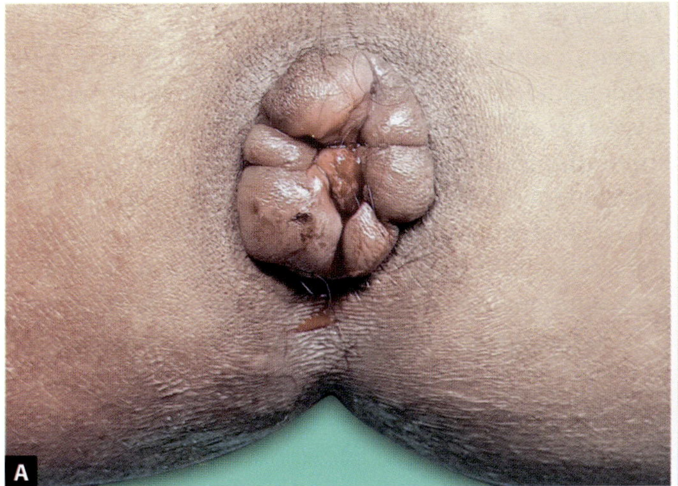

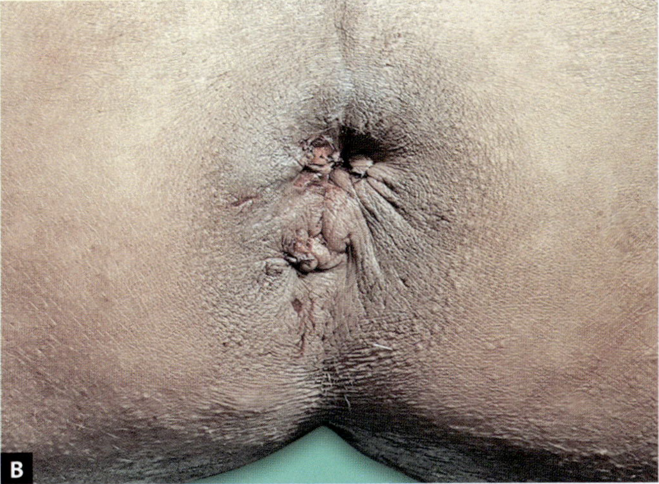

Figs. 24A and B: (A) Thrombosed external with prolapsed internal haemorrhoids; (B) Postoperative image after stapled haemorrhoidopexy with excision of haemorrhoids in the same patient.

TABLE 4: Management of internal haemorrhoids—decision often made on an individual case—basis.

Grade 1	• Only bleeding • No prolapse	• Diet and lifestyle modifications • Banding, laser and infrared therapy
Grade 2	• Bleeding • Prolapse with spontaneous reduction	• Diet and lifestyle modifications • Banding, laser • Excision/stapled haemorrhoidopexy
Grade 3	• Bleeding • Prolapse requiring manual reduction	• Excision/stapled haemorrhoidopexy • Laser
Grade 4	• Bleeding • Prolapsed cannot be reduced	Excision/stapled haemorrhoidopexy

Complications of surgery/procedure: Pain, retention of urine, reactionary/secondary haemorrhage, discharge, incontinence, anal stenosis and recurrence.

EXTERNAL PILE/HAEMORRHOIDS

It is single or multiple skin tags in perianal region and is often associated with internal haemorrhoids or chronic fissure in ano **(Fig. 25)**. It causes pain, perianal haematoma due venular oozing inside, infection and abscess formation. It is treated with excision under local anaesthesia. Associated conditions such as internal piles or chronic fissures are treated accordingly **(Table 5)**.

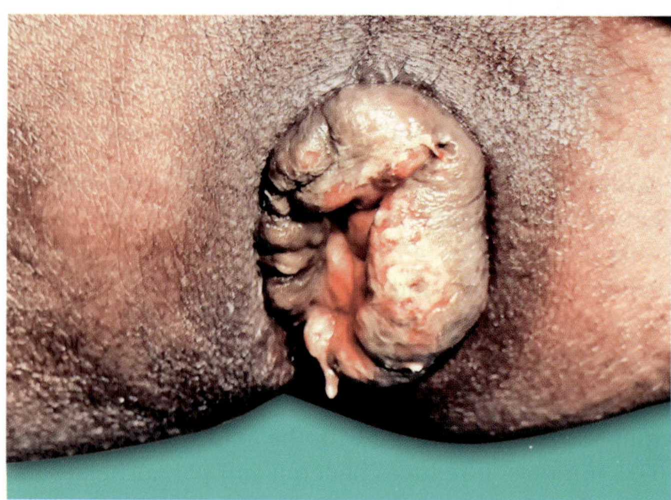

Fig. 25: Thrombosed external haemorrhoids.

TABLE 5: Management of external haemorrhoids.

External haemorrhoids		***Management***
Thrombosed	>72 hours	• Dietary modifications • Pain control • Sitz bath
	<72 hours	Consider surgical excision
Nonthrombosed		• Dietary modifications • Consider excision if large, poor hygiene and painful

ANORECTAL ABSCESS

Definition

It is an abscess in perianal region usually caused by infection of cryptoglands in perianal region. It is common in diabetics and immunosuppressed.

Causes

Cryptoglandular Infection (90%)

Other causes: Other causes include injury, postperianal surgery, skin infection, specific diseases such as Crohn's disease, ulcerative colitis, immunosuppression, perianal haematoma and bloodborn infections.

Causative Organisms

Escherichia coli is the main organism (60%); *Staphylococcus, Streptococcus* and *Proteus* are other organisms.

Classification (Figs. 26A and B)

(1) Perianal (60%), (2) ischiorectal, (3) submucous, (4) pelvirectal and (5) fissure abscess.

Features

Severe, excruciating, throbbing pain often with fever, tender, smooth, soft, tender and swelling at the specified sites such as perianal, ischiorectal or submucous. Brawny induration with localised swelling often with or without fluctuation is the typical presentation **(Fig. 27)**.

Ischiorectal abscess occurs in the pyramidal ischiorectal fossa, which is bounded by the rectum, skin, levator ani and obturator fascia covering obturator internus.

Digital rectal examination must be done to assess clinically the extent.

Differential Diagnoses

Differential diagnoses include periurethral abscess, Bartholin abscess and tuberculous cold abscess.

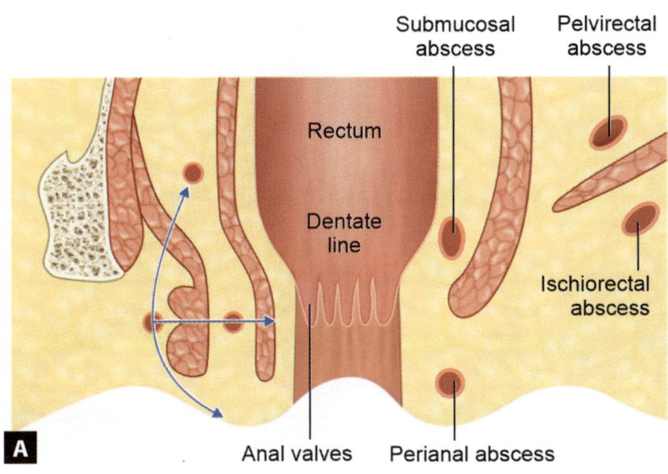

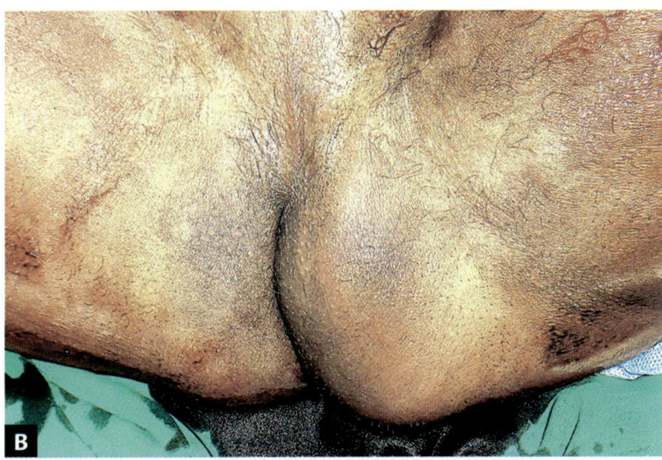

Figs. 26A and B: (A) Anorectal abscess—types; (B) Ischiorectal abscess—Left sided.

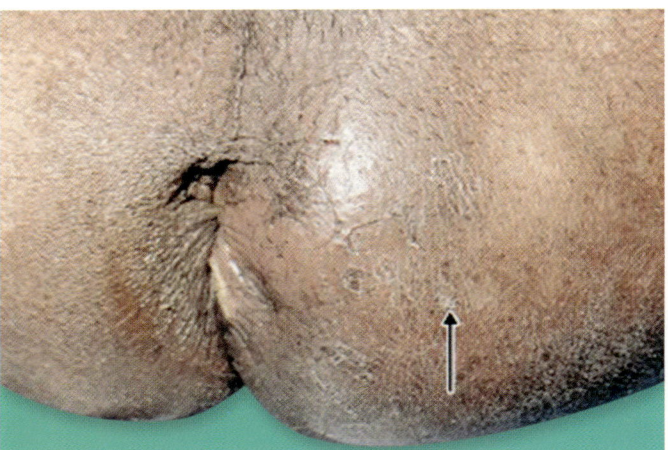

Fig. 27: Ischiorectal abscess (black arrow).

Evaluation

- Blood—haematocrit, blood sugar, HIV and other relevant tests
- Perianal ultrasound/MRI perineum
- Proctoscopy/sigmoidoscopy

Treatment

Incision and drainage under general or spinal anaesthesia should be done; pus should be sent for culture and sensitivity. Antibiotics should be started prior to drainage, and control of diabetes mellitus is also important. In severe cases, hospitalisation should be done for proper management.

Complications and Problems

Complications and problems can be septicaemia, recurrent abscess formation and fistula formation.

FISTULA-IN-ANO

It is fistula track which connects superficially outwards and below from skin to deeply into the anorectum. It usually occurs after anorectal abscess as a sequelae.

Types

- *Cryptoglandular*—90%
- *Non-cryptoglandular:* Tuberculosis, Crohn's disease, ulcerative colitis, trauma, carcinoma, lymphogranuloma venereum

Classification

- *Standard (Milligan Morgan) classification:* Subcutaneous, low anal; submucous, high, pelvirectal.
- *Park's classification:* Intersphincteric (70%), transphincteric (25%), suprasphincteric (supralevator) and extrasphincteric (1%) **(Figs. 28A to D)**.

Based on levels: Low and high levels.

It can be simple fistula without extensions; complex fistula with extensions. The term complex fistula means the track crosses >50% of the external sphincter, anterior in females, multiple tracks, recurrent or the patient has pre-existing incontinence, local irradiation, or Crohn's disease **(Figs. 29 and 30)**.

Features

It is common in males, common in diabetics and HIV patients.

It has a prevalence of 0.01% and is common in adult males (2:1, male to female). It presents with seropurulent discharge (65%), along with skin irritation and one or

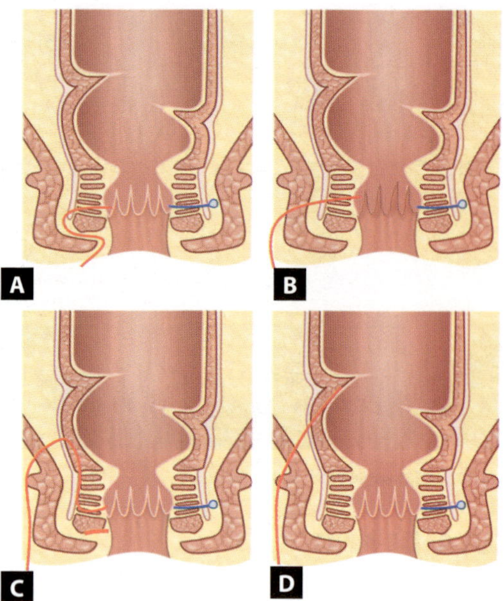

Figs. 28A to D: Fistula-in-ano—Park's classification. (A) Intersphincteric fistula; (B) Transphincteric fistula; (C) Supralevator fistula; (D) Extrasphincteric fistula.

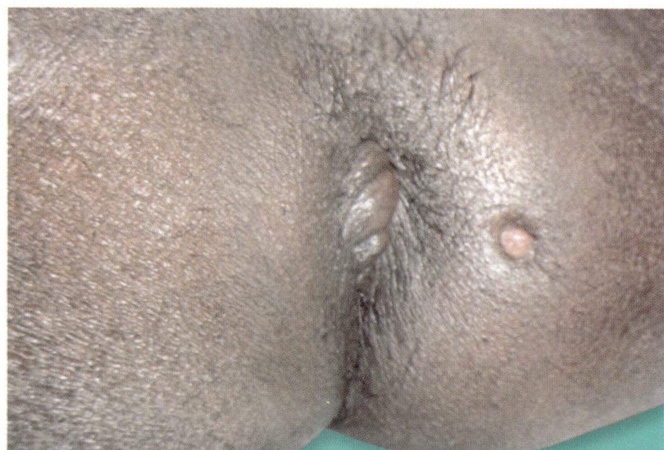

Fig. 29: Typical look of external opening in fistula-in-ano.

more external opening may be present with induration of the surrounding skin.

Often it may heal superficially but pus may collect beneath forming an abscess which again discharges through the same or new opening. Ischiorectal fossa on each side most often communicates with each other behind the anus causing a horseshoe fistula.

P/R examination shows an indurated internal opening usually in the midline posteriorly. Most of the fistulas are on posterior half of anus. Extent, extensions, to rule out carcinoma or to identify aetiology digital rectal examination is important.

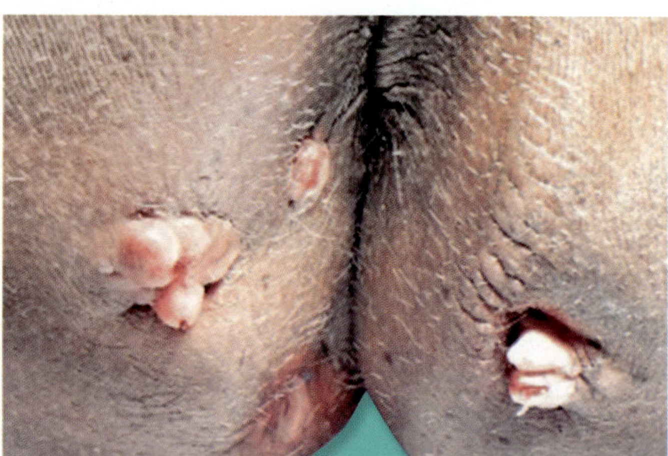

Fig. 30: Multiple fistulas in ano.

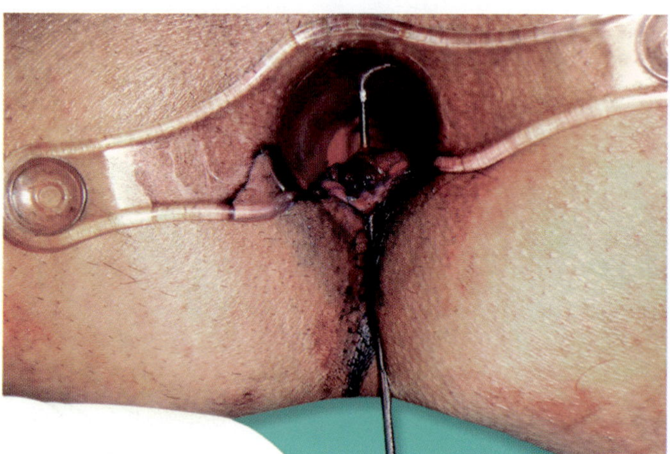

Fig. 31: Probing of fistula is done carefully under general anaesthesia.

Probing in the ward and fistulogram in the ward before surgery using Lipiodol is not advisable as it may cause recrudescence of inflammation. It can be done with adequate precaution. Probing is done under general anaesthesia gently with care without creating extensions **(Figs. 31 to 33)**.

Goodsall's rule: Anterior fistulas have a straight track. Posterior fistulas have curved track with internal opening in the posterior midline **(Fig. 34)**.

Differential diagnosis for fistula-in-ano: Urethral fistula in male, chronically infected Bartholin's gland, pilonidal sinus, Hidradenitis suppurativa, Carcinoma, Crohn's tuberculosis and ulcerative colitis.

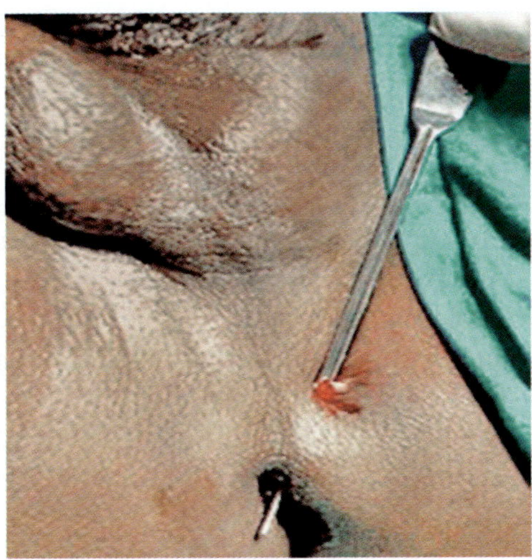

Fig. 32: Anterior fistula-in-ano with probe.

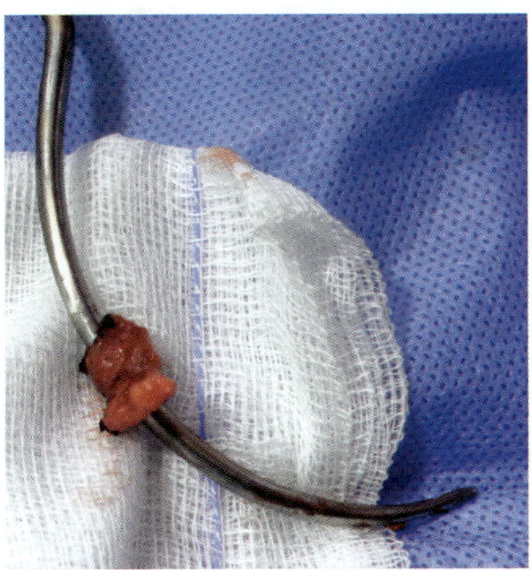

Fig. 33: Fistulectomy specimen with probe.

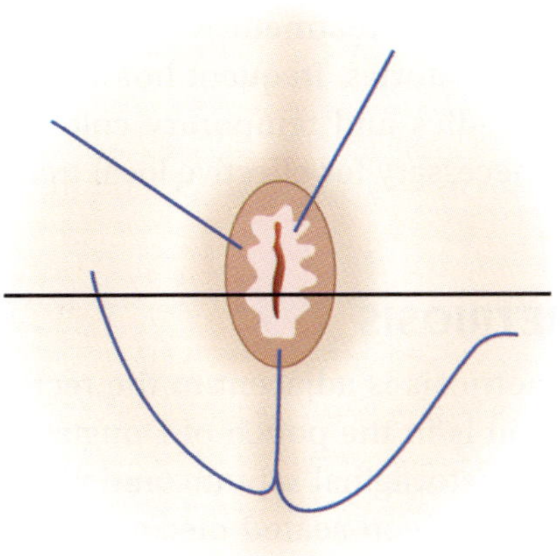

Fig. 34: Goodsall's rule.

Investigations

- Blood—erythrocyte sedimentation rate (ESR), specific relevant tests
- Chest X-ray, ESR and barium enema X-ray. If required, fistulogram is done only under anaesthesia.
- MRI/MRI fistulogram ideal
- Endorectal ultrasound (US perineum) is useful to assess the deeper plane.
- Discharge study, methylene blue dye study and biopsy
- Colonoscopy is often when ulcerative colitis/Crohn's is suspected. Specific blood test.

Treatment

Surgical procedures: Fistulotomy with lay opening for low fistula, fistulectomy with open wound and hybrid procedures with partial excision with laser or seton technique. Specimen should be sent for biopsy/histology. High fistula often may require hybrid procedures covering temporary diversion colostomy.

Newer methods: Gluing of the tract, anal fistula plug repair, ligation of intersphincteric fistula tract (LIFT), video-assisted anal fistula tract ligation (VAAFT), laser fulguration of the tract and hybrid procedures.

Under spinal anaesthesia (local anaesthesia is used for low, simple fistula-in-ano) with lithotomy or jackknife position surgery is done. Warm normal saline or hydrogen peroxide or dilute methylene blue solution is injected into the external opening to delineate the tract and extensions. Cryptoglands should be eradicated completely. Sphincter mechanism should be preserved. Procedure is decided in the table to prevent recurrence with optimum results **(Fig. 35 and Table 6)**.

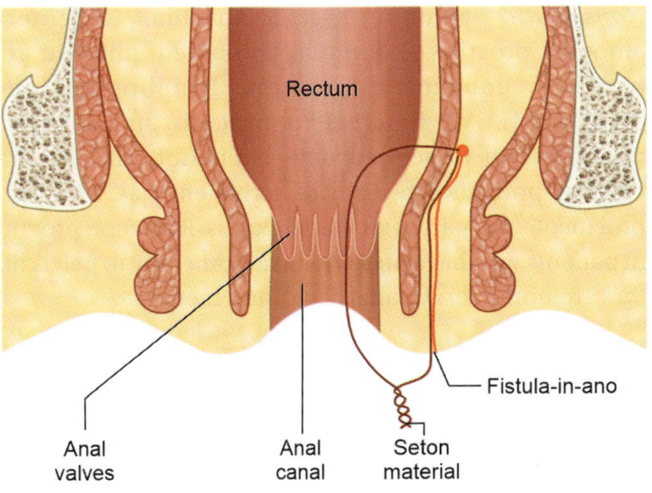

Fig. 35: Seton technique.

TABLE 6: Different procedures used for fistula-in-ano.

Principles of treatment	*Procedures*
• Identify the cause—cryptoglandular or other delineate exactly the fistula anatomy—MRI/EUS • Identify relation of fistula to anal sphincter • Drain all sites of infection • Eradicate track and secondary extensions • Preserve anal continence function • The primary objectives are to eradicate the tract and drain all associated sites of infection while simultaneously preserving anal continence	• Laying open the fistula—fistulotomy with curetting • Fistulectomy • Gluing of fistula—not very useful • Mucosal flap procedure • Fistulectomy with primary repair • Fistulectomy with primary repair with episiorectopexy • Fistulectomy with secondary repair • Anal fistula plug (AFP) repair • Ligation of intersphincteric fistula track (LIFT) technique • Seton technique (Latin—seta—a bristle) • Colostomy—lay open, fistulectomy and later closure of colostomy—for high type • Video-assisted anal fistula track ligation (VAAFT) procedure

(EUS: endoscopic ultrasound)

PROCTITIS

It is the inflammation of the rectal mucosa often with the inflammation of colon and anal canal.

Types

Acute or Chronic

Nonspecific—common, *specific*—bacillary dysentery, amoebic proctitis—common, combined amoebic and bacillary, gonococcal proctitis, lymphogranuloma inguinale (LGV), tuberculous proctitis and bilharzial proctitis due to schistosoma haematobium. Enema-induced proctitis especially of herbal enemas. Ulcerative proctocolitis as part of ulcerative colitis. Radiation proctitis in patients who have undergone radiotherapy to pelvis like for carcinoma cervix, anal canal, and rectum.

Features

- Pain per rectum and anum; tenesmus
- Passage of mucus and blood; frequent urge to pass stool
- Fever, loss of appetite; pain and tenderness in left lower abdomen
- P/R is tender.

Investigations

- Sigmoidoscopy is more relevant than just proctoscopy; stool study, stool culture, mucosal biopsy and serological tests.
- Relevant investigations such as ESR, blood smear and chest X-ray

Treatment

- Antibiotics, antiamoebic drugs such as metronidazole. In severe cases, retention enema using metronidazole, prednisolone and salazopyrin
- IV fluids, IV antibiotics and IV metronidazole are often required.
- Treating the specific causes such as tuberculosis, gonococcal infection and bilharzial infection.

Radiation Proctitis

Proctitis can be an immediate temporary reaction to radiation or can appear many months or years later. In the latter circumstance, it causes intense pain which is throbbing and sickening in character, deep-seated and sometimes referred to as the buttocks. This is accompanied by the passage of blood and pus when the lesion becomes ulcerated. On examination, the anterior rectal wall feels indurated and is fixed by adjacent cellulitis. It bleeds on examination and a frank ulcer may be seen or felt. The condition is thus often mistaken for a recurrence of malignancy.

Radiation proctitis is treated by keeping the motions soft and loose, local treatment with corticosteroids as enemas or suppositories, frequent hot baths, analgesics and antispasmodics and temporary colostomy, which may become necessary for effective local treatment to be carried out.

ENDOMETRIOSIS

When endometriosis is adjacent to the rectum—as it is when the lesion is in the pouch of Douglas, uterosacral ligaments and rectovaginal septum, and when it invades the rectal wall—a deep-seated discomfort results. This amounts to actual pain at the time of defaecation and is especially noticeable just before and at the time of menstruation. Endometriosis rarely penetrates the bowel mucosa and does not often cause rectal bleeding.

NEOPLASM OF THE ANAL CANAL

Carcinoma of the rectum, and carcinoma invading or approaching the rectum from any of the genital organs, invariably give rise to an incessant and deep-seated ache with a frequent desire to empty the bowel. Rectal spasm plays an important part in causing these sensations.

Condyloma Acuminata

- It is the most common sexually transmitted anal disease. It is common in homosexual men.
- Penile warts or female genital warts may be present.
- It is caused by human papillomavirus (HPV). Pruritus, discharge, pain and bleeding are the features. Large warts may block the anal canal orifice.
- Whitening occurs when acetic acid is on it. A biopsy confirms the diagnosis.
- Treatment is local application of 25% podophyllin cream, surgical excision of the wart and intralesional injection of interferon alfa-2b. Malignancy should be ruled out by histology.

Note: Buschke-Lowenstein disease (giant condyloma acuminata) is a slow growing, locally destructive verrucous plaque but seldom metastasizes that typically appears on the penis but may occur elsewhere in the anogenital region. It is commonly considered to be a regional variant of verrucous carcinoma. It is common in the penis but can also occur in the anal region, vagina and scrotum. It is common in males. HPV 6, 11 and HIV infections may commonly coexist. Biopsy and MRI confirm the diagnosis. Giant condyloma acuminatum is differentiated histologically from ordinary condyloma acuminata by its thicker stratum corneum and the presence of an endophytic downgrowth, along with a tendency to invade deeper.

Anal Intraepithelial Neoplasia

It is dysplasia of anal or perianal epidermis. It is seen in individuals with HIV infection, HPV infection (16, 18) and individuals who do anorectal intercourse.

Classification: Anal intraepithelial neoplasia I (AIN I)—absence of keratocyte maturation and cellular atypia observed in outer one third of epithelium—low grade. AIN II—cellular atypia observed in middle one third—low-grade squamous intraepithelial neoplasia. AIN III—cellular atypia full thickness—high-grade squamous intraepithelial neoplasia.

Thirty percent of anal warts will show AIN. It is a raised scaly white/pigmented/cracked lesion. Biopsy confirms the disease.

Treatment: Excision; topical imiquimod, 80% trichloroacetic acid and oral retinoids.

Malignant Tumours of Anal Area

Anal malignant tumours are <2% of large bowel tumours. It can be below the dentate line [squamous cell carcinoma (SCC), 80% of anal tumours] and above the dentate line (basaloid/transitional/cloacogenic).

Causes may be HPV infection, HIV infection, AIN, organ transplant recipients and immunosuppression.

Anal canal tumours arise from the anorectal ring proximally to the anal verge distally and include the anal transition zone and the nonhair or gland-bearing squamous tissue comprising the anoderm. The anal margin is defined as the hair and gland-bearing skin lateral and up to 5 cm away from the anal verge. This distinction between anal canal and anal margin malignancies is important as anal canal lesions are more aggressive and are treated differently. The incidence of anal canal lesions is significantly higher (five times) than that of anal margin lesions.

Squamous cell carcinoma is the most common type; predisposing causes: Papilloma, irradiation, dermatitis and long-standing fistula-in-ano. Basaloid carcinoma, basal cell carcinoma, mucoepidermoid carcinoma, melanoma and adenocarcinoma are other types.

Twenty to twenty-five percent of cases metastases occur to inguinal lymph node.

Anal canal tumours are common in females **(Fig. 36)**.

Features: Ulceration, bleeding, pain, pruritus and discharge; irregular indurated mass; anovaginal fistula in females; faecal incontinence in late cases and palpable inguinal node—hard, nontender; iliac nodes may be palpable. Later—late constipation—obstruction; sepsis, discomfort, foul smelling discharge and fungation develops.

Investigations: Biopsy from the anal region; fine needle aspiration cytology (FNAC) of inguinal node; US abdomen, CECT abdomen and pelvis and MRI perineum is very useful. Haematocrit, molecular study for HPV, CEA are needed;

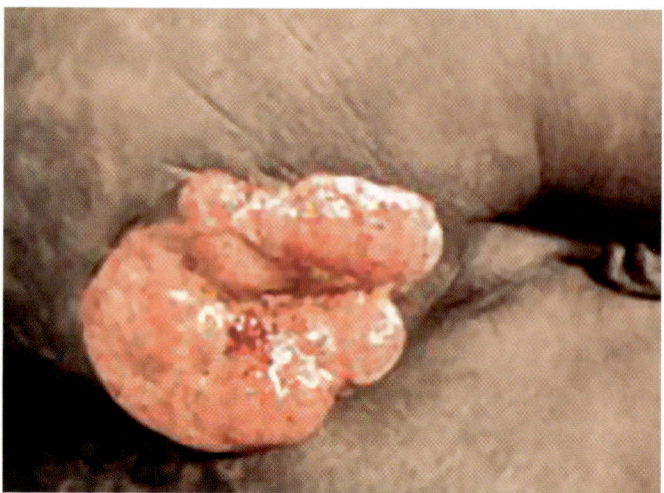

Fig. 36: SCC of anal canal; note the typical everted edge. (SCC: squamous cell carcinoma)

P/R is a must to assess the upper extent of the growth. American Joint Committee on Cancer (AJCC) staging of carcinoma anal canal (8th edition, 2018) is used.

Treatment: Wide local excision with unilateral/bilateral inguinal lymph node dissection if lesion is small; then adjuvant radiotherapy and chemotherapy. If the lesion is large, initial chemoradiotherapy is given; then abdominoperineal resection (APR) with permanent colostomy is done, later adjuvant chemotherapy (5-fluorouracil, mitomycin C, cisplatin and bleomycin) is continued (Nigro regime).

Rectal Spasm and Proctalgia Fugax

Although rectal spasm usually has an organic lesion as its basis, it does occur as a functional disorder. Its aetiology is then the same as for colonic spasm in the irritable bowel syndrome.

Rectal spasm causes deep-seated pelvic discomfort and a desire to evacuate the bowel. The rectum is tender, so dyspareunia is a common complaint and the findings on vaginal examination may mislead the observer into thinking that adnexal disease, cellulitis or retroversion is the cause of symptoms. The treatment of rectal spasms is the same as for the spastic colon of irritable bowel syndrome.

Proctalgia fugax is characterised by sudden, and sometimes severe, rectal pain that occurs at irregular intervals by day but more often by night. It is sudden severe recurring pain in the rectum of unknown cause with segmental pubococcygeal spasm. It can be easily diagnosed clinically. It is common in young people may be due to stress and straining. Common at night, starts suddenly, lasts for a few minutes and then subsides spontaneously. Pain is unbearable and severe with often constipation; gradually subsides on its own. Treatment may be difficult. Some patients may respond to the oral administration of nifedipine. Topical application of nitroglycerin has also been found to be useful. Occasionally, only cutting of puborectalis muscle is required but with danger of developing incontinence.

Vaginal Neuralgia and Vaginal Myalgia

For want of better names, these are devised to describe a complaint of deep-seated pain, usually unilateral and paravaginal, which is persistent for years. It is not relieved by sitting or lying. The pain is often at the level of the insertions of the pubovaginalis and puborectalis muscles, and these may appear to be in spasm. However, despite the fullest investigation and prolonged observation, the majority have no organic cause in the spine or the pelvic organs. The patient is usually of introspective and tense disposition, and sometimes has cancerophobia. It is, therefore, tempting to conclude that the syndrome has a psychogenic basis. This is supported by the fact that the pain, of which the patient complains bitterly, rarely keeps her awake.

The only treatment of any value consists of the elimination of background factors, placebos and reassurance. Pudendal nerve block sometimes gives temporary relief, but such an effect is probably psychological because, on repetition, the treatment is usually unsuccessful.

SUGGESTED READING

1. Elsebae MMA. A study of fecal incontinence in patients with chronic anal fissure: prospective, randomized, controlled trial of the extent of internal anal sphincter division during lateral sphincterotomy. World J Surg. 2007;31: 2052-7.
2. Gordon PH, Hoexter B. Complications of the Ripstein procedure. Dis Colon Rectum. 1978;21:277-80.
3. Rashid Z, Basson MD. Association of rectal prolapse with colorectal cancer. Surgery. 1996;119:51-5.
4. Thompson JR, Chen AH, Pettit PD, Bridges MD. Incidence of occult rectal prolapse in patients with clinical rectoceles and defecatory dysfunction. Am J Obstet Gynecol. 2002;187:1494-9.

62 CHAPTER

Preoperative and Postoperative Management and Postoperative Complications

Srirama Bhat M

Chapter Outline

- Fluid and Electrolytes
- Preoperative Management
- Postoperative Management
- Fast-track Protocol
- Postoperative Examination
- Postoperative Complications
- Deep Venous Thrombosis
- Pulmonary Embolism
- Pulmonary Complications

INTRODUCTION

Although minor procedures usually cause little disturbance, most major operations impose nervous and physical stresses, which result in metabolic and chemical changes in the body tissues and fluids. Many of these are brought about by 'stress' alterations in the functions of the adrenal cortex, but other mechanisms, some not fully explained, are also involved. Increased adrenal cortical activity is manifested by a rise in the excretion of 17-ketosteroids and by a fall in the eosinophil count (indicative of increased production of hydrocortisone) for 1 or 2 weeks after operation.

FLUID AND ELECTROLYTES

Water constitutes approximately 50–55% of the body weight of the average woman. Two-thirds of this water is contained in the intracellular compartment. One-third is contained in the extracellular compartment, of which one-fourth is contained in plasma, and the remaining three-fourths is in the interstitium.

Normal physiology total body water (TBW) is 60% of body weight in males, 50% of body weight in females, i.e. 30 litres. Intracellular water—20 litres (2/3). Extracellular water—10 litres (1/3); Plasma (1/4) (2.5 litres). Interstitial fluid (7.5 litres). Ion intracellular fluid (ICF), extra-cellular fluid (ECF) and plasma ECF volume and osmolality regulation are controlled by three hormones: (1) Aldosterone, (2) antidiuretic hormone (ADH) and (3) atrial natriuretic hormone **(Table 1)**.

TABLE 1: Osmolality of different ions and their ICF, ECF and plasma ECF volumes.

Ion	*ICF*	*ECF and plasma*
Sodium	10 mmol/L	140 mmol/L
Potassium	150 mmol/L	4.5 mmol/L
Chloride	Trace only	105 mmol/L

(ECF: extracellular fluid; ICF: intracellular fluid)

Osmolarity, or tonicity, is a property derived from the number of particles in a solution. Sodium and chloride are the primary electrolytes contributing to the osmolarity of the extracellular compartment. Potassium and, to a lesser extent, magnesium and phosphate are the major intracellular electrolytes. Water flows freely between the intracellular and the extracellular spaces to maintain osmotic neutrality throughout the body. Any shifts in osmolarity in any fluid spaces within the body are accompanied by corresponding shifts in free water from spaces of lower to higher osmolarity, thus maintaining equilibrium.

The average adult daily fluid maintenance requirement is approximately 30 mL/kg/day, or 2,000–3,000 mL/day. This is offset partially by insensible losses of 1,200 mL/day, which includes losses from the lungs (600 mL), skin (400 mL) and gastrointestinal tract (200 mL). Urinary output from the kidney will provide the remainder of the fluid loss, and this output will vary depending on total body intake of water and sodium. Both the lung and the kidney play integral roles in the maintenance of normal extracellular pH via retention or excretion of carbon dioxide and bicarbonate. Under conditions of alkalosis, minute ventilation decreases and renal excretion of bicarbonate increases to restore the normal ratio of bicarbonate to carbonic acid. The opposite occurs with acidosis. Ultimately, the kidney plays the most important role in fluid and electrolyte balance through excretion and retention of water and solute.

The main changes which immediately follow surgical procedures are as follows:

- Loss of blood and surface evaporation from exposed tissues during the operation reduces the volume of circulating fluid. This is gradually made good by water taken from the extracellular space, but in the meantime, haemoconcentration and vasoconstriction maintain blood pressure and conserve the blood supply to the brain and heart. The number of blood corpuscles is subsequently restored to normal by increased activity on the part of the bone marrow.

  A further loss of fluid from the circulation occurs by way of exudates into damaged tissues and from wounds during the early postoperative period.
- The volume of urine excreted is at first reduced, so the amount of extracellular fluid is kept constant or increased. A phase of diuresis follows 3–7 days after operation. In the meantime, the reduced urinary output is not to be interpreted as being due to an inadequate intake and as an indication for administering more fluids.
- Breakdown of tissue protein results in an increased excretion of urea, ammonia, and amino acids, and this, unless counteracted by a high intake, can cause a lowering of the plasma protein level. The excretion of nitrogen returns to normal, and the tissue proteins are restored, 1–2 weeks after operation.
- Sodium and chloride are retained within the body because of increased adrenal cortical activity and decreased excretion by the kidneys. Salt excretion returns to normal along with the diuresis after a few days. Unless sodium and chloride are being lost by other channels (for example as a result of vomiting), saline is rarely required in the early postoperative phase. This is true even though the blood level of sodium is low because this finding is accounted for by a shift from the extracellular to the intracellular compartment.
- Depletion of the potassium content of the tissues is caused by an increased excretion of potassium by the kidneys for a few days postoperatively; a loss of potassium-rich intestinal secretions by way of vomiting, diarrhoea and gastric suction, and the breakdown of tissue proteins. The blood level of potassium may not reveal this deficiency to the full. It tends to be kept at a constant level and can remain within normal limits no matter whether cellular potassium is being depleted or replenished. Muscle activity is very sensitive to potassium concentration in the tissues so one of the best methods to assess the latter is to study electrocardiographs, taken daily if required.

BOX 1: The bodily reactions to surgery.

The bodily reactions to surgery become pathological when they are exaggerated, inhibited or modified by factors such as:
- Excessive blood loss before, during or after operation which is not immediately replaced
- Artificial overloading of the patient with fluid and salt
- Starvation before and after operation
- Vomiting and diarrhoea (including purgation) before and after operation
- Operations affecting renal and intestinal function.
- Prolonged shock affecting the functions of endocrine and other organs
- Depression of haemopoiesis by disease or drugs

These and other changes are essentially protective and represent the normal response of the body to injury. The extent to which they occur after operation depends on the severity of the procedure, on its nature, and on the ability of the patients' organs to respond. The capacity of the adrenal cortex to react to stress is all important, and women with adrenal insufficiency (such as occurs in Sheehan's syndrome or after corticosteroid therapy) can die as a result of a minor operation or even of anaesthesia **(Box 1)**.

Fortunately, most gynaecological surgeries are relatively simple and do not disturb the alimentary and renal tracts. Moreover, it is usually carried out on women whose general health and capacity to react to stress are good. So metabolic and electrolyte disturbances rarely give rise to serious problems for the gynaecologist, unless the case is complicated or mishandled.

Hyponatraemia

Hyponatremia is defined as a serum sodium concentration <135 mEq/L. The normal serum sodium concentration is 135–145 mEq/L. It is the most common electrolyte disorder; incidence is 1%; prevalence is 2.5% (in surgical ward 4.4%; in ICU patients, it is 30%). It is more common in elderly, hepatic/cardiac/renal failures.

Classification of Hyponatraemia

- *According to serum sodium level:* Mild: 130–134 mmol/L; moderate: 125–129 mmol/L; and profound: 125 mmol/L. Often considered severe: Brain oedema, seizures, and coma.

- *According to volume status*: *Hypovolemic*: Decrease in TBW with more decrease in total body sodium. *Normovolemic/euvolemic*: Increase in total body water with normal body sodium. *Hypervolemic:* Great increase in total body water with an increase in total body sodium
- *According to the onset*: *Acute*: Onset in 48 hours; *Chronic*: Onset > 48 hours.
- *According to the osmolality*: *Hypotonic:* >280; *Isotonic:* 280-295—hyperlipidaemia; hyperproteinaemia (multiple myeloma); *Hypertonic:* >295—hyperglycaemia; mannitol or glycerol therapy. Urine sodium should be checked, and FeNa% (*Fractional excretion of sodium*) should be calculated. Low urine sodium (20) and high FeNa (>1%) imply the kidneys are not functioning properly.

Causes of Hypotonic Hyponatraemia

- *Hypovolemic:* When urinary (Na^+) >20 mEq/L: Diuretic use; salt-wasting nephropathy (renal tubular acidosis, chronic renal failure, interstitial nephritis); osmotic diuresis (glucose, urea, mannitol, and hyperproteinaemia); mineralocorticoid (aldosterone) deficiency (Addison's); cerebral salt syndrome.
- *When urinary (Na^+) <20 mEq:* Volume replacement with hypotonic fluids; GI loss (vomiting, diarrhoea, fistula, and tube suction); trauma; third-space loss (burns, haemorrhagic pancreatitis and peritonitis).
- *Hypervolemic*: Urinary (Na^+) >20 mEq/L: Renal failure (inability to excrete free water). Urinary (Na^+)<20 mEq/L: Congestive heart failure; nephrotic syndrome; cirrhosis.
- *Euvolemic:* Here urine [Na^+] is usually >20 mEq/L. SIADH (syndrome of inappropriate secretion of antidiuretic hormone). Hypothyroidism (possible increased ADH or decreased glomerular filtration rate). Pain, stress, nausea, psychosis (stimulates ADH). Drugs: ADH, nicotine, sulfonylureas, morphine, barbiturates, NSAIDs, acetaminophen, carbamazepine, phenothiazines, tricyclic antidepressants, colchicine, clofibrate, cyclophosphamide, isoproterenol, tolbutamide, vincristine, monoamine oxidase inhibitor. Water intoxication; glucocorticoid deficiency; positive pressure ventilation; porphyria; reset osmostat or sick cell syndrome—usually in the elderly.

Features of Hyponatraemia

- Nausea, vomiting, anorexia, headache, muscle cramps, confusion, disorientation, restlessness, convulsions, lethargy, tremors, and hypotension. Seizures and coma—seizures are quite likely at (Na^+) of 113 mEq/L or less. In acute hyponatraemia—brain oedema, tentorial herniation and sudden death can occur. In chronic hyponatraemia—brain adapts to keep the oedema within limits and rapid correction leads on to cell shrinkage and demyelination—Osmotic demyelination syndrome (ODS) with spastic/flaccid quadriplegia, dysarthria, dysphagia which can develop as late as 2 weeks after therapy (ODS/pontine demyelination).
- *Evaluation:* Serum electrolytes and urinary electrolytes estimation; evaluation for specified causes. Sodium deficit formula: (Desired change in Na) × TBW (Total body water); TBW is 0.6 × body weight in kg in men and 0.5 × body weight in kg in women.

Treatment

- Fluid restriction is the mainstay of treatment. In acute type, however, rapid correction is needed, but the rise in (Na^+) should not be >0.5–1.0 mEq/L/h. Hypertonic (3%) saline (containing 513 mEq Na/L) is used, but only with frequent (2–4 hourly) electrolyte determinations.
- Sodium correction should be 6 mmol/L per day and should not exceed 12 mmol/L per day. In hypovolemia, 0.9% normal saline (154 mEq Na/L) may be used as a slow gradual correction. Often, associated hypokalaemia needs to be corrected. The cause should be treated.
- Chronic hyponatraemia is treated by—water restriction; demeclocycline 300–600 mg tid (causes nephrogenic diabetes insipidus); lithium; oral urea; VAPTANS [vasopressin receptor antagonists (Arginine Vasopressin Antagonists)]. Chronic hyponatraemia, when present with seizures, should be treated using carefully monitored infusion of hypertonic saline 3%.

Hypernatraemia

It is raised in serum sodium concentration >145 mmol/L. It is a hyperosmolar condition related to TBW related to electrolyte content. It is common in aged, with impaired thirst, poor access to needed water and increased fluid loss. There is net water loss or sodium gain or both. Serum sodium concentration >160 mmol/L is severe hypernatraemia. *Acute hypernatraemia* occurs within 24 hours and should be corrected rapidly, whereas chronic type develops in >24 hours and should be corrected slowly otherwise, cerebral oedema develops.

Normal plasma osmolality (Posm) is 275–290 mOsm/kg. Calculated Posm is—2(Na) mEq/L + serum glucose (mg/dL)/18 + BUN (mg/dL/2.8). Posm and plasma sodium concentration is regulated by antidiuretic hormone [ADH/arginine vasopressin (AVP)] and thirst mechanism. When there is thirst raised Posm occurs with hypernatraemia, which draws water from cells dehydrating the neuronal cells, which stimulates ADH release initiating the thirst mechanism causing adequate water intake and thus correction of the hypernatraemia.

Causes

It is commonly observed in the ICU, in shock patients, in old aged, mental illness, uncontrolled diabetes mellitus, diabetes insipidus, polyuria, diuretic therapy, tube feeding, lactulose therapy, sedatives, and mechanical ventilation. Diabetes insipidus is due to deficiency of ADH. It can be central wherein pituitary gland cannot secrete adequate ADH causing diuresis. It can also be nephrogenic wherein there are systemic diseases involving kidneys, making kidney (nephrons) inability to response to ADH.

Features

- *Features of volume depletion*: Tachycardia, hypotension, dry skin.
- *Features of neuronal inactivity*: Irritability, seizures, lethargy, confusion.
- *General features:* Weakness, polyuria, polydipsia.
- *Investigations:* Serum electrolytes, blood glucose estimation, blood urea and serum creatinine, urine electrolytes. Plasma and urine osmolality, 24-hour urine volume, plasma AVP level estimation, tests relevant to suspected cause.

Treatment

In acute type (hypernatraemia <24 hours)—serum sodium correction rate is 3 mEq/L/h for 3 hours with maximum correction per day is 12 mEq/L. Serum and urine electrolytes, plasma and urine osmolality should be measured every two hours. In chronic hypernatraemia, correction rate is 0.5 mEq/L/h with total correction per day of 8 mEq/L. *Note*: Rapid correction may cause cerebral oedema and herniation of brain and myelinolysis.

Hypokalaemia

- It is defined as a plasma concentration of potassium <3.5 mEq/L. Normal value is 3.5–5.0/5.5 mEq/L.
- 98% of body potassium is intracellular. Gradient is maintained by sodium/potassium pump. Total body potassium store is 50 mEq/kg (3500 mEq in a 70 kg adult). Normal daily intake is 60 mEq/day. 90% of potassium excretion occurs through kidney, at cortical collecting duct with presence of adequate sodium in distal convoluted tubule with the effect of aldosterone. Aldosterone, insulin, alkalosis, beta adrenergic agents decrease the plasma potassium level whereas acidosis, alpha adrenergic agents, cell damage, succinylcholine increases the plasma potassium level.
- *Mild hypokalaemia*: 3.0–3.5 mEq/L—asymptomatic. *Moderate hypokalaemia*: <3.0 mEq/L—symptomatic. *Severe hypokalaemia*: <2.5 mEq/L.

Causes

Decreased intake. Redistribution into cells; metabolic alkalosis; hypothermia; hypomagnesemia (magnesium is essential for potassium absorption). Increased loss which may be either due to renal or extrarenal.

Renal causes are—diabetes insipidus, hyperaldosteronism (primary hyperaldosteronism/Conn's syndrome), hyperreninaemia, European licorice (liquorice) ingestion, Cushing's syndrome, and dialysis. Extrarenal causes are vomiting (pyloric stenosis, gastroenteritis); diarrhoea (villous tumour of the rectum, ulcerative colitis); duodenal/pancreatic fistula, ileostomy; after uretrosigmoidostomy; malabsorption syndrome; and laxative abuse.

Drugs such as frusemide, thiazides, steroids, amphotericin B, cisplatin, insulin excess, chloroquine, beta 2 agonist and alpha antagonist. Myocardial infarction and acute asthma are associated with hypokalaemia as there is activation of sympathetic (beta 2 adrenergic) system causing transcellular potassium shift. Rare hereditary defects like—Bartter and Gitelman syndrome (familial hypokalaemic alkalosis syndrome) wherein renal salt transportation is defective.

Hypokalaemic periodic paralysis: It is an autosomal dominant genetic disorder with sudden hypokalaemia during awakening, after exercise, after high carbohydrate or sodium meals, after change in temperature. There will be muscle weakness of one part or entirely which gradually recovers; occasionally muscle weakness may persist for days.

Thyrotoxic periodic paralysis is hypokalaemia causing muscle paralysis in thyrotoxic patient.

Pseudohypokalaemia can occur as seasonal in summer or in acute myeloid leukaemia due to increased white cell count or in stored blood with large quantity of leukocytes. Other causes—total parental nutrition (TPN); hypothermia; barium toxicity; trauma, post-surgery.

Features

Muscle weakness/cramps, constipation, hypoventilation, reduced reflexes and paralysis. Cardiac arrhythmias and heart blocks are known to occur. Hypokalaemia occurs in 20% of hospitalised patients. It shows 10-fold increase in mortality rates by its adverse effects on cardiac rhythm, blood pressure, respiratory depression. It precipitates hepatic encephalopathy in patients with liver disease. It worsens blood pressure in hypertension patients on treatment with diuretics. Prolonged hypokalaemia leads to acute kidney injury. Hypokalaemic myopathy often leads into rhabdomyolysis. It increases the risk of arrhythmias in patients who are on digitalis therapy.

Evaluation: Serum potassium, sodium and magnesium estimation. ECG changes (QRS prolongation, T wave inversion, presence of U wave); electromyography (EMG to assess muscle weakness); investigations for specific causes. Urine potassium excretion is best measured by a 24-hour urine collection. A spot urine potassium concentration can also be measured (less accurate, but easier to obtain) with a value of 15 mEq/L indicating renal potassium wasting.

Treatment

- *Prevention of potassium loss:* Avoiding diuretics/ laxatives; treat vomiting or diarrhoea; control hyperglycaemia.
- *Repletion of potassium loss:* Oral potassium (potassium chloride) syrup is ideal, safer and simpler way. But often it may not be tolerated by patients. Diet rich in potassium should be encouraged. Magnesium supplementation may be added along with oral therapy. In hypokalaemic patient with acidosis, potassium bicarbonate/citrate may be used. Oral potassium phosphate in patients with associated hypophosphatemia. Usually, dose of 20 mEq three to four times a day is given and should not exceed 200 mEq/day. In moderate and severe cases, intravenous potassium should be used. It should be given slowly in a normal saline bottle (not in dextrose) as 20–40 mEq (potassium chloride) in four hours under cardiac monitoring with a daily maximum total dose of 240 mEq. Correction should be done gradually over 4 days. Rapid infusion should be avoided as it will precipitate cardiac asystole. Phlebitis, thrombosis and cardiac arrhythmias are the complications of intravenous potassium therapy. Hourly potassium estimation should be done to avoid occurrence of hyperkalaemia. ACE inhibitors like captopril and enalapril, potassium-sparing diuretics such as amiloride, spironolactone and triamterene cause increased risk of hyperkalaemia. Concomitant use with corticosteroids and corticotropins is not recommended.
- *Hypokalaemia due to loop diuretics* is treated with potassium-sparing diuretics (amiloride, spironolactone, eplerenone), oral potassium supplements. In both familial and nonfamilial periodic paralysis (e.g. from thyrotoxicosis), hypokalaemia can be life-threatening. Oral propranolol (nonselective beta blocker) at the dose of 1–2 mg/kg is an effective treatment to treat an acute attack of thyrotoxic periodic paralysis. Patients who are receiving digitalis therapy and have hypokalaemia are prone to having serious cardiac arrhythmias (especially in overdose situations) and must be treated urgently.
- Patients with significant *magnesium deficiency* have renal potassium wasting and often must have their magnesium levels corrected before therapy for hypokalaemia is initiated.

Hyperkalaemia

- *Hyperkalaemia* is defined as serum potassium level more than the normal to the age; in adult it is >5.5 mEq/L. Level >7 causes significant haemodynamic and neurologic changes and level >8.5 will cause muscle paralysis, respiratory failure and cardiac arrest.
- *Hyperkalaemia: Mild:* 5.5–6.0 mEq/L; *moderate:* 6.1–7.0 mEq/L; *severe:* >7.0 mEq/L; *fatal:* >8.5 mEq/L.
- *Hyperkalaemia* can be acute, which is often critical and fatal needing emergency management; or it can also be chronic, which is not critical but needs ongoing management.

Causes

- *Excessive intake*: Intravenously or orally with compromised kidney function; packed red cell transfusion. Effect may not be significant if GFR is >60 mL/minute.
- *Decreased excretion*: Renal failure; renal tubular acidosis; metabolic acidosis; diabetic nephropathy;

hypoaldosteronism; drugs like potassium-sparing diuretics, ACE inhibitors, NSAIDs, cyclosporine, heparin, Septran, and ketoconazole; Addison's disease; and hyporeninaemic hypoaldosteronism.

- Shift from intracellular space to extracellular space: Hyperosmolality due to hyperglycaemia, mannitol, contrast agents, hypernatraemia; rhabdomyolysis; tumour lysis syndrome; propofol infusion syndrome; digitalis or fluoride intoxication; malignant hyperthermia; hyperkalaemic periodic paralysis with myotonia; and electric/thermal burns.
- *Pseudohyperkalaemia*: It occurs after drawing of blood due to haemolysis, which is found to be more if fisting is done; thrombocytosis and leucocytosis are other causes.

Features

- Often hyperkalaemia can be asymptomatic.
- Weakness, muscle pain and tenderness, paralysis, bradycardia, tachypnoea, arrhythmias and sudden cardiac arrest can occur.
- *Evaluation:*
  - *ECG changes:* Tall T wave, shortened QT interval, ST segment depression, and prolonged PR interval.
  - *Blood:* Serum electrolytes, blood sugar, blood urea, serum creatinine estimation, arterial and venous blood gas analysis; serum aldosterone and cortisol estimation; serum uric acid and phosphate level for tumour lysis; serum creatinine phosphokinase (CPK) and calcium measurement for rhabdomyolysis and crush injury. Urine analysis; urine myoglobin test, urine sodium, potassium and creatinine level estimation; TTKG (The transtubular potassium gradient) measurement.

Treatment

- Avoid potassium-rich diet and drugs causing hyperkalaemia. Intravenous calcium gluconate 10 mL 10% (contains 2.26 mmol of calcium) in 3–5 minutes or calcium chloride 10 mL 10% solution (contains 6.8 mmol of calcium); it protects the heart. Calcium chloride contains three times more elemental calcium than calcium gluconate and so calcium chloride is more effective in emergency cardiac situations due to hyperkalaemia. 6.8 mmol of elemental calcium is required to correct the ECG changes of hyperkalaemia.
- *Intravenous insulin* as 10 units in 50% of 50 mL glucose. Frusemide diuresis intravenously. Sodium polystyrene sulfonate ion (cation) exchange resin orally or rectally—30 gram in 33% sorbitol; Patiromer sorbitex calcium is a nonabsorbed, cation exchange polymer is also used.
- Albuterol/salbutamol nebulisation as beta adrenergic agent. Intravenous sodium bicarbonate in metabolic acidosis. In severe cases, haemodialysis is a must as a life-saving measure.

PREOPERATIVE MANAGEMENT

Preoperative Counselling

Personal exchange of information between physician and patient is essential before surgery. An informed written consent is to be taken after explaining to the patient the diagnosis, procedure, its benefits, risks, expected outcome, and alternative treatments. The only exception to this may be in times of medical emergencies or sometimes in the case of minors. In all cases, the physician must have a sound knowledge of the law of the land with regard to medical practice. Offering the patient a second opinion is wise in case of any doubt regarding diagnosis or management. If the patient refuses therapy, an informed refusal should be documented.

Preoperative Evaluation

Preoperative evaluation helps to detect any undiagnosed disease and to quantify the severity of known comorbidities so that adequate optimisation can be achieved. The extent of evaluation depends on the risk of the planned procedure (low, medium or high), anaesthetic technique, and postoperative condition of the patient (outpatient or inpatient, wards bed or intensive care). In case a significant underlying comorbidity is detected or poor control of a known comorbidity is known preoperatively, consultation with a medical subspecialist may help define realistic goals and expedite management **(Box 2)**.

BOX 2: The American Society of Anaesthesiologist classification for prediction of mortality.

Despite its subjectivity, the American Society of Anaesthesiologist classification is still regarded as a significant independent predictor of mortality. Patients are classified as follows:

- Normal healthy patient
- Patient with mild systemic disease
- Patient with severe systemic disease that limits activity, but is not incapacitating
- Patient who has an incapacitating disease that is a constant threat to life
- Moribund patient not expected to survive 24 hours with or without an operation

The letter 'E' is added for an emergency operation.

Surgery and Menstruation

Many gynaecologists prefer not to operate when a menstrual period is in progress. It is argued that the pelvic tissues are more vascular at this time that a high vaginal pH makes infection more likely, and that endometrial debris may become implanted in vaginal and perineal incisions to cause endometriosis. These arguments do not withstand critical inquiry: the tissues are more vascular premenstrually than intramenstrually; the raised pH is caused by the presence of blood alone and follows any vaginal operation at any time; endometrium spilled during menstruation, when it is relatively inactive, is less likely to become implanted than is endometrium at any other stage in the cycle.

Note: There is no contraindication to operating during menstruation except when tubal testing, hysteroscopy or a similar procedure which involves the risk of intravasation of gas or fluid is contemplated.

Prophylactic Antibiotics

The prophylactic use of antibiotics is recommended when the expected incidence of infection is in excess of 10%. Gynaecological procedures which carry a significant risk of infection include vaginal hysterectomy, abdominal hysterectomy, pelvic abscess drainage, radical surgery for gynaecological malignancies and selected cases of termination of pregnancy. Routine prophylaxis is desirable in all cases of vaginal hysterectomy. It may not always be necessary in the case of abdominal hysterectomy, but is certainly desirable in high-risk patients, e.g. those from a poor socioeconomic status, prolonged procedure (>2 hours), presence of malignancy, and combination of surgical procedures.

Antibiotic Prophylaxis for Obstetric and Gynaecologic Surgery (Table 2)

Drugs selected for prophylaxis are generally older agents which would not ordinarily be used to treat established infection; which have a broad spectrum of action; which are cost-effective; and which have a low risk of complications.

The antibiotic is administered prior to giving the skin incision for adequate concentrations to be present in the wound area when the incision is given and in the case of hysterectomy, when the vaginal cuff is opened. The drug remains effective for 3–4 hours. Depending on the agent selected, one to three doses are required, i.e. coverage for the first 24 hours. If surgery is prolonged and blood loss is significant, a second intraoperative dose may be required especially if an antibiotic with a short half-life is used.

There is a very thin line between prophylaxis and early treatment. Overuse of prophylactic antibiotics leads to the development of resistance. Cross-infection is also more likely; there is an increased incidence of superinfection due to *Pseudomonas* and *Candida* with cephalosporins. For optimal results, prophylactic antibiotics should be used as an adjunct to, and not in lieu of, sound surgical principles which include careful handling of tissues, meticulous haemostasis, avoidance of unnecessary tissue

TABLE 2: Antibiotic prophylaxis for obstetric and gynaecologic surgery.

Procedure	*Pathogens*	*Recommended antimicrobial*
Vaginal, abdominal or laparoscopic hysterectomy	Enteric Gram-negative bacilli, anaerobes, group B streptococci, enterococci	Cefoxitin *or* cefazolin 1–2 g intravenous (IV) or ampicillin-sulbactam 3 g IV (for patients allergic to penicillins and cephalosporins, clindamycin with gentamicin, ciprofloxacin, levofloxacin, or aztreonam is a reasonable alternative)
Caesarean section	Enteric Gram-negative bacilli, anaerobes, group B streptococci, enterococci	Cefazolin 1–2 g IV after cord clamping
Abortion	Enteric Gram-negative bacilli, anaerobes, group B streptococci, enterococci	• First trimester, high risk (patients with previous pelvic inflammatory disease, previous gonorrhoea, or multiple sex partners): Aqueous penicillin G 2 million U IV or doxycycline 300 mg PO (divided into 100 mg 1 hour before the abortion and 200 mg 1/2 hours after the abortion) • Second trimester: Cefazolin 1–2 g IV
Genitourinary	Enteric Gram-negative bacilli, enterococci	High risk (cultures unavailable): Ciprofloxacin 500 mg PO or 400 mg IV

pedicles in ligatures, minimal use of suture material and adequate drainage.

Preparation of the Bowel

The alimentary tract should be disturbed as little as possible. The evening meal before surgery should be light and easily digestible. Thereafter, the patient remains in the fasting state. For most gynaecological operations, all that is necessary is to make sure that the lower bowel is empty; this can be achieved by an enema or a stimulating suppository, such as one containing 10 mg bisacodyl given 6–12 hours before the operation.

In the case of operations involving the lower bowel such as the repair of a complete perineal tear or rectovaginal fistula, or if bowel injury is a possibility as in cases of severe endometriosis or advanced ovarian cancer, more vigorous and complete bowel preparation is required. The patient is advised to take a low residue diet for 3–4 days before surgery and only clear fluids for 1–2 days preoperatively. Oral gut lavage solution containing polyethylene glycol, sodium chloride, potassium chloride, and sodium bicarbonate is ingested at a rate of 1.5 L/h until the diarrhoeal effluent is clear. Usually about 4 L of fluid is required but the concomitant use of bisacodyl reduces the requirement to 2 L.

Rarely, in the case of inadvertent bowel injury with an unprepared bowel, intraoperative irrigation of the bowel with Hartmann's solution can be done through a 14 F Foley catheter inserted through a purse-string suture into the colon or rectum.

Antibiotics are generally used in addition to the mechanical methods described above for complete bowel preparation. Oral neomycin, alone or in combination with erythromycin reduces the gut flora; the addition of metronidazole is required for the elimination of anaerobes. Neomycin has now been replaced by ciprofloxacin. Oral antibiotics have the disadvantage of promoting antibiotic resistance and superinfection with staphylococci and yeasts. Systemic antibiotic therapy overcomes this disadvantage. Various combinations include metronidazole with ciprofloxacin, ceftriaxone or gentamicin.

Preparation of the Vagina

Although the attempt must be made, it is difficult if not impossible to sterilise the vagina with its irregular surface of rugae. Fortunately, organisms normally found within it are nonpathogenic or of low virulence. When it comes within the field of any operation, the vagina is prepared in the operating room after the patient is anaesthetised. This is done by swabbing out any discharge, washing with gauze or cotton wool pledgets soaked in antiseptic solution, and thereafter by painting it with povidone-iodine. One of the most efficient vaginal antiseptics is *Bonney's blue*—equal parts of crystal violet and brilliant green to make a 1.0% solution in 50% alcohol—but it stains everything with which it comes in contact. Some gynaecologists argue that this should be used because the colour permits identification of the vagina during total hysterectomy. If they need this help, they should not be doing this operation. Some gynaecologists regularly operate without any form of antiseptic treatment of the vagina. Certainly, if total hysterectomy becomes unexpectedly necessary when the vagina has not been previously prepared, the surgeon need not worry about subsequent infection. Obvious infection should, of course, be treated preoperatively.

Preparation of the Bladder

The bladder should, for reasons of safety and surgical access, always be empty at the time of a pelvic operation when performed by the abdominal route. But for vaginal procedures such as curettage, cervical biopsy, vaginal hysterectomy, and repair of prolapse, catheterisation is quite unnecessary. It is enough for the patient to void voluntarily a short time before anaesthesia is induced. If some urine remains in the bladder, it is of no consequence; it helps rather than hinders identification of the bladder during dissection and offers it protection from injury. The need for catheterisation should be judged in each case by the surgeon, and the catheter passed when the patient is anaesthetised. If by chance the bladder is full at laparotomy it is perfectly safe to suck out the contents with a syringe attached to a needle passed directly through the bladder wall.

Preparation of the Abdomen

Shaving of the abdomen and vulva are not essential, but if required can be done preoperatively just prior to surgery. The use of an epilator is recommended over razor or surgical blade in this situation. Excess pubic hair can be trimmed with scissors, and this is often more comfortable for the patient.

The abdomen is prepared by scrubbing for 5 minutes with povidone-iodine solution. The entire area from the rib cage to the mid-thigh and laterally up to the anterior axillary line must be cleaned. Special attention should be paid to cleaning the umbilicus with a sponge on a holder or a Q-tip applicator.

Universal Precautions

All patients may not have been screened for human immunodeficiency virus (HIV), hepatitis B, and other blood-borne pathogens, and it is safer that the entire surgical team observe universal precautions, treating all patients' blood and other body fluids as potentially infective. All members of the team should be vaccinated against hepatitis B infection.

Box 3 outlines the recommendations for universal precautions.

BOX 3: Recommendations for universal precautions.

- The routine use of gloves when handling blood and body fluids (or items soiled with these), mucous membranes, or broken skin
- Wearing double gloves while performing surgery
- Wearing a gown or plastic apron and gum boots if splashing of blood or other fluids is anticipated
- Wearing masks and eye protection if splashing or aerosolisation is expected
- Special care in handling and disposing of needles, blades and other sharp objects
- Prompt and thorough washing if accidental contamination occurs
- Relieving personnel with exudative skin lesions from patient care till treated
- In addition, emergency resuscitation devices should be available to minimise the need for mouth-to-mouth resuscitation

Blood Transfusion

The almost routine infusion of fluid replacement, which anaesthetists are prone to give, may have merit in helping the patients to recover. Blood replacement is, however, quite unnecessary for the straightforward hysterectomy or other operation carried out on a relatively fit woman. Even where necessary, the use of blood components is advocated. The risk of transmission of blood-borne infections such as hepatitis and HIV has led many centres to practice autotransfusion. A healthy woman can donate one unit of her own blood preoperatively, which is then set aside for her and transfused intraoperatively, if required. When large volume of blood loss is anticipated, the use of cell savers and prewarming units for transfusion are useful. The guidelines for the same are mentioned in **Box 4**.

BOX 4: Guidelines for blood transfusion in patients undergoing surgery.

Guidelines are as follows:

- Evaluate the risk for ischemia
- Estimate or anticipate the degree of blood loss. Less than 30% rapid volume loss probably does not require transfusion in a previously healthy individual
- *Measure the haemoglobin concentration*: Less than 6 g/dL, transfusion usually required; 6–10 g/dL, transfusion dictated by clinical circumstance and >10 g/dL, transfusion rarely required
- Measure vital signs and tissue oxygenation when haemoglobin is 6–10 g/dL and the extent of blood loss is unknown. Tachycardia and hypotension refractory to volume suggest the need for transfusion; O_2 extraction ratio <50% and decreased VO_2 suggest that transfusion is usually needed

Deep Vein Thrombosis Prophylaxis

Levels of risk and preventive strategy for deep vein thrombosis are shown in **Table 3**.

For moderate- and high-risk patients, initiate pharmacologic prophylaxis within 12–24 hours after procedure for 7–10 days. For very high-risk patients, initiate pharmacologic prophylaxis 2–12 hours before or 12–24 hours after procedure. Continue for at least 7–10 days.

Consideration should be given to continuing for 4 weeks postoperatively in those not requiring chronic anticoagulation. If the bleeding risk posed by the operation is high, consider placement of a removable inferior vena cava (IVC) filter preoperatively for patients with current deep venous thrombosis (DVT).

POSTOPERATIVE MANAGEMENT

Postanaesthesia Recovery

On return from the operating room to the recovery ward, the patient is put to bed and covered with blankets. Anaesthesiologists all over the world have been using the Aldrete scoring system and the Post Anaesthetic Discharge Scoring System (PADSS) in assessing postanaesthetic recovery **(Table 4)**. However, discharge criteria cannot replace sound medical judgement and common sense. Ultimately, it is the decision of the anaesthetist, who decides when a patient is ready for discharge. Both, the modified Aldrete system and PADSS, evaluate five key parameters to ensure safe transfer or discharge of the patient postoperatively. Patients achieving a total score of

TABLE 3: Levels of risk and preventive strategy for deep vein thrombosis.

Level of risk	***Definition of risk***	***Preventive strategy***
Low	Minor surgery in patients <40 years with no additional risk factors	Aggressive, early mobilisation
Moderate	Minor surgery in patients with additional risk factors; nonmajor surgery in patients 40–60 years with no additional risk factors; and major surgery in patients <40 years with no additional risk factors	Graded compression stockings; IPC; LDUH 5,000 U q 12 hours; LMWH—enoxaparin 40 mg/day SC; dalteparin 5,000 IU/day SC; and factor Xa inhibitor (fondaparinux, 2.5 mg/day SC)
High	Nonmajor surgery in patients >60 years or with additional risk factors; major surgery in patients >40 years or with additional risk factors	LDUH 5,000 U q 8 hours; LMWH—enoxaparin 40 mg/day SC; dalteparin 5,000 IU/day SC; factor Xa inhibitor (fondaparinux, 2.5 mg/day SC); and combined IPC plus anticoagulant strategy above
Very high risk	Major surgery in patients >40 years plus previous VTE, cancer, or molecular hypercoagulable state; hip or knee arthroplasty, hip fracture surgery, major trauma and spinal cord injury	LDUH 5,000 U q 8 hours; LMWH—enoxaparin 40 mg/day SC; dalteparin 5,000 IU/day SC; tinzaparin, 3,500 IU/day SC; and factor Xa inhibitor (fondaparinux, 2.5 mg/day SC), combined IPC plus anticoagulant strategy above

(IPC: intermittent pneumatic compression; LDUH: low-dose unfractionated heparin; LMWH: low-molecular-weight heparin; VTE: venous thromboembolism)

TABLE 4: Discharge scoring systems.

Modified Aldrete's scoring system		***PADSS***	
Oxygenation		*Vital signs*	
SpO_2 > 92% on room air	2	Within 20% of preoperative baseline	2
SpO_2 > 90% on oxygen	1	Within 20–40% of preoperative baseline	1
SpO_2 < 90% on oxygen	0	>40% of preoperative baseline	0
Respiration		*Activity*	
Breathes deeply and coughs freely	2	Steady gait, no dizziness at preoperative level	2
Dyspnoeic, shallow or limited breathing	1	Requires assistance	1
Apnoea	0	Unable to ambulate	0
Circulation		*Nausea and vomiting*	
Blood pressure ± 20 mm Hg of normal	2	Minimal, treated with oral medication	2
Blood pressure ± 20–50 mm Hg of normal	1	Moderate, treated with parenteral medications	1
Blood pressure > ± 50 mm Hg of normal	0	Continues after repeated medications	0
Consciousness		*Pain: Minimal or none, acceptable to patient, controlled with oral medications*	
Fully awake	2	Yes	2
Arousable on calling	1	No	1
Not responsive	0		
Activity		*Surgical bleeding*	
Moves all extremities	2	Minimal: No dressing change required	2
Moves two extremities	1	Moderate: Up to two dressing changes	1
No movement	0	Severe: Three or more dressing changes	0

(PADSS: Post Anaesthetic Discharge Scoring System)

9 or 10 are considered fit for transfer or discharge to the next phase of recovery, whether ward, intensive care unit (ICU), or home.

General

Deep breathing and simple arm, leg and foot exercises are commenced on the first day after operation. They should be carried out every hour when the patient is awake. Routine postoperative exercises reduce the incidence of fatal embolism. It is now established that it is advantageous to encourage ambulation as soon as possible. This is true for practically all types of gynaecological operations, including repair of the vagina and perineum although exceptions may have to be made when continuous gastric, intestinal or bladder drainage is employed. Early ambulation involves no risk of disruption of wounds in any site, even when the only buried suture material is thin catgut. It has the merits of reducing postoperative chest, bladder, and alimentary tract complications, of avoiding muscle wasting, and of ensuring rapid physical and mental recovery from the operation. Besides raising morale, it contributes to the patient's comfort in many ways, by soon freeing her from the need for bed pans and from dependence on others for all her minor wants. Early ambulation also lowers the incidence of thrombosis and embolism in those clinics where a physiotherapist is not available to see that exercises are performed in bed; but in those where postoperative exercises are conscientiously performed its value in this respect is not established.

Ambulation must be early if it is to be valuable. The usual plan is to allow the patient to sit on the edge of the bed, then stand and take a few steps on the first day; to walk round the bed on the second day; and thereafter to venture and walk at her will. Unfortunately, early ambulation as often practised is not ambulation. Having risen from bed, the woman sits in a chair, takes a few steps and sits again. Many hospitals are so planned that there is nowhere for her to walk. Sitting with flexed legs impedes the circulation of the lower legs more than any other posture. To obtain the best results from the standpoint of preventing thromboembolism, the patient should be either walking or in bed, not sitting.

The time of discharge from hospital depends on many factors, such as the type of surgical procedure, home conditions, and the amount of domestic help available. In some places, it is influenced by shortage of hospital beds or cost.

After minor surgery, the patient can be discharged in a few hours or days. In the case of biopsy or diathermy coagulation of the cervix, she must be warned of the possibility of secondary haemorrhage and told to report to the hospital if it occurs.

Ideally, after a major abdominal or vaginal operation, it is wise to keep the patient under observation in hospital for 3–5 days until she is fit and active. There is always a risk of thromboembolic complications in the first week and secondary haemorrhage up to 15 days postoperatively; she must be warned of these and explained the steps to be taken in such an eventuality.

The rising costs of hospital care have led to a situation in many countries where, even for major surgery, the patient is admitted on the morning of the surgery and may be discharged on the same or the next day. This practice is followed not only for endoscopic procedures, but also for vaginal hysterectomy. Excellent support systems are required if such practices are to be successfully implemented. Patients must receive clear verbal and written instructions, a home care support team must be functional and ambulance and flying squads should be available to rush the patient to hospital if any untoward complication ensues.

Analgesics and Hypnotics

While the operation site is painful, as it usually is for 2–5 days, analgesics should be given freely, not 'as a favour', and the patient should know that they are available whenever she thinks that she needs them. Pain is a symptom which can always be relieved, and there is no excuse for not doing so. Any respiratory depressant effect, which some analgesics may have, is of little consequence compared with their beneficial action. There is nothing more conducive to restricting respiratory excursion than a sore abdomen. Morphine in some form or pethidine is efficient, but can cause nausea and vomiting. These side effects can be prevented by the simultaneous administration of chlorpromazine or prochlorperazine; this also potentiates the sedation. The use of patient-controlled analgesia perhaps improves the quality of analgesia. Usually, the total dose of the agent is not exceeded by this method, but in-built controls are provided to prevent toxicity due to overdosage.

The use of opioids or fentanyl in epidural anaesthesia provides effective pain relief and should be considered in all patients with large abdominal incisions. A combination of opioids and local anaesthetics provides a synergistic effect. Here also, patient-controlled top-up administration improves analgesia. Long-acting anaesthetic agents injected into the incision are of doubtful value.

Once the acute pain subsides, injectable diclofenac and tramadol are suitable analgesics. After a few days, milder analgesics such as paracetamol are generally sufficient.

In addition to analgesics a hypnotic is usually desirable at night, initially. Sometimes, this may have to be continued even when the physical discomforts of the operation have passed. There is always a reaction to the mental stress of an operation, and the relatively inactive life in the strange atmosphere of the hospital is not conducive to sleep. There is little need to fear a drug habit; patients give up the hypnotic as soon as they are convalescent.

Epigastric and Shoulder Pain

One special type of pain commonly seen after abdominal operations is situated in the epigastrium, or referred to the shoulder tip, and it can be troublesome for 2–3 days. When injury to the brachial plexus has been excluded, it can be assumed that the pain is either due to a pneumoperitoneum or to the soiling of the diaphragm with blood and other fluids. The relationship of the shoulder pain to posture permits a distinction. In either case, the cure is spontaneous.

Fluid Replacement—Diet

If the blood loss during an operation is excessive, it should be replaced at the time or immediately afterwards. Nevertheless, many blood transfusions are given unnecessarily and without appreciation of the potential risk. One unit of blood is hardly ever required for haemorrhage; it needs at least 1–2 L or none at all! After operation, care is necessary not to overload the circulation with any sort of fluid.

In addition to the basal requirements, intraoperative losses, third-space losses and losses through sweat, bowel secretion, or effects of anaesthetics on effective blood volume need replacement. If a central venous line is in place, it provides an accurate guide to replacement.

The maintenance fluid requirement can be calculated in the following ways: (1) The body surface area is multiplied by 1,000 to get the daily fluid requirement in millilitres; or, (2) by the second method, a 60-kg patient need 100 mL/h. For every additional kilogram body weight, 1 mL/h is added.

Crystalloid solutions are used for perioperative fluid replacement. Ringer's lactate is preferred to normal saline, but in cases where there is hyponatraemia or in the presence of brain injury, normal saline is preferred.

Colloid solutions are used only when large amounts of crystalloids have already been infused, blood pressure is difficult to maintain, or in patients with low colloid oncotic pressure, e.g. in patients with carcinoma of the ovary with massive ascites. Albumin and starch are the most commonly used. Albumin, although a blood product, is free from infectious agents because of heat treatment, which is a part of the process of preparation. Dextran was popular earlier, but it causes problems in crossmatching of blood. Hetastarch is a synthetic colloidal agent, which is also free from infection but can affect the kidney and decrease coagulation so it needs to be used with caution. Packed cells are used when the haemoglobin level is <10 g/dL.

Most patients complain of a dry mouth or thirst during the first 24–48 hours after operation. This is due to the preoperative drugs used, by the anaesthetic, by insensible fluid loss from the lungs and skin, and sometimes by vomiting. Unless there is clear evidence of dehydration, thirst does not call for intravenous (IV) infusions and, moreover, the patient should be prevented from drinking large quantities of fluid. Frequent small sips and mouth washes are permissible, but large quantities tend to cause intestinal distension and vomiting.

Provided the operation has not involved the intestine, the patient should be encouraged to eat a few sweet biscuits or a finger of dry toast within 24 hours of operation. Thereafter, and despite the fact that anorexia is likely for 4–5 days, the diet is built-up gradually but quickly; the sooner it is back to normal the better. Foods containing protein and potassium are particularly required.

Total parenteral nutrition (TPN) is occasionally required in patients with cancer or impaired oral intake and bowel function. Any patient who cannot eat for more than a week should be put on TPN, and this decision should be made sooner rather than later. A peripheral or central access is used. TPN provides all the essential and trace element components of the diet, but may vary depending on the presence of other metabolic and endocrine conditions. The patient with acute blood loss needs replacement with appropriate isotonic fluid or blood or both. There are a wide range of plasma volume expanders, including albumin, dextran, and hetastarch solutions, which contain large molecular weight particles (>50,000 molecular weight). These particles are slow to exit the intravascular space, and about one-half of the particles remain after 24 hours. These solutions are expensive, however, and for most cases, simple replacement with 0.9 normal saline or lactated Ringer's solution will suffice. One-third of the volume of lactated Ringer's solution or normal saline typically will remain in the intravascular space, and the remainder goes to the interstitium.

Bowel Action

The intestinal function is usually disturbed to some extent by the operation, and it should be made a rule not to disturb it further by irritating laxatives and enemas. With a limited intake of food for a few days after operation, there is little residue and, in any case, it does not matter whether the bowel remains unmoved for 3–4 days.

To avoid inspissation of faeces, and provided the continuity of the intestine was not disturbed at operation, 15 mL of liquid paraffin or a preparation of mucilage may be given twice or thrice daily, commencing as soon as postoperative nausea and vomiting have subsided. This, with increasing activity of the patient, is usually followed by spontaneous evacuation within a few days. A simple enema or a mildly stimulating suppository may be given if no action occurs at the end of a week, and is occasionally indicated by the second or third day if intestinal distension or colic is troublesome. *No stimulating laxative should be given until a bowel action has already occurred.*

After perineorrhaphy, while it was customary to delay bowel action if possible until the fourth or fifth day, it is of no consequence if it occurs earlier.

After the repair of a complete perineal tear, many aim to delay bowel action for 7–8 days by giving a low residue diet. At the end of that time, an enema should never be given, because the nozzle can damage the operation site. A suppository together with a mild laxative should be enough.

Attention to Bladder—Urinary Retention

For the reasons, and by the mechanisms, urinary retention is common after any pelvic operation. Because of this many surgeons make it a rule to insert a catheter at the end of all except minor procedures and to leave it in place for 24 hours. The advantage is that it allows measurement of urinary output but it hinders movement, and almost invariably results in some urethritis and cystitis, so when the standard of supervision in the ward is high it can be omitted because 50–75% of women will void spontaneously. If, however, nursing supervision is inadequate then it is safer always to drain the bladder. Retention rarely follows vaginal operations if posterior colpoperineorrhaphy is omitted. There are certain procedures, such as radical hysterectomy, operations for urinary stress incontinence, and the repair of a fistula in which an indwelling catheter is essential for many days.

When a catheter is omitted, careful watch is kept and the output of urine measured. During the first 12 hours, and especially if the operation is a major one, very little urine may be secreted. But if none has been voided or if the woman's discomfort or percussion of the lower abdomen reveals a distended bladder, a self-retaining catheter should be passed and allowed to drain continuously for 48 hours or more; keeping the bladder empty allows it to recover tone.

After the initial catheterisation and with encouragement and relief of pain, the woman will usually void naturally.

When urine is being passed regularly, it can never be assumed that all is well, and ultrasound examination for residual urine should be made whenever it is uncertain that voiding is complete. The woman who, in the days following operation, passes small amounts of urine at very frequent intervals is not suffering from cystitis. She nearly always has overflow incontinence or incomplete emptying of the bladder. This is most likely to happen when initial retention is overlooked or not treated by prompt catheterisation. The neglect of retention and incomplete emptying is a serious matter, which sometimes leads to gangrenous cystitis.

Residual urine is a nidus for infection and the overdistended bladder, damaged possibly by ischaemia, is ill equipped to put up a good defence. The bladder which is emptied regularly has little difficulty in coping with bacterial invaders.

Initial postoperative retention in a nervous woman can sometimes be overcome by simple measures, such as encouragement, running a tap, use of a commode instead of a bed pan and by ensuring privacy. However, too much reliance should neither be placed on these, nor on cholinergic drugs. It is better to catheterise too soon than too late, and too often than too seldom.

When catheterisation becomes necessary, the risk of causing cystitis is minimised by:

- The use of a disposable, presterilised plastic or latex catheter
- The employment of a 'no touch' technique rather than 'scrubbing up' for insertion
- The application of chlorhexidine jelly to the urethra before inserting the catheter
- When an indwelling catheter is employed, it should drain into a closed sterile container, which is fitted with a 'no return' valve
- While the prophylactic use of antibiotics during continuous drainage is often advocated, it is better to reserve these agents for selective use if infection occurs.

FAST-TRACK PROTOCOL

Fast-track surgery (FTS) programs are also known as *enhanced recovery after surgery (ERAS)* or rapid or accelerated recovery after surgery programs. These programs derive their success from being multidisciplinary, with all the members of the team having an important function. Team members include all those involved in patient care: Surgeons, nurses, anaesthetist, pain specialists, ward nursing staff, social worker, occupational, and physical therapy staff. Evidence supporting FTS has been published in the colorectal literature and the same has translated into the gynaecological literature.

Many elements of the FTS programs are already practiced by surgeons, but few embrace the entirety to gain the maximum benefits in patient care. By minimising stress and maintaining normal physiology, the catabolic insults of surgery and anaesthesia can be minimised. Evidence indicates that completion of a FTS program is not only achievable, but is safe, and allows early discharge with a low risk of readmission and improved outcomes **(Box 5)**.

BOX 5: Goals of fast-track protocol.

Goals include:
- To reduce the risk of complications
- To shorten the hospital stays
- To reduce the medical costs
- To improve patient outcomes

Elements

- Preoperative patient assessment and counselling
- No premedication
- Pre-emptive analgesia
- Minimising fasting
- Avoidance of mechanical bowel preparation
- Venous thromboembolism (VTE) prophylaxis
- Intraoperative analgesia and regional anaesthesia
- Avoidance of nasogastric (NG) tubes
- Short acting anaesthetics
- Avoid fluid overload
- Early catheter removal
- Avoid drains
- Temperature regulation and intraoperative warming
- Postoperative care pathways
- Nonopioid analgesia and nonsteroidal anti-inflammatory drugs (NSAIDs)
- Early oral feeding
- Postoperative nausea and vomiting (PONV) protocol
- Incentive spirometry
- Early mobilisation
- Laxatives.
- Nurse led follow-up clinic
- Audit.

POSTOPERATIVE EXAMINATION

Full examination of the patient is essential prior to her discharge from the hospital. This includes the inspection of wounds to assess their state of healing. All unabsorbable sutures should have been removed (a nylon or silk suture in the perineum is easily overlooked), or in the event of an early discharge, a clear plan for removal of these sutures must be given to the patient. Vaginal examination is required if there is any suspicion of collection of blood or pus in the pelvis.

It is desirable for all patients to be seen 6–8 weeks after operation to ensure that progress is normal and that healing is complete. This is instructive to the surgeon as well as satisfying to the patient who often finds a few questions, which she has previously omitted to ask. Any light adhesions between anterior and posterior vaginal walls after colporrhaphy can be broken down **(Fig. 1)**.

Instructions to the patient should include advice about return to work. Women vary in the rapidity with which they recover. After a minor operation such as curettage, the patient requires 2–7 days convalescence at home before returning to work outside the house. After major abdominal and vaginal operations, light household duties can be resumed in 3–4 weeks but heavy physical effort and work outside the home should be avoided for 6–8 weeks. At that time, recovery is relatively complete, but most women find that it is 3–6 months before they

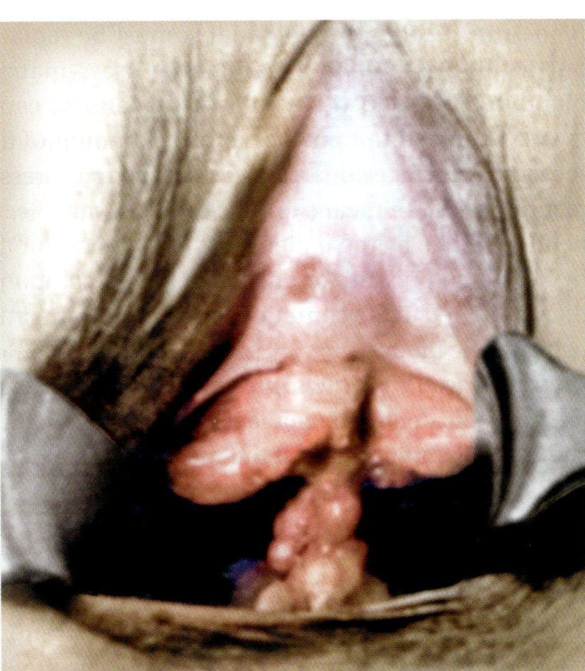

Fig. 1: Adhesions between the anterior and posterior walls of the vagina following colporrhaphy. Because these were not recognised and broken down 2–3 weeks after operation, they became so strong as to form a septum which required division under anaesthesia.

feel entirely well, mentally and physically, after a major operation.

One question which is uppermost in their minds, but which women hesitate to ask, concerns resumption of coitus. They should therefore be counselled, and this varies with the type of operation. Most will find that they have little sexual desire until they are physically fit, and this is in itself a good guide. Whenever the operation has involved the vaginal walls or cervix, coitus should be banned for 6–8 weeks; preferably until after the first follow-up visit. Premature attempts at coitus can cause breakdown of incisions and, if painful, may result in vaginismus with permanent dyspareunia. On the other hand, the avoidance of coitus for too long after vaginal operations may allow senile contracture to occur to such an extent as to produce permanent apareunia or dyspareunia.

POSTOPERATIVE COMPLICATIONS

Shock

A condition of shock may develop during or following major operations, especially if they are difficult and long lasting. The word shock in this context does not have a precise meaning, but can be defined as a severe circulatory disturbance which may progress to circulatory failure and death of the patient. The mechanical factors concerned are: The central venous pressure on the right side of the heart; cardiac efficiency; the resistance in the pulmonary circuit; and peripheral vascular resistance (arteriolar spasm).

The clinical picture of shock is variable. The causes of shock can broadly be categorised as hypovolaemic, intravascular volume depletion, cardiogenic, extracardiac and mixed.

The blood pressure is usually low but may be normal or high. The pulse can be rapid or slow, full or thready. The skin can be warm or cold, moist or dry, pale, cyanosed or pink. Two types are sometimes described as *warm hypotension* and *cold hypotension*; the former usually precedes the latter. In warm hypotension, the pulse volume is good, the skin is warm and pink. The underlying cause is often a state of infection. In cold hypotension, the cardiac output is poor and the peripheral vessels are in spasm. The pulse volume is poor and the patient is pale and cold. This is seen classically in conditions of blood loss or in advanced septic shock.

Causes

Hypovolaemic: Loss of volume may be due to loss of blood or loss of other body fluids.

- *Loss of blood:* The most common cause of shock and collapse during and immediately after operations is loss of blood, and the effect of this is accentuated if the anaesthesia results in anoxia. Unless steps are taken to measure it, the amount of bleeding that occurs during an operation is generally underestimated by the surgeon. Haemorrhage, revealed or concealed, may also occur after the operation, from a vessel insecurely ligatured. The clinical presentation varies depending on the rate and amount of blood loss.
- *Loss of fluids:* This may be the result of evaporation from exposed tissues, vomiting, diarrhoea or rapid drainage of ascitic fluid.

Intravascular Volume Depletion

In these cases, the total body water is normal or marginally decreased, but there is a shift of fluid from the intravascular compartment, leading to volume depletion.

- *Sepsis:* Peritonitis arising in the early postoperative period often does not cause the classical symptoms and signs. There may be distension and vomiting, but sometimes the picture is only that of warm hypotension. If the operation disturbs a focus of sepsis, evacuation of incomplete abortion, e.g. a sudden bacteraemia can produce a most alarming and serious state of shock.

- *Adrenal insufficiency:* Adrenal atrophy, possibly associated with previous corticosteroid therapy or with an incompetent anterior pituitary gland can also cause shock.
- *Drug sensitivity:* Allergic reactions to antibiotics and drugs can simulate shock and be fatal.
- *Posture:* Prolonged maintenance of the lithotomy or Trendelenburg position causes loss of vasomotor tone in the leg vessels, so when the patient is later put in a horizontal position, the volume of blood available for circulation outside the legs is considerably reduced.
- *Cardiogenic:* Myocardial infarction, cardiomyopathies, and dysrhythmias can all result in decreased cardiac output which further results in circulatory collapse.
- *Extracardiac:* Extracardiac lesions that have an obstructive effect include pulmonary embolism, constrictive pericarditis, severe pulmonary hypertension, cardiac tamponade and coarctation of the aorta. Here, a vicious cycle of progressively decreasing filling and decreasing cardiac output develops, leading to myocardial insufficiency and collapse.

Mixed Aetiology

Neurogenic: Sometimes, immediate postoperative collapse occurs, presumably caused by an autonomic nerve reflex, in patients who have stimulation of the genital tract without adequate anaesthesia. This has been seen in some patients in whom a pack was inserted into the uterus. Removal of the pack results in rapid recovery. A similar situation may occur in some patients undergoing dilatation and curettage under local anaesthesia and mild sedation.

Treatment

- *Position:* Lay the patient flat and elevate the foot of the bed to maintain the circulation to the brain.
- *Warmth:* Cover with blankets but do not apply heat. Pallor and coldness of the skin are manifestations of a protective mechanism whereby the peripheral circulation is reduced to maintain the blood supply to the vital organs. Warmth counteracts this and also involves serious risk of skin burns.
- *Oxygen:* Oxygen is administered through a mask or nasal catheter.
- *Blood transfusions:* Any blood lost must be replaced, but if there is a delay in obtaining cross-matched blood, a blood substitute (plasma expander) can be given. The need to transfuse and the amount of fluid required are best estimated by central venous pressure recordings. If the means for this are not available, it is better to judge by the patient's general condition than by her blood pressure or pulse rate. Blood component therapy suited to the condition is desirable, rather than using whole blood.
- *Inotropic agents and vasopressors:* Vasoactive agents are not indicated in the management of hypovolaemic shock. Dopamine is used if the mean arterial pressure is <60 mm Hg. In doses <3 mg/kg/min it produces vasodilation by increasing systemic perfusion, but at moderate doses of up to 10 mg/kg/min it has b_1-adrenergic inotropic effects which increase cardiac output. Dobutamine has b_1- and b_2-adrenergic effects and is the preferred agent in cardiogenic shock. Epinephrine and norepinephrine increase blood pressure, but their vasoconstrictor effect can precipitate myocardial ischaemia, so they need to be used with caution.
- *Antibiotics:* For the patient exhibiting the warm hypotension syndrome, it is wise to give large doses of antibiotics intravenously, on the assumption that the underlying cause is infection or septicaemia.
- *Glucocorticoids:* Glucocorticoids can be life-saving in anaphylactic shock, but have no role in treating other types of shock.
- *Morphine:* This is used only in patients with cardiogenic shock. As soon as restorative measures are instituted and the patient's general condition permits, she must be examined to exclude the possibility of haemorrhage from an insecurely ligated vessel at the site of operation. Once this is excluded, other causes are looked for and treated according to their nature.

Haemorrhage

Vaginal Site

Haemorrhage from the vaginal walls is commonly seen after operations such as colporrhaphy and vaginal hysterectomy, from the cervix after amputation, cone biopsy, cauterisation or trachelorrhaphy and from the vaginal vault after abdominal hysterectomy.

Primary: This type of haemorrhage is apparent within the first 24 hours after operation and is the result of failure to control one or more large vessels, often an artery. It can be so severe and persistent as to threaten the patient's life and should not be treated by packing the vagina. Effectual tamponade is impossible without anaesthetising the patient and is nearly always followed by infection and breakdown of incisions. It should therefore be made a rule to treat primary haemorrhage of any degree by taking the woman back to the operating room and by suturing the bleeding area, even if this means opening and reclosing perineorrhaphy incisions to obtain access. Vacillation rarely pays; it is worrying to the patient and attendants and means that ultimately the resuturing has to be carried out on an anaemic woman or be accompanied by blood transfusion.

In the case of bleeding from the vaginal vault after abdominal hysterectomy, the bleeding point can often be sutured by a vaginal approach.

Secondary: Secondary haemorrhage usually occurs between the 8th and 14th day or earlier after the first 24 hours after operation and is associated with the separation of a slough. It is nearly always the result of a low-grade infection in the wound, so whatever local measures are adopted, systemic treatment with antibiotics is also indicated. The amount of bleeding may be small, and the only treatments then necessary are recumbency, antibiotics and sedation. When the bleeding is more severe, the vagina can be packed tightly with an 8–10 cm wide gauze. This is left in place for 24–48 hours, and if bleeding recurs after its removal, another pack is inserted. Packing is done under general anaesthesia after carefully observing vault.

Suturing for *secondary* bleeding is usually unnecessary and is always difficult. The bleeding is rarely localised to one point and is more in the nature of an ooze; the tissues are infected and friable and sutures cut out unless they are deeply placed and mattress in type.

Intrapelvic Site

Haemorrhage occurring after an abdominal operation is nearly always the result of a slipped ligature on the ovarian or uterine vessels, more often the former. It requires laparotomy to secure the bleeding point. An ovarian vessel usually retracts retroperitoneally, so the haemorrhage is not within the peritoneal cavity and is difficult both to diagnose and to control. A bleeding uterine vessel causes so much extravasation into the cellular tissues that it can be impossible to find; in this case, the anterior branch of the internal iliac artery has to be tied. Remedies like intra-arterial embolisation are seldom helpful and usually result in wastage of time.

Haemorrhage from the cavity of the uterus after myomectomy or hysterotomy can occasionally be controlled by packing the uterus under general anaesthesia.

Pyrexia

Pyrexia of a slight or moderate degree during the first 48 hours after an operation is common and sometimes called 'reactionary'. It is probably caused by absorption of the products of tissue damage and blood clots and does not require treatment. Operations which inevitably involve some oozing and haematoma formation, separation of adhesions and myomectomy, e.g. are nearly always followed by a low-grade pyrexia which may persist for 7–10 days. This is never an indication for administering antibiotics. Nor is the occurrence of a slight rise in temperature 7–14 days after abdominal or vaginal total hysterectomy. This is nearly always caused by a small vaginal vault haematoma with or without low-grade secondary infection. The resulting pyrexia settles when the haematoma discharges itself vaginally, as it nearly always does.

More serious rises in temperature, especially when accompanied by tachycardia, systemic upset, or localising symptoms, call for investigation of their cause. Treatment is then planned according to the findings. The most common causes are urinary tract infection; infection in an abdominal wound, usually preceded by haematoma formation; peritonitis, pelvic or generalised; and pulmonary complications including embolism.

Retention of Urine

See above page 1253 for details.

Anuria

Anuria is not common after pelvic operations, but has to be excluded when the patient appears to be suffering from retention. Failure to secure urine on catheterisation is of serious concern and, if renal disease can be excluded, suggests obstruction of both ureters. Although the ureters are vulnerable during many operations, it is exceptional for both to be involved. Anuria may result from ligature of a one and only ureter, but bilateral ureteric obstruction has been reported following anterior colporrhaphy when the dissection and suturing have extended widely in front of the cervix. In such a case, the ureters are obstructed by distortion and oedema rather than by actual ligation, and if the colporrhaphy is immediately undone, urine begins to flow again. This simple and effective measure is always the best treatment for this complication. Nephrostomy or ureterostomy is sometimes advised but is unnecessary. Whenever a patient complains of one-sided ureteric pain after a gynaecological operation, the possibility of the ureter on that side being obstructed should be excluded by urography.

Incontinence of Urine

Through the Urethra

The cause of urethral incontinence after operation is either retention of urine with overflow or a failure of the sphincter mechanism. The latter is not uncommon after a self-retaining catheter has been in place for a long time; it is usually temporary and self-curative.

Through the Vagina

Escape of urine through the vagina is always due to a fistula between the urinary and genital tracts. If the leakage occurs immediately after operation, it causes a direct injury to the bladder or ureter. If it appears 7–14 days later, the cause is ischaemic necrosis of tissues. If the case is handled promptly and well, either type of bladder fistula may heal spontaneously.

Cystitis, Urethritis and Pyelonephritis

Cystitis is the most common complication of pelvic surgery. There may be an associated urethritis, but this is not easy to establish. The infection sometimes extends to cause pyelitis and pyelonephritis.

Causes

Bacteriology: The most common organism found is *Escherichia coli* but *Klebsiella*, *Streptococcus faecalis*, *Proteus vulgaris* and *Pseudomonas* are also prevalent. About 7% of all apparently healthy women carry these and other organisms in the form of bacteriuria.

Mechanism

- Residual urine in the bladder resulting from retention or incomplete emptying is an underlying aetiological factor. Stasis in the ureters associated with the hydroureter of prolapse favours pyelitis.
- Catheterisation

Clinical Features

The disease ordinarily makes itself manifest by dysuria, frequency and urgency, commencing 5–10 days after operation. Pyrexia is common, especially if the ureters are involved. The diagnosis is confirmed by the finding of pus cells, a significant number of bacteria and sometimes red blood corpuscles, in the urine. The organisms present should be identified and tested for sensitivity to antibiotics.

Treatment

- Make sure that the patient is emptying the bladder completely; if she is not, catheterise.
- Give large quantities of water or bland fluids, at least 2–3 L daily.
- Render the urine alkaline (pH 7.5) by administering large doses (2 g) of potassium citrate or sodium bicarbonate 2–4 hourly. Alkalinisation of the urine enhances the antibacterial activity of penicillins, erythromycin and aminoglycosides. This is especially useful in infections caused by *E. coli. Proteus* and some other coliforms, some diphtheroids and *Staphylococcus albus* give rise to alkaline urine. Acidification is ineffective in such cases.
- *Antibiotics*: The choice depends on the results of bacteriological examination. Pending the result of sensitivity tests, it is generally best to administer one of the quinolones as these offer the broadest spectrum of coverage.

Results

It is usually not difficult to eradicate the infection. Moreover, the cure is almost always complete and permanent. Follow-up studies show that, in women, infection rarely persists in chronic form after an episode of postoperative cystitis. If it does, there is some underlying anatomical or other defect in the urinary tract.

Postoperative Vomiting (PONV)

Nausea and vomiting are common after any operation, but usually subside within 12–24 hours.

Causes

- *Anaesthesia:* Vomiting is seen more often after general anaesthesia.
- *Operation and pain:* Abdominal operations are more likely than vaginal to be followed by vomiting. The more extensive the procedure and the greater the handling of the bowel, the more likely the vomiting.
- *Drugs:* Morphine and other opiates are very prone to cause sickness and should not be used for preoperative

medication. The use of morphine postoperatively should always be suspected as the cause of vomiting, which is more persistent than usual. Pethidine is less likely to cause this problem, but is by no means blameless.

- *Inherent tendency:* Certain individuals are more prone to vomit than others. The person who suffers from travel sickness is generally also subject to postanaesthetic vomiting.
- *Radiotherapy:* This causes nausea and vomiting by its effects on the gastrointestinal mucosa. When vomiting persists for longer than 24 hours and when it does not respond to simple measures, one of the following more serious causes should be suspected.
    - Acidosis resulting from starvation and vomiting.
    - Electrolyte disturbance (see paralytic ileus below).
    - Dilatation of the stomach. The stomach muscle is quiescent for at least 48 hours after abdominal surgery and can become distended with fluid and gas. The last is mostly air swallowed by the patient.
    - Paralytic ileus
    - Intestinal obstruction

Treatment

Postoperative vomiting is best treated by the administration of ondansetron, a highly selective 5-HT3 receptor antagonist, which acts on 5-HT receptors in the chemoreceptor trigger zone. At induction, 4 mg is administered IV or intramuscular (IM) and 4–8 mg repeated after 8 hours or as required. Ranitidine 50 mg IV 8 hourly can be administered to patients at risk for vomiting and stress ulcers.

The treatment of persistent vomiting is described below under 'ileus' and 'intestinal obstruction'.

Intestinal Distension and Colic

One of the most distressing features of any abdominal operation, and of certain vaginal operations as well, is the tendency to intestinal distension, which occurs in some degree approximately 48 hours after operation. This can be replaced or accompanied by intestinal cramps. These symptoms probably reflect returned activity of the large bowel which, unlike the small intestine, is generally quiescent for 2 or more days after operation. They generally subside within 24 hours of their onset and with the passage of flatus.

Postoperative distension or colic is less likely if the surgeon is gentle in handling viscera and pays scrupulous attention to haemostasis and asepsis; drinking of large quantities of fluid after operation is discouraged, and the eating of solid food is encouraged; and early ambulation is encouraged.

Distension causing more than minimal discomfort should be treated with analgesics and antispasmodics administered parenterally every 4–6 hours. A rectal tube can be passed, and sometimes a simple enema helps. On no account should a laxative or other bowel stimulant be given. A heat cradle over the abdomen for a few hours may give relief.

Sometimes, the distension fails to settle spontaneously or in response to simple measures, the abdomen becomes larger and tympanitic, and vomiting ensues. The late onset of vomiting or its persistence from the time of operation is always ominous. In association with distension, it betokens mechanical intestinal obstruction or paralysis of the bowel (ileus) and unless handled promptly and efficiently, can prove fatal.

Paralytic Ileus

Clinical Features

Distension and vomiting are the leading features of ileus, the vomit being profuse and foul. When the vomiting becomes feculent, it usually betokens mechanical intestinal obstruction. Intestinal colic is absent and auscultation fails to reveal the bowel sounds characteristic of peristalsis. The tense abdomen causes generalised discomfort and embarrasses respiration, increasing the risk of chest infection. The patient who suffers from ileus may be of anxious disposition, and if she is not, the condition itself arouses her anxiety; this makes matters worse.

The vomiting leads to acidosis, dehydration and depletion of potassium and sodium. Hypokalaemia has a paralysing effect on the gut and causes further distension. The facies become hippocratic, the pulse rate rises as the blood pressure falls, but death often occurs suddenly from myocardial failure associated with potassium deficiency.

Causes

Shock and injury to intestine: These, occasioned by prolonged operation, rough handling and traction on autonomic nerves were formerly regarded as the main causal agents but are now accepted as being unimportant **(Box 6)**.

BOX 6: The main known aetiological factors.

The factors include the following:

- *Haemoperitoneum*: Because of this, ileus is more common after myomectomy (where haemostasis is difficult) and after wide separation of adhesions, such as may be required during operations for pelvic infection and endometriosis.
- *Peritonitis*: This may be primary or may follow haemoperitoneum, but it can also be the end result of intestinal obstruction. The occurrence of ileus in the presence of peritonitis is considered by some to be a natural defence mechanism; it discourages spread of the infection.
- *Swallowed air:* This makes the distension worse

Treatment

A paralysed bowel should be left at rest, and the patient treated with analgesics and sedatives. With the onset of vomiting, a fine tube is passed down to the stomach or into the small intestine. Continuous or intermittent suction is then applied. Feeding is by IV drip infusion, starting with 5% dextrose saline but varying the solution according to the blood chemistry, care being taken not to overload the patient with sodium.

Records are kept of the IV fluid intake and the output by both tube and kidneys, and an attempt is made to achieve a proper balance. The blood electrolyte levels are studied before and during treatment. Hypokalaemia is corrected by adding potassium chloride to the IV infusion fluid or giving it by way of the gastric tube.

Bearing in mind the likelihood of underlying peritonitis, antibiotics are given intramuscularly or in the infusion, and as the days pass, a watch is kept for evidence of a collection of blood or pus in the pelvis or abdomen.

The above regimen is only discontinued when satisfactory bowel sounds return, when it is clear from the gastric suction records that fluid is passing along the alimentary tract, and when flatus is passed. The sensation of hunger is the best indication that normal bowel motility has returned.

Intestinal Obstruction

If intestinal function does not return to normal within a few days, or if the patient complains of attacks of colic unaccompanied by bowel action and exaggerated peristaltic waves can be heard through a stethoscope, it is practically certain that the intestine is mechanically obstructed. Adhesions which cause this can form within 2–3 days of operation.

Straight radiological examination of the abdomen with the patient in sitting and horizontal positions is of considerable assistance in diagnosis *(X-ray abdomen and chest in erect posture or in lateral decubitus)*. Many of these patients will respond to conservative measures such as restarting of IV fluids, nil per orally and continuous nasogastric suction. If the patient does not respond to these measures, the abdomen must be reopened. It is less dangerous to carry out laparotomy unnecessarily than to overlook a mechanical obstruction. In any case, it provides an opportunity to release adhesions and any collection of pus or blood.

Peritonitis

Types

General peritonitis makes itself manifest 2–3 days after operation and presents the clinical features described under 'ileus'. Pyrexia, tenderness in areas other than around the incision, rebound tenderness and hyperaesthesia may be present, but *the onset of the disease is often insidious and without the classical signs*. Distension and vomiting are the prominent features; muscle rigidity is slight or absent. The onset of shock may be the first warning.

After gynaecological operation, peritonitis is more often limited to the pelvis where an abscess may form. This is shown by the patient failing to recover as she should and by pyrexia, tachycardia and leucocytosis. The localising symptoms, however, are nearly all rectal—pain on defaecation, diarrhoea, frequent motions and colic. A rectal examination or ultrasound should be done to exclude a collection of blood or pus in the pelvis before diarrhoea, occurring a few days after operation, is blamed on the hospital food. It is remarkable that general peritonitis paralyses the bowel, whereas pelvic peritonitis tends to stimulate it. The diarrhoea, however, is often spurious in that the fluid is excessive mucus from the hyperaemic bowel rather than faeces.

Causes

- Inadequate haemostasis
- The use of unabsorbable nonirritant suture material in a healthy peritoneum can ordinarily cope with bacterial invaders, provided the invasion is arrested. The development of peritonitis after operation may mean contamination with organisms of unusual virulence but is *more often secondary to haemoperitoneum*; occasionally it results from an unsealed opening

in a viscus. The presence of a swab or instrument left behind at the time of operation should also be considered.

Treatment

This is primarily conservative and is the same as for ileus, with particular emphasis on antibiotic therapy. Surgery is indicated when an abscess forms or when there is a cause for peritonitis, which can be removed. A pelvic abscess is generally best drained through the vagina.

Wound Infection and Wound Disruption

Closed wounds do not become infected in the ward and can be left completely uncovered after 3 hours from the time of operation when fibrin seals the wound. This practice avoids much postoperative discomfort and reactions from adhesive strapping; it is economical and permits ready inspection of the incision.

Infection and breakdown of wounds are, in most cases, the results of an error in surgical techniques at the time of the operation, although blame is often attached to a particular batch of suture material or some other factor outside the surgeon's control. Of all the agents, which come into contact with the tissues during operation, the suture material as supplied by reputable firms is the least likely to be contaminated. The fault lies more often in the method of scrubbing up, of application of gloves and gowns, of sterilising and handling of instruments, of preparation of the skin and in the operative technique.

Asepsis is always relative, and it is inevitable that some organisms enter the operation field by one means or another. Their types and numbers can, however, be controlled by care; their survival and growth can be prevented by not damaging tissues and by not leaving dead spaces and collections of blood on which they thrive. The basis of nearly all wound breakdowns is haematoma formation and this can be avoided by conscientious haemostasis or, if oozing cannot be arrested, by drainage. It is more important to drain a bleeding than an infected operation field.

Causes

Errors in surgical technique:

- Breakdown in aseptic technique
- Contaminated dust and air in the operating room
- Operating in the presence of active infection
- Careless and inaccurate suturing
- Inadequate haemostasis
- The use of unabsorbable nonirritant suture material in the fascia makes dehiscence of abdominal wounds less likely. It is important to concentrate on haemostasis and technique in closing abdominal and vaginal incisions.
- Incisions in the upper abdomen are more likely to disrupt than those in the lower. In the lower abdomen, a vertical incision is more liable to serious breakdown than is the Pfannenstiel incision. The latter involves a greater likelihood of small haematoma formation, but I have never seen it break down to involve fascia and peritoneum. Except for removing large or ovarian tumours or undertaking radical surgery, it is always preferable for abdominal gynaecological procedures.

Inability to sterilise the operation field:

- Infection, e.g. peritonitis, may already be present and be the indication for operation.
- The vagina is practically impossible to sterilise (as discussed earlier), but this is of little importance.

Defects in the healing properties of tissues:

- *General debility:* Complete disruption of the wound is not uncommon after laparotomy for cancer and occurs without evidence of infection or haematoma.

  There appears to be a failure in the healing processes, yet it is extraordinary that when such a wound is immediately resutured after freshening the edges, it nearly always unites without further difficulty. The explanation of this is that the original suturing sets in motion a repair reaction in the tissues of which they take advantage of the second time.
- *Deficiency states:* Protein and vitamin C deficiencies are especially important.
- *An obese abdominal wall*: Leaving a drain inside markedly improves the chances of primary healing.
- Old age and senile tissues
- Diabetes mellitus

Associated postoperative complications:

- Haemoperitoneum
- Ileus causing abdominal distension and vomiting
- Severe coughing

Diagnosis

The diagnosis of wound infection and breakdown can be obvious, but the early recognition of dehiscence of abdominal incisions is not always easy. This is because it usually occurs from within outwards, that is, the peritoneal layer breaks first. Unexplained abdominal discomfort with malaise, distension, and colic can be the first warnings, while *the escape of a volume of lightly blood-stained fluid*, too large to represent the serum from a haematoma in the abdominal wall, is pathognomonic of a '*burst abdomen*'. Such fluid can only come from the peritoneal cavity.

Treatment

Rupture of an abdominal incision through to the peritoneum calls for immediate resuture of the *whole* incision, even though part of it appears secure. Accurate apposition in layers is inadvisable, even if it is possible, and the usual method is to place strong, unabsorbable sutures through all layers. The results are surprisingly good in that recurrent breakdown is rare. Incisional hernias, however, follow in 10% of cases.

Superficial breakdown and infection of abdominal wounds require antiseptic applications, and possibly treatment with antibiotics according to bacterial sensitivity.

Vaginal and perineal incisions often give way a little but, generally, it is only the surface layer which is involved, and there is rarely any need to worry that a prolapse might recur. Treatment consists of daily sitz baths and sometimes antiseptic douches, but the cure is mainly dependent on time and tissue resistance. The ultimate result is invariably good functionally and often anatomically as well.

Suppurative Thrombophlebitis

Thrombosis of the pelvic veins secondary to infection and sometimes resulting in pyaemia is an unusual complication of surgery.

Superficial Venous Thrombosis

Thrombosis of the superficial veins of the leg shows itself within 2–3 days of operation, often within 24 hours, and is the result of circulatory stasis caused by immobility before, during, and immediately after operation. Varicosities are important predisposing factors. The vein and surrounding cellular tissue become painful, hard and tender; the overlying skin is reddened.

This condition is not serious, for it hardly ever gives rise to embolism. It is treated by active movement of the leg within the limits allowed by the pain. Local applications soothe the patient's mind rather than the local disease; cure occurs spontaneously. Treatment with anticoagulants is unnecessary and unwise, unless there is evidence that the thrombosis is spreading and threatening to involve the deep veins.

DEEP VENOUS THROMBOSIS

Incidence and Site

Deep vein thrombosis occurs with equal frequency after any type of operation. Indeed, patients in medical as well as surgical wards of a hospital are prone to develop phlebothrombosis. It occurs in men as well as women and is not explained by the latter taking oral contraceptives.

In those gynaecological units where the medical team is on the alert to prevent and diagnose the condition, not <1% of patients develop *clinically evident* deep phlebothrombosis or pulmonary embolism or both, *after* admission to hospital. These diseases complicate 3–5% of major operations, irrespective of whether the abdominal or vaginal approach is employed. The figures may be higher in those units where reasonable prophylactic measures are not adopted. Hysterectomy and prolapse repair operations carry equal risk, but certain operations, notably radical vulvectomy and urethral sling operations, are particularly liable to be followed by thromboembolic episodes.

The above figures apply to thromboembolism that gives rise to symptoms and clinical signs of its presence. The use of sophisticated means for studying the venous circulation reveals evidence of some degree of *occult* thrombosis in the lower limbs following 30–60% of *major* operations and in one-third of all hospital inpatients, medical or surgical. About 40% of deaths following hysterectomy are due to pulmonary embolism.

Nevertheless, significant thrombosis found at autopsy has often given no sign of its presence during life. In some such cases it is probably only a terminal event.

There is always some degree of thrombosis in ligated veins and arteries at an operation site; haemostasis depends on this. It is difficult to say how far this has to extend before it is regarded as being beyond the normal reaction to injury. It is reported that asymptomatic pelvic vein thrombosis can be found following 2–4% of hysterectomy operations. Mostly *it starts in the venous plexuses in the soleus muscle of the calf.* From these it spreads upwards to affect the main venous trunks. Less common *primary* sites are the popliteal, anterior tibial, deep femoral, and external iliac veins.

Causes

- *Blood stasis*: Risk factors for this include:
  - Obesity, body weight over 80 kg
  - Immobility before operation for >4 days; during and after operation

- Impairment of the venous return at the time of operation by flexion of the knees or thighs, as in prolonged vaginal or laparoscopic procedures
- Direct pressure on the popliteal veins by pillows or pads used to support the knees during and after the operation
- Direct pressure by the operating table on the calves, the veins being even less protected when the muscles are paralysed by relaxant drugs.
- Shallow breathing during the days following operation; this is most likely with a painful abdominal wound and abdominal distension.
- Circulatory failure associated with shock
- Age over 45 years
- Compression of the left common iliac vein by the overlying artery; this normal anatomical feature explains why deep thrombosis is more often left-sided.
- Gross varicose veins

- *Hospital life:* As noted above, all women entering hospital are at risk, even if an operation is not performed. This is because of limitation of physical activity; sitting in chairs rather than walking; and lying in bed on their backs.
- *Dehydration:* This results from vomiting, diarrhoea and haemorrhage.
- *Anaemia:* This results from disease and haemorrhage before, during or after operation, without adequate replacement.
- *Injury to the vein walls by pressure or anoxia:* This is caused by compression of the popliteal veins in the lithotomy position, as noted above.
- *Blood changes:* Although the modern trend is to attach blame for postoperative thrombosis on blood stasis during the operation, this mostly results in only minor, asymptomatic degrees of thrombosis. It is the later extent of the thrombotic process in the leg or at the operation site, which causes trouble and this does not usually become manifest until 7–14 days after the operation. This development coincides with an increasing coagulability of the blood which reaches a maximum at 8–12 days. Changes in the blood are the most important of all factors in causing significant and dangerous thromboembolism and they include: A rise in the number of platelets; an increased adhesive property of platelets; and an increase in fibrinogen content. All these happenings are exaggerated when the operation is prolonged, difficult, or complicated by infection, so these must also be reckoned as aetiological factors.
- *Pregnancy:* Pregnancy alone is characterised by alterations in the blood clotting factors and by slowing of the venous circulation. It therefore involves a risk of the spontaneous occurrence of thromboembolism. Labour is followed by all the changes which occur after an operation, so *clinically evident* puerperal thromboembolism complicates 1 in 300 deliveries. Any operation on a pregnant woman, or delivery by caesarean section, doubles this incidence.
- *Oestrogens and progestogens:* The oestrogen-progestogen preparations used as contraceptives and in the treatment of endometriosis induce blood and circulatory changes similar to those of pregnancy. It may, therefore, be that women who have been on such therapy are at greater risk if subjected to surgery, but this is not proven. Oestrogens, especially natural oestrogens which a woman coming to surgery might be taking for climacteric symptoms, may not encourage venous thrombosis but, added to her age and potential immobility, the risk is greater. Also, women with deficiency of protein C, protein S, and antithrombin III are at greater risk.
- *Constitutional:* Certain individuals and certain families seem especially prone to this disease. A past history of phlebothrombosis or embolism is an ominous portent.
- *Malignant disease:* Advanced pelvic cancer often becomes complicated by deep venous phlebothrombosis in the legs and death from embolism is not uncommon. The aetiological factors concerned are: Interference with the venous return by the growth itself; cachexia and anaemia; and physical immobility.

Clinical Features

The first clinical evidence of DVT is usually pain, tenderness and stiffness or cramp in the back of the calf, which the patient tends to dismiss as a muscle ache caused by posture, inactivity or unaccustomed activity **(Fig. 2)**. It is wise, therefore, to apply Homan's test (dorsiflexion of the foot to put tension on the calf muscles causes pain if thrombosis is present) daily to all patients recovering from an operation. Those using sophisticated diagnostic methods say that Homan's sign is unreliable. This may be true for minor degrees of thrombosis in the lower leg, but the test is certainly valuable for thrombosis of clinical significance. Patients should also be instructed to report

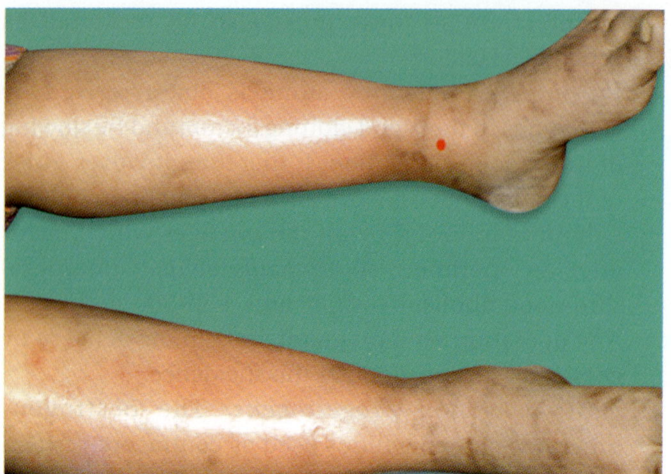

Fig. 2: Deep vein thrombosis in both legs.

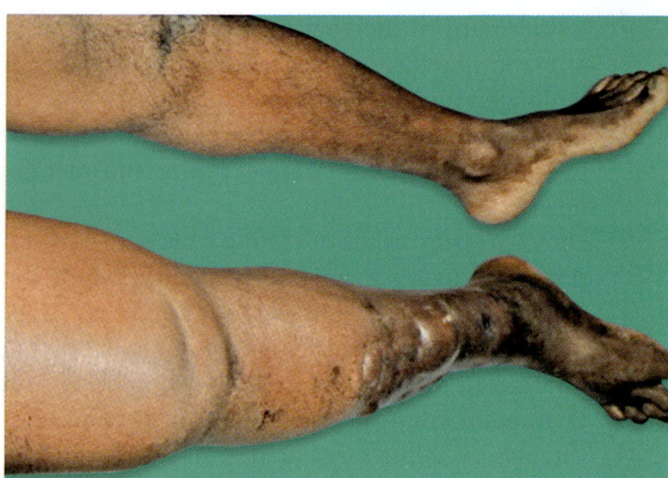

Fig. 3: Deep vein thrombosis with venous gangrene leg with discoloration and blebs.

immediately any discomfort in the leg, and if this is situated over any part of the course of the deep veins, it should always be regarded as a sign of thrombosis. Tenderness is present at the site of thrombosis (Moses' sign).

The first sign of deep thrombosis usually appears 7–14 days after operation, but may be earlier in patients who have been confined to bed preoperatively. Any leg pain which is reported during the second postoperative week should be regarded as being due to phlebothrombosis until proved to the contrary. Low-grade pyrexia often accompanies or precedes other evidence of thrombosis. This is the effect and not the cause of the disease; the thrombosis is not due to phlebitis.

Within 2–4 days of the onset of pain, the foot and ankle and sometimes the whole leg, begin to swell. Exceptionally, the first clinical evidence of phlebothrombosis is painless swelling of the leg. Otherwise, it is a mistake to wait for the appearance of oedema before making a diagnosis and starting treatment. By the time the lower leg is swollen, the venous system is extensively involved and permanent impairment of the circulation is the likely outcome **(Fig. 3)**.

It seems that to cause obvious enlargement of the leg the thrombosis must be as high as the iliofemoral junction. If it extends above this to the inferior vena cava, gross swelling of both legs results.

The typically swollen lower limb is traditionally called a 'white leg' or *phlegmasia alba dolens* although initially at least, the skin often looks slightly cyanosed. It is often associated with lymphangitis to a certain extent.

The much rarer condition of 'blue leg' or *phlegmasia cerulea dolens* is the result of total occlusion of the vein at a high level and associated obstruction of the artery by spasm or by pressure of the tense tissues. The consequence is cyanosis and ecchymosis as well as woody oedema and disappearance of the pulse at the ankle. A possible sequel to 'blue leg' is gangrene of the foot or leg. This condition can have a very acute onset and cause severe pain and even shock. It can develop postoperatively but its usual basis is advanced pelvic or abdominal malignant disease.

Investigations

To confirm clinical phlebothrombosis and to detect occult disease, the following procedures are described.

- The ultrasonic Doppler instrument can be applied over the main leg and groin veins to detect the flow of blood. This is simple and reasonably efficient, but it is not sensitive in detecting thrombosis in smaller veins, e.g. the soleal sinuses in the calf (accuracy <60%). It is also not effective as a screening test for higher-risk groups. *B mode Duplex Doppler imaging,* which combines Doppler examination with real-time ultrasound, is most accurate, allows direct visualisation of clots in the femoral system, assessment of venous collapsibility with the probe, is noninvasive, and has replaced venography as the gold standard for the diagnosis of DVT.
- *Venography*: The dorsal veins of the foot are injected with a radio-opaque medium, and its movement up the veins is studied with X-rays. A persisting filling

defect must be seen in at least two films for the diagnosis of thrombosis. Although it has been the 'gold standard', it involves hazards like allergic reactions and renal injury. About 5% of patients may develop phlebitis. Other noninvasive tests are usually preferred nowadays. Venography may have a role in cases in which embolectomy is under consideration.

- *Radioisotopes*: 125I-labelled fibrinogen is injected into the lower venous system, and its progress up the leg is studied by scanning. The discovery of a hold-up is said to be one of the most reliable methods of diagnosis. However, 72 hours may be required for a positive result. Moreover, it is unreliable in the upper thigh and pelvis because iodine excreted into the urinary bladder and the pelvic blood vessels generates 'noise'.
- *Impedance plethysmography:* It is a noninvasive bedside technique, which measures the change in electrical resistance in response to altered venous blood flow. It has a 95% correlation with venography in the larger veins (external iliac, femoral, and popliteal), but this falls to 50% for smaller veins, e.g. in the calf and also does not detect thrombi in the internal iliac venous system.
- *Magnetic resonance imaging:* It can demonstrate venous clots. It has the advantage of being noninvasive but is expensive.
- *Other methods:* Whole blood D-dimer assay and light reflection rheography (scatter of infrared light) have also been used, mainly in research protocols.

None of these procedures can be trusted to reveal thrombosis, which does not actually obstruct the vein to some extent, and even large thrombi in the iliofemoral segment do not always do so. Is it any wonder then that those who use them conclude that the only reliable clinical sign is oedema?

Complications

The *immediate* fear is spread of the thrombosis to involve the large veins at a higher level. With or without this, the main danger is the occurrence of pulmonary embolism, which can be lethal. Even when supervision and treatment are assiduous and prompt, clinically recognisable embolism can still occur, but is then hardly ever fatal.

Remote sequelae are rarely seen if efficient anticoagulant therapy is commenced within 12–24 hours of the first clinical evidence of thrombosis. This ordinarily results in complete cure without any damage to the veins.

Late diagnosis and neglect of phlebothrombosis can result in the following:

- Extension of the thrombotic process from the lower leg to involve the popliteal, femoral and iliac veins, even the inferior vena cava.
- Permanent occlusion of the main vein with consequent development of chronic oedema, superficial varicosities and gravitational ulcers.
- Even if the main veins do not become obstructed or if they become recanalised, their valves are damaged, so they function badly.
- Intractable menorrhagia is a rare sequel but happens when the iliac vein is obstructed and a collateral circulation develops through the uterus.

Treatment

Prevention (Box 7)

Measures under this heading include the correction of anaemia and blood loss; the avoidance of pressure on the calf and popliteal fossa; careful surgical technique; early movement and ambulation (*not* angulation) after operation; routine breathing and other exercises before and after operations; the avoidance of the dorsal position and 'foot drop' in bed; the omission of restrictive dressings on the abdomen; and the avoidance of the steep Trendelenburg and Fowler positions. It is also suggested that women confined to bed or hospital should compress their legs (to hurry the venous return) by wearing elastic or thromboembolism deterrent (TED) stockings routinely, but this cannot be very acceptable to most patients.

Special machines are designed to maintain a good venous circulation during and for 24 hours after

BOX 7: Prevention of DVT.

Categorise the patient as low/moderate and high risk:

- *Low risk*—young patients undergoing surgery for <30 minutes
- *Moderate risk*—patients above 40 years of age undergoing major surgery
- *High risk*—one who had existing cardiac diseases, stroke, previous history of DVT, suffering from malignancy

Methods:

- *Mechanical methods*—elastic compression bandage; elevation; external pneumatic bandage
- *Pharmacological*—low-molecular-weight heparin—once a day

(DVT: deep venous thrombosis)

major surgery. These include a motorised foot mover, leggings which are intermittently inflated by an electric pump and means for automatic electrical stimulation of the calf muscles. Such measures have been shown to improve the venous return and to prevent stasis, and perhaps their place is for cases in which the patient is known to be at special risk of developing thrombosis and in all major operations.

Low-risk patients, i.e. those who are young without any of the risk factors or those who have undergone only minor surgery can be advised early mobilisation and hydration.

Patients with any of the risk factors mentioned above are at moderate risk and should receive low-dose heparin 5,000 units administered subcutaneously 2 hours preoperatively and repeated every 12 hours postoperatively for 5–7 days. At this dose, there is no significant change in clotting time and therefore no increase in intraoperative or postoperative bleeding. Low-dose heparin binds to antithrombin III and inhibits the early stages of coagulation before the formation of thrombosis.

Low-molecular-weight (LMW) heparin, e.g. enoxaparin (20 mg/day) has been found to be nearly as effective as subcutaneous heparin in preventing thrombosis formation and is superior to dextran. Other LMW heparins are tinzaparin, dalteparin and reviparin.

Patients with three or more of the risk factors, those with a past or family history of thromboembolism or those who undergo radical surgery for gynaecological cancer are high-risk patients. They should receive 5,000 IU of heparin subcutaneously 8 hourly or LMW heparin 40 mg/day beginning at least 12 hours before surgery and should also be advised to wear graduated compression stockings.

The use of low-dose heparin has been associated with thrombocytopenia and an increased incidence of lymphocyst formation. Infusion of a solution of 6% dextran 70 (molecular weight 70,000) in saline, 1 L over 6–8 hours, provides protection akin to heparin for 5 days. Dextran 40 needs to be given continuously at 20 mL/h, because it is cleared rapidly or, alternatively, 500 mL of dextran 40 may be administered over a period of 4–6 hours daily.

Treatment in an Established Case of Deep Venous Thrombosis

General: As soon as thrombosis is diagnosed or suspected, the patient should be laid flat, and the foot of the bed raised to speed the venous return from the legs. Once anticoagulant therapy is established, and as soon as pain allows, active movement of the legs is to be encouraged. Walking (not standing still or sitting) is permissible and desirable within 1–3 days, as pain, tenderness and oedema disappear. Anticoagulants appear to relieve pain very quickly; the patient sometimes notices this within 1 hour of being given heparin intravenously.

Anticoagulants: Immediately, there is any evidence of deep venous thrombosis, treatment with anticoagulants is a matter of extreme urgency. It cannot wait until the next morning. These drugs save lives and prevent permanent disability. Only those who have seen thrombosis left untreated can appreciate how remarkable are the results of anticoagulant therapy.

If overdosage and consequent haematuria and haemorrhage from other sites are to be avoided, the administration of most anticoagulants requires strict laboratory control; even this cannot eliminate the dangers completely. The only really safe procedure is to give heparin *intravenously and in divided doses*. We have used this for years without strict laboratory control and without any problems. At the same time, complications occurred with all other anticoagulants and even with heparin given by continuous IV infusion.

Anticoagulants prevent the extension of thrombosis; it is the new and not the established thrombus, which is potentially embolic. It is doubtful whether they ever clear a vein already obstructed; this explains why they must be employed early in the disease, while the clot is attached to the vessel wall and not filling the lumen, if the circulation is not to be permanently affected.

When anticoagulant therapy is discontinued suddenly, *'rebound hypercoagulability'* of the blood may occur and result in a further episode of thrombosis or embolism. To avoid this, anticoagulants are given in full dosage while the clinical picture demands it (at least 7–10 days of treatment is required, no matter how satisfactory the patients' response is), followed by the administration of oral anticoagulants for at least 3 months.

Heparin: Heparin is an antithromboplastin, which acts by interfering with the conversion of prothrombin into thrombin; it may also interfere with the interaction of thrombin and fibrinogen. When given intravenously in a single dose, it is effective within minutes, but its action gradually wanes during the course of 4 hours. It is this short-lived effect which, although a nuisance from the practical standpoint, makes heparin safe. Even if an overdose is given and some haemorrhage results, the situation corrects itself in a short time and can meanwhile be controlled easily by the antidote protamine sulphate, given in solution intravenously; 1 mg neutralises 1,000 IU heparin.

In theory, the most efficient mode of administration is by continuous IV drip infusion, a 5,000 units bolus being followed by an infusion at the rate of 1,000 units per hour. This technique has the disadvantage that it makes ambulation more difficult; it also requires constant expert supervision of the rate of the infusion, and repeated laboratory checks if overdosage and underdosage are to be avoided. Heparin therapy should be monitored by estimating the activated partial thromboplastin time (APTT), 4 hours after such therapy is initiated. The aim is to maintain the APTT at 1.5–2.0 times the control value. If the APTT test is not available, clotting time is done; it should be maintained at not <12 minutes. Because of the difficulty in ensuring a constant delivery speed by day and night, an automatic delivery pump must be used, or else *continuous* IV heparin therapy can be either ineffective or cause haemorrhage.

Transistorised visual and audio alarm systems for monitoring the rate of infusion offer a degree of security. But, unless such equipment is available, it is better and safer in practice to give heparin by repeated IV injection, commencing with 10,000 IU and thereafter giving 5,000–8,000 IU 4 hourly by day and night. This puts great demands on the services of the resident medical staff, and in practice, good results can be obtained by giving 10,000 IU at 6–8 hourly intervals. The treatment needs no control by blood studies, because overdosage causes only temporary bleeding, the occurrence of which is a clear guide to reduce the next dose.

With this treatment, all evidence of early thrombosis usually disappears within 4–5 days, but heparin should be continued for a further 5 days during which time oral anticoagulant therapy is initiated, bringing the prothrombin time (PT) to 1.5 times the control value.

Heparin given intramuscularly is painful and dangerous and is very liable to cause a large haematoma at the site of the injection.

For pregnant women, all anticoagulants except heparin are dangerous, for they cross the placenta to cause foetal malformation in the early weeks and haemorrhages in the child at a later stage.

The introduction of reliable low-dose subcutaneous heparin has changed the management of women at risk. It can be given twice daily, and the woman can be trained to take the injections herself; the recommended dose is 5,000 IU every 12 hours.

Oral anticoagulants: Synthetic anticoagulants, e.g. warfarin sodium, phenindione and anisindione, are given orally. They compete with vitamin K and interfere with the liver's synthesis of factors V, VII, IX and X, thromboplastin components, and prothrombin. Their effects on coagulation, being indirect, are delayed in onset and slow to disappear. Depending on the particular drug, full anticoagulant action is established in 12–36 hours, and disappears completely in 36–72 hours from the start of medication. Thus, all these preparations require a supplement of heparin to cover the first 1–2 days of treatment. Their use also necessitates careful laboratory control with daily estimation of the PT.

Individual patients show wide variations in their response to the same dose. The effect of oral anticoagulants is influenced by renal competence, liver function and the vitamin K content of the diet. The simultaneous administration of sedatives and tranquillisers, including phenobarbitone, may call for an increased dose of salicylates and chlorpromazine, a decreased one.

Control of treatment is exacting; if overdosage occurs and haemorrhage commences from the operation site or elsewhere, it may be many hours before the situation can be controlled. The antidote is vitamin K1 (not a vitamin K analogue), and this can be given intravenously in a dose of 20–25 mg or orally in doses of 50–150 mg. It does not take effect for 6 hours; meanwhile, treatment is by repeated transfusions of fresh whole blood.

These agents are of particular benefit in cases of *suppurative* thrombophlebitis with recurrent embolism where it is difficult, if not impossible, to correct the situation by IV heparin alone.

The usual dose of warfarin sodium is 40 mg initially, followed by 30 mg on the next day and 5–15 mg daily thereafter. The comparable doses of phenindione are 200 mg, 100 mg, and 50–100 mg daily thereafter. In all cases, however, the daily dose depends on the PT.

*Thrombolysins (**Box 8**):* Thrombolysins/fibrinolysins are used mainly for free thrombus, which dissolves the thrombus rapidly to prevent pulmonary embolism. Once coagulation is arrested, the body is quite capable of dealing with all except the largest clots by the natural reactionary release of fibrinolysins. For massive thrombosis, however,

BOX 8: Thrombolysins.

Fibrinolysins/thrombolysins

- Tissue plasminogen activator—directly into the thrombus through popliteal/femoral vein
- Urokinase—1,20,000 to 2,50,000 units/h; derived from human urine
- Reptilase—0.5–1 unit/h
- Streptokinase—2.5–6 lakhs to start with, later 1 lakh hourly; derived from streptococci

streptokinase, an activator of plasminogen, has been tried in the hope of restoring the patency of a large vein. The dose is 600,000 IU intravenously for 30 minutes initially, followed by a continuous infusion of a 10% solution aimed to offer *a maximum* of 100,000 IU hourly for 3 days. The dose is gradually decreased over the next 4 days.

Strict laboratory control is essential, and this is difficult as well as critical. The stated aim is to reduce the thrombin time to two to four times less than the original reading, or the clot lysis time from 24 hours to 4 hours.

The treatment carries the hazard of precipitating haemorrhages and the antidote is epsilon-aminocaproic acid (EACA). The therapeutic value of thrombolysins is not established and they have little, if any place in the management of thromboembolism as seen in gynaecological practice.

Surgical intervention

- *Ligation of veins/thrombectomy:* Ligation of the common iliac vein or the inferior vena cava is hardly ever necessary in cases of phlebothrombosis but may have a small place in the treatment of suppurative thrombophlebitis with pyaemia or in some cases of pulmonary embolism (see further).
- *Thrombectomy:* Removal of the thrombus from the femoral or iliac veins, with or without ligation or plication of the vessel, is rarely required in gynaecological practice. Despite the enthusiasm of vascular surgeons, there is usually no need for such drastic measures. Complete occlusion of the vessel leading to acute iliofemoral thrombosis and phlegmasia caerulea dolens may require surgical treatment, otherwise as many as 50% cases can develop pulmonary embolism. Recurrent thrombosis and embolism, as well as permanent damage to and occlusion of, the main veins are common after thrombectomy, so anticoagulant therapy must be continued for 6–9 months.
- *Venous thrombectomy* is done using Fogarty venous balloon catheter. Special thrombectomy device of 7–9 French sheath is passed through the thrombosed segment to have partial mechanical thrombectomy and through that thrombolytics (tissue plasminogen activator) are infused. Thrombus can be removed nowadays through balloon angioplasty tube. Open venotomy and thrombectomy also can be done. Thrombotic emboli are prevented from reaching the heart by filtering it at IVC level using intracaval filters—Kim ray Greenfield filter, suture sieve plication, stapler plication, vena caval ligation and Mobin Uddin umbrella filter.
- *Palma operation:* In iliofemoral thrombosis, common femoral vein below the block is communicated to opposite femoral vein through opposite long saphenous vein. *May-Husni operation*: When blockage is in popliteal vein, popliteal vein below the block is anastomosed to a long saphenous vein (end-to-end) to bypass the blood across the popliteal block.

Treatment of residual oedema: Major degrees of venous thrombosis may leave the affected leg oedematous, or oedema may appear on standing. The best treatment of this is to apply a well-fitting elastic stocking *after the patient has been at rest* to reduce the swelling to a minimum. The stocking is then worn continuously. With time and with the establishment of a collateral circulation, the oedema usually gradually becomes less, and the leg then gives little trouble. The imperfection of the venous drainage, however, may continue to show by slight premenstrual swelling of the leg.

PULMONARY EMBOLISM

In gynaecological units, recognisable pulmonary embolism occurs once for every 300 operations of all kinds, much more frequently if only major surgery is considered. In 50% of cases, it is preceded or followed by clinical evidence of DVT in the leg; otherwise, it presents without warning. Small embolic accidents are probably extremely common but, being silent, pass unnoticed. Where preventive physiotherapy and early treatment of DVT and nonfatal embolism with anticoagulants are practised conscientiously, the incidence of fatal pulmonary embolism is reduced to 1 in 2,500–5,000 gynaecological operations, varying with the proportion of major to minor procedures. Following major surgery, the risk is approximately 1 in 1,000 cases.

Aetiology

The factors concerned in causing pulmonary embolism are the same as for deep venous phlebothrombosis (see above). Pulmonary embolism is often a recurrent disease; the woman who has one attack is liable to another within a few hours or days.

Pathology

The clot which shifts to enter the pulmonary arteries is not one which is established and giving evidence of its presence in the veins of the legs. It is an unstable one, newly formed or a new extension of the original. For this reason, embolism can occur before there is any sign of venous thrombosis.

Pulmonary infarction requires the lodgement of a large clot in one of the main branches of the pulmonary artery. This clot comes from the femoral or iliac vein in 70–80% of cases, from the pelvic veins in 10–15%. To kill, it is necessary for the embolus to put out of action at least 50% of all lung tissue (counting both lungs); this means that associated spasm of unblocked arteries plays an important role in fatal cases. Small emboli do not cause infarction of healthy lungs, only of those already diseased or congested by cardiac failure.

Note: A late sequel to the deposition of multiple and recurrent emboli can be *pulmonary hypertension.*

Clinical Features

Pulmonary embolism, like DVT, most often manifests itself 7–14 days after operation but can be earlier if the patient has spent some time in the hospital before operation. Massive embolism results in a dramatic picture in which the patient complains of sudden, violent pain in the chest; this is followed by shock and sometimes by death from ventricular fibrillation or cardiac arrest within a few minutes. Severe dyspnoea can be a leading symptom, but generally follows initial nonfatal pain and collapse. It is then accompanied by tachycardia, cyanosis and congestion of the neck veins; the patient may become mentally confused or comatose.

Minor degrees of embolism with peripheral infarction present by way of pain over one or other lung which quickly assumes the features of pleuritis, being made worse by deep breathing and by any movement of the chest wall. A cough develops, and within a day or two, the sputum is likely to be stained with blood. By that time, but not previously, there may be clinical signs of consolidation of the lung.

Pyrexia of varying degree is generally present, and this may persist for a considerable time if a pleural effusion develops, as it not infrequently does. Pyrexia is the result and not the cause of the disease.

The sequence of events and the findings make it clear how easy it is to mistake minor and moderate degrees of pulmonary embolism for a painful muscular condition, and for pleuritis and pneumonia.

Diagnostic Aids

The diagnosis is essentially a clinical one, particularly in the early stages of the disease, but ancillary aids described are:

- *Direct radiography:* This gives negative findings until consolidation of the lung, or a pleural effusion develops a few days later.
- *Electrocardiography:* This generally reveals no abnormality and never unless at least one half of a lung is out of action.
- *Arterial blood gas assessment:* This shows evidence of hypoxaemia consequent to hypoperfusion.
- *Ventilation perfusion lung scanning:* This shows decreased perfusion within areas of adequate ventilation, but very often the pictures are indeterminate.
- *Arteriography:* This has little place unless embolectomy is contemplated.

Table 5 outlines the Modified Well's Criteria for predicting pulmonary embolism.

TABLE 5

Modified Well's criteria for predicting PE	*Points*
Clinical symptoms and signs of DVT	3
Alternative diagnosis less likely PE	3
Heart rate >100 beats/min	1.5
Immobilisation >3 days or surgery within last 4 weeks	1.5
Previous DVT or PE	1.5
Haemoptysis	1.0
Malignancy in last 6 months	1.0

(DVT: deep venous thrombosis)
Note: Score <4 PE is unlikely; score >4 = suggestive of PE.

Treatment

In gynaecological practice, unlike obstetrics, the first embolic incident is rarely fatal; hence the importance of its recognition by constant vigilance. Its occurrence is a sure sign that there is deep venous thrombosis somewhere in the body and that a second embolus, possibly a fatal one, is imminent.

If left untreated, 25–30% of women who suffer one embolism will have a second, and one-fifth of these will die as a result. Prompt and efficient treatment of the first attack with anticoagulants usually prevents a recurrence.

General

Massive embolism calls for resuscitation, the administration of oxygen intratracheally and the treatment of shock. External cardiac massage can be carried out for cardiac arrest. Morphine, atropine, antispasmodics and digitalis given intravenously may help. Any electrolyte imbalance must be corrected.

For the ordinary nonfatal case, the main requirements are oxygen and relief of pain. When pyrexia develops, as it often does, antibiotics are not indicated; it settles of its own accord as the extravasated blood is absorbed. Nor should a pleural effusion be tapped; it will resolve spontaneously in the course of a few weeks.

Once the acute phase is under control and pain permits, active physiotherapy and ambulation are indicated.

Anticoagulants

As soon as there is any evidence of embolism, 20,000 IU of heparin should be injected intravenously; thereafter, treatment with this agent is continued for 7–10 days.

Embolectomy

This is only indicated if the situation is desperate and the patient shows no response to resuscitative measures. Even then, it is rarely practicable, because death occurs within 2 hours in two-thirds of the fatal cases; this gives no time to prepare for and carry out the operation. The results are not good and, where cardiac massage has been required, they are very bad. One of the problems attending successful embolectomy is a recurrence of embolism; this prompts some surgeons to say that it must always be combined with thrombectomy.

Thrombolysins

Pulmonary artery catheterisation with the administration of thrombolytic agents may be of help in patients with massive embolism.

Vena Cava Interruption

Usually, anticoagulant therapy will suffice to prevent the recurrence of thrombosis and embolism, while the pulmonary embolus is lysed by normal thrombolytic mechanisms. However, in some cases, repeated embolisation from the pelvic veins or lower extremities may require clipping of the vena cava or placement of a vena cava umbrella or filter.

Inferior vena cava *filter placement* is essential in recurrent DVT with anticoagulation, DVT with contraindication for anticoagulation and pulmonary hypertension. Greenfield IVC filter is ideal with 95% patency rate. Complications are—bleeding, haematoma, migration of filter into pulmonary artery, thrombosis at filter level and IVC perforation.

Retrievable IVC filters are newer method used to prevent long-term filter complications. It is used in young patients who are at risk of DVT and embolism, for a short, specified period only like—high-risk trauma with orthopaedic injuries, extensive iliofemoral thrombosis, during thrombolytic therapy. Recovery filter, Gunthur-Tulip filter and OptEase filters are used. They are deployed through IJV or femoral vein under angiographic or intravascular US guidance. Recovery and Gunthur-Tulip types are recovered through right IJV. OptEase is recovered from right femoral vein. Complications are same as nonretrievable IVC filters. Retrieval failure, retrieval site thrombosis and embolism are specific complications.

Venous Thromboembolism

- Venous thromboembolism (VTE) can be *provoked* (with identifiable causes) or *unprovoked* (no identifiable causes)
- Acute dyspnoea, chest pain, haemoptysis, later haemodynamic instability, shock, and RV dysfunction are the features. High, moderate and low risk groups are identified.
- Wells and modified Geneva criteria are used.
- CT angiogram is diagnostic. D dimer/duplex Doppler US of leg, MRI pelvis, coagulation profile, chest X-ray are other needed investigations.

- *Treatment modalities*—anticoagulants, thrombolysis, percutaneous interventions, surgery.
- *Anticoagulants* (heparin) are used in pulmonary embolism without haemodynamic instability or without right ventricular dysfunction.
- *Thrombolysis*—Indications: Pulmonary embolism with haemodynamic instability with right ventricular dysfunction or instability in spite of heparin therapy or with intracavitary right heart thrombi/massive embolism. Thrombolysis dissolves the thrombus obstructing the pulmonary artery; prevents the release of neurohumoral factors and serotonin which causes pulmonary arterial hypertension (PAH); reverses right heart failure; dissolves venous thrombus in periphery. Thrombolysins used are—streptokinase (loading dose is 2,50,000 units IV; continuous infusion of 1,00,000 units/hour for 24 hours), urokinase (loading dose 2,000 units/lb infused IV in 10 minutes, continuous infusion IV 2,000 units/lb/hour for 24 hours), tissue plasminogen activator (tPA is ideal)—alteplase continuous infusion 100 mg/2 hours, reteplase bolus IV 10 units in every 30 minutes, tenectplase and desmoteplase. Contraindications for thrombolysis—stroke, brain tumour, bleeding disorders, major trauma/surgery, recent GI bleed, pregnancy, endocarditis, and advanced liver disease.
- *Percutaneous catheter fragmentation* of clots and thrombolysis using pigtail catheter/clot buster/angio jet.
- *Retrievable IVC filters* are used commonly now. Permanent filters are used only in—high-risk group, risk of recurrent embolism and life expectancy <6 months

Venous thrombosis/VTE in pregnancy:

- Venous thrombosis/VTE in pregnancy is more common with 2/1,000 pregnancies with five times more in the postnatal period.
- It is 90% left side mainly proximal. Left calf asymmetry with >2 cm in first trimester with features of embolism.
- Calf and thigh US for leg DVT and MRI for pelvic DVT should be done. Echocardiography should be done to check embolism; chest X-ray with abdominal shield may be needed.
- LMWH should be given. Warfarin (crosses placenta) and rivaroxaban are avoided.
- TPA crosses the placenta but is used in massive pulmonary embolism with haemodynamic instability as lifesaving often along with embolectomy. LMWH is given throughout the pregnancy; stopped peridelivery period; continued postnatal period for 1 month with 75% of earlier dose; later compression stockings and warfarin for 6 months.
- Compression stockings, hydration, ambulation and left lateral position are preventive measures in pregnancy often along with LMWH, if needed/indicated.

ACCP guidelines 2012 for VTE therapy:

- *Initial phase* up to 7 days—UFH/LMWH/fondaparinux/rivaroxaban
- *Long-term* up to 3 months—LMWH/rivaroxaban/dabigatran/VKA with INR 2–3 range (optimum 2.5)
- *Extended* is beyond 3 months—VKA/rivaroxaban/dabigatran/LMWH, if needed

PULMONARY COMPLICATIONS

Inhalation of anaesthesia involves the risk of postoperative bronchitis, bronchopneumonia, pulmonary collapse, inhalation asphyxia and pneumonia. Prevention of these complications depends on good preoperative preparation and anaesthetic technique, and by encouraging the patient to perform deep-breathing exercises both before and after operation, as well as to stop smoking. Treatment consists of the administration of antibiotics and oxygen as required, together with breathing exercises and postural drainage. Incentive spirometry improves lung ventilation and prevents atelectasis. Suction bronchoscopy is occasionally necessary when an obstruction in a bronchus or one of its branches does not clear by itself.

The above conditions give evidence of their presence within the 2–3 days, in some cases hours, following operation. *Chest symptoms which commence after the first week are nearly always caused by embolism*, even if there is no evidence of venous thrombosis in the legs or pelvis. Failure to recognise this leads to many cases of minor embolism being overlooked, or being misdiagnosed as pleuritis and pneumonia.

Adult Respiratory Distress Syndrome

Adult respiratory distress syndrome (ARDS) is a relatively common pulmonary complication with a high mortality rate of about 50%. It is characterised by progressive hypoxaemia resistant to oxygen therapy. Criteria for the diagnosis of ARDS include acute dyspnoea, tachypnoea (<20 breaths per minute), cyanosis, absence of left ventricular failure, diffuse pulmonary infiltrates on chest

X-ray, partial pressure of oxygen (PaO_2), <50 mm Hg, increased dead space ventilation and decreased total respiratory compliance.

Adult respiratory distress syndrome has been associated with gastric aspiration, pneumonia, fat and amniotic fluid embolism and thoracic trauma. It is also seen in cases of eclampsia, disseminated intravascular coagulation, pancreatitis, infections, acute hepatic failure and massive transfusion.

Treatment is essentially supportive. Ventilatory support is the cornerstone of therapy. The use of steroids is controversial, but they may be used in the first 48 hours. Careful fluid administration and broad-spectrum antibiotics in a sophisticated intensive care setting are vital to a successful outcome.

Vaginal Discharge after Operations

Healing of Vaginal Incisions by Secondary Intention

Healing of the vaginal wall, and especially of the vaginal vault after total hysterectomy, is rarely completed by primary intention. As the wound granulates, it gives rise to a purulent and sometimes blood-stained discharge, which is maximum 10–14 days after operation. It gradually decreases and disappears 3–6 weeks after operation. The patient worries over this discharge unless she is warned that it is likely to occur. Treatment is necessary if infection is present.

Granulation Tissue

In 20–30% of cases of total hysterectomy, granulation tissue, often polypoidal, forms in the vaginal vault. Those who use chromic gut for closing the vagina can expect an incidence of 30–40%. Meticulous attention to accurate apposition of the cut vaginal surfaces reduces the chance of this development. The granulation tissue causes discharge, sometimes bloodstained, which can persist for months and even years after operation. The lesion is commonly mistaken for cancer or endometriosis, but is easily distinguished microscopically. It is treated by avulsing the redundant tissue and by cauterising the area with silver nitrate; it then rarely recurs.

Cellulitis

Prolonged vaginal discharge following total hysterectomy, vaginal or abdominal, is sometimes the result of cellulitis and haematoma formation at the vault. This is diagnosed by feeling the tender indurated area. Antibiotics and anti-inflammatory agents such as chymotrypsin may help.

Retained Foreign Body

Whenever an unusually profuse and offensive discharge occurs after operation, the possibility of an overlooked swab or tampon in the vagina should be investigated. It is a legal issue amount for negligence.

Vaginitis

Trichomonas, Candida or other kinds of vaginitis not infrequently date from an operation. It is explained by lowered resistance due to ill health; alteration in the vaginal flora by the administration of antibiotics; acquisition of the infection from another occupant of the ward; and inadequate sterilisation of gloves and instruments.

Cervical Discharge

After subtotal hysterectomy, the cervical stump is often responsible for leucorrhoea or for mucopurulent discharge at a later date. The best treatment is to excise the remainder of the cervix, preferably by the vaginal route. This operation involves considerable risk of injury to the bladder which is usually lying partly on top of the stump. To avoid this during the vaginal approach, the peritoneal cavity should be opened behind the stump at an early stage in the operation.

Rare Causes

Infrequent causes of a discharge following operation include a fistula between the Fallopian tube and the vaginal vault after hysterectomy, and endometriosis of the vagina.

Urinary and Faecal Fistulas

Urinary fistulas: Common cause for urinary fistulas in females is post hysterectomy. It can be vesicovaginal which is common or ureterovaginal which is not uncommon. Injury during dissection of urinary bladder is the common especially with previous Caesarean section patients. Often cautery dissection during bladder separation also can lead into the fistula. Often while closing the vault after hysterectomy if bladder is not pushed down adequately, inadvertent biting of the urinary bladder will lead into the same. Ureter injury occurs while dissecting and ligating the pedicles like uterine and Meckenrodt's ligament. This happens especially when there is an urgency to control undue bleeding from the pedicles wherein blind clamping of the bleeding area using haemostat has been undertaken. Continuous urinary discharge per vagina is typical. Small fistulas can close spontaneously. *Three swab test with cystoscopy* and vaginoscopy is diagnostic. Usually corrective surgery is deferred for three to four months as dissection and resuturing the walls of the urinary bladder and vagina are difficult as tissues will be very much friable. After 3–4 months, usually cystoscopy is done to identify the fistula track; a guidewire is passed through fistula track; often ureteric stenting may need to be placed one or both sides depending on the anatomical location of the fistula in relation to trigone area. Re-exploration of the abdomen using Pfannenstiel incision is done. Urinary bladder is opened away from the ureteric orifices; fistula track is dissected off; bladder wall is sutured separately off from the vaginal wall after secure closing the vaginal wall separately using polyglactin 910 (vicryl) suture material. Irrigating three way Foley's catheter is placed per urethrally. Often suprapubic cystostomy catheter is placed. Bladder wall is closed; suprapubic extraperitoneal drain is placed. Fistula with ureter is repaired after placing a ureteric stent. Often may require ureteric re-implantation over the dome of the urinary bladder. All these procedures can be undertaken through laparoscopically or robotically.

Faecal fistulas: Usually it is rectovaginal fistula. It can occur during rectal surgery or after sigmoid resection for sigmoid diverticula. It can also occur denova by involvement of the vagina by different diseases. Radiotherapy to pelvis for various conditions like carcinoma rectum or cervix may precipitate either by radiation itself or after post radiotherapy surgeries as a Neoadjuvant approach for carcinomas. Vaginoscopy/hysteroscopy and sigmoidoscopy with MRI pelvis is needed to assess the fistula and its severity. Treatment is often difficult. But needs initial diversion proximal colostomy usually through transverse colon. Later as second stage management of fistula with resection and repair after three months. Closure of colostomy further after three months is done once sigmoidoscopy confirms that fistula is closed and healed adequately. In resilient and resistant fistulas often in advanced terminal stage cancers, palliative permanent colostomy is the only choice left behind.

SUGGESTED READING

1. Carter J, Philp S, Arora A. Fast track gynaecologic surgery in the overweight and obese patient. Int J Clin Med. 2010;1:64-9.
2. Carter J, Philp S, Arora V. Discharge on postop day 2 after major gynaecological surgery. Is it possible? Bunker Bay, Western Australia: Annual Scientific Meeting Australian Society of Gynaecological Oncologists; 2010.
3. Carter J, Philp S, Arora V. Early discharge after major gynaecological surgery: advantages of fast track surgery. Open J Obstet Gynecol. 2011;1:1-5.
4. Carter J, Philp S, Arora V. Poster presentation. Extended experience with an enhanced surgical recovery program. European Union, Prague: International Gynecologic Cancer Society; 2010.
5. Carter J, Philp S. Assessing outcomes after fast track surgical management of corpus cancer. Open J Obstet Gynecol. 2011;1:139-43.
6. Carter J, Philp S. Development and Extended Experience with a Fast Track Surgery Program. Queenstown, New Zealand: Australian Society of Gynaecological Oncologists Annual Scientifc Meeting Millbrook Resort; 2011.
7. Carter J, Szabo R, Sim WW, Pather S, Philp S, Nattress K, et al. Fast track surgery in gynaecological oncology. A clinical audit. Aust N Z J Obstet Gynaecol. 2010;50: 159-63.
8. Geerts WH, Heit JA, Clagett GP, Pineo GF, Colwell CW, Anderson FA Jr, et al. Prevention of venous thrombo-embolism. Chest. 2001;119:132S-75S.
9. Lassen K, Soop M, Nygren J, Cox PB, Hendry PO, Spies C, et al. Consensus review of optimal perioperative care in colorectal surgery: enhanced Recovery after Surgery (ERAS) Group recommendations. Arch Surg. 2009;144:961-9.
10. Muntz JE, Michota FA. Prevention and management of venous thromboembolism in the surgical patient: options by surgery type and individual patient risk factors. Am J Surg. 2010;199 (1 Suppl):S11-20.
11. Simon TL, Alverson DC, AuBuchon J, Cooper ES, DeChristopher PJ, Glenn GC, et al: Practice parameters for the use of red blood cell transfusions: developed by the Red Blood Cell Administration Practice Guideline development task force of the College of American Pathologists. Arch Pathol Lab Med. 1998;122:130-8.
12. Varadhan K, Neal K, Dejong CHC, Fearon KC, Ljungqvist O, Lobo DN. The enhanced recovery after surgery (ERAS) pathway for patients undergoing major elective open colorectal surgery: a meta-analysis of randomised controlled trials. Clin Nutr. 2010;29:434-40.

63

CHAPTER

Nutrition and Exercise in Women

Vidya Thobbi

Chapter Outline

Nutrition in Women
- Maternal, Infant and Young Child Nutrition and Sustainable Goals
- Nutrition Basics
- Micronutrients
- Macronutrients
- Energy
- Adolescents Nutrition
- Nutrition during the Preconception Period
- Nutritional Requirements in Midlife

Exercise and Physiotherapy in Gynaecology
- Active Muscle Exercises
- Electrical Stimulation of Pelvic Muscles
- Short-wave Therapy
- Infrared Radiation
- Transcutaneous Electric Nerve Stimulation
- Ultrasound

NUTRITION IN WOMEN

INTRODUCTION

Nutrition constitutes the foundation of human development, required to achieve full physical and cognitive potential that further translates into enhanced learning capacities and increased productivity.

The term malnutrition encompasses both undernutrition and overnutrition. There is a vast magnitude of the many forms of nutritional deficiency, along with their associated mortality and morbidity in infants, young children and mothers. Poor maternal nutrition and continued low birth weight are indicative of the intergenerational transfer of undernutrition from the mother to the child. The low status of women and poor maternal nutrition pose major difficulties in improving child nutrition. Proper nutrition in women from childhood to menopause is very important not for the individual but for that matter for the whole family and for the health of whole nation. The first 1,000 days of life, which includes gestation and the first 2 years of life, are a vulnerable period in human development when poor nutrition can have short- and long-lasting consequences on human health and function. The nutritional status of the population has well-established, profound effects on health throughout the lifecycle and is closely associated with cognitive and social development, particularly in early childhood. Tackling malnutrition in all its forms requires that nutritional needs are addressed at key life stages through the entire life-course. Women's nutrition before and during pregnancy and through lactation is critical for optimal child growth and development as well as the well-being of mothers. This underscores the importance of adolescent nutrition. Securing optima nutrition during adolescence is important for the sound health of future offspring. This can be protected by promoting well-being and healthy nutritional practices in adolescence. Undernutrition in the womb owing to poor maternal nutrition manifests as intrauterine growth restriction prematurity, and low birth weight (LBW). Adolescence is an age of opportunity for attaining the maximum potential for growth

An adequate, well-balanced diet with a wide range of nutrients combined with regular physical activity is a cornerstone of good health.

Better nutrition is directly related to improved health across the lifespan, stronger immune systems, safer pregnancy and childbirth, and lower risk of noncommunicable diseases. Poor nutrition can lead to reduced immunity, increased susceptibility to disease, impaired physical and mental development, and reduced productivity.

Proper nutrition in women from childhood to menopause is very important not for the individual but for that matter for the whole family and for health of the whole nation.

MATERNAL, INFANT AND YOUNG CHILD NUTRITION AND SUSTAINABLE GOALS

As a global response to address nutrition, millennium development goals (MDGs-2000) initiated an era of global cooperation for result-based development and provided the basis for measuring the progress and extent of effectiveness of investments. To accelerate the pace of action to reduce malnutrition, in 2012, world health assembly (WHA) set up the targets for nutrition focusing on six areas: stunting, anaemia, exclusive breastfeeding, wasting, low birth weight, and overweight. In 2016, the declaration of 'Decade of Nutrition (2016–25)' by the UN General Assembly further strengthened efforts to advance the global agenda of ending all forms of malnutrition.

Sustainable development goals (SDGs) adopted by United Nations Member States in 2015 further enhanced focus on nutrition as a sustainable development agenda, and brought nutrition to the stage of development with the adopting resolution to end malnutrition in all its forms by the year 2030 as Goal 2 of SDG. Some of the WHA nutrition targets are adopted as targets for SDG-2.

World Health Assembly (WHA)—Nutrition Targets

World Health Assembly (WHA)—nutrition targets are shown in **Table 1**.

NUTRITION BASICS

Nutrition is a basic prerequisite to sustain life. Variety in food is not only the spice of life but also the essence of nutrition and health.

TABLE 1: World Health Assembly (WHA)—nutrition targets.

Nutrition target	***2030 global target***
1. Stunting	50% reduction in the number of children under five who are stunted
2. Anaemia	50% reduction of anaemia in women of reproductive age
3. Low birth weight	30% reduction of low birth weight
4. Overweight	Reduce and maintain childhood overweight to <3%
5. Breastfeeding	Increase the rate of exclusive breastfeeding in the first 6 months up to at least 70%
6. Wasting	Reduce and maintain childhood wasting to <3%

Source: WHO, 2014 and 2017.

A diet consisting of foods from several food groups provides all the required nutrients in proper amounts. The nutrients include proteins, fats, carbohydrates, vitamins and minerals. The foods from which we get these nutrients are classified:

- Cereals
- Legumes (pulses)
- Vegetables, fruits
- *Animal sources:* Milk and milk products, and flesh foods (fish meat and poultry)
- Nuts and oilseeds
  - Energy-yielding foods (carbohydrates and fats)
  - Bodybuilding foods (proteins)
  - Protective and regulatory foods (vitamins, minerals and other foods).

MICRONUTRIENTS

Vitamins and micronutrients are organic compounds essential for specific metabolic reactions and cannot be synthesised by human tissue cells from simple metabolites. Many act as coenzymes or as parts of enzymes responsible for promoting essential chemical reactions. Vitamin A and niacin can be formed in the body if their precursors are supplied. Vitamin K, biotin, folate and vitamin B_{12} are produced by microorganisms in the intestinal tract. Vitamin D is synthesised from a cholesterol precursor in the skin upon exposure to sunlight. Carbohydrates, fats and proteins are macronutrients, which are needed in large amounts. Vitamins and minerals constitute the micronutrients and are required in small amounts. These nutrients are necessary for physiological and biochemical processes by which the human body acquires, assimilates and utilises food to maintain health and activity.

MACRONUTRIENTS

Carbohydrates

Carbohydrates are either simple or complex, and are major sources of energy in all human diets **(Fig. 1)**. They provide energy of 4 Kcal/g. The simple carbohydrates, glucose and fructose are found in fruits, vegetables and honey, sucrose in sugar and lactose in milk, while the complex polysaccharides are starches in cereals, millets, pulses and root vegetables and glycogen in animal foods. The other complex carbohydrates which are resistant to digestion in the human digestive tract are cellulose in vegetables and whole grains, and gums and pectins in vegetables, fruits and cereals, which constitute the dietary fibre component. In India, 70–80% of total dietary calories are derived from

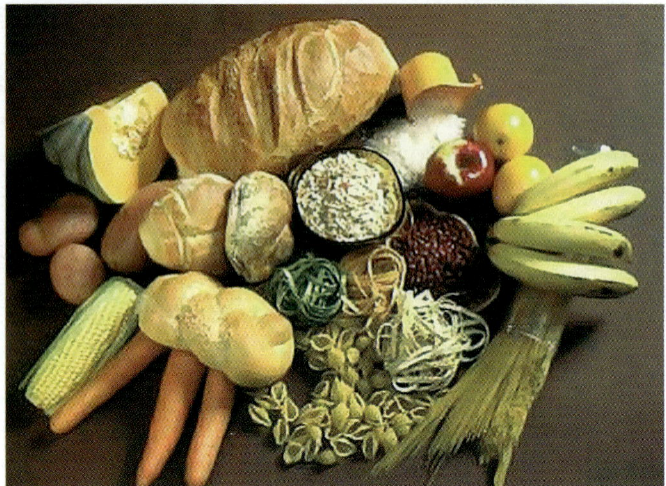

Fig. 1: Carbohydrate-rich food.

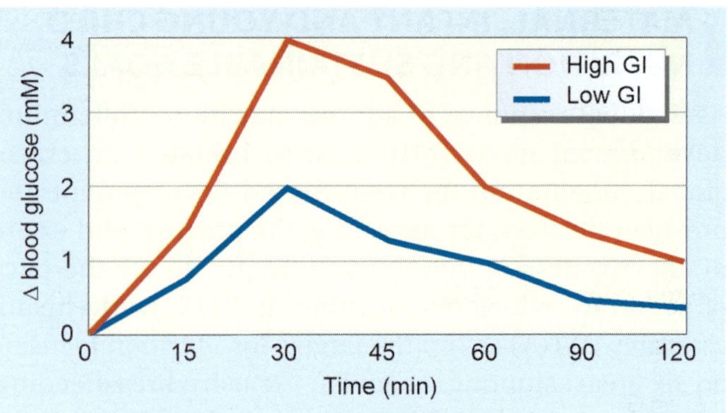

Fig. 2: Illustration of the changes in blood glucose over time following a high and low glycaemic index carbohydrate.

carbohydrates present in plant foods such as cereals, millets and pulses.

Dietary fibre delays and retards absorption of carbohydrates and fats and increases the satiety value. Diets rich in fibre reduce glucose and lipids in blood and increase the bulk of the stools. Diets rich in complex carbohydrates are healthier than low-fibre diets based on refined and processed foods.

Definition and Composition

Carbohydrates are a group of energy-yielding organic compounds that consist of carbon, hydrogen, and oxygen and in their simplest form formula are $C_nH_{2n}O_n$. Only hexoses (six carbon sugars) and pentoses (five carbon sugars) play important role in nutrition.

Classification

- Monosaccharides are the simplest form.
- Disaccharides can be hydrolysed to give two monosaccharides.
- Oligosaccharides yield from 3–10 monosaccharide units.
- Polysaccharides yield from 10–10,000 or more.
- Food ingredients, such as simple sugars, cane sugars, glucose and honey, are pure carbohydrates.
- Grain foods, roots and tubers are largely composed of starch, a complex carbohydrate. When eaten in a cooked form, they are completely digested in the gastrointestinal tract, and the released glucose is absorbed and metabolised in the body to yield energy.

What is the Glycaemic Index?

Glycaemic index (GI) is a ranking system for carbohydrates based on their immediate effect on blood glucose levels. It compares carbohydrates gram for gram in individual foods, providing a numerical, evidence-based index of postprandial (postmeal) glycaemia.

Carbohydrates that break down rapidly during digestion have the highest GIs. Such carbohydrates require less energy to be converted into glucose, which results in faster digestion and a quicker increase in blood glucose. Carbohydrates that break down slowly, releasing glucose gradually into the bloodstream, have a low GI. A lower GI suggests slower rates of digestion and absorption of the sugars and starches in the foods and may also indicate greater extraction from the liver and periphery of the products of carbohydrate digestion. Additionally, a lower glycaemic response equates to a lower insulin demand, better long-term blood glucose control and a reduction in blood lipids.

The GI of a food is defined by the area under the 2-hour blood glucose response curve (AUC) **(Fig. 2)** following the ingestion of a fixed portion of carbohydrate (usually 50 g). The AUC of the test food is divided by the AUC of the standard (either glucose or white bread) and multiplied by 100.

- *Low GI:* 55 or less
- *Moderate GI:* 56–69 inclusive
- *High GI:* 70 or more

Glycaemic Index of Foods

Glycaemic index values can be interpreted intuitively as percentages on an absolute scale and are commonly interpreted as indicated in **Table 2**.

TABLE 2: Classification of glycaemic index values.

Classification	*Glycaemic index range*	*Examples (glycaemic index value)*
Low GI	Below 55	Sourdough bread (54), apple juice (40), pumpernickel (50), oatmeal (48), pasta (54), Indian basmati rice (58)
Intermediate GI	56–69	Croissant (67), coca cola (63), raisin bran (61), wholemeal bread (65)
High GI	Above 70	White bread (70), corn flakes (80), doughnut (76), white rice (98)

Proteins

Proteins are the primary structural and functional components of every living cell.

Proteins are needed for various tissues and cells of the body:
- They are an important component of muscles and other proteins in the body in the form of enzymes and hormones, and are needed for metabolic processes.
- They supply building materials and make good for the loss that occurs due to wear and tear.
- As antibodies, proteins help to defend the body against infections.

Proteins are complex molecules composed of different amino acids. Certain amino acids, which are termed 'essential', have to be obtained from proteins in the diet since they are not synthesised in the human body. Other nonessential amino acids can be synthesised in the body to build proteins.

Protein requirements vary with age, physiological status and stress. More proteins are required by growing infants and children, pregnant women and individuals during infections and illness, or stress.

Animal foods such as milk, meat, fish and eggs and plant foods such as pulses and legumes are rich sources of proteins.

Animal proteins are of high quality as they provide all the essential amino acids in the right proportions, while plant or vegetable proteins are not of the same quality because of their low content of some of the essential amino acids. However, a combination of cereals, millets and pulses provides most of the amino acids, which complement each other to provide better quality proteins.

Sources of Proteins

Protein-rich foods are animal proteins—meat, fish, eggs, milk and milk products, plant foods such as pulses, oilseeds and nuts. Proteins from animal sources are rich sources, containing 20% proteins, and soya bean is the richest source, containing 40% proteins and cereals and millets are moderate sources containing 10% protein. Rice contains only 7% protein, but its quality is better. Leafy vegetables, fruits, roots and tubers are poor sources as they contain only about 2% protein.

Biological Values of Proteins

Nine amino acids are designated as essential amino acids since they cannot be synthesised in the body. These nine essential amino acids are threonine, tryptophan, histidine, lysine, leucine, isoleucine, methionine, valine, phenylalanine and possibly arginine. Nonessential amino acids can be synthesised in the body. Egg protein and human milk protein satisfy these criteria and are classified as high-quality proteins, which serve as a reference point for other proteins. Cereal proteins are poor in the amino acid lysine, whereas pulses and oilseeds are rich in lysine but poor in sulphur-containing amino acids, so individually they are incomplete proteins. But to improve the quality of incomplete proteins, they can be used in combinations so deficiency of one can be overcome by other. Combination of cereals and pulses in the ratio of 5:1 is the optimum combination.

Fats

Fat is a concentrated source of energy; it supplies per unit weight more than twice the energy furnished by either proteins or carbohydrates, 9 kcal/g of fat. It also provides the mechanism for absorption of the fat-soluble vitamins A, D, E and K, and carries flavour **(Fig. 3)**.

Sources of Fats

Fats can be of two types: Visible fat, i.e. derived from animal fats such as butter and ghee, which are solid fats or derived from vegetable fats such as groundnut oil, coconut oil, safflower oil, til oil, flaxseed oil, canola and soya bean oil, which are liquid fats. Hydrogenated oil, vanaspati is solid fat and is popular in India.

Second is invisible fat, which is present in food items such as cereals, pulses, oilseeds, milk, egg and meat. Dietary fat is predominantly triglycerides, which consist

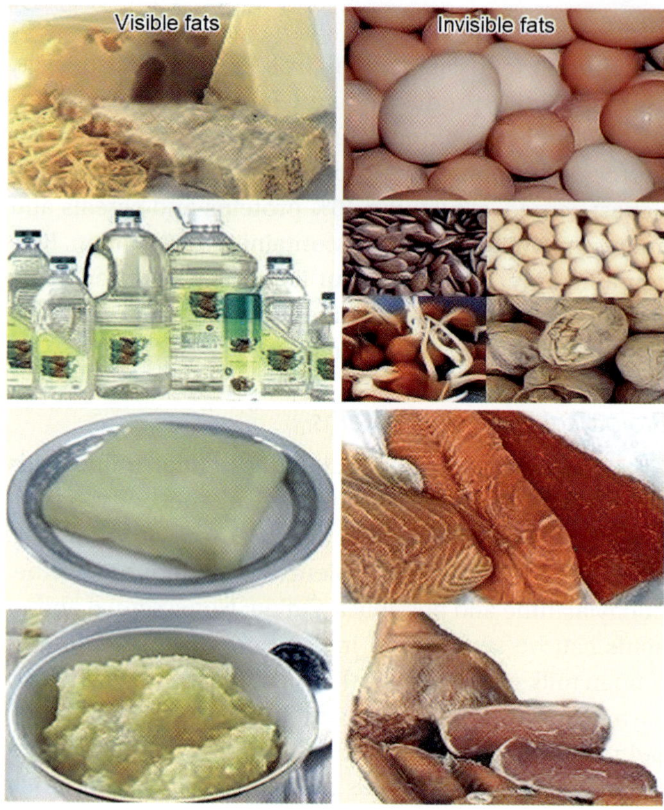

Fig. 3: Fat-rich foods.

of three fatty acids and one glycerol unit. Fatty acids can be classified into saturated, monounsaturated, trans and polyunsaturated fatty acids (PUFAs).

Saturated Fatty Acids

- Found in high amounts in animal products; also, in high amounts in coconut and palm kernel oils.
- Because saturated fats are stable at high temperatures, they are often used for deep-frying. Deep-fried foods should be avoided, but if you have to fry foods at high temperatures, palm oil, which is mostly saturated, may be the best choice for its stability.
- Many saturated fats raise the risk of heart disease.
- Saturated fatty acids predominate in animal fats, and unsaturated fatty acids predominate in vegetable oils. Animal fats, such as ghee and butter, contain vitamin A and D, which are not present in vegetable oils. However, these two vitamins can be added at a level of 700 IU and 50 IU, respectively to hydrogenated fats, i.e. vanaspati, which is derived from vegetable oil. Vegetable oil, on the other hand, contains vitamin E, which protects the oil from oxidation.

Trans Fatty Acids

Found mostly in foods made with hydrogenated or partially hydrogenated oils, including margarine, shortening, commercial frying fats, crackers, cookies and other snacks. One must check the label. Butter and animal fat can also contain trans fats from bacterial fermentation. The consensus among nutritional professionals is that large amounts of trans fats increase the risk of heart disease and many other diseases.

Monounsaturated Fats

Monounsaturated fats (MUFAs) are also known as omega-9 fats, n-9 or oleic acid. They improve cholesterol levels and are abundant in olive oil, canola oil, high-oleic sunflower oil, hazelnut oil, high-oleic safflower oil, and almond oil. Olive oil may be the best oil for cooking at moderate temperatures. It is not as refined as other oils, making it a reliable source of vitamin E and possibly other healthy components.

Avocados and many nuts (almonds, cashews, filberts/hazelnuts, macadamias, peanuts and pecans) are high in MUFA. Because nuts are high in nutrients and other protective compounds, one can benefit from eating them on a daily basis. In one study, eating nuts (including peanuts) five or more times per week reduced heart disease by about 50%.

Polyunsaturated Fats

There are two types of PUFA, (1) linoleic acid (LA) and (2) α-linolenic acid (ALA), which cannot be synthesised in the body and so have to be supplied in the food, and they belong to families: Omega-3s and omega-6s. **Table 3** lists the important ones. Individuals can use LA (omega-6) and ALA (omega-3) to make the long-chain polyunsaturated fatty acids (LCPUFAs)—arachidonic acid (AA), gamma-linolenic acid (GLA), eicosapentaenoic acid (EPA), docosahexaenoic acid (DHA) and docosapentaenoic acid (DPA).

Docosahexaenoic acid: It is found in seaweeds and fatty fish. DHA can be made from EPA. It is a major component of the grey matter of the brain, retina, testis, sperm and cell membranes. Low levels of DHA have been associated with depression.

Polyunsaturated fatty acids are known to prevent cardiovascular disease.

In addition to quantity and quality, the mode of consumption of fats appears important as smaller amounts of fats consumed frequently during the day causes less elevation of cholesterol.

TABLE 3: Dietary sources of essential and long-chain polyunsaturated fatty acids.

	Omega-6	*Sources*	*Omega-3*	*Sources*
Essential fatty acids	Linoleic acid (18:2, omega-6)	Corn, soya, safflower and sunflower oils, green leafy vegetables, nuts and seeds	α-linolenic acid (18:3, omega-3) (α-LNA)	Canola, flaxseed, walnut, soya bean oils, nuts and seeds
LCPUFA	• Arachidonic acid (20:4, omega-6) • Gamma-linolenic acid (22:5, omega-6)	Egg yolk, meats (particularly organ meats) evening primrose, blackcurrant, oils	• Eicosapentaenoic acid (20:5, omega-3) • Docosahexaenoic acid (22:6, omega-3) • Docosapentaenoic acid (22:6, omega-3)	• Fish oils, fish • Fish oils, fish

(LCPUFA: long-chain polyunsaturated fatty acids)

TABLE 4: Ratio of omega-6 to omega-3.

Omega-3 sources	*Approximate n-6:n-3 ratio*
Flaxseeds/flaxseed oil	1:4
Canola oil	2:1
English walnuts	4:1–5:1
Walnut oil	5:1
Soya bean oil	7.5:1
Black walnuts	10:1

Energy from fats should be 20–30%, EFA should be 3–6% of total energy intake and the ratio of omega-6 to omega-3 should be ideally 5:1 or 10:1.

Limit Omega-6 Fats

Limiting omega-6 intake is important for maximising the conversion of omega-3s into EPA and DHA. One should aim for an omega-6 to omega-3 ratio of 4:1 or less. The following sources of n-3s are followed by their approximate ratio of omega-6 to omega-3 **(Table 4)**.

Fibres

Besides starch and other digestible carbohydrates, many foods contain nondigestible carbohydrates such as cellulose, hemicellulose, gums, pectins and lignins. These undigestible carbohydrates are designated as 'dietary fibres'.

- Presence of fibre in the diet is necessary for the mechanism of digestion and elimination of waste. By contraction of the musculature of the digestive tract, they counteract the tendency to constipation.
- They increase transit time and reduce the time of release of ingested food in the colon. Adding fibre to diet decreases the chance of colon cancer.

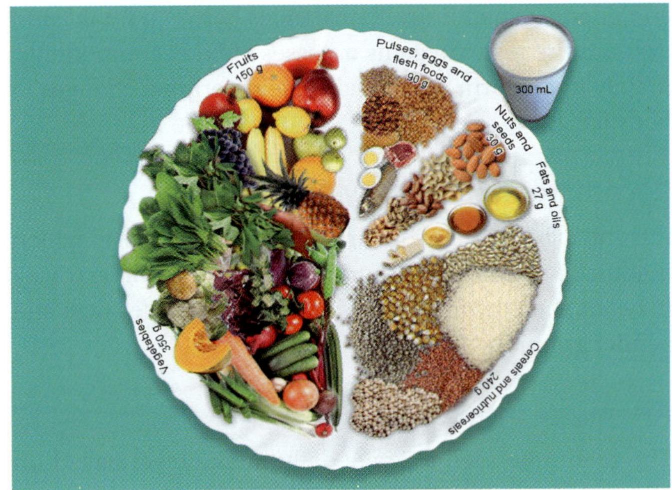

Fig. 4: My plate.

- Some of the dietary fibres such as gums and mucilage, in our diets have been shown to lower blood cholesterol in hypercholesterolaemic subjects.
- Lower blood glucose in diabetes.

Sources of Fibres

Vegetables, particularly the leafy ones, fruits, condiments, spices and unrefined cereals are comparatively rich in fibres and a generous inclusion of these provide a diet rich in fibre.

Recommended Dietary Allowance

Recommendation is 25–35 g/day. Excessive fibre may interfere with absorption of calcium and zinc, especially in children and elderly **(Fig. 4)**.

- *Eat sparingly:* Fat, oils and sugars
- *Eat moderately:* Meat and flesh foods

- *Eat liberally:* Vegetables and fruits
- *Eat adequately:* Cereals, pulses and milk

ENERGY

Energy is required to sustain the body's various functions, including respiration, circulation, physical work and maintenance of core body temperature. The energy in foods is released in the body by oxidation, yielding the chemical energy needed to sustain metabolism, nerve transmission, respiration, circulation, and physical work. The heat produced during these processes is used to maintain body temperature. Energy balance in an individual depends on his or her dietary energy intake and energy expenditure. Imbalances between intake and expenditure result in gains or losses of body components, mainly in the form of fat, and these determine changes in body weight.

Recommended Dietary Allowance

It is the average daily dietary nutrient intake level which is sufficient to meet the nutrient requirement of nearly all (97–98%) healthy individuals in a particular life stage and gender group.

Adequate Intake

The recommended average daily intake level based on observed or experimentally determined approximations or estimates of nutrient intake by a group (or groups) of apparently healthy people that are assumed to be adequately used when an RDA cannot be determined.

Tolerable Upper Intake Level

The highest average daily nutrient intake level that is likely to pose no risk of adverse health effects to almost all individuals in the general population. As intake increases above the upper limit, the potential risk of adverse effects may increase.

Epigenetics of Nutrition

Nutrition in early life induces long-term changes in DNA methylation that impact on individual health and age-related diseases throughout life.

Nutrients can either act directly by inhibiting epigenetic enzymes, such as DNA methyltransferase (DNMT), histone deacetylase (HDAC), or histone acetyltransferase (HAT), which are responsible for methylation or acetylation or by altering the availability of substrate necessary for those enzymatic reactions. This, in turn, modifies the expression of critical genes and impacts on our overall health and longevity.

ADOLESCENTS NUTRITION (TABLES 5 TO 8)

Definition of Adolescents

Adolescents are those who are aged between 10 and 19 years, young people between 10 and 24 years and youth between 15 and 24 years. The world's adolescent population—1,200 million persons of 10–19 years of age, or about 19% of the total world's population—faces a series of serious nutritional challenges not only affecting their growth and development but also their livelihood as adults.

Adolescence is a particularly unique period in life, because it is a time of intense physical, psychosocial and cognitive development. It has increased nutritional needs because:

- Adolescents gain up to 50% of their adult weight
- They gain >20% of their adult height
- About 50% of their adult skeletal mass is formed during this period
- Caloric and protein requirements are maximal
- Increased physical activity combined with poor eating habits changes their nutritional needs
- Pregnancy contributes to accentuating the potential risk for adolescents of poor nutrition.
- The term malnutrition encompasses both under-nutrition and overnutrition. Undernutrition is commonly measured by inadequate height-for-age (stunting), by inadequate weight-for-height (wasting), or by deficiencies in micronutrients, such as vitamin A, iodine, zinc and iron. Overnutrition is often measured as excessive weight-for-height (overweight and obesity) using growth reference standards for children and body mass index measurements (weight-for-height squared, or kg/m^2) for adults. Millions of adolescents, mothers and children in low and middle-income countries are experiencing the two extremes of malnutrition. Some are facing chronic undernourishment with high rates of micronutrient deficiency (such as anaemia), on the other hand rapid increases in obesity (driven by high caloric but poor-quality diets) as well as hypertension and diabetes is increasingly common; a dual burden where both types of malnutrition coexist simultaneously is also present in many cases.

TABLE 5: Dietary reference intakes (DRIs): Recommended intakes for individuals for vitamins.

Life stage group	Vitamin A (μg/day)	Vitamin C (mg/day)	Vitamin D (μg/day)	Vitamin E (mg/day)	Vitamin K (μg/day)	Thiamine (mg/day)
Females						
9–13 years	600	45	5*	11	60*	0.9
14–18 years	700	65	5*	15	75*	1.0
19–30 years	700	75	5*	15	90*	1.1
31–50 years	700	75	5*	15	90*	1.1
51–70 years	700	75	10*	15	90*	1.1
>70 years	700	75	15*	15	90*	1.1
Pregnancy						
14–18 years	750	80	5*	15	75*	1.4
19–30 years	770	85	5*	15	90*	1.4
31–50 years	770	85	5*	15	90*	1.4
Lactation						
14–18 years	1,200	115	5*	19	75*	1.4
19–30 years	1,300	120	5*	19	90*	1.4
31–50 years	1,300	120	5*	19	90*	1.4

Note: This table (taken from the DRI reports) presents recommended dietary allowances (RDAs) and adequate intakes (AIs) in ordinary type, followed by an asterisk (*). All individuals covered by this intake.
Source: Food and Nutrition Board, Institute of Medicine, and National Academies.

TABLE 6: Dietary reference intakes (DRIs): Recommended intakes for individuals for elements.

Life stage group	Calcium (mg/day)	Chromium (μg/day)	Copper (μg/day)	Fluoride (mg/day)	Iodine (μg/day)	Iron (mg/day)	Magnesium (mg/day)
Females							
9–13 years	1,300*	21*	700	2*	120	8	240
14–18 years	1,300*	24*	890	3*	150	15	360
19–30 years	1,000*	25*	900	3*	150	18	310
31–50 years	1,000*	25*	900	3*	150	18	320
51–70 years	1,200*	20*	900	3*	150	8	320
>70 years	1,200*	20*	900	3*	150	8	320
Pregnancy							
14–18 years	1,300*	29*	1,000	3*	220	27	400
19–30 years	1,000*	30*	1,000	3*	220	27	350
31–50 years	1,000*	30*	1,000	3*	220	27	360
Lactation							
14–18 years	1,300*	44*	1,300	3*	290	10	360
19–30 years	1,000*	45*	1,300	3*	290	9	310
31–50 years	1,000*	45*	1,300	3*	290	9	320

Note: This table presents recommended dietary allowances (RDAs) and adequate intakes (AIs) in ordinary type, followed by an asterisk (*).
Source: Food and Nutrition Board, Institute of Medicine, and National Academies.

TABLE 7: Dietary reference intakes (DRIs): Recommended intakes for individuals for total water and macronutrients.

Life stage group	*Total water (L/day)*	*Carbohydrate (g/day)*	*Total fibre (g/day)*	*Fat (g/day)*	*Linoleic acid (g/day)*	*α-linolenic acid (g/day)*	*Protein (g/day)*
Females							
9–13 years	2.1*	130	26*	ND	10*	1.0*	34
14–18 years	2.3*	130	26*	ND	11*	1.1*	46
19–30 years	2.7*	130	25*	ND	12*	1.1*	46
31–50 years	2.7*	130	25*	ND	12*	1.1*	46
51–70 years	2.7*	130	21*	ND	11*	1.1*	46
>70 years	2.7*	130	21*	ND	11*	1.1*	46
Pregnancy							
14–18 years	3.0*	175	28*	ND	13*	1.4*	71
19–30 years	3.0*	175	28*	ND	13*	1.4*	71
31–50 years	3.0*	175	28*	ND	13*	1.4*	71
Lactation							
14–18 years	3.8*	210	29*	ND	13*	1.3*	71
19–30 years	3.8*	210	29*	ND	13*	1.3*	71
31–50 years	3.8*	210	29*	ND	13*	1.3*	71

Note: This table presents recommended dietary allowances (RDAs) and adequate intakes (AIs) in ordinary type, followed by an asterisk (*). Total water includes all water contained in food, beverages, and drinking water.

TABLE 8: Dietary reference intakes (DRIs): Acceptable macronutrient distribution ranges.

Macronutrient	*Children, 1–3 years*	*Children, 4–18 years*	*Adults*
Fat	30–40	25–35	20–35
n-6 polyunsaturated fatty acids[a] (linoleic acid)	5–10	5–10	5–10
n-3 polyunsaturated fatty acids[a] (α-linolenic acid)	0.6–1.2	0.6–1.2	0.6–1.2
Carbohydrate	45–65	45–65	45–65
Protein	5–20	10–30	10–35

[a]Approximately 10% of the total can come from longer-chain n-3 or n-6 fatty acids.
Source: Food and Nutrition Board, Institute of Medicine, and National Academies.
Source: Dietary reference intakes for energy, carbohydrate, fibre, fat, fatty acids, cholesterol, protein and amino acids (2002/2005).

- In summary, the main nutrition problems affecting adolescent populations worldwide include:
  - Obesity
  - Undernutrition in terms of stunting and thinness, catch-up growth, and intrauterine growth restriction in pregnant adolescent girls
  - Iron deficiency and anaemia
  - Iodine deficiency
  - Vitamin A deficiency
  - Calcium deficiency
  - Specific nutrient deficiencies, e.g. zinc and folate.

Obesity in Adolescents

According to the World Health Organization (WHO) classification, an incidence of >15% means that there is epidemic, and worldwide incidence of obesity is much more, in the last 10 years, the incidence of obesity has doubled.

Parameters of Obesity

We use body mass index (BMI) as a predictor of obesity, i.e. weight in kg/height in m^2.

WHO classification for adults:

- BMI 20–25 kg/m^2 normal (for Asia 18–23 kg/m^2)
- BMI 25–30 kg/m^2 overweight
- BMI >30 kg/m^2, obese
- BMI >40 kg/m^2, morbidly obese.

Body mass index increases with increasing age, and also varies by pubertal stage and gender, so BMI percentiles are used to define degrees of overweight and obesity and normal weight in adolescents.

- BMI >85 percentile for the age is overweight
- BMI >95 percentile is obese.

Aetiology of Obesity

- Genetic factors explain a large part of the variation of body weight within a given population in a common environment.
- Environmental factors tend to explain changes in obesity over time in that population.
- Adaptive responses to environmental conditions in gestation are proposed to produce a 'thrifty phenotype' or metabolic programme that affords an individual a better chance for survival. However, when that individual is then exposed to plentiful nutrition after birth, the metabolic programme may be inappropriate for the new conditions and cause disease.

Other Factors

- High birth weight has been associated with overweight and obesity in children, adolescents and adults.
- Infants of high weight relative to length at birth [e.g. ponderal index (kg/m^3)] have a higher degree of overweight or obesity in childhood and in adulthood.
- Higher a child's or adolescent's BMI and the older the child, the more likely they would be an overweight or obese adult.
- The mother's and father's own birth weights have been reported to have significance for the infant's birth size.
- Height in adolescence is predicted by length and weight at birth and by parents' height, whereas BMI is predicted by birth weight and parents' BMI.
- Mother's higher prepregnant weight or obesity has also been associated with children having higher weight at 2, 3 and 5 years of age and is responsible for obesity later on also.

Environmental Influences on Obesity

Epidemiologists have used cohort studies and case-control designs to determine which environmental factors may contribute to obesity. Such studies have pointed to:

- Dietary trends
- Sedentary lifestyle
- Decreases in structured physical activity
- Psychosocial stressors as likely contributors to the obesity epidemic.

Prevention of Obesity in Adolescents

Nutritional:

- It should be a balanced diet with plenty of low GI cereals, vegetables, fruits, low calorie yoghurt or double tone milk, legumes, nuts, poultry, meat and fish
- Limited intake of salt and fats
- Plenty of fluids; sweetened beverages should be avoided
- No cold drinks such as Coke
- No television viewing with food
- Family should eat together
- No fast foods such as pizzas
- Meal skipping or inadequate meals (which often lead to out-of-control eating later in the day)
- 'Grazing' is bad; there should be meal-based eating habits
- *Physical activity:* 1 hour of intense physical activity, such as lawn tennis.

Anaemia in Adolescent Girls

Definition

Anaemia is a condition of low circulating haemoglobin (Hb) in which Hb concentration has fallen below the threshold lying two standard deviations below the median of a healthy population of the same age, sex, and same period of pregnancy. This is a statistical definition, and the WHO definition is <11 g% in pregnant and <12 g/dL in non-pregnant and haematocrit of <0.33 (CDC) **(Table 9)**.

Incidence

Globally, it is 30% and in developing countries it is 40–90%. Requirement of iron in adolescent girls is more as they are menstruating and iron stores are needed for future pregnancy and lactation.

Poor availability and lack of knowledge:

- Poor bioavailability of iron in a vegetarian diet
- Worm infestation

TABLE 9: Classification of anaemia.

Type of anaemia	*Haemoglobin (g/dL)*	*Haematocrit (%)*
Mild anaemia	7–11.9	24–37
Moderate anaemia	4–6.9	13–23
Severe anaemia	<4	<13

- Gender bias
- Chronic malaria

Bioavailability of Iron Absorption

Iron absorption is increased by:
- Ascorbic acid
- Haem proteins
- Fermentation, ferrous ions

Increase bioavailability of iron in vegetarian diets; citrus fruits and juices should be taken with meals. Adding vitamin C sources such as tomatoes, potatoes and amla to the diet in vegetarians would also increase the bioavailability of iron. Other recommendation is cooking food in iron utensils.

Folic Acid

Folic acid is required for the nucleic acid metabolism and for cell division and growth. Its deficiency causes megaloblastic anaemia, neural tube defects, homocysteinaemia. It also prevents isolated cleft lip congenital anomalies.

Sources of folic acid are green leafy vegetables, fruits, liver and kidney. RDA for adolescent girls is 500 μg/day.

Folic acid supplementation should be given to all adolescent girls preconceptionally. The 500 μg/day in low-risk cases and in the high-risk cases, with a history of previous neural tube defect, should be given in the dose of 5 mg/day, minimum 1 month before conception. Iron and folate should be given together.

Iodine Deficiency Disorders

Iodine is required for the synthesis of thyroid hormones, which are involved in regulating metabolic activities of all cells throughout the life cycle. In addition, it plays a key role in cell replication. This is particularly relevant for the brain since neural cells multiply mainly in utero and during the first 2 years of life. Iodine deficiency disorder (IDD) comprises all the effects of iodine deficiency.

Prevention and Control

Globally, 68% of households in countries with IDD now consume iodised salt. Iodisation rates are highest in the Americans at 90%. Africa has achieved a level of 63%.

Vitamin A Deficiency

Vitamin A is an essential micronutrient for the normal functioning of the visual system, growth and development, maintenance of epithelial cellular integrity, immune function, and reproduction.

Sources of Vitamin A

Vitamin A or retinol is present in some animal foods such as butter, ghee, whole milk, curds, egg yolk and liver. The liver oil of certain fish like cod, halibut, shark and sawfish is one of the richest known sources. The rich source of beta-carotene are green leafy vegetables, spinach, amaranth, coriander, drumstick leaves, curry leaves, mint, radish leaves, etc. and ripe yellow fruits such as mangoes, papaya, tomatoes, carrots and yellow pumpkin.

Prevention

- Vitamin A supplementation to all children
- Promotion of egg consumption
- Fortification of food like maize and sugar with vitamin A.

Calcium Requirements in Adolescents

- Recommended dietary allowance for calcium is 1,300 mg/day, but this varies and depends on many factors. Adequate calcium intakes are affected by many variable factors, including age, gender, physical activity and multiple dietary considerations. Genetic and ethnic variability are also important factors **(Table 10)**.
- The current dietary intake of calcium by children and adolescents is well below the recommended optimal levels. The available data support recent recommendations for calcium intakes of 1,200–1,500 mg/day beginning during the preteen years and continuing throughout adolescence.
- Optimising calcium intake is particularly important during adolescence. Peak calcium-accretion rate is attained at an average of 12.5 years of age in girls and 14.0 years of age in boys. During the 3- to 4-year period of increased bone mass acquisition that occurs during adolescence, 40% of total lifetime bone mass is accumulated.
- The efficiency of calcium absorption is increased during puberty, and the majority of bone formation occurs during this period.
- The largest source of dietary calcium for most persons is milk and other dairy products. Other sources of calcium are, however, important, especially for achieving calcium intakes of 1,200–1,500 mg/day.

TABLE 10: Approximate calcium contents of one serving of some common foods.

Food serving size	*Calcium content*
Milk 1 cup (240 mL)	300 mg
White beans 1/2 cup (110 g)	113 mg
Broccoli cooked 1/2 cup (71 g)	35 mg
Broccoli raw 1 cup (71 g)	35 mg
Cheddar cheese 1.5 oz (42 g)	300 mg
Low-fat yoghurt 8 oz (240 g)	300–415 mg
Spinach cooked 1/2 cup (90 g)	120 mg
Spinach raw 11/2 cup (90 g)	120 mg
Calcium-fortified orange juice 1 cup (240 mL)	300 mg
Orange 1 medium (1 medium)	50 mg
Sardines or salmon with bones: 20 sardines (240 g)	50 mg
Sweet potatoes 1/2 cup mashed (160)	44

Source: United Nations Subcommittee on Nutrition Fourth Report on the World Nutrition Situation, 2000—modified.

TABLE 11: Nutrition risk factors and effects on birth outcomes.

Nutrition risk factors	*Effect on birth outcomes*
Maternal age:	
Teenage pregnancy	50% increased risk of stillbirths and preterm births
Advanced maternal age	Increased risk of perinatal death by 44% and preterm birth by 29%. Increased risk of Down syndrome
Micronutrient deficiencies:	
Iron deficiency anaemia	Iron deficiency anaemia associated with increased risk of foetal growth retardation
Folate and multivitamin deficiency	Folate deficiency is associated with neural tube defects
Malnutrition:	
Underweight	Increased risk of preterm birth by 32%
Overweight	Increased risk of preeclampsia and GDM

- Physical activity, primarily weight-bearing exercise, is encouraged as part of an overall healthy bone programme.

NUTRITION DURING THE PRECONCEPTION PERIOD

The preconception period is defined as the period of 3 months before conception. Health and nutrition status of both men and women before conception is important not only for pregnancy outcomes but also for the lifelong health of their children and even the next generation.

Nutrition Risks During Preconception

The importance of nutrition before conception has been increasingly recognised. Recent research has established linkages of preconception and interventions with improved maternal, perinatal and neonatal health outcomes, and it has been suggested that several proven interventions recommended during pregnancy may be even more effective if implemented before conception.

Nutrition Risk Factors During Preconception, Effect on Birth Outcomes and Effect of Preconception Nutrition Interventions (Table 11)

Attaining optimal weight: For optimal weight gain, women should consume a balanced diet rich in fruits and vegetables, low-fat dairy products, whole grains and high-protein foods. A balanced diet will ensure that women acquire the recommended daily requirements for vitamins and minerals, and also adequate nutrient stores for pregnancy.

Diagnosis and treatment of anaemia: Anaemia among women is a major risk factor for maternal and birth outcomes. It is recommended that women in preconception period should be screened for anaemia, and if diagnosed with anaemia appropriate treatment strategy should be adopted for the treatment as per national guidelines. Iron and folic acid supplementation and consumption of iron and vitamin C-rich food stuff should be consumed by women to address anaemia.

NUTRITIONAL REQUIREMENTS IN MIDLIFE

Energy

Recommended dietary allowance for the elderly calls for a reduction in energy intake after 51 years of age, 600 kcal/day for men and 300 kcal for women. But it should not be less than 1,800 kcal/day, otherwise it would be deficient in protein, calcium, iron and vitamins, so nutrient-dense food should be planned for them.

Protein

Body protein in healthy elderly is 60–70% of that of young adults, but still protein intake of 1.0 g/kg daily is best for them for nitrogen balance.

Carbohydrates

Recommended dietary allowance for carbohydrates is at least 55% of calories and mainly from complex carbohydrates. Diminished lactase secretion frequently leads to lactose intolerance and in these cases lactase treated milk and fermented dairy products would alleviate the symptoms of flatulence, cramping and diarrhoea.

Fats

Approximately 30% of the calories should be from fats, and they should be in combination. One of the unfortunate consequences of the lower-fat diet message is that often the replacement for fat calories is calories from simple carbohydrates, which can elevate plasma triglyceride levels, resulting in lower high-density lipoprotein cholesterol concentrations, which has been shown to be an important determinant of coronary heart disease risk in the elderly. An additional effect of a low-fat, high-simple-carbohydrate diet is to increase the expression of low-density lipoprotein particles.

Minerals

Calcium requirement in menopausal women is 1,200–1,500 mg/day. As calcium absorption is decreased, it results in osteoporosis and hypochlorhydria. All these factors cause increased demand for calcium. But along with calcium, we have to advise weight-bearing exercises to decrease bone resorption and calcium deposition. In those taking diuretics for hypertension, sodium intake should be reduced to 2–4 mg/day and potassium and magnesium should be supplemented.

Vitamins

As the capacity of the skin to synthesise vitamin D is decreased in elderly, lesser exposure to sunlight especially in institutionalised and homebound, and some evidence suggests decreased capacity of aging kidney to convert vitamin D to the active $1,25(OH)_2D_3$ form so elderly women might develop deficiency of vitamin D. Vitamin D supplementation of 400 IU/day might be required. Lack of calcium and vitamin D would result in osteoporosis and osteomalacia. But most of the elderly use more vitamins than required, and that should be avoided.

Water

Proper fluid intake is very important for the elderly. Dehydration is the most common cause of fluid and electrolyte disturbances and can be because of:

- Reduced thirst sensation and diminished fluid intake
- Diminished water conservation by the kidneys
- Use of diuretics
- Diarrhoea or fever
- Incontinent patients

So, all these conditions must be monitored for proper fluid intake by the elderly.

CONCLUSION

For health from adolescent to menopause if we can do some lifestyle modifications such as increasing our daily routine activities, reducing sedentary lifestyle and making exercise an integral part of our life then it would go a long way in keeping us fit and our weight would be under control our diet should be roughly like the pyramid mentioned as follows **(Fig. 5)**:

- Our diet should have basically more of whole grains that is why we put them on the base of the pyramid. Oatmeal, brown rice and whole wheat have low GI, so they should be used more often.
- *Oils*: They should be mainly from vegetable oils such as canola, soya oil, sunflower oil and peanut oil. Whatever recommended daily requirements should not be substituted by carbohydrates.
- *Vegetables and fruits*: There should be three helpings of vegetables daily with two to three helpings of fresh fruits to give us our all vitamins, antioxidants and iron. They should be of different colours to add variability and taste.
- Fish, poultry and eggs to give us proteins and DHA, a type of LCPUFAs.
- *Nuts and legumes*: They are the source of fibre, protein, vitamins, minerals and fats. Daily 1–3 helpings are needed.
- Milk as a source of calcium is very essential for proper development of bones. One cup of milk gives 300 mg of calcium. It can be consumed as milk products also as yoghurt with fruit would make an ideal dessert. Always take low-fat milk and milk products.
- Red meat and butter should be in a minimum quantity.

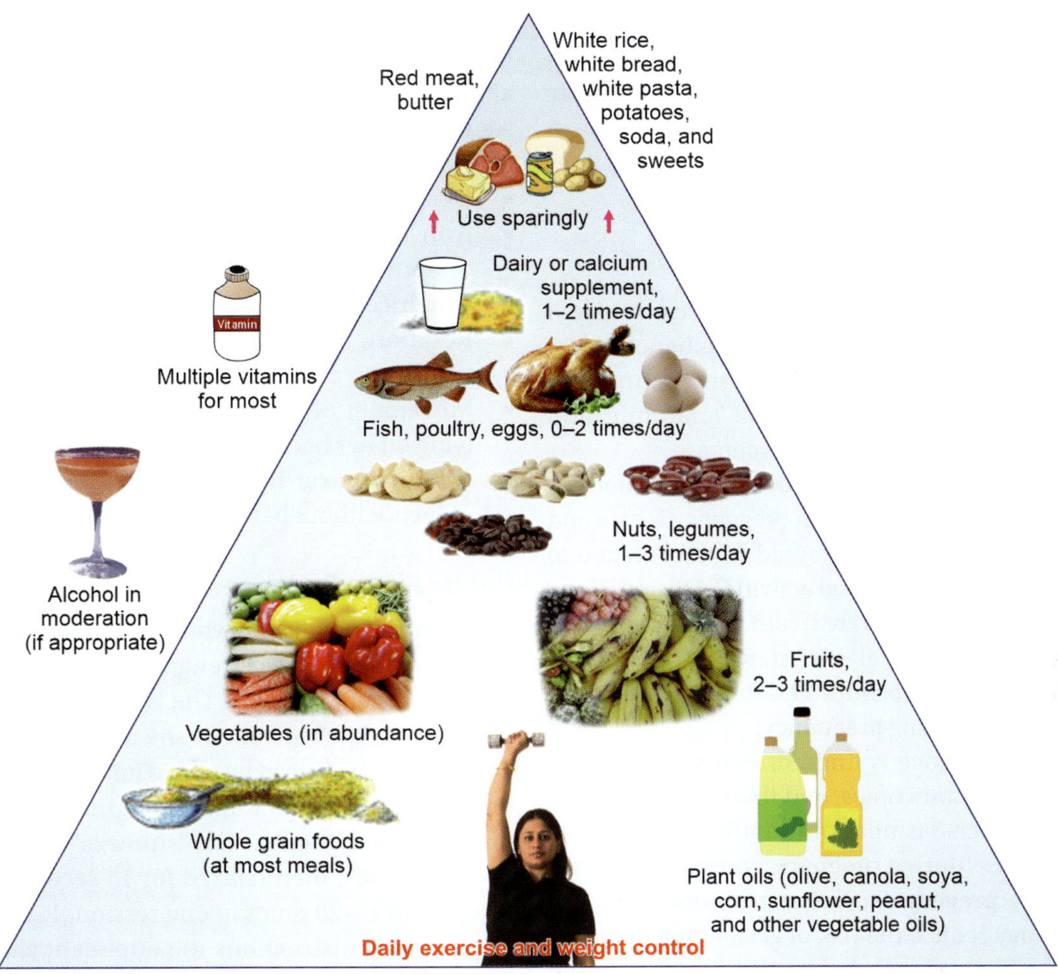

Fig. 5: Eat and exercise pyramid.

- Alcohol in moderation, just 1–2 drinks.
- Pasta, white bread, potatoes, white rice, sweets and aerated cold drinks should be used sparingly as they add to empty calories in the body.

EXERCISE AND PHYSIOTHERAPY IN GYNAECOLOGY

Regular physical activity provides numerous health benefits, which include the reduction in risks of coronary heart disease, hypertension, diabetes mellitus, obesity, colon cancer and mortality.

The American College of Sports Medicine and Centers for Disease Control and Prevention (CDC) both recommend a regular pattern of moderate intensity physical activity of 30 minutes or more, which can be accumulated throughout the day and should be performed on most days of the week. Despite this information and these recommendations, many women remain largely sedentary.

ACTIVE MUSCLE EXERCISES

Regular physical exercise is essential for health and maintaining good posture. A woman ordinarily has no need for specially planned exercises, because the movements carried out in the course of polishing, bending, lifting and running up and down stairs could hardly be improved upon. The woman unoccupied in this way, and doing sedentary work in a factory or office, should be encouraged to take up other activities such as games, dancing, gardening and walking. If she has no other opportunities, she can at least walk part of the way to work. The only muscles not exercised routinely in the course of domestic chores are those of the lower abdomen.

The pursuit of physical exercise may be of curative as well as prophylactic value in the treatment of certain cases of dysmenorrhoea, premenstrual syndrome, climacteric symptoms, constipation and other disorders with a background of introspection and overanxiety. It disciplines the mind as well as the body and satisfies the self.

Postnatal Exercises

Physical activity and exercise in pregnancy are associated with minimal risks and have been shown to benefit most women, although some modification to exercise routines may be necessary because of normal anatomic and physiologic changes and foetal requirements.

In the absence of obstetric or medical complications or contraindications, physical activity in pregnancy is safe and desirable, and pregnant women should be encouraged to continue or to initiate safe physical activities. Obstetrician-gynaecologists and other obstetric care providers should evaluate women with medical or obstetric complications carefully before making recommendations on physical activity participation during pregnancy.

Although the evidence is limited, exercise results in benefits to pregnancy outcomes, and there is no evidence of harm when exercise is not contraindicated. Physical activity and exercise during pregnancy promote physical fitness and may prevent excessive gestational weight gain. Exercise may reduce the risk of gestational diabetes, preeclampsia and caesarean birth. Additional research is needed to study the effects of exercise on pregnancy-specific conditions and outcomes and to clarify further effective behavioural counselling methods and the optimal type, frequency, and intensity of exercise. Similar research is needed to create an improved evidence base concerning the effects of occupational physical activity on maternal-foetal health.

Day-to-day activities, together with walking, are valuable during pregnancy. They help to make the muscles strong and supple, prevent constipation and varicose veins, preserve posture, and ensure a quick return to health after delivery. Their objectives are: Preservation or restoration of normal bladder and bowel functions; full expansion of the lungs after pregnancy and anaesthesia; maintenance of the circulation to reduce the risk of thrombosis and embolism; restoration of muscle tone, figure and posture; rapid and complete involution of pelvic organs and their supports; and prevention of prolapse.

Postnatal exercises are introduced gradually, commencing on the first day after delivery and continued for at least 3 months. Their exact details vary from clinic to clinic, but in principle, they help to return the pelvic floor and the abdominal wall as near as possible to the prepregnancy state. They consist of the following:

- Attention to posture when sitting, standing and walking
- Deep breathing—inspiration and expiration
- Arm, leg and foot movements of flexion, extension and rotation
- Quadriceps drill
- Rotation, flexion and extension movements of the trunk
- Movement of the legs as in cycling, with the patient lying on her back
- Instruction on how to lift the baby or other heavy objects without bending and injuring the back.

Pelvic Floor Exercises

These can be carried out while the patient is lying, standing or sitting; they aim to strengthen the levator ani and the pubococcygeal muscles. The woman is instructed to lift the anus and pelvic floor as she does at the conclusion of defaecation, or she can be told to imagine that she is voiding urine and then to go through the motion of interrupting the stream suddenly. The 'squeeze' is maintained for 10–12 seconds, then relaxed for 15 seconds. The process is repeated 15–20 times in one session, 1–3 sessions a day. When giving instructions the attendant should examine the patient vaginally to ensure that she is contracting the right muscles. The grip of the levators around the vagina is easily felt. The concurrent contraction of the gluteus maximus can also be perceived by a hand placed gently on the buttock. In order to encourage her to make stronger efforts, and to assure her that she is doing the right exercise, it can be of help to give her a Kegel's perineometer **(Fig. 6)**. This consists of a vaginal obturator with an air-containing sleeve connected to a manometer which measures the squeeze of the vaginal muscles. Vaginal cones of increasing weight have also been developed to assist the patient in biofeedback.

By pelvic floor exercises carried out for several months, a woman can develop considerable power in the muscles and can learn to control minor degrees of prolapse and urethral incompetence.

Preoperative Physiotherapy

Preoperative chest physiotherapy is especially beneficial in women with chronic lung disease, obesity, large

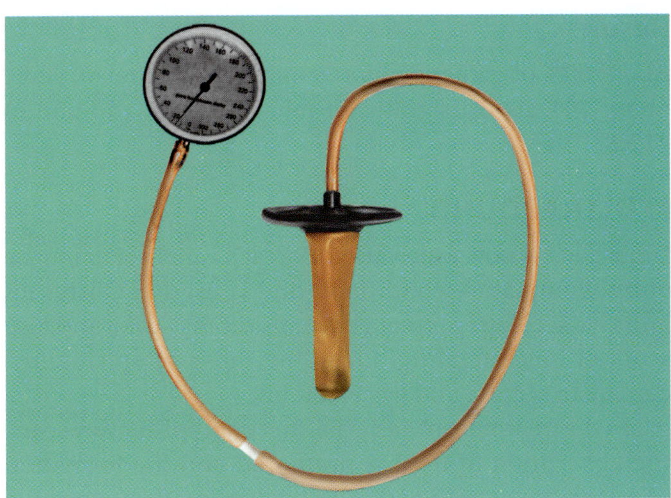

Fig. 6: Kegel's perineometer for pelvic floor exercises.

abdominal tumours or massive ascites, which can embarrass respiration, and in smokers. Deep breathing exercises can be better taught at this time. Devices such as the incentive spirometer are useful in high-risk cases as they demonstrate the depth of the breath taken and allow the patient to judge adequacy and improvement herself.

Postoperative Exercises

These should be carried out each morning and evening, commencing with simple manoeuvres such as deep breathing and leg and arm movements on the first day after the operation. Thereafter, the exercises are graduated according to the patient's speed of recovery. They are the same in principle as those advised for the postnatal period, with omissions and modifications according to the operation site. Deep breathing encourages expansion of the lungs, prevents atelectasis and improves venous return. Limb movements also help in preventing venous stasis and deep vein thrombosis.

ELECTRICAL STIMULATION OF PELVIC MUSCLES

Much work has been done on devising means for providing continuous or intermittent electrical stimulation of pelvic muscles. These are energised by a small generator attached to and controlled by the patient; their aim is the relief of faecal and urinary incontinence not caused by fistulas, and when surgery has failed.

By such means it is certainly possible to induce strong contractions of the voluntary muscles of the pelvic floor, including the external sphincters of the anus and urethra. So, rectal prolapse and faecal incontinence can be controlled to some extent. Stress incontinence of urine is, however, not benefited, probably because the involuntary internal sphincter is not stimulated, or, if it is, simultaneous stimulation of the bladder detrusor muscle (which is continuous with this sphincter) also occurs to counteract the effect.

SHORT-WAVE THERAPY

Short-wave therapy aims to raise the temperature of deeply situated tissues and to induce hyperaemia. This, in turn, promotes natural resistance to infection and encourages resolution of inflammatory processes, as well as the elimination of metabolic waste products.

Indications

Short-wave therapy can easily become a quack remedy, soothing to the mind rather than the body of the patient. It has been, and is, used in the treatment of almost all 'female complaints', and claims are made for its value in conditions such as dysmenorrhoea, cervical erosion, infertility and pelvic pain. All such claims are without scientific foundation.

The only acceptable indications for short-wave therapy are:

- Subacute and chronic cellulitis
- Subacute and chronic salpingo-oophoritis
- Late radiation effects characterised by ischaemia of the tissues in and around the vagina, uterus, bladder and rectum.

Short-wave therapy should not be used during the *acute* stages of pelvic inflammatory disease, nor in cases of tuberculous infection. In both these circumstances, it is likely to cause an exacerbation of the problem. When a patient believed to have chronic pyogenic salpingo-oophoritis fails to respond, or it gets worse after treatment, the diagnosis should be reviewed with the possibilities of endometriosis and tuberculosis in mind.

Techniques

Treatment is given every alternate day for a total of 15–18 exposures. The patient may lie on a couch or be semirecumbent in a special chair. Electrodes are placed on the lower abdomen and back and sometimes on the flexed thighs. The dose is small at first and is gradually increased according to the patient's reactions and progress.

Results

Usually, the patient suffering from chronic pelvic infection gets relief from pain during treatment, but some pain may persist for a short time afterwards. During the course of days or weeks, the inflammatory reaction in the pelvis tends to subside, masses get smaller and organs become less tender and fixed. This, however, is the natural history of pelvic inflammatory disease, and it is always difficult to decide how far pelvic heat assists spontaneous resolution.

INFRARED RADIATION

Infrared rays are electromagnetic waves with a wavelength of 750–400,000 nm. The penetration is only up to the deeper epidermis. They help in pain relief and muscle relaxation in much the same way as short-wave diathermy and are effective in relieving the pain of episiotomies and abdominal wounds.

TRANSCUTANEOUS ELECTRIC NERVE STIMULATION

Transcutaneous electric nerve stimulation (TENS) is a method of electroanalgesia, which stimulates the large-diameter afferent sensory fibres and produces an antinociceptive effect at the spinal or supraspinal level. It also decreases ischaemia by improving the blood flow and probably decreases the oxygen consumption. The latter effect is thought to be mediated by enkephalins, beta-endorphins and dynorphins, which are synthesised locally and which may serve a paracrine function. A segmental decrease in sympathetic activity may also contribute to decreased local oxygen consumption.

Indications

Transcutaneous electric nerve stimulation is ineffective for visceral pain of neurogenic and musculoskeletal origin, but is useful if the pain is secondary to local ischaemia, as in severe primary dysmenorrhoea and in some cases of chronic pelvic pain. It is used alone or as an adjuvant therapy to conventional pharmacological methods.

Technique

Commercially available TENS stimulators deliver current at 0.2 ms at a frequency of about 70–100 Hz. Electrodes applied to the lower abdomen and sacroiliac region deliver a high-intensity stimulation of 40–50 mA, which can be decreased if it causes discomfort.

Results

About 90% of patients report some degree of relief, while about 30% report significant relief with the addition of TENS.

ULTRASOUND

Ultrasound is now widely used to treat a variety of traumatic and inflammatory conditions, and is used in Obstetrics and Gynaecology to treat early episiotomy scars, and also scars of long-standing, including those of episiotomy, caesarean section and hysterectomy.

In the treatment of early (i.e. first day) episiotomy scars, the absorption of fluid is promoted and the formation of adhesions is reduced. The analgesic effect gives the patient relief from pain and discomfort, and increased blood supply aids tissue repair.

Long-standing scars, of whatever nature, are softened by the application of ultrasound, and it is of value both for superficial scars and others, up to a depth of approximately 3 cm, including induration following a haematoma.

Therapeutic ultrasound is administered through a transducer head which is kept moving and in contact with the part to be treated by means of a coupling gel, water bag or immersion in water. This ensures maximum contact and therefore maximum absorption. The device can be either pulsed or continuous, according to the depth of the area to be treated and the effect to be achieved.

SUGGESTED READING

1. Auerback VH, DiGeorge AM, Carpenter GG. Phenylalaninemia: A study of the diversity of disorders which produce elevation of blood concentrations of phenylalanine. In: Nyhan WL (Ed). Amino Acid Metabolism and Genetic Variation. New York: McGraw Hill; 1967.
2. Belza B, Warms CA. Physical activity and exercise in women's health. Nurs Clin North Am.2004;39(1):181-93.
3. Bhagat S. Asanas that help cure disease and symptoms. In: Bhagat S (Eds). Alternative Therapies. New Delhi: Jaypee Brothers Medical Publishers (P) Ltd.; 2004. pp. 18-82.
4. Borg GA. Psychophysical bases of perceived exertion. Med Sci Sports Exerc. 1982;14:377-81.
5. Brigelius-Flohe R, Kelly FJ, Salonen JT, Neuzil J, Zingg JM, Azzi A. The European perspective on vitamin E: current knowledge and future research. Am J Clin Nutr. 2002;76:703-16.
6. Bursch SG. Interrater reliability of diastasis recti abdominis measurement. Phys Ther. 1987;67(7):1077-9.
7. Centers for Disease Control and Prevention. Recommendations to prevent and control iron deficiency in the United States. MMWR. 1998;47 (No. RR-3):51.

8. Dallman PR, Ray Y, Johnson C. Prevalence and causes of anemia in the United States, 1976 to 1980. Am J Clin Nutr. 1984;39(3):437-45.
9. Das UN. Can perinatal supplementation of long-chain polyunsaturated fatty acids prevent atopy, bronchial asthma and other inflammatory conditions? Med Sci Monit. 2006;12(6):RA99-111.
10. Das UN. Can perinatal supplementation of long-chain polyunsaturated fatty acids prevent schizophrenia in adult life? Med Sci Monit. 2004;10(12):HY33-7.
11. Das UN. Perinatal supplementation of long-chain polyunsaturated fatty acids, immune response and adult diseases. Med Sci Monit. 2004;10(5):HY19-25.
12. Denke MA. Dietary fats, fatty acids, and their effects on lipoproteins. Curr Atheroscler Rep. 2006;8(6):466-71.
13. Farrell M, Ward J, Mattick R, Hall W, Stimson GV, des Jarlais D, et al. Methadone maintenance in opiate dependence: a review. BMJ. 1994;309:997-1001.
14. Food and Nutrition Board. Dietary reference intakes for energy, carbohydrate, fiber, fatty acids, cholesterol, protein and amino acids (macronutrients). Dietary fats: total fats and fatty acids. Washington: National Academic Press; 2005.
15. Ford ES, Cogswell ME. Diabetes and serum ferritin concentration among US adults. Diabetes Care. 1999; 22:1978-83.
16. Frieden TR, Blakeman DE. The dirty dozen: 12 myths that undermine tobacco control. Am J Public Health. 2005;95(9):1500-5.
17. Goodlett CR, Horn KH. Mechanisms of alcohol-induced damage to the developing nervous system. Alcohol Res Health. 2001;25(3):175-84.
18. Grundy SM. Monounsaturated fatty acids and cholesterol metabolism: Implications for dietary recommendations. J Nutr. 1989;119(4):529-33.
19. Haddad EH, Sabaté J, Whitten CG. Vegetarian food guide pyramid: a conceptual framework. Am J Clin Nutr. 1999;70(3):615S-9S.
20. Hellekson KL. NIH Consensus Statement on phenylketonuria. Am Fam Physician. 2001;63(7):1430-32.
21. Jiang R, Manson JE, Meigs JB, Ma J, Rifai N, Hu FB. Body iron stores in relation to risk of type 2 diabetes in apparently healthy women. JAMA. 2004;291:711-7.
22. Kapandji IA. Nutation and counter-nutation. The Physiology of the Joints: The trunk and the Vertebral Column. Oxford: Churchill Livingstone; 1974.
23. Kuczmarski RJ, Flegal KM, Campbell SM, Johnson CL. Increasing prevalence of overweight among US adults: the National Health and Nutrition Examination Surveys, 1960-1961. JAMA. 1994;272(3):205-11.
24. Kumar P, Raju P, Prasad V. Fundamentals of Physiotherapy. New Delhi: Jaypee Brothers Medical Publishers (P) Ltd.; 2005.
25. Kumar V, Cotran RS, Robbins SL. Cellular adaptations, cell injury, and cell death. Robbins Basic Pathology, 7th edition. Philadelphia: Lippincott Williams and Wilkins; 2005.
26. Lutz C, Karen P. Nutrition and Diet Therapy: Evidence-Based Applications, 4th edition. Philadelphia: FA Davis; 2008.
27. Michals K, Matalon R. Phenylalanine metabolites, attention span and hyperactivity. Am J Clin Nutr. 1985;42(2):361-5.
28. Mokdad AH, Ford ES, Bowman BA, Dietz WH, Vinicor F, Bales VS. Prevalence of obesity, diabetes, and obesity-related health risk factors. JAMA. 2001;289:76-9.
29. Monzillo LU, Hamdy O, Horton ES, Ledbury S, Mullooly C, Jarema C, et al. Effect of lifestyle modification on adipokine levels in obese subjects with insulin resistance. Obesity Res. 2003;11:1048-54.
30. Morgan MY, Ritson EB. Alcohol and Health: A Handbook for Students and Medical Practitioners, 4th edition. London: Medical Council on Alcohol; 2003.
31. Nair KM, Brahamam GN, Ranganathan S, Vijayaraghavan K, Sivakumar B, Krishnaswamy K. Impact evaluation of iron and iodine fortified salt. Indian J Med Res. 1998;108:203-11.
32. National Academy of Sciences: Institute of Medicine. Food and Nutrition Board (2004). US Department of Agriculture. [online] Available from https://www.nationalacademies.org/fnb/food-and-nutrition-board.
33. Owen AL, Owen GM. Twenty years of WIC: a review of some effects of the program. J Am Diet Assoc. 1997;97(7):777-82.
34. Pasceri V, Wu HD, Willerson JT, Yeh ET. Modulation of vascular inflammation in vitro and in vivo by peroxisome proliferator-activated receptor-gamma activators. Circulation. 2000;101:235-8.
35. Pietz J, Kreis R, Rupp A, Mayatepek E, Rating D, Boesch C. Large neutral amino acids block phenylalanine transport into brain tissue in patients with phenylketonuria. J Clin Invest. 1999;103(8):1169-78.
36. Rajala MW, Scherer PE. Minireview: the adipocyte—at the crossroads of energy homeostasis, inflammation, and atherosclerosis. Endocrinology. 2003;144(9):3765-73.
37. Savage DB, Petersen KF, Shulman GI. Mechanisms of insulin resistance in humans and possible links with inflammation. Hypertension. 2005;45(5):828-33.
38. Smith DE, Schwartz RH, Martin DM. Heavy cocaine use by adolescents. Paediatrics. 1989;83(4):539-42.
39. Takahashi HK, Iwagaki H, Hamano R, Yoshino T, Tanaka N, Nishibori M. Effect of nicotine on IL-18-initiated immune response in human monocytes. J Leukoc Biol. 2006;80(6):1388-94.
40. Vallee BL, Falchuck KH. The biochemical basis of zinc physiology. Physiol Rev. 1993;73:79-118.
41. Whittaker P, Tufaro PR, Rader JI. Iron and folate in fortified cereals. J Am Coll Nutr. 2001;20(3):247-54.
42. Wolsko PM, Eisenberg DM, Davis RB, Phillips RS. Use of mind-body medical therapies. J Gen Intern Med. 2004;19(1):43-50.

64

CHAPTER

Applications of Lasers in Gynaecology

Vidya Bhat, Mythreyi Kadambi

Chapter Outline

- History
- Laser Physics
- Types of Lasers
- Laser Safety
- Extraperitoneal Laser Surgery
- Clinical Applications of Lasers in Intra-abdominal Gynaecological Surgery
- Other Clinical Applications of Lasers in Gynaecology and Reproductive Medicine
- Novel Concepts—Lasers in Cosmetic Gynaecology

INTRODUCTION

The use of laser technology in gynaecology has greatly expanded since Kaplan and colleagues first employed the CO_2 laser in 1973 to treat cervical erosions. Since then, there have been significant advancements in laser technology, leading to the development of other types of lasers, such as the neodymium yttrium aluminium garnet (Nd:YAG), potassium-titanyl-phosphate (KTP) and argon lasers. Concurrently, lasers have become a favoured tool in laparoscopy, particularly in the field of infertility treatment.

HISTORY

The term 'laser' is an acronym for 'light amplification by the stimulated emission of radiation', a principle first introduced by Einstein in 1917. The first laser, created by Theodore Maiman in 1960, used a ruby as its active medium, and in 1961, the CO_2 laser was developed. In 1973, the CO_2 laser was first applied in gynaecology to treat cervical erosions and was later utilised by Bellina for treating cervical intraepithelial neoplasia (CIN) and performing microsurgery on the fallopian tubes. The use of KTP, argon and Nd:YAG lasers gained popularity in the early 1980s.

LASER PHYSICS

Lasers are classified according to the medium that is activated. Each medium produces light waves at a specific wavelength, giving it a distinct monochromatic colour.

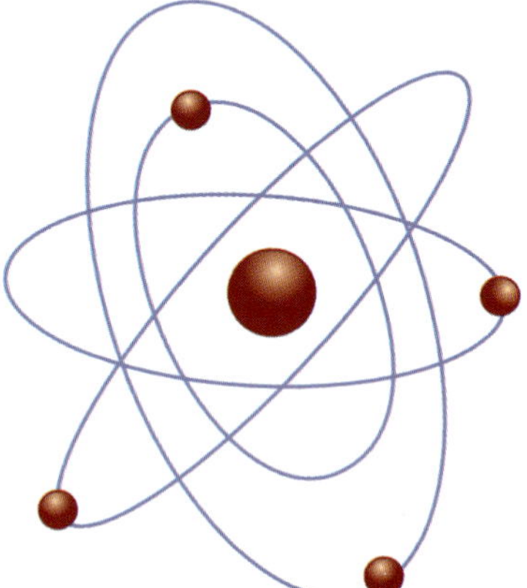

Fig. 1: Illustration of an atom with a nucleus and orbiting electrons.

A simple way to understand light emission is by examining an atom and its surrounding electrons **(Fig. 1)**. These electrons occupy specific orbits, which shift to higher levels when they absorb energy **(Fig. 2)**. When the laser medium is activated, the electrons move to higher energy orbits. In the case of a CO_2 laser, this activation is achieved by using an electrical wall current to energise the gas particles. The displaced electrons quickly return to their original orbits, releasing energy in the form of a photon during the process **(Fig. 3)**.

In a laser, these photons can stimulate an already excited atom along their path to emit an identical photon. This newly released photon is in phase (coherent), has the same wavelength and colour (monochromatic) and travels in the same direction without spreading out (collimated).

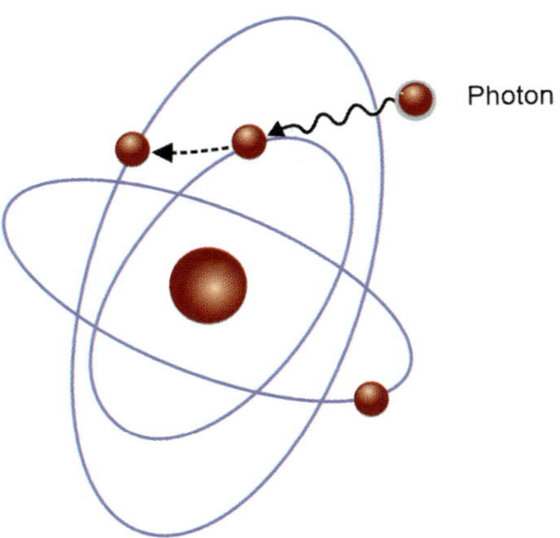

Fig. 2: Stimulated absorption occurs as a photon impacts an electron, driving it into a higher orbit.

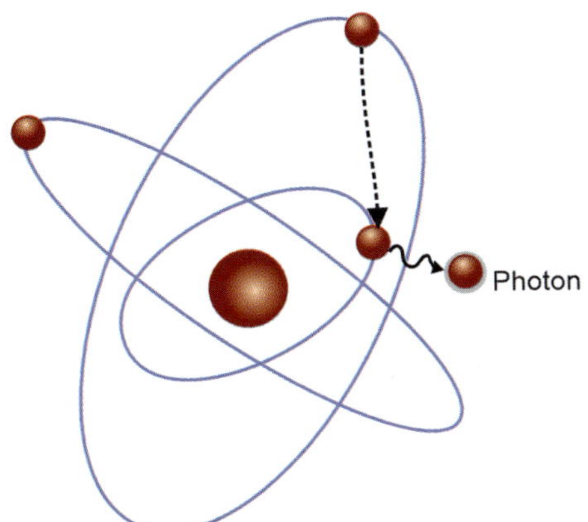

Spontaneous emission
$\Delta E = hf$
ΔE = *difference in energy between 2 orbits.*
η= *Planck's constant* 6.625×10^{-34} *Joule/sec.*
f= *frequency*

Fig. 3: Slow, natural decay causes an electron to drop into a lower orbit, resulting in a photon being emitted at a predicted frequency equal to the difference in energy between the two orbits.

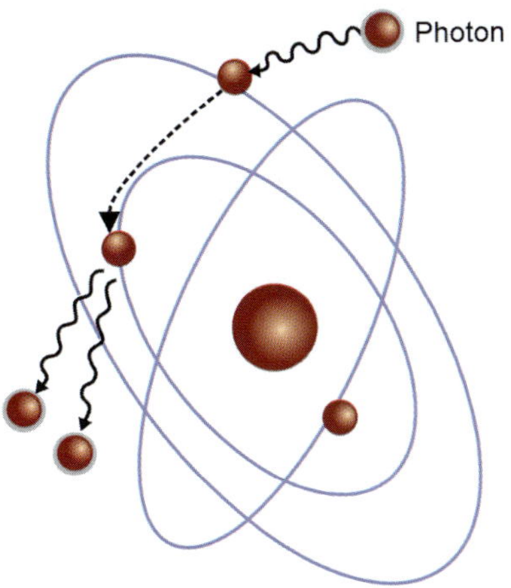

Fig. 4: The natural 'slow' decay process may be stimulated by collisional processes, resulting in many photons traveling at the same frequency as the inducing photons.

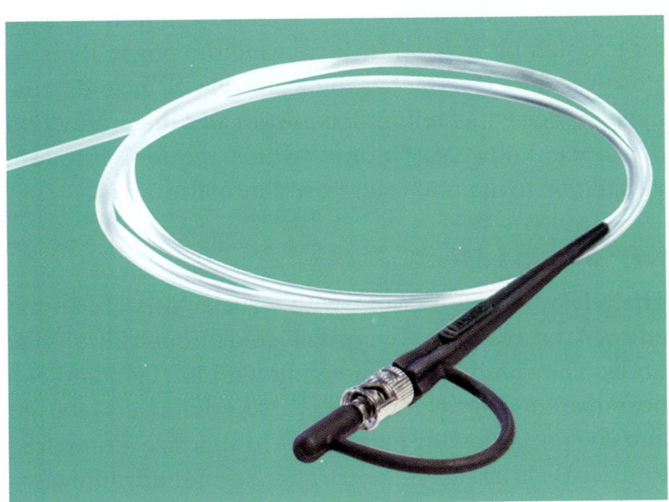

Fig. 5: Flexible fibres used for laser surgeries.

This phenomenon is known as stimulated emission **(Fig. 4)**.

Different lasers produce different colours of light. The argon laser emits a wavelength of 510 nm, resulting in blue-green light. The KTP laser produces a wavelength of 532 nm, giving off a green colour. In contrast, the CO_2 laser generates a wavelength of 10,800 nm, which falls within the nonvisible part of the electromagnetic spectrum. Therefore, a helium-neon laser, which emits red light, is used alongside it to indicate the location of the CO_2 beam. The laser beam initially exits the port as an unfocused beam, and a lens system is used to focus it to a specific point. Fine focusing can be done through a joystick or automatically with a coupler. Also, with the use of wave guides, one eliminates the problem of intermittent focusing of the beam that is associated with the joystick device. In contrast to the CO_2 laser, which is transmitted through long tubes and is reflected by mirrors, the argon, KTP, Nd:YAG and diode lasers are transmitted via a fibre **(Fig. 5)**.

TYPES OF LASERS

Table 1 highlights the various types of lasers used for gynaecology.

TABLE 1: Types of lasers used in gynaecology.

Type	*Wavelength (nm)*	*Colour*	*Fibre*	*Depth of penetration*
Argon	488–512	Blue-green	Yes	0.5 mm
KTP/532	532	Green	Yes	1–2 mm
Nd:YAG	1,064	Infrared	Yes	3–4 mm
CO_2	10,600	Infrared	No	0.1 mm

(Nd:YAG: neodymium yttrium aluminium garnet; KTP: potassium-titanyl-phosphate)

CO_2 Laser

Among the various lasers available, the CO_2 laser is the most versatile and extremely safe due to its shallow penetration depth (0.1–0.5 mm) and minimal lateral thermal damage (0.5 mm). This makes it suitable for use in delicate areas where cautery would be risky, such as the bladder, the lateral side wall near the ureter and the bowel serosa. In addition to vaporisation, the CO_2 laser can also be used for excision or incision by increasing the power density. However, the CO_2 laser has some drawbacks, including the need to focus the helium-neon beam and the production of smoke, known as 'plume,' which requires frequent evacuation to maintain clear visibility of the target.

KTP-argon Lasers

The KTP and argon lasers, with wavelengths of 532 nm and 514 nm, respectively, are delivered through fibre-optic fibres. They produce an intense green-blue light and can be transmitted through fibres of varying diameters (400 μm and 600 μm), allowing for changes in spot size. Compared to the CO_2 laser, these lasers offer several advantages—selective absorption by haemoglobin, reduced plume production and a convenient delivery system that operates at lower power settings, typically in the range of 5–10 W. However, a significant drawback is the requirement to wear special glasses, which can distort the view of the pelvis and make it challenging to see small endometriosis implants.

Nd:YAG Laser

Neodymium yttrium aluminium garnet lasers emit an invisible beam with a wavelength of 1,064 nm, which, like the CO_2 beam, must be guided using a helium-neon spot. The Nd:YAG beam is readily absorbed by tissue, with a deep penetration of 3–4 mm. Its energy is poorly absorbed by fluids, making it an ideal tool for hysteroscopic surgery. Additionally, the Nd:YAG beam can be transmitted through an operating hysteroscope. There are two delivery methods for the Nd:YAG laser—the bare quartz fibre and the quartz fibre equipped with a sapphire contact tip.

LASER SAFETY

Laser surgery in gynaecology has been practiced for 20 years with a strong safety record. However, like any surgical device, lasers carry the potential for serious injury. Gynaecologists seeking laser privileges must be certified for the specific laser type they plan to use. Certification requires attending didactic instruction and gaining practical experience with the laser in a laboratory setting before using it on patients. When operating the laser, a warning sign such as 'Laser in Use' should be posted on all operating room doors. Surgeons and operating room staff should always wear protective safety glasses appropriate for the laser in use. The laser should be kept in stand-by mode whenever it is not being actively fired. Surgical drapes near the operating field should be fire-retardant and, if possible, kept wet. Adequate suction must be available to remove any plume produced by the laser, as intact viral DNA and papillomavirus have been detected in the plume. Understanding the specific tissue interactions of various laser wavelengths is crucial to prevent unintended trauma.

EXTRAPERITONEAL LASER SURGERY

Cervix–Cervical Intraepithelial Neoplasia

Treatment for cervical intraepithelial neoplasia (CIN) can be carried out through vaporisation or excisional conisation using a laser instead of a scalpel, with the carbon dioxide (CO_2) laser being the preferred choice.

The CO_2 laser offers several benefits:

- High degree of clinical efficacy
- Bloodless field
- Microscopic precision
- Sparing of normal tissue
- Rapid healing with minimal scar formation
- Small number of complications
- Outpatient methodology

The main disadvantages of the CO_2 laser include the absence of a histologic sample when vaporisation is performed and the expense of the laser machine.

Condyloma Acuminata

The primary use of CO_2 laser surgery in the lower genital tract is for treating condyloma acuminata. Warts should

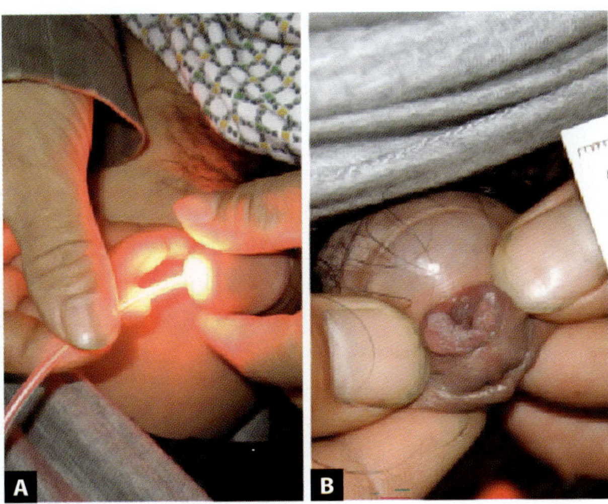

Figs. 6A and B: Laser treatment for urethral condyloma accuminata.

be vaporised to a depth no greater than the level of the surrounding skin **(Figs. 6A and B)**, using a power setting of 40–60 W and a beam diameter of 3 mm. Once the genital warts are fully vaporised, the area around each lesion, about 1-2 cm in diameter, should be treated with a 10 W power setting and a 2-mm diameter spot size. This additional treatment helps destroy subclinical HPV infection and reduces the likelihood of recurrence.

CLINICAL APPLICATIONS OF LASERS IN INTRA-ABDOMINAL GYNAECOLOGICAL SURGERY

Endometriosis

Endometriosis lesions can be treated with the CO_2 laser either by vaporisation or excision, depending on how deep the lesions penetrate. For superficial endometriosis in areas such as the cul-de-sac, uterosacral ligaments or the peritoneum, a wattage of 10–20 W with a 1-mm spot size is typically used for vaporisation. The CO_2 laser is the preferred choice for managing endometriosis from American Fertility Society (AFS) stage I to IV due to its excellent safety profile. Its limited peripheral tissue damage and shallow penetration make it especially suitable for excising adhesions close to sensitive structures, such as the ureters and bowel.

Adhesiolysis

Pelvic adhesions frequently result from prior pelvic infections and surgeries. While adhesiolysis is typically done using scissors or electrosurgery, lasers offer a valuable alternative. Lasers are particularly effective for lysis of vascular adhesions, because they allow for simultaneous excision and coagulation, while minimising damage to surrounding tissue. To prevent harm to adjacent normal tissue, the use of quartz rods, rods with backstops and irrigation is advised.

Ectopic Pregnancy

In the laparoscopic treatment of ectopic pregnancy, the CO_2 laser provides an alternative to electrosurgery and scissors. A linear incision is created on the antimesenteric side of the tube over the swollen area of the ectopic pregnancy using 30 W of energy with a precisely focused beam. To minimise intraoperative bleeding, a dilute solution of vasopressin can be injected into the mesosalpinx beneath the ectopic tissue and onto the serosa covering the ectopic pregnancy.

Uterine Fibroids

Laser energy can be applied through a handpiece during laparotomies or via a laparoscope. Small fibroids can be directly vaporised using 20–30 W of energy or completely removed, similar to conventional surgery. The CO_2 laser offers several benefits for fibroid removal compared to scissors and traditional electrosurgery, including better haemostasis, reduced tissue trauma and a lower risk of adhesion formation. Approximately 50–60% of patients who undergo laser myomectomy ultimately achieve pregnancy.

Ovarian Wedge Resection

Ovarian wedge resection via laparotomy, once a common treatment for patients unresponsive to clomiphene citrate, is now infrequently performed due to severe postoperative adhesion formation. However, with meticulous microsurgical techniques and the use of fine electrocautery needles or lasers, ovarian wedge resection can achieve pregnancy rates of 40%, likely due to reduced adhesion formation. In this procedure, each ovary may be cauterised with a unipolar needle electrode or treated with laser energy in multiple areas, creating small ovarian craters **(Fig. 7)**. Lasers such as CO_2, KTP, argon and Nd:YAG have been employed for treating polycystic ovaries, resulting in ovulation rates of 70% and pregnancy rates of 40%.

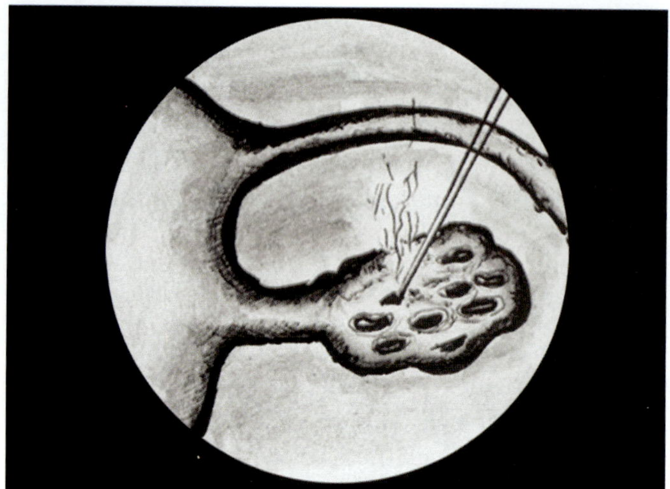

Fig. 7: Ovarian wedge craters produced by CO_2 laser.

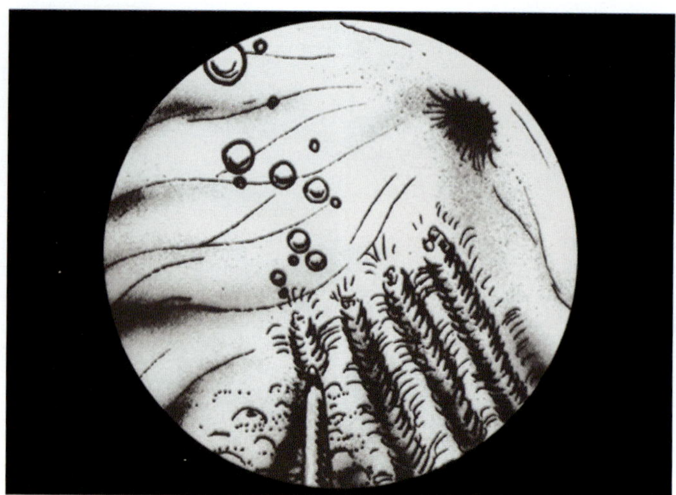

Fig. 8: Endometrial ablation with Nd:YAG laser fibre.

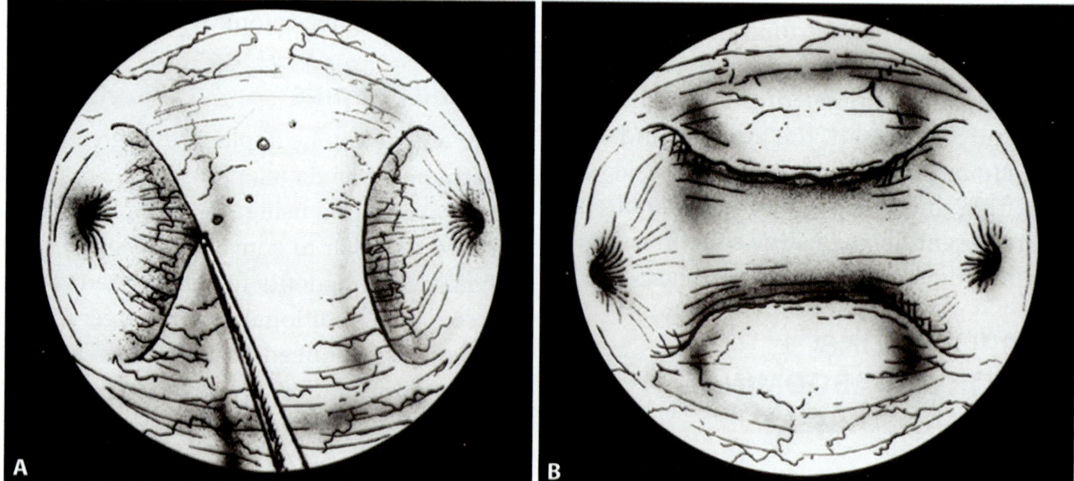

Figs. 9A and B: Uterine septum treated with Nd:YAG laser.

Endometrial Ablation

Endometrial ablation aims to destroy the entire endometrium to prevent its regeneration and eliminate menstrual bleeding. Patients are typically pretreated with a gonadotrophin-releasing hormone (GnRH) agonist or danazol for 4 weeks to thin the endometrial lining to a menopausal level, which helps the energy penetrate to the myometrium effectively.

Once the uterine cavity is adequately visualised, the laser fibre can be introduced through the hysteroscope's operating channel **(Fig. 8)**. The Nd:YAG laser fibre can be utilised using either a touch or no-touch technique.

Septate Uterus

Resection of a uterine septum can be carried out using various tools, including scissors, a resectoscope or an Nd:YAG laser. This procedure is typically performed with operative hysteroscopy and laparoscopy, allowing for a more consistent depth of incision across the septum and providing a warning if perforation is approaching. The Nd:YAG laser fibre is generally set to 40 W and applied using the touch technique, similar to a scalpel **(Figs. 9A and B)**. The laser incision is continued until uniform light transmission is observed throughout the fundus via laparoscopy, or until bleeding from the fundal myometrium is seen. The main advantage of using the laser fibre over scissors is reduced bleeding.

OTHER CLINICAL APPLICATIONS OF LASERS IN GYNAECOLOGY AND REPRODUCTIVE MEDICINE

- Genitourinary syndrome of menopause (GSM) is a chronic condition affecting approximately 40–60% of postmenopausal women. The first-line treatment is low-dose vaginal oestrogens. Intravaginal laser has potential when vaginal oestrogens are contraindicated or ineffective and for women who decline hormones. The safety of vaginal fractional CO_2 laser therapy has been proved in several randomised controlled trials (RCTs).
- Laser treatment for stress urinary incontinence (SUI) employs fractional CO_2 or Erbium:YAG lasers to induce controlled thermal microablation of the vaginal mucosa and submucosal tissues, promoting neocollagenesis and neoelastogenesis. This process results in the remodelling and fortification of the pelvic floor structures, enhancing the support of the urethrovesical junction and bladder neck, thereby mitigating urethral hypermobility and reducing the incidence of involuntary detrusor contractions.
- *Laser-assisted hatching:* Hatching of a blastocyst is a crucial step in the process leading up to implantation **(Figs. 10A to C)**. If hatching fails due to intrinsic abnormalities in the blastocyst or the zona pellucida (ZP), it can limit reproductive success. Assisted hatching (AH) involves artificially thinning or creating an opening in the ZP and is proposed as a method to enhance implantation and increase pregnancy rates following in vitro fertilisation (IVF).
  - Indications of assisted hatching:
    - *Age:* Woman is older than 37 years
    - Woman with poor ovarian reserve
    - Women with poor-quality embryos
    - Cases with thick zona pellucida
    - Previous failed IVF cycles

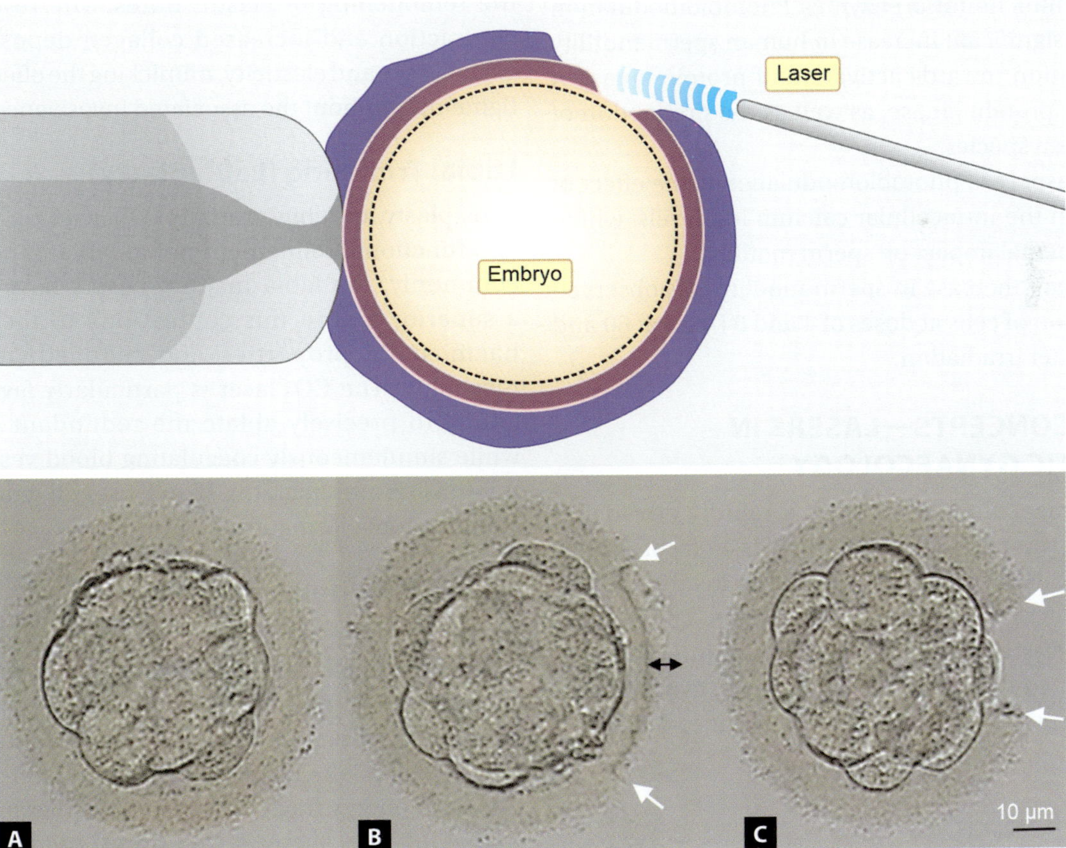

Figs. 10A to C: Laser-assisted embryo hatching.

- Complications of laser hatching:
  - Damage to the embryo
  - Damage to individual blastomeres with reduction of embryo viability
  - Monozygotic twinning
- *Laser acupuncture in female infertility:* Laser acupuncture activates the inferior parietal lobule, the primary somatosensory cortex, the precuneus of the parietal lobe and the medial and superior frontal gyri of the frontal lobe, which are associated with mood changes.

  Studies show the use of laser and needle acupunctures in ameliorating emotional distress in women undergoing infertility treatments. This intervention before and after embryo transfer has resulted in higher implantation rates and live birth rates.
- *Lasers in male infertility (low-level laser therapy):* Phototherapy with a low-level laser is referred to as photobiomodulation. This process would subsequently augment the sperm motility.

On the molecular level, the *low-level laser therapy* (LLLT) is mediated in the upregulation of genes coding for a number of mitochondrial enzymes. Photobiomodulation resulted in a significant increase in human sperm motility and capacitation towards activation of protein kinase A and sarcoma protein kinase, as well as the production of reactive oxygen species.

Another aspect of photobiomodulation is the effect of irradiation on the intracellular calcium ion levels, which has a fundamental impact on sperm motility.

A significant increase in sperm motility was observed with irradiation of cells at doses of 4 and 6 J/cm^2 at 60 and 45 minutes after irradiation.

NOVEL CONCEPTS—LASERS IN COSMETIC GYNAECOLOGY

Cosmetic gynaecology represents a rapidly advancing subspecialty, wherein the integration of laser technologies has significantly enhanced both the aesthetic and functional outcomes of various procedures. The precise, minimally invasive nature of laser-based interventions has transformed the landscape of cosmetic gynaecology, offering patients superior results with reduced morbidity and shorter recovery periods.

Vaginal Rejuvenation

Vaginal rejuvenation, an umbrella term encompassing a spectrum of procedures aimed at enhancing vaginal tightness, improving sexual function and ameliorating vaginal health, has been revolutionised by the advent of laser technology. The primary modalities employed are fractional CO_2 lasers and erbium lasers. These lasers induce controlled thermal injury to the vaginal mucosa and submucosa, leading to neocollagenesis and the remodelling of elastin fibres. The resultant tissue contraction and increased collagen deposition restore vaginal tone and elasticity, mimicking the effects of surgical tightening without the associated invasiveness **(Fig. 11)**.

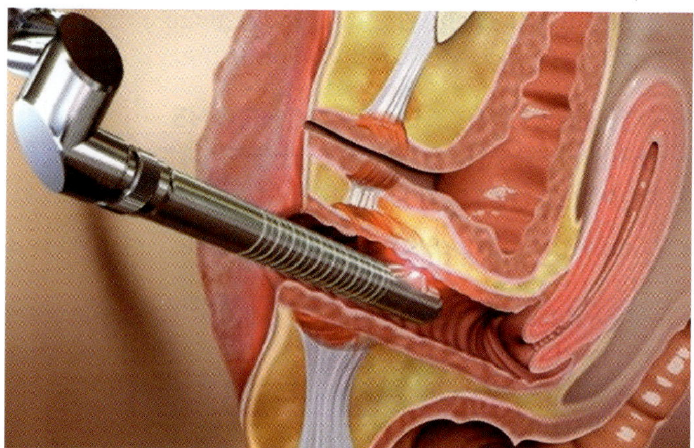

Fig. 11: Vaginal rejuvenation.

Labial Trimming (Labiaplasty)

Labiaplasty, or labial trimming, focuses on the aesthetic and functional refinement of the labia minora and, less commonly, the labia majora. Lasers have emerged as a superior tool in this context due to their precision, haemostatic properties and reduced postoperative morbidity. The CO_2 laser is particularly favoured for its ability to precisely ablate the redundant labial tissue while simultaneously coagulating blood vessels, thereby minimising intraoperative blood loss and reducing the risk of haematoma formation.

Vulvar Melanosis Treatment

Vulvar melanosis, characterised by benign hyperpigmented macules on the vulvar skin, often presents a cosmetic concern despite its benign nature.

These lasers specifically target melanin within the pigmented lesions, resulting in selective photothermolysis. The laser energy fragments the melanin granules without damaging the surrounding keratinocytes or dermal structures, allowing for a gradual lightening of the hyperpigmented areas.

Liposuction of the Pubic Mound (Mons Pubis)

The reduction of the mons pubis, particularly when characterised by excessive adiposity, is another area where laser-assisted techniques have gained popularity. Excess fatty tissue in this region can lead to discomfort, altered body image and difficulty with clothing fit. Traditional liposuction techniques, while effective, often result in significant tissue trauma and prolonged recovery.

SUGGESTED READING

1. Athanasiou S, Pitsouni E, Cardozo L, Zacharakis D, Petrakis E, Loutradis D, et al. Can pelvic organ prolapse in postmenopausal women be treated with laser therapy? Climacteric. 2021;24:101-6.
2. Borhani S, Salman Yazdi R. Clinical applications of low-level laser therapy in reproductive medicine: a literature review. Arch Reprod Med Sex Health. 2018;1(1): 14-21.
3. DeLeon FD, Baggish MS. Lasers in Gynecology. Glob Libr Women's Med. 2008.
4. Giarenis I, Tsiapakidou S, Zacche M, Mukhopadhyay S, Mahmood T. European Board and College of Obstetrics and Gynaecology (EBCOG) position statement on the use of laser vaginal devices for treatment of genitourinary syndrome of menopause, vaginal laxity, pelvic organ prolapse and stress urinary incontinence. Eur J Obstet Gynecol Reprod Biol. 2024;299:342-4.
5. Güneş A, Alinsod RM. A mini-review of aesthetic gynecology and leading gynecology associations' approaches to this issue. Turk J Obstet Gynecol. 2018;15(2):105-11.
6. Karu TI. Lasers in infertility treatment: irradiation of oocytes and spermatozoa. Photomed Laser Surg. 2012; 30(5):239-41.
7. Li FG, Maheux-Lacroix S, Deans R, Nesbitt-Hawes E, Budden A, Nguyen K, et al. Effect of fractional carbon dioxide laser vs sham treatment on symptom severity in women with postmenopausal vaginal symptoms: a randomized clinical trial. JAMA. 2021;326(14):1381-9.
8. O'Reilly BA, Viereck V, Phillips C, Toozs-Hobson P, Kuhn A, Athanasiou S, et al. Vaginal erbium laser treatment for stress urinary incontinence: a multicenter randomised sham-controlled clinical trial. Int J Gynaecol Obstet 2024;164(3):1184-94.
9. Ogrinc UB, Sencar S. Non-ablative vaginal erbium YAG laser for the treatment of cystocele. Ital J Gynaecol Obstet. 2017;29:19-25.
10. Page AS, Verbakel JY, Verhaeghe J, Latul YP, Housmans S, Deprest J. Laser versus sham for genitourinary syndrome of menopause: a randomised controlled trial. BJOG. 2023;130(3):312-9.
11. Practice Committee of the American Society for Reproductive Medicine. The role of assisted hatching in in vitro fertilization: a guideline. Fertil Steril. 2022;117(6): 1177-82.
12. Ruanphoo P, Bunyavejchevin S. Treatment for vaginal atrophy using microablative fractional CO2 laser: a randomized double-blinded sham-controlled trial. Menopause. 2020;27(8):858-63.

65

CHAPTER

Genetics in Gynaecology

Krupa Hitesh Shah, Muralidhar V Pai

Chapter Outline

- Genetics of Gynaecological Cancers
- Genetics of Common Benign Condition
- Genetic Testing
- Genetic Counselling

INTRODUCTION

It is all in deoxyribonucleic acid (DNA). The genotype, DNA of all genes, influences distinctive traits such as physical attributes (appearance, height, weight, eye and hair colour, etc.), susceptibility to diseases and response to a drug. Alteration or variation in genetic constitution explains the disease or other health effects. With the advances in genetics and technology, scientists are now capable of studying all genes. A similar effort of scientists created a project, named the Human Genome Project (HGP), has sequenced and mapped all the genes (human genotype) after international research collaboration.

In gynaecology, genetics also plays a pivotal role and it influences a woman's overall health and well-being. The key benign conditions wherein genetic component can be identified as a strong component are polycystic ovary syndrome (PCOS), endometriosis and fibroids. Genetic tests are valuable even for fertility management. It has a critical role in the genesis of hereditary cancers. It has improved our understanding of various gynaecological conditions and their treatment by providing personalised medicine.

There are currently over 7,000 genetic tests available for human conditions worldwide, which empowers the assessment of patients' risks for the acquisition of diseases and diagnose genetic conditions. Genetic testing is fundamental in oncology services including primary cancer prevention and treatment. Even medical treatments can be tailored to more effectively according to an individual's unique genetic code.

GENETICS OF GYNAECOLOGICAL CANCERS

Gynaecological cancers arise due to genetic mutation as one of the key aetiological factors. It may occur sporadically or have inherited susceptibility. Cervical, uterine and ovarian cancers are found in descending manner in the developing world. The very common cervical cancer is usually triggered by human papillomavirus (HPV) infection, resulting in somatic mutation. Germline mutation occurs in approximately 5% of all uterine cancers and 20% of all ovarian cancers. Here, cancer-causing genes are present in gametes; hence, mutation passes on from generation to generation, resulting in familial segregation. Gynaecological tumours can be a part of a genetic syndrome also. Genetics has a significant role in genesis, hence screening, diagnosis and management of cancer.

Genetic Basis of Cancer

Unregulated, uncontrolled proliferation of cells is a basic pathology of any neoplasm; it is the invasive propensity of the cell, which generates cancer (otherwise it is benign). Based on Knudson's hypothesis, two mutations are required within the genome of a cell to develop into cancer. In hereditary cancer, one among the two genomes of a gamete has already one mutation, and that is passed in every cell, hence, only one hit in the form of mutation is needed to damage the second gene allele within the genome of the cell and to disrupt cell cycle at any time in life. In sporadic cases, the cell must have both hits in the allele of single somatic cell for a neoplasm to develop. **Flowchart 1** explains normal homeostasis for cell division.

Proto-oncogenes are normal cellular genes for the growth and survival of cells. Gain-of-function mutation leads to the formation of oncogenes that stimulate the growth of cells and inhibit apoptosis, facilitating malignant transformation of cells. Thus, there are two main types of driver gene (mutation-containing gene), an activated oncogene and an inactivated tumour suppressor

Flowchart 1: Normal homeostasis for cell division.

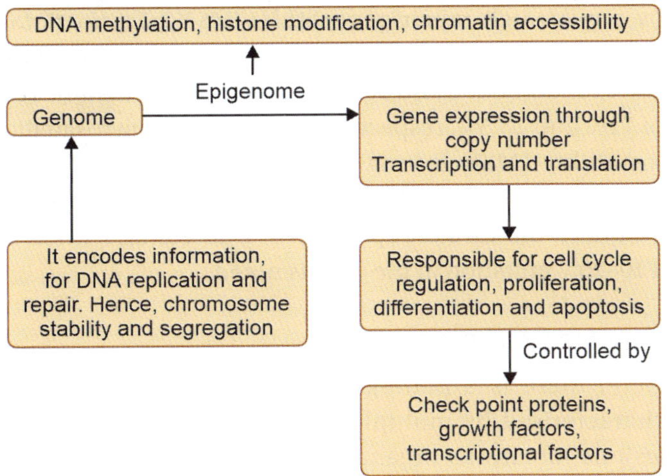

Flowchart 2: Cancer transformation.

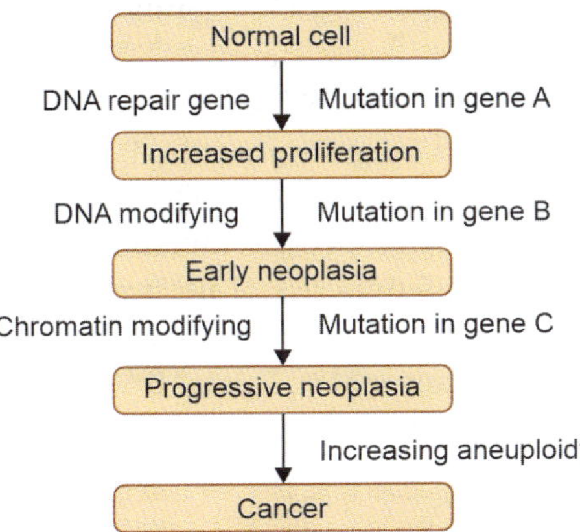

gene (TSG). A loss of function mutation or epi-genomic silencing in a TSG leads to disturbed regulatory control or aberrant gene mutation. **Flowchart 2** explains cancer transformation.

The other two types are familial and sporadic cancers. Sporadic ones are responsible for 75–85% of cancers. Familial cancer contributes to nearly 10–20%; herein, low-to-moderate-risk genes with shared environment and lifestyle also contribute. 5–10% are hereditary cancers, wherein high-risk genes are responsible for cancer.

Family History and Gynaecological Cancers

Many times, women present with a family history of different cancers such as ovarian, breast cancer, endometrial and bowel cancer. The family history and pedigree analysis help in cancer inheritance assessment.

Flowchart 3: Family history-driven testing and case-driven testing.

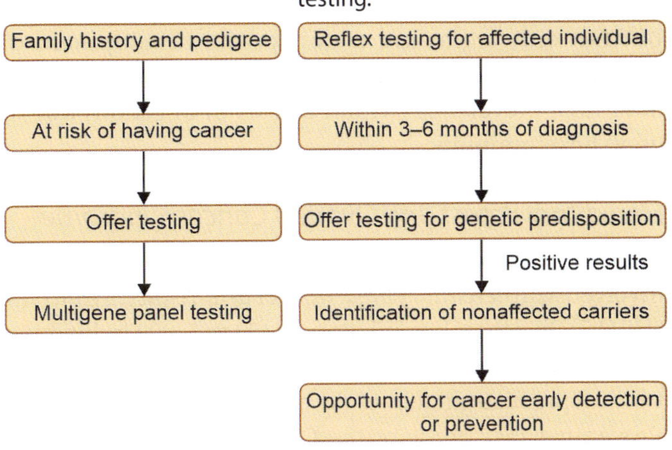

It illustrates the mode of inheritance when a three-generation pedigree analysis is noted down. Identification of families at risk requires workup to find carrier status.

Another way to identify families at risk is through reflex testing. If a woman is diagnosed with cancer, reflex testing for the diagnosis of germline or somatic mutation is done. Which is generally advised between 3 and 6 months of diagnosis of cancer. Family history-driven testing and case-driven testing increase chances of detection of predisposition genes **(Flowchart 3)**. Once that is identified, unaffected members of the family are offered the test after appropriate counselling.

Only one third of the cancers are familial; hence, other strategies for early detection of sporadic cancers or precancer conditions are still needed.

Sporadic Somatic Mutation in Cervical Malignancy

Cervical malignancy is multifactorial, but somatic mutation of the host genome by HPV is the key event. HPV is a nonenveloped, eight-gene containing double-stranded DNA virus, contained in a protein capsid. There are over 150 types of HPV identified, which cause almost all cases of cervical cancer and also oropharyngeal cancer, vulval, vaginal, penile and cancer of anal canal. High-risk HPV (HR-HPV) types, which include types 16, 18, 31, 33, 35, etc., are responsible for >70% of cervical cancers. They can integrate their DNA into the host genome, leading to unscheduled re-entry into the cell cycle, hence, unregulated cell proliferation, which is a key factor for cancer development. HPV E6/E7 oncoproteins induce not only host cell proliferation but also invasion, metastasis through their effect on tumour-related signalling pathway.

Low-risk HPV (LR-HPV) types are generally not cancer-causing types. Infection with HPV is an essential, but not only sufficient, factor for the development of cervical cancer. Many HPV lesions regress spontaneously after high prevalence (within 2 years of infection) due to good host immunity.

Hereditary Breast and Ovarian Cancer Syndrome

Mainly, breast cancer-associated (*BRCA*) genes 1 and 2 are involved with *hereditary breast and ovarian cancer syndrome* (HBOC). In general population, 1/400 to 1/800 individuals bear the *BRCA* gene; in the Ashkenazi population, it is 1/40. Clinical practice guidelines developed by the United States Preventive Task Force or the Center for Disease Control and Prevention for BRCA testing can be referred. Many national guidelines are available worldwide. Evaluation by genetic test is generally done for premenopausal breast cancer (BC), triple negative BC, bilateral BC, ovarian cancer, male BC, postmenopausal BC, with additional relatives with BC, and in women with known hereditary susceptibility syndromes. Online Manchester scoring systems, BOADICEA and BRCAPRO, are available, which can be used to calculate the probability of cancer. Mutation testing is recommended at a ≥10% probability.

About 15–20% of patients with ovarian cancers are *BRCA* 1/2 carriers. This increases the risk of ovarian cancers by 40% in *BRCA* 1 and 20% in *BRCA2* carriers in their life span. Estimates of the lifetime risk of *BRCA* 1/2 mutation carriers for breast carcinoma are 40–80%. Other genes in the homologous recombination pathway are *RAD51C, RAD51D, BRIP1, PALB2 and BARD1*, which influence HBOC. Genetic counselling and testing are recommended to affected and unaffected woman. A population-based approach to genetic testing identifies 50% more carriers at risk, which has been extensively investigated in the Ashkenazi Jewish population. High-risk women should have genetic counselling and testing.

Lynch Syndrome

It is recognised by familial clustering of cancer such as colorectal cancer, pancreatic, uterine, endometrial and urothelial malignancies in multiple generations. Nearly 5% of women with a diagnosis of uterine cancer carry a hereditary gene mutation, and 2–3% of women with endometrial cancer have Lynch syndrome. Carriers are at risk for cancer development, have early onset cancers, have multiple organ systems involvement or have increased risk for second primary cancer. It is caused by a mismatch repair gene *MLH1/MSH2/MSH6/PMS2* mutation. Women with these mutations have an increased risk of endometrial and ovarian cancers with a lifetime risk of 71% and 13.5%, respectively. Molecular [microsatellite instability (MSI) testing] analysis of tumour tissue is done here. *BRCA1/BRCA2* testing is recommended for all nonmucinous invasive epithelial ovarian cancers, wherein a 10–20% mutation in the gene is noted.

Cowden Syndrome

Here, there is a pathogenic mutation of PTEN. It is characterised by multiple hamartomas and cancerous lesions in various organs such as endometrial, breast, brain, thyroid, skin, mucous membrane, etc. Lifetime risk of BC is 25–50%. The risk of endometrial cancer is 30%. It is inherited as autosomal dominant pattern.

Peutz–Jeghers Syndrome

It is characterised by gastrointestinal polyps, mucocutaneous pigmentation, gastrointestinal (GI), breast and nonepithelial ovarian cancers. A mutation in *STK11/LKB1* gene produces a lifetime risk of BC from 8 to 45%, even cervical cancer is associated with it, with a lifetime risk of 10% and ovarian cancer 21%. This is HPV-negative variant; hence, conventional cytology is recommended. It is also an autosomal dominant condition.

Li-Fraumeni Syndrome

Li-Fraumeni syndrome is a rare hereditary cancer syndrome (HCS) associated with TP53 mutation. It is associated with a wide range of tumours; premenopausal BC is a part of the spectrum. This is also an autosomal recessive condition.

Table 1 narrates the above-mentioned conditions with the driver gene, resulting in malignancies and pathways.

GENETICS OF COMMON BENIGN CONDITION

Forty percent of fibroids bear some chromosomal abnormalities. Most common aberrations are of 6, 7, 12 and 14 numbered chromosomes. It is the Fumarate hydratase gene, which causes autosomal dominant syndromes, and fibroids are one of the components. Endometriosis is found to have a genetic aetiology, as it is found in close relatives, hence, disease clustering is seen in the population. It has

TABLE 1: Malignancies with driver genes and pathways.

Common	*Driver gene*	*Driver mutation*	*Pathways*
Hereditary breast ovarian cancer	*BRCA1* (Ch: 17) *BRCA2* (Ch: 13) *PAD51C, RAD51D, BRIP1* and *PALB2*	• 40% risk of ovarian carcinoma • 20% risk of ovarian carcinoma	Homologous recombination
Lynch syndrome	*MLH1, MSH2, MSSH6* and *PMS2*	• 60% risk for endometrial carcinoma • 20% ovarian carcinoma	DNA mismatch repair gene/loss of expression
Cowden syndrome	*PTEN, SDHB-D, Killin*	Endometrial carcinoma	Autosomal dominant, TSG
Peutz–Jeghers syndrome	*LKB1/STK11*	• Cervical adenocarcinoma (10%) • Ovarian carcinoma (20%)	Autosomal dominant, germline mutation
Li-Fraumeni syndrome	*P53*	Ovarian adenocarcinoma	Germline mutation

(TSG: tumour suppressor genes)

a polygenetic and multifactorial aetiology. Many gene variants are found to be associated with increased risk of endometriosis; however, the candidate gene is still being investigated. Linkage study, genome-wide association and single-nucleotide polymorphism (SNP) as a genetic marker, and a few epigenetic events are associated with it.

Follicular-stimulating Hormone Receptor Gene Polymorphism

Follicle-stimulating hormone (FSH) is essential for normal reproductive functions in both genders. It stimulates follicle to produce mature ovum in females and sperms in male. Thus, it has an impact on ovarian steroidogenesis and on the menstrual cycle. Any abnormality in the FSH receptor gene would make reproductive disturbances. Loss of function (inactivating) mutation in the follicular-stimulating hormone receptor (FSHR) gene leads to gonadal dysgenesis, amenorrhoea (primary or secondary), subfertility and premature ovarian failure. Gain-of-function (activating) mutation leads to ovarian hyperstimulation syndrome with exogenous FSH administration. FSH receptor is located at chromosome 2p. A homozygous missense mutation in the FSH receptor (identified genes are over 10, such as BMP15 and SPIDR) is responsible for ovarian dysgenesis.

Various SNPs at the FSHR coding region are studied, wherein Thr 307Ala and Asn680 Ser are the most common. They are located on the exome 10 of the FSHR gene. Polymorphisms and alternatively spliced variants are associated with poor ovarian response or hyperovarian response. Moreover, FSHR polymorphism is associated with gonadal cancer and benign conditions like 1° or 2° amenorrhoea, premature ovarian failure and polycystic ovarian condition. Premature ovarian aging occurs due to *FMR1* gene mutations.

Congenital Adrenal Hyperplasia

Congenital adrenal hyperplasia (CAH) is an inherited metabolic disorder caused by a deficiency of enzymes of cortisol biosynthesis. It has both clinical and genetic heterogeneity, generally passed on as an autosomal recessive disorder. The phenotypic heterogeneity depends on the underlying enzymatic defect. About 95% of cases are due to 21-hydroxylase gene impairment, wherein the gene is located on 6p21.33, namely *CYP21A2*, *CYP11B1*, etc. It is classified as: (1) Classic salt wasting, (2) simple virilising and (3) nonclassic CAH. The last group is most found. The genes are well characterised, and mutation analysis is also widely available, which is challenging due to complex rearrangements. Diagnosis is by 17-OH progesterone measurement. Genotyping helps in confirming the diagnosis, provides information on disease severity, identification of carrier status and genetic counselling.

Genetics of Human Hypogonadotropic Hypogonadism

Hypogonadotropic hypogonadism (HH) is characterised by irreversible pubertal delay, reproductive problems such as infertility, and low serum levels of FSH and luteinising hormone (LH). Genetically, it is largely unknown; however, 5–10% do have mutations. X-linked recessive HH is found with the KAL gene and AHC gene mutation. Autosomal recessive HH occurs due to the gonadotrophin-releasing hormone (GnRH) receptor, leptin and the leptin receptor gene mutation. Isolated deficiencies of the gonadotrophins, i.e. FSH and LH, are due to corresponding beta-subunit gene mutations. *PROP1* and *HESX* gene mutations also result in HH as one of the manifestations. There are clinical syndromes, e.g. Prader–Willi syndrome, which have features of widespread hypothalamic-pituitary dysfunction.

GENETIC TESTING

Genetic risk assessment starts with a detailed family and personal history and if testing criteria are met, then a decision for testing is taken. Informed consent is essential before any genetic test in a counselling session. If a hereditary predisposition/syndrome is identified, post-test counselling and relative testing after counselling are needed. This may help in improving quality of life. However, emotional burden, guilt sentiment and lack of desire to inform relatives are a few barriers to further testing in relatives/family.

Types of Tests

Mainly, two types of tests are available: (1) Diagnostic test and (2) predictive test. Predictive test includes screening test, presymptomatic tests and carrier testing. Testing is generally in the form of gene-specific testing, such as *BRCA* 1/2; however, multiplex testing is another option. Hereditary cancer multigene panel testing gives more robust cumulative results for high-risk women. The disadvantage is a higher rate of variances of unknown significance (VUS) and findings of delirious mutations in unexpected genes on a panel test.

The available molecular tests are based on microarray or sequencing. Multigene panels, targeted disease-specific panels and SNP-based panels are the recommended tests. Whole-exome and genome sequences provide information about the abnormality. They are examples of next-generation sequencing (NGS). Known mutations are studied by polymerase chain reaction (PCR) test, multiplex PCR, oligonucleotide hybridisation and genotypic microarray. Cytogenetic abnormalities can be identified by karyotype, fluorescence in situ hybridisation (FISH) and array comparative genomic hybridisation (CGH) again. New mutations and variants are being identified by exome and genome-wide association/sequencing.

Tumour expression and personalised medicine: The most advanced application of gene expression study is in predicting disease outcomes and treatment decisions. Personalised medicine is a kind of targeted therapy, wherein genes of tumor are taken into consideration, and matching treatment is provided. In short, it is tailoring health care to each person's unique genetic makeup.

Advantages of Testing

- Genetic testing helps in identifying genetic predispositions gene. Identifying high-risk genetic mutations allows for risk reduction strategies, for example, prophylactic surgeries or cancer surveillance at an earlier age, thus helps to prevent or detect the condition at an earlier (more treatable) stage. Early detection leads to better treatment outcomes and survival benefits.
- A personalised treatment plan based on genetic profile can optimise therapeutic interventions and hence, improve treatment efficacy and reduce adverse effects and relapses.

GENETIC COUNSELLING

Specific disease condition will decide specific screening or diagnostic test. The genetic counsellor's role is to provide as much information as possible to help make an informed choice about testing; however, one should never be pressured into having a test done.

If the patient chooses to have tests, they will help in taking informed consent, wherein risks, benefits and limitations of testing, including negative and positive results implications, are discussed. False negative results and uncertainties with unknown significant variants are discussed. They identify families at risk, analyses family history information, provide information about the condition or concern. Post-test counselling includes education on risk reduction strategies.

CONCLUSION

Since all the cancers and many diseases have a genetic aetiology, clinical history taking should be strong. Adequate personal history and three-generation family history are needed to confirm family clustering. Performing appropriate testing for a contributory or disease-causing gene, seeking specialist advice and planning for future reproductive and paediatric life are essential.

Applications of genetics and genomics are flooding into clinical medicine. The future is not so far when personal genotyping will influence many medical decisions. Even effective medical treatments with fewer side effects are anticipated with progressive understanding of genomic and molecular factors. However, certain genetic testing with unknown significance results produces some social implications. Otherwise, information provided by certain test results has legal and ethical considerations.

SUGGESTED READING

1. Amirthanayagam A, Crawford R. Genetics in gynaeoncology: Diagnostic and therapeutic implications. Obstet Gynaecol Reprod Med. 2022;32(2):1-6.
2. Comparetto C, Borruto F. The role of genetic counseling in gynecological oncology. OBM Genetics. 2019;3(4):1-45.
3. Josifova DJ. Genetics of gynaecological disorders. Best Pract Res Clin Obstet Gynaecol. 2017;42:100-13.
4. Laganà AS, Garzon S, Götte M, Viganò P, Franchi M, Ghezzi F, et al. The pathogenesis of endometriosis: molecular and cell biology insights. Int J Mol Sci. 2019;20(22):5615.
5. National Cancer Institute; National Institute of Health. Genetics of Breast and Gynecologic Cancers (PDQ®)–Health Professional Version. [online] Available from https://www.cancer.gov/types/breast/hp/breast-ovarian-genetics-pdq [Last accessed April, 2025].
6. Peshkin BN, Issac C. (2025). Genetic testing and management of individuals at risk of hereditary breast and ovarian cancer syndromes. [online] Available from https://www.uptodate.com/contents/genetic-testing-and-management-of-individuals-at-risk-of-hereditary-breast-and-ovarian-cancer-syndromes [Last accessed April, 2025].
7. Smith LP. The spectrum of genetic testing. Semin Oncol Nurs. 2019;35(1):11-21.
8. Wade KS, Estes JM, Kline RC. Genetics and the gynecologic patient. Ochsner J. 2020;20(4):446-51.

66

CHAPTER

Artificial Intelligence in Gynaecology

Sonal Panchal, Chaitanya Nagori

Chapter Outline

- How Artificial Intelligence Works?
- Artificial Intelligence Applications in Gynaecology
- Imaging
- Role of Artificial Intelligence in Benign Gynaecology
- Role of Artificial Intelligence in Gynaecological Cancers
- Role of Artificial Intelligence in Gynaecological Surgery
- Artificial Intelligence in In Vitro Fertilisation
- Embryology
- Urogynaecology
- Drug Research
- Artificial Intelligence Limitations
- Challenges

INTRODUCTION

Human intelligence was considered a superpower that could memorise and analyse tremendous amount of facts and use these for a just and logical decision making. But it has a very high chance of bias due to emotional and social factors affecting this decision making. Invention of computers brought a huge revolution in this by being able to analyse unbelievable large amount of data without biases mentioned above. This capability of it at a point of time during development got comparable with human intelligence and was named therefore as Artificial Intelligence (AI). So, basically AI is based on training the computer systems to simulate human intelligence in thinking process and decision making.

Application of AI started at a time in different fields including mechanics, electronics, engineering and brought changes in planning and execution of building bridges, making dams, making complicated machines, etc. These were chiefly by making mathematical models that can be designed on computers along with the help of human intelligence making them more accurate and flawless. This also gradually entered into the healthcare system, initially on the administration side of hospitals and healthcare organisations but then also later into the actual patient care. Use of AI on the administration side significantly improved the way patient's records were maintained, the execution of the orders that were given for the patients by medical experts and hospital management. A little later it started peeping into the actual patient care and now it has taken over the decision making in many branches of medicines and especially by crucial decision making. This was probably becoming too mechanical in taking decisions, especially because every patient, presentation of disease in every patient, and their response to treatment to different treatment protocols are different and therefore fixed protocols may not be an optimal approach. But still AI at present has become an integral part of all fields of medicine. As it infiltrated into other fields of medicine, it also did in gynaecology. AI has revolutionised the way healthcare professionals diagnose, treat and manage conditions affecting the female reproductive system. Increasing use of AI in different fields of medicine is the cause that will demand not only high investment on development of this field but will also demand trainings of the people employed in the healthcare field for successful implementation of AI.

One of the earliest examples of AI was the development of computer-aided diagnostic systems for ultrasound images in the 1970s and 1980s. These systems were designed to assist radiologists in identifying foetal anomalies and other conditions.

MYCIN was developed by a team at Stanford University led by Edward Shortliffe, and its success demonstrated the potential of AI in medical decision making. This was an AI program, which decided which antibiotic will work for a particular infection. In the 1980s, AI-based expert systems such as DXplain, developed at Massachusetts General Hospital, were used to assist in the diagnosis of diseases.

HOW ARTIFICIAL INTELLIGENCE WORKS?

A computer system based on digitalisation of data, which is designed to process the information and work like human brain, is termed artificial intelligence (AI). This intelligence system is systematised similarly in that the brain's neuron is arrayed with numerous neural nodes, which are known as neural networks.

Machine learning (ML) is a part of AI, which deals with the development of algorithms and statistical models based on huge datasets that enable computers to learn from and make predictions or decisions without being explicitly programmed to do so. ML is a subfield of AI that broadly defines the machine's capability for imitating intelligent human behaviour. Large datasets are processed with the help of computer systems, and algorithms are designed and learnt for speedy processing, which are the basis of ML and has brought a breakthrough in the medical field with computing systems **(Table 1)**.

Machine learning algorithms can be divided into three categories: Supervised learning, unsupervised learning and reinforcement learning. Supervised learning algorithms are trained on a labelled dataset, where the desired output (label) is already known. Unsupervised learning algorithms are trained on an unlabelled dataset and are used to discover patterns or relationships in the data. Reinforcement learning algorithms are trained using a trial-and-error approach, where the agent receives a reward or penalty for its actions. The goal of reinforcement learning is to learn a policy that maximises the expected reward over time.

Data mining (DM) is a technique for finding or establishing patterns in large databases by combination of AI and advanced statistics. DM finds and collects the needed data, it also searches for other factors that may influence the outcome, thus increasing the amount of available data that can be used for processing and establishing algorithms.

Analysis of the huge amount of data that needs to be done before coming to conclusions in which errors can be minimised, becomes even more intricated when there are multiple deciding factors. Such analysis is very difficult manually. Interpreting multifactorial data with mathematical systems has led to advancements in artificial neural network (ANNs) and rapid growth of AI.

These networks attain the most probable outcomes as the neurons are associated with numerous synapses that aid in transferring the data among the neurons back and forth. Assembling these manifold connections allows the computers to imitate cognitive functions of the human brain such as finding the appropriate solution to a problem and reasoning.

Deep learning (DL) is a subfield of ML that utilises neural networks with multiple layers, known as deep neural networks (DNNs), to learn from data. DNNs are inspired by the structure and function of the human brain and are capable of automatically learning high-level features from raw data, such as images, audio and text. DL has been very successful in various applications such as image and speech recognition, natural language processing and computer vision **(Table 2)**.

Application of AI includes monitoring patients, diagnosis, prognostication of disease, treatment planning and disease prevention. This is based on analysis of huge amount of data, making it evidence based and reliable.

ARTIFICIAL INTELLIGENCE APPLICATIONS IN GYNAECOLOGY

Artificial intelligence has now merged into daily practice in all fields of medicine including obstetrics and gynaecology. One of the primary areas in which AI and

TABLE 1: The three main machine learning techniques.

Supervised learning	***Unsupervised learning***	***Reinforcement learning***
Learning with a labelled training dataset	Discovering patterns in unlabelled data	Learning based on feedback or reward
Predict surgical site infection rates after caesarean section: Build a regression model by providing data on the patients' characteristics and surgical site infections to show variables that best correlate with infections	*Categorise ultrasound examination by normal or abnormal images:* Use deep learning techniques to build a model that learns different features of images to recognise different patterns	Allocate specialised medical services for various obstetric emergency patients

Source: Adapted from Seval MM, Varlı B. Current developments in artificial intelligence from obstetrics and gynecology to urogynecology. Front Med (Lausanne). 2023;10:1098205.

TABLE 2: Comparison of machine learning and deep learning.

Machine learning	***Deep learning***
A subfield of artificial intelligence	A subfield of machine learning
Considerable human intervention is needed to correct and learn	Learns by itself from experiences and prior failures
Able to learn with less data sets	Need a significant quantity of data
Shorter training time and lesser accuracy	Longer training and higher accuracy
Establishes basic, linear relationships	Generates complex, nonlinear relationships

Source: Adapted from Seval MM, Varlı B. Current developments in artificial intelligence from obstetrics and gynecology to urogynecology. Front Med (Lausanne). 2023;10:1098205.

ML are being used in obstetrics and gynaecology is in the analysis of imaging data, such as ultrasound and magnetic resonance imaging (MRI). AI algorithms can be trained to automatically identify and classify different structures in the images, such as the placenta or foetal organs, with high accuracy. By analysing large datasets of patient information and outcome, AI algorithms can identify patterns, correlations and trends within these datasets, and help to generate insights that improve understanding of gynaecologic conditions and apply into clinical practice.

Artificial intelligence algorithms can identify patterns and risk factors with a very high accuracy and is very fast in analysis. This can help to improve the prediction of gynaecological malignancies, and suggest protocols for individual cases. It helps to plan the treatment protocol based on the findings of individual patient, and this correlates and even competes with the decision making of human brain. It can be used to plan surgeries, execute these through robotics and assess prognosis. AI has proved its role in prognostication and planning of assisted reproductive technologies also.

IMAGING

Ultrasound and Magnetic Resonance Imaging

Ultrasound is one of the most important imaging modalities for patients with gynaecological complaints and infertility. It is for this reason that there is a huge data available for normal and abnormal images of the reproductive organs. This makes a strong database for the development of the AI basis. It is interesting to know that more larger the database is used for development of the AI algorithms, more accurate is the outcome/results of the AI techniques. Numerous ML techniques have been widely used for capturing distinct data pertaining to the prior scans.

When supported by AI, ultrasound becomes even more potent modality and is more easily and widely used by medical personnel.

Wu designed the artificial bee colony algorithm to process Doppler ultrasound from images that significantly improve the ultrasound images quality, by eliminating noise from the images, thus improving the clinical diagnoses.

Artificial intelligence also improves the workflow significantly. By the use of AI and the sensors, the probe selection and activation can be automatically done just by a touching the probe or the socket for that probe. As the scanning starts, AI identifies the parts and accordingly selects the preset. The images are automatically optimised when during the scanning, the operator achieves a nearly correct section. Based on the presets, the measurement callipers are automatically placed identifying the body parts. When Doppler is started, AI identifies the body part and makes relevant Doppler settings. Not only this, Doppler assistant determines the location and direction of the vessels. With the details of guidelines like International Ovarian Tumour Analysis (IOTA), International Endometrial Tumour Analysis (IETA), Morphological Uterine Sonographic Assessment (MUSA), European Society of Human Reproduction and Embryology/European Society for Gynaecological Endoscopy (ESHRE/ESGE) classification for müllerian abnormalities, fed in the system, AI assists in diagnosis of ovarian, endometrial, myometrial and müllerian abnormalities.

Magnetic resonance imaging systems are also loaded with AI, and these software help in autoalignment of body parts, and also help to decide the relevant body cuts in recommended modes (T1, T2, FatSat, etc), depending on the abnormalities identified by the AI, when these images are compared with normal images.

ROLE OF ARTIFICIAL INTELLIGENCE IN BENIGN GYNAECOLOGY

Benign gynaecology is a vast field and deals with several pathologies. Many of these have similar presentations and are difficult to diagnose in spite of wide use of imaging technologies such as ultrasound and MRI.

AI has an important role to play in pattern recognition and analysis. AI has made its place, especially in differential diagnosis of müllerian abnormalities, in fibroid mapping, endometriosis, IOTA-based differential diagnosis of adnexal lesions, etc.

Another area where AI and ML are being applied is in the management of fibroids. ML algorithms are being used to analyse imaging data and predict the growth and behaviour of fibroids, which can aid in the development of personalised treatment plans.

Development of computer-aided diagnostic systems have been used for endometriosis. These systems use ML algorithms to analyse ultrasound and MRI images of the pelvic region and identify the presence of endometrial tissue, which can be a sign of endometriosis. Not only diagnosis, AI is an important assistant for the planning and execution of the surgical management of these lesions. Robotics aid to AI. Another area where AI and ML are being used in surgery is in the development of robotic systems. These systems can be programmed to perform specific tasks, such as suturing or cutting tissue, with a high degree of precision and accuracy. For benign tumour surgeries, the application of AI and robotic systems must be evaluated against cost–benefit ratio unlike in cases of more complex or malignant cases.

ROLE OF ARTIFICIAL INTELLIGENCE IN GYNAECOLOGICAL CANCERS

Diagnosis

Gynaecological cancers are usually diagnosed late and therefore generally has poor prognosis. Correct and early diagnosis is the basis of better prognosis of these patients. This is based on the power of imaging, which is supported by AI and leads to better and timely diagnosis of malignancy also as mentioned earlier.

The conventional methods of diagnosis and grading and staging of malignancy are considered inadequate to decide management on an individualised basis. To predict invasion and correctly assess the tumour stage, a comprehensive diagnostic approach is required but should be noninvasive. One may use International Federation of Gynaecology and Obstetrics (FIGO) staging, lymphovascular space invasion (LVSI) and deep myometrial invasion (DMI) as significant prognostic factors for risk stratification.

Researchers at Brigham and Women's Hospital and Dana-Farber Cancer Institute used AI to manipulate vast volumes of microribonucleic acid (microRNA) data to build models capable of diagnosing early ovarian cancer.

In comparison to an ultrasound screening test, which detected abnormal results <5% of the time, the AI neural network could keep up with the intricate linkages between microRNA and accurately recognised nearly 100% of anomalies associated with ovarian cancer.

The third way of coming to the diagnosis and also assessing the extent and staging of high-level tumours with DMI and LVSI staging is by texture analysis and radiofrequency modelling-based MRI. The diagnostic outcome of AI system is equivalent to the most experienced radiologists.

The texture feature-based MRI used in computer-aided diagnosis (CAD) and MRI combined with AI, differentiates clinical and pathological prognosticators before treatment. For example, the myometrial invasion assessed by MRI, in a case of endometrial cancer, can be detected by AI, using DL with convolutional neural network (CNN), and thus it can assist radiologists to detect the myometrial invasion, depth of stage I endometrial carcinoma with fair reliability.

Three different AI-based approaches such as learning rate (LR), ANN and classification and regression tree (CART) are utilised for comparing the diagnostic efficiency of endometrial carcinoma among postmenopausal women with endometrial thickness of 5 mm with irregular vaginal bleeding. LR determines how far the neural network weights change within the context of optimisation while minimising the loss function. CART is a predictive model, which explains how an outcome variable's values can be predicted based on other values. DL has enhanced specificity and sensitivity, and is a useful and powerful tool for more accurate and early diagnosis of endometrial cancer. ANN can also predict which treatment will be most beneficial for each patient depending on their diagnosis.

Prognosis

Neural network models are used to estimate prognoses for patients with ovarian cancer. ANNs could predict survival with a 97% accuracy.

By the use of established patient parameters, repeating patterns and treatment algorithms, AI can forecast the outcome in these patients. This is very different from what is done during or after surgery, wherein several independent variables will interfere or play with the final decision.

The same technology can also be used for uterine sarcoma. ANN system can differentiate malignant/

diseased cervical tissue from normal based on a spectral database. Thus AI can be successfully used to diagnose carcinoma in situ (CIN) by differentiating it from normal cervical, therefore it can be used for screening preinvasive cervical lesions.

ROLE OF ARTIFICIAL INTELLIGENCE IN GYNAECOLOGICAL SURGERY

Preoperative planning is a fundamental phase in gynaecologic surgery, where accurate diagnosis, strategic planning and patient-specific simulation can significantly influence surgical outcomes. AI plays a crucial role in preoperative planning to enhance imaging diagnostics. AI and ML are being applied in image analysis in surgery. Algorithms can be used to automatically segment and identify structures in medical images, such as tumours or blood vessels. This can help surgeons plan procedures more accurately and reduce the risk of complications. By integrating AI models in traditional imaging modalities such as ultrasound, MRI and computerised tomography, more detailed anatomical and pathological information can be achieved. AI can be used both before and during surgery with better imaging information that it gives. By 3D computer reconstruction, the visual representation of the anatomy becomes more informative and makes it more useful. It has increased precision, safety and takes less time to execute tasks. Three-dimensional printing (3DP) produces images that exactly appear like the operation site and is far superior to two-dimensional (2D) printing.

Artificial intelligence improves precision and reduces operating time, thus decreasing surgical complications. AI-supported 3D printing techniques can further help minimise surgical errors. AI also helps to notify surgeons when vessels or vital organs are closely the surgical field and surgeon needs to be careful. AI may also recommend customised rehabilitation protocols, dietary adjustments and pain management strategies.

Preoperative 3D radiological images enable precise surgical planning, while adjustable augmented reality (AR) models and DL collectively optimise robotic surgery.

Artificial intelligence can process intraoperative data to predict potential complications before they arise. In gynaecologic surgery, this could mean identifying early signs of excessive bleeding, detecting subtle changes in patient vitals, or predicting the likelihood of injury to adjacent structures.

Artificial intelligence and ML are also being used to assist with postoperative care. For example, algorithms can be used to analyse patient data and predict which patients are at risk of complications, such as infection or bleeding, allowing surgeons to take preventative measures.

Artificial intelligence can predict the risk of wound dehiscence or surgical site infections based on factors such as preoperative health conditions, surgical duration and intraoperative blood loss.

In robotic-assisted surgeries, AI analyses instrument movements and complication rates and also analyses to identify techniques that maximise precision and minimise tissue damage. Apart from the accuracy of the surgical technique, AI with robotics can be efficiently used for teaching and learning surgical technique with simulators. These can be used to help individualised training for surgery on artificial human models and mannequins. Efficient algorithms can be developed with advancements in hardware capabilities, and improve data streaming and compression techniques. Moreover, as many algorithms operate as 'black boxes', it is challenging for clinicians to comprehend these. It may be difficult for expert surgeons to trust their recommendations.

Learning Surgeries/Education

Artificial intelligence-based tools can bridge the gap in surgical education as mentioned earlier by offering realistic simulations, personalised learning paths and real-time feedback. This ultimately results into better and safer treatment delivery (surgery) for patients with more precise and standardised care. Trainees can practice these procedures repeatedly, to master their skills without the pressure or risk associated with live patients. AI-based platforms can be used for customised trainings to improve specific skills or surgical techniques and can also be used to objectively evaluate trainee's decision-making and surgical proficiency. These insights can result into making of more proficient surgeons.

ARTIFICIAL INTELLIGENCE IN IN VITRO FERTILISATION

Increasing incidence of infertility has made assisted reproductive techniques very commonly used. There are lots of variables, in the indications for which in vitro fertilisation (IVF) is done, treatment protocols for ovulation induction, trigger agent, luteal support, etc. Moreover several new researches are coming up in this field every day, this being a developing field at this time. Standardisation is therefore very essential in this field, and therefore there is a high demand for AI-supported techniques and decision making in this field.

Genetic engineering is a new advancement in the field of IVF, and this has enhanced the role of AI in assisted reproductive technology. Moreover AI can also be used to estimate and predict the results for short term (single cycle) and for long term. AI-based algorithms help improve the performance and efficiency and by way of that helps sort out diagnostic challenges.

Guy and colleagues used DM and AI to create a computer model that can help clinicians in the prediction of pregnancy after IVF. All these make AI in IVF an essential component of the practice.

Artificial intelligence and ML algorithms can help identify patterns and predict outcomes that would be of ovarian reserve, predict ovulation timing and improve the efficiency and cost-effectiveness of fertility clinics. Prediction of result of IVF is a major judgement in assisted reproduction. AI when combined and integrated with omics, enhances the success rate of treatment. The quality of the sperm, oocyte and embryo and prediction of outcome of the cycle were assessed after studying and analysing demographic parameters, IVF cycle characteristics, transcriptomics, biomarkers and metabolomics by deep ML. Finally, the development of the ANN system is used for increasing objectivity and accuracy for prediction of IVF outcome.

Artificial intelligence and ML are also being used to improve the timing of embryo transfer during IVF by analysing data from patient medical histories. It has been expected that the evolution of the reproductive, simple and cheap system could be employed in the everyday practice in IVF units, particularly after the large-scale evaluation of metabolomics and transcriptomics that would reduce the cost of tests and make them obtainable in routine use.

EMBRYOLOGY

Artificial intelligence and ML algorithms can predict which embryos are most likely to result in a successful pregnancy. Another area where AI and ML have shown potential is in the optimisation of culture conditions for embryos. Manna et al. suggested to combine AI and ANNs to extract texture descriptors from oocyte or embryo images to identify the most viable oocytes and embryos with a high chance of pregnancy. The detailed study of the blastocyst structure viz. zona pellucida, trophectoderm, inner cell mass and blastocoel is done to evaluate the viability of blastocyst. This when done manually takes up a lot of effort and time. DL and semantic segmentation very efficiently does a detail study of these crucial human blastocyst components by the help of digitalisation and computer evaluations. An SSS-Net employed for the detection of blastocyst components for the analysis of embryology involves sprint convolutional block (SCB) that uses asymmetric kernel convolutions with depth-wise separable convolution.

This approach could be employed for verifying blastocysts' morphological properties for and reliably predict and plan success of the IVF procedure.

UROGYNAECOLOGY

Urinary incontinence is a common complaint in women with obstetric history. Because of macro- or microtrauma to the muscle fibres of the pelvic floor, there is decrease in the holding capacity of the pelvic floor leading to descent of the urethra, bladder, vaginal vault, uterus, or bowel. These lead to abnormalities in normal micturition, normal bowel evacuation and also at times sexual function, including prolapse vault or uterus. These all come under the urogynaecological umbrella. Regular monitoring may be required for assessment of residual bladder volume, monitoring on incontinence, maximum bladder volume, etc., and this has been now made possible by use of wearable devices like urine incontinence monitors and postvoid residual bladder volume scanners both for adults and children and could help telemedicine in urogynaecology.

To monitor patients with incontinence or over-distention, medical team at present works manually, but with AI, team may be able to access collected data remotely. Pelvic floor measurements are objective way of predicting the risk of these complaints, and this can be effectively done with 2D and 3D ultrasound and by MRI too. AI is used to do these measurements after selecting correct sections and also assists to achieve correct sections and not only prognosticate but also decide the line of treatment. Nekooeimehr et al. proposed a method for automatically monitoring and segmenting pelvic organs on dynamic MRI, followed by multiple-object trajectory classification, to aid in the understanding of pelvic organ prolapse (POP). Statistically significant associations between various radiomic markers and urodynamic findings were discovered by Keene et al. The authors concluded that CT texture analysis of the bladder wall could be a useful tool for identifying patients with high-risk urodynamic features in spina bifida and that it could be employed instead of or in addition to urodynamics in neurogenic patient populations in the future.

A more standardised urodynamic tract interpretation with least human interference was developed by

Wang et al. Detrusor overactivity (DO) has different patterns and depending on that the patients present with different symptoms and presentation. Wang et al. used manifold learning of ML technique as the data had multiple dimensions and also used dynamic time-warping techniques and reported an overall accuracy of 81.35%, a sensitivity of 76.92% and a specificity of 81.41% for their AI-based model for identifying the DO. Cullingsworth et al. evaluated low-amplitude rhythmic detrusor contractions (LARC) in patients with DO. In another study, the model was automatically constructed using a Fast Fourier Transform approach that yielded 100% specificity for DO when LARC was identified and documented independently of abdominal pressure traces. Niederhauser et al. used 'Wavelet' time-frequency analysis with AI-based algorithms to diagnose and classify overactive bladder (OAB) based on the amplitude and frequency of nonvoiding contractions. They also investigated the possibility of automatically detecting DO by ML-based urodynamic automation.

An externally validated prediction model was developed for anticholinergic response using an RF (random forest) algorithm by Sheyn et al. for a cohort of 559 female patients treated with anticholinergic drugs for OAB.

Evaluation of the diagnosis and follow-up progress after treatments seem to be promising using AI. AI may also assist to increase the accuracy of diagnosis and make the management more effective for patients with pelvic floor dysfunctions. This can be of great help in improving the quality-of-life for these patients.

In cases of pelvic floor repair or other gynaecologic procedures, AI can suggest individualised physical therapy exercises to strengthen pelvic muscles and prevent complications like urinary incontinence or prolapse recurrence.

DRUG RESEARCH

Artificial intelligence plays a vital role in drug research development. New compounds are characterised by spectral data like mass spectrometry (MS), fourier transform infrared spectroscopy (FTIR) and nucleomagnetic resonance (NMR). These compounds are tested in vitro by the A2780 cell line and were found to be biocompatible and were efficient as anticancerous drugs. A novel approach with the presence of the Hill function is employed for characterising the optimal anticancer activities of these new drugs, which include esters and amides. AI was also utilised and support vector machines (SVMs) were also used with pharmacodynamics modelling paradigm to verify the efficiency of anticancer compounds. These methods efficiently infer the in vitro outcome of the leading compounds produced in both the preclinical and in vivo research.

ARTIFICIAL INTELLIGENCE LIMITATIONS

There are several limitations to AI in medicine, including the following:

- *Lack of data:* AI models require large amounts of data to be effectively trained and tested.
- *Bias in data:* The data used to train AI models may be biased, leading to models that are not generalisable to certain populations or that make incorrect predictions for certain groups of patients.
- *Limited interpretability:* Many AI models are considered 'black boxes', because it can be difficult to understand how they arrived at a particular decision or prediction. This can make it difficult for doctors to trust and use the predictions made by the AI model.
- *Inability to handle uncertainty*: AI models can struggle to make predictions in cases where there is a lot of uncertainty or where multiple outcomes are possible. This can be particularly challenging in medicine where many diagnoses are based on patterns and symptoms.

CHALLENGES

Artificial intelligence models have been widely developed related to all the segments of health care that integrate imaging chiefly but also integrate electronic health record data to not only guide toward more accurate diagnosis and treatment but also to develop more reliable decision making in medical and surgical line of therapy. In this era of AI and ML, the most important issue is to gain trust in the decisions derived from this computerised analysis, especially because it relates to health and life of the human being.

The quantity and quality of the data used to generate the models is the fundamental constraint on the robustness of these methods. Small data may not derive reliable answers, and this is particularly true for rare disorders that have erratic or subjective symptoms. Moreover, the data though sophisticated, it is multidimensional, may be skewed, and may also be biased depending on its source and professional responsibility and liability of the medical staff and statistical assistance who played part in creating the model. This is especially important and may lead to wrong derivations if the people playing part in the development and implementation of the model are not adequately trained. Moreover nonmentioned clinical data are ignored by the AI model, because AI models can only account for data that were 'seen'.

When applying AI in clinical practice, it is also important to assess its applicability.

The ethical issues surrounding the usage of AI should also be taken into consideration. Professional liability for doctors who use AI!! Should hospitals and doctors be held liable for judgments made by AI software? However, it is important to note that AI is a complementary tool to the obstetrics and gynaecology specialist, and it is not meant to replace human expertise.

CONCLUSION

Over the past few decades, use of AI has been markedly increased in healthcare systems, because AI can potentially help clinicians and practitioners to take appropriate decisions to reach a diagnosis and manage cases. The subsets of AI, namely ML and DL methods, have aided in detecting complex patterns from huge datasets and using such patterns in making predictions. Computerised algorithms of AI can make predictions simple and accurate. But it is essential to know that AI is not an alternative for clinical knowledge and excellence. AI enhances diagnostic accuracy, improves surgical outcomes by personalising treatments and optimising education but is useful for commonly found diseased and not very complicated cases, where human expertise always supersedes.

Though significant achievements have been accomplished in the application of AI in gynaecology and obstetrics, it is still in its infancy, and further exploration and improvement are required to attain optimal effectiveness and universality. Various studies have explored several controversial aspects to solve the restricted accuracy, by developing ensemble algorithms by utilising time series data as a validation set or ultrasound videos or by focusing features in harmonising imaging modalities.

It is essential to eliminate subjective bias, to avoid misdiagnosis. Continuous modification and optimisation of algorithms are still required, because as mentioned a wiser decision requires wider data and over and above that, the technology is in its growing phase. It must be remembered that the ultimate goal is to achieve fair, unified and objective generalisation standards, to deliver best possible treatment to every individual and to achieve best results with optimal treatment. Medical professionals and algorithm developers have equal stakes. So far, AI is still immature, in its start-up stage, problems still need to be solved in the future as these get uncovered. Medical professionals are still suggested to use AI combined with their clinical knowledge to optimise their clinical practice.

Despite challenges such as data quality, algorithmic bias and ethical considerations, the future of AI in gynaecology holds great promise for further improving women's health.

SUGGESTED READING

1. Ajao MO, Clark NV, Kelil T, Cohen SL, Einarsson JI. Case report: three-dimensional printed model for deep infiltrating endometriosis. J Minim Invasive Gynecol. 2017;24:1239-42.
2. Alagapan S, Shin HW, Fröhlich F, Wu HT. Diffusion geometry approach to efficiently remove electrical stimulation artifacts in intracranial electroencephalography. J Neural Eng. 2019;16:036010.
3. Arsalan M, Haider A, Choi J, Park KR. Detecting blastocyst components by artificial intelligence for human embryological analysis to improve success rate of in vitro fertilization. J Pers Med. 2022;12:124.
4. Beam AL, Kohane IS. Big data and machine learning in health care. JAMA. 2018;319:1317-8.
5. Colhoun AF, Speich JE, Cooley LF, Bell ED III, Barbee RW, Guruli G, et al. Low amplitude rhythmic contraction frequency in human detrusor strips correlates with phasic intravesical pressure waves. World J Urol. 2017;35:1255-60.
6. Cullingsworth ZE, Kelly BB, Deebel NA, Colhoun AF, Nagle AS, Klausner AP, et al. Automated quantification of low amplitude rhythmic contractions (LARC) during real-world urodynamics identifies a potential detrusor overactivity subgroup. PLoS One. 2018;13:e0201594.
7. Desai GS. Artificial intelligence: the future of obstetrics and gynecology. J Obstet Gynaecol India. 2018;68:326-7.
8. Dirie NI, Wang Q, Wang, S. Two-dimensional versus three-dimensional laparoscopic Systems in Urology: a systematic review and meta-analysis. J Endourol. 2018;32:781-90.
9. Dong HC, Dong HK, Yu MH, Lin YH, Chang CC. Using deep learning with convolutional neural network approach to identify the invasion depth of endometrial cancer in myometrium using MR images: a pilot study. Int J Environ Res Public Health. 2020;17:5993.
10. Enshaei A, Robson CN, Edmondson RJ. Artificial intelligence systems as prognostic and predictive tools in ovarian cancer. Ann Surg Oncol. 2015;22:3970-5.
11. Garg P, Mohanty A, Ramisetty S, Kulkarni P, Horne D, Pisick E, et al. Artificial intelligence and allied subsets in early detection and preclusion of gynecological cancers. Biochim Biophys Acta Rev Cancer. 2023;1878:189026.
12. Guerin S, Huaulmé A, Lavoue V, Jannin P, Timoh KN. Review of automated performance metrics to assess surgical technical skills in robot-assisted laparoscopy. Surg Endosc. 2022;36:853-70.
13. Guh RS, Tsung-Chieh JW, Shao-Ping W. Integrating genetic algorithm and decision tree learning for assistance in

predicting in vitro fertilization outcomes. Expert Syst Appl. 2011;38:4437-49.
14. Gupta K, Balyan K, Lamba B, Puri M, Sengupta D, Kumar M. Ultrasound placental image texture analysis using artificial intelligence to predict hypertension in pregnancy. J Matern Fetal Neonatal Med. 2022;35:5587-94.
15. Iftikhar P, Kuijpers MV, Khayyat A, Iftikhar A, DeGouvia De Sa M. Artificial intelligence: a new paradigm in obstetrics and gynecology research and clinical practice. Cureus. 2020;12:e7124.
16. Jiang Y, Wang C, Zhou S. Artificial intelligence-based risk stratification, accurate diagnosis and treatment prediction in gynecologic oncology. Semin Cancer Biol. 2023;96:82-99.
17. Kannaiyan A, Bagchi S, Vijayan V, Georgiy P, Manickavasagam S, Kumar DS. Revolutionizing women's health: artificial intelligence's impact on obstetrics and gynecology. J South Asian Feder Obst Gynae. 2024;16:161-8.
18. Kann BH, Thompson R, Thomas CR Jr, Dicker A, Aneja S. Artificial intelligence in oncology: Current applications and future directions. Oncology (Williston Park). 2019;33: 46-53.
19. Khan I, Khare BK. Exploring the potential of machine learning in gynecological care: a review. Arch Gynecol Obstet. 2024;309:2347-2365.
20. Khene ZE, Richard C, Hascoet J, Gasmi A, Goujon A, Brochard C, et al. Contrast-enhanced CT texture parameters as predictive markers of high-risk urodynamic features in adult patients with spina bifida. Urology. 2019;134:84-9.
21. Malek M, Gity M, Alidoosti A, Oghabian Z, Rahimifar P, Seyed Ebrahimi SM, et al. A machine learning approach for distinguishing uterine sarcoma from leiomyomas based on perfusion weighted MRI parameters. Eur J Radiol. 2019;110:203-11.
22. Manna C, Nanni L, Lumini A, Pappalardo S. Artificial intelligence techniques for embryo and oocyte classification. Reprod Biomed Online. 2013;26:42-9.
23. Moawad G, Tyan P, Louie M. Artificial intelligence and augmented reality in gynecology. Curr Opin Obstet Gynecol. 2019;31:345-8.
24. Narayanan S, Ramakrishnan R, Durairaj E, Das A. Artificial intelligence revolutionizing the field of medical education. Cureus. 2023;15:e49604.
25. Nekooeimehr I, Lai-Yuen S, Bao P, Weitzenfeld A, Hart S. Automated contour tracking and trajectory classification of pelvic organs on dynamic MRI. J Med Imaging (Bellingham). 2018;5:014008.
26. Niederhauser T, Gafner ES, Cantieni T, Grämiger M, Haeberlin A, Obrist D, et al. Detection and quantification of overactive bladder activity in patients: can we make it better and automatic? Neurourol Urodyn. 2018;37: 823-31.
27. Roweis ST, Saul LK. Nonlinear dimensionality reduction by locally linear embedding. Science. 2000;290:2323-6.
28. Saeed H, El Naqa I. Artificial intelligence in clinical trials. In: El NaqaI, Murphy MJ (Eds). Machine and Deep Learning in Oncology, Medical Physics and Radiology. Cham: Springer International Publishing; 2022. pp. 453-501.
29. Seval MM, Varli B. Current developments in artificial intelligence from obstetrics and gynecology to urogynecology. Front Med (Lausanne). 2023;10:1098205.
30. Sherin L, Sohail A, Shujaat S. Time-dependent AI-Modeling of the anticancer efficacy of synthesized gallic acid analogues. Comput Biol Chem. 2019;79:137-46.
31. Sheyn D, Ju M, Zhang S, Anyaeche C, Hijaz A, Mangel J, et al. Development and validation of a machine learning algorithm for predicting response to anticholinergic medications for overactive bladder syndrome. Obstet Gynecol. 2019;134:946-57.
32. Shozu K, Komatsu M, Sakai A, Komatsu R, Dozen A, Machino H, et al. Model-agnostic method for thoracic wall segmentation in fetal ultrasound videos. Biomolecules. 2020;10(12):1691.
33. Siristatidis C, Stavros S, Drakeley A, Bettocchi S, Pouliakis A, Drakakis P, et al. Omics and artificial intelligence to improve in vitro fertilization (IVF) success: A proposed protocol. Diagnostics (Basel). 2021;11(5):743.
34. Smith VJ, Marshall A, Lie ML, Bidmead E, Beckwith B, Van Oudgaarden E, et al. Implementation of a fetal ultrasound telemedicine service: women's views and family costs. BMC Pregnancy Childbirth. 2021;21:38.
35. Torrents-Barrena J, Monill N, Piella G, Gratacós E, Eixarch E, Ceresa M, et al. Assessment of Radiomics and deep learning for the segmentation of fetal and maternal anatomy in magnetic resonance imaging and ultrasound. Acad Radiol. 2021;28:173-88.
36. Toscano M, Marini TJ, Drennan K, Baran TM, Kan J, Garra B, et al. Testing telediagnostic obstetric ultrasound in Peru: a new horizon in expanding access to prenatal ultrasound. BMC Pregnancy Childbirth. 2021;21(1):328.
37. Ueno Y, Forghani B, Forghani R, Dohan A, Zeng XZ, Chamming's F, et al. Endometrial carcinoma: MR imaging-based texture model for preoperative risk stratification-A preliminary analysis. Radiology. 2017;284(3):748-57.
38. van Leuteren PG, Nieuwhof-Leppink AJ, Dik P. SENS-U: clinical evaluation of a full-bladder notification - a pilot study. J Pediatr Urol. 2019;15:381.e1-5.
39. Wang HS, Cahill D, Panagides J, Nelson CP, Wu HT, Estrada C. Pattern recognition algorithm to identify detrusor overactivity on urodynamics. Neurourol Urodyn. 2021;40:428-34.
40. Xie HN, Wang N, He M, Zhang LH, Cai HM, Xian JB, et al. Using deep-learning algorithms to classify fetal brain ultrasound images as normal or abnormal: AI classifies fetal brain images. Ultrasound Obstet Gynecol. 2020;56(4):579-87.
41. Yin P, Wang H. Evaluation of nursing effect of pelvic floor rehabilitation training on pelvic organ prolapse in postpartum pregnant women under ultrasound imaging with artificial intelligence algorithm. Comput Math Methods Med. 2022;2022:1786994.

Index

Page numbers followed by *b* refer to box, *f* refer to figure, *fc* refer to flowchart, and *t* refer to table.

A

Abacavir 377
Abdomen 6, 1208
- contrast-enhanced computed tomography of 585*f*
- examination 420
- percussion of 7*f*
- preparation of 1248
- shaving of 1248

Abdominal incision 669
- closure of 1161
- rupture of 1262

Abdominal instrument set 888*f*
Abdominal pain
- acute 183
- cramping 1136

Abdominal procedures 1220
Abdominal scar 441
- endometriosis of 440*f*

Abdominal sling operations 344
Abdominal wall 59, 439, 1261
- lesions 440*f*
- muscle of 440*f*
- vessel injury 1036

Abdominocervicopexy 344
Abdominoperineal resection 1240
Aberrant ureter 284
Abnormal intrauterine pregnancy 190
Abnormal uterine bleeding 606, 743, 743*t*, 744, 749, 896, 911*f*, 934*f*, 1041, 1195
- causes of 744, 911*f*

Abnormal vaginal bleeding 117, 460, 814
Abortion 162, 271, 346, 351, 607, 854, 1134, 1139, 1247
- aneuploid 163
- causes of 351
- cervical 167
- complete 168, 187
- euploid 164
- first-trimester 1135
- incomplete 168, 187, 985*f*
- induced 1138
- inevitable 167
- mechanism of 162
- medical methods of 1135
- mid-trimester 1136
- missed 168, 187
- recurrent 780
  - spontaneous 381
- septic 169, 1092
- spontaneous 162, 163, 164*f*, 218
- threatened 163*f*, 167, 780
- tubal 185, 965*f*
- unsafe 1133, 1133*t*
- uterine causes of 272*f*

Abruptio placentae 616
Abscess 1214, 1228
- anorectal 1234
- appendix 655
- chronic 407*f*
- drainage of 373
- formation 408, 1228
  - recurrent 1235
- multiple tuberculous 383*f*
- paraurethral 552
- pelvic 655, 1224
- periurethral 1234

Absorbable sutures 323*f*, 891*f*, 1159, 1213
Absorption, complete 187
Acanthosis 378
- nigricans, development of 468

Acetaminophen 461
Acetic acid 502, 515, 519, 527, 576-578, 581
Acetylation 1280
Acid-fast bacilli 430
- examination of 421
- microscopy 386

Acne 472, 1111
- treatment of 472

Acquired immunodeficiency syndrome 366, 374, 376, 877, 1068, 1081, 1099
Acquired uterine
- abnormalities 975
- pathologies 910

Acromegaly 308
Actinomyces 1091
- *israelii* 389

Actinomycin D 222, 532
Actinomycosis 389, 395
Activated protein C 148
Activin 81
- levels 207

Acute pelvic inflammatory disease 417*b*
- oral therapy of 417*b*
- parenteral therapy of 418*b*
- severe 961*f*

Acute pelvic pain 962
- diagnosis of 457*t*

Acute respiratory distress syndrome 127
- diagnosis of 1271

Acyclic nucleoside analogue 393
Acyclovir 393
Adalimumab 710
Adaptive immune response 701
Addison's disease 1202
Adductor longus muscle 1158
Adenocarcinoma 436, 440*f*, 502, 503*fc*, 536, 542, 567, 574, 619, 942
- classification of 574
- endometrioid 619, 668, 936*f*
- in situ 503, 575*f*, 577, 578, 620*f*
- mucinous 619
- papillary serous 642
- primary 647*f*
- vaginal 567

Adenohypophysis 82
Adenoma 536, 559, 597
- cystic 338*f*
- liver 1102
- malignum 942, 943
- pituitary 145

Adenomyoma 978, 980*f*
- posterior wall 923*f*

Adenomyomectomy 640
Adenomyosis 383*f*, 433, 434*f*, 454, 457, 596, 636, 637, 637*b*, 637*f*, 745, 758, 788, 919, 978, 1112
- diagnosis of 637, 979, 980*f*
- diffuse 745*f*, 921*f*, 980*f*
- echo texture of 921*f*
- focal 922*f*
- label of 433
- location of 980
- management of 920*fc*
- non-cystic focal 981*f*
- treatment of 640, 745
- uteri 434*f*, 637
  - management of 638

Adenosine triphosphate 66*f*, 378
Adenosis 238, 559
Adhesiolysis 1043, 1049, 1295
Adhesions 350, 362, 432, 457, 986, 1043*f*, 1141
- formation, lower risk of 1295
- lysis of 739, 1027

Adipose tissue 474
ADNEX model 958*t*
- risk calculator 958*t*
- sensitivity of 958*t*
- specificity of 958*t*

Adnexa 8, 60, 457, 943, 947, 960*f*, 1001
- operations on 1029
- torsion of 360*f*, 362*f*
- tuberculosis of 384

Adnexal masses 47, 183, 191, 192*f*, 209
- chronic ectopic 185, 187
- diagnosis of 957
- evaluation of 956
- torsion of 188
- ultrasound evaluation of 947

Adnexum 42
Adoptive cell transfer 708
Adrenal androgens 135
Adrenal cortex 76*fc*, 729, 772
- androgenic tumours of 307
- forms, anlage of 261

Adrenal cortical
- activity 132
- adenoma 735

failure, signs of 723
hyperplasia 308
stimulators 308
tumour 730*f*
Adrenal failure, states of 785
Adrenal glands 306, 465
Adrenal hyperandrogenism 481
Adrenal hyperplasia
congenital 123, 138, 160, 236, 259, 295, 296*f*, 299, 300, 301*f*, 303*f*, 304, 305, 464, 481, 738, 739, 1303
nonclassic congenital 481
Adrenal insufficiency 1256
Adrenal neoplastic growths 464
Adrenal tumours 307, 481
Adrenal vein studies 236
Adrenalectomy, partial 308
Adrenocorticotropic hormone 83, 132, 235, 295, 465, 723, 862, 863
Adrenogenital syndrome 295, 308
Adriamycin 532
Adult respiratory distress syndrome 1271
Aerobic exercises 1197
Agalactia 232
Agenesis 259, 264279
Air, sound of 1033
Alanine
aminotransferase 375
transaminase 609
Albright syndrome 140*f*
Alcohol 232, 241, 601, 1150
Aldosterone 1241, 1243
antagonist 472
Aldrete's scoring system, modified 1250
Aldridge sling operation 1154*f*
Alendronate 118
Alimentary castration 730
Alimentary tract 606
complications 1251
Alkaline cervical mucus 32
Alkylating agents 532, 687
Alleged postmenopausal atrophy 615
Allergen immunotherapy 714
Allergic contact dermatitis 798, 805
Allergic reactions 769
Allergic rhinitis 714
Allergy 404, 769, 810
pelvic 769
Allis forceps, set of 884
Alloimmune factors 165
Alopecia 473, 688
Alpha-blockers 1150
Alpha-fetoprotein 657, 658, 703
Alpha-linolenic acid 1278, 1282
Alpha-methyl dopamine 145
Altemeier perineal rectosigmoidectomy 1221
Alternate current electrolysis 472
Alzheimer's disease 112, 775, 1198, 1201
Amastia 228
Amazia 228
unilateral 228*f*
Amenorrhoea 124, 137, 145, 183, 233, 275, 308, 385, 420, 482, 718, 722*f*, 723*f*, 727, 730*f*, 731*f*, 732, 733, 735, 775, 777, 780, 1078, 1091, 1103, 1113
division of 720
exercise-related 732
hypergonadotropic 724
hypothalamic 720, 736
incidence of 1103
management of 739*fc*
ovarian 724
pathological 719
physiological 718
pituitary 722
postpill 722, 736
primary 285*f*, 300, 721*fc*, 722*f*, 737
secondary 719*fc*, 722*f*, 737, 741*f*
true 718
uterine 729
Amikacin 387
Amiloride 1245
Amine odour 798
Amino acid 1277
cystathionine 118
essential 1277
nonessential 1277
sulphur-containing 1277
Aminoglycosides 1258
Aminosalicylate 716
Amiodarone 233
Amitriptyline, beneficial effect of 817
Amoebiasis 390
Amoxicillin 387
Amoxicillin-clavulanic acid 1177
Ampicillin 169, 232
Amprenavir 377
Ampulla 40, 181
Amsel's criteria 797
Anabolic drugs 482
Anaemia 218, 489, 1080, 1104, 1207, 1219, 1263, 1275, 1280, 1283
classification of 1283*t*
diagnosis of 1285
treatment of 1285
type of 811, 1283
Anaerobic streptococci 169, 415
Anaesthesia 838, 1032, 1128, 1258
general 1130, 1236*f*
inhalation of 1271
local 1130, 1237
regional 1130
spinal 1223, 1237
Anaesthetic agents, long-acting 1252
Anagen 479
Anal canal 1232
continence of 1223
lower 1228, 1229
neoplasm of 1239
stretching of 1233
surgical anatomy of 1216*f*
tumours 1239
Anal dilator 1225*f*
Anal epidermis, dysplasia of 1239
Anal fissure, chronic 1229*f*
Anal hygiene 1227
Anal intraepithelial neoplasia 1239
Anal manometry 1220
Anal orifice drains 57
Anal pruritus, causes of 1227, 1227*t*
Analgesia 1252
local 491
Analgesics 1251
drugs 233*t*
Anaplastic lymphoma kinase translocated tumours 689
Ancillary instruments 1022
Androblastoma 295, 735
Androgen 76*fc*, 86, 130, 295, 479, 479*t*, 783, 1202
action 290
administration of 307
biosynthesis defect 290
deficiency 305
excess of 290, 466*fc*
high levels of 726
insensitivity syndrome 138, 728, 728*f*, 729*f*
natural 783
overproduction of 724
physiology 479
production, removal of source of 484
secreting maternal tumour 297
stimulus, excessive 307
suppression 466
synthesis 290
defects 297
Androgenic adrenal cortical tumour 75*f*
Androstenedione 67, 72*f*, 136, 301, 307, 464, 465, 479, 1185
peripheral conversion of 87
Anechoic lacunae 637
Anechoic unilocular cyst 948*f*
Aneuploidy, focal 160
Angina 1194
Angioma 536, 559, 572
Angiotensin-converting enzyme 1150
inhibitors 1150
reduction of 112
Animal parasitic infections 810
Annual mammography, timing of 243
Anogenital warts, differential diagnosis of 368*b*
Anorectal abscess 1234
types 1235*f*
Anorectal manometry 1224
Anorexia nervosa 123, 720, 730, 731*f*, 733, 734
Anovulation 147, 464, 469*fc*
mechanism of 468
treatment of 863*fc*
Anoxia 1255
Antacids 1116
Antecedent gestational event 218
Anterior colporrhaphy 341, 344
steps of 343*f*
Anterior compartment defects 332
Anterior lobe hormones 81
Anterior prolapse repair 342
Anterior rectal
mucosal prolapse 1224
wall 961*f*
Anterior rectus fascia 1032, 1033
Anterior vaginal wall 559*f*, 1141
cyst 558, 558*f*
retractor 884, 887, 887*f*

Anthracyclines 687
Anthraquinones 232
Antiandrogens 309, 785
Antiangiogenic drugs 450
Antianxiety 837
Anti-beta 2-glycoprotein-1 antibody 171
Antibiotics 365*f*, 412, 769, 1175, 1177, 1235, 1256, 1258, 1260
- antitumour 532, 687
- prophylaxis 1178*t*, 1247, 1247*t*
- therapy 169, 1148, 1175, 1224
- use of 1247

Antibody 710, 842
- non-treponemal 369
- tests 369

Anticancer immune surveillance 702
Anti-chlamydia antibody 380
Anticholinergic effects 1227
Anticoagulants 1266, 1270, 1271
- oral 1267
- therapy 1266, 1270

Anticonvulsant drugs 1116
Anti-D gamma globulin 1139
Anti-D immunoglobulins 188
Antidepressants 837, 1187
- long-acting 824

Antidiuretic hormone 1241
Antidote 1267
Antifibrinolytic agents 746
Antigas gangrene 169
Antigens, tumour-associated 703, 703*f*
Antigonadotrophins 787
Antihistamines 232
Anti-inflammatory drugs 233*t*
Antimetabolites 532, 687
Antimicrobial agent 1176
Anti-Müllerian hormone 66*f*, 108, 111, 289, 290, 304, 464, 476
- abnormal 299
- elevated serum 464

Antinuclear antibodies 170
Antioestrogenic hormonal therapy 689
Antioestrogens 534, 778
Antioxidants 450
Antiphospholipid syndrome 170, 173
- immunotherapy in 711
- pathogenetic pathways in 711

Antiplatelet aggregation factors 112
Antiprogestins 447, 449
Antiprogestogens 782
Antiretroviral drugs 1116
Antiretroviral therapy 377
Antisepsis 1204
Antiseptics 405
Antispasmodics 1227
Antithrombin deficiency 1194
Anti-thyroid peroxidase antibody 174
Antitubercular therapy 425*f*, 430
Antitubercular treatment 388
Antitumour necrosis factor 174
Anti-vascular endothelial growth factor 593
Antral follicle count 992
Anuria 1257
Anus 48, 57
- constriction of 1225
- diseases of 810

Anxiety 110, 765, 824, 829, 833, 845
Aorta 252*f*
- focal 16
- peritoneum over bifurcation of 758*f*

Apareunia 845
- permanent 1255

Aplasia 229, 259, 290
Apocrine glands 391
Apocrine miliaria 810
Apoptosis 747
Appendicitis 188, 408, 411, 412
Arachidonic acid 1278
Arbor vitae 37, 37*f*
Arcus tendineus 1161*f*
- fascia pelvis 328*f*, 329

Areola, raised areas of 230
Areolar bud 225*f*
Arginine 1277
- vasopressin 1244

Argon 18
Aromatase 452
- deficiency 160, 290
- inhibitors 450, 632, 736
  - mechanism of action of 452, 453*fc*
  - surpass oestrogen production 450

Arrhythmia 1035
- cardiac 1245

Arterial blood gas assessment 1269
Arterial pressure 755
Arterial thrombosis 1101
Arteriography 1269
Arteriolar spasm 1255
Arteriovenous malformation 16*f*, 616, 926*f*
Arteriovenous shunts 604
Artery 53
- cerebral 16
- forceps 884, 885, 885*f*

Arthropathy, menopausal 112
Artificial intelligence 1306, 1308, 1310-1312
- applications of 1306, 1307
- based tools 241
- integration 1018
- limitations 1312
- role of 1308-1310

Artificial neural network 1307
Artificial reproductive techniques 476
Ascites 246, 614, 1008*f*
- massive 1289

Asherman's syndrome 166, 432, 729, 844, 939*f*, 1043
Asoprisnil 609
Aspartate aminotransferase 609
Aspirin 174, 233, 530, 755, 767
- low-dose 712

Assisted hatching 1297
- indications of 1297

Assisted reproductive technology 180, 453*fc*, 709, 865, 869
- complications of 880
- immunotherapy in 709

Asthenoterato-oligozoospermia 843
Asthenozoospermia 843
Athelia 228
- bilateral 228*f*

Atresia 75
- congenital 281, 407, 1166
- early stages of 75*f*

Atretic follicles 43, 72*f*, 73*f*-75*f*, 293
Atrial natriuretic hormone 1241
Atrophic epithelium 487*f*
Atrophic ovary 1007*f*
- normal 1006

Atrophic thin endometrium 1002*f*
Atrophic urethritis 1142
Atrophic vaginitis 397, 449, 752, 793, 796, 798, 805
Atrophy 615
- loss of 308

Atypia 509
Atypical endometrial hyperplasia, aspects of 511*f*
Atypical glandular cells 502, 503
Atypical smooth muscle tumours 614
Atypical squamous cell 502, 503, 517, 521, 577-579
- management of 576, 579*fc*

Augmentation mammoplasty 229
Augmentin 1177
Auramine 386
Autoimmune ovarian failure 138
Autoimmunisation 489
Autologous endometrial antigen 442
Automated volume count 993*f*
Autonomic nervous system 755
Autonomic neuropathy 533
Autoprime 84
Autopsy 365*f*
Autosomes, normal distribution of 288*fc*
Avelumab 708
Axilla, management of 248
Axillary hair 108, 297
- growth of 135
- lack of 139*f*

Axillary lymph node 248
- dissection 249
- status 245

Ayre's scrape technique 526
Ayre's spatula 526, 890, 890*f*
Azathioprine 716
Azithromycin 374, 1225
Azole 801, 808
Azoospermia 145, 843, 859, 860, 861
- classification 860
- evaluation of 862*fc*
- factor region 262
- nonobstructive 878
- obstructive 878
- post-testicular 861
- testicular 860
- treatment 860

Aztreonam 1247

B

Babcock's forceps 884
Bacilluria 810, 1141
Bacillus Calmette-guérin inoculations 714

Back pain
lower 605*f*
premenstrual low 350
Backache 118, 338
deep-seated causes of 458
low 351
Bacteraemia, sudden 1256
Bacterial flora 403*f*
Bacterial vaginosis 367, 380, 402, 417, 793, 794*f*, 798, 802, 807, 808, 1188
diagnosis of 797, 799
recommended regimens for 801
treatment for 800*t*
Bacteriology 1258
Bacteriuria 1258
asymptomatic 1172, 1173
Bacteroides 169, 365, 402, 808
Baden's system 329
Baden–Walker halfway system 329, 330*f*
Bagel's sign 190, 190*f*
Barbiturates 232
Bard-Parker knife handle 884
Barrier methods 1068, 1074, 1123
Bartholin's abscess 396, 396*f*, 396*t*, 536, 550, 551*f*, 1234
Bartholin's cyst 396, 396*t*, 536, 550, 550*f*
Bartholin's duct, cyst of 550*f*
Bartholin's gland 26, 29, 150, 256, 1236
carcinoma 542
duct of 29*f*
enlargement of 536
neoplasms of 551
tumours of 550
Bartholinitis 371*f*, 395, 536
Basal body temperature 844, 875, 1065
method 1065, 1066*f*
Basal cell carcinoma 542, 548
Basal hormonal evaluation, significance of 851
Basophil cells, predominance of 308
Basophilism, pituitary 308
Bazedoxifene 1193
Beak sign 984, 986*f*
Behçet's disease 393
Behçet's syndrome 373
Belimumab 712, 716
Bellagio's criteria 1067
Benign tumour 958, 958*t*, 1225
surgeries 1309
Benzalkonium chloride 1074
Benzoyl peroxide 472
Beta-carotene 845
Beta-human chorionic gonadotrophin 150, 193, 208, 897
assay 205
concentration 188
discriminatory zone of 189
evaluation 219*t*
Beta-subunit gene mutations 1304
Bevacizumab 534, 648, 692
Bicornis bicollis 909*f*
Bicornuate uterus 191*f*, 264, 267, 273*f*, 429*f*, 570*f*, 909*f*
rudimentary horn of 179
Bictegravir 377
Bifid clitoris 282, 282*f*
Bilaminar disc embryo 261
Bilateral cornual block 424*f*, 429*f*
Bilateral rigid pipeline tubes 424*f*
Bilateral salpingo-oophorectomy 313, 425*f*, 645, 932*f*, 935*f*
Bilateral salpingo-ovariectomy 665*f*, 669, 671
Bilateral tubal
ligation 427*f*
occlusion 872*fc*
ostia 1046*f*
Bilharzia 390
proctitis 1238
Bilirubin 375, 1173
Billings' method change 1064
Bilobed papilloma 554*f*
Biodegradable implant contraception 1109
Biological therapy 701
Biopsy
forceps 1039, 1049*f*
specimen 493*f*
testicular 850
Biotin 1275
Biphasic pills 1092
Bipolar circuit 1025*f*
Bipolar forceps 1025*f*
Birth
control pills 648
spacing 1063
weight, low 381, 1274, 1275
Bisphosphonates 118, 1193
Bivalve vaginal speculum 498
Bladder 30*f*, 43, 46, 57, 280, 438, 606, 943*f*, 1170, 1209
cancer 532
carcinoma of 752, 1142
catheterisation 1031
collapsed lower compartment of 1164*f*
detrusor 1166
muscle 1165
development of 257
diary 1189
diseases of 1141
displacement of 1141
dissection of 1208, 1210*f*
dysfunction 1140, 1153
causes of 1140
emptying, nervous control of 45*f*
endometriosis 439*f*
filling, nervous control of 45*f*
fistula, type of 1258
function of 44*f*
herniates 342
incomplete emptying of 1141, 1167
irritability of 456, 1140, 1163
muscle 1165
neck
identification of 1159
resection of 1167
sling 1157
suspension procedures 1161*f*
overactive 1312
over-distended 354
pillar
artery of 328
veins of 328
preparation of 1248
psychogenic 1143
sound 884
tenesmus 755
Blade scissors, straight and curved 1023*f*
Blaivas and Olsson classification 1144*f*
Blastocoel 1311
Blastocyst 153
compaction of 153
formation of 153
Bleeding 95, 97, 270, 775
abnormal 443, 744
acute 750
clinical types of 750
cyclical 121
disorders 749*b*
episodes of 97*f*
intraoperative 1049
intraperitoneal 3, 184
irregular 456, 658, 1041
management of 1196
nonmenstrual 750
painless 1231
pattern 1114
perimenopausal 751
postmenopausal 13, 420, 568*f*, 618*f*, 623*f*, 751, 932*f*, 933, 935*f*, 936*f*, 938*fc*, 1002, 1005*f*, 1196
postoperative 1049
prepubertal 750
pubertal 751
secondary 1257
uterine 94, 97*f*, 102, 738
Bleomycin 593, 692, 1240
cycles of 692
Blood 568, 965*f*
casts 759*f*
cells 1173
changes 1263
cholesterol, level of 80
cyst 440*f*
large 570*f*
diseases of 752
disorder, primary 770
dyscrasias 147, 208
exudate 203
glucose 1276*f*
group typing 188
loss of 1255
replacement 1249
stained fluid 1262
stasis 1262
sugar, fasting 375
supply 42*f*, 56*f*, 899, 901*f*, 946
test 387
theoretical concept of 97*f*
transfusion 169, 1204, 1249, 1249*b*, 1256
transmitted infections, screening for 322
urea 127, 375
vessels 46, 53, 56*f*, 616
Blood-born infections 1234
Bloodstream 575, 621
Blunts adrenocorticotropic hormone 126

Body
fluids 1241
mass index 111, 136, 175, 194, 473, 482, 851, 1033, 1081, 1101, 1108, 1282
tissues 1241
Bone 458
age 143
deformity 293
densitometry 1198
loss 1190
marrow
derived stem cells 636
suppression 688
mass of 1191*b*
mineral density 117, 1190, 1191*b*
morphogenetic protein 15 293
turnover 1191*f*
biochemical markers of 1191
Bonney's blue 1248
Bonney's hood technique 611, 611*f*
Bonney's myomectomy clamp 610, 610*f*, 888
Bonney's test 1151, 1151*f*
Bony pelvis 29
Borderline epithelial ovarian tumours 663, 665
Borderline malignancy, histological features of 665*f*
Borrelia burgdorferi 490
Botox therapy 837
Botulinum toxin
injection of 1229
therapy 837
Bowel
action 1253
injury 1036*f*
preparation of 1031, 1248
Bowen's disease 494
Brachial plexus injury 1036
Brachytherapy 566, 589, 593, 696, 699, 700
interstitial 591
Brain 737, 1186, 1302
development of 231
oedema 1243
Breadth 1081
Breakthrough bleeding 448, 1103
Breastfeeding 208, 231, 648, 717, 1103, 1275
exclusive 1275
Breasts 6, 78, 81, 115, 135, 139*f*, 225, 226*f*, 229, 233, 777, 782, 1080, 1302
absence of 138, 228
accessory 228*f*
anomalies, congenital 228
atrophy 232, 235
classification 235
late-onset 235
management of 237*fc*
secondary 236
cancer 241, 245, 1102, 1201
advanced 249, 529
bilateral 1302
diagnosis of 1196
early premenopausal 1102
history of 1196
male 1302
management of 246
postmenopausal 1302
premenopausal 243, 1201, 1302
radiotherapy for 933*f*
risk of 1102
screening methods 240*t*, 244
susceptibility gene 240
treatment of 246
triple negative 1302
carcinoma 245, 245*f*, 789
risk factors for 245*b*
conditions 776, 782
conservation therapy 248
delayed of development of 230
development 225, 776
stages of 225
developmental anomalies of 227
disease 231
benign 241, 244*f*
normal anatomy of 244*f*
screening for 240
disorders 1
enlargement of 226, 228*f*, 778*f*
failure of development of 230
function 225
imaging reporting and data system 243
increased erectility of 230
lump 117
mammography 242
masses 236
multiple 228
nodularity of 230
normal 245*f*
ovarian cancer, hereditary 1303
Paget's disease of 494*f*
preparation of 230
self-examination 241, 242*f*, 1196
side view of 225*f*
slight enlargement of 294*f*
small 236*t*
stimulation, persistent 235
supernumerary 229
tenderness 1065, 1096
tubular 230*f*
unit 229*t*
Breathing exercises 837
Bremelanotide 827
Brenner tumour 665, 666
Broad ligament 35*f*, 40, 40*f*, 49, 327, 564, 1213
cellulitis of 415
cyst of 649
fibroid 991
haematoma 312, 314, 651
leaves of 1209, 1210*f*
leiomyoma 602*f*, 651*f*, 652*t*
removal of 47
tumours 655
Bromocriptine 128, 232, 768
Bronchial asthma 755
Bronchospasm 755, 1136
Brucella 164
Bulbocavernosus muscle 29, 835
Bulbospongiosus muscle 29, 34
Bulbourethral glands 258
Bulimia nervosa 731
Bulldog clamps 884
Bupropion 827
Burch procedure 1156
Buschke–Lowenstein disease 1239
Buserelin 447, 449
Buspirone 827

C

Cabergoline 450
Cabotegravir 377
Cachexia 529
Caesarean delivery, emergency 324
Caesarean scar pregnancy 179, 202
Caesarean section 612, 1247
classic 439
lower segment 316, 414, 606
previous 1209
Caffeine 165, 232, 601
Calcification
endometrium of 939*f*
evidence of 244*f*
Calcitonin 1193
Calcium 1281, 1285*t*
absorption 1279
efficiency of 1284
accretion rate 1284
channel blockers 757, 1150
elemental 450
gluconate, intravenous 1246
requirement 1284, 1286
Call–Exner bodies 68, 676, 676*f*
Calvert formula 700
Calymmatobacterium granulomatis 365
Cancer 778, 1226
age 522
antigen 125 525, 658
cells 495, 707
cervical 523, 525, 943*f*
cervix 583
chemotherapy, effect of 686
colon 112
colorectal 1201
detection of 576
development of 109, 594
diagnosis of 1300, 1301
endometrial 217, 525, 616, 627, 629, 688, 752, 777*f*, 1017*f*, 1045*f*, 1051, 1102, 1104, 1201
endometrium 934*f*, 935*f*
epithelial 657
gastrointestinal 657
genetic basis of 1300
genome atlas research 704
gonadal 1303
immunotherapies 705*f*
invasive 487*f*, 490, 503*fc*, 574*t*
liver 1102
management of 1300
microinvasive 592
mucinous 657
ovarian 523, 525, 646, 672, 1102, 1201, 1302
pelvic 781
phobia 4

risk of 1102
screening 1196
surveillance 1304
testicular 532
therapy 702
transformation 1301*fc*
tubal 644
tumour-node-metastasis staging of 544*t*
uterine 523, 706*fc*
vaginal 523
vulva 544*t*
vulvar 523, 523*f*, 805
Candida 8, 367, 402, 403, 489, 752, 807, 1247, 1272
albicans 365, 394, 400, 400*f*, 490, 794*f*, 795, 798
balanitis 489
cultures 799
infection 394, 401*f*, 493*f*, 795
diagnosis of 402
treatment for 402
vaginitis 400, 401, 500, 811*f*
vulvitis 1101
Candidiasis 375, 394, 806
treatment of recurrent 801
Cannula 1020*f*
Capillary, diseases of 752
Capreomycin 387
Capronor 1109
Carbamazepine 232, 1104
Carbenicillin 232
Carbohydrate 1275, 1276*f*, 1277, 1282, 1286
complex 1276
nondigestible 1279
Carbon dioxide 495
insufflation 1033, 1034
laser 508, 1294, 1296*f*
laser vaporisation 562
Carboplatin 532, 646, 671, 687, 688, 691, 693, 700, 706
Carboprost 1136
Carcinoembryonic antigen 657, 658, 703, 1229
Carcinoma 459, 498, 596, 597, 619, 697, 933, 949, 1142, 1236, 1239
adenosquamous 570
corporis 407
embryonal 658, 659, 679
endometrial 42*f*, 596, 627, 688, 1004, 1005, 1042
endometrioid 619, 624, 625*f*, 626*f*, 642, 668, 945*f*
in situ 500, 810, 1102, 1310
invasive 567
mixed 619
ovarian 954*f*
papillary serous 619
peritoneal 652
serous 619, 697, 935*f*
specimen of 564*f*
stage of 250*t*
stump 594
Carcinosarcoma 619, 630, 658, 682, 697
Cardiac malformation 293
Cardinal ligaments 47, 1204, 1208, 1213
Cardiomyopathy 1256
Cardiopulmonary dysfunction, severe 1131
Cardiotoxicity 688
Cardiovascular disease 1031, 1080, 1190
Cardiovascular system 822
Carnett test 460
Caruncle 536
Catagen 479
Catechol oestrogens 82
Catechol-O-methyltransferase encoding gene 600
Catheters 1039
Causative organisms 1234
Cavitated uterine mass 759
Cavity
abdominal 179, 187
normal 1038*f*
Cefixime 373
Cefotaxime 417
Cefotetan 418
Cefoxitin 417, 418
Ceftizoxime 417
Ceftriaxone 373, 374, 389, 417, 418, 1248
Celebrex 714
Cell
adhesion molecule 626*f*
antigen-presenting 703*f*
cervical smear of 501*f*
cleavage 153
clusters 253
cycle 686, 1301
division 155
normal homeostasis for 1300, 1301*fc*
embolism 441
growth cycle 531
irradiation of 1298
malignant 524
survival of 1300
types of 291, 474
Cellular potassium 1242
Cellular therapies 174
Cellular tissue 52, 1257
Cellulitis 1272
acute 414
chronic 415
pelvic 407*f*, 414
subacute 414
Centchroman 1117
Central endometrial echo 16*f*
Central nervous system 45*f*, 61, 141, 142, 146, 231, 235, 368, 822, 823, 1186
diseases of 1142
Central venous pressure 169
Cephalexin 1072, 1177
Cephalopelvic disproportion 315
Cephaloridine 232
Cephalosporin 169, 1247
parenteral third-generation 417
Cerebral cortex influences 720
Cerebrospinal fluid 370
Cerebrovascular accidents 1100
Ceritinib 689
Cervical anomaly 905
Cervical aplasia 266
Cervical atresia 273
Cervical biopsy 528, 751, 1195
Cervical canal 264, 273, 427*f*, 428*f*, 910*f*
anomalies, classification of 975
dilatation of 427*f*
Cervical cancer 523, 525, 943*f*
immunotherapy in 704
management of 579*f*
parametrial
extension of 16
invasion of 943*f*
prevention of 579*f*
screening for 576
staging 584*t*
treatment of 687
Cervical cap 1072, 1072*f*
removal of 1073*f*
Cervical cerclage 175
Cervical cone biopsy 507*f*
Cervical conisation 509
Cervical cycle 99
Cervical cytology 502, 541, 576
classification systems for 502*t*
management of 579
sampling devices for 526*f*
Cervical diaphragm 1070*f*
types of 1070*f*
Cervical dilatation 429*f*
Cervical discharge 1272
Cervical duplication 908*f*
Cervical epithelial abnormality, screening for 527
Cervical erosion 1289, 1292
Cervical fibroid 570, 919*f*
posterior 941*f*
Cervical hoods 268
Cervical insufficiency 166, 171
physical examination-based 166
Cervical intraepithelial neoplasia 493*f*, 496, 500, 501, 501*f*, 502, 503, 504, 516, 517, 520, 521, 573, 577-579, 1102, 1292, 1294
treatment for 1294
Cervical irritation 573
Cervical lesion 944*f*, 975
evaluation of 16
Cervical mucous polyp 570, 570*f*
Cervical mucus 38, 121, 125, 1083, 1113
crystallisation of 122*f*
method 1064, 1066*f*
postcoital testing of 857
progesterone-dominant 1066*f*
Cervical pathology 941
Cervical polyp 570, 797, 940*f*
removal of 800
simple removal of 797
simulating prolapse 338*f*
small 941*f*
Cervical precancers, detection of 576
Cervical pregnancy 202, 202*f*
diagnosis of 202
ultrasound for 202*b*
Cervical punch biopsy forceps 891, 891*f*, 893
Cervical repair 315

Cervical secretion 792
Cervical smear 498, 501*f*
  interpretation of 504
  significance of positive 504
Cervical stenosis 844, 931
Cervical stroma, invasion of 624
Cervical stump 338*f*
  development of 594
Cervical tears 314
  deep 315
Cervicitis 404, 414, 940*f*, 942
  acute 404
  chronic 404, 405, 456, 793, 796, 1141
  forms of 406
Cervicography 528
Cervicovaginal junction 327
Cervicovaginal ligament 1210
Cervix 8, 32*f*, 37, 38*f*, 40, 40*f*, 57, 179, 364, 383, 432, 441, 497, 500*f*, 507*f*, 522, 693, 939, 941, 944*f*, 977*f*, 1082, 1141, 1195, 1204, 1208, 1294
  abnormal 527
  acute anteflexion of 276*f*, 278*f*, 351
  adenocarcinoma of 504, 575*f*
  adenomatous 405
  advanced cancer of 590*f*
  amputation of 346, 456
  anterior lips of 1213
  atresia of 275
  benign
    lesion of 942
    neoplasms of 570
    tumours of 570
  bicollis 909*f*
  cancer of 934, 944*f*, 1102
  carcinoma of 73*f*, 335, 445, 522*f*, 572, 588, 594, 593, 617, 696, 699, 700, 1141, 1225
  columnar epithelium of 498
  congenital hypertrophy of 279
  decubital ulceration of 334*f*, 752
  dilatation of 865, 893
  early invasive cancer of 574*f*
  elimination of 429*f*
  endometriosis of 454*f*, 456*f*, 1139
  enlarged 940*f*
  expansion of 429*f*
  functional closure of 364
  funnelling of 167*f*
  hypertrophy of 334
  incarceration of 340
  invasive cancer of 574*t*, 586, 587*t*
  laceration of 312, 314
  level of 275
  malignant
    disease of 617
    neoplasms of 570
    tumours of 595
  mechanical stimulation of 85
  microinvasive cancer of 574*f*
  multiple
    condylomas of 571*f*
    nabothian cysts of 571*f*
  normal 940*f*
  oedematous 333*f*
  overt tuberculosis of 384
  posterior lips of 1213
  postradiated cancer of 586*f*
  single normal 977*f*
  stage of cancer of 524
  strawberry patches on 795*f*
  stump of 344
  unilateral 266
  uteri, tumours of 570
  vaginal aspect of 525
Cetirizine 1187
Chancroid 366, 373, 373*f*, 393
Charged-coupled device camera 1022*f*
Chemical
  factors 260
  reactions, essential 1275
  substances 804
Chemoradiation 592, 700
Chemoreceptor trigger zone 581
Chemotherapeutic agents 531, 673
  development of 523
Chemotherapy 222*t*, 531, 533, 534, 593, 629, 646, 672, 686, 693, 737, 860, 1181
  adjuvant 672
  concurrent 566
  drugs, classification of 532*fc*
  first-line 706
  intraperitoneal 673
  neoadjuvant 673, 691
  platinum-based 676
  prophylactic 219
  toxicity 688
  type of 672
Chest
  lesions 235
  pain 1270
  radiograph 421
  symptoms 1271
Chiari–Frommel syndrome 124, 226*f*, 736
Chimeric antigen receptor T-cell therapy 703, 708
Chimerism 291
Chinese hamster ovary cells 786
Chlamydia 8, 180, 367, 380, 405, 752, 807, 857, 1075, 1116
  infection 857, 868
  ophthalmia neonatorum 379
  tests for 800
  trachomatis 164, 365, 396, 793, 795, 796*f*, 798, 808, 857, 1116
    infections 378
    screening for 857
Chloasma 777, 1100
Chloramphenicol 374
Chlordiazepoxide 232
Chlorhexidine jelly 1254
Chloride 1241, 1242
Chloroquine 232
Chlorpromazine 232
Chocolate cyst 851*f*
Cholestasis, history of 1080
Cholesterol 76*fc*
  precursor 1275
Chorioadenoma destruens 217
Chorioamnionitis, preterm premature rupture of 381
Choriocarcinoma 183, 214, 217, 218*f*, 222, 596, 597, 642, 658, 659, 679, 690
  incidence of 218, 218*t*
Chorionic gonadotrophins 43, 158, 786
Chorionic villi 157, 164*f*
Chromium 1281
Chromopertubation 1027
Chromosomal abnormalities 163, 259
Chromosomal anomalies 162
Chromosomal formation, mechanism of abnormal 290
Chromosomal microarray 173
Chromosomal sex 287
Chromosome 602, 1303
  abnormal division of 291*f*
  complement 292
  pairs of 287*f*
  studies 734
Chromotubation, laparoscopic 14
Chronic cellulitis 415
  diagnosis of 416
Chronic non-neoplastic epithelial disorders 546
Chronic pelvic pain 433, 448, 459
  diagnosis of 457*t*
  incidence of 459
  step-wise evaluation of 460
Chronic vulvar epithelial disorder 488*f*, 776*f*
  hyperkeratotic form of 487*f*
Cimetidine 232, 485
Cinedefaecography 1219
  films 1221*f*
  suite 1220*f*
Ciprofloxacillin 373
Ciprofloxacin 1176, 1177, 1247, 1248
Circulatory thyroid hormone 791
Cisplatin 532, 593, 687, 692, 706, 1240
Citalopram 824
Clavicle, top of 242*f*
Clavulanic acid 387
Clear cell
  carcinoma 619, 642, 697
    endometrium 621*f*
  tumours 665, 668
Cleavage vesicovaginal space, line of 342
Cleft lip congenital anomalies 1284
Climacteric symptoms 110, 110*f*, 112, 1288
Clindamycin 389, 403, 418, 472, 801, 1247
Clitoral cysts 536, 538
Clitoral devices 831
Clitoral function 324
Clitoral glans 319
  removal of 319
Clitoral jewellery 831
Clitoral lesions 830
Clitoral massagers 831
Clitoral pulsators 831
Clitoral reconstruction 324
  role of 324
Clitoral stimulating gels 831
Clitoral suction devices 831

Clitoral tissue removed 324
Clitoral vibrators 831
Clitoris 27, 303*f*, 391*f*, 557, 897
  carcinoma of 542*f*
  enlargement of 785
  enlarges 307
  hypertrophy of 283, 536
  root of 29
  total removal of 319
Clitoromegaly 728*f*
Clitoroplasty 302
Cloaca, partition of 256*f*
Cloacal membrane 261, 303*f*
Clofazimine 387
Clomiphene 124, 126, 127, 736, 860
  antioestrogenic action of 125
  citrate 473
    challenge test 865, 882
    cis and trans isomers of 124
Clomipramine 824
  on-demand use of 824
Clonidine hydrochloride 114
Clostridium
  difficile infection 1175
  tetani 365
  welchii 365, 365*f*
Clotrimazole 402, 801, 808
Clumps 253, 676
Clutton's joints 369
Coagulated uterine vessel, level of 1209
Coagulation
  abnormality, screening for 749
  electrodes 1039
  failure 881
  studies 127
Coagulopathy 748
Cobalt machine 696
Codeine 232
Coelomic cells 253
Coelomic epithelium 261, 288
Coelomic metaplasia 441
Coenzymes 1275
Cognitive behavioural therapy 765, 817
Coital difficulties 821
  correction of 859
Coital errors 845
Coital function, penile adequacy for 302
Coitus 5, 346, 572, 776, 782, 819
  frequency of 820, 845
  interruptus 1067
  painful 6
  regular 32
  timing of 845
  voluntary 819
Cold abscess, tuberculous 1234
Colic artery 48
Coliform bacteria 1188
Collagen 1188
Colloid
  degeneration 74
  oncotic pressure 1252
  solutions 1252
Colloidal degeneration, evidence of 158
Colon
  cancer 112
    chance of 1279
  carcinoma of 683*f*, 1226
  descending 1226
Colonic spasm 1226
Colonoscopy 1230
Colostomy, temporary diversion 1237
Colour Doppler 16, 915, 922
  assessment 994
  examination 192
Colpitis cystica 404
Colpomicroscopy 505
Colpoperineorrhaphy, posterior 342, 344, 1213
Colporrhaphy 346, 1255*f*
Colposcopy 405, 505, 528, 580, 581*t*, 894, 1195
  interpretation of 580*t*
  triage 577*fc*
Colpotomy 14, 1213*f*
Columnar epithelium 29*f*, 498, 499*f*
Combined chemotherapy regimens 646
Combined hormonal contraceptive 1064, 1092, 1100
  pills 1092
Combined oral contraceptive 747, 1094, 1098, 1101
  newer 1094
  pills 472, 639, 749, 1064, 1092, 1094, 1099
    efficacy of 1099
Common iliac artery 54
Communication skills 837
Comparative genomic hybridisation 1304
Complement inflammatory pathway 712
Complete androgen insensitivity syndrome 290, 297, 298*f*, 304, 305
Complete blood count 148, 188, 194, 219, 250, 323, 375, 458, 875
Complete gonadal dysgenesis 290
Complete mole 215, 216, 216*f*
  treatment of 218
Computed tomography 21, 142, 146, 250, 421, 584, 1172, 1174
  abdominal 21
  cystourethrography 1148, 1149*f*
  scan 21, 244, 623
Computer axial tomographic scan 236
Concentric rectal musculature 1223
Conception 150, 152, 776, 780
  cycles 127
  genetic testing of products of 173, 174
  products of 1138
Concomitant multiple hormone therapy 1202
Condom 1062, 1068, 1096, 1120
  applications of 1068*f*
  average failure rate of 1069
  female 1069*f*, 1070, 1074
  latex 1068, 1069
  male 1068, 1068*f*, 1069, 1069*f*
  rupture 1063
  silicone 1068*f*, 1070
  synthetic nonlatex 1069
  types of 1068
  use 1069
Condyloma 378, 570, 571
  acuminata 368, 378, 378*f*, 394*f*, 536, 539, 539*f*, 1239, 1294
  syphilitic 536
Condylomatous reactions 505
Cone biopsy 507, 507*f*
Congenital adrenal hyperplasia 123, 138, 160, 236, 259, 295, 296*f*, 299, 300, 301*f*, 303*f*, 304, 305, 464, 481, 738, 739, 1303
Congenital anomalies 227, 901, 1092
Congenital uterine abnormalities 971, 972*f*
  diagnosis of 1042
Congestion 334
Conical cervix 278
Conn's syndrome 1244
Connective tissue 650
  cells 36
  scar 74*f*
  secondary leucocytic infiltration of 553*f*
Conservative laparoscopic surgery 205
Constipation 1215-1217, 1225, 1226, 1228, 1245, 1288
Constituent cells 90*f*
Continual incontinence 1149
Continuous oestrogen therapy 1003
Contraceptive 776, 780, 846, 1061, 1073, 1106*t*, 1111, 1113, 1124
  action 1117
  adolescent's choice of 1123
  advantages 1082
  barrier methods of 1074
  choice of 1119, 1124
  education 1123
  efficacy of 1062
  emergency 1063, 1115
    postcoital 1115
  failure 1063, 1131
  implant 1108
    subdermal 780, 1105
  indications of 1063
  injectable 1106
  method 367, 1064, 1064*b*, 1064*t*, 1096, 1117, 1119, 1131
    hormonal 1064, 1092, 1097
  patch, transdermal 484
  pills 1103, 1119
  postpartum choice of 1119
  practice of 1135
  sponge 1073
  steroids, transfer of 1103
  vaginal ring 1095, 1095*f*
Contrast-enhanced spectral mammography 242
Controlled ovarian
  hyperstimulation 451, 869, 871*f*
  stimulation protocols 869*b*
Conventional laparoscopic ports 1053
Convolutional neural network 1309
Cooper's ligament 1157, 1161*f*
Copper 1281
  alloys of 1075
  intrauterine contraceptive devices 1083, 1085
  T 1081, 1088*f*-1090*f*

Core biopsy 238
Cornual rudimentary horn 182*f*
Cornual tubal blockage, management of 1044
Corona radiata 68*f*, 152*f*
Coronary artery disease 775
  incidence of 111
Coronary thrombosis, incidence of 80
Coronavirus infection 2019 (COVID-19) 419
Corpora lutea 73*f*
Corpus 36, 40, 40*f*, 901*b*
  albicans 74*f*, 661
  fibrosum 661
Corpus luteum 72*f*-74*f*, 158, 160, 181, 300*f*, 661, 984, 985, 986*f*, 997, 998*f*
  cyst 73*f*, 445, 658, 660, 947
  degenerates 74
  haematoma 411, 760
  life cycle of 74
  ruptured 188
Corpus uteri 38, 57
  tumours of 596
Corticosteroids 126, 308, 309, 491, 735, 769
Corticotrophin-releasing hormone 83, 791
Cortisol 226, 231, 825
  biosynthesis 1303
  low level of 295
Corynebacterium minutissimum 489
Cosmetic 309
  gynaecology 1298
    landscape of 1298
Cough
  chronic 1216
  persistent 575
  stress test 1156
Couple's therapy 837
Cowden's syndrome 1302, 1303
Cowper's glands 29, 258
Cramps, intestinal 1259
Craniopharyngioma 145, 235, 722*f*
Creatinine phosphokinase 1246
Crizotinib 689
Crohn's disease 1228, 1229, 1234, 1235
Crohn's tuberculosis 1236
Cryomyolysis, laparoscopic 613
Cryopreservation 873
Cryotherapy 405, 508
  gun 508*f*
Cryptococcus 375
Cryptoglandular infection 1234
Cryptomenorrhoea 274
  diagnosis of 275
Cryptorchidism 306, 786, 789
Cryptosporidium 375
Crystalloid solutions 1252
Cubitus valgus 292
Cuff infection 1214
Cul-de-sac, deep 344
Culdocentesis 14
Culdotomy 14
Cullen's sign 3, 185
Curative punch biopsy 508
Cusco's speculum 9*f*, 887, 887*f*
Cushing's disease 236, 481
Cushing's syndrome 145, 307, 308, 464, 481
  part of 730*f*
  screening for 484
CuT 1081, 1088*f*-1090*f*
CuT 200 1077, 1091
CuT 380 1077
CuT 380A 1091
Cutaneous nerves, division of 491
Cycle progesterone 749
Cyclebeads 1066, 1067*f*
Cyclofem 1106
Cyclo-oxygenase-2 inhibitors 713, 714
Cyclophosphamide 532, 687, 690, 716
Cycloserine 387
Cyclosporine 482, 716
Cyproterone acetate 309, 484, 1200
  pills 484
Cyst 75*f*, 443, 536, 558*f*-560*f*, 570, 596, 660, 656, 984
  excision of 550
  fimbrial 992*f*
  formation 550
  haemorrhagic 947, 949*f*, 951, 952*f*, 984, 985, 987*f*
  hymeneal 536, 538
  laparoscopic removal of 461
  lifting up 559*f*
  mesenteric 655
  myometrial 637, 980
  neoplastic 445
  nonseptated clear 984
  paraurethral 1142
  peritoneal 410
  periurethral 339
  retention 405*f*, 536, 537
  rupture of 685
  sebaceous 536, 537
  small follicle-like thin-walled 1006
  unilateral 950
  wall of 437, 559*f*
Cystadenocarcinoma
  mucinous 663
  papillary serous 668
Cystadenoma
  mucinous 295, 664, 664*f*, 953*f*
  serous 949*fc*
  typical of 665*f*
Cystectomy 73*f*
Cystic degeneration 615, 919*f*
Cystic fibrosis 862
  transmembrane conductance regulator gene 861
Cystic focal adenomyosis 981*f*
Cystic spaces 920
Cystitis 411, 1141, 1171, 1171*t*, 1172, 1173, 1258
  acute 1141
    bacterial 1176*t*
  haemorrhagic 687
  interstitial 459, 813
  recurrent 399
Cystocele 332, 332*f*
Cystometry 1146
  normal 1147*f*
Cystourethrocele 1213
Cystourethroscopy 1148
Cytochrome p450 system 452, 485
Cytogenetic abnormalities 1304
Cytokeratin 674
Cytological atypia, moderate 511*f*
Cytomegalovirus 173, 375
Cytoreductive surgery, secondary 648
Cytotoxic T-lymphocyte-associated antigen 4 703*f*
Cytotrophoblast 157

D

da Vinci surgical system 1011, 1012*f*
  parts of 20
Dacarbazine 532
Dactinomycin 690
Daefecography 1219
Damage-associated molecular pattern molecules 701
Danazol 130, 447, 449, 482, 638
Dapoxetine
  hydrochloride 824
  on-demand use of 824
Deafness 369
Death, causes of 293
Debulking surgery 671
Deep rectosigmoidal endometriosis 452
Deep rectovaginal endometriosis 452
Deep venous thrombosis 1249, 1250*t*, 1262, 1264*f*, 1265, 1266, 1269
  prevention of 1265*b*
  prophylaxis 1031, 1249, 1269
Deeply infiltrating endometriosis 442, 452
  classification 452
Defaecation 5, 362
  pain on 443
Defaecography 1224
Defibulation 318
Degeneration, types of 915
Dehydration 301, 1263
  hyponatraemic 296
Dehydroepiandrosterone 66*f*, 135, 301, 307, 453, 479, 480, 825, 1184*f*
  sulphate 142, 143, 301, 479, 480, 484, 740, 1184*f*, 1185
Deinfibulation, technique of 323*f*
Delancey 329
Delavirdine 377
Delayed puberty 135*f*, 137
  causes of 138*t*
Delorme procedure 1222
Dementia 1198, 1201
Denosumab 118
Deoxycorticosteroid 304
Deoxycorticosterone 297
  serum 737
Deoxycortisol 297
Deoxyribonucleic acid 170, 375, 703, 795, 1300
  methyltransferase 1280
  mismatch repair protein deficiency 627
  replication errors 707
Depoprovera 1110, 1120

Depot medroxyprogesterone acetate 719, 757, 1105-1107
  injection of 448
Depressants 308
Depression 111, 114, 448, 829, 841, 1081, 1100, 1143
  diagnosis of 111
Dermal fibroblasts 80
Dermatitis 1239
  vulval 793
Dermatofibrosarcoma protuberans 549
Dermis, atrophy of 488
Dermoid 952*f*, 988, 989*f*
  cyst 656, 656*f*, 660, 678*f*, 679*f*, 680, 951
    cut section of 678*f*
    large 1028*f*
Descending perineal syndrome 1223
Desipramine 232
Desmopressin 148, 1164
Desogestrel 116, 1105, 1200
Desquamation 369
Desquamative inflammatory vaginitis 793, 796
Detrusor
  dysfunction 1148
  incontinence 1151
  muscle 46, 1166*f*
    automatic contraction of 45
  overactivity 1162, 1312
  sphincter dyssynergia 1145
Developmental breast hypoplasia 235, 236
Dexamethasone 126
Diabetes mellitus 164, 469, 617, 1002, 1031, 1080, 1123
  diagnosis of 810
  non-insulin-dependent 476
Diabetic vulvitis 394
Diagnostic hysteroscopy 1038*f*
  contraindications of 1051*b*
Diaphanography 244
Diaphragm 1070-1072, 1074
  care of 1071
  removal of 1071*f*
  types of 1070, 1070*f*, 1071
  urogenital 27*f*, 29, 49, 329
Diarrhoea 1136, 1216, 1217, 1223, 1224, 1243, 1244, 1260, 1286
Diathermy 475
  coagulation 548, 554
Diazepam 233
Diazoxide 478, 482
Dichloralphenazone 232
Diclofenac 714
Didanosine 377
Dienogest 447, 449, 639, 781, 1093
  dosage of 1095
  structural formula of 781*f*
Diet 147, 241, 845
  fibre-rich 1229
Dietary calcium, source of 1284
Dietary fibre 1276, 1279
Diethylstilbestrol 124, 207, 268, 436, 573, 1198
Diffuse adenomyosis 745*f*, 921*f*, 980*f*
  diagnosis of 638*f*
Digital breast tomosynthesis 242
Digital rectal examination 1234
Digoxin 232
Dihydrotestosterone 304, 479, 728
  influence of 289
Dilatation and curettage 344, 414, 885*f*
Dilated tubular structure 960*f*
Dilator set 887*f*
Dilator therapy 836
Diltiazem 1229
Dilute vasopressin 610
Diminished sphincter tone 1219
Dinoprostone 1136
Diphallus 282
Diphtheria 395
Diplotene stage 71
Dipstick test 1174
Direct intraperitoneal insemination 878
Direct oocyte transfer 878
Directly-observed treatment short-course strategy 387
  treatment 387
Disc lesions 761
Discharge scoring systems 1250*t*
Disorders of sex development 290, 295, 304
  classification of 290*t*
  clinical features of 304*t*
  investigations of 304*t*
Dispermy 291
Displaced muscle fibres 976
Dissecting vesicovaginal space 1209
Disseminated intravascular coagulation 200
Disseminated metastatic disease 629
Distant metastasis 583
Distension machines 1041
Distension media 1039, 1051
  types of 1039
Diuretics, use of 1286
Diverticulitis 408, 411, 414, 1226
Diverticulum, excision of 552
Dizziness 118, 1100
Docosahexaenoic acid 1278
Docosapentaenoic acid 1278
Döderlein's bacilli 31, 792
Dolutegravir 377
Donor insemination 877, 877*b*
Donovan bodies 381*f*
Donovanosis 381
Dopamine receptor blocking agents, use of 145
Dopamine-depleting agents 145
Doppler guided haemorrhoidal artery ligation 1233
Doppler imaging 930
Doppler waveforms 192
Dorsal fissurectomy 1230
Dorsal lithotomy position 1207
Dostarlimab 688, 707
Double cervix 266, 909*f*
Double uterus, cavity of 271
Double vagina 268*f*, 282
Double-coiled mahua ring 1077*f*
Doughnut's sign 190
Douglas pouch 8, 14, 34, 35, 185, 351, 408, 437, 440, 962*f*, 1006
Doxorubicin 532, 687, 688
Doxycycline 370, 389, 417, 1225
Driver gene 1303, 1303*t*
Driver mutation 1303
Drospirenone 1093, 1200
Drugs 130, 232, 233, 306, 308, 403, 755, 757
  enzyme-inducing 1116
  interactions 1116
  research 1312
  sensitivity 404, 810, 1256
  therapy 460
  types of 232, 532
Dsenonvillier's fascia 1220
Duct
  complete obstruction of 550
  ectasia 239, 239*f*
  sudden obstruction of 550
  system 227, 289
Ductal proliferation 238
Ductography 244
Duloxetine 1155
Dummy transfer 872
Durvalumab 688
Dutch cap 1070
Dwarfed uterine bilateral cornual block 429*f*
Dydrogesterone 447, 448, 1200
Dye, intravasation of 427*f*
Dynorphins 82
Dyschezia 6
Dysfunctional uterine bleeding 148, 188, 233, 744, 752, 775, 780, 784, 789, 1104
Dysgerminoma 658, 677, 679, 680*f*
Dyskeratosis 568*f*
Dysmenorrhoea 5, 6, 14, 420, 442, 445, 754, 759*f*, 760, 761, 775, 788, 1091, 1104, 1288-1290
  congestive 350, 412
  endometriosis associated 448
  management of 756*fc*, 758
  membranous 760
  menstrual type of 5
  primary 457, 754
  role in 755
  secondary 457, 754, 758, 760
  spasmodic 270, 350, 606, 754, 759*f*, 780
  types of 5
  up-to-date treatment of 755
Dyspareunia 5, 6, 270, 346, 350, 351, 443, 445, 456, 821, 845, 1081, 1162, 1189, 1255
Dysplasia 500, 1102, 1239
  cervical 704
  mild 502
  moderate 502
Dyspnoea
  acute 1270
  severe 1269
Dystocia
  cervical 346
  focal 265
Dysuria 5

E

Early pregnancy
  hormonal control of 158
  loss 606

Eccentric gestational sac 205
Echinococcal cysts 655
Echogenic subendometrial lines 745*f*
Ectocervix, multilayered squamous epithelium of 32*f*
Ectopia vesicae 282*f*, 284
Ectopic endometrium 433, 434
Ectopic gestation 208, 966
Ectopic glands 455
Ectopic menstruation 5
Ectopic pregnancy 12, 179, 181, 184*f*, 185, 189, 190, 191*f*, 193, 200, 206, 208, 218, 385, 411, 412, 443, 655, 965, 1089, 1090, 1104, 1111, 1139, 1295
  aetiology of 180
  ampullary 183*f*
  chronic 184
  complications of 200
  cornual 191*f*
  course of 186*f*, 186*fc*
  diagnosis of 191*t*
  early 183*f*
  expectant management of 194*b*
  frequency of 179
  high-risk factors for 207*t*
  incidence of 420
  intramural 204
  medical treatment of 194*b*
  risk of 1114
  ruptured 191, 200
  sites of 179
  surgery for 411
  treatment of 192, 193*fc*, 208, 1027, 1295
Ectopy 497
  cervical 498
Eculizumab 712
Eczema 806, 811
Efavirenz 377
Effluvium seminis 845
Eflornithine hydrochloride 485
Eggshell calcification 919*f*
Eicosapentaenoic acid 1278
Ejaculation, premature 822, 859
Ejaculatory ducts, bilateral obstruction of 842
Elagolix 787
Elastin fibres, remodelling of 1298
Elastography 238
Electrocardiogram 250, 1031
Electrolyte 127, 219, 1241
  balance 282*f*
  disturbance 1259
  free distension media 1041
  imbalance 127, 299, 881
  studies 308
Electromechanical morcellator 1022, 1025*f*
Electromyography 1148, 1224
Electronic insufflator, high-flow 1020*f*
Electrostimulation devices 831
Electrosurgery 1023
Electrosurgical system 1040
Elephantiasis 380*f*, 395, 419*f*, 536
Elvitegravir 377
Embolectomy 1270
Embolism 853, 1139
  minor degrees of 1269
  pulmonary 1268
  risk of 363
Embryo 154*f*, 162*f*, 172*f*, 1311
  development of 156*f*
  donation 874
  implantation 710
  intrafallopian transfer 878
  loading of 872
  poor-quality 1297
  transfer 453, 869, 872, 874*f*, 994
    surgical 878
  viability, reduction of 1298
Embryoblast 156
Embryonal cell carcinoma 677
Embryonic chromosomal abnormalities 171
Embryonic disc 252
Embryonic tissues, cyst of 570
Emergency contraceptive 1063, 1115
  efficacy of 1116
  pills 1116
    hormonal 1116
    repeated use of 1116
Emotional burden 1304
Emotional instability 765
Emotional upsets 720
Emphysematous bullae, rupture of 771
Empty sella syndrome 235
Empty uterine cavity 203*f*, 205
Endo tip reusable visual access cannula 1021*f*
Endocervical canal 14, 1045, 1046
Endocervical curettage 503
Endocervical cytobrush 526*f*
Endocervical epithelium 498
Endocervical mass, large 945*f*
Endocervical mucosa 797, 1042, 1046*f*
Endocervical mucus-secreting epithelium 32*f*
Endocervical polyp 1046*f*
Endocervix 370, 402*f*, 525
Endocrinal tests 234
Endocrine 236
  abnormalities 164
  disorders 232, 729
    types of 729*fc*
  disrupting chemicals 241
  system 78, 81
Endocrinopathies, immune mediated 688
Endoderm 257
Endodermal sinus 658
  tumour 549
Endometria, secretory 92*f*
Endometrial ablation 1043, 1296, 1296*f*
Endometrial aspiration 13, 386, 609, 622
  cannula 13*f*
Endometrial biopsy 13, 386, 387, 844, 852, 893, 1049*f*
  curette 890, 890*f*
  examination of 618*f*, 623*f*
Endometrial calcification 983, 985*f*
Endometrial cancer 217, 525, 616, 627, 629, 688, 752, 777*f*, 1017*f*, 1045*f*, 1051, 1102, 1104, 1201
  diagnosis of 1309
  immunotherapy in 704
  low-risk 629
  radiotherapy in 697
  risk of 1302
  staging of 623
Endometrial carcinoma 42*f*, 596, 627, 688, 1004, 1005, 1042
  classification of 619*b*
  high risk of 1004*f*
  histological types of 619
  radiation in 697
Endometrial cavity 422*f*, 631*f*, 929*f*, 939*f*, 943*f*, 982, 985*f*
  distortion of 914*f*
  evaluation of 750
  fluid 934
Endometrial cells 442
Endometrial changes 121, 900*f*
Endometrial cycle 88, 927
  correction of 92
  hormonal control of 95*f*
Endometrial cytology 751
Endometrial destruction 420
Endometrial glandular hyperplasia 510*f*
Endometrial hyperplasia 117, 509, 510*f*, 596, 618*f*, 929, 933*fc*, 934, 981, 982, 982*f*, 1004, 1042, 1093, 1113
Endometrial intraepithelial neoplasia 617, 618*f*
Endometrial lesions 975, 983
  diagnosis of 983
  treatment of 749
Endometrial lining, destruction of 934
Endometrial maturation 994
Endometrial metaplasia 512
Endometrial morphology, abnormal 1002
Endometrial myometrial border 637
Endometrial polyp 457, 596, 597*f*, 930, 937*f*, 941*f*, 982, 983*f*, 1005*f*, 1042
  large 938*f*
Endometrial sampling 421, 748, 1195
  procedures 13
  suction devices 13
Endometrial serous carcinoma 625*f*
Endometrial spill 440
Endometrial stroma 961
Endometrial stromal sarcoma 630, 632*f*
  low-grade 632, 682
Endometrial stromal tumours 632
Endometrial thickness 94*f*, 1001, 1003
Endometrial tissue sampling 525
Endometrial ulceration 432
Endometrial vascularity 927*f*, 928*f*, 929
Endometrioid
  benign 665
  borderline tumours 666
  carcinoma 619, 624, 625*f*, 626*f*, 642, 668, 945*f*
    endometrium stage 697*fc*
    low-grade 624
    treatment schema for 697
Endometrioma 23*f*, 951, 952*f*, 985, 986, 987*f*
  bilateral 961*f*
  encapsulation of 434
Endometrio-myometrial junction 982

Endometriosis 5, 47, 177, 183, 188, 200, 351, 433, 437, 438, 440*f*, 441, 443, 446, 447*f*, 451, 452, 452*t*, 457, 655, 781, 784, 788, 960, 1104, 1202, 1225, 1238, 1247, 1295, 1300
cervical 455, 456, 942
deep 961*f*, 962*f*
infiltrating 962*f*
immunotherapeutic methods for 713*fc*
immunotherapy in 712
lesions 1295
mass of 435*f*
mild 450
pathological lesions in 435*f*
progression 450
propagation of 441
prophylaxis 1104
resection 1016
risk of 436
severe 453, 1031, 1248
sign of 1309
sites of 437
superficial 961*f*, 1295
theories of sites of 441*t*
treatment of 446, 450, 452, 1027
ultrasound evaluation of 962
ureteric 439*f*
Endometriotic cysts 435*f*, 438*f*, 440*f*, 446*f*, 558, 662
rupture of 411, 435
Endometriotic deposits 536
Endometriotic lesion 433, 439
Endometriotic tissue 442
atrophy of 449
Endometritis 388, 402*f*, 406, 407, 414, 752, 793, 931, 981, 982, 982*f*, 1091
acute 406
chronic 406
puerperal 407
tuberculous 407, 843
Endometrium 36, 81*f*, 94*f*, 96, 97, 97*f*, 402*f*, 431, 510, 511*f*, 512, 926, 927, 931*f*, 995, 996, 996*f*, 997, 1002, 1005, 1195
adenocarcinoma of 620*f*
air in 933
atrophy 1003
basal layer of 432
cancer of 115, 934, 934*f*, 935*f*
carcinoma of 616, 617*f*
columnar epithelium of 512
dating of 122*f*
early proliferative 89*f*
ectopic 433, 434
evaluation of 750
hyperplastic 932*f*
infection of 931
inflammation of 931
invasive carcinoma of 619
irregular 934
midsecretory 91*f*
normal 926
periodic shedding of surface 364
postmenopausal 935*f*
preovulatory 995
roller ball ablation of 1047*f*
secretory 37*f*, 92*f*
shrinkage of 92
thick 932*f*, 933*fc*, 1007*f*
thin 1002*f*
transcervical resection of 1043, 1047*f*
ultrasound evaluation of 1002
volume histogram of 997*f*
Endomyometrial ablation 639
Endomyometrial junction 637, 899*f*, 923*f*
Endopelvic fascia 327
attachment of 1161*f*
deep 329
Endorphin 82
Endosalpingiosis 455
Endosalpinx 408
higher magnification of 41*f*
Endoscopic techniques 387
Endoscopy 17, 421
cart 1025*f*
type of 1019
Endothelins 755
End-to-end technique 313
Enema 1225
Energy 591, 1280, 1285
Enfuvirtide 377
Engorgement, painful 229
Enseal 1023
Entamoeba histolytica 390
Enterobacteriaceae 408
Enterobius 810
Enterocele 330, 342
repair 342
types of 333
Enterococci 1173
Entrectinib 689
Enuresis 1163
treatment of 1163
Environmental toxins 165
Enzymatic reactions 1280
Enzyme 158, 1173
deficiency of 1303
immunoassay 393
parts of 1275
Enzyme-linked immunosorbent assay 372, 387
Ephedrine 1155
Epidermal growth factor 441
Epidermis, atrophy of 488
Epidermoid cyst 536, 537, 538*f*, 558
Epididymis
bilateral obstruction of 842
obstruction of 861
Epigastric vessels 1036
Epigenetic theory 637
Epilepsy 771
menstrual 771
Epiphyseal closure 775, 785
Epipodophyllotoxins 533
Episiotomy
requirement for 324
scar 439, 441, 1290
selective 323
Epispadias 284
Epithelial abnormalities 487, 496
oral 492
Epithelial cellular integrity 1284
Epithelial membrane antigen 674
Epithelial ovarian cancer 667, 686, 691, 1129, 1302
advanced-stage 671
early stage 691
lower incidence of 1130
Epithelial ovarian tumours 658, 663, 674
Epithelial tumours 574, 988, 989
benign 664, 665
malignant 666, 692
Epithelial vulvar disease, classification of 488*b*
Epithelioid 630
granuloma 430
trophoblastic tumours 217
Epithelium 31, 489
atrophies 32
lined tract 1228
thickened 505*f*
transitional 553*f*
Eplerenone 1245
Epoophoron 50, 254*f*, 649
Epsilon-aminocaproic acid 1268
Epstein-Barr virus 703
Equine oestrogen, conjugated 1193, 1198
Erectile dysfunction 821, 822, 823*f*, 824
psychogenic 823*t*
treatment for 822
Erosive lichen planus 793
Erythema ab igne 723
Erythrocyte sedimentation rate 139, 875
Erythromycin 232, 370, 374, 389, 472, 1177, 1225, 1248, 1258
Escherichia coli 169, 365, 395, 808, 1075, 1173, 1175, 1176, 1179, 1234
infection 805
Ethacridine 1137
lactate 1137
Ethambutol 387, 388, 430
Ethanolamine oleate 1233
Ethinyloestradiol 115, 130, 1092, 1094, 1198
Ethionamide 387
Ethosuximide 1104
Ethylene vinyl
acetate copolyme 1095
alcohol 1161
Ethynodiol diacetate 1105
Etidronate 118
Etonogestrel implant 1111
Etoposide 222, 690, 692
active principle 533
Evra patch 1097
Exacerbation 460
Excisional procedures 508, 564
Exenteration 534
Exercise 145, 1274, 1287
isotonic resistance 1192
postnatal 1288
postoperative 1289
prescription of 1197
techniques 765
Exogenous oestrogen 1103
Expulsion 1090
faulty powers of 1225
rate 1091

Extensive iliofemoral thrombosis 1270
Extensive proliferative cancer 543*f*
External beam radiotherapy 588, 589, 593, 686, 697
  treatment volumes for 697
External cervical muscle 37
External genital organs, anatomy of 28*f*
External genitalia 257*f*, 287, 289, 292, 292*t*, 294, 312
  deformity of 303*f*
  examination of 301
External iliac
  artery 54
  nodes 40
External pudendal arteries 55
Extracellular fluid 1241
Extracervical adhesions 456
Extracorporeal knot-tying and suturing technique 1026, 1027*f*
Extraovarian cystic lesion 990
Extraperitoneal laser surgery 1294
Extraperitoneal lymphadenectomy, bilateral 588
Extrauterine echogenic ring 190
Extrauterine endometriosis 433
  classical symptom of 442
  operative diagnosis of 435
Extrauterine leiomyomas 602
Extrauterine mass 655*f*
Extreme glandular coiling 91*f*

F

Faecal fistula 314, 1272, 1273
  types of 314*fc*
Faecal incontinence 531, 805, 1216, 1223, 1224, 1224*t*
  major 1223
  minor 1223
Faeculent discharges 793
Fainting attack 418
Fallopian tubes 40, 49, 57, 60, 77, 179, 181, 192*f*, 201*f*, 277, 360, 361*f*, 383, 402*f*, 420, 431, 432, 438, 512, 642, 645, 959, 959*f*, 960*f*, 970, 1113, 1129, 1292
  abnormal 970
  bilateral 428*f*
    adenocarcinomas of 645*f*
  blood supply of 42*f*
  cancer 523, 691
    histopathology of 645
    prevention of 648
    screening test for 645
  carcinoma of 646*t*
  diverticulum of 181, 183*f*
  end of 72
  endometriosis of 181
  inflammation of 989
  laparoscopic visualisation of 1030*f*
  malignancy, primary 644*t*
  mucosa of 41*f*
  secretion 792
  sperm perfusion 878
  torsion of 361*f*
  tumours of 642
Falope ring 1030*f*, 1053, 1129
  applications of 1030*f*
Family planning 896
Fascia 32
Fast-track protocol 1254
  goals of 1254*b*
Fast-track surgery 1254
Fat 1275, 1277, 1282, 1286
  distribution 1189
  emulsions, intravenous 710
  monounsaturated 1278
  necrosis 239, 239*f*
    histology of 240*f*
  polyunsaturated 1278
  sources of 1277
Fatty acids
  essential 764, 1279
  polyunsaturated 1278
  saturated 1278
  unsaturated 231
Fatty degeneration, calcification 615
Fatty tissue 1299
Faulty sexual development 228, 230
Feedback loops 84, 84*f*
Feeding vessel 983*f*
Feig's imaging protocol 245*t*
Fellatio 819
Fem cap 1073
Female arousal disorder 826
Female breast
  development of 133*f*, 227*t*
  endocrine control of 226
  function 227*t*
Female genital mutilation 318, 319*f*, 320
  classification of 318, 319*f*, 319*t*
  prevalence of 318, 319*f*
Female genital tract 792
  development of 261*t*
  injuries 312
  malformations 264, 265*f*
    classification of 263, 264*t*
    complications of 264*t*
  physiology of 1
Female genital tuberculosis 419
  hysteroscopic evidence of 430
  incidence of 382
  laparoscopic evidence of 430
  management 430
  multidrug-resistant 388
  signs of 420, 420*t*
  stepwise decision 430
  symptoms of 420, 420*t*
Female genitalia 319
  removal of external 318
Female hypoactive desire disorder 821
Female infertility 840, 1298
  assessment of 851
  causes of 473*f*
  prevention of 868
  unexplained 858*fc*
Female orgasmic disorder 821, 829
  evaluation of 830
  treatment of 830
Female pelvic
  anatomy, normal 897
  organ prolapse 331*f*
Female reproductive cycle 96*t*
Female reproductive system
  benign disease of 433
  embryonic formation of 263*f*
  parts of 898*f*
Female sexual dysfunction 821*t*
  prevalence of 826
  type of 833
Female sexual function index 830
Female sterilisation 1129
  complications of 1132*t*
  techniques of 1131*t*
Female urethra 1142*f*
Female urogenital anatomy, normal 805*f*
Feminine reconstructive surgeries 302
Feminism 303, 304
  causes of 306
Femoral neck fractures 593
Femoral node 563
Femoral veins 1268
Femovan 1106
Fern test 122*f*
Ferning pattern 1066*f*
Ferriman-Gallwey score, modified 464, 482
Fertile period 151, 1065*f*
Fertilisation 151*f*, 288*fc*
  rates, lower 879
Fertilised ovum, development of 153*f*
Fertility 656, 781, 845, 976, 1103
  awareness-based methods 152, 1064
  concept of 840
  issue 654
  male 847
  management 476
  rate, free 1062
  return of 1109, 1114
  sparing 587
Fesoterodin 1155
Fever 1286
Fibre 1279, 1294
  sources of 1279
Fibre-optic fibres 1294
Fibrinolysins 1267, 1268
Fibrinolysis 112
Fibroadenoma 238, 238*f*
Fibroadenosis 784
Fibroblasts 287*f*
Fibrocystic breast changes 1202
Fibrocystic disease 112, 238
Fibroids 457, 597, 599*f*, 609, 952*f*, 975, 976, 978, 1112, 1202, 1204, 1300
  cervical 570, 919*f*
  classification of 978*f*
  clinical symptoms of 606*b*
  colour Doppler 978*f*
  degenerated 188, 915
  growth of 747
  hysterectomy specimen of 600*f*
  intracavitary 599*f*
  intramural 976
  management of 608*fc*
  mapping 915

medical therapy for 608
multiple 600*f*, 914*f*, 978*f*
polyps 599*f*, 745, 752, 917*f*
small 1295
sonographic evaluation of 915*fc*
uterus 600*f*
Fibroma 555, 559, 642, 658, 674, 952*f*, 988
Fibromatosis, diffuse 918*f*
Fibromyalgia 813
Fibromyoma 117, 536, 597
Fibromyomatous tissue reaction 454
Fibrositis 112, 457
Fibrous tissue 598*f*
Figure-of-eight sutures 1208
Fimbria, disappearance of 409*f*
Fimbrial salpingoscopy 14
Fimbriolysis 866
Finasteride 309, 472, 485
Fine-needle aspiration 238, 862
cytology 246
Finger pressure 353
Fissure 369, 752, 1229, 1229*f*, 1230
Fissure-in-Ano 1228
acute 1229
chronic 1229, 1229*f*
Fistula 340, 384, 1236, 1243, 1273
complicated 316
extrasphincteric 1236*f*
formation 564, 1235
obstetric 315
pregnancy after cure of 316
prevention of 316
probing of 1236*f*
types of 314, 314*fc*
urethrorectal 315, 1149*f*
Fistula-in-Ano 1235, 1236*f*
anterior 1237*f*
differential diagnosis of 1236
long-standing 1239
multiple 1236*f*
used for 1238*t*
Fistulectomy specimen 1237
Fitz-Hugh-Curtis syndrome 379, 380, 1028*f*
Flatulence 460
Flatus, incontinence of 1224*t*
Flexible plastic petals 1077*f*
Flibanserin 828, 829
contraindications of 829
Floridiform 1219
Fluconazole 402, 801, 802, 808
Flufenamic acid 757
Fluid 1006, 1241
collection, irregular areas of 939*f*
elimination of 765
endometrial 934
fluid level 987*f*
globules of 31
loss of 1255
premenstrual restriction of 768
removal of 127
replacement 1252
retention 785
therapy 169
thrill 7
Fluorescence in situ hybridisation 1304
Fluorescent
antibody 393
dyes 386
treponemal antibody absorption test 369
Fluoride 1281
Fluorodeoxyglucose positron emission tomography 542
Fluoroquinolones 1175, 1177
Fluorouracil 222, 532, 562, 686, 1240
Fluoxetine 824
Flutamide 309, 472, 485
Foam 1096
Foetal adrenal insufficiency
primary 160
secondary 160
Foetal anomalies 175
Foetal aromatase deficiency 295
Foetal blood 157
Foetal distress 368
Foetal growth restriction 175, 216
Foetal loss, proposed mechanisms of 163*f*
Foetal medicine 1
Foetal ovarian stroma differentiates 262
Foetal tissue 216
Foetal vessels 216
Foetoplacental unit secretes 207
Foetus
formation of 155
malposition of 607
malpresentation of 607
Folate 1275
antagonists 532
Foley's catheter 198
Folic acid 118, 208, 232, 489, 490, 1284
sources of 1284
supplementation 1284
Folinic acid 222
Follicle
cyst 660
mature 68
rupture of 71
Follicle-stimulating hormone 70*f*, 82, 83, 84*f*, 95*f*, 101*f*, 113, 120, 125*f*, 127*f*, 129, 130, 141, 143, 236, 294, 304, 464, 465, 469, 482, 721, 738*f*, 739, 740, 786, 842, 844, 859, 862-865, 870*f*, 875, 993, 1096, 1184*f*, 1303
elevated 740*fc*
high 106
levels of 86*f*
plasma levels of 82*f*
receptor 1303
gene polymorphism 1303
release of 449
Follicular 5 alfa-reductase inhibitor 309
Follicular assessment 995
Follicular atresia 74
delayed 1114
Follicular cyst 510, 510*f*, 661, 947, 948*f*, 949*fc*, 984
wall of 662*f*
Follicular development, inhibition of 1105
Follicular dysfunction 145
Follicular fluid escapes 72
Follicular phase 61, 67
Follicular recruitment fails 1001
Follicular ring sign 963, 988*f*
Follistatin 81
Forbes-Albright syndrome 235
Forkhead box protein 658, 674
Fosfomycin 1177
tromethamine 1176
Fothergill's operation 343, 1130
Fourchette epidermoid cyst 538*f*
Fourier transform infrared spectroscopy 1312
Fox-Fordyce disease 810
Fracture, common sites of 1192*f*
Frank's dilators 728
Frank's non-surgical method 281
Frank's procedure 281
Frazee operative laparoscope 1056*f*
Free testosterone 483, 825
levels 465
Free thyroxine 739
levels 138
Frohlich syndrome 841
Frusemide 232, 1244
Fundal leiomyoma 269*f*, 357*f*
Fundamental radiographic sign 46
Fungal infection 810
sites for 492
Fungicides 491
Fungus infection 490*f*
Furunculosis 391
Fusion inhibitor 377
Fusobacterium 394

G

Gabapentin 461, 816
Gadolinium enhancement 733*f*
Galactography 244, 245*f*
Galactokinesis 230, 231
Galactopoiesis reflex 234*f*
Galactorrhoea 145, 232, 233, 482, 1111
causes of 233, 235*t*
evidence of 733
pathophysiology of 233
Galactosemia 138
Gallbladder disease 115, 1080, 1201
Galvanic electrolysis 472
Gamete intrafallopian transfer 858, 878
Gamma-aminobutyric acid 234*f*
Gamma-linolenic acid 1278
Ganglion-blocking agents 720
Gangrene 360*f*
Gardnerella vaginalis 365, 367, 402, 794*f*, 798, 808
Gartner's cyst 339
Gartner's duct 42*f*, 559, 650
cyst of 552
rudimentary 254
vestigial 50
Gas embolism 853, 1035, 1051
Gaseous distension medium 1039
Gastric
suction 1242

tube 1260
ulceration 450
Gastroenteritis 188, 1244
Gastrointestinal tract 457, 458, 1241
Gatifloxacin 1176
Gemcitabine 692
Gemeprost 1135, 1136
Gene
deletions 262
mutation, hereditary 1302
polymorphism 600
Genetic
anomalies 172*f*
applications of 1304
counselling 1304
counsellor's role 1304
engineering 1311
factors 163, 768, 1283
sex 287
testing 174, 302, 1300, 1304
GeneXpert 430
Genital anomalies 834
Genital cancer 522, 523*b*, 534
significance of 522
Genital cosmetic surgery, female 320
Genital crisis 751
Genital discharge 367*b*
Genital diseases 392
Genital ducts, development of 300*f*
Genital examination 825, 830
Genital fistula 314
Genital herpes 366, 392
Genital human papillomavirus 377
Genital infection 321
screening 322
Genital Koch's, typical of 426*f*
Genital mesentery 252*f*
Genital molluscum contagiosum 366
Genital mycoplasmas 312, 366, 380
Genital organs
external 28*f*
internal 36*f*
supports of 52
Genital prolapse 335, 1195
Genital ridge 253
Genital scabies 366
Genital scarring 320
Genital schistosomiasis 390
Genital sexual syndrome 112
Genital suspension operations, laparoscopy for 1029
Genital system, female 31*f*
Genital tract 80, 364, 456, 777
epithelial abnormalities of 487
female 792
fistula 312
lower 1294
maldevelopments of 259
malformations of 259
natural defences of 364
obstruction 436
Genital tuberculosis 382, 419, 1195
female 419
investigation of 387*b*
Genital ulcer
diseases 373
differential diagnosis of 373*b*
recurrent 393
Genital urinary syndrome 112
Genital vitiligo 821
Genital wart therapies 540
Genitalia 136
ambiguous 299
atypical 300
external 257*f*, 287, 289, 292, 292*t*, 294, 312
female 319
feminine external 298*f*
internal 304
Genito-pelvic penetration disorder 821, 832
Genitourinary syndrome 112, 1189, 1297
Genome-wide association 1303
Genomic, applications of 1304
Gentamicin 232, 1247, 1248
Genuine stress incontinence 1150
diagnosis of 1152
Germ cells 289, 294
sex cord-stromal tumours 660, 681
tumours 642, 659, 677-679
Gestation, ectopic 208, 966
Gestational sac 191*f*
embryonic 162
implantation of 202
Gestational trophoblastic disease 214
classification of 214*t*, 221
low-risk 220*fc*
staging of 221
Gestational trophoblastic neoplasia 214, 221, 222, 523, 689
immunotherapy in 708
low-risk 708
prognostic scoring index for 690*t*
Gestational trophoblastic tumour
exception of 534
high-risk 222, 223
low-risk 222*t*
treatment of 222
Gestodene 447, 449, 787, 1094, 1200
Giant condyloma acuminata 1239
Giemsa stain plus trypsin 287*f*
Glairy fluid, secretion of 230
Glands 230
acini of 550*f*
atrophy of 1083
ectopic 455
endometrial 38, 88, 97*f*, 961, 1113
paraurethral 43
sebaceous 27
secretion of 29, 89*f*
Glandular elements 447*f*
Glandular hypertrophy 334
Glandular tissue 229
excision of 230*f*
Glans clitoris, oedema of 536
Global tuberculosis report 419
Global vaginismus 835
Globular uterine enlargement 637, 919
Glucocorticoid-induced tumour necrosis factor receptor-related protein 703*f*
Glucocorticoids 174, 715, 1256
agents 485
Glucose 1173, 1243
oxidation of 474
tolerance 777
impaired 469
transporter 474
Glutaraldehyde 1155, 1161
Gluteus maximus 1288
Glycaemia 1276
Glycaemic index 1276, 1276*f*
range 1277
values, classification of 1277*t*
Glycine 1040
Glycoproteins 68, 158
Glycosuria 391
Glycyrrhizin 714
Golaris classification 881
Gonadal development 904*fc*
disorders of 262, 290
Gonadal dysgenesis 276, 290
partial 290
Gonadal regression 290
Gonadal sex 287
Gonadal size 143
Gonadectomy 303, 305
Gonadoblastoma 681
Gonadomimetic agents 1202
Gonadomimetic synthetic steroid 117
Gonadotrophin 85, 107, 126-128, 135, 301, 305, 736, 870*f*, 871*f*, 994, 1303
analogues 145
levels 138
measurement of 141
normal release of 137
outpouring of 86
pituitary 785
production of 111
recombinant 786
release 309
secretion of 294
therapy 126, 475, 787, 862
types of 785
very low-dose 475
Gonadotrophin-releasing hormone 70*f*, 74, 83, 84, 84*f*, 125*f*, 128, 135, 138, 141-143, 447, 453, 464, 465, 608, 652, 738*f*, 747, 758, 764, 791, 860, 871*f*, 872, 874*f*, 1031, 1067, 1119, 1184, 1184*f*, 1296, 1303
agonists 128, 129*fc*, 309, 449, 453, 608, 638, 736, 748, 765, 788-790, 871*f*, 1031
indications of 789*t*
analogue 272, 639, 977
antagonists 128, 129, 787, 871*f*
associated protein 234*f*
production 309
secretion 720
stimulation 234
Gonadotrophin-resistant testis 299
Gonads 253, 293, 304
appears, primordium of 261
influence of 300*f*
removed 728*f*

Gonococcal proctitis 1238
Gonococcal tonsillitis 371
Gonococci 370
Gonocytes 261
Gonorrhoea 366, 367, 370, 370*f*, 405, 798, 800, 1075
  acute 371*f*
  diplococci 372*f*
  elimination of 868
Goodsall's ligature 1218, 1218*f*
Goodsall's rule 1236, 1237*f*
Goserelin 447, 449, 693, 748
Graafian follicle 15, 68*f*, 69*f*, 75*f*, 82, 661
Gracilis muscle, tendon of 1224
Gräfenberg ring 1084*f*, 1085*f*
  broken 1086*f*
  extrauterine 1086*f*
  extrauterine position of 1086*f*
  intrauterine position of 1085*f*
Gram staining 798
Granulation tissue 1272
Granulocyte colony-stimulating factor 709
Granuloma 560
  inguinale 366, 373, 381, 381*f*, 394, 394*f*, 1225
  primary 369
Granulomatous caruncle 553
Granulosa
  cells 67, 67*f*, 72*f*, 662*f*
    corona radiata of 68*f*
    luteinisation of 676
    tumour 510, 658, 674, 675, 675*f*, 676, 676*f*
  lutein cells 72*f*
  single layer of 63
Grasping forceps, types of 1042*f*
Gravid uterus 358*f*
Gravigard 1077*f*
Grey-Turner artery forceps, set of 884
Griseofulvin 1104, 1116
Groin
  nodes 563
  pain 342
Groove sign 379
Growth 479
  cycle 531
  factor 444
    macrophage-derived 441
  hormone 83, 132, 231, 862, 863
    releasing hormone 83
  primary 547
  ulceroproliferative 551*f*
Guanethidine 232
Guilt sentiment 1304
Gunshot lesions 446
Gunthur-Tulip filter 1270
Gut, mesentery of 252*f*
Gynaecological brachytherapy, radioactive sources for 591*t*
Gynaecological cancer 1300, 1301, 1309
  genetics of 1300
  immunotherapy in 702
  surgery 1017
  treatment of 687
Gynaecological diseases 188
Gynaecological emergencies 962
Gynaecological examination 322
  part of 7
Gynaecological malignancies 686, 688, 703*f*, 1207
  management of 1017
  radiotherapy in 695
Gynaecological oncology 1
Gynaecological operation 457, 888, 1260
  types of 1251
Gynaecological problems 3*fc*
Gynaecological procedures 884, 892
Gynaecological resectoscope 1052
Gynaecological surgery 1247
Gynaecological urology 1
Gynaecology 772, 896, 1019, 1056*b*, 1287, 1292, 1300, 1306, 1307
  lasers in 1297
Gynaecomastia 294, 300, 304, 305, 305*f*, 778*f*, 787
Gynandroblastomas 480, 481
Gynefix 1081-1083, 1083*f*
  device 1081
  insertion of 1083*f*

H

Haemangioma 642
Haemangiopericytoma 634
Haematocele, pelvic 414, 1224
Haematocolpos 274, 348
  unilateral 273*f*
Haematocrit 1283
Haematoma 536
  formation 1036, 1229, 1261, 1272, 1298
  intrauterine 864
  management of 312*fc*
  vulvar 312
Haematometra 273*f*, 619, 619*f*, 1052
  seat of 759*f*
Haematosalpinx 191, 361*f*, 570*f*, 960
Haematoxylin and eosin-stained section 626*f*
Haemi-uterus 266, 974
  rudimentary contralateral 268*f*
Haemoglobin 148, 375, 1283, 1294
  concentration 1249
Haemoperitoneum 184*f*, 1260
Haemophilus
  ducreyi 365
  influenzae 416
Haemorrhage 270*f*, 322, 530, 614, 656, 1092, 1138, 1162, 1214, 1255-1257
  active intra-abdominal 208
  intractable 580, 675*f*
  intraperitoneal 188
  postoperative 1036
  postpartum 175, 263, 606, 749
  secondary 1251, 1257
  type of 1256
Haemorrhoidal cushions 1230
Haemorrhoidopexy, stapled 1233, 1233*f*
Haemorrhoids 752, 1230, 1232, 1233*f*, 1234
  complications of 1232
  degrees of 1231
  external 1234, 1234*f*, 1234*t*
  internal 1234*t*
  internoexternal 1233*f*
  overenthusiastic treatment for 1225
Haemostasis 1295
Haemostatic instruments 1023
Haemothorax, cyclical 770
Hair 306
  abdominal 1032
  follicles 27
  growth 108, 306
    physiology of 478
  terminal 478
  tuft of 1228
  types of 478
  unwanted 478
Hair-bearing skin 26
Halogen light 1022*f*
Haloperidol 145
Hanging drop test 1033
Harbouring metastasis 672
Harmonic scalpel 1023, 1210
Haultain's operation 357
Hay–Ison criteria 798
Headache 118, 1096, 1100, 1143
  severe vascular 1104
Healthcare 110
Heaney clamp 1208
Hearing loss 532
Heart
  disease
    coronary 1194, 1286
    risk of 1278
Heavy menstrual bleeding 420, 749
  treatment of 1095
Helium-neon beam 1294
Hematometra 945*f*
Hemizona assay 850
Heparin 232, 712, 1266, 1271
  low-dose 1250, 1266
Heparinisation 127
Hepatic metastasis 223
Hepatitis 688
  B
    core 874
    infections 321
    surface antigen 874, 875
    virus 366, 703
  C 321
    virus 703, 875
Hepatocellular adenomas 1102
Herbal therapies 119
Hereditary breast cancer syndrome 1302
Hereditary nonpolyposis colorectal cancer 616
Hereditary ovarian cancer syndrome 1302
Hernia 340
  diaphragmatic 259
  incisional 1036
  inguinal 299, 536, 555
  tentorial 1243
  uterine inguinale 299, 300
Heroin 232

Herpes
genitalis 392
infection, severe manifestations of 392
simplex
genitalis, primary 393
virus 173, 365, 373, 392
Heterosexual impulses 306
Heterosexual libido 784
Hidradenitis suppurativa 392, 1236
Hidradenoma 536, 538*f*
High-density lipoproteins 80, 111
levels of 470
High-grade squamous intraepithelial lesion 492, 503, 540, 579, 580
Hilus cell tumours 481
Hinged spring circumference 340
Hip
abduction 1037
fractures 112
Hirsutism 233, 306, 307, 464, 472, 473*f*, 478, 482, 727, 789
cosmetic treatment of 485
grading severity of 483*f*
treatment of 472
Histidine 1277
Histiocytes 122
Histone
acetyltransferase 1280
deacetylase 1280
Histopathological examination 220, 421, 568*f*, 933
Histoplasma 375
Hodge pessary 352*f*
Holmium 18
Homan's sign 1263
Homan's test 1263
Homeobox gene 293
Homocysteinaemia 1284
Homogeneous hyaline tissue, corpus albicans of 74*f*
Homogeneous radiation beam 696
Homosexuality 825
Hormonal assay 304
Hormonal assessment 825, 850
Hormonal changes 96, 834, 1183
Hormonal contraception
methods 1064, 1092, 1097
pill 1116
types of 1092
Hormonal drugs, side effects of 749
Hormonal fluctuations 764
Hormonal imbalances 826
Hormonal influence 769, 900*f*
Hormonal pharmacological agents, types of 1198
Hormonal profile 1189
Hormonal treatments 832
Hormone 148, 226, 231, 241, 260, 769
administration, method of 1199*t*
agonist 1117
analysis 460
antagonist 1117
assays 122, 308, 733, 852
delivery system 1199
disturbances 145
dosage of 1095*t*
hypothalamic 83, 790
imbalance 754
influences 488
levels 70*f*, 86, 159*f*
pituitary 81
placental 158
posterior lobe 81
receptor assays 534
replacement therapy 112, 114, 117, 302, 482, 752, 764, 781, 933, 1002, 1003
therapy 106, 139, 447, 534, 629, 638, 735, 757, 766, 772, 861, 1187, 1201
Horseshoe kidney 285, 286
Host immune system 702
Hot flushes 1186, 1199
differential diagnosis of 1187
physiology of 1186
Hulka clip 1130
Human chorionic gonadotrophin 74, 113, 125*f*, 127*f*, 129, 130, 139, 141, 158, 194, 195, 208, 209, 216, 219-221, 304, 476, 482, 596, 657, 658, 690, 708, 786, 858, 870, 870*f*, 871*f*, 874*f*, 1081, 1108, 1118
clinical application of 159
Human corpus luteum 160
Human digestive tract 1275
Human epididymis protein 657, 658
Human gonadotrophins 127*f*
Human hypogonadotropic hypogonadism, genetics of 1303
Human immunodeficiency virus 8, 173, 231, 321, 365, 374, 376, 518-521, 578, 795, 807, 819, 872, 874, 1062, 1098, 1099, 1228, 1249
infection 374, 394, 518, 541, 1080, 1123
status 514, 518
Human leucocyte antigen 170
Human menopausal gonadotrophin 844
Human papillomavirus 365, 373, 487, 488, 502, 503, 514-516, 518-520, 525, 540, 551*f*, 576-579, 703, 1239, 1300
infection 505, 572
testing 527
high-risk 504, 527
Human placental
gonadotrophin 785
lactogen 159, 217
Human sperm motility 1298
Human spermatozoa 151
Human tissue cells 1275
Hutchison's incisors 369
Hyaline degeneration 615, 915
Hydatid cysts 655
Hydatidiform mole 183, 689
complete 216*t*
partial 216*t*
Hydrocele 536
Hydrocortisone 1241
Hydrogenated fats 1278
Hydronephrosis 341
Hydrops 292, 368
tubae profluens 642
Hydrosalpinges 409*f*
Hydrosalpingography 427*f*, 428*f*
bilateral terminal 427*f*
Hydrosalpinx 14, 361*f*, 408, 409*f*, 410*f*, 655, 952*f*, 959, 960*f*, 990*f*
bilateral 425*f*, 426*f*
pathogenesis of 409
Hydroxy steroid dehydrogenase, expression of 442
Hydroxychloroquine 174, 711*f*, 712
Hydroxyindoleacetic acid 1187
Hydroxylase deficiency 296
Hydroxypregnenolone 465
Hydroxyprogesterone 483, 1200
Hydroxysteroid dehydrogenase deficiency 66*f*, 297
Hygroma, cystic 292
Hymen 28, 274
abnormalities of 283
Hymenal edges 819
Hymenal laceration 331
Hyperaemia 498
Hyperandrogenic insulin-resistant acanthosis nigricans syndrome 480
Hyperandrogenism 464, 465, 478
biochemical 463
causes of 480
clinical 463
diagnosis of 482
worsening 464
Hyperchromatic tumour cells 676
Hyperconvex nails 292
Hyperechoic islands 637, 745*f*
Hyperhomocysteinaemia 173
Hyperinsulinaemia 465
compensatory 467
Hyperkalaemia 1245, 1246
Hyperkalaemic acidosis 296
Hyperkeratotic vulvar epithelial disorder 811*f*
Hyperlipidaemia 1243
Hypernatraemia 1243, 1244
acute 1243
chronic 1244
Hyperosmolar urea 1137
Hyperpigmentation 301
Hyperpigmented macules, benign 1298
Hyperplasia 238, 509, 510
atypical 509
simple 510*f*, 930*f*
types of 929
Hyperplastic prickle cell layer 378
Hyperprolactinaemia 144
clinical features of 145*t*
management of 146*fc*
Hyperproteinaemia 1243
Hyperreactio luteinalis 660
Hyperreninaemia 1244
Hypersecretion, persistent 475
Hypersensitivity 755
Hyperstimulation syndrome 474, 874*f*
Hypertension 601, 782, 881, 1031, 1101, 1136, 1202
pregnancy-induced 234*f*
pulmonary 1269

Hyperthermic intraperitoneal chemotherapy 647, 673
Hyperthyroidism 306
Hypertonic saline 1137
Hypertrichosis 478
Hypertriglyceridaemia 1201
Hypertrophied granulosa cells 72*f*
Hypertrophy 510*f*, 596
Hypnotics 1251
Hypoaldosteronism 1246
Hypoechoic stroma 990
Hypoestrogenic states 734
Hypogastric nerves 58
Hypogastric pain, periodic 133
Hypogonadism
  hypergonadotropic 138, 738*f*
  hypogonadotropic 138, 1303
Hypointense uterine
  fundal leiomyoma, large 22*f*
  posterior wall leiomyoma 23*f*
Hypokalaemia 1244, 1245, 1260
  mild 1244
  moderate 1244
  severe 1244
Hypokalaemic periodic paralysis 1244
Hypomagnesemia 1244
Hypomenorrhoea 137, 420, 718, 738
Hyponatraemia 1242
  acute 1243
  chronic 1243
  classification of 1242
  features of 1243
Hypo-osmotic swelling test 850
Hypoplasia 229, 277, 282, 742
  types 277
Hypoproteinaemia 881
Hypospadias repair 303
Hypotension, cold 1255
Hypotensive agents 114
Hypothalamic-pituitary
  compartment 465*fc*
  dysfunction 123
  failure 123
  ovarian axis 132
Hypothalamic-releasing factors 128
  analogues of 131
  control of 790
Hypothalamic-releasing hormone 83
Hypothalamus 84, 86, 306, 308
  agents influencing 736
  inhibition of 722*f*, 777
  part of 83*f*
Hypothyroidism 145, 164, 235
Hypotonic bladder 1143
Hypotonic hyponatraemia, causes of 1243
Hypoventilation 1245
Hypoxaemia, progressive 1271
Hypoxic cells 695
Hysterectomy 202*f*, 219, 339, 344, 406, 414, 423*f*, 439, 452, 613, 639, 665*f*, 748, 1016, 1029, 1053, 1204, 1205, 1214
  abdominal 1204, 1207, 1247, 1257
  clamps 884
  classes of 1205*t*
  complications of 1214
  extended 587
  extrafascial 1205
  indications of 222*b*
  laparoscopic 614, 1029, 1208, 1247
  specimen 507*f*, 600*f*
  subtotal 1272
  total 509, 639, 671, 1204
    laparoscopic 1212
  types of 1204, 1205, 1205*f*
  underwent 426*f*
Hystero-cervicography 166
Hysterography 203*f*, 359*f*
Hysteromat of Hamou 1041*f*
Hysterosalpingography 14, 268*f*, 387, 421, 423*f*, 426*f*, 600*f*, 760, 846, 852, 856*f*, 1086*f*, 1088*f*
  cornual block 853*f*
  mid-tubal block 853*f*
  unicornuate uterus 853*f*
Hysteroscope 1037, 1294
  inside uterine cavity 1038*f*
  operative 1039*f*
Hysteroscopic morcellator 1052
Hysteroscopic myomectomy 612
  complications of 613
  techniques of 612
Hysteroscopic resectoscope 1052
Hysteroscopic scissors, types of 1041
Hysteroscopic surgery 1037
Hysteroscopic transcervical cannulation 867
Hysteroscopic tubal cannulation 050*f*
Hysteroscopic-guided targeted endometrial biopsy 749
Hysteroscopy 14, 19, 20, 622, 855, 894, 1044, 1195
  complications of 1051*b*
  set 894*f*
Hysterotomy 169, 1138

I

Iatrogenic enterocele 333
Ibalizumab 377
Ibuprofen 757, 1044
Ichthyosis uteri 512
Idiopathic hirsutism, mild-to-moderate 785
Ifosfamide 532, 593, 687
Ileal loop bladder 534
Iliac fossa 1087*f*
Iliac veins 1268
Iliococcygeus muscle 836
Ilioinguinal nerves 755
Iliopectineal ligaments 1161*f*
Imipramine 232, 1155
Imiquimod 562
Immature teratoma 659, 679
Immediate postpartum intrauterine contraceptive device insertion 1121
Immune checkpoint
  inhibitors 534, 704
  pathways 702
Immune factors 442
Immune modulating therapies 714
Immune pathway 687
Immune response modulator 562
Immune system 701
  deficiency 572
  dysregulation of 709
Immunodeficiency 208
Immunoglobulin
  A 231
  G 170
  intravenous 709, 710
  M 170
Immunological disorder 769
Immunological method 1117
Immunomodulatory drugs 450
Immuno-oncology 702
Immunosuppression 702, 1234
Immunotherapy 647, 687, 701, 707, 711, 715*f*, 717
Impaired cellular immune 442
Imperforate anus 259
Imperforate cervix 570*f*
Imperforate vagina 274
Implantation 154
  dermoid 537, 558
  preparation for 92
Impotence 859
In vitro cross-over sperm-cervical mucus contact test 849
In vitro fertilisation 123, 180, 388, 452, 453, 476, 709, 842, 848, 858, 864, 869, 876, 1128, 1297, 1310
  protocols 871*f*
In vitro sperm penetration tests 849
Incision, abdominal 669
Incomplete androgen insensitivity syndrome 300
Incontinence pessaries 340
Indinavir 377
Indocyanine green fluorescence imaging-guided sentinel lymph node dissection 1017*f*
Indoleamine 2,3-dioxygenase 703*f*
Indomethacin 232, 233, 757
Induced abortions 1138
  complications of 1138
Infarction 1035
  pulmonary 1269
Infection 164, 356*f*, 370*f*, 489, 498, 536, 614, 656, 798*t*, 805, 1051, 1121, 1139, 1148, 1261
  cervical 573, 872, 1103
  chronic interdigital 490*f*
  genital 321
  gonococcal 180, 409*f*, 410
  opportunistic 375
  postabortal 410
  puerperal 410, 855*f*
  recurrent 1228
  risk factors of 798*t*
  secondary 813*f*
  spread of 1178
  stricture following 1225
  transfer of 401
  tubercular 410
  vulvovaginal 1081

Inferior epigastric vessels 1034*f*
Inferior mesenteric artery 48
Inferior vena cava 56, 1249, 1270
  retrievable 1270, 1271
Inferior vesical artery 47
Infertility 1, 145, 207, 233, 271, 300, 321, 346, 351, 385, 443, 473, 780, 789, 840, 841*fc*, 896, 1139, 1289
  causes of 841, 1041
  female 840, 1298
  investigation of 846
  male 840
  management of 872*fc*
  secondary 840
  treatment of 846*fc*
  ultrasound in 970
  unexplained 858, 998
Infestations 805
Inflammatory dermatoses, noninfectious 809
Inflammatory reactions
  acute 414
  chronic 433
Infra-colic omentectomy 645
Infundibulopelvic ligament 1208
  separation of 1210
Infundibulum 40
Inguinal canal, tumours of 555
Inguinal hernia 299, 536, 555, 555*f*
  sacs of 267
Inguinal nodes 47
Injury 312, 1259
  cervical 1091, 1138
  electrical 1051
  intestinal 1036
  local 391
  surgical 336
  traumatic 1049
  types of 312
  urologic 1036
  visceral 1162
Innate immune
  cells 701
  response 562, 701
Inner cell mass 1311
Inner circular muscle layer 961*f*
Inotropic agents 1256
Insemination 870, 876
Insomnia 1141
Insufflation test 14
Insulin 226, 231, 465*f*, 468
  concentrations, high 474
  function 483
    assessment of 483
  intravenous 1246
  sensitivity 474
Insulin-like growth factor 62, 134, 466, 469, 601
  binding protein 467
  release of 471
Integrase inhibitor 377
Intelligent tissue monitoring 1026
Intensity-modulated radiation therapy 566, 629, 697
Interconception period 166
Interleukin 442, 701, 713
Intermenstrual discharge 386
Internal anatomical sex 287
Internal genital organs
  anatomy of 36*f*
  blood supply of 56*f*
  development of 289*fc*
Internal genitalia 304
  roots, autonomic innervation of 59*f*
Internal iliac
  artery 30, 54
  nodes 40, 47
  veins 856*f*
Internal pelvic organs, lymphatic drainage of 47*f*
Internal piles, typical location of 1231*f*
Internal pudendal artery 55
Internal sphincter
  interference of 1165
  opening of 46, 1165
  plication operation 1154*f*
Intersphincteric fistula 1236*f*
  tract, ligation of 1237
Interstitial cells 261
  large islands of 298*f*
Interstitial cervical leiomyoma 602*f*
Interstitial fluid 1241
Interstitial line sign 205
Interstitial tubal blockage, management of 1044
Intertrigo 391
Interureteric bar 43
Intestinal distension 1259
Intestinal tract, lower 1216
Intestine 438, 1259
  loops of 35
  small 1036
Intra-abdominal bleeding, severe 188
Intra-abdominal gynaecological surgery 1295
Intra-abdominal pressure 348, 1020, 1223
  measurement of 1033
Intra-abdominal procedure 1019, 1035
Intra-amniotic injection 1136
Intracavernous injection test 822
Intracavitary brachytherapy application 588, 591*f*
Intracavitary radiotherapy 566
Intracellular electrolytes 1241
Intracellular fluid 1241
Intracorporeal knot-tying and suturing technique 1026, 1026*f*
Intracytoplasmic sperm injection 476, 842, 848, 864, 876, 878
  indications of 878*fc*
Intraepithelial neoplasia 368
Intrafallopian insemination 878
Intrafascial supracervical hysterectomy, classic 1204
Intramural calcification 919*f*
Intramural myoma 746
Intramuscular injection 1136
Intramuscular prostaglandin 1136
Intramyometrial intravasation 424*f*
Intraovarian lesion 986*f*
Intrapelvic adhesions 14
  diagnosis of 855*f*
Intraperitoneal placement 1035
Intrauterine adhesions 173*f*, 420, 844
Intrauterine aspiration techniques 526
Intrauterine ball 1078
Intrauterine contraceptive devices 180, 207, 273, 312, 368, 447, 757, 780, 896, 1045*f*, 1062, 1064, 1075, 1075*f*-1077*f*, 1078, 1078*f*, 1079, 1081, 1086*f*, 1090*f*, 1092, 1120, 1123
  adverse effects of 1091
  complications of 1091
  displaced 1091
  efficacy of 1090
  extrauterine site of 1090*f*
  first-generation 1078*f*
  fourth-generation 1079*f*
  levonorgestrel 511
  misplaced 19
  nonmedicated 1083
  postpartum 1120
  progesterone-releasing 1083
  types of 1075, 1075*f*, 1079, 1083*f*
  use of 180, 1118*t*
  varieties of 1075*f*
Intrauterine foetal death 1137
Intrauterine growth
  restriction prematurity 1274
  retardation 606
Intrauterine hormonal contraceptive system 1112
Intrauterine insemination 152, 451, 842, 848, 858, 862, 864, 875, 875*b*, 876, 877, 994
  indications of 875*b*
  steps of 875*b*
Intrauterine pregnancy 180, 206
  signs of 190
Intrauterine system 1078, 1081, 1082*t*, 1105
  type of 1081
Intravaginal culture 878
Intravascular volume depletion 1255
Intravenous immunoglobulin 709, 710
  use of 174
Intrinsic muscle, involuntary 45*f*
Intrinsic sphincter deficiency 1143
Invasive cancer 487*f*, 490, 503*fc*, 574*t*
  incidence of 527
Invasive carcinoma 567
Invasive trophoblastic antigen 220
Invasive tumour, histopathological examination of 568*f*
Inversion
  acute 355
  degrees of 355*f*
  spontaneous cure of 356
Involuntary detrusor contractions 1297
Iodine 281, 1280
  deficiency disorder 1284
  supplementation, role of 238
Ion 1241
  intracellular fluid 1241
Ionising radiation 241, 260
Ipriflavone 608
Iron 232, 1280, 1281

absorption, bioavailability of 1284
consumption of 1285
deficiency 489
anaemia 1231
Irradiation 130, 1239, 1298
Irritable bowel syndrome 459, 789, 1143, 1226
diagnosis of 1226
Irritant contact dermatitis 798
Ischaemia 1035, 1290
Ischiocavernosus muscle 836
Ischiorectal abscess 1234, 1235*f*
Isoflavones 1203
Isolated pituitary gonadotropin deficiency syndrome 722
Isoleucine 1277
Isoniazid 232, 387, 430, 431
Isthmo-isthmic anastomosis 1129
Isthmus 37, 40, 46, 181
mucous membrane of 37
Itching 1189
Itraconazole 801

J

Jarisch–Herxheimer reaction 370
Jeffcoate's theory 196*f*
Joint
aches 114
lesions 458
pain 112, 118
Juvenile granulosa cell tumour 676

K

Kallman's syndrome 123, 138
Kaltenbach chart 740*f*
Kanamycin 232, 387
Kaolin clotting time test 173
Karl Storz resectoscope 1039, 1040*t*
Karman's cannula 13*f*, 421, 527
Karman's syringe 889, 889*f*
Karyotype 216
analysis 138
Kegel's balls 831
Kegel's exercises 1149, 1153
Kegel's perineometer 1288, 1289*f*
Kelley's forceps 1120
Keratinocytes 1298
Keratosis, seborrhoeic 368
Ketoconazole 485
Ketone bodies 1173
Ketoprofen 757
Khanna's sling 344
operation 345*f*
surgery 345*f*
Kidney 1170
disease 208, 459
failure 881
function test 250
fusion of 285
pelvic 275, 285, 286
system, middle 263
Kim ray greenfield filter 1268
Kissing fallopian tubes 439*f*
Kissing ovaries 437*f*
Klebsiella 1173, 1258
Klinefelter syndrome 138, 262, 290, 292, 294, 294*f*, 304, 305, 860
Knee-chest position 11
Knudson's hypothesis 1300
Kobelt's tubules 50, 354, 650, 650*f*
Kocher's clamps 884
Koilocytes 378
Kremer test 849
Krukenberg tumour 246, 295, 683, 683*f*
Kyphosis 459, 1191, 1192*f*
back exercises of 1192

L

Labia 830
divarication of 282*f*
majora 26, 29, 281, 319, 897, 1189, 1298
mass in 546*f*
oedema of 419*f*
minora 27, 29, 281, 295, 319, 419*f*, 897, 1189, 1298
asymmetry of 283
atresia of 283
development of 284*f*
hypertrophy of 283, 283*f*
Labial fusion, partial 728*f*
Labial kiss ulcers 542
Labial tears 324
Labiaplasty 302, 1298
Labiovaginal flaps 281
Labium majus 549*f*
tumour of 555*f*
Labium minus 536, 550*f*
sebaceous cyst of 538*f*
Labour
obstructed 271, 607
pain of 59
precipitate 346
premature 271, 346, 607, 1139
preterm 368, 606, 1092
Lactate dehydrogenase 630, 657, 658
Lactation 228*f*, 230-232, 236
failure of 231
inhibition of 776
probable safe drugs in 232*t*
suppression of 232
Lactational amenorrhoea method 1067
use of 1067*fc*
Lactobacillus 31, 402, 403, 792
Lactobacteria 403*f*
Lactoferrin 231
Lactogenesis 230
Laminaria 1136
Lamivudine 377
Lamont and Pacik's
classification 834
grading system 835
Lane's toothed dissecting forceps 884
Lanugo 478
Laparoendoscopic single-site
surgery, indications of 1056*b*
surgical techniques 1055
Laparoscope insertion, technique of 1032
Laparoscopic access equipment 2020
types of 1020
Laparoscopic access instruments
first-generation 1020
second-generation 1021
Laparoscopic bipolar forceps, types of 1024*f*
Laparoscopic detorsion 361
Laparoscopic hand instruments 892*f*
Laparoscopic ovarian
diathermy 868, 868*b*
drilling 475, 475*f*, 1029
Laparoscopic posterior mesh rectopexy 1220
Laparoscopic sterilisation 1130
steps of 1030*f*
Laparoscopic supracervical hysterectomy 1029
Laparoscopic surgery 198, 198*b*, 1015*t*, 1019, 1020, 1035, 1220
advantages of 198*b*
Laparoscopic suturing techniques 1026
types of 1026
Laparoscopic telescope 1021, 1021*f*, 1034
Laparoscopic tubal ligation 1029
Laparoscopic ultrasound nerve ablation 17, 758
Laparoscopy 17, 18*f*, 73*f*, 734, 757, 760, 855, 895, 1019, 1026, 1027, 1030
chromotubation 14
surgery 1015
therapeutic 1027
Laparotomy 198, 204, 452, 1088*f*
indications of 199*b*
time of 199, 724*f*
Large-scale screening programmes 528
Larotrectinib 689
Laser
ablation 405, 406
acupuncture 1298
applications of 1292, 1295
hatching, complications of 1298
injuries 1051
physics 1292
safety 1294
surgeries 1293*f*
technology, use of 1292
therapy, low-level 1298
treatment 1297
types of 1293, 1294*t*
Laser-assisted hatching 897, 1297, 1297*f*
Latzko's triad 643*f*
Lavage, abdominal 475
Lax protuberant abdominal wall 5
Le Fort's operation 344
Learning
deep 1307, 1308, 1308*t*
surgeries 1310
Leech–Wilkinson's cannula 889
Lee–Huang point 1209
Leflunomide 717
Leg, swelling of 531
Leiomyomas 571, 596-598, 602-604, 607, 610, 615*f*, 616, 617*f*, 642, 651, 745, 747, 788, 912, 913, 922, 942
cervical 571*f*

complications of 614
intramural 912
medical treatment of 609*fc*
parasitic 615*f*
small 854*f*
subclassification of 747*f*
uterine 433, 436, 445, 595, 655, 784, 844, 1202
Leiomyomatosis 978*f*
diffuse 913, 978
Leiomyosarcomas 630, 631*f*, 689, 924
prognosis of 631
treatment of 631
two-thirds of 630
uterine 922
Leptin receptor gene mutation 1303
Lesions 950
adnexal 983
benign neoplastic 953*f*
complex 988
description of 950*f*
digital 489
malignant 942
mimicking tubal malignancy 643
multifocal high-grade 564
muscular 457
myometrial 975
nonmolar 217
size of 981
solid 986
tumour-like 660
Letrozole 125, 474, 693, 736
Leucine 1277
Leucocytes 881
Leucoderma 543*f*
Leucoplakia 487*f*, 505*f*, 542*f*, 543*f*, 813*f*
Leucorrhoea 283, 350, 792, 1096
Leucovorin 690
Leukaemia 549
Leukotrienes 755
Leuprolide 447, 693
acetate 309, 748
Leuprorelin 449
Levator ani 49*f*, 51
muscles 45*f*
Levator plate, assessment of 333
Levofloxacin 1176, 1247
Levonorgestrel 447, 448, 1075, 1105
Levonorgestrel intrauterine contraceptive
device 511
system 455, 639, 1078, 1200
advantages of 1082*b*
use of 1080*t*
Leydig cell 255, 289, 674, 676
agenesis 300
hypoplasia 290
tumour 480, 481, 658, 674, 675
Libido 304, 306, 778, 782
loss of 308, 1100
Lichen planus 806, 809
Lichen sclerosus 488, 806, 809
treatment of 491
Lidocaine 824
Li-Fraumeni syndrome 1302, 1303
Ligamentary lesions 457
Ligaments 49, 255, 1208, 1211
Ligand chain reaction 795
Ligasure 1023
Ligating uterine vessels 1209
Light emitting diode 386
Lignocaine gel application 1225
Lincomycin 232
Lincosamides 389
Linea nigra 132
Linoleic acid 1282
Lipogenesis 474
Lipoid cell tumour 668
Lipoma 536, 559
Lipoprotein
high-density 80, 111
low-density 80
Lippes loop 1077*f*, 1084*f*, 1087*f*, 1088*f*, 1091
extrauterine 1087*f*
intrauterine position of 1087*f*
Liquid biopsy 244
Liquor folliculi 67*f*
Liquorice 1244
Listeria monocytogenes 164
vaccine 704
Lithium 233
Lithopaedion 204*f*
Lithotomy 1230*f*
position 11, 12*f*
Litigation 1124
Liver
adenomas 1102
cancer 1102
cirrhosis of 145
disease 208
advanced 1271
chronic 1201
dullness, loss of 1033
dysfunction 117, 449
enlargement 246
failure 881
function test 139, 219, 250
metabolic capacity 1104
metastases 575
synthesis 1267
Lloyd-Davis needle holder 884
Lobular cancer in situ 243
Lobuloalveolar system 230
Local oestrogen therapy 1199
Localised vulvar pain syndrome 814
Long protocol-controlled ovarian stimulation 870*f*
Long-armed X isochromosomes 291
Long-chain polyunsaturated fatty acids 1278, 1279, 1279*t*
Loop electrosurgical excision procedure 313, 503, 508, 509*f*, 514-521, 577-579
Loop-mediated isothermal amplification 387
Lord's eight-finger dilatation 1230, 1233
Low cuboidal cells, single layer of 75
Low-amplitude rhythmic detrusor contractions 1312
Low-density lipoprotein 80
cholesterol levels 112
particles 1286
Low-dose oral contraceptive pills 1093, 1099*t*, 1101
benefits of 1104
Löwenstein-Jensen medium 421
Lower abdominal wall, defects of 282*f*
Lower anogenital squamous terminology 540
Lower vagina 58
disease 566
Low-molecular-weight heparin 1250, 1266
Low-risk gestational trophoblastic
disease 220*fc*
neoplasia 708
tumour 222*t*
Lubricants 845
Ludwig visual scales 464
Lugol's iodine 496, 505, 527
Lukewarm water 816
Lumbago 458
Lumbar vertebra 459
Lumbosacral plexopathy 593
Lumina 262
Lung 439
cancer 525
disease, chronic 1288
metastasis 223
Lupus anticoagulant 171
testing for 165
Luteal cysts 662
Luteal phase defect 145, 233, 998
treatment of 160
Luteinised follicle cyst 660
Luteinised unruptured follicle 436, 985, 987*f*, 998
Luteinising hormone 70*f*, 82*f*, 83, 84, 84*f*, 86*f*, 95*f*, 101*f*, 111, 120, 125*f*, 141-143, 152, 236, 294, 304, 449, 465, 465*f*, 466*f*, 469, 471, 721, 738*f*, 739, 740, 844, 862, 868, 870, 870*f*, 875, 993, 1067, 1184, 1184*f*, 1303
elevated 740*fc*
increased sensitivity of 135
influence of 783
sensitivity of 135
release of 111
Luteoma 295
Lycopene 845
Lymph node 441, 567*f*, 586, 644
enlarged 672
evaluation 583
femoral 379
metastasis 248
pelvic 589*f*
Lymphadenomatous growth 634
Lymphangioma 536
Lymphatic
drainage 57
embolism 441, 575
permeation 575
regional 590
spread 568
Lymphocytes 287*f*
Lymphoedema 292

Lymphogranuloma
inguinale 1238
venereum 366, 373, 379, 380*f*, 393, 394, 1125
Lymphoid tumours 660
Lymphoma 634, 642
Lymphovascular space invasion 587, 592, 623, 625, 696, 1309
Lynch syndrome 1302, 1303
Lynestrenol 447, 1105
Lysine 1277

M

Machine learning 1307, 1308, 1308*t*
techniques 1307*t*
Mackenrodt's ligament 328, 1272
Macrodantin 1177
Macrolides 389
Macrometastasis 624
Macronutrient 1275, 1282
Macrophage colony-stimulating factor 657, 709
Madlener operation 1129, 1130*f*
Maffucci syndrome 676
Magnesium 1281
deficiency 1245
Magnetic resonance-guided focused ultrasound 639
Major histocompatibility complex 703*f*
Malabsorption syndrome 730, 812
Male breast cancer 1302
Male contraceptive pill 1119
Male external genitalia, development of 289*fc*
Male fertility, assessment of 847
Male infertility 840
lasers in 1298
prevention of 861
Male sterilisation 1131
Malformation 266
causes of 259
Malignancy 24*f*, 368, 643*f*, 656, 667, 748, 1303*t*
cervical 1195, 1301
endometrial 981
evidence of 685
grading of 1309
index, risk of 956, 957
low-grade 689
risk of 956
second 688
staging of 1309
suspicion of 1005*f*
Malignant disease 415, 1263
signs of 504
stages of 644*t*
symptoms of 504
Malignant epithelial tumours 666, 692
pathology of 667
treatment of 681
Malignant neoplasms
primary 642, 647*fc*
secondary 648
Malignant ovarian tumours
metastases of 668
primary treatment of 669
Malignant sex cord stromal tumours 692
surgical treatment of 674
Malignant tumour 958, 958*t*
Malleable probes 889, 889*f*
Malnutrition 1274
Mammary dysplasia 787
Mammary gland 225, 230
Mammary prosthesis 229
Mammogenesis 230
hormones responsible for 231
Mammography 242
screening 241, 242
Manchester operation 343, 344
principles of 342*f*
Manchester system 699*f*
Mannequins 1310
Mantoux test 387
Manual clitoral stimulators 831
Manual vacuum aspiration 1137
Marshall-Marchetti-Krantz procedure 333, 1161
Marsupialisation, technique of 396
Marvelon 1106
Masculine reconstruction 302
Mass
palpable 896
per abdomen, examination of 7
Mastalgia 1100, 1202
bilateral 1110
cyclical 768
premenstrual 121, 767, 784
Mastectomy 246
radical 246
Mastitis 229, 239, 239*f*
Masturbation 831
Maternal androgen-producing tumours 295
Maternal serum alpha-fetoprotein, levels of 160
Matrix metalloproteinases 814
Maturation index 99
Mature cystic teratoma 655*f*, 678
wall of 679*f*
Maxilla, short 369
Mayer-Rokitansky-Küster-Hauser syndrome 727, 727*f*
May-Husni operation 1268
Mayo scissors 884, 885*f*
McCall's culdoplasty 1214*f*
McIndoe vaginoplasty 728
Meatus, external 43
Medical therapy 305, 452, 638
Meditation 837
Mediterranean races 306
Medroxyprogesterone acetate 116, 148, 309, 447, 448, 484, 608, 1200
Mefenamic acid 232, 233, 746, 757
Megestrol acetate 447
Meigs syndrome 674
Melanin granules 1298
Melanocortin receptor agonist 827
Melanocyte
stimulating hormone 104, 132
tumours of 805
Melanoma 536, 549, 549*f*, 567, 634
malignant 549
origin of 567
Melena 755
Membrana granulosa 69*f*
Membranes
formation of 155
premature rupture of 381, 606, 931
Membranous expression 626*f*
Memory loss 111
Menarche, early 245
Mendelian inheritance pattern 436
Menfegol 1074
Menopausal hormone therapy 114, 1187, 1196, 1197, 1200
additional benefits of 1197
advantages of 1198
indications of 1196
informed consent for 1198
use, temporal implications of 1202
Menopause 43, 106, 109, 120, 719, 1001, 1085, 1181, 1184*f*, 1185, 1188, 1189, 1191*f*, 1192*f*, 1196, 1202
abnormal 119
alternative therapy for 118
artificial 119, 767
diagnosis of 113
effect of 1189
factors influencing age of 1183
genitourinary syndrome of 112, 1297
late 119, 245
management of 112, 1196
normal uterus in 1001
physiology of 1183
premature 119, 1183, 1193
staging of 1182, 1182*t*
surgical 119
symptoms of 109*f*, 1181
ultrasound in 1001
urogenital syndrome of 1188
vasomotor symptoms of 118
Menorrhagia 14, 37*f*, 270, 350, 416, 434*f*, 443, 445, 639, 1041, 1113, 1204
anovulatory 1195
idiopathic 1112, 1113
puberty 146, 420
reduction of 1113
treatment of 787
Menstrual bleeding 102, 421, 606, 1121
heavy 420, 749
irregular 604*f*
outflow of 275
Menstrual cups 104
Menstrual cycle 32, 86, 97*f*, 123*f*, 472*f*, 482, 900*f*, 947*f*
clinical dimensions of 102, 911
features of 93*t*
irregular 464
misinterpretation of 5*f*
normal 88, 101, 472*f*
shortening of 751
Menstrual difficulties 321
Menstrual discharge 434
Menstrual disorders 137
Menstrual disturbance 385, 606, 658, 782, 1139

Menstrual endometrium 88, 89*f*
  low-power view of 89*f*
Menstrual epilepsy 771
Menstrual fluid 754
Menstrual function 5, 107
Menstrual irregularities 445, 471, 718, 1108
Menstrual migraine 766
  aetiology of 766
Menstrual molimina 275
Menstrual parameters in mid-reproductive years 102*t*, 911*t*
Menstrual period 5, 108, 1030
  postponement of 776, 780
Menstrual phenomena 762
Menstrual problems 103, 1195
Menstrual products, types of 104
Menstrual symptoms 5
Menstrual vaginal tampon 270*f*
Menstruation 2, 4, 88, 95, 97*f*, 101, 101*f*, 102, 103, 740*f*, 1247
  abnormal 443
  advancement of 105
  anovular 97
  clinical dimensions of 102, 911
  disorders of 6, 775, 780
  ectopic 5
  normal 104
  retrograde 441
  vicarious 770
Mental development 1274
Mental disorder, diagnostic and statistical manual of 821
Mercier's bar 43
Merkel cell carcinoma 549
Mersilene mesh 345
Mesenchymal stroma 676
Mesenchyme 261
  invades 157
Mesenteric thrombosis 188
Mesigyna 1106
Mesonephric duct 255, 289
  lower parts of 257*f*
Mesonephric tubules 252*f*
Mesonephroid tumours 666, 668
Mesonephroma 567
Mesonephros 253
Mesorectal basins 700
Mesosalpinx 200
Mesotheliomas 653
  peritoneal malignant 653
Mesterolone 784
Metabolic waste products 1289
Metabolism 782
Metabolite 716
Metanephros 253
Metaplasia 499
Metastases 568, 621, 648, 1301
  management of 223
  site of 221, 690
Metastatic disease 248
  low-risk 222
Metastatic ovarian tumours 682
Metformin 474, 474*f*
  mechanism of action of 474
Methionine 1277
Methotrexate 188, 205, 207, 208, 222, 593, 686, 687, 690, 716, 1135
  single-dose 208*t*
    protocol of 208*t*
  therapy 195*b*
  use of 208
Methyl cyanoacrylate 20
Methylation 1280
Methyldopa 232, 306
Methylergometrine 232
Methyltestosterone 482
Metoclopramide 145
Metritis 407
Metronidazole 232, 400, 403, 404, 417, 554, 800, 801, 1248
Michael applebaum 929
Mickey mouse configuration 1056
Miconazole 402, 808
Microadenoma, pituitary 733*f*
Microepididymal sperm aspiration 842, 862
Micromastia 235
Micronutrients 1275
Microribonucleic acid 1309
Microsatellite instability 625, 689
  hypermutated 704
  status of 707
  testing 1302
Microstix-Candida medium 799
Microsurgical epididymal sperm aspiration 877
Microtip pressure transducers 1146
Micturition 5, 362, 1164
  end of 46
  process of 46
  voluntary arrest of 46*f*
Midbrain 308
Mid-luteal phase plasma progesterone level 122
Midproliferative endometrium 89*f*
Midurethra 1157
Mifepristone 450, 609, 748, 782, 1117
Migraine 1188
  headache 103, 1104, 1202
  menstrual 766, 767
Milk
  secretion of 230
  synthesis of 230
Milligan Morgan classification 1235
Mindfulness 837
Minerals 1286
Minilaparotomy 1088*f*, 1090*f*
Minimally invasive
  hysterectomy procedures 1208
  slings 1161
  surgery 193
  techniques 1011, 1014
Minipill 1105
Minoxidil 478
Mirena 1081*t*, 1082, 1091, 1113*f*
  fundal positioning of 1115
Miscarriage 368
  recurrent 170
  spontaneous 1092
  sporadic 171
Misoprostol 1135-1137
Misplaced pluripotent Müllerian remnants 636
Mitogenic hormone 468
Mitomycin C 532, 1240
Mitosis 90
  phase of 532
Mitoxantrone 533
Mittelschmerz 121, 457, 760, 1104
Mixed antiglobulin reaction test 850
Mixed germ cell 681
  tumour 659, 680
Mixed gonadal dysgenesis 290, 304
Mixed non-neoplastic epithelial disorders 488
Mobile health applications 241
Mock transfer 872
Modern contraception, use of 1062
Molar gestation 218
Molar pregnancy 215, 217, 222
  aetiopathogenesis of 217*f*
  complications of 218*b*
Molar tissue filling uterus, typical 15*f*
Mole
  malignant 217
  partial 216, 216*f*, 689
Molecular classification 624, 625*t*
Molluscum contagiosum 368
Monoclonal antibody ovarian 657
Monodermal teratoma 660, 680
Monophasic pills 1094*t*
Monopolar circuit 1025*f*
Monosomy X 163
Monozygotic twinning 1298
Mons
  pubis 1299
  veneris 26
Montogomery's tubercle 230
Mood
  changes 1188
  lability 114
Morgagni hydatid 50, 254, 254*f*
Morphine 232, 233, 1256, 1258
Morphological uterus sonographic assessment 638, 745, 911, 979, 980*f*, 1308
Morula 153
Mosaicism, type of 291
Moses' sign 1264
Moth-Eaten appearance 424*f*
Motile spermatozoa 849
Mouth, neurotic ulcers of 769
Moxifloxacin 417
M-rules 957
Mucin 557
Mucinous borderline tumours 666
Mucinous ovarian
  malignancy 657
  tumour 665*f*
Mucoid discharge 1232
Mucoid fluid 274*f*
Mucosa 1219
Mucosal abrasion 340
Mucosal immune response 364
Mucous membrane 35, 1302
  form of 36

Mucus, collection of 274
Müllerian adenosarcoma 633
Müllerian agenesis 727
 laparoscopic view of 727*f*
Müllerian anomalies 901
 causes of 269
 types of 255
Müllerian buds 273
Müllerian ducts 252*f*, 254*f*, 255, 261, 264, 266-268, 273, 289, 300*f*
 development of 255*f*
 diverticula of 273
 duplication of 273
 fusion deformity 359
 imperfect fusion of 267
 incomplete canalization of 273
 malfusion deformity, types of 269*f*
 syndrome, persistent 290, 299
 system 255
Müllerian epithelium, spill of 439
Müllerian hypoplasia, segmental 264
Müllerian inhibiting factor 288, 289, 904
 substance 289, 674
Müllerian malformations 269, 270
Müllerian mesenchymal cells 633
Müllerian tubercle 257, 261, 268
Müllerian tumour, mixed 597, 633
Multicystic structure 650*f*
Multiload Cu 250 1077
Multilocular cyst 950, 950*f*
Multipigmented nevi 292
Multiple burnt match head spots 437
Multiple cystic spaces 940*f*
Multiple gestation, higher order 880
Multiple organ systems 1302
Multiple small tarry cysts 454*f*
Multi-port technique 1055
Mumps orchitis 860
Musa criteria 745*f*
Muscle 32
 abdominal 12
 cramps 1145
 deep 836
 exercises, active 1287
 fibres 981, 1311
  involuntary 35
 layers 961*f*
 mass
  weight gain of 1189
  weight loss of 1189
 paralysis 1244
 pelvic 33*f*
 relaxation 838
 superficial 835
 weakness 1245
Mutation 1300
 analysis 1303
Mycobacterium
 growth indicator tube 386
 tuberculosis 365, 419
  infection, spectrum of 420*f*
Mycophenolate 717
Mycoplasma 380, 402
 group 380
 hominis 380
Myeloid tumours 660
Myeloid-derived suppressor cell 703*f*
Myeloma, multiple 1243
Myelosuppression 532
Myoblastoma 536
Myocardial infarction 111, 470, 1100, 1101, 1194, 1201, 1244, 1256
 phase of 117
 risk of 1101
Myocardial ischaemia 1256
Myohyperplasia 596
Myoma 597
 classification of 746
 multiple 73*f*
 pedunculated 613
 resected 612
 screw 889, 889*f*
 STEPW classification of 747*t*
Myomectomy 439, 610, 610*f*, 748, 1016, 1029, 1257
 abdominal 610
 clamp 889*f*
 laparoscopic 612, 748
 procedures 1049
Myometrial basalis, invagination of 636
Myometrial cycle 98
Myometrial invasion 623, 697, 1006*f*
Myometrial islands 745*f*
Myometrial linear striations 637
Myometrial pathology 913*f*
Myometrium 16*f*, 427*f*, 433, 510, 637*f*, 911, 976, 978, 979*f*, 1002, 1089*f*, 1297
 deep invasion of 619*f*
 layers of 899*f*
 outer 981*f*
Myopathy, proximal 377
Myositis 112
Myxoid
 leiomyosarcomas 630
 soft-tissue tumours 559
Myxomatous degeneration 615

N

Nabothian cyst 570
 multiple 940*f*
Nabothian follicles 405, 405*f*, 570
Nafarelin 447, 449
Nalidixic acid 232
Naproxen 714
 sodium 757
Natural family planning method 1064
 advantages of 1067
 disadvantages of 1068
Natural fertility awareness methods 1064
Natural killer cells 171
 role of 709
Natural language processing 1307
Natural orifice transluminal endoscopic surgery 1053
Nausea 688, 1096, 1100, 1258
Neck, spontaneous fracture of 731*f*
Necrotic tissue
 infection of 575
 liquefaction of 615*f*
Negative sexual scripts 833
Neisseria gonorrhoeae 365, 396, 793, 795, 798, 808
Nelfinavir 377
Neocollagenesis 1297
Neodymium-doped yttrium aluminum garnet laser 1292, 1294, 1296*f*
Neoelastogenesis 1297
Neonatal intensive care unit 175
Neoplasms
 benign 536, 538, 557, 558, 596, 597, 642
 malignant 536, 557, 563, 596, 616
Neoplastic epithelial disorders 488
Neoplastic ovarian tumours 663
Nephritis 688
Nerve 606
 block 416, 491
 growth factors 814
 impulses 85
 injuries 1036, 1162
Nervous exhaustion 1143
Nervous stress, periods of 1226
Nestorone 1093
Neural tissue 61
Neuroendocrinology 61
Neurofibroma 536
Neurohormonal connections 85
Neurokinin 3 receptors 118
Neurological disease 1142
Neurological disorders 1225
Neuroma 536
Neuronal inactivity 1244
Neuropathy, peripheral 533
Neurotransmitter abnormalities 764
Neurotrophic tyrosine receptor kinase
 fusion 689
 gene 689
Nevirapine 377
Next-generation sequencing 1304
Niacin 1275
Nickerson medium 799
Nipple
 absence of 228
 breast 230
 development of 776
 discharge 232, 245
  history of 245*f*
 multiple 228
 retracted 227, 228*f*
 stimulation 145
Niraparib 534
Nitrazepam 232
Nitric oxide 112
Nitrofurantoin 232, 1177
 macrocrystals 1176
 monohydrate 1176
Nitrogen balance 1286
Nitroglycerine 1229
Nocturnal enuresis 1143
Nocturnal penile tumescence 822
Nodal metastasis, evidence of 547*f*
Nodosa 425*f*
Nomegestrol 1093
Nonabsorbable sutures 892*f*

Nonallergic silicone rubber 1073
Noncommunicable diseases, lower risk of 1274
Nonepithelial ovarian tumours 674
Nonfertility management 476
Nonfertility sparing 587
Non-Hodgkin's lymphoma 549
Nonhormonal medications 1187
Nonhormonal pharmacological agents, types of 1198
Nonhormone replacement therapy regimens 118
Non-neoplastic epithelial disorders 488
Non-neoplastic tumours 660*b*
  management of 663
Nonnucleoside reverse transcriptase inhibitor 377
Nonoxynol-9 1074
Nonsexually transmitted infections 793
Nonspecific serological tests 387
Nonsteroidal anti-inflammatory drugs 127, 450, 453, 530, 638, 745, 757, 757*t*, 758, 767, 1044
Nontoothed dissecting forceps 884
Norepinephrine 1155
  reuptake inhibitors 118, 765, 1187
Norethindrone 1093, 1200
  pellet 1109
Norethisterone 116, 1105, 1200
  acetate 609
  enanthate 1106
Norfloxacin 1176
Norgestimate 1200
Norgestrel 1105, 1200
Norplant 1109*f*
  subdermal insertion of 1110*f*
Norsteroids 779
Nortestosterone derivatives 779
No-scalpel vasectomy 1133
  technique of 1133
Novel 19-nortestosterone derivative 639
N-telopeptides-collagen 1191
Nuck canal 536
Nuclear factor kappa-B ligand 118
Nuclear magnetic resonance, property of 22
Nuclear pleomorphism 217
Nucleic acid amplification test 372, 387, 396, 421
Nucleoside reverse transcriptase inhibitor 377
Nucleus 632*f*
Nugent score 798
Nulliparity 245, 436
Nulliparous uterovaginal prolapse 336*f*
Nutrition 164, 730, 1274, 1280, 1285
  basics 1275
  constitutes 1274
  epigenetics of 1280
  risk factors 1285, 1285*t*
  target 1275, 1275*t*

O

Obesity 2, 136, 241, 467*fc*, 468*f*, 732, 851, 1035, 1143, 1202, 1282, 1283
  aetiology of 1283
  childhood 136, 137*fc*
  parameters of 1282
  prevention of 1283
Obstetric anal sphincter injuries 313
Obstetric complications 321
  absence of 1288
Obstetric diseases 187
Obstetric surgery 1247
Obstruction
  chronic lymphatic 380
  intestinal 411, 425*f*, 580, 656, 1260
  surgical 180
  ureteric 583
Obturator internus fascia 1161*f*, 1234
Obturator nodes 40
Octoxynol-9 1074
Oedema 334, 373, 537, 615, 1243
Oedematous chorionic villi 215
Oesophageal atresia 259
Oestradiol 76, 111, 115, 136, 143, 160, 739, 763, 772, 780, 844, 863, 870*f*, 875, 1184, 1185, 1198
  concentrations 111
  critical blood level of 112
  micronisation of 1198
  ovarian production of 136
  plasma levels of 77*f*
  releasing vaginal silicon ring, low-dose 116
  ring 1199
  serum 1113
  vaginal tablets of 1199
  valerate 1198
    dosage of 1095
Oestriol 608, 763, 1198
Oestrogen 71, 72*f*, 76-79, 86, 103, 112, 114-116, 130, 145, 152, 160, 246, 309, 337, 397, 447, 491, 617, 632, 724, 736, 763, 772, 773*f*, 775*f*, 776*f*, 778, 778*f*, 1092, 1102, 1115, 1155, 1188, 1191, 1193, 1199, 1202, 1263
  absence of 1186
  actions of 79*f*
  bleeding threshold level of 95
  conjugated 1103
  continuous production of 724
  deficiency 112, 307, 1191
    effect of 1186
  depot 148
  dominant cervical mucus 1066*f*
  dosage of 1199
  effect of 772
  excretion of 86
  indiscriminate use of 752
  influences 766
  inhibitory action of 79*f*
  levels of 109
  long-acting 774
  low-dose 1200
  micronised 1198
  mixed 117
  natural 118, 772, 1198
  pregnancy levels of 1119
  producing tumours 752
  production 67
    age-related 1184*fc*
  progestogen
    antiovulatory preparations, effect of 447*f*
    contraceptive pill 722, 722*f*
    preparation 440*f*
    therapy 448
  receptor 78, 689, 1186
    beta 76, 442
    loss of 625
  replacement therapy 245, 1157
  role of 160
  secretion 1188
  semisynthetic 1198
  sequential 1003, 1004
  suppression 466
  synthetic 772, 1198
  therapy 225*f*, 752, 832
  topical 1154
  underproduction of 724
  vaginal 1199, 1297
  withdrawal bleeding 94
Oestrone 763, 772, 1185, 1198
  levels 1184
  sulphate 1198
Oestrone-3-glucuronide 1067
Ofloxacin 387
Olaparib 534
Olendalizumab 712
Oligo-anovulation 864*fc*
Oligomenorrhoea 137, 145, 233, 300, 307, 385, 420, 464, 482, 718, 741, 1113
  causes of 741*f*
  treatment of 742
Oligonucleotide hybridisation 1304
Oligospermia, severe 299
Oligozoospermia 786, 843, 878
Oliguria 881
Ollier syndrome 676
Olsen visual scales 464
Omega-3 1279, 1279*t*
Omega-6 1279, 1279*t*
Omental cake 6
Omentectomy 671
Omentum
  piece of 1088*f*
  portion of 1088*f*
Onapristone 782
Oncosurgeries 1214
Oocyte 1311
  depletion of 1181
  donation 873
    indications of 874*b*
  maturation, phase of 67*f*
  mature 151*f*
  meiotic arrest of 71
  recipient, evaluation of 874*b*
  retrieval 870
Oogenesis 63*f*
Oogonia 71
Oophorectomy 452, 1029, 1128
  bilateral 1202, 1204
Oophoritis 413, 662, 990
Open laparoscopy 1032

Operative hysteroscopy 1037, 1046, 1053
steps of 1046
Operative telescope 1022*f*
Opiates 145
Opioids 461, 1252
use of 1251
Opportunistic salpingectomy salpingo-oophorectomy 1214
Optima nutrition 1274
Optimal cytoreduction 673, 691
Oral anticoagulants 1267
effect of 1267
Oral antimicrobial treatment 1175
Oral contraceptive 114, 220, 232, 1062, 1093*fc*, 1102-1104, 1119, 1123, 1124
fourth-generation 1093
long-term 1102
pills 148, 447, 573, 757, 764, 874*f*, 933, 1094
conventional combined 1098*t*
low-dose 1093, 1099*t*, 1101
switching 1099*t*
use of 145, 745
preparations 484
use of 482
previous 1102
second-generation 1093
third-generation 1093
ultra-low-dose 1094*t*
Oral estrogen-progestogen 1202
Oral pills, long-term use of 241
Oral probiotic therapy 403
Orchidectomy 303
Organic disease 1163
Organic erectile dysfunction 823*t*
Organs
abdominal 1130
unusual mobility of 361
Orgasm 845
absent of 829
delayed 829
Orgasmic sensations, reduced intensity of 829
Origami male condom 1070
Ormeloxifene 1117
Orthopaedic injuries 1270
Osmotic demyelination syndrome 1243
Osteitis pubis 1161, 1162
Osteoarthritis, development of 112
Osteomalacia 1286
Osteopenia 1190*f*
Osteoporosis 112, 118, 233, 1190, 1190*f*, 1191
family history of 1197
management of 1192
prevalence of 1190*t*
prevention of 114, 1192
senile 112
spinal complications of 1191
Osteoprotegerin 1191, 1194
Outer longitudinal muscle layer 961*f*
Ova, production of 62
Ovarian abnormalities 971
Ovarian abscess 952*f*
endometrium aspiration 451*f*
Ovarian activity, suppression of 1117
Ovarian anatomy 943
Ovarian antral follicle count 111
Ovarian artery 39, 47, 53
branches 53
Ovarian cancer 523, 525, 646, 672, 1102, 1201, 1302
advanced 1248
history of 1196
immunotherapy in 705
incidence of 666
marker for 444
prognosis of 668
screening 1006
surgical staging of 669*t*
treatment 707*f*
Ovarian capsule 954*f*
Ovarian cortex, slice of 725*f*
Ovarian cycle 784
correction of 92
hormonal control of 95*f*
phases of 61
Ovarian cyst 275, 595, 1008*f*, 1100, 1111
axial torsion of pedicle of 655*f*
rupture of 411
unilateral 949*fc*
Ovarian cystectomy 363, 451, 1016, 1029
Ovarian development, disorders of 290
Ovarian diameters 992
Ovarian diathermy, risk of 475
Ovarian disorder 865*fc*
Ovarian drilling 1029
Ovarian dysfunction 123
Ovarian endometrioma 437*f*, 451*f*, 952*f*
Ovarian endometriosis superficial ovarian lesions 451
Ovarian failure
premature 1303
primary 138
Ovarian fibroma 988*f*
Ovarian follicles 661
synchronise development of 874*f*
Ovarian fossa 42, 946, 946*f*
Ovarian function 61, 120, 946, 1113
Ovarian hormones 75
effect of 32
Ovarian hyperstimulation syndrome 126, 475, 662, 868, 872, 873, 880, 992
early 881, 881*t*
Golaris classification of 881
late 881, 881*t*
Ovarian hyperthecosis 464
Ovarian Krukenberg tumour 684
Ovarian lesions 951, 984
classification of 984
Ovarian ligament 51, 1213
Ovarian malignant lesions 953
Ovarian mass
categorisation of 956*t*
complications of 655
Ovarian neoplasms 457, 658
Ovarian neoplastic growths 464
Ovarian origin, menstrual pain of 760
Ovarian parameters 993
Ovarian parenchymal blood flow 990
Ovarian peritoneal carcinoma 644*f*
Ovarian pregnancy 200, 201*f*, 662
diagnosis 200
Spiegelberg criteria for 201*b*
Ovarian response, predictors of 992
Ovarian steroid secretion 1184
Ovarian stimulation 874*f*
Ovarian stromal hyperthecosis 480
Ovarian structure, normal 947*f*
Ovarian tissue 440*f*
Ovarian torsion 360, 962, 963*f*, 988
transvaginal sonography 964*f*
Ovarian transposition 566
Ovarian tumours 17, 236, 360, 412, 654, 656, 657*f*, 682, 683, 752
benign 656
classification of 659*t*
clinical diagnosis of 654
complications of 655
malignant 668
non-neoplastic 658
occurrence of 654
pathology of 658
positions of 661*f*
secondary 683*f*
Ovarian vein 40, 236
Ovarian wedge
craters 1296*f*
resection 1295
Ovary 41, 57, 60, 76*fc*, 96, 179, 252*f*, 276, 308, 384, 432, 437, 445, 465, 522, 725*f*, 947, 970, 992, 1001, 1006, 1008*f*, 1225
accessory 277
androblastoma of 735
androgen producing tumours of 481
appearance of 1001
blood supply of 42*f*
carcinoma of 670*t*
cut section of 73*f*
dermoid cyst of 678*f*
development of 288
endocrine activity of 75
endometriosis of 434*f*, 435*f*, 440*f*
enlargement of 127*f*
lacks follicles 1006
mucinous carcinoma of 687
nondominant 998
normal 463*f*, 469*f*, 947*f*
ovulating 76
peritoneum 445
prepubertal 139*f*
prolapse of 347
radiograph of 54*f*
removal of 665*f*
reserve 993
response of 993*t*
serous cystadenoma of 438*f*
simple cyst of 984
substance of 54
supernumerary 277, 228
surface endometriosis of 436*f*
syndrome 457
torsion of 360, 362*f*
tuberculosis of 384*f*
tumours of 295, 654

vascular connections of 43*fc*
wedge resection of 130
Overlap technique 313
Oversuppressive syndrome 722
Overweight 1275
Ovulation 61, 62*f*, 63, 120, 151*f*, 188, 1105
abnormal 970
assessment of 844*fc*
bleeding 121, 750
clinical aspects of 101
control of 85
diagnosis of 121
disorders of 775, 780
estimation of time of 851
induction of 124, 473
marks 92
pain 121, 411, 760, 761, 775
prediction of 123
signs of 1065
spontaneous 120
suppression of 130
symptoms of 1065
tablets, mechanism of 125*f*
Ovulatory cycles 123
Ovulatory disorders, treatment of 749
Ovulatory dysfunction 463, 749
Ovum
division of 288*fc*
early development of 152
external migration of 181
fertilisation of 152*f*
high-power view of 68*f*
holding forceps 890, 890*f*
maturation of 71, 151*f*, 152*f*
overdevelopment of 181
pick-up 870*f*
Oxaliplatin 687
Oxybutynin 118
Oxygen 1256
Oxytetracycline 370
Oxytocics 1139
Oxytocin infusion 169

P

Paclitaxel 533, 646, 671, 688, 692, 693
Paget's cells, large 494*f*
Paget's disease 494, 805
extramammary 542
Pain 4, 386, 657, 660, 1121
abdominal 420, 443, 755, 1065, 1081
distension 881
anal 1228
chest 1270
chronic suprapubic 1162
colicky 183
cyclic 457
diffuse suprapubic 350
endometriosis associated 447*t*, 453*fc*, 788
epigastric 1252
fear of 833
genito-pelvic 821, 832
intermenstrual 1091
management 815, 1138
mid-cycle 760
modifiers 816, 817
noncyclic 457
ovulation 121, 411, 760, 761, 775
persists 1229
rectal 275, 1228
reduction 838
relief of 412, 530
shoulder 1252
sudden onset of 4
type of 459
ureteric 1258
vulvar 813, 814
Painkillers 1175
Palatial arch, high 369
Palliative therapy 248
Palma operation 1268
PALM-COEIN, classification of 744, 744*f*, 911*f*
Palmer's point 1033, 1209
Palmer's test 1033
Pamidronate 118
Pampiniform plexus 40
Pancreas 729
Pancreatitis, haemorrhagic 1243
Panty vibrators 831
Pap smear 322, 525, 527
abnormal 576, 579*fc*
cytology 576
Pap test 525
Papillary lesion, basis of 954*f*
Papillary protrusion 954*f*
Papilloma 536, 559, 571, 752, 1142, 1239
urethral 554
Papular warts 378
Papules 369
Para-aminosalicylic acid 387
Para-aortic basin 700
Para-aortic lymph node 47, 590, 624, 856*f*
enlargement 1008
sampling 671
Para-aortic nodal basin irradiation 697
Para-aortic radiotherapy 697
Paracervical node 47*f*
Paracervical plexus 40
Paracetamol 232, 530
Paralytic ileus 1259
Paramesonephric duct system 255, 289
Parametria 698
Paraovarian cyst 649, 649*f*, 650*f*, 983, 991, 992*f*
Paraphimosis 536
Pararectal defects 329
Parasitic mature cystic teratoma 656*f*
Parathyroid hormone 1193
Paraurethral implants 1155
Paraurethral tubules 370, 552, 552*f*
Paravaginal defect 329, 332*f*
Paravaginal fibromyxoma 562*f*
Paravaginal lipoma 558
Paravaginal tissue 698, 700
Park's classification 1235, 1236*f*
Paroophoron 50, 254*f*, 649
Paroxetine 824
Partial androgen insensitivity syndrome 290, 297, 300, 304, 305
Partial mole 216, 216*f*, 689
picture of 217*f*
treatment of 218
Partial rectal prolapse 1217, 1217*f*
treatment of 1218
Partial thromboplastin time 1267
Patent tube 853*f*
Peak systolic velocity 936*f*, 993
Pearl index 1062
Pedicle, torsion of 655, 656
Pediculocides 395
Pediculosis 810
pubis 366, 394
Pegylated liposomal doxorubicin 692
Pellagra 489
Pellets 784
Pelvic adhesions 37*f*, 866*f*, 1295
risk of 1091
Pelvic adhesive disease 47
Pelvic anatomy 47
Pelvic cancer 781
advanced 529, 531, 534
prevention of 523, 524*fc*
Pelvic cellular tissue 327
Pelvic congestion syndrome 350, 457
Pelvic diaphragm, relaxation of 46
Pelvic discomfort 275
Pelvic endometriosis 274, 412, 438*f*
removal of 439
sites of 961*f*
Pelvic examination 7, 12, 281, 459, 637
position of patient for 10
Pelvic fascia 52
Pelvic floor 51, 1145, 1149, 1223, 1311
disorders 834
dysfunction 331*f*, 833
exercises 1288, 1289*f*
measurements 1311
muscle 816, 838
training 1153
myofascial syndrome 459
physical therapy 462, 816, 833, 836
physiotherapy 1149
relaxation exercises 836
repair 1312
training devices 831
Pelvic infection 1295
chronic 386
tuberculous 382*f*
Pelvic inflammatory disease 5, 153, 180, 321, 402*f*, 416, 795, 807, 897, 989, 991*f*, 1072, 1082, 1099
acute 417*b*
chronic 758
incidence of 375
lower incidence of 1130
part of 989
risk of 1114
Pelvic lesions 457, 758
Pelvic ligaments
neoplasms of 650
tumours of 649
Pelvic lymph node
dissection 595
sampling 671

Pelvic mass 259
Pelvic muscles 33*f*
  electrical stimulation of 1289
Pelvic musculature 51
  weakness of 1216
Pelvic nerves, invasion of 443
Pelvic operation 1141
Pelvic organ 50*f*
  innervation of 57
  inspection of 266
  pathology of 431
  prolapse 327, 1162, 1311
    female 331*f*
    quantification staging system 331, 332*f*
    repair 1017
    stages of 331
  torsion of 359, 362, 362*fc*, 363
  ultrasound imaging of 899
Pelvic pain 342, 351, 420, 448, 630, 896, 910, 1081, 1289
  acute 962
  chronic 433, 448, 459
  nonmenstrual 788
  spasmodic 642
  ultrasound diagnosis of 897*fc*
Pelvic peritoneum 49, 437, 441, 653
  pyogenic infection of 408
Pelvic peritonitis 413, 415, 1224
Pelvic plexus 49, 59
Pelvic radiation 1181
  external 696*t*
Pelvic structures 986
Pelvic surgery 648, 1141, 1295
Pelvic tissues 441
Pelvic tuberculosis, diagnosis of 386
Pelvic tumour 1141, 1225
Pelvic ultrasound 174, 301, 760
  advanced 962
Pelvic vaginal examination 655*f*
Pelvic varicocele 457
Pelvic veins
  suppurative thrombophlebitis of 417
  thrombosis of 1262
Pelvic viscera, anatomy of 898*f*
Pelvis 42, 337, 384*f*, 965*f*, 1027, 1087*f*, 1089*f*
  anterior 1161
  blood vessels of 53
  bones of 30*f*
  floor of 675*f*
  frontal projection 422*f*
  normal 22*f*
  right side of 49*f*, 902*f*
  side wall of 385*f*
  transabdominal sonography transverse section of 910*f*
  veins of 55
  view of 1027*f*
Pembrolizumab 534, 689, 707
Penetration 747
  depth of 1294
Penicillamine 478
Penicillin 232, 370, 1258
Penile anomalies 824
Penis
  duplex ultrasound of 822
  manipulation of 819
Pentazocine 232, 233, 1138
Peptic ulcer 208
Peptostreptococcus 365, 402, 416
Percutaneous catheter fragmentation 1271
Percutaneous epididymal sperm aspiration 877
Percutaneous tibial nerve stimulation 1155
Perianal epidermis, dysplasia of 1239
Perianal haematoma 1234
Pericarditis 688
Pericervical ring 327
Perifimbrial paratubal cysts 269
Perifollicular flow 994*f*, 995*f*
Perimenopause 1182
  diagnosis of 113
Perineal anus 283, 284*f*
Perineal body descent 333
Perineal laceration, chronic 331
Perineal muscles 52
Perineal procedures 1220
Perineal tear 312, 313, 316
  classification of 313*t*
  fourth-degree 313
  old complete 316
  third-degree 313
Perineorrhaphy 316
Perineum 26, 27, 57, 380*f*, 830
  nerves of 56*f*
Periodic acid-Schiff 494
Periovarian adhesions 475
Peripheral mononuclear cells 710
Peripheral smear 148
Peripheral stem cell therapy 223
Peripheral vascularisation 746*f*
Peripheral vessels, short-coursed 987*f*
Peristalsis 990
Peritoneal blebs 961*f*
Peritoneal carcinoma, primary 644*f*, 691
Peritoneal cavity 127, 364, 613, 1027*f*, 1036, 1090*f*, 1257
Peritoneal inclusion cyst 952*f*, 983, 991, 992*f*
Peritoneal irritation, signs of 183
Peritoneal metastasis, abdominal 624
Peritoneal oocyte sperm transfer 878
Peritoneal pouch 49
Peritoneal reaction 854
Peritoneal sac 1219
Peritoneal serous carcinomas 653
Peritoneal surface 444, 672
Peritoneum 46, 402*f*, 1209, 1220, 1295
  neoplasms of 652
  redundant 344
  uterovesical fold of 1209
Peritonitis 402*f*, 1243, 1260
  general 371, 413
  tuberculous 275
Peritubal adhesions dating 855*f*
Periurethral bulking
  agents, use of 1161
  injections 1155
Perivascular predecidual reaction 91*f*
Permanent detrusor dysfunction 1141
Permissive hormones 227
Persistent trophoblastic disease 218, 219
  evaluation of 221*b*
Persistent vulvar pain, classification of 813*b*
Pessary
  insertion of 352
  management of 353
  size of 353
  test 352
  treatment 339
Pethidine 232
Peutz-Jeghers syndrome 1302, 1303
Pfannenstiel incision 1208*f*
Pflüger's tubules 253
pH 793, 798
Phallus, coronary sulcus of 261
Phantom tumours 655
Pharyngitis 371
Phenindione 233
Phenothiazine 145, 232
  derivatives 720
Phenotype 1171
Phenylalanine 1277
Phenylbutazone 232, 233
Phenytoin 478, 1104
Phimosis 536
Phlebothrombosis 417
Phlegmasia
  alba Dolens 1264
  cerulea dolens 1264
Phosphodiesterase 823*f*
  type 5 inhibitors 824, 827
Photobiomodulation 1298
Photons 1293*f*
Phyllodes tumour 238, 238*f*
Physiotherapy 339, 1287
  preoperative 1288
Phytoestrogens 119, 1203
  classes of 118
Pigment-laden lining cells 435
Piles
  differential diagnosis of 1232*f*
  mass 1233
  parts of 1231*f*
  position of 1231*f*
  second-degree 1233
  strangulated 1232*f*
  third-degree 1219
Pills 1094-1096
  missed 1097
  morning after 1115
  placebo 1096, 1187
Pilonidal sinus 1228, 1228*f*, 1236
Pinhole ostium 278
Pinworms 805
Pipelle device 421
Piriformis muscle, pelvic part of 52
Piroxicam 757
Pituitary gland, anterior lobe of 733*f*
Pituitary receptors, loss of 449
Pituitary-hypothalamic hormones 83*t*
Pituitary-ovarian relations 85
Piver-Rutledge-Smith classification 587, 1204

Placenta 1136
  delivery of 230
  transforms foetal adrenal dehydroepiandrosterone sulphate 158
Placental site trophoblastic tumour 217, 220, 222, 689
Plasma 232*t*, 1241
  androstenedione 236
  extracellular fluid volumes 1241*t*
  osmolality, normal 1243
  proopiomelanocortin peptides 1187
  protein 1242
    pregnancy-associated 160
Plasminogen, activator of 1268
Platelet-activating factor 163*f*
Platinum 706
  agents 687
Plethysmography 1265
Pleura 439
Pleural cavities 127
Pleural effusion 246
Pleuritic pain, cyclical development of 439
Plexus
  vertebral 40
  vesical 46
Pneumococcus 365, 397
Pneumocystis carinii pneumonia 375
Pneumocystography 244
Pneumonitis 688
Pneumoperitoneum 1020, 1209, 1212
Pneumothorax, cyclical 770
Point-of-care tests 799
Poly polymerase inhibitors 534
Polyacrylamide hydrogel injection 1155
Polycarbonate 1130
Polycystic nephropathy 1172
Polycystic ovary 17, 128, 463*f*, 464, 469*f*, 470*f*, 475, 475*f*, 662, 663, 725*f*, 734, 734*f*, 843*f*, 953, 993*f*, 995, 1028*f*
  bilateral 953*f*
  disease 236
  hyperstimulated 470*f*
  syndrome 69, 171, 308, 463, 463*f*, 465*fc*, 468, 468*f*, 471, 471*fc*, 472*f*, 473*f*, 476, 480, 510, 511*f*, 720, 721, 725*f*, 726*f*, 734*f*, 738-740, 741*f*, 785, 864, 864*fc*, 868, 1002, 1300
    biochemical features of 466*f*, 469
    clinical features of 466*f*, 469
    diagnostic pathway for 476*fc*
    endocrine aspects of 465
    metabolic component of 467
    metabolic features of 466*f*, 469
    typical of 724*f*
  uterine artery Doppler in 470*f*
Polycythaemia 604
Polydimethylsiloxane 1113, 1161
Polyethylene 1077
  glycol 393, 1248
Polyhydramnios 368
Polymastia 228, 229*f*
Polymenorrhagia 350, 443
Polymenorrhoea 443
Polymerase chain reaction 421, 795, 879
  test 369, 1304
Polymorphic sites 1183
Polyp 642, 744, 942, 981, 984, 1043*f*
  mucosal 642
  multiple 597, 744*f*
  pedicle of 357, 983*f*, 984*f*
Polypectomy 12, 609, 1043
Polypoidal endometrial hyperplasia 1044*f*
Polyposis, endometrial 675*f*
Polypropylene sutures 1220
Polytetrafluoroethylene 1161
Polythelia 228, 229*f*
  areolaris 228
Polyunsaturated fatty acids 1278
  types of 1278
Polyuria 1140
Pomeroy operation 1129, 1130*f*
Poor ovarian reserve 1297
Port site endometriosis 455*f*
Positron emission tomography scan 23, 387, 565, 586, 586*f*
Postanaesthetic discharge scoring system 1250
Postchemotherapy surveillance 223
Postcoital test 857
Posterior cervix, endometriosis of 456
Posterior compartment defects 333
Posterior urethrovesical angles, types of 1145*f*
Posterior vaginal fornix 440*f*
Posterior vaginal wall
  anatomy of 961*f*
  lower part of 558*f*
Postgastrectomy syndrome 812
Postmenopausal bleeding 13, 420, 568*f*, 618*f*, 623*f*, 751, 932*f*, 933, 935*f*, 936*f*, 938*fc*, 1002, 1005*f*, 1196
  causes of 752
Postmenopausal endometrium 935*f*
  evaluation of 1003*fc*
Postmenopausal hormone therapy 1124
Postmolar surveillance 219
Postnatal adrenogenital syndrome 307*f*
Postoperative radiation therapy 627
Postpartum intrauterine contraceptive device 1120
  insertion 1120, 1120*f*, 1121
Postperianal surgery 1234
Postradiation ulceration 752
Post-therapy beta human chorionic gonadotrophin evaluation 222*t*
Potassium 1241
  chloride 205, 1245, 1248
  iodide 232
  loss
    prevention of 1245
    repletion of 1245
  serum 1245
  titanyl phosphate 18, 1292, 1294
Potency 772
Potentially pathogenic micro-organisms 804
Pouch of Douglas 8, 14, 34, 185, 351, 408, 437, 440, 962*f*, 1006
  peritoneum of 437
Powder-burn
  lesions 444
  typical 446
Preantral follicle 65
Precancerous lesions, management of 541, 561
Precocious pseudopuberty 140
  causes of 141
Precocious puberty 140, 140*f*, 141*f*, 142*fc*, 143*f*, 144, 750, 788
  central 140
  gonadotrophin
    dependent 141, 141*t*
    independent 141, 141*t*
  true 144
  types of 141
Pre-eclampsia 537*f*
Pre-existing tubal damage 873
Pregabalin 461, 816
Pregnancy 34, 125, 228*f*, 230, 236, 346, 361, 457, 596, 683, 718, 776, 780, 1092, 1140, 1201, 1225, 1263
  abdominal 183, 187, 203, 203*f*
  antecedent 221, 690
  associated plasma protein A, biological function of 160
  category 1177
  cervical 202, 202*f*
  cornual 201, 271
  corpus luteum of 158
  ectopic 12, 179, 181, 184*f*, 185, 189, 190, 191*f*, 193, 200, 206, 208, 218, 385, 411, 412, 443, 655, 965, 1089, 1090, 1104, 1111, 1139, 1295
  effect of 607
  fear of 110
  heterotopic 179
  immunotherapy in 714
  interstitial 204, 205
  intraligamentary 205
  loss
    early 606
    prediction of 207
    recurrent 169, 170, 606, 709
  luteoma of 480, 481, 662
  medical termination of 220
  molar 215, 217, 222
  morbidity 171
  normal 218
  of unknown location 189, 205, 207
    management of 207, 209*fc*
  ovarian 200, 201*f*, 662
  pelvic congestion of 1230
  prepubertal stage to 227*t*
  progresses 157
  rate 1091
    clinical 451
    higher 995
  recurrent 169
  reflects, sodium balance in 160
  signs of 183
  symptoms 183
    regression of 168
  termination of 127, 162, 1128, 1133, 1133*b*, 1134*t*, 1137, 1247
  test 719*fc*, 733
    positive 205

tubal 184*f*, 204
tumour found in
first trimester of 684
third trimester of 684
unplanned 1134
Pregnanediol, excretion of 86
Pregnanetriol 86
Preimplantation genetic diagnosis 877, 879
Premature ejaculation 822, 859
acquired 823
Premenstrual dysphoric disorder 762, 763*t*
Premenstrual mastalgia 121, 767, 784
aetiology of 767
Premenstrual syndrome 457, 762, 764*t*, 780, 1226, 1288
signs of 103*f*
symptoms of 103*f*
Presacral nerves 758*f*
Presacral neurectomy 758
operation of 758*f*
Presacral plexus 50*f*
Preterm labour 368, 606, 1092
Prevagina 1005
Prilocaine 824
Primary abdominal pregnancy, diagnosis of 203*b*
Primary broad ligament tumours 651
Primary cytology screening 577*fc*
Primidone 1104
Primordial follicle 64*f*, 65, 262, 1183
number 106*f*
Primordial germ cells 261
arrival of 253
migrate 253
originate 62, 288
Procidentia 330*f*, 1218
complete 329, 334*f*
Proctalgia fugax 1240
Proctitis 1238
tuberculous 1238
Proctoscopy 1232
Progestasert 1079, 1090, 1091
Progesterone 76*fc*, 80, 86, 148, 159, 465*f*, 609, 724, 745, 780, 870*f*, 1075, 1093, 1117
action of 79*f*, 1117, 1096
analogues 1200
antagonist 450, 1117
comparative doses of 1200*t*
competes 160
continuous production of 724
daily production of 159
deficiency 164
derivatives 779
fluid retaining effects of 81
generation 1200
halogenated 1200
high levels of 81
micronised 116
natural 1200
plasma levels of 77*f*
pregnancy levels of 1119
receptor 246, 534, 625
modulator 609, 609*fc*
relaxes smooth muscle 81
resistance 442
secretion 1188
stereoisomers of 779
therapy 1003, 1004
regimes of 1200
types of 1105, 1200
underproduction of 724
use of 1200
withdrawal bleeding 94
Progestin 1093, 1094, 1115
low-dose 115
serum concentration of 1083
structural formula of 781*f*
therapy 1195
Progestogen 127, 130, 308, 447, 448, 491, 534, 629, 639, 736, 779, 1092, 1093, 1105*t*, 1187, 1199, 1202, 1263
first-generation 1093
intrauterine system 1112
natural 779
newest 1093
preparations 116
synthetic 779
therapy 440*f*
third-generation 1093
Progestogen-only
contraceptive pill 747, 1064, 1105, 1109
use of 1107*b*
implants 1108
injectables 1105
minipill 1119
Progressive disease 671
Progynova 148
Prolactin 113, 144, 226, 234*f*, 235, 482, 739, 825, 844, 864
inhibiting factor 83, 234, 235
levels 144*t*, 235, 740*fc*
lower 823
management 144*t*
releasing hormone 230*f*
secretion
control of 234*f*
dopaminergic inhibition of 768
Prolapse 350, 456, 1204
congenital 335
favours pyelitis 1258
incarceration of 335
recurrent 357*f*
second-degree 350*f*
third-degree 330*f*
Proliferative endometrium 37*f*
late 90*f*, 929*f*
Proliferative phase gland 90
Promethazine 1138
Promiscuity 367
Promiscuous sexual behaviour 1172
Pronephric duct 254
Propantheline 232
Prophylactic antibiotics 1031, 1247
use of 1031
Prophylactic surgeries 1304
Propiverine 1155
Prostacyclin 112, 163*f*
Prostaglandin 168, 444, 754, 1135, 1136
analogues 1137
metabolism 764
synthesis, clomiphene-induced inhibition of 125
synthetase inhibitors 746, 755
Prostate
carcinoma of 789
diseases 824
Protease inhibitor 377
Protein 158, 1173, 1275, 1277, 1282, 1286
biological values of 1277
C 1194
rich foods 1277
S 1194
sources of 1277
Proteus
mirabilis 1173
vulgaris 1258
Proton pump inhibitors 1116
Pruritus 490*f*, 805, 1232, 1239
ani 305*f*, 1227
causes of 805
differential diagnosis of 807
general 809
vulvae 804, 806*t*, 811*f*, 812*f*
aetiological classification of 805
Pseudocyesis 655, 720
Pseudocysts 410
Pseudogestational sac 190
Pseudohyperkalaemia 1246
Pseudohyphae 799
Pseudohypokalaemia 1244
Pseudo-Meigs' syndrome 127, 614
Pseudomenopause 449
Pseudomonas 1173, 1247, 1258
Pseudopuberty, precocious 140
Pseudosac, uterine of 190*f*
Psoriasis 806
Psychological sequelae 321
Psychoses 720
Psychosomatic medicine 2
Pthirus pubis 394
Puberty 34, 132, 134, 135, 226*f*, 236, 471, 1191*f*
abnormalities of 136
delayed 135*f*, 137
menorrhagia 146, 420
causes of 147, 147*t*
management of 147, 148*fc*
precocious 140, 140*f*, 141*f*, 142*fc*, 143*f*, 144, 750, 788
Pubic bone 543*f*, 1157, 1159
back of 1160
Pubic hair 108, 135, 297, 1032
development of 134*f*, 138
growth of 135
lack of 139*f*
Pubic mound, liposuction of 1299
Pubic symphysis, periosteum of 1161*f*
Pubocervical fascia 52, 341, 342, 344
Pubocervical ligament 328, 342
Pubococcygeus muscle 51, 836, 1145, 1157, 1288
Puborectalis 44
muscle 836
tone 1220

Pubourethral ligaments 1157
Pubovaginal sling surgery 1158, 1160*f*
Pubovesicocervical fascia 1213
Pudendal block, anatomy of 58*f*
Pudendal nerve 58
Puerperium 339
Pulmonary artery catheterisation 1270
Pulsatile growth hormone secretion 471
Pulsatility index 16, 932*f*, 936*f*, 955*f*
Pulsion enterocele 333
Puppy fat, development of 137
Purandare's cervicopexy 344
Pure sex cord tumours 659
Pure stromal tumours 659
Purgatives, abuse of 1226
Purine antagonists 532
Purulent discharge 844
Pustular dermatitis 371
Pyaemia, portal 1233
Pyelitis 411
Pyelogram, intravenous 268*f*, 285*f*
Pyelography 286
  intravenous 335*f*
Pyelonephritis 1171, 1171*t*, 1172, 1173, 1258
  mild 1171
  moderate 1171
  severe 1171
Pyloric stenosis 1244
Pyogenic infections 391
Pyohaematometra 407, 619*f*
Pyometra 407, 530, 580, 619
Pyosalpinx 410*f*, 655, 960
  3D ultrasound 408*f*
  bilateral 961*f*
  tuberculous 431*f*
Pyrazinamide 387, 388, 430
Pyrexia 1257, 1258
  postpartum 380
Pyridoxine 232
Pyrimidine antagonists 532
Pyuria 810

Q

Q-tip test 1151
Querleu-Morrow classification 1205-1207
Quinacrine 20
Quinestrol 1198
Quinine 232

R

Radiation 165, 460, 566, 737
  dosage 695
  exposure 245
  high-dose of 242
  kills cells 695
  menopause 120
  proctitis 1238, 1238
  therapy 250, 587, 590*t*, 647, 860
    sequelae of 593
  vaginitis 593
Radical hysterectomy 587*f*, 595, 696*t*, 1165, 1206
  classic 1206
  modified 1206
Radical operation 529
Radical surgery 534, 593
  mortality of 588
Radioimmunoassay techniques 307
Radioisotopes 1265
Radiotherapy
  adjuvant 592, 592*t*
  conventional 589
  machines 696
  primary 535
  role of 673
  treatment, biological basis of 695
  volumes 699
Raloxifene 76, 117, 452, 608, 779
Raltegravir 377
Randomised controlled trials 1297
Ranitidine 145
Rapamycin pathways, mammalian target of 230
Rapid plasma regain test 369
Reactive oxygen species, production of 573
Reactive squamous cell hyperplasia 499*f*
Reconstructive clitoral surgery 324
Reconstructive surgeries 302
Rectal examination 10, 301
Rectal polyp 1219, 1232, 1232*f*
Rectal prolapse 1216, 1218*f*, 1219*f*, 1220, 1222*t*, 1232
  acute management of 1220
  complete 1218, 1218*f*
  complications of 1219
  defecographic grading of 1219
  partial 1217, 1217*f*
  types of 1217*f*
Rectal spasm 1239, 1240
Rectocele 333, 1225
  small 333*f*
Rectosigmoid intussusception 1219
Rectouterine muscle 328
Rectovaginal examination 312, 460
Rectovaginal fascia 32
Rectovaginal fistula 314, 580
Rectovaginal septum 328, 329, 435*f*, 438, 456
  umbilicus 441
Rectum 48, 57, 280, 1226
  carcinoma of 752, 1225, 1230, 1232, 1239, 1273
  circumferential incision of 1221
  constriction of 1225
  diseases of 459, 810
  funnel-shaped 1219
  villous tumour of 1244
Rectus fascia, harvesting strip of 1158, 1160*f*
Recurrent pregnancy loss 170, 606, 709
  aetiology of 171*f*
Recurrent urinary tract infection 112, 1178*fc*
  evaluation of 1174*fc*
Reductase deficiency 304, 305
Regulatory T-cell 703*f*
Reiter's disease 371
Relaxation techniques 765, 837
Remote sequelae 1265
Remote surgery 1018
Renal abnormalities 970
Renal anomalies 266
Renal artery 47
Renal disease 235, 1136
Renal failure 145
  chronic 785
  infection of 334
Renal function test 219
Renal insufficiency 1172
Renal pelvis, diseases of 1141
Renal receptor sites, aldosterone for 160
Renal scarring 1177
Reproductive aging workshop, stages of 108*t*
Reproductive cycle, female 96*t*
Reproductive development, stages of 793*t*
Reproductive health 711
Reproductive medicine 1297
  immunotherapy in 709
Reproductive problems 901
Reproductive system, female 433
Resectoscope 1039*f*
  sheath 1039*f*, 1042*f*
Reserpine 145, 232, 720
Residual oedema, treatment of 1268
Residual pelvic adhesions 414
Residual urine 1253, 1258
Resistive index 932*f*, 936*f*, 945*f*, 955*f*
Respiratory distress syndrome 218, 1272
Rete ovarii, tumours of 660
Rete testis 261
  aspiration 878
Retention
  acute 1164
  causes of 1164
  mechanisms of 1164
Retina fields, examination of 733
Retinol 845
Retroflexion 349
Retrograde endometrial spill 441
Retroperitoneal fat deposits 1035
Retroperitoneal vessel 1020
  injury 1036
Retropronation 349
Retropubic bladder neck colposuspension 1161
Retropubic procedures, types of 1161*t*
Retroversion 349, 437, 456
  correction of 352*f*
Retroverted gravid uterus 353, 1164*f*, 1225
Retroviral therapy, highly affective 375
Retzius space 46, 1159
Rhabdomyosarcomas 633
Rhabdomyosarcomatous elements 633*f*
Rhesus 874
  factor 1128
  isoimmunisation 1139
  isoimmunisation, severe 877
Rheumatic diseases 1080
Rhodamine 386
Rhythm method 1064
Riboflavin 489, 491
Ribonucleic acid 375, 687, 703
Richardson technique 1208

Rifabutin 387
Rifampicin 387, 388, 430, 1104
Rifampin 1116
Rigid hymen 821
Rigidity test 822
Rim sign 984
Ringer's lactate 1040
Ringer's solution 1253
Ringworm 394
Ripening Graafian follicle 67*f*
Risedronate 118
Ritonavir 377
Rituximab 711*f*, 712, 716
  use of 712
Robotic surgery 20, 1011, 1013-1015, 1015*t*, 1016, 1018, 1057
  future of 1018
  innovation 1018
Robotic systems 1309
Robotic-assisted laparoscopy 612, 1058*f*
  uses of 1058
Rosenmuller organ 50
Rotterdam criteria 864
Round ligament 51, 327, 438, 1213
  division of 1209, 1210*f*
  endometriosis of 555
  insertion of 201
Rubella 173
Rubin's insufflation cannula 889
Rubin's test 14
Rucaparib 534
Rudimentary cavity 266
Ruptured tubal ectopic gestation 965

S

Sacral colpopexy, abdominal 345
Sacral nodes 40
Sacrospinous ligament fixation 345
Sacrum, promontory of 758*f*
Safe periods 1065*f*
Saf-T-coil 1077, 1077*f*
Saint John's wort 1116
Salicylate 232, 716
Saline
  infusion sonography 622
  instillation of 16
  laxatives 1226
Salmonella typhi 365, 403
Salpingectomy 192, 195, 199, 361, 1128
  indications of 199*b*
  Jeffcoate's theory of different effects of 196*f*
  opportunistic 648
  partial 199
  procedure of 199
Salpingitis 180, 402*f*, 1104
  acute 188
  isthmica nodosa 180, 181, 424*f*
    severe form of 425*f*
  subacute 188
  tubercular 388, 431*f*
Salpingography 650*f*
Salpingolysis 413, 866, 866*f*
Salpingo-oophorectomy 196*f*, 1053
  risk of reduction 648
Salpingo-oophoritis 407, 414, 457, 595, 663
  acute 411, 412, 415, 1091
  chronic 407*f*, 411, 412, 445, 1091
  subacute 411, 412
Salpingo-ovariectomy, unilateral 670
Salpingoscopy, ampullary 14
Salpingostomy 192, 195, 196*b*, 413, 866
  laparoscopic 196
  tube-sparing 199
Salpingotomy 195, 199
  laparoscopic 197*f*
Salt-and-pepper appearance 978
Sampson's runs, small artery of 1208
Sampson's theory 440
Sanitary pads 104
Saprophytes 575
Saquinavir 377
Sarcoidosis 389, 413
Sarcoma 536, 549, 568, 596, 597, 633, 642
  botryoides 568, 634
  progression to 614
Sarcomatoid 574
Sarcopenia 1189
Sarcoptes scabiei hominis 805
Saucer-shaped rubber diaphragm 1070
Scabies 805
Scar
  abdominal 441
  endometriosis 439
Schistosoma haematobium 365, 390
Schistosomiasis 390, 1080
  genital 390
Scissors 884, 1022, 1039
  types of 1041*f*
Sclerosants, percutaneous injection of 1133
Sclerosing chemicals 20
Scoliosis 459
Scrotum 262
Sebaceous balls 678*f*
Sebaceous contents, leakage of 656
Secondary sex characteristics 287, 304
  development of 135*t*
Secondary sex organ 77, 80
Secretory cells, single-layered lining of 664*f*
Sedatives 1150
Seizures 375
Selective oestrogen receptor
  down regulators 534
  modulator 76, 117, 452, 779, 1117, 1193
    development of 117
Selective progesterone receptor modulator 450, 608, 609, 747
Selective serotonin reuptake inhibitors 118, 461, 764, 824
Sella turcica
  imaging techniques of 236*t*
  lateral coned-down view of 236
Semen
  analysis 847
    abnormalities, evaluation of 848*fc*
    guidelines 843*t*
  defects, severe 877
  preparation 876, 876*b*
    density gradient for 876*b*
    methods for 876*b*
  quality
    abnormal 843
    severe deficits in 878
  volume 843
Seminal fluid 150
Seminal plasma 710
  factors 150
Seminiferous tubule 253, 262
  dysgenesis 294
Senile
  atrophy 487
  inversion 357
  pyometra 752
  vaginitis 397, 775*f*
  vulvitis 392
Sensate focus 837
  exercises 832
Sensitivity, rates of 638
Sensory loss 1224
Sensual awareness training 824
Sentinel lymph node biopsy 248, 249, 586
Sepsis 1255
  immunotherapy for 715*f*
Sepsis-induced immunological dysregulation, immunotherapy in 714
Septae, partial 960*f*
Septal dystocia 265
Septate cervix 266, 909*f*
Septate uterus 264, 266, 267, 269*f*, 908*f*, 973, 1042, 1296
  bicorporeal 974, 975*f*
  complete septum 908*f*
Septate vagina 267, 270*f*, 271, 281
  imperforate 273*f*
Septicaemia 1233, 1235
Septum 977*f*
  complete 974, 974*f*
  incomplete 951
  longitudinal 279
  partial 908*f*, 974, 974*f*
Serological tests 369
Serosa 981*f*
Serosanguinous discharge 793
Serotonin reuptake inhibitors 118, 765, 1187
Serous cyst adenoma 951
Serous papillary tubal carcinoma, stained slide of 646*f*
Serous tubal intraepithelial carcinoma 645
Serous tumours 658
  benign 664
Serratia 1173
Sertoli-Leydig cell tumours 480, 481, 658, 675-677
Sertraline 824
Serum B-human chorionic gonadotrophin levels 188
Serum cancer antigen-125 623, 657
Serum creatinine 127, 375
Serum dehydroepiandrosterone concentration, measurement of 138
Serum glutamic-pyruvic transaminase 375
Serum human chorionic gonadotrophin levels 189
Serum progesterone levels 191
Serum prolactin levels 138, 144

Serum testosterone
levels 138
measurement of 308
Serum thyroid-stimulating hormone 483, 763
measurement of 138
Serum total testosterone 482
Sessile leiomyoma 539*f*
Seton technique 1237*f*
Severe dysplasia carcinoma in situ 502
Sex chromosome 288*fc*, 293*f*
aberrations of 295
component, abnormal 292
disorders 290
distribution 290
division 290
pattern arise 291
polysomy 163
Sex cord 253
budding 261
free ends of 261
mesenchymal tumour with annular tubules 677
stromal tumours 481, 658, 659, 674, 681
Sex development 290
disorders of 290, 295, 304
ovotesticular disorders of 299, 300
XX disorders of 290, 295
XY disorders of 290, 297
Sex hormone 29
binding
globulin 308, 466, 466*f*, 449, 467, 480, 825
hormone concentration 465
female 309
Sex organs 304, 306
Sex steroid 71, 1119, 1189
active 1185
secretion 85
Sex therapy 833
Sex-determining region Y 288, 289
chromosome 262
Sexual aversion disorder 821
Sexual contact 819
Sexual desire 828
inventory 830
Sexual development
normal 288*fc*
stages of 793*t*
Sexual dysfunction 145, 821, 825
classification of 821
disorders 821
female 821*t*
Sexual education 136, 830, 837
lack of 834
Sexual function, impaired 321
Sexual functioning questionnaire 830
Sexual health screening 322
Sexual intercourse 819, 1116
unprotected 372, 1115
Sexual maturity 34
Sexual satisfaction 818, 828
Sexual unresponsiveness 784
Sexually transmitted
disease 136, 364, 366, 396, 572, 1062, 1099, 1132
types of 366
infections 366, 366*f*, 573, 793, 807, 809
Shaw's classification 330*f*
Sheehan's syndrome 123, 723, 733, 774*f*
Shirodkar's abdominal sling 344
Shirodkar's methods 1130
Shock 1138, 1255, 1259
treatment of 193
uroseptic 1171
Short stature 292
Short-armed X isochromosomes 291
Short-wave therapy 1289
Sigmoid colon 47, 57
Sigmoidoscopy 1226, 1230
Silver nitrate 20
Simple ovarian cyst 949*fc*
Simple plastic procedure 283*f*
Simple serous cyst 952*f*
Simpson uterine sound 884
Sims' double-bladed posterior vaginal speculum 886
Sims' position, modified 11
Sims' semiprone position 10, 11*f*
Sims' speculum 9*f*, 280*f*, 887*f*
Sims' vaginal speculum 884
Single incision
laparoscopic surgery, port devices for 1054*f*
technique 1056*f*
Single intramural leiomyoma 600*f*
Single subserous leiomyoma 615*f*
Single vagina 268*f*
Single-agent therapy 534
Single-nucleotide polymorphism 1303
Single-port laparoscopic surgery 1053
Singular access device, use of 1056
Sinus 384
primary 1228
secondary 1228
tract formation 1162
Sitz bath 1229, 1229*f*, 1233
Skeletal system 78
Skene's tubules 43, 258, 552
cyst of 536, 552, 552*f*, 558
Skin 777, 1302
haemorrhagic 777
infection 1234
irritation 1235
lichenification of 489
lies, squamous epithelium of 434*f*
manifestations 472
preparation 1032
resistance 1186
sensitivity 810
tests 490
tags, multiple 1234
vulvar 1298
Skull, base of 308
Sleep disturbances 111, 114
Slim resectoscope 1052, 1052*f*
Smegma concretion 391, 391*f*
Smell, absence of 799
Smith-Lemli-Opitz syndrome 160
Smooth muscle
growth, inhibition of 112
interlacing bonds of 598*f*
internal 1145
minimal 328
tumours 614
Snoopy' breasts 230
Social medicine 2
Sodium 1241, 1242
chloride 1248
fractional excretion of 1243
fusidate 232
serum 1242
tetradecyl sulphate 1233
Soft sore 373*f*
Solid mass 950, 1007*f*
Solid ovarian tumour, torsion of 360*f*
Solid papillary projection 950
Solifenacin 1155
Somatic copy-number alteration low 625
Somatic mutation 1301
Somatic nerves 57
Somatotropin-releasing hormone 83
Sonography, abdominal 341
Sonohysterography 983, 984*f*
Sonohysterosalpingography 897
Sonosalpingography 14, 387
Soonawala's sling 344
Sorbitol-mannitol solution 1041
Spaniel ear nymphae 283
Sparfloxacin 387
Spasmodic vaginismus 835
Spectral Doppler of perifollicular flow 994*f*
Speculum 559*f*
examination 8, 892
size of 8
Sperm
agglutinins 842
antibodies 850
function tests 849
granulomas 1132
head 423*f*, 426*f*
penetration 1083
assay 849
test 849
retrieval 879
semen consists of 150
wash 876
Spermatogenesis 859
Spermatozoa 125, 150, 710, 841, 1132
active 1132
immature forms of 848
maturation of 294
Spermatozoon 288*fc*
Spermicide 1073, 1074, 1120
Sphincter
dysfunction 1149
vaginae muscle 29, 34
weakness 1224
Spinnbarkeit test 1066*f*
Spiral fibres 60*f*
Spironolactone 309, 472, 485, 1245
therapy 484

Split pelvis 282*f*
Sponge 1074
  holding forceps 884
Spontaneous abortion 162, 163, 164*f*, 218
  clinical varieties of 167
  pathology of 162
Sporadic cancers 1301
  detection of 1301
Sporadic somatic mutation 1301
Squamocolumnar junction 32*f*, 497*f*, 581
Squamous cell 502
  carcinoma 507*f*, 536, 542, 543*f*, 557, 564, 568*f*, 573, 574, 942, 944*f*, 1239, 1240*f*
    classification of 573
  hyperplasia 499, 502, 512
  malignant 568*f*
Squamous epithelium 496, 498
Squamous intraepithelial
  lesion 561
    low-grade 503, 540, 577, 579
  neoplasia 492
Squamous metaplasia 498, 502
Squamous vulvar carcinoma 541
Staphylococcus 365, 395, 397
  aureus 104
    methicillin-resistant 1175
  saprophyticus 1173
Stapled transnational rectal resection 1218
Starch test 14
Starvation 730
Statins 714
Stavudine 377
Stem cell
  mesenchymal 714
  rescue 692
Sterilisation 1128
  female 1129
  hysteroscopic 1048*f*
  indications of 1129*b*
  laparoscopic 1130
  male 1131
  procedure 1128, 1131
  routes of 1129
  techniques of 1130
  timing of 1129*t*
  tubal 207, 1027
Sterility 840
Steroid 1244
  biosynthesis, pathway for 295*fc*
  cell
    malignant 674
    tumours 480, 481, 677
  hormones 76*fc*, 86, 295
    higher concentrations of 600
Steroidogenesis, multiple enzymes of 449
Stimulation test 483
Stratified squamous epithelium 370
Stratum compactum 88
Streptococcal infection 805, 1176
Streptococcus 397
  faecalis 395, 1258
  pneumoniae 395
Streptomycin 232, 374
Streptothrix organisms 365
Stress 145
  hormone levels 233
  incontinence 112, 345, 1145, 1150, 1151, 1151*f*, 1155, 1156
    demonstration of 1151
    surgery for 1149
  urinary incontinence 338, 347, 1143, 1150, 1189
    grading of 1144
String problems 1122
Stroke 1031, 1101, 1194
Stroma 230
  swollen 1113
Stromal cells 90
Stromal invasion 592, 668, 696
Stromal oedema 91*f*, 963
Stromal sarcoma, high-flow 632
Struma ovarii 660, 681*f*
Styrene-ethylene-butylene-styrene 1069
Subendometrial halo thickening 637
Subendometrial myometrium 636
Subfertility 660
Sublingual allergen immunotherapy 714
Submucosal fibroids 976, 1042
  types of 977*f*
Submucosal leiomyoma 913
Submucosal tissues 1297
Submucous fibroid 745, 746*f*, 917*f*, 918*f*, 1044*f*
Submucous polyp 844
Subnormal bladder capacity 1163
Subnuclear vacuolation 90*f*
Subnuclear vacuoles 91*f*
Subsequent axillary lymph node dissection 249
Subserosal fibroid 976, 977*f*
  presence of 746*f*
Subserosal leiomyoma 913
Substances, production of 443
Substantial overlap 1191
Suburethral sling 1155, 1157
Suburethral vaginal tissues 1157
Suction pipette 526*f*
Sulpha antibiotic 716
Sulphamethoxazole 1176, 1177
Sulphapyridine 716
Sulphasalazine 716
Sulphonamides 232, 365*f*, 374
Sulprostone 1135
Superficial abdominal wall 1036
Superficial peritoneal endometriosis 961*f*
Superficial transverse perineal muscle 836
Superficial venous thrombosis 1262
Superior rectal veins 1230
Suppurative thrombophlebitis 417, 1262
Supraclavicular lymph node 246
Supralevator fistula 1236*f*
Suprapubic mini-laparotomy incision 1130
Supravaginal cervix 37, 46, 202*f*
  elimination of 334
Surgery 1247
  abdominal 1035
  aims of 1156
  conventional 1295
  endoscopic 1019
  hysteroscopic-guided 1052
  indications of 389, 1156
  types of 1157
Surgical procedure 130, 199, 208, 1237
  type of 1251
Surgical simulation 1018
Surgical sperm recovery 878
Surgical therapy 452
  indications of 195*b*
Surgical treatment 412, 413, 455, 736, 757
Surrogacy 874
Suture materials 891
Swallowed air 1260
Sweat gland 27
  tumour 536, 538*f*
Sweating phenomenon 31
Swede score 507*t*
  interpretation of 580
Swelling
  abdominal 667
  sensation of 337
Swim-up technique 876, 876*b*
Swyer syndrome 290
Symmastia 228
Sympathetic nerves 758*f*
Symphysis pubis 1164*f*, 1165, 1166*f*
Symptothermal method 1065, 1066*f*
Syncytiotrophoblast cells 217, 711
Synechiae 19, 432, 981, 983, 984*f*
  formation 387
  intrauterine 1043*f*
  treatment for 739
Syosalpinges, tuberculous 383*f*, 384*f*
Syphilis 366-368, 373, 393
  chancre 367*f*
  congenital 368, 369
  early 370
  latent 368, 370
  secondary 368
  serological tests for 393
  tertiary 368
  treatment of 369
  ulcer 392*f*
Syphilitic lesions, secondary 368*f*
Systemic inflammatory response syndrome 1172
Systemic lupus erythematosus 1080, 1123

T

Tachycardia 1249, 1257
Tacrolimus 710
Tamoxifen 76, 117, 125, 534, 618, 693, 933*f*, 1003, 1004
Tampons 104
Tanner's staging 226, 227*f*
Tarry cysts 437
Taxane 687, 706
T-cell
  immune response 708
  receptor 703*f*
  proliferation of tumour-specific 703
Tear, grade of 313
Teflon mesh 345

Teleoperation 1018
Telescope 1037, 1038*f*, 1040
Telogen 479
Tenaculum 890, 890*f*
Tenderness 657
Tenesmus 5
Tenofovir 377
Tension-free
 manner, placing sling in 1160
 obturator tape 1159*f*
 vaginal tape surgery 1158*f*
Teratoma 678
 mature 23*f*
Teratozoospermia 843
Teriparatide 1193
Terminal hair 478
 growth 464
Termination of pregnancy 127, 162, 1128, 1133, 1133*b*, 1134*t*, 1137, 1247
 methods for 1135*t*
 techniques of 1135
Testicular
 activity, depression of 841
 biosynthesis defect 300
 feminisation syndrome 298*f*
 sperm
  aspiration 842
  extraction 862, 877
 torsion 860
Testis 76*fc*, 728*f*, 777
 absence of 300*f*
 descend 262
 determining factor 262, 288, 904
 undescended 301
Testosterone 86, 143, 304, 307, 465, 479, 784, 1185
 analogues 1200
 biosynthesis 298*fc*
  defect 304, 305
  inborn errors of 297
 derivatives 779
 free 464
 intratesticular 1119
 metabolism 299
 production of 728
 replacement therapy 825
 therapy 832
 total 464
Tetracycline 232, 374, 389
Thalidomide 270
Theca
 cell
  luteinisation of 676
  tumours 510
 interna 67*f*
 lutein
  cells 72*f*, 662*f*
  cyst 15*f*, 662
Thecoma 658, 674
Therapeutic cancer vaccines 708
Therapeutic tests 734
Thermocoagulation 508, 613
Thermography 244
Thermolysis 472
Thiacetazone 387
Thiamine 1281
Thiazide 1244
 diuretics 232
Thick in-homogeneous endometrium 1004*f*
Thoracic kyphosis 1192
Threadworms 810
Three-dimensional
 printing 1310
 ultrasound septate 172*f*
 vision technology 1014
Threonine 1277
Thrombectomy 1268
Thromboembolic diseases 1031
Thromboembolism 115, 777, 782, 1265
Thrombolysins 1267, 1268, 1268*b*, 1270
Thrombolysis 1271
Thrombophilia 165
Thrombophlebitis, superficial 238
Thromboprophylaxis 1032
Thrombosis 117, 881, 1139, 1264
Thrombotic events 711
Thromboxane
 A2 163*f*
 B2 711*f*
Thyroid 729, 735, 1302
 disorder 738, 1080
  characteristics of 738*t*
 enlargement of 132
 examination, abnormal 738, 738*t*
 function tests 141
 gland, typical structure of 681*f*
 hormone
  replacement therapy 140
  synthesis of 1284
 storm 218
 temporary enlargement of 135
Thyroid-stimulating hormone 83, 107, 113, 132, 142, 146, 158, 170, 219, 460, 482, 723, 739, 740, 790, 823, 844, 862-864, 875
 elevated 740*fc*
Thyrotoxic periodic paralysis 1244
Thyrotoxicosis 841, 1245
Thyrotrophin-releasing hormone 83, 234*f*, 235, 791
 stimulation 234
Thyroxine 231, 226, 232, 719
Tibolone 117, 608, 784, 832, 1187, 1193, 1194
Tinea cruris 394
Tinidazole 400, 403, 800
Tinnitus 532
Tipranavir 377
Tissue
 clamps 885, 886*f*
 factor 163*f*, 711*f*
 healing properties of 1261
 injury induced 637
 new growth of 654
 plasminogen activator 1268
 trauma 1295
Today's sponge 1073, 1074*f*
 applications of 1074*f*
Tolbutamide 232
Toll-like receptor 703*f*
Tolterodin 1155
Topography 747
Torsion 359
 pedicle of 963
Total abdominal hysterectomy 654, 932*f*, 935*f*, 1204, 1214
Total parental nutrition 1245, 1252
Toxic shock syndrome 104, 1068
Toxicity 776, 782, 785
 immunotherapy-associated 688
 pulmonary 532
Toxoplasma gondii 260, 375
Toxoplasmosis, others, rubella, cytomegalovirus, herpes screening 173
Trachelorrhaphy 406
Traction enterocele 333
Traditional liposuction techniques 1299
Tramadol, on-demand use of 824
Tranexamic acid 747
Trans fatty acids 1278
Transabdominal sonography 896, 908*f*, 932*f*, 955*f*
Transcervical dye instillation 1027
Transcutaneous electric nerve stimulation 758, 1290
Transdermal delivery system 1199
Transdermal oestradiol gels 115, 1198, 1199
Transdermal patch 757
 contraceptive 1095
Transdermal testosterone gels 1202
Transformation zone, large loop excision of 577, 578
Transient ischaemic attack 1194
Transitional cell carcinoma 542, 642
Transobturator tapes 1156
Transperitoneal transvesical approach 315
Transphincteric fistula 1236*f*
Transrectal sonography 16
Trans-tubular potassium gradient 1246
Transvaginal colour Doppler 971, 992
Transvaginal falloposcopy 14
Transvaginal natural orifice transluminal endoscopic surgery 1208
Transvaginal probes 970
Transvaginal scan 208, 843*f*, 971
Transvaginal sonography 16, 193, 194, 206*f*, 209, 637, 920, 926*f*, 932*f*, 933, 938, 949, 955*f*, 971, 1003, 1051, 1195
 transducer orientation for 903*f*
Transvaginal ultrasonography 189, 454, 1001
 ultrasound on 965
Transvaginal ultrasound 444, 622, 623*f*, 1004*f*
Transverse cervical ligaments 52
Transverse vaginal septum 266
Trastuzumab 688, 689
Trauma 1142
 cervical 1051
Treponema pallidum 365
 haemagglutination assay 369
 immunoblot 369
 particle agglutination assay 369
Treponema pertenue 369

Treponemal chemiluminescence immunoassay 369
Treponemal enzyme immunoassay 369
Triangular ligament 27*f*, 29, 52
  lower layer of 29
Triazole 808
Tricarboxylic acid 601
Trichloroacetic acid 540
Trichomonads 404, 799
Trichomonas 8, 367, 402, 403, 752, 1272
  endocervicitis 399
  group 398
  infection 371, 398, 401, 808
  infestation 399, 553
  organisms 809
  urethritis 399
  vaginalis 395, 401*f*, 490, 795*f*, 798, 800*t*, 802, 808
    diagnosis of 799
    organisms 398*f*, 553, 819
    parasite 365
  vaginitis 398-401, 793, 795, 844
Trichomoniasis 366, 398, 798
  recommended regimens for 800
  recurrent 801
  treatment for 800
Tricyclic antidepressants 461
Triglycerides 1277
Trigonitis 1142
Trimegestone 1093
Trimethoprim 374, 1176, 1177
Triphasic pills 1092
Triple X syndrome 293
Triploidy 163
Triptorelin 447, 449
Trisomy 159
Trocar 1020
  cannula 1022
  insertion 1036*f*, 1057
  secondary 1034
Troglitazone 1104
Tromethamine 1136
Trophectoderm 1311
Trophoblast 181
  hyperplasia of 216
Trophoblastic cells 157
Trophoblastic proliferation 220*b*
Trophoblastic tissue 214
Trophoblastic tumour 215
  intermediate 691
Trospium 1155
Troublesome 404
Tryptophan 177
Tubal corrective surgery 207
Tubal damage 180
Tubal ectopic gestation 965*f*, 966*f*
Tubal embryo transfer 878
Tubal inflammation 991
  sonographic markers for 991*t*
Tubal insufflation 865
Tubal lesions 971, 989
Tubal ligation, site of 1129
Tubal mole 187
Tubal musculature 424*f*
Tubal occlusion 1129
  incidence of 1129
Tubal patency
  normal 854*f*
  test 14, 852, 855
    cannulas 889*f*
Tubal pregnancy 184*f*, 204
  management of 195
  unruptured 183*f*, 208
Tubal resection 1129
  noncontraceptive benefits of 1130
  sterilisation procedures, types of 1130*f*
Tubal ring 965
  sign 965
Tubal rupture 185, 187, 208
Tubal surgery 180, 181
Tubal-ostia, assessment of 1042
Tube
  atrophy of 783
  mechanical blockage of 1029
  reactions of 181
  reconstruction operations on 865
  reimplantation of 413, 866
  resection of 1129
  sarcoidosis of 389*f*
  suction 1243
  terminal ends of 428*f*
  torsion of 361
Tubectomy 426*f*
Tubercle bacillus 419
  invades pelvic organs 382*f*
Tuberculosis 13, 413, 419, 420*f*, 431*fc*
  extensively drug-resistant 431
  extrapulmonary 430
  genital 382, 419, 1195
  infection 430
    active 421*t*
    latent 421*t*
  management of 430
  multidrug-resistant 431
  preoperative diagnosis of 384*f*
  pulmonary 420, 430
Tubo-ovarian
  abscess 990
    bilateral 408*f*
  anatomy contraindicates 453
  ligament, division of 1209
  mass 410
Tuboretroperitoneal fistula 385*f*
Tumour 22, 145, 350, 362, 440*f*, 456, 480, 606, 658, 685, 723
  abdominal 354*f*, 383*f*, 456, 1141, 1289
  adenomatoid 642
  anal malignant 1239
  androgenic 308
  axial torsion of 685
  benign 616, 958*t*, 1225
  cavities 611
  cells
    clumps of 676
    staining in 625*f*
  characteristics 657
  classification 488*t*
  cystic 656, 668
  deep-seated 696
  endometrioid 668, 988
  expression 1304
  formation 443
  gynaecological 1300
  interstitial 611
  intra-abdominal 1145
  intrinsic signalling pathway inhibitors 534
  malignant 958*t*
    mucinous 668
    serous 667
  marker 528, 657, 658, 658*t*, 1008
  mesenchymal 658, 682
  metastatic 549
  mixed mesodermal 596
  mixed type of 677
  mucinous 658
  mutation burden 689
  necrosis factor 713
    alpha 710, 712
    secretion of 441
  neuroendocrine 570
  node-metastasis 544, 584, 646, 670
    classification 544
  non-broad ligament origin of 651*t*
  nonepithelial 574
  ovarian 17, 236, 360, 412, 654, 656, 657*f*, 682, 683, 752
  paravaginal 348
  primary cervical 590
  regression 671
  resection of 675
  retroperitoneal 655
  sebaceous 660
  serous 658
    borderline 666
  size 245, 582, 592, 684, 696
  somatic-type 680
  suppressor gene 1300, 1303
    expression of 215
  tissue, analysis of 1302
  trophoblastic 215
  types of 214, 659
  uterine 634
  vulvar 338
  wide range of 1302
Tunica albuginea 253
Turner's syndrome 138, 290, 292, 292*f*, 293, 293*f*, 300, 304, 305, 738*f*, 1202
Twins 880
Two-gonadotrophin theory 67

U

Ulcer 356*f*, 369, 380*f*, 392*f*, 1228
  acute simple 392
  aphthous 768
  chronic 1229
  decubitus 332*f*, 334, 752
  gastrointestinal 755
Ulcerative colitis 1229, 1234, 1236, 1244
Ulcerative squamous cell carcinoma, early 543*f*
Ulipristal acetate 609, 748, 1115
  use of 1116

Ultra-low-dose oral contraceptives 1094*t*
advantages of 1094*b*
disadvantages of 1094*b*
Ultrasonic scalpel tool 1025*f*
Ultrasonography 15, 148, 250, 458, 525, 596, 721, 851, 870*f*, 875, 896, 897, 920, 933, 949, 1191
field of 896
guided transfer 872
translabial 897
transperineal 897
transrectal 897
transvaginal 189, 454, 1001
scan 745
Ultrasound 123, 528, 734, 970, 971, 1148, 1290, 1308
applications of 901
endoscopic 1238
methods, sensitivity and specificity of 971*t*
therapeutic 1290
transabdominal 1001
transrectal 859
types of 896
Umbilical artery 16
Umbilical cord 157
Unilocular solid cyst 950
Unique genetic code 1300
United Nations Children's Fund 231, 318
Unruptured follicle, luteinisation of 436
Upper urinary tract infections 1173
Upper vagina 352, 698
disease 566
carcinoma of 564
Uraemia 580
Ureaplasma 808
infection 381
urealyticum 164, 380
Ureter 47, 438, 1170, 1204, 1273
accessory 284
bilateral aberrant 285*f*
diseases of 459, 1141
injury 1272
Ureteric buds 261
Ureteric fistula 315
Ureteric obstruction 583, 943*f*
Ureteroneocystostomy 672
Urethra 30*f*, 43, 44, 45*f*, 46, 57, 295, 370, 557, 1170
angulation of 1167
bulking agents, injection of 1161
carcinoma of 554, 554*f*
closure of 295
development of 257
dilatation of 46
diseases of 1142
diverticulum 536, 552, 552*f*, 558
diagnosis of 552
elimination of 1164*f*
female 1142*f*
function of 44*f*
lessen angulation of 1167*f*
lower end of 44*f*
normal development of 303*f*
obstruction of 1161, 1166
opens 1144*f*
prolapse of 536, 551
proximal 1145, 1157
unwanted 1166
Urethral caruncle 553, 752
Urethral catheter 1146
Urethral condyloma acuminata, laser treatment for 1295*f*
Urethral diverticulectomy 1156
Urethral incompetence 338
form of 1151*f*
Urethral length 1145
Urethral loss 1156
Urethral meatus 552*f*, 554*f*, 830
drains, external 47
Urethral plug 1155
Urethral profilometry 1148
Urethral prolapse 552, 1142
Urethral sling 1160
Urethral sphincter 1143, 1145
dysfunction 1143, 1150
muscle weakness 1145
Urethral tumours 551, 1142
Urethritis 398, 1142, 1258
Urethrocele 332, 552
Urethrocystogram 1166*f*
tracings of 1153*f*, 1167*f*
Urethrocystography, lateral 44*f*, 1164
Urethrocystopexy, effect of 1166*f*
Urethroplasty 1154*f*
Urethrovaginal junction 1152
Urethrovesical angle, posterior 1154*f*
Urethrovesical junction 30*f*, 60, 1151, 1154*f*, 1164*f*
anatomy of 30*f*
Urge incontinence 1150, 1151, 1155
diagnosis of 1150
surgery for 1156
Urinalysis 733
Urinary bladder, dissection of 1272
Urinary calculus 1142*f*
Urinary discharges 793
Urinary diversion 1149
Urinary fistula 315, 1272
types of 315*fc*
Urinary flow rate 1146
Urinary incontinence 805, 1140, 1151*t*, 1311
investigation of 1151
management of 1152*fc*
Urinary obstruction, nonresolvable 1172
Urinary problems
investigation of 1145
treatment of 1148
Urinary retention 323, 838, 1164, 1253
acute 1164*f*
diagnosis of 1164*t*
treatment of 1167
Urinary stasis 1141
Urinary stress test 1156
Urinary symptoms 337, 1140, 1189
Urinary tract 78, 1150, 1162
complications 321
conditions of 810
infection 341, 334, 458, 897, 1072, 1162, 1170, 1172-1174, 1188
adverse effects of 1178
classification of 1170, 1172*f*
complicated 1175
lower 1173
prevalence of 1170*fc*
recurrent 112, 1178*fc*
risk factors for 1171*t*, 1173*t*
treatment of 1175, 1177
types of 1173*t*
uncomplicated 1175
malformations of 284
medications affect 1150*t*
obstructive lesions of 334
symptoms 531
Urine 188
alkaline 1258
constant leakage of 391
culture 1173
examination of 1146
incontinence of 285, 810, 1149, 1258
microscopy 1146
midstream sample of 1152, 1172
outflow of 1164
postdelivery 312
retention of 354*f*, 1165*f*, 1166, 1166*f*, 1257
routine 375, 1173
volume of 1242
Uroflowmetry 1146
Urogenital fistula 1162
Urogenital membrane 257
Urogenital mesentery 252*f*
Urogenital ridge 252*f*, 253, 288
Urogenital sinus 257, 257*f*, 258, 283, 303*f*
part of 257
tissues 498
Urogenital system 254*f*
development of 252
Urogenital triangle 27
Urogynaecological umbrella 1311
Urorectal septum 261
Urosepsis 1171, 1171*t*, 1172
Uterine abnormalities 971
congenital 971, 972*f*
Uterine adhesions, lysis of 1046
Uterine anomalies 263, 268*f*, 902, 905
Uterine arteriovenous malformations 925
Uterine artery 39, 40*f*, 47, 55, 328, 994, 997, 1204, 1211*f*, 1212*f*
embolisation 205, 613, 639
laparoscopic occlusion of 613
ligation 1211*f*
terminal part of 42*f*
vaginal occlusion of 613
Uterine aspiration, vacuum for 1137
Uterine bleeding 94, 97*f*, 102, 738
abnormal 606, 743, 743*t*, 744, 749, 896, 911*f*, 934*f*, 1041, 1195
excessive 743
mild 360
phenomenon of 94
Uterine cancer 523, 706*fc*
diagnosis of 1302

Uterine cannula 1027
Uterine cavity 312, 355, 422*f*, 973, 1209
  carcinoma in situ of 1102
  inner lining of 424*f*
  outside of 1089*f*
Uterine colic 1091
Uterine contractions 457, 1122
  expulsive 457
Uterine cornu 179
Uterine corpus 509
Uterine factors 843
Uterine fibroids 165, 598, 599*fc*, 1295
  driver mutations 601
  multiple 22*f*
Uterine flexion 349*f*
Uterine hernia syndrome 299
Uterine hyperactivity 754
Uterine hyperperistalsis 637
Uterine hypoplasia, diagnosis of 278
Uterine inertia 265
Uterine ischemia develops 755
Uterine isthmus 1046
Uterine layer
  infiltration 981*f*
  involvement 981
Uterine leiomyoma 433, 436, 445, 595, 655, 784, 844, 1202
  sites of 602*f*
  small 606*f*
Uterine lesions 922
Uterine lipoleiomyoma 925*f*
Uterine malformation 359*f*
  accessory cavitated 911
  congenital 171
Uterine manipulator 891, 891*f*, 1024*f*, 1209
Uterine mass 655*f*
  examination of 631*f*
Uterine musculature 60*f*
Uterine natural killer 155
Uterine origin, pain of 4
Uterine perforation 218, 1051
Uterine polyps 597
Uterine position 899
  correction of 867
Uterine prolapse 327, 329, 333*f*, 536, 1219*f*
  degrees of 329*f*
Uterine retroflexion 351
Uterine retroversion 351
Uterine rupture 1052
Uterine sarcoma 596, 630, 689, 922, 924*f*, 1309
  classification of 630*fc*
Uterine secretion 792
Uterine segment, lower 1210*f*
Uterine septum 1045*f*, 1296*f*
  hysteroscopic resection of 1048*f*
Uterine serosa, invasion of 624
Uterine serosal layer 611
Uterine size 901*b*
Uterine smooth muscle tumours 924
Uterine softening 183
Uterine sound 886, 886*f*, 1087*f*, 1089*f*
Uterine submucosal fibroids 173*f*
Uterine synechiae 166, 938
Uterine trauma 636
  causes of 636
Uterine tumours 634
Uterine vein 40, 56, 328
Uterine wall 407*f*
  distended 1041*f*
  invasion of 215
  thickening 905*f*, 920
Uterocervical length 994*f*
Utero-ovarian ligaments 1208
Uterosacral ligament 49, 51, 52, 328, 438, 452, 564, 653, 1204, 1208, 1210, 1211, 1213
  endometriosis of 435*f*
Uterosacral plexus, portion of 328
Uterotubal junction 1044
Uterovaginal prolapse 329, 332*f*, 334*f*, 335*f*, 342*f*
Uterovesical fistula 315
Uterovesical fold separation 1210*f*
Uterovesical pouch 437, 1141
Uterus 16*f*, 21*f*, 35, 35*f*, 38, 52, 77, 266, 277, 328, 351, 364, 383, 384, 429*f*, 431, 522, 637, 655*f*, 782, 897, 970, 994, 1001, 1008*f*, 1083, 1208, 1209, 1213, 1225
  abnormalities of 284
  absence of 259, 285
  acute puerperal inversion of 356*f*
  anteflexed 34*f*
  anteverted 34*f*
  aplasia 975
  appearance of 1001
  arcuatus 264, 268*f*
  assessment of 912*f*
  asymmetrical enlargement of 201
  backward displacement of 349
  bicornis unicollis 269*f*, 270*f*
  bicornuate 191*f*, 264, 267, 273*f*, 429*f*, 570*f*, 909*f*
  bicorporeal 266, 974
  bimanual manipulation of 352
  body of 8, 278*f*
  broad-topped 273*f*
  capacity of 354
  cardinal ligaments of 47
  cavity of 35, 619*f*
  classes of 263, 267*f*
  cochleate 276*f*, 278
  complete bicorporeal 974, 975*f*
  congenital retroflexion of 278
  contour of 912*f*
  descends 350
  didelphys 264, 267, 268*f*-270*f*, 273*f*, 910*f*
  dimorphic 266
  displacement of 348
  drainage of 406
  duplex 264, 268*f*
    bicollis 264
    unicollis 268*f*
  dysmorphic 973, 974*f*
  early carcinoma of 753
  enlargement of 454, 596, 596*t*
  forward displacement of 348
  generalised myohyperplasia of 510*f*
  hypertrophies 39
  hypoplasia of 277, 742
  hypoplastic 973*f*
  impaction of 354
  infantilis 973
  inversion of 355, 357*f*, 536
  inverted fundus of 356*f*
  isthmus of 46
  laparotomy 777*f*
  lateral deviation of 349*f*
  leiomyomas of 598*f*
  ligaments of 51*f*
  Lippes loop in 1086*f*
  longitudinal section of 970*f*, 971*f*
  major support of 328*t*
  malformation of 14
  melanoma of 634
  multiple leiomyomas in 436*f*
  myohyperplasia of 675*f*
  normal 359, 899*f*, 973, 973*f*
  operation on 1029
  outer coat of 437
  partial bicorporeal 975*f*
  parts of 913*f*
  perforation of 313, 1091, 1139
  permanent retrodisplacement of 350
  position of 39, 901*f*
  postpartum 1120, 1120*f*
  prepubertal 139*f*
  radiograph of 54*f*
  reactions of 181
  relations of 39
  replacement of 352
  retrodisplacement of 349, 351
  rudimentary horn of 179, 976*f*
  rupture of 312, 313, 1139
  sacculation of 271, 355
  sections of 904*f*
  septus 264, 268*f*
  size of 38*f*, 901*b*, 912*f*
  spontaneous correction of 353
  subseptate 267
  subseptus 264, 268*f*
  supports of 327, 328*f*
  symmetrical enlargement of 600*f*
  transverse section of 907*f*, 970*f*
  T-shaped 973, 1042
  tumours of 597
  type of 263, 266*b*, 349*f*
  unicornis 264, 268*f*
  unicornuate 264, 266, 268*f*, 300*f*, 427*f*, 907*f*, 976*f*
  upward displacement of 348

V

Vabra aspirator 13
Vacuum aspiration 1138
Vagina 8, 30, 32, 40*f*, 53, 57, 77, 150, 264, 274, 279, 295, 312, 337, 355, 364, 383, 432, 439, 441, 496, 522, 693, 1002, 1160, 1204, 1225
  absence of 279
  acidity of 32
  agenesis of 279
  anterior wall of 567*f*, 1255*f*

anterolateral wall of 557*f*
artificial 280, 280*f*
atresia of 275, 821
benign neoplasms of 558, 752
canalises 262
carcinoma of 335, 445, 564
cuff of 440*f*
development of 256*f*, 257
different ages 33*f*
diseases of 1142
endometriosis of 1139
epithelial abnormalities of 496
eversion of 344
following colporrhaphy, posterior walls of 1255*f*
hypoplasia of 742
invasive cancer of 563
keratinisation of 334
length of 351
lower 58
lymphatic drainage of 563
malignant neoplasms of 752
melanomas of 563
normal development of 303*f*
preparation of 1248
prevention of carcinoma of 560
relations of 34
subseptate 267, 281
superficial ulceration of 593
supports of 329
swellings of 557
transverse axis of 9*f*
tuberculosis of 384
tumours of 557
upper compartment of 280*f*
Vaginal acidity 364
Vaginal adenosis 496, 497
benign 268
Vaginal agenesis 279, 727*f*
Vaginal anomalies 457, 905, 975
Vaginal anus 283
Vaginal aplasia 266
Vaginal approach repair 315
Vaginal artery 55
Vaginal atresia 273
Vaginal atrophy 1145, 1189*f*, 1200
Vaginal attachment 37
Vaginal bleeding 167, 183, 184, 205, 207, 1201
abnormal 460, 814
severe 962
Vaginal brachytherapy 697
Vaginal burns 313
Vaginal cancer 523
diagnosis of 563
radiotherapy in 700
staging systems for 565*t*
Vaginal candidiasis 489, 794*f*, 799, 800*t*, 802, 807
diagnosis of 799
recommended regimens for 801
Vaginal cell
adenocarcinoma 269
normal mature 403*f*
Vaginal cones 339, 1288
Vaginal contraceptive
film 1074, 1074*f*
ring 484
Vaginal creams 1199
Vaginal cuff 1208
closure 21*f*
Vaginal cycle 99
Vaginal cyst 339, 557
simulating prolapse 339*f*
Vaginal cytology 405, 525
Vaginal diaphragm 1070
Vaginal dilatation 303
Vaginal dilator 889*f*, 890
Vaginal discharge 8, 420, 792, 807, 807*fc*, 1272
after operations 1272
cultures of 398*f*, 400*f*
infective causes of 793*f*
mucopurulent 411
noninfective causes of 793, 793*f*
offensive 169
Vaginal discomfort 1189
Vaginal dissection 1159
Vaginal dryness 787
Vaginal epithelium 32, 557
Vaginal eversion 344
Vaginal examination 8, 892, 1254
Vaginal factors 844
Vaginal faecal fistula 531
Vaginal flaps 1213
Vaginal flora 364, 401, 792
Vaginal growth 568*f*
punch biopsy 568*f*
Vaginal haematoma 312
Vaginal hypoplasia 281
Vaginal hysterectomy 342, 344, 1212, 1247
laparoscopy-assisted 748, 1029
Vaginal incision
closure of 1161
healing of 1272
Vaginal infection 401, 403, 834, 1145
Vaginal injury 834
Vaginal intraepithelial neoplasia 496, 561, 563
Vaginal introitus 323
infibulation of 323*f*
Vaginal irritation 834
Vaginal itching 551*f*
Vaginal length, total 331
Vaginal membrane, incomplete 274
Vaginal micronised 1200
Vaginal mucosa 314, 342, 566, 830, 1297
Vaginal muscle 1070, 1240, 1288
tightening 832
Vaginal myalgia 1240
Vaginal myomectomy 609
Vaginal oestrogen 1199, 1297
therapy 346, 1199
Vaginal operation 1130
Vaginal orifice tends 29
Vaginal outlet 264
Vaginal palpation 10
Vaginal parameters 34*t*
Vaginal penetration, avoidance of 832
Vaginal pessaries 1136
Vaginal plexus 40, 46
Vaginal prolapse 284*f*, 327, 332, 344, 830
Vaginal pruritus, causes of 809
Vaginal rejuvenation 1298, 1298*f*
Vaginal rhabdomyosarcomas 634
Vaginal rings 757, 774
Vaginal secretions, culture of 799
Vaginal septum
longitudinal non-obstructing 266
longitudinal obstructing 266
Vaginal site 1256
Vaginal smear 121, 775*f*
Vaginal sonography 941*f*
Vaginal spasm 830
Vaginal speculum 351
Vaginal stenosis 593
Vaginal support 329
Vaginal suppositories 1136
Vaginal swabs 799
examination of 490
high 800
Vaginal thrush 400
classical patch of 401*f*
Vaginal tightness 1298
Vaginal total hysterectomy 1257
Vaginal transcutaneous electrical nerve stimulation 816
Vaginal trauma 834
Vaginal tumour 348, 557, 563, 844
Vaginal vault 32, 39, 46, 339, 345, 440*f*, 525, 585*f*
Vaginal wall
healing of 1272
lower anterior 552*f*
prolapse of 334*f*
stretching of 32
upper
anterior 46
posterior 564*f*
Vaginismus 821, 832, 833, 837
causes of 833
idiopathic 835
Lamont and Pacik's classification of 834
muscles involved in 835
prevalence of 833
primary 834
secondary 835
severity of 835
situational 835
treatment of 836
Vaginitis 396, 752, 1096, 1101, 1272
emphysematosa 401*f*, 404
kinds of 1272
noninfective 404
part of 498
recurrent 1189
types of 401*f*, 798
Vaginograms 301*f*
Vaginoplasty 266, 302
Vague pains 4
Valine 1277
Valsalva's manoeuvre 1156
Varicocele assessment 850
Varicose veins 339, 536, 537
severe degree of 537*f*

Vas deferens
bilateral obstruction of 842
congenital bilateral absence of 859, 862
Vascular adhesions, lysis of 1295
Vascular apparatus 183
Vascular changes 536, 812
Vascular corpus luteum 948*f*
Vascular embolism 441
Vascular endothelial growth factor 450, 706, 713
antibody 647
Vascular microthrombus formation 420
Vascular thrombosis 171
Vascularity 930
Vasectomy 1132
adverse effects of 1132
reliability of 1132
Vasomotor symptoms 1196
Vasopressin 200, 755
dilute solution of 1295
Vault 1211
closure of 1211
suturing 1214*f*
Veins 55, 606
ligation of 1268
plexus of 35, 56
Vellus hair 478
Vena cava interruption 1270
Venereal disease research laboratory 874, 875
slide test 369
Venlafaxine 1187
Venn diagram 463*f*
Venography 1264
Venom immunotherapy 714
Venous thrombectomy 1268
Venous thromboembolism 1100, 1101, 1250, 1270
Venous thrombosis 1271
history of 1201
Ventilation perfusion lung scanning 1269
Ventrofixation 439
Veress needle 18*f*, 19, 1020, 1020*f*
insertion 1032, 1033
Verrucous carcinoma 542, 574
Vertebral wedging 1191
Verumotanum 1149*f*
Vesical calculus 1142
Vesicovaginal fistula 10, 315, 534
Vestibular bulb 28
Vestibular glands 29
Vestibulectomy
modified 816
posterior 816*f*
Vestigial structures 42*f*
Vicryl sutures 342
Video-assisted anal fistula tract ligation 1237
Videocystourethrography 1146
Villoglandular variant 945*f*
Villous choriocarcinoma 217
Vincristine 690
Virginal vulva 26*f*
Virilisation 300, 478
type of 295
Virilism 236, 303, 306, 782, 785
causes of 308
cutaneous 306
manifestations of 307
signs of 306
Virkud sling 344
Virus infection 769
Viscera, abdominal 441
Vision 1188
system 1014
Visual fields, examination of 733
Visual inspection 515, 527, 576-578
Vital disease 260
Vital signs, observation for 169
Vitamin 491, 765, 1187, 1275, 1286
A 1275, 1280, 1281, 1284
deficiency 1284
sources of 1284
supplements 147
B_{12} 118, 490, 1275
deficiencies 490
B_6 118, 765
C 147, 1281
consumption of 1285
D 714, 1281, 1286
deficiency of 600, 1286
metabolism 600
E 118, 765, 1278, 1281
supplements 147
K 1275, 1281
analogue 1267
K_1 1267
Vitiligo, genital 821
Voice, irreversible deepening of 449
Voiding dysfunction 1162
Volumetric modulated arc therapy techniques 629
Voluntary external urethral sphincter, spasm of 1166
Voluntary urethral sphincter muscles 1149
Vomiting 688, 1100, 1243, 1258
postoperative 1258
severe 1136
von Willebrand's disease 748
Vulsellum forceps 884, 888, 888*f*
Vulva 8, 26, 29, 30, 57, 77, 276, 282, 312, 364, 368*f*, 383, 493*f*, 397, 432, 439, 487*f*, 522, 693
benign neoplasms of 752
Bowen's disease of 494
candida infection of 394
carcinoma of 554
condyloma acuminatum of 394*f*, 539*f*
cyst of 550
development of 257
diseases of 699, 1142
duplication of 282*f*
endometriosis of 434*f*
exfoliative dermatitis of 811*f*
fungal infection of 394
hidradenoma of 538*f*
hypertrophic tuberculosis of 419*f*
invasive squamous carcinoma, parts of 488*f*
malignant neoplasms of 542, 752
melanoma of 549*f*
multiple
carcinomatous lesions of 542*f*
warts of 539*f*
nerves of 56*f*
normal development of 303*f*
oedema of 537*f*
Paget's disease of 494, 494*f*, 549, 810
pedunculated fibroma of 539*f*
psoriasis of 395*f*
recurrent cancer of 548
shaving of 1248
swellings of 536
tissues of 30*f*, 543*f*
tuberculosis of 384
tumours of 536
varicosities of 537*f*
Vulval cancer tumour-node-metastasis classification 545
Vulval growth biopsy 551*f*
Vulvar abnormalities 492
Vulvar acanthosis 493
Vulvar anaesthesia, local 58*f*
Vulvar cancer 523, 523*f*, 805
immunotherapy in 708
radiotherapy in 698
types of 542
Vulvar candidiasis 489, 808
Vulvar carcinoma 547*f*
Vulvar epithelial disorder 490, 492*f*, 775, 784
Vulvar epithelium, dysplasia of 523
Vulvar hair follicles, infection of 391
Vulvar high-grade squamous intraepithelial lesion 492
Vulvar intraepithelial neoplasia 488, 490, 492, 492*f*, 493, 493*f*, 494, 805, 806
treatment of 532
Vulvar malignancy 549
Vulvar melanosis 1298
treatment 1298
Vulvar oedema 799
Vulvar pruritus, diagnosis of 805
Vulvar swabs, examination of 490
Vulvar tissues 548
Vulvar ulceration, recurrent 768
Vulvectomy 491, 523
radical 548*f*
three-incision technique of 547*f*
Vulvitis 391
acute 536
infantile 392
Vulvodynia 804, 813, 813*b*, 815*b*
aetiology of 814*fc*
localised provoked 814, 815
unprovoked 814, 817
Vulvovaginal candidiasis 366, 793, 794, 798
Vulvovaginal haematoma, formation of 312
Vulvovaginitis 396, 774

W

Wamsteker classification 746
Wandering cells 157
Warfarin 232, 1271

Warm hypotension 1255
Warts 536
keratotic 378
macular 378
vulvar 539
Wearable clitoral stimulators 831
Weight gain, prevention of 1190
Weight loss 473, 484, 575
Wertheim's operation 73*f*, 1206
Whiff test 798
Whirlpool sign 963, 988*f*
White blood cell 122, 195, 396, 798, 848, 1171, 1173
Whitish collar fibers 1230
Whole-breast ultrasound 244
Withdrawal method 1067
Wolffian duct 252*f*, 254, 255, 257*f*, 261, 262, 289, 557, 557*f*
development of 255*f*, 296
origin 567
adenoma of 536
Wolffian system 253
Wolffian tumour 660
Womb stone 615, 615*f*
Wound
abdominal 1262
disruption 1261
healing, delayed 1230
infection 1162, 1261
diagnosis of 1261
Wuchereria bancrofti 395

X

X chromosome 262, 290, 293
X sperm fertilising XX ovum 293
Xeromammography 242
X-linked ichthyosis 160
XX gonadal dysgenesis 277
XXX chromosome makeup 293

Y

Y cell line 733
Y chromosome 262, 289, 292, 294
material 733
microdeletion of 860
Yaws, treatment for 369
Yeast vaginitis 1188
Yolk sac 162*f*, 261, 658
endoderm of 288
tumour 659, 679
Yuzpe's regimen 1115
YY syndrome 294

Z

Zalcitabine 377
Zidovudine 377
Ziehl-Neelsen staining 386
Zinc 1280
absorption of 1279
oxide 491
Zirconium, carbon coated 1161
Zoledronic acid 1194
Zona pellucida 68, 68*f*, 155, 1119, 1311
thick 879
Zona thinning 879
Zygote 153
cytoplasm of 153
intrafallopian transfer 878